MANAGEMENT OF ANAPHYLACTIC REACTIONS

1. **Discontinue suspected drug.**
   (stop IV, tourniquet IM, or SC site).
2. **Maintain airway.** Aminophylline or other bronchodilators may be required for severe respiratory distress.
3. **Administer *epinephrine*.**
   SC (Adults): 0.2–0.5 mg, may repeat q 5–15 min.
   SC (Children): 0.01 mg/kg or 0.1 mg, may repeat q 5–15 min.
   IV (Adults): 0.3–0.5 mg over 5 min, may repeat q 15 min, or 0.1 mg over 5–10 min, *or* 1–4 mcg/min infusion.
   IV (Children): 0.01 mg/kg/dose or 0.1–0.2 mg over 5 min, may repeat q 30 min or 0.1–1.5 mcg (maximum)/kg/min infusion.
4. **Administer *antihistamines*.** May prevent recurrence and decrease intensity of reaction.
   ***diphenhydramine* (Benadryl)**
   IM, IV (Adults): 50–100 mg single dose, may follow with oral therapy for 1–2 days.
   IM, IV (Children): 5 mg/kg/day or 150 mg/m^2 in divided doses q 6–8 hr (not to exceed 300 mg/day), may follow with oral therapy for 1–2 days.
   ***cimetidine* (Tagamet)**
   IV (Adults): 300 mg q 6 hr.
   IV (Children): 25–30 mg/kg/day in 6 divided doses.
5. **Support blood pressure.** If necessary use fluids and/or vasopressors.
6. **Administer *glucocorticoids*.** May decrease intensity of reaction.
   ***hydrocortisone* (Solu-Cortef)**
   IV (Adults and Children): 100–1000 mg, may follow with 7 mg/kg/day IV or oral therapy for 1–2 days.
7. **Document reaction** in medical record, inform patient/family to carry identification.

—*Davis's*—
DRUG
GUIDE
for Nurses

Davis's
DRUG GUIDE
forNurses

Fourth Edition

JUDITH HOPFER DEGLIN, PharmD
Consultant Pharmacist
United Community Services-Hospice
Norwich, Connecticut

Formerly
University of Connecticut
Schools of Pharmacy and Nursing
Storrs, Connecticut

APRIL HAZARD VALLERAND, MSN, RN
University of Pennsylvania
School of Nursing
Philadelphia, Pennsylvania

 F. A. DAVIS COMPANY • Philadelphia

F. A. Davis Company
1915 Arch Street
Philadelphia, PA 19103

Printed in the United States of America

Last digit indicates print number 10 9 8 7 6 5 4 3 2 1

NOTE: As new scientific information becomes available through basic and clinical research, recommended treatments and drug therapies undergo changes. The authors and publisher have done everything possible to make this book accurate, up to date, and in accord with accepted standards at the time of publication. However, the reader is advised always to check product information (package inserts) for changes and new information regarding dose and contraindications before administering any drug. Caution is especially urged when using new or infrequently ordered drugs.

Library of Congress Cataloging-in-Publication Data

Deglin, Judith Hopfer, 1950–
   Davis's drug guide for nurses / Judith Hopfer Deglin, April Hazard Vallerand.—4th ed.
      p.   cm.
   Includes bibliographical references and index.
   ISBN 0-8036-2458-1 (pbk. : alk. paper)
   1. Drugs—Handbooks, manuals, etc.   2. Nursing—Handbooks, manuals, etc.   I. Vallerand, April Hazard.   II. Title.   III. Title: Drug guide for nurses.
   [DNLM: 1. Drugs—handbooks.   2. Drugs—nurses' instruction.   QV 39 D318d   1995]
   RM301.12.D44   1995
   615'.1'024613—dc20
   DNLM/DLC
   for Library of Congress   93-48230
                                                                        CIP

CONSULTANTS

ACKNOWLEDGMENTS

We offer our thanks and gratitude to our families, whose support and patience with our endless computer time and phone calls gave us the time and strength to complete this manuscript.

To those at F. A. Davis, especially Bob Martone, Ruth De George, Herb Powell, and Crystal McNichol, who saw our projects through to completion.

Judi and April

NEW FEATURES AT A GLANCE

- At least 66 new drug monographs have been added.

- New and enhanced **life span dosing considerations** for adult, geriatric, pediatric, and neonatal patients are included.

- Newly approved drug indications as well as new unlabeled uses are identified.

- All drugs now include an **Availability** section identifying all available dosage forms with respective strengths.

- A unique section, **Medication Misadventures: The Nurse's Role in Detecting, Preventing, and Documenting Adverse Drug Reactions and Medication Errors,** is included.

- MEDWATCH, the new Food and Drug Administration (FDA) form for reporting serious adverse reactions and product defects associated with medications, devices, and nutritional products, is now included.

- A new classification—**Antiulcer Agents**—has been added, for a total of 49 drug classifications.

- **IV therapy** data has been completely updated, and **IV rate** information has been expanded to include the implications of drug administration at incorrect rates. This vital information is unique to *Davis's Drug Guide for Nurses,* fourth edition.

- 100 more combination drugs have be added, for a total of 500 such drugs.

- For quick clinical look-ups, a pull-out chart identifying **syringe compatibilities,** as well as **opioid analgesics** with dosage forms and equivalence, is included.

WHAT'S NEW IN THE FOURTH EDITION

The fourth edition of *Davis's Drug Guide for Nurses* again sets new standards for nursing drug references. While providing the most comprehensive, up-to-date, and practical information available to nurses, it also makes available the most relevant information required for the safe and effective administration and monitoring of drug therapy. Its consistent, easy-to-follow format ensures that once the nurse is familiar with the layout of drug monographs, finding specific facts for individual drugs becomes a very efficient process.

Once again, this new edition reflects the authors' commitment to providing the most up-to-date material available. At least 66 new pharmacologic entities and more than 100 combination drugs have been added. Some new drugs added include a new agent for migraine headaches, 7 new anti-infectives, 3 new agents for use in patients with AIDS, a benzodiazepine antidote, 2 new antidepressants, and a variety of other new agents.

A useful new clinical feature entitled "Availability" identifies available dosage forms and their respective strengths.

Existing monographs have been updated to include newly approved indications and unlabeled uses, as well as interactions with recently released drugs.

Nursing implications have been streamlined to afford better accessibility to data, and IV administration information is more clearly delineated to facilitate rapid retrieval.

The dosage information includes the ranges recommended by manufacturers and approved by the Food and Drug Administration (FDA). Because special dosing considerations are usually required depending on the age, size, condition, and tolerance of the patient, more extensive neonatal, pediatric, and geriatric dosing information is provided in the fourth edition, as are more details on dosage modification in hepatic/renal disease. The book's information on contraindications, precautions, adverse reactions, interactions, and side effects is condensed to a level essential to responsible clinical practice.

This reference not only provides the pharmacologic profile of what each drug does and how it works, it also links essential nursing data—such as what parameters to assess in the patient taking the drug, how to administer the medication, and how to evaluate the drug's effectiveness—while incorporating the nursing diagnoses applicable to its administration. In addition, the necessary information to provide appropriate patient and family teaching is covered.

The fourth edition of *Davis's Drug Guide for Nurses* should fill the drug information needs of every student and practicing nurse and facilitate the safe and efficacious use of medications.

No other drug reference presents such depth of pharmacologic content within the framework of the nursing process and does it in such a convenient size and format.

From THE PUBLISHER

TABLE OF CONTENTS

HOW TO USE *DAVIS'S DRUG GUIDE FOR NURSES*

The purpose of *Davis's Drug Guide for Nurses* is to provide readily accessible, easy to understand drug information for the most commonly prescribed drugs for clinical use. The sections below describe the organization of the book and the information provided for each drug.

Special Dosing Considerations

In many clinical situations, the average dosing range can be inappropriate. This section presents general guidelines for conditions in which special considerations must be made to assure optimum therapeutic outcome.

Classifications

Brief summaries of the major therapeutic classifications are provided along with a listing of those drugs included in *Davis's Drug Guide for Nurses* and the page numbers on which those monographs may be found.

Drug Monographs

The following information appears for each drug:

Generic/Trade Name: The generic name appears first, with a pronunciation key. This is followed by an alphabetical listing of trade names. The generic name is the official name of the drug assigned by the United States Adopted Names (USAN) Council in the United States and by the World Health Organization (WHO) in other countries. In many institutions, drugs are labeled generically. Canadian trade names appear in brackets. Common names, abbreviations, and selected foreign names are also included. For users who do not know the generic name, a color-coded Comprehensive Drug and Agent Index, which contains entries for both trade names and generic names, as well as classifications, provides this information quickly and easily.

Classification: The most common classification is listed first followed by other classification(s) according to the use(s) of the drug. For example, propranolol (Inderal) is classified first as an antihypertensive but is also used as an antianginal and an antiarrhythmic. For a better explanation of drug classifications, refer to the Classifications section of the book (pages C1–C78), which provides brief summaries of the classifications, lists the drugs contained in each classification, and identifies the page numbers on which the drugs can be found.

Controlled Substance Schedule: If a drug is a controlled substance, its legal status or schedule is listed. This information alerts the reader to observe the necessary regulations when handling these drugs and should help instruct the patient regarding refill allotments. (See Appendix C for a description of the Schedule of Controlled Substances and a list of controlled substances included in *Davis's Drug Guide for Nurses*.)

Pregnancy Category: If the Food and Drug Administration (FDA) assigned pregnancy category is known, it is listed in this part of the monograph. A more detailed explanation of these categories (A, B, C, D, and X) is found in Appendix E. These categories allow for some assessment of risk to the fetus when a drug is used in the pregnant patient or in the patient who may be trying to conceive while receiving the drug.

Indications: The most common FDA uses of the drug are listed. Significant unlabeled uses are also included.

Action: This section contains a concise description of how a drug is known or believed to act in producing the desired therapeutic effect.

Pharmacokinetics: This information describes what happens to a drug following administration and includes an analysis of the absorption, distribution, metabolism, excretion, and half-life (amount of time for drug level to decrease by 50%).

> **Absorption:** Absorption describes the process that follows drug administration and its subsequent delivery to systemic circulation. If only a small fraction is absorbed following oral administration (diminished bioavailability), then the oral dose will be much larger than the parenteral dose. Absorption into systemic circulation also follows other routes of administration such as topical, transdermal, intramuscular, subcutaneous, rectal, and ophthalmic routes. Drugs administered intravenously are usually 100% bioavailable.

> **Distribution:** Following absorption, drugs are distributed, sometimes selectively, to various body tissues and fluids. These factors become important in choosing one drug over another, as in selecting antibiotics that may need to penetrate the central nervous system in the treatment of meningitis, or avoiding drugs that cross the placenta in pregnancy or concentrate in breast milk during lactation. During distribution many drugs interact with specific receptors and exert their pharmacologic effect. Binding to proteins, including albumin, occurs as well. Only the free or unbound portion of the drug is available for activity at receptor sites.

> **Metabolism and Excretion:** Following their intended action, drugs leave the body by either being converted to inactive compounds by the liver (metabolism or biotransformation), which are then excreted by the kidneys, or by renal elimination of unchanged drug. In addition, some drugs may be eliminated by other pathways such as biliary excretion, sweat, feces, and breath. If drugs are extensively liver-metabolized, then patients with severe liver disease may require dosage reduction. If the kidney is the major organ of elimination, then dosage adjustment may be necessary in the face of renal impairment. The very young (premature infants and neonates) and the elderly (over 60 years old) have diminished renal excretory and hepatic metabolic capacity. These patients may require dosage reduction or increased dosing intervals.

> **Half-Life:** The half-life of a drug is useful to know in planning effective regimens, since it correlates roughly with the duration of action. Half-lives are given for patients with normal renal or hepatic function. Other conditions that may alter the half-life are noted.

Contraindications and Precautions: Situations in which drug use should be avoided or alternatives strongly considered are listed as contraindications. In general, most drugs are contraindicated in pregnancy or lactation, unless the potential benefits outweigh the possible risks to the mother or baby (for example, anticonvulsants and antihypertensives). Contraindications may be absolute (i.e., the drug in question should be avoided completely) or relative where certain clinical situations may allow cautious use of the drug. The precautions portion includes disease states or clinical situations in which drug use involves particular risks or in which dosage modification may be necessary.

Adverse Reactions and Side Effects: In order to simplify long lists of possible reactions, a systems approach to side effects and adverse reactions has been taken. The order is such that these reactions have been listed in head-to-toe order for systems amenable to noting in this manner (CNS, EENT, Resp, CV, GI, GU). Other systems follow in alphabetical order (Endo, F and E, Hemat, Metab, MS, Local, Neuro), ending with a miscellaneous section. Although it is not possible to include all reported reactions, an effort has been made to include major side effects. Life-threatening adverse reactions or side effects are CAPITALIZED, while the most commonly encountered problems are underlined. In general, those underlined have an incidence of 10% or greater. Those not underlined occur in less than 10%, but more than 1%, of patients. Although life-threatening reactions may be rare (less than 1%), they are included because of their significance. The following abbreviations are used for body systems.

CNS: central nervous system
EENT: eye, ear, nose, and throat
Resp: respiratory
CV: cardiovascular
GI: gastrointestinal
GU: genitourinary
Derm: dermatologic
Endo: endocrinologic
F and E: fluid and electrolyte
Hemat: hematologic
Local: local
Metab: metabolic
MS: musculoskeletal
Neuro: neurologic
Misc: miscellaneous

Interactions: As the number of medications a patient receives increases, so does the likelihood of experiencing a drug–drug interaction. The most important drug–drug interactions and their results are explained. Significant drug–food interactions also are noted.

Route and Dosage: The usual routes of administration are grouped together and include recommended dosages for adults, children, and other more specific age groups if available. Dosage units are given in the terms in which they will most likely be prescribed. (For example, penicillin G dosage is given in units rather than milligrams.) Dosing intervals also are mentioned in the manner in which they are most likely to be ordered. Although antibiotics and antiarrhythmics should be given at regular intervals around the clock, it is neither necessary nor practical to give other medications, such as oral antihypertensives, in this manner. In situations in which dosage or interval is different from that commonly encountered, these indications are listed separately for clarification.

Availability: This section lists what strengths and concentrations of various dosage forms are available. Such information is useful in planning more convenient regimens (fewer tablets/capsules, less injection volume) and in determining whether certain dosing forms are available (suppositories, oral concentrates).

Time/Action Profile: This information is provided so that the onset of drug action, its peak effect, and its duration of activity can be anticipated and considered in planning administration schedules. The pharmacodynamics of each route of administration have been tabulated so that the reader may appreciate differences achieved by choosing one route over another. Durations of action of anti-infective agents generally have not been included. Most regimens for these agents are designed to avoid toxicity while ensuring high peak levels necessary for anti-infective action. Because of this, duration of action and blood level information are not necessarily comparable.

Nursing Implications: This section has been developed to help the nurse apply the nursing process to pharmacotherapeutics. It is divided into subsections which give the nurse a step-by-step guide to clinical assessment, implementation, and evaluation as they relate to medication administration.

Assessment: This subsection includes parameters for patient history and physical data that should be assessed before and during drug therapy. The **General Info** section describes assessment that is pertinent to all patients taking the medication. Other sections also are identified to specify assessments based on the drug's various indications. **Lab Test Considerations** provide the nurse with information regarding which laboratory tests to monitor and how the results may be effected by the medication. **Toxicity and Overdose** discusses therapeutic serum drug levels and signs and symptoms of toxicity. The antidote and treatment for toxicity or overdose of appropriate medications also are included.

Potential Nursing Diagnoses: The nursing diagnoses approved by the North American Nursing Diagnosis Association (NANDA) are used. The three most pertinent diagnoses that apply to a patient receiving the medication are listed. Following each diagnosis, the location of the information from which the diagnosis has been developed is listed in parentheses to provide a reference for the nursing diagnosis—for example, Infection, high risk for (indications, side effects). All of the NANDA diagnostic labels are listed in Appendix O.

Implementation: Guidelines specific for medication administration are discussed in this subsection. The information listed under the **General Info** heading applies to all routes of administration and includes timing of administration and details for patient care. Other headings in this section provide data regarding routes of administration. **PO** describes when and how to administer the drug, whether tablets may be crushed or capsules opened, and when to administer the medication in relation to food. **IV** provides details for reconstitution and dilution. **Direct IV** (IV Push), **Intermittent Infusion,** and **Continuous Infusion** specify amount and type of further dilution. **Rate** includes infusion time for each type of administration. **Syringe Compatibility/Incompatibility** identifies the medications each drug is compatible or incompatible with when mixed in a syringe. This type of compatibility is usually limited to 15 minutes after mixing. **Y-Site Compatibility/ Incompatibility** identifies those medications that are compatible or incompatible with each drug when administered via Y-injection site or 3-way stopcock in IV tubing. **Additive Compatibility/Incompatibility** identifies those medications that are compatible or incompatible when admixed in solution. This type of compatiblity is usually limited to 24 hours. Compatibility information is compiled from Trissel's *Supplement to Handbook of Injectable Drugs,* ed 7. (See Bibliography, page 1305.)

Patient/Family Teaching: This subsection includes material that should be taught to patients and/or families of patients. Side effects that should be reported, information on how to minimize side effects, details on administration, and follow-up requirements are presented. The nurse also should refer to the **Adverse Reactions and Side Effects** and **Interactions** sections for additional data to complete the patient/family teaching plan. **Home Care Issues** discusses aspects to be considered for medications taken in the home setting.

Evaluation: Outcome criteria for determination of the effectiveness of the medication are provided.

SPECIAL DOSING CONSIDERATIONS

For almost every drug there is an average dosing range. There are many situations, however, when this average range can be either toxic or ineffective. The purpose of this section is to describe situations in which special dosing considerations must be made to ensure a successful therapeutic outcome. The guidelines presented are general but should lead to a finer appreciation of individual dosing parameters. When these clinical situations are encountered, the doses of drugs ordered should be reviewed and the necessary adjustments made.

The Pediatric Patient

The most obvious reason for adjusting dosages in pediatric patients is size. Most drug dosages for this population are given on a mg/kg basis, or even more specifically on the basis of body surface area (BSA). Body surface area is determined by using a Body Surface Area Nomogram (see Appendix G) or calculated by using formulas (Appendix F).

The neonate and the premature infant require additional adjustments besides those made on the basis of size. In this population, absorption following oral administration may be incomplete or altered because of changes in gastric pH or GI motility, distribution may be altered because of varying amounts of total body water, and metabolism and excretion may be delayed because liver and kidney function have not yet matured. Progressive hepatic and renal function maturation may necessitate frequent dosage adjustments during the course of therapy to reflect improved drug handling in the premature infant or neonate. Rapid weight changes in this age group require that additional frequent adjustments be made.

In addition to pharmacokinetic variables, other nursing considerations should be addressed. The route of administration chosen in pediatric patients often reflects the seriousness of the illness. The nurse should consider the child's developmental level and ability to understand the situation. Medications that must be administered intravenously or by intramuscular injection may seem frightening to a young child or cause concern to the parents. The nurse should allay these fears by educating the parents and comforting the child. Intramuscular or subcutaneous injection sites should be carefully chosen in this age group to prevent possible nerve or tissue damage.

The Geriatric Patient

In patients more than 55–60 years of age, the pharmacokinetic behavior of drugs changes. Drug absorption may be delayed secondary to diminished GI motility (from age or other drugs) or passive congestion of abdominal blood vessels as seen in congestive heart failure. Distribution may be altered because of low plasma proteins, particularly in malnourished patients. Because plasma proteins are decreased, a larger proportion of free or unbound drug will result in an increase in drug action. The result may be a patient becoming toxic while receiving a standard dose of a drug. Metabolism performed by the liver and excretion handled by the kidneys are both slowed as part of the aging process and may result in prolonged and exaggerated drug action. Body composition also changes with age. There is an increase in fatty tissue and a decrease in skeletal muscle and total body water. Height and weight usually decrease. A dosage of medication that was acceptable for the robust 50-year-old patient may be excessive in the same patient 20 years later.

An additional concern is that most elderly patients are receiving numerous drugs. With increasing numbers of drugs being used, there is an increased risk of one drug negating, potentiating, or otherwise altering the effects of another drug (drug–drug interaction). In general, doses of most medications should be decreased in the geriatric population. Drugs to be specifically concerned about are the cardiac glycosides (digoxin and digitoxin), sedatives/hypnotics, oral anticoagulants, nonsteroidal anti-inflammatory agents, and antihypertensives.

Dosing regimens should be kept simple in this patient population, because many of these patients are taking multiple drugs. Doses should be scheduled so that the patient's day is not interrupted multiple times to take medications. The use of fixed-dose combination drugs may help to simplify dosing regimens. However, some of these combinations are more expensive than the individual components.

In explaining medication regimens to elderly patients, the nurse should remember that hearing deficits are common in this group. Patients may find it embarrassing to disclose this information, and full compliance may be hindered.

The Obstetric Patient

During pregnancy, both the mother and the fetus must be considered. The placenta, once thought to be a protective barrier, is simply a membrane that is capable only of protecting the fetus from extremely large molecules. Transfer of drugs through the placenta to the fetus occurs by both passive and active processes. The fetus is particularly vulnerable during the first trimester and the last trimester of pregnancy. During the first trimester, the vital organs are being formed. Ingestion of drugs that cause harm (potential teratogens) during this stage of pregnancy may lead to fetal malformation or cause miscarriage. Unfortunately, this is the time when a woman is least likely to know that she is pregnant. Therefore, it is wise to inform all patients of child-bearing age of potential harm to an unborn child. In the third trimester the major concern is that drugs that are administered to the mother and transferred to the fetus may not be safely metabolized and excreted by the fetus. This is especially true of drugs administered near term. After the infant is delivered, he or she no longer has the placenta available to help with drug excretion. If drugs administered before delivery are allowed to accumulate, toxicity may result.

The possibility of medications altering sperm quality and quantity in potential fathers also is becoming an area of increasing concern. Male patients should be informed of this risk when taking any medications known to have this potential.

There are situations in which, for the sake of the mother's health and to protect the fetus, drug administration is required throughout pregnancy. Two examples of this are the epileptic patient and the hypertensive patient. In these circumstances, the safest drug in the smallest effective dose is chosen. Because of changes in the behavior of drugs that may occur throughout pregnancy, dosage adjustments may be required during the progression of pregnancy and after delivery. A special situation related to drug behavior in pregnancy is the mother who abuses drugs. Infants born to mothers addicted to alcohol, sedatives (including benzodiazepines), heroin, and cocaine may be of low birth weight, may experience drug withdrawal after birth, and may display developmental delay. A careful history should alert the nurse to these possibilities.

Renal Disease

The kidneys are the major organ of drug elimination. Some drugs are excreted only after being metabolized or biotransformed by the liver. Others may be eliminated unchanged by the kidneys. The premature infant has immature renal function. Elderly patients have an age-related decrease in renal function. In order to make dosage adjustments in patients with renal dysfunction, assessment of the degree of renal impairment in the individual patient and the percentage of drug eliminated by the kidneys must be made. The degree of renal function can be measured by laboratory testing, most commonly by the creatinine clearance (CCr or Ccr), which also can be approximated by calculation (Appendix F). The percentage of each drug excreted by the kidneys can be determined from references on pharmacokinetics. In addition, the dosage frequently can be optimized by measuring blood levels of the drug in the individual patient and making any further necessary changes. Two types of drugs for which this type of dosage adjustment are commonly used are digoxin and the aminoglycoside antibiotics (amikacin, gentamicin, and tobramycin).

Liver Disease

The liver is the major organ for metabolism of drugs. For most drugs this is an inactivation step. The inactive metabolites are subsequently excreted by the kidneys. The conversion process usually changes the drug from a relatively lipid or fat-soluble compound to a more water-soluble substance. Liver function is not as easily quantified as renal function; therefore, it is difficult to predict the correct dosage for a patient with liver dysfunction based on laboratory tests alone. In addition, it appears that only minimal liver function may be required for complete drug metabolism.

A patient who is severely jaundiced or who has very low serum proteins (particularly albumin) may be expected to have some problems metabolizing drugs. Chronic alcoholic patients are at risk of developing this type of situation. In advanced liver disease, drug absorption also may be impaired secondary to portal vascular congestion. Decreased levels of serum proteins also affect the amount of drug that may be bound. If less drug is bound to proteins, then more drug is unbound (free drug) and available to exert its pharmacologic effect. Examples of drugs that should be carefully dosed in patients with liver disease include theophylline, diuretics, and sedatives that are liver-metabolized. Some drugs require the liver for activation (such as sulindac or cyclophosphamide) and should be avoided in patients with severely compromised liver function.

Congestive Heart Failure

Patients with congestive heart failure also require dosage modifications. In these patients, drug absorption may be impaired because of passive congestion of blood vessels feeding the GI tract. This same passive congestion slows drug delivery to the liver and delays metabolism. In addition, renal function may be compromised, leading to delayed elimination and prolonged drug action. Many patients who have congestive heart failure are already in a special dosing category because of their age. Dosages of drugs that are mainly metabolized by the liver or mainly excreted by the kidneys should be decreased in patients with apparent congestive heart failure.

Body Size

In most situations, drug dosing is based on total body weight. Some drugs selectively penetrate fatty tissues. If the drug is known not to penetrate fatty tissues and the patient is obese, dosage should be determined by ideal body weight or estimated lean body mass (e.g., digoxin, gentamicin). These quantities may be determined from tables of desirable weights or may be estimated using formulas for lean body mass when the patient's height and weight are known (see Appendix F). If this type of adjustment is not made, considerable toxicity may result.

Body size also should be appreciated in patients who are grossly underweight. Elderly patients, chronic alcoholics, AIDS patients, and patients who are terminally ill from cancer or other chronic, debilitating illness may need careful attention to dosing, which may be based on the size of a normal adult (70 kg) patient. Patients who have had a major limb amputated also need to have this change in body size taken into account.

Delivery to Sites of Action

In order to have a successful therapeutic outcome, the drug must reach its intended site of action. Under the most desirable of conditions, the drug will have only a minimal effect on other tissues or body systems. A good example is drugs that are applied topically for skin conditions and are only minimally absorbed. In many diseases this arrangement is neither achievable nor practical. Often unusual routes of administration must be used to guarantee the presence of drug at the intended site of response. In patients with bacterial meningitis, administering drugs parenterally may not produce high enough levels in the cerebrospinal fluid. Intrathecal administration may be required in addition to parenteral therapy, as is the case with the aminoglycoside antibiotics (amikacin, gentamicin, and tobramycin). The eye represents another barrier that is relatively impermeable to many drugs. To overcome this barrier, local instillation or injection may be required.

In some cases local absorption may not occur, and the desired systemic effect will not happen. Drugs may not be absorbed into systemic circulation from subcutaneous sites in patients with shock or poor tissue perfusion due to other causes.

When considering the route of administration, identify the site at which the drug is intended to have its primary action. In order to achieve its maximal effect it must be delivered to its intended site of action.

Drug Interactions

The presence of additional drugs may also necessitate dosage adjustments. Drugs highly bound to plasma proteins, such as warfarin and phenytoin, may be displaced by other highly protein bound drugs. When this phenomenon occurs, the drug that has been displaced exhibits an increase in its activity because the free or unbound drug is active.

Some agents decrease the ability of the liver to metabolize other drugs. Drugs capable of doing this include cimetidine and chloramphenicol. Concurrently administered drugs that are highly metabolized by the liver may need to be administered in decreased dosages. Other agents, such as phenobarbital, other barbiturates, and rifampin are capable of stimulating (inducing) the liver to metabolize drugs more rapidly, requiring larger doses to be administered.

Drugs that significantly alter urine pH can affect excretion of other drugs for which the excretory process is pH dependent. Alkalinizing the urine will hasten the excretion of acidic drugs. Acidification of the urine will enhance reabsorption of acidic drugs, prolonging and enhancing drug action. In the reverse situation, drugs that acidify the urine will hasten the excretion of alkaline drugs. An example of this is administering sodium bicarbonate in cases of aspirin overdose. Alkalinizing the urine promotes renal excretion of aspirin.

Some drugs compete for enzyme systems with other drugs. Allopurinol inhibits the enzyme involved in uric acid production, but it also inhibits the metabolism (inactivation) of 6-mercaptopurine, greatly increasing its toxicity. The dosage of mercaptopurine needs to be significantly reduced when coadministered with allopurinol.

Dosage Forms

The nurse frequently encounters problems that relate to the dosage form itself. Some medications may not be commercially available in liquid or chewable dosage forms. The pharmacist may have to compound such dosage forms for an individual patient. It may be necessary to disguise the taste or appearance of a medication in food or a beverage in order for the patient to fully comply with a given regimen. Finally, some dosage forms, such as aerosol inhalers, may not be suitable for very young patients because use of the form requires cooperation beyond the patient's developmental level.

Before altering dosage forms (crushing tablets or opening capsules) or using them by routes for which they were not intended, check to be sure that the effect of the drug will not be altered by doing so. In general, neither extended- nor sustained-release dosage forms should be crushed, nor should capsules containing beads of medication be opened. Altering these dosage forms may shorten and intensify their intended action. Others (sprinkle preparations) are designed to be opened. Enteric-coated tablets, which may appear to be sugar-coated or candy-coated, also should not be crushed. This coating may be designed to protect the stomach from the irritating effects of these drugs. Crushing the tablets will expose the stomach lining to these agents and increase GI irritation. If a dosage form needs to be crushed, it should be ingested right away. A glass of water should be taken before administration of powders or crushed tablets to wet the esophagus and prevent the material from sticking to upper GI mucosal surfaces.

Environmental Factors

Cigarette smoke is capable of inducing liver enzymes to metabolize drugs more rapidly. Patients who smoke may need larger doses of liver-metabolized drugs to compensate for this. Patients who are passively exposed to cigarette smoke also may exhibit otherwise unexplained needs for larger doses of medications. The effect of cigarette smoke on drug metabolism may persist for months.

Nutritional Factors

Certain foods can alter the dosing requirement for some medications. Dietary calcium found in high concentrations in dairy products combines (chelates) with tetracycline and prevents its absorption. Many antibiotics are absorbed better if taken when the stomach is empty. Foods high in pyridoxine (vitamin B_6) content can negate the antiparkinson effect of levodopa (this is counteracted with coadministration of carbidopa). Foods capable of altering urine pH may effect the excretion patterns of medications, enhancing or diminishing their effectiveness. There are no general guidelines for nutritional factors. It is prudent to check if these problems exist, or if they may explain therapeutic failures, and to make the necessary dosage adjustments.

Summary

The average dosing range for drugs is intended for an average patient. However, every patient is an individual with specific drug-handling capabilities. Taking into account these special dosing considerations allows the planning of an individualized drug regimen that results in a desired therapeutic outcome while minimizing the risk of toxicity.

KEY TO COMMONLY USED ABBREVIATIONS

ABGs	arterial blood gases
ac	before meals
ACE	angiotensin converting enzyme
AD	right ear
ADD	attention deficit disorder
AIDS	acquired immunodeficiency syndrome
ANC	absolute neutrophil count
AS	left ear
AU	both ears
bid	two times a day
BP	blood pressure
c̄	with
cap	capsule
CBC	complete blood count
CCr (or Ccr)	creatinine clearance
CNS	central nervous system
COPD	chronic obstructive pulmonary disease
CR	controlled-release
CSF	colony-stimulating factor; cerebrospinal fluid
CV	cardiovascular
CVP	central venous pressure
D5/LR	5% dextrose and lactated Ringer's solution
D5/0.9% NaCl	5% dextrose and 0.9% NaCl; 5% dextrose and normal saline
D5/0.25% NaCl	5% dextrose and 0.25% NaCl; 5% dextrose and quarter normal saline
D5/0.45% NaCl	5% dextrose and 0.45% NaCl; 5% dextrose and half normal saline
D5W	5% dextrose in water
D10W	10% dextrose in water
Derm	dermatologic
dl	deciliter
DNA	deoxyribonucleic acid
ECG	electrocardiogram
EENT	eye, ear, nose, and throat
Endo	endocrinologic
ER	extended-release
F and E	fluid and electrolyte
g	gram(s)
GERD	gastroesophageal reflux disease
GFR	glomerular filtration rate
GI	gastrointestinal
gr	grain(s)
G6-PD	glucose-6-phosphate dehydrogenase
gtt	drop(s)
GU	genitourinary

HDL	high-density lipoproteins
Hemat	hematologic
HIV	human immunodeficiency virus
hr(s)	hour(s)
hs	hour of sleep (bed time)
IA	intra-articular
IL	intralesional
IM	intramuscular
in.	inch(es)
Inhaln	inhalation
IPPB	intermittent positive pressure breathing
IS	intrasynovial
IT	intrathecal
IU	international unit
IV	intravenous
K	potassium
KCl	potassium chloride
kg	kilogram
LDL	low-density lipoproteins
LR	lactated Ringer's solution
MAO	monoamine oxidase
Metab	metabolic
mcg	microgram(s)
mg	milligram(s)
min(s)	minute(s)
Misc	miscellaneous
ml	milliliter(s)
mo(s)	month(s)
MS	musculoskeletal; morphine sulfate
Na	sodium
NaCl	sodium chloride
0.9% NaCl	0.9% sodium chloride, normal saline
Neuro	neurologic
ng	nanogram(s)
NS	sodium chloride, normal saline (0.9% NaCl)
NSAIAs (or NSAIDs)	nonsteroidal anti-inflammatory agents/drugs
OCD	obsessive-compulsive disorder
OD	right eye
Oint	ointment
Ophth	ophthalmic
OS	left eye
OTC	over-the-counter
OU	both eyes
oz	ounce(s)
pc	after meals
PCA	patient-controlled analgesia
PO	by mouth, orally
prn	as needed
q	every
qd	every day
qh	every hour
qid	four times a day

qod	every other day
qwk	every week
q 2 h	every 2 hours
q 3 h	every 3 hours
q 4 h	every 4 hours
RBC	red blood cell count
Rect	rectally or rectal
REM	rapid eye movement
Resp	respiratory
RNA	ribonucleic acid
s̄	without
SC	subcutaneous
sec(s)	second(s)
SL	sublingual
SR	sustained-release
s̄s̄	one half
stat	immediately
supp	suppository
tab	tablet
tbs	tablespoon(s)
tid	three times a day
Top	topically or topical
tsp	teaspoon(s)
UK	unknown
Vag	vaginal
VLDL	very low-density lipoproteins
WBC	white blood cell count
wk(s)	week(s)
yr(s)	year(s)

MEDICATION MISADVENTURES: The Nurse's Role in Detecting, Preventing, and Documenting Adverse Drug Reactions and Medication Errors

Medication misadventures include all drug experiences that result in an unwanted or unintended response to drug therapy. The term includes both adverse drug reactions and medication errors.[1] The nurse should be familiar with the varied aspects of such misadventures and be knowledgeable in how to detect, prevent (if possible), and document these events. Tantamount to this task and as the first step in this process, a detailed and accurate medication history should be obtained, and it should include questions about over-the-counter (nonprescription) medications, dietary or social habits (smoking, alcohol, or drug abuse), and any previous reactions patients have had to medications (allergic and nonallergic).

Adverse Drug Reactions

Unwanted or undesired drug effects fall into several categories. An appreciation of these categories can protect patients from subsequent misadventures when receiving the same drug or drugs in related chemical or pharmacologic categories. Before administering drugs, especially for the first time, it is wise to become familiar with the most commonly encountered adverse drug reactions (underlined in the **Adverse Reactions and Side Effects** section of each monograph). When they manifest, the nurse should know what measures should be taken and how to prioritize them. In addition to commonly encountered reactions, the nurse also should be aware of those more rarely encountered but more disastrous reactions (CAPITALIZED in the **Adverse Reactions and Side Effects** section of each monograph). These may require immediate intervention at the time of the reaction or preparation prior to administering the drug in case they occur.

Adverse drug reactions should be suspected whenever there is a change in a patient's condition not interpreted as a therapeutic response to drugs being administered, particularly when a new drug has been introduced. Although intercurrent or progressive illness also may explain the appearance of new or worsening symptoms, adverse drug reactions and side effects should be strongly considered as a cause.

Dose-Related Reactions (Toxic Reactions): These reactions may mean several different things, but basically the dose prescribed for the patient is excessive. Some of the obvious reasons for this type of reaction include failure to take into account the patient's size (cachectic, elderly, or debilitated patients); failure to appreciate the distributive characteristics of the drug (some drugs do not enter fatty tissue well, basing dose on actual weight rather than ideal body weight may result in toxicity); failure to evaluate excretory/metabolic ability (renal or hepatic impairment from underlying disease or age); failure to determine the effect of other drugs being taken (displacement of drugs for protein binding sites); or increased sensitivity to a drug as a result of underlying illness (hypo-thyroid patients are very sensitive to the effects of digoxin). In any event, the clear course of action is to temporarily discontinue the drug and then to reduce the dose or increase the dosing interval, depending on the drug. In evaluating these reactions, the use of blood level monitoring may take the guesswork out of the situation. Patients should be taught that this type of reaction means that they may still receive the drug in question, despite the occurrence of the effect. They should not be under the misconception that they are "allergic" to the drug. Documentation of reactions as being dose-related is important because it does not preclude use of the drug in question and may lend an appreciation for pa-tient parameters that could determine doses of other drugs.

Side Effects: Side effects are usually considered to be symptoms that occur as a consequence of drug administration and are unrelated to the intended or de-sired action of the drug. Although they are undesirable and may be bothersome, they occur commonly enough at usual doses that patients should be aware of their occurrence and know how to deal with their presence. Certain side effects are so minimal that continued administration of the offending agent is allowed. An example of this type of situation is the headache that usually accompanies nitroglycerin administration. With chronic administration, this side effect dissi-pates and may be managed initially with acetaminophen. Other side effects re-quire dosage alteration, the addition of another agent, or drug discontinuation, depending on patient response or severity of the reaction. Some antihyperten-sives may cause male impotence. If patients find this unacceptable, alternative agents should be sought. Opioid analgesics commonly cause constipation; however, the addition of a laxative to the medication regimen or simple dietary changes can eliminate or prevent this side effect. Appearance of neuroleptic malignant syndrome, a potentially life-threatening reaction that may occur as a consequence of phenothiazine therapy, precludes further use of the offending agent.

Documentation of side effects should identify the agent in question and time of occurrence, and it may help to avoid choosing the offending agent again if the side effect was serious or serve as an aid to patient education if the drug is to be used again.

Idiosyncratic Reactions: These reactions occur without relation to dose. Their occurrence is unpredictable and sporadic. Reactions of this type may manifest in many different ways including fever, blood dyscrasias, cardiovascu-lar effects, or unwanted mental status changes. The time frame between the oc-currence of a problem and initiation of therapy is sometimes the only clue link-ing drug to symptom. Several issues remain puzzling regarding these types of reactions. One is that this reaction may or may not recur when the patient is re-challenged with the same drug. The decision to proceed with rechallenge obvi-ously depends on the necessity of continued therapy and choice of alternatives. Another issue is whether or not the same reaction will occur when similar drugs are given. Again, such decisions are made on an individual basis. Some idio-syncratic reactions may be explained by genetic differences in drug metaboliz-ing enzymes. Patient education is very important, as there needs to be clear un-derstanding of the unpredictability of such events. Patients need to understand that the prescriber has taken into consideration the potential benefits of a par-ticular drug and weighed them against any risks of therapy. When idiosyncratic reactions occur, they may not preclude further treatment with similar agents, but their occurrence should be documented so that the planning of future regi-mens may take them into account.

Hypersensitivity Reactions: Generally speaking, hypersensitivity reactions are usually allergic in nature and imply that there has been previous exposure to the agent. Manifestations of hypersensitivity reactions may range from mild rashes of all types, to nephritis, pneumonitis, or hemolytic anemia, to the potentially life-threatening manifestations of anaphylaxis. Drugs that are proteins (vaccines, enzymes) are more likely to induce hypersensitivity reactions on subsequent exposures. In many instances, antibody formation is involved in the process. In the case of these reactions, it is necessary to consider cross-sensitivity. The best example of this is hypersensitivity to penicillin. If a patient has a history of such a reaction to penicillin, then similar reactions may be expected with related anti-infectives (other penicillins and/or cephalosporins). Because of this, documenting hypersensitivity reactions is very important. Future regimens should avoid related agents, or if they are required, pretreatment (with antihistamines and/or glucocorticoids) or desensitization may be necessary.

Reactions that Occur as a Consequence of a Second (or Third or Fourth) Drug Being Added to the Regimen (Drug–Drug Interactions): Some adverse reactions or side effects may not manifest unless the presence of another drug initiates the process. Neither drug alone can be blamed for the problem, but nonetheless an adverse reaction has occurred. The management of these situations requires careful attention to which drug was started first, when the second agent was added, and how long it took for the reaction to manifest. An example is the interaction between digoxin and quinidine. When quinidine is added to the regimen of a patient who has been stabilized on an appropriate dose of digoxin, in the first several days, many patients experience gastrointestinal complaints (nausea, vomiting). Initially, it would appear that because the quinidine was just started, the quinidine is to blame. However, it has been documented that the presence of quinidine increases serum digoxin levels significantly within the first few days of therapy. In anticipation of this interaction, digoxin dosing may need to be decreased by as much as 50%, and then quinidine may be safely added to the regimen. If a drug–drug interaction occurs or is suspected, the continued need for both agents should be assessed, and appropriate changes in agents or doses should be made. Documenting such events should help to prevent their recurrence in the future. Certain classes of drugs are more likely to result in serious drug–drug interactions, and patients receiving these agents should be monitored carefully. In addition, it is useful to inform patients receiving these drugs to beware of the addition of new agents and to always check with a physician or pharmacist before taking any additional nonprescription drugs. Medications that may produce potentially serious drug–drug interactions are oral anticoagulants, oral hypoglycemic agents, nonsteroidal anti-inflammatory agents, theophylline, monoamine oxidase inhibitors, antihypertensives, anticonvulsants, cimetidine, lithium, and cardiac glycosides.

Food and Drug Administration MedWatch Program

Because of the demand for new drug entities, the time between drug development and marketing is becoming shorter. Consequently, there is a need to continuously survey the occurrence of adverse reactions after marketing has begun. In an effort to monitor and assess the occurrence of adverse reactions, the Food and Drug Administration (FDA) has launched MedWatch, a new program that gives health care practitioners the opportunity to report *serious* adverse reactions or product defects encountered from medications, medical devices, special nutritional products, or other FDA-regulated items. Through this reporting program, products may be withdrawn from the market if reporting is sufficient to warrant it. The FDA considers serious those reactions that may result in death, life-threatening illness or injury, hospitalization, disability, or congenital anomaly or those that may require medical/surgical intervention. In addition to reporting serious adverse reactions, health care providers should also report product problems including suspected contamination, questionable stability, defective components, or poor packaging/labeling. The FDA encourages all physicians, nurses, dentists, and pharmacists to become familiar with this program and to report serious adverse reactions or product problems using the Med-Watch reporting form. Reports should be submitted even if there is some uncertainty about the cause/effect relationship or if some details are missing. This form may be found in this edition of *Davis's Drug Guide for Nurses* and may be photocopied. Reports may also be faxed to the FDA (1-800-FDA-0178) or sent via computer modem (1-800-FDA-7737). If a reaction to a vaccine is suspected, it should be reported to the Vaccine Adverse Event Reporting System (VAERS; 1-800-822-7967). If a report is submitted, the FDA will hold the identity of the patient in strict confidence. Nurses, in addition to other health care providers, have the responsibility for reporting adverse reactions and are encouraged to participate in the MedWatch program.

Medication Errors

Preventing Medication Errors: The most striking difference between adverse drug reactions and medication errors lies in the preventability of the latter. If the goal of optimal drug therapy is to provide the right drug, for the right patient, in the right dose, by the right route, at the right time, and for the right indication, then one can appreciate the many opportunities for potential errors in the process. There are also many checkpoints in the medication process, and the many people located along such checkpoints each play a role in detecting potential errors, preventing their occurrence, and documenting any effects that may occur as a consequence. Because nurses are responsible for administering medications, they are often the last and probably the most important checkpoint in the system. Although errors may take place at this point, they may also be detected and ultimately prevented. The following additional recommendations for nurses have been suggested.[2]

- Become familiar with the institutional medication order process and administration system (floor stock versus unit dose).
- Know where to go for drug information. Resources include physicians, pharmacists, libraries, and drug references.
- Verify orders as much as possible. The transcription process is fraught with places for potential error.
- Use standard drug administration times. This helps to avoid confusion, particularly when lab test monitoring must be performed at a certain time following administration.
- When administering medications, inspect products for possible defects (cracks in capsules, cloudy injections, sediment in solutions). Report these as soon as possible. Verify the identity of the patient before administration. Keep medications clearly labeled as long as possible (leave in unit dose packaging right up to the bedside). Document administration in appropriate records. If a medication is unavailable for administration, resist the temptation to borrow from another patient's supply. Investigate why the drug is not there. There may be compelling reasons for the drug not to be administered pending confirmation of the order (potential interaction, history of previous reaction).
- Observe for any and all drug effects, including the presence of adverse reac-

tions. It is just as important to document the desired therapeutic outcome as it is to report a rash.

- If any drug calculations are necessary, it is wise to check them with another person (pharmacist or nurse). The use of standard concentrations or infusion rate tables may be useful (see Appendix D).
- Be familiar with administration devices before using them and understand their benefits as well as potential disadvantages. The wide variety of high technology delivery systems (infusion pumps, inhalers, patches) requires attention to their proper use.
- Teach patients as much as possible about their medications. Present this information in a format that the patient will understand. Use large print information, translators, pictures, or whatever it takes to produce an informed consumer. Initiate teaching with the first dose and reinforce the information with subsequent doses.
- If a medication is not given as ordered, for whatever reason, this must be documented.

Handling Medication Orders: In handling medication orders, care should be taken to avoid some of these common pitfalls, which may lead to medication errors.

Abbreviations: The use of abbreviations for names of drugs or direction for administration should be discouraged. For example, "AZT" could mean azathioprine, zidovudine, or aztreonam. Generic or brand names should be used. Another example is the direction "qd" (every day), which could be misread as "qid" (four times a day) or "qod" (every other day). The use of standard names (generic/brand) should be encouraged.

Ambiguous Directions: Directions for medication administration should be clearly stated. Avoid "take as directed." Additional directions should be transcribed if they will alter the response to treatment or prevent an adverse reaction. This might include directions to take with food or on an empty stomach.

Dosage Problems: Write doses in strengths rather than dosage units (i.e., in mg, not tablets or half tablets). Make sure to clearly write strengths that may be confused, such as milligrams and micrograms. Abbreviating these could also cause further confusion (mg; mcg). One possible exception to this might be combination drug products. When the strength is specified in units, the word "units" should be spelled out. Using "U" as an abbreviation may be confused with the number "0."

Decimal Problems: Leading zeros should always appear in numbers less than 1 (such as 0.3), whereas terminal zeros to the right of the decimal point should not appear, as they may lead to tenfold dosage errors (misreading 5.0 as 50).

Which Measurement System? If at all possible use the metric system. Older apothecary measurements are not only poorly standardized, their abbreviations are easily confused with other units of measurement.

What's in a Name? Many drugs have similar names. A few prominent examples of this phenomenon are vincristine and vinblastine, carboplatin and cisplatin, digoxin and digitoxin, ranitidine and rimantadine. When there may be doubt, the brand name and generic name may be written together to clarify the identity of the medication, and of course, the dosage should be appropriate for the drug in question.

Verbal Orders: Orders given verbally or over the phone should be put in writing as soon as possible. In doing so, the nurse should repeat the order clearly and make sure that numerical values are understood. This is especially problematic with numbers that end in "teen" (fourteen may be easily confused with forty).

Hold Orders: Orders for temporarily stopping a medication should be clear as to what parameters should be observed in reinstituting therapy. Institutional hold policies should specify a certain period of time in order to avoid confusion. It may make more sense for many types of medication to be discontinued and therapy reinstituted at a later time.

Common Sense: Any order that just does not make sense, would result in a large number of tablets or large injection volume, or is geared toward a disease or problem the patient does not have should be reconfirmed. This includes administration by routes not necessary, as in an order for an intramuscular drug in a patient who is able to take solids.

What If an Error Does Occur?

If, after all preventative steps fail and a medication error occurs, it is vital that the incident be documented, even if no harm comes to the patient. Institutional reporting policies are designed to evaluate where the problem lies and to seek measures that should prevent its recurrence.

References

1. Manasse, HR Jr: Medication use in an imperfect world: Drug misadventuring as an issue of public policy, Part 1. Am J Hosp Pharm 46:929–944, 1989.
2. ASHP Report: ASHP guidelines for preventing medication errors in hospitals. Am J Hosp Pharm 50:305–314, 1993.

CLASSIFICATIONS

▪ ALPHA-ADRENERGIC BLOCKING AGENTS

Pharmacologic Profile

General Use: Used in situations of adrenergic (sympathetic) excess such as pheochromocytoma or hypertensive crises associated with excessive sympathomimetic amines (interaction between monoamine oxidase [MAO] inhibitors and foods containing tyramine).

General Action and Information: Alpha-adrenergic blocking agents noncompetitively block alpha-adrenergic receptors, inhibiting the normal excitatory response to epinephrine and norepinephrine. Receptors primarily affected are located in vascular smooth muscle and exocrine glands.

Contraindications: Conditions in which a precipitous fall in blood pressure could be dangerous.

Precautions: Cardiovascular effects may be severe and require intervention and supportive treatment. Use cautiously in patients with history of peptic ulcer.

Interactions: Any drugs that stimulate alpha-adrenergic receptors will be antagonized. Alpha-adrenergic and beta-adrenergic amines in combination with alpha blockers will result in exaggerated hypotension and arrhythmias.

Nursing Implications

ASSESSMENT
▪ Monitor blood pressure and pulse frequently during initial or IV administration and periodically throughout therapy.

POTENTIAL NURSING DIAGNOSES
▪ Tissue perfusion, altered (indications).
▪ Injury, high risk for (side effects).
▪ Knowledge deficit related to medication regimen (patient/family teaching).

IMPLEMENTATION
▪ **PO:** May be administered with meals or milk if GI irritation becomes a problem.
▪ **IV:** Patient should remain supine throughout parenteral administration.

PATIENT/FAMILY TEACHING
▪ Advise patient to make position changes slowly to minimize orthostatic hypotension.

EVALUATION
Effectiveness of therapy can be demonstrated by: ▪ Decrease in blood pressure.

Alpha-adrenergic Blockers Included in *Davis's Drug Guide for Nurses*
phenoxybenzamine, 925
phentolamine, 926

▪ ANESTHETICS/GENERAL AND LOCAL

Pharmacologic Profile

General Use: Ketamine and thiopental are used as intravenous general anesthetic agents. Other agents that have been used alone or as adjuncts include diazepam, midazolam, propofol, and droperidol/fentanyl. Benzocaine, butamben, dibucaine, dyclonine, lidocaine, pramoxime, prilocaine, and tetracaine are available in a variety of dosage forms for local use.

General Action and Information: General anesthetics provide sufficient CNS depression to allow invasive procedures and are frequently used with sedative/hypnotics, opioid analgesics, and neuromuscular blocking agents. Local anesthetics produce limited and brief effects by decreasing nerve transmission only in the area of injection or application; used in situations when generalized CNS depression is not warranted.

Contraindications: Hypersensitivity.

Precautions: General anesthesia requires skilled personnel and facilities to support respiration. Choose agents and doses carefully in pediatric, geriatric, cardiac, and obstetric patients. Cross-sensitivity may exist for local anesthetics.

Interactions: Many general anesthetics increase cardiac irritability. Risk of arrhythmias may be increased by concurrent cardiac glycoside, beta blocker, or antiarrhythmic therapy. Degree of respiratory depression may be increased by concurrent use of sedative/hypnotics, opioid analgesics, antihistamines, or antidepressants. Concurrent injection of epinephrine with local anesthetics helps to localize and prolong effects.

Nursing Implications—General Anesthetics

ASSESSMENT
▪ Assess level of consciousness frequently throughout therapy.
▪ Monitor blood pressure, ECG, and respiratory status frequently throughout therapy.

POTENTIAL NURSING DIAGNOSES
▪ Injury, high risk for (side effects).
▪ Knowledge deficit related to medication regimen (patient/family teaching).

IMPLEMENTATION
▪ Administer on an empty stomach to prevent vomiting and aspiration.

PATIENT/FAMILY TEACHING
▪ Psychomotor impairment may last for 24 hr following anesthesia. Caution patient to avoid driving or other activities requiring alertness until response to medication is known.
▪ Advise patient to avoid alcohol or other CNS depressants for 24 hr following anesthesia.

EVALUATION
Effectiveness of therapy can be demonstrated by: ▪ General anesthesia.

Nursing Implications—Local Anesthetics

ASSESSMENT
- Assess type, location, and intensity of pain or feeling prior to and a few minutes following administration.
- Assess integrity of involved skin and mucous membranes prior to and periodically throughout course of therapy.

POTENTIAL NURSING DIAGNOSES
- Pain (indications).
- Knowledge deficit related to medication regimen (patient/family teaching).

IMPLEMENTATION
- **Throat Spray:** Ensure gag reflex is intact before allowing patient to eat or drink.
- **Infiltration:** Lidocaine may be combined with epinephrine to minimize systemic absorption and prolong local anesthesia.

PATIENT/FAMILY TEACHING
- Instruct patient on correct application technique. Emphasize the need to avoid contact with the eyes.
- Advise patient to discontinue use if erythema, rash, or irritation at site of administration occurs.

EVALUATION
Effectiveness of therapy can be demonstrated by: ▪ Temporary relief of discomfort associated with minor irritations of the skin or mucous membranes ▪ Local anesthesia.

Anesthetics Included in *Davis's Drug Guide for Nurses*

general anesthetics/adjuncts	local anesthetics
diazepam, 326	benzocaine, 1173
droperidol/fentanyl, 391	butamben, 1173
ketamine, 619	dibucaine, 1173
midazolam, 758	dyclonine, 1173
propofol, 1010	lidocaine, 644
thiopental, 1141	lidocaine/prilocaine, 647
	pramoxime, 1174
	tetracaine, 1174

▪ ANTIANEMICS

Pharmacologic Profile

General Uses: Prevention and treatment of anemias.

General Action and Information: Iron (ferrous fumarate, ferrous gluconate, ferrous sulfate, iron dextran) is required for production of hemoglobin, which is necessary for oxygen transport to cells. Cyanocobalamin and hydroxocobalamin (vitamin B_{12}) and folic acid (vitamin B_9) are water-soluble vitamins that are required for red blood cell production.

Contraindications: Undiagnosed anemias. Hemochromatosis, hemosiderosis, hemolytic anemia (iron).

Precautions: Use parenteral iron cautiously in patients with a history of allergy or hypersensitivity reactions.

Interactions: Iron can decrease the absorption of tetracycline, fluoroquinolones, or penicillamine. Vitamin E may impair the therapeutic response to iron. Phenytoin and other anticonvulsants may decrease the absorption of folic acid. Response to vitamin B_{12} or folic acid may be delayed by chloramphenicol.

Nursing Implications

ASSESSMENT
- Assess patient's nutritional status and dietary history to determine possible cause of anemia and need for patient teaching.
- **Lab Test Considerations:** Monitor hemoglobin, hematocrit, reticulocyte, and indices values before and periodically throughout therapy.

POTENTIAL NURSING DIAGNOSES
- Activity intolerance (indications).
- Nutrition, altered: less than body requirement (indications).
- Knowledge deficit related to medication regimen (patient/family teaching).

IMPLEMENTATION
- Available in combination with many vitamins and minerals (see Appendix A).

PATIENT/FAMILY TEACHING
- Encourage patients to comply with diet recommendations of physician. Explain that the best source of vitamins and minerals is a well-balanced diet with foods from the 4 basic food groups.
- Patients self-medicating with vitamin and mineral supplements should be cautioned not to exceed RDA (see Appendix L). The effectiveness of megadoses for treatment of various medical conditions is unproven and may cause side effects.

EVALUATION
Clinical response is indicated by: ▪ Resolution of anemia.

Antianemics Included in *Davis's Drug Guide for Nurses*

iron (ferrous) salts
- ferrous fumarate, 462
- ferrous gluconate, 463
- ferrous sulfate, 463
- iron dextran, 602

water–soluble vitamins
- cyanocobalamin, 1231
- folic acid, 497
- hydroxocobalamin, 1231

▪ ANTIANGINALS

Pharmacologic Profile

General Uses: Nitrates are used to treat and prevent attacks of angina. Only nitrates (sublingual, lingual spray, or intravenous) may be used in the acute treatment of attacks of angina pectoris. Calcium channel blockers and beta-adrenergic blockers are used prophylactically in long-term management of angina.

General Action and Information: Several different groups of medications are used in the treatment of angina pectoris. The nitrates (isosorbide dinitrate, isosorbide mononitrate, and nitroglycerin) are available as a lingual spray, sublingual tablets, parenterals, transdermal systems, and sustained-release oral dosage forms. Nitrates dilate coronary arteries and cause systemic vasodilation (decreased preload). Calcium channel blockers dilate coronary arteries. Beta-adrenergic blocking agents decrease myocardial oxygen consumption via a decrease in heart rate. Therapy may be combined if selection is designed to minimize side effects or adverse reactions.

Contraindications: Hypersensitivity. Avoid use of beta blockers or calcium channel blockers in advanced heart block, cardiogenic shock, or untreated congestive heart failure.

Precautions: Beta-adrenergic blockers should be used cautiously in patients with diabetes mellitus, pulmonary disease, or hypothyroidism.

Interactions: Nitrates, calcium channel blockers, and beta-adrenergic blockers may cause hypotension with other antihypertensive agents or acute ingestion of alcohol. Verapamil, diltiazem, and beta-adrenergic blockers may have additive myocardial depressant effects when used with other agents that affect cardiac function.

Nursing Implications

ASSESSMENT
- Assess location, duration, intensity, and precipitating factors of patient's anginal pain.
- Monitor blood pressure and pulse periodically throughout therapy.

POTENTIAL NURSING DIAGNOSES
- Pain (indications).
- Tissue perfusion, altered (indications).
- Knowledge deficit related to medication regimen (patient/family teaching).

IMPLEMENTATION
- Available in various dose forms. See specific drugs for information on administration.

PATIENT/FAMILY TEACHING
- Instruct patient on concurrent nitrate therapy and prophylactic antianginal agents to continue taking both medications as ordered and using SL nitroglycerin as needed for anginal attacks.
- Advise patient to contact physician immediately if chest pain does not improve, worsens after therapy, or is accompanied by diaphoresis or shortness of breath, or if severe, persistent headache occurs.
- Caution patient to make position changes slowly to minimize orthostatic hypotension.
- Advise patient to avoid concurrent use of alcohol with these medications.

EVALUATION
Effectiveness of therapy can be demonstrated by: - Decrease in frequency and severity of anginal attacks - Increase in activity tolerance.

C6

Antianginals Included in *Davis's Drug Guide for Nurses*

beta-adrenergic blockers
atenolol, 84
metoprolol, 747
nadolol, 794
propranolol, 1014

calcium channel blockers
amlodipine, 50
bepridil, 112
diltiazem, 351

nicardipine, 814
nifedipine, 819
verapamil, 1219

nitrates and nitrites
amyl nitrite, 69
isosorbide dinitrate, 609
isosorbide mononitrate, 609
nitroglycerin, 825

■ ANTIARRHYTHMICS

Pharmacologic Profile

General Use: Suppression of cardiac arrhythmias.

General Action and Information: Correct cardiac arrhythmias by a variety of mechanisms, depending on the group used. The therapeutic goal is decreased symptomatology and increased hemodynamic performance. Choice of agent depends on etiology of arrhythmia and individual patient characteristics. Treatable causes of arrhythmias should be corrected before therapy is initiated (e.g., electrolyte disturbances). Major antiarrhythmics are generally classified by their effects on cardiac conduction tissue (see Table below). Adenosine, atropine, cardiac glycosides (digitoxin, digoxin), edrophonium, and isoproterenol are also used as antiarrhythmics.

MECHANISM OF ACTION OF MAJOR ANTIARRHYTHMIC DRUGS

GROUP	DRUGS	MECHANISM
I	moricizine	Shares properties of IA, IB and IC agents
IA	quinidine, procainamide, disopyramide	Depress Na conductance, increase APD and ERP, decrease membrane responsiveness
IB	tocainide, lidocaine, phenytoin, mexiletine	Increase K conductance, decrease APD and ERP
IC	flecainide, propafenone	Profound slowing of conduction, markedly depress phase 0
II	acebutolol, esmolol, propranolol, sotalol	Interfere with Na conductance, depress cell membrane, decrease automaticity and increase ERP of the AV node, block excess sympathetic activity
III	amiodarone, bretylium, sotalol	Interfere with norepinephrine, increase APD and ERP
IV	diltiazem, verapamil	Increase AV nodal ERP, Ca channel blocker

Na = sodium; K = potassium; Ca = calcium; ERP = effective refractory period; APD = action-potential duration.

Contraindications: Differ greatly among various agents. See individual drugs.

Precautions: Differ greatly among agents used. Appropriate dosage adjustments should be made in the elderly and those with renal or hepatic impairment, depending on agent chosen. See individual drugs.

Interactions: Differ greatly among agents used. See individual drugs.

Nursing Implications

ASSESSMENT
- Monitor ECG, pulse, and blood pressure continuously throughout IV administration and periodically throughout oral administration.

POTENTIAL NURSING DIAGNOSES
- Cardiac output, decreased (indications).
- Knowledge deficit related to medication regimen (patient/family teaching).

IMPLEMENTATION
- Take apical pulse before administration of oral doses. Withhold dose and notify physician if heart rate is <50 bpm.
- Administer oral doses with a full glass of water. Sustained-release preparations should be swallowed whole. Do not crush, break, or chew tablets or open capsules.

PATIENT/FAMILY TEACHING
- Instruct patient to take oral doses around the clock, as directed, even if feeling better.
- Instruct patient or family member on how to take pulse. Advise patient to report changes in pulse rate or rhythm to physician.
- Caution patient to avoid taking over-the-counter medications without consulting physician or pharmacist.
- Advise patient to carry identification describing disease process and medication regimen at all times.
- Emphasize the importance of follow-up examinations to monitor progress.

EVALUATION
Effectiveness of therapy can be demonstrated by: - Resolution of cardiac arrhythmias without detrimental side effects.

Antiarrhythmics Included in *Davis's Drug Guide for Nurses*

ANTICHOLINERGICS

Pharmacologic Profile

General Uses: Atropine—Bradyarrhythmias. **Scopolamine**—Nausea and vomiting related to motion sickness and vertigo. **Propantheline and glycopyrrolate**—Decreasing gastric secretory activity and increasing esophageal sphincter tone. **Benztropine and trihexyphenidyl**—Management of dyskinesias, including the Parkinsonian syndrome. Atropine, scopolamine, and cyclopentolate are also used as ophthalmic mydriatics.

General Action and Information: Competitively inhibit the action of acetylcholine. In addition, atropine, glycopyrrolate, propantheline, and scopolamine are antimuscarinic in that they inhibit the action of acetylcholine at sites innervated by postganglionic cholinergic nerves.

Contraindications: Hypersensitivity, narrow-angle glaucoma, severe hemorrhage, tachycardia (due to thyrotoxicosis or cardiac insufficiency), or myasthenia gravis.

Precautions: Elderly and pediatric patients are more susceptible to adverse effects. Use cautiously in patients with urinary tract pathology, those at risk for GI obstruction, and those with chronic renal, hepatic, pulmonary, or cardiac disease.

Interactions: Additive anticholinergic effects (dry mouth, dry eyes, blurred vision, constipation) with other agents possessing anticholinergic activity, including antihistamines, antidepressants, quinidine, and disopyramide. May alter GI absorption of other drugs by inhibiting GI motility and increasing transit time. Antacids may decrease absorption of anticholinergics.

Nursing Implications

ASSESSMENT
- Assess vital signs and ECG tracings frequently during the course of IV drug therapy. Report any significant changes in heart rate or blood pressure, or increased ventricular ectopy or angina to physician promptly.
- Monitor intake and output ratios in elderly or surgical patients; may cause urinary retention.
- Assess patient regularly for abdominal distension and auscultate for bowel sounds. Constipation may become a problem. Increasing fluids and adding bulk to the diet may help alleviate constipation.

POTENTIAL NURSING DIAGNOSIS
- Cardiac output, decreased (indications).
- Oral mucous membranes, altered (side effects).
- Constipation (side effects).

IMPLEMENTATION
- **PO:** Administer oral doses of atropine, glycopyrrolate, propantheline, or scopolamine 30 min before meals. Benztropine and trihexyphenidyl should be administered with or immediately after meals.
- Scopolamine transdermal patch should be applied at least 4 hr before travel.

PATIENT/FAMILY TEACHING
- **General Info:** Instruct patient that frequent rinses, sugarless gum or candy, and good oral hygiene may help relieve dry mouth.
- May cause drowsiness. Caution patient to avoid driving or other activities requiring alertness until response to medication is known.
- **Ophth:** Advise patients that ophthalmic preparations may temporarily blur vision and impair ability to judge distances. Dark glasses may be needed to protect eyes from bright light.

EVALUATION
Effectiveness of therapy can be demonstrated by: ▪ Increase in heart rate ▪ Decrease in nausea and vomiting related to motion sickness or vertigo ▪ Dryness of mouth ▪ Dilation of pupils ▪ Decrease in GI motility ▪ Resolution of signs and symptoms of Parkinson's disease.

Anticholinergics included in *Davis's Drug Guide for Nurses*

atropine, 89	propantheline, 1007
benztropine, 110	scopolamine, 1058
cyclopentolate (ophth only), 847	trihexyphenidyl, 1193
glycopyrrolate, 519	

▪ ANTICOAGULANTS/ANTIPLATELET AGENTS

Pharmacologic Profile

General Uses: Prevention and treatment of thromboembolic disorders including deep vein thrombosis, pulmonary embolism, and atrial fibrillation with embolization. Antiplatelet agents are used in a variety of settings to prevent thromboembolic events including stroke and myocardial infarction. Aspirin is used to prevent strokes and myocardial infarction. Dipyridamole is commonly used after cardiac surgery. Ticlopidine is used to prevent thrombotic strokes.

General Action and Information: Anticoagulants are used to prevent clot extension and formation. They do not dissolve clots. The two types of anticoagulants in common use are parenteral heparin and oral warfarin. Therapy is usually initiated with heparin because of its rapid onset of action, while maintenance therapy consists of warfarin. Warfarin takes several days to produce therapeutic anticoagulation. In serious or severe thromboembolic events, heparin therapy may be preceded by thrombolytic therapy (alteplase, anistreplase, streptokinase, or urokinase). Enoxaparin, an anticoagulant similar to heparin, is used only to prevent deep vein thrombosis after hip surgery. Aspirin, dipyridamole, and ticlopidine have antiplatelet activity and are used to prevent myocardial infarction or stroke.

Contraindications: Underlying coagulation disorders, ulcer disease, malignancy, recent surgery, or active bleeding.

Precautions: Anticoagulation should be undertaken cautiously in any patient with a potential site for bleeding. Pregnant or lactating patients should not receive warfarin. Heparin does not cross the placenta.

Interactions: Oral anticoagulants are highly protein-bound and may displace or be displaced by other highly protein-bound drugs. The resultant interactions depend on which drug is displaced. Bleeding may be potentiated by aspirin or large doses of penicillins or penicillin-like drugs, cefamandole, cefotetan, cefoperazone, plicamycin, or valproic acid.

Nursing Implications

ASSESSMENT

- Assess patient for signs of bleeding and hemorrhage (bleeding gums, nose bleed, unusual bruising; tarry, black stools, hematuria, fall in hematocrit or blood pressure; guaiac-positive stools, urine, or nasogastric aspirate).
- Assess patient for evidence of additional or increased thrombosis. Symptoms will depend on area of involvement.
- **Lab Test Considerations:** Monitor activated partial thromboplastin time (aPTT) with heparin therapy, prothrombin time (PT) with warfarin therapy, and hematocrit and other clotting factors frequently during therapy.
- **Toxicity and Overdose:** If overdose occurs or anticoagulation needs to be immediately reversed, the antidote for heparin is protamine sulfate; for warfarin the antidote is vitamin K (phytonadione [AquaMEPHYTON]). Administration of whole blood or plasma may also be required in severe bleeding due to warfarin because of the delayed onset of vitamin K.

POTENTIAL NURSING DIAGNOSES

- Tissue perfusion, altered (indications).
- Injury, high risk for (side effects).
- Knowledge deficit related to medication regimen (patient/family teaching).

IMPLEMENTATION

- Inform all personnel caring for patient of anticoagulant therapy. Venipunctures and injection sites require application of pressure to prevent bleeding or hematoma formation.
- Use an infusion pump with continuous infusions to ensure accurate dosage.

PATIENT/FAMILY TEACHING

- Caution patient to avoid activities leading to injury, to use a soft toothbrush and electric razor, and to report any symptoms of unusual bleeding or bruising to physician immediately.
- Instruct patient not to take over-the-counter medications, especially those containing aspirin, ibuprofen, or alcohol without advice of physician or pharmacist.
- Review foods high in vitamin K (see Appendix K) with patients on warfarin. Patient should have consistent limited intake of these foods, as vitamin K is the antidote for warfarin and alternating intake of these foods will cause PT levels to fluctuate.
- Emphasize the importance of frequent lab tests to monitor coagulation factors.
- Instruct patient to carry identification describing medication regimen at all times and to inform all health care personnel caring for patient of anticoagulant therapy before laboratory tests, treatment, or surgery.

EVALUATION

Clinical response can be evaluated by: ▪ Prevention of undesired clotting without signs of hemorrhage.

Anticoagulants Included in *Davis's Drug Guide for Nurses*

anticoagulants	antiplatelet agents
enoxaparin, 403	aspirin, 80
heparin, 543	dipyridamole, 364
warfarin, 1235	ticlopidine, 1155

■ ANTICONVULSANTS

Pharmacologic Profile

General Uses: See Table below.

General Action and Information: Anticonvulsants include a variety of agents, all capable of depressing abnormal neuronal discharges in the CNS that may result in seizures. They may work by preventing the spread of seizure activity, depressing the motor cortex, raising seizure threshold, or altering levels of neurotransmitters, depending on the group. See individual drugs.

MAJOR ANTICONVULSANT CLASSES, DRUGS, AND MOST COMMON USES

CLASS	DRUGS	TYPE OF SEIZURE CONTROLLED
Barbiturates	amobarbital	Status epilepticus
	phenobarbital	Tonic-clonic seizures, partial seizures, prophylaxis of febrile seizures
	primidone	Prophylaxis of partial seizures with complex symptomatology
Benzodiazepines	clonazepam	Absence seizures, akinetic seizures, myoclonic seizures
	clorazepate	Partial seizures
	diazepam (IV)	Status epilepticus, tonic-clonic seizures
Hydantoins	phenytoin	Tonic-clonic seizures, partial seizures with complex symptomatology
Succinimides	ethosuximide	Absence seizures
Miscellaneous	acetazolamide	Refractory seizures
	carbamazepine	Tonic-clonic seizures, complex partial seizures, mixed seizures
	felbamate	Partial seizures, Lennox-Gastaut syndrome
	magnesium sulfate	Eclamptic seizures
	valproates	Simple and complex partial seizures

Contraindications: Previous hypersensitivity.

Precautions: Use cautiously in patients with severe hepatic or renal disease; dosage adjustment may be required. Choose agents carefully in pregnant and lactating women. Fetal hydantoin syndrome may occur in offspring of patients who receive phenytoin during pregnancy.

Interactions: Barbiturates stimulate the metabolism of other drugs that are metabolized by the liver, decreasing their effectiveness. Hydantoins are highly protein-bound and may displace or be displaced by other highly protein-bound drugs. For more specific interactions, see individual drugs. Many drugs are capable of lowering seizure threshold and may decrease the effectiveness of anticonvulsants, including tricyclic antidepressants and phenothiazines.

Nursing Implications

ASSESSMENT
- Assess location, duration, and characteristics of seizure activity.
- **Toxicity and Overdose:** Monitor serum drug levels routinely throughout anticonvulsant therapy.

C L A S S I F I C A T I O N S

POTENTIAL NURSING DIAGNOSES

- Injury, high risk for (indications, side effects).
- Knowledge deficit related to medication regimen (patient/family teaching).

IMPLEMENTATION

- Administer anticonvulsants around-the-clock. Abrupt discontinuation may precipitate status epilepticus.
- Implement seizure precautions.

PATIENT/FAMILY TEACHING

- Instruct patient to take medication every day, exactly as directed.
- May cause drowsiness. Caution patient to avoid driving or other activities requiring alertness until response to medication is known. Do not resume driving until physician gives clearance based on control of seizures.
- Advise patient to avoid taking alcohol or other CNS depressants concurrently with these medications.
- Advise patient to carry identification describing disease process and medication regimen at all times.

EVALUATION

Effectiveness of therapy can be demonstrated by: ▪ Decrease or cessation of seizures without excessive sedation.

Anticonvulsants Included in *Davis's Drug Guide for Nurses*

barbiturates
  amobarbital, 52
  phenobarbital, 920
  primidone, 985
  thiopental, 1140

benzodiazepines
  clonazepam, 263
  clorazepate, 267
  diazepam, 326

hydantoins
  phenytoin, 933

succinamides
  ethosuximide, 436

valproates
  valproic acid, 1210
  divalproex sodium, 1210

miscellaneous
  acetazolamide, 170
  carbamazepine, 164
  felbamate, 453
  magnesium sulfate, 680

▪ ANTIDEPRESSANTS

Pharmacologic Profile

General Uses: Used in the treatment of various forms of endogenous depression, often in conjunction with psychotherapy. Other uses include: ▫ Treatment of anxiety (doxepin) ▫ Enuresis (imipramine) ▫ Chronic pain syndromes (amitriptyline, doxepin, imipramine, and nortriptyline).

General Action and Information: Antidepressant activity most likely due to preventing the reuptake of dopamine, norepinephrine, and serotonin by presynaptic neurons resulting in accumulation of these neurotransmitters. Most possess significant anticholinergic and sedative properties, which explain many of their side effects (except bupropion, sertraline, paroxetine, and fluoxetine).

Contraindications: Hypersensitivity. Should not be used in narrow-angle glaucoma. Should not be used in pregnancy or lactation or immediately after myocardial infarction.

Precautions: Use cautiously in older patients and those with pre-existing cardiovascular disease. Elderly men with prostatic enlargement may be more susceptible to urinary retention. Anticholinergic side effects (dry eyes, dry mouth, blurred vision, and constipation) may require dosage modification or drug discontinuation. Dosage requires slow titration; onset of therapeutic response may be 2–4 wk. May decrease seizure threshold, especially bupropion.

Interactions: Tricyclic antidepressants—May cause hypertension, tachycardia, and convulsions when used with monoamine oxidase (MAO) inhibitors. May prevent therapeutic response to some antihypertensives. Additive CNS depression with other CNS depressants. Sympathomimetic activity may be enhanced when used with other sympathomimetics. Additive anticholinergic effects with other drugs possessing anticholinergic properties. **MAO inhibitors**—Hypertensive crisis may occur with concurrent use of MAO inhibitors and amphetamines, methyldopa, levodopa, dopamine, epinephrine, norepinephrine, desipramine, imipramine, guanethidine, reserpine, vasoconstrictors, or ingestion of tyramine-containing foods. Hypertension or hypotension, coma, convulsions, and death may occur with meperidine or other opioid analgesics and MAO inhibitors. Additive hypotension with antihypertensives or spinal anesthesia and MAO inhibitors. Additive hypoglycemia with insulin or oral hypoglycemic agents and MAO inhibitors. **Fluoxetine, bupropion, paroxetine,** or **sertraline** should not be used in combination with or within weeks of MAO inhibitors (see individual monographs).

Nursing Implications

ASSESSMENT
- Monitor mental status and affect. Assess for suicidal tendencies, especially during early therapy. Restrict amount of drug available to patient.
- **Toxicity and Overdose:** Concurrent ingestion of monamine oxidase inhibitors and tyramine-containing foods may lead to hypertensive crisis. Symptoms include chest pain, severe headache, nuchal rigidity, nausea and vomiting, photosensitivity, and enlarged pupils. Treatment includes IV phentolamine.

POTENTIAL NURSING DIAGNOSES
- Coping, ineffective individual (indications).
- Injury, high risk for (side effects).
- Knowledge deficit related to medication regimen (patient/family teaching).

IMPLEMENTATION
- Administer drugs that are sedating at bedtime to avoid excessive drowsiness during waking hours and drugs that cause insomnia (fluoxetine, paroxetine, monamine oxidase inhibitors) in the morning. Bupropion must be given in divided doses.

PATIENT/FAMILY TEACHING
- Caution patient to avoid alcohol and other CNS depressants. Patients receiving monamine oxidase inhibitors should also avoid over-the-counter drugs and foods or beverages containing tyramine (see Appendix K for foods included) during and for at least 2 wk after therapy has been discontinued, as they may precipitate a hypertensive crisis. Physician should be contacted immediately if symptoms of hypertensive crisis develop.
- Inform patient that dizziness or drowsiness may occur. Caution patient to

avoid driving and other activities requiring alertness until response to the drug is known.
- Caution patient to make position changes slowly to minimize orthostatic hypotension.
- Advise patient to notify physician if dry mouth, urinary retention, or constipation occurs. Frequent rinses, good oral hygiene, and sugarless candy or gum may diminish dry mouth. An increase in fluid intake, fiber, and exercise may prevent constipation.
- Advise patient to notify physician or dentist of medication regimen before treatment or surgery. Monamine oxidase inhibitor therapy usually needs to be withdrawn at least 2 wk before use of anesthetic agents.
- Emphasize the importance of participation in psychotherapy and follow-up examinations to evaluate progress.

EVALUATION
Effectiveness of therapy can be demonstrated by: ■ Resolution of depression ■ Decrease in anxiety ■ Control of bedwetting in children over 6 yr of age ■ Management of chronic neurogenic pain.

Antidepressants Included in *Davis's Drug Guide for Nurses*

tricyclic antidepressants	*miscellaneous antidepressants*	*monoamine oxidase (MAO) inhibitors*
amitriptyline, 48	bupropion, 143	isocarboxazid, 780
amoxapine, 54	fluoxetine, 488	phenelzine, 780
doxepin, 380	maprotiline, 684	tranylcypromine, 780
imipramine, 579	paroxetine, 884	
nortriptyline, 835	sertraline, 1065	
	trazadone, 1181	

■ ANTIDIABETIC AGENTS

Pharmacologic Profile

General Use: Insulin is used in the management of insulin-dependent diabetes mellitus (IDDM, type I, juvenile-onset). It may also be used in adult-onset non–insulin-dependent diabetes mellitus (NIDDM, type II, adult-onset) when diet and/or oral hypoglycemic therapy fails to adequately control blood sugar. The choice of insulin preparation (rapid-acting, intermediate-acting, long-acting) and source (beef, beef/pork, pork, semisynthetic, human-recombinant DNA) depends on the degree of control desired, daily blood sugar fluctuations, and history of previous reactions. Oral hypoglycemics can only be used in adult-onset non–insulin-dependent diabetes mellitus (NIDDM, type II, adult-onset). Oral agents are used when diet therapy alone fails to control blood sugar or symptoms or when patients are not amenable to using insulin.

General Action and Information: Insulin, a hormone produced by the pancreas, lowers blood glucose by increasing transport of glucose into cells and promotes the conversion of glucose to glycogen. It also promotes the conversion of amino acids to proteins in muscle, stimulates triglyceride formation, and inhibits the release of free fatty acids. Oral hypoglycemic agents lower blood sugar by stimulating endogenous insulin secretion by beta cells of the pancreas and by increasing sensitivity to insulin at intracellular receptor sites. Intact pancreatic function is required for oral agents. Chemically, oral hypoglycemics are referred to as sulfonylureas.

Contraindications: Insulin—Hypoglycemia. **Oral hypoglycemic agents—** Hypersensitivity (cross-sensitivity with other sulfonylureas and sulfonamides may exist). Hypoglycemia. Insulin-dependent diabetes mellitus (IDDM, type I, juvenile-onset, brittle). Avoid use in patients with severe kidney, liver, thyroid, and other endocrine dysfunction. Should not be used in pregnancy or lactation.

Precautions: Insulin—Infection, stress, or changes in diet may alter requirements. **Oral hypoglycemic agents**—Use cautiously in the elderly—dosage reduction may be necessary. Infection, stress, or changes in diet may alter requirements. Use with caution in patients with a history of cardiovascular disease.

Interactions: Insulin—Additive hypoglycemic effects with oral hypoglycemic agents. **Oral hypoglycemic agents**—Ingestion of alcohol may result in disulfiram-like reaction. Alcohol, glucocorticoids, rifampin, glucagon, and thiazide diuretics may decrease effectiveness. Anabolic steroids, chloramphenicol, clofibrate, MAO inhibitors, most nonsteroidal anti-inflammatory agents, salicylates, sulfonamides, and oral anticoagulants may increase hypoglycemic effect. Beta-adrenergic blocking agents may produce hypoglycemia and mask signs and symptoms.

Nursing Implications

ASSESSMENT
- Observe patient for signs and symptoms of hypoglycemic reactions.

POTENTIAL NURSING DIAGNOSES
- Nutrition, altered: more than body requirements (indications).
- Knowledge deficit related to medication regimen (patient/family teaching).
- Noncompliance (patient/family teaching).

IMPLEMENTATION
- **General Info:** Patients stabilized on a diabetic regimen who are exposed to stress, fever, trauma, infection, or surgery may require sliding scale insulin.
- Patients switching from daily insulin dose may require gradual conversion to oral hypoglycemics.
- **Insulin:** Available in different types and strengths and from different species. Check type, species' source, dose, and expiration date with another licensed nurse. Do not interchange insulins without physician's order. Use only insulin syringes to draw-up dose.

PATIENT/FAMILY TEACHING
- **General Info:** Explain to patient that medication controls hyperglycemia but does not cure diabetes. Therapy is long term.
- Review signs of hypoglycemia and hyperglycemia with patient. If hypoglycemia occurs, advise patient to take a glass of orange juice or 2–3 tsp of sugar, honey, or corn syrup dissolved in water, and notify physician.
- Encourage patient to follow prescribed diet, medication, and exercise regimen to prevent hypoglycemic or hyperglycemic episodes.
- Instruct patient in proper testing of serum glucose or urine glucose and ketones.
- Advise patient to notify physician if nausea, vomiting, or fever develops; if unable to eat usual diet; or if blood sugar levels are not controlled.
- Advise patient to carry sugar and identification describing medication regimen at all times.

- **Insulin:** Instruct patient on proper technique for administration; include type of insulin, equipment (syringe and cartridge pens), storage, and where to discard syringes. Discuss the importance of not changing brands of insulin or syringes, selection and rotation of injection sites, and compliance with therapeutic regimen.
- **Oral Hypoglycemic Agents:** Advise patient that concurrent use of alcohol may cause a disulfiram-like reaction (abdominal cramps, nausea, flushing, headaches, and hypoglycemia).

EVALUATION

Effectiveness of therapy can be demonstrated by: ▪ Control of blood glucose levels without the appearance of hypoglycemic or hyperglycemic episodes.

Antidiabetic Agents Included in *Davis's Drug Guide for Nurses*

oral hypoglycemic agents
acetohexamide, 855
chlorpropamide, 855
glipizide, 855
glyburide, 855
tolazamide, 855
tolbutamide, 855

insulins, 589
rapid-acting insulin
regular insulin
prompt zinc suspension

intermediate-acting insulin
isophane suspension,
NPH insulin
zinc suspension, lente insulin

long-acting insulin
extended zinc suspension,
ultra lente insulin

insulin mixture
regular plus NPH insulin

▪ ANTIDIARRHEALS

Pharmacologic Profile

General Use: For the control and symptomatic relief of acute and chronic nonspecific diarrhea.

General Action and Information: Diphenoxylate/atropine, difenoxin/atropine, loperamide, and paregoric slow intestinal motility and propulsion. Attapulgite, kaolin/pectin, and bismuth subsalicylate affect fluid content of the stool. Polycarbophil acts as an antidiarrheal by taking on water within the bowel lumen to create a formed stool. Octreotide is used specifically for diarrhea associated with gastrointestinal endocrine tumors.

Contraindications: Previous hypersensitivity. Severe abdominal pain of unknown cause, especially when associated with fever.

Precautions: Use cautiously in patients with severe liver disease or inflammatory bowel disease. Safety in pregnancy and lactation not established (diphenoxylate/atropine and loperamide). Octreotide may aggravate gall bladder disease.

Interactions: Kaolin may decrease absorption of digoxin. Polycarbophil decreases the absorption of tetracycline. Octreotide may alter the response to insulin or oral hypoglycemic agents. Attapulgite may decrease absorption of medications administered orally within 3 hr before or 4 hr after.

Nursing Implications

ASSESSMENT
- Assess the frequency and consistency of stools and bowel sounds before and throughout course of therapy.
- Assess patient's fluid and electrolyte status and skin turgor for dehydration.

POTENTIAL NURSING DIAGNOSES
- Diarrhea (indications).
- Constipation (side effects).
- Knowledge deficit related to medication regimen (patient/family teaching).

IMPLEMENTATION
- Shake liquid preparations before administration.

PATIENT/FAMILY TEACHING
- Instruct patient to notify physician if diarrhea persists; or if fever, abdominal pain, or palpitations occur.

EVALUATION
Effectiveness of therapy can be demonstrated by: ▪ Decrease in diarrhea.

Antidiarrheals Included in *Davis's Drug Guide for Nurses*

▪ ANTIDOTES

Pharmacologic Profile

General Use: See Table below.

General Action and Information: Antidotes are employed in accidental and intentional overdoses of medications or toxic substances. The goal of antidotal therapy is to decrease systemic complications of the overdosage while supporting vital functions. Obtaining a precise history will determine aggressiveness of therapy, choice, and dose of agent. Some antidotes are designed to aid removal of the offending agent before systemic absorption occurs, or speed elimination (activated charcoal). Other agents are more specific and require more detailed history as to type and amount of agent ingested.

POISONS AND SPECIFIC ANTIDOTES

POISON	ANTIDOTE
acetaminophen	acetylcysteine
anticholinesterases	atropine, pralidoxime
benzodiazepines	flumazenil
cyanide	amyl nitrite, sodium nitrite, sodium thiosulfate
digoxin, digitoxin	digoxin immune Fab
fluorouracil	leucovorin calcium
heparin	protamine sulfate

C
L
A
S
S
I
F
I
C
A
T
I
O
N
S

POISON	ANTIDOTE
iron	deferoxamine
lead	edetate calcium disodium, dimercaprol, succimer
methotrexate	leucovorin calcium
opioid analgesics, heroin	naloxone
tricyclic antidepressants	physostigmine
warfarin	phytonadione (vitamin K_1)

Contraindications: See individual drugs.

Precautions: See individual drugs.

Interactions: See individual drugs.

Nursing Implications

ASSESSMENT
- Inquire as to the type of drug or poison and time of ingestion.
- Consult reference, poison control center, or physician for symptoms of toxicity of ingested agent(s) and antidote. Monitor vital signs, affected systems, and serum levels closely.
- Monitor for suicidal ideation; institute suicide precautions as necessary.

POTENTIAL NURSING DIAGNOSIS
- Ineffective coping, individual (indications).
- Injury, high risk for: poisoning (patient/family teaching).
- Knowledge deficit related to medication regimen (patient/family teaching).

IMPLEMENTATION
- May be used in conjunction with induction of emesis or gastric aspiration and lavage, cathartics, agents to modify urine pH, and supportive measures for respiratory and cardiac effects of overdose or poisoning.

PATIENT/FAMILY TEACHING
- When counseling about poisoning in the home, discuss methods of prevention and the need to confer with poison control center, physician, or emergency department prior to administering syrup of ipecac, and the need to bring ingested substance to the hospital for identification. Reinforce need to keep all medications and hazardous substances out of the reach of children.

EVALUATION
Effectiveness of therapy is demonstrated by: ▪ Prevention or resolution of toxic side effects of ingested agent.

Antidotes Included in *Davis's Drug Guide for Nurses*

acetylcysteine, 4
amyl nitrite, 69
atropine, 89
deferoxamine, 310
digoxin immune Fab, 348
dimercaprol, 355
edetate calcium disodium, 395
flumazenil, 480

leucovorin calcium, 633
naloxone, 802
physostigmine, 937
phytonadione (vitamin K_1), 939
pralidoxime, 973
protamine sulfate, 1019
succimer, 1097

▪ ANTIEMETICS

Pharmacologic Profile

General Use: Phenothiazines, benzquinamide, metoclopramide, trimethoben-zamide, and ondansetron are used to manage nausea and vomiting of many causes, including surgery, anesthesia, and antineoplastic therapy. Dimenhydrinate, scopolamine, and meclizine are used almost exclusively to prevent motion sickness. Dronabinol is used for short-term management of nausea and vomiting associated with antineoplastics and to stimulate appetite in patients with AIDS.

General Action and Information: Phenothiazines and benzquinamide act on the chemoreceptor trigger zone to inhibit nausea and vomiting. Dimenhydrinate, scopolamine, and meclizine act as antiemetics mainly by diminishing motion sickness. Metoclopramide decreases nausea and vomiting by its effects on gastric emptying. Dronabinol acts centrally to decrease nausea and vomiting. Ondansetron blocks the effects of serotonin.

Contraindications: Previous hypersensitivity.

Precautions: Use phenothiazines cautiously in children who may have viral illnesses. Choose agents carefully in pregnant patients (no agents are approved for safe use).

Interactions: Additive CNS depression with other CNS depressants including antidepressants, antihistamines, opioid analgesics, and sedative/hypnotics. Phenothiazines may produce hypotension when used with antihypertensives, nitrates, or acute ingestion of alcohol.

Nursing Implications

ASSESSMENT
▪ Assess nausea, vomiting, bowel sounds, and abdominal pain before and following administration.
▪ Monitor hydration status and intake and output. Patients with severe nausea and vomiting may require IV fluids in addition to antiemetics.

POTENTIAL NURSING DIAGNOSES
▪ Fluid volume deficit (indications).
▪ Nutrition, altered: less than body requirements (indications).
▪ Injury, high risk for (side effects).

IMPLEMENTATION
▪ For prophylactic administration, follow directions for specific drugs so that peak effect corresponds to time of anticipated nausea.

PATIENT/FAMILY TEACHING
▪ Advise patient and family to use general measures to decrease nausea (begin with sips of liquids and small nongreasy meals, provide oral hygiene, and remove noxious stimuli from environment).
▪ May cause drowsiness. Advise patient to call for assistance when ambulating and to avoid driving or other activities requiring alertness until response to medication is known.

- Advise patient to make position changes slowly to minimize orthostatic hypotension.

EVALUATION
Effectiveness of therapy can be demonstrated by: ■ Prevention of, or decrease in, nausea and vomiting.

Antiemetics Included in *Davis's Drug Guide for Nurses*

anticholinergic
scopolamine, 1058

antihistamines
dimenhydrinate, 354
meclizine, 693

phenothiazines
chlorpromazine, 235
perphenazine, 917
prochlorperazine, 995

promethazine, 1003
thiethylperazine, 1136
trifluoperazine, 1191

miscellaneous
benzquinamide, 108
dronabinol, 387
metoclopramide, 741
ondansetron, 845
trimethobenzamide, 1197

■ ANTIFUNGALS

Pharmacologic Profile

General Use: Treatment of fungal infections. Infections of skin or mucous membranes may be treated with topical or vaginal preparations. Deep-seated or systemic infections require oral or parenteral therapy.

General Action and Information: Kill (fungicidal) or stop growth of (fungistatic) susceptible fungi by affecting the permeability of the fungal cell membrane or protein synthesis within the fungal cell itself.

Contraindications: Previous hypersensitivity.

Precautions: Since most systemic antifungals may have adverse effects on bone marrow function, use cautiously in patients with depressed bone marrow reserve. Amphotericin B commonly causes renal impairment. Flucytosine and fluconazole require dosage adjustment in the presence of renal impairment. Adverse reactions to fluconazole may be more severe in HIV-positive patients.

Interactions: Differ greatly among various agents. See individual drugs.

Nursing Implications

ASSESSMENT
- Assess patient for signs of infection and assess involved areas of skin and mucous membranes before and throughout therapy.

POTENTIAL NURSING DIAGNOSES
- Infection, high risk for (indications).
- Skin integrity, impairment of (indications).
- Knowledge deficit related to medication regimen (patient/family teaching).

IMPLEMENTATION
- **General Info:** Available in various dosage forms. Refer to specific drugs for directions for administration.
- **Topical:** Consult physician for cleansing technique before applying medication. Wear gloves during application. Do not use occlusive dressings unless specified by physician.

PATIENT/FAMILY TEACHING
- Instruct patient on proper use of medication form.
- Advise patient to report increased skin irritation or lack of therapeutic response to physician.

EVALUATION
Effectiveness of therapy can be demonstrated by: ▪ Resolution of signs and symptoms of infection. Length of time for complete resolution depends on organism and site of infection. Deep-seated fungal infections may require prolonged therapy (weeks–months).

Antifungals Included in *Davis's Drug Guide for Nurses*

ophthalmic antifungals
natamycin, 847

systemic antifungals
amphotericin B, 61
fluconazole, 473
flucytosine, 474
griseofulvin, 529
itraconazole, 615
ketoconazole, 621
miconazole, 757

topical antifungals
amphotericin B, 1167
ciclopirox, 1167
clioquinol, 1167
clotrimazole, 1167
econazole, 1167
haloprogin, 1167

ketoconazole, 1167
miconazole, 1167
naftifine, 1167
nystatin, 1167
oxiconazole, 1167
sulconazole, 1167
terbinafine, 1167
tolnafate, 1167
triacetin, 1167
undecylenic acid, 1167

vaginal antifungals
butoconazole, 1208
clotrimazole, 1208
miconazole, 1208
nystatin, 1208
terconazole, 1208
tioconazole, 1208

▪ ANTIGLAUCOMA AGENTS

Pharmacologic Profile

General Use: Management of glaucoma. Open-angle glaucoma is usually treated with medications. Other forms of glaucoma may require surgery.

General Action and Information: Agents used in the management of glaucoma decrease intraocular pressure by either decreasing the formation of aqueous humor or increasing the outflow of aqueous humor. Ophthalmic beta blockers and orally administered carbonic anhydrase inhibitors decrease the production of aqueous humor. Direct-acting miotics, cholinesterase inhibitors, and sympathomimetics increase aqueous humor outflow.

Contraindications: Avoid use in patients with hypersensitivity to medications themselves, additives, or preservatives. Miotics should be avoided in patients with narrow-angle glaucoma.

Precautions: Use cautiously in patients with underlying cardiovascular disease, diabetes mellitus, or severe pulmonary disease.

Interactions: Beta blockers and carbonic anhydrase inhibitors have additive effects on intraocular pressure with other agents. Miotics and sympathomimetics also have additive effects and are frequently used together. Cholinesterase inhibitors may prolong the action of neuromuscular blocking agents.

Nursing Implications

ASSESSMENT
- Monitor patient for changes in vision, eye irritation, and persistent headache.
- Monitor patient for signs of systemic side effects. Notify physician if these signs occur.

POTENTIAL NURSING DIAGNOSES
- Sensory-perceptual alteration: visual (indications, side effects).
- Knowledge deficit related to medication regimen (patient/family teaching).

IMPLEMENTATION
- When instilling eyedrops, have patient tilt head back, pull down on the lower lid, and instill drops into the conjunctival sac. Apply pressure to the inner canthus for 1 minute following instillation to prevent systemic absorption.

PATIENT/FAMILY TEACHING
- Instruct patient to take as directed and not to discontinue without physician's approval. Lifelong therapy may be required.
- Instruct patient on correct technique for administration of ophthalmic medication. Emphasize the importance of not touching tip of container to eye, finger, or any other surface, and of preventing systemic absorption by placing pressure on the inner canthus.
- Explain to patient that temporary stinging and blurring of vision may occur. Physician should be notified if blurred vision or brow ache persists.
- Caution patient that night vision may be impaired. Advise patient not to drive at night until response to medication is known. To prevent injury at night, patient should use a night-light and keep environment uncluttered.
- Advise patient of the need for regular eye examinations to monitor intraocular pressure and visual fields.

EVALUATION
Effectiveness of therapy can be demonstrated by: - Control of elevated intraocular pressure.

Antiglaucoma Agents Included in *Davis's Drug Guide for Nurses*

beta blockers (ophthalmic)	carbonic anhydrase inhibitors
betaxolol, 119	acetazolamide, 170
carteolol, 179	dichlorphenamide, 170
levobunolol, 847	methazolamide, 170
metipranolol, 847	
timolol, 1157	

miotic (cholinesterase inhibitors)
demecarium, 847
echothiophate, 847
isoflurophate, 847
physostigmine, 937

miotics (direct-acting)
carbachol, 847
pilocarpine, 847

sympathomimetics
apraclonidine, 847
epinephrine, 407

miscellaneous
glycerin, 517

▪ ANTIGOUT AGENTS

Pharmacologic Profile

General Use: In the treatment of active gout (colchicine) and prevention of recurrent attacks (allopurinol, probenecid). Allopurinol and probenecid are also used to treat secondary hyperuricemia.

General Action and Information: Reduce the inflammatory response (colchicine) or lower serum uric acid either by enhancing its renal excretion (probenecid, sulfinpyrazone) or decreasing its production (allopurinol). Sulfinpyrazone also has antiplatelet activity.

Contraindications: Hypersensitivity. Allopurinol should be avoided during acute attacks of gout.

Precautions: Akalinizing the urine enhances uricosuric effects. Rapid lowering of uric acid may cause precipitation of urate cystals in soft tissue.

Interactions: Probenecid promotes reabsorption and increases blood levels of many drugs including penicillins and cephalosporins. This interaction may be used to produce higher and more sustained blood levels of these drugs. Allopurinol increases toxicity from several antineoplastic agents (6-mercaptopurine, azathioprine). When allopurinol and ampicillin are used concurrently, the incidence of skin rash is greatly increased. Small doses of aspirin ($<$2 g/day) elevate serum uric acid and may interfere with the management of gout. Sulfinpyrazone may increase the risk of bleeding with other agents that affect hemostasis (aspirin, anticoagulants).

Nursing Implications

ASSESSMENT
▪ Assess for joint pain and swelling throughout therapy.
▪ Monitor intake and output ratios. Ensure that patient maintains adequate fluid intake (minimum 2500–3000 ml/day) to minimize risk of kidney stone formation.

POTENTIAL NURSING DIAGNOSES
▪ Pain (indications).
▪ Knowledge deficit related to medication regimen (patient/family teaching).

IMPLEMENTATION
▪ Administer with or after meals to minimize gastric irritation.

PATIENT/FAMILY TEACHING
- Inform patient of the need for increased fluid intake.
- Advise patient to follow physician's recommendations regarding weight loss, diet, and alcohol consumption.

EVALUATION
Effectiveness of therapy can be demonstrated by: ▪ Prevention or treatment of gout.

Antigout Agents Included in *Davis's Drug Guide for Nurses*
allopurinol, 20   probenecid, 987
colchicine, 275   sulfinpyrazone, 1107

▪ ANTIHISTAMINES

Pharmacologic Profile

General Uses: Relief of symptoms associated with allergies, including rhinitis, urticaria, and angioedema, and as adjunctive therapy in anaphylactic reactions. Some antihistamines are used to treat motion sickness (dimenhydrinate and meclizine); insomnia (diphenhydramine); Parkinson-like reactions (diphenhydramine); and other nonallergic conditions.

General Action and Information: Antihistamines block the effects of histamine at the H_1 receptor. They do not block histamine release, antibody production, or antigen-antibody reactions. Most antihistamines have anticholinergic properties and may cause constipation, dry eyes, dry mouth, and blurred vision. In addition, many antihistamines cause sedation. Some phenothiazines have strong antihistaminic properties (hydroxyzine and promethazine).

Contraindications: Hypersensitivity and narrow-angle glaucoma. Should not be used in premature or newborn infants.

Precautions: Elderly patients may be more susceptible to adverse anticholinergic effects of antihistamines. Use cautiously in patients with pyloric obstruction, prostatic hypertrophy, hyperthyroidism, cardiovascular disease, or severe liver disease. Use cautiously in pregnancy and lactation.

Interactions: Additive sedation when used with other CNS depressants, including alcohol, antidepressants, opioid analgesics, and sedative/hypnotics. MAO inhibitors prolong and intensify the anticholinergic properties of antihistamines. Erythromycin, ketoconazole, and itraconazole increase the risk of serious cardiac arrhythmias with astemizole and terfenadine.

Nursing Implications

ASSESSMENT
- **General Info:** Assess allergy symptoms (rhinitis, conjunctivitis, hives) before and periodically throughout course of therapy.
- Monitor pulse and blood pressure before initiating and throughout IV therapy.
- Assess lung sounds and character of bronchial secretions. Maintain fluid intake of 1500–2000 ml/day to decrease viscosity of secretions.

- **Nausea and Vomiting:** Assess degree of nausea and frequency and amount of emesis when administering for nausea and vomiting.
- **Anxiety:** Assess mental status, mood, and behavior when administering for anxiety.
- **Pruritus:** Observe the character, location, and size of affected area when administering for pruritic skin conditions.

POTENTIAL NURSING DIAGNOSES
- Airway clearance, ineffective (indications).
- Injury, high risk for (adverse reactions).
- Knowledge deficit related to medication regimen (patient/family teaching).

IMPLEMENTATION
- When used for prophylaxis of motion sickness administer at least 30 min and preferably 1–2 hr before exposure to conditions that may precipitate motion sickness.
- When administering concurrently with opioid analgesics (hydroxyzine, promethazine) supervise ambulation closely to prevent injury secondary to increased sedation.

PATIENT/FAMILY TEACHING
- Inform patient that drowsiness may occur. Avoid driving or other activities requiring alertness until response to drug is known.
- Drowsiness is less likely to occur with astemizole and terfenadine.
- Caution patient to avoid using concurrent alcohol or CNS depressants.
- Advise patient that good oral hygiene, frequent rinsing of mouth with water, and sugarless gum or candy may help relieve dryness of mouth.
- Instruct patient to contact physician if symptoms persist.

EVALUATION
Effectiveness of therapy can be demonstrated by: ▪ Decrease in allergic symptoms ▪ Prevention or decreased severity of nausea and vomiting ▪ Decrease in anxiety ▪ Relief of pruritus ▪ Sedation when used as a sedative/hypnotic.

Antihistamines Included in *Davis's Drug Guide for Nurses*

astemizole,	82	diphenhydramine,	359
azatadine,	96	hydroxyzine,	568
brompheniramine,	138	loratidine,	665
chlorpheniramine,	233	meclizine,	693
clemastine,	253	promethazine,	1003
cyproheptadine,	294	terfenadine,	1125
dimenhydrinate,	354	triprolidine,	1203

▪ ANTIHYPERTENSIVE AGENTS

Pharmacologic Profile

General Use: Treatment of hypertension of many causes; most commonly essential hypertension. Parenteral products are used in the treatment of hypertensive emergencies. Oral treatment should be initiated as soon as possible and individualized to assure compliance for long-term therapy. Therapy is initiated with agents having minimal side effects. When such therapy fails, more potent drugs with different side effects are added in an effort to control blood pressure while causing minimal patient discomfort.

General Action and Information: As a group, the antihypertensives are used to lower blood pressure to a normal level (<90 mmHg diastolic) or to the lowest level tolerated. Antihypertensives are classified into groups according to their site of action. These include peripherally acting antiadrenergics, centrally acting alpha adrenergics, beta-adrenergic blockers, vasodilators, angiotensin converting enzyme (ACE) inhibitors, calcium channel blockers, diuretics, and indapamide, a diuretic with vasodilatory properties. Hypertensive emergencies may be managed with parenteral vasodilators such as diazoxide, nitroprusside, or enalaprilat.

Contraindications: Hypersensitivity to individual agents.

Precautions: Choose agents carefully in pregnancy, lactation, or patients receiving cardiac glycosides. ACE inhibitors should be avoided during pregnancy. Alpha-adrenergic agonists and beta-adrenergic blockers should be used only in patients who will comply with regimen, because abrupt discontinuation of these agents may result in rapid and excessive rise in blood pressure (rebound phenomenon). Thiazide diuretics may increase the requirement for insulin, diet therapy, or oral hypoglycemic agents in diabetic patients. Vasodilators may cause tachycardia if used alone and are commonly used in combination with beta-adrenergic blocking agents. Most antihypertensives (except for beta-adrenergic blockers, angiotensin converting enzyme [ACE] inhibitors, and calcium channel blockers) cause sodium and water retention and are usually combined with a diuretic.

Interactions: Many drugs can negate the therapeutic effectiveness of antihypertensives, including antihistamines, nonsteroidal anti-inflammatory agents, sympathomimetic bronchodilators, decongestants, appetite suppressants, antidepressants, and MAO inhibitors. Hypokalemia from diuretics may increase the risk of cardiac glycoside toxicity. Potassium supplements and potassium-sparing diuretics may cause hyperkalemia when used with angiotensin coverting enzyme (ACE) inhibitors.

Nursing Implications

ASSESSMENT
- Monitor blood pressure and pulse frequently during dosage adjustment and periodically throughout therapy.
- Monitor intake and output ratios and daily weight.

POTENTIAL NURSING DIAGNOSES
- Tissue perfusion, altered (indications).
- Knowledge deficit related to medication regimen (patient/family teaching).
- Noncompliance (patient/family teaching).

IMPLEMENTATION
- Many antihypertensive agents are available as combination products to enhance compliance (see Appendix A).

PATIENT/FAMILY TEACHING
- Instruct patient to continue taking medication, even if feeling well. Abrupt

withdrawal may cause rebound hypertension. Medication controls but does not cure hypertension.
- Encourage patient to comply with additional interventions for hypertension (weight reduction, low-sodium diet, regular exercise, discontinuation of smoking, moderation of alcohol consumption, and stress management).
- Instruct patient and family on proper technique for monitoring blood pressure. Advise them to check blood pressure weekly and report significant changes to physician.
- Caution patient to make position changes slowly to minimize orthostatic hypotension. Advise patient that exercising or hot weather may enhance hypotensive effects.
- Advise patient to consult physician or pharmacist before taking any over-the-counter medications, especially cold remedies. Patients should also avoid excessive amounts of tea, coffee, or cola.
- Advise patient to inform physician or dentist of medication regimen before treatment or surgery.
- Patients taking ACE inhibitors should notify physician if pregnancy is planned or suspected.
- Emphasize the importance of follow-up examinations to monitor progress.

EVALUATION
Effectiveness of therapy can be demonstrated by: ▪ Decrease in blood pressure.

Antihypertensive Agents Included in *Davis's Drug Guide for Nurses*

angiotensin converting enzyme (ACE) inhibitors
benazepril, 107
captopril, 161
enalapril, enalaprilat, 399
fosinopril, 501
lisinopril, 654
quinapril, 1032
ramipril, 1039

beta-adrenergic blockers
acebutolol, 1
atenolol, 84
betaxolol, 118
carteolol, 179
labetalol, 627
metoprolol, 747
nadolol, 794
penbutolol, 888
pindolol, 941
propranolol, 1014
timolol, 1157

calcium channel blockers
amlodipine, 50
diltiazem, 351
felodipine, 454
isradipine, 613
nicardipine, 814
nifedipine, 819
verapamil, 1219

centrally acting adrenergics
clonidine, 264
guanabenz, 532
guanfacine, 538
methyldopa, 732
methyldopate, 732

diuretics
chlorthalidone, 238
furosemide, 502
hydrochlorothiazide, 553
indapamide, 584
metolazone, 745

ganglionic blockers
trimethaphan, 1195

peripherally acting antiadrenergics
doxazosin, 379
guanadrel, 534
guanethidine, 536
prazosin, 978
reserpine, 1042
terazosin, 1120

vasodilators
diazoxide, 329
hydralazine, 551
minoxidil, 765
nitroprusside, 832

▪ ANTI-INFECTIVES

Pharmacologic Profile

General Use: Treatment and prophylaxis of various bacterial infections. See specific drugs for spectrum and indications. Some infections may require additional surgical intervention and supportive therapy.

General Action and Information: Kill (bactericidal) or inhibit the growth of (bacteriostatic) susceptible pathogenic bacteria. Not active against viruses or fungi. Anti-infectives are subdivided into categories depending on chemical similarities and antimicrobial spectrum.

Contraindications: Known hypersensitivity to individual agents. Cross-sensitivity among related agents may occur.

Precautions: Culture and susceptibility testing is desirable to optimize therapy. Dosage modification may be required in patients with hepatic or renal insufficiency. Use cautiously in pregnant and lactating women. Prolonged inappropriate use of broad spectrum anti-infectives may lead to superinfection with fungi or resistant bacteria.

Interactions: Penicillins and aminoglycosides chemically inactivate each other and should not be physically admixed. Erythromycins may decrease hepatic metabolism of other drugs. Probenecid increases serum levels of penicillins and related compounds. Highly protein-bound anti-infectives such as sulfonamides may displace or be displaced by other highly bound drugs. See individual drugs. Extended-spectrum penicillins (mezlocillin, ticarcillin, piperacillin) and some cephalosporins (cefamandole, cefoperazone, cefotetan) may increase the risk of bleeding with anticoagulants, antiplatelet agents, or nonsteroidal anti-inflammatory agents.

Nursing Implications

ASSESSMENT
- Assess patient for signs and symptoms of infection prior to and throughout course of therapy.
- Determine previous hypersensitivities in patients receiving penicillins or cephalosporins.
- Obtain specimens for culture and sensitivity prior to initiating therapy. First dose may be given before receiving results.

POTENTIAL NURSING DIAGNOSES
- Infection, high risk for (indications).
- Knowledge deficit related to medication regimen (patient/family teaching).
- Noncompliance (patient/family teaching).

IMPLEMENTATION
- Most anti-infectives should be administered around the clock to maintain therapeutic serum drug levels.

PATIENT/FAMILY TEACHING
- Instruct patient to continue taking medication around the clock until finished completely, even if feeling better.
- Advise patient to report the signs of superinfection (black, furry overgrowth on the tongue, vaginal itching or discharge, loose or foul-smelling stools) and allergy to physician.

Instruct patient to notify physician if fever and diarrhea develop, especially if stool contains pus, blood, or mucus. Advise patient not to treat diarrhea without consulting physician or pharmacist.
- Instruct patient to notify physician if symptoms do not improve.

EVALUATION
Effectiveness of therapy can be demonstrated by: ▪ Resolution of the signs and symptoms of infection. Length of time for complete resolution depends on organism and site of infection.

Anti-Infectives Included in *Davis's Drug Guide for Nurses*

aminoglycosides
amikacin, 35
gentamicin, 511
kanamycin, 616
neomycin, 806
netilmicin, 810
streptomycin, 1090
tobramycin, 1159

antiprotozoal
atovaquone, 86
pentamidine, 902

carbapenam
imipenem/cilastatin, 577

cephalosporins—first generation
cefadroxil, 184
cefazolin, 188
cephalexin, 215
cephalothin, 216
cephapirin, 219
cephradine, 220

cephalosporins—second generation
cefaclor, 182
cefamandole, 186
cefmetazole, 191
cefonicid, 193
cefotetan, 199
cefoxitin, 201
cefpodoxime, 203
cefuroxime, 213
loracarbef, 664

cephalosporins—third generation
cefixime, 190
cefoperazone, 195
cefotaxime, 197

ceftazidime, 207
ceftizoxime, 209
ceftriaxone, 211

extended-spectrum penicillins
carbenicillin, 166
mezlocillin, 754
piperacillin, 945
piperacillin/tazobactam, 945
ticarcillin, 1151
ticarcillin/clavulanate, 1154

fluoroquinolones
ciprofloxacin, 246
enoxacin, 401
lomefloxacin, 659
norfloxacin, 833
ofloxacin, 840

macrolides
azithromycin, 99
clarithromycin, 252
erythromycin, 419

monobactam
aztreonam, 101

penicillins
amoxicillin, 56
amoxicillin/clavulanate, 58
ampicillin, 63
penicillin G benzathine, 892
penicillin G potassium, 894
penicillin G procaine, 897
penicillin G sodium, 898
penicillin V, 901

pencillinase-resistant pencillins
cloxacillin, 269
dicloxacillin, 333
methicillin, 719
nafcillin, 798
oxacillin, 859

continued

sulfonamides
sulfacetamide, 847
sulfamethoxazole, 1104
sulfasalazine, 1105
sulfisoxazole, 1109
trimethoprim/sulfamethoxazole, 1200

tetracyclines
doxycycline, 385
minocycline, 763
tetracycline, 1128

miscellaneous
chloramphenicol, 226
clindamycin, 255
metronidazole, 750
nitrofurantoin, 823
spectinomycin, 1084
trimethoprim, 1198
vancomycin, 1212

▪ ANTINEOPLASTICS

Pharmacologic Profile

General Use: Used in the treatment of various solid tumors, lymphomas, and leukemias. Also used in some autoimmune disorders such as rheumatoid arthritis (cyclophosamide, methotrexate). Often used in combinations to minimize individual toxicities and increase response. Chemotherapy may be combined with other treatment modalities such as surgery and radiation therapy. Dosages vary greatly depending on extent of disease, other agents used, and patient's condition.

General Action and Information: Act by many different mechanisms (see Table below). Most commonly affect DNA synthesis or function. Action may not be limited to neoplastic cells.

MECHANISM OF ACTION OF VARIOUS ANTINEOPLASTIC AGENTS

MECHANISM OF ACTION	AGENT	EFFECTS ON CELL CYCLE
ALKYLATING AGENTS Cause cross-linking of DNA	busulfan carboplatin chlorambucil cisplatin cyclophosphamide dacarbazine estramustine ifosfamide mechlorethamine melphelan procarbazine thiotepa	Cell cycle—nonspecific
ANTHRACYCLINES Interfere with DNA and RNA synthesis	daunorubicin doxorubicin idarubicin	Cell cycle—nonspecific
ANTITUMOR ANTIBIOTICS Interfere with DNA and RNA synthesis	bleomycin dactinomycin mitomycin mitoxantrone plicamycin streptozocin	Cell cycle—nonspecific (except bleomycin)
ANTIMETABOLITES Take the place of normal proteins	cytarabine fludarabine fluorouracil hydroxyurea mercaptopurine methotrexate thioguanine	Cell cycle—specific, work mostly in S phase (DNA syn- thesis)

MECHANISM OF ACTION	AGENT	EFFECTS ON CELL CYCLE
ENZYME (Depletes asparagine)	asparaginase	Cell cycle—phase specific
HORMONAL AGENTS Alter hormonal status in tumors that are sensitive	diethylstilbestrol (estrogens) estramustine flutamide leuprolide megestrol tamoxifen testosterone (androgens)	Unknown
PODOPHYLLOTOXIN DERIVATIVE (Damages DNA before mitosis)	etoposide teniposide	Cell cycle—phase specific
VINCA ALKALOIDS Interfere with mitosis	vinblastine vincristine	Cell cycle—specific, work during M phase (mitosis)
ANTIPROLIFERATIVE	interferon alfa-2A interferon alfa-2B	Unknown
ADRENAL SUPPRESSANT	mitotane	Unknown
IMMUNE MODULATOR	aldesleukin BCG levamisole	Unknown Unknown Unknown
MISCELLANEOUS	altretamine paclitaxel pentostatin	Unknown Affects interphase and mitosis Unknown

Contraindications: Previous bone marrow depression or hypersensitivity. Contraindicated in pregnancy and lactation.

Precautions: Use cautiously in patients with active infections, decreased bone marrow reserve, radiation therapy, or other debilitating illnesses. Use cautiously in patients with childbearing potential.

Interactions: Allopurinol decreases metabolism of mercaptopurine. Toxicity from methotrexate may be increased by other nephrotoxic drugs or larger doses of aspirin or nonsteroidal anti-inflammatory agents. Bone marrow depression is additive. See individual drugs.

Nursing Implications

ASSESSMENT

- Assess for fever, chills, sore throat, and signs of infection. Notify physician if these symptoms occur.
- Monitor platelet count throughout therapy. Assess for bleeding (bleeding gums, bruising, petichiae; guaiac stools, urine, and emesis). If thrombocytopenia occurs, avoid IM injections and rectal temperatures, and apply pressure to venipuncture sites for 10 min.
- Monitor intake and output ratios, appetite, and nutritional intake. Confer with physician regarding administration of an antiemetic. Adjusting diet as tolerated may help maintain fluid and electrolyte balance and nutritional status.
- Anemia may occur. Monitor for increased fatigue, dyspnea, and orthostatic hypotension.
- Monitor IV site carefully and ensure patency. Discontinue infusion immedi-

ately if discomfort, erythema along vein, or infiltration occurs. Tissue ulceration and necrosis may result from infiltration. Notify physician.
- Monitor for symptoms of gout (increased uric acid, joint pain, and edema). Encourage patient to drink at least 2 liters of fluid each day. Allopurinol may be given to decrease uric acid levels. Alkalinization of urine may be ordered to increase excretion of uric acid.

POTENTIAL NURSING DIAGNOSES
- Infection, high risk for (side effects).
- Nutrition, altered: less than body requirements (adverse reactions).
- Knowledge deficit related to medication regimen (patient/family teaching).

IMPLEMENTATION
- Solutions for injection should be prepared in a biologic cabinet. Wear gloves, gown, and mask while handling medication. Discard equipment in designated containers (see Appendix I for guidelines for safe handling).

PATIENT/FAMILY TEACHING
- Caution patient to avoid crowds and persons with known infections. Physician should be informed immediately if symptoms of infection occur.
- Instruct patient to report unusual bleeding. Advise patient of thrombocytopenia precautions.
- These drugs may cause gonadal suppression; however, patient should still use birth control, as most antineoplastics are teratogenic. Advise patient to inform physician immediately if pregnancy is suspected.
- Discuss with patient the possibility of hair loss. Explore methods of coping.
- Instruct patient to inspect oral mucosa for erythema and ulceration. If ulceration occurs advise patient to use sponge brush, rinse mouth with water after eating and drinking, and confer with physician if mouth pain interferes with eating.
- Instruct patient not to receive any vaccinations without advice of physician.
- Advise patient of need for medical follow-up and frequent lab tests.

EVALUATION
Effectiveness of therapy can be demonstrated by: ▪ Decrease in size and spread of tumor ▪ Improvement in hematologic status in patients with leukemia.

Antineoplastics Included in *Davis's Drug Guide for Nurses*

alkylating agents
busulfan, 146
carboplatin, 172
chlorambucil, 224
cisplatin, 249
cyclophosphamide, 288
dacarbazine, 299
estramustine, 428
ifosfamide, 575
mechlorethamine, 691
melphalan, 699
procarbazine, 992
thiotepa, 1145

anthracyclines
daunorubicin, 307
doxorubicin, 382
idarubicin, 573

antimetabolites
cytarabine, 295
floxuridine, 471
fludarabine, 476
fluorouracil, 485
hydroxyurea, 566
mercaptopurine, 708
methotrexate, 726
thioguanine, 1138

antitumor antibiotics
bleomycin, 132
dactinomycin, 301
mitomycin, 769
mitoxantrone, 773
plicamycin, 953
streptozocin, 1093

enzyme
asparaginase, 77

hormonal agents
diethylstilbestrol, 338
estramustine, 428
flutamide, 496
leuprolide, 634
megestrol, 698
tamoxifen, 1116
testosterone, 1126

podophyllotoxin derivative
etoposide, 441
teniposide, 1118

vinca alkaloids
vinblastine, 1223
vincristine, 1226

miscellaneous
aldesleukin, 16
altretamine, 28
interferon alfa-2A, 591
interferon alfa-2B, 594
levamisole, 636
mitotane, 771
paclitaxel, 874

▪ ANTIPARKINSON AGENTS

Pharmacologic Profile

General Use: Used in the treatment of parkinsonism of various causes: degenerative, toxic, infective, neoplastic, or drug-induced.

General Action and Information: Drugs used in the treatment of the Parkinsonian syndrome and other dyskinesias are aimed at restoring the natural balance of two major neurotransmitters in the CNS: acetylcholine and dopamine. The imbalance is a deficiency in dopamine that results in excessive cholinergic activity. Drugs used are either anticholinergics (benztropine, biperiden, orphenadrine, and trihexyphenidyl) or dopaminergic agonists (amantadine, bromocriptine, levodopa, and pergolide). Selegiline inhibits the enzyme that degrades dopamine, augmenting its effects.

Contraindications: Anticholinergics should be avoided in patients with narrow-angle glaucoma.

Precautions: Use cautiously in patients with severe cardiac disease, pyloric obstruction, or prostatic enlargement.

Interactions: Pyridoxine, MAO inhibitors, benzodiazepines, phenytoin, phenothiazines, and haloperidol may antagonize the effects of levodopa. Concurrent use of selegiline with opioid analgesics may result in two potentially fatal reactions (excitation, sweating, rigidity, and hypertension; or hypotension and coma). Doses of selegiline >10 mg/day may produce reactions with tyramine-containing foods.

Nursing Implications

ASSESSMENT
▪ Assess parkinsonian and extrapyramidal symptoms (akinesia, rigidity, tremors, pill rolling, mask facies, shuffling gait, muscle spasms, twisting motions,

and drooling) before and throughout course of therapy. On-off phenomena may cause symptoms to appear or improve suddenly.
- Monitor blood pressure frequently during therapy. Instruct patient to remain supine during and for several hours after first dose of bromocriptine, as severe hypotension may occur.

POTENTIAL NURSING DIAGNOSES
- Physical mobility, impaired (indications).
- Injury, high risk for (indications).
- Knowledge deficit related to medication regimen (patient/family teaching).

IMPLEMENTATION
- In the carbidopa/levodopa combination the number following the drug name represents the milligram of each respective drug.

PATIENT/FAMILY TEACHING
- May cause drowsiness or dizziness. Advise patient to avoid driving or other activities that require alertness until response to medication is known.
- Caution patient to make position changes slowly to minimize orthostatic hypotension.
- Instruct patient that frequent rinsing of mouth, good oral hygiene, and sugarless gum or candy may decrease dry mouth. Patient should notify physician if dryness persists (saliva substitutes may be used). Also notify the dentist if dryness interferes with use of dentures.
- Advise patient to confer with physician or pharmacist before taking over-the-counter medications, especially cold remedies, or drinking alcoholic beverages. Patients receiving levodopa should avoid multivitamins. Vitamin B$_6$ (pyridoxine) may interfere with levodopa's action.
- Caution patient that decreased perspiration may occur. Overheating may occur during hot weather. Patients should remain indoors in an air-conditioned environment during hot weather.
- Advise patient to increase activity, bulk, and fluid in diet to minimize constipating effects of medication.
- Advise patient to notify physician if confusion, rash, urinary retention, severe constipation, visual changes, or worsening of parkinsonian symptoms occur.

EVALUATION
Effectiveness of therapy can be demonstrated by: ▪ Resolution of parkinsonian signs and symptoms ▪ Resolution of drug-induced extrapyramidal symptoms.

Antiparkinson Agents Included in *Davis's Drug Guide for Nurses*

anticholinergics
    benztropine, 110
    biperiden, 124
    trihexyphenidyl, 1193

dopamine agonist
    amantadine, 33
    bromocriptine, 136

carbidopa/levodopa, 167
levodopa, 638
pergolide, 913

monoamine oxidase type B inhibitor
    selegiline, 1062

▪ ANTIPSYCHOTIC AGENTS

Pharmacologic Profile

General Use: Treatment of acute and chronic psychoses, particularly when accompanied by increased psychomotor activity. Clomipramine is only used for obsessive-compulsive disorder (OCD). Use of clozapine is limited to schizophrenia unresponsive to conventional therapy. Selected agents are also used as antihistamines or antiemetics. Chlorpromazine is also used in the treatment of intractable hiccups.

General Action and Information: Block dopamine receptors in the brain, also alter dopamine release and turnover. Peripheral effects include anticholinergic properties and alpha-adrenergic blockade. Most antipsychotics are phenothiazines except for haloperidol, which is a butyrophenone; molindone, which resembles a phenothiazine in its action; clomipramine, which resembles tricyclic antidepressants; and loxapine and clozapine, which are miscellaneous compounds. Phenothiazines differ in their ability to produce sedation (greatest with chlorpromazine, promazine, thioridazine, and thiothixine), extrapyramidal reactions (greatest with fluphenazine, perphenazine, prochlorperazine, and trifluoperazine), and anticholinergic effects (greatest with chlorpromazine, promazine).

Contraindications: Hypersensitivity. Cross-sensitivity may exist among phenothiazines. Should not be used in narrow-angle glaucoma. Should not be used in patients who have CNS depression.

Precautions: Safety in pregnancy and lactation not established. Use cautiously in patients with symptomatic cardiac disease. Avoid exposure to extremes in temperature. Use cautiously in severely ill or debilitated patients, diabetics, and patients with respiratory insufficiency, prostatic hypertrophy, or intestinal obstruction. May lower seizure threshold. Clozapine may cause agranulocytosis. Most agents are capable of causing neuroleptic malignant syndrome.

Interactions: Additive hypotension with acute ingestion of alcohol, antihypertensives, or nitrates. Antacids may decrease absorption. Phenobarbital may increase metabolism and decrease effectiveness. Additive CNS depression with other CNS depressants, including alcohol, antihistamines, antidepressants, opioid analgesics, or sedative/hypnotics. Lithium may decrease blood levels and effectiveness of phenothiazines. May decrease the therapeutic response to levodopa. May increase the risk of agranulocytosis with antithyroid agents.

Nursing Implications

ASSESSMENT
▪ Assess patient's mental status (orientation, mood, behavior) before and periodically throughout therapy.
▪ Monitor blood pressure (sitting, standing, lying), pulse, and respiratory rate before and frequently during the period of dosage adjustment.
▪ Observe patient carefully when administering medication to ensure medication is actually taken and not hoarded.
▪ Observe patient carefully for extrapyramidal symptoms (akathisia—restless-

ness; dystonia—muscle spasms and twisting motions; pseudoparkinsonism—mask facies, rigidity, tremors, drooling, shuffling gait, dysphagia, pill-rolling motions); tardive dyskinesia (uncontrolled movements of face, mouth, tongue, or jaw, and involuntary movements of extremities); and neuroleptic malignant syndrome (pale skin, hyperthermia, skeletal muscle rigidity, autonomic dysfunction, altered consciousness, leukocytosis, elevated liver function tests, and elevated CPK). Notify physician immediately at the onset of these symptoms.

POTENTIAL NURSING DIAGNOSES
- Thought processes, altered (indications).
- Knowledge deficit related to medication regimen (patient/family teaching).
- Noncompliance (patient/family teaching).

IMPLEMENTATION
- **General Info:** Keep patient recumbent for at least 30 min following parenteral administration to minimize hypotensive effects.
- To prevent contact dermatitis avoid getting solution on hands.
- Phenothiazines should be discontinued 48 hr before and not resumed for 24 hr following metrizamide myelography, as they lower the seizure threshold.
- **PO:** Administer with food, milk, or a full glass of water to minimize gastric irritation.
- Dilute most concentrates in 120 ml of distilled or acidified tap water or fruit juice just before administration.

PATIENT/FAMILY TEACHING
- Advise patient to take medication exactly as directed and not to skip doses or double up on missed doses. Abrupt withdrawal may lead to gastritis, nausea, vomiting, dizziness, headache, tachycardia, and insomnia.
- Advise patient to make position changes slowly to minimize orthostatic hypotension.
- Medication may cause drowsiness. Caution patient to avoid driving or other activities requiring alertness until response to the medication is known.
- Caution patient to avoid taking alcohol or other CNS depressants concurrently with this medication.
- Advise patient to use sunscreen and protective clothing when exposed to the sun to prevent photosensitivity reactions. Extremes of temperature should also be avoided, as these drugs impair body temperature regulation.
- Advise patient that increasing activity, bulk, and fluids in the diet help minimize the constipating effects of this medication.
- Instruct patient to use frequent mouth rinses, good oral hygiene, and sugarless gum or candy to minimize dry mouth.
- Advise patient to notify physician or dentist of medication regimen before treatment or surgery.
- Emphasize the importance of routine follow-up examinations and continued participation in psychotherapy as indicated.

EVALUATION
Effectiveness of therapy can be demonstrated by: ▪ Decrease in excitable, paranoic, or withdrawn behavior ▪ Relief of nausea and vomiting ▪ Relief of intractable hiccups.

Antipsychotic Agents Included in *Davis's Drug Guide for Nurses*

phenothiazines

chlorpromazine, 235
fluphenazine, 490
mesoridazine, 712
perphenazine, 916
prochlorperazine, 995
promazine, 1000
thioridazine, 1142
thiothixine, 1147
trifluoperazine, 1191

butyrophenone

haloperidol, 541

miscellaneous

clomipramine, 261
clozapine, 270
loxapine, 670
molindone, 777

▪ ANTIPYRETICS

Pharmacologic Profile

General Use: Used to lower fever of many causes (infection, inflammation, and neoplasms).

General Action and Information: Antipyretics lower fever by affecting thermoregulation in the CNS and by inhibiting the action of prostaglandins peripherally.

Contraindications: Avoid aspirin or ibuprofen in patients with bleeding disorder (risk of bleeding is less with other salicylates). Aspirin and other salicylates should be avoided in children and adolescents.

Precautions: Use aspirin or ibuprofen cautiously in patients with ulcer disease. Avoid chronic use of large doses of acetaminophen.

Interactions: Large doses of aspirin may displace other highly protein-bound drugs. Additive GI irritation with ibuprofen, aspirin, and other nonsteroidal anti-inflammatory agents or glucocorticoids. Aspirin or ibuprofen may increase the risk of bleeding with other agents affecting hemostasis (anticoagulants, thrombolytics, antineoplastics, and certain anti-infectives).

Nursing Implications

ASSESSMENT
▪ Assess fever; note presence of associated symptoms (diaphoresis, tachycardia, and malaise).

POTENTIAL NURSING DIAGNOSES
▪ Body temperature, altered, high risk for (indications).
▪ Knowledge deficit related to medication regimen (patient/family teaching).

IMPLEMENTATION
▪ Administration with food or antacids may minimize GI irritation (aspirin and ibuprofen).
▪ Available in oral and rectal dosage forms and in combination with other drugs.

PATIENT/FAMILY TEACHING

- Advise patient to consult physician if fever is not relieved by routine doses or if greater than 39.5°C (103°F) or lasts longer than 3 days.
- Centers for Disease Control warn against giving aspirin to children or adolescents with varicella (chickenpox), or influenza-like or viral illnesses because of a possible association with Reye's syndrome.

EVALUATION

Effectiveness of therapy can be demonstrated by: ▪ Reduction of fever.

Antipyretics Included in *Davis's Drug Guide for Nurses*

acetaminophen, 3	choline salicylate, 242
aspirin, 80	ibuprofen, 570
choline and magnesium salicylates, 241	salsalate, 1055

▪ ANTITHYROID AGENTS

Pharmacologic Profile

General Use: Used in the treatment of hyperthyroidism of various causes (Graves' disease, multinodular goiter, thyroiditis, and thyrotoxic crisis) in children, pregnant women, and other patients in whom hyperthyroidism is not expected to be permanent. These agents are also used to prepare patients for thyroidectomy or those in whom thryoidectomy is contraindicated. Beta-adrenergic blockers (propranolol) are sometimes used in conjunction with antithyroid agents to control symptoms (tachycardia and tremor) but have no effect on thyroid status. Iodine and iodides are also used as radiation protectants.

General Action and Information: Inhibit thyroid hormone formation (iodine) or inhibit oxidation of iodine (methimazole and propylthiouracil).

Contraindications: Hypersensitivity. Previous bone marrow depression.

Precautions: Use methimazole cautiously in patients with decreased bone marrow reserve.

Interactions: Lithium may cause thyroid abnormalities and interfere with the response to antithyroid therapy. Phenothiazines may increase the risk of agranulocytosis.

Nursing Implications

ASSESSMENT

- **General Info:** Monitor response of symptoms of hyperthyroidism or thyrotoxicosis (tachycardia, palpitations, nervousness, insomnia, fever, diaphoresis, heat intolerance, tremors, weight loss, diarrhea).
- Assess patient for development of hypothyroidism (intolerance to cold, constipation, dry skin, headache, listlessness, tiredness, or weakness). Dosage adjustment may be required.
- Assess patient for skin rash or swelling of cervical lymph nodes. Treatment may be discontinued if this occurs.
- Monitor thyroid function studies before and periodically throughout therapy.
- **Iodides:** Assess for signs and symptoms of iodism (metallic taste, stomatitis,

skin lesions, cold symptoms, severe GI upset) or anaphylaxis. Report these symptoms promptly to physician.

POTENTIAL NURSING DIAGNOSES
- Knowledge deficit related to medication regimen (patient/family teaching).

IMPLEMENTATION
- Mix iodide solutions in a full glass of fruit juice, water, or milk. Administer after meals to minimize GI irritation.

PATIENT/FAMILY TEACHING
- Instruct patient to take medication exactly as directed. Missing doses may precipitate hyperthyroidism.
- Advise patient to consult physician regarding dietary sources of iodine (iodized salt, shellfish, cabbage, kale, turnips).
- Advise patient to carry identification describing medication regimen at all times and to notify physician or dentist of medical regimen before treatment or surgery.
- Emphasize the importance of routine examinations to monitor progress and check for side effects.

EVALUATION
Effectiveness of therapy can be demonstrated by: ▪ Decrease in severity of symptoms of hyperthyroidism ▪ Decrease in vascularity and friability of the thyroid gland before preparation for surgery ▪ Protection of the thyroid gland during radiation emergencies.

Antithyroid Agents Included in *Davis's Drug Guide for Nurses*
methimazole, 721	propylthiouracil, 1017
potassium iodide, 968	strong iodine solution, 1094

▪ ANTITUBERCULARS

Pharmacologic Profile

General Use: Used in the treatment and prevention of tuberculosis and other diseases caused by mycobacterium. Combinations are used in the treatment of active disease to rapidly decrease the infectious state and delay or prevent the emergence of resistant strains. In selected situations, intermittent (twice weekly) regimens may be employed. Streptomycin is also used as an antitubercular.

General Action and Information: Kill (tuberculocidal) or inhibit the growth of (tuberculostatic) mycobacterium responsible for causing tuberculosis. Combination therapy with two or more agents is required, unless used as prophylaxis (isoniazid alone).

Contraindications: Hypersensitivity. Severe liver disease.

Precautions: Use cautiously in patients with a history of liver disease; elderly or debilitated patients. Ethambutol requires ophthalmologic follow-up. Safety in pregnancy and lactation not established, although selected agents have been used without adverse effects on the fetus. Compliance is required for optimal response.

Interactions: Isoniazid inhibits the metabolism of phenytoin. Rifampin stimulates hepatic drug-metabolizing enzymes and may decrease the effects of drugs that are metabolized by the liver.

Nursing Implications

ASSESSMENT
- Mycobacterial studies and susceptibility tests should be performed prior to and periodically throughout therapy to detect possible resistance.

POTENTIAL NURSING DIAGNOSES
- Infection, high risk for (indications).
- Knowledge deficit related to medication regimen (patient/family teaching).
- Noncompliance (patient/family teaching).

IMPLEMENTATION
- Most medications can be administered with food or antacids if GI irritation occurs.

PATIENT/FAMILY TEACHING
- Advise patient of the importance of continuing therapy even after symptoms have subsided.
- Emphasize the importance of regular follow-up examinations to monitor progress and check for side effects.

EVALUATION
Effectiveness of therapy can be demonstrated by: ▪ Resolution of the signs and symptoms of tuberculosis ▪ Negative sputum cultures.

Antituberculars Included in *Davis's Drug Guide for Nurses*
ethambutol, 434

isoniazid, 605

pyrazinamide, 1024

rifampin, 1051

streptomycin, 1090

▪ ANTITUSSIVES/EXPECTORANTS

Pharmacologic Profile

General Use: Used for the symptomatic relief of cough due to various causes including viral upper respiratory infections. Not intended for chronic use.

General Action and Information: Antitussives (codeine, dextromethorphan, diphenhydramine, hydrocodone, and hydromorphone) suppress cough by central mechanisms. Expectorants (acetylcysteine and guaifenesin) aid in mobilizing pulmonary secretions. Productive cough should not be suppressed unless it interferes with sleeping or other activities of daily living. Increasing fluid intake probably serves as the best expectorant, decreasing the viscosity of secretions so that they may be more easily mobilized.

Contraindications: Hypersensitivity.

Precautions: Use cautiously in children. Should not be used for prolonged periods unless under the advice of a physician.

Interactions: Centrally acting antitussives may have additive CNS depression with other CNS depressants.

Nursing Implications

ASSESSMENT
- Assess frequency and nature of cough, lung sounds, and amount and type of sputum produced.

POTENTIAL NURSING DIAGNOSES
- Airway clearance, ineffective (indications).
- Knowledge deficit related to medication regimen (patient/family teaching).

IMPLEMENTATION
- Unless contraindicated, maintain fluid intake of 1500–2000 ml to decrease viscosity of bronchial secretions.

PATIENT/FAMILY TEACHING
- Instruct patient to cough effectively, sit upright, and take several deep breaths before attempting to cough.
- Advise patient to minimize cough by avoiding irritants (cigarette smoke, fumes, dust). Humidification of environmental air, frequent sips of water, and sugarless hard candy may also decrease the frequency of dry, irritating cough.
- Caution patient to avoid taking concurrent alcohol or CNS depressants.
- May cause dizziness or drowsiness. Caution patient to avoid driving or other activities requiring alertness until response to medication is known.
- Advise patient that any cough lasting over 1 wk or accompanied by fever, chest pain, persistent headache, or skin rash warrants medical attention.

EVALUATION
Effectiveness of therapy can be demonstrated by: ▪ Decrease in frequency and intensity of cough without eliminating patient's cough reflex.

Antitussives Included in *Davis's Drug Guide for Nurses*
codeine, 273
dextromethorphan, 321
diphenhydramine, 359
hydrocodone, 555
hydromorphone, 560

Expectorants Included in *Davis's Drug Guide for Nurses*
acetylcysteine, 4
guaifenesin, 530

▪ ANTIULCER AGENTS

Pharmacologic Profile

General Uses: Treatment and prophylaxis of peptic ulcer and gastric hypersecretory conditions such as Zollinger-Ellison Syndrome. Histamine H_2 receptor antagonists and omeprazole are also used in the management of gastroesophageal reflux disease (GERD).

General Action and Information: Medications used in the management of gastric/duodenal ulcer disease are aimed at neutralizing gastric acid (antacids), decreasing acid secretion (histamine H_2 antagonists, misoprostol, omeprazole) or protecting the ulcer surface from further damage (misoprostol, sucralfate). Histamine H_2 receptor antagonists (blockers) competitively inhibit the action of histamine at the H_2 receptor, located primarily in gastric parietal cells, resulting in inhibition of gastric acid secretion. Misoprostol decreases gastric acid secretion and increases production of protective mucus. Omeprazole prevents the transport of hydrogen ions into the gastric lumen.

Contraindications: Hypersensitivity. Misoprostol should be avoided in women with child-bearing potential.

Precautions: Most histamine H_2 antagonists require dosage reduction in renal impairment and in the elderly. Safety of agents besides misoprostol in pregnancy, lactation, and children not established. Magnesium-containing antacids should be used cautiously in patients with renal impairment.

Interactions: Calcium and magnesium-containing antacids decrease the absorption of tetracyline and fluoroquinolones. Cimetidine inhibits the ability of the liver to metabolize several drugs, increasing the risk of toxicity from oral anticoagulants, tricyclic antidepressants, theophylline, metoprolol, phenytoin, propranolol, and lidocaine. Omeprazole decreases metabolism of phenytoin, diazepam, and warfarin. Histamine H_2 antagonists and omeprazole decrease the absorption of ketoconazole.

Nursing Implications

Assessment
- **General Info:** Assess patient routinely for epigastric or abdominal pain and frank or occult blood in the stool, emesis, or gastric aspirate.
- **Antacids:** Assess for heartburn and indigestion as well as the location, duration, character, and precipitating factors of gastric pain.
- **Histamine H_2 Antagonists:** Assess elderly and severely ill patients for confusion routinely. Notify physician promptly should this occur.
- **Misoprostol:** Assess women of child-bearing age for pregnancy. Medication is usually begun on second or third day of menstrual period following a negative serum pregnancy test within 2 wks of beginning therapy.

Lab Test Considerations:
- **Histamine H_2 Antagonists:** Antagonize the effects of pentagastrin and histamine during gastric acid secretion test. Avoid administration during the 24 hr preceding the test.
- May cause false-negative results in skin tests using allergen extracts. These drugs should be discontinued 24 hr prior to the test.

Potential Nursing Diagnoses
- Pain (indications).
- Knowledge deficit related to medication regimen (patient/family teaching).

Implementation
- **Antacids:** Antacids cause premature dissolution and absorption of enteric-

coated tablets and may interfere with absorption of other oral medications. Separate administration of antacids and other oral medications by at least 1 hr.
- Shake liquid preparations well before pouring. Follow administration with water to assure passage to stomach. Liquid and powder dosage forms are considered to be more effective than chewable tablets.
- Chewable tablets must be chewed thoroughly before swallowing. Follow with ½ glass of water.
- Administer 1 and 3 hr after meals and at bedtime for maximum antacid effect.
- **Misoprostol:** Administer with meals and at bedtime to reduce the severity of diarrhea.
- **Omeprazole:** Administer before meals, preferably in the morning. Capsules should be swallowed whole; do not open, crush, or chew.
- May be administered concurrently with antacids.
- **Sucralfate:** Administer on an empty stomach 1 hr before meals and at bedtime. Do not crush or chew tablets. If nasogastric administration is required, consult pharmacist for diluent, as sucralfate is relatively insoluble and may form a bezoar.

PATIENT/FAMILY TEACHING
- **General Info:** Instruct patient to take medication as directed for the full course of therapy, even if feeling better. If a dose is missed, it should be taken as soon as remembered but not if almost time for next dose. Do not double doses.
- Advise patient to avoid alcohol, products containing aspirin or ibuprofen, and foods that may cause an increase in GI irritation.
- Advise patient to report onset of black, tarry stools to the physician promptly.
- Inform patient that cessation of smoking may help prevent the recurrence of duodenal ulcers.
- **Antacids:** Caution patient to consult physician before taking antacids for more than 2 wk or if problem is recurring. Advise patient to consult physician if relief is not obtained or if symptoms of gastric bleeding (black, tarry stools, coffee-ground emesis) occur.
- **Misoprostol:** Emphasize that sharing of this medication may be dangerous.
- Inform patient that misoprostol may cause spontaneous abortion. Women of child-bearing age must be informed of this effect through verbal and written information and must use contraception throughout course of therapy. If pregnancy is suspected, the woman should stop taking misoprostol and immediately notify her physician.
- **Sucralfate:** Advise patient to continue with course of therapy for 4–8 wk, even if feeling better, to ensure ulcer healing.
- Advise patient that an increase in fluid intake, dietary bulk, and exercise may prevent drug-induced constipation.

EVALUATION
Effectiveness of therapy can be demonstrated by: ■ Decrease in GI pain and irritation ■ Prevention of gastric irritation and bleeding. Healing of duodenal ulcers can be seen by x-rays or endoscopy. Therapy with Histamine H_2 antagonists is continued for at least 6 wk after initial episode ■ Decreased symptoms of gastroesophageal reflux disease ■ Increase in the pH of gastric secretions (antacids) ■ Prevention of gastric ulcers in patients receiving chronic nonsteroidal antiinflammatory drug therapy (misoprostol only).

Antiulcer Agents Included in *Davis's Drug Guide for Nurses*

antacids
aluminum hydroxide, 31
calcium carbonate, 157
magaldrate, 674
magnesium hydroxide, 677
magnesium hydroxide/
aluminum hydroxide, 679
sodium bicarbonate, 1070

**histamine H₂ receptor
antagonists**
cimetidine, 244
famotidine, 448

nizatidine, 830
ranitidine, 1040

*miscellaneous antiulcer
agents*
misoprostol, 768
omeprazole, 843
sucralfate, 1101

■ ANTIVIRALS

Pharmacologic Profile

General Uses: Acyclovir and vidarabine are used in the management of serious herpes virus infections. Acyclovir also is used in the management of chickenpox. Amantadine and rimantadine are used primarily in the prevention of influenza A viral infections. Didanosine, zalcitabine, and zidovudine slow the progression of AIDS. Idoxuridine and trifluridine are used for ophthalmic viral infections. Ribavirin is used in the management of respiratory syncitial virus (RSV). Ganciclovir and foscarnet are used in the treatment of cytomegalovirus (CMV) retinitis.

General Action and Information: Acyclovir, didanosine, foscarnet, ganciclovir, idoxuridine, ribavirin, trifluridine, vidarabine, and zidovudine inhibit viral replication. Amantadine prevents penetration of the virus into host cells.

Contraindications: Previous hypersensitivity.

Precautions: All require dosage adjustment in renal impairment. Acyclovir may cause renal impairment. Acyclovir and amantadine may cause CNS toxicity. Vidarabine commonly causes GI adverse reactions. Zidovudine should be used cautiously in patients with bone marrow depression. Didanosine and foscarnet increase risk of seizures.

Interactions: Acyclovir may have additive CNS and nephrotoxicity with drugs causing similar adverse reactions. Amantadine may have additive anticholinergic properties with other drugs causing anticholinergic side effects. Adverse reactions to vidarabine may be potentiated by concurrent allopurinol. Zidovudine toxicity may be increased by amphotericin B, acyclovir, chronic acetaminophen, cimetidine, indomethacin, interferon, pentamidine, sulfonamides, or probenecid. Food significantly decreases absorption of didanosine. Didanosine may alter requirements for oral anticoagulants, insulin, or oral hypoglycemic agents. Risk of neuropathy from zalcitabine is increased by other neurotoxic agents. Risk of pancreatitis from zalcitabine is increased by other agents causing pancreatitis. Aminoglycosides, amphotericin, and foscarnet increase risk of toxicity from zalcitabine.

Nursing Implications

ASSESSMENT
- **General Info:** Assess patient for signs and symptoms of infection before and throughout course of therapy.
- **Ophth:** Assess eye lesions before and daily during therapy.
- **Topical:** Assess lesions before and daily during therapy.

POTENTIAL NURSING DIAGNOSES
- Infection, high risk for (indications).
- Skin integrity, impairment of (indications).
- Knowledge deficit related to medication regimen (patient/family teaching).

IMPLEMENTATION
- Most systemic antiviral agents should be administered around the clock to maintain therapeutic serum drug levels.

PATIENT/FAMILY TEACHING
- Instruct patient to continue taking medication around the clock for full course of therapy, even if feeling better.
- Instruct patient in correct technique for topical or ophthalmic preparations.
- Instruct patient to notify physician if symptoms do not improve.

EVALUATION
Effectiveness of therapy can be demonstrated by: ▪ Prevention or resolution of the signs and symptoms of viral infection. Length of time for complete resolution depends on organism and site of infection.

Antivirals Included in *Davis's Drug Guide for Nurses*

acyclovir,	8	ribavirin,	1046
amantadine,	33	rimantadine,	1052
didanosine,	334	trifluridine,	847
foscarnet,	499	vidarabine,	1221
ganciclovir,	508	zalcitabine,	1237
idoxuridine,	847	zidovudine,	1239

▪ BETA-ADRENERGIC BLOCKING AGENTS

Pharmacologic Profile

General Uses: Used in the management of hypertension, angina pectoris, tachyarrhythmias, hypertrophic subaortic stenosis, migraine headache (prophylaxis), myocardial infarction (prevention), glaucoma (betaxolol, levobunolol, metipranalol, and timolol), pheochromocytoma, tremors (propranolol only), and hyperthyroidism (management of symptoms only).

General Action and Information: Beta-adrenergic receptor blocking agents compete with adrenergic (sympathetic) neurotransmitters (epinephrine and norepinephrine) for beta-adrenergic receptor sites. Beta$_1$-adrenergic receptor sites are located chiefly in the heart, where stimulation results in increased heart rate, contractility, and AV conduction. Beta$_2$-adrenergic receptors are found mainly in bronchial and vascular smooth muscle and the uterus. Stimulation of beta$_2$-adrenergic receptors produces vasodilation, bronchodilation, and uterine relaxation. Blockade of these receptors antagonizes the effect of the neurotransmitters. Beta blockers may be relatively *selective* for beta$_1$-adrenergic receptors (acebutolol, atenolol, betaxolol, esmolol, and metoprolol) or *nonselective* (carteolol, labetalol, levobunolol, nadolol, penbutolol, pindolol, propranolol, sotalol, and timolol) blocking both beta$_1$- and beta$_2$-adrenergic receptors. Labetalol has additional alpha-adrenergic blocking action. Acebutolol, carteolol, penbutolol, and pindolol possess *intrinsic sympathomimetic action (ISA)* which may result in less bradycardia than other agents. Ophthalmic beta blockers decrease production of aqueous humor.

Contraindications: Congestive heart failure, acute bronchospasm, some forms of valvular heart disease, bradyarrhythmias, and heart block.

Precautions: Use cautiously in pregnant and lactating females (may cause fetal bradycardia and hypoglycemia). Use cautiously in any form of lung disease, bradyarrhythmias, or underlying compensated congestive heart failure. Use cautiously in diabetics and patients with severe liver disease. Beta-adrenergic blockers should not be discontinued abruptly in patients with cardiovascular disease.

Interactions: May cause additive myocardial depression and bradycardia when used with other agents having this effect (cardiac glycosides and selected antiarrhythmics). May antagonize the therapeutic effect of bronchodilators. May alter insulin dosage requirements. Cimetidine may decrease metabolism and increase the effect of certain beta blockers.

Nursing Implications

ASSESSMENT
- **General Info:** Monitor blood pressure and pulse frequently during dosage adjustment and periodically throughout therapy.
- Monitor intake and output ratios and daily weight. Assess patient routinely for signs and symptoms of congestive heart failure (dyspnea, rales/crackles, weight gain, peripheral edema, and jugular venous distension).
- **Angina:** Assess frequency and severity of episodes of chest pain periodically throughout therapy.
- **Migraine Prophylaxis:** Assess frequency and severity of migraine headaches periodically throughout therapy.

POTENTIAL NURSING DIAGNOSES
- Tissue perfusion, altered (indications).
- Knowledge deficit related to medication regimen (patient/family teaching).
- Noncompliance (patient/family teaching).

IMPLEMENTATION
- Take apical pulse before administering. If heart rate is <50 bpm or if arrhythmias occur, hold medication and notify physician.
- Many beta-adrenergic blockers are available as combination products to enhance compliance (see Appendix A).

PATIENT/FAMILY TEACHING

- **General Info:** Instruct patient to continue taking medication, even if feeling well. Abrupt withdrawal may cause life-threatening arrhythmias, hypertension, or myocardial ischemia. Medication controls but does not cure hypertension.
- Encourage patient to comply with additional interventions for hypertension (weight reduction, low-sodium diet, regular exercise, discontinuation of smoking, moderation of alcohol consumption, and stress management).
- Instruct patient and family on proper technique for monitoring blood pressure. Advise them to check blood pressure weekly and report significant changes to physician.
- Caution patient to make position changes slowly to minimize orthostatic hypotension. Advise patient that exercising or hot weather may enhance hypotensive effects.
- Advise patient to consult physician or pharmacist before taking any over-the-counter medication, especially cold remedies. Patients should also avoid excessive amounts of tea, coffee, or cola.
- Caution patient that these medications may cause increased sensitivity to cold.
- Diabetics should monitor blood sugar closely, especially if weakness, malaise, irritability, or fatigue occurs. May mask tachycardia and increased blood pressure as signs of hypoglycemia, but dizziness and sweating may still occur.
- Advise patient to inform physician or dentist of medication regimen before treatment or surgery.
- Advise patient to carry identification describing disease process and medication regimen at all times.
- Emphasize the importance of follow-up examinations to monitor progress.
- **Ophth:** Instruct patient in correct technique for administration of ophthalmic preparations.

EVALUATION

Effectiveness of therapy can be demonstrated by: ■ Decrease in blood pressure ■ Decrease in frequency and severity of anginal attacks ■ Control of arrhythmias ■ Prevention of myocardial reinfarction ■ Prevention of migraine headaches ■ Decrease in tremors ■ Lowering of intraocular pressure.

Beta-Adrenergic Blocking Agents
Included in *Davis's Drug Guide for Nurses*

C
L
A
S
S
I
F
I
C
A
T
I
O
N
S

▪ BRONCHODILATORS

Pharmacologic Profile

General Uses: Used in the treatment of reversible airway obstruction due to asthma or COPD.

General Action and Information: Beta-adrenergic agonists (albuterol, epinephrine, isoproterenol, metaproterenol, and terbutaline) produce bronchodilation by stimulating the production of cyclic adenosine monophosphate (cAMP). Newer agents (albuterol, bitolterol, metaproterenol, pirbuterol, and terbutaline) are relatively selective for pulmonary (beta$_1$) receptors, whereas older agents produce cardiac stimulation (beta$_2$-adrenergic effects) in addition to bronchodilation. Ephedrine also has alpha-adrenergic effects. Phosphodiesterase inhibitors (aminophylline, dyphylline, oxtriphylline, and theophylline) inhibit the breakdown of cAMP. Ipratropium is an anticholinergic compound that produces bronchodilation by blocking the action of acetylcholine in the respiratory tract.

Contraindications: Hypersensitivity to agents, preservatives (bisulfites), or propellants used in their formulation. Avoid use in uncontrolled cardiac arrhythmias.

Precautions: Use cautiously in patients with diabetes, cardiovascular disease, or hyperthyroidism.

Interactions: Therapeutic effectiveness may be antagonized by concurrent use of beta-adrenergic blocking agents. Additive sympathomimetic effects with other adrenergic (sympathetic) drugs, including vasopressors and decongestants. Cardiovascular effects may be potentiated by antidepressants and MAO inhibitors.

Nursing Implications

ASSESSMENT
- Assess blood pressure, pulse, respiration, lung sounds, and character of secretions before and throughout therapy.
- Patients with a history of cardiovascular problems should be monitored for ECG changes and chest pain.

POTENTIAL NURSING DIAGNOSES
- Airway clearance, ineffective (indications).
- Activity intolerance (indications).
- Knowledge deficit related to medication regimen (patient/family teaching).

IMPLEMENTATION
- Administer around the clock to maintain therapeutic plasma levels.

PATIENT/FAMILY TEACHING
- Emphasize the importance of taking only the prescribed dose at the prescribed time intervals.
- Encourage the patient to drink adequate liquids (2000 ml/day minimum) to decrease the viscosity of the airway secretions.
- Advise patient to avoid over-the-counter cough, cold, or breathing preparations without consulting physician or pharmacist and to minimize intake

of xanthine-containing foods or beverages (colas, coffee, and chocolate), as these may increase side effects and cause arrhythmias.
- Caution patient to avoid smoking and other respiratory irritants.
- Instruct patient on proper use of metered-dose inhaler.
- Advise patient to contact physician promptly if the usual dose of medication fails to produce the desired results, symptoms worsen after treatment, or toxic effects occur.
- Patients using other inhalation medications and bronchodilators should be advised to use bronchodilator first and allow 5 min to elapse before administering the other medication, unless otherwise directed by physician.

EVALUATION
Effectiveness of therapy can be demonstrated by: ■ Decreased bronchospasm ■ Increased ease of breathing.

Bronchodilators Included in *Davis's Drug Guide for Nurses*

alpha- and beta-adrenergic agonists
ephedrine, 404

beta-adrenergic agonists
albuterol, 14
bitolterol, 130
epinephrine, 407
isoproterenol, 606
metaproterenol, 715
pirbuterol, 948
terbutaline, 1122

phosphodiesterase inhibitors
aminophylline, 43
dyphylline, 394
oxtriphylline, 864
theophylline, 1131

anticholinergic agents
ipratropium, 601

■ CALCIUM CHANNEL BLOCKERS

Pharmacologic Profile

General Uses: Used in the treatment of hypertension (amlodipine, diltiazem, felodipine, isradipine, nicardipine, nifedipine, verapamil), treatment and prophylaxis of angina pectoris or coronary artery spasm (amlodipine, bepridil, diltiazem, nicardipine, verapamil). Verapamil and diltiazem are also used for control of arrhythmias. Nimodipine is used to prevent neurologic damage due to certain types of cerebral vasospasm.

General Action and Information: Block calcium entry into cells of vascular smooth muscle and myocardium. Dilate coronary arteries in both normal and ischemic myocardium and inhibit coronary artery spasm. Decrease AV conduction (verapamil and diltiazem). Nimodipine appears to have a relatively selective effect on cerebral blood vessels.

Contraindications: Hypersensitivity. Contraindicated in bradycardia, second and third degree heart block, or uncompensated congestive heart failure (bepridil, verapamil).

Precautions: Safety in pregnancy and lactation not established. Use cautiously in patients with liver disease or uncontrolled arrhythmias. Bepridil has been associated with serious arrythmias and agranulocytosis.

Interactions: Additive myocardial depression with beta-adrenergic blocking agents and disopyramide (verapamil and diltiazem). Effectiveness may be decreased by phenobarbital or phenytoin; increased by propranolol or cimetidine. Verapamil and diltiazem may increase serum digoxin levels and cause toxicity.

Nursing Implications

ASSESSMENT
- **General Info:** Monitor blood pressure and pulse before and periodically during therapy.
- Monitor intake and output ratios and daily weight. Assess patient routinely for signs and symptoms of congestive heart failure (dyspnea, rales/crackles, weight gain, peripheral edema, jugular venous distension).
- **Angina:** Assess frequency and severity of episodes of chest pain periodically throughout therapy.
- **Arrhythmias:** ECG should be monitored continuously during IV therapy and periodically during long-term therapy with verapamil.
- **Cerebral Vasospasm:** Assess patient's neurologic status (level of consciousness, movement) before and periodically during therapy with nimodipine.
- **Lab Test Considerations:** Patients receiving cardiac glycosides concurrently with verapamil or diltiazem should have routine serum digitalis levels and be monitored for signs and symptoms of cardiac glycoside toxicity.

POTENTIAL NURSING DIAGNOSES
- Tissue perfusion, altered (indications).
- Pain (indications).
- Knowledge deficit related to medication regimen (patient/family teaching).

IMPLEMENTATION
- Do not crush, break, chew, or open sustained-release tablets or capsules.

PATIENT/FAMILY TEACHING
- **General Info:** Caution patient to make position changes slowly to minimize orthostatic hypotension.
- May cause dizziness or drowsiness. Caution patient to avoid driving or other activities requiring alertness until response to medication is known.
- Instruct patient to avoid concurrent use of alcohol or over-the-counter medications without consulting physician or pharmacist.
- Advise patient to inform physician or dentist of medication regimen before treatment or surgery.
- Advise patient to carry identification describing disease process and medication regimen at all times.
- Emphasize the importance of follow-up examinations to monitor progress.
- **Angina:** Instruct patients on concurrent nitrate therapy to continue taking both medications as ordered and using SL nitroglycerin as needed for anginal attacks.
- Advise patient to contact physician if chest pain worsens or does not improve after therapy or is accompanied by diaphoresis or shortness of breath, or if severe, persistent headache occurs.
- Advise patient to discuss activity limitations with physician.
- **Hypertension:** Encourage patient to comply with additional interventions for hypertension (weight reduction, low-sodium diet, regular exercise, discontinuation of smoking, moderation of alcohol consumption, stress management). Medication controls but does not cure hypertension.

- Instruct patient and family on proper technique for monitoring blood pressure. Advise them to check blood pressure weekly and report significant changes to physician.

EVALUATION
Effectiveness of therapy can be demonstrated by: ■ Decreased frequency and severity of anginal attacks ■ Decreased need for nitrate therapy ■ Increase in activity tolerance and sense of well-being ■ Decreased blood pressure ■ Resolution and prevention of supraventricular tachyarrhythmias ■ Improvement in neurologic deficits due to vasospasm, which may follow subarachnoid hemorrhage due to ruptured intracranial aneurysms (nimodipine).

Calcium Channel Blockers Included in *Davis's Drug Guide for Nurses*

amlodipine, 50	nicardipine, 814
bepridil, 112	nifedipine, 819
diltiazem, 351	nimodipine, 821
felodipine, 454	verapamil, 1219
isradipine, 613	

■ CENTRAL NERVOUS SYSTEM STIMULANTS

Pharmacologic Profile

General Use: Used in the treatment of narcolepsy and as adjunctive treatment in the management of attention deficit disorder (ADD).

General Action and Information: Produce CNS stimulation by increasing levels of neurotransmitters in the CNS. Produce CNS and respiratory stimulation, dilated pupils, increased motor activity and mental alertness, diminished sense of fatigue, and brighter spirits. In children with ADD these agents decrease restlessness and increase attention span.

Contraindications: Hypersensitivity. Should not be used in pregnant or lactating women. Should not be used in hyperexcitable states. Avoid use in patients with psychotic personalities or suicidal or homicidal tendencies. Contraindicated in glaucoma and severe cardiovascular disease.

Precautions: Use cautiously in patients with a history of cardiovascular disease, hypertension, or diabetes mellitus, or in elderly or debilitated patients. Continual use may result in psychological dependence or addiction.

Interactions: Additive sympathomimetic effects. Use with MAO inhibitors can result in hypertensive crisis. Alkalinizing the urine (sodium bicarbonate and acetazolamide) decreases excretion and enhances effect of amphetamines. Acidification of urine (ammonium chloride and ascorbic acid) decreases effect of amphetamines. Phenothiazines may also decrease effect. Methylphenidate may decrease the metabolism of other drugs.

Nursing Implications

ASSESSMENT
- **General Info:** Monitor blood pressure, pulse, and respiration before administering and periodically throughout course of therapy.
- Monitor weight biweekly and inform physician of significant loss.

- Monitor height periodically in children; inform physician if growth inhibition occurs.
- May produce a false sense of euphoria and well-being. Provide frequent rest periods and observe patient for rebound depression after the effects of the medication have worn off.
- **Attention Deficit Disorders:** Assess attention span, impulse control, and interactions with others in children. Therapy may be interrupted at intervals to determine if symptoms are sufficient to warrant continued therapy.
- **Narcolepsy:** Observe and document frequency of episodes.

POTENTIAL NURSING DIAGNOSES
- Thought processes, altered (side effects).
- Knowledge deficit related to medication regimen (patient/family teaching).

IMPLEMENTATION
- Medication should be administered at least 6 hr before bedtime to minimize sleep disturbances.

PATIENT/FAMILY TEACHING
- Instruct patient not to alter dose without consulting physician. These medications have a high dependence and abuse potential. Abrupt cessation with high doses may cause extreme fatigue and mental depression.
- Inform patient that the effects of drug-induced dry mouth can be minimized by rinsing frequently with water or chewing sugarless gum or candies.
- Advise patient to avoid the intake of large amounts of caffeine.
- Medication may impair judgment. Advise patients to use caution when driving or during other activities requiring alertness until response to medication is known.
- Inform patient that physician may order periodic holidays from the drug to assess progress and decrease dependence.

EVALUATION
Effectiveness of therapy can be demonstrated by: ▪ Decreased frequency of narcoleptic episodes ▪ Improved attention span and social interactions.

Central Nervous System Stimulants
Included in *Davis's Drug Guide for Nurses*

amphetamine, 60	methylphenidate, 735
dextroamphetamine, 319	pemoline, 886

▪ CHOLINERGICS

Pharmacologic Profile

General Use: Used in the treatment of nonobstructive urinary retention (bethanechol), and the diagnosis (edrophonium) and treatment (neostigmine and pyridostigmine) of myasthenia gravis. Physostigmine is used in the diagnosis and management of cholinergic excess, which occurs following antidepressant overdosage. Cholinesterase inhibitors may be used to reverse nondepolarizing neuromusclar blocking agents. Edrophonium has been used in the treatment of supraventricular tachyarrhythmias. Acetylcholine is administered as an eye drop to produce miosis during ophthalmic surgery.

General Action and Information: Cholinergics intensify and prolong the action of acetylcholine by either mimicking its effects at cholinergic receptor sites (bethanechol) or preventing the breakdown of acetylcholine by inhibiting cholinesterases (edrophonium, neostigmine, physostigmine, and pyridostigmine). Effects include increased tone in GU and skeletal muscle, decreased intraocular pressure, increased secretions, and decreased bladder capacity.

Contraindications: Hypersensitivity. Avoid use in patients with possible obstruction of the GI or GU tract.

Precautions: Use with extreme caution in patients with a history of asthma, peptic ulcer disease, cardiovascular disease, epilepsy, or hyperthyroidism. Safety in pregnancy and lactation not established. Atropine should be available to treat excessive dosage.

Interactions: Additive cholinergic effects. Do not use with depolarizing neuromuscular blocking agents. Use with ganglionic blocking agents may result in severe hypotension.

Nursing Implications

ASSESSMENT

- **General Info:** Monitor pulse, respiratory rate, and blood pressure frequently throughout parenteral administration.
- **Myasthenia Gravis:** Assess neuromuscular status (ptosis, diplopia, vital capacity, ability to swallow, and extremity strength) before and at time of peak effect.
- Assess patient for overdosage and underdosage or resistance. Both have similar symptoms (muscle weakness, dyspnea, and dysphagia), but symptoms of overdosage usually occur within 1 hr of administration, while underdosage symptoms occur 3 hr or more after administration. A Tensilon test (edrophonium chloride) may be used to distinguish between overdosage and underdosage.
- **Antidote to Nondepolarizing Neuromuscular Blocking Agents:** Monitor reversal of effects of neuromuscular blocking agents with a peripheral nerve stimulator.
- **Urinary Retention:** Monitor intake and output ratios. Palpate abdomen for bladder distention. Physician may order catheterization to assess postvoid residual.
- **Glaucoma:** Monitor patient for changes in vision, eye irritation, and persistent headache.
- **Toxicity and Overdose:** Atropine is the specific antidote.

POTENTIAL NURSING DIAGNOSES

- Urinary elimination, altered (indications).
- Breathing pattern, ineffective (indications).
- Knowledge deficit related to medication regimen (patient/family teaching).

IMPLEMENTATION

- **Myasthenia Gravis:** For patients who have difficulty chewing, medication may be administered 30 min before meals.

PATIENT/FAMILY TEACHING

- **General Info:** Instruct patients with myasthenia gravis to take medication exactly as ordered. Taking the dose late may result in myasthenic crisis. Taking the dose early may result in a cholinergic crisis. This regimen must be continued as a lifelong therapy.

- **Ophth:** Instruct patient on correct method of application of drops or ointment (see Appendix H).
- Explain to patient that pupil constriction and temporary stinging and blurring of vision is expected. Physician should be notified if blurred vision and brow ache persist.
- Caution patient that night vision may be impaired.
- Advise patient of the need for regular eye examinations to monitor intraocular pressure and visual fields.

EVALUATION

Effectiveness of therapy can be demonstrated by: ▪ Reversal of CNS symptoms secondary to anticholinergic excess resulting from drug overdosage or ingestion of poisonous plants ▪ Control of elevated intraocular pressure ▪ Increase in bladder function and tone ▪ Decrease in abdominal distention ▪ Relief of myasthenic symptoms ▪ Differentiation of myasthenic from cholinergic crisis ▪ Reversal of paralysis after anesthesia ▪ Resolution of supraventricular tachycardia.

Cholinergic Agents Included in *Davis's Drug Guide for Nurses*

cholinomimetic
bethanechol, 120

cholinesterase inhibitors
demecarium, 847
echothiophate, 847

edrophonium, 397
neostigmine, 807
physostigmine, 937
pyridostigmine, 1025

▪ DIURETICS

Pharmacologic Profile

General Use: Thiazide and loop diuretics are used alone or in combination in the treatment of hypertension or edema due to congestive heart failure or other causes. Potassium-sparing diuretics have weak diuretic and antihypertensive properties and are used mainly to conserve potassium in patients receiving thiazide or loop diuretics. Osmotic diuretics are often used in the management of cerebral edema.

General Action and Information: Enhance the selective excretion of various electrolytes and water by affecting renal mechanisms for tubular secretion and reabsorption. Groups commonly used are thiazide diuretics and thiazide-like diuretics (chlorthalidone, hydrochlorothiazide, indapamide, and metolazone); loop diuretics (bumetanide, ethacrynic acid, and furosemide); potassium-sparing diuretics (amiloride, spironolactone, and triamterene); and osmotic diuretics (mannitol). Mechanisms vary depending on agent.

Contraindications: Hypersensitivity. Thiazide diuretics may exhibit cross-sensitivity with other sulfonamides.

Precautions: Use with caution in patients with renal or hepatic disease. Safety in pregnancy and lactation not established.

Interactions: Additive hypokalemia with glucocorticoids, amphotericin B, mezlocillin, piperacillin, or ticarcillin. Hypokalemia enhances cardiac glycoside toxicity. Potassium-losing diuretics decrease lithium excretion and may cause toxicity. Additive hypotension with other antihypertensives or nitrates. Potassium-sparing diuretics may cause hyperkalemia when used with potassium supplements or angiotensin converting enzyme (ACE) inhibitors.

Nursing Implications

ASSESSMENT

- **General Info:** Assess fluid status throughout therapy. Monitor daily weight, intake and output ratios, amount and location of edema, lung sounds, skin turgor, and mucous membranes.
- Assess patient for anorexia, muscle weakness, numbness, tingling, paresthesia, confusion, and excessive thirst. Notify physician promptly if these signs of electrolyte imbalance occur.
- **Increased Intracranial Pressure:** Monitor neurologic status and intracranial pressure readings in patients receiving osmotic diuretics to decrease cerebral edema.
- **Increased Intraocular Pressure:** Monitor for persistent or increased eye pain or decreased visual acuity.
- **Lab Test Considerations:** Monitor electrolytes (especially potassium), blood glucose, BUN, and serum uric acid levels before and periodically throughout course of therapy.
- Thiazide diuretics may cause increased serum cholesterol, low-density lipoprotein (LDL), and triglyceride concentrations.

POTENTIAL NURSING DIAGNOSES

- Fluid volume excess (indications).
- Knowledge deficit related to medication regimen (patient/family teaching).

IMPLEMENTATION

- Administer oral diuretics in the morning to prevent disruption of sleep cycle.
- Many diuretics are available in combination with antihypertensives or potassium-sparing diuretics.

PATIENT/FAMILY TEACHING

- **General Info:** Caution patient to make position changes slowly to minimize orthostatic hypotension. Caution patient that the use of alcohol, exercise during hot weather, or standing for long periods during therapy may enhance orthostatic hypotension.
- Instruct patient to consult physician regarding dietary potassium guidelines.
- Instruct patient to monitor weight weekly and notify physician of significant changes. Instruct patients with hypertension in the correct technique for monitoring weekly blood pressure.
- Caution patient to use sunscreen and protective clothing to prevent photosensitivity reactions.
- Advise patient to consult physician or pharmacist before taking over-the-counter medication concurrently with this therapy.
- Instruct patient to notify physician or dentist of medication regimen before treatment or surgery.
- Advise patient to contact physician immediately if muscle weakness, cramps, nausea, dizziness, or numbness or tingling of extremities occur.
- Emphasize the importance of routine follow-up.

- **Hypertension:** Reinforce the need to continue additional therapies for hypertension (weight loss, regular exercise, restricted sodium intake, stress reduction, moderation of alcohol consumption, and cessation of smoking).

EVALUATION
Effectiveness of therapy can be demonstrated by: ▪ Decreased blood pressure ▪ Increased urine output ▪ Decreased edema ▪ Reduced intracranial pressure ▪ Prevention of hypokalemia in patients taking diuretics ▪ Treatment of hyperaldosteronism.

Diuretics Included in *Davis's Drug Guide for Nurses*

loop diuretics
 bumetanide, 139
 furosemide, 502

osmotic diuretics
 mannitol, 683

potassium-sparing diuretics
 amiloride, 37
 spironolactone, 1085
 triamterene, 1187

thiazide and thiazide-like diuretics
 chlorthalidone, 238
 hydrochlorothiazide, 553
 indapamide, 584
 metolazone, 745

▪ ELECTROLYTES/ELECTROLYTE MODIFIERS

Pharmacologic Profile

General Use: Use to prevent or treat deficiencies or excesses of electrolytes. Acidifiers and alkalinizers are used to increase solubility and promote renal excretion of substances that accumulate in certain disease states (kidney stones and uric acid).

General Action and Information: Electrolytes are essential for homeostasis. Maintenance of electrolyte levels within normal levels is required for many physiologic processes such as cardiac, nerve, and muscle function; bone growth and stability; and other processes. Electrolytes may also serve as catalysts in many enzymatic reactions.

Contraindications: Contraindicated in situations in which replacement would cause excess or when risk factors for retention are present.

Precautions: Use cautiously in disease states in which electrolyte imbalances are common, such as hepatic or renal disease, adrenal disorders, pituitary disorders, and diabetes mellitus.

Interactions: Depend on individual agents. Akalinizers and acidifiers can alter excretion of drugs whose renal elimination is pH-dependent. See specific entries.

Nursing Implications

ASSESSMENT
- Observe patient carefully for evidence of electrolyte excess or insufficiency. Monitor lab values before and periodically throughout therapy.

POTENTIAL NURSING DIAGNOSES
- Nutrition, altered: less than body requirements (indications).
- Knowledge deficit related to medication and dietary regimens (patient/family teaching).

IMPLEMENTATION
- **Potassium chloride:** Do not administer parenteral potassium chloride undiluted.

PATIENT/FAMILY TEACHING
- Review diet modifications with patients with chronic electrolyte disturbances.

EVALUATION
Effectiveness of therapy can be demonstrated by: ▪ Return to normal serum electrolyte concentrations and resolution of clinical symptoms of electrolyte imbalance ▪ Changes in pH or composition of urine, which prevent formation of renal calculi.

Electrolytes/Electrolyte Modifiers
Included in *Davis's Drug Guide for Nurses*

alkalinizing agents
  sodium bicarbonate, 1070

calcium salts
  calcium carbonate, 157
  calcium chloride, 157
  calcium gluceptate, 157
  calcium gluconate, 157
  calcium lactate, 157

hypocalcemic agents
  calcitonin, 153
  etidronate, 437
  gallium nitrate, 507
  pamidronate, 876
  plicamycin, 953

hypophosphatemic
  aluminum hydroxide, 31

magnesium salts
  magnesium citrate, 676
  magnesium sulfate, 680

phosphates
  monobasic potassium and
    sodium phosphates, 960

potassium and sodium
  phosphates, 960

potassium exhange resin
  sodium polystyrene
    sulfonate, 1078

potassium salts
  potassium bicarbonate/
    citrate, 963
  potassium chloride, 964
  potassium gluconate, 967

replacement solutions
  sodium chloride, 1073

urinary acidifiers
  potassium and sodium
    phosphates, 960
  monobasic potassium and
    sodium phosphates, 960

urinary alkalinizer
  sodium citrate and citric
    acid, 1075

▪ GLUCOCORTICOIDS

Pharmacologic Profile

General Use: Used in replacement doses (20 mg of hydrocortisone or equivalent) to treat adrenocortical insufficiency. Larger doses are usually used for their anti-inflammatory, immunosuppressive, or antineoplastic activity. Used adjunctively in many other situations including hypercalcemia and autoimmune diseases. Topical glucocorticoids are used in a variety of inflammatory and allergic conditions.

General Action and Information: Produce profound and varied metabolic effects in addition to modifying the normal immune response and suppressing inflammation. Available in a variety of dosage forms including oral, injectable, topical, and inhalation. Prolonged use of large amounts of topical or inhaled agents may result in systemic absorption and/or adrenal suppression.

Contraindications: Serious infections (except for certain forms of meningitis). Do not administer live vaccines to patients on larger doses.

Precautions: Chronic treatment will result in adrenal suppression. Do not discontinue abruptly. Additional doses may be needed during stress (surgery and infection). Safety in pregnancy and lactation not established. Chronic use in children will result in decreased growth. May mask signs of infection. Use lowest dose possible for shortest time possible. Alternate day therapy is preferable during chronic treatment.

Interactions: Additive hypokalemia with amphotericin B, potassium-losing diuretics, mezlocillin, piperacillin, and ticarcillin. Hypokalemia may increase the risk of cardiac glycoside toxicity. May increase requirements for insulin or oral hypoglycemic agents. Phenytoin, phenobarbital, and rifampin stimulate metabolism and may decrease effectiveness. Oral contraceptives may block metabolism. Cholestyramine and colestipol may decrease absorption.

Nursing Implications

ASSESSMENT
- These drugs are indicated for many conditions. Assess involved systems before and periodically throughout course of therapy.
- Assess patient for signs of adrenal insufficiency (hypotension, weight loss, weakness, nausea, vomiting, anorexia, lethargy, confusion, restlessness) prior to and periodically throughout course of therapy.
- Children should also have periodic evaluations of growth.

POTENTIAL NURSING DIAGNOSES
- Infection, high risk for (side effects).
- Knowledge deficit related to medication regimen (patient/family teaching).
- Body image disturbance (side effects).

IMPLEMENTATION
- **General Info:** If dose is ordered daily or every other day, administer in the morning to coincide with the body's normal secretion of cortisol.
- **PO:** Administer with meals to minimize gastric irritation.

PATIENT/FAMILY TEACHING
- Emphasize need to take medication exactly as directed. Review symptoms of adrenal insufficiency that may occur upon stopping the medication and that may be life-threatening.
- Encourage patients on long-term therapy to eat a diet high in protein, calcium, and potassium and low in sodium and carbohydrates.
- These drugs cause immunosuppression and may mask symptoms of infec-

tion. Instruct patient to avoid people with known contagious illnesses and to report possible infections. Advise patient to consult physician before receiving any vaccinations.

- Discuss possible effects on body image. Explore coping mechanisms.
- Advise patient to carry identification in the event of an emergency in which patient cannot relate medical history.

EVALUATION

Effectiveness of therapy can be demonstrated by: ▪ Suppression of the inflammatory and immune responses in autoimmune disorders, allergic reactions, and organ transplants ▪ Replacement therapy in adrenal insufficiency ▪ Resolution of skin inflammation, pruritus, or other dermatologic conditions.

Glucocorticoids Included in *Davis's Drug Guide for Nurses*

topical glucocorticoids, 1170

short-acting glucocorticoids
cortisone, 284
hydrocortisone, 557

intermediate-acting glucocorticoids
methylprednisolone, 737
prednisolone, 979
prednisone, 982
triamcinolone, 1184

long-acting glucocorticoids
beclomethasone, 105
betamethasone, 115
dexamethasone, 316
flunisolide, 481

topical glucocorticoids
aclometasone, 1170
amcinonide, 1170
betamethasone, 1170
clobetasol, 1170
clocortolone, 1170
desonide, 1170
desoximethasone, 1170
dexamethasone, 1170
diflorasone, 1170
fluocinolone, 1170
fluocinonide, 1171
flurandrenolide, 1171
fluticasone, 1171
halcinonide, 1171
halobetasol, 1171
hydrocortisone, 1171
mometasone, 1171
prednicarbate, 1171
triamcinolone, 1171

▪ HORMONES

Pharmacologic Profile

General Use: Used in the treatment of deficiency states including diabetes (insulin), diabetes insipidus (desmopressin), hypothyroidism (thyroid hormone), and menopause (estrogens). Combinations of hormones (estrogens and progestins) are used as oral contraceptive agents. Hormones may be used to treat hormonally sensitive tumors (androgens and estrogens) and in other selected situations. See individual drugs.

General Action and Information: Natural or synthetic substances that have a specific effect on target tissue. Differ greatly in their effects, depending on individual agent and function of target tissue.

Contraindications: Differ greatly among agents. See individual entries.

Precautions: Use cautiously in patients with severe cardiac, hepatic, or renal disease. When used in deficiency states, appropriate laboratory monitoring is necessary to adjust dosages and monitor progress.

Interactions: Differ greatly among agents. See individual entries.

Nursing Implications

ASSESSMENT
- **General Info:** Monitor patient for symptoms of hormonal excess or insufficiency.
- **Sex hormones:** Blood pressure and hepatic function tests should be monitored periodically throughout therapy.
- **Epoetin Alpha:** Monitor blood pressure, hematocrit, hemoglobin, reticulocyte count, and RBC, as well as symptoms of anemia throughout therapy. Uncontrolled hypertension is contraindicated.

POTENTIAL NURSING DIAGNOSES
- Sexual dysfunction (indications).
- Body image disturbance (indications, side effects).
- Knowledge deficit related to medication regimen (patient/family teaching).

IMPLEMENTATION
- **Sex hormones:** Continue to administer according to schedule followed prior to hospitalization.

PATIENT/FAMILY TEACHING
- **General Info:** Explain dosage schedule (and withdrawal bleeding with female sex hormones).
- Emphasize importance of follow-up examinations to monitor effectiveness of therapy and to ensure proper development of children and early detection of possible side effects.
- **Female sex hormones:** Advise patient to report signs and symptoms of fluid retention, thromboembolic disorders, mental depression, or hepatic dysfunction to physician.

EVALUATION
Effectiveness of therapy can be demonstrated by: ▪ Resolution of clinical symptoms of hormone imbalance including menopausal symptoms and effective contraception ▪ Correction of fluid and electrolyte imbalances ▪ Control of the spread of advanced metastatic breast or prostate cancer ▪ Slowed progression of postmenopausal osteoporosis ▪ Increase in hematocrit (epoetin alpha) ▪ Induction of ovulation in women with primary hypothalmic amenorrhea (gonadorelin) ▪ Resolution of the signs of precocious puberty (histrelin, nafarelin).

Hormones Included in *Davis's Drug Guide for Nurses*

■ IMMUNOSUPPRESSANTS

Pharmacologic Profile

General Use: Azathioprine and cyclosporine are used with glucocorticoids in the prevention of transplantation rejection reactions. Muromonab-CD3 is used to manage rejection reactions not controlled by other agents. Azathioprine, cyclophosphamide, and methotrexate are used in the management of selected autoimmune diseases (nephrotic syndrome of childhood and severe rheumatoid arthritis).

General Action and Information: Inhibit cell-mediated immune responses by different mechanisms. In addition to azathioprine and cyclosporine, which are used primarily for their immunomodulating properties, cyclophosphamide and methotrexate are used to suppress the immune responses in certain disease states (nephrotic syndrome of childhood and severe rheumatoid arthritis). Muromonab-CD3 is a recombinant immunoglobulin antibody that alters T cell function.

Contraindications: Hypersensitivity to drug or vehicle.

Precautions: Use cautiously in patients with infections. Safety in pregnancy and lactation not established.

Interactions: Allopurinol inhibits the metabolism of azathioprine. Drugs that alter liver metabolizing processes may change the effect of cyclosporine. The risk of toxicity of methotrexate may be increased by other nephrotoxic drugs, large doses of aspirin, or nonsteroidal anti-inflammatory agents. Muromonab-CD3 has additive immunosuppressive properties; concurrent immunosuppressive doses should be decreased or eliminated.

Nursing Implications

ASSESSMENT

■ **General Info:** Monitor for infection (vital signs, sputum, urine, stool, WBC). Notify physician immediately if symptoms occur.

C
L
A
S
S
I
F
I
C
A
T
I
O
N
S

- **Organ Transplant:** Assess for symptoms of organ rejection throughout therapy.
- **Lab Test Considerations:** Monitor CBC and differential throughout course of therapy.

POTENTIAL NURSING DIAGNOSES
- Infection, high risk for (side effects).
- Knowledge deficit related to medication regimen (patient/family teaching).

IMPLEMENTATION
- Protect transplant patients from staff and visitors who may carry infection.
- Maintain protective isolation as indicated.

PATIENT/FAMILY TEACHING
- Reinforce the need for lifelong therapy to prevent transplant rejection. Review symptoms of rejection for transplanted organ and stress need to notify physician immediately if they occur.
- Advise patient to avoid contact with contagious persons and those who have recently taken oral poliovirus vaccine. Patients should not receive vaccinations without first consulting with physician.
- Emphasize the importance of follow-up examinations and lab tests.

EVALUATION
Effectiveness of therapy can be demonstrated by: ▪ Prevention or reversal of rejection of organ transplants or decrease in symptoms of autoimmune disorders.

Immunosuppressants Included in *Davis's Drug Guide for Nurses*
azathioprine, 97
cyclophosphamide, 288
cyclosporine, 291
methotrexate, 726
muromonab-CD3, 790

▪ INOTROPIC AGENTS

Pharmacologic Profile

General Use: Management of congestive heart failure or cardiac decompensation unresponsive to conventional therapy with cardiac glycosides, diuretics, or vasodilators. Also used during cardiac surgery.

General Action and Information: Increase cardiac output mainly by direct myocardial effects and some peripheral vascular effects. Cardiac glycosides (deslanoside, digoxin, and digitoxin) act by direct effects on the myocardium.

Contraindications: Hypersensitivity. Avoid use in patients with hypertrophic cardiomyopathy.

Precautions: Safety in pregnancy and lactation not established.

Interactions: Beta-adrenergic blockers may negate the effects of dobutamine or dopamine. Several drugs may increase the arrhythmogenic and hypertensive effects of dobutamine or dopamine. Amrinone may produce excessive hypotension when given with disopyramide. Agents that cause hypokalemia, hypomagnesemia, or hypercalcemia increase the risk of cardiac glycoside toxicity. Bradycardia from beta blockers may be additive with cardiac glycosides. Quinidine increases serum digoxin levels.

Nursing Implications

ASSESSMENT

- Monitor pulse, blood pressure, ECG, and hemodynamic parameters frequently during parenteral administration and periodically throughout oral administration.
- Monitor intake and output ratios and daily weights. Assess patient for signs and symptoms of congestive heart failure (peripheral edema, rales/crackles, dyspnea, weight gain, and jugular venous distension) throughout therapy.
- Before administering initial loading dose, determine if patient has taken any cardiac glycoside preparations in the preceding 2–3 wk.
- **Lab Test Considerations:** Serum electrolyte levels, especially potassium, magnesium, and calcium, and renal and hepatic function should be evaluated periodically during course of therapy.
- **Toxicity and Overdose:** Patients taking cardiac glycosides should have serum levels measured regularly.

POTENTIAL NURSING DIAGNOSES

- Cardiac output, decreased (indications).
- Knowledge deficit related to medication regimen (patient/family teaching).

IMPLEMENTATION

- Hypokalemia should be corrected before administration of amrinone, milrinone, digoxin, or digitoxin.
- Hypovolemia should be corrected with volume expanders before administration.

PATIENT/FAMILY TEACHING

- Advise patient to notify physician if symptoms are not relieved or worsen.
- Instruct patient to notify nurse immediately if pain or discomfort at the insertion site occurs during IV administration.

EVALUATION

Effectiveness of therapy can be demonstrated by: ▪ Increased cardiac output ▪ Decrease in severity of congestive heart failure ▪ Increased urine output.

Inotropic Agents Included in *Davis's Drug Guide for Nurses*

amrinone, 68
digitoxin, 342
digoxin, 344
dobutamine, 370

dopamine, 373
isoproterenol, 606
milrinone, 760

▪ LAXATIVES

Pharmacologic Profile

General Uses: Used to treat or prevent constipation or to prepare the bowel for radiologic or endoscopic procedures.

General Action and Information: Induce one or more bowel movements per day. Groups include stimulants (bisacodyl, cascara and its derivatives, phenolphthalein, and senna); saline laxatives (magnesium salts and phosphates); stool softeners (docusate); bulk-forming agents (polycarbophil and psyllium); lubricants (mineral oil); and osmotic cathartics (glycerin, lactulose, polyethylene glycol/electrolyte). Increasing fluid intake, exercise, and adding more dietary fiber are also useful in the management of chronic constipation.

Contraindications: Hypersensitivity. Contraindicated in persistant abdominal pain, nausea, or vomiting of unknown cause, especially if accompanied by fever or other signs of an acute abdomen.

Precautions: Excessive or prolonged use may lead to dependence. Should not be used in children unless advised by a physician.

Interactions: Theoretically may decrease the absorption of other orally administered drugs by decreasing transit time.

Nursing Implications

ASSESSMENT
- Assess patient for abdominal distention, presence of bowel sounds, and usual pattern of bowel function.
- Assess color, consistency, and amount of stool produced.

POTENTIAL NURSING DIAGNOSES
- Constipation (indications).
- Knowledge deficit related to medication regimen (patient/family teaching).

IMPLEMENTATION
- Many laxatives may be administered at bedtime for morning results.
- Taking oral doses on an empty stomach will usually produce more rapid results.
- Do not crush or chew enteric-coated tablets. Take with a full glass of water or juice.
- Stool softeners and bulk laxatives may take several days for results.

PATIENT/FAMILY TEACHING
- Advise patients, other than those with spinal cord injuries, that laxatives should be used only for short-term therapy. Long-term therapy may cause electrolyte imbalance and dependence.
- Advise patient to increase fluid intake to a minimum of 1500–2000 ml/day during therapy to prevent dehydration.
- Encourage patients to utilize other forms of bowel regulation: increasing bulk in the diet, increasing fluid intake, and increasing mobility. Normal bowel habits are individualized and may vary from 3 times/day to 3 times/wk.
- Instruct patients with cardiac disease to avoid straining during bowel movements (Valsalva maneuver).
- Advise patient that laxatives should not be used when constipation is accompanied by abdominal pain, fever, nausea, or vomiting.

EVALUATION
Effectiveness of therapy can be demonstrated by: ▪ The patient having a soft, formed bowel movement ▪ Evacuation of the colon.

Laxatives Included in *Davis's Drug Guide for Nurses*

bulk-forming agents
polycarbophil, 955
psyllium, 1022

lubricant
mineral oil, 761

osmotic agents
glycerin, 517
lactulose, 630
poleythylene
glycol/electrolyte, 957

saline laxatives
magensium citrate, 676

magnesium hydroxide, 677
magnesium sulfate, 680
phosphate/biphosphate, 936

stimulants
bisacodyl, 126
casanthranol, 181
cascara sagrada, 181
phenolphthalein, 923
senna, 1063

stool softeners
docusate, 371

■ LIPID-LOWERING AGENTS

Pharmacologic Profile

General Use: Used as a part of a total plan including diet and exercise to reduce blood lipids in an effort to reduce the morbidity and mortality of atherosclerotic cardiovascular disease.

General Action and Information: HMG-CoA reductase inhibitors (lovastatin, simvastatin, pravastatin) inhibit an enzyme involved in cholesterol synthesis. Bile acid sequestrants (cholestyramine, colestipol) bind cholesterol in the GI tract. Niacin, probucol, and gemfibrozil act by other mechanisms (see individual monographs).

Contraindications: Hypersensitivity.

Precautions: Safety in pregnancy, lactation, and children not established. See individual drugs. Dietary therapy should be given a 2–3 mo trial before drug therapy is initiated.

Interactions: Bile acid sequestrants (cholestyramine and colestipol) may bind lipid-soluble vitamins (A, D, E, and K) and other concurrently administered drugs in the GI tract. The risk of myopathy from HMG-CoA reductase inhibitors is increased by niacin, erthromycin, gemfibrozil, and cyclosporine.

Nursing Implications

ASSESSMENT
- Obtain a diet history, especially in regard to fat and alcohol consumption.
- **Lab Test Considerations:** Serum cholesterol and triglyceride levels should be evaluated before initiating and periodically throughout course of therapy. Medication should be discontinued if paradoxical increase in cholesterol level occurs.
- Liver function tests should be assessed before and periodically throughout therapy. May cause an increase in levels.

POTENTIAL NURSING DIAGNOSES
- Knowledge deficit related to medication regimen (patient/family teaching).
- Noncompliance (patient/family teaching).

IMPLEMENTATION
- See specific medications to determine timing of doses in relation to meals.

PATIENT/FAMILY TEACHING
- Advise patient that these medications should be used in conjunction with diet restrictions (fat, cholesterol, carbohydrates, and alcohol), exercise, and cessation of smoking.

EVALUATION
Effectiveness of therapy can be demonstrated by: ▪ Decreased serum triglyceride and low-density lipoprotein (LDL) cholesterol levels and improved high-density lipoprotein (HDL) cholesterol ratios. Therapy is usually discontinued if the clinical response is not evident after 3 mo of therapy.

Lipid-Lowering Agents Included in *Davis's Drug Guide for Nurses*

  bile acid sequestrants
    cholestyramine, 122
    colestipol, 122

  HMG-CoA reductase inhibitors
    gemfibrozil, 510
    lovastatin, 669

  niacin, nicotinic acid, 812
  pravastatin, 975
  probucol, 988
  simvastatin, 1069

▪ NEUROMUSCULAR BLOCKING AGENTS

Pharmacologic Profile

General Use: Used to facilitate mechanical ventilation or as adjuncts with general anesthesia to allow skeletal muscle paralysis, which may be required during surgical procedures.

General Action and Information: Paralyze muscular function by inhibiting neuromuscular transmission. These agents act as agonists of acetylcholine, producing initial fasciculation then neuromuscular blockade. Blockade from depolarizing agents resists the action of cholinesterase and is more prolonged than that of nondepolarizing agents. Neuromuscular blocking agents have no analgesic properties.

Contraindications: Products may contain iodides, bromides, parabens, or sulfites. Select agents carefully in patients with known hypersensitivity. Avoid use of succinylcholine in patients with a history of malignant hyperthermia or fractures.

Precautions: Use with caution in the very young or elderly patients (increased sensitivity). Provide adequate analgesia/anesthesia as required. Use cautiously in patients with cardiovascular or pulmonary disease.

Interactions: Additive respiratory depression with opioid analgesics and other CNS depressants. Increased risk of adverse cardiovascular reactions with antihypertensives, cardiac glycosides, or antiarrhythmics. Neuromuscular blockade may be enhanced by nonpenicillin anti-infectives, diuretics, antiarrhythmics, anticholinesterases, or local anesthetics. Avoid concurrent use of succinylcholine with any agents that may act as cholinesterase inhibitors (results in prolonged neuromuscular blockade).

Nursing Implications

ASSESSMENT

- Assess respiratory status continuously throughout therapy. Neuromuscular blocking agents should be used only for intubated patients. Assess patient for increased respiratory secretions; suction as necessary.
- Neuromuscular response to these medications should be monitored with a peripheral nerve stimulator intraoperatively. Monitor deep tendon reflexes during prolonged administration. Paralysis is initially selective and usually occurs consecutively in the following muscles: levator muscles of eyelids, muscles of mastication, limb muscles, abdominal muscles, muscles of the glottis, intercostal muscles, and the diaphragm. Recovery of muscle function usually occurs in reverse order.
- Monitor heart rate, ECG, and blood pressure periodically throughout therapy. May cause a slight increase in heart rate and blood pressure.
- Observe the patient for residual muscle weakness and respiratory distress during the recovery period.
- **Toxicity and Overdose:** If overdose occurs, use peripheral nerve stimulator to determine the degree of neuromuscular blockade. Maintain airway patency and ventilation until recovery of normal respirations occurs.
- Administration of anticholinesterase agents (edrophonium, neostigmine, and pyridostigmine) may be used to antagonize the action of nondepolarizing neuromuscular blocking agents. Atropine is usually administered before or concurrently with anticholinesterase agents.

POTENTIAL NURSING DIAGNOSES

- Breathing pattern, ineffective (indications).
- Communication, impaired verbal (side effects).
- Fear (patient/family teaching).

IMPLEMENTATION

- Neuromuscular blocking agents have no effect on consciousness or the pain threshold. Adequate anesthesia should *always* be used when these agents are used as an adjunct to surgical procedures or when painful procedures are performed. Benzodiazepines and/or analgesics should be administered concurrently when prolonged therapy is used for ventilator patients; patient is awake and able to feel all sensations.
- If eyes remain open throughout prolonged administration, protect corneas with artificial tears.

PATIENT/FAMILY TEACHING

- Explain all procedures to patient receiving neuromuscular-blocking agents without anesthesia; consciousness is not affected by these agents alone. Provide emotional support.
- Reassure patient that communication abilities will return as the medication wears off.

EVALUATION

Effectiveness of therapy can be demonstrated by: ■ Adequate suppression of the twitch response when tested with peripheral nerve stimulation and subsequent muscle paralysis.

▪ NONOPIOID ANALGESICS/NONSTEROIDAL ANTI-INFLAMMATORY AGENTS

Pharmacologic Profile

General Use: Most agents in this group are used to control mild to moderate pain, fever, and various inflammatory conditions, such as rheumatoid arthritis and osteoarthritis. Acetaminophen has analgesic and antipyretic properties but is not effective as an anti-inflammatory agent. Phenazopyridine is used as a urinary tract analgesic only. Methotrimeprazine is a phenothiazine with analgesic properties; however, excessive hypotension precludes routine use.

General Action and Information: The largest group of nonopioid analgesics are the nonsteroidal anti-inflammatory agents (NSAIAs, NSAIDs). Although not labeled for all actions, NSAIAs and salicylates have analgesic, antipyretic, and anti-inflammatory properties. The mechanism for analgesia is probably due to inhibition of prostaglandin synthesis. Antipyretic action is due to prostaglandin synthesis inhibition in the CNS and vasodilation. Prostaglandin synthesis inhibition also explains the ability to suppress inflammation. Acetaminophen possesses antipyretic and analgesic action but has no anti-inflammatory properties.

Contraindications: Hypersensitivity to aspirin is a contraindication for the whole class of NSAIAs. Only acetaminophen is safe for occasional use in pregnancy or lactation.

Precautions: Use NSAIAs cautiously in patients with a history of bleeding disorders or gastrointestinal bleeding (effect may be less with nonaspirin salicylates), and in severe hepatic, renal, or cardiovascular disease. Safety of NSAIAs in pregnancy is not established.

Interactions: NSAIAs prolong bleeding time and potentiate the effect of anticoagulants, thrombolytic agents, plicamycin, some cephalosporins, and valproic acid. Chronic use of NSAIAs with aspirin may result in increased GI side effects and decreased effectiveness. NSAIAs may decrease the response to diuretics or antihypertensive therapy. Chronic use of acetaminophen with NSAIAs may increase the risk of adverse renal reactions. Methotrimeprazine will produce additive hypotension with other agents that lower blood pressure.

Nursing Implications

ASSESSMENT
▪ **General Info:** Patients who have asthma, aspirin-induced allergy, and nasal

polyps are at increased risk for developing hypersensitivity reactions. Assess for rhinitis, asthma, and urticaria.
- **Arthritis:** Assess pain and range of motion before and 1–2 hr following administration.
- **Pain:** Assess pain (note type, location, and intensity) before and 1–2 hr following administration.
- **Fever:** Monitor temperature; note signs associated with fever (diaphoresis, tachycardia, and malaise).
- **Lab Test Considerations:** May cause prolonged bleeding time, which may persist following discontinuation of therapy.

POTENTIAL NURSING DIAGNOSES
- Pain (indications).
- Physical mobility, impaired (indications).
- Knowledge deficit related to medication regimen (patient/family teaching).

IMPLEMENTATION
- **General Info:** Coadministration with opioid analgesics may have additive analgesic effects and may permit lower opioid doses.
- **PO:** For rapid initial effect, administer 30 min before or 2 hr after meals. May be administered with food, milk, or antacids to decrease GI irritation. Food slows but does not reduce the extent of absorption.
- **Dysmenorrhea:** Administer as soon as possible after the onset of menses. Prophylactic treatment has not been shown to be effective.

PATIENT/FAMILY TEACHING
- Advise patients to take these medications with a full glass of water and to remain in an upright position for 15–30 min after administration.
- These medications may occasionally cause drowsiness or dizziness. Advise patient to avoid driving or other activities requiring alertness until response to medication is known.
- Caution patient to avoid the concurrent use of alcohol, aspirin, ibuprofen, acetaminophen, or other over-the-counter medications without consultation with physician or pharmacist.
- Advise patient to inform physician or dentist of medication regimen before treatment or surgery.

EVALUATION
Effectiveness of therapy can be demonstrated by: ■ Improved joint mobility ■ Decrease in severity of pain ■ Reduction in fever. Patients who do not respond to one nonsteroidal anti-inflammatory agent may respond to another.

Nonopioid Analgesics/Nonsteroidal Anti-inflammatory Agents Included in *Davis's Drug Guide for Nurses*

nonsteroidal anti-inflammatory agents
- aspirin, 80
- choline and magnesium salicylates, 241
- choline salicylate, 242
- diclofenac, 331
- etodolac, 440
- fenoprofen, 456

- flurbiprofen, 494
- ibuprofen, 570
- indomethacin, 586
- ketoprofen, 623
- ketorolac, 625
- meclofenamate, 694
- nabumetone, 792

continued

▪ OPIOID ANALGESICS

Pharmacologic Profile

General Uses: Management of moderate to severe pain. Some agents used as general anesthetic adjuncts (alfentanil, fentanyl, and sufentanil).

General Action and Information: Opioids bind to opiate receptors in the CNS, where they act as agonists of endogenously occurring opioid peptides (eukephalins and endorphins). The result is alteration to the perception of and response to pain.

Contraindications: Hypersensitivity to individual agents.

Precautions: Use cautiously in patients with undiagnosed abdominal pain, head trauma or pathology, liver disease, or history of addiction to opioids. Use smaller doses initially in the elderly and those with respiratory diseases. Chronic use may result in tolerance and the need for larger doses to relieve pain. Psychological or physical dependence may occur.

Interactions: Increases the CNS depressant properties of other drugs, including alcohol, antihistamines, antidepressants, sedative/hypnotics, phenothiazines, and MAO inhibitors. Use of partial-antagonist opioid analgesics (buprenorphine, butorphanol, dezocine, nalbuphine, and pentazocine) may precipitate opioid withdrawal in physically dependent patients. Use with MAO inhibitors or procarbazine may result in severe paradoxical reactions (especially with meperidine). Nalbuphine or pentazocine may decrease the analgesic effects of other concurrently administered opioid analgesics.

Nursing Implications

ASSESSMENT
- Assess type, location, and intensity of pain prior to and at peak following administration.
- Assess blood pressure, pulse, and respiratory rate before and periodically during administration.
- Prolonged use may lead to physical and psychological dependence and tolerance. This should not prevent patient from receiving adequate analgesia. Most patients who receive opioid analgesics for medical reasons do not develop psychological dependence. Progressively higher doses may be required to relieve pain with long-term therapy.

- Assess bowel function routinely. Increased intake of fluids and bulk, stool softeners, and laxatives may minimize constipating effects.
- Monitor intake and output ratios. If significant discrepancies occur, assess for urinary retention and inform physician.
- **Toxicity and Overdose:** If overdose occurs, naloxone (Narcan) is the antidote. Monitor patient closely; dose may need to be repeated or may need to be administered as an infusion.

POTENTIAL NURSING DIAGNOSES
- Pain (indications).
- Sensory-perceptual alteration: visual, auditory (side effects).
- Injury, high risk for (side effects).
- Knowledge deficit related to medication regimen (patient/family teaching).

IMPLEMENTATION
- Explain therapeutic value of medication before administration to enhance the analgesic effect.
- Regularly administered doses may be more effective than prn administration. Analgesic is more effective if given before pain becomes severe.
- Co-administration with nonopioid analgesics may have additive analgesic effects and may permit lower doses.
- Medication should be discontinued gradually after long-term use to prevent withdrawal symptoms.

PATIENT/FAMILY TEACHING
- Instruct patient on how and when to ask for pain medication.
- Medication may cause drowsiness or dizziness. Caution patient to call for assistance when ambulating or smoking and to avoid driving or other activities requiring alertness until response to medication is known.
- Advise patient to make position changes slowly to minimize orthostatic hypotension.
- Caution patient to avoid concurrent use of alcohol or other CNS depressants with this medication.
- Encourage patient to turn, cough, and breathe deeply every 2 hr to prevent atelectasis.

EVALUATION
Effectiveness of therapy can be demonstrated by: • Decreased severity of pain without a significant alteration in level of consciousness, respiratory status, or blood pressure.

Opioid Analgesics Included in *Davis's Drug Guide for Nurses*

opioid agonists
alfentanil, 18
codeine, 272
fentanyl, 458
fentanyl transdermal, 460
hydrocodone, 555
hydromorphone, 560
levorphanol, 640
meperidine, 704
methadone, 717
morphine, 784
oxycodone, 868
oxymorphone, 870
propoxyphene, 1012
sufentanil, 1102

opioid agonist/antagonists
buprenorphine, 142
butorphanol, 150
dezocine, 324
nalbuphine, 800
pentazocine, 905

▪ SEDATIVE/HYPNOTICS

Pharmacologic Profile

General Use: Sedatives are used in the treatment of various anxiety states. Hypnotics are used to treat insomnia. Selected agents are useful as anticonvulsants (clorazepate, diazepam, and phenobarbital); as skeletal muscle relaxants (diazepam); as adjuncts in the treatment of the alcohol withdrawal syndrome (chlordiazepoxide, clorazepate, diazepam, and oxazepam); and as general anesthetic adjuncts or amnesics. Some phenothiazines are also used as sedatives.

General Action and Information: Cause generalized CNS depression. May produce tolerance with chronic use and the potential for psychological or physical dependence. These agents have no analgesic properties.

Contraindications: Hypersensitivity. Should not be used in comatose patients or those with pre-existing CNS depression. Should not be used in patients with uncontrolled severe pain. Avoid use during pregnancy or lactation.

Precautions: Use cautiously in patients with hepatic dysfunction, severe renal impairment, or severe underlying pulmonary disease. Use with caution in patients who may be suicidal or who may have been addicted to drugs previously. Hypnotic use should be short-term. Elderly patients may be more sensitive to CNS depressants effects (initial dosage reduction may be required).

Interactions: Additive CNS depression with alcohol, antihistamines, antidepressants, opioid analgesics, or phenothiazines. Barbiturates induce hepatic drug-metabolizing enzymes and can decrease the effectiveness of drugs metabolized by the liver. Should not be used with MAO inhibitors.

Nursing Implications

ASSESSMENT

- **General Info:** Monitor blood pressure, pulse, and respiratory status frequently throughout IV administration.
- Prolonged high-dose therapy may lead to psychological or physical dependence. Restrict the amount of drug available to patient, especially if patient is depressed, suicidal, or has a history of addiction.
- **Insomnia:** Assess sleep patterns before and periodically throughout course of therapy.
- **Anxiety:** Assess degree of anxiety and level of sedation (ataxia, dizziness, and slurred speech) before and periodically throughout therapy.
- **Seizures:** Observe and record intensity, duration, and characterisitics of seizure activity. Institute seizure precautions.
- **Muscle Spasms:** Assess muscle spasms, associated pain, and limitation of movement before and throughout therapy.
- **Alcohol Withdrawal:** Assess patient experiencing alcohol withdrawal for tremors, agitation, delirium, and hallucinations. Protect patient from injury.

POTENTIAL NURSING DIAGNOSES

- Sleep pattern disturbance (indications).
- Injury, high risk for (side effects).
- Knowledge deficit related to medication regimen (patient/family teaching).

IMPLEMENTATION
- Supervise ambulation and transfer of patients following administration of hypnotic doses. Remove cigarettes. Side rails should be raised and call bell within reach at all times. Keep bed in low position.

PATIENT/FAMILY TEACHING
- Discuss the importance of preparing environment for sleep (dark room, quiet, avoidance of nicotine and caffeine). If less effective after a few weeks, consult physician; do not increase dose. Gradual withdrawal may be required to prevent reactions following prolonged therapy.
- May cause daytime drowsiness. Caution patient to avoid driving or other activities requiring alertness until response to medication is known.
- Advise patient to avoid the use of alchol and other CNS depressants concurrently with these medications.
- Advise patient to inform physician if pregnancy is planned or suspected.

EVALUATION
Effectiveness of therapy can be demonstrated by: ▪ Improvement in sleep patterns ▪ Decrease in anxiety level ▪ Control of seizures ▪ Decrease in muscle spasm ▪ Decreased tremulousness ▪ More rational ideation when used for alcohol withdrawal.

Sedative/Hypnotics Included in *Davis's Drug Guide for Nurses*

antihistamines
diphenhydramine, 359
hyroxyzine, 568
promethazine, 1003

barbiturates
amobarbital, 52
butalbital compound, 148
pentobarbital, 907
phenobarbital, 920
secobarbital, 1060
thiopental, 1140

benzodiazepines
alprazolam, 22
chlordiazepoxide, 228
clorazepate, 267
diazepam, 326
estazolam, 424

flurazepam, 493
halazepam, 593
lorazepam, 667
midazolam, 758
oxazepam, 863
prazepam, 976
quazepam, 1031
temazepam, 1117
triazolam, 1189

miscellaneous
buspirone, 145
chloral hydrate, 222
glutethimide, 516
meprobamate, 706
propiomazine, 1008
zolpidem, 1242

▪ SKELETAL MUSCLE RELAXANTS

Pharmacologic Profile

General Use: Two major uses are spasticity associated with spinal cord diseases or lesions (baclofen and dantrolene) or adjunctive therapy in the symptomatic relief of acute painful musculoskeletal conditions (cyclobenzaprine, diazepam, and methocarbamol). IV dantrolene is also used to treat and prevent malignant hyperthermia.

General Action and Information: Act either centrally (baclofen, carisoprodol, cyclobenzaprine, diazepam, and methocarbamol) or directly (dantrolene).

Contraindications: Baclofen and oral dantrolene should not be used in patients in whom spasticity is used to maintain posture and balance.

Precautions: Safety in pregnancy and lactation not established. Use cautiously in patients with a previous history of liver disease.

Interactions: Additive CNS depression with other CNS depressants, including alcohol, antihistamines, antidepressants, opioid analgesics, and sedative/hypnotics.

Nursing Implications

ASSESSMENT
- Assess patient for pain, muscle stiffness, and range of motion before and periodically throughout therapy.

POTENTIAL NURSING DIAGNOSES
- Pain (indications).
- Physical mobility, impaired (indications).
- Injury, high risk for (side effects).

IMPLEMENTATION
- Provide safety measures as indicated. Supervise ambulation and transfer of patients.

PATIENT/FAMILY TEACHING
- Encourage patient to comply with additional therapies prescribed for muscle spasm (rest, physical therapy, heat).
- Medication may cause drowsiness. Caution patient to avoid driving or other activities requiring alertness until response to drug is known.
- Advise patient to avoid concurrent use of alcohol or other CNS depressants with these medications.

EVALUATION
Effectiveness of therapy can be demonstrated by: ▪ Decreased musculoskeletal pain ▪ Decreased muscle spasticity ▪ Increased range of motion.

Skeletal Muscle Relaxants Included in *Davis's Drug Guide for Nurses*
centrally acting
baclofen, 103
carisoprodol, 176
cyclobenzaprine, 287

diazepam, 326
methocarbamol, 722

direct-acting
dantrolene, 305

▪ THROMBOLYTIC AGENTS

Pharmacologic Profile

General Use: Used in the treatment of acute massive pulmonary emboli and deep vein thromboses. Also used to lyse coronary artery thrombi following myocardial infarction and arterial thrombi, and to clear IV catheters and arteriovenous cannulae.

General Action and Information: Activate plasminogen by converting it to plasmin, which subsequently degrades fibrin clots, fibrinogen, and other plasma proteins. Alteplase stimulates the conversion to plasmin by binding to fibrin. Anistreplase produces local fibrinolysis at the site of new thrombus.

Contraindications: Hypersensitivity. Recent streptococcal infection (strepto-kinase only). Contraindicated in active internal bleeding, recent cerebrovascular accident, surgery, or intracranial neoplasm.

Precautions: Safety in pregnancy, lactation, and children not established. Use with extreme caution postpartum or in patients currently taking oral anticoagulants. Use cautiously in patients who have risk of left heart thrombus or have had recent minor trauma, cerebrovascular disease, or diabetic hemorrhagic retinopathy.

Interactions: Concurrent use with other anticoagulants, including aspirin, NSAIAs, and other antiplatelet agents, some cephalosporins, plicamycin, or valproic acid may increase the risk of bleeding.

Nursing Implications

ASSESSMENT
- **General Info:** Assess patients for signs of bleeding and hemorrhage. Monitor all previous puncture sites. May cause internal bleeding including intracranial hemorrhage. Guaiac all body fluids and stools. Monitor neurologic status. Assess peripheral pulses.
- Therapy should be administered as soon as possible after onset of symptoms.
- **Coronary Thrombosis:** Monitor ECG continuously. Notify physician if significant arrhythmias or chest pain occur. Cardiac enzymes should be monitored.
- **Pulmonary Embolism:** Monitor pulse, blood pressure, hemodynamics, and respiratory status (rate, degree of dyspnea, ABGs).
- **Deep Vein Thrombosis/Acute Arterial Occlusion:** Observe extremities and palpate pulses of affected extremities every hour. Notify physician immediately if circulatory impairment occurs.
- **Cannula/Catheter Occulsion:** Monitor ability to aspirate blood as indicator of patency. Ensure patient exhales and holds breath when connecting and disconnecting IV syringe to prevent air embolism.
- **Toxicity and Overdose:** Aminocaproic acid (Amicar) may be used as an antidote.

POTENTIAL NURSING DIAGNOSES
- Tissue perfusion, altered (indications).
- Injury, high risk for (side effects).

IMPLEMENTATION
- These medications should only be used in settings in which hematologic function and clinical response can be adequately monitored.
- Invasive procedures, such as IM injections or arterial punctures, should be avoided with this therapy.
- Obtain type and cross-match and have blood available at all times in case of hemorrhage.
- Systemic anticoagulation with heparin is usually begun several hours after the completion of thrombolytic therapy.

PATIENT/FAMILY TEACHING

- Explain purpose of the medication. Instruct patient to report hypersensitivity reactions (rash, dyspnea) or bleeding or bruising.
- Explain need for bed rest and minimal handling during therapy to avoid injury.

EVALUATION

Effectiveness of therapy can be demonstrated by: ▪ Lysis of thrombi or emboli ▪ Restoration of blood flow ▪ Cannula or catheter patency.

Thrombolytic Agents Included in *Davis's Drug Guide for Nurses*

alteplase, 26
anistreplase, 71
streptokinase, 1087
urokinase, 1206

▪ VASOPRESSORS

Pharmacologic Profile

General Use: Used to correct the hemodynamic imbalances that may persist despite adequate fluid replacement in the treatment of shock. Phenylephrine is also used as a topical decongestant and mydriatic. Isoproterenol is used as a bronchodilator.

General Action and Information: Stimulate adrenergic receptors, resulting in vasoconstriction (alpha-adrenergic effects) and/or myocardial stimulation (beta-adrenergic effects).

Contraindications: Contraindicated in occlusive vascular diseases, uncorrected arrhythmias, or hypotension secondary to fluid deficit.

Precautions: Use cautiously in patients with underlying cardiovascular disease. Safety in pregnancy and lactation not established.

Interactions: Use with MAO inhibitors may result in severe hypertension. Beta-adrenergic blockers may block therapeutic effectiveness.

Nursing Implications

ASSESSMENT

- Monitor blood pressure, pulse, respiration, ECG, and hemodynamic parameters every 5–15 min during and after administration. Notify physician if significant changes in vital signs or arrhythmias occur. Consult physician for parameters for pulse, blood pressure, or ECG changes for adjusting dosage or discontinuing medication.
- Monitor urine output frequently throughout administration. Notify physician promptly if urine output decreases.
- Assess IV site frequently throughout infusion. Administer into a large vein to minimize the risk of extravasation. Extravasation of dopamine, norepinephrine, or phenylephrine may cause severe irritation, necrosis, and sloughing of tissue. If extravasation occurs, affected area should be infiltrated with 10–15 ml of 0.9% NaCl containing 5–10 mg of phentolamine.

POTENTIAL NURSING DIAGNOSES

- Cardiac output, decreased (indications).
- Tissue perfusion, altered (indications).

IMPLEMENTATION
- Hypovolemia should be corrected before administration of vasopressors.
- Infusions must be administered via infusion pump to ensure precise amount delivered. Rate of administration is titrated according to patient response (blood pressure, heart rate, urine flow, peripheral perfusion, presence of ectopic activity, and cardiac output).

PATIENT/FAMILY TEACHING
- Instruct patient to inform nurse immediately if chest pain, dyspnea, or pain at infusion site occurs.

EVALUATION
Effectiveness of therapy can be demonstrated by: ▪ Increase in blood pressure ▪ Increase in peripheral circulation ▪ Increase in urine output.

Vasopressors Included in *Davis's Drug Guide for Nurses*

▪ VITAMINS

Pharmacologic Profile

General Use: Used in the prevention and treatment of vitamin deficiencies and as supplements in various metabolic disorders.

General Action and Information: Serve as components of enzyme systems that catalyze numerous varied metabolic reactions. Necessary for homeostasis. Water-soluble vitamins (B-vitamins, vitamin C, and pantothenic acid) rarely cause toxicity. Fat-soluble vitamins (vitamins A, D, E, and K) may accumulate and cause toxicity.

Contraindications: Hypersensitivity to additives, preservatives, or colorants.

Precautions: Dosage should be adjusted to avoid toxicity, especially for fat-soluble vitamins.

Interactions: Pyridoxine in large amounts may interfere with the effectiveness of levodopa. Cholestyramine, colestipol, and mineral oil decrease absorption of fat-soluble vitamins.

Nursing Implications

ASSESSMENT
- Assess patient for signs of vitamin deficiency before and periodically throughout therapy.
- Assess nutritional status through 24 hr diet recall. Determine frequency of consumption of vitamin-rich foods.

POTENTIAL NURSING DIAGNOSES
- Nutrition, altered: less than body requirements (indications).
- Knowledge deficit related to medication regimen (patient/family teaching).

C
L
A
S
S
I
F
I
C
A
T
I
O
N
S

IMPLEMENTATION
- Because of infrequency of single vitamin deficiencies, combinations are commonly administered.

PATIENT/FAMILY TEACHING
- Encourage patients to comply with diet recommendations of physician. Explain that the best source of vitamins is a well-balanced diet with foods from the 4 basic food groups.
- Patients self-medicating with vitamin supplements should be cautioned not to exceed RDA (see Appendix L). The effectiveness of megadoses for treatment of various medical conditions is unproven and may cause side effects and toxicity.

EVALUATION
Effectiveness of therapy may be demonstrated by: - Prevention of or decrease in the symptoms of vitamin deficiencies.

Vitamins Included in *Davis's Drug Guide for Nurses*

fat-soluble vitamins
vitamin A, 1228
vitamin D
  calcitriol (vitamin D_3), 155
  dihydrotachysterol (vitamin D analogue), 349
  ergocalciferol (vitamin D_2), 412
vitamin E (alpha-tocopherol), 1233
vitamin K
  phytonadione (vitamin K_1), 939

water-soluble vitamins
vitamin B
  cyanocobalamin (vitamin B_{12}), 1231

folic acid (vitamin B_9), 497
hydroxocobalamin (vitamin B_{12}), 1231
niacin (vitamin B_3), 812
niacinamide, 812
pyridoxine (vitamin B_6), 1028
riboflavin (vitamin B_2), 1047
thiamine (vitamin B_1), 1134
vitamin C (ascorbic acid), 75

miscellaneous
multiple vitamins (oral and parenteral), 787
vitamin B complex with C (oral and parenteral), 1230

ACEBUTOLOL
(ace-**byoo**-toe-lole)
{Monitan}, Sectral

CLASSIFICATION(S):
Antihypertensive, Beta-adrenergic blocker (selective), Antiarrhythmic (group II)
Pregnancy Category B

INDICATIONS

■ Treatment of hypertension (single agent or with other antihypertensives) ■ Treatment of ventricular tachyarrhythmias. **Unlabeled Uses:** ■ Prophylaxis of myocardial infarction, treatment of angina pectoris, anxiety, tremors, thyrotoxicosis, mitral valve prolapse, idiopathic hypertrophic subaortic stenosis.

ACTION

■ Blocks stimulation of beta$_1$ (myocardial) adrenergic receptors. Does not usually effect beta$_2$ (pulmonary, vascular, or uterine) receptor sites. **Therapeutic Effects:** ■ Decreased heart rate ■ Decreased AV conduction ■ Decreased blood pressure.

PHARMACOKINETICS

Absorption: Well absorbed following oral administration.
Distribution: Minimal penetration of the CNS. Crosses the placenta and enters breast milk in small amounts.
Metabolism and Excretion: Mostly metabolized to diacetolol, which is also a beta blocker.
Half-life: 3–4 hr (8–13 hr for diacetolol).

CONTRAINDICATIONS AND PRECAUTIONS

Contraindicated in: ■ Uncompensated congestive heart failure ■ Pulmonary edema ■ Cardiogenic shock ■ Bradycardia or heart block.
Use Cautiously in: ■ Renal impairment (dosage reduction recommended if CCr <50 ml/min/1.73m^2) ■ Elderly

patients (increased sensitivity to the effects of beta-adrenergic blockers) ■ Thyrotoxicosis (may mask symptoms) ■ Diabetes mellitus (may mask symptoms of hypoglycemia) ■ Pregnancy, lactation, or children (safety not established; neonatal bradycardia, hypotension, hypoglycemia, and respiratory depression may occur rarely) ■ Patients with a history of severe allergic reactions (intensity of reactions may be increased).

ADVERSE REACTIONS AND SIDE EFFECTS*

CNS: fatigue, weakness, dizziness, depression, insomnia, memory loss, mental changes, nightmares, anxiety, nervousness, drowsiness.
EENT: blurred vision, stuffy nose.
CV: BRADYCARDIA, CONGESTIVE HEART FAILURE, PULMONARY EDEMA, peripheral vasoconstriction, hypotension.
Resp: bronchospasm, wheezing.
GI: constipation, diarrhea, nausea, vomiting.
GU: impotence, diminished libido, urinary frequency.
Derm: rashes.
Endo: hyperglycemia, hypoglycemia.
MS: joint pain, athralgia.

INTERACTIONS

Drug–Drug: ■ **General anesthesia, IV phenytoin,** and **verapamil** may cause additive myocardial depression ■ Concurrent use with **cardiac glycosides** may increase bradycardia ■ **Antihypertensive agents,** acute ingestion of **alcohol,** or **nitrates** may cause additive hypotension ■ Use with **epinephrine** may result in unapposed alpha-adrenergic stimulation ■ Concurrent **thyroid** may decrease effectiveness ■ Concurrent use with **insulin** may result in prolonged hypoglycemia ■ May decrease effectiveness of **theophylline.**

ROUTE AND DOSAGE

■ **PO (Adults):** 400–800 mg/day—single dose or twice daily (up to 1200 mg/day).

AVAILABILITY

▪ *Capsules:* 200, 400 mg ▪ {*Tablets:* 200, 400 mg}.

TIME/ACTION PROFILE

	ONSET	PEAK	DURATION
Antihypertensive effect			
PO	1–1.5 hr	2–8 hr	12–24 hr
Antiarrhythmic effect			
PO	1 hr	4–6 hr	up to 10 hr

NURSING IMPLICATIONS

ASSESSMENT

▫ Monitor blood pressure, ECG, and pulse frequently during dosage adjustment period and periodically throughout therapy.

▫ Monitor intake and output ratios and daily weights. Assess routinely for signs and symptoms of congestive heart failure (dyspnea, rales/crackles, weight gain, peripheral edema, jugular venous distension).

▪ **Lab Test Considerations:** May alter serum lipoproteins, potassium, triglyceride, and uric acid levels.

▫ May cause >20% decrease in blood glucose when tested with Chemstrip bG, Dextrostix, and Visidex II.

POTENTIAL NURSING DIAGNOSES

▪ Cardiac output, decreased (side effects).

▪ Knowledge deficit related to medication regimen (patient/family teaching).

▪ Noncompliance related to medication regimen (patient/family teaching).

IMPLEMENTATION

▪ **PO:** Take apical pulse prior to administering. If <50 bpm or if arrhythmia occurs, withhold medication and notify physician.

▫ May be administered with food or on an empty stomach.

PATIENT/FAMILY TEACHING

▫ Instruct patient to take medication exactly as prescribed even if feeling well; do not skip or double up on missed doses. If a dose is missed, it should be taken as soon as remembered up to 4 hr before next dose. Abrupt withdrawal may precipitate life-threatening arrhythmias, hypertension, or myocardial ischemia.

▫ Teach patient and family how to check pulse and blood pressure. Instruct them to check pulse daily and blood pressure biweekly and to report significant changes to physician.

▫ May occasionally cause drowsiness. Caution patients to avoid driving or other activities that require alertness until response to the drug is known.

▫ Reinforce the need to continue additional therapies for hypertension (weight loss, sodium restriction, stress reduction, regular exercise, moderation of alcohol consumption, and smoking cessation). Acebutolol controls but does not cure hypertension.

▫ Caution patient that this medication may increase sensitivity to cold.

▫ Instruct patient to consult physician or pharmacist before taking any over-the-counter medications concurrently with this medication.

▫ Diabetics should closely monitor blood sugar, especially if weakness, malaise, irritability, or fatigue occur.

▫ Advise patient to notify physician if slow pulse, dizziness, lightheadedness, confusion, depression, rash, fever, sore throat, unusual bleeding, or bruising occurs.

▫ Instruct patient to inform physician or dentist of medication regimen prior to treatment or surgery.

▫ Advise patient to carry identification describing disease process and medication regimen at all times.

EVALUATION

Effectiveness of therapy can be demonstrated by: ▪ Decrease in blood pressure ▪ Control of arrhythmias without appearance of detrimental side effects.

ACETAMINOPHEN

(a-seat-a-**min**-oh-fen)
{Abenol}, Aceta, Actamin, Aminofen, Anacin-3, Apacet, APAP, {Apo-Acetaminophen}, Arthritis Pain Formula Aspirin-Free, Atasol, Banesin, Dapa, Datril, Dolanex, Dorcol Children's Fever and Pain Reducer, {Exdol}, Feverall, Genapap, Genebs, Halenol, Liquiprin, Meda Cap, Myapap, Neopap, Oraphen, Panadol, Panex, paracetamol, Phenaphen, Redutemp, Ridenol, {Robigesic}, {Rounox}, Snaplets-FR, St. Joseph's Aspirin-Free, Suppap, Tapanol, Tempra, Tenol, Tylenol, Ty-Pap, Ty-Tab, Valadol, Valorin

CLASSIFICATION(S):
Nonopioid analgesic,
Antipyretic
Pregnancy Category B

INDICATIONS

▪ Mild to moderate pain ▪ Fever.

ACTION

▪ Inhibits the synthesis of prostaglandins that may serve as mediators of pain and fever. **Therapeutic Effects:** ▪ Analgesia (due to peripheral prostaglandin inhibition) ▪ Antipyresis (lowers fever); due to inhibition of prostaglandins in the CNS ▪ No significant anti-inflammatory properties.

PHARMACOKINETICS

Absorption: Well absorbed following oral administration. Rectal absorption is variable.
Distribution: Widely distributed. Crosses the placenta; enters breast milk.
Metabolism and Excretion: 85–95% metabolized by the liver. Metabolites may be toxic in overdose situation. Metabolites excreted by the kidneys.
Half-life: 1–4 hr.

CONTRAINDICATIONS AND PRECAUTIONS

Contraindicated in: ▪ Previous hypersensitivity ▪ Products containing alcohol, aspartame, saccharin, sugar, or tartrazine (FDC yellow dye #5) should be avoided in patients who have hypersensitivity or intolerance to these compounds.
Use Cautiously in: ▪ Severe hepatic disease ▪ Renal disease ▪ Chronic alcohol abuse ▪ Malnutrition ▪ Pregnancy and lactation.

ADVERSE REACTIONS AND SIDE EFFECTS*

GI: HEPATIC NECROSIS (overdose).
Derm: rash, urticaria.

INTERACTIONS

Drug–Drug: ▪ **Antipyretics** may cause severe hypothermia when used with phenothiazine antipsychotics ▪ Hepatotoxicity may be additive with other **hepatotoxic substances** including **alcohol**. ▪ **Phenobarbital** may increase liver toxicity in acetaminophen overdosage ▪ **Cholestyramine** and **colestipol** decrease absorption and may decrease effectiveness.

ROUTE AND DOSAGE

Children ≤12 yr should not receive >5 doses/24 hr without notifying physician.

▪ **PO (Adults and Children >12 yr):** 325–1000 mg q 4–6 hr as needed (not to exceed 4 g/day, or 2.6 g/day chronically)
▪ **PO/Rect (Children 11–12 yr):** 480 mg q 4–6 hr as needed.
▪ **PO/Rect (Children 9–11 yr):** 400 mg q 4–6 hr as needed.
▪ **PO/Rect (Children 6–9 yr):** 320 mg q 4–6 hr as needed.
▪ **PO/Rect (Children 4–6 yr):** 240 mg q 4–6 hr as needed.
▪ **PO/Rect (Children 2–4 yr):** 160 mg q 4–6 hr as needed.
▪ **PO (Children 1–2 yr):** 120 mg q 4–6 hr as needed.

{} = Available in Canada only.
*Underlines indicate most frequent; **CAPITALS** indicate life-threatening.

- **PO (Children 4–12 mo):** 80 mg q 4–6 hr as needed.
- **PO (Children <3 mo):** 40 mg q 4–6 hr as needed.
- **Rect (Adults and Children >12 yr):** 325–650 mg q 4 hr as needed (not to exceed 6 suppositories/24 hr).

AVAILABILITY

- *Chewable tablets:* 80, 160 mg
- *Granules:* ▪ 80 mg/packet, 80 mg/capsule ▪ *Tablets:* 160, 325, 500, 650 mg
- *Capsules:* 500 mg ▪ *Solution:* 100 mg/ml, 120 mg/2.5 ml ▪ *Liquid:* 120 mg/5 ml, 160 mg/5 ml, 500 mg/15 ml
- *Elixir:* 120 mg/5 ml, 130 mg/5 ml, 160 mg/5 ml, 325 mg/5 ml ▪ *Suppositories:* 120, 125, 300, 650 mg ▪ *In combination with:* many other medications. See Appendix A.

TIME/ACTION PROFILE (analgesia and antipyresis)

	ONSET	PEAK	DURATION
PO	0.5–1 hr	1–3 hr	3–4 hr
Rect	0.5–1 hr	1–3 hr	3–4 hr

NURSING IMPLICATIONS

ASSESSMENT

- **General Info:** Assess overall health status and alcohol usage before administering acetaminophen. Malnourished patients or chronic alcohol abusers are at higher risk of developing hepatotoxicity with chronic use of usual doses of this drug.
- **Pain:** Assess type, location, and intensity prior to and 30–60 min following administration.
- **Fever:** Assess fever; note presence of associated signs (diaphoresis, tachycardia, and malaise).
- **Lab Test Considerations:** Hepatic, hematologic, and renal function should be evaluated periodically throughout prolonged, high-dose therapy.
  - Increased serum bilirubin, LDH, AST (SGOT), ALT (SGPT), and prothrombin time may indicate hepatotoxicity.

- **Toxicity and Overdose:** If overdose occurs, acetylcysteine (Mucomyst) is the antidote.

POTENTIAL NURSING DIAGNOSES

- Pain (indications).
- Body temperature, altered, high risk for (indications).
- Knowledge deficit related to medication regimen (patient/family teaching).

IMPLEMENTATION

- **PO:** Administer with a full glass of water.
  - May be taken with food or on an empty stomach.

PATIENT/FAMILY TEACHING

- Advise patient to take medication exactly as directed and not to take more than the recommended amount. Severe and permanent liver damage may result from prolonged use or high doses of acetaminophen. Adults should not take acetaminophen longer than 10 days and children not longer than 5 days unless directed by physician.
- Advise patient to consult the physician if discomfort or fever is not relieved by routine dosages of this drug or if fever is greater than 39.5°C (103°F) or lasts longer than 3 days.

EVALUATION

Effectiveness of therapy can be demonstrated by: ▪ Relief of mild to moderate discomfort ▪ Reduction of fever.

ACETYLCYSTEINE
(a-se-til-**sis**-teen)
{Airbron}, Mucomyst, Mucosil

CLASSIFICATION(S):
Antidote (acetaminophen),
Mucolytic
Pregnancy Category B

INDICATIONS

- **PO:** Overdosage of acetaminophen.
- **Inhalation:** Mucolytic.

ACTION

- **PO:** Decreases the build-up of a hepatotoxic metabolite in acetaminophen overdosage ■ **Inhalation:** Degrades mucus, allowing easier mobilization and expectoration. **Therapeutic Effects:** ■ *PO:* Prevention of liver damage following acetaminophen overdose by decreasing the build-up of a hepatotoxic metabolite ■ *Inhalation:* Lowers the viscosity of mucus.

PHARMACOKINETICS

Absorption: Absorbed from the GI tract following oral administration. Action is local following inhalation; remainder may be absorbed from pulmonary epithelium.

Distribution: Not known.

Metabolism and Excretion: Metabolized by the liver.

Half-life: UK.

CONTRAINDICATIONS AND PRECAUTIONS

Contraindicated in: ■ Hypersensitivity.

Use Cautiously in: ■ Severe respiratory insufficiency or asthma ■ Elderly or debilitated patients ■ Pregnancy or lactation (safety not established).

ADVERSE REACTION AND SIDE EFFECTS*

CNS: drowsiness.

EENT: rhinorrhea, stomatitis.

Resp: increased secretions.

GI: nausea, vomiting.

Derm: urticaria.

Misc: fever, chills.

INTERACTIONS

Drug–Drug: ■ **Activated charcoal** may adsorb acetylcysteine and decrease its effectiveness as an antidote.

ROUTE AND DOSAGE

Acetaminophen Overdose

- **PO (Adults and Children):** 140 mg/kg initially followed by 70 mg/kg q 4 hr for 17 additional doses.

Mucolytic

- **Inhalation (Adults and Children):** 1–10 ml of 20% solution or 2–20 ml of 10% solution q 2–6 hr.

AVAILABILITY

- *Solution:* 10%, 20%.

TIME/ACTION PROFILE

	ONSET	PEAK	DURATION
PO (antidote)	UK	UK	4 hr
Inhaln (mucolytic)	1 min	5–10 min	short

NURSING IMPLICATIONS

ASSESSMENT

- **Antidote in Acetaminophen Overdose:** Monitor AST (SGOT), ALT (SGPT), bilirubin, prothrombin time, creatinine, BUN, serum glucose, electrolytes, and acetaminophen levels. Initial levels are drawn 4 hr after ingestion of acetaminophen. Do not wait for results to administer dose.
- □ Assess patient for nausea, vomiting, and urticaria. Notify physician if these occur. Maintain fluid and electrolyte balance.
- **Mucolytic:** Assess respiratory function (lung sounds, dyspnea) and color, amount, and consistency of secretions before and immediately following treatment to determine effectiveness of therapy.

POTENTIAL NURSING DIAGNOSES

- Violence, high risk for: directed at self (indications).
- Airway clearance, ineffective (indications).
- Knowledge deficit related to medication regimen (patient/family teaching).

IMPLEMENTATION

- **General Info:** After opening, may turn light purple; does not alter potency. Refrigerate open vials and discard after 96 hr.
- □ Drug reacts with rubber and metals

(iron, nickel, copper); avoid contact with these substances.

- **PO: Acetaminophen Overdose**—first empty stomach contents by inducing emesis or lavage. Dilute 20% solution with cola, water, or juice to a final concentration of 1 : 3 to increase palatability. May be administered by duodenal tube if patient unable to swallow. If patient vomits loading dose or maintenance doses within 1 hr of administration, readminister dose.
- **Inhalation: Mucolytic**—encourage adequate fluid intake (2000–3000 ml/day) to decrease viscosity of secretions.
- For aerosol use, the 20% solution may be diluted with 0.9% NaCl for injection or inhalation or Sterile Water for Injection or inhalation. May use 10% solution undiluted. May be administered by nebulization, or 1–2 ml may be instilled directly into airway. During administration, when 25% of medication remains in nebulizer, dilute with equal amount of 0.9% NaCl or sterile water.
- An increased volume of liquified bronchial secretions may occur following administration. Have suction equipment available for patients unable to effectively clear airways.
- If bronchospasm occurs during treatment, discontinue and consult physician regarding possible addition of bronchodilator to therapy.
- Rinse patient's mouth and wash face following treatment as drug leaves a sticky residue on surfaces.

PATIENT/FAMILY TEACHING
- **Inhalation:** Instruct patient to clear airway by coughing deeply before taking aerosol treatment.
- Inform patient that unpleasant odor of this drug becomes less noticeable as treatment progresses.

EVALUATION
Effectiveness of therapy can be demonstrated by: ▪ Decreased acetaminophen

levels □ No further increase in hepatic damage during acetaminophen overdose therapy ▪ Decreased dyspnea and clearing of lung sounds when used as a mucolytic.

ACTIVATED CHARCOAL
Acta-Char, Acta-Char Liquid-A, Actidose-Aqua, {Aqueous Charcodote}, {Charac-50}, Insta-Char, Insta-Char Aqueous Suspension, Liqui-Char, SuperChar, Super-Char Aqueous

CLASSIFICATION(S):
Antidote (adsorbent)
Pregnancy Category C

INDICATIONS
- Acute management of many oral poisonings following emesis/lavage.

ACTION
- Binds drugs and chemicals within the GI tract. **Therapeutic Effect:** ▪ Decreased intestinal absorption of drugs or chemicals in the overdose situation, thereby preventing toxicity.

PHARMACOKINETICS
Absorption: None.
Distribution: None.
Metabolism and Excretion: Excreted unchanged in the feces.
Half-life: UK.

CONTRAINDICATIONS AND PRECAUTIONS
Contraindicated in: ▪ No known contraindications.
Use Cautiously in: ▪ Poisonings due to cyanide, corrosives, ethanol, methanol, petroleum distillates, organic solvents, mineral acids, or iron ▪ Endoscopic examination (observation will be obscured).

ADVERSE REACTIONS AND SIDE EFFECTS*

GI: vomiting, constipation, diarrhea, black stools.

INTERACTIONS

Drug–Drug: ▪ **Other drugs** including **ipecac** and **laxatives** will be adsorbed by charcoal and as a result will not be systemically absorbed from the GI tract.
Drug–Food: ▪ **Milk, ice cream,** and **sherbet** will decrease the ability of charcoal to absorb other agents.

ROUTE AND DOSAGE

Antidote
▪ **PO (Adults):** 25–100 g.
▪ **PO (Children):** 1 g/kg.

Antiflatulent
▪ **PO (Adults):** 1.04–3.9 g tid.

AVAILABILITY

▪ *Powder:* 15-, 30-, 40-, 120-, 125-, 240-g containers ▪ *Oral suspension:* 12.5 g/60 ml, 15 g/72 ml, 15 g/120 ml, 25 g/120 ml, 30 g/120 ml, 50 g/240 ml, {15 g/120 ml}, {25 g/125 ml}, {50 g/225 ml}, {50 g/250 ml}.

TIME/ACTION PROFILE (antidote)

	ONSET	PEAK	DURATION
PO	within min	UK	4–12 hr

NURSING IMPLICATIONS

ASSESSMENT
▪ **General Info:** Assess neurologic status; administer only if patient is alert (unless airway is protected).
□ Consult reference, poison control center, or physician for symptoms of toxicity of ingested agent(s).
□ Monitor blood pressure, pulse, respiratory and neurologic status, and urine output as indicated by toxicity of agent(s). Notify physician if symptoms persist or worsen.
▪ **Poisoning:** Inquire as to the type of drug or poison and time of ingestion.
▪ **Lab Test Considerations:** Chronic use may impair absorption of essen-

tial nutrients. This may result in decreased mineral or electrolyte levels.

POTENTIAL NURSING DIAGNOSES
▪ Violence, high risk for, directed at self (indications).
▪ Injury, high risk for (indications).

IMPLEMENTATION
▪ **Treatment of Poisoning:** Activated charcoal is most effective if administered within 30 min of ingestion of drug or poison. Dosage may be repeated for drugs subjected to enterohepatic elimination to minimize further absorption.
□ Administer syrup of ipecac first and wait until emesis occurs before administering activated charcoal.
□ Powder is the most effective form and should be the form used. Tablets and capsules should not be used in the treatment of poisoning.
▪ **PO:** Mix dose in 6–8 oz of water, administer as a slurry. May be flavored with juice, cocoa, or chocolate powder to make more palatable. Do not administer with milk products (milk, ice cream, or sherbet). May need to be diluted with additional water to be thin enough to administer through a nasogastric tube.
□ Rapid ingestion may cause vomiting. If vomiting occurs shortly after administering dose, confer with physician about repeating dose.
□ Do not administer other oral drugs for 2 hr before or after administering activated charcoal.
□ Slurry is constipating; physician may order a laxative to speed removal of the drug. Sorbitol or magnesium citrate are commonly used for this purpose and may cause diarrhea. Some products contain sorbitol.

PATIENT/FAMILY TEACHING
▪ **General Info:** Inform patient that stools will turn black.
▪ **Poisoning:** When counseling, discuss methods of prevention, need to confer with poison control center, physician, or emergency department prior to administering, and need to bring in-

gested substance to emergency room for identification.

EVALUATION
Effectiveness of therapy can be demonstrated by: ▪ Prevention or resolution of toxic side effects of ingested agent.

ACYCLOVIR
(ay-**sye**-kloe-veer)
Zovirax

CLASSIFICATION(S)
Antiviral
Pregnancy Category C

INDICATIONS

▪ **PO:** Treatment of initial and prophylaxis of recurrent genital herpes infections ▪ **PO:** Treatment of localized cutaneous herpes zoster infections (shingles) and chickenpox (varicella) ▪ **IV:** Used in the treatment of severe initial episodes of genital herpes in nonimmunosuppressed patients ▪ **IV:** Management of initial or recurrent mucosal or cutaneous herpes simplex infections in immunosuppressed patients ▪ **IV:** Treatment of herpes simplex encephalitis in patients > 6 mo ▪ **Top:** Treatment of herpes genitalis infections.

ACTION

▪ Interferes with viral DNA synthesis. **Therapeutic Effect:** ▪ Inhibition of viral replication, decreased viral shedding, and reduced time to healing of lesions.

PHARMACOKINETICS

Absorption: Oral absorption is poor (15–30%), although therapeutic blood levels are achieved.
Distribution: Widely distributed. CSF concentrations are 50% of plasma. Crosses the placenta.
Metabolism and Excretion: >90% eliminated unchanged by the kidneys; remainder metabolized by the liver.
Half-life: 2.1–3.5 hr (increased in renal failure).

CONTRAINDICATIONS AND PRECAUTIONS

Contraindicated in: ▪ Hypersensitivity.
Use Cautiously in: ▪ Pre-existing serious neurologic, hepatic, pulmonary, or fluid and electrolyte abnormalities ▪ Renal impairment (dosage reduction required) ▪ Pregnancy and lactation (safety not established).

ADVERSE REACTIONS AND SIDE EFFECTS*

CNS: dizziness, headache, hallucinations, trembling, SEIZURES.
EENT: gingival hyperplasia.
GI: diarrhea, nausea, vomiting, anorexia, abdominal pain.
GU: RENAL FAILURE, hematuria, crystalluria.
Derm: acne, unusual sweating, skin rashes, hives.
Endo: changes in menstrual cycle.
Local: pain, phlebitis.
MS: joint pain.
Misc: polydypsia.

INTERACTIONS

▪ **Probenecid** increases blood levels of acyclovir ▪ Concurrent use of other **nephrotoxic drugs** increases the risk of adverse renal effects ▪ Intrathecal **methotrexate** increases the risk of CNS side effects.

ROUTE AND DOSAGE

Dosage should be decreased in renal impairment.

Initial Genital Herpes
▪ **PO (Adults):** 200 mg q 4 hr while awake (5 times a day) for 10 days.
▪ **IV (Adults):** 5 mg/kg q 8 hr for 5 days.

Chronic Suppressive Therapy for Recurrent Genital Herpes
▪ **PO (Adults):** 400 mg twice daily for up to 12 mo.

Intermittent Therapy for Recurrent Genital Herpes
▪ **PO (Adults):** 200 mg q 4 hr while awake (5 times a day) for 5 days, initiated at first sign of symptoms.

*Underlines indicate most frequent; **CAPITALS** indicate life-threatening.

Acute Treatment of Herpes Zoster
- **PO (Adults):** 800 mg q 4 hr while awake (5 times a day) for 7–10 days.

Chickenpox
- **PO (Adults and Children):** 20 mg/kg (not to exceed 800 mg/dose) qid for 5 days.

Mucosal and Cutaneous Herpes Simplex Infections in Immunosuppressed Patients
- **IV (Adults and Children >12 yr):** 5 mg/kg q 8 hr for 7 days.
- **IV (Children <12 yr):** 250 mg/m^2 q 8 hr for 7 days.
- **Top (Adults):** ½-in. ribbon of 5% ointment for every 4-square-in. area q 3 hr 6 times/day for 7 days.

Herpes Simplex Encephalitis
- **IV (Adults):** 10 mg/kg q 8 hr for 10 days.
- **IV (Children <12 yr):** 500 mg/m^2 q 8 hr for 10 days.

Varicella Zoster Infections in Immunosuppressed Patients
- **IV (Adults):** 10 mg/kg q 8 hr for 7 days.
- **IV (Children <12 yr):** 500 mg/m^2 q 8 hr for 7 days.

AVAILABILITY
- *Capsules:* 200 mg ▪ *Tablets:* ▪ *Suspension:* 200 mg/5 ml ▪ *Injection:* 500-, 1000-mg vials.

TIME/ACTION PROFILE (antiviral blood levels)

	ONSET	PEAK
PO	UK	1.5–2.5 hr
IV	prompt	end of infusion

NURSING IMPLICATIONS

ASSESSMENT
- ▢ Assess lesions prior to and daily during therapy.
- ▢ Monitor neurologic status in patients with herpes encephalitis.
- ▪ **Lab Test Considerations:** Monitor BUN, serum creatinine, and creatinine clearance before and during therapy. Increased BUN and serum creatinine levels or decreased creatinine clearance may indicate renal failure.

POTENTIAL NURSING DIAGNOSES
- ▪ Skin integrity, impaired (indications).
- ▪ Infection transmission, high risk for (indications, patient/family teaching).
- ▪ Knowledge deficit related to medication regimen (patient/family teaching).

IMPLEMENTATION
- ▪ **General Info:** Acyclovir treatment should be started as soon as possible after herpes symptoms appear.
- ▪ **PO:** Acyclovir may be administered with food or on an empty stomach.
- ▪ **IV:** Maintain adequate hydration (2000–3000 ml/day), especially during first 2 hr following IV infusion, to prevent crystalluria.
- ▢ Observe infusion site for phlebitis. Rotate infusion site to prevent phlebitis.
- ▢ Acyclovir sodium should not be administered topically, IM, SC, PO, or in the eye.
- ▪ **Intermittent Infusion:** Reconstitute 500-mg or 1000-mg vial with 10 ml or 20 ml, respectively, of Sterile Water for Injection for a concentration of 50 mg/ml. Do not reconstitute with bacteriostatic water with benzyl alcohol or parabens. Shake well to dissolve completely. Dilute in D5W, D5/0.25% NaCl, D5/0.45% NaCl, D5/0.9% NaCl, 0.9% NaCl, or lactated Ringer's solution for a concentration not to exceed 7 mg/ml. Use reconstituted solution within 12 hr. Once diluted for infusion, should be used within 24 hr. Refrigeration results in precipitation, which dissolves at room temperature.
- ▪ *Rate:* Administer via infusion pump, over at least 1 hr to minimize renal tubular damage.
- ▪ **Y-Site Compatibility:** ▪ amikacin ▪ ampicillin ▪ cefamandole ▪ cefazolin ▪ cefonicid ▪ cefoperazone ▪ ceforanide ▪ cefotaxime ▪ cefoxitin ▪ ceftazidime ▪ ceftizoxime ▪ ceftriaxone ▪ cefuroxime ▪ cephapirin ▪ chloramphenicol ▪ cimetidine ▪ clinda-

mycin ▪ dexamethasone sodium phosphate ▪ dimenhydrinate ▪ diphenhydramine ▪ doxycycline ▪ erythromycin lactobionate ▪ fluconazole ▪ gentamicin ▪ heparin ▪ hydrocortisone sodium succinate ▪ hydromorphone ▪ imipenem/cilastatin ▪ lorazepam ▪ magnesium sulfate ▪ methylprednisolone sodium succinate ▪ metoclopramide ▪ metronidazole ▪ multivitamin infusion ▪ nafcillin ▪ oxacillin ▪ penicillin G potassium ▪ piperacillin ▪ potassium chloride ▪ ranitidine ▪ sodium bicarbonate ▪ theophylline ▪ ticarcillin ▪ tobramycin ▪ trimethoprim-sulfamethoxazole ▪ vancomycin ▪ zidovudine.

▪ **Y-Site Incompatibility:** ▪ dobutamine ▪ dopamine ▪ fludarabine ▪ foscarnet ▪ ondansetron ▪ sargramostim ▪ verapamil.

▪ **Additive Incompatibility:** ▪ blood products ▪ protein-containing solutions.

▪ **Top:** Apply to skin lesions only; do not use in the eye.

PATIENT/FAMILY TEACHING

▪ **General Info:** Advise patient to take medication exactly as directed for the full course of therapy. If a dose is missed take as soon as remembered but not just before next dose is due; do not double doses. Acyclovir should not be used more frequently or longer than prescribed.

▫ Advise patients that the additional use of over-the-counter creams, lotions, and ointments can delay healing and may cause spreading of lesions.

▫ Inform patient that acyclovir is not a cure, as the virus lays dormant in the ganglia, and will not prevent the spread of infection to others.

▫ Advise patient that condoms should be used during sexual contact and that no sexual contact should be made while lesions are present.

▫ Instruct patient on the importance of maintaining good dental hygiene and seeing a dentist for teeth cleaning regularly to prevent tenderness, bleeding, and gingival hyperplasia.

▫ Patient should consult the physician if symptoms are not relieved following 7 days of topical therapy or if oral acyclovir docs not decrease the frequency and severity of recurrences.

▫ Instruct women with genital herpes to have yearly Pap smears because they may be more likely to develop cervical cancer.

▪ **Top:** Instruct patient to apply ointment in sufficient quantity to cover all lesions every 3 hr, 6 times/day for 7 days. One ½-in. ribbon of ointment covers approximately 4 square in. Use a finger cot or glove when applying to prevent inoculation of other areas or spread to other people. Keep affected areas clean and dry. Loose fitting clothing should be worn to prevent irritation.

▫ Avoid drug contact in or around eyes. Report any unexplained eye symptoms to the physician immediately, as ocular herpetic infection can lead to blindness.

EVALUATION

Effectiveness of therapy can be demonstrated by: ▪ Crusting over and healing of skin lesions ▪ Decrease in frequency and severity of recurrences ▪ Shortening of time to complete healing and cessation of pain in herpes zoster ▪ Decrease in intensity of chickenpox.

ADENOSINE
(a-**den**-oh-seen)
Adenocard

CLASSIFICATION(S):
Antiarrhythmic
Pregnancy Category C

INDICATIONS

▪ Conversion of paroxysmal supraventricular tachycardia to normal sinus rhythm when vagal manuevers have been unsuccessful.

ACTION

▪ Restores normal sinus rhythm by interrupting re-entrant pathways in the

AV node ▪ Slows conduction time through the AV node. **Therapeutic Effect:** ▪ Restoration of normal sinus rhythm.

PHARMACOKINETICS

Absorption: Following IV administration absorption is essentially complete.

Distribution: Taken up by erythrocytes and vascular endothelium.

Metabolism and Excretion: Rapidly converted to inosine and adenosine monophosphate.

Half-life: <10 sec.

CONTRAINDICATIONS AND PRECAUTIONS

Contraindicated in: ▪ Hypersensitivity ▪ 2nd- or 3rd-degree AV block or sick sinus syndrome, unless a functional artificial pacemaker is present.

Use Cautiously in: ▪ Patients with a history of asthma (may induce bronchospasm) ▪ Pregnancy, lactation, or children (safety not established).

ADVERSE REACTIONS AND SIDE EFFECTS*

CNS: headache, lightheadedness, dizziness, apprehension, head pressure.

EENT: blurred vision, throat tightness.

Resp: shortness of breath, chest pressure, hyperventilation.

CV: facial flushing, transient arrhythmias, palpitations, chest pain, hypotension.

GI: nausea, metallic taste.

Derm: sweating, burning sensation, facial flushing.

MS: neck and back pain.

Neuro: tingling, numbness.

Misc: pressure sensation in groin, heaviness in arms.

INTERACTIONS

Drug–Drug: ▪ **Carbamazepine** may increase the likelihood of progressive heart block ▪ **Dipyridamole** potentiates the effects of adenosine (dosage reduction of adenosine recommended) ▪ Effects of adenosine may be decreased by **theophylline** or **caffeine** (larger doses of

adenosine may be required) ▪ **Nicotine** (in cigarette smoke or nicotine gum) may increase risk of tachycardia.

ROUTE AND DOSAGE

▪ **IV (Adults):** 6 mg by rapid IV bolus, if no results repeat 1–2 min later as 12 mg rapid bolus. This dose may be repeated. (Single dose not to exceed 12 mg).

AVAILABILITY

▪ *Injection:* 6 mg/2 ml vial.

TIME/ACTION PROFILE
(antiarrhythmic effect)

	ONSET	PEAK	DURATION
IV	immediate	UK	1–2 min

NURSING IMPLICATIONS

ASSESSMENT

▫ Monitor heart rate frequently (every 15–30 sec) and ECG continuously throughout therapy. Once conversion to normal sinus rhythm is achieved, transient arrhythmias (premature ventricular contractions, atrial premature contractions, sinus tachycardia, sinus bradycardia, skipped beats, AV nodal block) may occur, but generally last a few seconds.

▫ Monitor blood pressure during therapy.

▫ Assess respiratory status (breath sounds, rate) following administration. Patients with history of asthma may experience bronchospasm.

POTENTIAL NURSING DIAGNOSES

▪ Cardiac output, decreased (indications).

▪ Knowledge deficit related to medication regimen (patient/family teaching).

IMPLEMENTATION

▪ **General Info:** Crystals may occur if adenosine is refrigerated. Warm to room temperature to dissolve crystals. Solution must be clear before use. Discard unused portions.

▪ **Direct IV:** Administer undiluted over

1–2 sec via direct IV or into proximal IV line. Follow with rapid saline flush to ensure injection reaches systemic circulation. Slow administration may cause increased heart rate in response to vasodilation.

PATIENT/FAMILY TEACHING

- Caution patient to make position changes slowly to minimize orthostatic hypotension. Doses >12 mg decrease blood pressure by decreasing peripheral vascular resistance.
- Instruct patient to report facial flushing, shortness of breath, or dizziness.

EVALUATION

Effectiveness of therapy can be demonstrated by: ▪ Conversion of supraventricular tachycardia to normal sinus rhythm.

ALBUMIN, Human

(al-**byoo**-min)
Albuminar, Albutein, Buminate, Normal Human Serum Albumin, Plasbumin

CLASSIFICATION(S):
Volume expander
Pregnancy Category C

INDICATIONS

▪ Expansion of plasma volume and maintenance of cardiac output in situations associated with fluid volume deficit including shock, hemorrhage and burns ▪ Temporary replacement of albumin in diseases associated with low levels of plasma proteins such as nephrotic syndrome or end stage liver disease resulting in relief or reduction of associated edema.

ACTION

▪ Provides colloidal oncotic pressure, which serves to mobilize fluid from extravascular tissues back into the intravascular space. **Therapeutic Effect:** ▪ Mobilization of fluid from extravascular tissue into intravascular space.

PHARMACOKINETICS

Absorption: Following IV administration absorption is essentially complete.
Distribution: Confined to the intravascular space, unless capillary permeability is increased.
Metabolism and Excretion: Probably degraded by the liver.
Half-life: UK.

CONTRAINDICATIONS AND PRECAUTIONS

Contraindicated in: ▪ Allergic reactions to albumin ▪ Severe anemia ▪ Congestive heart failure ▪ Normal or increased intravascular volume.

Use Cautiously in: ▪ Severe hepatic or renal disease ▪ Dehydration (additional fluids may be required).

ADVERSE REACTIONS AND SIDE EFFECTS*

CNS: headache.
CV: hypertension, hypotension, fluid overload, PULMONARY EDEMA, tachycardia.
GI: nausea, vomiting, increased salivation.
Derm: urticaria, rash.
MS: back pain.
Misc: fever, chills, flushing.

INTERACTIONS

Drug–Drug: ▪ None significant.

ROUTE AND DOSAGE

Dose is highly individualized and depends on condition being treated.

- **IV (Adults):** 25 g, may be repeated in 15–30 min, not to exceed 125 g in 24 hr or 250 g in 48 hr.
- **IV (Children):** 25 g or 25–50% of the adult dose.
- **IV (Premature Infants):** 1 g/kg as 25% solution administered prior to necessary transfusion.

AVAILABILITY

- *Injection:* 5%, 25%.

---

*Underlines indicate most frequent; **CAPITALS** indicate life-threatening.

TIME/ACTION PROFILE (oncotic effect)

	ONSET	PEAK	DURATION
IV	15–30 min	UK	UK

NURSING IMPLICATIONS

ASSESSMENT

- **General Info:** Monitor vital signs, CVP, and intake and output prior to and frequently throughout therapy. If fever, tachycardia, or hypotension occur, stop infusion and notify physician immediately. Antihistamines may be required to suppress this hypersensitivity response. Hypotension may also result from infusing too rapidly.
- □ Assess for signs of vascular overload (elevated CVP, rales/crackles, dyspnea, hypertension, jugular venous distention) during and following administration.
- **Surgical Patients:** Assess for increased bleeding following administration caused by increased blood pressure and circulating blood volume. Albumin does not contain clotting factors.
- **Lab Test Considerations:** Serum protein levels should increase with albumin therapy.
- □ Monitor serum sodium; may cause increased concentrations.
- □ Infusions of normal serum albumin may cause false elevation of alkaline phosphatase levels.
- **Hemorrhage:** Monitor hemoglobin and hematocrit. These values may decrease due to hemodilution.

POTENTIAL NURSING DIAGNOSES

- Cardiac output, decreased (indications).
- Fluid volume deficit, [active loss] (indications).
- Fluid volume excess (side effects).

IMPLEMENTATION

- **General Info:** Follow manufacturer's recommendations for administration and use set provided. Administer through a large gauge (at least 20 g) needle or catheter.
- □ Solution should be clear amber; do not administer cloudy solution or one containing a precipitate. Store at room temperature.
- □ There is no danger of serum hepatitis or HIV infection from normal serum albumin. Crossmatching is not required.
- □ 25 g of normal serum albumin are osmotically equivalent to 2 units of fresh frozen plasma; 100 ml of normal serum albumin 25% provides the plasma protein of 500 ml of plasma or 2 pt of whole blood. Normal serum albumin 5% is isotonic and osmotically equivalent to an equal amount of plasma. The 25% albumin solution is equal to 5 times the osmotic value of plasma. Each liter of normal serum albumin contains 130–160 mEq of sodium and are thus no longer labeled "salt-poor" albumin.
- □ Administration of large quantities of normal serum albumin may need to be supplemented with whole blood to prevent anemia. If more than 1000 ml of 5% normal serum albumin are given or if hemorrhage has occurred, the administration of whole blood or packed red blood cells may be needed. Hydration status should be monitored and maintained with additional fluids.
- **Continuous Infusion:** Administer 5% normal serum albumin undiluted. Normal serum albumin 25% may be administered undiluted or diluted in 0.9% NaCl or D5W. Infusion must be completed within 4 hr.
- **Rate:** Rate of administration is determined by concentration of solution, blood volume, indication, and patient response. In patients with normal blood volume, 5% normal serum albumin should be administered at 2–4 ml/min and 25% normal serum albumin at a rate of 1 ml/min. The rate for children is usually ¼–½ the adult rate.
- □ *Shock with Associated Hypovolemia:* 5% or 25% normal serum al-

bumin may be administered as rapidly as tolerated and repeated in 15–30 min if necessary.

□ *Burns:* Rate after the first 24 hr should be set to maintain a plasma albumin level of 2.5 g/100 ml or a total serum protein level of 5.2 g/100 ml.

□ *Hypoproteinemia:* Normal serum albumin 25% is the preferred solution due to the increased concentration of protein. The rate should not exceed 3 ml/min of 25% or 5–10 ml/min of 5% solution to prevent circulatory overload and pulmonary edema. This treatment provides a temporary rise in plasma protein until the hypoproteinemia is corrected.

▪ **Additive Compatibility:** Normal serum albumin is compatible with 0.9%, NaCl, D5W, D5/0.9% NaCl, D5/0.45% NaCl, D5/LR, and lactated Ringer's solution.

PATIENT/FAMILY TEACHING

□ Explain the purpose of this solution to the patient.

□ Instruct patient to report signs and symptoms of hypersensitivity reaction.

EVALUATION

Effectiveness of therapy can be demonstrated by: ▪ Increase in blood pressure and blood volume when used to treat shock and burns ▪ Increased urinary output reflects the mobilization of fluid from extravascular tissues ▪ Elevated serum plasma protein in patients with hypoproteinemia.

ALBUTEROL
(al-**byoo**-ter-ole)
{Novosalmol}, Proventil, salbutamol, Ventolin

CLASSIFICATION(S):
Bronchodilator (beta-adrenergic agonist)
Pregnancy Category C

INDICATIONS

▪ **PO, Inhalation:** Used as a bronchodilator in reversible airway obstruction due to asthma or COPD ▪ **Inhalation:** Prevention of exercise-induced bronchospasm.

ACTION

▪ Results in the accumulation of cyclic adenosine monophosphate (cAMP) at beta-adrenergic receptors ▪ Produces bronchodilation ▪ Relatively selective for beta$_2$ (pulmonary) receptors. **Therapeutic Effect:** ▪ Bronchodilation.

PHARMACOKINETICS

Absorption: Well absorbed following oral administration, but rapidly undergoes extensive metabolism.
Distribution: Not well known. Small amounts appear in breast milk.
Metabolism and Excretion: Extensively metabolized by the liver and other tissues.
Half-life: 3.8 hr.

CONTRAINDICATIONS AND PRECAUTIONS

Contraindicated in: ▪ Hypersensitivity to adrenergic amines ▪ Hypersensitivity to fluorocarbons (inhaler).
Use Cautiously in: ▪ Cardiac disease ▪ Hypertension ▪ Hyperthyroidism ▪ Diabetes ▪ Glaucoma ▪ Elderly patients (more susceptible to adverse reactions; may require dosage reduction) ▪ Pregnancy (near term), lactation, and children <2 yr (safety not established) ▪ Excessive use may lead to tolerance and paradoxical bronchospasm (inhaler).

ADVERSE REACTIONS AND SIDE EFFECTS*

CNS: <u>nervousness</u>, <u>restlessness</u>, insomnia, <u>tremor</u>, headache.
CV: hypertension, arrhythmias, angina.
Endo: hyperglycemia.
GI: nausea, vomiting.

INTERACTIONS

Drug–Drug: ▪ Concurrent use with other **adrenergic (sympathomimetic) agents** will have additive adrenergic side effects ▪ Use with **MAO inhibitors** may lead to hypertensive crisis ▪ **Beta-adrenergic blockers** may negate therapeutic effect.

ROUTE AND DOSAGE

▪ **PO (Adults and Children ≥12 yr):** 2–6 mg 3–4 times daily (not to exceed 32 mg/day) or 4–8 mg of extended-release tablets (Proventil Repetabs) twice daily.

▪ **PO (Children 6–14 yr):** 2 mg 3–4 times daily. May be carefully increased as needed (not to exceed 24 mg/day).

▪ **PO (Children 2–6 yr):** 0.1 mg/kg 3 times daily (not to exceed 2 mg 3 times daily initially), may be carefully increased to 0.2 mg/kg 3 times daily (not to exceed 4 mg 3 times daily).

▪ **Inhalation (Adults and Children ≥12 yr):** via metered-dose inhaler— 2 inhalations q 4–6 hr or 2 inhalations 15 min prior to exercise.

▪ **Inhalation (Adults and Children >5 yr):** via nebulization or IPPB— 1.25–5 mg 3–4 times daily.

AVAILABILITY

▪ *Tablets:* 2 mg, 4 mg ▪ *Extended-release tablets:* 4 mg ▪ {*Oral solution:* 2 mg/5 ml} ▪ *Metered dose aerosol:* 90 mcg/spray, {100 mcg/spray}, {200 inhalations/canister} ▪ *Inhalation solution:* 0.83 mg/ml, {1 mg/ml}, 5 mg/ml ▪ *Capsules for inhalation (Rotacaps):* 200 mcg.

TIME/ACTION PROFILE
(bronchodilation)

	ONSET	PEAK	DURATION
PO	30 min	2–3 hr	6 hr or more
PO–ER	30 min	2–3 hr	12 hr
Inhaln	5–15 min	60–90 min	4–6 hr

NURSING IMPLICATIONS

ASSESSMENT
▫ Assess lung sounds, pulse, and blood pressure before administration and during peak of medication.

▫ Monitor pulmonary function tests before initiating therapy and periodically throughout course to determine effectiveness of medication.

▫ Observe for paradoxical bronchospasm (wheezing). If condition occurs, withhold medication and notify physician immediately.

POTENTIAL NURSING DIAGNOSES
▪ Airway clearance, ineffective (indications).
▪ Knowledge deficit related to medication regimen (patient/family teaching).

IMPLEMENTATION
▪ **PO:** Administer oral medication with meals to minimize gastric irritation.
▪ **Inhalation:** Allow at least 1 min between inhalations of aerosol medication.

PATIENT/FAMILY TEACHING
▫ Instruct patient to take albuterol exactly as directed. If on a scheduled dosing regimen, take a missed dose as soon as remembered, spacing remaining doses at regular intervals. Do not double doses. Caution patient not to exceed recommended dose; may cause adverse effects, paradoxical bronchospasm, or loss of effectiveness of medication.

▫ Instruct patient to contact physician immediately if shortness of breath is not relieved by medication or is accompanied by diaphoresis, dizziness, palpitations, or chest pain.

▫ Advise patient to consult physician or pharmacist before taking any over-the-counter medications or alcohol concurrently with this therapy. Caution patient to also avoid smoking and other respiratory irritants.

▪ **Inhalation:** Instruct patient in the proper use of the metered-dose inhaler or Rotahaler (see Appendix H).

▫ Advise patients to use albuterol first if using other inhalation medications, and allow 5 min to elapse before administering other inhalant medications, unless otherwise directed.

□ Advise patient to rinse mouth with water after each inhalation dose to minimize dry mouth.

EVALUATION

Effectiveness of therapy can be demonstrated by: ▪ Prevention or relief of bronchospasm.

ALDESLEUKIN
(al-dess-**loo**-kin)
interleukin-2, IL-2, Proleukin

CLASSIFICATION(S):
Antineoplastic (modified recombinant interleukin)
Pregnancy Category C

INDICATIONS

▪ Management of renal cell carcinoma.

ACTION

▪ Increases cellular immunity (noted as lymphocytosis and eosinophilia), increases the production of cytokines (including tumor necrosis factor, interleukin-1 and gamma interferon) and inhibits tumor growth. **Therapeutic Effects:** ▪ Regression of renal cell carcinoma.

PHARMACOKINETICS

Absorption: IV administration results in complete bioavailability.

Distribution: Rapidly distributes to intravascular, extracellular space. 70% is taken up by the liver, kidneys, and lungs.

Metabolism and Excretion: Metabolized to amino acids by cells lining the proximal convoluted tubules of the kidneys.

Half-life: 85 min.

CONTRAINDICATIONS AND PRECAUTIONS

Contraindicated in: ▪ Hypersensitivity to aldesleukin or mannitol ▪ Patients with any history of cardiac or pulmonary disease as assessed by abnormal thallium stress testing or abnormal pulmonary function testing ▪ Patients who have experienced any of the following toxicities during previous courses of aldesleukin—sustained ventricular tachycardia (≥5 beats), angina pectoris or myocardial infarction as indicated by ECG changes, respiratory problems requiring more than 72 hr of intubation, pericardial tamponade, renal toxicity requiring more than 72 hr of dialysis, CNS dysfunction consisting of more than 48 hr of coma or psychosis, intractable seizures, bowel perforation or ischemia, GI bleeding requiring surgical intervention ▪ Patients who have had allograft organ transplantation (increased risk of rejection).

Use Cautiously in: ▪ Patients with a history of cardiovascular, respiratory, hepatic, or renal disease ▪ Patients with a history of seizures or suspected CNS metastases (symptoms may be exaggerated, and seizures may occur) ▪ Pregnancy, lactation, or children <18 yr (safety not established) ▪ Patients with child-bearing potential.

ADVERSE REACTIONS AND SIDE EFFECTS*

Resp: <u>pulmonary congestion</u>, dyspnea, <u>pulmonary edema</u>, RESPIRATORY FAILURE, APNEA, tachypnea, pleural effusion, wheezing, pneumothorax, hemoptysis.

CV: MYOCARDIAL INFARCTION, CARDIAC ARREST, CONGESTIVE HEART FAILURE, STROKE, <u>hypotension</u>, <u>tachycardia</u>, <u>arrhythmias</u>, myocardial ischemia, pericardial effusion, thrombosis.

GI: BOWEL PERFORATION, <u>jaundice</u>, ascites, hepatomegaly.

GU: <u>oliguria/anuria</u>, <u>proteinuria</u>, hematuria, dysuria, renal failure.

Derm: <u>pruritus</u>.

F and E: <u>hypocalcemia</u>, <u>hypomagnesemia</u>, <u>hypophosphatemia</u>, <u>hypokalemia</u>, acidosis, hyperuricemia, hyponatremia, hyperkalemia, alkalosis.

Hemat: <u>anemia</u>, <u>leukopenia</u>, <u>thrombocytopenia</u>, <u>coagulation disorders</u>, leukocytosis, eosinophilia.

---

*Underlines indicate most frequent; **CAPITALS** indicate life-threatening.

Misc: CAPILLARY LEAK SYNDROME, fever, chills, weight gain, weight loss.

INTERACTIONS

Drug–Drug: ▪ **Glucocorticoids** decrease antineoplastic effectiveness. Avoid concurrent use ▪ Additive hypotension may occur with **antihypertensives** ▪ Concurrent **cardiotoxic, hepatotoxic, myelotoxic,** or **nephrotoxic drug therapy** increases the risk of toxicity in these organs.

ROUTE AND DOSAGE

▪ **IV (Adults):** 600,000 IU/kg (0.037 mg/kg) every 8 hr for 14 doses. Cycle is repeated once after a 9-day rest period to a total of 28 doses. After a rest period of 7 wk, patients who have had a beneficial response may be evaluated for additional courses.

AVAILABILITY

▪ *Vials:* containing 22×10^6 IU.

TIME/ACTION PROFILE (tumor regression after completion of first course)

	ONSET	PEAK	DURATION
IV	4 wk	UK	12 mo

NURSING IMPLICATIONS

ASSESSMENT

▫ Monitor ECG continuously during infusion. Monitor respiratory status frequently. Pulmonary function tests and chest x-ray should be monitored prior to and periodically throughout therapy.

▪ Monitor vital signs and weight daily. Assess patient for the development of capillary leak syndrome (hypotension, hypovolemia, edema, ascites, pleural effusions). This initially manifests as a drop in arterial blood pressure beginning 2–12 hr from start of administration. Hypotensive patients should have ECG monitored continuously and CVP monitored throughout therapy.

▫ Monitor for changes in mental status. Hold administration if patient devel-

ops moderate-to-severe lethargy or somnolence. May progress to coma.

▫ Assess frequently for signs of infection, particularly sepsis and bacterial endocarditis. Antibiotic prophylaxis directed against *Staphylococcus aureus* is recommended for all patients with central lines. Any intercurrent infections should be managed aggressively. Aldesleukin impairs the function of white blood cells.

▪ Assess for signs of anemia and bleeding. Transfusions of red blood cells and/or platelets may be required.

▪ **Lab Test Considerations:** Monitor CBC, differential, platelet count, blood chemistries including electrolytes, and renal and hepatic function prior to and daily throughout therapy. May cause elevated bilirubin, BUN, serum creatinine, transaminase, and alkaline phosphatase. May cause hypomagnesemia, acidosis, hypocalcemia, hypophosphatemia, hypokalemia, hyperuricemia, hypoalbuminemia, and hypoproteinemia.

POTENTIAL NURSING DIAGNOSES

▪ Infection, high risk for (side effects).

▪ Knowledge deficit related to medication regimen (patient/family teaching).

IMPLEMENTATION

▪ **Intermittent Infusion:** Reconstitute each vial with 1.2 ml of Sterile Water for Injection for a concentration of 18 million IU (1.1 mg)/ml. Direct the sterile water during reconstitution at the side of the vial and swirl contents gently to prevent excess foaming. Do not shake. Solution should be clear and colorless to slightly yellow. Administer within 48 hr of reconstitution. Discard unused portion.

▫ Dilute reconstituted dose in 50 ml of D5W. Do not reconstitute or dilute with Bacteriostatic Water for Injection, 0.9% NaCl, or albumin.

▪ *Rate:* Infuse each dose over 15 min.

▪ **Additive Incompatibility:** Do not mix with other drugs.

PATIENT/FAMILY TEACHING

▫ Instruct patient to notify physician if

dyspnea, sore throat, fever, chills, yellow skin, unusual bleeding or bruising, or fatigue occur.
▫ Advise patient to use a nonhormonal method of contraception throughout therapy.

EVALUATION

Effectiveness of therapy can be determined by: ▪ Decrease in size or spread of renal cell carcinoma.

ALFENTANIL
(al-**fen**-ta-nil)
Alfenta, {Rapifen}

CLASSIFICATION(S):
Opioid analgesic (agonist)
Schedule II
Pregnancy Category C

INDICATIONS

▪ Analgesic adjunct when given in increasing doses in the maintenance of anesthesia with barbiturate/nitrous oxide/oxygen ▪ Analgesic when administered by continuous IV infusion with nitrous oxide/oxygen while maintaining general anesthesia ▪ Primary induction of anesthesia when endotracheal intubation and mechanical ventilation are required.

ACTION

▪ Binds to opiate receptors in the CNS, altering the response to and perception of pain while causing generalized CNS depression. **Therapeutic Effects:** ▪ Relief of moderate to severe pain ▪ Anesthesia.

PHARMACOKINETICS

Absorption: Following IV administration absorption is essentially complete.
Distribution: Does not readily penetrate adipose tissue. Crosses the placenta, enters breast milk.
Metabolism and Excretion: >95% metabolized by the liver.
Half-life: 60–130 min.

CONTRAINDICATIONS AND PRECAUTIONS

Contraindicated in: ▪ Hypersensitivity ▪ Known intolerance.
Use Cautiously in: ▪ Elderly patients ▪ Debilitated or severely ill patients ▪ Diabetics ▪ Severe pulmonary or hepatic disease ▪ CNS tumors ▪ Increased intracranial pressure ▪ Head trauma ▪ Adrenal insufficiency ▪ Undiagnosed abdominal pain ▪ Hypothyroidism ▪ Alcoholism ▪ Cardiac disease (arrhythmias) ▪ Pregnancy, lactation, and children <12 yr (safety not established).

ADVERSE REACTIONS AND SIDE EFFECTS*

CNS: dizziness, sleepiness.
EENT: blurred vision.
CV: <u>bradycardia</u>, <u>tachycardia</u>, <u>hypotension</u>, <u>hypertension</u>, arrhythmias.
Resp: apnea.
GI: <u>nausea</u>, <u>vomiting</u>.
MS: <u>thoracic muscle rigidity</u>, skeletal muscle rigidity.

INTERACTIONS

Drug–Drug: ▪ **Alcohol, antihistamines, antidepressants,** and other **sedative/hypnotics**—concurrent use results in additive CNS depression ▪ **MAO inhibitors** should be avoided for 14 days prior to use ▪ **Cimetidine** or **erythromycin** may prolong duration of recovery ▪ Concurrent use with **benzodiazepines** may increase the risk of hypotension ▪ **Nalbuphine** or **pentazocine** may decrease analgesia.

ROUTE AND DOSAGE

Incremental Injection (Duration of Anesthesia <30 min)

Induction Period
▪ **IV (Adults):** 8–20 mcg/kg.

Maintenance Period
▪ **IV (Adults):** 3–5 mcg/kg increments or 0.5–1.0 mcg/kg/min (total dose 8–40 mcg/kg).

{} = Available in Canada only.
*<u>Underlines</u> indicate most frequent; **CAPITALS** indicate life-threatening.

Incremental Injection (Duration of Anesthesia 30–60 min)

Induction Period

▪ IV (Adults): 20–50 mcg/kg.

Maintenance Period

▪ IV (Adults): 5–15 mcg/kg increments (up to total dose of 75 mg/kg).

Continuous Infusion (Duration of Anesthesia >45 min)

Induction

▪ IV (Adults): 50–75 mcg/kg.

Maintenance

▪ IV (Adults): 0.5–3.0 mcg/kg/min (average infusion rate 1–1.5 mcg/kg/min). Infusion rate should be decreased by 30–50% after first hour of maintenance. If lightening occurs, infusion rate may be increased up to 4 mcg/kg/min or boluses of 7 mg/kg may be administered.

Anesthetic Induction (Duration of Anesthesia >45 min)

▪ IV (Adults): 130–245 mcg/kg followed by 0.5–1.5 mcg/kg/min or general anesthesia.

AVAILABILITY

▪ *Injection:* 500 mg/ml.

TIME/ACTION PROFILE (analgesia and respiratory depression)

	ONSET	PEAK	DURATION
IV	immediate	1–1.5 min	5–10 min*

*Longer in children.

NURSING IMPLICATIONS

ASSESSMENT

□ Assess vital signs, especially respiratory status and ECG, frequently throughout and following administration. Notify physician immediately of significant changes.

▪ **Lab Test Considerations:** May cause elevated serum amylase and lipase concentrations.

▪ **Toxicity and Overdose:** Symptoms of toxicity include respiratory depression, hypotension, arrhythmias, bradycardia, and asystole. Respiratory depression may be reversed with naloxone. Bradycardia may be treated with atropine. Opioid antagonist, oxygen, and resuscitative equipment should be readily available during the administration of alfentanil.

POTENTIAL NURSING DIAGNOSES

▪ Pain [acute] (indications).

▪ Sensory–perceptual alteration: visual, auditory (side effects).

▪ Breathing pattern, ineffective (side effects).

IMPLEMENTATION

▪ **General Info:** Benzodiazepines may be administered prior to administration of alfentanil to reduce the induction dose requirements and decrease the time to loss of consciousness. This combination may also increase the risk of hypotension.

□ Alfentanil's duration of action is short, therefore postoperative pain may require treatment relatively early in the recovery period.

▪ **Direct IV:** Administer small volumes for direct IV use via tuberculin syringe for accuracy.

▪ *Rate:* Injections should be administered slowly over 90 sec–3 min. Slow IV administration may reduce the incidence and severity of muscle rigidity, bradycardia, or hypotension. Neuromuscular blocking agents may be administered concurrently to decrease muscle rigidity.

▪ **Continuous Infusion:** For continuous IV infusion dilute to a concentration of 25–80 mcg/ml (20 ml of alfentanil in 230 ml of diluent provides a 40 mcg/ml solution) with 0.9% NaCl, D5W, D5/0.9% NaCl, or lactated Ringer's solution.

□ IV infusion should be discontinued at least 10–15 min prior to the end of surgery.

PATIENT/FAMILY TEACHING

□ Discuss the use of anesthetic agents and the sensations to expect with the patient prior to surgery.

□ Alfentanil may cause drowsiness and dizziness. Advise patient to call for assistance when ambulating or smoking.

□ Advise patient to make position

changes slowly to minimize orthostatic hypotension.
□ Following outpatient surgery instruct patients to avoid alcohol or other CNS depressants for 24 hr after the administration of alfentanil.

EVALUATION

Effectiveness of therapy can be demonstrated by: ▪ General quiescence □ Reduced motor activity ▪ Pronounced analgesia.

ALLOPURINOL
(al-oh-**pure**-i-nole)
{Alloprin}, {Apo Allopurinol}, Lopurin, {Novo-purol}, {Purinol}, Zyloprim

CLASSIFICATION(S):
Antigout agent (xanthene oxidase inhibitor)
Pregnancy Category C

INDICATIONS

▪ Prevention of attack of gouty arthritis and nephropathy ▪ Treatment of secondary hyperuricemia, which may occur during treatment of tumors or leukemias.

ACTION

▪ Inhibits the production of uric acid.
Therapeutic Effect: ▪ Lowering of serum uric acid levels.

PHARMACOKINETICS

Absorption: Well absorbed (80%) following oral administration.
Distribution: Widely distributed in tissue water.
Metabolism and Excretion: Metabolized to oxypurinol, an active compound with a long half-life. Both allopurinol and oxypurinol are excreted mainly by the kidneys.
Half-life: 2–3 hr (oxypurinol 24 hr).

CONTRAINDICATIONS AND PRECAUTIONS

Contraindicated in: ▪ Hypersensitivity ▪ Pregnancy or lactation.
Use Cautiously in: ▪ Acute attacks of gout ▪ Renal insufficiency (dosage reduction required if CCr <20 ml/min) ▪ Dehydration (adequate hydration necessary).

ADVERSE REACTIONS AND SIDE EFFECTS*

CNS: drowsiness.
Derm: <u>rash</u>, urticaria.
GI: nausea, vomiting, diarrhea, hepatitis.
GU: renal failure.
Hemat: bone marrow depression.
Misc: hypersensitivity reactions.

INTERACTIONS

Drug–Drug: ▪ Use with **mercaptopurine** and **azathioprine** increases bone marrow depressant properties—dosages of these drugs should be reduced ▪ Use with **ampicillin** increases the risk of rash ▪ Use with **oral hypoglycemics** and **oral anticoagulants** increases the effects of these drugs ▪ Use with **thiazide diuretics** increases the risk of hypersensitivity reactions.

ROUTE AND DOSAGE

▪ **PO (Adults):** 200–800 mg/day (doses >300 mg should be divided and given twice a day).
▪ **PO (Children 6–10 yr):** 300 mg/day as a single dose or 100 mg tid.
▪ **PO (Children <6 yr):** 50 mg tid.

AVAILABILITY

▪ *Tablets:* 100 mg, {200 mg}, 300 mg.

TIME/ACTION PROFILE
(hypouricemic effect)

	ONSET	PEAK	DURATION*
PO	2–3 days	1–3 wk	1–2 wk

*Duration after discontinuation of allopurinol.

{} = Available in Canada only.
*<u>Underlines</u> indicate most frequent; **CAPITALS** indicate life-threatening.

NURSING IMPLICATIONS

ASSESSMENT

□ Monitor for joint pain and swelling. Addition of colchicine or nonsteroidal anti-inflammatory agents may be necessary for acute attacks. The incidence of acute attacks may increase during the initial months of therapy.

□ Monitor intake and output ratios. Decreased kidney function can cause drug accumulation and toxic effects. Ensure that patient maintains adequate fluid intake (minimum 2500–3000 ml/day) to minimize risk of kidney stone formation.

■ Lab Test Considerations: Serum and urine uric acid levels usually begin to decrease 2–3 days after initiation of therapy.

□ Monitor blood glucose in patients receiving oral hypoglycemic agents. May cause hypoglycemia.

□ Hematologic, renal, and liver function tests should be monitored prior to and periodically throughout therapy. May cause elevation of serum alkaline phosphatase, AST (SGOT), and ALT (SGPT) levels. Decreased CBC and platelets may indicate bone marrow depression. Elevated BUN, serum creatinine, and creatinine clearance may indicate nephrotoxicity. These are usually reversed with discontinuation of therapy.

POTENTIAL NURSING DIAGNOSES

■ Pain (indications).

■ Knowledge deficit related to medication regimen (patient/family teaching).

IMPLEMENTATION

■ PO: May be administered with milk or meals to minimize gastric irritation. May be crushed and given with fluid or mixed with food for patients who have difficulty swallowing.

PATIENT/FAMILY TEACHING

□ Instruct patient to take allopurinol exactly as directed. If a dose is missed, take as soon as remembered. If dosing schedule is once daily, do not take if remembered the next day. If dosing schedule is more than once a day, take up to 300 mg for the next dose.

□ Alkaline diet may be ordered. Urinary acidification with large doses of vitamin C or other acids may increase kidney stone formation (see Appendix K). Advise patient of need for increased fluid intake.

□ May occasionally cause drowsiness. Caution patient to avoid driving or other activities requiring alertness until response to drug is known.

□ Instruct patient to report itching, skin rash, chills, fever, nausea, or vomiting to physician promptly.

□ Advise patient that large amounts of alcohol increase uric acid concentrations and may decrease the effectiveness of allopurinol.

□ Emphasize the importance of follow-up examinations to monitor effectiveness and side effects.

EVALUATION

Effectiveness of therapy can be determined by: ■ Decreased serum and urinary uric acid levels. May take 2–6 wk to observe clinical improvement.

ALPHA₁-PROTEINASE INHIBITOR
alpha₁-antitrypsin, Prolastin

CLASSIFICATION(S):
Enzyme inhibitor
Pregnancy Category C

INDICATIONS

■ Replacement therapy (chronic) in patients with demonstrated panacinar emphysema associated with alpha-antitrypsin deficiency.

ACTION

■ Prevents the destructive action of elastase on alveolar tissue in patients who have alpha₁-antitrypsin deficiency. **Therapeutic Effect:** ■ Slowing of the destructive process on lung tissue.

PHARMACOKINETICS

Absorption: Following IV administration absorption is essentially complete.

Distribution: Achieves high concentration in epithelial fluid of lungs.
Metabolism and Excretion: Broken down in the intravascular space.
Half-life: 4.5–5.2 days.

CONTRAINDICATIONS AND PRECAUTIONS

Contraindicated in: ▪ Hypersensitivity to polyethylene glycol ▪ Emphysema associated with alpha₁-antitrypsin deficiency where risk of panacinar emphysema is small (PiMZ and PiMS phenotype).
Use Cautiously in: ▪ Patients with irreversible destruction of lung tissue secondary to alpha₁-antitrypsin deficiency ▪ Pregnancy, lactation, and children (safety not established).

ADVERSE REACTIONS AND SIDE EFFECTS*

CNS: lightheadedness, dizziness.
Hemat: transient leukocytosis.
Misc: delayed fever.

INTERACTIONS

Drug–Drug: ▪ None known.

ROUTE AND DOSAGE

▪ **IV (Adults):** 60 mg/kg once weekly.

AVAILABILITY

▪ *Injection:* 500-mg, 1000-mg vials.

TIME/ACTION PROFILE (increased serum levels of alpha₁-proteinase inhibitor)

	ONSET	PEAK	DURATION
IV	2–6 days	several wk	UK

NURSING IMPLICATIONS

ASSESSMENT

▫ Monitor respiratory status (rate, lung sounds, dyspnea) prior to and weekly throughout course of therapy.
▪ **Lab Test Considerations:** Monitor serum alpha₁-proteinase inhibitor levels to determine response to therapy. Minimum serum concentration should be 80 mg/100 ml.

▫ May cause transient mild increase in leukocytes.

POTENTIAL NURSING DIAGNOSES

▪ Gas exchange, impaired (indications).
▪ Knowledge deficit related to medication regimen (patient/family teaching).

IMPLEMENTATION

▪ **Direct IV:** Bring bottles to room temperature. Reconstitute with provided Sterile Water for Injection to yield a concentration of 20 mg/ml. May be diluted in 0.9% NaCl if necessary. Do not refrigerate after reconstitution. Use within 3 hr.
▪ *Rate:* Administer direct IV at a rate of 0.08 ml/kg/min or greater.

PATIENT/FAMILY TEACHING

▫ Explain purpose of medication and need for chronic weekly therapy to patient. Patient should avoid smoking and notify physician of any changes in breathing pattern or sputum production.
▫ Advise patient of need for periodic pulmonary function tests.
▫ Explain purpose of hepatitis B vaccine prior to beginning therapy. A small risk of hepatitis is caused by the manufacturing process, and vaccination is recommended to ensure prevention of hepatitis.

EVALUATION

Effectiveness of therapy can be demonstrated by: ▪ Slowing of the destructive process on lung tissue as measured by increased serum alpha₁-proteinase inhibitor levels.

ALPRAZOLAM
(al-**pray**-zoe-lam)
{Apo-Alpraz}, {Novo-Alprazol}, {Nu-Alpraz}, Xanax

CLASSIFICATION(S):
Sedative/hypnotic (benzodiazepine)
Schedule IV
Pregnancy Category D

INDICATIONS
▪ Treatment of anxiety ▪ Adjunct in the treatment of depression ▪ Management of panic attacks.

ACTION
▪ Acts at many levels in the CNS to produce anxiolytic effect ▪ Depresses the CNS, probably by potentiating gamma aminobutyric acid (GABA), an inhibitory neurotransmitter. **Therapeutic Effect:** ▪ Relief of anxiety.

PHARMACOKINETICS
Absorption: Slowly but completely absorbed from the GI tract.
Distribution: Widely distributed, crosses blood–brain barrier.
Metabolism and Excretion: Metabolized by the liver to an active compound that is subsequently rapidly metabolized. Accumulation is minimal.
Half-life: 12–15 hr.

CONTRAINDICATIONS AND PRECAUTIONS
Contraindicated in: ▪ Hypersensitivity ▪ Cross-sensitivity with other benzodiazepines may exist ▪ Patients with pre-existing CNS depression ▪ Severe uncontrolled pain ▪ Narrow-angle glaucoma ▪ Pregnancy and lactation.
Use Cautiously in: ▪ Hepatic dysfunction (dosage reduction required) ▪ Patients who may be suicidal or have been addicted to drugs previously ▪ Elderly or debilitated patients (dosage reduction required).

ADVERSE REACTIONS AND SIDE EFFECTS*
CNS: <u>dizziness</u>, <u>drowsiness</u>, <u>lethargy</u>, hangover, paradoxical excitation, confusion, mental depression, headache.
EENT: blurred vision.
GI: nausea, vomiting, diarrhea, constipation.
Derm: rashes.
Misc: tolerance, psychologic dependence, physical dependence.

INTERACTIONS
Drug–Drug: ▪ Alcohol, antidepressants, antihistamines, and opioid analgesics—concurrent use results in additive CNS depression ▪ Cimetidine, oral contraceptives, disulfiram, erythromycin, fluoxetine, isoniazid, ketoconazole, metoprolol, propoxyphene, propranolol, or valproic acid may decrease the metabolism of alprazolam, enhancing its actions ▪ May decrease efficacy of levodopa ▪ Rifampin or barbiturates may increase the metabolism and decrease effectiveness ▪ Sedative effects may be decreased by theophylline.

ROUTE AND DOSAGE

Anxiety
▪ **PO (Adults):** 0.25–0.5 mg 2–3 times daily as needed (not >4 mg/day; begin with 0.25 mg 2–3 times daily in elderly/debilitated patients).

Panic Attacks
▪ **PO (Adults):** 0.5 mg tid, may be increased as needed (not >10 mg/day).

AVAILABILITY
▪ *Tablets:* 0.25 mg, 0.5 mg, 1 mg, 2 mg.

TIME/ACTION PROFILE (sedation)

	ONSET	PEAK	DURATION
PO	1–2 hr	1–2 hr	up to 24 hr

NURSING IMPLICATIONS

ASSESSMENT
▫ Assess degree and manifestations of anxiety and mental status prior to and periodically throughout therapy.
▫ Assess patient for drowsiness, lightheadedness, and dizziness. These symptoms usually disappear as therapy progresses. Dosage should be reduced if these symptoms persist.
▫ Prolonged high-dose therapy may lead to psychological or physical dependence. Restrict the amount of drug available to patient.
▪ **Lab Test Considerations:** Monitor CBC and liver and renal function periodically during long-term therapy. May cause decreased hematocrit and neutropenia.

*<u>Underlines</u> indicate most frequent; **CAPITALS** indicate life-threatening.

POTENTIAL NURSING DIAGNOSES
- Anxiety (indications).
- Injury, high risk for (side effects).
- Knowledge deficit related to medication regimen (patient/family teaching).

IMPLEMENTATION
- **PO:** May be administered with food if GI upset occurs.
  - Tablets may be crushed and taken with food or fluids if patient has difficulty swallowing.

PATIENT/FAMILY TEACHING
- Instruct patient to take medication exactly as directed; do not skip or double up on missed doses. If a dose is missed it can be taken within 1 hr, otherwise skip the dose and return to the regular schedule. If medication is less effective after a few weeks, check with physician; do not increase dose. Abrupt withdrawal of alprazolam may cause sweating, vomiting, muscle cramps, tremors, and convulsions.
- May cause drowsiness or dizziness. Caution patient to avoid driving and other activities requiring alertness until response to the medication is known.
- Advise patient to avoid the use of alcohol or other CNS depressants concurrently with this medication. Instruct patient to consult physician or pharmacist before taking over-the-counter medications concurrently with this medication.

EVALUATION
Effectiveness of therapy can be demonstrated by: ▪ Decreased sense of anxiety and an increased ability to cope. Treatment with this medication should not exceed 4 mo without re-evaluation of the patient's need for the drug.

ALPROSTADIL
(al-**pros**-ta-dil)
prostaglandin E₁, Prostin VR Pediatric, {Prostin VR}

CLASSIFICATION(S):
Hormone (prostaglandin)
Pregnancy Category UK

INDICATIONS
- Temporary maintenance of patent ductus arteriosus in neonates who depend on patency until surgery can be performed.

ACTION
- Directly relaxes smooth muscle of the ductus arteriosus. **Therapeutic Effect:** ▪ Short-term maintenance of patent ductus arteriosus in neonates born with congenital heart defects who require patency to maintain blood oxygenation and perfusion of the lower body.

PHARMACOKINETICS
Absorption: Following IV administration absorption is essentially complete.
Distribution: UK.
Metabolism and Excretion: Up to 80% rapidly metabolized in the lungs.
Half-life: 5–10 min.

CONTRAINDICATIONS AND PRECAUTIONS
Contraindicated in: ▪ Respiratory distress syndrome.
Use Cautiously in: ▪ Neonates with bleeding tendencies.

ADVERSE REACTIONS AND SIDE EFFECTS*
CNS: SEIZURES, cerebral bleeding, irritability, jitteriness, lethargy.
CV: bradycardia, hypotension.
Resp: APNEA, wheezing, hypercapnea, respiratory depression, altered respiratory rate (slow and fast).
GI: diarrhea, gastric regurgitation, hyperbilirubinemia.
GU: anuria, hematuria.
Derm: flushing.
F and E: hypokalemia.
Hemat: disseminated intravascular coagulation, anemia, thrombocytopenia, bleeding.

{} = Available in Canada only.
*Underlines indicate most frequent; **CAPITALS** indicate life-threatening.

Metab: hypoglycemia.
MS: neck hyperextension, stiffness.
Misc: fever, hypothermia, sepsis, peritonitis.

INTERACTIONS

Drug–Drug: ▪ None known.

ROUTE AND DOSAGE

▪ **IV, Intra-Arterial (Neonates):** 0.05–0.1 mcg/kg/min initially until satisfactory response, then decrease to maintenance dose by halving. (Initial dose may be increased up to 0.4 mcg/kg/min.)

AVAILABILITY

▪ *Injection:* 500 mg/ml.

TIME/ACTION PROFILE (improvement in blood gases, pulmonary blood flow)

	ONSET	PEAK	DURATION
IV (achd)*	1.5–3 hr	15 min– 11 hr	duration of infusion
IV (cghd)†	15–30 min	30 min	duration of infusion

*Acyanotic congenital heart disease.
†Cyanotic congenital heart disease.

NURSING IMPLICATIONS

ASSESSMENT

▢ Monitor rectal temperature, respiratory rate, pulse, blood pressure, and ECG continuously during therapy.

▢ In neonates with aortic arch anomalies also monitor pulmonary artery and descending aorta pressures, and urinary output. Palpate femoral pulse frequently to assess circulation to lower extremities. Blood pressure may be monitored in a lower and upper extremity simultaneously.

▢ Assess lung sounds and heart sounds frequently. Monitor neurologic status closely. Neonates less than 2 kg are at higher risk of developing respiratory, cardiovascular, and neurologic side effects. A ventilator should be readily available. Monitor for the development of congestive heart failure. Observe for seizure activity.

▢ During intra-arterial administration, assess frequently for facial or arm

flushing; may indicate catheter displacement and necessitate repositioning of the catheter.

▪ **Lab Test Considerations:** Monitor arterial blood gases prior to and periodically throughout therapy. In cyanotic defects, PaO_2 should increase within 30 min. In noncyanotic defects, correction of metabolic acidosis should occur within 4–11 hr.

▢ May rarely cause decreased serum glucose or increased serum bilirubin levels. May increase or decrease serum potassium levels.

▪ **Toxicity and Overdose:** Symptoms of overdose include flushing, hypotension, bradycardia, fever, and decreased respiratory rate or apnea. Infusion should be discontinued if apnea or bradycardia occurs.

POTENTIAL NURSING DIAGNOSES

▪ Cardiac output, decreased (indications).
▪ Tissue perfusion, altered: (indications).

IMPLEMENTATION

▪ **General Info:** May be administered intravenously through a peripheral or central line; intra-arterially through an umbilical artery catheter or pulmonary artery catheter; or by intra-aortic infusion.

▢ Duration of therapy is usually limited to 24–48 hr. Closure of the ductus arteriosus usually begins within 1 or 2 hr after discontinuing therapy.

▢ Notify physician if fever or hypotension occur. These side effects may resolve with a decrease in infusion rate.

▪ **Continuous Infusion:** Dilute further in 0.9% NaCl or D5W. Diluting 1 ml (500 mcg) of alprostadil in 250 ml of IV fluid will yield a final concentration of 2 mcg/ml; in 100 ml of IV fluid will yield 5 mcg/ml; in 50 ml of IV fluid will yield 10 mcg/ml; in 25 ml of IV fluid will yield 20 mcg/ml. Do not use solution containing benzyl alcohol as a diluent. Stable for 24 hr at room temperature.

▪ *Rate:* Administer the 2 mcg/ml solution at 0.05 ml/kg/min, the 5 mcg/ml solution at 0.02 ml/kg/min, the 10 mcg/ml solution at 0.01 ml/kg/min and the 20 mcg/ml solution at 0.005 ml/kg/min for a dose of 0.1 mcg/kg/min.

□ Administer via infusion pump to ensure precise dose delivered.

▪ **Additive Incompatibility:** Do not admix.

PATIENT/FAMILY TEACHING

□ Explain the purpose of alprostadil and the need for continuous monitoring to the parents.

EVALUATION

Effectiveness of therapy in the neonate with congenital heart disease may be demonstrated by: ▪ Maintained patency of the ductus arteriosus as evidenced by improved oxygenation in cyanotic disorders ▪ Improved circulation to the lower extremities □ Correction of metabolic acidosis □ Improved urine output in noncyanotic disorders.

ALTEPLASE
(al-te-plase)
Activase, {Activase rt-PA}, tissue plasminogen activator, t-PA

CLASSIFICATION(S):
Thrombolytic
Pregnancy Category C

INDICATIONS

▪ Acute (within 4–6 hr from onset of chest pain) management of myocardial infarction ▪ Management of acute massive pulmonary embolism associated with obstructed pulmonary blood flow or unstable hemodynamics.

ACTION

▪ Stimulates the conversion of plasminogen trapped in thrombi to plasmin by binding to fibrin. **Therapeutic Effects:** ▪ Lysis of coronary thrombi and subsequent limitation of infarct size ▪ Lysis of life-threatening pulmonary emboli.

PHARMACOKINETICS

Absorption: Following IV administration absorption is essentially complete.
Distribution: Not known.
Metabolism and Excretion: >80% rapidly metabolized by the liver.
Half-life: 35 min.

CONTRAINDICATIONS AND PRECAUTIONS

Contraindicated in: ▪ Active internal bleeding ▪ History of cerebrovascular accident ▪ Recent (within 2 mo) intracranial or intraspinal trauma or surgery ▪ Intracranial neoplasm ▪ Severe uncontrolled hypertension ▪ Arteriovenous malformation ▪ Bleeding tendencies.
Use Cautiously in: ▪ Recent (within 10 days) major surgery, trauma, GI or GU bleeding ▪ Cerebrovascular disease ▪ Uncontrolled hypertension ▪ Left heart thrombus ▪ Severe hepatic or renal disease ▪ Hemorrhagic ophthalmic conditions ▪ Septic phlebitis ▪ Elderly patients (>75 yr) ▪ Children, pregnancy, or lactation (safety not established).
Extreme Caution in: ▪ Early postpartum period (10 days) ▪ Patients receiving oral anticoagulant therapy.

ADVERSE REACTIONS AND SIDE EFFECTS*

CNS: INTRACRANIAL BLEEDING, headache.
CV: arrhythmias (due to reperfusion), hypotension.
EENT: epistaxis, gingival bleeding.
GI: GASTROINTESTINAL BLEEDING, RETROPERITONEAL BLEEDING, nausea, vomiting.
GU: GENITOURINARY TRACT BLEEDING.
Derm: ecchymoses, urticaria, itching, flushing.
Hemat: BLEEDING.
MS: musculoskeletal pain.
Misc: fever, hypersensitivity reactions.

INTERACTIONS

Drug–Drug: ▪ **Aspirin, oral anticoagulants, heparin, nonsteroidal anti-**

---

inflammatory agents, **dipyridamole**, or some **cephalosporins**, **plicamycin**, or **valproic acid**—concurrent use may increase the risk of bleeding, although these agents are frequently used together or in sequence.

ROUTE AND DOSAGE

Acute Myocardial Infarction

See infusion rate chart in Appendix D. Doses greater than 150 mg have been associated with an increased risk of intracranial bleeding.

- **IV (Adults >65 kg):** 60 mg over the first hr (6–10 mg of this given as a bolus over the first 1–2 min), 20 mg over the second hr and 20 mg over the third hr for a total of 100 mg.
- **IV (Adults <65 kg):** 1.25 mg/kg total dose over 3 hr given as 0.75 mg/kg over the first hr (0.075–0.125 mg/kg of this given as a bolus over the first 1–2 min), 0.25 mg/kg over the second hr and 0.25 mg/kg over the third hr.

Pulmonary Embolism

- **IV (Adults):** 100 mg over 2 hr (followed by heparin therapy).

AVAILABILITY

- *Injection:* 20-mg, 50-mg vials.

TIME/ACTION PROFILE (reperfusion)

	ONSET	PEAK	DURATION
IV	UK	20 min–2 hr	UK

NURSING IMPLICATIONS

ASSESSMENT

- Monitor vital signs every 15 min until stable then hourly. Notify physician if systolic BP >180 mmHg or diastolic BP >110 mmHg. Inform physician if hypotension occurs. Hypotension may result from the drug, hemorrhage, or cardiogenic shock.
- Monitor ECG continuously. Document segment changes. Notify physician of arrhythmias. Accelerated idioventricular rhythm, bradycardia, asystole, and ventricular arrhythmias due to reperfusion have been reported. Prophylactic antiarrhythmic therapy may be ordered during and following alteplase.
- Assess intensity, character, location, and radiation of chest pain. Note presence of associated symptoms (nausea, vomiting, diaphoresis). Administer analgesics as ordered by physician. Notify physician if chest pain is unrelieved or recurs.
- Monitor heart and breath sounds frequently. Inform physician of signs of congestive heart failure (rales/crackles, dyspnea, S_3 heart sound, jugular venous distension, elevated CVP).
- Assess patients for bleeding and hemorrhage. Monitor puncture sites every 15 min. May cause internal bleeding including intracranial hemorrhage. Guaiac all body fluids and stools. Monitor neurologic status. Assess peripheral pulses.
- Assess patient for development of urticaria, which may indicate hypersensitivity reaction. Inform physician promptly if this occurs.
- **Lab Test Considerations:** Monitor prothrombin time, partial thromboplastin time, fibrinogen, fibrin degradation products, CBC and platelets, and CPK-MB to assess effectiveness of therapy and prevent hemorrhage. CPK-MB may rise from washout of reperfused area. Confer with physician about type and crossmatch of blood in the event of hemorrhage.
- **Toxicity and Overdose:** Alteplase is rapidly cleared from the body; discontinue immediately if serious bleeding occurs.

POTENTIAL NURSING DIAGNOSES

- Pain [acute] (indications).
- Tissue perfusion, altered (indications).
- Injury, high risk for (side effects).

IMPLEMENTATION

- **General Info:** Avoid IM injections and unnecessary venipunctures. Apply pressure to all arterial and venous punctures for at least 30 min. Avoid venipunctures at noncompressable sites (e.g., jugular and subclavian sites).

□ Maintain patient on bedrest. Avoid unnecessary procedures such as shaving and vigorous toothbrushing for 24 hr.

□ Heparin and/or aspirin therapy may be ordered concurrently and following alteplase administration.

▪ **IV:** Prior to therapy start 2 IV lines: one for alteplase, the other for any additional IV infusions.

□ Vials are packaged with Sterile Water for Injection (without preservatives) to be used as diluent. Do not use Bacteriostatic Water for Injection. Reconstitute 20-mg vials with 20 ml and 50-mg vials with 50 ml using 18-g needle. Avoid excess agitation during dilution; swirl or invert gently to mix. Solution may foam upon reconstitution. Bubbles will resolve upon standing a few minutes. Solution will be clear to pale yellow. Stable for 8 hr at room temperature.

▪ **Intermittent Infusion:** May be administered as reconstituted (1 mg/ml) or may be further diluted immediately prior to use in equal amount of 0.9% NaCl or D5W. Do not admix.

□ *Myocardial Infarction:* Standard dose is given over 3 hr. Infuse 60% of the total dose via infusion pump for the first hour, 20% of the total dose over the second hour, and 20% over the third hour. Flush line with 25–30 ml of saline at completion of infusion to ensure entire dose is received.

□ *Pulmonary Emboli:* Administer over 2 hr.

▪ **Y-Site Compatibility:** ▪ lidocaine.

▪ **Y-Site Incompatibility:** ▪ dobutamine ▪ dopamine ▪ heparin ▪ nitroglycerin.

PATIENT/FAMILY TEACHING

□ Explain purpose of alteplase and the need for close monitoring to patient and family.

□ Instruct patient to report signs of hypersensitivity and bleeding promptly.

EVALUATION
Effectiveness of therapy can be demonstrated by: ▪ Restoration of coronary perfusion as demonstrated by cardiac catherization ▪ Decreased incidence of congestive heart failure without the occurrence of bleeding ▪ Lysis of pulmonary emboli with improvement of hemodynamic status.

ALTRETAMINE
(al-**tret**-a-meen)
hexamethylmelamine, Hexalen, {Hexastat}

CLASSIFICATION(S):
Antineoplastic agent
Pregnancy Category D

INDICATIONS
▪ Management of ovarian cancer unresponsive to treatment with other agents.

ACTION
▪ Mechanism unknown, but may disrupt DNA and RNA synthesis. **Therapeutic Effect:** ▪ Death of rapidly replicating cells, particularly malignant ones.

PHARMACOKINETICS
Absorption: Well absorbed following oral administration.
Distribution: Reaches high concentrations in liver, kidney, and small intestine. Poor penetration into brain.
Metabolism and Excretion: Mostly metabolized by the liver to compounds with antineoplastic activity.
Half-life: 4.7–10.2 hr.

CONTRAINDICATIONS AND PRECAUTIONS
Contraindicated in: ▪ Hypersensitivity ▪ Pregnancy or lactation.
Use Cautiously in: ▪ Children (safety not established) ▪ Pre-existing neurologic diseases ▪ Patients with childbearing potential ▪ Infections ▪ Decreased bone marrow reserve ▪ Other chronic debilitating illnesses.

{} = Available in Canada only.

ADVERSE REACTIONS AND SIDE EFFECTS*

CNS: SEIZURES, fatigue.

GI: nausea, vomiting, anorexia, hepatic toxicity.

GU: renal toxicity, gonadal suppression.

Derm: alopecia (<1%), skin rash, pruritus.

Endo: gonadal suppression.

Hemat: anemia, leukopenia, thrombocytopenia.

Neuro: peripheral neuropathy.

INTERACTIONS

Drug–Drug: ▪ Concurrent use with **MAO inhibitors** may produce orthostatic hypotension ▪ May decrease antibody response and increase risk of adverse reactions from **live virus vaccines** ▪ Additive bone marrow depression may occur with other **antineoplastic agents** or **radiation therapy**.

ROUTE AND DOSAGE

▪ **PO (Adults):** 260 mg/m^2/day in 4 divided doses for 14 or 21 days of each 28-day cycle. Dosage reduction to 200 mg/m^2/day in 4 divided doses after meals and at bedtime recommended after 14 or more day rest for any of the following: GI intolerance, severe bone marrow depression, or progressive neurologic toxicity.

AVAILABILITY

▪ **Tablets:** 50 mg, {100 mg}.

TIME/ACTION PROFILE (effects on blood counts)

	ONSET	PEAK	DURATION
PO	UK	3–4 wk	6 wk

NURSING IMPLICATIONS

ASSESSMENT

▢ Nausea and vomiting of gradual onset frequently occurs. Tolerance may develop after several weeks of therapy. Treatment includes antiemetics or dosage reduction, and rarely, discontinuation. Monitor amount of emesis and notify physician if emesis exceeds guidelines to prevent dehydration.

▢ Assess for signs of anemia (increased fatigue, dyspnea, orthostatic hypotension) throughout therapy.

▢ Assess for fever, chills, sore throat, and signs of infection. Notify physician if these symptoms occur.

▢ Assess for signs of bleeding (bleeding gums, bruising, petechiae; guaiac stools, urine, and emesis). Avoid IM injections and rectal temperatures. Apply pressure to venipuncture sites for 10 min.

▢ Assess patient for signs of peripheral neuropathy (numbness, tingling, paresthesia) prior to initiation of each course and routinely throughout therapy. Pyridoxine may minimize peripheral neuropathy. Peripheral neuropathy is usually reversible on discontinuation of medication.

▪ **Lab Test Considerations:** Monitor CBC and platelets prior to each course of therapy, monthly, and as clinically indicated. The nadir of leukopenia and thrombocytopenia occur in 3–4 wk with 21-day therapy and recover in 6 wk. Dose should be held for 14 or more days and resumed at 200 mg/m^2/day in 4 divided doses for any of the following: GI intolerance unresponsive to conventional therapy, WBC <2000 mm^3, granulocytes <1000 mm^3, platelet count <75,000 mm^3, or progressive neurologic toxicity.

POTENTIAL NURSING DIAGNOSES

▪ Infection, high risk for (adverse reactions).

▪ Injury, high risk for (side effects).

▪ Knowledge deficit related to medication regimen (patient/family teaching).

IMPLEMENTATION

▪ **PO:** Administer doses after meals and at bedtime.

PATIENT/FAMILY TEACHING

- Instruct patient to notify physician promptly if fever, sore throat, signs of infection, bleeding gums, bruising, petechiae; blood in stools, urine, or emesis; increased fatigue, dyspnea, or orthostatic hypotension occur. Caution patient to avoid crowds and persons with known infections. Instruct patient to use soft toothbrush and electric razor and to avoid falls. Caution patient not to drink alcoholic beverages or take medications containing aspirin or ibuprofen, as these may precipitate gastric bleeding.
- Instruct patient to report promptly any numbness or tingling in extremities.
- Instruct patient not to receive any vaccinations without advice of physician.
- Advise patient of the need for contraception.
- Emphasize the need for periodic lab tests to monitor for side effects.

EVALUATION

Effectiveness of therapy can be demonstrated by: ■ Decrease in size or spread of malignancy.

ALUMINUM ACETATE

Bluboro, Boropak, Burow's Solution, Modified Burow's Solution, Domeboro, Pedi-Boro

CLASSIFICATION(S):
Astringent (topical)
Pregnancy Category C

INDICATIONS

■ Minor skin inflammation.

ACTION

■ Astringent; soothing effect results from cooling and vasoconstriction. **Therapeutic Effect:** ■ Relief of painful inflammation of the skin.

PHARMACOKINETICS

Absorption: Small amounts may be systemically absorbed.
Distribution: UK.
Metabolism and Excretion: UK.
Half-life: UK.

CONTRAINDICATIONS AND PRECAUTIONS

Contraindicated in: ■ Hypersensitivity ■ For external use only, avoid using near eyes.
Use Cautiously in: ■ Skin conditions in which irritation continues to spread.

ADVERSE REACTIONS AND SIDE EFFECTS*

Misc: hypersensitivity.

INTERACTIONS

Drug–Drug: ■ May inactivate concurrently applied **collagenase**.

ROUTE AND DOSAGE

■ **Top (Adults and Children):** 1 : 20 or 1 : 40 solution as wet dressing every 15–30 min for 4–8 hr or soak for 15–30 min 3 times daily.

AVAILABILITY

■ *Packets:* yielding a 1 : 40 solution
■ *Tablets:* yielding 1 : 20 or 1 : 40 solution.

TIME/ACTION PROFILE (relief of inflammation)

	ONSET	PEAK	DURATION
Top	upon application	UK	during application

NURSING IMPLICATIONS

ASSESSMENT

- Inspect skin for erythema, excoriation, vesicles, maceration, and drainage.

POTENTIAL NURSING DIAGNOSES

■ Pain (indications).
■ Infection, high risk for (indications).
■ Knowledge deficit related to medication regimen (patient/family teaching).

---

*Underlines indicate most frequent; **CAPITALS** indicate life-threatening.

IMPLEMENTATION

- **Topical:** Prepare solution by mixing one packet or tablet in 1 pt lukewarm water (or per manufacturer's directions). Use only clear portion. Do not apply precipitate to skin.
- □ Do not apply occlusive dressing; will hinder evaporation and may cause maceration.
- □ To prevent chilling and hypothermia, do not apply to more than ⅓ of the body at one time. Position patient away from drafts.
- □ Clear, unprecipitated solution is stable for 7 days at room temperature.

PATIENT/FAMILY TEACHING

- □ Instruct patient on preparation of solution and application of soaks.
- □ Instruct patient not to apply solution near eyes or to mucous membranes.
- □ Advise patient to notify physician if area of skin irritation spreads or worsens.

EVALUATION

Effectiveness of therapy can be demonstrated by: ▪ Relief of skin irritation.

ALUMINUM HYDROXIDE
AlternaGEL, Alucap, {Alugel}, Aluminet, Alu-tab, Amphojel, Basalgel, Dialume, Nephrox

CLASSIFICATION(S):
Antacid, Electrolyte modifier (hypophosphatemic)
Pregnancy Category UK

INDICATIONS

▪ Lowering of phosphate levels in patients with chronic renal failure ▪ Adjunctive therapy in the treatment of peptic, duodenal, and gastric ulcers ▪ Hyperacidity, indigestion, reflux esophagitis.

ACTION

▪ Binds phosphate in the GI tract ▪ Neutralizes gastric acid and inactivates pepsin. **Therapeutic Effects:** ▪ Lowering of serum phosphate levels ▪ Healing of ulcers and decreased pain associated with ulcers or gastric hyperacidity ▪ Constipation limits use alone in the treatment of ulcer disease ▪ Frequently found in combination with magnesium-containing compounds.

PHARMACOKINETICS

Absorption: With chronic use, small amounts of aluminum are systemically absorbed.
Distribution: If absorbed, aluminum is widely distributed, crosses the placenta, enters breast milk and, with chronic use, concentrates in the CNS.
Metabolism and Excretion: Mostly excreted in feces. Small amounts absorbed are excreted by the kidneys.
Half-life: UK.

CONTRAINDICATIONS AND PRECAUTIONS

Contraindicated in: ▪ Severe abdominal pain of unknown cause.
Use Cautiously in: ▪ Hypercalcemia ▪ Hypophosphatemia ▪ Pregnancy (generally considered safe; chronic high-dose therapy should be avoided).

ADVERSE REACTIONS AND SIDE EFFECTS*

GI: constipation.
F and E: hypophosphatemia.

INTERACTIONS

Drug–Drug: ▪ Absorption of **tetracyclines, chlorpromazine, iron salts, isoniazid,** or **fluoroquinolones** may be decreased ▪ **Salicylate** blood levels may be decreased ▪ **Quinidine, mexiletine,** and **amphetamine** levels may be increased if enough antacid is ingested such that urine pH is increased.

ROUTE AND DOSAGE

Hypophosphatemic
▪ **PO (Adults):** 1.9–4.8 g 3–4 times daily.

{} = Available in Canada only.
*Underlines indicate most frequent; **CAPITALS** indicate life-threatening.

- **PO (Children):** 50–150 mg/kg/24 hr— titrate to normal serum phosphate levels.

Antacid
- **PO (Adults):** 500–1800 mg (5–30 ml) 3–6 times daily.

AVAILABILITY

- *Capsules:* 475 mg, 500 mg • *Tablets:* 300 mg, 600 mg • *Suspension:* 320 mg/5 ml, 450 mg/5 ml, 600 mg/5 ml, 675 mg/5 ml.

TIME/ACTION PROFILE

	ONSET	PEAK	DURATION
PO*	hr–days	days–wks	days
PO†	15–30 min	30 min	30 min–3 hr

*Hypophasphatemic effect.
†Antacid effect.

NURSING IMPLICATIONS

ASSESSMENT
- Assess location, duration, character, and precipitating factors of gastric pain.
- **Lab Test Considerations:** Monitor serum phosphate and calcium levels periodically during chronic use of aluminum hydroxide.
- May cause increased serum gastrin and decreased serum phosphate concentrations.
- In treatment of severe ulcer disease, guaiac stools and emesis and monitor pH of gastric secretions.

POTENTIAL NURSING DIAGNOSES
- Pain (indications).
- Constipation (side effects).
- Knowledge deficit related to medication regimen (patient/family teaching).

IMPLEMENTATION
- **General Info:** Antacids cause premature dissolution and absorption of enteric-coated tablets and may interfere with absorption of other oral medications. Separate administration of aluminum hydroxide and oral medications by at least 1 hr.
- Tablets must be chewed thoroughly before swallowing to prevent entering small intestine in undissolved form.

Follow with a glass of water.
- Shake liquid preparations well before pouring. Follow administration with water to assure passage into stomach.
- Liquid and powder dosage forms are considered to be more effective than tablets.
- **Hypophosphatemic:** For phosphate lowering, follow dose with full glass of water or fruit juice.
- **Antacid:** May be given in conjunction with magnesium-containing antacids to minimize constipation, except in patients with renal failure. Administer 1 and 3 hr after meals and at bedtime for maximum antacid effect.
- For treatment of peptic ulcer, aluminum hydroxide may be administered every 1–2 hr while awake or diluted with 2–3 parts of water and administered intragastrically every 30 min for 12 or more hr per day. Physician may order nasogastric tube clamped following administration.
- For reflux esophagitis, administer 15 ml 20–40 min after meals and at bedtime.

PATIENT/FAMILY TEACHING
- **General Info:** Instruct patient to take aluminum hydroxide exactly as directed. If on a regular dosing schedule and a dose is missed, take as soon as remembered if not almost time for next dose; do not double doses.
- Advise patients to check label for sodium content. Patients with congestive heart failure, hypertension, or those on a sodium restriction should use low-sodium preparations.
- Inform patients of potential for constipation from aluminum hydroxide.
- **Hypophosphatemic:** Patients taking aluminum hydroxide for hyperphosphatemia should be taught the importance of a low-phosphate diet.
- **Antacid:** Caution patient to consult physician before taking antacids for more than 2 wk if problem is recurring or if taking other medications. Advise patient to consult physician if relief is not obtained or if symptoms of gastric bleeding (black tarry stools, coffee ground emesis) occur.

EVALUATION

Effectiveness of therapy can be demonstrated by: ▪ Decrease in serum phosphate levels ▪ Decrease in GI pain and irritation □ Increase in the pH of gastric secretions. In treatment of peptic ulcer, antacid therapy should be continued for at least 4–6 wk after symptoms have disappeared, since there is no correlation between disappearance of symptoms and healing of ulcers.

AMANTADINE
(a-**man**-ta-deen)
Symmetrel, Symadine

CLASSIFICATION(S):
Antiparkinson agent, Antiviral
Pregnancy Category C

INDICATIONS

▪ Symptomatic initial and adjunct treatment of Parkinson's disease ▪ Prophylaxis and treatment of influenza A viral infections.

ACTION

▪ Potentiates the action of dopamine in the CNS ▪ Prevents penetration of influenza A virus into host cell. **Therapeutic Effects:** ▪ Relief of Parkinsonian symptoms ▪ Prevention and decreased symptoms of influenza virus A infection.

PHARMACOKINETICS

Absorption: Well absorbed from the GI tract.
Distribution: Distributed to various body tissues and fluids. Crosses blood–brain barrier and enters breast milk.
Metabolism and Excretion: Excreted unchanged in the urine.
Half-life: 24 hr.

CONTRAINDICATIONS AND PRECAUTIONS

Contraindicated in: ▪ Hypersensitivity.

Use Cautiously in: ▪ Seizure disorders ▪ Liver disease ▪ Psychiatric problems ▪ Cardiac disease ▪ Renal impairment (dosage reduction required if CCr <60 ml/min) ▪ May increase susceptibility to rubella infections ▪ Pregnancy and lactation (safety not established) ▪ Elderly.

ADVERSE REACTIONS AND SIDE EFFECTS*

CNS: <u>dizziness</u>, <u>ataxia</u>, <u>insomnia</u>, depression, psychosis, anxiety, drowsiness, confusion.
CV: <u>hypotension</u>, congestive heart failure, edema.
EENT: dry mouth, blurred vision.
GU: urinary retention.
Derm: rashes, <u>mottling</u>.
Hemat: leukopenia, neutropenia.
Resp: dyspnea.

INTERACTIONS

Drug–Drug: ▪ Concurrent use of **antihistamines, phenothiazines, quinidine, disopyramide,** and **tricyclic antidepressants** may increase anticholinergic effects (dry mouth, blurred vision, constipation).

ROUTE AND DOSAGE

Parkinson's Disease
▪ PO (Adults): 100 mg 1–2 times daily.

Influenza A Viral Infection
▪ **PO (Adults and Children >9 yr):** 200 mg/day as a single dose or 100 mg bid (not >100 mg/day in elderly patients).
▪ **PO (Children 1–9 yr):** 4.4–8.8 mg/kg/day up to 150 mg/day as a single daily dose or 2 divided doses.

AVAILABILITY

▪ *Capsules:* 100 mg ▪ *Syrup:* 50 mg/5 ml.

TIME/ACTION PROFILE
(antiparkinson effect)

	ONSET	PEAK	DURATION
PO	within 48 hr	up to 2 wk	UK

---

*<u>Underlines</u> indicate most frequent; **CAPITALS** indicate life-threatening.

NURSING IMPLICATIONS

ASSESSMENT

- **General Info:** Monitor blood pressure periodically. Assess patient for drug-induced orthostatic hypotension.
- Monitor intake and output closely in the elderly. May cause urinary retention. Notify physician of significant discrepancy or bladder distention.
- Monitor vital signs and mental status periodically during first few days of dosage adjustment in patients receiving more than 200 mg daily, as side effects are more likely.
- Assess for congestive heart failure (peripheral edema, weight gain, dyspnea, rales/crackles, jugular venous distension) especially in patients with chronic therapy or history of congestive heart failure.
- Assess patient for the appearance of a diffuse red mottling of the skin (livedo reticularis), especially in the lower extremities or on exposure to cold. Disappears with continued therapy but may not completely resolve until several weeks after therapy has been discontinued.
- **Parkinson's Disease:** Assess akinesia, rigidity, tremors, and gait disturbances prior to and throughout course of therapy.
- **Influenza Prophylaxis or Treatment:** Monitor respiratory status (rate, breath sounds, sputum) and temperature periodically. Supportive treatment is indicated if symptoms occur.
- **Toxicity and Overdose:** Symptoms of toxicity include CNS stimulation (confusion, mood changes, tremors, seizures, arrhythmias, and hypotension). There is no specific antidote, although physostigmine has been used to reverse CNS effects.

POTENTIAL NURSING DIAGNOSES

- Physical mobility, impaired (indications).
- Infection, high risk for (indications).
- Knowledge deficit related to medication regimen (patient/family teaching).

IMPLEMENTATION

- **PO:** Do not administer last dose of medication near bedtime; may produce insomnia in some patients.
- Administering amantadine in divided doses may decrease CNS side effects.
- The contents of capsules may be mixed with food or fluids if the patient has difficulty swallowing pills.

PATIENT/FAMILY TEACHING

- **General Info:** Advise patient to take medication around the clock as directed and not to skip doses or double up on missed doses. If a dose is missed, do not take within 4 hr of the next dose.
- May cause dizziness or blurred vision. Advise patient to avoid driving or other activities that require alertness until response to the drug is known.
- Advise patient to make position changes slowly to minimize orthostatic hypotension.
- Inform patient that frequent mouth rinses, good oral hygiene, and sugarless gum or candy may decrease dry mouth.
- Advise patient to confer with physician or pharmacist prior to taking over-the-counter medications, especially cold remedies, or drinking alcoholic beverages.
- Instruct patient and family to notify physician if influenza symptoms occur (when used as prophylaxis) or if confusion, mood changes, difficulty with urination, edema and shortness of breath, or worsening of Parkinson's disease symptoms occur.
- **Parkinson's Disease:** Amantadine should be tapered gradually; abrupt withdrawal may precipitate a parkinsonian crisis.

EVALUATION

Effectiveness of therapy can be demonstrated by: ■ Decrease in akinesia and rigidity. Full therapeutic effects may require 2 wk of therapy ▪ Absence or reduction of influenza A symptoms.

AMIKACIN
(am-i-**kay**-sin)
Amikin

CLASSIFICATION(S):
Anti-infective (aminoglycoside)
Pregnancy Category D

INDICATIONS
▪ Treatment of serious gram-negative bacillary infections and infections due to staphylococci when penicillins or other less toxic drugs are contraindicated.

ACTION
▪ Inhibits protein synthesis in bacteria at the level of the 30S ribosome. **Therapeutic Effect:** ▪ Bactericidal action against susceptible bacteria. **Spectrum:** ▪ Notable for activity against: ▫ *Pseudomonas aeruginosa* ▫ *Klebsiella pneumoniae* ▫ *Escherichia coli* ▫ *Proteus* ▫ *Serratia* and *Acinetobacter* where resistance to gentamicin or tobramycin has occurred ▫ *Staphylococcus aureus* ▪ In the treatment of enterococcal infections, synergy with a penicillin is required.

PHARMACOKINETICS
Absorption: Well absorbed after IM administration.
Distribution: Widely distributed throughout extracellular fluid. Crosses the placenta. Poor penetration into CSF.
Metabolism and Excretion: Excretion is mainly (>90%) renal. Minimal amounts metabolized by the liver.
Half-life: 2–3 hr (increased in renal impairment).

CONTRAINDICATIONS AND PRECAUTIONS
Contraindicated in: ▪ Hypersensitivity to amikacin or bisulfites ▪ Cross-sensitivity with other aminoglycosides may occur.

Use Cautiously in: ▪ Renal impairment of any kind (dosage adjustments necessary—blood level monitoring useful in preventing ototoxicity and nephrotoxicity) ▪ Pregnancy, lactation, infants, and neonates (safety not established) ▪ Neuromuscular diseases such as myasthenia gravis.

ADVERSE REACTIONS AND SIDE EFFECTS*
EENT: ototoxicity (vestibular and cochlear).
GU: nephrotoxicity.
Neuro: enhanced neuromuscular blockade.
Misc: hypersensitivity reactions.

INTERACTIONS
Drug–Drug: ▪ Inactivated by **penicillins** when coadministered to patients with renal insufficiency ▪ Possible respiratory paralysis after **inhalation anesthetics** or **neuromuscular blockers** ▪ Increased incidence of ototoxicity with **loop diuretics** ▪ Increased incidence of nephrotoxicity with other **nephrotoxic drugs**.

ROUTE AND DOSAGE
▪ **IM, IV (Adults, Children, and Older Infants):** 15 mg/kg/day in divided doses every 8–12 hr.
▪ **IM, IV (Younger Infants and Neonates):** 10 mg/kg initially, 7.5 mg/kg every 12 hr.

AVAILABILITY
▪ *Injection:* 50 mg/ml, 250 mg/ml.

TIME/ACTION PROFILE (peak blood levels)

	ONSET	PEAK
IM	rapid	0.75–1.5 hr
IV	rapid	end of infusion

NURSING IMPLICATIONS
ASSESSMENT
▫ Assess patient for infection (vital signs; wound appearance, sputum,

---

*Underlines indicate most frequent; **CAPITALS** indicate life-threatening.

urine, and stool; WBC) at beginning and throughout course of therapy.

□ Obtain specimens for culture and sensitivity prior to initiating therapy. First dose may be given before receiving results.

□ Evaluate eighth cranial nerve function by audiometry prior to and throughout course of therapy. Hearing loss is usually in the high-frequency range. Prompt recognition and intervention is essential in preventing permanent damage. Also monitor for vestibular dysfunction (vertigo, ataxia, nausea, vomiting). Eighth cranial nerve dysfunction is associated with persistently elevated peak amikacin levels. Amikacin should be discontinued if tinnitus or subjective hearing loss occurs.

□ Monitor intake and output and daily weight to assess hydration status and renal function.

□ Assess patient for signs of superinfection (fever, upper respiratory infection, vaginal itching or discharge, increasing malaise, diarrhea).

■ **Lab Test Considerations:** Monitor renal function by urinalysis, specific gravity, BUN, creatinine, and creatinine clearance prior to and throughout therapy.

□ May cause increased BUN, AST (SGOT), ALT (SGPT), serum alkaline phosphatase, bilirubin, creatinine, and LDH concentrations.

□ May cause decreased serum calcium, magnesium, potassium, and sodium concentrations.

■ **Toxicity and Overdose:** Therapeutic blood levels should be monitored periodically during therapy. Timing of blood levels is important in interpreting results. Draw blood for peak levels 1 hr after IM injection and 15–30 min after IV infusion is completed. Trough levels should be drawn just prior to next dose. Acceptable peak level is 30–35 mcg/ml; trough level should not exceed 5–10 mcg/ml.

POTENTIAL NURSING DIAGNOSES
■ Infection, high risk for (indications).

■ Sensory–perceptual alteration: auditory (side effects).

IMPLEMENTATION
■ **General Info:** Keep patient well hydrated (1500–2000 ml/day) during therapy.

■ **Intermittent Infusion:** Dilute 500 mg of amikacin in 100–200 ml of D5W, D10W, 0.9% NaCl, D5/0.9% NaCl, D5/0.45% NaCl, D5/0.25% NaCl, or lactated Ringer's solution. Solution may be pale yellow without decreased potency. Stable for 24 hr at room temperature. Flush IV line with D5W or 0.9% NaCl following administration.

■ *Rate:* Infuse over 30–60 min (over 1–2 hr for infants).

■ **Syringe Incompatibility:** ■ heparin.

■ **Y-Site Compatibility:** ■ acyclovir ■ cyclophosphamide ■ enalaprilat ■ esmolol ■ fluconazole ■ fludarabine ■ foscarnet ■ furosemide ■ labetalol ■ magnesium sulfate ■ morphine ■ ondansetron ■ perphenazine ■ sargramostim ■ zidovudine.

■ **Y-Site Incompatibility:** ■ hetastarch.

■ **Additive Incompatibility:** Manufacturer does not recommend admixing. If aminoglycosides and penicillins or cephalosporins must be administered concurrently, administer in separate sites.

PATIENT/FAMILY TEACHING
□ Instruct patient to report signs of hypersensitivity, tinnitus, vertigo, or hearing loss.

EVALUATION
Clinical response can be evaluated by:
■ Resolution of the signs and symptoms of infection. If no response is seen within 3–5 days, new cultures should be taken.

AMILORIDE
(a-**mill**-oh-ride)
Midamor

CLASSIFICATION(S):
Diuretic (potassium-sparing)
Pregnancy Category B

INDICATIONS

■ Counteracts potassium loss induced by other diuretics ■ Commonly used in combination with other agents to treat: □ Edema □ Hypertension □ Hyperaldosteronism.

ACTION

■ Causes excretion of sodium bicarbonate and calcium while conserving potassium and hydrogen ions. **Therapeutic Effects:** ■ Weak diuretic and antihypertensive response when compared to other diuretics ■ Conservation of potassium.

PHARMACOKINETICS

Absorption: Variable absorption from the GI tract (15–50%).
Distribution: Not known.
Metabolism and Excretion: 50% eliminated unchanged by the kidneys, 40% excreted unabsorbed in the feces.
Half-life: 6–9 hr.

CONTRAINDICATIONS AND PRECAUTIONS

Contraindicated in: ■ Hypersensitivity ■ Renal insufficiency.
Use Cautiously in: ■ Hepatic dysfunction ■ Elderly patients ■ Debilitated patients ■ Pregnancy, lactation, or children (safety not established).

ADVERSE REACTIONS AND SIDE EFFECTS*

CNS: headache, dizziness.
CV: arrhythmias.
GI: <u>nausea</u>, <u>vomiting</u>, <u>anorexia</u>, <u>diarrhea</u>, cramps, constipation, flatulence.
GU: impotence.
F and E: <u>hyperkalemia</u>, hyponatremia, hypochloremia.
Hemat: dyscrasias, megaloblastic anemia.
MS: muscle cramps.

INTERACTIONS

Drug–Drug: ■ Additive hypotension with acute ingestion of **alcohol,** other **antihypertensive agents,** or **nitrates** ■ Use with **angiotensin converting enzyme (ACE) inhibitors, indomethacin,** or **potassium supplements,** or **cyclosporine** may lead to hyperkalemia. ■ Decreases **lithium** excretion; may lead to toxicity ■ Effectiveness may be decreased by **NSAIDs.**

ROUTE AND DOSAGE

■ **PO (Adults):** 5–10 mg/day (up to 20 mg).

AVAILABILITY

■ *Tablets:* 5 mg ■ *In combination with:* hydrochlorothiazide (Moduretic). See Appendix A.

TIME/ACTION PROFILE (effects on electrolyte excretion)

	ONSET	PEAK	DURATION
PO	2 hr	6–10 hr	24 hr

NURSING IMPLICATIONS

ASSESSMENT

□ Monitor intake and output ratios and daily weight throughout therapy.
□ If medication is given as an adjunct to antihypertensive therapy, blood pressure should be evaluated before administering.
□ Periodic ECGs are recommended in patients receiving prolonged therapy.
□ Assess patient frequently for hyperkalemia (fatigue, muscle weakness, paresthesia, flaccid paralysis, cardiac arrhythmias). Patients who have diabetes mellitus, kidney disease, or who are elderly are at an increased risk of hyperkalemia.
■ **Lab Test Considerations:** Monitor serum electrolytes, glucose, BUN, and creatinine periodically throughout therapy. Withhold drug and notify physician if patient becomes hyperkalemic. Patients with elevated BUN and creatinine may be at an increased risk for developing hyperkalemia. May cause elevated magnesium and uric acid levels. May cause decreased serum sodium and chloride levels.

*Underlines indicate most frequent; **CAPITALS** indicate life-threatening.

□ May cause increased serum glucose in patients with diabetes. Discontinue amiloride 3 days prior to a glucose tolerance test.

POTENTIAL NURSING DIAGNOSES
- Fluid volume excess (indications).
- Knowledge deficit related to medication regimen (patient/family teaching).

IMPLEMENTATION
- **PO:** Administer in AM to avoid interrupting sleep pattern.
□ Administer with food or milk to minimize gastric irritation.

PATIENT/FAMILY TEACHING
□ Instruct patient to take medication exactly as directed, even if feeling well. If dose is missed, take as soon as remembered unless almost time for next dose; do not double doses.
□ Teach hypertensive patients how to check blood pressure weekly.
□ Caution patients to avoid salt substitutes and foods that contain high levels of potassium unless directed by physician (see Appendix K).
□ Reinforce need to continue additional therapies for hypertension (weight loss, restricted sodium intake, stress reduction, regular exercise, moderation of alcohol consumption, and cessation of smoking). Amiloride controls but does not cure hypertension.
□ Advise patient to consult with physician or pharmacist before taking any over-the-counter decongestants, cough or cold preparations, or appetite suppressants concurrently with this medication because of potential for increased blood pressure.
□ May cause dizziness. Caution patient to avoid driving or other activities requiring alertness until response to medication is known.
□ Instruct patient to notify physician or dentist of medication regimen prior to treatment or surgery.
□ Advise patient to notify physician if muscle weakness or cramps, fatigue, or weakness occur.

EVALUATION
Effectiveness of therapy can be demonstrated by: ■ Lowering of blood pressure and increase in diuresis while maintaining serum potassium level in an acceptable range.

AMINO ACIDS
Aminess, Aminosyn, Branch-Amin, FreAmine, HepatAmine, NeprAmine, Novamine, Procal-Amine, RenAmin, Travasol, Trophamine

CLASSIFICATION(S):
Caloric agent (protein source)
Pregnancy Category C

INDICATIONS
■ Provides protein to patients who are unable to ingest enough protein by mouth to maintain positive nitrogen balance. □ Used perioperatively in patients who are unable to ingest protein, as in GI disorders, or to provide an extra source of protein in patients with large requirements who are unable to ingest enough, as seen in extensive burns, severe trauma, or overwhelming sepsis. □ Usually used with a carbohydrate source (dextrose) and a fat source as part of a total parenteral nutrition (TPN, hyperalimentation) program or protein-sparing regimen. Electrolytes, minerals, trace elements, and vitamins are also included. **Treatment must be individualized for each patient and requires facilities and personnel skilled in its use.**

ACTION
■ Promotes protein synthesis by acting as a protein calorie source, decreases rate of protein breakdown (catabolism). **Therapeutic Effect:** ■ Maintenance of positive nitrogen balance.

PHARMACOKINETICS
Absorption: Following IV administration absorption is essentially complete.
Distribution: Widely distributed.
Metabolism and Excretion: Metabolized as part of anabolic processes, then excreted in urine as urea nitrogen.
Half-life: UK.

CONTRAINDICATIONS AND PRECAUTIONS

Contraindicated in: ▪ No known contraindications.

Use Cautiously in: ▪ Uncontrolled sepsis ▪ Advanced cardiac, renal, and hepatic disease (specific formulations may be required).

ADVERSE REACTIONS AND SIDE EFFECTS*

CNS: headache, confusion.
CV: congestive heart failure, hypotension, hypertension.
GI: nausea, vomiting.
F and E: hypervolemia, hypovolemia, electrolyte disturbances.
Metab: hyperglycemia, hypoglycemia, azotemia, fatty acid deficiency, hyperammonemia.
Misc: INFECTION.

INTERACTIONS

Drug–Drug: ▪ **Glucocorticoids, diuretics,** or **tetracyclines** may exaggerate negative nitrogen balance.

ROUTE AND DOSAGE

Doses must be individualized to meet metabolic needs. If amino acids are part of total parenteral nutrition (hyperalimentation), then additional calories (dextrose and lipid emulsions) must be provided with electrolytes, vitamins, trace minerals, and other micronutrients.

▪ **IV (Adults):** 1–2 g protein/kg/day.
▪ **IV (Children):** 2–3 g protein/kg/day.
▪ **IV (Neonates):** 2–3 g protein/kg/day.

AVAILABILITY

▪ *Injection:* 2.75%, 3.5%, 4.25%, 5%, 5.5%, 6%, 8.5%, 10%, 11.4%, 15% amino acids.

TIME/ACTION PROFILE

	ONSET	PEAK	DURATION
IV	UK	UK	UK

NURSING IMPLICATIONS

ASSESSMENT

□ Nutritional status must be assessed prior to and periodically throughout therapy because amino acids are most commonly used as a component of total parenteral nutrition. Parameters to assess include height, weight, skinfold thickness, arm circumference, total protein, serum albumin, CBC, electrolytes, nitrogen balance, function of gastrointestinal tract, and caloric need.
□ Monitor intake and output; assess for fluid overload (rales/crackles, dyspnea, peripheral edema).
□ Monitor for infection (fever, chills, diaphoresis). If sepsis occurs, physician may order changing site, culturing catheter tip, hanging new solution and tubing, and obtaining blood cultures.
▪ **Lab Test Considerations:** May cause increased BUN. A 10–15% increase for 3 consecutive days may necessitate discontinuing therapy or altering formulation.
□ May cause increased ammonia and ketone levels.

POTENTIAL NURSING DIAGNOSES

▪ Nutrition, altered: less than body requirements (indications).
▪ Infection, high risk for (side effects).
▪ Knowledge deficit related to medication regimen (patient/family teaching).

IMPLEMENTATION

▪ **General Info:** Component of total parenteral nutrition. Usually given in conjunction with hypertonic dextrose. Trace elements, vitamins, electrolytes, and insulin are usually incorporated into formulation.
□ Special formulas available for patients with hepatic or renal dysfunction, patients under extreme stress (trauma, sepsis), and children.
▪ **Continuous Infusion:** Do not add anything to solution without conferring with pharmacist. Total parenteral nu-

trition solutions should be prepared aseptically in a biologic cabinet.

□ Solution should be clear. Addition of multivitamins will result in bright yellow color.

□ Infuse through 0.22-micron filter unless mixed with dextrose and fat emulsion in a 3-in-1 admixture. Control rate with pump or controller.

□ If administered peripherally, change peripheral site every 48–72 hr or according to institutional policy. Monitor for thrombophlebitis. Avoid infiltration; may cause tissue necrosis.

□ Peripheral line may be used to administer protein-sparing regimen using dilute amino acid solution (3.5%) with or without D5W or D10W and fat emulsion. Central line must be used to administer more concentrated solution when mixed with hypertonic glucose.

□ Use aseptic technique with central line. Change dressing every 48 hr or according to institutional policy. Auscultate breath sounds and assess site for erythema, edema, and leakage.

■ **Y-Site Compatibility:** ■ cefamandole ■ cefazolin ■ cefoperazone ■ cefotaxime ■ cefoxitin ■ cephalothin ■ cephapirin ■ chloramphenicol ■ clindamycin ■ digoxin ■ dobutamine ■ dopamine ■ doxycycline ■ erythromycin lactobionate ■ fat emulsion ■ foscarnet ■ furosemide ■ gentamicin ■ isoproterenol ■ kanamycin ■ lidocaine ■ meperidine ■ methicillin ■ mezlocillin ■ miconazole ■ morphine ■ nafcillin ■ netilmicin ■ norepinephrine ■ oxacillin ■ penicillin G potassium ■ piperacillin ■ sargramostim ■ ticarcillin ■ tobramycin ■ urokinase ■ vancomycin.

■ **Y-Site Incompatibility:** ■ cephradine.

PATIENT/FAMILY TEACHING

□ If used as a component of total parenteral nutrition, assure patient that solution is capable of fulfilling all nutritional needs.

□ Instruct patient to report fever, chills, or swelling, pain, and leakage at infusion site immediately.

■ **Home Care Issues:** Patients receiving total parenteral nutrition at home may receive infusion only at night. Prior to discharge the patient and family must understand rationale for therapy, procedures, and symptoms to report to physician. Patients must correctly demonstrate aseptic technique in caring for site, spiking bag, and priming tubing, and regulating infusion pump. Discharge planning should be coordinated with home care agency that will provide equipment, solutions, and professional support to the patient and family.

EVALUATION
Effectiveness of therapy can be demonstrated by: ■ Increased weight □ Improvement of nutritional parameters □ Improved healing.

AMINOCAPROIC ACID
(a-mee-noe-ka-**proe**-ik)
Amicar, epsilon aminocaproic acid

CLASSIFICATION(S):
Hemostatic
Pregnancy Category UK

INDICATIONS

■ Management of acute, life-threatening hemorrhage due to systemic hyperfibrinolysis or urinary fibrinolysis. **Unlabeled Use:** ■ Prevention of recurrent subarachnoid hemorrhage.

ACTION

■ Inhibits activation of plasminogen. **Therapeutic Effects:** ■ Inhibition of fibrinolysis ■ Stabilization of clot formation.

PHARMACOKINETICS

Absorption: Well absorbed following oral administration.
Distribution: Widely distributed.
Metabolism and Excretion: Mostly eliminated unchanged by the kidneys.
Half-life: UK.

CONTRAINDICATIONS AND PRECAUTIONS

Contraindicated in: ▪ Active intravascular clotting.

Use Cautiously in: ▪ Upper urinary tract bleeding ▪ Cardiac, renal, or liver disease (dosage reduction may be required) ▪ Pregnancy and lactation (safety not established) ▪ Disseminated intravascular coagulation (should be used concurrently with heparin).

ADVERSE REACTIONS AND SIDE EFFECTS*

CNS: dizziness, malaise.
CV: arrhythmias, hypotension (IV only).
EENT: tinnitus, nasal stuffiness.
GI: nausea, cramping, diarrhea, anorexia, bloating.
GU: diuresis, renal failure.
MS: myopathy.

INTERACTIONS

Drug–Drug: ▪ None significant.

ROUTE AND DOSAGE

Acute Bleeding Syndromes due to Elevated Fibrinolytic Activity

▪ **PO (Adults):** 5 g first hr, followed by 1–1.25 g q hr for 8 hr or until hemorrhage is controlled or 6 g/24 hr after prostate surgery.
▪ **IV (Adults):** 4–5 g over first hr, followed by 1 g/hr for 8 hr or until hemorrhage is controlled or 6 g/24 hr after prostate surgery (not >30 g/day).
▪ **PO, IV (Children):** 100 mg/kg or 3 g/m² over first hr, followed by continuous infusion of 33.3 mg/kg/hr or 1 g/m²/hr; (total dosage not >18 g/m²/24 hr).

Subarachnoid Hemorrhage

▪ **PO (Adults):** 3 g q 24 hr (36 g/day). If no surgery is performed, continue for 21 days after bleeding stops, then decrease to 2 g q 2 hr (24 g/day) for 3 days, then 1 g q 2 hr (12 g/day) for 3 days.

AVAILABILITY

▪ **Tablets:** 500 mg ▪ **Syrup:** 1.25 g/5 ml
▪ **Injection:** 250 mg/ml.

TIME/ACTION PROFILE (peak blood levels)

	ONSET	PEAK
PO	UK	2 hr
IV	UK	2 hr

NURSING IMPLICATIONS

ASSESSMENT

□ Monitor blood pressure, pulse, and respiratory status as indicated by severity of bleeding.
□ Monitor for overt bleeding every 15–30 min.
□ Monitor neurologic status (pupils, level of consciousness, motor activity) in patients with subarachnoid hemorrhage.
□ Monitor intake and output ratios frequently; notify physician if significant discrepancies occur.
□ Assess for thromboembolic complications (especially in patients with history). Notify physician of positive Homans' sign, leg pain and edema, hemoptysis, dyspnea, or chest pain.
▪ **Lab Test Considerations:** Monitor platelet count and clotting factors prior to and periodically throughout therapy in patients with systemic fibrinolysis.
□ Increased CPK, AST (SGOT), and serum aldolase may indicate myopathy.
□ May elevate serum potassium.

POTENTIAL NURSING DIAGNOSES

▪ Tissue perfusion, altered (indications).
▪ Injury, high risk for (indications, side effects).
▪ Knowledge deficit related to medication regimen (patient/family teaching).

IMPLEMENTATION

▪ **IV:** Stabilize IV catheter to minimize thrombophlebitis. Monitor site closely.

*Underlines indicate most frequent; **CAPITALS** indicate life-threatening.

- **Intermittent Infusion:** Do not administer undiluted. Dilute initial 4–5 g dose in 250 ml of Sterile Water for Injection, 0.9% NaCl, D5W, or lactated Ringer's solution. Do not dilute with sterile water in patients with subarachnoid hemorrhage.
- *Rate:* Administer over 1 hr.
- **Continuous Infusion:** Initial dose may be followed by a continuous infusion of 1 g/hr, in 50 ml of diluent.
- *Rate:* Administer IV solution using infusion pump to ensure accurate dose. Administer via slow IV infusion. Rapid infusion rate may cause hypotension, bradycardia, or other arrhythmias.
- **Additive Incompatibility:** Do not admix.

PATIENT/FAMILY TEACHING
- **General Info:** Instruct patient to notify the nurse immediately if bleeding recurs, or if thromboembolic symptoms develop.
- **IV:** Caution patient to make position changes slowly to avoid orthostatic hypotension.

EVALUATION
Effectiveness of therapy can be demonstrated by: ■ Cessation of bleeding ■ Prevention of rebleeding in subarachnoid hemorrhage, without occurrence of undesired clotting.

AMINOGLUTETHIMIDE
(a-meen-oh-gloo-**teth**-i-mide)
Cytadren

CLASSIFICATION(S):
Antineoplastic agent
Pregnancy Category D

INDICATIONS
- Short-term adrenal suppression of adrenal function in patients with Cushing's syndrome. **Unlabeled Uses:** ■ Advanced metastatic postmenopausal breast or prostate cancer.

ACTION
- Inhibits the synthesis of adrenal hormones including glucocorticoids, mineralocorticoids, estrogens, and androgens. **Therapeutic Effects:** ■ Decreased production of adrenal hormones in Cushing's disease ■ Decreased spread of postmenopausal breast or prostate cancer.

PHARMACOKINETICS
Absorption: Well absorbed following oral administration.
Distribution: Distribution not known.
Metabolism and Excretion: 50% metabolized by the liver. 50% excreted unchanged by the kidneys.
Half-life: 11–16 hr initially, drops to 2–9 hr after 2 wk of therapy.

CONTRAINDICATIONS AND PRECAUTIONS
Contraindicated in: ■ Hypersensitivity to glutethimide or aminoglutethimide.
Use Cautiously in: ■ Pregnancy (although normal pregnancies have occurred, may cause fetal harm) ■ Lactation or children (safety not established) ■ Stress (trauma, surgery, or acute illness); additional mineralocorticoid; and hydrocortisone may be required.

ADVERSE REACTIONS AND SIDE EFFECTS*
CNS: drowsiness, headache, dizziness, weakness.
CV: hypotension.
GI: nausea, anorexia, vomiting, drug-induced hepatitis.
Derm: morbilliform rash, pruritus, urticaria.
Hemat: AGRANULOCYTOSIS, leukopenia, thrombocytopenia.
Endo: adrenal suppression, adrenal insufficiency, hypothyroidism, masculinization in females, hirsutism in females.
MS: myalgia.
Misc: fever.

INTERACTIONS
Drug–Drug: ■ Increases metabolism and decreases effectiveness of **dexa-**

methasone ■ Decreases the effects of **warfarin, theophylline, digitoxin,** and **medroxyprogesterone** ■ **Alcohol** potentiates the effects of aminoglutethimide.

ROUTE AND DOSAGE
■ **PO (Adults):** 250 mg q 6 hr may be increased by 250 mg/day at 1–2 wk intervals, up to a daily total of 2 g.

AVAILABILITY
■ *Tablets:* 250 mg.

TIME/ACTION PROFILE (adrenal suppression)

	ONSET	PEAK	DURATION
PO	3–5 days	UK	36–72 hr*

*Recovery of adrenal function following discontinuation of short-term therapy; may take longer (up to 1 yr) after chronic therapy.

NURSING IMPLICATIONS
ASSESSMENT
□ Monitor patient for changes in signs of Cushing's syndrome (moon face, buffalo hump, hypertension, fragility, hirsutism, mood swings, increased susceptibility to infections) throughout therapy.
□ Monitor blood pressure periodically throughout therapy.
□ Assess patient for rash throughout therapy. Dose reduction or temporary discontinuation may be required if severe skin rash occurs.
■ **Lab Test Considerations:** Monitor plasma cortisol levels throughout therapy. Dose may be titrated according to levels.
□ May cause hypothyroidism. Monitor thyroid function tests periodically during therapy.
□ May cause elevated AST (SGOT), alkaline phosphatase, and bilirubin concentrations.
□ Monitor CBC and serum electrolytes periodically during therapy.

POTENTIAL NURSING DIAGNOSES
■ Injury, high risk for (side effects).
■ Knowledge deficit related to medication regimen (patient/family teaching).

IMPLEMENTATION
■ **General Info:** Therapy should be initiated in a hospital setting until a stable dosing regimen has been achieved.
□ Mineralocorticoid replacement (fludrocortisone) or glucocorticoid replacement (hydrocortisone) may be necessary.
■ **PO:** Administer around the clock, every 6 hr.

PATIENT/FAMILY TEACHING
□ May cause drowsiness or dizziness. Caution patient to avoid driving or other activities requiring alertness until response to medication is known.
□ Instruct patient to notify physician if rash, fainting, weakness, or headache become pronounced.
□ Advise patient that nausea and loss of appetite may occur during first 2 wk of therapy. Physician should be notified if these persist or become pronounced.
□ Advise patient to avoid concurrent use of alcohol while taking aminoglutethimide.

EVALUATION
Effectiveness of therapy can be demonstrated by: ■ Suppression of adrenal function in patients with Cushing's syndrome ■ Decreased spread of malignancy in advanced postmenopausal or prostate cancer.

AMINOPHYLLINE
(am-in-**off**-i-lin)
{Corophyllin}, {Palaron}, Phyllocontin, Truphylline

CLASSIFICATION(S):
Bronchodilator (phosphodiesterase inhibitor)
Pregnancy Category C

INDICATIONS

- Bronchodilator in reversible airway obstruction due to asthma or COPD. **Unlabeled Use:** ▪ Respiratory and myocardial stimulant in apnea of infancy.

ACTION

▪ Inhibits phosphodiesterase, producing increased tissue concentrations of cyclic adenosine monophosphate (cAMP). Increased levels of cAMP result in: □ Bronchodilation □ CNS stimulation □ Positive inotropic and chronotropic effects □ Diuresis □ Gastric acid secretion. Aminophylline is a salt of theophylline and releases free theophylline following administration. **Therapeutic Effect:** ▪ Bronchodilation.

PHARMACOKINETICS

Absorption: Well absorbed from oral dosage forms. Absorption from extended-release dosage forms is slow but complete. Absorption from rectal suppositories is erratic and unreliable.

Distribution: Widely distributed as theophylline. Crosses the placenta. Breast milk concentrations 70% of plasma levels.

Metabolism and Excretion: Metabolized by the liver to caffeine, which may accumulate in neonates. Metabolites are renally excreted.

Half-life: 3–13 hr (theophylline). Increased in the elderly (>60 yr), neonates, and in patients with congestive heart failure or liver disease. Shortened in cigarette smokers and children.

CONTRAINDICATIONS AND PRECAUTIONS

Contraindicated in: ▪ Uncontrolled arrhythmias ▪ Hyperthyroidism.

Use Cautiously in: ▪ Elderly patients (>60 yr), CHF, or liver disease (dosage reduction required) ▪ Has been used safely in pregnancy.

ADVERSE REACTIONS AND SIDE EFFECTS*

CNS: <u>nervousness</u>, <u>anxiety</u>, headache, insomnia, SEIZURES.

CV: <u>tachycardia</u>, palpitations, arrhythmias, angina pectoris.

GI: <u>nausea</u>, <u>vomiting</u>, anorexia, cramps.

Neuro: tremor.

INTERACTIONS

Drug–Drug: ▪ Additive CV and CNS side effects with **adrenergic (sympathomimetic) agents** ▪ May decrease the therapeutic effect of **lithium** ▪ **Smoking, adrenergic agents, barbiturates, phenytoin, ketoconazole,** and **rifampin** may increase metabolism and may decrease effectiveness ▪ **Erythromycin, beta blockers, cimetidine, influenza vaccination, oral contraceptives, glucocorticoids, disulfiram, interferon, mexiletine, thiabendazol, flouroquinolones,** and large doses of **allopurinol** decrease metabolism and may lead to toxicity ▪ Increased risk of arrhythmias with **halothane** ▪ **Isoniazid, carbamazepine,** and **loop diuretics** may increase or decrease theophylline levels.

Drug–Food: ▪ Excessive regular intake of **charcoal-broiled foods** may decrease effectiveness ▪ Excessive intake of **xanthine-containing foods** or **beverages (colas, coffee, chocolate)** may increase the risk of CV and CNS side effects.

ROUTE AND DOSAGE

Dosage should be determined by theophylline serum level monitoring. Loading dose should be decreased or eliminated if theophylline preparation has been used in preceding 24 hr. Aminophylline is 86% theophylline.

- **PO (Adults):** Loading dose—500 mg, followed by 250–500 mg q 6–8 hr.
- **PO (Children):** Loading dose—7.5 mg/kg, followed by 3–6 mg/kg q 6–8 hr.
- **IV (Adults):** Loading dose—5.6 mg/kg infused over 30 min, followed by 0.1–0.8 mg/kg/hr continuous infusion.
- **IV (Children):** Loading dose—5.6 mg/kg, followed by 0.8–1.2 mg/kg/hr continuous infusion.
- **IV, PO (Neonates >8 wk):** Ini-

*<u>Underlines</u> indicate most frequent; CAPITALS indicate life-threatening.

tial dose—1 mg/kg (theophylline) for each 2 mcg/ml increase in plasma level desired, then 1–3 mg/kg (theophylline) q 6 hr.

- **IV, PO (Neonates 4–8 wk):** Initial dose—1 mg/kg (theophylline) for each 2 mcg/ml increase in plasma level desired, then 1–2 mg/kg (theophylline) q 8 hr.
- **IV, PO (Term Neonates <4 wk):** Initial dose—1 mg/kg (theophylline) for each 2 mcg/ml increase in plasma level desired, then 1–2 mg/kg (theophylline) q 12 hr.
- **IV, PO (Premature Neonates):** Initial dose—1 mg/kg (theophylline) for each 2 mcg/ml increase in plasma level desired, then 1 mg/kg (theophylline) q 12 hr.

AVAILABILITY

- ***Tablets:*** 100 mg, 200 mg ▪ ***Controlled-release tablets:*** 225 mg ▪ ***Liquid:*** 105 mg/5 ml ▪ ***Suppositories:*** 250 mg, 500 mg ▪ ***Injection:*** 250 mg/10 ml.

TIME/ACTION PROFILE
(bronchodilation)

	ONSET	PEAK*	DURATION
PO	15–60 min	1–2 hr	6–8 hr
PO-ER	UK	4–7 hr	8–12 hr
IV	rapid	end of infusion	6–8 hr

*Peak plasma levels.

NURSING IMPLICATIONS

ASSESSMENT

- **General Info:** Assess blood pressure, pulse, respiration, and lung sounds before and throughout therapy.
- □ Patients with a history of cardiovascular problems should be monitored for chest pain and ECG changes (PACs, supraventricular tachycardia, PVCs, ventricular tachycardia). Resuscitative equipment should be readily available.
- **Respiratory Stimulant:** Monitor neonate for apnea, bradycardia, and cyanosis.
- **Toxicity and Overdose:** Monitor drug

levels routinely. Therapeutic plasma levels range from 10–20 mcg/ml. Drug levels in excess of 20 mcg/ml are associated with toxicity.

- □ Observe patient for symptoms of drug toxicity (anorexia, nausea, vomiting, restlessness, insomnia, tachycardia, arrhythmias, seizures). Notify physician immediately if these occur.

POTENTIAL NURSING DIAGNOSES

- Airway clearance, ineffective (indications).
- Activity intolerance (indications).
- Knowledge deficit related to medication regimen (patient/family teaching).

IMPLEMENTATION

- **General Info:** Administer around the clock to maintain therapeutic plasma levels.
- □ Determine if patient has had any form of theophylline within 24 hr prior to administering loading dose.
- □ Wait at least 4 hr after stopping IV therapy to begin immediate-release oral dosage; for extended-release oral dosage form, give first oral dose at time of IV discontinuation.
- **PO:** Administer oral preparations with food or a full glass of water to minimize GI irritation. Food slows but does not reduce the extent of absorption. Once-a-day tablets should be given in the morning, after fasting overnight, and 1 hr before eating. Do not crush, break, or chew enteric-coated or extended-release tablets.
- **IV:** May be diluted in D5W, D10W, D20W, 0.9% NaCl, 0.45% NaCl, D5/0.9% NaCl, D5/0.45% NaCl, D5/0.25% NaCl, or lactated Ringer's solution. Mixture is stable for 24 hr if refrigerated.
- □ Do not administer discolored or precipitated solution. Flush main IV line prior to administration. Admixing infusion is not recommended due to many incompatibilities.
- □ If extravasation occurs, local injection of 1% procaine and application of heat may relieve pain and promote vasodilation.

- **Direct IV:** Do not administer at a rate faster than 25 mg/min.
- **Intermittent Infusion:** Dilute in 100–200 ml of compatible IV solution.
- *Rate:* Do not exceed 25 mg/min. Administer via infusion pump to ensure accurate dosage. Rapid administration may cause hypotension, arrhythmias, syncope, and death.
- **Continuous Infusion:** Usually given as a loading dose in a small volume followed by continuous infusion in larger volume.
- **Syringe Compatibility:** ▪ heparin ▪ metoclopramide.
- **Syringe Incompatibility:** ▪ doxapram.
- **Y-Site Compatibility:** ▪ amrinone ▪ atracurium ▪ cimetidine ▪ enalaprilat ▪ esmolol ▪ famotidine ▪ fluconazole ▪ fludarabine ▪ foscarnet ▪ labetalol ▪ morphine ▪ neticmicin ▪ pancuronium ▪ potassium chloride ▪ ranitidine ▪ sargramostim ▪ tolazoline ▪ vecuronium.
- **Y-Site Incompatibility:** ▪ dobutamine ▪ hydralazine ▪ ondansetron.
- **Additive Compatibility:** ▪ calcium gluconate ▪ chloramphenicol ▪ cimetidine ▪ dexamethasone ▪ diphenhydramine ▪ erythromycin lactobionate ▪ esmolol ▪ furosemide ▪ heparin ▪ hydrocortisone ▪ methicillin ▪ methyldopate ▪ metronidazole ▪ potassium chloride ▪ ranitidine ▪ terbutaline.
- **Additive Incompatibility:** ▪ ascorbic acid ▪ bleomycin ▪ cephalothin ▪ cefotaxime ▪ chlorpromazine ▪ clindamycin ▪ codeine ▪ dimenhydrinate ▪ doxorubicin ▪ doxycycline ▪ erythromycin glucceptate ▪ hydralazine ▪ hydroxyzine ▪ insulin ▪ meperidine ▪ morphine ▪ penicillin G potassium ▪ pentazocine ▪ phenytoin ▪ prochlorperazine.

PATIENT/FAMILY TEACHING
▫ Emphasize the importance of taking only the prescribed dose at the prescribed time intervals. Missed doses should be taken as soon as remembered or omitted if close to next dose.
▫ Encourage the patient to drink adequate liquids (2000 ml/day minimum) to decrease the viscosity of the airway secretions.
▫ Advise patient to avoid over-the-counter cough, cold, or breathing preparations without consulting physician or pharmacist. These medications may increase side effects and cause arrhythmias.
▫ Encourage patients not to smoke. A change in smoking habits may necessitate a change in dosage.
▫ Advise patient to minimize intake of xanthine-containing foods or beverages (colas, coffee, chocolate) and not to eat charcoal-broiled foods daily.
▫ Instruct patient not to change brands or dosage forms without consulting physician.
▫ Advise patient to contact physician promptly if the usual dose of medication fails to produce the desired results, symptoms worsen after treatment, or toxic effects occur.
▫ Emphasize the importance of having serum levels routinely tested every 6–12 mo.

EVALUATION
Effectiveness of therapy can be demonstrated by: ▪ Increased ease in breathing ▫ Clearing of lung fields on auscultation ▪ Respiratory and myocardial stimulation in apnea of infancy.

AMIODARONE
(am-ee-**oh**-da-rone)
Cordarone

CLASSIFICATION(S):
Antiarrhythmic (group III)
Pregnancy Category C

INDICATIONS
▪ Management/prophylaxis of life-threatening ventricular arrhythmias unresponsive to less toxic agents.

ACTION
▪ Prolongs the action potential and refractory period in myocardial tissue ▪ Inhibits adrenergic stimulation

- Slows the sinus rate, increases PR and QT intervals, and decreases peripheral vascular resistance. **Therapeutic Effect:** ▪ Suppression of ventricular arrhythmias.

PHARMACOKINETICS

Absorption: Slowly and variably absorbed from the GI tract (35–65%).
Distribution: Distributed to and accumulates slowly in body tissues. Crosses the placenta; enters breast milk.
Metabolism and Excretion: Metabolized by the liver, excreted into bile. Minimal renal excretion.
Half-life: 13–107 days.

CONTRAINDICATIONS AND PRECAUTIONS

Contraindicated in: ▪ Severe sinus node dysfunction ▪ 2nd- and 3rd-degree AV block ▪ Bradycardia (has caused syncope unless a pacemaker is in place) ▪ Pregnancy and lactation.
Use Cautiously in: ▪ Thyroid disorders ▪ Severe pulmonary or liver disease ▪ Children (safety not established).

ADVERSE REACTIONS AND SIDE EFFECTS*

CNS: malaise, fatigue, dizziness, insomnia, headache.
Resp: PULMONARY FIBROSIS.
CV: congestive heart failure, bradycardia, WORSENING OF ARRHYTHMIAS.
Derm: photosensitivity.
EENT: corneal microdeposits, photophobia, dry eyes, abnormal taste, abnormal smell.
Endo: hypothyroidism, hyperthyroidism.
GI: nausea, vomiting, constipation, anorexia, LIVER DAMAGE, abdominal pain.
GU: decreased libido.
Neuro: tremor, involuntary movement, poor coordination, peripheral neuropathy, paresthesia.

INTERACTIONS

Drug–Drug: ▪ Increases blood levels and may lead to toxicity from **digoxin** (decrease dose by 50%) ▪ Increases

blood levels and may lead to toxicity from other **group I antiarrhthymics** (**quinidine, procainamide, mexiletine,** or **flecainide**—decrease doses by 30–50%) ▪ Increases blood levels of **phenytoin** ▪ Increases the activity of **warfarin** (decrease dose by 33–50%) ▪ Increased risk of bradyarrhythmias, sinus arrest, or AV heart block with **beta blockers** or **calcium channel blockers** ▪ Concentrated **oxygen** administered postoperatively may increase the risk of pulmonary fibrosis.

ROUTE AND DOSAGE

- **PO (Adults):** 800–1600 mg/day in 1–2 doses for 1–3 wk, then 600–800 mg/day in 1–2 doses for 1 mo, then 400 mg/day maintenance dose.
- **PO (Children):** 10 mg/kg/day (800/1.72 m²/day) for 1 wk or until response or adverse reaction occurs, then 5 mg/kg/day (400 mg/1.72 m²/day) for several weeks, then decreased to 2.5 mg/kg/day (200 mg/1.72 m²/day) or lowest effect dose.

AVAILABILITY

- **Tablets:** 200 mg.

TIME/ACTION PROFILE (suppression of ventricular arrhythmias)

	ONSET	PEAK	DURATION
PO	1–3 wk	UK	wks–mos

NURSING IMPLICATIONS

ASSESSMENT

- ECG should be monitored continuously during initiation of therapy. Monitor heart rate and rhythm throughout therapy. PR prolongation, slight QRS widening, T-wave amplitude reduction with T-wave widening and bifurcation, and U-waves may occur. QT prolongation may be associated with worsening of arrhythmias. Report bradycardia or increase in arrhythmias promptly.
- Assess patient for signs of pulmonary toxicity (rales/crackles, decreased

breath sounds, pleuritic friction rub, fatigue, dyspnea, cough, pleuritic pain, fever). May need to discontinue therapy.

□ Ophthalmic examinations should be performed prior to therapy and if visual changes (photophobia, halos around lights, decreased acuity) occur.

□ Assess patient for signs of thyroid dysfunction, especially during initial therapy. Lethargy, edema of the hands, feet, and periorbital region and cool, pale skin suggest hypothyroidism and may require decrease in dosage or discontinuation of therapy and supplementation of thyroid hormone. Tachycardia, weight loss, and warm, flushed, moist skin suggest hyperthyroidism and may require discontinuation of therapy and treatment with antithyroid agents.

■ **Lab Test Considerations:** Monitor liver, lung, thyroid, and neurologic functions prior to and periodically throughout therapy. Drug effects persist long after adjustment or discontinuation.

□ May cause increased AST (SGOT), ALT (SGPT), and serum alkaline phosphatase concentrations.

POTENTIAL NURSING DIAGNOSES

■ Cardiac output, decreased (indications).
■ Gas exchange, impaired (side effects).
■ Knowledge deficit related to medication regimen (patient/family teaching).

IMPLEMENTATION

■ **General Info:** Patients should be hospitalized and monitored closely during the initiation of therapy.
□ Hypokalemia may decrease effectiveness of amiodarone or may cause additional arrhythmias and should be corrected prior to therapy.
□ Assist patient during ambulation to prevent falls from neurologic deficits. Peripheral neuropathy (proximal muscle weakness, tingling, numb-

ness), tremors, and abnormal gait are common during initial therapy.
■ **PO:** May be administered with meals and in divided doses if GI intolerance occurs.

PATIENT/FAMILY TEACHING

□ Instruct patient to take this medication exactly as directed. If a dose is missed, do not take at all. Consult physician if more than two doses are missed.
□ Teach patients to monitor pulse daily and report abnormalities.
□ Advise patients that photosensitivity reactions may occur through window glass, thin clothing, and with sunscreens. Protective clothing and sunblock are recommended during and for 4 mo following therapy.
□ Inform patients that bluish discoloration of the face, neck, and arms is a possible side effect of this drug following prolonged use. This is usually reversible and will fade over several mos. Notify physician if this occurs.
□ Instruct patient to notify physician or dentist of medication regimen prior to treatment or surgery.
□ Emphasize the importance of follow-up examinations, including chest x-ray and pulmonary function tests every 3–6 mo and ophthalmic examinations after 6 mo of therapy, and then annually.

EVALUATION

Effectiveness of therapy can be demonstrated by: ■ Cessation of life-threatening ventricular arrhythmias. Pharmacologic effects may not be seen for 1–3 wk. Adverse effects may take up to 4 mo to resolve.

AMITRIPTYLINE
(a-mee-**trip**-ti-leen)
{Apo-Amitriptyline}, Elavil, Emitrip, Endep, Enovil, {Levate}, {Meravil}, {Novotriptyn}

CLASSIFICATION(S):
Antidepressant (tricyclic)

INDICATIONS

- Treatment of depression, often in conjunction with psychotherapy. **Unlabeled Use:** ■ Chronic pain syndromes.

ACTION

- Potentiates the effect of serotonin and norepinephrine in the CNS ■ Has significant anticholinergic properties. **Therapeutic Effect:** ■ Antidepressant action (may only develop over several weeks).

PHARMACOKINETICS

Absorption: Well absorbed from the GI tract.
Distribution: Widely distributed.
Metabolism and Excretion: Extensively metabolized by the liver. Some metabolites are pharmacologically active. Undergoes enterohepatic recirculation and secretion into gastric juices. Probably crosses the placenta and enters breast milk.
Half-life: 10–50 hr.

CONTRAINDICATIONS AND PRECAUTIONS

Contraindicated in: ■ Narrow-angle glaucoma ■ Pregnancy and lactation.
Use Cautiously in: ■ Elderly patients ■ Patients with pre-existing cardiovascular disease ■ Prostatic hypertrophy (increased susceptibility to urinary retention) ■ History of seizures (threshold may be lowered).

ADVERSE REACTIONS AND SIDE EFFECTS*

CNS: <u>drowsiness</u>, <u>sedation</u>, <u>lethargy</u>, <u>fatigue</u>.
EENT: <u>dry mouth</u>, <u>dry eyes</u>, <u>blurred vision</u>.
CV: <u>hypotension</u>, ECG changes, **ARRHYTHMIAS**.
Derm: photosensitivity.
Endo: gynecomastia, changes in blood glucose.
GI: <u>constipation</u>, paralytic ileus, hepatitis.
GU: urinary retention.
Hemat: blood dyscrasias.

INTERACTIONS

Drug–Drug: ■ May cause hypotension, tachycardia, and potentially fatal reactions when used with **MAO inhibitors** (avoid concurrent use—discontinue 2 wk prior to amitriptyline) ■ May prevent the therapeutic response to most **antihypertensives** ■ May cause severe hypertension when used with **clonidine** (avoid concurrent use) ■ Additive CNS depression with other **CNS depressants** including **alcohol, antihistamines, opioid analgesics,** and **sedative/hypnotics** ■ **Adrenergic** and **anticholinergic** side effects may be additive with other **agents having these properties** ■ **Cimetidine, fluoxetine, phenothiazines,** or **oral contraceptives** increase levels and may cause toxicity ■ May produce transient delirium with **disulfiram** ■ **Smoking** may increase metabolism and decrease effectiveness.

ROUTE AND DOSAGE

- **PO (Adults):** 30–100 mg/day single bedtime dose or divided doses. Dose may be gradually increased up to 150–300 mg/day.
- **PO (Children 6–12 yr):** 10–30 mg/day (1–5 mg/kg/day in 2 divided doses.
- **PO (Adolescents):** 10 mg tid and 20 mg at hs. May be slowly increased to 100 mg/day given as a single dose at hs.
- **PO (Elderly):** 25 mg at hs. May be slowly increased up to 10 mg tid and 20 mg at hs (daily dose not to exceed 100 mg).
- **IM (Adults):** 20–30 mg 4 times daily.

AVAILABILITY

- *Tablets:* 10 mg, 25 mg, 50 mg, 75 mg, 100 mg, 150 mg ■ {*Syrup:* 10 mg/5 ml}
- *Injection:* 10 mg/ml.

TIME/ACTION PROFILE
(antidepressant effect)

	ONSET	PEAK	DURATION
PO	2–3 wk	2–6 wk	days–wks
IM	2–3 wk	2–6 wk	days–wks

*<u>Underlines</u> indicate most frequent; **CAPITALS** indicate life-threatening.

NURSING IMPLICATIONS

ASSESSMENT

◻ Monitor mental status and affect. Assess for suicidal tendencies, especially during early therapy. Restrict amount of drug available to patient.

◻ Monitor blood pressure and pulse prior to and during initial therapy. Notify physician of decreases in blood pressure (10–20 mmHg) or sudden increase in pulse rate.

▪ **Lab Test Considerations:** Assess leukocyte and differential blood counts, liver function, and serum glucose periodically. May cause an elevated serum bilirubin and alkaline phosphatase. May cause bone marrow depression. Serum glucose may be increased or decreased.

POTENTIAL NURSING DIAGNOSES

▪ Coping, ineffective individual (indications).

▪ Injury, high risk for (side effects).

▪ Knowledge deficit related to medication regimen (patient/family teaching).

IMPLEMENTATION

▪ **General Info:** Dose increases should be made at bedtime because of sedation. Dose titration is a slow process; may take weeks to months. May give entire dose at bedtime.

▪ **PO:** Administer medication with or immediately after a meal to minimize gastric upset. Tablet may be crushed and given with food or fluids.

▪ **IM:** For short-term IM administration only. Do not administer IV

PATIENT/FAMILY TEACHING

◻ Instruct patient to take medication exactly as directed. Advise patient that drug effects may not be noticed for at least 2 wk. Abrupt discontinuation may cause nausea, headache, and malaise.

◻ May cause drowsiness and blurred vision. Caution patient to avoid driving and other activities requiring alertness until response to drug is known.

◻ Orthostatic hypotension, sedation, and confusion are common during early therapy, especially in the elderly. Protect patient from falls and advise patient to make position changes slowly.

◻ Advise patient to avoid alcohol or other CNS depressant drugs during and for 3–7 days after therapy has been discontinued.

◻ Instruct patient to notify physician if urinary retention occurs or if dry mouth or constipation persist. Sugarless candy or gum may diminish dry mouth and an increase in fluid intake or bulk may prevent constipation. If symptoms persist, dose reduction or discontinuation may be necessary.

◻ Caution patient to use sunscreen and protective clothing to prevent photosensitivity reactions.

◻ Inform patient of need to monitor dietary intake. Increase in appetite may lead to undesired weight gain.

◻ Inform patient that urine may turn a blue-green color.

◻ Advise patient to notify physician or dentist of medication regimen prior to treatment or surgery.

◻ Therapy for depression is usually prolonged. Emphasize the importance of follow-up examinations to monitor effectiveness and side effects.

EVALUATION

Effectiveness of therapy can be demonstrated by: ▪ Increased sense of well-being ◻ Renewed interest in surroundings ◻ Increased appetite ◻ Improved energy level ◻ Improved sleep ▪ Decrease in chronic pain symptoms ▪ Full therapeutic effects may be seen 2 wk to 1 mo after initiating therapy.

AMLODIPINE
(am-**loe**-di-peen)
Norvasc

CLASSIFICATION(S):
Antihypertensive (calcium channel blocker), Antianginal
Pregnancy Category C

INDICATIONS

▪ Alone or with other agents in the management of hypertension, angina pectoris, and vasospastic (Prinzmetal's) angina.

ACTION

- Inhibits the transport of calcium into myocardial and vascular smooth muscle cells, resulting in inhibition of excitation-contraction coupling and subsequent contraction. **Therapeutic Effects:** • Systemic vasodilation resulting in decreased blood pressure • Coronary vasodilation resulting in decreased frequency and severity of attacks of angina.

PHARMACOKINETICS

Absorption: Well absorbed following oral administration (64–90%).
Distribution: Probably crosses the placenta.
Metabolism and Excretion: Mostly metabolized by the liver.
Half-life: 30–50 hr.

CONTRAINDICATIONS AND PRECAUTIONS

Contraindicated in: ▪ Hypersensitivity.
Use Cautiously in: ▪ Severe hepatic impairment or elderly patients (dosage reduction recommended) ▪ Pregnancy, lactation, or children (safety not established.

ADVERSE REACTIONS AND SIDE EFFECTS*

CNS: drowsiness, lightheadedness, headache, weakness, fatigue, tremor, vertigo, insomnia, nervousness, depression.
EENT: abnormal vision, conjunctivitis, diplopia, tinnitus.
Resp: shortness of breath, dyspnea, wheezing, epistaxis.
CV: peripheral edema, palpitations, syncope, arrhythmias, bradycardia, tachycardia, hypotension, chest pain, cardiac failure.
GI: nausea, abdominal discomfort, anorexia, constipation, dyspepsia, dry mouth.

GU: sexual dysfunction, urinary frequency, malodorous urine, nocturia.
Derm: rash, dermatitis, pruritus, urticaria, flushing, increased sweating.
MS: muscle cramps.
Neuro: paresthesia.
Misc: weight gain, rigors.

INTERACTIONS

Drug–Drug: ▪ Additive hypotension may occur when used concurrently with **fentanyl, other antihypertensives, nitrates,** and acute ingestion of **alcohol.**

ROUTE AND DOSAGE

- **PO (Adults):** 5–10 mg as a single dose (range 2.5–10 mg).

AVAILABILITY

- *Tablets:* 2.5 mg, 5 mg, 10 mg.

TIME/ACTION PROFILE
(antihypertensive effect)

	ONSET	PEAK	DURATION
PO	UK	UK	24 hr

NURSING IMPLICATIONS

ASSESSMENT

- **General Info:** Monitor blood pressure and pulse prior to and periodically throughout therapy. Monitor ECG periodically during prolonged therapy.
  □ Monitor intake and output ratios and daily weight. Assess for signs of congestive heart failure (peripheral edema, rales/crackles, dyspnea, weight gain, jugular venous distention).
- **Angina:** Assess location, duration, intensity, and precipitating factors of patient's anginal pain.
- **Lab Test Considerations:** Monitor hepatic function periodically during chronic therapy. May cause elevated liver function tests.

POTENTIAL NURSING DIAGNOSES

- Cardiac output, decreased (indications).
- Pain (indications).

---

*Underlines indicate most frequent; **CAPITALS** indicate life-threatening.

- Knowledge deficit related to medication regimen (patient/family teaching).

IMPLEMENTATION

- **PO:** May be administered without regard to meals.

PATIENT/FAMILY TEACHING

- **General Info:** Advise patient to take medication exactly as directed, not to skip or double up on missed doses. May need to be discontinued gradually.
- □ Caution patient to make position changes slowly to minimize orthostatic hypotension.
- □ May cause drowsiness. Advise patient to avoid driving or other activities requiring alertness until response to the medication is known.
- □ Instruct patient to avoid concurrent use of alcohol or over-the-counter medications without consulting physician or pharmacist.
- □ Advise patient to notify physician if irregular heart beats, dyspnea, swelling of hands and feet, pronounced dizziness, nausea, constipation, or hypotension occur.
- **Angina:** Instruct patient on concurrent nitrate or beta-blocker therapy to continue taking both medications as ordered and use SL nitroglycerin as needed for anginal attacks.
- □ Advise patient to contact physician if chest pain does not improve or worsens after therapy or occurs with diaphoresis or shortness of breath or if severe, persistent headache occurs.
- **Hypertension:** Encourage patient to comply with other interventions for hypertension (weight reduction, low-sodium diet, smoking cessation, moderation of alcohol consumption, regular exercise, and stress management).

EVALUATION

Effectiveness of therapy can be demonstrated by: ▪ Decrease in blood pressure ▪ Decrease in frequency and severity of anginal attacks □ Decrease in need for nitrate therapy □ Increase in activity tolerance and sense of well-being.

AMOBARBITAL
(ah-mo-**bar**-bi-tal)
Amytal

CLASSIFICATION(S):
Sedative/hypnotic (barbiturate),
Anticonvulsant
Schedule II
Pregnancy Category D

INDICATIONS

- Preoperative sedative and in other situations where sedation may be required
- Hypnotic.

ACTION

- Produces all levels of CNS depression:
□ Depresses sensory cortex □ Decreases motor activity □ Alters cerebral function
- Inhibits transmission in the CNS and raises seizure threshold. **Therapeutic Effects:** ▪ Anticonvulsant action ▪ Sedation.

PHARMACOKINETICS

Absorption: Well absorbed following oral or IM administration.

Distribution: Rapidly and widely distributed, concentrates in brain, liver, and kidneys. Readily crosses placenta, small amounts enter breast milk.

Metabolism and Excretion: Mostly metabolized by the liver.

Half-life: 16–40 hr.

CONTRAINDICATIONS AND PRECAUTIONS

Contraindicated in: ▪ Hypersensitivity ▪ Comatose patients ▪ Pre-existing CNS depression ▪ Severe uncontrolled pain ▪ Pregnancy and lactation.

Use Cautiously in: ▪ Suicidal patients ▪ Patients previously addicted to barbiturates ▪ Elderly or debilitated patients ▪ Patients with hepatic or renal impairment (dosage should be reduced).

ADVERSE REACTIONS AND SIDE EFFECTS*

CNS: <u>drowsiness</u>, lethargy, vertigo, depression, <u>hangover</u>, excitation, delerium, syncope.

Resp: respiratory depression, LARYNGOSPASM (IV ONLY), BRONCHOSPASM (IV ONLY).

CV: hypotension, bradycardia.

GI: nausea, vomiting, diarrhea, constipation.

Derm: rashes, urticaria, photosensitivity, exfoliative dermatitis.

Local: phlebitis at IV site, pain or sterile abscess at IM site.

Misc: hypersensitivity reactions including STEVENS JOHNSON SYNDROME.

MS: mylagia, arthralgia.

INTERACTIONS

Drug–Drug: ▪ Additive CNS depression with other **CNS depressants** including **alcohol, antidepressants, antihistamines, opioid analgesics,** and **other sedative/hypnotics** ▪ Sedation may be prolonged with **MAO inhibitors** ▪ Induces hepatic enzymes that metabolize other drugs, decreasing their effectiveness, including **oral contraceptives, chloramphenicol, acebutolol, propranolol, metoprolol, timolol, doxycycline, glucocorticoids, tricyclic antidepressants, phenothiazines,** and **quinidine.**

ROUTE AND DOSAGE

▪ **IM/IV (Adults):** Sedative—30–50 mg 2–3 times daily. Hypnotic—65–200 mg.

▪ **IV (Children 6–12 yr):** 65–500 mg, depending on response.

AVAILABILITY

▪ *Injection:* 250-mg, 500-mg vials.

TIME/ACTION PROFILE (sedation)

	ONSET	PEAK	DURATION
IM	30–45 min	UK	6–8 hr
IV	several min	UK	6–8 hr

NURSING IMPLICATIONS

ASSESSMENT

▪ **General Info:** Monitor respiratory status, pulse, and blood pressure frequently in patients receiving amobarbital IV.

▫ Prolonged therapy may lead to psychological or physical dependence. Restrict amount of drug available to patient, especially if depressed, suicidal, or having a history of addiction.

▪ **Hypnotic:** Assess sleep patterns prior to and periodically throughout therapy. Hypnotic doses of amobarbital suppress REM sleep. Patient may experience an increase in dreaming upon discontinuation of medication.

POTENTIAL NURSING DIAGNOSES

▪ Sleep pattern disturbance (indications).

▪ Injury, high risk for (side effects).

▪ Knowledge deficit related to medication regimen (patient/family teaching).

IMPLEMENTATION

▪ **General Info:** Remove cigarettes and monitor ambulation following administration.

▪ **IM/IV:** Reconstitute with Sterile Water for Injection for a concentration of 100 mg/ml. Rotate vial to mix; do not shake. May be further diluted in D5W, D10W, D20W, D5/0.9% NaCl, D5/LR, 0.9% NaCl, 3% NaCl, or lactated Ringer's injection. Solution should be used within 30 min of reconstitution. Do not use if solution does not become absolutely clear within 5 min following reconstitution or if precipitate forms after the solution clears.

▪ **IM:** Do not administer SC. Administer IM injections deep into gluteal muscle to minimize tissue irritation.

▪ **Direct IV:** Use the largest vein possible to prevent thrombosis. Solution is highly alkaline; avoid extravasation, which may cause tissue damage and necrosis. If extravasation occurs, infiltration of 5% procaine solution into affected area and application of moist heat may be ordered.

- **Rate:** Do not exceed the rate of 50 mg/min. Titrate slowly for desired response. Rapid administration may result in respiratory depression, apnea, laryngospasm, bronchospasm, or hypotension. Equipment for resuscitation should be readily available.

PATIENT/FAMILY TEACHING

□ Advise patient to take medication exactly as directed. Do not increase the dose of the drug without consulting physician. Advise patients on prolonged therapy not to discontinue medication without consulting physician. May need to be gradually discontinued over 5–6 days to prevent withdrawal symptoms.

□ Discuss the importance of preparing environment for sleep (dark room, quiet, avoidance of nicotine and caffeine).

□ May cause daytime drowsiness. Caution patient to avoid driving and other activities requiring alertness until response to medication is known.

□ Advise patient to make position changes slowly to minimize orthostatic hypotension.

□ Caution patients to avoid taking alcohol or other CNS depressants concurrently with this medication.

□ Instruct patient to contact physician immediately if pregnancy is suspected or if sore throat, fever, mouth sores, unusual bleeding or bruising, or petechiae occur.

EVALUATION

Effectiveness of therapy can be demonstrated by: ▪ Improvement in sleep pattern without excessive daytime sedation. May take 2 days for effects to become evident. Therapy is usually limited to a 2-wk period ▪ Sedation ▪ Control of seizures.

AMOXAPINE
(a-**mox**-a-peen)
Asendin

CLASSIFICATION(S):
Antidepressant (tricyclic)
Pregnancy Category C

INDICATIONS

▪ Treatment of depression accompanied by anxiety, often with psychotherapy.

ACTION

▪ Potentiates the effects of serotonin and norepinephrine in the CNS ▪ Has significant anticholinergic properties ▪ Also has antianxiety effect related to sedative properties. **Therapeutic Effect:** ▪ Antidepressant action that may only develop slowly over several weeks.

PHARMACOKINETICS

Absorption: Well absorbed following oral administration.
Distribution: Widely distributed. Enters breast milk.
Metabolism and Excretion: Extensively metabolized by the liver. Some metabolites have antidepressant activity.
Half-life: Amoxapine—8 hr.

CONTRAINDICATIONS AND PRECAUTIONS

Contraindicated in: ▪ Narrow-angle glaucoma ▪ Pregnancy and lactation.
Use Cautiously in: ▪ Elderly patients (dosage reduction required) ▪ History of cardiovascular disease ▪ Elderly men (increased susceptibility to urinary retention) ▪ History of seizures (threshold may be lowered) ▪ Children <16 yr (safety not established).

ADVERSE REACTIONS AND SIDE EFFECTS*

CNS: <u>drowsiness</u>, <u>lethargy</u>, <u>sedation</u>, <u>fatigue</u>, extrapyramidal reactions, tardive dyskinesia, NEUROLEPTIC MALIGNANT SYNDROME.

---

*<u>Underlines</u> indicate most frequent; **CAPITALS** indicate life-threatening.

CV: hypotension, ECG changes, AR-RHYTHMIAS.
EENT: dry mouth, dry eyes, blurred vision.
GI: constipation, paralytic ileus.
GU: urinary retention, testicular swelling.
Derm: photosensitivity, rash.
Endo: gynecomastia, sexual dysfunction.
Hemat: blood dyscrasias.
Misc: fever, weight gain.

INTERACTIONS

Drug–Drug: ■ May cause hypotension, tachycardia, and potentially fatal reactions when used with **MAO inhibitors** (avoid concurrent use—discontinue 2 wk prior to amoxapine) ■ May prevent the therapeutic response to most **antihypertensives** ■ May cause severe hypertension when used with **clonidine** (avoid concurrent use) ■ Additive CNS depression with other **CNS depressants** including **alcohol, antihistamines, opioid analgesics,** and **sedative/hypnotics** ■ **Adrenergic** and **anticholinergic** side effects may be additive with other **agents having these properties** ■ **Cimetidine, fluoxetine, phenothiazines,** or **oral contraceptives** increase levels and may cause toxicity ■ May produce transient delirium with **disulfiram** ■ **Smoking** may increase metabolism and decrease effectiveness.

ROUTE AND DOSAGE

■ **PO (Adults):** 100–150 mg daily initially in divided doses, increase to 200–300 mg daily by end of first week (not to exceed 300 mg daily in outpatients, 600 mg daily in divided doses in hospitalized patients). Once optimal dose is achieved, may be given as a single bedtime dose; no single dose to exceed 300 mg.
■ **PO (Elderly):** 25 mg 2–3 times daily, may be increased to 50 mg 2–3 times daily (not >300 mg/day).

AVAILABILITY

■ **Tablets:** 25 mg, 50 mg, 100 mg, 150 mg.

TIME/ACTION PROFILE
(antidepressant effect)

	ONSET	PEAK	DURATION
PO	1–2 wk	2–6 wk	days–wks

NURSING IMPLICATIONS

ASSESSMENT

□ Monitor mental status and affect. Assess for suicidal tendencies, especially during early therapy. Restrict amount of drug available to patient.
□ Observe for onset of extrapyramidal side effects (akathisia—restlessness; dystonia—muscle spasms and twisting motions; pseudoparkinsonism—mask facies, rigidity, tremors, drooling, shuffling gait, dysphagia, pill-rolling motions). Dosage reduction or discontinuation may be necessary. Physician may order trihexyphenidyl or diphenhydramine to control these symptoms.
□ Monitor for tardive dyskinesia (rhythmic movement of mouth, face, and extremities). Notify physician immediately if these symptoms occur, as they may be irreversible.
□ Monitor for development of neuroleptic malignant syndrome (fever, respiratory distress, tachycardia, convulsions, diaphoresis, hypertension or hypotension, pallor, tiredness). Notify physician immediately if these symptoms occur.
□ Monitor for drug rash or fever. Notify physician if these symptoms of hypersensitivity reaction occur.
■ **Lab Test Considerations:** May cause elevated serum prolactin levels.
□ Monitor CBC and differential during chronic therapy. May rarely cause bone marrow suppression.
□ In chronic therapy periodically monitor hepatic, pancreatic, and renal function.

POTENTIAL NURSING DIAGNOSES

■ Coping, ineffective individual (indications).
■ Injury, high risk for (side effects).
■ Knowledge deficit related to medica-

tion regimen (patient/family teaching).

IMPLEMENTATION

- **General Info:** Dose increases should be made at bedtime because of sedation. Dosage titration is a slow process; may take weeks to months. May give entire dose (if <300 mg) at bedtime, when dose is stabilized.
- **PO:** Administer medication with or immediately following a meal to minimize gastric irritation.

PATIENT/FAMILY TEACHING

- Instruct patient to take medication exactly as directed. Abrupt discontinuation may cause nausea, headache, and malaise.
- May cause drowsiness and blurred vision. Caution patient to avoid driving and other activities requiring alertness until response to drug is known.
- Advise patient to avoid alcohol or other CNS depressant drugs during and for 3–7 days after therapy.
- Instruct patient to notify physician if dry mouth or constipation persists or if urinary retention, uncontrolled movements, or rigidity occur. Sugarless candy or gum may diminish dry mouth, and an increase in fluid intake or bulk may prevent constipation. If these symptoms persist, dosage reduction or discontinuation may be necessary.
- Advise patient to inform physician if breast enlargement or sexual dysfunction occurs.
- Caution patient to use sunscreen and protective clothing to prevent photosensitivity reactions.
- Instruct patient to monitor dietary intake. Increased appetite may lead to undesired weight gain.
- Advise patient to notify physician or dentist of medication regimen prior to treatment or surgery.
- Therapy for depression is usually prolonged. Emphasize the importance of follow-up examinations to monitor effectiveness and side effects.

EVALUATION

Effectiveness of therapy can be demonstrated by: ■ Increased sense of well-being □ Renewed interest in surroundings □ Increased appetite □ Improved energy level □ Improved sleep □ Decreased anxiety. Initial response may be noted in 4–7 days in some patients. Most patients respond within 2 wk.

AMOXICILLIN
(a-mox-i-**sill**-in)
Amoxil, {Apo-Amoxi}, Biomox, {Novamoxin}, {Nu-Amoxi}, Polymox, Sumox, Trimox, Wymox

CLASSIFICATION(S):
Anti-infective (extended-spectrum penicillin)
Pregnancy Category B

INDICATIONS

- Treatment of the following infections:
  □ Skin and skin structure infections
  □ Otitis media □ Sinusitis □ Respiratory infections □ Genitourinary infections □ Meningitis □ Septicemia ■ Endocarditis prophylaxis. **Unlabeled Use:** ■ Lyme disease.

ACTION

- Binds to bacterial cell wall, causing cell death. **Therapeutic Effect:** ■ Bactericidal action. Resists action of beta-lactamase, an enzyme produced by bacteria that is capable of inactivating some penicillins. **Spectrum:** ■ Active against: □ Streptococci □ Pneumococci □ Enterococci □ *Hemophilus influenzae* □ *Escherichia coli* □ *Proteus mirabilis* □ *Neisseria menigitidis* □ *Neisseria gonorrhea* □ *Shigella* □ *Salmonella* □ *Borrelia burgdoferi*.

PHARMACOKINETICS

Absorption: Well absorbed from the duodenum (75–90%). More resistant to acid inactivation than other penicillins.
Distribution: Diffuses readily into most body tissues and fluids. CSF pen-

etration is increased when meninges are inflamed. Crosses the placenta; enters breast milk in small amounts.
Metabolism and Excretion: 70% excreted unchanged in the urine. 30% metabolized by the liver.
Half-life: 1–1.3 hr.

CONTRAINDICATIONS AND PRECAUTIONS

Contraindicated in: ■ Hypersensitivity to penicillins.
Use Cautiously in: ■ Severe renal insufficiency (dosage reduction necessary) ■ Has been used during pregnancy and lactation ■ Infectious mononucleosis (increased incidence of rash).

ADVERSE REACTIONS AND SIDE EFFECTS*

CNS: SEIZURES (high doses).
Derm: <u>rashes</u>, urticaria.
GI: nausea, vomiting, <u>diarrhea</u>.
Hemat: blood dyscrasias.
Misc: superinfection, allergic reactions including serum sickness.

INTERACTIONS

Drug–Drug: ■ **Probenecid** decreases renal excretion and increases blood levels of amoxicillin—therapy may be combined for this purpose ■ May potentiate the effect of **warfarin** ■ May decrease the effectiveness of **oral contraceptive agents**.

ROUTE AND DOSAGE

■ **PO (Adults and Children >20 kg):** 250–500 mg q 8 hr.
■ **PO (Children 8–20 kg):** 6.7–13.3 mg/kg q 8 hr.
■ **PO (Children 6–8 kg):** 50–100 mg q 8 hr.
■ **PO (Children <6 kg):** 25–50 mg q 8 hr.

Gonorrhea
■ **PO (Adults):** 3 g plus 1 g probenecid single dose.
■ **PO (Children >2 yr):** 50 mg/kg plus 25 mg/kg probenecid single dose.

AVAILABILITY

■ **Chewable tablets:** 125 mg, 250 mg
■ **Capsules:** 250 mg, 500 mg ■ **Suspension:** 50 mg/ml, 125 mg/5 ml, 250 mg/5 ml.

TIME/ACTION PROFILE (blood levels)

	ONSET	PEAK
PO	30 min	1–2 hr

NURSING IMPLICATIONS

ASSESSMENT

☐ Assess patient for infection (vital signs; appearance of wound, sputum, urine, and stool; WBC) at beginning and throughout course of therapy.
☐ Obtain a history before initiating therapy to determine previous use of and reactions to penicillins or cephalosporins. Persons with a negative history of penicillin sensitivity may still have an allergic response.
☐ Observe for signs and symptoms of anaphylaxis (rash, pruritus, laryngeal edema, wheezing). Notify the physician immediately if these occur.
☐ Obtain specimens for culture and sensitivity prior to therapy. First dose may be given before receiving results.
■ **Lab Test Considerations:** May cause false-positive reactions with copper sulfate urine glucose tests (Clinitest). Use Clinistix or Tes-Tape to monitor urine glucose.
☐ May cause increased AST (SGOT) and ALT (SGPT) concentrations.

POTENTIAL NURSING DIAGNOSES

■ Infection, high risk for (indications, side effects).
■ Knowledge deficit related to medication regimen (patient/family teaching).
■ Noncompliance related to medication regimen (patient/family teaching).

IMPLEMENTATION

■ **PO:** Administer around the clock. May be given without regard to meals. May

---

be given with meals to decrease GI side effects. Capsule contents may be emptied and swallowed with liquids. Chewable tablets should be crushed or chewed before swallowing with liquids. Discard refrigerated reconstituted suspension after 10 days.

PATIENT/FAMILY TEACHING

□ Instruct patients to take medication around the clock and to finish the drug completely as directed, even if feeling better. Advise patients that sharing of this medication may be dangerous.

□ Advise patient to report the signs of superinfection (furry overgrowth on the tongue, vaginal itching or discharge, loose or foul-smelling stools) and allergy.

□ Instruct the patient to notify the physician if symptoms do not improve or if nausea or diarrhea persist when drug is administered with food.

□ Teach patients with a history of rheumatic heart disease or valve replacement the importance of using antimicrobial prophylaxis before invasive medical or dental procedures.

EVALUATION

Clinical response can be evaluated by: ▪ Resolution of the signs and symptoms of infection. Length of time for complete resolution depends on the organism and site of infection ▪ Endocarditis prophylaxis.

AMOXICILLIN/ CLAVULANATE

(a-mox-i-**sill**-in/klav-yoo-**lan**-ate)
Augmentin, {Clavulin}

CLASSIFICATION(S):
Anti-infective (extended-spectrum penicillin)
Pregnancy Category B

INDICATIONS

▪ Treatment of a variety of infections including: □ Skin and skin structure infections □ Otitis media □ Sinusitis □ Respiratory tract infections □ Genitourinary tract infections □ Meningitis □ Septicemia.

ACTION

▪ Binds to bacterial cell wall, causing cell death. Resists action of beta-lactamase, an enzyme produced by bacteria that is capable of inactivating some penicillins. Combination with clavulanate enhances this resistance. **Therapeutic Effect:** ▪ Bactericidal action against susceptible bacteria. **Spectrum:** ▪ Active against: □ Streptococci □ Pneumococci □ Enterococci □ *Hemophilus influenzae* □ *Escherichia coli* □ *Proteus mirabilis* □ *Neisseria menigitidis* □ *Neisseri gonorrhea* □ *Shigella* □ *Salmonella*.

PHARMACOKINETICS

Absorption: Well absorbed from the duodenum (75–90%). More resistant to acid inactivation than other penicillins.
Distribution: Diffuses readily into most body tissues and fluids. CSF penetration is increased in the presence of inflamed meninges. Crosses the placenta and enters breast milk in small amounts.
Metabolism and Excretion: 70% excreted unchanged in the urine. 30% metabolized by the liver.
Half-life: 1–1.3 hr.

CONTRAINDICATIONS AND PRECAUTIONS

Contraindicated in: ▪ Hypersensitivity to penicillins ▪ Hypersensitivity to clavulanate.
Use Cautiously in: ▪ Severe renal insufficiency (dosage reduction necessary) ▪ Infectious mononucleosis (increased incidence of rash).

ADVERSE REACTIONS AND SIDE EFFECTS*

CNS: SEIZURES (high doses).
Derm: rashes, urticaria.
GI: nausea, vomiting, diarrhea.

{} = Available in Canada only.
*Underlines indicate most frequent; **CAPITALS** indicate life-threatening.

Hemat: blood dyscrasias.
Misc: superinfection, allergic reactions including serum sickness.

INTERACTIONS

Drug–Drug: ▪ **Probenecid** decreases renal excretion and increases blood levels of amoxicillin—therapy may be combined for this purpose ▪ May potentiate the effect of **oral anticoagulants**. ▪ Concurrent **allopurinol** therapy increases risk of rash ▪ May decrease the effectiveness of **oral contraceptive agents**.

ROUTE AND DOSAGE

▪ **PO (Adults):** 250–500 mg amoxicillin with 125 mg clavulanate q 8 hr.
▪ **PO (Children ≤40 kg):** 6.7–13.3 mg/kg amoxicillin equivalent q 8 hr.

AVAILABILITY

▪ *Tablets:* 250 mg amoxicillin with 125 mg clavulanic acid; 500 mg amoxicillin with 125 mg clavulanate ▪ *Chewable tablets:* 125 mg amoxicillin with 31.25 mg clavulanate, 250 mg amoxicillin with 62.5 mg clavulanate ▪ *Suspension:* 125 mg amoxicillin with 31.25 mg clavulanic acid/5 ml, 250 mg amoxicillin with 62.5 mg clavulanate/5 ml.

TIME/ACTION PROFILE (peak blood levels)

	ONSET	PEAK
PO	30 min	1–2 hr

NURSING IMPLICATIONS

ASSESSMENT

▫ Assess patient for infection (vital signs; appearance of wound, sputum, urine, and stool; WBC) at beginning and throughout course of therapy.
▫ Obtain a history before initiating therapy to determine previous use of and reactions to penicillins or cephalosporins. Persons with a negative history of penicillin sensitivity may still have an allergic response.
▫ Observe for signs and symptoms of anaphylaxis (rash, pruritus, laryngeal edema, wheezing). Notify the physician immediately if these occur.
▫ Obtain specimens for culture and sensitivity prior to therapy. First dose may be given before receiving results.
▪ **Lab Test Considerations:** May cause false-positive reactions with copper sulfate urine glucose tests (Clinitest). Use Clinistix or Tes-Tape to monitor urine glucose.
▫ May cause increased AST (SGOT) and ALT (SGPT) concentrations.

POTENTIAL NURSING DIAGNOSES

▪ Infection, high risk for (indications, side effects).
▪ Knowledge deficit related to medication regimen (patient/family teaching).
▪ Noncompliance related to medication regimen (patient/family teaching).

IMPLEMENTATION

▪ **PO:** Administer around the clock. May be given without regard to meals. May be given with meals to decrease GI side effects. Capsule contents may be emptied and swallowed with liquids. Chewable tablets should be crushed or chewed before swallowing with liquids. Available as a powder for reconstitution to an oral suspension. Refrigerated reconstituted suspension should be discarded after 10 days.

PATIENT/FAMILY TEACHING

▫ Instruct patients to take medication around the clock and to finish the drug completely as directed, even if feeling better. Advise patients that sharing of this medication may be dangerous.
▫ Advise patient to report the signs of superinfection (furry overgrowth on the tongue, vaginal itching or discharge, loose or foul-smelling stools) and allergy.
▫ Instruct the patient to notify the physician if symptoms do not improve or if nausea or diarrhea persist when drug is administered with food.

EVALUATION

Clinical response can be evaluated by:
▪ Resolution of the signs and symptoms of infection. Length of time for complete

resolution depends on the organism and site of infection.

AMPHETAMINE
(am-**fet**-a-meen)

CLASSIFICATION(S):
CNS stimulant
Schedule II
Pregnancy Category C

INDICATIONS

■ Treatment of narcolepsy ■ Adjunct in the management of attention deficit disorder (ADD).

ACTION

■ Causes release of norepinephrine from nerve endings. Pharmacologic effects are: □ CNS and respiratory stimulation □ Vasoconstriction □ Mydriasis (pupillary dilation). **Therapeutic Effects:** ■ Increased motor activity, mental alertness, and decreased fatigue in narcoleptic patients ■ Increased attention span in attention deficit disorder.

PHARMACOKINETICS

Absorption: Well absorbed following oral administration.
Distribution: Widely distributed in body tissues with high concentrations in the brain and CSF. Crosses the placenta and enters breast milk.
Metabolism and Excretion: Some metabolism by the liver. Urinary excretion is pH dependent. Alkaline urine promotes reabsorption and prolongs action.
Half-life: 10–30 hr (depends on urine pH).

CONTRAINDICATIONS AND PRECAUTIONS

Contraindicated in: ■ Pregnancy or lactation (potentially embryotoxic) ■ Hyperexcitable states including hyperthyroidism ■ Psychotic personalities ■ Suicidal or homicidal tendencies ■ Chemical dependence ■ Glaucoma.

Use Cautiously in: ■ Cardiovascular disease ■ Hypertension ■ Diabetes mellitus ■ Elderly or debilitated patients.

ADVERSE REACTIONS AND SIDE EFFECTS*

CNS: restlessness, tremor, hyperactivity, insomnia, irritability, dizziness, headache.
CV: tachycardia, palpitations, hypertension, hypotension.
Derm: urticaria.
GI: nausea, vomiting, anorexia, dry mouth, cramps, diarrhea, constipation, metallic taste.
GU: impotence, increased libido.
Misc: psychological dependence.

INTERACTIONS

Drug–Drug: ■ Additive effects with other **adrenergic (sympathomimetic) agents** or **thyroid** ■ Use with **MAO inhibitors** or **meperidine** can result in hypertensive crisis ■ **Alkalinizing urine (sodium bicarbonate, acetazolamide)** decreases excretion, enhances effect ■ **Acidification of urine (ammonium chloride,** large doses of **ascorbic acid)** decreases effect ■ Increased risk of hypertension and bradycardia with **beta blockers** ■ Increased risk of arrhythmias with **cardiac glycosides** ■ **Tricyclic antidepressants** may enhance the effect of amphetamine but increase risk of arrhythmias, hypertension, or hyperpyrexia.
Drug–Food: Foods that alkalinize the urine (cranberry juice) can enhance the effect of amphetamine.

ROUTE AND DOSAGE

Narcolepsy
■ **PO (Adult):** 5–60 mg/day in 1–3 divided doses.
■ **PO (Children >12 yr):** 10 mg/day in 2 divided doses. May decrease by 10 mg/day at weekly intervals.
■ **PO (Children 6–12 yr):** 5 mg/day in 2 divided doses, increase by 5 mg at weekly intervals.

---

*Underlines indicate most frequent; **CAPITALS** indicate life-threatening.

Attention Deficit Disorder

- **PO (Children >6 yr):** 5 mg/day 1–2 times daily, increase by 5 mg at weekly intervals.
- **PO (Children 3–6 yr):** 2.5 mg/day, increase by 2.5 mg at weekly intervals.

AVAILABILITY

- **Tablets:** 5 mg, 10 mg.

TIME/ACTION PROFILE (stimulation)

	ONSET	PEAK	DURATION
PO	1–2 hr	UK	4–10 hr

NURSING IMPLICATIONS

ASSESSMENT

- Monitor blood pressure, pulse, and respiration before and periodically during therapy.
- Monitor weight biweekly and inform physician of significant loss. Monitor height periodically in children; inform physician of growth inhibition.
- Observe and document frequency of narcoleptic episodes.
- Assess attention span, impulse control, and interactions with others in children with attention-deficit disorders.
- May produce a false sense of euphoria and well-being. Provide frequent rest periods and observe patient for rebound depression after the effects of the medication have worn off.
- Has high dependence and abuse potential. Tolerance to medication occurs rapidly; do not increase dose.

POTENTIAL NURSING DIAGNOSES

- Thought processes, altered (side effects).
- Knowledge deficit related to medication regimen (patient/family teaching).

IMPLEMENTATION

- **PO:** Use the lowest effective dose.

PATIENT/FAMILY TEACHING

- Instruct patient to take medication at least 6 hr before bedtime to avoid sleep disturbances. Missed doses should be taken as soon as remembered up to 6 hr before bedtime. Do not double doses. Instruct patient not to alter dosage without consulting physician. Abrupt cessation with high doses may cause extreme fatigue and mental depression.
- Inform patient that the effects of drug-induced dry mouth can be minimized by rinsing frequently with water or chewing sugarless gum or candies.
- Advise patient to limit caffeine intake.
- May impair judgment. Advise patient to use caution when driving or during other activities requiring alertness.
- Inform patient that periodic holidays from the drug may be used to assess progress and decrease dependence.
- Advise patient to notify physician if nervousness, restlessness, insomnia, dizziness, anorexia, or dry mouth becomes severe.

EVALUATION

Effectiveness of therapy can be demonstrated by: ■ Decrease in narcoleptic symptoms ■ Improved attention span.

AMPHOTERICIN B
(am-foe-**ter**-i-sin)
Fungizone

CLASSIFICATION(S):
Antifungal
Pregnancy Category B

INDICATIONS

- **IV:** Treatment of active, progressive, potentially fatal fungal infections.
- **Top:** Treatment of superficial fungal infections.

ACTION

- Binds to fungal cell membrane, allowing leakage of cellular contents. **Therapeutic Effect:** ■ Fungistatic action. **Spectrum:** ■ Active against: □ Aspergillosis □ Blastomycosis □ Candida □ Coccidioidomycosis □ Histoplasmosis □ Mucormycosis.

PHARMACOKINETICS

Absorption: Not active orally. Topical

preparations are not significantly absorbed.

Distribution: Following administration, distributed to body tissues and fluids. Poor penetration into CSF.

Metabolism and Excretion: Elimination is very prolonged. Detectable in urine up to 7 wk after discontinuation.

Half-life: Biphasic—initial phase, 24–48 hr; terminal phase, 15 days.

CONTRAINDICATIONS AND PRECAUTIONS

Contraindicated in: ▪ Hypersensitivity. **Use Cautiously in:** ▪ Renal impairment ▪ Electrolyte abnormalities ▪ Pregnancy and lactation (safety not established).

ADVERSE REACTIONS AND SIDE EFFECTS*

CNS: headache.
CV: hypotension, arrhythmias.
F and E: hypokalemia.
GI: nausea, vomiting, diarrhea.
GU: nephrotoxicity, hematuria.
Hemat: anemia, dyscrasias.
Local: phlebitis.
Misc: fever, chills, HYPERSENSITIVITY REACTIONS.
MS: mylagia, arthralgia.
Neuro: peripheral neuropathy.
Resp: dyspnea, wheezing.

INTERACTIONS

Drug–Drug: ▪ Increased risk of nephrotoxicity with other **nephrotoxic agents** ▪ **Diuretics, glucocorticoids, mezlocillin, piperacillin,** or **ticarcillin** may potentiate hypokalemia.

ROUTE AND DOSAGE

▪ **IV (Adults):** Give test dose of 1 mg, then initial dose of 0.25 mg/kg, slowly; increase daily doses slowly to 0.5 mg/kg (can give up to 1 mg/kg/day or 1.5 mg/kg every other day).
▪ **IV (Children):** 0.25 mg/kg infused slowly initially; increase by 0.25 mg/kg every other day to maximum of 1 mg/kg/day.
▪ **Top:** Apply 2–4 times daily.

AVAILABILITY

▪ *Injection:* 50-mg vial ▪ *Cream, lotion, ointment:* 3%.

TIME/ACTION PROFILE (blood levels)

	ONSET	PEAK
IV	rapid	end of infusion

NURSING IMPLICATIONS

ASSESSMENT

▢ This drug should be administered IV only to hospitalized patients or those under close supervision. Diagnosis should be confirmed prior to administration.

▢ Monitor patient closely during test dose and the first 1–2 hr of each dose for fever, chills, headache, anorexia, nausea, or vomiting. Premedication with antipyretics, corticosteroids, antihistamines, and antiemetics and maintaining sodium balance may decrease these reactions. Febrile reaction usually subsides within 4 hr after the infusion is completed.

▢ Assess injection site frequently for thrombophlebitis or leakage. Drug is very irritating to tissues. Adding heparin to IV solution may decrease the likelihood of thrombophlebitis.

▢ Monitor pulse and blood pressure every 15–30 min during test dose and initial therapy. Assess respiratory status (lung sounds, dyspnea) daily. Notify physician of changes.

▢ Monitor intake and output and weigh daily. Adequate hydration (2000–3000 ml/day) may minimize nephrotoxicity.

▪ **Lab Test Considerations:** Monitor weekly hemoglobin and hematocrit, magnesium, BUN, and serum creatinine and biweekly potassium levels. Life-threatening hypokalemia may occur following each dose. If BUN exceeds 40 mg/100 ml or serum creatinine exceeds 3 mg/100 ml, dosage should be decreased or discontinued until renal function improves. May

---

*Underlines indicate most frequent; **CAPITALS** indicate life-threatening.

cause decreased hemoglobin, hematocrit, and magnesium levels.

□ Liver function tests should be monitored periodically throughout therapy. Elevated bromsulphalein, alkaline phosphatase, and bilirubin may require discontinuation of therapy.

POTENTIAL NURSING DIAGNOSES

- Infection, high risk for (indications).
- Knowledge deficit related to medication regimen (patient/family teaching).

IMPLEMENTATION

- **IV:** Reconstitute 50-mg vial with 10 ml of Sterile Water for Injection without bacteriostatic agent. Concentration equals 5 mg/ml. Shake until clear. Further dilute each 1 mg with at least 10 ml of D5W (pH>4.2) for a concentration of 100 mcg/ml. Do not use other diluents. Avoid use of precipitated solution. Use 20-gauge needle; change for each step of dilution. Wear gloves while handling.

□ Store in dark area. Reconstituted solution is stable for 24 hr at room temperature and 1 wk if refrigerated.

- **Test Dose:** Administer 1 mg in 20 ml of D5W over 10–30 min to determine patient tolerance. If medication is withheld for 7 days, restart at lowest dose level. In severe, life-threatening infections test dose may be omitted.
- **Intermittent Infusion:** Administer preferably through central line. If peripheral site is used, change site with each dose to prevent phlebitis. If an in-line filter is used, the mean pore diameter should be no less than 1 micron. Agitate hanging solution to mix every ½ hr. Short-term exposure to light (8 hr) does not alter potency.
- **Rate:** Administer slowly via infusion pump over 6 hr.
- **Syringe Compatibility:** ▪ heparin.
- **Y-Site Compatibility:** ▪ zidovudine.
- **Y-Site Incompatibility:** ▪ enalaprilat ▪ fludarabine ▪ foscarnet ▪ ondansetron.
- **Additive Compatibility:** ▪ heparin

- hydrocortisone ▪ methylprednisolone ▪ sodium bicarbonate.

- **Top:** While wearing gloves, apply topical preparations liberally and rub in well. Do not use occlusive dressings. Discontinue if lesions worsen or signs of hypersensitivity develop.

PATIENT/FAMILY TEACHING

- **General Info:** Explain need for long duration of IV or topical therapy.
- **IV:** Inform patient of potential side effects and discomfort at IV site.
- **Top:** Advise patient that topical preparations may stain clothing. Cream or lotion may be removed with soap and warm water; ointment may be removed with cleaning fluid.

EVALUATION

Effectiveness of therapy may be determined by: ▪ Resolution of signs and symptoms of infection. Several weeks to months of therapy may be required to prevent relapse.

AMPICILLIN

(am-pi-**sill**-in)
{Ampicin}, {D-Amp}, {Apo-Ampi}, {Nu-Ampi}, {NovoAmpicillin}, Omnipen, Penbritin, Principen, Polycillin, Supen, Totacillin

CLASSIFICATION(S):
Anti-infective (penicillin)
Pregnancy Category B

INDICATIONS

- Treatment of the following infections: □ Skin and skin structure infections, soft tissue infections □ Otitis media □ Sinusitis □ Respiratory infections □ Genitourinary infections □ Meningitis □ Septicemia ▪ Endocarditis prophylaxis.

ACTION

- Binds to bacterial cell wall, resulting in cell death. **Therapeutic Effect:** ▪ Bactericidal action. Resists action of beta-lactamase, an enzyme produced by bacteria that is capable of inactivating some penicillins. **Spectrum:** ▪ Active against: ▫ Streptococci ▫ Pneumococci ▫ Enterococci ▫ *Hemophilus influenzae* ▫ *Escherichia coli* ▫ *Proteus mirabilis* ▫ *Neisseria menigitidis* ▫ *Neisseria gonorrhea* ▫ *Shigella* ▫ *Salmonella*.

PHARMACOKINETICS

Absorption: Moderately absorbed from the duodenum (30–50%).
Distribution: Diffuses readily into body tissues and fluids. CSF penetration is increased in the presence of inflamed meninges. Crosses the placenta; enters breast milk in small amounts.
Metabolism and Excretion: Variably metabolized by the liver (12–50%). Renal excretion is variable (25–60% after oral dosing; 50–85% following IM administration).
Half-life: 1–1.5 hr.

CONTRAINDICATIONS AND PRECAUTIONS

Contraindicated in: ▪ Hypersensitivity to penicillins.
Use Cautiously in: ▪ Severe renal insufficiency (dosage reduction required if CCr ≤10 ml/min) ▪ Has been used during pregnancy and lactation ▪ Infectious mononucleosis (increased incidence of rash).

ADVERSE REACTIONS AND SIDE EFFECTS*

CNS: SEIZURES (high doses).
Derm: rashes, urticaria.
GI: nausea, vomiting, diarrhea.
Hemat: blood dyscrasias.
Misc: superinfection, allergic reactions including ANAPHYLAXIS and serum sickness.

INTERACTIONS

Drug–Drug: ▪ **Probenecid** decreases renal excretion and increases blood levels of ampicillin—therapy may be combined for this purpose ▪ May potentiate

the effect of **warfarin** ▪ Incidence of rash increases with concurrent **allopurinol** therapy ▪ May decrease the effectiveness of **oral contraceptives**.

ROUTE AND DOSAGE

▪ **PO, IM, IV (Adults):** 1–2 g/day in divided doses q 4–6 hr.
▪ **PO, IM, IV (Children):** 50–200 mg/kg/day in divided doses q 4–6 hr.
▪ **PO, IM, IV (Infants >7 days and >2000 g):** 100–200 mg/kg/day in divided doses q 6 hr.
▪ **PO, IM, IV (Infants >7 days and <2000 g or <7 days and >2000 g):** 75–150 mg/kg/day in divided doses q 8 hr.
▪ **PO, IM, IV (Infants <7 days and <2000 g):** 50–100 mg/kg/day in divided doses q 12 hr.

AVAILABILITY

▪ *Capsules:* 250 mg, 500 mg ▪ *Suspension:* 100 mg/ml, 125 mg/5 ml, 250 mg/5 ml, 500 mg/5 ml ▪ *Injection:* 125 mg, 250 mg, 1-g, 2-g, 10-g vials.

TIME/ACTION PROFILE (blood levels)

	ONSET	PEAK
PO	rapid	1.5–2 hr
IM	rapid	1 hr
IV	rapid	end of infusion

NURSING IMPLICATIONS

ASSESSMENT

▫ Assess patient for infection (vital signs; wound appearance, sputum, urine, and stool; WBC) at beginning and throughout course of therapy.
▫ Obtain a history before initiating therapy to determine previous use and reactions to penicillins or cephalosporins. Persons with a negative history of penicillin sensitivity may still have an allergic response.
▫ Obtain specimens for culture and sensitivity prior to therapy. First dose may be given before receiving results.
▫ Observe patient for signs and symp-

toms of anaphylaxis (rash, pruritus, laryngeal edema, wheezing). Discontinue the drug and notify the physician immediately if these occur. Keep epinephrine, an antihistamine, and resuscitation equipment close by in the event of an anaphylactic reaction.

□ Assess skin for "ampicillin rash," a nonallergic, dull red, macular or maculopapular, mildly pruritic rash.

■ **Lab Test Considerations:** May cause false-positive copper sulfate urine glucose tests (Clinitest); test urine with glucose enzymatic tests (Ketodiastix or Tes-Tape).

□ May cause increased AST (SGOT) and ALT (SGPT).

POTENTIAL NURSING DIAGNOSES

■ Infection, high risk for (indications, side effects).

■ Knowledge deficit related to medication regimen (patient/family teaching).

■ Noncompliance related to medication regimen (patient/family teaching).

IMPLEMENTATION

■ **PO:** Administer around the clock on an empty stomach at least 1 hr before or 2 hr after meals with a full glass of water. Tablets may be crushed and capsules may be opened and mixed with water. Reconstituted oral suspensions retain potency for 7 days at room temperature and 14 days if refrigerated. Combination with probenecid should be used immediately after reconstitution.

■ **IM, IV:** Reconstitute for IM or IV use by adding Sterile Water for Injection 0.9–1.2 ml to the 125-mg vial, 0.9–1.9 ml to the 250-mg vial, 1.2–1.8 ml to the 500-mg vial, 2.4–7.4 ml to the 1-g vial, and 6.8 ml to the 2-g vial.

■ **Direct IV:** May be given over 3–5 min (125–500 mg) or over 10–15 min (1–2 g) within 1 hr of reconstitution. Rapid administration may cause seizures.

■ **Intermittent Infusion:** Dilute in 50 ml or more of 0.9% NaCl, D5W, D5/0.45% NaCl, or lactated Ringer's solution for a concentration of no more than 30 mg/ml; administer within 4 hr.

■ **Syringe Compatibility:** ■ chloramphenicol ■ heparin ■ procaine.

■ **Syringe Incompatibility:** ■ erythromycin lactobionate ■ gentamicin ■ kanamycin ■ metoclopramide.

■ **Y-Site Compatibility:** ■ acyclovir ■ cyclophosphamide ■ enalaprilat ■ esmolol ■ famotidine ■ fludarabine ■ foscarnet hydromorphone ■ insulin, regular ■ labetalol ■ magnesium sulfate ■ meperidine ■ morphine ■ perphenazine ■ phytonadione ■ potassium chloride ■ tolazoline.

■ **Y-Site Incompatibility:** ■ epinephrine ■ fluconazole ■ hydralazine ■ ondansetron ■ sargramostim.

■ **Additive Incompatibility:** ■ amikacin ■ gentamicin ■ kanamycin. If aminoglycosides and penicillins must be administered concurrently, administer in separate sites.

PATIENT/FAMILY TEACHING

■ **General Info:** Instruct patient to take medication around the clock and to finish the drug completely as directed, even if feeling better. Advise patients that sharing of this medication can be dangerous.

□ Advise patient to report the signs of superinfection (furry overgrowth on the tongue, vaginal itching or discharge, loose or foul-smelling stools) and allergy.

□ Advise patient to use a nonhormonal method of contraception while taking ampicillin.

□ Instruct the patient to notify the physician if symptoms do not improve.

□ Patients with a history of rheumatic heart disease or valve replacement need to be taught the importance of using antimicrobial prophylaxis before invasive medical or dental procedures.

EVALUATION

Clinical response can be evaluated by:
■ Resolution of the signs and symptoms of infection. Length of time for complete resolution depends on the organism and site of infection ■ Endocarditis prophylaxis.

AMPICILLIN/SULBACTAM
(am-pi-**sill**-in/sul-**bak**-tam)
Unasyn

CLASSIFICATION(S):
Anti-infective (penicillin)
Pregnancy Category B (Ampicillin)

INDICATIONS

- Treatment of the following infections:
  □ Skin and skin structure infections, soft tissue infections □ Otitis media □ Sinusitis □ Respiratory infections □ Genitourinary infections □ Meningitis □ Septicemia.

ACTION

- Binds to bacterial cell wall, resulting in cell death. Addition of sulbactam increases resistance to beta-lactamases, enzymes produced by bacteria that may inactivate ampicillin. **Therapeutic Effect:** ■ Bactericidal action. **Spectrum:** ■ Active against: □ Streptococci □ Pneumococci □ Enterococci □ *Hemophilus influenzae* □ *Escherichia coli* □ *Proteus mirabilis* □ *Neisseria menigitidis* □ *Neisseria gonorrhea* □ *Shigella* □ *Salmonella* ■ Use should be reserved for infections caused by beta-lactamase producing strains.

PHARMACOKINETICS

Absorption: Well absorbed from IM sites.
Distribution: Ampicillin diffuses readily into body tissues and fluids. CSF penetration is increased when meninges are inflamed. Crosses the placenta; enters breast milk in small amounts.
Metabolism and Excretion: Ampicillin is variably metabolized by the liver (12–50%). Renal excretion of unchanged drug is variable (25–60% after oral dosing; 50–85% following IM administration).
Half-life: 1.5 hr (ampicillin).

CONTRAINDICATIONS AND PRECAUTIONS

Contraindicated in: ■ Hypersensitivity to penicillins or sulbactam.
Use Cautiously in: ■ Severe renal insufficiency (dosage reduction required if CCr <30 ml/min) ■ Has been used during pregnancy and lactation (ampicillin) ■ Infectious mononucleosis (increased incidence of rash) ■ Children <12 yr (safety not established).

ADVERSE REACTIONS AND SIDE EFFECTS*

CNS: SEIZURES (high doses).
Derm: rashes, urticaria.
GI: nausea, vomiting, diarrhea.
Hemat: blood dyscrasias.
Local: pain at IM site, pain at IV site.
Misc: superinfection, allergic reactions including ANAPHYLAXIS and serum sickness.

INTERACTIONS

Drug–Drug: ■ **Probenecid** decreases renal excretion and increases blood levels of ampicillin—therapy may be combined for this purpose ■ May potentiate the effect of **warfarin** ■ Concurrent **allopurinol** therapy (increased incidence of rash) ■ May decrease the effectiveness of **oral contraceptives.**

ROUTE AND DOSAGE

- **IM, IV (Adults):** 1.5–3 g (1 g ampicillin plus 0.5 g sulbactam–2 g ampicillin plus 1 g sulbactam) q 6–8 hr (not to exceed 4 g sulbactam/day).

AVAILABILITY

- *Injection:* 1 g ampicillin with 500 mg sulbactam; 2 g ampicillin with 1 g sulbactam.

TIME/ACTION PROFILE (blood levels)

	ONSET	PEAK
IM	rapid	1 hr
IV	immediate	end of infusion

*Underlines indicate most frequent; **CAPITALS** indicate life-threatening.

NURSING IMPLICATIONS

ASSESSMENT

□ Assess patient for infection (vital signs; wound appearance, sputum, urine, and stool; WBC) at beginning and throughout course of therapy.

□ Obtain a history before initiating therapy to determine previous use and reactions to penicillins or cephalosporins. Persons with a negative history of penicillin sensitivity may still have an allergic response.

□ Obtain specimens for culture and sensitivity prior to therapy. First dose may be given before receiving results.

□ Observe patient for signs and symptoms of anaphylaxis (rash, pruritus, laryngeal edema, wheezing). Discontinue the drug and notify the physician immediately if these occur. Keep epinephrine, an antihistamine, and resuscitation equipment close by in the event of an anaphylactic reaction.

■ **Lab Test Considerations:** May cause false-positive copper sulfate urine glucose tests (Clinitest); test urine with glucose enzymatic tests (Ketodiastix or Tes-Tape).

□ May cause increased AST (SGOT), ALT (SGPT), LDH, alkaline phosphatase, monocytes, basophils, eosinophils, BUN, and creatinine. May also cause presence of RBCs and hyaline casts in the urine.

□ May cause decreased hemoglobin, hematocrit, RBC, WBC, neutrophils, lymphocytes, platelets, serum albumin, and total proteins.

POTENTIAL NURSING DIAGNOSES

■ Infection, high risk for (indications, side effects).

■ Knowledge deficit related to medication regimen (patient/family teaching).

IMPLEMENTATION

■ **IM:** Reconstitute for IM use by adding 3.2 ml of sterile water or 0.5% or 2% lidocaine HCl to the 1.5-g vial or 6.4

ml to the 3-g vial. Administer within 1 hr of preparation, deep IM into well-developed muscle.

■ **IV:** For IV use reconstitute each 1.5 g with at least 4 ml of sterile water for a concentration of 375 mg/ml (250 mg ampicillin/125 mg sulbactam). Foaming should dissipate upon standing. Administer only clear solutions.

■ **Direct IV:** May be administered over 10–15 min (1–2 g) within 1 hr of reconstitution. More rapid administration may cause seizures.

■ **Intermittent Infusion:** Dilute immediately for infusion in 50–100 ml or more of 0.9% NaCl, D5W, D5/0.45% NaCl, or lactated Ringer's solution. Stability of solution varies from 2–8 hr at room temperature or 3–72 hr if refrigerated, depending on concentration and diluent.

■ *Rate:* Administer over 15–30 min.

■ **Y-Site Compatibility:** ■ enalaprilat ■ famotidine ■ fluconazole ■ fludarabine ■ insulin, regular ■ meperidine ■ morphine.

■ **Y-Site Incompatibility:** ■ ondansetron ■ sargramostim.

■ **Additive Incompatibilities:** If aminoglycosides and penicillins must be administered concurrently, administer in separate sites.

PATIENT/FAMILY TEACHING

□ Advise patient to report the signs of superinfection (furry overgrowth on the tongue, vaginal itching or discharge, loose or foul-smelling stools) and allergy.

□ Advise patient to use a nonhormonal method of contraception while taking ampicillin/sulbactam.

□ Instruct the patient to notify the physician if symptoms do not improve.

EVALUATION

Clinical response can be evaluated by:

■ Resolution of the signs and symptoms of infection. Length of time for complete resolution depends on the organism and site of infection.

AMRINONE
(am-ri-none)
Inocor

CLASSIFICATION(S):
Inotropic agent
Pregnancy Category C

INDICATIONS
- Short-term treatment of congestive heart failure unresponsive to cardiac glycosides, diuretics, and vasodilators.

ACTION
- Increases myocardial contractility
- Decreases preload and afterload by a direct dilating effect on vascular smooth muscle. **Therapeutic Effect:**
- Increased cardiac output (inotropic effect).

PHARMACOKINETICS
Absorption: Administered IV only, resulting in complete bioavailability.
Distribution: Distribution not known.
Metabolism and Excretion: 50% metabolized by the liver. 10–40% excreted unchanged by the kidneys.
Half-life: 3.6–5.8 hr (increased in congestive heart failure).

CONTRAINDICATIONS AND PRECAUTIONS
Contraindicated in: • Hypersensitivity to amrinone or bisulfites • Idiopathic hypertrophic subaortic stenosis.
Use Cautiously in: • Atrial fibrillation or flutter (may increase ventricular response; pretreatment with cardiac glycosides may be necessary) • Children <18 yr (safety not established).

ADVERSE REACTIONS AND SIDE EFFECTS*

CV: <u>arrhythmias</u>, <u>hypotension</u>.
Resp: dyspnea.
GI: nausea, vomiting, diarrhea, hepatotoxicity.
F and E: hypokalemia.
Hemat: <u>thrombocytopenia</u>.
Misc: hypersensitivity reactions, fever.

INTERACTIONS
Drug–Drug: • Inotropic effects may be additive with **cardiac glycosides** • Hypotension may be exaggerated by **disopyramide**.

ROUTE AND DOSAGE
See infusion rate chart in Appendix D.
- **IV (Adults):** 0.75 mg/kg loading dose; may be repeated in 30 min if necessary, then 5–10 mcg/kg/min infusion (total daily dose should not exceed 10 mg/kg).
- **IV (Infants):** 3–4.5 mg/kg in divided doses followed by infusion at 10 mcg/kg/min.
- **IV (Neonates):** 3–4.5 mg/kg in divided doses followed by infusion at 3–5 mcg/kg/min.

AVAILABILITY
- *Injection:* 5 mg/ml.

TIME/ACTION PROFILE (inotropic effect)

	ONSET	PEAK	DURATION*
IV	2–5 min	10 min	0.5–2 hr

*After infusion is discontinued.

NURSING IMPLICATIONS

ASSESSMENT
- Monitor blood pressure, pulse, ECG, respiratory rate, cardiac index, pulmonary capillary wedge pressure, and central venous pressure frequently during administration. Notify physician promptly if hypotension occurs.
- Monitor intake and output and weigh daily. Assess for resolution of signs of congestive heart failure (peripheral edema, dyspnea, rales/crackles, weight gain). Fluid intake may need to be increased cautiously to ensure adequate cardiac filling pressure.
- Observe for hypersensitivity reactions (pleuritis, pericarditis, ascites). Withhold drug and notify physician immediately if a reaction occurs.
- **Lab Test Considerations:** Platelet counts, serum electrolytes, liver en-

*<u>Underlines</u> indicate most frequent; **CAPITALS** indicate life-threatening.

zymes, and renal function should be evaluated periodically throughout the course of therapy. If platelet count is <150,000/mm^3 notify physician promptly. Increased liver enzymes may indicate hepatotoxicity. May cause decreased potassium levels.

POTENTIAL NURSING DIAGNOSES

- Cardiac output, decreased (indications).
- Activity intolerance (indications).
- Fluid volume excess (indications).

IMPLEMENTATION

- **General Info:** Hypokalemia should be corrected prior to administration.
- Patients with atrial fibrillation/flutter may require cardiac glycoside therapy prior to treatment; amrinone enhances atrioventricular conduction.
- **Direct IV:** Administer loading dose over 2–3 min. An additional loading dose may be given in 30 min.
- **Continuous Infusion:** Dilute amrinone with 0.9% NaCl or 0.45% NaCl only, for a concentration of 1–3 mg/ml. Dilution with dextrose products may lead to decomposition of amrinone, but may be administered through Y-tubing or directly into tubing of a running dextrose solution. Administer via infusion pump to ensure accurate dosage. Change tubing whenever concentration of solution is changed. Solution should be clear yellow. Use reconstituted solution within 24 hr of preparation.
- *Rate:* Rate is titrated according to patient response.
- **Syringe Compatibility:** ▪ propranolol ▪ verapamil.
- **Y-Site Compatibility:** ▪ aminophylline ▪ atropine ▪ bretylium ▪ calcium chloride ▪ cimetidine ▪ digoxin ▪ dobutamine ▪ dopamine ▪ epinephrine ▪ famotidine ▪ hydrocortisone sodium succinate ▪ isoproterenol ▪ lidocaine ▪ metaraminol bitartrate ▪ methylprednisolone sodium succinate ▪ nitroglycerin ▪ nitroprusside ▪ norepinephrine ▪ phenylephrine ▪ potassium chloride ▪ propranolol ▪ verapamil.

- **Y-Site Incompatibility:** ▪ furosemide ▪ sodium bicarbonate.

PATIENT/FAMILY TEACHING

- Advise patient to report an increase in dyspnea or chest pain, or the onset of hypersensitivity reactions promptly.
- Advise patient to make position changes slowly to minimize any drug-induced postural hypotension.

EVALUATION

Effectiveness of therapy may be determined by: ▪ Increase in cardiac index and diuresis ▫ Decrease in pulmonary capillary wedge pressure, dyspnea, and edema.

AMYL NITRITE
(**am**-il **nye**-trite)

CLASSIFICATION(S):
Antianginal, Antidote (cyanide poisoning)
Pregnancy Category X

INDICATIONS

- Acute treatment of angina pectoris. **Unlabeled Uses:** ▪ Acute management of cyanide poisoning ▪ Diagnosis of cardiac murmurs.

ACTION

- Reduces systemic arterial pressure (reduces afterload) ▪ Forms methemoglobin, which combines with cyanide, forming a nontoxic compound (cyanmethemoglobin). **Therapeutic Effects:** ▪ Relief of angina pectoris ▪ Prevention of fatal outcome in cyanide poisoning.

PHARMACOKINETICS

Absorption: Amyl nitrite is well absorbed through nasal mucosa.
Distribution: Widely distributed.
Metabolism and Excretion: Combines to form methemoglobin.
Half-life: UK.

CONTRAINDICATIONS AND PRECAUTIONS

Contraindicated in: ▪ Hypersensitivity ▪ Increased intracranial pressure ▪ Severe anemia ▪ No contraindications in cyanide poisoning.

Use Cautiously in: ▪ Hypotension ▪ Hypovolemia ▪ Constrictive pericarditis or cardiac tamponade ▪ Glaucoma ▪ Hyperthyroidism ▪ Recent head trauma ▪ Cerebral hemorrhage ▪ Recent myocardial infarction ▪ Cyanide poisoning in children (titrate doses based on methemoglobin levels).

ADVERSE REACTIONS AND SIDE EFFECTS*

CNS: headache, dizziness, fainting, weakness.
Resp: shortness of breath.
CV: hypotension, tachycardia.
Derm: cyanosis of lips, fingernail, or palms (indicates methemoglobinemia).

INTERACTIONS

Drug–Drug: ▪ Additive hypotension with **antihypertensive agents** ▪ Decreases the effects of **histamine, acetylcholine,** and **norepinephrine** ▪ Antianginal activity decreased by **adrenergic (sympathomimetic) agents** including **epinephrine, ephedrine,** and **phenylephrine** ▪ Blocks the alpha-adrenergic effects of **epinephrine,** resulting in hypotension and tachycardia.

ROUTE AND DOSAGE

Antianginal
▪ **Inhalation (Adults):** 1 ampule (aspirol, vaporole) crushed and inhaled, may be repeated in 3–5 min (1–6 inhalations).

Cyanide Poisoning
▪ **Inhalation (Adults and Children):** Inhale for 15–30 sec of each minute until sodium nitrite is prepared.

AVAILABILITY

▪ *Ampules for inhalation:* 0.18 ml, 0.3 ml.

TIME/ACTION PROFILE (antianginal)

	ONSET	PEAK	DURATION
Inhaln	30 sec	UK	3–5 min

NURSING IMPLICATIONS

ASSESSMENT
▪ **General Info:** Assess heart rate and blood pressure prior to and periodically throughout therapy.
▪ **Angina:** Assess patient for location, duration, intensity, and cause of chest pains prior to and following administration.
▪ **Cyanide Poisoning:** Determine source of cyanide and assess patient for signs of cyanide poisoning (tachycardia, headache, drowsiness, hypotension, coma, convulsions).
▪ **Heart Murmurs:** Assess heart rate prior to and throughout administration.

POTENTIAL NURSING DIAGNOSES
▪ Pain [acute] (indications).
▪ Injury, high risk for (side effects).
▪ Knowledge deficit related to medication regimen (patient/family teaching).

IMPLEMENTATION
▪ **General Info:** Ampule is wrapped in woven, absorbent covering. Do not remove covering. Crush ampule between fingers and hold to patient's nostrils for inhalation. Patient should be sitting during and immediately after administration.
▪ **Angina:** Titrate dose according to patient's response.
▪ **Cyanide Poisoning:** Begin treatment at the first sign of toxicity if cyanide exposure is known or strongly suspected.
□ *For Adults or Children*—Crush a 0.3 ml ampule every minute and have the patient inhale the vapors for 15–30 sec until IV sodium nitrate infusion is available.
▪ **Heart Murmurs:** Amyl nitrite should be inhaled until reflex tachycardia begins, then stop immediately.

PATIENT/FAMILY TEACHING
□ Explain purpose and procedure for therapy to patient.
□ Caution patient to change positions

---

*Underlines indicate most frequent; **CAPITALS** indicate life-threatening.

slowly to minimize orthostatic hypotension.

EVALUATION
Effectiveness of therapy can be demonstrated by: ■ Relief of angina pectoris ■ Relief of signs and symptoms of cyanide poisoning ■ Change in intensity of heart murmurs.

ANISTREPLASE
(an-**eye**-strep-lase)
aniosoylated plasminogen (streptokinase activator complex), APSAC, Eminase

CLASSIFICATION(S):
Thrombolytic agent
Pregnancy Category C

INDICATIONS

■ Acute management of myocardial infarction, in order to lyse thrombi in coronary arteries and thereby preserve ventricular function.

ACTION

■ Consists of an inactive complex of plasminogen and streptokinase. Following administration, controlled activation of the complex occurs, allowing the conversion of plasminogen to plasmin and subsequent fibrinolysis. **Therapeutic Effect:** ■ Lysis of thrombi in coronary arteries with preservation of ventricular function.

PHARMACOKINETICS

Absorption: Following IV administration absorption is essentially complete.
Distribution: Distribution not known.
Metabolism and Excretion: Inactivated by binding to plasmin inactivators.
Half-life: 70–120 min.

CONTRAINDICATIONS AND PRECAUTIONS

Contraindicated in: ■ Active internal bleeding ■ History of cerebrovascular accident ■ Recent (within 2 mo) intra-cranial or intraspinal trauma ■ Intracranial neoplasm ■ Severe uncontrolled hypertension ■ Arteriovenous malformation ■ Bleeding tendencies ■ Hypersensitivity to anistreplase or streptokinase

Use Cautiously in: ■ Recent (within 10 days) major surgery, trauma, GI or GU bleeding ■ Uncontrolled hypertension ■ Left heart thrombus ■ Severe hepatic or renal disease ■ Hemorrhagic ophthalmic conditions ■ Septic phlebitis ■ Elderly patients (>75 yr) ■ Pregnancy, lactation, or children (safety not established) ■ Recent streptococcal infection or previous therapy with anistreplase or streptokinase (from 5 days–6 mo)—may produce resistance due to antibody formation; increased dosage requirements may be encountered ■ Endocarditis ■ Pericarditis ■ Cerebrovascular disease.

Extreme Caution in: ■ Early postpartum period (10 days) ■ Patients receiving oral anticoagulant therapy.

ADVERSE REACTIONS AND SIDE EFFECTS*

CNS: INTRACRANIAL HEMORRHAGE.
EENT: epistaxis, gingival bleeding.
RESP: hemoptysis.
CV: arrhythmias, hypotension.
GI: GASTROINTESTINAL BLEEDING, RETROPERITONEAL BLEEDING.
GU: GENITOURINARY TRACT BLEEDING.
Hemat: BLEEDING.
Misc: allergic reactions including ANAPHYLAXIS, fever.

INTERACTIONS

Drug–Drug: ■ Aspirin, nonsteroidal anti-inflammatory agents, oral anticoagulants, heparin, or dipyridamole—concurrent use may increase the risk of bleeding, although these agents are frequently used together or in sequence.

ROUTE AND DOSAGE

■ **IV (Adults):** 30 units over 2–5 min.

AVAILABILITY

■ *Injection:* 30 units/vial.

---

*Underlines indicate most frequent; **CAPITALS** indicate life-threatening.

TIME/ACTION PROFILE (fibrinolysis)

	ONSET	PEAK	DURATION
IV	UK	45 min	6 hr*

*Systemic hyperfibrinolytic state may persist for 2 days.

NURSING IMPLICATIONS

ASSESSMENT

- **General Info:** Therapy should be administered as soon as possible after the onset of symptoms.
- ◻ Monitor vital signs, including temperature, closely following therapy.
- ◻ Assess patient carefully for bleeding. Frank bleeding may occur from invasive sites or body orifices. Internal bleeding may also occur (decreased neurologic status, abdominal pain with coffee ground emesis or black tarry stools, joint pain). If bleeding occurs, stop medication and notify physician immediately.
- ◻ Inquire about previous reaction to anistreplase or streptokinase therapy. Assess patient for hypersensitivity reaction (changes in facial skin color, rash, dyspnea, swelling around eyes, wheezing). If these occur, inform physician promptly. Keep epinephrine, an antihistamine, and resuscitation equipment close by in the event of an anaphylactic reaction.
- ◻ Inquire about recent streptococcal infection. Anistreplase may be less effective if administered within 5 days–6 mo of a streptococcal infection.
- **Coronary Thrombosis:** Monitor ECG continuously. Notify physician if significant arrhythmias occur. Cardiac enzymes should be monitored. Radionucleotide myocardial scanning and/or coronary angiography may be ordered 7–10 days following therapy.
- **Lab Test Considerations:** Hematocrit, hemoglobin, platelet count, prothrombin time, thrombin time, bleeding time, and activated partial thromboplastin time should be evaluated prior to and frequently throughout therapy. Fibrinogen degradation products (FDPs) may also be monitored prior to and following therapy.
- ◻ Obtain type and crossmatch and have blood available at all times in case of hemorrhage.
- **Toxicity and Overdose:** If local bleeding occurs, apply pressure to site. If severe or internal bleeding occurs, clotting factors and/or blood volume may be restored through infusions of whole blood, packed red blood cells, fresh frozen plasma, cryoprecipitate, platelets, and/or desmopressin. Do not administer dextran as it has antiplatelet activity. If heparin is being administered, discontinue and consider administration of protamine. Aminocaproic acid (Amicar) may be used as an antidote.

POTENTIAL NURSING DIAGNOSES

- Tissue perfusion, altered (indications).
- Injury, high risk for (side effects).
- Knowledge deficit related to medication regimen (patient/family teaching).

IMPLEMENTATION

- **General Info:** Invasive procedures, such as IM injections or arterial punctures, should be avoided with this therapy. If such procedures must be performed, apply pressure to IV puncture sites for at least 15 min and to arterial puncture sites for at least 30 min.
- ◻ Systemic anticoagulation with heparin is usually begun several hours after the completion of thrombolytic therapy. Aspirin may also be used to inhibit platelet aggregation.
- ◻ Acetaminophen may be ordered to control fever.
- **Direct IV:** Reconstitute with 5 ml of Sterile Water for Injection (direct to sides of vial) and swirl gently; do not shake to minimize foaming. Do not dilute further. Solution is colorless to transparent pale yellow. Use reconstituted solution within 30 min of preparation.
- *Rate:* Administer via IV line or vein over 2–5 min.

- **Y-Site/Additive Incompatibility:** Do not admix or administer via Y-site injection with any other medication.

PATIENT/FAMILY TEACHING

□ Explain purpose of the medication. Instruct patient to report hypersensitivity reactions (rash, dyspnea), bleeding, or bruising.
□ Explain need for bedrest and minimal handling during therapy to avoid injury.

EVALUATION

Effectiveness of therapy may be determined by: ▪ Lysis of thrombi with restoration of coronary blood flow.

ANTIHEMOPHILIC FACTOR
AHF-M, Factor VIII S.D., Hemofil M, Humate P, Koate HP, Kogenate, Monoclate P, Profilate OSD, Recombinate

CLASSIFICATION(S):
Hemostatic, Blood derivative
Pregnancy Category C

INDICATIONS

- Management of hemophilia A associated with a deficiency of factor VIII.

ACTION

- An essential clotting factor required for the conversion of prothrombin to thrombin. **Therapeutic Effect:** ▪ Correction of deficiency states with resultant control of excessive bleeding.

PHARMACOKINETICS

Absorption: Following IV administration absorption is essentially complete.
Distribution: Rapidly cleared from plasma. Does not cross the placenta.
Metabolism and Excretion: Used up in the clotting process.
Half-life: 4–24 hr (12 hr average).

CONTRAINDICATIONS AND PRECAUTIONS

Contraindicated in: ▪ Hypersensitivity to hamster protein (Kogenate, Recombinate only).
Use Cautiously in: ▪ Pregnancy (safety not established).

ADVERSE REACTIONS AND SIDE EFFECTS*

CNS: headache, somnolence, lethargy, loss of consciousness.
EENT: visual disturbances.
CV: tachycardia, hypotension, chest tightness.
GI: nausea, vomiting.
Hemat: intravascular hemolysis.
Derm: flushing, urticaria.
MS: back pain.
Neuro: paresthesia.
Misc: rigor, jaundice, allergic reactions, hepatitis B or HIV virus infection (small risk from frequent use of large amounts).

INTERACTIONS

Drug–Drug: ▪ None significant.

ROUTE AND DOSAGE

Dosage is determined by levels of antihemophilic factor.

Joint Hemorrhage

- **IV (Adults and Children):** 5–10 units/kg q 8–12 hr for 1 or more days.

Minor Hemorrhage into Nonvital Areas

- **IV (Adults and Children):** 8–10 units/kg q 24 hr for 2–3 days or 8 units/kg q 12 hr for 2 days, then q 24 hr for 2 more days.

Hemorrhage into Muscles near Vital Organs

- **IV (Adults and Children):** 15 units/kg initially, then 8 units/kg q 8 hr for 48 hr, then 4 units/kg q 8 hr for 48 hr.

Overt Bleeding

- **IV (Adults and Children):** 15–25 units/kg initially, then 8–15 units/kg q 8–12 hr for 3–4 days.

Hemorrhage from Massive Wounds or Vital Organs

- **IV (Adults and Children):** 40–50 units/kg initially, then 20–25 units/kg q 8–12 hr.

*Underlines indicate most frequent; **CAPITALS** indicate life-threatening.

Major Surgical Procedures
- IV (Adults and Children): 26–30 units/kg before surgery, then 15 units/kg q 5–8 hr postoperatively.

Prophylaxis of Hemophilia A
- IV (Patients >50 kg): 500 units daily.
- IV (Patients <50 kg): 250 units daily.

AVAILABILITY
- *Injection:* 250-unit, 500-unit, 750-unit, 1000-unit, 1500-unit vials.

TIME/ACTION PROFILE (levels of factor VIII)

	ONSET	PEAK	DURATION
IV	rapid	UK	8–12 hr

NURSING IMPLICATIONS

Assessment
- □ Monitor blood pressure, pulse, and respirations. If tachycardia occurs, slow or stop infusion rate and notify physician.
- □ Obtain history of current trauma; estimate amount of blood loss.
- □ Monitor for renewed bleeding every 15–30 min. Immobilize and apply ice to affected joints.
- □ Monitor intake and output ratios; note color of urine. Notify physician of significant discrepancy or if urine becomes red or orange. Patients with types A, B, and AB blood are particularly at risk for hemolytic reaction.
- □ Assess for allergic reaction (wheezing, tachycardia, urticaria, hives, chest tightness, stinging at IV site, nausea and vomiting, lethargy). Stop infusion, notify physician.
- Lab Test Considerations: Obtain baseline and periodic CBC, direct Coombs', urinalysis, partial thromboplastin time (PTT), thromboplastin generation test, and prothrombin generation test. Decreased hematocrit and increased Coombs' test may indicate hemolytic anemia.
- □ Monitor coagulation studies before, during, and after therapy to assess effectiveness of therapy.

- □ Patients with increased inhibitor levels may not respond or may require increased doses.

Potential Nursing Diagnoses
- Tissue perfusion, altered (indications).
- Injury, high risk for (indications).
- Knowledge deficit related to medication regimen (patient/family teaching).

Implementation
- General Info: Inform all personnel of bleeding tendency to prevent further trauma. Apply pressure to all venipuncture sites for at least 5 min; avoid all IM injections.
- □ Premedication with diphenhydramine (Benadryl) may prevent acute reactions.
- □ Dosage varies with degree of clotting factor deficit, desired level of clotting factors, and weight.
- □ Obtain type and crossmatch of blood in case a transfusion is necessary.
- □ To prevent spontaneous bleeding, at least 5% of the normal Factor VIII level must be present. To control moderate bleeding or prior to minor surgery, 30–50% must be present. For severe bleeding associated with trauma, or patient undergoing major surgery, 80–100% of the normal Factor VIII level must be present.
- □ The first dose of antihemophilic factor is given 1 hr before surgery. The second dose (half of the first dose) is given 5–8 hr postoperatively. Factor VIII level must be maintained at 30% of the normal level for 10–14 days postoperatively.
- IV: Administer IV only. Refrigerate concentrate until just prior to reconstitution. Warm concentrate and diluent (provided by manufacturer) to room temperature before reconstituting. Use plastic syringe for preparation and administration. Use an additional needle as an air vent to the vial when reconstituting. After adding diluent rotate vial gently until completely dissolved. Solution may vary

in color from light yellow to clear with a bluish tint. Do not refrigerate after reconstitution; use within 3 hr. Preparations should be filtered prior to administration.

■ **Direct IV:** May be administered by slow IV push (see Intermittent Infusion for rates).

■ **Intermittent Infusion:** Administration rate is based on antihemophilic factor (AHF) units/ml and patient response. Monoclate-P or Humate-P should be administered at 2 or 4 ml/min respectively. Antihemophilic Factor (Human), Hemofil M, and Profilate should be administered at a rate not to exceed 10 ml/min. Concentrations of less than 34 AHF units/ml may be administered at a rate of 10–20 ml over 3 min. Infusion rate should not exceed 10 ml/min.

■ **Additive Incompatibility:** ■ Do not admix.

PATIENT/FAMILY TEACHING

□ Instruct patient to notify nurse immediately if bleeding recurs.

□ Advise patient to observe for bleeding of gums, skin, urine, stool, or emesis.

□ Advise patient to carry identification describing disease process at all times.

□ Caution patient to avoid aspirin- or ibuprofen-containing products as they may further impair clotting.

□ Review prevention of bleeding with patient (use of soft toothbrush, avoid IM and SC injections, avoid potentially traumatic activities).

□ Advise patient that the risk of hepatitis or AIDS transmission may be diminished by the use of heat-treated or monoclonal antibody preparations. Current screening programs should decrease the risk.

EVALUATION

Effectiveness of therapy can be demonstrated by: ■ Prevention of spontaneous bleeding ■ Cessation of bleeding.

ASCORBIC ACID
(as-**kor**-bik **as**-id)
{Apo-C}, Ascorbicap, Cecon, Cemill, Cetane, Cevalin, Ce-Vi-Sol, Flavorcee, {Kamu-Jay}, Sunkist Vitamin C

CLASSIFICATION(S):
Vitamin (water-soluble)
Pregnancy Category C

INDICATIONS

■ Treatment/prevention of vitamin C deficiency (scurvy) with dietary supplementation ■ Supplemental therapy in some GI diseases, during long-term parenteral nutrition or chronic hemodialysis ■ States of increased requirements such as: □ Pregnancy □ Lactation □ Stress □ Hyperthyroidism □ Trauma □ Burns □ Infancy. **Unlabeled Uses:** ■ Urinary acidification ■ Prevention of the common cold.

ACTION

■ Necessary for collagen formation and tissue repair ■ Involved in oxidation-reduction reactions; tyrosine, folic acid, iron, and carbohydrate metabolism; lipid and protein synthesis; cellular respiration; and resisting infection. **Therapeutic Effect:** ■ Replacement in deficiency states ■ Supplementation during increased requirements.

PHARMACOKINETICS

Absorption: Actively absorbed following oral administration by a saturable process.
Distribution: Widely distributed. Crosses the placenta; enters breast milk.
Metabolism and Excretion: Oxidized to inactive compounds that are excreted by the kidneys. When serum levels are high, unchanged ascorbic acid is excreted by the kidneys.
Half-life: UK.

{} = Available in Canada only.

CONTRAINDICATIONS AND PRECAUTIONS

Contraindicated in: ▪ Tartrazine hypersensitivity (some products contain tartrazine—FDC yellow dye #5).
Use Cautiously in: ▪ Recurrent kidney stones ▪ Avoid chronic use of large doses in pregnant women.

ADVERSE REACTIONS AND SIDE EFFECTS*

CNS: fatigue, headache, insomnia, drowsiness.
GI: nausea, vomiting, heartburn, cramps, diarrhea.
GU: kidney stones.
Derm: flushing.
Hemat: deep vein thrombosis, sickle cell crises, hemolysis (in G6-PD deficiency).
Local: pain at SC or IM sites.

INTERACTIONS

Drug–Drug: ▪ If urinary acidification occurs, may increase excretion and decrease effects of **mexiletine, amphetamines,** or **tricyclic antidepressants** ▪ May decrease response to **oral anticoagulants** (large doses only) ▪ **Smoking, salicylates,** and **primidone** may increase requirements for ascorbic acid ▪ Increases iron toxicity when given concurrently with **deferoxamine.**

ROUTE AND DOSAGE

Scurvy
▪ **PO, IV, IM, SC (Adults):** 100–250 mg 1–3 times daily.
▪ **PO, IV, IM, SC (Children):** 100–300 mg/day in divided doses.

Supplementation
▪ **PO (Adults):** 45–60 mg/day.

Chronic Hemodialysis
▪ **PO (Adults):** 100–200 mg/day.

Pregnancy and Lactation
▪ **PO (Adults):** 60–80 mg/day.

Other States of Increased Requirements
▪ **PO (Adults):** 150–500 mg/day.

AVAILABILITY

▪ *Chewable tablets:* 60 mg, 100 mg, 250 mg, 500 mg, 1 g ▪ *Tablets:* 50 mg, 100 mg, 250 mg, 500 mg, 1 g, 1.5 g ▪ *Extended-release tablets:* {100 mg}, {200 mg}, 500 mg, 1 g, 1.5 g ▪ *Extended-release capsules:* 500 mg ▪ *Solution:* 35 mg/0.6 ml, 100 mg/ml ▪ *Syrup:* 500 mg/5 ml ▪ *Injection:* 100 mg/ml, {200 mg/ml}, 250 mg/ml, 500 mg/ml ▪ *In combination with:* other vitamins and minerals in multivitamin preparations.

TIME/ACTION PROFILE (response to skeletal and hemorrhagic changes in scurvy)

	ONSET	PEAK	DURATION
PO, IM, IV, SC	2 days–3 wk	UK	UK

NURSING IMPLICATIONS

ASSESSMENT
▪ **Vitamin C Deficiency:** Assess for signs of vitamin C deficiency (faulty bone and tooth development, gingivitis, bleeding gums, loosened teeth) before and during therapy. Vitamin C deficiency is also called scurvy.
▪ **Lab Test Considerations:** Megadoses of ascorbic acid (>10 times the RDA requirement) may cause false-negative results for occult blood in the stool, false-positive urine glucose test results with copper sulfate method (Clinitest), and false-negative urine glucose test results with glucose enzymatic tests (Tes-Tape).
  □ May cause decreased serum bilirubin and increased urine oxalate, urate, and cysteine levels.
  □ *Urinary Acidification*—Monitor the urinary pH of patients receiving ascorbic acid for urinary acidification periodically throughout therapy.

POTENTIAL NURSING DIAGNOSES
▪ Nutrition, altered: less than body requirements (indications).
▪ Knowledge deficit related to medica-

---

*Underlines indicate most frequent; **CAPITALS** indicate life-threatening.

tion regimen (patient/family teaching).

IMPLEMENTATION

- **General Info:** Often ordered as a part of multivitamin supplementation, because inadequate diet often results in multiple-vitamin deficiency.
- **PO:** Extended-release tablets and capsules should be swallowed whole without crushing, breaking, or chewing; contents of capsules may be mixed with jelly or jam. Chewable tablets should be chewed well or crushed before swallowing. Oral solution may be mixed with fruit juice, cereal, or other food.
- **IM:** May be preferred route due to increased absorption and utilization.
- **Direct IV:** Ascorbic acid may be administered IV undiluted at a rate of 100 mg over at least 1 min. Rapid IV administration may result in temporary dizziness and fainting.
- **Intermittent Infusion:** Dilute with D5W, D10W, 0.9% NaCl, 0.45% NaCl, lactated Ringer's or Ringer's solution, dextrose/saline or dextrose/Ringer's combinations. At room temperature, pressure in ampules may increase; wrap with protective cover before breaking.
- **Syringe Compatibility:** • metoclopramide.
- **Syringe Incompatibility:** • cefazolin • doxapram.
- **Additive Compatibility:** • amikacin • calcium chloride • calcium gluceptate • calcium gluconate • cephalothin • chloramphenicol • chlorpromazine • colistimethate • cyanocobalamin • diphenhydramine • heparin • kanamycin • methicillin • methyldopate • penicillin G potassium • polymyxin B • prednisolone • procaine • prochlorperazine • promethazine • verapamil.
- **Additive Incompatibility:** • bleomycin • cephapirin • nafcillin • sodium bicarbonate.

PATIENT/FAMILY TEACHING

- **General Info:** Advise patient to take this medication as directed and not to exceed dose prescribed. Excess dosage may lead to urinary stone formation. If a dose is missed, skip dose and return to dosage schedule.
- **Vitamin C Deficiency:** Encourage patient to comply with physician's diet recommendations. Explain that the best source of vitamins is a well-balanced diet.
  □ Foods high in ascorbic acid include citrus fruits, tomatoes, strawberries, cantaloupe, and raw peppers. Gradual loss of ascorbic acid occurs when fresh food is stored, but not when frozen. Rapid loss is caused by drying, salting, and cooking.
  □ Patients self-medicating with vitamin supplements should be cautioned not to exceed RDA (see Appendix L). The effectiveness of megadoses of vitamins for treatment of various medical conditions is unproven and may cause side effects. Abrupt withdrawal of megadoses of ascorbic acid may cause rebound deficiency.
- **Urinary Acidification:** Teach patients taking vitamin C for urinary acidification how to check urine pH.

EVALUATION

Effectiveness of therapy may be determined by: • Decrease in the symptoms of ascorbic acid deficiency • Acidification of the urine.

ASPARAGINASE
(a-**spare**-a-gin-ase)
colaspase, Elspar, {Kidrolase}

CLASSIFICATION(S):
Antineoplastic (enzyme)
Pregnancy Category C

INDICATIONS

- Part of combination chemotherapy in the treatment of acute lymphocytic leukemia (ALL) unresponsive to first-line agents.

ACTION

▪ Catalyst in the conversion of asparagine (an amino acid) to aspartic acid and ammonia ▪ Depletes asparagine in leukemic cells. **Therapeutic Effect:** ▪ Death of leukemic cells.

PHARMACOKINETICS

Absorption: Not absorbed from the GI tract. Is absorbed from IM sites.
Distribution: Mostly remains in the intravascular space. Poor penetration into the CSF.
Metabolism and Excretion: Slowly sequestered in the reticuloendothelial system.
Half-life: IV—8–30 hr; IM—39–49 hr.

CONTRAINDICATIONS AND PRECAUTIONS

Contraindicated in: ▪ Previous hypersensitivity.
Use Cautiously in: ▪ History of hypersensitivity reactions ▪ Severe liver disease ▪ Renal disease ▪ Pancreatic disease ▪ CNS depression ▪ Clotting abnormalities ▪ Patients with child-bearing potential ▪ Chronic debilitating illnesses.

ADVERSE REACTIONS AND SIDE EFFECTS*

CNS: depression, somnolence, fatigue, SEIZURES, coma, headache, confusion, irritability, agitation, dizziness, hallucinations.
GI: nausea, vomiting, anorexia, cramps, weight loss, pancreatitis, hepatotoxicity.
Derm: rashes, urticaria.
Endo: hyperglycemia.
Hemat: coagulation abnormalities, transient bone marrow depression.
Metab: hyperuricemia, hyperammonemia.
Misc: hypersensitivity reactions including ANAPHYLAXIS.

INTERACTIONS

Drug–Drug: ▪ May negate the antineoplastic activity of **methotrexate** ▪ May enhance the hepatotoxicity of other **hepatotoxic drugs** ▪ Additive hyperglycemia with **glucocorticoids** ▪ Concurrent IV use with or immediately preceding **vincristine** may result in increased neurotoxicity.

ROUTE AND DOSAGE

Various other regimens may be used.

Multiple Agent Induction Regimen (in combination with vincristine and prednisone)
▪ **IV (Children):** 1000 IU/kg/day for 10 successive days beginning on day 22 of regimen.
▪ **IM (Children):** 6000 IU/m^2 on days 4, 7, 10, 13, 16, 19, 22, 25, 28.

Single-Agent Therapy for Acute Lymphocytic Leukemia
▪ **IV (Adults and Children):** 200 IU/kg daily for 28 days.

Desensitization Regimen
▪ **IV (Adults and Children):** Administer 1 IU then double dose every 10 min until total dose for that day has been given or reaction occurs.

Test Dose
▪ **Intradermal (Adults and Children):** 2 IU.

AVAILABILITY

▪ *Injection:* 10,000 IU-vial.

TIME/ACTION PROFILE (depletion of asparagine)

	ONSET	PEAK*	DURATION
IM	immediate	14–24 hr	23–33 days
IV	immediate	UK	23–33 days

*Plasma levels of asparaginase.

NURSING IMPLICATIONS

ASSESSMENT
□ Monitor vital signs prior to and fre-

---

quently during therapy. Inform physician if fever or chills occur.

□ Monitor intake and output. Notify physician of significant discrepancies. Encourage patient to drink 2000–3000 ml/day to promote excretion of uric acid. Allopurinol and alkalinization of the urine may be used to prevent urate stone formation.

□ Monitor for hypersensitivity reaction (urticaria, diaphoresis, facial swelling, joint pain, hypotension, bronchospasm). Epinephrine and resuscitation equipment should be readily available. Reaction may occur up to 2 hr after administration.

□ Assess nausea, vomiting, and appetite. Weigh weekly. Confer with physician regarding an antiemetic prior to administration.

□ Monitor affect and neurologic status. Notify physician if depression, drowsiness, or hallucinations occur. Symptoms usually resolve 2–3 days after drug is discontinued.

■ **Lab Test Considerations:** Monitor CBC prior to and periodically throughout therapy. May alter coagulation studies. Platelets, PT, PTT, and thrombin time may be increased. May cause elevated BUN.

□ Hepatotoxity may be manifested by increased AST (SGOT), ALT (SGPT), alkaline phosphatase, bilirubin, or cholesterol. Liver function tests usually return to normal after therapy. May cause pancreatitis; monitor for elevated amylase or glucose.

□ May cause decreased serum calcium.

□ May cause elevated serum and urine uric acid concentrations.

□ May interfere with thyroid function tests.

POTENTIAL NURSING DIAGNOSES

■ Injury, high risk for (side effects).
■ Infection, high risk for (side effects).
■ Knowledge deficit related to medication regimen (patient/family teaching).

IMPLEMENTATION

■ **General Info:** Solution should be prepared in a biologic cabinet. Wear gloves, gown, and mask while handling medication. Discard equipment in specially designated containers (see Appendix I).

□ If coagulopathy develops, apply pressure to venipuncture sites; avoid IM injections.

■ **Test Dose:** Intradermal test dose must be performed prior to initial dose, and doses must be separated by more than 1 wk. Reconstitute vial with 5 ml of Sterile Water for Injection or 0.9% NaCl for injection (without preservatives). Add 0.1 ml of this 2000 IU/ml solution to 9.9 ml additional diluent to yield a 20 IU/ml solution. Inject 0.1 ml (2 IU) intradermally. Observe site for 1 hr for formation of wheal. Wheal is indicative of a positive reaction. Desensitization therapy may be used.

■ **Desensitization Therapy:** Begin by administering 1 IU every 10 min IV. Double dose every 10 min if hypersensitivity does not occur until full daily dose is administered.

■ **IM:** Prepare for IM dose by adding 2 ml of 0.9% NaCl for injection (without preservatives) to the 10,000-IU vial. Shake vial gently. Administer no more than 2 ml per injection site.

■ **Direct IV:** Prepare IV dose by diluting 10,000-IU vial with 5 ml of Sterile Water for Injection or 0.9% NaCl (without preservatives). If gelatinous fibers are present, administration through a 5-micron filter will not alter potency. Administration through a 0.2-micron filter may cause loss of potency. Solution should be clear after reconstitution. Discard if cloudy. Stable for 8 hr if refrigerated.

■ *Rate:* Administer through Y-site of rapidly flowing IV of D5W or 0.9% NaCl over at least 30 min. Maintain IV infusion for 2 hr after dose.

PATIENT/FAMILY TEACHING

□ Instruct patient to notify physician if abdominal pain, severe nausea and vomiting, jaundice, fever, chills, sore throat, bleeding or bruising, excess thirst or urination, or mouth sores occur. Caution patient to avoid crowds

and persons with known infections. Instruct patient to use soft toothbrush, electric razor, and to avoid falls. Patients should also be cautioned not to drink alcoholic beverages or take medication containing aspirin or ibuprofen, because these may precipitate gastric bleeding.
□ Advise patient of the need for contraception.
□ Instruct patient not to receive any vaccinations without advice of physician. Advise parents that this may alter immunization schedule.
□ Emphasize need for periodic lab test to monitor for side effects.

EVALUATION
Effectiveness of therapy can be demonstrated by: ▪ Improvement of hematologic status in patients with leukemia.

ASPIRIN
(as-pir-in)
acetylsalicylic acid, {Apo-ASA}, {Apo-Asen}, {Arthrinol}, {Arthrisin}, {Artria S.R., Aspirgum, ASA, {Astrin}, Bayer Aspirin, Bayer Timed-Release Arthritic Pain Formula {Coryphen}, Easprin, Ecotrin, 8-Hour Bayer Timed-Release, Empirin, {Entrophen} Genprin, Halfprin, {Headstart}, Measurin, Norwich Aspirin, {Riphen}, {Sal-Adult}, {Sal-Infant}, St. Joseph Adult Chewable Aspirin, Therapy Bayer, ZORprin

CLASSIFICATION(S):
Nonopioid analgesic, Nonsteroidal anti-inflammatory agent, Antipyretic, Antiplatelet agent
Pregnancy Category D

INDICATIONS
▪ Management of inflammatory disorders including: □ Rheumatoid arthritis □ Osteoarthritis ▪ Treatment of mild to moderate pain ▪ Treatment of fever ▪ Prophylaxis of transient ischemic attacks ▪ Prophylaxis of myocardial infarction.

ACTION
▪ Produces analgesia and reduces inflammation and fever by inhibiting the production of prostaglandins. ▪ Decreases platelet aggregation. **Therapeutic Effects:** ▪ Analgesia ▪ Reduction of inflammation ▪ Reduction of fever ▪ Decreased incidence of transient ischemic attacks and myocardial infarction

PHARMACOKINETICS
Absorption: Well absorbed from the upper small intestine. Absorption from enteric-coated preparations may be unreliable. Rectal absorption is slow and variable.
Distribution: Rapidly and widely distributed. Crosses the placenta and enters breast milk.
Metabolism and Excretion: Extensively metabolized by the liver. Inactive metabolites excreted by the kidneys.
Half-life: 2–3 hr for low doses (up to 15–30 hr with large doses).

CONTRAINDICATIONS AND PRECAUTIONS
Contraindicated in: ▪ Hypersensitivity to aspirin, tartrazine (FDC yellow dye #5), or other salicylates ▪ Cross-sensitivity with other nonsteroidal anti-inflammatory agents may exist ▪ Bleeding disorders or thrombocytopenia.
Use Cautiously in: ▪ History of GI bleeding or ulcer disease ▪ Severe renal or hepatic disease ▪ Pregnancy (may have adverse effects on fetus and mother) ▪ Lactation (safety not established) ▪ Self-medication for more than 10 days in adults or 5 days in children without medical supervision.

ADVERSE REACTIONS AND SIDE EFFECTS*
EENT: tinnitus, hearing loss.
GI: dyspepsia, heartburn, epigastric distress, nausea, vomiting, anorexia, abdominal pain, GI bleeding, hepatotoxicity.

{} = Available in Canada only.
*Underlines indicate most frequent; **CAPITALS** indicate life-threatening.

Hemat: anemia, hemolysis.
Misc: noncardiogenic pulmonary edema, allergic reactions including ANAPHYLAXIS and LARYNGEAL EDEMA.

INTERACTIONS

Drug–Drug: ▪ May potentiate oral anticoagulants, heparin, or thrombolytic agents ▪ May enhance the activity of penicillins, phenytoin, methotrexate, valproic acid, oral hypoglycemic agents, and sulfonamides ▪ May antagonize the beneficial effects of probenecid or sulfinpyrazone ▪ Glucocorticoids may decrease serum salicylate levels ▪ Urinary acidification enhances reabsorption and may increase serum salicylate levels ▪ Alkalinization of the urine or the ingestion of large amounts of antacids promotes excretion and decreases serum salicylate levels ▪ May blunt the therapeutic response to diuretics, antihypertensives, or nonsteroidal anti-inflammatory agents ▪ May increase the risk of bleeding with cefamandole, cefoperazone, cefotetan, valproic acid, or plicamycin ▪ Increased risk of gastrointestinal irritation with nonsteroidal anti-inflammatory agents ▪ Increased risk of ototoxicity with vancomycin.

Drug–Food: ▪ Foods capable of acidifying the urine (see Appendix K) may increase serum salicylate levels.

ROUTE AND DOSAGE

Analgesia and Antipyresis
▪ **PO, Rect (Adults):** 325–1000 mg q 4–6 hr as needed (not to exceed 4 g/day).
▪ **PO, Rect (Children 2–11 yr):** 60–80 mg/kg/day in 4–6 divided doses.

Anti-inflammatory
▪ **PO (Adults):** 2.6–6.2 g/day in divided doses.
▪ **PO (Children):** 60–110 mg/kg/day in divided doses (smaller doses have been used).

Prevention of Transient Ischemic Attacks
▪ **PO (Adults):** 1.3 g daily in 2–4 divided doses.

Prevention of Myocardial Infarction
▪ **PO (Adults):** 300–325 mg/day (smaller doses have been used).

Kawasaki Disease
▪ **PO (Children):** 80–180 mg/kg/day.

AVAILABILITY
▪ *Tablets:* 325 mg, 500 mg, 650 mg, {975 mg} ▪ *Chewing gum:* 227 mg ▪ {*Dispersible tablets:* 325 mg, 500 mg} ▪ *Enteric-coated (delayed-release) tablets:* 80 mg, 165 mg, {300 mg}, 325 mg, 500 mg, {600 mg}, 650 mg, 975 mg ▪ *Timed-release tablets:* 650 mg ▪ *Controlled-release tablets:* 800 mg ▪ {*Delayed-release capsules:* 325 mg, 500 mg} ▪ *Suppositories:* 60 mg, 120 mg, 125 mg, 130 mg, {150 mg}, {160 mg}, 195 mg, 200 mg, 300 mg, {320 mg}, 325 mg, 600 mg, {640 mg}, 650 mg, 1.2 g ▪ *In combination with:* antihistamines, decongestants, cough suppressants. See Appendix A.

TIME/ACTION PROFILE

	ONSET	PEAK	DURATION
PO	5–30 min	1–3 hr	3–6 hr
Rect	1–2 hr	4–5 hr	7 hr

NURSING IMPLICATIONS

ASSESSMENT
▪ **General Info:** Patients who have asthma, allergies, and nasal polyps or who are allergic to tartrazine are at an increased risk for developing hypersensitivity reactions.
▪ **Pain:** Assess pain and limitation of movement; note type, location, and intensity prior to and 30–60 min following administration.
▪ **Fever:** Assess fever and note associated signs (diaphoresis, tachycardia, malaise, chills).
▪ **Lab Test Considerations:** Aspirin prolongs bleeding time for 4–7 days and, in large doses, may cause prolonged prothrombin time, false-negative urine glucose test results with glucose enzymatic tests (Clinistix, Tes-Tape), and false-positive urine

glucose test results with copper sulfate method (Clinitest).

- **Toxicity and Overdose:** Monitor patient for the onset of tinnitus, hyperventilation, agitation, mental confusion, lethargy, diarrhea, and sweating. If these symptoms appear, withhold medication and notify physician immediately.

POTENTIAL NURSING DIAGNOSES

- Pain (indications).
- Physical mobility, impaired (indications).
- Knowledge deficit related to medication regimen (patient/family teaching).

IMPLEMENTATION

- **PO:** Administer aspirin after meals or with food or an antacid to minimize gastric irritation. Food slows but will not alter the total amount absorbed.
- Do not crush or chew enteric-coated tablets. Do not take antacids within 1–2 hr of enteric-coated tablets. Chewable tablets may be chewed, dissolved in liquid, or swallowed whole. Some extended-release tablets may be broken or crumbled but must not be ground up before swallowing. See manufacturer's prescribing information for individual products.

PATIENT/FAMILY TEACHING

- **General Info:** Instruct patient to take aspirin with a full glass of water and to remain in an upright position for 15–30 min after administration.
- Advise patient to report tinnitus, unusual bleeding of gums, bruising, black, tarry stools, or fever lasting longer than 3 days.
- Caution patient to avoid concurrent use of alcohol with this medication to minimize possible gastric irritation.
- Teach patients on a sodium-restricted diet to avoid effervescent tablets or buffered-aspirin preparations.
- Tablets with an acetic (vinegar-like) odor should be discarded.
- Advise patients on long-term therapy to inform physician or dentist of medication regimen prior to surgery. Aspirin may need to be withheld for 1 wk prior to surgery.
- Centers for Disease Control warn against giving aspirin to children or adolescents with varicella (chickenpox), or influenza-like or viral illnesses because of a possible association with Reye's syndrome.
- **Transient Ischemic Attacks or Myocardial Infarction:** Advise patients receiving aspirin prophylactically to take only prescribed dosage. Increasing the dosage has not been found to provide additional benefits.

EVALUATION

Effectiveness of therapy can be demonstrated by: ▪ Relief of mild to moderate discomfort ▪ Increased ease of joint movement ▪ Reduction of fever ▪ Prevention of transient ischemic attacks ▪ Prevention of myocardial infarction.

ASTEMIZOLE
(a-**stem**-mi-zole)
Hismanyl

CLASSIFICATION(S):
Antihistamine
Pregnancy Category C

INDICATIONS

- Symptomatic relief of allergic symptoms (rhinitis, urticaria) caused by histamine release ▪ May be less sedating than other antihistamines.

ACTION

- Blocks the following effects of histamine: □ Vasodilation □ Increased GI tract secretions □ Increased heart rate □ Hypotension. **Therapeutic Effect:** ▪ Relief of symptoms associated with histamine excess usually seen in allergic conditions. Does not block the release of histamine.

PHARMACOKINETICS

Absorption: Well absorbed following oral administration.
Distribution: Distribution not known.

A

Metabolism and Excretion: Extensively metabolized by the liver, partially converted to desmethylastemizole, which has antihistaminic activity. **Half-life:** 100 hr—astemizole; 12 days —desmethylastemizole.

CONTRAINDICATIONS AND PRECAUTIONS

Contraindicated in: ▪ Hypersensitivity ▪ Acute attacks of asthma ▪ Lactation (avoid use) ▪ Significant hepatic dysfunction ▪ Patients taking ketoconazole, itraconazole, or erythromycin ▪ History of synape during previous astemizole therapy.

Use Cautiously in: ▪ Narrow-angle glaucoma ▪ Liver disease ▪ Elderly patients (more susceptible to adverse reactions) ▪ Pregnancy or children <12 yr (safety not established) ▪ Underlying cardiovascular disease.

ADVERSE REACTIONS AND SIDE EFFECTS*

CNS: drowsiness, ataxia, dizziness, inability to concentrate, headache, fatigue, stimulation, syncope.
CVS: arrhythmias.
EENT: conjunctivitis, pharyngitis.
Resp: cough.
GI: dry mouth, nausea, diarrhea, abdominal pain, flatulence, increased appetite.
Derm: rash, eczema.
MS: joint pain.
Misc: weight gain.

INTERACTIONS

Drug–Drug: ▪ Concurrent **ketoconazole, itraconazole, clarithromycin, azithromycin,** or **erythromycin** increases the risk of cardiac arrhythmias ▪ Additive CNS depression with other **CNS depressants** including **alcohol, opioid analgesics,** and **sedative/hypnotics** ▪ **MAO inhibitors** intensify and prolong the anticholinergic effects of antihistamines.
Drug–Food: ▪ **Food** decreases the absorption of astemizole.

ROUTE AND DOSAGE
▪ **PO (Adults):** 10 mg/day.

AVAILABILITY
▪ **Tablets:** 10 mg.

TIME/ACTION PROFILE
(antihistaminic effects)

	ONSET	PEAK	DURATION
PO	2–3 days	UK	up to several wk

NURSING IMPLICATIONS

ASSESSMENT
▫ Assess allergy symptoms (rhinitis, conjunctivitis, hives) prior to and periodically throughout therapy.
▫ Assess lung sounds and character of bronchial secretions. Maintain fluid intake of 1500–2000 ml/day to decrease viscosity of secretions.
▪ **Lab Test Considerations:** May cause false-negative allergy skin testing.

POTENTIAL NURSING DIAGNOSES
▪ Airway clearance, ineffective (indications).
▪ Injury, high risk for (adverse reactions).
▪ Knowledge deficit related to medication regimen (patient/family teaching).

IMPLEMENTATION
▪ **PO:** Administer on an empty stomach.

PATIENT/FAMILY TEACHING
▫ Instruct patient to take medication at least 1 hr before or 2 hr after eating.
▫ May cause drowsiness. Caution patient to avoid driving or other activities requiring alertness until response to medication is known.
▫ Discuss possibility of increased appetite. Patients on chronic therapy may need to limit caloric intake and increase activity to avoid undesired weight gain.
▫ Advise patient that good oral hygiene, frequent rinsing of mouth with water, and sugarless gum or candy may minimize dry mouth. Patient should no-

tify dentist if dry mouth persists >2 wk.
- □ Instruct patient to contact physician if symptoms persist.

EVALUATION
Effectiveness of therapy may be determined by: ▪ Decrease in allergic symptoms.

ATENOLOL
(a-**ten**-oh-lole)
{Apo-Atenolol}, Tenormin

CLASSIFICATION(S):
Antihypertensive (beta-adrenergic blocker), Beta-adrenergic blocker (selective), Antianginal
Pregnancy Category C

INDICATIONS

▪ **PO:** Treatment of hypertension, alone or with other agents ▪ Management of angina pectoris ▪ **PO, IV:** Prevention of myocardial infarction. **Unlabeled Uses:** ▪ Management of arrhythmias, hypertrophic cardiomyopathy, mitral valve prolapse, pheochromocytoma, vascular headache, tremors, thyrotoxicosis.

ACTION

▪ Blocks stimulation of $beta_1$ (myocardial) adrenergic receptors. Does not usually effect $beta_2$ (pulmonary, vascular, or uterine) receptor sites. **Therapeutic Effects:** ▪ Decreased heart rate ▪ Decreased blood pressure ▪ Prevention of myocardial infarction.

PHARMACOKINETICS

Absorption: Incompletely absorbed from the GI tract (50–60%).
Distribution: Does not significantly cross the blood–brain barrier. Crosses the placenta and enters breast milk.
Metabolism and Excretion: 40–50% excreted unchanged by the kidneys. Remainder excreted in the feces as unabsorbed drug.
Half-life: 6–9 hr.

CONTRAINDICATIONS AND PRECAUTIONS

Contraindicated in: ▪ Uncompensated congestive heart failure ▪ Pulmonary edema ▪ Cardiogenic shock ▪ Bradycardia ▪ Heart block ▪ Lactation.
Use Cautiously in: ▪ Thyrotoxicosis (may mask symptoms) ▪ Diabetes mellitus (may mask symptoms of hypoglycemia) ▪ Renal impairment (dosage reduction required if creatinine clearance <35 ml/min/1.73 m^2) ▪ Pregnancy and children—neonatal, bradycardia, hypotension, hypoglycemia, and respiratory depression may occur (safety not established) ▪ Patients with a history of severe allergic reactions (intensity of reactions may be increased).

ADVERSE REACTIONS AND SIDE EFFECTS*

CNS: <u>fatigue</u>, <u>weakness</u>, dizziness, depression, memory loss, mental changes, nightmares, drowsiness.
EENT: dry eyes, blurred vision.
Resp: bronchospasm, wheezing.
CV: BRADYCARDIA, CONGESTIVE HEART FAILURE, PULMONARY EDEMA, peripheral vasoconstriction, hypotension.
GI: constipation, diarrhea, nausea.
GU: impotence, diminished libido.
Endo: hyperglycemia.

INTERACTIONS

Drug–Drug: ▪ **General anesthesia, IV phenytoin,** and **verapamil** may cause additive myocardial depression ▪ Additive bradycardia may occur with concurrent use of **cardiac glycosides** ▪ Additive hypotension may occur with other **antihypertensive agents** or **nitrates** ▪ Use with **epinephrine** may result in unopposed alpha-adrenergic stimulation ▪ Concurrent **thyroid** administration may decrease effectiveness.

ROUTE AND DOSAGE

▪ **PO (Adults):** 50–150 mg once daily (up to 200 mg/day).

{} = Available in Canada only.
*<u>Underlines</u> indicate most frequent: **CAPITALS** indicate life-threatening.

A

- **IV (Adults):** 5 mg initially, wait 10 min then give another 5 mg.

AVAILABILITY

- **Tablets:** 25 mg, 50 mg, 100 mg ▪ **Injection:** 5 mg/10 ml ▪ **In combination with:** Chlorthalidone (Tenoretic). See Appendix A.

TIME/ACTION PROFILE
(antihypertensive response)

	ONSET	PEAK	DURATION
PO	60 min	2–4 hr	24 hr
IV	UK	UK	UK

NURSING IMPLICATIONS

ASSESSMENT

- ◻ Monitor blood pressure and pulse frequently during dosage adjustment and periodically throughout therapy.
- ◻ Monitor intake and output ratios and weigh daily. Assess patient routinely for signs and symptoms of fluid overload (peripheral edema, dyspnea, rales/crackles, weight gain, jugular venous distension).
- ▪ **Lab Test Considerations:** May cause elevated serum uric acid, BUN, lipoproteins, and triglyceride levels.

POTENTIAL NURSING DIAGNOSES

- ▪ Activity intolerance (indications).
- ▪ Cardiac output, decreased (adverse reactions).
- ▪ Knowledge deficit related to medication regimen (patient/family teaching).

IMPLEMENTATION

- ▪ **General Info:** Take apical pulse prior to administration. If <50 bpm, withhold medication and notify physician.
- ▪ **PO:** Atenolol may be administered without regard to meals. Tablets may be crushed and mixed with fluids if the patient has difficulty swallowing.
- ▪ **Direct IV:** IV therapy for acute myocardial infarction should be initiated as soon as possible after patient arrives in the hosptial.
- ◻ May be diluted in D5W, 0.9% NaCl, or D5/0.9% NaCl. Stable for 48 hr.
- ▪ **Rate:** Administer 5 mg over 5 min, followed by another 5 mg 10 min later.
- ◻ If patient tolerates 10 mg IV dose, administer 50 mg orally 10 min after last IV dose and give another 50 mg oral dose 12 hr later.
- ▪ **Y-Site Compatibility:** ▪ meperidine ▪ morphine.

PATIENT/FAMILY TEACHING

- ◻ Instruct patient to take atenolol as directed, even if feeling well; do not skip or double up on missed doses. A missed dose may be taken as soon as remembered up to 8 hr before next dose. Abrupt withdrawal may precipitate life-threatening arrhythmias, hypertension, or myocardial ischemia.
- ◻ Teach patient and family how to check pulse and blood pressure. Advise them to take pulse daily and blood pressure weekly, and to report any significant changes to physician.
- ◻ May occasionally cause drowsiness. Caution patient to avoid driving or other activities that require alertness until response to drug is known.
- ◻ Advise patients to make position changes slowly to minimize orthostatic hypotension.
- ◻ Reinforce need to continue additional therapies for hypertension (weight loss, restricted sodium intake, stress reduction, regular exercise, moderation of alcohol consumption, and cessation of smoking). Atenolol controls but does not cure hypertension.
- ◻ Caution patient that atenolol may cause increased sensitivity to cold.
- ◻ Advise patient to consult physician or pharmacist before taking any over-the-counter drugs concurrently with this medication.
- ◻ Diabetics should closely monitor blood sugar, especially if weakness, malaise, irritability, or fatigue occur.
- ◻ Instruct patient to inform physician or dentist of this therapy prior to treatment or surgery.
- ◻ Advise patients to carry identification describing disease process and medication regimen at all times.
- ◻ Instruct patient to notify physician of

symptoms of fluid overload, slow pulse rate, dizziness, confusion, depression, skin rash, fever, sore throat, or unusual bleeding or bruising.

EVALUATION

Effectiveness of therapy can be demonstrated by: ▪ Decrease in blood pressure ▪ Decrease in anginal attacks □ Increase in activity tolerance ▪ Prevention of myocardial infarction.

ATOVAQUONE
(a-toe-va-kwone)
Mepron

CLASSIFICATION(S):
Antiprotozoal
Pregnancy Category C

INDICATIONS

▪ Used in the treatment of mild to moderate *Pneumocystis carinii* pneumonia (PCP) in patients who are unable to tolerate trimethoprim/sulfamethoxazole.

ACTION

▪ Inhibits the action of enzymes necessary to nucleic acid and ATP synthesis in protozoa. **Therapeutic Effect:** ▪ Antiprotozoal action against *Pneumocystis carinii.*

PHARMACOKINETICS

Absorption: Absorption is relatively poor but is greatly enhanced by food, particularly fat.
Distribution: Enters CSF in very low concentrations (less than 1% of plasma levels).
Metabolism and Excretion: Undergoes enterohepatic recycling. Elimination occurs in feces.
Half-life: 2.2–2.9 days.

CONTRAINDICATIONS AND PRECAUTIONS

Contraindicated in: ▪ Hypersensitivity.
Use Cautiously in: ▪ Patients with GI

disorders (absorption may be limited) ▪ Pregnancy, lactation, or children (safety not established) ▪ Patients with decreased hepatic, renal, or cardiac function (dosage modification may be necessary).

ADVERSE REACTIONS AND SIDE EFFECTS*

CNS: <u>headache</u>, <u>insomnia</u>, <u>weakness</u>, dizziness, anxiety.
EENT: sinusitis, rhinitis.
GI: <u>nausea</u>, <u>diarrhea</u>, <u>vomiting</u>, abdominal pain, constipation, abnormal liver function studies, anorexia, abnormal taste.
Derm: <u>rash</u>, pruritus.
Endo: hypoglycemia, hyperglycemia.
F and E: hyponatremia.
Hemat: anemia, neutropenia.
MS: <u>fever</u>.
Misc: moniliasis, sweating, pain.

INTERACTIONS

Drug–Drug: ▪ May interact with **drugs that are highly bound to plasma proteins** but does not appear to interact with phenytoin.
Drug–Food: ▪ Food enhances absorption.

ROUTE AND DOSAGE

▪ **PO (Adults):** 750 mg 3 times a day for 21 days.

AVAILABILITY

▪ *Tablets:* 250 mg.

TIME/ACTION PROFILE (blood levels)

	ONSET	PEAK*
PO	UK	1–8 hr 24–96 hr

*Two peaks are due to enterohepatic recycling.

NURSING IMPLICATIONS

ASSESSMENT

□ Assess patient for signs of *Pneumocystis carinii* pneumonia (vital signs, lung sounds, sputum, WBC) at beginning and throughout therapy.
□ Obtain specimens prior to initiating

---

*<u>Underlines</u> indicate most frequent; **CAPITALS** indicate life-threatening.

therapy. First dose may be given before receiving results.
- **Lab Test Considerations:** Monitor hematologic and hepatic functions. May cause anemia and neutropenia. May also cause elevated serum AST (SGOT), ALT (SGPT), and alkaline phosphatase.
- Monitor electrolytes. May cause hyponatremia.
- May cause alterations in serum glucose. Monitor in diabetic patients.

POTENTIAL NURSING DIAGNOSES
- Infection, high risk for (indications, side effects).
- Knowledge deficit related to medication regimen (patient/family teaching).

IMPLEMENTATION
- **PO:** Administer with food 3 times daily for 21 days.

PATIENT/FAMILY TEACHING
- Instruct patient to take atovaquone exactly as directed. Emphasize the importance of taking atovaquone with food, especially foods high in fat; taking without food may decrease plasma concentrations and effectiveness.
- Advise patient to notify physician if rash occurs.

EVALUATION
Clinical response to therapy can be demonstrated by: ■ Resolution of the signs and symptoms of *Pneumocystis carinii* pneumonia.

ATRACURIUM
(a-tra-**cure**-ee-um)
Tracrium

CLASSIFICATION(S):
Neuromuscular blocking agent (nondepolarizing)
Pregnancy Category C

INDICATIONS
- Production of skeletal muscle paralysis, after induction of anesthesia.

ACTION
- Prevents neuromuscular transmission by blocking the effect of acetylcholine at the myoneural junction. **Therapeutic Effect:** ■ Skeletal muscle paralysis.

PHARMACOKINETICS
Absorption: Following IV administration absorption is essentially complete.
Distribution: Distributes into extracellular space. Crosses the placenta.
Metabolism and Excretion: Metabolized in plasma.
Half-life: 20 min.

CONTRAINDICATIONS AND PRECAUTIONS
Contraindicated in: ■ Hypersensitivity to atracurium, benzenesulfonic acid, or benzyl alcohol.
Use Cautiously in: ■ History of pulmonary disease, cardiovascular disease, asthma, or severe allergies ■ Renal or liver impairment ■ Elderly or debilitated patients ■ Electrolyte disturbances ■ Patients receiving cardiac glycosides ■ Myasthenia gravis or myasthenic syndromes (extreme caution) ■ Has been used in pregnant women undergoing cesarean section.

ADVERSE REACTIONS AND SIDE EFFECTS*
CV: bradycardia, hypotension.
Resp: wheezing, increased bronchial secretions.
Derm: skin flush, erythema, pruritus, urticaria.
Misc: allergic reactions, including ANAPHYLAXIS.

INTERACTIONS
Drug–Drug: ■ Intensity and duration of paralysis may be prolonged by pretreatment with **succinylcholine, general anesthesia, aminoglycosides, polymyxin B, colistin, clindamycin, lidocaine, quinidine, procainamide, beta-adrenergic blocking agents, potassium-losing diuretics,** or **magnesium.**

*Underlines indicate most frequent; **CAPITALS** indicate life-threatening.

ROUTE AND DOSAGE

- **IV (Adults and Children >2 yr):** 0.4–0.5 mg/kg initially (0.25–0.35 mg/kg if administered after steady-state anesthesia with enflurane or isoflurane or 0.3–0.4 mg/kg following succinylcholine) then by continuous infusion (at 2–15 mcg/kg/min).
- **IV (Children 1 mo–2 yr):** 0.3–0.4 mg/kg initially (while under halothane anesthesia).

AVAILABILITY

- *Injection:* 10 mg/ml.

TIME/ACTION PROFILE
(neuromuscular blockade)

	ONSET	PEAK	DURATION
IV	2–2.5 min	5 min	30–40 min

NURSING IMPLICATIONS

ASSESSMENT

- □ Assess respiratory status continuously throughout atracurium therapy. Atracurium should be used only by individuals experienced in endotracheal intubation, and equipment for this procedure should be readily available.
- □ Neuromuscular response to atracurium should be monitored with a peripheral nerve stimulator intraoperatively. Paralysis is initially selective and usually occurs sequentially in the following muscles: levator muscles of eyelids, muscles of mastication, limb muscles, abdominal muscles, muscles of the glottis, intercostal muscles, and the diaphragm. Recovery of muscle function usually occurs in reverse order.
- □ Observe the patient for residual muscle weakness and respiratory distress during the recovery period.
- **Toxicity and Overdose:** If overdose occurs, use peripheral nerve stimulator to determine the degree of neuromuscular blockade. Maintain airway patency and ventilation until recovery of normal respirations occurs.
- □ Administration of anticholinesterase agents (edrophonium, neostigmine, pyridostigmine) may be used to antagonize the action of atracurium. Atropine is usually administered prior to or concurrently with anticholinesterase agents to counteract the muscarinic effects.
- □ Administration of fluids and vasopressors may be necessary to treat severe hypotension or shock.

POTENTIAL NURSING DIAGNOSES

- Breathing pattern, ineffective (indications).
- Communication, impaired verbal (side effects).
- Fear (side effects).

IMPLEMENTATION

- **General Info:** Dose is titrated to patient response.
- □ Atracurium has no effect on consciousness or the pain threshold. Adequate anesthesia/analgesia should *always* be used when atracurium is used as an adjunct to surgical procedures.
- □ Store in refrigerator.
- **Direct IV:** Administer initial IV dose as a bolus over 1 min.
- **Intermittent Infusion:** Maintenance dose is usually required 20–45 min following initial dose.
- □ Dilute further in D5W, 0.9% NaCl, or D5/0.9% NaCl and administer every 15–25 min or by continuous infusion.
- **Continuous Infusion:** Maintenance dose is administered by infusion. Titrate according to patient response.
- **Y-Site Compatibility:** ■ aminophylline ■ cefazolin ■ cefuroxime ■ cimetidine ■ dopamine ■ esmolol ■ fentanyl ■ gentamicin ■ heparin ■ hydrocortisone sodium succinate ■ isoproterenol ■ lorazepam ■ midazolam ■ morphine ■ ranitidine ■ trimethoprim/sulfamethoxazole ■ vancomycin.
- **Y-Site Incompatibility:** ■ diazepam.
- **Additive Incompatibility:** Incompatible with most barbiturates and sodium bicarbonate; do not administer in the same syringe or through the same needle during infusion.

PATIENT/FAMILY TEACHING
□ Explain all procedures to patient receiving atracurium therapy without general anesthesia, because consciousness is not affected by atracurium alone.
□ Reassure patient that communication abilities will return as the medication wears off.

EVALUATION
Effectiveness of atracurium can be demonstrated by: ■ Adequate suppression of the twitch response when tested with peripheral nerve stimulation and subsequent muscle paralysis.

ATROPINE
(at-ro-peen)
Atropair, Atro-Pen, Atropisol, Isopto-Atropine, I-Tropine, {Minims Atropine}, Ocu-Tropine

CLASSIFICATION(S):
Anticholinergic (antimuscarinic), Antiarrhythmic, Ophthalmic (mydriatic)
Pregnancy Category C

INDICATIONS
■ IM: Given preoperatively to decrease oral and respiratory secretions ■ IV: Treatment of sinus bradycardia ■ PO: Adjunctive therapy in the management of peptic ulcer and the irritable bowel syndrome ■ Ophth: Produces mydriasis, allows cycloplegic refraction, and used in the treatment of certain inflammatory conditions of the iris and uvea ■ IV: Reversal of adverse muscarinic effects of anticholinesterase agents (neostigmine, physostigmine, or pyridostigmine) ■ IM, IV: Treatment of anticholinesterase (organophosphate pesticide) poisoning.

ACTION
■ Inhibits the action of acetylcholine at postganglionic sites located in: □ Smooth muscle □ Secretory glands □ CNS (antimuscarinic activity). ■ Low doses decrease: □ Sweating □ Salivation □ Respiratory secretions. ■ Intermediate doses result in: □ Mydriasis (pupillary dilation) □ Cycloplegia (loss of visual accommodation) □ Increased heart rate ■ GI and GU tract motility are decreased at larger doses. **Therapeutic Effects:** ■ Increased heart rate ■ Decreased GI and respiratory secretions ■ Reversal of muscarinic effects ■ May have a spasmolytic action on the biliary and genitourinary tract.

PHARMACOKINETICS
Absorption: Well absorbed following oral, SC, or IM administration.
Distribution: Readily crosses the blood–brain barrier. Crosses the placenta and enters breast milk.
Metabolism and Excretion: Mostly metabolized by the liver; 30–50% excreted unchanged by the kidneys.
Half-life: 13–38 hr.

CONTRAINDICATIONS AND PRECAUTIONS
Contraindicated in: ■ Hypersensitivity ■ Narrow-angle glaucoma ■ Acute hemorrhage ■ Tachycardia secondary to cardiac insufficiency or thyrotoxicosis.
Use Cautiously in: ■ Elderly and the very young (increased susceptibility to adverse reactions) ■ Intra-abdominal infections ■ Prostatic hypertrophy ■ Chronic renal, hepatic, pulmonary, or cardiac disease ■ Pregnancy and lactation (safety not established; IV administration may produce fetal tachycardia).

ADVERSE REACTIONS AND SIDE EFFECTS*
CNS: drowsiness, confusion.
EENT: dry eyes, blurred vision, mydriasis, cycloplegia.
CV: palpitations, tachycardia.
GI: dry mouth, constipation.
GU: urinary hesitancy, retention.
Misc: decreased sweating.

{} = Available in Canada only.
*Underlines indicate most frequent; CAPITALS indicate life-threatening.

INTERACTIONS

Drug–Drug: ▪ Additive anticholinergic effects with other **anticholinergic compounds,** including **antihistamines, tricyclic antidepressants, quinidine,** and **disopyramide** ▪ Anticholinergics may alter the absorption of other **orally administered drugs** by slowing motility of the GI tract ▪ **Antacids** decrease the absorption of anticholinergics ▪ May increase GI mucosal lesions in patients taking **oral potassium chloride tablets.**

ROUTE AND DOSAGE

Preanesthesia

▪ **IM, SC (Adults):** 0.4–0.6 mg 30–60 min preop.
▪ **IM, SC (Children >20 kg):** 0.4 mg 30–60 min preop.
▪ **IM, SC (Children 12–16 kg):** 0.3 mg 30–60 min preop.
▪ **IM, SC (Children 7–9 kg):** 0.2 mg 30–60 min preop.
▪ **IM, SC (Children 3 kg):** 0.1 mg 30–60 min preop.

Bradycardia

▪ **IV (Adults):** 0.5–1.0 mg; may repeat as needed q 5 min or 0.4–1 mg q 1–2 hr to a total of 2 mg (total vagolytic dose).
▪ **IV (Children):** 0.01–0.03 mg/kg (maximum dose 0.4 mg); repeat as needed q 4–6 hr.

Adjunctive Therapy of GI Disorders

▪ **PO (Adults):** 0.3–1.2 mg q 4–6 hr (antimuscarinic dose).

Cycloplegic Refraction

▪ **Ophth (Adults):** 1–2 drops of 1% solution 1 hr before examination.
▪ **Ophth (Children):** 1–2 drops of 0.5% solution 2–3 times/day for 1–3 days before and 1 hr after examination.

Reversal of Adverse Muscarinic Effects of Anticholinesterases

▪ **IV (Adults):** 0.6–1.2 mg for each 0.5–2.5 mg of neostigmine methylsulfate or 10–20 mg of pyridostigmine bromide concurrently with anticholinesterase.

Organophosphate Poisoning

▪ **IM, IV (Adults):** 1–2 mg initially, then 1–2 mg q 20–30 min as needed. In severe cases 2–6 mg may be used initially and repeated every 5–60 min as needed. May be followed by oral therapy.
▪ **IM, IV (Children):** 0.05 mg/kg q 10–30 min as needed.

AVAILABILITY

▪ **Tablets:** 0.4 mg ▪ **Soluble Tablets:** 0.4 mg, 0.6 mg ▪ **Injection:** 0.05 mg/ml, 0.1 mg/ml, 0.3 mg/ml, 0.4 mg/ml, 0.5 mg/ml, 0.8 mg/ml, 1 mg/ml, 2 mg/0.7 ml Auto-injector ▪ **Ophthalmic solution:** 0.5%, 1%, 2%, 3% ▪ **Ophthalmic oint:** 0.5%, 1% ▪ **In combination with:** barbiturates and opioid analgesics (see Appendix A).

TIME/ACTION PROFILE (PO, IM, SC, IV = inhibition of salivation, Ophth = mydriasis)

	ONSET	PEAK	DURATION
PO	30 min	30–60 min	4–6 hr
IM, SC	rapid	15–50 min	4–6 hr
IV	immediate	2–4 min	4–6 hr
Ophth	30–40 min	up to 24 hr	1–2 wk

NURSING IMPLICATIONS

ASSESSMENT

▪ **General Info:** Assess vital signs and ECG tracings frequently during IV drug therapy. Report any significant changes in heart rate or blood pressure, or increased ventricular ectopy or angina to physician promptly.
□ Monitor intake and output ratios in elderly or surgical patients because atropine may cause urinary retention.
□ Assess patients routinely for abdominal distention and auscultate for bowel sounds. If constipation becomes a problem, increasing fluids and adding bulk to the diet may help alleviate constipation.
▪ **Toxicity and Overdose:** If overdose occurs, physostigmine is the antidote.

POTENTIAL NURSING DIAGNOSES

▪ Cardiac output, decreased (indications).

- Oral mucous membranes, altered (side effects).
- Constipation (side effects).

IMPLEMENTATION
- **PO:** Oral doses of atropine are usually given 30 min before meals.
- **IM:** Intense flushing of the face and trunk may occur 15–20 min following IM administration. In children, this response is called "atropine flush" and is not harmful.
- **Direct IV:** Give IV undiluted or dilute in 10 ml of sterile water.
- *Rate:* Administer at a rate of 0.6 mg over 1 min. Do not add to IV solution. Inject through Y-tubing or 3-way stopcock. When given IV in doses less than 0.4 mg or over more than 1 min, atropine may cause paradoxical bradycardia, which usually resolves in approximately 2 min.
- **Syringe Compatibility:** • benzquinamide • butorphanol • chlorpromazine • cimetidine • dimenhydrinate • diphenhydramine • droperidol • fentanyl • glycopyrrolate • heparin • hydromorphone • hydroxyzine • meperidine • metoclopramide • midazolam • milrinone • morphine • nalbuphine • pentazocine • perphenazine • prochlorperazine • promazine • promethazine • propiomazine • ranitidine • scopolamine.
- **Y-Site Compatibility:** • amrinone • famotidine • heparin • hydrocortisone sodium succinate • nafcillin • potassium chloride.
- **Ophth:** See Appendix H for administration of ophthalmic medications.

PATIENT/FAMILY TEACHING
- **General Info:** Instruct patient to take exactly as directed. If a dose is missed, take as soon as remembered unless almost time for next dose. Do not double doses.
- May cause drowsiness. Caution patients to avoid driving or other activities requiring alertness until response to medication is known.
- Instruct patient that oral rinses, sugarless gum or candy, and frequent oral hygiene may help relieve dry mouth.
- Caution patients that atropine impairs heat regulation. Strenuous activity in a hot environment may cause heat stroke.
- Instruct patient to consult physician or pharmacist before taking any over-the-counter medications concurrently with this medication.
- Inform male patients with benign prostatic hypertrophy that atropine may cause urinary hesitancy and retention. Changes in urinary stream should be reported to the physician.
- **Ophth:** Advise patients that ophthalmic preparations may temporarily blur vision and impair ability to judge distances. Dark glasses may be needed to protect eyes from bright light.

EVALUATION
Effectiveness of therapy can be demonstrated by: • Increase in heart rate • Dryness of mouth • Dilation of pupils • Decrease in GI motility • Reversal of muscarinic effects • Bronchodilation.

ATTAPULGITE
(at-a-**pull**-gite)
Diar-Aid, Diasorb, {Fowler's Diarrhea Tablets}, hydrated magnesium silicate, Kaopectate, Kaopectate Advanced Formula, Kaopectate Maximum Strength, Parepectolin, Rheaban, St. Joseph Antidiarrheal

CLASSIFICATION(S):
Antidiarrheal (adsorbent)
Pregnancy Category UK

INDICATIONS
- Adjunct in the symptomatic management of mild-to-moderate acute diarrhea.

ACTION
- Appears to act by adsorbing bacteria and toxins and decreasing loss of water.

{} = Available in Canada only.

Therapeutic Effect: ▪ Decreased number and water content of stools.

PHARMACOKINETICS

Absorption: Action is local. Attapulgite is not absorbed.
Distribution: UK.
Metabolism and Excretion: UK.
Half-life: UK.

CONTRAINDICATIONS AND PRECAUTIONS

Contraindicated in: ▪ Severe dehydration ▪ Diarrhea that may be caused by parasites ▪ Dysentary.
Use Cautiously in: ▪ Children <3 yr or elderly patients (increased risk of dehydration).

ADVERSE REACTIONS AND SIDE EFFECTS*

GI: constipation.

INTERACTIONS

Drug–Drug: ▪ May decrease the gastrointestinal absorption of concurrently administered medications (administer 2–3 hr before or 2–4 hr after attapulgite).

ROUTE AND DOSAGE

▪ **PO (Adults):** 1.2–1.5 g after each loose stool (not to exceed 9 g/24 hr).
▪ **PO (Children 6–12 yr):** 600 mg after each loose stool (not to exceed 4.2 g/24 hr).
▪ **PO (Children 3–6 yr):** 300 mg after each loose stool (not to exceed 2.1 g/24 hr).

AVAILABILITY

▪ *Oral suspension:* 600 mg/15 ml, 750 mg/15 ml ▪ *Tablets:* {630 mg}, 750 mg ▪ *Chewable tablets:* 300 mg.

TIME/ACTION PROFILE (antidiarrheal effect)

	ONSET	PEAK	DURATION
PO	UK	UK	UK

NURSING IMPLICATIONS

ASSESSMENT
▫ Assess the frequency and consistency of stools and bowel sounds prior to and throughout course of therapy.
▫ Assess fluid and electrolyte balance and skin turgor for dehydration.

POTENTIAL NURSING DIAGNOSES
▪ Diarrhea (indications).
▪ Constipation (side effects).
▪ Knowledge deficit related to medication regimen (patient/family teaching).

IMPLEMENTATION
▪ **General Info:** Administer after each loose bowel movement until diarrhea is controlled.
▪ **PO:** Shake suspension well prior to administration.

PATIENT/FAMILY TEACHING
▫ Instruct patient to notify physician if diarrhea persists longer than 48 hr or if fever or abdominal pain develops.

EVALUATION
Effectiveness of therapy can be demonstrated by: ▪ Decrease in frequency of loose stools ▫ Return to soft, formed stools.

AURANOFIN
(au-**rane**-oh-fin)
Ridaura

CLASSIFICATION(S):
Anti-inflammatory agent (gold compound)
Pregnancy Category C

INDICATIONS
▪ Treatment of progressive rheumatoid arthritis resistant to conventional therapy.

ACTION
▪ Inhibits the inflammatory process
▪ Has immunomodulating properties.

---

*Underlines indicate most frequent; **CAPITALS** indicate life-threatening.

Therapeutic Effects: ▪ Relief of pain and inflammation ▪ Slowing of the disease process in rheumatoid arthritis.

PHARMACOKINETICS

Absorption: 20–25% absorbed from the GI tract.
Distribution: Widely distributed. Appears to concentrate in arthritic joints. Enters breast milk.
Metabolism and Excretion: 60–90% slowly excreted by the kidneys (up to 15 mo). 10–40% excreted in the feces.
Half-life: Gold—26 days in blood, 40–128 days in tissue.

CONTRAINDICATIONS AND PRECAUTIONS

Contraindicated in: ▪ Hypersensitivity ▪ Severe hepatic or renal dysfunction ▪ Previous heavy metal toxicity ▪ Previous adverse reaction to gold therapy ▪ History of colitis or exfoliative dermatitis ▪ Uncontrolled diabetes mellitus ▪ Tuberculosis ▪ Congestive heart failure ▪ Systemic lupus erythematosus ▪ Recent radiation therapy ▪ Pregnancy or lactation ▪ Debilitated patients.
Use Cautiously in: ▪ History of blood dyscrasias ▪ Hypertension ▪ Rashes ▪ Discontinue at first sign of toxicity, skin rash, proteinuria, or stomatitis.

ADVERSE REACTIONS AND SIDE EFFECTS*

EENT: corneal gold deposition, corneal ulcerations.
CNS: <u>dizziness</u>, syncope, headache.
CV: bradycardia.
Resp: pneumonitis.
GI: <u>metallic taste</u>, stomatitis, diarrhea.
GU: <u>proteinuria</u>, nephrotoxicity.
Derm: <u>rash</u>, <u>dermatitis</u>, pruritus, photosensitivity reactions.
Hemat: <u>thrombocytopenia</u>, APLASTIC ANEMIA, AGRANULOCYTOSIS, leukopenia, eosinophilia.
Misc: allergic reactions including anaphylaxis, angioneurotic edema, nitritoid reactions.

INTERACTIONS

Drug–Drug: ▪ Bone marrow toxicity may be additive with other **agents causing bone marrow depression (antineoplastics, radiation therapy)** ▪ Risk of adverse reactions is greatly increased by concurrent **penicillamine.**

ROUTE AND DOSAGE

▪ **PO (Adults):** 6 mg/day in 1–2 doses; up to 9 mg/day in 3 divided doses.

AVAILABILITY

▪ *Capsules:* 3 mg.

TIME/ACTION PROFILE (anti-inflammatory activity)

	ONSET	PEAK	DURATION
PO	3–6 mo	UK	mos

NURSING IMPLICATIONS

ASSESSMENT

▫ Assess patient's range of motion and degree of swelling and pain in affected joints prior to and periodically throughout therapy.

▪ **Lab Test Considerations:** Monitor renal, hepatic, and hematologic function and urinalysis prior to and monthly during therapy. Notify physician immediately if WBC <4000/mm³, eosinophils >5%, granulocytes <1500/mm³, or platelets <100,000/mm³. These values may indicate hypersensitivity reactions and should improve upon discontinuation. Proteinuria or hematuria may necessitate discontinuation of therapy.

▫ May cause false-positive tuberculin skin test.

▪ **Toxicity and Overdose:** If signs of overdose occur, glucocorticoids are usually used to reverse effects. A chelating agent dimercaprol (BAL) may be given to enhance gold excretion when glucocorticoids are ineffective.

*<u>Underlines</u> indicate most frequent; **CAPITALS** indicate life-threatening.

POTENTIAL NURSING DIAGNOSES

- Physical mobility, impaired (indications).
- Diarrhea (adverse effects).
- Knowledge deficit related to medication regimen (patient/family teaching).

IMPLEMENTATION

- **PO:** Administer oral doses with meals to minimize gastric irritation.

PATIENT/FAMILY TEACHING

- Instruct patient to take medication exactly as directed, do not skip or double doses. Take missed dose as soon as remembered except if next dose almost due. Concurrent therapy with salicylates or other nonsteroidal anti-inflammatory agents or adrenocorticoids is usually necessary, especially during the first few months of gold therapy. Patients should continue physical therapy and ensure adequate rest. Explain that joint damage will not be reversed; the goal is to slow or stop disease process.
- Emphasize the importance of good oral hygiene to reduce the incidence of stomatitis.
- Caution patient to use sunscreen and protective clothing to prevent photosensitivity reactions.
- Instruct patient to report symptoms of leukopenia (fever, sore throat, signs of infection), thrombocytopenia (bleeding gums, bruising, petechiae, blood in stools, urine, or emesis) or gold toxicity (pruritus, skin rash, metallic taste in mouth, stomatitis, diarrhea) immediately. Diarrhea may be resolved by decreasing the dose.
- Discuss the need for contraception while receiving this medication. Advise patient to notify physician promptly if pregnancy is suspected.
- Emphasize the importance of regular visits to physician to monitor progress and evaluate blood and urine tests for side effects.

EVALUATION

Effectiveness of therapy can be demonstrated by: ▪ Decrease in swelling, pain, and stiffness of joints □ Increase in mobility. Continuous therapy for 3–6 mo may be required before therapeutic effects are seen.

AUROTHIOGLUCOSE
(aur-oh-thye-oh-**gloo**-kose)
Solganol

CLASSIFICATION(S):
Anti-inflammatory agent (gold compound)
Pregnancy Category C

INDICATIONS

- Treatment of progressive rheumatoid arthritis resistant to conventional therapy.

ACTION

- Inhibits the inflammatory process.
- Has immunomodulating properties.
Therapeutic Effects: ▪ Relief of pain and inflammation ▪ Slowing of the destructive process in rheumatoid arthritis.

PHARMACOKINETICS

Absorption: Slowly and irregularly absorbed following IM administration.
Distribution: Widely distributed. Appears to concentrate in arthritic joints. Enters breast milk.
Metabolism and Excretion: 60–90% slowly excreted by the kidneys (up to 15 mo); 10–40% excreted in the feces.
Half-life: Gold—26 days in blood, 40–128 days in tissue.

CONTRAINDICATIONS AND PRECAUTIONS

Contraindicated in: ▪ Hypersensitivity ▪ Severe hepatic or renal dysfunction ▪ Previous heavy metal toxicity ▪ Previous adverse reaction to gold therapy ▪ History of colitis ▪ History of exfoliative dermatitis ▪ Uncontrolled diabetes mellitus ▪ Tuberculosis ▪ Congestive heart failure ▪ Systemic lupus erythematosus ▪ Recent radiation therapy ▪ Pregnancy or lactation ▪ Debilitated patients.

Use Cautiously in: ▪ History of blood dyscrasias ▪ Hypertension ▪ Rashes

- Discontinue at first sign of toxicity, skin rash, proteinuria, or stomatitis
- Children <6 yr (safety not established).

ADVERSE REACTIONS AND SIDE EFFECTS*

CNS: dizziness, syncope, headache.
EENT: corneal gold deposition, corneal ulcerations.
CV: bradycardia.
Resp: pneumonitis.
GI: metallic taste, difficulty swallowing, stomatitis, nausea, vomiting, diarrhea, abdominal pain, cramping, anorexia, dyspepsia, flatulence, hepatitis.
GU: proteinuria, nephrotoxicity.
Derm: rash, dermatitis, pruritus, photosensitivity reactions.
Hemat: thrombocytopenia, APLASTIC ANEMIA, AGRANULOCYTOSIS, leukopenia, eosinophilia.
Neuro: neuropathy.
Misc: allergic reactions including ANAPHYLAXIS, angioneurotic edema, nitritoid reaction.

INTERACTIONS

Drug–Drug: ▪ Bone marrow toxicity may be additive with other **agents causing bone marrow depression (antineoplastics, radiation therapy)** ▪ Risk of adverse reactions is greatly increased by concurrent penicillamine.

ROUTE AND DOSAGE

- **IM (Adults):** 10 mg first week, 25 mg second and third week, then 25–50 mg weekly until 800 mg–1 g has been given; then maintenance dose of 25–50 mg q week for 2–20 wk, then 25–50 mg q 3–4 wk.
- **IM (Children 6–12 yr):** 2.5 mg first week, 6.25 mg second and third weeks, then 12.5 mg weekly until 200–250 mg has been given; then maintenance dose of 6.25–12.5 mg q 3–4 wk or 1 mg/kg/wk for 20 wk.

AVAILABILITY

- *Injection:* 50 mg/ml.

TIME/ACTION PROFILE (anti-inflammatory effect)

	ONSET	PEAK	DURATION
IM	6–8 wk	UK	mos

NURSING IMPLICATIONS

ASSESSMENT

▫ Assess patient's range of motion and degree of swelling and pain in affected joints prior to and periodically throughout therapy.

▫ Monitor patient for nitritoid reaction (flushing, fainting, dizziness, sweating, nausea, vomiting, headache, blurred vision, weakness, malaise) that may occur immediately to 10 min following injection. Reaction is transient and does not usually require discontinuation of therapy.

- **Lab Test Considerations:** Monitor renal, hepatic, and hematologic function and urinalysis prior to and periodically during therapy. Obtain urinalysis prior to each injection. Proteinuria or hematuria may necessitate discontinuation of therapy. Monitor CBC and platelets prior to every other injection or every 2–4 wk. Notify physician immediately if WBC <4000/mm^3, eosinophils >5%, granulocytes <1500/mm^3, or platelets <100,000/mm^3. These values may indicate hypersensitivity reactions and should improve upon discontinuation.

- **Toxicity and Overdose:** If signs of overdose occur, glucocorticoids are usually used to reverse effects. A chelating agent dimercaprol (BAL') may be given to enhance gold excretion when glucocorticoids are ineffective.

POTENTIAL NURSING DIAGNOSES

- Physical mobility, impaired (indications).
- Diarrhea (adverse effects).
- Knowledge deficit related to medication regimen (patient/family teaching).

*Underlines indicate most frequent; CAPITALS indicate life-threatening.

Implementation
- **IM:** Immerse vial in warm water bath and shake suspension well for ease of withdrawal. Use 1½–2 in., 20-gauge needle. Administer into the gluteal muscle only. Do not administer IV. Patient should remain supine for 10 min after injection and should be closely monitored for development of nitritoid reaction for 15 min.

PATIENT/FAMILY TEACHING
- Discuss need for continued therapy. Initially injections are given weekly. Later injections are spaced 3–4 wk apart. Concurrent therapy with salicylates, nonsteroidal anti-inflammatory agents, or glucocorticoids may be necessary. Patient should continue physical therapy and ensure adequate rest. Explain that joint damage will not be reversed; the goal is to slow or stop disease process.
- Emphasize the importance of good oral hygiene to reduce the incidence of stomatitis.
- Caution patient to use sunscreen and protective clothing to prevent photosensitivity reactions.
- Instruct patient to report symptoms of leukopenia (fever, sore throat, signs of infection), thrombocytopenia (bleeding gums, bruising, petechiae, blood in stools, urine, or emesis), or gold toxicity (pruritus, skin rash, metallic taste in mouth, stomatitis, diarrhea) immediately to physician.
- Discuss the need for contraception while receiving this medication. Advise patient to notify physician promptly if pregnancy is suspected.
- Instruct patient to notify physician immediately of symptoms of gold toxicity (pruritus, skin rash, metallic taste in mouth, stomatitis, diarrhea).
- Emphasize the importance of regular visits to physician to monitor progress and evaluate blood and urine tests for side effects.

EVALUATION
Effectiveness of therapy can be demonstrated by: ■ Decrease in swelling, pain, and stiffness of joints □ Increase in mobility. Continuous therapy for 3–6 mo may be required before therapeutic effects are seen.

AZATADINE
(a-**za**-ta-deen)
Optimine

CLASSIFICATION(S):
Antihistamine
Pregnancy Category B

INDICATIONS
- Symptomatic relief of allergic symptoms (rhinitis, urticaria) caused by histamine release.

ACTION
- Blocks the following effects of histamine: □ Vasodilation □ Increased heart rate □ Hypotension ■ Also has antiserotonin properties. **Therapeutic Effect:** ■ Relief of symptoms associated with histamine excess usually seen in allergic conditions. Does not block the release of histamine.

PHARMACOKINETICS
Absorption: Well absorbed following oral administration.
Distribution: Probably crosses the placenta.
Metabolism and Excretion: Extensively metabolized by the liver; 20% excreted unchanged by the kidneys.
Half-life: 12 hr.

CONTRAINDICATIONS AND PRECAUTIONS
Contraindicated in: ■ Hypersensitivity ■ Acute attacks of asthma ■ Lactation (avoid use).
Use Cautiously in: ■ Narrow-angle glaucoma ■ Liver disease ■ Elderly patients (more susceptible to adverse reactions) ■ Pregnancy or children <12 yr (safety not established) ■ Hyperthyroidism ■ Hypertension.

ADVERSE REACTIONS AND SIDE EFFECTS*

CNS: <u>drowsiness</u>, <u>sedation</u>, <u>dizziness</u>, headache, excitation, seizures.
CV: hypotension, <u>hypertension</u>, palpitations, arrhythmias, tachycardia, chest tightness.
EENT: blurred vision, <u>tinnitus</u>, nasal stuffiness.
Resp: <u>thickened bronchial secretions</u>, wheezing.
GI: dry mouth, vomiting, diarrhea, constipation, <u>epigastric distress</u>, anorexia.
GU: urinary hesitancy, retention, <u>early menses</u>.
Hemat: anemia, thrombocytopenia, agranulocytosis.
Derm: sweating.

INTERACTIONS

Drug–Drug: ▪ Additive CNS depression with other **CNS depressants** including **alcohol, narcotic analgesics,** and **sedative/hypnotics** ▪ **MAO inhibitors** intensify and prolong the anticholinergic effects of antihistamines.

ROUTE AND DOSAGE
▪ **PO (Adults and Children >12 yr):** 1–2 mg twice daily.

AVAILABILITY

▪ *Tablets:* 1 mg ▪ *In combination with:* pseudoephedrine (Trinalin). See Appendix A.

TIME/ACTION PROFILE
(antihistaminic effects)

	ONSET	PEAK	DURATION
PO	15–60 min	UK	12 hr

NURSING IMPLICATIONS

ASSESSMENT
□ Assess allergy symptoms (rhinitis, conjunctivitis, hives) prior to and periodically throughout therapy.
□ Assess lung sounds and character of bronchial secretions. Maintain fluid intake of 1500–2000 ml/day to decrease viscosity of secretions.

▪ **Lab Test Considerations:** May cause false-negative allergy skin testing. Discontinue antihistamines at least 72 hr before testing.

POTENTIAL NURSING DIAGNOSES
▪ Airway clearance, ineffective (indications).
▪ Injury, high risk for (adverse reactions).
▪ Knowledge deficit related to medication regimen (patient/family teaching).

IMPLEMENTATION
▪ **PO:** Administer oral doses with food or milk to decrease GI irritation.

PATIENT/FAMILY TEACHING
□ Instruct patient to take azatadine exactly as directed.
□ May cause drowsiness. Caution patient to avoid driving or other activities requiring alertness until effects of the medication are known.
□ Advise patient to avoid taking alcohol or other CNS depressants concurrently with this drug.
□ Advise patient that good oral hygiene, frequent rinsing of mouth, and sugarless gum or candy may help relieve dry mouth. Patient should notify dentist if dry mouth persists >2 wk.
□ Elderly patients are at risk for orthostatic hypotension. Advise patient to make position changes slowly.
□ Instruct patient to contact physician if symptoms persist.

EVALUATION
Effectiveness of therapy may be determined by: ▪ Decrease in allergic symptoms.

AZATHIOPRINE
(ay-za-**thye**-oh-preen)
Imuran

CLASSIFICATION(S):
Immunosuppressant
Pregnancy Category UK

---

*<u>Underlines</u> indicate most frequent; **CAPITALS** indicate life-threatening.

INDICATIONS
■ Adjunct with corticosteroids, local radiations, or other cytotoxic agents in the prevention of renal transplant rejection ■ Treatment of severe, active, erosive rheumatoid arthritis unresponsive to more conventional therapy with or without disease-modifying agents such as gold salts.

ACTION
■ Antagonizes purine metabolism with subsequent inhibition of DNA and RNA synthesis. **Therapeutic Effects:** ■ Suppression of cell-mediated immunity and altered antibody formation.

PHARMACOKINETICS
Absorption: Readily absorbed following oral administration.
Distribution: Crosses the placenta.
Metabolism and Excretion: Metabolized to mercaptopurine, which is further metabolized. Minimal renal excretion of unchanged drug.
Half-life: 3 hr.

CONTRAINDICATIONS AND PRECAUTIONS
Contraindicated in: ■ Hypersensitivity ■ Pregnancy or lactation.
Use Cautiously in: ■ Infections ■ Malignancies ■ Decreased bone marrow reserve ■ Previous or concurrent radiation therapy ■ Other chronic debilitating illnesses ■ Patients with childbearing potential.

ADVERSE REACTIONS AND SIDE EFFECTS*
EENT: retinopathy.
GI: nausea, vomiting, diarrhea, anorexia, mucositis, hepatotoxicity, pancreatitis.
Derm: rash, alopecia.
Hemat: leukopenia, anemia, pancytopenia, thrombocytopenia.
MS: arthralgia.
Resp: pulmonary edema.
Misc: fever, chills, serum sickness, retinopathy, Raynaud's phenomenon.

INTERACTIONS
Drug–Drug: ■ Additive myelosuppression with **antineoplastics, cyclosporine,** and **myelosuppressive agents** ■ **Allopurinol** inhibits the metabolism of azathioprine increasing toxicity. Dosage of azathioprine should be decreased by 25–33% with concurrent allopurinol.

ROUTE AND DOSAGE
Renal Allograft Rejection Prevention
■ **PO, IV (Adults and Children):** 3–5 mg/kg/day initially; maintenance dose 1–2 mg/kg/day.

Rheumatoid Arthritis
■ **PO (Adults):** 1 mg/kg/day for 6–8 wk, increase by 0.5 mg/kg q 4 wk until response or up to 2.5 mg/kg/day, then decrease q 4–8 wk to minimum effective dose.

AVAILABILITY
■ *Tablets:* 50 mg ■ *Injection:* 100-mg vial.

TIME/ACTION PROFILE

	ONSET	PEAK	DURATION
PO (anti-inflammatory)	6–8 wk	12 wk	UK
IV (immuno-suppression)	days–wks	UK	days–wks

NURSING IMPLICATIONS
ASSESSMENT
■ **General Info:** Assess for infection (vital signs; sputum, urine, stool, WBC) throughout therapy.
□ Monitor intake and output and daily weight. Decreased urine output may lead to toxicity with this medication.
■ **Rheumatoid Arthritis:** Assess range of motion, degree of swelling, pain and strength in affected joints, and ability to perform activities of daily living prior to and periodically throughout therapy.
■ **Lab Test Considerations:** Renal, hepatic, and hematologic functions

should be monitored prior to beginning course of therapy, weekly during the first month, bimonthly for the next 2–3 mo, and monthly thereafter.

□ Notify physician if leukocyte count is <3000 or platelet count is <100,000/ mm³; these may necessitate a reduction in dosage.

□ A decrease in hemoglobin may indicate bone marrow suppression.

□ Hepatotoxicity may be manifested by increased alkaline phosphatase, bilirubin, AST (SGOT), ALT (SGPT), and amylase.

□ May decrease serum and urine acid and plasma albumin.

POTENTIAL NURSING DIAGNOSES

- Infection, high risk for (indications).
- Knowledge deficit related to medication regimen (patient/family teaching).

IMPLEMENTATION

- **General Info:** Protect transplant patients from staff and visitors who may carry infection. Maintain protective isolation as indicated.
- **PO:** May be administered with or after meals or in divided dose to minimize nausea.
- **IV:** Reconstitute 100 mg with 10 ml of Sterile Water for Injection. Swirl vial gently until completely dissolved. Reconstituted solution may be administered up to 24 hr after preparation.
- **Intermittent Infusion:** Solution may be further diluted in 50 ml of 0.9% NaCl, 0.45% NaCl, or D5W. Do not admix.
- **Rate:** Infuse over at least 30 min.

PATIENT/FAMILY TEACHING

- **General Info:** Instruct patient to take azathioprine exactly as directed. If a dose is missed on a once-daily regimen, skip the dose; if on several-times-a-day dosing, take as soon as remembered or double next dose. Consult physician if more than 1 dose is missed or if vomiting occurs shortly after dose taken. Do not discontinue without consulting physician.
- □ Advise patient to report the onset of infection, bleeding gums, bruising, or

signs and symptoms of hepatic dysfunction (abdominal pain, pruritus, clay-colored stools) or transplant rejection to the physician immediately.

□ Reinforce the need for life-long therapy to prevent transplant rejection.

□ Instruct the patient to consult with physician or pharmacist before taking any over-the-counter medications or receiving any vaccinations while taking this medication.

□ Advise patient to avoid contact with persons with contagious diseases and persons who have recently taken oral poliovirus vaccine.

□ This drug may have teratogenic properties. Advise patient to use contraception during and for at least 4 mo after therapy is completed.

□ Emphasize the importance of follow-up examination and lab tests.

- **Rheumatoid Arthritis:** Concurrent therapy with salicylates, nonsteroidal anti-inflammatory agents, or glucocorticoids may be necessary. Patient should continue physical therapy and adequate rest. Explain that joint damage will not be reversed; goal is to slow or stop disease process.

EVALUATION

Effectiveness of therapy may be determined by: ■ Prevention of transplant rejection ■ Decreased stiffness, pain, and swelling in affected joints in 6–8 wk in rheumatoid arthritis. Therapy is discontinued if no improvement in 12 wk.

AZITHROMYCIN
(aye-**zith**-row-my-sin)
Zithromax

CLASSIFICATION(S):
Anti-infective (macrolide)
Pregnancy Category B

INDICATIONS

- Treatment of the following infections due to susceptible organisms □ Upper respiratory tract infections, including *Streptococcal pharyngitis* and tonsillitis □ Lower respiratory tract infections,

including bronchitis and pneumonia
□ Skin and skin structure infections
□ Nongonococcal urethritis and cervicitis.

ACTION

■ Inhibits protein synthesis at the level of the 50S bacterial ribosome. **Therapeutic Effect:** ■ Bacteriostatic action against susceptible bacteria. **Spectrum:** ■ Active against the following gram-positive aerobic bacteria □ *Staphylococcus aureus* □ *Streptococcus pneumoniae* □ *Streptococcus pyogenes* (group A strep) ■ Active against these gram-negative aerobic bacteria □ *Haemophilis influenzae* □ *Moraxella catarrhalis* ■ Also active against □ *Mycoplasma* □ *Legionella* □ *Chlamydia trachomatis* ■ Not active against methicillin-resistant *Staphylococcus aureus.*

PHARMACOKINETICS

Absorption: Rapidly absorbed (40%) following oral administration.
Distribution: Widely distributed to body tissues and fluids. Intracellular and tissue levels exceed those in serum. CSF levels very low.
Metabolism and Excretion: Mostly excreted unchanged in bile. 4.5% excreted unchanged in urine.
Half-life: 68 hr.

CONTRAINDICATIONS AND PRECAUTIONS

Contraindicated in: ■ Hypersensitivity to azithromycin, erythromycin, or other macrolide anti-infectives.
Use Cautiously in: ■ Pregnancy, lactation, and children <16 yr (safety not established) ■ Severe liver impairment (dosage adjustment may be required).

ADVERSE REACTIONS AND SIDE EFFECTS*

CNS: headache, dizziness, vertigo, drowsiness, fatigue.
CV: paliptations, chest pain.
GI: <u>diarrhea</u>, <u>nausea</u>, <u>abdominal pain</u>,

dypepsia, flatulence, melena, cholestatic jaundice.
GU: vaginitis, nephritis.
Derm: rashes, photosensitivity.
Endo: hyperglycemia.
F and E: hyperkalemia.
Misc: ANGIOEDEMA.

INTERACTIONS

Drug–Drug: ■ **Aluminum-** and **magnesium-containing antacids** decrease peak serum levels of azithromycin ■ May increase serum levels and the risk of toxicity from **theophylline, terfenadine, astemizole,** or **carbamazepine** ■ May increase the effect of **oral anticoagulants.**
Drug–Food: ■ Food decreases absorption by 43%.

ROUTE AND DOSAGE

Respiratory and Skin Infections
■ **PO (Adults):** 500 mg on first day, then 250 mg/day for 4 more days (total dose of 1.5 g).

Non-gonococcal Urethritis or Cervicitis
■ **PO (Adults):** single 1-g dose.

AVAILABILITY

■ *Capsules:* 250 mg.

TIME/ACTION PROFILE (serum levels)

	ONSET	PEAK
PO	UK	2.5–3.2 hr

NURSING IMPLICATIONS

ASSESSMENT
□ Assess patient for infection (vital signs; appearance of wound, sputum, urine, and stool; WBC) at beginning and throughout course of therapy.
□ Obtain specimens for culture and sensitivity prior to initiating therapy. First dose may be given before receiving results.
■ **Lab Test Considerations:** May cause increased serum bilirubin, AST (SGOT), ALT (SGPT), LDH, and alkaline phosphatase concentrations.

*<u>Underlines</u> indicate most frequent; **CAPITALS** indicate life-threatening.

□ May cause elevated creatine phosphokinase, potassium, prothrombin time, BUN, serum creatinine, and blood glucose concentrations.

□ May occasionally cause decreased WBC and platelet count.

POTENTIAL NURSING DIAGNOSES

■ Infection, high risk for (indications, side effects).

■ Knowledge deficit related to medication regimen (patient/family teaching).

■ Noncompliance related to medication regimen (patient/family teaching).

IMPLEMENTATION

■ **PO:** Administer 1 hr before or 2 hr after meals.

PATIENT/FAMILY TEACHING

□ Instruct patient to take medication as directed and to finish the drug completely, even if they are feeling better. Missed doses should be taken as soon as possible unless almost time for next dose; do not double doses. Advise patients that sharing of this medication may be dangerous.

□ Instruct patient not to take azithromycin with food or antacids.

□ May cause drowsiness. Caution patient to avoid driving or other activities requiring alertness until response to medication is known.

□ Advise patient to use sunscreen and protective clothing to prevent photosensitivity reactions.

□ Advise patient to report the signs of superinfection (black, furry overgrowth on the tongue, vaginal itching or discharge, loose or foul-smelling stools).

□ Instruct patient to notify the physician if fever and diarrhea develop, especially if stool contains blood, pus, or mucus.

□ Advise patient to notify physician if pregnancy is planned or suspected.

□ Instruct patient to notify physician if symptoms do not improve.

EVALUATION

Clinical response to therapy can be determined by: ■ Resolution of the signs and symptoms of infection. Length of time for complete resolution depends on the organism and site of infection.

A

AZTREONAM
(az-**tree**-oh-nam)
Azactam

CLASSIFICATION(S):
Anti-infective (monobactam)
Pregnancy Category B

INDICATIONS

■ Treatment of serious gram-negative infections including: □ Bone and joint infections □ Septicemia □ Skin and skin structure infections □ Intra-abdominal infections □ Gynecologic infections □ Respiratory tract infections □ Urinary tract infections.

ACTION

■ Binds to the bacterial cell wall membrane, causing cell death. **Therapeutic Effect:** ■ Bactericidal action against susceptible bacteria. **Spectrum:** ■ Displays significant activity against gram-negative aerobic organisms only: □ *Escherichia coli* □ *Serratia* □ *Klebsiella* □ *Enterobacter* □ *Shigella* □ *Providencia* □ *Salmonella* □ *Neisseria gonorrhea* □ *Haemophilus influenzae* ■ Has good activity against *Pseudomonas aeruginosa,* including strains resistant to other drugs ■ Not active against: □ *Staphylococcus aureus* □ *Enterococcus* □ *Bacteroides fragilis.*

PHARMACOKINETICS

Absorption: Well absorbed following IM administration.

Distribution: Widely distributed. Crosses the placenta and enters breast milk in low concentrations.

Metabolism and Excretion: 65–75% excreted unchanged by the kidneys. Small amounts metabolized by the liver.

Half-life: 1.5–2.2 hr (increased in renal impairment).

CONTRAINDICATIONS AND PRECAUTIONS

Contraindicated in: ▪ Hypersensitivity ▪ Cross-sensitivity with penicillins or cephalosporins may occur.

Use Cautiously in: ▪ Renal impairment (dosage reduction required if CCr <30 ml/min/1.73 m^2) ▪ Pregnancy, lactation, and young children (safety not established).

ADVERSE REACTIONS AND SIDE EFFECTS*

CNS: SEIZURES.

GI: altered taste (IV only), diarrhea, nausea, vomiting.

Derm: rashes.

Local: phlebitis at IV site, <u>pain</u> at IM site.

Misc: superinfection, allergic reactions including ANAPHYLAXIS.

INTERACTIONS

Drug–Drug: ▪ Concurrent use with **cefoxitin** or **imipenem** may antagonize effectiveness of aztreonam ▪ Serum levels are increased by **furosemide** or **probenecid**.

ROUTE AND DOSAGE

▪ **IM, IV (Adults):** 0.5–2.0 g q 6–12 hr.

AVAILABILITY

▪ *Injection:* 0.5-g, 1-g, 2-g vials and infusion bottles.

TIME/ACTION PROFILE (blood levels)

	ONSET	PEAK
IM	rapid	60 min
IV	rapid	end of infusion

NURSING IMPLICATIONS

ASSESSMENT

▪ **General Info:** Assess patient for infection (vital signs; wound appearance, sputum, urine, and stool; WBC) at beginning and throughout therapy.

▫ Obtain a history before initiating therapy to determine previous use of and reactions to penicillins and cephalosporins. Patients allergic to these drugs may exhibit hypersensitivity reactions to aztreonam.

▫ Obtain specimens for culture and sensitivity prior to initiating therapy. First dose may be given before receiving results.

▪ **Lab Test Considerations:** May cause elevations in AST (SGOT), ALT (SGPT), alkaline phosphatase, LDH, and serum creatinine. May cause increased prothrombin and partial thromboplastin times, eosinophilia, and positive Coombs' test.

POTENTIAL NURSING DIAGNOSES

▪ Infection, high risk for (indications).
▪ Knowledge deficit related to medication regimen (patient/family teaching).

IMPLEMENTATION

▪ **General Info:** After adding diluent to vial, shake immediately and vigorously. Not for multidose use; discard unused solution.

▪ **IM:** Use 15-ml vial and dilute each g of aztreonam with at least 3 ml of 0.9% NaCl, Sterile Water for Injection, or Bacteriostatic Water for Injection. Stable at room temperature for 48 hr or 7 days if refrigerated.

▫ Administer into large, well-developed muscle.

▪ **Direct IV:** For direct IV use add 6–10 ml of sterile water to each 15-ml vial.

▪ *Rate:* Administer slowly over 3–5 min by direct injection or into tubing of a compatible solution.

▪ **Intermittent Infusion:** Dilute 15-ml vial with at least 3 ml of sterile water for each g aztreonam. Dilute further with 50–100 ml of 0.9% NaCl, Ringer's or lactated Ringer's solution, D5W, D10W, D5/0.9% NaCl, D5/0.45% NaCl, D5/0.25% NaCl, sodium lactate, 5% or 10% Mannitol. Final concentration should not exceed 20 mg/ml. Solution is stable for 48 hr at room temperature and 7 days if refrigerated. Solutions range from colorless to light, straw yellow, or may develop a pink tint upon standing; this does not affect potency.

---

*<u>Underlines</u> indicate most frequent; **CAPITALS** indicate life-threatening.

- *Rate:* Infuse over 20–60 min.
- **Syringe Compatibility:** ▪ clindamycin.
- **Y-Site Compatibility:** ▪ ciprofloxacin ▪ enalaprilat ▪ fluconazole ▪ fludarabine ▪ foscarnet ▪ regular insulin ▪ meperidine ▪ morphine ▪ ondansetron ▪ sargramostim ▪ zidovudine.
- **Y-Site Incompatibility:** ▪ vancomycin.
- **Additive Compatibility:** ▪ cefazolin ▪ ciprofloxacin ▪ clindamycin ▪ gentamicin ▪ tobramycin.
- ▫ May be admixed with ampicillin in 0.9% NaCl; stable for 24 hr at room temperature and 48 hr if refrigerated.
- **Additive Incompatibility:** ▪ nafcillin ▪ cephradine ▪ metronidazole.

PATIENT/FAMILY TEACHING
- ▫ Warn patient that IV infusion may cause mild taste alteration.
- ◻ Advise patient to report the signs of superinfection (furry overgrowth on the tongue, vaginal itching or discharge, loose or foul-smelling stools) and allergy.

EVALUATION
Effectiveness of therapy can be demonstrated by: ▪ Resolution of signs and symptoms of infection. Length of time for complete resolution depends on the organism and site of infection.

BACLOFEN
(bak-loe-fen)
Lioresal

CLASSIFICATION(S):
Skeletal muscle relaxant
(centrally acting)
Pregnancy Category C

INDICATIONS

▪ **PO:** Treatment of reversible spasticity associated with multiple sclerosis or spinal cord lesions. ▪ **IT:** Treatment of severe spasticity originating in the spinal cord. **Unlabeled Use:** ▪ Management of pain in trigeminal neuralgia.

ACTION

▪ Inhibits reflexes at the spinal level. **Therapeutic Effect:** ▪ Relief of muscle spasticity; bowel and bladder function may also be improved.

PHARMACOKINETICS

Absorption: Rapidly and almost completely absorbed following oral administration.
Distribution: Widely distributed, crosses the placenta.
Metabolism and Excretion: 70–80% eliminated unchanged by the kidneys.
Half-life: 2.5–4 hr.

CONTRAINDICATIONS AND PRECAUTIONS

Contraindicated in: ▪ Hypersensitivity.
Use Cautiously in: ▪ Patients in whom spasticity is used to maintain posture and balance ▪ Pregnancy, lactation, and children (safety not established) ▪ Epileptics (may lower seizure threshold) ▪ Elderly (increased susceptibility to CNS side effects) ▪ Renal impairment (dosage reduction may be required).

ADVERSE REACTIONS AND SIDE EFFECTS*

CNS: <u>drowsiness</u>, <u>dizziness</u>, <u>weakness</u>, <u>fatigue</u>, headache, confusion, insomnia, ataxia, depression, SEIZURES (IT).
EENT: nasal congestion, tinnitus.
CV: hypotension, edema.
GI: <u>nausea</u>, constipation.
GU: frequency.
Derm: rash, pruritus.
Metab: hyperglycemia, weight gain.
Misc: hypersensitivity reactions, sweating.

INTERACTIONS

Drug–Drug: ▪ Additive CNS depression with other **CNS depressants** including **alcohol, antihistamines, opioid analgesics,** and **sedative/hypnotics** ▪ Use with **MAO inhibitors** may lead to increased CNS depression or hypotension.

ROUTE AND DOSAGE

- **PO (Adults):** 5 mg 3 times daily. May increase q 3 days by 5 mg/dose to maximum of 80 mg/day (total daily dose may also be given in divided doses 4 times daily).
- **IT:** 300–800 mcg/day. Dose is determined during screening phase.

AVAILABILITY

- **Tablets:** 10 mg, 20 mg ▪ **Intrathecal injection:** 10 mg/20 ml, 10 mg/5 ml.

TIME/ACTION PROFILE (effects on spasticity)

	ONSET	PEAK	DURATION
PO	hrs–wks	UK	UK
IT	0.5–1 hr	4 hr	4–8 hr

NURSING IMPLICATIONS

ASSESSMENT

- **General Info:** ▪ Assess muscle spasticity prior to and periodically throughout course of therapy.
- □ Observe patient for drowsiness, dizziness, or ataxia. A change in dose may alleviate these problems.
- **IT:** Monitor patient closely during test dose and titration. Resuscitative equipment should be immediately available for life-threatening or intolerable side effects.
- **Lab Test Considerations:** May cause increase in serum glucose, alkaline, phosphatase, AST (SGOT), and ALT (SGPT) levels.

POTENTIAL NURSING DIAGNOSES

- Physical mobility, impaired (indications).
- Injury, high risk for (adverse reactions).
- Knowledge deficit related to medication regimen (patient/family teaching).

IMPLEMENTATION

- **PO:** May be administered with milk or food to minimize gastric irritation.
- **IT:** For *test dose* dilute for a concentration of 50 mcg/ml with Sterile Preservative Free NaCl for Injection. Test dose should be administered over at least 1 min. Patient should be observed for a significant decrease in muscle tone or frequency or severity of spasm. If response is inadequate, 2 additional test doses, each 24 hr apart, 75 mcg/1.5 ml and 100 mcg/2 ml respectively, may be administered. Patients with an inadequate response should not receive chronic IT therapy.
- □ Dose titration for implantable IT pumps is based on patient response. If no substantive response after dose increase, check pump function and catheter patency.

PATIENT/FAMILY TEACHING

- □ Instruct patient to take baclofen as directed. Take a missed dose within 1 hr; do not double doses. Caution patient to avoid abrupt withdrawal of this medication as it may precipitate an acute withdrawal reaction (hallucinations, increased spasticity, seizures, mental changes, restlessness).
- □ May cause dizziness and drowsiness. Advise patient to avoid driving or other activities requiring alertness until response to drug is known.
- □ Instruct patient to make position changes slowly to minimize orthostatic hypotension.
- □ Advise patient to avoid concurrent use of alcohol or other CNS depressants while taking this medication.
- □ Instruct patient to notify physician if frequent urge to urinate or painful urination, constipation, nausea, headache, insomnia, tinnitus, depression, or confusion persist. Advise patient to report signs and symptoms of hypersensitivity (rash, itching) promptly.

EVALUATION

Effectiveness of therapy can be demonstrated by: ▪ Decrease in muscle spasticity and associated musculoskeletal pain with an increased ability to perform activities of daily living ▪ Decreased pain in patients with trigeminal neuralgia. May take weeks to obtain optimal effect.

BECLOMETHASONE
(be-kloe-**meth**-a-sone)
Beclovent, Beconase, Beconase
AQ Nasal, Vancenase, Vancenase AQ Nasal, Vanceril

B

CLASSIFICATION(S):
Glucocorticoid (long-acting)
Pregnancy Category C

INDICATIONS

- **Inhalation:** Anti-inflammatory and immunosuppressant in the treatment of chronic steroid-dependent asthma. May decrease requirement for or avoid use of systemic glucocorticoids ■ **Intranasal:** Used in the management of allergic rhinitis and other chronic nasal inflammatory conditions, including nasal polyps.

ACTION

- Potent, locally acting anti-inflammatory and immune modifier. **Therapeutic Effect:** Decrease in symptoms of chronic asthma and allergic rhinitis.

PHARMACOKINETICS

Absorption: Action is mostly local. Additional drug may be swallowed, but systemic absorption is minimal at recommended doses.
Distribution: Action is local; 10–25% of inhaled dose is deposited at sites of action in respiratory tract.
Metabolism and Excretion: Elimination is mainly fecal; remainder is rapidly metabolized. Crosses the placenta.
Half-life: 15 hr.

CONTRAINDICATIONS AND PRECAUTIONS

Contraindicated in: ■ Allergy to fluorocarbon propellants.
Use Cautiously in: ■ Chronic treatment at higher than recommended doses may lead to adrenal suppression ■ Systemic glucocorticoid therapy (should not be abruptly discontinued when inhalable or intranasal therapy is started).

ADVERSE REACTIONS AND SIDE EFFECTS*

EENT: nasal burning, nasal irritation, nasal bleeding, sneezing attacks (following intranasal administration), oropharyngeal fungal infections (following inhalation).
Resp: wheezing, bronchospasm (following inhalation).

INTERACTIONS

Drug–Drug: ■ None significant at recommended doses.

ROUTE AND DOSAGE

- **Inhalation (Adults):** 2–4 inhalations 3–4 times daily (not to exceed 20 inhalations/day).
- **Inhalation (Children 6–11 yr):** 1–2 inhalations 3–4 times daily (not to exceed 10 inhalations/day).
- **Intranasal (Adults):** 1 spray in each nostril 2–4 times daily.
- **Intranasal (Children 6–11 yr):** 1 spray in each nostril 3 times daily.

AVAILABILITY

- *Aerosol for inhalation:* Delivers 42 mcg/activation, 200 metered doses/16.8 g cannister ■ *Aerosol for nasal inhalation:* Delivers 42 mcg/activation, 200 metered doses/16.8-g cannister ■ *Aerosol solution for nasal inhalation:* 0.042% solution, 200 metered doses/25-g bottle.

TIME/ACTION PROFILE (anti-inflammatory activity)

	ONSET	PEAK	DURATION
Inhaln	days–wks	1–4 wk	UK
Intranasal	days–wks	1–4 wk	UK

NURSING IMPLICATIONS

ASSESSMENT

- **General Info:** When changing from systemic glucocorticoids or discontinuing beclomethasone, monitor patient for signs of glucocorticoid withdrawal (muscle and joint pain, fatigue, dizziness, hypotension). Notify physician immediately should these symptoms occur.

*Underlines indicate most frequent; **CAPITALS** indicate life-threatening.

- **Inhalation:** Assess respiratory status, (rate, ease of breathing, lung sounds) periodically throughout therapy. Inspect oral membranes frequently for signs of candida infection (white patches; red, sore mucous membranes). Report sore throat, hoarseness, and cough to physician.
- **Nasal:** Assess degree of nasal stuffiness and character of discharge. Nasal burning and irritation may follow administration.

POTENTIAL NURSING DIAGNOSES

- Airway clearance, ineffective (indications).
- Oral mucous membranes, altered (side effects).
- Knowledge deficit related to medication regimen (patient/family teaching).

IMPLEMENTATION

- **Inhalation:** Administer inhalation bronchodilators, if used, several minutes before beclomethasone to open airways and allow delivery of steroid to site of action. Wait 5 min before using other inhalation medications.
- **Nasal Spray:** Decongestant or antihistamine may be ordered prior to instillation of nasal spray if secretions are present.

PATIENT/FAMILY TEACHING

- **General Info:** Advise patient to carry identification describing disease process and medication regimen at all times.
- □ Instruct patient to notify physician immediately if symptoms of oral or nasal infection occur, because therapy may need to be discontinued.
- **Inhalation:** Instruct patient in the proper use of the metered-dose inhaler. See Appendix H for instructions.
- □ Caution patient not to use higher than recommended doses or to increase frequency. Maximum of 20 inhalations/day for adults, 10/day for children aged 6–12. Notify physician if prescribed dose is ineffective. Doses >1600 mcg/day may result in adrenal insufficiency.
- □ Caution patient that medication is for

prophylactic use only. During an acute asthma attack supplemental systemic glucocorticoids may be needed.
- □ Rinsing mouth and gargling with warm water or mouthwash may reduce dry mouth and hoarseness.
- **Nasal:** See Appendix H for Nasal Spray administration.

EVALUATION
Effectiveness of therapy can be demonstrated by: ■ Improved pulmonary function in chronic bronchial asthma ■ Relief of symptoms of seasonal or perennial rhinitis ■ Prevention of recurrence of nasal polyps. In patients not receiving systemic steroids, 1–4 wk may be required before effects are seen.

BENAZEPRIL
(ben-**az**-e-pril)
Lotensin

CLASSIFICATION(S):
Antihypertensive (angiotensin converting enzyme [ACE] inhibitor)
Pregnancy Category C (first trimester), D (second and third trimester)

INDICATIONS

- Alone or in combination with thiazide diuretics in the management of hypertension.

ACTION

- Prevents the production of angiotensin II, a potent vasoconstrictor that stimulates the production of aldosterone by blocking its conversion to the active form—result is systemic vasodilation. **Therapeutic Effect:** ■ Lowering of blood pressure in hypertensive patients.

PHARMACOKINETICS

Absorption: 37% absorbed following oral administration.
Distribution: Much of the distribution not known. Crosses the placenta. Trace amounts enter breast milk.

Metabolism and Excretion: Metabolized by the liver to the benazaprilate, its active metabolite.
Half-life: 10–11 hr (benzaprilate); increased in renal impairment.

CONTRAINDICATIONS AND PRECAUTIONS

Contraindicated in: ▪ Hypersensitivity ▪ Cross-sensitivity with other ACE inhibitors may exist ▪ Pregnancy (may cause fetal malformation or death; hypotension, oliguria, or hypokalemia may occur in newborn).
Use Cautiously in: ▪ Renal impairment, hypovolemia, hyponatremia, elderly patients (dosage reduction required if CCr <30 ml/min/1.73 m^2) ▪ Aortic stenosis ▪ Collagen vascular disorders (increased risk of adverse renal effects) ▪ Cerebrovascular or cardiac insufficiency ▪ Lactation and children (safety not established) ▪ Surgery/anesthesia (hypotension may be exaggerated).
Extreme Caution in: Family history of hereditary angioedema.

ADVERSE REACTIONS AND SIDE EFFECTS*

CNS: dizziness, headache, fatigue.
Resp: cough.
CV: hypotension, tachycardia, angina pectoris.
GI: anorexia, loss of taste, nausea.
GU: proteinuria, renal failure.
Derm: rashes, pruritus.
F and E: hyperkalemia.
Hemat: LEUKOPENIA, AGRANULOCYTOSIS.
Misc: fever, edema of face or lips.

INTERACTIONS

Drug–Drug: ▪ Additive hypotension with other **antihypertensives, nitrates, phenothiazines,** and acute ingestion of **alcohol** ▪ Hyperkalemia may result from concurrent use of **potassium supplements, potassium-sparing diuretics** or **cyclosporine** ▪ Antihypertensive response may be blunted by **nonsteroidal anti-inflammatory agents** ▪ May in-

crease serum **digoxin** levels ▪ May increase the risk of **lithium** toxicity ▪ Increased risk of hypersensitivity reactions with **allopurinal** ▪ **Capsaicin** may increase the incidence of cough.

ROUTE AND DOSAGE

Hypertension
▪ **PO (Adults):** 5–10 mg once daily initially, increased gradually to maintenance dose of 20–40 mg/day as a single dose or 2 divided doses.

AVAILABILITY
▪ *Tablets:* 5 mg, 10 mg, 20 mg, 40 mg.

TIME/ACTION PROFILE (effect on blood pressure*)

	ONSET	PEAK	DURATION
PO	1 hr	2–4 hr	12–24 hr

*Full effects may not be noted until several weeks of therapy.

NURSING IMPLICATIONS

ASSESSMENT
☐ Monitor blood pressure and pulse frequently during initial dosage adjustment and periodically throughout course of therapy. Notify physician of significant changes.
▪ **Lab Test Considerations:** Monitor BUN, creatinine, and electrolyte levels periodically. Serum potassium may be increased and BUN and creatinine transiently increased while sodium levels may be decreased.
☐ May cause ECG changes.
☐ Monitor CBC periodically during therapy. May cause decrease in hemoglobin and hematocrit.
☐ May cause elevated liver enzymes, serum billirubin, uric acid, and glucose.
☐ Periodic assessments of urine protein may be ordered because proteinuria and nephrotic syndrome may occur.

POTENTIAL NURSING DIAGNOSES
▪ Cardiac output, decreased (indications, side effects).
▪ Knowledge deficit related to medica-

tion regimen (patient/family teaching).

- Noncompliance (patient/family teaching).

IMPLEMENTATION

- **PO:** Precipitous drop in blood pressure following first dose may occur. Discontinuing diuretic therapy 2–3 days prior to initiation of benazepril may decrease risk of hypotension. Resume diuretics if blood pressure is not controlled with benazepril.

PATIENT/FAMILY TEACHING

□ Instruct patient to take benazepril exactly as directed, even if feeling better. Missed doses should be taken as soon as remembered but not if almost time for next dose. Do not double doses. Medication controls but does not cure hypertension. Warn patients not to discontinue benazepril therapy unless directed by the physician.

□ Encourage patients to comply with additional interventions for hypertension (weight reduction, discontinuation of smoking, moderation of alcohol consumption, regular exercise, and stress management).

□ Instruct patient and family on proper technique for blood pressure monitoring. Advise them to check blood pressure at least weekly and report significantly changes to physician.

□ Caution patient to avoid salt substitutes or foods containing high levels of potassium or sodium unless directed by physician (see Appendix K).

□ Caution patient to change positions slowly to minimize orthostatic hypotension, particularly after initial dose. Patients should also be advised that exercising or hot weather may increase hypotensive effects.

□ Advise patients to consult physician or pharmacist before taking any over-the-counter medications, especially cold remedies. Patients should also avoid excessive amounts of tea, coffee, or cola.

□ May cause dizziness. Caution patient to avoid driving and other activities requiring alertness until response to medication is known.

□ Advise patient to inform physician or dentist of medication regimen prior to treatment or surgery.

□ Instruct patient to notify physician if rash, mouth sores, sore throat, fever, swelling of hands or feet, irregular heart beat, chest pain, dry cough, swelling of face, eyes, lips, or tongue, or difficulty breathing occurs or if taste impairment persists.

□ Advise patient to notify physician if pregnancy is planned or suspected.

□ Emphasize the importance of follow-up examinations to monitor progress.

EVALUATION

Effectiveness of therapy can be demonstrated by: ■ Decrease in blood pressure without appearance of side effects.

BENZQUINAMIDE
(benz-**kwin**-a-mide)
Emete-con

CLASSIFICATION(S):
Antiemetic
Pregnancy Category UK

INDICATIONS

- Prevention and treatment of nausea and vomiting associated with anesthesia and surgery.

ACTION

- Depresses the chemoreceptor trigger zone in the CNS. **Therapeutic Effect:**
- Relief of nausea and vomiting.

PHARMACOKINETICS

Absorption: Rapidly absorbed following IM administration.
Distribution: Widely distributed.
Metabolism and Excretion: Mostly metabolized by the liver. Minimal amounts excreted unchanged in the urine.
Half-life: 30–40 min.

CONTRAINDICATIONS AND PRECAUTIONS

Contraindicated in: ▪ Hypersensitivity ▪ Pregnancy (avoid use).

Use Cautiously in: ▪ History of cardiovascular disease ▪ Lactation and children (safety not established).

ADVERSE REACTIONS AND SIDE EFFECTS*

CNS: drowsiness, insomnia, restlessness, tremor.
EENT: blurred vision, increased salivation.
CV: hypotension, hypertension, arrhythmias.
GI: nausea, vomiting, cramps, dry mouth.

INTERACTIONS

Drug–Drug: ▪ Additive CNS depression with other **CNS depressants** including **alcohol, antihistamines, opioid analgesics,** and **sedative/hypnotics** ▪ May cause hypertension in patients receiving **vasopressors** or **epinephrine.**

ROUTE AND DOSAGE

▪ **IM (Adults):** 50 mg (0.5–1.0 mg/kg), may be repeated in 1 hr, then q 3–4 hr as needed.
▪ **IV (Adults):** 25 mg (0.2–0.4 mg/kg).

AVAILABILITY

▪ *Injection:* 50 mg/vial.

TIME/ACTION PROFILE (antiemetic effect)

	ONSET	PEAK	DURATION
IM	15 min	30 min	3–4 hr
IV	15 min	UK	3–4 hr

NURSING IMPLICATIONS

ASSESSMENT

▫ Assess nausea, vomiting, bowel sounds, and abdominal pain prior to and following administration. Benzquinamide may mask the signs of an acute abdomen.
▫ Monitor hydration status and intake and output. Patients with severe nausea and vomiting may require IV fluids in addition to antiemetics.
▫ Following IV administration, monitor patient for arrhythmias and changes in blood pressure.

POTENTIAL NURSING DIAGNOSES

▪ Fluid volume deficit (indications).
▪ Nutrition, altered: less than body requirements (indications).
▪ Injury, high risk for (side effects).

IMPLEMENTATION

▪ **General Info:** May be administered prophylactically at least 15 min prior to emergence from anesthesia.
▫ Reconstitute with 2.2 ml of Sterile or Bacteriostatic Water for Injection. Results in 2 ml solution with concentration of 25 mg/ml. Do not use 0.9% NaCl for reconstitution as solution may form a precipitate. Reconstituted solution is stable at room temperature for 14 days if protected from light. Do not refrigerate.
▪ **IM:** IM injection should be made deep into muscle mass. Use deltoid site only if well developed. IM route is preferred because of arrhythmias resulting from IV administration. Aspirate carefully to prevent inadvertent IV administration.
▪ **Direct IV:** Do not administer through an IV line containing saline.
▪ ***Rate:*** Administer slowly, 1 ml (25 mg) over 30–60 sec, through Y-tubing or 3-way stopcock.
▪ **Syringe Compatibility:** ▪ atropine ▪ droperidol/fentanyl ▪ glycopyrrolate ▪ hydroxyzine ▪ ketamine ▪ meperidine ▪ midazolam ▪ morphine ▪ naloxone ▪ pentazocine ▪ propranolol ▪ scopolamine.
▪ **Syringe Incompatibility:** ▪ chlordiazepoxide ▪ diazepam ▪ pentobarbital ▪ phenobarbital ▪ secobarbital ▪ sodium chloride ▪ thiopental.
▪ **Y-Site Compatibility:** foscarnet.

PATIENT/FAMILY TEACHING

▫ Advise patient to call for assistance when ambulating, because this drug may cause drowsiness and sedation.

B

*Underlines indicate most frequent; **CAPITALS** indicate life-threatening.

□ Instruct patient to make position changes slowly to minimize orthostatic hypotension.

□ Inform patient that this drug may cause dry mouth. Frequent oral rinses, good oral hygiene, and sugarless gum or candy may minimize this effect.

□ Advise patient and family to use general measures to decrease nausea (begin with sips of liquids, small non-greasy meals, provide oral hygiene, remove noxious stimuli from environment).

EVALUATION

Effectiveness of therapy may be determined by: ▪ Decreased nausea and vomiting within 15–30 min following administration.

BENZTROPINE
(**benz**-troe-peen)
{Apo-benztropin}, {Bensylate},
benzatropine, Cogentin

CLASSIFICATION(S):
Anticholinergic, Antiparkinson agent
Pregnancy Category C

INDICATIONS

▪ Adjunctive treatment of all forms of Parkinson's disease, including drug-induced extrapyramidal effects and acute dystonic reactions.

ACTION

▪ Blocks cholinergic activity in the CNS, which is partially responsible for the symptoms of Parkinson's disease ▪ Restores the natural balance of neurotransmitters in the CNS. **Therapeutic Effect:** ▪ Reduction of rigidity and tremors.

PHARMACOKINETICS

Absorption: Rapidly and completely absorbed following oral and IM administration.

Distribution: UK.
Metabolism and Excretion: UK.
Half-life: UK.

CONTRAINDICATIONS AND PRECAUTIONS

Contraindicated in: ▪ Hypersensitivity ▪ Children <3 yr ▪ Narrow-angle glaucoma ▪ Tardive dyskinesia.
Use Cautiously in: ▪ Elderly patients (increased risk of adverse reactions) ▪ Pregnancy and lactation (safety not established).

ADVERSE REACTIONS AND SIDE EFFECTS*

CNS: confusion, weakness, hallucinations, headache, sedation, depression, dizziness.
EENT: <u>dry eyes</u>, <u>blurred vision</u>, mydriasis.
CV: tachycardia, arrhythmias, palpitations, hypotension.
GI: <u>constipation</u>, <u>dry mouth</u>, nausea, ileus.
GU: urinary retention, hesitancy.
Misc: decreased sweating.

INTERACTIONS

Drug–Drug: ▪ Additive anticholinergic affects with **drugs sharing anticholinergic properties** such as **antihistamines, phenothiazines, quinidine, disopyramide,** and **tricyclic antidepressants** ▪ Counteracts the cholinergic effects of **bethanechol** ▪ **Antacids** and **antidiarrheals** may decrease absorption.

ROUTE AND DOSAGE

Parkinsonism
▪ **PO (Adults):** 0.5–6 mg/day in 1–2 divided doses.

Acute Dystonic Reactions
▪ **IM, IV (Adults):** 1–2 mg initially, then 1–2 mg PO bid.

Drug-Induced Extrapyramidal Reactions
▪ **PO, IM, IV (Adults):** 1–4 mg given once or twice daily.

{} = Available in Canada only.
*Underlines indicate most frequent; **CAPITALS** indicate life-threatening.

AVAILABILITY

- **Tablets:** 0.5 mg, 1 mg, 2 mg **Injection:** 1 mg/ml.

TIME/ACTION PROFILE
(antidyskinetic activity)

	ONSET	PEAK	DURATION
PO	1–2 hr	several days	24 hr
IM, IV	within mins	UK	24 hr

NURSING IMPLICATIONS

ASSESSMENT

- **General Info:** Assess parkinson and extrapyramidal symptoms (akinesia, rigidity, tremors, pill rolling, mask facies, shuffling gait, muscle spasms, twisting motions, and drooling) prior to and throughout course of therapy.
- Assess bowel function daily. Monitor for constipation, abdominal pain, distention, or the absence of bowel sounds.
- Monitor intake and output ratios and assess patient for urinary retention (dysuria, distended abdomen, infrequent voiding of small amounts, overflow incontinence).
- Patients with mental illness are at risk of developing exaggerated symptoms of their disorder during early therapy with this medication. Withhold drug and notify physician if significant behavioral changes occur.
- **Parenteral Administration:** Monitor pulse and blood pressure closely and maintain bedrest for 1 hr after administration. Advise patients to make position changes slowly to minimize orthostatic hypotension.

POTENTIAL NURSING DIAGNOSES

- Physical mobility, impaired (indications).
- Injury, high risk for (indications).
- Knowledge deficit related to medication regimen (patient/family teaching).

IMPLEMENTATION

- **PO:** Administer with food or immediately after meals to minimize gastric irritation. May be crushed and administered with food if patient has difficulty swallowing.
- **IM:** Parenteral route is only used for dystonic reactions.
- **Direct IV:** IV route is rarely used because onset is same as with IM route.
- **Rate:** Administer at a rate of 1 mg over 1 min.
- **Syringe Compatibility:** metoclopramide.
- **Y-Site Compatibility:** fluconazole.

PATIENT/FAMILY TEACHING

- Encourage patient to take this drug as directed. Missed doses should be taken as soon as remembered up to 2 hr before the next dose. Taper gradually when discontinuing or a withdrawal reaction may occur (anxiety, tachycardia, insomnia, return of parkinson or extrapyramidal symptoms).
- May cause drowsiness or dizziness. Advise patient to avoid driving or other activities that require alertness until response to the drug is known.
- Instruct patient that frequent rinsing of mouth, good oral hygiene, and sugarless gum or candy may decrease dry mouth. Patient should notify physician if dryness persists (saliva substitutes may be used). Also notify the dentist if dryness interferes with use of dentures.
- Caution patient to make position changes slowly to minimize orthostatic hypotension.
- Instruct patient to notify physician if difficulty with urination, constipation, abdominal discomfort, rapid or pounding heartbeat, confusion, eye pain, or rash occur.
- Advise patient to confer with physician or pharmacist prior to taking over-the-counter medications, especially cold remedies, or drinking alcoholic beverages.
- Caution patient that this medication decreases perspiration. Overheating may occur during hot weather. Patients should notify physician if they cannot remain indoors in an air-conditioned environment during hot weather.

B

□ Advise patient to avoid taking antacids or antidiarrheals within 1–2 hr of this medication.
□ Emphasize the importance of routine follow-up examinations.

EVALUATION
Effectiveness of therapy can be demonstrated by: ▪ Decrease in drooling, tremors, and rigidity and an improvement in gait and balance. Therapeutic effects are usually seen 2–3 days after the initiation of therapy.

BEPRIDIL
(be-pri-dil)
Vascor

CLASSIFICATION(S):
Calcium channel blocker, Antianginal, Coronary vasodilator
Pregnancy Category C

INDICATIONS

▪ Management of effort-induced angina pectoris due to coronary insufficiency in patients who fail to respond to conventional therapy. Has been used with beta blockers or nitrates.

ACTION

▪ Inhibits the transport of calcium into myocardial and vascular smooth muscle cells, resulting in inhibition of excitation-contraction coupling and subsequent contraction. ▪ May decrease SA and AV node conduction. **Therapeutic Effect:** ▪ Coronary vasodilation with subsequent decrease in frequency and severity of attacks of angina pectoris.

PHARMACOKINETICS

Absorption: Well absorbed following oral administration.
Distribution: Crosses the placenta and enters breast milk, remainder of distribution not known.
Metabolism and Excretion: Mostly metabolized by the liver. Inactive metabolites excreted by the kidneys.

Half-life: 42 hr (following cessation of multiple dosing).

CONTRAINDICATIONS AND PRECAUTIONS

Contraindicated in: ▪ Hypersensitivity ▪ Serious ventricular arrhythmias (may be proarrhythmic) ▪ Hypotension ▪ Cardiac insufficiency ▪ Sick sinus syndrome (unless a pacemaker is placed) ▪ 2nd- and 3rd-degree heart block ▪ Congenital or drug-induced prolongation of the QT interval on ECG ▪ Recent (within 3 mo) myocardial infarction.
Use Cautiously in: ▪ Hepatic or renal impairment ▪ Left bundle branch block ▪ Sinus bradycardia (<50 bpm) ▪ Pregnancy, lactation, or children (safety not established).

ADVERSE REACTIONS AND SIDE EFFECTS*

CNS: <u>headache</u>, <u>weakness</u>, <u>dizziness</u>, drowsiness, insomnia, nervousness.
EENT: dry mouth, tinnitus.
Resp: dyspnea, respiratory infection.
CV: CONGESTIVE HEART FAILURE, VENTRICULAR ARRHYTHMIAS, <u>prolonged QT interval</u>, palpitations.
GI: <u>nausea</u>, dyspepsia, anorexia, <u>diarrhea</u>, abdominal pain, constipation.
F and E: hypokalemia.
Hemat: AGRANULOCYTOSIS.
Neuro: tremor, paresthesia.
Misc: flu-like syndrome.

INTERACTIONS

Drug–Drug: ▪ **Antiarrhythmics, antidepressants,** and **cardiac glycosides** may increase the likelihood of ventricular arrhythmias ▪ Increases serum **digoxin** levels.

ROUTE AND DOSAGE

▪ **PO (Adults):** 200 mg once daily, may increase after 10 days to 300 mg/day (not to exceed 400 mg/day).

AVAILABILITY

▪ *Tablet:* 200 mg, 300 mg, 400 mg.

---

*<u>Underlines</u> indicate most frequent; **CAPITALS** indicate life-threatening.

TIME/ACTION PROFILE

	ONSET	PEAK	DURATION
PO	8 days*	UK	24 hr

*Onset of steady state antianginal effects with chronic dosing.

NURSING IMPLICATIONS

ASSESSMENT

□ Assess location, duration, intensity, and precipitating factors of patient's anginal pain.

□ Monitor pulse before administering medication. Monitor ECG periodically in patients receiving prolonged therapy.

□ Monitor intake and output ratios and daily weight. Assess patient for signs of congestive heart failure (peripheral edema, rales/crackles, dyspnea, weight gain, jugular venous distention).

□ Patients receiving cardiac glycosides concurrently with bepridil should have routine serum cardiac glycoside levels and be monitored for signs and symptoms of digitalis glycoside toxicity.

■ **Lab Test Considerations:** Monitor WBC periodically in patients receiving long-term therapy.

□ May cause elevated ALT (SGPT).

□ Monitor serum potassium periodically. May cause hypokalemia.

POTENTIAL NURSING DIAGNOSES

■ Cardiac output, decreased (indications).

■ Pain (indications).

■ Knowledge deficit related to medication regimen (patient/family teaching).

IMPLEMENTATION

■ **PO:** May be administered with meals if GI irritation becomes a problem.

PATIENT/FAMILY TEACHING

□ Advise patient to take medication exactly as directed, not to skip or double up on missed doses. Bepridil may need to be discontinued gradually.

□ Instruct patients on concurrent nitrate or beta-blocker therapy to continue taking both medications as ordered and using SL nitroglycerin as needed for anginal attacks.

□ May cause dizziness. Advise patient to avoid driving or other activities requiring alertness until response to the medication is known.

□ Instruct patient to avoid concurrent use of alcohol or over-the-counter medications without consulting physician or pharmacist.

□ Advise patient to contact physician if chest pain does not improve or worsens after therapy, or is accompanied by diaphoresis, or shortness of breath, or if severe, persistent headache occurs. Also notify the physician if irregular heart beats, dyspnea, swelling of hands and feet, pronounced dizziness, nausea, or constipation occur.

EVALUATION

Effectiveness of therapy can be demonstrated by: ■ Decrease in frequency and severity of anginal attacks □ Decreased need for nitrate therapy □ Increase in activity tolerance and sense of well-being.

BERACTANT
(be-**rak**-tant)
Survanta

CLASSIFICATION(S):
Natural lung surfactant
Pregnancy Category UK

INDICATIONS

■ Treatment and prophylaxis of respiratory distress syndrome (RDS, hyaline membrane disease) in premature infants.

ACTION

■ Replaces endogenous pulmonary surfactant in premature infants, allowing normal surface activity in alveoli ■ Consists of natural bovine lung extract. **Therapeutic Effects:** ■ Decreased incidence, mortality, and complications from RDS.

PHARMACOKINETICS

Absorption: Administered directly to site of action. Systemic absorption not known.
Distribution: Rapidly distributes to lung tissue.
Metabolism and Excretion: Enters surfactant pathways where recycling and reutilization occur.
Half-life: UK.

CONTRAINDICATIONS AND PRECAUTIONS

Contraindicated in: ▪ No known contraindications.
Use Cautiously in: ▪ No known cautions. Nosocomial infections may be more common.

ADVERSE REACTIONS AND SIDE EFFECTS*

Resp: <u>oxygen desaturation</u> (as a result of administration process).
CV: <u>transient bradycardia</u>.

INTERACTIONS

Drug–Drug: ▪ None known.

ROUTE AND DOSAGE

▪ **Intratracheal (Premature Infants):** 100 mg phospholipids/kg (4 ml/kg), give 4 doses in first 48 hr of life, no closer than q 6 hr apart.

AVAILABILITY

▪ *Intratracheal suspension:* 25 mg phospholipid/ml—8-ml vials.

TIME/ACTION PROFILE (improved oxygenation)

	ONSET	PEAK	DURATION
intratracheal	within min	UK	UK

NURSING IMPLICATIONS

ASSESSMENT

▫ Monitor ECG, heart rate, color, chest expansion, facial expression, transcutaneous oxygen saturation, and endotracheal tube patency continuously during dosing. Continuous bedside monitoring should continue for at least 30 min following dosing.
▫ If bradycardia and decreased oxygen saturation occur during dosing, stop the dosing procedure and initiate measures to alleviate the condition. Then resume dosing.
▪ **Lab Test Considerations:** Monitor arterial blood gases frequently to prevent hyperoxia or hypocarbia.

POTENTIAL NURSING DIAGNOSES

▪ Impaired gas exchange (indications).

IMPLEMENTATION

▪ **General Info:** Only trained medical personnel with experience in airway and clinical management of unstable neonates should perform beractant instillation. Audiovisual instructional materials are available from the manufacturer.
▪ **Inhalation:** Does not require reconstitution. Inspect for discoloration prior to administration. Color should be off-white to light brown. If settling occurs, swirl gently, do not shake. Beractant must be refrigerated. Warm before administering by standing at room temperature for 20 min or warm in the hand for at least 8 min. Do not use artificial warming methods. Unopened vials that have been warmed may be refrigerated for 8 hr. Do not warm and re-refrigerate more than once. Discard unused doses.
▫ Administer intratracheally through a 5 French end-hole catheter inserted into the infant's endotracheal tube with the tip protruding just beyond the end of the endotracheal tube above the infant's carina. Shorten the length of the catheter before insertion to avoid instillation into main-stem bronchus.
▫ Determine dose and withdraw entire contents of vial into a plastic syringe with a large-gauge (at least 20 g) needle. Do not filter or shake. Attach catheter to end of syringe. Fill catheter with beractant and discard excess through catheter so that only the total dose remains in the syringe.

*<u>Underlines</u> indicate most frequent; **CAPITALS** indicate life-threatening.

□ Suction the infant endotracheally prior to instillation. Check position of endotracheal tube prior to instillation. Do not suction for 1 hr after instillation unless clinically necessary.

■ **Rate:** To ensure homogenous distribution, each ¼ dose should be administered gently over 2–3 sec with the infant in a different position. Sequence of positions is head and body inclined slightly down, head turned to the right; head and body inclined slightly down, head turned to the left; head and body inclined slightly up, head turned to the right; head and body inclined slightly up, head turned to the left. Ventilate the infant for at least 30 sec or until stable between each ¼ dose. After instillation of the last ¼ dose, remove the catheter without flushing it.

■ **Prevention Strategy:** Administer within 15 min of birth, if possible. Between each ¼ dose, manually ventilate with a handbag with sufficient oxygen to prevent cyanosis, at a rate of 60 breaths/min, and sufficient positive pressure for adequate air exchange and chest wall excursion.

■ **Rescue Strategy:** Administer as soon as possible after infant is placed on the ventilator for management of RDS. Immediately prior to instillation of first ¼ dose and between each ¼ dose, ventilate with ventilator settings at 60/min, inspiratory time 0.5 sec, and FiO₂ 1.

■ **Repeat Doses:** Obtain radiologic confirmation of RDS prior to repeat dose. FiO₂ may be increased by 0.2 or amount sufficient to prevent cyanosis. Rate may be set at 30/min with an inspiratory time of <1 sec. If pretreatment rate was ≥30 it may be unchanged during repeat dose. Do not use manual hand-bag ventilation during repeat doses.

PATIENT/FAMILY TEACHING
□ Explain purpose of medication to parents.

EVALUATION
Effectiveness of therapy may be determined by: ■ Prevention of RDS ■ Improvement in lung compliance □ Improved oxygenation □ Normalization of arterial blood gases.

B

BETAMETHASONE
(bay-ta-**meth**-a-sone)
Alphatrex, {Betacort}, {Betaderm}, Betatrex, Beta-Val, {Betnelan}, {Betnesol}, {Betnovate}, Celestone, Cel-U-Jec, Dermabet, Diprolene, Diprosone, {Ectosone}, {Metaderm}, {Novabetamet}, Selestoject, Uticort, Valisone, Valnac

CLASSIFICATION(S):
Glucocorticoid (long-acting)
**Pregnancy Category C (topical),
UK (systemic)**

INDICATIONS
■ Used systemically and locally in a wide variety of chronic inflammatory, allergic, hematologic, neoplastic, and autoimmune diseases ■ Not suitable for alternate-day therapy.

ACTION
■ Suppresses inflammation and normal immune response. Has numerous intense metabolic effects (see *Adverse Reactions and Side Effects*). Suppresses adrenal function at chronic oral doses of 0.6 mg/day. **Therapeutic Effects:** ■ Suppression of inflammation and modification of normal immune response.

PHARMACOKINETICS
Absorption: Well absorbed following oral administrations. Sodium phosphate salt is rapidly absorbed following IM administration. Acetate suspension is slowly absorbed. When injected locally, absorption is slow but complete.

Systemic absorption also follows topical administration.
Distribution: Crosses the placenta. Small amounts enter breast milk.
Metabolism and Excretion: Mostly metabolized by the liver.
Half-life: 3–5 hr (plasma), 36–54 hr (tissue); adrenal suppression lasts 3.25 days.

CONTRAINDICATIONS AND PRECAUTIONS

Contraindicated in: ▪ Acute untreated infections except for some forms of meningitis ▪ Lactation (avoid chronic use) ▪ Avoid abrupt discontinuation.
Use Cautiously in: ▪ Chronic treatment (leads to adrenal suppression) ▪ Stress (supplemental doses necessary) ▪ Glaucoma ▪ Diabetes mellitus ▪ Pregnancy (safety not established) ▪ Children (chronic treatment results in decreased growth; use of short- or intermediate-acting glucocorticoids is recommended) ▪ Use lowest dose for shortest period of time ▪ Some products contain bisulfites and/or tartrazine—use with caution in hypersensitive patients.

ADVERSE REACTIONS AND SIDE EFFECTS*

CNS: headache, restlessness, psychoses, depression, euphoria, personality changes, increased intracranial pressure (children only).
EENT: cataracts, increased intraocular pressure.
CV: hypertension.
GI: nausea, vomiting, anorexia, peptic ulceration, increased appetite.
Derm: impaired wound healing, petechiae, ecchymoses, skin fragility, hirsutism, acne.
Endo: adrenal suppression, hyperglycemia.
F and E: hypokalemia, hypokalemic alkalosis, fluid retention.
Hemat: thromboembolism, thrombophlebitis.
MS: muscle wasting, muscle pain, aseptic necrosis of joints, osteoporosis.

Misc: increased susceptibility to infection, cushingoid appearance (moon face, buffalo hump).

INTERACTIONS

Drug–Drug: ▪ Additive hypokalemia with **diuretics, amphotercin B, mezlocillin,** or **ticarcillin** ▪ Hypokalemia may increase the risk of **cardiac glycoside** toxicity ▪ **Barbiturates, phenytoin,** and **rifampin** increase metabolism and may decrease effectiveness ▪ May increase the need for **insulin** or **hypoglycemic agents**.

ROUTE AND DOSAGE

Adrenocortical Insufficiency
▪ **PO (Children):** 17.5 mcg/kg (500 mcg/m²) daily in 3 divided doses.
▪ **IM (Children):** 17.5 mcg/kg (500 mcg/m²) daily in 3 divided doses every third day; or 5.8–8.75 mcg/kg (166–250 mcg/m²) daily as a single dose.

Other Oral Uses
▪ **PO (Adults):** 0.6 mg–7.2 mg/day as single daily dose or in divided doses.
▪ **PO (Children):** 17.5–250 mcg/kg (1.875–7.5 mg/m²) daily in 3 divided doses.

Betamethasone Sodium Phosphate
▪ **IM, IV (Adults):** Up to 9 mg of betamethsone base (12 mg of betamethasone phosphate); given as needed.
▪ **IM (Children):** 17.5–125 mcg/kg (0.625–3.75 mg/m²) of the base q 12–24 hr.
▪ **IA, IL (Adults):** Up to 9 mg of betamethasone base (12 mg of betamethasone phosphate); given as needed.

Betamethasone Sodium Phosphate/ Betamethasone Acetate Suspension
▪ **IM (Adults):** 0.5–9 mg/day.
▪ **IA (Adults):** 1.5–12 mg (dose depends on joint); may be repeated as needed.
▪ **IL (Adults):** 1.2 mg/m² of affected skin (not to exceed 6 mg); may be repeated weekly.

*Underlines indicate most frequent; **CAPITALS** indicate life-threatening.

Topical (Betamethasone benzoate, dipropionate, valerate)

- **Top (Adults):** Apply 1–3 times daily.
- **Top (Children):** Apply once daily.
- **Ophth;** 1–2 drops q 1–2 hr, decrease as needed.

AVAILABILITY

- *Tablets:* 0.6 mg ▪ *Syrup:* 0.6 mg/5 ml
- {*Extended-release tablets:* 1 mg}
- *Injection (solution):* 3 mg/ml ▪ *Injection (suspension):* 6 mg (total)/ml
- *Cream:* 0.01%, 0.025%, 0.05%, 0.1%
- *Ointment:* 0.05%, 0.1% ▪ *Lotion:* 0.05%, 0.1% ▪ *Gel:* 0.025% ▪ *Aerosol:* 0.1% ▪ *Ophth solution:* 0.1%.

TIME/ACTION PROFILE (anti-inflammatory activity)

	ONSET	PEAK	DURATION
PO	UK	1–2 hr	3.25 days
IV	rapid	UK	UK
IM (phosphate)	rapid	UK	UK
IM (acetate/ phosphate)	1–3 hr	UK	1 wk
IA	UK	UK	1–2 wk
IL	UK	UK	1 wk
Top	hrs	UK	8–24 hr

NURSING IMPLICATIONS

ASSESSMENT

- **General Info:** Assess patient for signs of adrenal insufficiency prior to and periodically throughout therapy.
- ▫ Monitor intake and output ratios and daily weight. Assess for fluid overload (edema, steady weight gain, rales/crackles, or dyspnea).
- **IA:** Monitor pain, edema, and range of motion of affected joints.
- **Top:** Assess affected skin prior to and daily during therapy. Note degree of inflammation and pruritus.
- **Lab Test Considerations:** *Systemic*—Monitor serum electrolytes and glucose. May cause hyperglycemia, especially in persons with diabetes. May cause hypokalemia.
- ▫ Guaiac stools. Promptly report presence of guaiac-positive stools.
- ▫ Periodic adrenal function tests may be ordered to assess degree of hypothalamic-pituitary-adrenal axis suppression in systemic and chronic topical therapy.

POTENTIAL NURSING DIAGNOSES

- Skin integrity, impaired (indications).
- Infection, high risk for (side effects).
- Knowledge deficit related to medication regimen (patient/family teaching).

IMPLEMENTATION

- **General Info:** Suspension of betamethasone sodium phosphate and betamethasone acetate may be combined with 1% or 2% lidocaine without preservatives for injection into joint, tendon, or bursa.
- **PO:** Administer with meals to minimize GI irritation. For daily dose, give in AM to coincide with body's normal secretion of cortisol.
- **Direct IV:** Only betamethasone sodium phosphate may be given IV.
- **Rate:** Administer over at least 1 min.
- **Intermittent Infusion:** May be administered as infusion in D5W, 0.9% NaCl, Ringer's solution, D5/Ringer's solution, or D5/LR.
- **Y-Site Compatibility:** ▪ heparin ▪ hydrocortisone sodium succinate ▪ potassium chloride.
- **Top:** Apply to clean, slightly moist skin. Wear gloves. Do not apply occlusive dressing.
- ▫ Apply aerosol form from a distance of 15 cm for 3 sec.
- **Ophth:** See Appendix H for instillation of ophthalmic medications.

PATIENT/FAMILY TEACHING

- **General Info:** Instruct patient on correct technique of medication administration. Emphasize importance of avoiding the eyes. Advise patient to take medication as directed. Take missed doses as soon as remembered unless almost time for next dose. Do not double doses. Stopping the medication suddenly may result in adrenal insufficiency (anorexia, nausea, weakness, fatigue, hypotension, hypoglycemia). If these signs appear notify physician immediately. This can be life-threatening.

□ This drug causes immunosuppression and may mask symptoms of infection. Instruct patient to avoid persons with known contagious illnesses and to notify physician if infection occurs.

□ Caution patient to avoid vaccinations without first consulting with physician.

□ Instruct patient to notify physician if severe abdominal pain, tarry stools, unusual pain, swelling, weight gain, tiredness, bone pain, bruising, nonhealing sores, visual disturbances, or behavior changes occur.

□ Explain need for continued medical follow-up to assess effectiveness and possible side effects of medication. Physician may order periodic lab tests and eye examinations.

□ Instruct patient to inform physician if symptoms of underlying disease return or worsen.

□ Advise patient to carry identification describing disease process and medication regimen in the event of emergency in which patient cannot relate medical history.

■ **Long-term Therapy:** Encourage patient to eat a diet high in protein, calcium, and potassium, and low in sodium and carbohydrates (see Appendix K). Alcohol should be avoided during therapy.

EVALUATION
Effectiveness of therapy can be demonstrated by: ■ Decrease in presenting symptoms with minimal systemic side effects.

BETAXOLOL
(be-**tax**-oh-lol)
Betoptic, Betoptic S, Kerlone

CLASSIFICATION(S):
Antiglaucoma agent, Beta-adrenergic blocker (selective), Antihypertensive
Pregnancy Category C

INDICATIONS

■ **PO:** Used alone or in combination with other agents in the treatment of hypertension ■ **Ophth:** Decreases intraocular pressure in patients with chronic open-angle glaucoma.

ACTION

■ **PO:** Blocks stimulation of $beta_1$ (myocardial) receptors ■ **Ophth:** Decreases the production of aqueous humor. **Therapeutic Effect:** ■ **PO:** Decreased blood pressure ■ **Ophth:** Decreased intraocular pressure.

PHARMACOKINETICS

Absorption: Well absorbed following oral administration. Systemic absorption is minimal following ophthalmic administration.
Distribution: Widely distributed when administered systemically.
Metabolism and Excretion: Mostly metabolized by the liver; 20% excreted unchanged by the kidneys following systemic administration.
Half-life: 15–20 hr.

CONTRAINDICATIONS AND PRECAUTIONS

Contraindicated in: ■ Hypersensitivity to benzalkonium chloride or edetate disodium (ophthalmic preparation only) ■ Uncompensated congestive heart failure ■ Pulmonary edema ■ Cardiogenic shock ■ Bradycardia ■ Heart block ■ Patients with a history of severe allergic reactions (intensity of reaction may be increased).
Use Cautiously in: ■ Cardiac failure ■ Diabetes mellitus (may block some symptoms of hypoglycemia) ■ Pulmonary disease including asthma ■ Thyrotoxicosis ■ Children, pregnancy, or lactation (safety not established) ■ Renal impairment (dosage reduction recommended for oral dosage form) ■ Ophthalmic administration (systemic effects may occur) ■ Elderly patients (use small initial dose).

ADVERSE REACTIONS AND SIDE EFFECTS*

CNS: *Ophth*—insomnia, depressive neurosis; *PO*—dizziness, anxiety, nervousness, nightmares, vivid dreams, tiredness, weakness, confusion.

EENT: *Ophth*—ocular stinging, tearing, erythema, itching, keratitis, corneal staining, unequal pupil size, photophobia; *PO*—dry eyes, sore eyes, stuffy nose.

Resp: *Ophth* and *PO*—bronchospasm.

CV: *PO*—bradycardia, CONGESTIVE HEART FAILURE.

GI: *PO*—diarrhea, nausea, vomiting.

GU: *PO*—impotence.

Derm: rash.

Hemat: *PO*—thrombocytopenia.

MS: *PO*—back pain, joint pain.

Misc: Raynaud's phenomenon.

INTERACTIONS

Drug–Drug: ▪ **PO: General anesthesia, IV phenytoin,** and **verapamil** may cause additive myocardial depression ▪ Additive bradycardia may occur with concurrent use of **cardiac glycosides** ▪ Additive hypotension may occur with other **antihypertensive agents,** acute ingestion of **alcohol,** or **nitrates** ▪ Concurrent use with **amphetamines, cocaine, ephedrine, epinephrine, norepinephrine, phenylephrine,** or **pseudoephedrine** may result in excess alpha-adrenergic stimulation, hypertension, and bradycardia ▪ May negate the beneficial beta$_1$ cardiac effects of **dopamine** or **dobutamine** ▪ Concurrent **thyroid** administration may decrease effectiveness ▪ Concurrent use with **insulin** may result in prolonged hypoglycemia. ▪ **Ophth:** Additive beta-adrenergic blockade may occur with concurrent **systemic beta-adrenergic blocking agents** ▪ Use cautiously in patients receiving **reserpine** or **adrenergic psychotropic agents** ▪ Effectiveness of **theophylline** may be decreased.

ROUTE AND DOSAGE

▪ **PO (Adults):** 10 mg once daily, may be increased to 20 mg/day after 7–14 days of therapy. Start with 5 mg/day in elderly patients.

▪ **Ophth (Adults):** 1 drop twice daily.

AVAILABILITY

▪ *Tablets:* 10 mg, 20 mg ▪ *Ophth solution:* 0.5% ▪ *Ophth suspension:* 0.25%.

TIME/ACTION PROFILE

	ONSET	PEAK	DURATION
PO	3–4 hr	7–14 days*	24 hr
Ophth	30 min	2 hr	12 hr

*With multiple dosing.

NURSING IMPLICATIONS

ASSESSMENT

▪ **PO:** Monitor blood pressure and pulse frequently during period of dose adjustment and periodically during therapy. Confer with physician before giving drug if pulse is <50 bpm.

▫ Monitor intake and output ratios and daily weights. Assess routinely for signs and symptoms of congestive heart failure (dyspnea, rales/crackles, weight gain, peripheral edema, jugular venous distension).

▪ **Ophth:** Intraocular pressure should be monitored during the first month of therapy and periodically thereafter.

▪ **Lab Test Considerations:** May cause increased serum lipoprotein, triglyceride, potassium, and uric acid concentrations.

POTENTIAL NURSING DIAGNOSES

▪ Cardiac output, decreased (indications).

▪ Knowledge deficit related to medication regimen (patient/family teaching).

IMPLEMENTATION

▪ **PO:** May be administered concurrently with diuretic therapy.

▪ **Ophth:** See Appendix H for instillation of ophthalmic medications.

---

*Underlines indicate most frequent; **CAPITALS** indicate life-threatening.

□ When using betaxolol to replace other antiglaucoma agents, continue administration of all medications on the first day of betaxolol therapy. Decrease use of other medications weekly, one at a time, based on patient response.

□ To control intraocular pressure, betaxolol may be used concurrently with muscarinic agonists (pilocarpine, echothiophate, carbachol), beta-agonists (ophthalmic epinephrine, dipivefrin), or systemic carbonic anhydrase inhibitors (acetazolamide).

PATIENT/FAMILY TEACHING

▪ **General Info:** Advise patient to take medication exactly as directed. Missed doses should be administered as soon as remembered unless almost time for the next dose; administer next dose at scheduled time.

□ Inform diabetic patients that betaxolol may mask some signs of hypoglycemia.

□ Advise patient to inform physician or dentist of medication regimen prior to treatment or surgery. Gradual withdrawal of betaxolol may be necessary.

□ Instruct patient to notify physician if confusion, depression, sleep disturbance, weakness, wheezing, or dyspnea, dizziness, rash, sore throat, fever, unusual bleeding or bruising occur.

□ Emphasize the importance of regular follow-up examinations to monitor progress.

▪ **PO:** Teach patient and family how to check blood pressure and pulse. Instruct them to take pulse daily and blood pressure biweekly. Advise patient to hold dose and contact physician if pulse is <50 bpm or blood pressure changes significantly.

□ Reinforce need to continue additional therapies for hypertension (weight loss, restricted sodium intake, stress reduction, regular exercise, moderation of alcohol consumption, cessation of smoking). Betaxolol controls but does not cure hypertension.

□ Caution patient that this medication may cause increased sensitivity to cold.

□ Advise patient to consult physician before taking any over-the-counter drugs, especially cold remedies, concurrently with this medication. Patient should also avoid excessive amounts of coffee, tea, and cola.

□ Advise patient to carry identification describing medication regimen at all times.

▪ **Ophth:** Instruct patient in proper technique for instillation of ophthalmic medications. Emphasize the importance of not touching the applicator tip to any surface.

□ Advise patient to wear sunglasses and avoid exposure to bright light to prevent photophobia.

EVALUATION

Effectiveness of therapy can be demonstrated by: ▪ Decreased blood pressure ▪ Decreased intraocular pressure.

BETHANECHOL
(be-**than**-e-kole)
Duvoid, Myotonochol, Urebeth, Urecholine, Urolax

CLASSIFICATION(S):
Cholinergic (direct-acting)
Pregnancy Category C

INDICATIONS

▪ Postpartum and postoperative nonobstructive urinary retention or urinary retention due to neurogenic bladder.

ACTION

▪ Stimulates cholinergic receptors. Effects include: □ Contraction of the urinary bladder □ Decreased bladder capacity □ Increased frequency of ureteral periostaltic waves □ Increased tone and peristalsis in the GI tract □ Increased pressure in the lower esophageal sphincter □ Increased gastric secretions. **Therapeutic Effect:** ▪ Bladder emptying.

PHARMACOKINETICS

Absorption: Poorly absorbed following

oral administration, requiring larger doses by mouth than subcutaneously.
Distribution: Does not cross the blood–brain barrier.
Metabolism and Excretion: UK.
Half-life: UK.

CONTRAINDICATIONS AND PRECAUTIONS

Contraindicated in: ▪ Hypersensitivity ▪ Mechanical obstruction of the GI or GU tract ▪ Some products contain tartrazine and should be avoided in patients with known intolerance.
Use Cautiously in: ▪ History of asthma ▪ Ulcer disease ▪ Cardiovascular disease ▪ Epilepsy ▪ Hyperthyroidism ▪ Children, pregnancy, and lactation (safety not established) ▪ Sensitivity to cholinergic agents or effects.

ADVERSE REACTIONS AND SIDE EFFECTS*

CNS: malaise, headache.
EENT: lacrimation, miosis.
Resp: bronchospasm.
CV: hypotension, bradycardia, SYNCOPE/CARDIAC ARREST, heart block.
GI: abdominal discomfort, diarrhea, nausea, vomiting, salivation.
GU: urgency.
Misc: hypothermia, flushing, sweating.

INTERACTIONS

Drug–Drug: ▪ Quinidine and procainamide may antagonize cholinergic effects ▪ Additive cholinergic effects with cholinesterase inhibitors ▪ Use with ganglionic blocking agents may result in severe hypotension ▪ Do not use with depolarizing neuromuscular blocking agents ▪ Effectiveness will be decreased by anticholinergic agents.

ROUTE AND DOSAGE

▪ **PO (Adults):** Initially dose may be determined by administering 5–10 mg q 1–2 hr until response obtained or total of 50 mg administered. Maintenance dose is 10–50 mg 3 times daily (doses up to 50–100 mg 4 times daily have been used).

▪ **SC (Adults):** Initially dose may be determined by administering 2.5 mg q 15–30 min until response obtained or total of 4 doses administered. Maintenance dose is 2.5–5 mg 3–4 times daily, up to 7.5–10 mg q 4 hr for neurogenic bladder.

AVAILABILITY

▪ **Tablets:** 5 mg, 10 mg, 25 mg, 50 mg
▪ **Injection:** 5 mg/ml.

TIME/ACTION PROFILE (response on bladder muscle)

	ONSET	PEAK	DURATION
PO	30–90	1 hr	6 hr
SC	5–15	15–30 min	2 hr

NURSING IMPLICATIONS

ASSESSMENT

▫ Monitor blood pressure, pulse, and respirations before administering and for at least 1 hr following SC administration.

▫ Monitor intake and output ratios. Palpate abdomen for bladder distention. Notify physician if drug fails to relieve condition for which it was prescribed. Physician may order catheterization to assess postvoid residual.

▪ **Lab Test Considerations:** May cause an increase in serum amylase and lipase, AST (SGOT), and serum bilirubin.

▪ **Toxicity and Overdose:** Observe patient for drug toxicity (sweating, flushing, abdominal cramps, nausea, salivation). If overdosage occurs, treatment includes atropine sulfate (specific antidote).

POTENTIAL NURSING DIAGNOSES

▪ Urinary elimination, altered patterns of (indications).
▪ Knowledge deficit related to medication regimen (patient/family teaching).

IMPLEMENTATION

▪ **General Info:** A test dose is usually used prior to maintenance.

*Underlines indicate most frequent; CAPITALS indicate life-threatening

▫ Oral and SC doses are *not* interchangeable.

■ **PO:** Administer medication on an empty stomach, 1 hr before or 2 hr after meals, to prevent nausea and vomiting.

■ **SC:** Parenteral solution is intended only for subcutaneous administration. Do not give IM or IV. Inadvertent IM or IV administration may cause cholinergic overstimulation (circulatory collapse, drop in blood pressure, abdominal cramps, bloody diarrhea, shock, and cardiac arrest).

▫ Do not use if solution is discolored or contains a precipitate.

PATIENT/FAMILY TEACHING

▫ Instruct patient to take medication exactly as directed. Missed doses should be taken as soon as remembered within 1 hr; otherwise, return to regular dosing schedule. Do not double doses.

▫ Caution patient to make position changes slowly to minimize orthostatic hypotension.

▫ Advise patient to report abdominal discomfort, salivation, or flushing to physician.

EVALUATION

Effectiveness of therapy can be demonstrated by: ■ Increase in bladder function and tone ■ Decrease in abdominal distention.

BILE ACID SEQUESTRANTS

cholestyramine
(koe-less-**tear**-a-meen)
Cholybar, Questran, Questran Light

colestipol
(koe-**less**-tip-ole)
Colestid

CLASSIFICATION(S):
Lipid lowering agents
Pregnancy Category UK

INDICATIONS

■ Adjunct in the management of primary hypercholesterolemia ■ Relief of pruritus associated with elevated levels of bile acids.

ACTION

■ Bind bile acids in the GI tract, forming an insoluble complex. Result is increased clearance of cholesterol. **Therapeutic Effect:** ■ Decreased plasma cholesterol and low density lipoproteins.

PHARMACOKINETICS

Absorption: Action takes place in the GI tract. No absorption occurs.
Distribution: No distribution.
Metabolism and Excretion: After binding bile acids, insoluble complex is eliminated in the feces.
Half-life: UK.

CONTRAINDICATIONS AND PRECAUTIONS

Contraindicated in: ■ Hypersensitivity ■ Complete biliary obstruction ■ Hypersensitivity to propylene glycol (Questran) or aspartame (Questran Light) ■ Phenylketonuria (Questran Light).
Use Cautiously in: ■ History of constipation (causes severe constipation) ■ Other concurrently administered oral medications (may interfere with absorption).

ADVERSE REACTIONS AND SIDE EFFECTS*

EENT: irritation of the tongue.
GI: <u>nausea</u>, vomiting, <u>constipation</u>, impaction, hemorrhoids, flatulence, perianal irritation, steatorrhea, <u>abdominal discomfort</u>.
Derm: rashes, irritation.
F and E: hyperchloremic acidosis.
Hemat: bleeding.
Metab: vitamin A, D, and K deficiency.

INTERACTIONS

Drug–Drug: ■ May decrease absorption of orally administered **acetaminophen, amiodarone, glucocorticoids, cardiac glycosides, methotrexate, na-**

---

*<u>Underlines</u> indicate most frequent; **CAPITALS** indicate life-threatening.

proxen, phenylbutazone, piroxicam, propranolol, thiazide diuretics, thyroid, ursodiol, oral anticoagulants, and fat soluble vitamins (A, D, E, and K)
- May decrease absorption of other orally administered medications.

ROUTE AND DOSAGE

Cholestyramine
- **PO (Adults):** 4 g 1–6 times daily.
- **PO (Children):** 80 mg/kg 3 times daily.

Colestipol
- **PO (Adults):** 5 g once or twice daily initially. Gradually increase up to 30 g/day as a single dose or divided doses.

AVAILABILITY

Cholestyramine
Questran Light ▪ **Powder for suspension (with aspartame):** 5-g packets or bulk container with 5-g scoop. 5 g powder contains 4 g cholestryamine. *Questran* ▪ **Powder for suspension:** 9-g packets or bulk container with 9-g scoop. 9 g powder contains 4 g cholestyramine. *Cholybar* ▪ **Chewable bar (with sucrose and sorbitol):** 4 g cholestyramine/bar.

Cholestipol
□ **Granules for suspension:** 5-g packets or bulk container with 5-g scoop.

TIME/ACTION PROFILE
(hypocholesterolemic effects)

	ONSET	PEAK	DURATION
cholestyramine	24–48 hr	1–3 wk	2–4 wk
colestipol	24–48 hr	1 mo	1 mo

NURSING IMPLICATIONS

ASSESSMENT
- **Hypercholesterolemia:** Obtain a diet history, especially in regard to fat consumption.
- **Pruritus:** Asses severity of itching and skin integrity.
- **Lab Test Considerations:** Serum cholesterol and triglyceride levels should be evaluated before initiating and periodically throughout therapy. Discontinue medication if paradoxical increase in cholesterol level occurs.
□ May cause an increase in AST (SGOT), phosphate, chloride, and alkaline phosphatase and a decrease in serum calcium, sodium, and potassium levels.

POTENTIAL NURSING DIAGNOSES
- Constipation (side effects).
- Knowledge deficit related to medication regimen (patient/family teaching).
- Noncompliance (patient/family teaching).

IMPLEMENTATION
- **General Info:** Physician may order parenteral or water-miscible forms of fat-soluble vitamins (A, D, K) and folic acid for patients on chronic therapy.
- **PO:** Administer other medications 1 hr before or 4–6 hr after the administration of this medication.

PATIENT/FAMILY TEACHING
□ Instruct patient to take medication exactly as directed, do not skip doses or double up on missed doses.
□ Instruct patient to take medication before meals. Mix cholestyramine with 4–6 oz of water, milk, fruit juice, or other noncarbonated beverages. Colestipol can be mixed with water, juice, or carbonated beverges. Slowly stir in a large glass. Rinse glass with small amount of additional beverage to ensure all medication is taken. May also mix with highly fluid soups, cereals, or pulpy fruits (applesauce, crushed pineapple). Allow powder to sit on fluid and hydrate for 1–2 min prior to mixing. Do not take dry. Variations in the color of cholestyramine do not alter stability.
□ Advise patient that this medication should be used in conjunction with diet restrictions (fat, cholesterol, carbohydrates, alcohol), exercise, and cessation of smoking.
□ Explain that constipation may occur. Increasing fluids and bulk in diet, exercise, stool softeners, and laxatives may be required to minimize the

constipating effects. Instruct patient to notify physician if constipation, nausea, flatulence, and heartburn persist or if stools become frothy and foul smelling.

☐ Advise patient to notify physician if unusual bleeding or bruising, petechiae, or black, tarry stools occur. Treatment with vitamin K may be necessary.

EVALUATION
Effectiveness of therapy can be demonstrated by: ▪ Decrease in serum low-density lipoprotein (LDL) cholesterol levels. Cholesterol levels should begin to decrease in 48 hr but may take 1 yr to stabilize. Therapy is usually discontinued if the clinical response remains poor after 3 mo of therapy ▪ Decrease in severity of pruritus. Relief usually occurs 1–3 wk after therapy is initiated.

BIPERIDIN
(by-**per**-i-den)
Akineton

CLASSIFICATION(S):
Antiparkinson agent (anticholinergic)
Pregnancy Category C

INDICATIONS
▪ Adjunctive treatment of all forms of Parkinson's disease, including drug-induced extrapyramidal effects and acute dystonic reactions.

ACTION
▪ Blocks cholinergic activity in the CNS, which is partially responsible for the symptoms of Parkinson's disease ▪ Restores the natural balance of neurotransmitters in the CNS. **Therapeutic Effect:** ▪ Reduction of rigidity and tremors.

PHARMACOKINETICS
Absorption: Well absorbed following oral or IM administration.

Distribution: UK.
Metabolism and Excretion: UK.
Half-life: UK.

CONTRAINDICATIONS AND PRECAUTIONS
Contraindicated in: ▪ Hypersensitivity ▪ Narrow-angle glaucoma ▪ Bowel obstruction ▪ Megacolon ▪ Tardive dyskinesia.
Use Cautiously in: ▪ Elderly patients (increased risk of adverse reactions) ▪ Prostatic enlargement ▪ Seizure disorders ▪ Cardiac arrhythmias ▪ Pregnancy and lactation (safety not established).

ADVERSE REACTIONS AND SIDE EFFECTS*
CNS: confusion, weakness, hallucinations, headache, sedation, depression, dizziness.
EENT: dry eyes, blurred vision, mydriasis.
CV: tachycardia, arrhythmias, palpitations, hypotension.
GI: constipation, dry mouth, nausea, ileus.
GU: urinary retention, hesitancy.
Misc: decreased sweating.

INTERACTIONS
Drug–Drug: ▪ Additive anticholinergic affects with **drugs sharing anticholinergic properties** such as **antihistamines, phenothiazines, quinidine, disopyramide,** and **tricyclic antidepressants** ▪ Counteracts the cholinergic effects of **bethanecol** ▪ **Antacids** or **antidiarrheals** may decrease absorption.

ROUTE AND DOSAGE
Parkinsonism
▪ **PO (Adults):** 2 mg 3–4 times daily initially (not to exceed 16 mg/day).

Extrapyramidal Reactions
▪ **PO (Adults):** 2 mg 1–3 times daily.
▪ **IM, IV (Adults):** 2 mg, may repeat q 30 min (not to exceed 8 mg in 24 hr).

AVAILABILITY
▪ *Tablets:* 2 mg ▪ *Injection:* 5 mg/ml.

*Underlines indicate most frequent; **CAPITALS** indicate life-threatening.

TIME/ACTION PROFILE (relief of symptoms)

	ONSET	PEAK	DURATION
PO	UK	UK	UK
IM, IV	UK	UK	UK

NURSING IMPLICATIONS

ASSESSMENT

- **General Info:** Assess parkinson and extrapyramidal symptoms (akinesia, rigidity, tremors, pill rolling, mask facies, shuffling gait, muscle spasms, twisting motions, and drooling) prior to and throughout course of therapy.
- Assess bowel function daily. Monitor for constipation, abdominal pain, distention, or the absence of bowel sounds.
- Monitor intake and output ratios and assess patient for urinary retention (dysuria, distended abdomen, infrequent voiding of small amounts, overflow incontinence).
- After parenteral administration, monitor pulse and blood pressure closely and maintain bedrest for 1 hr. Advise patients to make position changes slowly to minimize orthostatic hypotension.

POTENTIAL NURSING DIAGNOSES

- Physical mobility impaired (indications).
- Knowledge deficit related to medication regimen (patient/family teaching).

IMPLEMENTATION

- **PO:** Administer with food or immediately after meals to minimize gastric irritation.
- **Direct IV:** Administer each dose over at least 1 min to minimize hypotension and mild bradycardia.

PATIENT/FAMILY TEACHING

- Advise patient to take medication exactly as directed. Missed doses should be taken as soon as remembered up to 2 hr before the next dose. Drug should be tapered gradually when discontinuing or a withdrawal reaction may occur (anxiety, tachycardia, insomnia, return of parkinson or extrapyramidal symptoms).
- May cause drowsiness, dizziness, or blurred vision. Advise patient to avoid driving or other activities that require alertness until response to the drug is known.
- Advise patient to make position changes slowly to minimize orthostatic hypotension.
- Advise patient that frequent mouth rinses, good oral hygiene, and sugarless gum or candy may decrease dry mouth. Patient should notify physician if dry mouth persists (saliva substitutes may be used). Also notify the dentist if dry mouth interferes with use of dentures.
- Instruct patient/family to notify physician if difficulty with urination, persistent constipation, persistent visual changes, or altered mental status occur.
- Advise patient to confer with physician or pharmacist prior to taking over-the-counter medications, especially cold remedies, or drinking alcoholic beverages.
- Caution patient that this medication decreases perspiration. Overheating may occur during hot weather. Patients should notify physician if they cannot remain indoors in an air-conditioned environment during hot weather.
- Advise patient to avoid antacids or antidiarrheals within 1–2 hr of this medication.
- Emphasize the importance of routine follow-up examinations.

EVALUATION

Effectiveness of therapy can be demonstrated by: ■ Decrease in drooling, tremors, and rigidity in Parkinson's disease ■ Resolution of drug-induced extrapyramidal reactions.

BISACODYL
(bis-a-**koe**-dill)
{Bisacolax}, Bisco-Lax, Carter's Little Pills, Dacodyl, Deficol, Dulcogen, Dulcolax, Fleet Laxative, {Laxit}, Theralax

CLASSIFICATION(S):
Laxative (stimulant)
Pregnancy Category UK

INDICATIONS

- Treatment of constipation, particularly when associated with: □ Prolonged bed rest □ Constipating drugs □ Slow transit time □ Irritable bowel syndrome - Evacuation of the bowel prior to radiologic studies or surgery - Used as part of a bowel regimen in patients with spinal cord injury.

ACTION

- Stimulates peristalsis - Alters fluid and electrolyte transport, producing fluid accumulation in the colon. **Therapeutic Effect:** - Evacuation of the colon.

PHARMACOKINETICS

Absorption: Minimal absorption following oral administration. Action is local in the colon.
Distribution: Small amounts of metabolites excreted in breast milk.
Metabolism and Excretion: Small amounts absorbed are metabolized by the liver.
Half-life: UK.

CONTRAINDICATIONS AND PRECAUTIONS

Contraindicated in: - Hypersensitivity - Abdominal pain - Obstruction - Nausea or vomiting, especially when associated with fever or other signs of an acute abdomen.
Use Cautiously in: - Severe cardiovascular disease - Anal or rectal fissures - Excess or prolonged use (may result in dependence) - Has been used during pregnancy and lactation.

ADVERSE REACTIONS AND SIDE EFFECTS*

GI: <u>nausea,</u> <u>abdominal cramps,</u> diarrhea, rectal burning.
MS: muscle weakness (chronic use).
F and E: hypokalemia (with chronic use).
Misc: protein losing enteropathy, tetany (with chronic use).

INTERACTIONS

Drug–Drug: - **Antacids** may remove enteric coating of tablets - May decrease the absorption of other **orally administered drugs** because of increased motility and decreased transit time.

ROUTE AND DOSAGE

- **PO (Adults):** 5–15 mg (up to 30 mg).
- **PO (Children >6 yr):** 5–10 mg.
- **Rect (Adults):** 10 mg.
- **Rect (Children 2–12 yr):** 5–10 mg.
- **Rect (Children <2 yr and Infants):** 5 mg.

AVAILABILITY

- *Enteric-coated tablets:* 5 mg - *Suppositories:* 5 mg, 10 mg.

TIME/ACTION PROFILE (evacuation of bowel)

	ONSET	PEAK	DURATION
PO	6–12 hr	UK	UK
Rect	15–60 min	UK	UK

NURSING IMPLICATIONS

ASSESSMENT

- **General Info:** Assess patient for abdominal distention, presence of bowel sounds, and usual pattern of bowel function.
- □ Assess color, consistency, and amount of stool produced.

POTENTIAL NURSING DIAGNOSES

- Constipation (indications).
- Knowledge deficit related to medication regimen (patient/family teaching).

{} = Available in Canada only.
*<u>Underlines</u> indicate most frequent; **CAPITALS** indicate life-threatening.

IMPLEMENTATION

- **General Info:** May be administered at bedtime for morning results.
- **PO:** Taking on an empty stomach will produce more rapid results.
- □ Do not crush or chew enteric-coated tablets. Take with a full glass of water or juice.
- □ Do not administer oral doses within 1 hr of milk or antacids; this may lead to premature dissolution of tablet and gastric or duodenal irritation.
- **Rect:** Suppository or enema can be given at the time a bowel movement is desired. Lubricate suppositories with water or water-soluble lubricant prior to insertion. Encourage patient to retain the suppository or enema 15–30 min before expelling.

PATIENT/FAMILY TEACHING

- □ Advise patients, other than those with spinal cord injuries, that laxatives should be used only for short-term therapy. Prolonged therapy may cause electrolyte imbalance and dependence.
- □ Advise patient to increase fluid intake to at least 1500–2000 ml/day during therapy to prevent dehydration.
- □ Encourage patients to utilize other forms of bowel regulation (increasing bulk in the diet, increasing fluid intake, or increasing mobility). Normal bowel habits may vary from 3 times/day to 3 times/wk.
- □ Instruct patients with cardiac disease to avoid straining during bowel movements (Valsalva maneuver).
- □ Advise patient that bisacodyl should not be used when constipation is accompanied by abdominal pain, fever, nausea, or vomiting.

EVALUATION

Effectiveness of therapy can be demonstrated by: ■ The patient having a soft, formed bowel movement when used for constipation ■ Evacuation of colon before surgery or radiologic studies, or for patients with spinal cord injury.

BISMUTH SUBSALICYLATE
(**bis**-muth sub-sa-li-si-late)
Bismtral, Pepto-Bismol, Pink Bismuth

B

CLASSIFICATION(S):
Antidiarrheal
Pregnancy Category UK

INDICATIONS

■ Adjunctive therapy in the treatment of mild to moderate diarrhea ■ Treatment of nausea, abdominal cramping, heartburn, and indigestion that may accompany diarrheal illnesses. **Unlabeled Use:** ■ Treatment and prevention of traveler's (enterotoxigenic *Escherichia coli*) diarrhea.

ACTION

■ Promotes intestinal adsorption of fluids and electrolytes ■ Decreases synthesis of intestinal prostaglandins. **Therapeutic Effect:** ■ Relief of diarrhea.

PHARMACOKINETICS

Absorption: Not absorbed.
Distribution: None.
Metabolism and Excretion: Excreted unchanged in the feces.
Half-life: UK.

CONTRAINDICATIONS AND PRECAUTIONS

Contraindicated in: ■ Elderly patients who may be impacted ■ Children or teenagers during or after recovery from chickenpox or flu-like illness (contains salicylate) ■ Aspirin hypersensitivity. **Use Cautiously in:** ■ Infants, elderly or debilitated patients (impaction may occur) ■ Patients undergoing radiologic examination of the GI tract (bismuth is radiopaque) ■ Pregnancy or lactation (safety not established) ■ Diabetes mellitus ■ Gout.

ADVERSE REACTIONS AND SIDE EFFECTS*

GI: constipation, impaction, gray-black stools.

*Underlines indicate most frequent; **CAPITALS** indicate life-threatening.

INTERACTIONS

Drug–Drug: ▪ If taken with **aspirin,** may potentiate signs of salicylate toxicity ▪ May decrease the absorption of **tetracycline** or **enoxacin** ▪ May alter the effect of **oral anticoagulants.**

ROUTE AND DOSAGE

- **PO (Adults):** 2 tablets or 30 ml; may repeat q 30 min–1 hr, up to 8 doses/24 hr.
- **PO (Children 9–12 yr):** 1 tablet or 15 ml; may repeat q 30 min–1 hr, up to 8 doses/24 hr.
- **PO (Children 6–9 yr):** ⅔ tablet or 10 ml; may repeat q 30 min–1 hr, up to 8 doses/24 hr.
- **PO (Children 3–6 yr):** ⅓ tablet or 5 ml; may repeat q 30 min–1 hr, up to 8 doses/24 hr.
- **PO (Children <3 yr weighing 28 lb or more):** 5 ml; may repeat q 4 hr, up to 6 doses/24 hr.
- **PO (Children <3 yr weighing 14–18 lb):** 2.5 ml; may repeat q 4 hr, up to 6 doses/24 hr.

AVAILABILITY

- *Chewable tablets:* 262 mg ▪ *Liquid:* 262 mg/15 ml, 524 mg/15 ml.

TIME/ACTION PROFILE (relief of diarrhea and other GI symptoms)

	ONSET	PEAK	DURATION
PO	within 24 hr	UK	UK

NURSING IMPLICATIONS

ASSESSMENT

- ☐ Assess the frequency and consistency of stools, presence of nausea and indigestion, and bowel sounds prior to and throughout course of therapy.
- ☐ Assess patient's fluid and electrolyte balance and skin turgor for dehydration if diarrhea is prolonged.

POTENTIAL NURSING DIAGNOSES

- ▪ Diarrhea (indications).
- ▪ Constipation (side effects).
- ▪ Knowledge deficit related to medication regimen (patient/family teaching).

IMPLEMENTATION

- ▪ **PO:** Shake liquid before using. Chewable tablets may be chewed or allowed to dissolve before swallowing.

PATIENT/FAMILY TEACHING

- ☐ Instruct patient to take medication exactly as directed.
- ☐ Inform patient that medication may temporarily cause stools and tongue to appear gray-black.
- ☐ Advise patient taking concurrent aspirin products that bismuth subsalicylate should be discontinued if ringing in the ears occurs.
- ☐ Instruct patient to notify physician if diarrhea persists for more than 2 days or if accompanied by a high fever.
- ☐ Centers for Disease Control warn against giving salicylates to children or adolescents with varicella (chickenpox) or influenza-ike or viral illnesses because of a possible association with Reye's syndrome.

EVALUATION

Effectiveness of therapy may be determined by: ▪ Decrease in diarrhea ▪ Decrease in symptoms of indigestion ▪ Prevention of traveler's diarrhea.

BISOPROLOL
(biss-**op**-proe-lol)
Zebeta

CLASSIFICATION(S):
Antihypertensive, Beta-adrenergic blocker (selective)
Pregnancy Category C

INDICATIONS

▪ Used alone or in combination with other agents in the management of hypertension. **Unlabeled Use:** ▪ Management of angina pectoris.

ACTION

▪ Blocks stimulation of beta$_1$ (myocardial) adrenergic receptors with less effect on beta$_2$ (pulmonary, vascular, uterine) receptor sites **Therapeutic Effects:** ▪ Decreased blood pressure. Heart rate is also lowered.

PHARMACOKINETICS

Absorption: Well absorbed following oral administration. Some (20%) first-pass metabolism occurs.

Distribution: Does not appear to enter CSF. Remainder of distribution not known.

Metabolism and Excretion: 50% excreted unchanged in urine; remainder as inactive metabolites. 2% eliminated in feces.

Half-life: 9–12 hr.

CONTRAINDICATIONS AND PRECAUTIONS

Contraindicated in: ▪ Uncompensated congestive heart failure ▪ Pulmonary edema ▪ Cardiogenic shock ▪ Bradycardia or heart block.

Use Cautiously in: ▪ Renal/hepatic impairment (initial dose reduction recommended if CCr <40 ml/min) ▪ Pregnancy or lactation (may cause apnea, low apgar scores, bradycardia, and hypoglycemia in the newborn) ▪ Hyperthroidism (may mask symptoms) ▪ Diabetes mellitus (may mask symptoms of hypoglycemia) ▪ Children (safety not established) ▪ Patients with a history of severe allergic reactions (intensity of reaction may be increased).

ADVERSE REACTIONS AND SIDE EFFECTS*

CNS: fatigue, weakness, dizziness, depression, memory loss, mental changes, nightmares, drowsiness.

EENT: blurred vision.

Resp: bronchospasm, wheezing.

CV: BRADYCARDIA, CONGESTIVE HEART FAILURE, PULMONARY EDEMA, peripheral vasoconstriction, hypotension.

GI: constipation, diarrhea, nausea, liver function abnormalities.

GU: impotence, diminished libido.

Endo: hyperglycemia, hypoglycemia.

INTERACTIONS

Drug–Drug: ▪ **General anesthesia, IV phenytoin,** and **verapamil** may cause additive myocardial depression ▪ Additive bradycardia may occur with concurrent use of **cardiac glycosides.** ▪ Additive hypotension may occur with other **antihypertensive agents,** acute ingestion of **alcohol, nitrates** or **haloperidol** ▪ Concurrent use with **amphetamines, cocaine, ephedrine, epinephrine, norepinephrine, phenylephrine** or **pseudoephedrine** may result in excess alpha adrenergic stimulation, hypertension, and bradycardia ▪ May negate the beneficial beta$_1$ cardiac effects of **dopamine** or **dobutamine** ▪ Concurrent **thyroid** administration may decrease effectiveness ▪ Use with **insulin** may result in prolonged hypoglycemia ▪ May produce hypertension within 14 days of **MAO inhibitor** therapy ▪ The risk of cardiovascular reactions may be increased by concurrent use of other **cardioactive agents** ▪ May decrease the effectiveness of **theophylline** ▪ **Cocaine** may decrease the antihypertensive effect of bisoprolol.

ROUTE AND DOSAGE

▪ **PO (Adults):** 5 mg once daily (range 2.5–20 mg). Start with 2.5 mg/day in renal impairment.

AVAILABILITY

▪ *Tablets:* 5 mg, 10 mg.

TIME/ACTION PROFILE
(antihypertensive effect)

	ONSET	PEAK	DURATION
PO	UK	UK	24 hr

NURSING IMPLICATIONS

ASSESSMENT

▫ Monitor blood pressure and pulse frequently during dosage adjustment and periodically throughout therapy.

▫ Monitor intake and output ratios and weigh daily. Assess patient routinely for signs and symptoms of fluid overload (peripheral edema, dyspnea, rales/crackles, weight gain, jugular venous distension).

*Underlines indicate most frequent; **CAPITALS** indicate life-threatening.

- **Lab Test Considerations:** May cause elevated AST (SGOT) and ALT (SGPT) concentrations.

POTENTIAL NURSING DIAGNOSES
- Activity intolerance (indications).
- Cardiac output, decreased (adverse reactions).
- Knowledge deficit related to medication regimen (patient/family teaching).

IMPLEMENTATION
- **General Info:** Take apical pulse prior to administration. If <50 bpm, withhold medication and notify physician.
- **PO:** Bisoprolol may be administered without regard to meals.

PATIENT/FAMILY TEACHING
- Instruct patient to take medication exactly as directed, even if feeling well; do not skip or double up on missed doses. Abrupt withdrawal may precipitate life-threatening arrhythmias, hypertension, or myocardial ischemia.
- Teach patient and family how to check pulse and blood pressure. Advise them to take pulse daily and blood pressure weekly and to report any significant change to physician.
- May occasionally cause dizziness. Caution patient to avoid driving or other activities that require alertness until response to drug is known.
- Advise patient to make position changes slowly to minimize orthostatic hypotension.
- Reinforce need to continue additional therapies for hypertension (weight loss, restricted sodium intake, stress reduction, regular exercise, moderation of alcohol consumption, and cessation of smoking). Bisoprolol controls but does not cure hypertension.
- Caution patient that bisoprolol may cause increased sensitivity to cold.
- Advise patient to consult physician or pharmacist before taking any over-the-counter drugs concurrently with this medication.
- Diabetics should closely monitor blood sugar, especially if weakness,

malaise, irritability, or fatigue occur.
- Instruct patient to notify physician if symptoms of fluid overload, slow pulse rate, dizziness, confusion, or depression occur.
- Instruct patient to inform physician or dentist of this therapy prior to treatment or surgery.
- Advise patients to carry identification describing disease process and medication regimen at all times.

EVALUATION
Effectiveness of therapy can be demonstrated by: ■ Decrease in blood pressure ■ Decrease in anginal attacks □ Increase in activity tolerance.

BITOLTEROL
(bye-**tol**-te-role)
Tornalate

CLASSIFICATION(S):
Bronchodilator (beta-adrenergic agonist)
Pregnancy Category C

INDICATIONS
- Used as a bronchodilator in the prevention and treatment of reversible airway obstruction due to asthma or COPD.

ACTION
- Results in the accumulation of cyclic adenosine monophosphate (cAMP) at beta-adrenergic receptors **Therapeutic Effect:** ■ Bronchodilation.

PHARMACOKINETICS
Absorption: Some absorption follows inhalation.
Distribution: Distribution not known.
Metabolism and Excretion: Converted in lungs to colterol, the active compound.
Half-life: UK.

CONTRAINDICATIONS AND PRECAUTIONS
Contraindicated in: ■ Hypersensitivity to adrenergic amines ■ Known alcohol intolerance.

B

Use Cautiously in: ▪ Cardiac disease ▪ Hypertension ▪ Hyperthyroidism ▪ Diabetes ▪ Glaucoma ▪ Elderly patients (more susceptible to adverse reactions; may require dosage reduction) ▪ Pregnancy (near term), lactation, and children <12 yr (safety not established) ▪ Excessive use may lead to tolerance and paradoxical bronchospasm.

ADVERSE REACTIONS AND SIDE EFFECTS*

EENT: dry throat.
CNS: <u>tremor</u>, dizziness, shakiness, nervousness, headache.
Resp: cough.
CV: palpitations, arrhythmias.
GI: nausea, vomiting.

INTERACTIONS

Drug–Drug: ▪ Concurrent use with other **sympathomimetic (adrenergic) agents** will have additive adrenergic side effects ▪ Use with **MAO inhibitors** may lead to hypertensive crisis ▪ **Beta adrenergic blockers** may negate therapeutic effect.

ROUTE AND DOSAGE

Metered Dose Inhaler

▪ **Inhalation (Adults and Children >12 yr):** 2–3 inhalations for acute treatment, 2 inhalations q 8 hr for prevention (not to exceed 3 inhalations every 6 hr or 2 inhalations q 4 hr).

Nebulization

▪ **Inhalation (Adults and Children >12 yr):** 0.5 ml (1 mg) tid by intermittent flow or 1.25 mg tid by continuous flow.

AVAILABILITY

▪ *Aerosol inhaler:* 0.37 mg/actuation (≥300 inhalations/15 ml-canister) ▪ *Inhalation solution:* 0.2%.

TIME/ACTION PROFILE
(bronchodilation)

	ONSET	PEAK	DURATION
inhalation	3–4 min	30–60 min	5–8 hr

NURSING IMPLICATIONS

ASSESSMENT

▫ Assess lung sounds, pulse, and blood pressure before administration and during peak of medication.
▫ Monitor pulmonary function tests before initiating therapy and periodically throughout course to determine effectiveness of medication.
▫ Observe for paradoxical bronchospasm (wheezing). If condition occurs, withhold medication and notify physician immediately.

POTENTIAL NURSING DIAGNOSES

▪ Airway clearance, ineffective (indications).
▪ Knowledge deficit related to medication regimen (patient/family teaching).

IMPLEMENTATION

▪ **Inhalation:** Allow at least 1 min between inhalations of aerosol medication.

PATIENT/FAMILY TEACHING

▫ Instruct patient to take bitolterol exactly as directed. If on a scheduled dosing regimen, take a missed dose as soon as remembered, spacing remaining doses at regular intervals. Do not double doses. Caution patient not to exceed recommended dose; may cause adverse effects, paradoxical bronchospasm, or loss of effectiveness of medication.
▫ Instruct patient in the proper use of the metered-dose inhaler. See Appendix H for use of inhalation medications.
▫ Advise patients to use bitolterol first if using other inhalation medications and to allow 5 min to elapse before administering other inhalation medications, unless otherwise directed by physician.
▫ Instruct patient to contact physician immediately if shortness of breath is not relieved by medication or is accompanied by diaphoresis, dizziness, palpitations, or chest pain.

---

*<u>Underlines</u> indicate most frequent; **CAPITALS** indicate life threatening.

▫ Advise patient to rinse mouth with water after each inhalation dose to minimize dry mouth.

▫ Advise patient to consult physician or pharmacist before taking any over-the-counter medications or alcoholic beverages concurrently with this therapy. Caution patient also to avoid smoking and other respiratory irritants.

EVALUATION

Effectiveness of therapy can be demonstrated by: ▪ Prevention or relief of bronchospasm.

BLEOMYCIN

(blee-oh-**mye**-sin)
Blenoxane

CLASSIFICATION(S):
Antineoplastic (antitumor antibiotic)
Pregnancy Category UK

INDICATIONS

▪ Used alone or in combination with other antineoplastic agents in the treatment of: ▫ Lymphomas ▫ Squamous cell carcinoma ▫ Testicular embryonal cell carcinoma ▫ Choriocarcinoma ▫ Teratocarcinoma. **Unlabeled Use:** ▪ Intrapleural/intraperitoneal administration to prevent the reaccumulation of malignant effusions.

ACTION

▪ Inhibits DNA and RNA synthesis. **Therapeutic Effect:** ▪ Death of rapidly replicating cells, particularly malignant ones.

PHARMACOKINETICS

Absorption: Not absorbed from the GI tract. Well absorbed from IM and SC sites. Absorption also occurs following intrapleural and intraperitoneal administration.

Distribution: Widely distributed, concentrates mainly in skin, lung, peritoneum, kidneys, and lymphatics.

Metabolism and Excretion: 60–70% excreted unchanged by the kidneys.

Half-life: 2 hr (increased in renal impairment).

CONTRAINDICATIONS AND PRECAUTIONS

Contraindicated in: ▪ Hypersensitivity ▪ Pregnancy or lactation.

Use Cautiously in: ▪ Renal impairment (dosage reduction required if creatinine clearance <35 ml/min) ▪ Pulmonary impairment ▪ Patients with childbearing potential ▪ Nonmalignant chronic debilitating illness ▪ Elderly patients (increased risk of pulmonary toxicity).

ADVERSE REACTIONS AND SIDE EFFECTS*

CNS: weakness, disorientation, aggressive behavior.

Resp: pneumonitis, PULMONARY FIBROSIS.

CV: hypotension, peripheral vasoconstriction.

GI: nausea, vomiting, anorexia, stomatitis.

Derm: mucocutaneous toxicity, urticaria, erythema, hyperpigmentation, alopecia, rashes, vesiculation, alopecia.

Hemat: thrombocytopenia, leukopenia, anemia.

Local: pain at tumor site, phlebitis at IV site.

Metab: weight loss.

Misc: fever, chills, ANAPHYLACTOID REACTIONS.

INTERACTIONS

Drug–Drug: ▪ Hematologic toxicity increased with concurrent use of **radiation therapy** and other **antineoplastic agents** ▪ Concurrent use with **cisplatin** decreases elimination of bleomycin and may increase toxicity ▪ Increased risk of pulmonary toxicity with other **antineoplastic agents** or thoracic **radiation**.

ROUTE AND DOSAGE

Lymphoma patients should receive initial test doses of 2 units or less for the first 2 doses.

*Underlines indicate most frequent; **CAPITALS** indicate life-threatening.

- **IV, IM, SC (Adults):** 0.25–0.5 units/kg (10–20 units/m²) weekly or twice weekly initially. If favorable response occurs, lower maintenance doses are employed (1 unit/day or 5 units/wk).

AVAILABILITY

- *Injection:* 15 units/vial.

TIME/ACTION PROFILE (tumor response)

	ONSET	PEAK	DURATION
IV, IM, SC	2–3 wk	UK	UK

NURSING IMPLICATIONS

ASSESSMENT

□ Monitor vital signs prior to and frequently during therapy.

□ Assess for fever and chills. May occur 2–6 hr after administration and last 4–6 hr. Confer with physician regarding antipyretic therapy.

□ Monitor for anaphylactic reaction (fever, chills, hypotension, and wheezing). Keep resuscitation equipment and medications on hand. Lymphoma patients are at particular risk.

□ Assess respiratory status for dyspnea and rales/crackles. Pulmonary toxicity occurs primarily in elderly patients (age 70 or older) who have received 400 or more units. May occur 4–10 wk after therapy. Physician may order periodic pulmonary function tests and carbon monoxide diffusion capacity for early detection of pulmonary toxicity. Pulmonary toxicity may occur at lower doses in patients also having received other antineoplastics or thoracic radiation.

□ Assess nausea, vomiting, and appetite. Weigh weekly. Modify diet as tolerated. Confer with physician regarding an antiemetic prior to administration.

- **Lab Test Considerations:** Monitor CBC prior to and periodically throughout therapy. May cause mild thrombocytopenia and leukopenia (nadir occurs in 2 wk).

□ Monitor baseline and periodic renal and hepatic function.

POTENTIAL NURSING DIAGNOSES

- Injury, high risk for (side effects).
- Body image disturbance (side effects).
- Knowledge deficit related to medication regimen (patient/family teaching).

IMPLEMENTATION

- **General Info:** Solution should be prepared in a biologic cabinet. Wear gloves, gown, and mask while handling medication. Discard equipment in specially designated containers (see Appendix I).

◻ Physician may order lymphoma patients to receive 2 test doses of 2 units initially. Monitor closely for anaphylactic reaction.

□ May be administered through thoracostomy tube by physician. Position patient as directed.

□ Reconstituted solution is stable for 24 hr at room temperature and 14 days if refrigerated.

- **IM/SC:** Reconstitute vial with 1–5 ml of Sterile Water for Injection, 0.9% NaCl, D5W, or Bacteriostatic Water for Injection. Do not reconstitute with diluents containing benzyl alcohol when used for neonates.

- **Direct IV:** Prepare IV and intra-arterial doses by diluting 15-unit vial with 5 ml of D5W or 0.9% NaCl.

- *Rate:* Administer slowly over 10 min.

- **Intermittent Infusion:** May be further diluted in 50–100 ml of D5W or 0.9% NaCl.

- **Syringe Compatibility:** ■ cisplatin ■ cyclophosphamide ■ doxorubicin ■ droperidol ■ fluorouracil ■ furosemide ■ heparin ■ leucovorin calcium ■ methotrexate ■ metoclopramide ■ mitomycin ■ vinblastine ■ vincristine.

- **Y-Site Compatibility:** ■ cisplatin ■ cyclophosphamide ■ doxorubicin ■ droperidol ■ fludarabine ■ fluorouracil ■ heparin ■ leucovorin calcium ■ methotrexate ■ metoclopramide ■ mitomycin ■ ondansetron ■ sargramostim ■ vinblastine ■ vincristine.

PATIENT/FAMILY TEACHING

- Instruct patient to notify physician if fever, chills, wheezing, faintness, diaphoresis, shortness of breath, prolonged nausea and vomiting, or mouth sores occur.
- Encourage patient not to smoke as this may worsen pulmonary toxicity.
- Explain to the patient that skin toxicity may manifest itself as skin sensitivity, hyperpigmentation (especially at skin folds and points of skin irritation), and skin rashes and thickening.
- Instruct patient to inspect oral mucosa for erythema and ulceration. If ulceration occurs, advise patient to use sponge brush and rinse mouth with water after eating and drinking. Physician may order viscous lidocaine swishes if pain interferes with eating.
- Discuss with patient the possibility of hair loss. Explore coping strategies.
- Advise patient of the need for contraception.
- Instruct patient not to receive any vaccinations without advice of physician.
- Emphasize need for periodic lab tests to monitor for side effects.

EVALUATION

Effectiveness of therapy can be demonstrated by: ▪ Decrease in tumor size without evidence of hypersensitivity or pulmonary toxicity.

BRETYLIUM
(bre-till-ee-yum)
{Bretylate}, Bretylol

CLASSIFICATION(S):
Antiarrhythmic (group III)
Pregnancy Category UK

INDICATIONS

▪ Treatment of ventricular tachycardia and prophylaxis against ventricular fibrillation ▪ Treatment of other serious ventricular arrhythmias resistant to lidocaine.

ACTION

▪ Initially releases norepinephrine, then blocks its release. **Therapeutic Effect:** ▪ Suppression of ventricular tachycardia and fibrillation.

PHARMACOKINETICS

Absorption: Well absorbed following IM administration.
Distribution: Reaches high concentration in areas of adrenergic innervation.
Metabolism and Excretion: Eliminated entirely unchanged by the kidneys.
Half-life: 5–10 hr (increased in renal impairment).

CONTRAINDICATIONS AND PRECAUTIONS

Contraindicated in: ▪ No significant contraindications.
Use Cautiously in: ▪ Suspected cardiac glycoside toxicity (increased risk of arrhythmias) ▪ Patients with fixed cardiac output (may produce severe hypotension requiring supportive therapy) ▪ Renal insufficiency (dosage reduction required) ▪ Pregnancy, lactation, and children (safety not established).

ADVERSE REACTIONS AND SIDE EFFECTS*

CNS: syncope, faintness, vertigo, dizziness.
EENT: nasal stuffiness.
CV: <u>postural hypotension</u>, transient hypertension, bradycardia, angina.
GI: <u>nausea</u>, <u>vomiting</u> (rapid IV administration to conscious patients), diarrhea.

INTERACTIONS

Drug–Drug: ▪ Combination with other **antiarrhythmics** may be additive or antagonistic ▪ Avoid using in suspected **cardiac glycoside** toxicity (initial release of norepinephrine may aggravate arrhythmias) ▪ Enhances actions of adrenergic vasopressors (dopamine, norepinephrine).

{} = Available in Canada only.
*<u>Underlines</u> indicate most frequent; **CAPITALS** indicate life-threatening.

ROUTE AND DOSAGE
See infusion rate table in Appendix D.

Ventricular Fibrillation
- **IV (Adults):** 5 mg/kg bolus over 15–30 sec initially; if no response, increase to 10 mg/kg, repeat as necessary (not to exceed 30 mg/kg/24 hr). For maintenance: 5–10 mg/kg q 6 hr or 1–2 mg/min continuous infusion.

Other Ventricular Arrhythmias
- **IV (Adults):** Dilute and infuse 5–10 mg/kg q 6–8 hr.
- **IM (Adults):** 5–10 mg/kg, repeat q 1–2 hr if arrhythmia persists, then q 6–8 hr.

AVAILABILITY
- *Injection:* 50 mg/ml.

TIME/ACTION PROFILE (suppression of arrhythmias)

	ONSET	PEAK	DURATION
IM	15 min–1 hr (fibrillation) 20 min–6 hr (VT, PVCs)	UK	6–24 hr
IV	within min (fibrillation) 20 min–6 hr (VT, PVCs)	end of infusion	6–24 hr

NURSING IMPLICATIONS

ASSESSMENT
- Patients receiving this medication should be hospitalized in a unit where ECG and blood pressure can be constantly monitored. Assess patient for arrhythmias and changes in blood pressure frequently. A transient increase in arrhythmias and hypertension may occur within 1 hr after initial administration.
- Assess patient frequently for orthostatic hypotension, keep supine until tolerance to hypotension develops. Instruct patient to make position changes slowly, assist with ambulation. If systolic blood pressure <75 mmHg or symptomatic notify physician. Dopamine, dobutamine, or norepinephrine, and volume replacement may be necessary.

POTENTIAL NURSING DIAGNOSES
- Cardiac output, decreased (indications).
- Injury, high risk for (adverse reactions).

IMPLEMENTATION
- **General Info:** Dosage should be reduced gradually and discontinued over 3–5 days with close ECG monitoring. Maintenance with an oral antiarrhythmic may be initiated.
- Available in premixed solution with 5% dextrose.
- **IM:** Do not dilute bretylium for IM injection. Rotate injection sites frequently during IM injection to prevent atrophy and necrosis of muscle tissue caused by repeated injections. May repeat injection at 1–2 hr intervals if arrhythmia persists.
- **Direct IV:** For ventricular fibrillation, give IV undiluted; arrhythmia usually resolves within minutes. Repeat in 15–30 min if arrhythmia persists. Do not exceed 30 mg/kg/24 hr. Employ usual resusitative procedures, including CPR and electrical cardioversion, prior to and following injection.
- *Rate:* Administer over 15–30 sec.
- **Intermittent Infusion:** For other ventricular arrhythmias, dilute 500 mg in at least 50 ml of D5W, 0.9% NaCl, D5/0.45% NaCl, D5/0.9% NaCl, D5/LR, ⅙ M sodium lactate, or lactated Ringer's solution.
- *Rate:* Administer over more than 8 min. More rapid infusion in the alert patient may cause nausea and vomiting. May repeat after 1–2 hr if necessary. Ventricular tachycardia usually resolves within 20 min.
- **Continuous Infusion:** Bretylium can be diluted in any amount of solution (1 g in 1000 ml equals 1 mg/ml).
- *Rate:* Infuse at 1–2 mg of diluted solution/min. Administer via infusion pump to ensure accurate dosage. (See Appendix D for Infusion Rate Table.)
- **Y-Site Compatibility:** ▪ amrinone ▪ dobutamine ▪ famotidine ▪ isoproterenol ▪ ranitidine.

PATIENT/FAMILY TEACHING

□ Instruct patient to make position changes slowly to minimize the effects of drug-induced orthostatic hypotension.

EVALUATION

Clinical response can be demonstrated by: ▪ Suppression of existing ventricular arrhythmias ▪ Prevention of additional arrhythmias.

BROMOCRIPTINE
(broe-moe-**krip**-teen)
Parlodel

CLASSIFICATION(S):
Antiparkinson agent
Pregnancy Category UK

INDICATIONS

▪ Adjunct to levodopa in the treatment of Parkinsonism ▪ Treatment of hyperprolactinemia (amenorrhea/galactorrhea) including associated female infertility ▪ Suppression of lactation ▪ Treatment of acromegaly.

ACTION

▪ Activates dopamine receptors in the CNS ▪ Decreases prolactin secretion. **Therapeutic Effects:** ▪ Relief of rigidity and tremor in Parkinsonism ▪ Restoration of fertility in hyperprolactinemia ▪ Suppression of lactation ▪ Decreased growth hormone in acromegaly.

PHARMACOKINETICS

Absorption: Poorly absorbed (30%) from the GI tract.
Distribution: Distribution not known.
Metabolism and Excretion: Completely metabolized by the liver.
Half-life: Biphasic—initial phase 4–4.5 hr, terminal phase 45–50 hr.

CONTRAINDICATIONS AND PRECAUTIONS

Contraindicated in: ▪ Hypersensitivity to bromocriptine, ergot alkaloids, or bi-

sulfites (capsules only) ▪ Children <15 yr ▪ Lactation.
Use Cautiously in: ▪ Cardiac disease ▪ Mental disturbances ▪ May restore fertility (additional contraception may be required if pregnancy is undesirable) ▪ Pregnancy (safety not established) ▪ Severe liver impairment (dosage reduction required).

ADVERSE REACTIONS AND SIDE EFFECTS*

CNS: headache, dizziness, drowsiness, insomnia, confusion, hallucinations, nightmares.
EENT: burning eyes, visual disturbances, nasal stuffiness.
Resp: pulmonary infiltrates, effusions.
CV: hypotension.
GI: nausea, vomiting, anorexia, abdominal pain, dry mouth, metallic taste.
Derm: urticaria.
MS: leg cramps.
Misc: digital vasospasm (acromegaly only).

INTERACTIONS

Drug–Drug: ▪ Additive hypotension with **antihypertensives** ▪ Additive **CNS depression** with **antihistamines, alcohol, opioid analgesics,** and **sedative/hypnotics** ▪ Additive neurologic effects with **levodopa** ▪ Effective on prolactin levels, may be antagonized by **phenothiazines, haloperidol, methyldopa, tricyclic antidepressants,** and **reserpine.**

ROUTE AND DOSAGE

Parkinsonism
▪ **PO (Adults):** 1.25 mg twice daily, increased by 2.5 mg/day in 2–4 wk intervals (usual dose range is 10–40 mg/day in 3 divided doses).

Hyperprolactinemia
▪ **PO (Adults):** 1.25–2.5 mg/day initially, may be gradually increased up to 30 mg/day (usual dose 5–7.5 mg/day).

Postpartum Lactation
▪ **PO (Adults):** 2.5 mg 1–3 times daily for 14–21 days.

---

*Underlines indicate most frequent; **CAPITALS** indicate life-threatening.

Acromegaly

- **PO (Adults):** 1.25–2.5 mg/day for 3 days, increase by 1.25–2.5 mg q 3–7 days until optimal response is obtained (usual range 20–30 mg/day; not to exceed 100 mg/day).

AVAILABILITY

- **Tablets:** 2.5 mg ▪ **Capsules:** 5 mg.

TIME/ACTION PROFILE (suppression of tremor in Parkinson's disease)

	ONSET	PEAK	DURATION
PO	30–90 min	1–2 hr	8–12 hr

NURSING IMPLICATIONS

ASSESSMENT

- **General Info:** Assess patient for allergy to ergot derivatives.
- ▫ Monitor blood pressure prior to and frequently during drug therapy. Instruct patient to remain supine during and for several hours after first dose, because severe hypotension may occur. Supervise ambulation and transfer during initial dosing to prevent injury from hypotension.
- **Parkinson's Disease:** Assess symptoms (akinesia, rigidity, tremors, pill rolling, mask facies, shuffling gait, muscle spasms, twisting motions, drooling) prior to and throughout course of therapy.
- **Lactation Suppression:** Assess breasts for firmness, discomfort, and milk production.
- **Lab Test Considerations:** May cause elevated serum BUN, ALT (SGOT), AST (SGPT), CPK, alkaline phosphatase, and uric acid levels. Elevations are usually transient and not clinically significant.

POTENTIAL NURSING DIAGNOSES

- Physical mobility, impaired (indications).
- Injury, high risk for (indications, side effects).
- Knowledge deficit related to medication regimen (patient/family teaching).

IMPLEMENTATION

- **General Info:** This medication is often given concurrently with levodopa or a levodopa-carbidopa combination in the treatment of Parkinson's disease.
- **PO:** Administer with food or milk to minimize gastric distress. Tablets may be crushed if patient has difficulty swallowing.

PATIENT/FAMILY TEACHING

- **General Info:** Instruct patient to take medication exactly as directed. If a dose is missed it should be taken within 4 hr of the scheduled dose or omitted. Do not double doses.
- ▫ May cause drowsiness and dizziness. Caution patients to avoid driving and other activities requiring alertness until response to medication is known.
- ▫ Caution patient to avoid concurrent use of alcohol during the course of therapy.
- ▫ Instruct patient to inform physician if increasing shortness of breath is noted; pulmonary infiltrates and pleural effusions may occur with long-term therapy.
- ▫ Advise women to consult with physician regarding a nonhormonal method of birth control. Women should contact the physician promptly if pregnancy is suspected.
- ▫ Emphasize the importance of regular follow-up examinations to determine effectiveness and monitor side effects.
- **Pituitary Tumors:** Instruct patients taking bromocriptine for pituitary tumors to inform physician immediately if signs of tumor enlargement (blurred vision, sudden headache, severe nausea, and vomiting) occur.
- **Infertility:** Instruct women treated for infertility to obtain daily basal body temperatures to determine when ovulation occurs.
- **Lactation Suppression:** Explain that course of therapy usually lasts 2–3 wk. Mild to moderate breast engorgement may occur after therapy is discontinued.

B

EVALUATION
Effectiveness of therapy can be demonstrated by: ■ Decrease in tremor, rigidity, and bradykinesia □ Improvement in balance and gait in patients with Parkinson's disease ■ Resumption of normal ovulatory menstrual cycles with restoration of fertility. In patients with amenorrhea and galactorrhea, menses usually resume within 6–8 wk, and galactorrhea subsides within 8–12 wk ■ Decreased breast engorgement and galactorrhea ■ Decreased serum levels of growth hormone in patients with acromegaly.

BROMPHENIRAMINE
(brome-fen-**eer**-a-meen)
Bromphen, Codimal-A, Conjec-B, Cophene-B, Dehist, Diamine, Dimetane, Histaject, Nasahist B, ND Stat, Oraminic II, Sinusol-B, Veltane

CLASSIFICATION(S):
Antihistamine
Pregnancy Category B

INDICATIONS
■ Symptomatic relief of allergic symptoms caused by histamine release; most useful for nasal allergies and allergic dermatoses ■ Severe allergic or hypersensitivity reactions, including anaphylaxis and transfusion reactions.

ACTION
■ Blocks the following effects of histamine: □ Vasodilation □ Increased GI tract secretions □ Increased heart rate □ Hypotension. **Therapeutic Effect:** ■ Relief of symptoms associated with histamine excess usually seen in allergic conditions. Does not block the release of histamine.

PHARMACOKINETICS
Absorption: Well absorbed following oral and IM administration.
Distribution: Widely distributed. Minimal amounts excreted in breast milk. Crosses the blood–brain barrier.
Metabolism and Excretion: Extensively metabolized by the liver.
Half-life: 12–35 hr.

CONTRAINDICATIONS AND PRECAUTIONS
Contraindicated in: ■ Hypersensitivity ■ Acute attacks of asthma ■ Lactation (avoid use) ■ Known alcohol intolerance (some elixirs).
Use Cautiously in: ■ Narrow-angle glaucoma ■ Liver disease ■ Elderly patients (more susceptible to adverse reaction) ■ Pregnancy (safety not established).

ADVERSE REACTIONS AND SIDE EFFECTS*
CNS: <u>drowsiness</u>, <u>sedation</u>, excitation (in children), dizziness.
CV: hypotension, <u>hypertension</u>, palpitations, arrhythmias.
EENT: <u>blurred vision</u>.
GI: <u>dry mouth</u>, obstruction, constipation.
GU: urinary hesitancy, retention.
Derm: sweating.
Misc: hypersensitivity reaction (IV use).

INTERACTIONS
Drug–Drug: ■ Additive CNS depression with other **CNS depressants** including **alcohol, opioids,** and **sedative/ hypnotics** ■ **MAO inhibitors** intensify and prolong the anticholinergic effects of antihistamines.

ROUTE AND DOSAGE
■ **PO (Adults):** 4 mg q 4–8 hr daily (not to exceed 24 mg/day), or 8 mg q 8–12 hr of extended-release form or 12 mg q 12 hr of extended-release form.
■ **PO (Children 6–12 yr):** 2 mg q 4–6 hr (not to exceed 12 mg/day) or 8–12 mg of extended-release form q 12 hr.
■ **PO (Children 2–6 yr):** 1 mg q 4–6 hr (not to exceed 6 mg/day).
■ **SC, IM, IV (Adults):** 10 mg q 8–12 hr (not to exceed 40 mg/day).

<u>Underlines</u> indicate most frequent; **CAPITALS indicate life-threatening.*

- **SC, IM, IV (Children):** 0.125 mg/kg
or 3.75 mg/m^2 3–4 times daily.

AVAILABILITY

- **Tablets:** 4 mg, 8mg, 12 mg ▪ **Timed-released tablets:** 8 mg, 12 mg ▪ **Elixir:** 2 mg/5 ml ▪ **Injection:** 10 mg/ml, 100 mg/ml.

TIME/ACTION PROFILE (relief of allergic symptoms)

	ONSET	PEAK	DURATION
PO	15–30 min	1–2 hr	6–8 hr*
SC	20–30 min	UK	8–12 hr
IM	20–30 min	UK	8–12 hr
IV	rapid	UK	8–12 hr

*Duration is longer (8–12 hr) for sustained-release oral preparations.

NURSING IMPLICATIONS

ASSESSMENT

- **Allergy:** Assess allergy symptoms (rhinitis, conjunctivitis, hives) prior to and periodically throughout course of therapy.
- Assess lung sounds and character of bronchial secretions. Maintain fluid intake of 1500–2000 ml/day to decrease viscosity of secretions.
- **Transfusion Reaction or Anaphylaxis:** Monitor for resolution of symptoms of allergic transfusion reaction or anaphylaxis (urticaria, wheezing, bronchospasm, hypotension). Monitor pulse and blood pressure prior to and throughout therapy.
- **IV:** Observe patient for sweating, hypotension, dizziness, drowsiness, or hypersensitivity reactions when administering medication intravenously. Elderly patients are more susceptible to side effects with this medication.
- **Lab Test Considerations:** May cause false negatives in allergy skin testing. Discontinue antihistamines at least 72 hr before testing.

POTENTIAL NURSING DIAGNOSES

- Airway clearance, ineffective (indications).
- Injury, high risk for (adverse reactions).
- Knowledge deficit related to medication regimen (patient/family teaching).

IMPLEMENTATION

- **PO:** Administer oral doses with food or milk to decrease GI irritation. Extended-release tablets should be swallowed whole; do not crush, break, or chew.
- **Direct IV:** May be given IV undiluted, but further dilution of each ml of 10 mg/ml solution with 10 ml of 0.9% NaCl for injection is recommended to reduce side effects.
- **Rate:** Administer each single dose slowly over at least 1 min.
- **Intermittent Infusion:** May be further diluted in 0.9% NaCl, D5W, or whole blood for IV infusion. The 100 mg/ml concentration is not recommended for IV use.

PATIENT/FAMILY TEACHING

- Instruct patient to take medication as directed; do not double doses.
- Commonly causes drowsiness. Caution patient to avoid driving or other activities requiring alertness until response to the medication is known.
- Advise patient to avoid taking alcohol or other CNS depressants concurrently with this drug.
- Frequent oral rinses, good oral hygiene, and sugarless gum or candy may help relieve dry mouth.
- Instruct patient to contact physician if symptoms persist.

EVALUATION

Effectiveness of therapy may be determined by: ▪ Decrease in allergic symptoms.

BUMETANIDE
(byoo-**met**-a-nide)
Bumex

CLASSIFICATION(S):
Diuretic (loop)
Pregnancy Category C

INDICATIONS

- Edema secondary to congestive heart failure or hepatic or renal disease. **Unlabeled Use:** ▪ Used alone or in combination with antihypertensives in the treatment of hypertension.

ACTION

- Inhibits the reabsorption of sodium and chloride from the loop of Henle and distal renal tubule ▪ Increases renal excretion of water, sodium, chloride, magnesium, hydrogen, and calcium ▪ Has renal and peripheral vasodilatory effects ▪ Effectiveness persists in impaired renal function. **Therapeutic Effects:** ▪ Diuresis with mobilization of excess fluid (edema, pleural effusions); also lowers blood pressure.

PHARMACOKINETICS

Absorption: Rapidly and completely absorbed after oral or IM administration.
Distribution: Distribution not known.
Metabolism and Excretion: Partially metabolized by the liver. 50% eliminated unchanged by the kidneys. 20% excreted in the feces.
Half-life: 1–1.5 hr.

CONTRAINDICATIONS AND PRECAUTIONS

Contraindicated in: ▪ Hypersensitivity ▪ Cross-sensitivity with sulfonamides may exist ▪ Pregnancy or lactation ▪ Anuria or increasing azotemia.
Use Cautiously in: ▪ Severe liver disease ▪ Electrolyte depletion ▪ Diabetes mellitus.

ADVERSE REACTIONS AND SIDE EFFECTS*

CNS: dizziness, headache, encephalopathy.
CV: hypotension.
Derm: rashes.
EENT: hearing loss, tinnitus.
F and E: metabolic alkalosis, hypovolemia, dehydration, hyponatremia, hypokalemia, hypochloremia, hypomagnesemia.
GI: nausea, vomiting, diarrhea, constipation, dry mouth.
GU: frequency.
Metab: hyperglycemia, hyperuricemia.
MS: muscle cramps.

INTERACTIONS

Drug–Drug: ▪ Additive hypotension with **antihypertensives**, acute ingestion of **alcohol** or **nitrates** ▪ Additive hypokalemia with other **diuretics, ticarcillin, mezlocillin, piperacillin, amphotericin B**, and **glucocorticoids** ▪ Hypokalemia may increase **cardiac glycoside** toxicity ▪ Decreases **lithium** excretion, may cause toxicity ▪ Increased risk of ototoxicity with **aminoglycosides**.

ROUTE AND DOSAGE

- **PO (Adults):** 0.5–2 mg/day (up to 10 mg/day; larger doses may be required in renal insufficiency).
- **IM, IV (Adults):** 0.5–1.0 mg; may give 1–2 more doses q 2–3 hr (not to exceed 10 mg/24 hr). In severe renal impairment, an infusion of 12 mg over 12 hr has been used.

AVAILABILITY

- **Tablets:** 0.5 mg, 1 mg, 2 mg ▪ **Injection:** 0.25 mg/ml.

TIME/ACTION PROFILE (onset of diuresis)

	ONSET	PEAK	DURATION
PO	30–60 min	1–2 hr	3–6 hr
IM	40 min	1–2 hr	4–6 hr
IV	within mins	15–45 min	3–6 hr

NURSING IMPLICATIONS

ASSESSMENT

▫ Assess fluid status throughout therapy. Monitor daily weight, intake and output ratios, amount and location of edema, lung sounds, skin turgor, and mucous membranes. Notify physician if thirst, dry mouth, lethargy, weak-

---

*Underlines indicate most frequent; **CAPITALS** indicate life-threatening.

ness, hypotension, or oliguria occur.

□ Monitor blood pressure and pulse before and during administration.

□ Assess patients receiving cardiac glycosides for anorexia, nausea, vomiting, muscle cramps, paresthesia, confusion. Notify physician if these symptoms occur.

□ Assess patient for hearing loss. Audiometry is recommended for patients receiving prolonged therapy. Hearing loss is most common following rapid or high-dose IV administration in patients with decreased renal function or those taking other ototoxic drugs.

□ Assess for allergy to sulfonamides.

▪ **Lab Test Considerations:** Monitor electrolytes, renal and hepatic function, glucose, and uric acid prior to and periodically throughout course of therapy. May cause decreased electrolyte levels (especially potassium). May cause elevated blood glucose, BUN, uric acid, and urinary phosphate levels.

POTENTIAL NURSING DIAGNOSES

▪ Fluid volume excess (indications).

▪ Fluid volume deficit (side effects).

▪ Knowledge deficit related to medication regimen (patient/family teaching).

IMPLEMENTATION

▪ **General Info:** Administer medication in the morning to prevent disruption of sleep cycle.

□ Intermittent dose, given on alternate days or for 3–4 days with rest periods of 1–2 days in between, may be used for continued control of edema.

□ 1 mg bumetanide is approximately equivalent to 40 mg furosemide.

▪ **PO:** Administer orally with food or milk to minimize gastric irritation.

▪ **Direct IV:** Administer over 1–2 min. May repeat at 2–3 hr intervals, not to exceed 10 mg/day.

▪ **Intermittent Infusion:** Dilute in D5W, 0.9% NaCl, or lactated Ringer's solution, and administer through Y-tubing or 3-way stopcock. Use reconstituted solution within 24 hr.

▪ *Rate:* May be administered over 12 hr for patients with renal impairment.

▪ **Y-Site Compatibility:** ▪ meperidine ▪ morphine.

PATIENT/FAMILY TEACHING

▪ **General Info:** Instruct patient to take bumetanide exactly as directed. Missed doses should be taken as soon as possible; do not double doses. Advise patients on antihypertensive regimen to continue taking medication, even if feeling better. Bumetanide controls but does not cure hypertension.

□ Caution patient to make position changes slowly to minimize orthostatic hypotension. Caution patient that the use of alcohol, exercise during hot weather, or standing for long periods during therapy may enhance orthostatic hypotension.

□ Instruct patient to consult physician regarding a diet high in potassium (see Appendix K).

□ Advise patient to consult physician or pharmacist before taking over-the-counter medication concurrently with this therapy.

□ Instruct patient to notify physician or dentist of medication regimen prior to treatment or surgery.

□ Advise patient to contact physician immediately if muscle weakness, cramps, nausea, dizziness, numbness, or tingling of extremities occur.

□ Emphasize the importance of routine follow-up examinations.

▪ **Hypertension:** Reinforce the need to continue additional therapies for hypertension (weight loss, exercise, restricted sodium intake, stress reduction, regular exercise, moderation of alcohol consumption, cessation of smoking).

EVALUATION

Effectiveness of therapy can be demonstrated by: ▪ Decrease in edema □ Decrease in abdominal girth □ Increase in urinary output ▪ Decrease in blood pressure.

BUPRENORPHINE
(byoo-pre-**nor**-feen)
Buprenex

CLASSIFICATION(S):
Opioid analgesic (agonist/ antagonist)
Schedule V
Pregnancy Category C

INDICATIONS

- Management of moderate to severe pain.

ACTION

- Binds to opiate receptors in the CNS
- Alters the perception of and response to painful stimuli, while producing generalized CNS depression
- Has partial antagonist properties that may result in opioid withdrawal in physically dependent patients. **Therapeutic Effect:**
- Decreased severity of pain.

PHARMACOKINETICS

Absorption: Well absorbed from IM sites.
Distribution: Crosses the placenta and enters breast milk.
Metabolism and Excretion: Mostly metabolized by the liver.
Half-life: 2–3 hr.

CONTRAINDICATIONS AND PRECAUTIONS

Contraindicated in: ▪ Hypersensitivity. **Use Cautiously in:** ▪ Increased intracranial pressure ▪ Severe renal, hepatic, or pulmonary disease ▪ Hypothyroidism ▪ Adrenal insufficiency ▪ Alcoholism ▪ Elderly or debilitated patients (dosage reduction required) ▪ Undiagnosed abdominal pain ▪ Prostatic hypertrophy ▪ Pregnancy, labor, lactation, or children <13 yr (safety not established).

ADVERSE REACTIONS AND SIDE EFFECTS*

CNS: sedation, confusion, headache, euphoria, floating feeling, unusual dreams, hallucinations, dysphoria, dizziness.
EENT: miosis (high doses), blurred vision, diplopia.
Resp: respiratory depression.
CV: hypotension, hypertension, palpitations.
GI: nausea, vomiting, constipation, ileus, dry mouth.
GU: urinary retention.
Derm: sweating, clammy feeling.
Misc: sweating, tolerance, physical dependence, psychological dependence.

INTERACTIONS

Drug–Drug: ▪ Use with caution in patients receiving **MAO inhibitors** (increased CNS and respiratory depression and hypotension; decrease buprenorphine dose by 50%, may need to decrease MAO inhibitor dose) ▪ Additive CNS depression with **alcohol, antihistamines, antidepressants,** and **sedative/hypnotics** ▪ May decrease effectiveness of other **opioid analgesics.**

ROUTE AND DOSAGE

- **IM, IV (Adults):** 0.3 mg q 4–6 hr as needed. May repeat initial dose after 30 min (up to 0.3 mg q 4 hr or 0.6 mg q 6 hr).

AVAILABILITY

- *Injection:* 0.3 mg/ml.

TIME/ACTION PROFILE (analgesia)

	ONSET	PEAK	DURATION
IM	15 min	60 min	6 hr
IV	rapid	rapid	6 hr

NURSING IMPLICATIONS

ASSESSMENT

▫ Assess type, location, and intensity of pain prior to and 15 min following IM and 5 min following IV administration.
▫ Assess blood pressure, pulse, and respirations before and periodically during administration. Buprenorphine 0.3 mg has approximately

---

*Underlines indicate most frequent; **CAPITALS** indicate life-threatening.

equal respiratory depression with morphine 10 mg.

- While this drug has a low potential for dependence, prolonged use may lead to physical and psychological dependence and tolerance. This should not prevent patient from receiving adequate analgesia. Most patients receiving buprenorphine for medical reasons do not develop psychological dependence. If tolerance develops, changing to an opioid agonist may be required to relieve pain.
- Assess prior analgesic history. Antagonistic properties may induce withdrawal symptoms (vomiting, restlessness, abdominal cramps, increased blood pressure and temperature) in opioid-dependent patients. Symptoms may occur up to 15 days after discontinuation and persist for 1–2 wk.
- **Lab Test Considerations:** May cause elevated serum amylase and lipase levels.
- **Toxicity and Overdose:** If overdose occurs, respiratory depression may be partially reversed by naloxone (Narcan). Doxapram may also be ordered as a respiratory stimulant.

POTENTIAL NURSING DIAGNOSES

- Pain (indications).
- Injury, high risk for (side effects).

IMPLEMENTATION

- **General Info:** Explain therapeutic value of medication prior to administration to enhance the analgesic effect.
- Regularly administered doses may be more effective than prn administration. Analgesic is more effective if given before pain becomes severe.
- Coadministration with nonopioid analgesics may have additive effects and permit lower opioid doses.
- **IM:** Administer IM injections deep into well-developed muscle. Rotate sites of injections.
- **Direct IV:** May give IV undiluted. Administer slowly. Rapid administra-

tion may cause respiratory depression, hypotension, and cardiac arrest.

- **Syringe Compatibility:** ▪ midazolam.
- **Additive Compatibility:** ▪ 0.9% NaCl ▪ D5W ▪ D5/0.9% NaCl ▪ lactated Ringer's solution ▪ atropine ▪ diphenhydramine ▪ droperidol ▪ glycopyrrolate ▪ haloperidol ▪ hydroxyzine ▪ promethazine ▪ scopolamine.
- **Additive Incompatibility:** ▪ diazepam ▪ lorazepam.

PATIENT/FAMILY TEACHING

- Instruct patient on how and when to ask for pain medication.
- Medication may cause drowsiness or dizziness. Advise patient to call for assistance when ambulating and to avoid driving or other activities requiring alertness until response to medication is known.
- Encourage patient to turn, cough, and deep breathe every 2 hr to prevent atelectasis.
- Advise patient that good oral hygiene, frequent mouth rinses, and sugarless gum or candy may decrease dry mouth.
- Instruct patient to change positions slowly to minimize orthostatic hypotension.
- Advise patient to avoid concurrent use of alcohol or other CNS depressants.

EVALUATION

Effectiveness of therapy can be demonstrated by: ▪ Decrease in severity of pain without a significant alteration in level of consciousness or respiratory status.

BUPROPION
(byoo-**proe**-pee-on)
Wellbutrin

CLASSIFICATION(S):
Antidepressant
Pregnancy Category B

INDICATIONS

- Treatment of depression, often in conjunction with psychotherapy.

ACTION

■ Decreases neuronal reuptake of dopamine in the CNS ■ Diminished neuronal uptake of serotonin and norepinephrine (less than tricyclic antidepressants). **Therapeutic Effect:** ■ Diminished depression.

PHARMACOKINETICS

Absorption: Although well absorbed, bioavailability appears to be low due to extensive rapid metabolic clearance by the liver.
Distribution: Distribution not known.
Metabolism and Excretion: Extensively metabolized by the liver. Some conversion to active metabolites.
Half-life: 14 hr (active metabolites may have longer half-lives).

CONTRAINDICATIONS AND PRECAUTIONS

Contraindicated in: ■ Hypersensitivity ■ History of seizures, bullemia, and anorexia nervosa ■ Concurrent MAO inhibitor therapy.
Use Cautiously in: ■ History of cranial trauma ■ Renal or hepatic impairment (dosage reduction recommended) ■ Pregnancy, lactation, or children (safety not established) ■ Recent history of myocardial infarction ■ Unstable cardiovascular status.

ADVERSE REACTIONS AND SIDE EFFECTS*

CNS: SEIZURES, agitation, insomnia, psychoses, mania, headache.
GI: dry mouth, nausea, vomiting, change in appetite, weight gain, weight loss.
Neuro: tremor.

INTERACTIONS

Drug–Drug: ■ Increased risk of adverse reactions when used with **levodopa** or **MAO inhibitors** ■ Increased risk of seizures with **phenothiazines, antidepressants**, cessation of **benzodiazepines**, or cessation of **alcohol**.

ROUTE AND DOSAGE

■ **PO (Adults):** 100 mg twice daily (morning and evening) initially; after 3 days may be increased to 100 mg 3 times daily after 4 wk of therapy, may increase to a maximum daily dose of 450 mg/day in divided doses. (No single dose to exceed 150 mg, wait at least 6 hr between doses at the 300 mg/day dose, or at least 4 hr between doses at the 450 mg/day dose).

AVAILABILITY

■ *Tablets:* 75 mg, 100 mg.

TIME/ACTION PROFILE
(antidepressant effect)

	ONSET	PEAK	DURATION
PO	up to 4 wk	UK	UK

NURSING IMPLICATIONS

ASSESSMENT

□ Monitor mood changes. Inform physician if patient demonstrates significant increase in anxiety, nervousness, or insomnia.
□ Assess for suicidal tendencies, especially during early therapy. Restrict amount of drug available to patient.

POTENTIAL NURSING DIAGNOSES

■ Coping, ineffective individual (indications).
■ Knowledge deficit related to medication regimen (patient/family teaching).

IMPLEMENTATION

■ **PO:** Administer doses in equally spaced time increments throughout day to minimize the risk of seizures.
□ May be initially administered concurrently with sedatives to minimize agitation. This is not usually required after the first week of therapy.
□ Insomnia may be decreased by avoiding bedtime doses.

PATIENT/FAMILY TEACHING

□ Instruct patient to take bupropion ex-

---

*Underlines indicate most frequent; **CAPITALS** indicate life-threatening.

actly as directed. If a dose is missed, omit dose and return to regular dosing schedule. Do not double doses.

□ Bupropion may impair judgment or motor and cognitive skills. Caution patient to avoid driving and other activities requiring alertness until response to medication is known.

□ Advise patient to avoid alcohol during therapy and to consult with physician before taking other medications with bupropion.

□ Inform patient that frequent mouth rinses, good oral hygiene, and sugarless gum or candy may minimize dry mouth. If dry mouth persists for more than 2 wk consult physician or dentist regarding use of saliva substitute.

□ Instruct female patients to inform physician if pregnancy is planned or suspected.

◻ Emphasize the importance of follow-up examinations to monitor progress. Encourage patient participation in psychotherapy.

EVALUATION
Effectiveness of therapy can be demonstrated by: ▪ Increased sense of well-being □ Renewed interest in surroundings. Acute episodes of depression may require several months of treatment.

BUSPIRONE
(byoo-**spye**-rone)
BuSpar

CLASSIFICATION(S):
Antianxiety agent
Pregnancy Category B

INDICATIONS

▪ Management of anxiety.

ACTION

▪ Binds to serotonin and dopamine receptors in the brain ▪ Increases norepinephrine metabolism in the brain. **Therapeutic Effect:** ▪ Relief of anxiety.

PHARMACOKINETICS

Absorption: Rapidly absorbed.
Distribution: Distribution not known.
Metabolism and Excretion: Extensively metabolized by the liver. 20–40% excreted in feces.
Half-life: 2–3 hr.

CONTRAINDICATIONS AND PRECAUTIONS

Contraindicated in: ▪ Hypersensitivity. **Use Cautiously in:** ▪ Patients receiving other antianxiety agents (other agents should be slowly withdrawn to prevent withdrawal or rebound phenomenon) ▪ Severe liver disease ▪ Pregnancy, lactation, and children (safety not established) ▪ Patients receiving other psychoactive drugs.

ADVERSE REACTIONS AND SIDE EFFECTS*

CNS: dizziness, insomnia, nervousness, drowsiness, light-headedness, excitement, headache, personality changes, fatigue, weakness.
EENT: tinnitus, sore throat, blurred vision, nasal congestion, altered taste or smell, conjunctivitis.
Resp: hyperventilation, shortness of breath, chest congestion.
CV: chest pain, palpitations, tachycardia, syncope, hypotension, hypertension.
GI: nausea, dry mouth, diarrhea, constipation, abdominal pain, vomiting.
GU: frequency, hesitancy, dysuria, changes in libido.
Derm: rashes, pruritis, edema, flushing, easy bruising, hair loss, dry skin, blisters.
Endo: irregular menses.
MS: myalgia.
Neuro: paresthesia, numbness, incoordination, tremor.
Misc: sweating, clamminess, fever.

INTERACTIONS

Drug–Drug: ▪ Use with **MAO inhibitors** may result in hypertension ▪ May

*Underlines indicate most frequent; **CAPITALS** indicate life-threatening.

increase the risk of hepatic effects from **trazadone** ▪ Avoid concurrent use with **alcohol**.

ROUTE AND DOSAGE

▪ **PO (Adults):** 15 mg/day in 3 divided doses, increase by 5 mg/day at 2–3-day intervals (not to exceed 60 mg/day). Usual dose is 20–30 mg/day.

AVAILABILITY

▪ *Tablets:* 5 mg, 10 mg.

TIME/ACTION PROFILE (relief of anxiety)

	ONSET	PEAK	DURATION
PO	7–10 days	3–4 wk	UK

NURSING IMPLICATIONS

ASSESSMENT

▪ **General Info:** Assess degree and manifestations of anxiety prior to and periodically throughout therapy.
▫ Buspirone does not appear to cause physical or psychological dependence or tolerance. However, patients with a history of drug abuse should be assessed for tolerance or dependence, and the amount of drug available to these patients should be restricted.

POTENTIAL NURSING DIAGNOSES

▪ Anxiety (indications).
▪ Injury, high risk for (side effects).
▪ Knowledge deficit related to medication regimen (patient/family teaching).

IMPLEMENTATION

▪ **General Info:** Patients changing from other antianxiety agents should receive gradually decreasing doses because buspirone will not prevent withdrawal symptoms.
▪ **PO:** May be administered with food to minimize gastric irritation. Food slows but does not alter extent of absorption.

PATIENT/FAMILY TEACHING

▫ Instruct patient to take buspirone exactly as directed. If a dose is missed, take as soon as remembered if not just before next dose; do not double doses. Do not take more than amount prescribed; 1–2 wk of therapy may be required before antianxiety effect is noticeable.
▫ May cause dizziness or drowsiness. Caution patient to avoid driving or other activities requiring alertness until response to the medication is known.
▫ Advise patient to avoid concurrent use of alcohol or other CNS depressants with this medication.
▫ Advise patient to consult physician or pharmacist before taking over-the-counter medications with this drug.
▫ Instruct patient to notify the physician if any chronic abnormal movements occur (dystonia, motor restlessness, involuntary movements of facial or cervical muscles) or if pregnancy is suspected.
▫ Emphasize the importance of follow-up examinations to determine effectiveness of this medication.

EVALUATION

Effectiveness of therapy can be demonstrated by: ▪ Increase in well-being ▫ Decrease in subjective feelings of anxiety. Some improvement may be seen in 7–10 days. Optimal results take 3–4 wk of therapy. Buspirone is usually used for short-term therapy (3–4 wk). If prescribed for long-term therapy, efficacy should be periodically assessed.

BUSULFAN
(byoo-**sul**-fan)
Myleran

CLASSIFICATION(S):
Antineoplastic (alkylating agent)
Pregnancy Category D

INDICATIONS

▪ Treatment of chronic myelogenous leukemia and bone marrow disorders.

ACTION

▪ Disrupts nucleic acid function and protein synthesis (cell cycle-

B

phase nonspecific). **Therapeutic Effect:**
▪ Death of rapidly growing cells, especially malignant ones.

PHARMACOKINETICS

Absorption: Rapidly absorbed from the GI tract.
Distribution: Distribution not known.
Metabolism and Excretion: Extensively metabolized by the liver.
Half-life: UK.

CONTRAINDICATIONS AND PRECAUTIONS

Contraindicated in: ▪ Hypersensitivity ▪ Failure to respond to previous courses ▪ Pregnancy or lactation.
Use Cautiously in: ▪ Patients with childbearing potential ▪ Active infections ▪ Decreased bone marrow reserve ▪ Other chronic debilitating diseases.

ADVERSE REACTIONS AND SIDE EFFECTS*

Resp: PULMONARY FIBROSIS.
GI: nausea, vomiting, hepatitis.
Derm: alopecia.
Endo: gynecomastia, gonadal suppression.
Hemat: bone marrow depression.
Metab: hyperuricemia.

INTERACTIONS

Drug–Drug: ▪ Additive bone marrow suppression with other **antineoplastic agents** or **radiation therapy**.

ROUTE AND DOSAGE

▪ **PO (Adults):** 4–8 mg/day initially; maintenance 1–3 mg/day.
▪ **PO (Children):** 0.06–0.12 mg/kg/day or 1.8–4.6 mg/m^2/day initially.

AVAILABILITY

▪ *Tablets:* 2 mg.

TIME/ACTION PROFILE (effects on blood counts)

	ONSET	PEAK	DURATION
PO	10–15 days	wks	up to 1 mo*

*Complete recovery may take up to 20 mo.

NURSING IMPLICATIONS

ASSESSMENT

▢ Assess for fever, sore throat, and signs of infection. If these symptoms occur, notify physician immediately.
▢ Assess for bleeding (bleeding gums, bruising, petechiae; guaiac stools, urine, emesis). Avoid IM injections and rectal temperatures or products containing aspirin or ibuprofen. Hold pressure on all venipuncture sites for at least 10 min.
▢ Monitor intake and output ratios and daily weights. Notify physician if significant changes in totals occur.
▢ Monitor for symptoms of gout (increased uric acid, joint pain, swelling). Encourage patient to drink at least 2 liters of fluid each day. Allopurinol may be given to decrease uric acid levels. Alkalinization of urine may be ordered to increase excretion of uric acid.
▢ Anemia may occur. Monitor for increased fatigue, dyspnea, and orthostatic hypotension.
▪ **Lab Test Considerations:** Monitor CBC and differential prior to and weekly during course of therapy. The nadir of leukopenia occurs within 10–30 days. Recovery usually occurs within 12–20 wk. Notify physician if WBC is <15,000 mm^3 or if a precipitous drop occurs. Institute thrombocytopenia precautions if platelet count is <150,000/mm^3.
▢ Monitor liver function tests, BUN, serum creatinine, and uric acid prior to and periodically during course of therapy.
▢ May cause false-positive cytology results of breast, bladder, cervix, and lung tissues.

POTENTIAL NURSING DIAGNOSES

▪ Body image disturbance (side effects).
▪ Injury, high risk for (side effects).
▪ Infection, high risk for (side effects).

IMPLEMENTATION

▪ **PO:** Administer either 1 hr before or 2 hr after meals.

*Underlines indicate most frequent; **CAPITALS** indicate life-threatening.

PATIENT/FAMILY TEACHING

- Instruct patient to take medication exactly as directed, at the same time each day, even if nausea and vomiting is a problem. Consult physician if vomiting occurs shortly after dose is taken. If a dose is missed do not take at all; do not double doses.
- Instruct patient to report unusual bleeding. Advise patient of thrombocytopenia precautions (use soft tooth brush, electric razor, and avoid falls). Do not drink alcoholic beverages or take medication containing aspirin or ibuprofen, as these may precipitate gastric bleeding.
- Caution patient to avoid crowds and persons with known infections. Physician should be informed immediately if symptoms of infection occur.
- Discuss with patient the possibility of hair loss. Explore methods of coping.
- Review with patient the need for contraception during therapy. Women need to use contraception even if amenorrhea occurs.
- Instruct patient not to receive any vaccinations without advice of physician.
- Advise patient to notify physician if unusual bleeding or bruising, or flank, stomach, or joint pain occurs. Advise patients on long-term therapy to notify physician immediately if cough, shortness of breath, and fever occur. Patients should also notify physician if darkening of skin, diarrhea, dizziness, fatigue, anorexia, confusion, or nausea and vomiting become pronounced.

EVALUATION

Effectiveness of therapy can be demonstrated by: ■ Decrease in leukocyte count to within normal limits □ Decreased night sweats □ Increase in appetite □ Increased sense of well-being. Therapy is resumed when leukocyte count reaches 50,000/mm^3.

BUTALBITAL COMPOUND
(byoo-**tal**-bi-tal)

butalbital, acetaminophen
Bancap, Phrenilin, Phrenilin Forte, Sedapap-10, Triaprin

butalbital, acetaminophen, caffeine
Amaphen, Anoquan, Arcet, Butace, Endolor, Esgic, Esgic Plus, Femcet, Fioricet, G-1, Medigesic Plus, Repan, Two-Dyne

butalbital, aspirin
Axotal

butalbital, aspirin, caffeine
B-A-C, Fiorgan PF, Fiorinal, Isollyl Improved, Lanorinal, Marnal, {Tecanl}

CLASSIFICATION(S):
Nonopioid analgesics with barbiturates
Schedule III
Pregnancy Category D

INDICATIONS

■ Management of mild to moderate pain.

ACTION

■ Contains an analgesic (aspirin or acetaminophen) for relief of pain, a barbiturate (butalbital) for its sedative effect, and some contain caffeine, which may be of benefit in vascular headaches. **Therapeutic Effect:** ■ Decreased severity of pain with some sedation.

PHARMACOKINETICS

Absorption: All components are well absorbed.
Distribution: All components are widely distributed, cross the placenta, and enter breast milk.
Metabolism and Excretion: All components are mostly metabolized by the liver.
Half-life: Aspirin, 2–3 hr (low doses); acetaminophen, 1–4 hr; butalbital, UK.

{} = Available in Canada only.

CONTRAINDICATIONS AND PRECAUTIONS

Contraindicated in: ▪ Hypersensitivity to aspirin, acetaminophen, or butalbital ▪ Cross-sensitivity may exist with other nonsteroidal anti-inflammatory agents or barbiturates ▪ Aspirin should be avoided in patients with bleeding disorders or thrombocytopenia ▪ Acetaminophen should be avoided in patients with severe hepatic or renal disease ▪ Butalbital should not be used in comatose patients or those with pre-existing CNS depression ▪ Uncontrolled severe pain ▪ Pregnancy or lactation ▪ Caffeine should be avoided in patients with severe cardiovascular disease.

Use Cautiously in: ▪ Patients who may be suicidal or who may have been addicted to drugs previously ▪ Elderly patients (dosage reduction required) ▪ Use should be short-term only ▪ Children (safety not established).

ADVERSE REACTIONS AND SIDE EFFECTS*

CNS: *caffeine*—nervousness, irritability, insomnia; *butalbital*—drowsiness, lethargy, vertigo, depression, hangover, excitation, delerium.

EENT: *aspirin*—tinnitus, hearing loss.

Resp: *butalbital*—respiratory depression.

CV: *caffeine*—tachycardia, palpitations.

GI: *acetaminophen*—HEPATIC NECROSIS (overdose); *aspirin*—dyspepsia, heartburn, epigastric distress, nausea, vomiting, anorexia, abdominal pain, GI BLEEDING, hepatotoxicity; *caffeine*—heartburn, epigastric distress; *butalbital*—nausea, vomiting, diarrhea, constipation.

Derm: *acetaminophen*—rash, dermatitis.

Hemat: *aspirin*—increased bleeding time, anemia, hemolysis.

Misc: *aspirin*—noncardiogenic pulmonary edema, allergic reactions including ANAPHYLAXIS and LARYNGOSPASM; *butalbital*—hypersensitivity reactions including ANGIOEDEMA and serum sickness, physical dependence, psychological dependence.

INTERACTIONS

Drug–Drug: ▪ *Aspirin*—May potentiate **oral anticoagulants** ▪ May enhance the activity of **penicillins, phenytoin, methotrexate, valproic acid, oral hypoglycemic agents,** and **sulfonamides** ▪ May antagonize the beneficial effects of **uricosuric agents** ▪ May decrease effects of most nonsteroidal anti-inflammatory agents ▪ **Glucocorticoids** may decrease salicylate levels ▪ **Urinary acidification** may increase salicylate levels ▪ **Alkalinization** may decrease salicylate levels ▪ May blunt the therapeutic response to **diuretics** ▪ *Acetaminophen*—Hepatotoxicity may be additive with other **hepatotoxic agents** including **alcohol** ▪ **Phenobarbital** may potentiate hepatotoxicity in overdosage ▪ **Cholestyramine** and **colestipol** may decrease absorption ▪ *Butalbital*—Additive CNS depression with other **CNS depressants,** including **alcohol, antihistamines, antidepressants, opioid analgesics,** and **sedative/hypnotics** ▪ May increase the liver metabolism and decrease the effectiveness of other drugs including **oral contraceptives, chloramphenicol, acebutolol, propranolol, metoprolol, timolol, doxycycline, glucocorticoids, tricyclic antidepressants, phenothiazines, phenylbutazone,** and **quinidine.** ▪ **MAO inhibitors, primidone,** and **valproic acid** may prevent metabolism and increase the effectiveness of butalbital ▪ May enhance the hematologic toxicity of **cyclophosphamide.**

ROUTE AND DOSAGE

▪ **PO (Adults):** 1–2 capsules or tablets (50–100 mg butalbital) every 2–6 hr as needed for pain.

AVAILABILITY

■ *Tablets and capsules:* In combination with aspirin, acetaminophen, caffeine, and codeine. See Appendix A.

TIME/ACTION PROFILE

	ONSET	PEAK	DURATION
PO	15–30 min	1–2 hr	2–6 hr

NURSING IMPLICATIONS

ASSESSMENT

□ Assess type, location, and intensity of pain prior to and 60 min following administration.

□ Prolonged use may lead to physical and psychological dependence and tolerance. This should not prevent patient from receiving adequate analgesia. Most patients who receive butalbital compound for medical reasons do not develop psychological dependence.

■ **Lab Test Considerations:** Aspirin prolongs bleeding time for 4–7 days and, in large doses, may cause prolonged prothrombin time.

□ False-negative urine glucose test results with glucose oxidase method (Clinistix, Tes-Tape), and false-positive urine glucose test results with copper sulfate method (Clinitest).

POTENTIAL NURSING DIAGNOSES

■ Pain (indications).

■ Injury, high risk for (side effects).

IMPLEMENTATION

■ **General Info:** Explain therapeutic value of medication prior to administration to enhance the analgesic effect.

□ Regularly administered doses may be more effective than prn administration. Analgesic is more effective if given before pain becomes severe.

□ Medication should be discontinued gradually after long-term use to prevent withdrawal symptoms.

■ **PO:** Oral doses may be administered with food or milk to minimize GI irritation.

PATIENT/FAMILY TEACHING

□ Instruct patient to take medication exactly as directed. Do not increase dose due to the habit-forming potential of butalbital. If medication appears less effective after a few weeks, consult physician.

□ Instruct patient on how and when to ask for pain medication.

□ Medication may cause drowsiness or dizziness. Advise patient to avoid driving and other activities requiring alertness until response to medication is known.

□ Caution patient to avoid concurrent use of alcohol or other CNS depressants.

□ Tablets containing aspirin that have an acetic (vinegar-like) odor should be discarded.

□ Centers for Disease Control warn against giving aspirin to children or adolescents with varicella (chickenpox) or influenza-like or viral illnesses because of a possible association with Reye's syndrome.

EVALUATION

Effectiveness of therapy can be demonstrated by: ■ Decrease in severity of pain without a significant alteration in level of consciousness.

BUTORPHANOL
(byoo-**tor**-fa-nole)
Stadol, Stadol NS

CLASSIFICATION(S):
Opioid analgesic (agonist/ antagonist)
Pregnancy Category UK

INDICATIONS

■ Management of moderate to severe pain ■ Analgesia during labor ■ Sedation prior to surgery ■ Supplement in balanced anesthesia.

ACTION

■ Binds to opiate receptors in the CNS ■ Alters the perception of and response to painful stimuli, while producing generalized CNS depression ■ Has partial antagonist properties that may result

in opioid withdrawal in physically dependent patients. **Therapeutic Effect:**
▪ Decreased severity of pain.

PHARMACOKINETICS

Absorption: Well absorbed from IM sites and nasal mucosa .
Distribution: Crosses the placenta and enters breast milk.
Metabolism and Excretion: Mostly metabolized by the liver; 11–14% excreted in the feces. Minimal amounts excreted unchanged by the kidneys.
Half-life: 3–4 hr.

CONTRAINDICATIONS AND PRECAUTIONS

Contraindicated in: ▪ Hypersensitivity ▪ Opioid-dependent patients who have not been detoxified (may precipitate withdrawal).
Use Cautiously in: ▪ Head trauma ▪ Increased intracranial pressure ▪ Severe renal, hepatic, or pulmonary disease (increase interval in hepatic/renal impairment) ▪ Hypothyroidism ▪ Adrenal insufficiency ▪ Alcoholism ▪ Elderly or debilitated patients (dosage reduction required) ▪ Undiagnosed abdominal pain ▪ Prostatic hypertrophy ▪ Pregnancy, lactation, or children (safety not established, but has been used during labor—may cause respiratory depression in the newborn).

ADVERSE REACTIONS AND SIDE EFFECTS*

CNS: sedation, confusion, headache, euphoria, floating feeling, unusual dreams, hallucinations, dysphoria.
EENT: miosis (high doses), blurred vision, diplopia.
Resp: respiratory depression.
CV: hypotension, hypertension, palpitations.
GI: nausea, vomiting, constipation, ileus, dry mouth.
GU: urinary retention.
Derm: sweating, clammy feeling.
Misc: tolerance, physical dependence, psychological dependence.

INTERACTIONS

Drug–Drug: ▪ Use with extreme caution in patients receiving **MAO inhibitors** (may produce severe, potentially fatal reactions—reduce initial dose of butorphanol to 25% of usual dose) ▪ Additive CNS depression with **alcohol, antihistamines, antidepressants,** and **sedative/hypnotics** ▪ May precipitate withdrawal in patients who are physically dependent on opioid analgesics and have not been detoxified ▪ May decrease effects of concurrently administered **opioid analgesics**.

ROUTE AND DOSAGE

▪ **IM (Adults):** 2 mg q 3–4 hr as needed (range 1–4 mg).
▪ **IV (Adults):** 0.5–2.0 mg q 3–4 hr as needed (range 0.5–2 mg).
▪ **Intranasal (Adults):** 1 mg (1 spray in one nostril) initially. An additional dose may be given 60–90 min later. This sequence may be repeated in 3–4 hr. If pain is severe, an initial dose of 2 mg (1 spray in each nostril) may be given. May be repeated in 3–4 hr.

AVAILABILITY

▪ *Injection:* 1 mg/ml, 2 mg/ml ▪ *Intranasal solution:* 10 mg/ml, in 2.5-ml–metered dose spray pump (14–15 doses).

TIME/ACTION PROFILE (analgesia)

	ONSET	PEAK	DURATION
IM	1–30 min	30–60 min	3–4 hr
IV	1 min	4–5 min	2–4 hr
IN	within 15 min	1–2 hr	4–5 hr

NURSING IMPLICATIONS

ASSESSMENT

▫ Assess type, location, and intensity of pain prior to and 30–60 min following IM, 5 min following IV, and 60–90 min following intranasal administration.
▫ Assess blood pressure, pulse, and

---

*Underlines indicate most frequent; **CAPITALS** indicate life-threatening.

respirations before and periodically during administration. Respiratory depression does not increase in severity, only in duration, with increased dosage.

□ While this drug has a low potential for dependence, prolonged use may lead to physical and psychological dependence and tolerance. This should not prevent patient from receiving adequate analgesia. Most patients who receive butorphanol for medical reasons do not develop psychological dependence. If tolerance develops, changing to an opioid agonist may be required to relieve pain.

□ Assess prior analgesic history. Antagonistic properties may induce withdrawal symptoms (vomiting, restlessness, abdominal cramps, increased blood pressure and temperature) in opioid-dependent patients.

▪ **Lab Test Considerations:** May cause elevated serum amylase and lipase levels.

▪ **Toxicity and Overdose:** If overdose occurs, respiratory depression may be partially reversed by naloxone (Narcan), the antidote.

POTENTIAL NURSING DIAGNOSES
▪ Pain (indications).
▪ Injury, high risk for (side effects).
▪ Sensory-perceptual alteration: visual, auditory (side effects).
▪ Knowledge deficit related to medication regimen (patient/family teaching).

IMPLEMENTATION
▪ **General Info:** Explain therapeutic value of medication prior to administration to enhance the analgesic effect.

□ Regularly administered doses may be more effective than prn administration. Analgesic is more effective if given before pain becomes severe.

□ Coadministration with nonopioid analgesics may have additive analgesic effects and permit lower opioid doses.

▪ **IM:** Administer IM injections deep into well-developed muscle. Rotate sites of injections.

▪ **Direct IV:** May give IV undiluted.
▪ **Rate:** Administer over 3–5 min. Rapid administration may cause respiratory depression, hypotension, and cardiac arrest.
▪ **Syringe Compatibility:** ▪ atropine ▪ chlorpromazine ▪ cimetidine ▪ diphenhydramine ▪ droperidol ▪ fentanyl ▪ hydroxyzine ▪ meperidine ▪ midazolam ▪ morphine ▪ pentazocine ▪ perphenazine ▪ prochlorperazine ▪ promethazine ▪ scopolamine ▪ thiethylperazine.
▪ **Syringe Incompatibility:** ▪ dimenhydrinate ▪ pentobarbital.
▪ **Y-Site Compatibility:** ▪ enalaprilat ▪ esmolol ▪ fludarabine ▪ sargramostim.
▪ **Intranasal:** Administer 1 spray in nostril.

PATIENT/FAMILY TEACHING
□ Instruct patient on how and when to ask for pain medication.
□ Medication may cause drowsiness or dizziness. Advise patient to call for assistance when ambulating and to avoid driving or other activities requiring alertness until response to the medication is known.
□ Encourage patient to turn, cough, and breathe deeply every 2 hr to prevent atelectasis.
□ Instruct patient to change positions slowly to minimize orthostatic hypotension.
□ Caution patient to avoid concurrent use of alcohol or other CNS depressants with this medication.
▪ **Intranasal:** Instruct patient on proper use of nasal spray. Blow nose gently to clear both nostrils. Pull off clear dust cover and remove protective clip from neck of pump unit. Prior to initial use spray unit must be primed. Hold unit with thumb on bottom of bottle and spray tip between first and second fingers and push down. Pump firmly and quickly until fine spray appears (may require 7–8 strokes). If pump unit is not used within 48 hr, must be reprimed (requires only 1–2 strokes). Each repriming reduces

number of effective doses per bottle. Insert tip of spray unit into nostril approximately 1 cm (width of small finger), pointing tip toward back of nose. Close the other nostril with forefinger and tilt head slightly forward. Pump spray unit once, firmly and quickly. Sniff gently with mouth closed. After spraying remove pump unit, tilt head backwards; sniff gently a few more seconds.

□ If 2-mg dose is prescribed, administer additional spray in other nostril. Patient should remain recumbent following administration of 2-mg dose until response to medication is known.

□ Instruct patient to replace protective clip and clear cover following use and to store the unit in the child-resistant container. Caution patient that medication should not be used by anyone other than for whom it was prescribed. Excess medication should be disposed of as soon as it is no longer needed. To dispose of, unscrew cap, rinse bottle and pump with water, and dispose of in waste can.

EVALUATION
Effectiveness of therapy can be demonstrated by: ▪ Decrease in severity of pain without a significant alteration in level of consciousness or respiratory status.

CALCITONIN—salmon
(kal-si-**toe**-nin)
Calcimar, Miacalcin
CALCITONIN—human
Cibacalcin

CLASSIFICATION(S):
Hormone, Electrolyte modifier
(hypocalcemic)
Pregnancy Category C

INDICATIONS
▪ Treatment of Paget's disease of bone (human and salmon) ▪ Adjunctive therapy for hypercalcemia (salmon only) ▪ Management of postmenopausal osteoporosis (salmon only).

ACTION
▪ Decreases serum calcium by a direct effect on bone, kidney, and GI tract ▪ Promotes renal excretion of calcium. ▪ Salmon source is more potent on a weight basis and has a longer duration of action. **Therapeutic Effects:** ▪ Decreased rate of bone turnover ▪ Lowering of serum calcium.

PHARMACOKINETICS
Absorption: Destroyed in GI tract, necessitating parenteral administration. Completely absorbed from IM and SC sites.
Distribution: Distribution not known. Does not appear to cross the placenta.
Metabolism and Excretion: Rapidly metabolized in kidneys, blood, and tissues.
Half-life: Human, 60 min; salmon, 70–90 min.

CONTRAINDICATIONS AND PRECAUTIONS
Contraindicated in: ▪ Hypersensitivity to salmon protein or gelatin diluent (salmon product) ▪ Pregnancy or lactation (use not recommended).
Use Cautiously in: Children (safety not established).

ADVERSE REACTIONS AND SIDE EFFECTS*
CNS: headaches.
GI: nausea, vomiting, diarrhea, strange taste.
GU: urinary frequency.
Derm: rashes.
Local: injection site reactions.
Misc: allergic reactions including ANA-PHYLAXIS (more common with salmon product), swelling, tingling, and tenderness in the hands, facial flushing.

INTERACTIONS
Drug–Drug: ▪ None significant.

---

*Underlines indicate most frequent; **CAPITALS** indicate life-threatening.

ROUTE AND DOSAGE

Calcitonin—Salmon

Precede therapy with 1-IU intradermal skin test. 1 IU = 1 MRC unit.

Paget's Disease

- **IM, SC (Adults):** 100 IU/day initially, 50 IU/day or 50–100 IU q 1–3 days maintenance dose.

Hypercalcemia

- **IM, SC (Adults):** initially 4 IU/kg q 12 hr, can increase up to 8 IU/kg q 6 hr.

Osteoporosis

- **IM, SC (Adults):** 100 IU q 1–3 days.

Calcitonin—Human

Paget's Disease

- **SC (Adults):** 0.25–0.5 mg daily or 2–3 times weekly as single daily dose, up to 1.0 mg/day in 2 divided doses.

AVAILABILITY

Calcitonin—salmon

- *Injecton:* 200 IU/ml.

Calcitonin—human

- *Injection:* 500-mg vial.

TIME/ACTION PROFILE (Effects on serum calcium)

	ONSET	PEAK	DURATION
IM	15 min	4 hr	8–24
SC	15 min	4 hr	8–24

NURSING IMPLICATIONS

ASSESSMENT

- Observe patient for signs of hypersensitivity (skin rash, fever, hives, anaphylaxis, serum sickness). Keep epinephrine, antihistamines, and oxygen nearby in the event of a reaction.
- Assess patient for signs of hypocalcemic tetany (nervousness, irritability, paresthesia, muscle twitching, tetanic spasms, convulsions) during the first several doses of calcitonin. Parenteral calcium, such as calcium gluconate, should be available in case of this event.
- **Lab Test Considerations:** Serum calcium and alkaline phosphatase should be monitored periodically throughout therapy. These levels should normalize within a few months of initiation of therapy.
- Urine sediment should be monitored for the presence of casts periodically during the course of therapy.

POTENTIAL NURSING DIAGNOSES

- Pain (indications).
- Injury, high risk for (indications, side effects).
- Knowledge deficit related to medication regimen (patient/family teaching).

IMPLEMENTATION

- **General Info:** Assess for sensitivity to calcitonin–salmon by administering an intradermal test dose on the inner aspect of the forearm prior to initiating therapy. Test dose is prepared in a dilution of 10 IU/ml by withdrawing 0.05 ml in a tuberculin syringe and filling to 1 ml with 0.9% NaCl for injection. Mix well and discard 0.9 ml. Administer 0.1 ml and observe site for 15 min. More than mild erythema or wheal constitutes positive response.
- Store solution in refrigerator.
- **IM/SC:** Inspect injection site for the appearance of redness, swelling, or pain. Rotate injection sites. SC is the preferred route. Use IM route if dose exceeds 2 ml in volume. Use multiple sites to minimize inflammatory reaction.

PATIENT/FAMILY TEACHING

- **General Info:** Advise patient to take medication exactly as directed. If dose is missed and medication is scheduled for twice a day, take only if remembered within 2 hr of correct time. If scheduled for daily dose, take only if remembered that day. If scheduled for every other day, take when remembered and restart alternate day schedule. Do not double doses.
- Instruct patient in the proper method of self-injection.
- Advise patient to report signs of hypercalcemic relapse (deep bone or flank pain, renal calculi, anorexia, nausea, vomiting, thirst, lethargy) or allergic response to the physician promptly.

□ Reassure patient that flushing and warmth following injection is transient and usually lasts about 1 hr.
□ Explain that nausea following injection tends to decrease even with continued therapy.
□ Instruct patient to follow low-calcium diet if ordered by physician (see Appendix K). Women with postmenopausal osteoporosis should adhere to diet high in calcium and vitamin D.
■ **Osteoporosis:** Advise patients receiving calcitonin for the treatment of osteoporosis that exercise has been found to arrest and reverse bone loss. The patient should discuss any exercise limitations with physician before beginning program.

EVALUATION
Effectiveness of therapy can be measured by: ■ Lowered serum calcium levels ■ Decreased bone pain ■ Slowed progression of postmenopausal osteoporosis.

CALCITRIOL
(kal-si-**trye**-ole)
1,25 dihydroxycholecalciferol, Calcijex, Rocaltrol, vitamin D_3

CLASSIFICATION(S):
Vitamin (fat-soluble)
Pregnancy Category C

INDICATIONS
■ Management of hypocalcemia in chronic renal failure patients ■ Treatment of hypoparathyroidism or pseudohypoparathyroidism.

ACTION
■ Synthetic active form of vitamin D_3 ■ Promotes the absorption of calcium from the GI tract ■ Regulates calcium homeostasis in conjunction with parathyroid hormone and calcitonin. **Therapeutic Effect:** ■ Normalization of serum calcium levels in hypocalcemic chronic renal failure patients receiving dialysis.

May also reduce elevated parathyroid hormone levels.

PHARMACOKINETICS
Absorption: Well absorbed following oral administration.
Distribution: Primarily stored in liver. Crosses the placenta.
Metabolism and Excretion: Metabolized by the liver, excreted primarily in bile.
Half-life: 3–8 hr.

CONTRAINDICATIONS AND PRECAUTIONS
Contraindicated in: ■ Hypercalcemia ■ Any other evidence of vitamin D toxicity.
Use Cautiously in: ■ Sarcoidosis ■ Hyperparathyroidism ■ Pregnancy, lactation, or children (safety not established).

ADVERSE REACTIONS AND SIDE EFFECTS*
Seen primarily as manifestations of toxicity (hypercalcemia).
CNS: weakness, headache, somnolence.
EENT: photophobia, conjunctivitis, rhinorrhea.
CV: hypertension, arrhythmias.
GI: nausea, vomiting, dry mouth, constipation, metallic taste, polydipsia, anorexia, weight loss.
GU: polyuria, nocturia, decreased libido, albuminuria.
Derm: pruritus.
F and E: hypercalcemia.
Metab: hyperthermia.
MS: muscle pain, bone pain.

INTERACTIONS
Drug–Drug: ■ Use with caution in patients receiving **cardiac glycosides, magnesium-containing antacids,** or **thiazide diuretics** ■ Absorption may be decreased by concurrent administration of **cholestyramine** or **colestipol** ■ **Glucocorticoids** may antagonize the effects of calcitriol.

Drug–Food: ▪ Ingestion of foods high in **calcium** content (see Appendix K) may lead to hypercalcemia.

ROUTE AND DOSAGE

Hypocalcemia in Chronic Renal Failure Patients

▪ **PO (Adults):** 0.25 mcg/day initially, increase by 0.25 mcg/day at 4–8 wk intervals. Usual dose 0.5–1.0 mcg/day.
▪ **PO (Children):** 0.25–2 mcg/day.
▪ **IV (Adults):** 0.5 mcg (0.01 mcg/kg) 3 times weekly. May be increased by 0.25–0.5 mcg/dose at 2–4 wk intervals. Usual dose is 0.5–3.0 mcg 3 times weekly (0.01–0.05 mcg/kg 3 times weekly).

Hypoparathyroidism or Pseudohypoparathyroidism

▪ **PO (Adults):** 0.25 mcg/day, may be increased at 2–4 wk intervals (usual range, 0.5–2.0 mcg/day).
▪ **PO (Children 1–5 yr):** 0.25–0.75 mcg/day (0.04–0.08 mcg/kg/day).

AVAILABILITY

▪ *Capsules:* 0.25 mcg, 0.5 mcg ▪ *Injection:* 1 mcg/ml, 2 mcg/ml.

TIME/ACTION PROFILE (effect on calcium)

	ONSET	PEAK	DURATION
PO	2–6 hr	2–6 hr	1–5 days
IV	UK	UK	UK

NURSING IMPLICATIONS

Assessment

□ Assess patient for bone pain and weakness prior to and throughout course of therapy.
□ Observe patient carefully for evidence of hypocalcemia (paresthesia, muscle twitching, laryngospasm, colic, cardiac arrhythmias, and Chvostek's or Trousseau's sign). Protect symptomatic patient by raising and padding side rails; keep bed in low position.
▪ **Lab Test Considerations:** Serum calcium levels should be drawn weekly during initial therapy.
□ Monitor BUN, serum creatinine, alkaline phosphatase parathyroid hormone levels, creatine clearance, 24–hr urinary calcium periodically.
□ Monitor serum phosphorous levels prior to and periodically throughout course of therapy. Serum phosphorous must be controlled prior to initiating calcitriol. Aluminum carbonate or aluminum hydroxide is used for this purpose in dialysis patients.
□ A fall in alkaline phosphatase levels may signal onset of hypercalcemia. Overdosage is associated with a serum calcium times phosphate (Ca × P) level of greater than 70 and elevated BUN, AST (SGOT), and ALT (SGPT).
□ May cause false elevated cholesterol levels.
▪ **Toxicity and Overdose:** Toxicity is manifested as hypercalcemia, hypercalciuria, and hyperphosphatemia. Assess patient for appearance of nausea, vomiting, anorexia, weakness, constipation, headache, bone pain, and metallic taste. Later symptoms include polyuria, polydipsia, photophobia, rhinorrhea, pruritus, and cardiac arrhythmias. Notify physician immediately if these signs of hypervitaminosis D occur. Treatment usually consists of discontinuation of calcitriol, low calcium diet, and use of low calcium dialysate in dialysis patients.

Potential Nursing Diagnoses

▪ Nutrition, altered: less than body requirements (indications).
▪ Knowledge deficit related to medication regimen (patient/family teaching).

Implementation

▪ **PO:** May be administered without regard to meals.
▪ **Direct IV:** Administer by rapid injection through the catheter at the end of a period of hemodialysis.

Patient/Family Teaching

□ Advise patient to take calcitriol exactly as directed. If dose is missed take as soon as remembered; do not double up on doses.

▫ Review diet modifications with patient. See Appendix K for foods high in calcium and vitamin D. Renal patients must still consider renal failure diet in food selection. Physician may order concurrent calcium supplement.

▫ Review symptoms of overdosage and instruct patient to report these promptly to physician.

EVALUATION
Effectiveness of therapy can be demonstrated by: ▪ Normalization of serum calcium and parathyroid hormone levels ▪ Decreased bone pain and weakness in patients with renal osteodystrophy.

CALCIUM SALTS
calcim acetate (25% Ca or 12.6 mEq/g)
(**kal**-see-um **ass**-e-tate)
Phos-Ex, PhosLo

calcium carbonate (40% Ca or 20 mEq/g)
(**kal**-see-um **kar**-boh-nate)
Cal Carb-HD, Calciday, Cal-Sup, Caltrate, Gencalc, Nephro-calci, Os-cal, Oysco, Oystcal, Titrilac, Tums

calcium chloride (27% Ca or 13.6 mEq/g)
(**kal**-see-um **kloh**-ride)

calcium citrate (21% Ca or 12 mEq/g)
(**kal**-see-um **si**-trate)
Citrical, Citrical Liquitab

calcium glubionate (6.4% Ca or 3.2 mEq/g)
(**kal**-see-um gloo-**bye**-oh-nate)
Neo-Calglucon

calcium gluceptate (8.2% Ca or 4.1 mEq/g)
(**kal**-see-um **gloo**-sep-tate)

calcium gluconate (9% Ca or 4.5 mEq/g)
(**kal**-see-um **gloo**-koh-nate)
Kalcinate

calcium lactate (13% Ca or 6.5 mEq/g)
(**kal**-see-um **lak**-tate)

tricalcium phosphate (39% Ca or 19.5 mEq/g)
(trye-**kal**-see-um **foss**-fate)

calcium phosphate, tribasic; Posture

CLASSIFICATION(S):
Electrolyte
Pregnancy Category C

C

INDICATIONS
▪ Treatment and prevention of hypocalcemia, which may be associated with hypoparathyroidism, achlorhydria, chronic diarrhea, pancreatitis, vitamin D deficiency, and hyperphosphatemia ▪ Adjunct in the prevention of postmenopausal osteoporosis ▪ Treatment of some heavy metal poisonings ▪ Has been used as an antacid (PO calcium carbonate) ▪ *Calcium acetate:* Control of hyperphosphatemia in end-stage renal disease.

ACTION
▪ Essential for nervous, muscular, and skeletal systems ▪ Maintains cell membrane and capillary permeability ▪ Acts as an activator in the transmission of nerve impulses and contraction of cardiac, skeletal, and smooth muscle ▪ Essential for bone formation and blood coagulation. **Therapeutic Effect:** ▪ Replacement of calcium in deficiency states. Control of hyperphosphatemia in end-stage renal disease without promoting aluminum absorption (calcium acetate).

PHARMACOKINETICS
Absorption: Absorption from the GI tract requires vitamin D. IV administration results in complete bioavailability.
Distribution: Readily enters extracellular fluid. Crosses the placenta and enters breast milk.
Metabolism and Excretion: Excreted mostly in the feces. 20% eliminated by the kidneys.

Half-life: UK.

CONTRAINDICATIONS AND PRECAUTIONS

Contraindicated in: ▪ Hypercalcemia ▪ Renal calculi ▪ Ventricular fibrillation. **Use Cautiously in:** ▪ Patients receiving cardiac glycosides ▪ Severe respiratory insufficiency ▪ Renal disease ▪ Cardiac disease.

ADVERSE REACTIONS AND SIDE EFFECTS*

CNS: tingling, syncope (IV). **CV:** bradycardia, <u>arrhythmias</u>, <u>cardiac arrest</u> (IV). **GI:** nausea, vomiting, <u>constipation</u>. **GU:** hypercalcuria, calculi. **Local:** <u>phlebitis</u> at IV site.

INTERACTIONS

Drug–Drug: ▪ Hypercalcemia increases the risk of **cardiac glycoside** toxicity ▪ Chronic use with **antacids** in renal insufficiency may lead to milk–alkali syndrome ▪ Ingestion by mouth decreases the absorption of orally administered **tetracycline, fluoroquinolones,** or **iron salts** ▪ May decrease the effects of **verapamil** or **atenolol** ▪ Concurrent use with **thiazide diuretics** may result in hypercalcemia. **Drug–Food:** ▪ Cereals, spinach, or rhubarb may decrease the absorption of calcium supplements ▪ Calcium acetate should not be given concurrently with other calcium supplements.

ROUTE AND DOSAGE

Doses are expressed as elemental calcium.

Prevention of Hypocalcemia, Treatment of Depletion, Osteoporosis
▪ PO (Adults): 1–2 g/day.

Supplementation
▪ PO (Children): 45–65 mg/kg/day.

Neonatal Hypocalcemia
▪ PO (Infants): 50–150 mg/kg (not to exceed 1 g).

Emergency Treatment of Hypocalcemia
▪ IV (Adult): 7–14 mEq.
▪ IV (Children): 1–7 mEq.
▪ IV (Infants): <1 mEq.

Hypocalcemic Tetany
▪ IV (Adults): 4.5–16 mEq repeat until symptoms are controlled.
▪ IV (Children): 0.5–0.7 mEq/kg 3–4 times daily.
▪ IV (Neonates): 2.4 mEq/kg/day in divided doses.

Cardiac Standstill
▪ IV (Adults): 7–14 mEq.

Hyperphosphatemia in End-Stage Renal Disease (Calcium Acetate)
▪ PO (Adults): Amount necessary to control serum phosphate and calcium.

AVAILABILITY

Calcium Acetate
▪ *Tablets:* 250 mg, 667 mg, 668 mg, 1 g
▪ *Capsules:* 500 mg.

Calcium Carbonate
▪ *Tablets:* 650 mg, 667 mg, 1.25 g, 1.5 g
▪ *Chewable tablets:* 750 mg, 1.25 g.
▪ *Capsules:* 1.25 g ▪ *Oral suspension:* 1.25 g/5 ml ▪ *Powder:* 6.5 g/packet.

Calcium Chloride
▪ *Injection:* 10%.

Calcium Gluceptate
▪ *Injection:* 1.1 g/5 ml (4.5 mEq/5 ml).

Calcium Gluconate
▪ *Tablets:* 500 mg, 650 mg, 975 mg, 1 g
▪ *Injection:* 10% (0.45 mEq/ml).

Calcium Lactate
▪ *Tablets:* 325 mg, 650 mg.

TIME/ACTION PROFILE (effects on serum calcium)

	ONSET	PEAK	DURATION
PO	UK	UK	UK
IV	immediate	immediate	0.5–2 hr

NURSING IMPLICATIONS

ASSESSMENT
▪ **Calcium Supplement/Replacement:** Observe patient closely for symptoms

*<u>Underlines</u> indicate most frequent; **CAPITALS** indicate life-threatening.

of hypocalcemia (paresthesia, muscle twitching, laryngospasm, colic, cardiac arrhythmias, Chvostek's or Trousseau's sign). Notify physician if these occur. Protect symptomatic patients by elevating and padding side rails and keeping bed in low position.

□ Monitor blood pressure, pulse, and ECG frequently throughout therapy. May cause vasodilation with resulting hypotension, bradycardia, arrhythmias, and cardiac arrest.

□ Assess IV site for patency. Extravasation may cause cellulitis, necrosis, and sloughing.

□ Monitor patient on cardiac glycosides for signs of toxicity.

- **Antacid:** When used as an antacid, assess for heartburn, indigestion, and abdominal pain. Inspect abdomen; auscultate bowel sounds.

- **Lab Test Considerations:** Monitor calcium, chloride, sodium, potassium, magnesium, and albumin levels prior to and periodically throughout therapy. May cause false decreased serum and urine magnesium levels.

□ Digitalis levels should be monitored in patients receiving calcium and digitalis glycosides concurrently, as hypercalcemia increases the risk of cardiac toxicity.

□ When used to treat hyperphosphatemia in renal failure patients monitor phosphate levels.

- **Toxicity and Overdose:** Observe patient for appearance of nausea, vomiting, anorexia, thirst, severe constipation, paralytic ileus, and bradycardia. Contact physician immediately if these signs of hypercalcemia occur.

POTENTIAL NURSING DIAGNOSES

- Nutrition, altered: less than body requirements (indications).
- Injury, high risk for, related to osteoporosis or electrolyte imbalance (indications).
- Knowledge deficit related to medication and dietary regimes (patient/family teaching).

IMPLEMENTATION

- **General Info:** Milligram doses of calcium chloride, calcium gluconate, and calcium gluceptate are not equal. Chloride and gluconate forms are stocked on most hospital crash carts. Physician should specify form of calcium desired. Doses should be expressed in mEq.

□ In arrest situations, the use of calcium chloride is now limited to patients with hyperkalemia, hypocalcemia, and calcium channel blocker toxicity.

- **PO:** Administer with or 1 hr after meals and at bedtime. Chewable tablets should be well chewed before swallowing; follow with a full glass of water. Administer with meals for patients with hyperphosphatemia.

- **IM:** IM administration of calcium gluconate and calcium gluceptate may be tolerated in an emergency if IV administration is not feasible. For child administer only in thigh. For adult administer only in gluteal region. Do not administer calcium chloride IM.

- **IV:** IV solution should be warmed to body temperature and given through a small-bore needle in a large vein to minimize phlebitis. Do not administer through a scalp vein. May cause cutaneous burning sensation, peripheral vasodilation, and a drop in blood pressure. Patient should remain recumbent for 30–60 min following IV administration. Administer slowly. High concentrations may cause cardiac arrest.

□ If infiltration occurs, discontinue IV. Confer with physician about local infiltration of 1% procaine HCl or hyaluronidase, or application of heat.

□ Rapid administration may cause tingling, sensation of warmth, and a metallic taste. Halt infusion if these symptoms occur, and resume infusion at a slower rate when they subside.

□ Do not administer solutions that are not clear or that contain a precipitate.

C

Calcium Chloride

- **Direct IV:** May be administered undiluted by IV push.
- **Intermittent/Continuous Infusion:** May be diluted with D5W, D10W, 0.9% NaCl, D5/0.25% NaCl, D5/0.45% NaCl, D5/0.9% NaCl, or D5/LR.
- **Rate:** Maximum rate for adults is 0.7–1.4 mEq/min (0.5–1 ml of 10% solution); for children 0.5 ml/min.
- **Syringe Compatibility:** ▪ milrinone.
- **Y-Site Compatibility:** ▪ amrinone ▪ dobutamine ▪ epinephrine ▪ esmolol ▪ morphine.
- **Y-Site Incompatibility:** ▪ sodium bicarbonate.

Calcium Gluceptate

- **Direct IV:** May be administered undiluted.
- **Rate:** Administer at a rate not to exceed 2 ml/(1.8 mEq)/min for adults; 0.5 ml/(0.45 mEq)/min for children. In exchange transfusion for neonates, 0.5 ml (0.45 mEq) is given after each 100 ml of citrated blood.
- **Intermittent Infusion:** May be further diluted in D5W, D10W, 0.9% NaCl, 0.45% NaCl, D5/LR, or lactated Ringer's solution. Solution should be clear; do not use if crystals are present.
- **Rate:** Do not exceed 200 mg/min.

Calcium Gluconate

- **Direct IV:** Administer slowly by direct IV push.
- **Rate:** Maximum administration rate for adults is 1.5–2 ml/min.
- **Continuous Infusion:** May be further diluted in 1000 ml of D5W, D10W, D20W, D5/0.9% NaCl, 0.9% NaCl, D5/LR, or lactated Ringer's solution.
- **Rate:** Administer over 12–24 hr.
- **Syringe Incompatibility:** ▪ metoclopramide.
- **Y-Site Compatibility:** ▪ cefazolin ▪ dobutamine ▪ enalaprilat ▪ epinephrine ▪ famotidine ▪ labetalol ▪ netilmicin ▪ potassium chloride ▪ sargramostim ▪ tolazoline.

PATIENT/FAMILY TEACHING

- **General Info:** Instruct patient not to take enteric-coated tablets within 1 hr of calcium carbonate as this will result in premature dissolution of the tablets.
- ▢ Do not administer concurrently with foods containing large amounts of oxalic acid (spinach, rhubarb); phytic acid (brans, cereals); or phosphorus (milk or daily products). Administration with milk products may lead to milk-alkali syndrome (nausea, vomiting, confusion, headache).
- ▢ Advise patient that calcium carbonate may cause constipation. Review methods of preventing constipation (increasing bulk in diet, increasing fluid intake, increasing mobility). Patient may need to discuss use of laxatives with the physician. Severe constipation may indicate toxicity.
- **Calcium Supplement:** Encourage patients to maintain a diet adequate in vitamin D (see Appendix K).
- **Osteoporosis:** Advise patients that exercise has been found to arrest and reverse bone loss. The patient should discuss any exercise limitations with physician before beginning program.

EVALUATION

Effectiveness of therapy can be demonstrated by: ▪ Increase in serum calcium levels ▪ Decrease in the signs and symptoms of hypocalcemia ▪ Resolution of indigestion ▪ Control of hyperphosphatemia in patients with renal failure (calcium acetate only).

CAPSAICIN
(cap-**say**-sin)
{Axsain}, Zostrix, Zostrix-HP

CLASSIFICATION(S):
Analgesic (topical)
Pregnancy Category UK

{} = Available in Canada only.

INDICATIONS

- Temporary management of pain due to rheumatoid arthritis and osteoarthritis
- Treatment of pain associated with neuralgias (shingles or diabetic neuropathy).

ACTION

- May deplete and prevent the reaccumulation of a chemical (substance P) responsible for transmitting painful impulses from peripheral sites to the central nervous system. **Therapeutic Effect:**
- Relief of discomfort associated with peripheral painful syndromes.

PHARMACOKINETICS

Absorption: Absorption not known.
Distribution: Distribution not known.
Metabolism and Excretion: Metabolism and excretion not known.
Half-life: Half-life not known.

CONTRAINDICATIONS AND PRECAUTIONS

Contraindicated in: ■ Hypersensitivity ■ Not for use near eyes or on open or broken skin.
Use Cautiously in: ■ Pregnancy, lactation, or children <2 yr (safety not established).

ADVERSE REACTIONS AND SIDE EFFECTS*

Resp: cough.
Derm: transient burning.
Misc: Hypersensitivity to capsaicin, hot peppers, or components in preparations.

INTERACTIONS

Drug–Drug: ■ Concurrent use may increase the incidence of cough from ACE inhibitors.

ROUTE AND DOSAGE

- **Top:** Apply to affected areas not more than 3–4 times/day.

AVAILABILITY

- *Cream:* 0.025%, 0.075%.

TIME/ACTION PROFILE

	ONSET	PEAK	DURATION
Top	days	UK	UK

NURSING IMPLICATIONS

ASSESSMENT
□ Assess pain intensity and location prior to and periodically throughout therapy.

POTENTIAL NURSING DIAGNOSES
- Pain, chronic (indications).
- Knowledge deficit related to medication regimen (patient/family teaching).

IMPLEMENTATION
- **Top:** Apply to affected area not more than 3–4 times daily. Avoid getting medication into eyes or broken or irritated skin. Do not bandage tightly.

PATIENT/FAMILY TEACHING
□ Instruct patient on the correct method for application of capsaicin. Gloves should be worn during application or hands should be washed immediately after application.
□ Advise patient that transient burning may occur with application, especially if applied less than 3–4 times daily.
□ Advise patient to discontinue use and notify physician if pain persists longer than 14–28 days or clears up and recurs within a few days or if signs of infection are present.

EVALUATION
Effectiveness of therapy can be demonstrated by: ■ Decrease in discomfort associated with: □ Postherpetic neuropathy □ Diabetic neuropathy □ Rheumatoid arthritis □ Osteoarthritis.

CAPTOPRIL
(**kap**-toe-pril)
Capoten

INDICATIONS

▪ Alone or in combination with other antihypertensives in the management of hypertension ▪ Used in combination with other drugs in the treatment of congestive heart failure.

ACTION

▪ Prevents the production of angiotensin II, a potent vasoconstrictor that stimulates the production of aldosterone, by blocking its conversion to the active form. Result is systemic vasodilation. **Therapeutic Effects:** ▪ Lowering of blood pressure in hypertensive patients ▪ Decreased preload and afterload in patients with congestive heart failure.

PHARMACOKINETICS

Absorption: Rapidly absorbed (75%) from the GI tract. Food decreases absorption.

Distribution: Widely distributed but does not cross blood–brain barrier. Crosses the placenta. Small amounts enter breast milk.

Metabolism and Excretion: 50% metabolized by the liver. 50% excreted unchanged by the kidneys.

Half-life: <2 hr.

CONTRAINDICATIONS AND PRECAUTIONS

Contraindicated in: ▪ Hypersensitivity ▪ Cross-sensitivity with other ACE inhibitors may exist ▪ Pregnancy (may cause fetal malformation or death; hypotension, oliguria, or hypokalemia may occur in newborns).

Use Cautiously in: ▪ Renal impairment (dosage reduction required) ▪ Aortic stenosis ▪ Cerebrovascular or cardiac insufficiency ▪ Lactation and children (safety not established) ▪ Surgery/anesthesia (hypotension may be exaggerated) ▪ Patients with child-bearing potential.

Extreme Caution in: Family history of hereditary angioedema.

ADVERSE REACTIONS AND SIDE EFFECTS*

CNS: dizziness.
Resp: cough.
CV: hypotension, tachycardia, angina pectoris.
GI: anorexia, loss of taste perception.
GU: proteinuria, renal failure.
Derm: rashes.
Hemat: LEUKOPENIA, AGRANULOCYTOSIS.
Misc: fever.

INTERACTIONS

Drug–Drug: ▪ Additive hypotension with other **antihypertensives, phenothiazines,** acute ingestion of **alcohol,** and **vasodilators** ▪ Hyperkalemia may result from concurrent use of **potassium supplements, potassium-sparing diuretics,** or **cyclosporine** ▪ Antihypertensive response may be blunted by **nonsteroidal anti-inflammatory agents** ▪ Absorption may be decreased by **antacids** ▪ Increases levels and may increase risk of **digoxin** or **lithium** toxicity ▪ **Probenecid** decreases elimination and increases levels of captopril ▪ Risk of hypersensitivity reactions increased by concurrent **allopurinol** ▪ **Capsaicin** may increase the incidence of cough.

ROUTE AND DOSAGE

▪ **PO (Adults):** *Hypertension*—Initial dose 12.5–25 mg 2–3 times daily, may be increased at 1–2 week intervals up to 150 mg 3 times daily (usual dose 50 mg 3 times daily). *Congestive heart failure*—6.25–12.5 mg 3 times daily, may be increased up to 50–100 mg 3 times daily (range 12.5–450 mg/day). *Post–myocardial infarction*—6.25 mg test dose, followed by 12.5 mg 3 times daily, may be increased up to 50 mg 3 times daily.

*Underlines indicate most frequent; **CAPITALS** indicate life-threatening.

AVAILABILITY

■ *Tablets:* 12.5 mg, 25 mg, 50 mg, 100 mg ■ *In combination with:* hydrochlorathrazide (Capozide). See Appendix A.

TIME/ACTION PROFILE (effect on blood pressure)*

	ONSET	PEAK	DURATION
PO	15–60 min	60–90 min	6–12 hr

*Full effects may not be noted until several wks of therapy.

NURSING IMPLICATIONS

ASSESSMENT

□ Monitor blood pressure and pulse frequently during initial dosage adjustment and periodically throughout course of therapy. Notify physician of significant changes.

□ Monitor weight and assess patient routinely for resolution of fluid overload (peripheral edema, rales/crackles, dyspnea, weight gain, jugular venous distension) if on concurrent diuretic therapy.

■ Lab Test Considerations: Periodic assessments of urine protein may be ordered, because proteinuria and nephrotic syndrome may occur with patients on captopril therapy.

□ Monitor BUN, creatinine, and electrolyte levels periodically. Serum potassium may be increased and BUN and creatinine transiently increased, while sodium levels may be decreased.

□ WBC with differential should be monitored prior to initiation of therapy, every 2 wk for the first 3 mo, and periodically thereafter during the course of therapy.

□ May cause false-positive test results for urine acetone.

POTENTIAL NURSING DIAGNOSES

■ Cardiac output, decreased (indications, side effects).

■ Knowledge deficit related to medication regimen (patient/family teaching).

■ Noncompliance (patient/family teaching).

IMPLEMENTATION

■ General Info: Precipitous drop in blood pressure during first 1–3 hr following first dose may require volume expansion with normal saline, but is not normally considered an indication for stopping therapy.

■ PO: Administer 1 hr before or 2 hr after meals, because food reduces absorption by 30–40%. May be crushed if patient has difficulty swallowing. Tablets may have a sulfurous odor.

□ An oral solution may be prepared by crushing a 25-mg tablet and dissolving it in 25–100 ml of water. Shake for at least 5 min and administer within 30 min.

PATIENT/FAMILY TEACHING

□ Instruct patient to take captopril exactly as directed, even if feeling better. Missed doses should be taken as soon as remembered but not if almost time for next dose. Do not double doses. Medication controls but does not cure hypertension. Warn patients not to discontinue captopril therapy unless directed by the physician.

□ Encourage patient to comply with additional interventions for hypertension (weight reduction, discontinuation of smoking, moderation of alcohol consumption, regular exercise, and stress management).

□ Instruct patient and family on proper technique for blood pressure monitoring. Advise them to check blood pressure at least weekly and report significant changes to physician.

□ Caution patient to avoid salt substitutes or foods containing high levels of potassium or sodium unless directed by physician (see Appendix K).

□ Advise patient that captopril may cause an impairment of taste that generally reverses itself within 8–12 wk, even with continued therapy.

□ Caution patient to change positions slowly to minimize orthostatic hypotension, particularly after initial dose. Patients should also be advised that exercising in hot weather may increase hypotensive effects.

□ Advise patient to consult physician or pharmacist before taking any over-the-counter medications, especially cold remedies. Patients should also avoid excessive amounts of tea, coffee, or cola.

□ Captopril may cause dizziness. Caution patient to avoid driving and other activities requiring alertness until response to medication is known.

□ Advise patient to inform physician or dentist of medication regimen prior to treatment or surgery.

□ Instruct patient to notify physician if cough, rash, sore throat, fever, irregular heart beat, chest pain, swelling of face, eyes, lips, or tongue, or difficulty breathing occurs.

□ Advise patient to notify physician if pregnancy is planned or suspected.

□ Emphasize the importance of follow-up examinations to monitor progress.

EVALUATION
Effectiveness of therapy can be demonstrated by: ▪ Decrease in blood pressure without appearance of side effects ▪ Decrease in signs and symptoms of congestive heart failure. Several weeks may be necessary before full effects of the drug are recognized.

CARBAMAZEPINE
(kar-ba-**maz**-e-peen)
{Apo-Carbamazepine}, Epitol, {Mazepine}, {Novo Carbamaz}, Tegretol

CLASSIFICATION(S):
Anticonvulsant
Pregnancy Category C

INDICATIONS
▪ Prophylaxis of tonic–clonic, mixed, and complex–partial seizures ▪ Management of pain in trigeminal neuralgia. **Unlabeled Uses:** ▪ Other forms of neurogenic pain.

ACTION
▪ Decreases synaptic transmission in the CNS. **Therapeutic Effects:** ▪ Prevention of seizures ▪ Decreased severity of pain in trigeminal neuralgia.

PHARMACOKINETICS
Absorption: Slowly but completely absorbed from the GI tract. Absorption of suspension results in earlier and higher peak and lower trough levels than tablets.
Distribution: Widely distributed. Crosses the blood–brain barrier. Crosses the placenta and enters breast milk.
Metabolism and Excretion: Extensively metabolized by the liver.
Half-life: 14–30 hr or longer.

CONTRAINDICATIONS AND PRECAUTIONS
Contraindicated in: ▪ Hypersensitivity ▪ Bone marrow depression.
Use Cautiously in: ▪ Cardiac disease ▪ Hepatic disease ▪ Elderly men with prostatic hypertrophy ▪ Increased intraocular pressure ▪ Pregnancy and lactation (safety not established).

ADVERSE REACTIONS AND SIDE EFFECTS*
CNS: vertigo, drowsiness, fatigue, ataxia, psychosis.
EENT: blurred vision, corneal opacities.
Resp: pneumonitis.
CV: congestive heart failure, syncope, hypertension, hypotension.
GI: hepatitis.
GU: hesitancy, urinary retention.
Derm: rashes, urticaria, photosensitivity.
Hemat: APLASTIC ANEMIA, AGRANULOCYTOSIS, THROMBOCYTOPENIA, leukopenia, leukocytosis, eosinophilia.
Misc: fever, chills, lymphadenopathy.

INTERACTIONS
Drug–Drug: ▪ May decrease effectiveness of **glucocorticoids, doxycycline,**

felbamate, quinidine, warfarin, oral contraceptives, barbiturates, benzodiazepines, and other anticonvulsants ▪ Concurrent use (within 2 wk) of MAO inhibitors may result in hyperpyrexia, hypertension, seizures, and death ▪ Verapamil, diltiazem, propoxyphene, or erythromycin increase levels and may cause toxicity ▪ May increase risk of hepatotoxicity from isoniazid ▪ Cimetidine increases blood levels and the risk of toxicity ▪ Felbamate decreases carbamazepine levels but increases levels of active metabolite.

ROUTE AND DOSAGE
Anticonvulsant
▪ PO (Adults): Start with 200 mg bid (tablets) or 100 mg qid (suspension); increase by 200 mg/day until therapeutic levels are achieved. Range is 800–1200 mg/day in divided doses q 6–8 hr. Not to exceed 1 g/day in 12–15 yr olds. Extended-release tablets are given 1–2 times daily.
▪ PO (Children 6–12 yr): 100 mg bid (tablets) or 50 mg qid (suspension) increased until therapeutic levels are obtained (range 400–800 mg/day; not to exceed 1 g/day). Extended-release tablets are given 1–2 times daily.

Trigeminal Neuralgia
▪ PO (Adults): 200 mg/day in 2–4 divided doses; increase until pain is relieved. Range 200–1200 mg/day.

AVAILABILITY
▪ Tablets: 200 mg ▪ Chewable tablets: 100 mg, 200 mg ▪ {Extended-release tablets: 200 mg, 400 mg} ▪ Oral suspension: 100 mg/5 ml.

TIME/ACTION PROFILE
(anticonvulsant activity)

	ONSET	PEAK	DURATION
PO	2–4 days	2–12 hr	UK hr

NURSING IMPLICATIONS
ASSESSMENT
▪ Seizures: Assess location, duration, and characteristics of seizure activity.
▪ Trigeminal Neuralgia: Assess for fa-

cial pain. Ask patient to identify stimuli that may precipitate facial pain (hot or cold foods, bed clothes, touching face).
▪ Lab Test Considerations: Monitor CBC, including platelet count, reticulocyte count, and serum iron, weekly during the first 3 mo and monthly thereafter, for evidence of potentially fatal blood cell abnormalities. Medication should be discontinued if bone marrow depression occurs.
▫ Liver function tests, urinalysis, and BUN should be routinely performed. May cause elevated AST (SGOT), ALT (SGPT), serum bilirubin, BUN, urine protein, and urine glucose levels.
▫ Thyroid function tests and serum calcium concentrations may be decreased.
▫ May cause false-negative pregnancy test results with tests that determine human chorionic gonadotropin.
▪ Toxicity and Overdose: Serum blood levels should be routinely monitored throughout course of therapy. Therapeutic levels range from 6–12 mcg/ml.

POTENTIAL NURSING DIAGNOSES
▪ Injury, high risk for (indications, side effects).
▪ Pain, chronic (indications).
▪ Knowledge deficit related to medication regimen (patient/family teaching).

IMPLEMENTATION
▪ General Info: Implement seizure precautions as indicated.
▪ PO: Administer medication with food to minimize gastric irritation. Tablets may be crushed if patient has difficulty swallowing.

PATIENT/FAMILY TEACHING
▪ General Info: Instruct patient to take carbamazepine around the clock, exactly as directed. If a dose is missed, take as soon as remembered but not just before next dose; do not double doses. Notify physician if more than one dose is missed. Medication should be gradually discontinued to prevent seizures and status epilepticus.

□ May cause dizziness or drowsiness. Advise patients to avoid driving or other activities requiring alertness until response to medication is known.

□ Instruct patients that fever, sore throat, mouth ulcers, easy bruising, petechiae, unusual bleeding, abdominal pain, chills, pale stools, dark urine, or jaundice should be reported to the physician immediately.

□ Advise patient not to take alcohol or other CNS depressants concurrently with this medication.

□ Caution patients to use sunscreen and protective clothing to prevent photosensitivity reactions.

□ Inform patient that frequent mouth rinses, good oral hygiene, and sugarless gum or candy may help reduce dry mouth. Saliva substitute may be used. Consult dentist if dry mouth persists >2 wk.

□ Advise patients to use a nonhormonal form of contraception while taking carbamazepine.

□ Instruct patient to notify physician or dentist of medication regimen prior to treatment or surgery.

□ Emphasize the importance of follow-up lab tests and eye examinations to monitor for side effects.

■ Seizures: Advise patients to carry identification describing disease and medication regimen at all times.

EVALUATION

Clinical response to therapy can be indicated by: ■ Absence or reduction of seizure activity ■ Decrease in trigeminal neuralgia pain. Patients with trigeminal neuralgia should be re-evaluated every 3 mo to determine minimum effective dose.

CARBENICILLIN
(kar-ben-i-**sill**-in)
Geocillin

> *CLASSIFICATION(S):*
> *Anti-infective (extended-spectrum penicillin)*
> **Pregnancy Category B**

INDICATIONS
■ Treatment of urinary tract infections or prostatitis due to susceptible organisms.

ACTION
■ Binds to bacterial cell wall membrane, causing cell death. **Therapeutic Effect:** ■ Bactericidal against susceptible bacteria. Spectrum is broader than other penicillins. **Spectrum:** ■ Active against: □ *Pseudomas aeruginosa* □ *Escherichia coli* □ *Proteus mirabilis* □ *Proteus vulgaris* □ *Morganella morganii* □ *Enterobacter* □ *Enterococci* ■ Not active against penicillinase-producing staphylococci.

PHARMACOKINETICS
Absorption: Oral form is rapidly but incompletely absorbed.
Distribution: Widely distributed. Enters CSF well only when meninges are inflamed. Crosses the placenta and enters breast milk in low concentrations.
Metabolism and Excretion: Metabolized by plasma and tissues to yield free carbenicillin. 80–99% excreted unchanged by the kidneys.
Half-life: 0.8–1 hr (increased in renal impairment).

CONTRAINDICATIONS AND PRECAUTIONS
Contraindicated in: ■ Hypersensitivity to penicillins or cephalosporins.
Use Cautiously in: ■ Renal impairment (dosage reduction required) ■ Severe liver disease ■ Pregnancy or lactation (safety not established).

ADVERSE REACTIONS AND SIDE EFFECTS*
GI: nausea, <u>diarrhea</u>.
Derm: <u>rashes</u>, urticaria.
Hemat: blood dyscrasias.

---

*<u>Underlines</u> indicate most frequent; **CAPITALS** indicate life-threatening.

CARBIDOPA/LEVODOPA   167

Misc: superinfection, hypersensitivity reactions including ANAPHYLAXIS and serum sickness.

INTERACTIONS

Drug–Drug: ▪ **Probenecid** decreases renal excretion and increases blood levels.

ROUTE AND DOSAGE

▪ **PO (Adults):** 382–764 mg (1–2 tablets) every 6 hr.

AVAILABILITY

▪ *Tablets:* 382 mg.

TIME/ACTION PROFILE (blood levels)

	ONSET	PEAK
PO	30 min	30–120 min

NURSING IMPLICATIONS

ASSESSMENT

□ Assess patient for infection (vital signs; appearance of wound, sputum, urine, and stool; WBC) at beginning and throughout course of therapy.

□ Obtain a history before initiating therapy to determine previous use and reactions to penicillins or cephalosporins. Persons with a negative history of penicillin sensitivity may still have an allergic response.

□ Obtain specimens for culture and sensitivity prior to initiating therapy. First dose may be given before receiving results.

□ Observe patient for signs and symptoms of anaphylaxis (rash, pruritus, laryngeal edema, wheezing). Discontinue the drug and notify the physician immediately if these occur. Keep epinephrine, an antihistamine, and resuscitation equipment close by in the event of an anaphylactic reaction.

▪ **Lab Test Considerations:** Renal and hepatic function, CBC, serum potassium, and bleeding times should be evaluated prior to and routinely throughout therapy.

□ May cause elevated AST (SGOT) and ALT (SGPT) levels.

POTENTIAL NURSING DIAGNOSES

▪ Infection, high risk for (indications, side effects).
▪ Knowledge deficit related to medication regimen (patient/family teaching).
▪ Noncompliance related to medication regimen (patient/family teaching).

IMPLEMENTATION

▪ **PO:** Administer around the clock on an empty stomach at least 1 hr before or 2 hr after meals, with a full glass of water.

PATIENT/FAMILY TEACHING

□ Instruct patient to take medication around the clock and to finish the drug completely as directed, even if feeling better. Advise patient that sharing of this medication may be dangerous.

□ Advise patient to report the signs of superinfection (furry overgrowth on the tongue, vaginal itching or discharge, loose or foul smelling stools) and allergy.

□ Instruct the patient to notify the physician if symptoms do not improve.

EVALUATION

Clinical response to therapy may be determined by: ▪ Resolution of the signs and symptoms of infection. Length of time for complete resolution depends on the organism and site of infection.

CARBIDOPA/LEVODOPA

(**kar**-bi-doe-pa/**lee**-voe-doe-pa)
Sinemet, Sinemet CR

CLASSIFICATION(S):
Antiparkinson (decarboxylase inhibitor/dopamine agonist)
Pregnancy Category C

INDICATIONS

▪ Treatment of Parkinson's disease and other forms of parkinsonism. Not useful for drug-induced extrapyramidal reactions.

ACTION

- Levodopa is converted to dopamine in the CNS where it serves as a neurotransmitter. Carbidopa prevents peripheral destruction of levodopa so more is available to the CNS. **Therapeutic Effect:** ▪ Relief of tremor and rigidity in parkinsonian syndrome.

PHARMACOKINETICS

Absorption: Both agents are well absorbed following oral administration. CR dosage form is absorbed more slowly and produces less fluctuation in blood levels.

Distribution: Both agents are widely distributed. Levodopa administered alone enters the CNS in small concentrations. Carbidopa does not cross the blood–brain barrier, but does cross the placenta and enter breast milk.

Metabolism and Excretion: Levodopa is mostly metabolized by the GI tract and liver. 30% of carbidopa is excreted unchanged by the kidneys.

Half-life: Levodopa—1 hr; carbidopa—1–2 hr.

CONTRAINDICATIONS AND PRECAUTIONS

Contraindicated in: ▪ Hypersensitivity ▪ Narrow-angle glaucoma ▪ Patients receiving MAO inhibitors ▪ Malignant melanoma ▪ Undiagnosed skin lesions ▪ Lactation.

Use Cautiously in: ▪ History of cardiac, psychiatric, or ulcer disease ▪ Pregnancy or children <18 yr (safety not established).

ADVERSE REACTIONS AND SIDE EFFECTS*

CNS: <u>involuntary movements</u>, memory loss, anxiety, psychiatric problems, hallucinations, dizziness, drowsiness.

EENT: mydriasis, blurred vision.

CV: hypertension, hypotension.

GI: <u>nausea</u>, <u>vomiting</u>, anorexia, dry mouth, hepatotoxicity.

Derm: melanoma.

Hemat: hemolytic anemia, leukopenia.

INTERACTIONS

Drug–Drug: ▪ Concurrent use with **MAO inhibitors** (within 14 days) may result in hypertensive crisis ▪ **Phenothiazines, haloperidol, papaverine, phenytoin, reserpine,** and large doses of **pyridoxine** may antagonize the beneficial effect of levodopa ▪ Additive hypotension with **methyldopa, quanethidine,** or **tricyclic antidepressants**.

Drug–Food: Ingestion of food containing high amounts of **pyridoxine** may reverse the beneficial effect of levodopa ▪ Peak levels of extended-release tablets are increased when administered with food.

ROUTE AND DOSAGE

Sinemet
- **PO (Adults):** 75/300–150/1500 mg/day in 3 to 4 divided doses, can increase up to 200/2000 mg/day.

Sinemet CR
- **PO (Adults):** Usual dose 1 tablet bid at intervals of not less than 6 hr. Doses of 2–8 tablets/day in divided doses at intervals of 4–8 hr while awake have been used. Wait 3 days between dosage adjustments.

AVAILABILITY

- *Tablets:* 10 mg carbidopa/100 mg levodopa, 25 mg carbidopa/100 mg levodopa, 25 mg carbidopa/250 mg levodopa ▪ *Extended-release tablets:* 50 mg carbidopa/200 mg levodopa.

TIME/ACTION PROFILE
(antiparkinson effect)

	ONSET	PEAK*	DURATION
PO	UK	0.7 hr	5–24 hr
PO-CR	UK	2.4 hr	UK

*Plasma levels.

NURSING IMPLICATIONS

ASSESSMENT

□ Assess symptoms of parkinsonism (akinesia, rigidity, tremors, pill rolling, shuffling gait, mask facies, twist-

---

*<u>Underlines</u> indicate most frequent; **CAPITALS** indicate life-threatening.

ing motions, and drooling) prior to and throughout course of therapy.

□ Assess blood pressure and pulse frequently during period of dose adjustment.

□ Assess for signs of toxicity (involuntary muscle twitching, facial grimacing, spasmodic eye winking, exaggerated protrusion of tongue, or behavioral changes). Consult physician promptly if these symptoms occur.

■ **Lab Test Considerations:** May cause false-positive Coombs' test, serum and urine uric acid, serum gonadotropin, urine norepinephrine, and urine protein concentrations.

□ May interfere with results of urine glucose and urine ketone tests. Copper reduction method of testing urine glucose (Clinitest) and dipstick for urine ketones may reveal false-positive results. Glucose enzymatic urine glucose tests (Tes-Tape) may yield false-negative results.

□ Patients on long-term therapy should have hepatic and renal function and CBC monitored periodically. May cause elevated BUN, AST (SGOT), ALT (SGPT), bilirubin, alkaline phosphatase, LDH, and serum protein-bound iodine concentrations.

POTENTIAL NURSING DIAGNOSES

■ Physical mobility, impaired (indications).

■ Injury, high risk for (indications).

■ Knowledge deficit related to medication regimen (patient/family teaching).

IMPLEMENTATION

■ **General Info:** In the carbidopa/levodopa combination, the numbers following the drug name represent the mg of each respective drug.

□ Wait 8 hr after last levodopa dose before switching patient to carbidopa/levodopa. Addition of carbidopa reduces the need for levodopa by 75%. Administering carbidopa shortly after a full dose of levodopa may result in toxicity.

□ To change from Sinemet to Sinemet

CR, administer an amount of Sinemet CR that provides approximately 10% more levodopa per day; may need to be increased to provide up to 30% more levodopa per day.

□ In preoperative patients or patients that are NPO, confer with physician regarding continuing medication administration.

■ **PO:** Administer food shortly after medication to minimize gastric irritation; taking food before or concurrently may retard levodopa's effects.

□ Controlled-release tablets may be administered as whole or half tablets, but should not be crushed or chewed.

PATIENT/FAMILY TEACHING

□ Instruct patient to take this drug exactly as prescribed. If a dose is missed, take as soon as remembered unless next scheduled dose is within 2 hr; do not double doses.

□ Explain that gastric irritation may be decreased by taking medication with or after meals, but that high-protein meals may impair levodopa's effects. Dividing the daily protein intake between all the meals may help ensure adequate protein intake and drug effectiveness.

□ May cause drowsiness or dizziness. Advise patient to avoid driving or other activities that require alertness until response to the drug is known.

□ Caution patient to make position changes slowly to minimize orthostatic hypotension.

□ Instruct patient that frequent rinsing of mouth, good oral hygiene, and sugarless gum or candy may decrease dry mouth.

□ Caution patient to monitor skin lesions for any changes. Physician should be notified promptly as carbidopa/levodopa may activate a malignant melanoma.

□ Advise patient to confer with physician or pharmacist prior to taking over-the-counter medications, especially cold remedies.

□ Inform patient that harmless darkening of urine or sweat may occur.

□ Advise patient to notify physician if palpitations, urinary retention, involuntary movements, behavioral changes, or severe nausea and vomiting occur.

EVALUATION
Effectiveness of therapy can be demonstrated by: ▪ Resolution of parkinsonian signs and symptoms. Therapeutic effects usually become evident after 2 to 3 wk of therapy, but may require up to 6 mo. Patients who take this medication for several years may experience a decrease in the effectiveness of this drug. An increased response to the drug may occur after a drug holiday.

CARBONIC ANHYDRASE INHIBITORS

acetazolamide
(a-set-a-**zole**-a-mide)
{Acetazolam}, AK-Zol, Dazamide, Diamox

dichlorphenamide
(dye-klor-**fen**-a-mide)
Daranide

methazolamide
(meth-a-**zole**-a-mide)
Naptazane

CLASSIFICATION(S):
Antiglaucoma agents, Diuretics
Pregnancy Category C

INDICATIONS
▪ Lower intraocular pressure in the treatment of glaucoma ▪ Adjunct treatment of refractory seizures (acetazolamide) ▪ Acute altitude sickness (acetazolamide). **Unlabeled Use:** ▪ Prevention of renal calculi composed of uric acid or cystine.

ACTION
▪ Inhibition of carbonic anhydrase in the eye results in decreased secretion of aqueous humor ▪ Inhibits renal carbonic anhydrase, resulting in self-limit-

ing urinary excretion of sodium, potassium, bicarbonate, and water ▪ CNS inhibition of carbonic anhydrase and resultant diuresis may decrease abnormal neuronal firing ▪ Alkaline diuresis prevents precipitation of uric acid or cystine in the urinary tract. **Therapeutic Effects:** ▪ Lowering of intraocular pressure ▪ Diuresis ▪ Control of some types of seizures ▪ Prevention and treatment of acute altitude sickness ▪ Prevention of uric acid or cystine renal calculi.

PHARMACOKINETICS
Absorption: Well absorbed following oral administration. IV administration results in complete bioavailability.
Distribution: Cross the placenta. Acetazolamide enters breast milk.
Metabolism and Excretion: *Acetazolamide*—excreted mostly unchanged in urine. *Dichlorphenamide*—Metabolism and excretion not known. *Methazolamide*—15–30% excreted unchanged in urine. 2.4–5.8 hr excreted mostly unchanged in urine. *Dichlorphenamide*—UK. *Methazolamide*—14 hr.

CONTRAINDICATIONS AND PRECAUTIONS
Contraindicated in: ▪ Hypersensitivity. Cross-sensitivity with sulfomanides may occur. Avoid during first trimester of pregnancy.
Use Cautiously in: ▪ Chronic respiratory disease ▪ Electrolyte abnormalities ▪ Renal or hepatic disease ▪ Diabetes mellitus ▪ Second and third trimester of pregnancy or lactation (safety not established).

ADVERSE REACTIONS AND SIDE EFFECTS*
CNS: drowsiness, <u>tiredness</u>, <u>weakness</u>, <u>depression</u>.
EENT: transient nearsightedness.
GI: <u>metallic taste</u>, nausea, vomiting, <u>anorexia</u>.
GU: crystalluria, renal calculi.
Derm: rashes.

Endo: hyperglycemia.
F and E: hyperchloremic acidosis, hypokalemia.
Hemat: APLASTIC ANEMIA, HEMOLYTIC ANEMIA, LEUKOPENIA.
Metab: weight loss, hyperuricemia.
Neuro: paresthesias.
Misc: allergic reactions.

INTERACTIONS

Drug–Drug: ▪ Excretion of **barbiturates, aspirin** and **lithium** is decreased and may lead to decreased effectiveness ▪ Excretion of **amphetamines, quinidine, procainamide,** and possibly **tricyclic antidepressants** is decreased and may lead to toxicity.

ROUTE AND DOSAGE

Acetazolamide

- **PO (Adults):** *Glaucoma*—250–1000 mg/day in 1–4 divided doses or 500 mg extended-release capsules twice daily. *Epilepsy*—4–30 mg/kg/day in 1–4 divided doses. *Altitude sickness*—250 mg 2–4 times daily. *Antiurolithic*—250 mg at bedtime.
- **IM, IV (Adults):** 250–500 mg, may repeat in 2–4 hr.
- **IM, IV (Children):** 5–10 mg/kg q 6 hr.
- **PO (Children):** 8–30 mg/kg/day in divided doses.

Dichlorphenamide

- **PO (Adults):** 100–200 mg followed by 100 mg q 12 hr initially, then maintenance dose of 25–50 mg 1–3 times daily.

Methazolamide

- **PO (Adults):** 25–100 mg 2–3 times daily.

AVAILABILITY

Acetazolamide

- ▪ **Tablets:** 125 mg, 250 mg ▪ **Extended-release capsules:** 500 mg ▪ **Injection:** 500 mg/vial.

Dichlorphenamide

- ▪ **Tablets:** 25 mg, 50 mg.

Methazolamide

- ▪ **Tablets:** 25 mg, 50 mg.

TIME/ACTION PROFILE (lowering of intraocular pressure)

	ONSET	PEAK	DURATION
acetazolamide PO	1 hr	2–4 hr	8–12 hr
acetazolamide PO-ER	2 hr	8–18 hr	18–24 hr
acetazolamide IV	2 min	15 min	4–5 hr
dichlorphen-amide PO	0.5–1 hr	2–4 hr	6–12 hr
methazola-mide PO	2–4 hr	6–8 hr	10–18 hr

C

NURSING IMPLICATIONS

ASSESSMENT

- ▪ **General Info:** Observe patient for signs of hypokalemia (muscle weakness, malaise, fatigue, ECG changes, vomiting).
- ▫ Assess for allergy to sulfonamides.
- ▪ **Intraocular Pressure:** Assess for eye discomfort or decrease in visual acuity.
- ▪ **Seizures:** Monitor neurologic status in patients receiving acetazolamide for seizures. Initiate seizure precautions.
- ▪ **Altitude Sickness:** Monitor for decrease in severity of symptoms (headache, nausea, vomiting, fatigue, dizziness, drowsiness, shortness of breath). Notify physician immediately if neurologic symptoms worsen or patient becomes more dyspneic and rales/crackles develop.
- ▪ **Lab Test Considerations:** Serum electrolytes, complete blood counts, and platelet counts should be evaluated initially and periodically throughout prolonged therapy. May cause decreased potassium, bicarbonate, WBCs, and RBCs. May cause increased serum chloride.
- ▫ May cause increase in serum glucose; monitor serum and urine glucose carefully in diabetic patients.
- ▫ May cause false-positive results for urine protein and 17-hydroxysteroid tests.
- ▫ May cause increased blood ammonia, bilirubin, uric acid, and increased

urine urobilinogen and calcium. May decrease urine citrate.

POTENTIAL NURSING DIAGNOSES
- Sensory-perceptual alteration: visual (indications).
- Knowledge deficit related to medication regimen (patient/family teaching).

IMPLEMENTATION
- **General Info:** Encourage fluids to 2000–3000 ml/day, unless contraindicated, to prevent crystalluria and stone formation.
- **PO:** Give with food to minimize GI irritation. Tablets may be crushed and mixed with fruit-flavored syrup to minimize bitter taste for patients with difficulty swallowing. Long-acting capsules may be opened and sprinkled on soft food, but do not crush, chew, or swallow contents dry.
- **IM:** Extremely painful; avoid if possible.
- **Direct IV:** Dilute 500 mg of acetazolamide in at least 5 ml of Sterile Water for Injection. Use reconstituted solution within 24 hr.
- *Rate:* Administer over at least 1 min.
- **Intermittent Infusion:** Further dilute in D5W, D10W, 0.45% NaCl, 0.9%, NaCl, Ringer's or lactated Ringer's solution, or combinations of dextrose and saline or dextrose and Ringer's solution.
- *Rate:* Infuse over 4–8 hr.
- **Additive Compatibility:** ▪ cimetidine.
- **Additive Incompatibility:** ▪ multiple vitamins.

PATIENT/FAMILY TEACHING
- **General Info:** Instruct patient to take exactly as directed. If a dose is missed, take as soon as remembered unless almost time for next dose. Do not double doses. Patients on anticonvulsant therapy may need to gradually reduce dose prior to discontinuation.
- Advise patient to report numbness or tingling of extremities, weakness, rash, sore throat, unusual bleeding or bruising, or fever to the physician.
- May occasionally cause drowsiness.

Caution patient to avoid driving and other activities that require alertness until response to the drug is known.
- Caution patient to use sunscreen and wear protective clothing to prevent photosensitivity reactions.
- **Intraocular Pressure:** Advise patient of the need for periodic ophthalmologic examinations; loss of vision may be gradual and painless.

EVALUATION
Effectiveness of therapy can be demonstrated by: ▪ Decrease in intraocular pressure when used for glaucoma ▪ Decrease in the frequency of seizures ▪ Prevention of altitude sickness ▪ Prevention of uric acid or cystine stones in the urinary tract.

CARBOPLATIN
(kar-boe-**pla**-tin)
Paraplatin

CLASSIFICATION(S):
Antineoplastic agent (alkylating agent)
Pregnancy Category D

INDICATIONS
- Treatment of ovarian carcinoma alone or in combination with cyclophosphamide.

ACTION
- Inhibits DNA synthesis by producing cross-linking of parent DNA strands (cell cycle-phase nonspecific). **Therapeutic Effect:** ▪ Death of rapidly replicating cells, particularly malignant cells.

PHARMACOKINETICS
Absorption: Administered IV only, resulting in complete bioavailability.
Distribution: Distribution not known.
Metabolism and Excretion: Excreted mostly by the kidneys.
Half-life: 2.6–5.9 hr (increased in renal impairment).

CONTRAINDICATIONS AND PRECAUTIONS

Contraindicated in: ▪ Hypersensitivity to carboplatin, cisplatin, or mannitol ▪ Pregnancy or lactation.

Use Cautiously in: ▪ Hearing loss ▪ Electrolyte abnormalities ▪ Patients with childbearing potential ▪ Active infections ▪ Diminished bone marrow reserve (dosage reduction recommended) ▪ Other chronic debilitating illnesses ▪ Renal impairment (dosage reduction recommended if creatinine <60 ml/min).

ADVERSE REACTIONS AND SIDE EFFECTS*

CNS: weakness.
EENT: ototoxicity.
GI: <u>vomiting</u>, <u>nausea</u>, <u>abdominal pain</u>, diarrhea, constipation, hepatitis, stomatitis.
GU: nephrotoxicity, gonadal suppression.
Derm: rash, alopecia.
F and E: <u>hyponatremia</u>, <u>hypocalcemia</u>, <u>hypomagnesemia</u>, <u>hypokalemia</u>.
Hemat: <u>leukopenia</u>, <u>thrombocytopenia</u>, <u>anemia</u>.
Neuro: peripheral neuropathy.
Misc: hypersensitivity reactions including ANAPHYLAXIS.

INTERACTIONS

Drug–Drug: ▪ Additive nephrotoxicity and ototoxicity with other **nephro-** and **ototoxic drugs (aminoglycosides, loop diuretics)** ▪ Additive bone marrow depression with other **bone-marrow-depressing drugs** or **radiation therapy.**

ROUTE AND DOSAGE

▪ **IV (Adults):** 360 mg/m^2 as a single dose; may be repeated at 4-wk intervals depending on response, or 300 mg/m^2 with cyclophosphamide at 4-wk intervals.

AVAILABILITY

▪ *Injection:* 50 mg-, 150 mg-, 450 mg-vials.

TIME/ACTION PROFILE (effects on blood counts)

	ONSET	PEAK	DURATION
IV	UK	21 days	28 days

NURSING IMPLICATIONS

ASSESSMENT

▫ Assess for nausea and vomiting. Mild to moderately severe nausea and vomiting often occur 6–12 hr after therapy and may persist for 24 hr. Confer with physician about prophylactic use of antiemetics. Adjust diet as tolerated to maintain fluid and electrolyte balance and ensure adequate nutritional intake.

▫ Monitor platelet count throughout therapy. Assess for bleeding (bleeding gums, bruising, petechiae, guaiac stools, urine, and emesis). Avoid IM injections and rectal temperatures. Apply pressure to venipuncture sites for 10 min.

▫ Assess for fever, chills, sore throat, and signs of infection. Notify physician if these symptoms occur.

▫ Anemia may occur. Monitor for increased fatigue, dyspnea, and orthostatic hypotension.

▫ Monitor for signs of anaphylaxis (rash, urticaria, pruritus, wheezing, tachycardia, hypotension). Discontinue medication immediately and notify physician if these occur. Epinephrine and resuscitation equipment should be readily available.

▪ **Lab Test Considerations:** CBC, differential, and clotting studies should be monitored prior to and routinely throughout course of therapy. The nadir of thrombocytopenia occurs within 14–28 days. Withhold subsequent doses until neutrophil count is >2,000/mm^3 and platelet count is >100,000/mm^3.

▫ Monitor renal and hepatic function prior to and periodically throughout course of therapy.

*<u>Underlines</u> indicate most frequent; **CAPITALS** indicate life-threatening.

POTENTIAL NURSING DIAGNOSES
- Infection, high risk for (adverse reactions).
- Injury, high risk for (side effects).
- Knowledge deficit related to medication regimen (patient/family teaching).

IMPLEMENTATION
- **General Info:** Do not use aluminum needles or equipment during preparation or administration, because aluminum reacts with the drug.
- Solution should be prepared in a biologic cabinet. Wear gloves, gown, and mask while handling medication. Discard equipment in specially designated containers (see Appendix I).
- **Intermittent Infusion:** Reconstitute to a concentration of 10 mg/ml with Sterile Water for Injection, D5W, or 0.9% NaCl for injection. May be further diluted in D5W or 0.9% NaCl to a concentration of 0.5 mg/ml. Stable for 8 hr at room temperature.
- *Rate:* Administer over 15–60 min.
- **Y-Site Compatibility:** ▪ fludarabine ▪ ondansetron ▪ sargramostim.

PATIENT/FAMILY TEACHING
- Instruct patient to notify physician promptly if fever, sore throat, signs of infection, bleeding gums, bruising, petechiae; blood in stools, urine or emesis; increased fatigue, dyspnea, or orthostatic hypotension occur. Caution patient to avoid crowds and persons with known infections. Instruct patient to use soft toothbrush and electric razor and to avoid falls. Patients should be cautioned not to drink alcoholic beverages or take medication containing aspirin or ibuprofen, because these may precipitate gastric bleeding.
- Instruct patient to promptly report any numbness or tingling in extremities or face, decreased coordination, difficulty with hearing or tinnitus, unusual swelling or weight gain to physician. The risks of ototoxicity, neurotoxicity, and nephrotoxicity are less than with cisplatin.
- Instruct patient not to receive any vaccinations without advice of physician.
- Advise patient of the need for contraception (if patient is not infertile as a result of surgical or radiation therapy).
- Instruct patient to inspect oral mucosa for erythema and ulceration. If ulceration occurs advise patient to notify physician, rinse mouth with water after eating, and use sponge brush. Physician may order viscous lidocaine swishes if mouth pain interferes with eating.
- Discuss with patient the possibility of hair loss. Explore methods of coping.
- Emphasize the need for periodic lab tests to monitor for side effects.

EVALUATION
Effectiveness of therapy can be demonstrated by: ▪ Decrease in size or spread of ovarian carcinoma.

CARBOPROST
(**kar**-bo-prost)
Hemabate, {Prostin/15M}

CLASSIFICATION(S):
Abortifacient (prostaglandin),
Oxytocic
Pregnancy Category C

INDICATIONS
- Induction of midtrimester abortion
- Treatment of postpartum hemorrhage that has not responded to conventional therapy.

ACTION
- Causes uterine contractions by directly stimulating the myometrium. Also produces cervical softening and dilation. **Therapeutic Effects:** ▪ Expulsion of fetus ▪ Control of postpartum bleeding.

PHARMACOKINETICS
Absorption: Well absorbed following IM administration.

{} = Available in Canada only.

Distribution: UK.
Metabolism and Excretion: Metabolized by tissue enzymes.
Half-life: UK.

CONTRAINDICATIONS AND PRECAUTIONS

Contraindicated in: ▪ Hypersensitivity ▪ Acute pelvic inflammatory disease ▪ Active pulmonary, renal, or hepatic disease.
Use Cautiously in: ▪ Uterine scarring ▪ Asthma ▪ Hypotension ▪ Hypertension ▪ Cardiac disease ▪ Adrenal disease ▪ Anemia ▪ Jaundice ▪ Diabetes mellitus.

ADVERSE REACTIONS AND SIDE EFFECTS*

CNS: headache.
Resp: wheezing.
GI: diarrhea, vomiting, nausea, abdominal pain, cramps.
GU: UTERINE RUPTURE.
Derm: flushing, redness of the face.
Misc: fever, chills, shivering.

INTERACTIONS

Drug–Drug: ▪ Augments the effects of other **oxytocics**.

ROUTE AND DOSAGE

Test Dose
▪ **IM (Adults):** 100 mcg.

Abortifacient
▪ **IM (Adults):** 250 mcg every 1.5–3.5 hr may be increased to 500 mcg if doses of 250 mcg produce inadequate response (not to exceed 2 days of continuous therapy or total dose of 12 mg).

Oxytocic
▪ **IM (Adults):** 250 mcg; may be repeated every 15–90 min (total dose not to exceed 2 mg).

AVAILABILITY

▪ *Injection:* 250 mcg/ml.

TIME/ACTION PROFILE (peak noted as mean abortion time)

	ONSET	PEAK	DURATION
IM	UK	16 hr	UK

NURSING IMPLICATIONS

ASSESSMENT

▫ Monitor frequency, duration, and force of contractions and uterine resting tone. Notify physician if contractions are absent or last more than 1 min.
▫ Monitor temperature, pulse, and blood pressure periodically throughout course of therapy. Large dose may cause hypertension. Temperature elevation beginning 1 to 16 hr after initiation of therapy and lasting for several hours is not unusual.
▫ Auscultate breath sounds. Wheezing and sensation of chest tightness may indicate hypersensitivity reaction.
▫ Assess for nausea, vomiting, and diarrhea. Vomiting and diarrhea occur in approximately ⅔ of patients. Premedication with antiemetic and antidiarrheal may be ordered.
▫ Monitor amount and type of vaginal discharge. Notify physician immediately if symptoms of hemorrhage (increased bleeding, hypotension, pallor, tachycardia) occur.

POTENTIAL NURSING DIAGNOSES

▪ Knowledge deficit related to medication regimen (patient/family teaching).

IMPLEMENTATION

▪ **General Info:** Avoid contact with skin. Thoroughly wash skin immediately after spillage.
▫ Premedication with an analgesic may be ordered for uterine cramping.
▫ Store in refrigerator.
▪ **IM:** Administer deep IM. Dose may be repeated every 1½–3½ hr. Rotate sites.

---

*Underlines indicate most frequent; **CAPITALS** indicate life-threatening.

PATIENT/FAMILY TEACHING
- **General Info:** Explain purpose of vaginal examinations (to assess for trauma to cervix).
- Instruct patient to notify physician immediately if fever and chills, foul-smelling vaginal discharge, lower abdominal pain, or increased bleeding occurs.

EVALUATION
Effectiveness of therapy can be demonstrated by: ■ Complete abortion ■ Control of postpartum or postabortal hemorrhage.

CARISOPRODOL
(kar-i-soe-**proe**-dole)
Rela, Sodol, Soma, Soprodol, Soridol

CLASSIFICATION(S):
Skeletal muscle relaxant (centrally acting)
Pregnancy Category UK

INDICATIONS
■ Adjunct to rest and physical therapy in the treatment of muscle spasm associated with acute painful musculoskeletal conditions.

ACTION
■ Skeletal muscle relaxation, probably due to CNS depression. **Therapeutic Effect:** ■ Skeletal muscle relaxation.

PHARMACOKINETICS
Absorption: Appears to be well absorbed following oral administration.
Distribution: Crosses the placenta. High concentrations in breast milk.
Metabolism and Excretion: Mostly metabolized by the liver.
Half-life: 8 hr.

CONTRAINDICATIONS AND PRECAUTIONS
Contraindicated in: ■ Hypersensitivity to carisoprodol or to meprobamate ■ Porphyria or suspected porphyria.

Use Cautiously in: ■ Severe liver or kidney disease ■ Pregnancy, lactation, or children <12 yr (safety not established) ■ Some products may contain tartrazine; use cautiously in patients with tartrazine sensitivity.

ADVERSE REACTIONS AND SIDE EFFECTS*
CNS: <u>dizziness</u>, <u>drowsiness</u>, ataxia, vertigo, agitation, irritability, headache, depression, syncope, insomnia.
Resp: asthmatic attacks.
CV: tachycardia, hypotension.
GI: nausea, vomiting, hiccups, epigastric distress.
Derm: rashes, flushing.
Hemat: eosinophilia, leukopenia.
Misc: severe idiosyncratic reaction, fever, ANAPHYLACTIC SHOCK.

INTERACTIONS
Drug–Drug: ■ Additive CNS depression with other **CNS depressants** including **alcohol, antihistamines, opioid analgesics,** and **sedative/hypnotics.**

ROUTE AND DOSAGE
■ **PO (Adults):** 350 mg 3–4 times daily.

AVAILABILITY
■ *Tablets:* 350 mg ■ *In combination with:* aspirin (Soma compound) and codeine. See Appendix A.

TIME/ACTION PROFILE (skeletal muscle relaxation)

	ONSET	PEAK	DURATION
PO	30 min	UK	4–6 hr

NURSING IMPLICATIONS
ASSESSMENT
- Assess patient for pain, muscle stiffness, and range of motion prior to and periodically throughout therapy.
- Observe patient for idiosyncratic symptoms that may appear within minutes or hours of administration during the first dose. Symptoms include extreme weakness, quadriplegia, dizziness, ataxia, dysarthria, visual disturbances, agitation, eu-

*Underlines indicate most frequent; **CAPITALS** indicate life-threatening.

phoria, confusion, and disorientation. Usually subsides over several hours.

POTENTIAL NURSING DIAGNOSES
- Pain (indications).
- Physical mobility, impaired (indications).
- Injury, high risk for (side effects).

IMPLEMENTATION
- **General Info:** Provide safety measures as indicated. Supervise ambulation and transfer of patients.
- **PO:** Administer with food to minimize GI irritation. Last dose should be given at bedtime.

PATIENT/FAMILY TEACHING
□ Instruct patient to take medication exactly as directed. Missed doses should be taken within 1 hr; if not, return to regular dosing schedule. Do not double doses.
□ Encourage patient to comply with additional therapies prescribed for muscle spasm (rest, physical therapy, heat, etc).
□ May cause dizziness or drowsiness. Advise patient to avoid driving or other activities requiring alertness until response to drug is known.
□ Instruct patient to make position changes slowly to minimize orthostatic hypotension.
□ Advise patient to avoid concurrent use of alcohol and other CNS depressants while taking this medication.
□ Instruct patient to notify physician if signs of allergy (rash, hives, swelling of tongue or lips, dyspnea) or idiosyncratic reaction occur.

EVALUATION
Effectiveness of therapy can be demonstrated by: ■ Decreased musculoskeletal pain and muscle spasticity □ Increased range of motion.

CARMUSTINE
(kar-**mus**-teen)
BCNU, BiCNU

CLASSIFICATION(S):
Antineoplastic (alkylating agent)
Pregnancy Category D

INDICATIONS
■ Alone or in combination with other treatment modalities (surgery, radiation) in the treatment of: □ Brain tumors □ Multiple myeloma □ Hodgkin's disease □ Other lymphomas.

ACTION
■ Inhibits DNA and RNA synthesis (cell cycle-phase nonspecific). **Therapeutic Effect:** ■ Death of rapidly replicating cells, especially malignant ones.

PHARMACOKINETICS
Absorption: Following IV administration absorption is essentially complete. **Distribution:** Highly lipid-soluble, readily penetrates CSF. Enters breast milk. **Metabolism and Excretion:** Rapidly metabolized. Some metabolites have antineoplastic activity. **Half-life:** UK.

CONTRAINDICATIONS AND PRECAUTIONS
Contraindicated in: ■ Hypersensitivity ■ Pregnancy or lactation. **Use Cautiously in:** ■ Patients with childbearing potential ■ Infections ■ Depressed bone-marrow reserve ■ Other chronic debilitating illnesses.

ADVERSE REACTIONS AND SIDE EFFECTS*
Resp: pulmonary infiltrates, pulmonary fibrosis. **GI:** nausea, vomiting, diarrhea, esophagitis, anorexia, hepatotoxicity. **GU:** renal failure. **Derm:** alopecia. **Hemat:** leukopenia, thrombocytopenia, anemia. **Local:** pain at IV site.

INTERACTIONS
Drug–Drug: ■ Additive bone marrow

depression with other **antineoplastics** or **radiation therapy** ▪ **Smoking** increases the risk of pulmonary toxicity.

ROUTE AND DOSAGE

▪ **IV (Adults and Children):** 150–200 mg/m^2 every 6 wk. Give as a single dose or as 75–100 mg/m^2/day for 2 days.

AVAILABILITY

▪ *Injection:* 100-mg vial.

TIME/ACTION PROFILE (effect on platelet counts)

	ONSET	PEAK	DURATION
IV	days	4–5 wk	6 wk

NURSING IMPLICATIONS

Assessment

▫ Monitor vital signs prior to and frequently during therapy.

▫ Assess for fever, chills, sore throat, and signs of infection. Notify physician if these symptoms occur.

▫ Assess respiratory status for dyspnea or cough. Pulmonary toxicity usually occurs after high cumulative doses or several courses of therapy. Notify physician promptly if these symptoms occur.

▫ Monitor platelet count throughout therapy. Assess for bleeding (bleeding gums, bruising, petechiae, guaiac stools, urine, and emesis). Avoid IM injections, rectal temperatures, and aspirin- or ibuprofen-containing products. Apply pressure to venipuncture sites for 10 min.

▫ Anemia may occur. Monitor for increased fatigue, dyspnea, and orthostatic hypotension.

▫ Monitor IV site closely. Carmustine is an irritant. Instruct patient to notify nurse immediately if discomfort at IV site occurs. Discontinue IV immediately if infiltration occurs. Confer with physician about application of ice to site. May cause hyperpigmentation of skin along vein.

▫ Monitor intake and output, appetite, and nutritional intake. Assess for nausea and vomiting, which may occur within 2 hr of administration and persist for 6 hr. Administration of an antiemetic prior to and during therapy and adjusting diet as tolerated may help maintain fluid and electrolyte balance and nutritional status.

▪ **Lab Test Considerations:** Monitor CBC and differential prior to and throughout therapy. The nadir of thrombocytopenia occurs in 4–5 wk; the nadir of leukopenia in 5–6 wk. Withhold dose and notify physician if platelet count is <100,000/mm^3 or leukocyte count is <4000/mm^3. Anemia is usually mild.

▫ May cause mild, reversible increase in AST (SGOT), alkaline phosphatase, and bilirubin.

▫ Monitor renal studies; notify physician if BUN is elevated.

Potential Nursing Diagnoses

▪ Injury, high risk for (side effects).

▪ Body image disturbance (side effects).

▪ Knowledge deficit related to medication regimen (patient/family teaching).

Implementation

▪ **General Info:** Solution should be prepared in a biologic cabinet. Wear gloves, gown, and mask while handling medication. Discard equipment in designated containers. Contact with skin may cause transient hyperpigmentation (see Appendix I).

▪ **Intermittent Infusion:** Dilute contents of each 100-mg vial with 3 ml of absolute ethyl alcohol provided as a diluent. Dilute this solution with 27 ml of Sterile Water for Injection. Further dilute with 500 ml of D5W or 0.9% NaCl in a glass container.

▫ Solution is clear and colorless. Do not use vials that contain an oily film, which indicates decomposition. Reconstituted solution is stable for 24 hr when refrigerated and protected from light. Solution contains no preserva-

tives; do not use as a multi-dose vial.
- ◻ IV lines may be flushed with 5–10 ml of 0.9% NaCl prior to and following carmustine infusion.
- ■ **Rate:** Administer dose over 1–2 hr. Rapid infusion rate may cause local pain, burning at site, and flushing. Facial flushing may persist for 4 hr.
- ■ **Y-Site Compatibility:** ■ fludarabine ■ ondansetron ■ saragramostim.
- ■ **Additive Incompatibility:** ■ sodium bicarbonate.

PATIENT/FAMILY TEACHING
- ◻ Instruct patient to notify physician if fever, chills, sore throat, signs of infection, bleeding gums, bruising, petechiae, or blood in urine, stool, or emesis occur. Caution patient to avoid crowds and persons with known infections. Instruct patient to use soft toothbrush and electric razor. Patients should be cautioned not to drink alcoholic beverages or take products containing aspirin or ibuprofen.
- ◻ Instruct patient to notify physician if shortness of breath or increased cough occurs. Encourage patient not to smoke, because smokers are at greater risk for pulmonary toxicity.
- ◻ Instruct patient to inspect oral mucosa for redness and ulceration. If mouth sores occur advise patient to use sponge brush and rinse mouth with water after eating and drinking. Consult physician if pain interferes with eating.
- ◻ Discuss with patient the possibility of hair loss. Explore coping strategies.
- ◻ Advise patient of the need for contraception.
- ◻ Instruct patient not to receive any vaccinations without advice of physician.
- ◻ Emphasize need for periodic lab tests to monitor for side effects.

EVALUATION
Effectiveness of therapy can be demonstrated by: ■ Decrease in size and spread of tumor ◻ Improvement in hematologic parameters in nonsolid cancers.

CARTEOLOL
(kar-tee-oh-lole)
Cartrol, Ocupress

CLASSIFICATION(S):
Beta-adrenergic blocking agent (nonselective), Antihypertensive
Pregnancy Category C

INDICATIONS
- ■ **PO:** Alone or with other agents in the management of hypertension
- ■ **Ophth:** Decreases intraocular pressure in chronic open-angle glaucoma and intraocular hypertension.

ACTION
- ■ Blocks stimulation of beta$_1$ (myocardial) and beta$_2$ (pulmonary, vascular, or uterine) receptor sites ■ Possesses mild intrinsic sympathomimetic (ISA) activity ■ **Ophth:** Decreases the production of aqueous humor. **Therapeutic Effects:**
- ■ **PO:** Decreased heart rate and blood pressure ■ **Ophth:** Decreased intraocular pressure.

PHARMACOKINETICS
Absorption: 85% absorbed following oral administration. Systemic absorption is minimal after ophthalmic administration.
Distribution: Distribution not known.
Metabolism and Excretion: Some metabolism by the liver, with conversion to at least 1 active compound (8-hydroxycarteolol). 50–70% excreted unchanged by the kidneys.
Half-life: Carteolol 6–8 hr, 8-hydroxycarteolol 8–12 hr (both increased in renal impairment).

CONTRAINDICATIONS AND PRECAUTIONS
Contraindicated in: ■ Uncompensated congestive heart failure ■ Pulmonary edema ■ Cardiogenic shock ■ Bradycardia ■ Heart block ■ COPD or asthma.
Use Cautiously in: ■ Thyrotoxicosis or hypoglycemia (may mask symptoms) ■ Diabetes mellitus (may mask symptoms of hypoglycemia) ■ Renal impair-

ment (increased dose interval suggested if creatinine clearance ≤60 ml/min) ▪ Pregnancy or lactation (safety not established) ▪ Children (safety not established) ▪ Patients with a history of severe allergic reactions (intensity of reactions may be increased).

ADVERSE REACTIONS AND SIDE EFFECTS*

CNS: <u>fatigue</u>, <u>weakness</u>, drowsiness, depression, memory loss.
EENT: dry eyes, blurred vision, nasal stuffiness, <u>eye irritation</u> (ophth only).
Resp: bronchospasm, wheezing.
CV: BRADYCARDIA, CONGESTIVE HEART FAILURE, PULMONARY EDEMA, hypotension, peripheral vasoconstriction, chest pain.
GI: diarrhea, nausea.
GU: impotence, diminished libido.
Derm: rash, itching.
Endo: hyperglycemia, hypoglycemia.
MS: muscle cramps, back pain.
Neuro: paresthesia.
Misc: Raynaud's phenomenon.

INTERACTIONS

Drug–Drug: ▪ **General anesthesia, IV phenytoin,** and **verapamil** may cause additive myocardial depression ▪ Additive bradycardia may occur with concurrent use of **cardiac glycosides** ▪ Additive hypotension may occur with other **antihypertensive agents,** acute ingestion of **alcohol,** or **nitrates** ▪ Concurrent use with **amphetamines, cocaine, ephedrine, epinephrine, norepinephrine, phenylephrine,** or **pseudoephedrine** may result in excess alpha-adrenergic stimulation, hypertension, and bradycardia ▪ May negate the beneficial beta$_1$ cardiac effects of **dopamine** or **dobutamine** ▪ Concurrent **thyroid** administration may decrease effectiveness ▪ Use with **insulin** may result in prolonged hypoglycemia ▪ May decrease beneficial effects of **theophylline.**

ROUTE AND DOSAGE

▪ **PO (Adults):** 2.5 mg/day as a single

dose; may be increased up to 10 mg/day (usual dose 2.5–5.0 mg/day).
▪ **Ophth (Adults):** 1 drop bid.

AVAILABILITY

▪ *Tablets:* 2.5 mg, 5 mg. ▪ *Ophthalmic solution:* 1%.

TIME/ACTION PROFILE (pressure-lowering effect)

	ONSET	PEAK	DURATION
PO	UK	1–3 hr	UK
Ophth	UK	UK	12 hr

NURSING IMPLICATIONS

ASSESSMENT
▪ **PO:** Monitor blood pressure and pulse frequently during dosage adjustment period and periodically throughout therapy. Confer with physician prior to giving drug if pulse is <50 bpm.
▫ Monitor intake and output ratios and daily weight. Assess patient routinely for evidence of fluid overload (peripheral edema, dyspnea, rales/crackles, fatigue, weight gain, jugular venous distension).
▪ **Ophth:** Monitor intraocular pressure periodically during therapy.

POTENTIAL NURSING DIAGNOSES
▪ Cardiac output, decreased (side effects).
▪ Knowledge deficit related to medication regimen (patient/family teaching).
▪ Noncompliance related to medication regimen (patient/family teaching).

IMPLEMENTATION
▪ **PO:** Administered as a single daily dose. Doses >10 mg do not usually increase effectiveness and may decrease response.
▪ **Ophth:** See Appendix H for instillation of ophthalmic medications.

PATIENT/FAMILY TEACHING
▪ **PO:** Instruct patient to take medication exactly as directed, even if feeling well. If a dose is missed, it may be

*<u>Underlines</u> indicate most frequent; **CAPITALS** indicate life-threatening.

taken as soon as remembered up to 4 hr before next dose. Abrupt withdrawal may result in life-threatening arrhythmias, hypertension, or myocardial ischemia.

□ Teach patient and family how to check pulse and blood pressure. Instruct them to take pulse daily and blood pressure biweekly. Advise patient to withhold dose and contact physician if pulse is <50 bpm or blood pressure changes significantly.

□ May occasionally cause drowsiness. Caution patients to avoid driving or other activities that require alertness until response to medication is known.

□ Reinforce the need to continue additional therapies for hypertension (weight loss, exercise, restricted sodium intake, stress reduction, regular exercise, moderation of alcohol consumption, and cessation of smoking). Carteolol controls but does not cure hypertension.

□ Caution patient that this medication may cause increased sensitivity to cold.

□ Advise patient to consult physician or pharmacist before taking any over-the-counter medications, especially cold remedies, concurrently with this medication. Patients on antihypertensive therapy should also avoid excessive amounts of coffee, tea, and cola.

□ Diabetics should closely monitor blood sugar, especially if weakness, malaise, irritability, or fatigue occur.

□ Advise patient to notify physician if slow pulse rate, fever, dizziness, light-headedness, confusion, or depression, skin rash, sore throat, or unusual bleeding or bruising occur.

□ Instruct patient to inform physician or dentist of medication regimen prior to treatment or surgery.

□ Advise patient to carry identification describing disease process and medication regimen at all times.

▪ **Ophth:** Instruct patient in proper technique for instillation of ophthalmic medications. Emphasize the importance of not touching the applicator tip to any surface.

□ Advise patient to wear sunglasses and avoid exposure to bright light to prevent photophobia.

EVALUATION
Effectiveness of therapy can be demonstrated by: ▪ Decrease in blood pressure ▪ Decreased intraocular pressure.

C

CASANTHRANOL
(ka-**san**-thra-nole)
CASCARA SAGRADA
(kas-**kar**-a sa-**grad**-a)

CLASSIFICATION(S):
Laxative (stimulant)
Pregnancy Category UK

INDICATIONS

▪ Treatment of constipation. Particularly useful when constipation is secondary to prolonged bed rest or constipating drugs.

ACTION

▪ Stimulates peristalsis ▪ Alters fluid and electrolyte transport, producing fluid accumulation in the colon. **Therapeutic Effect:** ▪ Evacuation of the colon. Cascara is another name for cascara sagrada, which is naturally derived from the bark of the Buckhorn tree. Casanthranol is the active ingredient that has been extracted from cascara.

PHARMACOKINETICS

Absorption: Minimally absorbed. Converted in the colon to active drug.
Distribution: Distribution not known.
Metabolism and Excretion: Small amounts absorbed are metabolized by the liver.
Half-life: Unknown.

CONTRAINDICATIONS AND PRECAUTIONS

Contraindicated in: ▪ Hypersensitivity ▪ Abdominal pain, obstruction, nausea or vomiting, especially when associated

with fever or other signs of acute abdomen ▪ Pregnancy or lactation.
Use Cautiously in: ▪ Severe cardiovascular disease ▪ Anal or rectal fissures ▪ Excessive or prolonged use may lead to dependence.

ADVERSE REACTIONS AND SIDE EFFECTS*

GI: nausea, abdominal cramps, diarrhea.
GU: discoloration of urine.
F and E: hypokalemia (with chronic use).

INTERACTIONS

Drug–Drug: ▪ May decrease the absorption of concurrently administered **oral medications** due to increased motility and decreased transit time.

ROUTE AND DOSAGE

Casanthranol
▪ **PO (Adults):** 30–90 mg once daily.
▪ **PO (Children 2–11 yr):** 50% of adult dose.
▪ **PO (Younger Children and Infants):** 25% of adult dose.

AVAILABILITY

▪ *Tablets, extracts, and fluid extracts:* alone and in combination with other laxatives. See Appendix A.

TIME/ACTION PROFILE (evacuation of colon)

	ONSET	PEAK	DURATION
PO	6–12 hr	UK	UK

NURSING IMPLICATIONS

ASSESSMENT
▫ Assess patient for abdominal distention, presence of bowel sounds, and usual pattern of bowel function.
▫ Assess color, consistency, and amount of stool produced.

POTENTIAL NURSING DIAGNOSES
▪ Constipation (indications).
▪ Diarrhea (side effects).
▪ Knowledge deficit related to medica-

tion regimen (patient/family teaching).

IMPLEMENTATION
▪ **PO:** Administer with full glass of water. Administer at bedtime for evacuation 6–12 hr later. Administer on an empty stomach for more rapid results.

PATIENT/FAMILY TEACHING
▫ Advise patients that laxatives should be used only for short-term therapy. Long-term therapy may cause electrolyte imbalance and dependence.
▫ Encourage patient to utilize other forms of bowel regulation such as increasing bulk in the diet, increasing fluid intake, increasing mobility. Normal bowel habits are individualized and may vary from 3 times/day to 3 times/wk.
▫ Inform patients that this medication may cause a change in urine color to a pink, red, violet, or brown color.
▫ Instruct patients with cardiac disease to avoid straining during bowel movements (Valsalva maneuver).
▫ Advise patients not to use laxatives when abdominal pain, nausea, vomiting, or fever are present.

EVALUATION
Effectiveness of therapy can be demonstrated by: ▪ The patient having a soft, formed bowel movement.

CEFACLOR
(**sef**-a-klor)
Ceclor

CLASSIFICATION(S):
Anti-infective (second generation cephalosporin)
Pregnancy Category B

INDICATIONS

▪ Useful in the treatment of the following infections due to susceptible organisms: ▫ Otitis media ▫ Respiratory tract infections ▫ Skin and skin structure infections ▫ Bone and joint infections

---

*Underlines indicate most frequent; **CAPITALS** indicate life-threatening.

□ Urinary tract and gynecologic infections □ Septicemia.

ACTION

■ Binds to bacterial cell wall membrane, causing cell death. **Therapeutic Effect:** ■ Bactericidal action against susceptible bacteria. **Spectrum:** ■ Many gram-positive cocci including: □ *Streptococcus pneumoniae* □ Group A beta-hemolytic streptococci □ Penicillinase-producing staphylococci ■ Has increased activity against several other important gram-negative pathogens including: □ *Haemophilus influenzae* □ Acinetobacter □ Enterobacter □ *Escherichia coli* □ *Klebsiella pneumoniae* □ *Neisseria gonorrhea* (including penicillinase-producing strains) □ Providencia □ Proteus □ Serratia ■ Has no activity against: □ Methicillin-resistant staphylococci □ Enterococcus.

PHARMACOKINETICS

Absorption: Well absorbed following oral administration.

Distribution: Widely distributed. Penetration into CSF is poor. Crosses the placenta and enters breast milk in low concentrations.

Metabolism and Excretion: Excreted primarily unchanged by the kidneys.

Half-life: 0.6–0.9 hr (increased in renal impairment).

CONTRAINDICATIONS AND PRECAUTIONS

Contraindicated in: ■ Hypersensitivity to cephalosporins ■ Serious hypersensitivity to penicillins.

Use Cautiously in: ■ Renal impairment (dosage reduction required if severe) ■ Pregnancy and lactation (safety not established, but has been used in obstetric surgery).

ADVERSE REACTIONS AND SIDE EFFECTS*

GI: nausea, vomiting, cramps, diarrhea, PSEUDOMEMBRANOUS COLITIS.

Derm: rashes, urticaria.

Hemat: blood dyscrasias, hemolytic anemia.

Misc: superinfection, allergic reactions including ANAPHYLAXIS and serum sickness.

INTERACTIONS

Drug–Drug: ■ **Probenecid** decreases excretion and increases blood levels.

ROUTE AND DOSAGE

Cefaclor

■ **PO (Adults):** 250–500 mg q 8 hr.
■ **PO (Children >1 mo):** 20–40 mg/kg/day in divided doses q 8–12 hr.

AVAILABILITY

■ *Capsules:* 250 mg, 500 mg ■ *Oral suspension:* 125 mg/5 ml, 187 mg/5 ml, 250 mg/5 ml, 375 mg/5 ml.

TIME/ACTION PROFILE (blood levels)

	ONSET	PEAK
PO	rapid	30–60 min

NURSING IMPLICATIONS

ASSESSMENT

□ Assess patient for infection (vital signs; appearance of wound, sputum, urine, and stool; WBC; earache) at beginning and throughout therapy.

□ Obtain a history before initiating therapy to determine previous use of and reactions to penicillins or cephalosporins. Persons with a negative history of penicillin sensitivity may still have an allergic response.

□ Obtain specimens for culture and sensitivity prior to initiating therapy. First dose may be given before receiving results.

□ Observe patient for signs and symptoms of anaphylaxis (rash, pruritus, laryngeal edema, wheezing). Discontinue the drug and notify the physician immediately if these occur. Keep epinephrine, an antihistamine, and resuscitation equipment close by in the event of an anaphylactic reaction.

- **Lab Test Considerations:** May cause false-positive results for Coombs' test and urine glucose when tested with copper sulfate method (Clinitest). Use glucose enzymatic tests (Clinistix or Tes-Tape) to test urine glucose.
- □ May cause elevated BUN, serum creatinine, AST (SGOT), ALT (SGPT), billirubin and alkaline phosphatase levels.

POTENTIAL NURSING DIAGNOSES
- Infection, high risk for (indications, side effects).
- Diarrhea (adverse reactions).
- Knowledge deficit related to medication regimen (patient/family teaching).

IMPLEMENTATION
- **PO:** Administer around the clock. May be administered without regard to meals. If gastric irritation occurs administer with food. Food slows but does not effect amount absorbed.
- □ Shake suspension well before administering. Suspension is stable for 14 days if refrigerated.

PATIENT/FAMILY TEACHING
- □ Instruct patient to take cefaclor around the clock and to finish the drug completely, even if feeling better. Advise patient that sharing of this medication may be dangerous.
- □ Instruct patients receiving suspension on the correct method for measuring liquid.
- □ Advise patient to report the signs of superinfection (furry overgrowth on the tongue, vaginal itching or discharge, loose or foul-smelling stools) and allergy.
- □ Instruct patient to notify physician if fever and diarrhea develop, especially if stool contains blood, pus, or mucus. Advise patient not to treat diarrhea without consulting physician or pharmacist.

EVALUATION
Clinical response to therapy can be evaluated by: ■ Resolution of the signs and symptoms of infection. Length of time for complete resolution depends on the organism and site of infection.

CEFADROXIL
(sef-a-**drox**-ill)
Duricef, Ultracef

CLASSIFICATION(S):
Anti-infective (first generation cephalosporin)
Pregnancy Category B

INDICATIONS
■ Treatment of: □ Serious skin and skin structure infections □ Urinary tract infections □ Bone and joint infections □ Septicemia □ Group A beta-hemolytic streptococcal pharyngitis.

ACTION
■ Binds to bacterial cell wall membrane, causing cell death. **Therapeutic Effect:** ■ Bactericidal action against susceptible bacteria. **Spectrum:** ■ Active against many gram-positive cocci including: □ *Streptococcus pneumoniae* □ Group A beta-hemolytic streptococci □ Penicillinase-producing staphylococci ■ Has limited activity against some gram-negative rods: □ *Klebsiella pneumoniae* □ *Proteus mirabilis* □ *Escherichia coli* ■ Not active against: □ Methicillin-resistant staphylococci □ *Bacteroides fragilis* □ Enterococcus.

PHARMACOKINETICS
Absorption: Well absorbed following oral administration.
Distribution: Widely distributed. Crosses the placenta and enters breast milk in low concentrations. Minimal penetration into CSF.
Metabolism and Excretion: Excreted almost entirely unchanged by the kidneys.
Half-life: Cefadroxil 1.1–2 hr.

CONTRAINDICATIONS AND PRECAUTIONS
Contraindicated in: ■ Hypersensitivity to cephalosporins ■ Serious hypersensitivity to penicillins.
Use Cautiously in: ■ Renal impairment (dosage reduction required if creatinine clearance ≤50 ml/min)

- Pregnancy or lactation (safety not established).

ADVERSE REACTIONS AND SIDE EFFECTS*

GI: nausea, vomiting, cramps, diarrhea, PSEUDOMEMBRANOUS COLITIS.
Derm: rashes, urticaria.
GU: interstitial nephritis.
Hemat: dyscrasias, hemolytic anemia.
Misc: superinfection, allergic reactions including ANAPHYLAXIS and serum sickness.

INTERACTIONS

Drug–Drug: ■ Probenecid decreases excretion and increases blood levels.

ROUTE AND DOSAGE

- **PO (Adults):** 1–2 g/day single dose or divided doses q 12 hr.
- **PO (Children):** 30 mg/kg/day single dose or divided doses q 12 hr.

AVAILABILITY

- *Capsules:* 500 mg ■ *Tablets:* 1 g
- *Oral suspension:* 125 mg/5 ml, 250 mg/5 ml, 500 mg/5 ml.

TIME/ACTION PROFILE (blood levels)

	ONSET	PEAK
PO	rapid	1.5–2 hr

NURSING IMPLICATIONS

ASSESSMENT

- Assess patient for infection (vital signs; appearance of wound, sputum, urine, and stool; WBC) at beginning and throughout course of therapy.
- Obtain a history before initiating therapy to determine previous use of and reactions to penicillins or cephalosporins. Persons with a negative history of penicillin sensitivity may still have an allergic response.
- Obtain specimens for culture and sensitivity prior to initiating therapy. First dose may be given before receiving results.
- Observe patient for signs and symptoms of anaphylaxis (rash, pruritus, laryngeal edema, wheezing). Discontinue the drug and notify the physician immediately if these occur. Keep epinephrine, an antihistamine, and resuscitation equipment close by in the event of an anaphylactic reaction.

- **Lab Test Considerations:** May cause false-positive results for Coombs' test and urine glucose when tested with copper sulfate method (Clinitest). Use glucose enzymatic tests (Clinistix or Tes-Tape) to test urine glucose.
- May cause transient increase in AST (SGOT), ALT (SGPT), and alkaline phosphatase.

POTENTIAL NURSING DIAGNOSES

- Infection, high risk for (indications, side effects).
- Knowledge deficit related to medication regimen (patient/family teaching).
- Noncompliance related to medication regimen (patient/family teaching).

IMPLEMENTATION

- **PO:** Administer around the clock. May be administered without regard to food or meals. If gastric irritation occurs, administer with food.
- Shake suspensions well before administering. Suspension is stable for 14 days if refrigerated.

PATIENT/FAMILY TEACHING

- Instruct patient to take cefadroxil around the clock and to finish the drug completely, even if feeling better. Advise patients that sharing of this medication may be dangerous.
- Instruct patients receiving suspension on correct method for measuring liquid.
- Advise patient to report the signs of superinfection (furry overgrowth on the tongue, vaginal itching or discharge, loose or foul-smelling stools) and allergy.
- Instruct patient to notify physician if fever and diarrhea develop, especially if stool contains blood, mucus, or pus. Advise patient not to treat diarrhea without consulting physician or pharmacist.

---

*Underlines indicate most frequent; **CAPITALS** indicate life-threatening.

Clinical response to therapy can be evaluated by: ▪ Resolution of the signs and symptoms of infection. Length of time for complete resolution depends on the organism and site of infection.

CEFAMANDOLE
(sef-a-**man**-dole)
Mandol

CLASSIFICATION(S):
Anti-infective (second generation cephalosporin)
Pregnancy Category B

INDICATIONS
▪ Treatment of the following infections: ▢ Respiratory tract infections ▢ Skin and skin structure infections ▢ Bone and joint infections ▢ Urinary tract and gynecologic infections ▢ Septicemia ▢ Intra-abdominal and biliary tract infections ▪ Has also been used as a perioperative prophylactic anti-infective.

ACTION
▪ Binds to bacterial cell wall membrane, causing cell death. **Therapeutic Effect:** ▪ Bactericidal action against susceptible bacteria. **Spectrum:** ▪ Many gram-positive cocci including: ▢ *Streptococcus pneumoniae* ▢ Group A beta-hemolytic streptococci ▢ Penicillinase-producing staphylococci ▪ Increased activity against several other important gram-negative pathogens including: ▢ *Haemophilus influenzae* ▢ Acinetobacter ▢ Enterobacter ▢ *Escherichia coli* ▢ *Klebsiella pneumoniae* ▢ *Neisseria gonorrhea* (including penicillinase-producing strains) ▢ Providencia ▢ Proteus ▢ Serratia ▪ Also active against *Bacteroides fragilis* ▪ Has no activity against: ▢ Methicillin-resistant staphylococci ▢ Enterococcus.

PHARMACOKINETICS
Absorption: Well absorbed following IM administration.

Distribution: Widely distributed. Penetration into CSF is poor. Crosses the placenta and enters breast milk in low concentrations.
Metabolism and Excretion: Excreted primarily unchanged by the kidneys.
Half-life: 0.5–1.2 hr (increased in renal impairment).

CONTRAINDICATIONS AND PRECAUTIONS
Contraindicated in: ▪ Hypersensitivity to cephalosporins ▪ Serious hypersensitivity to penicillins.
Use Cautiously in: ▪ Renal impairment (dosage reduction required if creatinine clearance <80 ml/min) ▪ Pregnancy and lactation (safety not established, but has been used in obstetric surgery).

ADVERSE REACTIONS AND SIDE EFFECTS*
GI: <u>nausea</u>, <u>vomiting</u>, cramps, <u>diarrhea</u>, PSEUDOMEMBRANOUS COLITIS.
Derm: <u>rashes</u>, urticaria.
Hemat: blood dyscrasias, hemolytic anemia, bleeding.
Local: <u>phlebitis</u> at IV site, <u>pain</u> at IM site.
Misc: superinfection, allergic reactions including ANAPHYLAXIS and serum sickness.

INTERACTIONS
Drug–Drug: ▪ **Probenecid** decreases excretion and increases blood levels ▪ If **alcohol** is ingested within 48–72 hr, a disulfiram-like reaction may occur ▪ May increase risk of bleeding with **oral anticoagulants, thrombolytics, nonsteroidal anti-inflammatory agents, plicamycin,** or **valproic acid**.

ROUTE AND DOSAGE
▪ **IM, IV (Adults):** 0.5–2 g q 6 hr (up to 2 g q 4 hr).
▪ **IM, IV (Children >1 mo):** 50–100 mg/kg/day in divided doses q 4–8 hr.

AVAILABILITY
▪ *Injection:* 1 g, 2 g, 10 g.

---

*<u>Underlines</u> indicate most frequent; **CAPITALS** indicate life-threatening.

TIME/ACTION PROFILE (blood levels)

	ONSET	PEAK
IM	rapid	30–120 min
IV	rapid	end of infusion

NURSING IMPLICATIONS

ASSESSMENT

- **General Info:** Assess patient for infection (vital signs; appearance of wound, sputum, urine, and stool; WBC) at beginning and throughout course of therapy.
- Obtain a history before initiating therapy to determine previous use of and reactions to penicillins or cephalosporins. Persons with a negative history of penicillin sensitivity may still have an allergic response.
- Obtain specimens for culture and sensitivity prior to initiating therapy. First dose may be given before receiving results.
- Observe patient for signs and symptoms of anaphylaxis (rash, pruritus, laryngeal edema, wheezing). Discontinue the drug and notify the physician immediately if these occur. Keep epinephrine, an antihistamine, and resuscitation equipment close by in the event of an anaphylactic reaction.
- **Lab Test Considerations:** Monitor prothrombin time and assess for bleeding (guaiac stools; check for hematuria, bleeding gums, ecchymosis) daily in patients receiving cefamandole, because it may cause hypoprothrombinemia. Elderly or debilitated patients are at increased risk for hypoprothrombinemia. If bleeding occurs, it can be reversed with vitamin K, or prophylactic vitamin K 10 mg/wk may be given.
- May cause transient increase in BUN, creatinine, AST (SGOT), ALT (SGPT), LDH, and alkaline phosphatase.
- May cause false-positive proteinuria, Coombs' test, and urine glucose when tested with copper sulfate method (Clinitest). Use glucose enzymatic tests (Clinistix or Tes-Tape) to test urine glucose.

POTENTIAL NURSING DIAGNOSES

- Infection, high risk for (indications, side effects).
- Diarrhea (adverse reactions).
- Knowledge deficit related to medication regimen (patient/family teaching).

IMPLEMENTATION

- **General Info:** Solution ranges in color from light yellow to amber. Do not use if solution is a different color or contains a precipitate.
- Reconstitution causes gas to form. Vial can be vented prior to withdrawal, or use gas to assist in withdrawal of the solution by inverting the vial over the syringe needle, allowing the solution to flow into the needle.
- Powder is difficult to dissolve. Reconstitute by keeping powder at stopper end of vial and adding diluent to other end of vial. Shake vigorously to dissolve.
- **IM:** Reconstitute IM doses with 3 ml of Sterile or Bacteriostatic Water for Injection or 0.9% NaCl for injection. Physician may order dilution with 0.5–2.0% lidocaine HCl to minimize injection discomfort. Inject deep into a well-developed muscle mass; massage well.
- **IV:** Change IV sites every 48–72 hr to prevent phlebitis.
- **Direct IV:** Dilute each g with 10 ml of Sterile Water for Injection, D5W, or 0.9% NaCl.
- **Rate:** Administer slowly over 3–5 min. Monitor for phlebitis.
- **Intermittent Infusion:** Reconstituted solution may be further diluted in 100 ml of 0.9% NaCl, D5W, D10W, D5/0.25% NaCl, D5/0.45% NaCl, D5/0.9% NaCl, or D5/LR. Solution is stable for 24 hr at room temperature and 96 hr if refrigerated.
- **Rate:** Administer over 15–30 min.
- **Continuous Infusion:** May be diluted in up to 1000 ml for continuous infusion.
- **Syringe Compatibility:** ▪ heparin.
- **Syringe Incompatibility:** ▪ cimetidine ▪ gentamicin ▪ tobramycin.

- **Y-Site Compatibility:** ▪ acyclovir ▪ cyclophosphamide ▪ hydromorphone ▪ magnesium sulfate ▪ meperidine ▪ morphine ▪ perphenazine.
- **Y-Site Incompatibility:** ▪ hetastarch.
- **Additive Incompatibility:** ▪ lactated Ringer's solution ▪ Ringer's solution.
- Do not admix with aminoglycosides; if administered concurrently, administer in separate sites.

PATIENT/FAMILY TEACHING

- Advise patient to report the signs of superinfection (furry overgrowth on the tongue, vaginal itching or discharge, loose or foul-smelling stools) and allergy.
- Caution patient that concurrent use of alcohol with cefamandole may cause a disulfiram-like reaction (abdominal cramps, nausea, vomiting, hypotension, palpitations, dyspnea, tachycardia, sweating, flushing). Alcohol and medications containing alcohol should be avoided during and for several days after therapy.
- Instruct patient to notify physician if fever and diarrhea develop, especially if stool contains blood, pus, or mucus. Advise patient not to treat diarrhea without consulting physician or pharmacist.

EVALUATION

Clinical response to therapy can be evaluated by: ▪ Resolution of the signs and symptoms of infection. Length of time for complete resolution depends on the organism and site of infection.

CEFAZOLIN
(sef-**a**-zoe-lin)
Ancef, Kefzol, Zolicef

CLASSIFICATION(S):
Anti-infective (first generation cephalosporin)
Pregnancy Category B

INDICATIONS

- Treatment of: □ Serious skin and skin structure infections □ Urinary tract infections □ Bone and joint infections □ Septicemia ▪ Has been used to treat intra-abdominal and biliary tract infections and as a perioperative prophylactic anti-infective.

ACTION

▪ Binds to bacterial cell wall membrane, causing cell death. **Therapeutic Effect:** ▪ Bactericidal action against susceptible bacteria. **Spectrum:** ▪ Active against many gram-positive cocci including: □ *Streptococcus pneumoniae* □ Group A beta-hemolytic streptococci □ Penicillinase-producing staphylococci ▪ Limited activity against some gram-negative rods including: □ *Klebsiella pneumoniae* □ *Proteus mirabilis* □ *Escherichia coli* ▪ Not active against: □ Methicillin-resistant staphylococci □ *Bacteroides fragilis* □ Enterococcus.

PHARMACOKINETICS

Absorption: Well absorbed following IM administration.
Distribution: Widely distributed. Crosses the placenta and enters breast milk in low concentrations. Minimal penetration into CSF.
Metabolism and Excretion: Excreted almost entirely unchanged by the kidneys.
Half-life: 1.2–2.2 hr.

CONTRAINDICATIONS AND PRECAUTIONS

Contraindicated in: ▪ Hypersensitivity to cephalosporins ▪ Serious hypersensitivity to penicillins.
Use Cautiously in: ▪ Renal impairment (dosage reduction required if creatinine clearance <55 ml/min) ▪ Pregnancy or lactation (safety not established).

ADVERSE REACTIONS AND SIDE EFFECTS*

CNS: SEIZURES (high doses).
GI: <u>nausea</u>, <u>vomiting</u>, cramps, <u>diarrhea</u>, PSEUDOMEMBRANOUS COLITIS.
GU: nephrotoxicity.

*<u>Underlines</u> indicate most frequent; **CAPITALS** indicate life-threatening.

Derm: <u>rashes</u>, urticaria.
Hemat: blood dyscrasias, hemolytic anemia.
Local: <u>phlebitis</u> at IV site, <u>pain</u> at IM site.
Misc: superinfection, allergic reactions including ANAPHYLAXIS and serum sickness.

INTERACTIONS

Drug–Drug: ■ **Probenecid** decreases excretion and increases blood levels.

ROUTE AND DOSAGE

- **IM, IV (Adults):** 0.25–2 g q 6–8 hr (up to 12 g/day).
- **IM, IV (Children and Infants >1 mo):** 25–50 mg/kg/day in divided doses every 6–8 hr (up to 100 mg/kg/day).

AVAILABILITY

- ***Injection:*** 500 mg, 1 g, 5 g, 10 g, 20 g.

TIME/ACTION PROFILE (blood levels)

	ONSET	PEAK
IM	rapid	1–2 hr
IV	rapid	end of infusion

NURSING IMPLICATIONS

ASSESSMENT

- ▫ Assess patient for infection (vital signs; appearance of wound, sputum, urine, and stool; WBC) at beginning and throughout course of therapy.
- ▫ Obtain a history before initiating therapy to determine previous use of and reactions to penicillins or cephalosporins. Persons with a negative history of penicillin sensitivity may still have an allergic response.
- ▫ Obtain specimens for culture and sensitivity prior to initiating therapy. First dose may be given before receiving results.
- ▫ Observe patient for signs and symptoms of anaphylaxis (rash, pruritus, laryngeal edema, wheezing). Discontinue the drug and notify the physician immediately if these occur. Keep epinephrine, an antihistamine, and resuscitation equipment close by in the event of an anaphylactic reaction.

- **Lab Test Considerations:** May cause false-positive results for Coombs' test and urine glucose when tested with copper sulfate method (Clinitest). Use glucose enzymatic tests (Clinistix or Tes-Tape) to test urine glucose.
- ▫ May cause transient elevation in BUN, AST (SGOT), ALT (SGPT), and alkaline phosphatase.

POTENTIAL NURSING DIAGNOSES

- Infection, high risk for (indications, side effects)
- Diarrhea (adverse reactions).
- Knowledge deficit related to medication regimen (patient/family teaching).

IMPLEMENTATION

- **General Info:** Do not use solution that is cloudy or contains a precipitate.
- **IM:** Reconstitute IM doses with 2 ml of Sterile or Bacteriostatic Water for Injection or 0.9% NaCl for Injection in the 250-mg or 500-mg vial and 2.5 ml in the 1-g vial for concentrations of 125, 225, or 330 mg/ml, respectively. Inject deep into a well-developed muscle mass, massage well.
- **IV:** Change IV sites every 48–72 hr to prevent phlebitis.
- **Direct IV:** For direct IV administration dilute in 10 ml of Sterile Water for Injection.
- ***Rate:*** Administer slowly over 3–5 min. Monitor for phlebitis.
- **Intermittent Infusion:** Reconstituted 500-mg or 1-g solution may be diluted in 50–100 ml of 0.9% NaCl, D5W, D10W, D5/0.25% NaCl, D5/0.45% NaCl, D5/0.9% NaCl, D5/LR, or lactated Ringer's solution. Solution is stable for 24 hr at room temperature and 96 hr if refrigerated.
- ***Rate:*** Administer over 30–60 min.
- **Syringe Compatibility:** ■ heparin ■ vitamin B complex.
- **Syringe Incompatibility:** ■ ascorbic acid injection ■ cimetidine ■ lidocaine.
- **Y-Site Compatibility:** ■ acyclovir ■ atracurium ■ calcium gluconate ■ cyclophosphamide ■ enalaprilat

- esmolol ■ famotidine ■ fluconazole ■ fludarabine ■ foscarnet ■ hydromorphone ■ insulin ■ labetalol ■ lidocaine ■ magnesium sulfate ■ meperidine ■ morphine ■ multivitamins ■ ondansetron ■ pancuronium ■ perphenazine ■ sargramostim ■ vecuronium.
- **Additive Incompatibility:** Do not admix with aminoglycosides; if administered concurrently, administer in separate sites.

PATIENT/FAMILY TEACHING
□ Advise patient to report the signs of superinfection (furry overgrowth on the tongue, vaginal itching or discharge, loose or foul-smelling stools) and allergy.
□ Instruct patient to notify physician if fever and diarrhea develop, especially if stool contains blood, mucus, or pus. Advise patient not to treat diarrhea without consulting physician or pharmacist.

EVALUATION
Clinical response to therapy can be evaluated by: ■ Resolution of the signs and symptoms of infection. Length of time for complete resolution depends on the organism and site of infection.

CEFIXIME
(se-fix-eem)
Suprax

CLASSIFICATION(S):
Anti-infective (third generation cephalosporin)
Pregnancy Category B

INDICATIONS
- Treatment of the following infections:
□ Uncomplicated urinary tract infections □ Otitis media □ Bronchitis (acute and exacerbations) □ Pharyngitis or tonsillitis.

ACTION
- Binds to the bacterial cell wall membrane causing cell death. **Therapeutic**

Effect: ■ Bactericidal action against susceptible bacteria. **Spectrum:** ■ Spectrum is similar to that of second generation cephalosporins; however, activity against streptococci staphylococci is diminished in comparison, while activity against gram-negative pathogens is enhanced, even for organisms resistant to first and second generation agents ■ Notable for activity against: □ *Hemophilus influenzae* (including β-lactamase-producing strains) □ *Escherichia coli* □ *Branhamella catarrhalis* □ *Proteus mirabilis.*

PHARMACOKINETICS
Absorption: 40–50% absorbed following oral administration (suspension produces higher blood levels than tablets).
Distribution: Widely distributed.
Metabolism and Excretion: 50% excreted unchanged by the kidneys, >10% excreted in bile.
Half-life: 180–240 min (increased in renal impairment).

CONTRAINDICATIONS AND PRECAUTIONS
Contraindicated in: ■ Hypersensitivity to cephalosporins ■ Serious hypersensitivity to penicillins.
Use Cautiously in: ■ Renal impairment (dosage reduction recommended if creatinine clearance <60 ml/min) ■ Pregnancy or lactation (safety not established).

ADVERSE REACTIONS AND SIDE EFFECTS*
CNS: headache, dizziness.
GI: diarrhea, abdominal pain, nausea, dyspepsia, flatulence, PSEUDOMEMBRANOUS COLITIS.
Derm: rashes, urticaria.
Misc: superinfection, allergic reactions including ANAPHYLAXIS, fever.

INTERACTIONS
Drug–Drug: ■ **Probenecid** increases serum levels.

*Underlines indicate most frequent; CAPITALS indicate life-threatening.

ROUTE AND DOSAGE

- **PO (Adults, Children >12 yr or >50 kg):** 400 mg/day as a single dose or 200 mg q 12 hr.
- **PO (Children):** 8 mg/kg/day as a single dose or in 2 divided doses q 12 hr; when treating otitis media use only suspension.

AVAILABILITY

- **Tablets:** 200 mg, 400 mg ▪ **Oral suspension:** 100 mg/5 ml.

TIME/ACTION PROFILE (blood levels)

	ONSET	PEAK
PO	rapid	2–6 hr

NURSING IMPLICATIONS

ASSESSMENT

- ▢ Assess patient for infection (vital signs; appearance of wound, sputum, urine, and stool; WBC; earache) at beginning and throughout therapy.
- ▢ Obtain a history before initiating therapy to determine previous use of and reactions to penicillins or cephalosporins. Persons with a negative history of penicillin sensitivity may still have an allergic response.
- ▢ Obtain specimens for culture and sensitivity prior to initiating therapy. First dose may be given before receiving results.
- ▢ Observe patient for signs and symptoms of anaphylaxis (rash, pruritus, laryngeal edema, wheezing). Discontinue the drug and notify the physician immediately if these occur. Keep epinephrine, an antihistamine, and resuscitation equipment close by in the event of an anaphylactic reaction.
- ▪ **Lab Test Considerations:** May cause false-positive results for Coombs' test and urine glucose when tested with copper sulfate method (Clinitest). Use glucose enzymatic tests (Clinistix or Tes-Tape) to test urine glucose.
- ▢ May cause elevated BUN, creatinine, AST (SGOT), ALT (SGPT), and alkaline phosphatase levels.

POTENTIAL NURSING DIAGNOSES

- ▪ Infection, high risk for (indications, side effects).
- ▪ Diarrhea (adverse reactions).
- ▪ Knowledge deficit related to medication regimen (patient/family teaching).

IMPLEMENTATION

- ▪ **PO:** Administer around the clock. Shake suspension well before administering.

PATIENT/FAMILY TEACHING

- ▢ Instruct patient to take cefixime around the clock and to finish the drug completely, even if feeling better. Advise patient that sharing of this medication may be dangerous.
- ▢ Instruct patients receiving suspension on the correct method for measuring liquid.
- ▢ Advise patient to report the signs of superinfection (furry overgrowth on the tongue, vaginal itching or discharge, loose or foul-smelling stools) and allergy.
- ▢ Instruct patient to notify physician if fever and diarrhea develop, especially if stool contains blood, pus, or mucus. Advise patient not to treat diarrhea without consulting physician or pharmacist.

EVALUATION

Clinical response to therapy can be evaluated by: ▪ Resolution of the signs and symptoms of infection. Length of time for complete resolution depends on the organism and site of infection.

CEFMETAZOLE
(sef-**met**-a-zole)
Zefazone

CLASSIFICATION(S):
Anti-infective (second generation cephalosporin)
Pregnancy Category B

INDICATIONS

- ▪ Treatment of the following infections:
- ▢ Lower respiratory tract infections

□ Skin and skin structure infections □ Urinary tract and intra-abdominal infections □ Has also been used as a perioperative prophylactic anti-infective in patients undergoing: □ Cesarean section □ Abdominal or vaginal hysterectomy □ Cholecystectomy □ Colorectal surgery.

ACTION

▪ Binds to bacterial cell wall membrane, causing cell death. **Therapeutic Effect:** ▪ Bactericidal action against susceptible bacteria. **Spectrum:** ▪ Many gram-positive cocci including: □ *Streptococcus pneumoniae* □ Group A beta-hemolytic streptococci □ Penicillinase-producing staphylococci ▪ In addition has increased activity against several other important gram-negative pathogens including: □ *Haemophilus influenzae* □ Acinetobacter □ Enterobacter ▪ *Escherichia coli* □ *Klebsiella sp* □ *Neisseria gonorrhea* (including penicillinase-producing strains) □ Providencia □ Proteus □ Serratia ▪ Also active against *Bacteroides fragilis* ▪ Has no activity against: □ Methicillin-resistant staphylococci □ Enterococcus.

PHARMACOKINETICS

Absorption: Following IV administration absorption is essentially complete. **Distribution:** Widely distributed. Penetration into CSF is poor. Crosses the placenta and enters breast milk in low concentrations. **Metabolism and Excretion:** 85% excreted unchanged by the kidneys. **Half-life:** 0.8–1.8 (increased in renal impairment).

CONTRAINDICATIONS AND PRECAUTIONS

Contraindicated in: ▪ Hypersensitivity to cephalosporins ▪ Serious hypersensitivity to penicillins. **Use Cautiously in:** ▪ Renal impairment (dosage reduction required if creatinine clearance <50 ml/min) ▪ Pregnancy, lactation, and children (safety not established, but has been used in obstetrical surgery).

ADVERSE REACTIONS AND SIDE EFFECTS*

GI: <u>nausea</u>, <u>vomiting</u>, cramps, <u>diarrhea</u>, PSEUDOMEMBRANOUS COLITIS. **Derm:** <u>rashes</u>, urticaria. **Hemat:** blood dyscrasias, hemolytic anemia, bleeding, bruising. **Local:** <u>phlebitis</u> at IV site. **Misc:** superinfection, allergic reactions including ANAPHYLAXIS and serum sickness.

INTERACTIONS

Drug–Drug: ▪ **Probenecid** decreases excretion and increases blood levels ▪ If **alcohol** is ingested within 48–72 hr a disulfiram-like reaction may occur ▪ May increase risk of bleeding with **anticoagulants, thrombolytics, nonsteroidal anti-inflammatory agents, plicamycin,** or **valproic acid**.

ROUTE AND DOSAGE

▪ **IV (Adults):** 1–2 g q 6–12 hr.

AVAILABILITY

▪ *Injection:* 1 g, 2 g.

TIME/ACTION PROFILE

	ONSET	PEAK
IV	rapid	end of infusion

NURSING IMPLICATIONS

ASSESSMENT

□ Assess patient for infection (vital signs; appearance of wound, sputum, urine, and stool; WBC) at beginning and throughout course of therapy.
□ Obtain a history before initiating therapy to determine previous use of and reactions to penicillins or cephalosporins. Persons with a negative history of penicillin sensitivity may still have an allergic response.
□ Obtain specimens for culture and sensitivity prior to initiating therapy. First dose may be given before receiving results.

---

*<u>Underlines</u> indicate most frequent; **CAPITALS** indicate life-threatening.

□ Observe patient for signs and symptoms of anaphylaxis (rash, pruritus, laryngeal edema, wheezing). Discontinue the drug and notify the physician immediately if these occur. Keep epinephrine, an antihistamine, and resuscitation equipment close by in the event of an anaphylactic reaction.

■ **Lab Test Considerations:** Monitor prothrombin time and assess patient for bleeding (guaiac stools; check for hematuria, bleeding gums, ecchymosis) daily in patient receiving cefmetazole as it may cause hypoprothrombinemia. Elderly or debilitated patients are at increased risk for hypoprothrombinemia. If bleeding occurs, it can be reversed with vitamin K, or prophylactic vitamin K 10 mg/wk may be given.

□ May cause false-positive results for Coombs' test and urine glucose when tested with copper sulfate method (Clinitest). Use glucose enzymatic tests (Tes-Tape, Clinistix) to test urine glucose.

□ May cause transient elevation in BUN, AST (SGOT), ALT (SGPT), and alkaline phosphatase.

POTENTIAL NURSING DIAGNOSES

■ Infection, high risk for (indications, side effects).
■ Diarrhea (adverse reactions).
■ Knowledge deficit related to medication regimen (patient/family teaching).

IMPLEMENTATION

■ **IV:** Change IV sites every 48–72 hr to prevent phlebitis.
■ **Intermittent Infusion:** Reconstitute with Sterile Water, Bacteriostatic Water, or 0.9% NaCl for Injection. Reconstituted solution may be further diluted to concentrations of 1–20 mg/ml in 0.9% NaCl, D5W, or LR. Solution is stable for 24 hr at room temperature and 7 days if refrigerated.
■ *Rate:* Administer over 30–60 min.
■ **Additive Incompatibility:** Do not admix with aminoglycosides; if administered concurrently, administer in separate sites.

PATIENT/FAMILY TEACHING

□ Advise patient to report the signs of superinfection (furry overgrowth on the tongue, vaginal itching or discharge, loose or foul-smelling stools) and allergy.
□ Caution patient that concurrent use of alcohol with cefmetazole may cause a disulfiram-like reaction (abdominal cramps, nausea, vomiting, hypotension, palpitations, dyspnea, tachycardia sweating, flushing). Alcohol and medications containing alcohol should be avoided during and for several days after therapy.
□ Instruct patient to notify physician if fever and diarrhea develop, especially if stool contains blood, pus, or mucus. Advise patient not to treat diarrhea without consulting physician or pharmacist.

EVALUATION

Effectiveness of therapy can be demonstrated by: ■ Resolution of the signs and symptoms of infection. Length of time for complete resolution depends on the organism and site of infection.

CEFONICID
(se-**fon**-i-sid)
Monocid

CLASSIFICATION(S):
Anti-infective (second generation cephalosporin)
Pregnancy Category B

INDICATIONS

■ Treatment of the following infections:
□ Respiratory tract infections □ Skin and skin structure infections □ Bone and joint infections □ Urinary tract and gynecologic infections □ Septicemia ■ Has also been used as a perioperative prophylactic anti-infective.

ACTION

■ Binds to bacterial cell wall membrane, causing cell death. **Therapeutic Effect:** ■ Bactericidal action against susceptible bacteria. **Spectrum:** ■ Many gram-positive cocci, including: □ *Streptococcus pneumoniae* □ Group A beta-hemolytic streptococci □ Penicillinase-producing staphylococci ■ Increased activity against several other important gram-negative pathogens, including: □ *Haemophilus influenzae* □ Acinetobacter □ Enterobacter □ *Escherichia coli* □ *Klebsiella pneumoniae* □ *Neisseria gonorrhea* (including penicillinase-producing strains) □ Providencia □ Proteus □ Serratia ■ Also active against *Bacteroides fragilis* ■ Has no activity against: □ Methicillin-resistant staphylococci □ Enterococcus.

PHARMACOKINETICS

Absorption: Well absorbed following IM administration.

Distribution: Widely distributed. Penetration into CSF is poor. Crosses the placenta and enters breast milk in low concentrations.

Metabolism and Excretion: Excreted primarily unchanged by the kidneys.

Half-life: 4.5 hr (increased in renal impairment).

CONTRAINDICATIONS AND PRECAUTIONS

Contraindicated in: ■ Hypersensitivity to cephalosporins ■ Serious hypersensitivity to penicillins.

Use Cautiously in: ■ Renal impairment (dosage reduction required if creatinine clearance <80 ml/min) ■ Pregnancy and lactation (safety not established, but has been used in obstetric surgery).

ADVERSE REACTIONS AND SIDE EFFECTS*

Derm: rashes, urticaria.

GI: nausea, vomiting, cramps, diarrhea, PSEUDOMEMBRANOUS COLITIS.

Hemat: blood dyscrasias, hemolytic anemia.

Local: phlebitis at IV site, pain at IM site.

Misc: superinfection, allergic reactions including ANAPHYLAXIS and serum sickness.

INTERACTIONS

Drug–Drug: ■ **Probenecid** decreases excretion and increases blood levels.

ROUTE AND DOSAGE

■ **IM, IV (Adults):** 0.5–2 g/day—single dose.

AVAILABILITY

■ *Injection:* 500 mg, 1 g, 10 g.

TIME/ACTION PROFILE (blood levels)

	ONSET	PEAK
IM	rapid	60 min
IV	rapid	end of infusion

NURSING IMPLICATIONS

ASSESSMENT

■ **General Info:** Assess patient for infection (vital signs; appearance of wound, sputum, urine, and stool; WBC) at beginning and throughout course of therapy.

□ Obtain a history before initiating therapy to determine previous use of and reactions to penicillins or cephalosporins. Persons with a negative history of penicillin sensitivity may still have an allergic response.

□ Obtain specimens for culture and sensitivity prior to initiating therapy. First dose may be given before receiving results.

□ Observe patient for signs and symptoms of anaphylaxis (rash, pruritus, laryngeal edema, wheezing). Discontinue the drug and notify the physician immediately if these occur. Keep epinephrine, an antihistamine, and resuscitation equipment close by in the event of an anaphylactic reaction.

■ **Lab Test Considerations:** May cause false-positive results for Coombs' test and urine glucose when tested with the copper sulfate method (Clinitest). Use glucose enzymatic tests (Clinistix, Tes-Tape) to test urine glucose.

□ May cause increase in AST (SGOT), ALT (SGPT), LDH, and alkaline phosphatase levels.

*Underlines indicate most frequent; CAPITALS indicate life-threatening.

POTENTIAL NURSING DIAGNOSES
- Infection, high risk for (indications, side effects).
- Diarrhea (adverse reactions).
- Knowledge deficit related to medication regimen (patient/family teaching).

IMPLEMENTATION
- **General Info:** Reconstitute IM and IV doses with 2 ml of Sterile Water for Injection to each 500-mg vial and 2.5 ml to each 1-g vial for concentrations of 220 and 325 mg/ml, respectively. Solution may be colorless to light amber.
- **IM:** Administer IM doses deep into a well-developed muscle mass; massage well. When administering 2-g dose, divide in half and inject into 2 large muscle mass sites.
- **IV:** Change IV sites every 48–72 hr to prevent phlebitis.
- **Direct IV:** Direct IV administration can be administered slowly over 3–5 min. Monitor for phlebitis.
- **Intermittent Infusion:** Reconstituted solution may be further diluted in 50–100 ml of D5W, D10W, D5/LR, D5/0.25% NaCl, D5/0.45% NaCl, D5/0.9% NaCl, 0.9% NaCl, or Ringer's or lactated Ringer's solution. Stable for 24 hr at room temperature and 72 hr if refrigerated.
- *Rate:* Administer over 20–30 min.
- **Y-Site Compatibility:** ▪ acyclovir.
- **Y-Site Incompatibility:** ▪ sargramostim.
- **Additive Incompatibility:** Do not admix with aminoglycosides; if administered concurrently, administer in separate sites.

PATIENT/FAMILY TEACHING
- □ Advise patient to report the signs of superinfection (furry overgrowth on the tongue, vaginal itching or discharge, loose or foul-smelling stools) and allergy.
- □ Instruct patient to notify physician if fever and diarrhea develop, especially if stool contains blood, pus, or mucus. Advise patient not to treat diarrhea without consulting physician or pharmacist.

EVALUATION
Clinical response to therapy can be evaluated by: ▪ Resolution of the signs and symptoms of infection. Length of time for complete resolution depends on the organism and site of infection.

C

CEFOPERAZONE
(sef-oh-**per**-a-zone)
Cefobid

CLASSIFICATION(S):
Anti-infective (third generation cephalosporin)
Pregnancy Category B

INDICATIONS
▪ Treatment of: □ Skin and skin structure infections □ Bone and joint infections □ Urinary and gynecologic infections □ Respiratory tract infections □ Intra-abdominal infections □ Septicemia.

ACTION
▪ Binds to the bacterial cell wall membrane causing cell death. **Therapeutic Effect:** ▪ Bactericidal action against susceptible bacteria. **Spectrum:** ▪ Activity against staphylococci is diminished in comparison to second generation cephalosporins, while action against gram-negative pathogens is enhanced, even for organisms resistant to first and second generation agents ▪ Notable is increased action against: □ Citrobacter □ Enterobacter □ *Escherichia coli* □ *Klebsiella pneumoniae* □ Neisseria □ Proteus □ Providencia □ Serratia □ *Pseudomonas aeruginosa* □ Hemophilus influenzae ▪ Has some activity against anaerobes including *Bacteroides fragilis.*

PHARMACOKINETICS
Absorption: Well absorbed following IM administration.
Distribution: Widely distributed.

Crosses the placenta and enters breast milk in low concentrations.
Metabolism and Excretion: Excreted in the bile.
Half-life: 1.6–2 hr.

CONTRAINDICATIONS AND PRECAUTIONS

Contraindicated in: ▪ Hypersensitivity to cephalosporins ▪ Serious hypersensitivity to penicillins.
Use Cautiously in: ▪ Severe hepatic and renal impairment (dosage reduction required) ▪ Pregnancy, lactation, or children <12 yr (safety not established).

ADVERSE REACTIONS AND SIDE EFFECTS*

Derm: <u>rashes</u>, urticaria.
GI: <u>nausea</u>, <u>vomiting</u>, <u>diarrhea</u>, cramps, PSEUDOMEMBRANOUS COLITIS.
Hemat: blood dyscrasias, hemolytic anemia, bleeding.
Local: <u>phlebitis</u> at IV site, <u>pain</u> at IM site.
Misc: superinfection, allergic reactions including ANAPHYLAXIS and serum sickness.

INTERACTIONS

Drug–Drug: ▪ Ingestion of **alcohol** within 48–72 hr may result in a disulfiram-like reaction ▪ May increase risk of bleeding with **anticoagulants, thrombolytics, nonsteroidal anti-inflammatory agents, plicamycin,** or **valproic acid.**

ROUTE AND DOSAGE

▪ **IM, IV (Adults):** 2–12 g/day in divided doses q 8–12 hr.

AVAILABILITY

▪ *Injection:* 1 g, 2 g.

TIME/ACTION PROFILE (blood levels)

	ONSET	PEAK
IM	rapid	1–2 hr
IV	rapid	end of infusion

NURSING IMPLICATIONS

ASSESSMENT

▪ **General Info:** Assess patient for infection (vital signs; appearance of wound, sputum, urine, and stool; WBC) at beginning and throughout course of therapy.
▫ Obtain a history before initiating therapy to determine previous use of and reactions to penicillins or cephalosporins. Persons with a negative history of penicillin sensitivity may still have an allergic response.
▫ Obtain specimens for culture and sensitivity prior to initiating therapy. First dose may be given before receiving results.
▫ Observe patient for signs and symptoms of anaphylaxis (rash, pruritus, laryngeal edema, wheezing). Discontinue the drug and notify the physician immediately if these occur. Keep epinephrine, an antihistamine, and resuscitation equipment close by in the event of an anaphylactic reaction.
▪ **Lab Test Considerations:** Monitor prothrombin time and assess for bleeding (guaiac stools; check for hematuria, bleeding gums, ecchymosis) daily in patients receiving cefoperazone, because it may cause hypoprothrombinemia. Elderly or debilitated patients are at greater risk of hypoprothrombinemia. If bleeding occurs, it can be reversed with vitamin K, or prophylactic vitamin K 10 mg/wk may be given.
▫ May cause false-positive results for Coombs' test and urine glucose when tested with copper sulfate method (Clinitest). Use glucose enzymatic tests (Clinistix or Tes-Tape) to test urine glucose.
▫ May cause elevated BUN, creatinine, AST (SGOT), ALT (SGPT), and alkaline phosphatase levels. Peak and trough blood levels should be drawn periodically on patients with hepatic, biliary, or renal dysfunction.

---

*<u>Underlines</u> indicate most frequent; **CAPITALS** indicate life-threatening.

POTENTIAL NURSING DIAGNOSES
- Infection, high risk for (indications, side effects).
- Diarrhea (adverse reactions).
- Knowledge deficit related to medication regimen (patient/family teaching).

IMPLEMENTATION
- **General Info:** Solution may be colorless to straw-colored.
- **IM:** Reconstitute IM doses with 2.8 ml of Sterile or Bacteriostatic Water for Injection to each 1-g vial or 5.4 ml to each 2-g vial. Physician may order additional dilution of 1 ml or 1.8 ml of 2% lidocaine, respectively, to minimize injection discomfort. Allow vial to stand so that foaming may dissipate.
- Inject deep into a well-developed muscle mass; massage well.
- **IV:** Change IV sites every 48–72 hr to prevent phlebitis.
- **Direct IV:** Manufacturer does not recommend direct IV administration.
- **Intermittent Infusion:** For IV administration, reconstitute each g with at least 2.8 ml of Sterile or Bacteriostatic Water for Injection or 0.9% NaCl. Do not use preparations containing benzyl alcohol when used for neonates. Shake vigorously and allow to stand following reconstitution for visualization of clarity.
- Each g in solution should be further diluted in 20–40 ml of 0.9% NaCl, D5W, D10W, D5/0.25% NaCl, D5/0.9% NaCl, D5/LR, or lactated Ringer's solution. Solution is stable for 24 hr at room temperature and 5 days if refrigerated.
- *Rate:* Administer intermittent infusions over 15–30 min. Monitor for phlebitis.
- **Continuous Infusion:** For continuous infusion, concentration should be 2–25 mg/ml.
- **Syringe Compatibility:** ▪ heparin.
- **Y-Site Compatibility:** ▪ acyclovir ▪ cyclophosphamide ▪ enalaprilat ▪ esmolol ▪ famotidine ▪ fludarabine

▪ foscarnet ▪ hydromorphone ▪ magnesium sulfate ▪ morphine.
- **Y-Site Incompatibility:** ▪ hetastarch ▪ labetalol ▪ meperidine ▪ ondansetron ▪ perphenazine ▪ promethazine ▪ sargramostim.
- **Additive Incompatibility:** Do not admix with aminoglycosides or other medications; if aminoglycosides are administered concurrently, administer separate sites.

PATIENT/FAMILY TEACHING
- Advise patient to report the signs of superinfection (furry overgrowth on the tongue, vaginal itching or discharge, loose or foul-smelling stools) and allergy.
- Caution patient that concurrent use of alcohol with cefoperazone may cause a disulfiram-like reaction (abdominal cramps, nausea, vomiting, hypotension, palpitations, dyspnea, tachycardia, sweating, flushing). Alcohol and medications containing alcohol should be avoided during and for several days after therapy.
- Instruct patient to notify physician if fever and diarrhea develop, especially if stool contains blood, pus, or mucus. Advise patient not to treat diarrhea without consulting physician or pharmacist.

EVALUATION
Clinical response to therapy can be evaluated by: ▪ Resolution of the signs and symptoms of infection. Length of time for complete resolution depends on the organism and site of infection.

CEFOTAXIME
(sef-oh-**tax**-eem)
Claforan

CLASSIFICATION(S):
Anti-infective (third generation cephalosporin)
Pregnancy Category B

INDICATIONS

- Treatment of: □ Skin and skin structure infections □ Bone and joint infections □ Urinary and gynecologic infections □ Respiratory tract infections □ Intra-abdominal infections □ Septicemia and meningitis ■ Has also been used as a perioperative prophylatic anti-infective.

ACTION

- Binds to the bacterial cell wall membrane, causing cell death. **Therapeutic Effect:** ■ Bactericidal action against susceptible bacteria. **Spectrum:** ■ Activity against staphylococci is diminished in comparison to second generation cephalosporins, while action against gram-negative pathogens is enhanced, even for organisms resistant to first and second generation agents ■ Notable is increased action against: □ Citrobacter □ Enterobacter □ *Escherichia coli* □ *Klebsiella pneumoniae* □ Neisseria □ Proteus □ Providencia □ Serratia □ *Pseudomonas aeruginosa* □ Hemophilus influenzae ■ Has some activity against anaerobes including *Bacteroides fragilis*.

PHARMACOKINETICS

Absorption: Well absorbed following IM administration.
Distribution: Widely distributed. Crosses the placenta and enters breast milk in low concentrations. CSF penetration sufficient to treat meningitis.
Metabolism and Excretion: Partly metabolized and partly excreted in the urine.
Half-life: 0.9–1.7 hr.

CONTRAINDICATIONS AND PRECAUTIONS

Contraindicated in: ■ Hypersensitivity to cephalosporins ■ Serious hypersensitivity to penicillins.
Use Cautiously in: ■ Pregnancy or lactation (safety not established) ■ Renal impairment (dosage reduction required if creatinine ≤20 ml/min).

ADVERSE REACTIONS AND SIDE EFFECTS*

Derm: <u>rashes</u>, urticaria.
GI: <u>nausea</u>, <u>vomiting</u>, <u>diarrhea</u>, cramps, PSEUDOMEMBRANOUS COLITIS.
Hemat: blood dyscrasias, hemolytic anemia.
Local: <u>phlebitis</u> at IV site, <u>pain</u> at IM site.
Misc: superinfection, allergic reactions including ANAPHYLAXIS and serum sickness.

INTERACTIONS

Drug–Drug: ■ **Probenecid** decreases excretion and increases serum levels.

ROUTE AND DOSAGE

- **IM, IV (Adults):** 1–2 g q 6–12 hr (up to 2 g q 4 hr).
- **IM, IV (Children >1 mo):** 50–180 mg/kg/day in divided doses q 4–6 hr.
- **IV (Infants 1–4 wk):** 50 mg/kg q 8 hr.
- **IV (Infants 0–1 wk):** 50 mg/kg q 12 hr.

AVAILABILITY

- *Injection:* 1 g, 2 g, 10 g.

TIME/ACTION PROFILE (blood levels)

	ONSET	PEAK
IM	rapid	0.5 hr
IV	rapid	end of infusion

NURSING IMPLICATIONS

ASSESSMENT

- □ Assess patient for infection (vital signs; appearance of wound, sputum, urine, and stool; WBC) at beginning and throughout course of therapy.
- □ Obtain a history before initiating therapy to determine previous use of and reactions to penicillins or cephalosporins. Persons with a negative history of penicillin sensitivity may still have an allergic response.
- □ Obtain specimens for culture and sensitivity prior to initiating therapy. First dose may be given before receiving results.

*<u>Underlines</u> indicate most frequent; **CAPITALS** indicate life-threatening.

□ Observe patient for signs and symptoms of anaphylaxis (rash, pruritus, laryngeal edema, wheezing). Discontinue the drug and notify the physician immediately if these occur. Keep epinephrine, an antihistamine, and resuscitation equipment close by in the event of an anaphylactic reaction.

■ **Lab Test Considerations:** May cause false-positive Coombs' test and urine glucose when tested with copper sulfate method (Clinitest). Use glucose enzymatic tests (Clinistix, Tes-Tape) to test urine.

□ May cause transient increase in BUN, AST (SGOT), ALT (SGPT), LDH, and alkaline phosphatase levels.

POTENTIAL NURSING DIAGNOSES

■ Infection, high risk for (indications, side effects).
■ Diarrhea (adverse reactions).
■ Knowledge deficit related to medication regimen (patient/family teaching).

IMPLEMENTATION

■ **General Info:** Reconstituted solution may range in color from light yellow to amber.
□ Change IV sites every 48–72 hr to prevent phlebitis.
■ **IM:** Reconstitute IM doses with 2, 3, or 5 ml of Sterile or Bacteriostatic Water for Injection in the 500-mg, 1-g, and 2-g vials, respectively. Shake well to dissolve.
□ Inject deep into well-developed muscle mass, massage well.
■ **Direct IV:** Dilute in 10 ml of Sterile or Bacteriostatic Water for Injection. Do not use preparations containing benzyl alcohol when used for neonates.
■ *Rate:* Administer slowly over 3–5 min. Monitor for phlebitis.
■ **Intermittent Infusion:** Reconstituted solution may be further diluted in 50–100 ml of D5W, D10W, lactated Ringer's solution, D5/0.25% NaCl, D5/0.45% NaCl, D5/0.9% NaCl, or 0.9% NaCl. Stable for 24 hr at room temperature and 5 days if refrigerated.
■ *Rate:* Administer over 30 min.

■ **Syringe Compatibility:** ■ heparin.
■ **Y-Site Compatibility:** ■ acyclovir, cyclophosphamide ■ famotidine ■ fludarabine ■ hydromorphone ■ magnesium sulfate ■ meperidine ■ morphine ■ ondansetron ■ perphenazine ■ sargramostim ■ tolazoline.
■ **Y-Site Incompatibility:** ■ fluconazole ■ hetastarch.
■ **Additive Incompatibility:** Do not admix with aminoglycosides; if administered concurrently, administer in separate sites.

PATIENT/FAMILY TEACHING

□ Advise patient to report the signs of superinfection (furry overgrowth on the tongue, vaginal itching or discharge, loose or foul-smelling stools) and allergy.
□ Instruct patient to notify physician if fever and diarrhea develop, especially if stool contains blood, pus, or mucus. Advise patient not to treat diarrhea without consulting physician or pharmacist.

EVALUATION

Clinical response to therapy can be evaluated by: ■ Resolution of the signs and symptoms of infection. Length of time for complete resolution depends on the organism and site of infection.

CEFOTETAN
(sef-oh-**tee**-tan)
Cefotan

CLASSIFICATION(S):
Anti-infective (second generation cephalosporin)
Pregnancy Category B

INDICATIONS

■ Treatment of the following infections: □ Respiratory tract infections □ Skin and skin structure infections □ Bone and joint infections □ Urinary tract and gynecologic infections □ Septicemia □ Intra-abdominal and biliary tract infections ■ Has also been used as a perioperative prophylactic anti-infective.

ACTION

- Binds to bacterial cell wall membrane, causing cell death. **Therapeutic Effect:** • Bactericidal action against susceptible bacteria. **Spectrum:** • Many gram-positive cocci including: □ *Streptococcus pneumoniae* □ group A beta-hemolytic streptococci □ penicillinase-producing staphylococci • Increased activity against several other important gram-negative pathogens including: □ *Haemophilus influenzae* □ Acinetobacter □ Enterobacter □ *Escherichia coli* □ *Klebsiella pneumoniae* □ *Neisseria gonorrhea* (including penicillinase-producing strains) □ Providencia □ Proteus □ Serratia • Also active against *Bacteroides fragilis* • Has no activity against: □ Methicillin-resistant staphylococci □ Enterococcus.

PHARMACOKINETICS

Absorption: Well absorbed following IM administration.

Distribution: Widely distributed. Penetration into CSF is poor. Crosses the placenta and enters breast milk in low concentrations.

Metabolism and Excretion: Excreted primarily unchanged by the kidneys.

Half-life: 3–4.6 hr (increased in renal impairment).

CONTRAINDICATIONS AND PRECAUTIONS

Contraindicated in: • Hypersensitivity to cephalosporins • Serious hypersensitivity to penicillins.

Use Cautiously in: • Renal impairment (increased dose interval recommended if creatinine clearance ≤30 ml/min) • Pregnancy and lactation (safety not established, but has been used in obstetrical surgery).

ADVERSE REACTIONS AND SIDE EFFECTS*

Derm: rashes, urticaria.

GI: nausea, vomiting, cramps, diarrhea, PSEUDOMEMBRANOUS COLITIS.

Hemat: blood dyscrasias, hemolytic anemia, bleeding.

Local: phlebitis at IV site, pain at IM site.

Misc: superinfection, allergic reactions including ANAPHYLAXIS and serum sickness.

INTERACTIONS

Drug–Drug: • **Probenecid** decreases excretion and increases blood levels • If **alcohol** is ingested within 48–72 hr, a disulfiram-like reaction may occur • May increase risk of bleeding with **anticoagulants, thrombolytics, nonsteroidal anti-inflammatory agents, plicamycin,** or **valproic acid.**

ROUTE AND DOSAGE

- **IM, IV (Adults):** 1–6 g/day in divided doses q 12 hr (1–2 g may be given q 24 hr for urinary tract infections).

AVAILABILITY

- *Injection:* 1 g, 2 g, 10 g.

TIME/ACTION PROFILE (blood levels)

	ONSET	PEAK
IM	rapid	1–3 hr
IV	rapid	end of infusion

NURSING IMPLICATIONS

ASSESSMENT

- **General Info:** Assess patient for infection (vital signs; appearance of wound, sputum, urine, and stool; WBC) at beginning and throughout course of therapy.
- □ Obtain a history before initiating therapy to determine previous use of and reactions to penicillins or cephalosporins. Persons with a negative history of penicillin sensitivity may still have an allergic response.
- □ Obtain specimens for culture and sensitivity prior to initiating therapy. First dose may be given before receiving results.
- □ Observe patient for signs and symptoms of anaphylaxis (rash, pruritus, laryngeal edema, wheezing). Discontinue the drug and notify the physi-

*Underlines indicate most frequent; CAPITALS indicate life-threatening.

cian immediately if these occur. Keep epinephrine, an antihistamine, and resuscitation equipment close by in the event of an anaphylactic reaction.

- **Lab Test Considerations:** Monitor prothrombin time and assess patient for bleeding (guaiac stools; check for hematuria, bleeding gums, ecchymosis) daily in patients receiving cefotetan as it may cause hypoprothrombinemia. Elderly or debilitated patients are at greater risk of developing hypoprothrombinemia. If bleeding occurs, it can be reversed with vitamin K, or prophylactic vitamin K 10 mg/wk can be given.
- □ May cause false-positive results for Coombs' test and urine glucose when tested with copper sulfate method (Clinitest). Use glucose enzymatic tests (Clinistix or Tes-Tape) to test urine glucose.
- □ May cause transient elevations in AST (SGOT), ALT (SGPT), LDH, and alkaline phosphatase concentrations.
- □ May cause falsely elevated serum and urine creatinine concentrations. Do not draw serum samples within 2 hr of administration.

POTENTIAL NURSING DIAGNOSES
- Infection, high risk for (indications, side effects).
- Diarrhea (adverse reactions).
- Knowledge deficit related to medication regimen (patient/family teaching).

IMPLEMENTATION
- **General Info:** Reconstituted solution may range from colorless to yellow in color.
- **IM:** Reconstitute IM doses with 2 ml of Sterile or Bacteriostatic Water for Injection or 0.9% NaCl for Injection for each 1-g vial, and 3 ml for each 2-g vial. Physician may order dilution with 0.5% or 1% lidocaine to minimize injection discomfort.
- □ Inject deep into a well-developed muscle mass, massage well.
- **IV:** Change IV sites every 48–72 hr to prevent phlebitis.
- **Direct IV:** Dilute in at least 1 g/10 ml.

- **Rate:** Administer slowly over 3–5 min. Monitor for phlebitis.
- **Intermittent Infusion:** Dilute further in 50–100 ml of D5W or 0.9% NaCl. Solution is stable for 24 hr at room temperature and 96 hr if refrigerated.
- **Rate:** Administer over 30–60 min.
- **Y-Site Compatibility:** ■ famotidine ■ fluconazole ■ fludarabine ■ insulin ■ meperidine ■ morphine ■ sargramastim.
- **Additive Incompatibility:** Do not admix with aminoglycosides; if administered concurrently, administer in separate sites.

PATIENT/FAMILY TEACHING
- **General Info:** Advise patient to report the signs of superinfection (furry overgrowth on the tongue, vaginal itching or discharge, loose or foul-smelling stools) and allergy.
- □ Caution patient that concurrent use of alcohol with cefotetan may cause a disulfiram-like reaction (abdominal cramps, nausea, vomiting, hypotension, palpitations, dyspnea, tachycardia, sweating, flushing). Alcohol and medications containing alcohol should be avoided during and for several days after therapy.
- □ Instruct patient to notify physician if fever and diarrhea develop, especially if stool contains blood, pus, or mucus. Advise patient not to treat diarrhea without consulting physician or pharmacist.

EVALUATION
Clinical response to therapy can be evaluated by: ■ Resolution of the signs and symptoms of infection. Length of time for complete resolution depends on the organism and site of infection.

CEFOXITIN
(se-**fox**-i-tin)
Mefoxin

CLASSIFICATION(S):
Anti-infective (second generation cephalosporin)
Pregnancy Category B

INDICATIONS

■ Treatment of the following infections: □ Respiratory tract infections □ Skin and skin structure infections □ Bone and joint infections □ Urinary tract and gynecologic infections □ Septicemia ■ Also used as a perioperative prophylactic anti-infective.

ACTION

■ Binds to bacterial cell wall membrane, causing cell death. **Therapeutic Effect:** ■ Bactericidal action against susceptible bacteria. **Spectrum:** ■ Many gram-positive cocci including: □ *Streptococcus pneumoniae* □ Group A beta-hemolytic streptococci □ Penicillinase-producing staphylococci ■ Increased activity against several other important gram-negative pathogens including: □ *Haemophilus influenzae* □ Acinetobacter □ Enterobacter □ *Escherichia coli* □ *Klebsiella pneumoniae* □ *Neisseria gonorrhea* (including penicillinase-producing strains) □ Providencia □ Proteus □ Serratia ■ Also active against *Bacteroides fragilis* ■ Has no activity against: □ Methicillin-resistant staphylococci □ Enterococcus.

PHARMACOKINETICS

Absorption: Well absorbed following IM administration.
Distribution: Widely distributed. Penetration into CSF is poor. Crosses the placenta and enters breast milk in low concentrations.
Metabolism and Excretion: Excreted primarily unchanged by the kidneys.
Half-life: 0.7–1.1 hr (increased in renal impairment).

CONTRAINDICATIONS AND PRECAUTIONS

Contraindicated in: ■ Hypersensitivity to cephalosporins ■ Serious hypersensitivity to penicillins.
Use Cautiously in: ■ Renal impairment (dosage reduction required if creatinine clearance <50 ml/min) ■ Pregnancy and lactation (safety not

established, but has been used in obstetric surgery).

ADVERSE REACTIONS AND SIDE EFFECTS*

Derm: <u>rashes</u>, urticaria.
GI: <u>nausea</u>, <u>vomiting</u>, cramps, <u>diarrhea</u>, PSEUDOMEMBRANOUS COLITIS.
Hemat: blood dyscrasias, hemolytic anemia.
Local: <u>phlebitis</u> at IV site, <u>pain</u> at IM site.
Misc: superinfection, allergic reactions including ANAPHYLAXIS and serum sickness.

INTERACTIONS

Drug–Drug: ■ **Probenecid** decreases excretion and increases blood levels.

ROUTE AND DOSAGE

■ **IM, IV (Adults):** 1–2 g q 6–8 hr (up to 12 g/day). For uncomplicated gonorrhea, 2 g IM single dose with 1 g probenecid PO.
■ **IM, IV (Children and Infants >3 mo):** 80–160 mg/kg/day in divided doses q 4–6 hr.

AVAILABILITY

■ *Injection:* 1 g, 2 g, 10 g.

TIME/ACTION PROFILE (blood levels)

	ONSET	PEAK
IM	rapid	30 min
IV	rapid	end of infusion

NURSING IMPLICATIONS

ASSESSMENT

□ Assess patient for infection (vital signs; appearance of wound, sputum, urine, and stool; WBC) at beginning and throughout course of therapy.
□ Obtain a history before initiating therapy to determine previous use of and reactions to penicillins or cephalosporins. Persons with a negative history of penicillin sensitivity may still have an allergic response.
□ Obtain specimens for culture and

---

*<u>Underlines</u> indicate most frequent; **CAPITALS** indicate life-threatening.

sensitivity prior to initiating therapy. First dose may be given before receiving results.

□ Observe patient for signs and symptoms of anaphylaxis (rash, pruritus, laryngeal edema, wheezing). Discontinue the drug and notify the physician immediately if these occur. Keep epinephrine, an antihistamine, and resuscitation equipment close by in the event of an anaphylactic reaction.

▪ **Lab Test Considerations:** May cause false-positive results for Coombs' test and urine glucose when tested with copper sulfate method (Clinitest). Use glucose enzymatic tests (Clinistix or Tes-Tape) to test urine glucose.

□ May cause transient increase in BUN, AST (SGOT), ALT (SGPT), LDH, and alkaline phosphatase levels.

□ May cause falsely elevated serum and urine creatinine concentrations. Do not draw serum samples within 2 hr of administration.

POTENTIAL NURSING DIAGNOSES

▪ Infection, high risk for (indications, side effects).
▪ Diarrhea (adverse reactions).
▪ Knowledge deficit related to medication regimen (patient/family teaching).

IMPLEMENTATION

▪ **General Info:** Darkened powder does not alter potency.
▪ **IM:** Reconstitute IM doses with 2 ml of Sterile Water for Injection to each 1-g vial. Physician may order dilution with 0.5% or 1% lidocaine HCl to minimize injection discomfort.

□ Inject deep into a well-developed muscle mass, massage well. IM injection is painful.
▪ **IV:** Change IV sites every 48–72 hr to prevent phlebitis.
▪ **Direct IV:** Dilute with 10 ml of Sterile Water for Injection to each 1-g vial and 20 ml to each 2-g vial. Shake well and allow to stand until solution becomes clear.
▪ *Rate:* Administer slowly over 3–5 min.
▪ **Intermittent Infusion:** Dilute further

with 50–100 ml of D5W, D10W, D5/0.25% NaCl, D5/0.45% NaCl, D5/0.9% NaCl, 0.9% NaCl, D5/LR, D5/0.02%, sodium bicarbonate, or Ringer's or lactated Ringer's solution. Stable for 24 hr at room temperature and 1 wk if refrigerated.

▪ *Rate:* Administer infusion over 15–30 min. Monitor for phlebitis.
▪ **Continuous Infusion:** May be diluted in 500–1000 ml.
▪ **Syringe Compatibility:** ▪ heparin.
▪ **Y-Site Compatibility:** ▪ acyclovir ▪ cyclophasphamide ▪ famotidine ▪ fluconazole ▪ foscarnet ▪ hydromorphone ▪ magnesium sulfate ▪ meperidine ▪ morphine ▪ ondansetron ▪ perphenazine.
▪ **Y-Site Incompatibility:** ▪ hetastarch.
▪ **Additive Incompatibility:** Do not admix with aminoglycosides; if administered concurrently, administer in separate sites.

PATIENT/FAMILY TEACHING

□ Advise patient to report the signs of superinfection (furry overgrowth on the tongue, vaginal itching or discharge, loose or foul-smelling stools) and allergy.
□ Instruct patient to notify physician if fever and diarrhea develop, especially if stool contains blood, pus, or mucus. Advise patient not to treat diarrhea without consulting physician or pharmacist.

EVALUATION

Clinical response to therapy can be evaluated by: ▪ Resolution of the signs and symptoms of infection. Length of time for complete resolution depends on the organism and site of infection.

CEFPODOXIME
(seff-poe-**dox**-eem)
Vantin

CLASSIFICATION(S):
Anti-infective (second generation cephalosporin)
Pregnancy Category B

INDICATIONS

- Useful in the treatment of the following infections due to susceptible organisms: □ Acute otitis media □ Pharyngitis/tonsillitis □ Acute uncomplicated urethral and cervical gonorrhea □ Anorectal gonorrhea in women □ Skin and skin structure □ Urinary tract infections.

ACTION

- Binds to bacterial cell wall membrane, causing cell death. **Therapeutic Effects:** ▪ Bactericidal action against susceptible bacteria. **Spectrum:** ▪ Many gram-positive cocci including: □ *Streptococcus pneumoniae*, group A beta-hemolytic streptococci and penicillinase-producing staphylococci ▪ In addition has increased activity against several other important gram-negative pathogens including: *Haemophilus influenzae, Escherichia coli, Klebsiella* sp, *Moraxella* sp, *Neisseria gonorrhea* (including penicillinase-producing strains), *Proteus sp and Serratia* sp ▪ Anaerobic spectrum includes Peptostreptococci ▪ Has no activity against methicillin-resistant staphylococci or enterococcus.

PHARMACOKINETICS

Absorption: Well absorbed following oral administration. Hydrolyzed in the intestinal wall to its active component.
Distribution: Widely distributed. Penetration into CSF is poor. Crosses the placenta and enters breast milk in low concentrations.
Metabolism and Excretion: 30% excreted unchanged by the kidneys.
Half-life: 2.1–2.8 hr (increased in renal impairment).

CONTRAINDICATIONS AND PRECAUTIONS

Contraindicated in: ▪ Hypersensitivity to cephalosporins ▪ Serious hypersensitivity to penicillins.
Use Cautiously in: ▪ Renal impairment (dosage modification required if creatinine clearance <30 ml/min—in-crease dose interval to q 24 hr) ▪ Patients >50 yr (increased risk of nephrotoxicity) ▪ Pregnancy, lactation, and children <6 mo (safety not established).

ADVERSE REACTIONS AND SIDE EFFECTS*

GI: <u>nausea</u>, <u>vomiting</u>, cramps, <u>diarrhea</u>, PSEUDOMEMBRANOUS COLITIS.
Derm: <u>rashes</u>, urticaria.
Hemat: blood dyscrasias, hemolytic anemia.
Misc: superinfection, allergic reactions including ANAPHYLAXIS and serum sickness.

INTERACTIONS

Drug–Drug: ▪ **Probenecid** increases serum levels ▪ **Antacids** decrease absorption.
Drug–Food: Absorption is increased by food.

ROUTE AND DOSAGE

- **PO (Adults):** 200–800 mg/day in divided doses q 12 hr.
- **PO (Children 6 mo–12 yr):** 10 mg/kg/day in divided doses q 12 hr (not to exceed 200 mg/day for pharyngitis/tonsillitis or 400 mg/day for acute otitis media).

AVAILABILITY

- *Tablets:* 200 mg ▪ *Oral suspension:* 50 mg/5 ml, 100 mg/5 ml

TIME/ACTION PROFILE (blood levels)

	ONSET	PEAK
PO	UK	UK

NURSING IMPLICATIONS

ASSESSMENT

- □ Assess patient for infection (vital signs; appearance of wound, sputum, urine, and stool; WBC; earache) at beginning and throughout therapy.
- □ Obtain a history before initiating therapy to determine previous use of and reactions to penicillins or cephalo-

---

*<u>Underlines</u> indicate most frequent; **CAPITALS** indicate life-threatening.

sporins. Persons with a negative history of penicillin sensitivity may still have an allergic response.

□ Obtain specimens for culture and sensitivity prior to initiating therapy. First dose may be given before receiving results.

□ Observe patient for signs and symptoms of anaphylaxis (rash, pruritus, laryngeal edema, wheezing). Discontinue the drug and notify the physician immediately if these occur. Keep epinephrine, an antihistamine, and resuscitation equipment close by in the event of an anaphylactic reaction.

▪ **Lab Test Considerations:** May cause false positive results for Coombs' test and urine glucose when tested with copper sulfate method (Clinitest). Use glucose enzymatic tests (Clinistix or Tes-Tape) to test urine glucose.

□ May cause elevated BUN, creatinine, AST (SGOT), ALT (SGPT), and alkaline phosphatase levels.

POTENTIAL NURSING DIAGNOSES

▪ Infection, high risk for (indications, side effects).
▪ Diarrhea (adverse reactions).
▪ Knowledge deficit related to medication regimen (patient/family teaching).

IMPLEMENTATION

▪ **PO:** Administer around the clock. Administer with food to enhance absorption.

□ Shake suspension well before administering. Suspension is stable for 14 days if refrigerated.

PATIENT/FAMILY TEACHING

□ Instruct patient to take cefpodoxime around the clock with food and to finish the drug completely, even if feeling better. Advise patient that sharing of this medication may be dangerous.

□ Instruct patients receiving suspension on the correct method for measuring liquid.

□ Advise patient to report the signs of superinfection (furry overgrowth on the tongue, vaginal itching or discharge, loose or foul-smelling stools) and allergy.

□ Instruct patient to notify physician if fever and diarrhea develop, especially if stool contains blood, pus, or mucus. Advise patient not to treat diarrhea without consulting physician or pharmacist.

EVALUATION

Clinical response to therapy can be evaluated by: ▪ Resolution of the signs and symptoms of infection. Length of time for complete resolution depends on the organism and site of infection.

CEFPROZIL
(seff-**proe**-zill)
Cefzil

CLASSIFICATION(S):
Anti-infective (second generation cephalosporin)
Pregnancy Category B

INDICATIONS

▪ Useful in the treatment of the following infections due to susceptible organisms: □ Acute otitis media □ Pharyngitis/tonsillitis □ Skin and skin structure infections □ Respiratory tract infections (bacterial exacerbations of acute/chronic bronchitis).

ACTION

▪ Binds to bacterial cell wall membrane, causing cell death. **Therapeutic Effects:** ▪ Bactericidal action against susceptible bacteria. **Spectrum:** ▪ Many gram-positive cocci including: *Streptococcus pneumoniae,* group A beta-hemolytic streptococci and penicillinase-producing-staphylococci ▪ In addition has increased activity against several other important gram-negative pathogens including: *Haemophilus influenzae, Escherichia coli, Klebsiella* sp, *Moraxella* sp, *Neisseria gonorrhea* (including penicillinase-producing strains) *Proteus mirabilis* ▪ Anaerobic spectrum includes Peptostreptococci, Fusibacterium, Clostridium and Bacteroides ■ Has no activity against methicillin-resistant staphylococci or enterococcus.

PHARMACOKINETICS

Absorption: Well absorbed following oral administration.
Distribution: Widely distributed. Penetration into CSF is poor. Crosses the placenta and enters breast milk in low concentrations.
Metabolism and Excretion: 60% excreted unchanged by the kidneys.
Half-life: 78 min (increased in renal impairment).

CONTRAINDICATIONS AND PRECAUTIONS

Contraindicated in: ■ Hypersensitivity to cephalosporins ■ Serious hypersensitivity to penicillins ■ Patients with phenylketonuria (suspension contains phenylalanine).
Use Cautiously in: ■ Renal impairment (dosage reduction required if creatinine clearance <30 ml/min) ■ Patients >50 yr (increased risk of nephrotoxicity) ■ Pregnancy, lactation, and children <6 mo (safety not established).

ADVERSE REACTIONS AND SIDE EFFECTS*

GI: <u>nausea</u>, <u>vomiting</u>, cramps, <u>diarrhea</u>, PSEUDOMEMBRANOUS COLITIS.
Derm: <u>rashes</u>, urticaria.
Hemat: blood dyscrasias, hemolytic anemia.
Misc: superinfection, allergic reactions including ANAPHYLAXIS and serum sickness.

INTERACTIONS

Drug–Drug: ■ **Probenecid** increases serum levels.

ROUTE AND DOSAGE

■ **PO (Adults):** 250–500 mg q 12 hr or 500 mg q 24 hr.
■ **PO (Children 6 mo–12 yrs):** 15 mg/kg/day q 12 hr.

AVAILABILITY

■ *Tablets:* 250 mg, 500 mg ■ *Oral suspension:* 125 mg/5 ml, 250 mg/5 ml.

TIME/ACTION PROFILE (blood levels)

	ONSET	PEAK
PO	UK	1.5

NURSING IMPLICATIONS

ASSESSMENT

□ Assess patient for infection (vital signs; appearance of wound, sputum, urine, and stool; WBC; earache) at beginning and throughout therapy.
□ Obtain a history before initiating therapy to determine previous use of and reactions to penicillins or cephalosporins. Persons with a negative history of penicillin sensitivity may still have an allergic response.
□ Obtain specimens for culture and sensitivity prior to initiating therapy. First dose may be given before receiving results.
□ Observe patient for signs and symptoms of anaphylaxis (rash, pruritus, laryngeal edema, wheezing). Discontinue the drug and notify the physician immediately if these occur. Keep epinephrine, an antihistamine, and resuscitation equipment close by in the event of an anaphylactic reaction.
■ **Lab Test Considerations:** May cause false-positive results for Coombs' test and urine glucose when tested with copper sulfate method (Clinitest). Use glucose enzymatic tests (Clinistix or Tes-Tape) to test urine glucose.
□ May cause elevated BUN, creatinine, AST (SGOT), ALT (SGPT), and alkaline phosphatase levels.

POTENTIAL NURSING DIAGNOSES

■ Infection, high risk for (indications, side effects).
■ Knowledge deficit related to medication regimen (patient/family teaching).
■ Noncompliance related to medication regimen (patient/family teaching).

---

*<u>Underlines</u> indicate most frequent; **CAPITALS** indicate life-threatening.

C

IMPLEMENTATION

- **PO:** Administer with food or milk to minimize GI irritation. Food slows but does not decrease absorption.
- □ Refrigerate oral suspension.

PATIENT/FAMILY TEACHING

- □ Instruct patient to finish the medication completely as directed, even if feeling better. Advise patient that sharing of this medication may be dangerous.
- □ Advise patient to report the signs of superinfection (furry overgrowth on the tongue, vaginal itching or discharge, loose or foul-smelling stools) and allergy.
- □ Instruct patient to notify physician if fever and diarrhea develop, especially if stool contains blood, mucus, or pus. Advise patient not to treat diarrhea without consulting physician or pharmacist.

EVALUATION

Clinical response to therapy can be evaluated by: ▪ Resolution of the signs and symptoms of infection. Length of time for complete resolution depends on the organism and site of infection.

CEFTAZIDIME
(sef-**tay**-zi-deem)
Ceptaz, Fortaz, {Magnacef}, Pentacef, Tazicef, Tazidime

CLASSIFICATION(S):
Anti-infective (third generation cephalosporin)
Pregnancy Category B

INDICATIONS

- ▪ Treatment of: □ Skin and skin structure infections ⊔ Bone and joint infections □ Urinary and gynecologic infections □ Respiratory tract infections □ Intra-abdominal infections □ Septicemia and meningitis due to susceptible organisms.

ACTION

- ▪ Binds to the bacterial cell wall membrane, causing cell death. **Therapeutic Effect:** ▪ Bactericidal action against susceptible bacteria. **Spectrum:** ▪ Activity against staphylococci is diminished in comparison to second generation cephalosporins, while action against gram-negative pathogens is enhanced, even for organisms resistant to first and second generation agents ▪ Notable is increased action against: □ Citrobacter □ Enterobacter □ *Escherichia coli* □ *Klebsiella pneumoniae* □ Neisseria □ Proteus □ Providencia □ Serratia □ *Pseudomonas aeruginosa* □ *Hemophilus influenzae* ▪ Has some activity against anaerobes including *Bacteroides fragilis.*

PHARMACOKINETICS

Absorption: Well absorbed following IM administration.
Distribution: Widely distributed. Crosses the placenta and enters breast milk in low concentrations. CSF penetration sufficient to treat meningitis.
Metabolism and Excretion: >90% excreted unchanged by the kidneys.
Half-life: 1.4–2 hr (increased in renal impairment).

CONTRAINDICATIONS AND PRECAUTIONS

Contraindicated in: ▪ Hypersensitivity to cephalosporins ▪ Serious hypersensitivity to penicillins ▪ Hypersensitivity to L-Arginine (Ceptaz and Pentacef formulations only).
Use Cautiously in: ▪ Renal impairment (dosage reduction required if creatinine clearance <50 ml/min) ▪ Pregnancy or lactation (safety not established).

ADVERSE REACTIONS AND SIDE EFFECTS*

Derm: <u>rashes</u>, urticaria.
GI: <u>nausea</u>, <u>vomiting</u>, <u>diarrhea</u>, cramps, PSEUDOMEMBRANOUS COLITIS.

{} = Available in Canada only.
*<u>Underlines</u> indicate most frequent; **CAPITALS** indicate life-threatening.

Hemat: blood dyscrasias, hemolytic anemia.
Local: phlebitis at IV site, pain at IM site.
Misc: superinfection, allergic reactions including ANAPHYLAXIS and serum sickness.

INTERACTIONS

Drug–Drug: ▪ **Probenecid** decreases excretion and increases serum levels.

ROUTE AND DOSAGE

▪ **IM, IV (Adults):** 0.5–2 g q 8–12 hr (250–500 mg q 12 hr for urinary tract infections).
▪ **IM, IV (Children 1 mo–12 yr):** 30–50 mg/kg q 8 hr (up to 6 g/day).
▪ **IV (Neonates <4 wk):** 30 mg/kg q 12 hr.

AVAILABILITY

▪ *Injection:* 500 mg, 1 g, 2 g, 6 g.

TIME/ACTION PROFILE (blood levels)

	ONSET	PEAK
IM	rapid	1 hr
IV	rapid	end of infusion

NURSING IMPLICATIONS

ASSESSMENT

□ Assess patient for infection (vital signs; appearance of wound, sputum, urine, and stool; WBC) at beginning and throughout course of therapy.
□ Obtain a history before initiating therapy to determine previous use of and reactions to penicillins or cephalosporins. Persons with a negative history of penicillin sensitivity may still have an allergic response.
□ Obtain specimens for culture and sensitivity prior to initiating therapy. First dose may be given before receiving results.
□ Observe patient for signs and symptoms of anaphylaxis (rash, pruritus, laryngeal edema, wheezing). Discontinue the drug and notify the physician immediately if these occur. Keep epinephrine, an antihistamine, and resuscitation equipment close by in the event of an anaphylactic reaction.

▪ **Lab Test Considerations:** May cause false-positive results for Coombs' test and urine glucose when tested with copper sulfate method (Clinitest). Use glucose enzymatic tests (Clinistix or Tes-Tape) to test urine glucose.
□ May cause increased BUN, creatinine, AST (SGOT), ALT (SGPT), LDH, and alkaline phosphatase levels.

POTENTIAL NURSING DIAGNOSES

▪ Infection, high risk for (indications, side effects).
▪ Diarrhea (adverse reactions).
▪ Knowledge deficit related to medication regimen (patient/family teaching).

IMPLEMENTATION

▪ **General Info:** Dilution causes carbon dioxide to form inside vial resulting in positive pressure; vial may require venting after dissolution to preserve sterility of vial. Not required with L-Arginine formulation (Ceptaz, Pentacef).
□ Solution may range from light yellow to amber; darkened solution or powder does not alter potency.
▪ **IM:** Reconstitute IM doses with 1.5 ml of Sterile or Bacteriostatic Water for Injection in each 500-mg vial and 3 ml in each 1 g-vial. Physician may order dilution with 0.5% or 1% lidocaine HCl to minimize injection discomfort.
□ Inject deep into a well-developed muscle mass; massage well.
▪ **IV:** Change IV sites every 48–72 hr to prevent phlebitis.
▪ **Direct IV:** Add 5 ml of Sterile Water for Injection to each 500-mg vial or 10 ml to each 1- or 2-g vial. Do not use preparations with benzyl alcohol when used for neonates.
▪ *Rate:* Administer slowly over 3–5 min.
▪ **Intermittent Infusion:** Reconstituted solution may be further diluted in at least 1 g/10 ml of 0.9% NaCl, D5W, D10W, D5/0.25% NaCl, D5/0.45% NaCl, D5/0.9% NaCl, or lactated Ringer's solution. Stable for 18 hr at

room temperature and 7 days if refrigerated.

- *Rate:* Administer over 30–60 min. Monitor for phlebitis.
- **Y-Site Compatibility:** ▪ acyclovir ▪ ciprofloxacin ▪ enalaprilat ▪ esmolol ▪ famotidine ▪ fludarabine ▪ foscarnet ▪ labetolol ▪ meperidine ▪ morphine ▪ ondansetron ▪ zidovudine.
- **Y-Site Incompatibility:** ▪ fluconazole ▪ sargramostim.
- **Additive Incompatibility:** Do not admix with aminoglycosides or sodium bicarbonate; if administered concurrently with aminoglycosides, administer in separate sites.

PATIENT/FAMILY TEACHING
- Advise patient to report the signs of superinfection (furry overgrowth on the tongue, vaginal itching or discharge, loose or foul-smelling stools) and allergy.
- Instruct patient to notify physician if fever and diarrhea develop, especially if stool contains blood, pus, or mucus. Advise patient not to treat diarrhea without consulting physician or pharmacist.

EVALUATION
Clinical response to therapy can be evaluated by: ▪ Resolution of the signs and symptoms of infection. Length of time for complete resolution depends on the organism and site of infection.

CEFTIZOXIME
(sef-ti-**zox**-eem)
Cefizox

CLASSIFICATION(S):
Anti-infective (third generation cephalosporin)
Pregnancy Category B

INDICATIONS
- Treatment of: □ Skin and skin structure infections □ Bone and joint infections □ Urinary and gynecologic infections □ Respiratory tract infections □ Intra-abdominal infections □ Septicemia and meningitis.

ACTION
- Binds to the bacterial cell wall membrane, causing cell death. **Therapeutic Effect:** ▪ Bactericidal action against susceptible bacteria. **Spectrum:** ▪ Activity against staphylococci is diminished in comparison to second generation cephalosporins, while action against gram-negative pathogens is enhanced, even for organisms resistant to first and second generation agents ▪ Notable is increased action against: □ Citrobacter □ Enterobacter □ *Escherichia coli* □ *Klebsiella pneumoniae* □ Neisseria □ Proteus □ Providencia □ Serratia □ *Pseudomonas aeruginosa* □ Hemophilus influenzae ▪ Has some activity against anaerobes including *Bacteroides fragilis.*

PHARMACOKINETICS
Absorption: Well absorbed following IM administration.
Distribution: Widely distributed. Crosses the placenta and enters breast milk in low concentrations. CSF penetration sufficient to treat meningitis.
Metabolism and Excretion: >90% excreted unchanged by the kidneys.
Half-life: 1.4–1.9 hr.

CONTRAINDICATIONS AND PRECAUTIONS
Contraindicated in: ▪ Hypersensitivity to cephalosporins ▪ Serious hypersensitivity to penicillins.
Use Cautiously in: ▪ Renal impairment (dosage reduction recommended if creatinine clearance <80 ml/min) ▪ Pregnancy or lactation (safety not established).

ADVERSE REACTIONS AND SIDE EFFECTS*
GI: <u>nausea</u>, <u>vomiting</u>, <u>diarrhea</u>, cramps, PSEUDOMEMBRANOUS COLITIS.
Derm: <u>rashes</u>, urticaria.
Hemat: blood dyscrasias, hemolytic anemia.

---

*<u>Underlines</u> indicate most frequent; CAPITALS indicate life-threatening.

Local: phlebitis at IV site, pain at IM site.

Misc: superinfection, allergic reactions including ANAPHYLAXIS and serum sickness.

INTERACTIONS

Drug–Drug: ▪ **Probenecid** decreases excretion and increases serum levels.

ROUTE AND DOSAGE

- **IM, IV (Adults):** 0.5–4 g q 8–12 hr.
- **IM, IV (Children >6 mo):** 50 mg/kg q 6–8 hr (not to exceed 200 mg/kg/day).

AVAILABILITY

- *Injection:* 1 g, 2 g, 10 g.

TIME/ACTION PROFILE (blood levels)

	ONSET	PEAK
IM	rapid	0.5–1.5 hr
IV	rapid	end of infusion

NURSING IMPLICATIONS

ASSESSMENT

- ▫ Assess patient for infection (vital signs; appearance of wound, sputum, urine, and stool; WBC) at beginning and throughout course of therapy.
- ▫ Obtain a history before initiating therapy to determine previous use of and reactions to penicillins or cephalosporins. Persons with a negative history of penicillin sensitivity may still have an allergic response.
- ▫ Obtain specimens for culture and sensitivity prior to initiating therapy. First dose may be given before receiving results.
- ▫ Observe patient for signs and symptoms of anaphylaxis (rash, pruritus, laryngeal edema, wheezing). Discontinue the drug and notify the physician immediately if these occur. Keep epinephrine, an antihistamine, and resuscitation equipment close by in the event of an anaphylactic reaction.
- ▪ **Lab Test Considerations:** May cause false-positive results for Coombs' test and urine glucose when tested with copper sulfate method (Clinitest).

Use glucose enzymatic tests (Clinistix, Tes-Tape) to test urine glucose.
- ▫ May cause increased BUN, creatinine, AST (SGOT), ALT (SGPT), and alkaline phosphatase levels.

POTENTIAL NURSING DIAGNOSES

- ▪ Infection, high risk for (indications, side effects).
- ▪ Diarrhea (adverse reactions).
- ▪ Knowledge deficit related to medication regimen (patient/family teaching).

IMPLEMENTATION

- ▪ **General Info:** Solution varies in color from yellow to amber.
- ▪ **IM:** Reconstitute IM doses with 3 ml of Sterile Water for Injection in each 1-g vial or 6 ml in each 2-g vial for a concentration of 270 mg/ml.
- ▫ Inject deep into a well-developed muscle mass; massage well.
- ▪ **IV:** Change IV sites every 48–72 hr to prevent phlebitis.
- ▪ **Direct IV:** For direct IV administration dilute with 10 ml of Sterile Water for Injection in each 1-g vial or 20 ml in each 2-g vial.
- ▪ *Rate:* Administer slowly over 3–5 min.
- ▪ **Intermittent Infusion:** May be further diluted in 50–100 ml of D5W, D10W, 0.9% NaCl, D5/0.25% NaCl, D5/0.45% NaCl, D5/0.9% NaCl, or lactated Ringer's solution. Stable for 8 hr at room temperature and 48 hr if refrigerated.
- ▪ *Rate:* Administer over 30 min. Monitor for phlebitis.
- ▪ **Y-Site Compatibility:** ▪ acyclovir ▪ enalaprilat ▪ esmolol ▪ famotidine ▪ fludarabine ▪ foscarnet ▪ hydromorphone ▪ labetalol ▪ meperidine ▪ morphine ▪ ondansetron ▪ sargramostim.
- ▪ **Additive Incompatibility:** Do not admix with aminoglycosides; if administered concurrently, administer in separate sites.

PATIENT/FAMILY TEACHING

- ▫ Advise patient to report the signs of superinfection (furry overgrowth on the tongue, vaginal itching or discharge, loose or foul-smelling stools) and allergy.

□ Instruct patient to notify physician if fever and diarrhea develop, especially if stool contains blood, pus, or mucus. Advise patient not to treat diarrhea without consulting physician or pharmacist.

EVALUATION

Clinical response to therapy can be evaluated by: ■ Resolution of the signs and symptoms of infection. Length of time for complete resolution depends on the organism and site of infection.

CEFTRIAXONE
(cef-try-**ax**-one)
Rocephin

CLASSIFICATION(S):
Anti-infective (third generation cephalosporin)
Pregnancy Category B

INDICATIONS

■ Treatment of: □ Skin and skin structure infections □ Bone and joint infections □ Urinary and gynecologic infections (including chancroid, gonorrhea, and acute pelvic inflammatory disease) □ Respiratory tract infections □ Intra-abdominal infections □ Meningitis ■ Has also been used as a perioperative prophylactic anti-infective.

ACTION

■ Binds to the bacterial cell wall membrane, causing cell death. **Therapeutic Effect:** ■ Bactericidal action against susceptible bacteria. **Spectrum:** ■ Activity against staphylococci is diminished in comparison to second generation cephalosporins, while action against gram-negative pathogens is enhanced, even for organisms resistant to first and second generation agents ■ Notable is increased action against: □ Citrobacter □ Enterobacter □ *Escherichia coli* □ *Klebsiella pneumoniae* □ Neisseria □ Proteus □ Providencia □ Serratia □ Hemophilus influenzae □ *Pseudomonas aeruginosa* ■ Has some activity against anaerobes including *Bacteroides fragilis*.

PHARMACOKINETICS

Absorption: Well absorbed following IM administation.

Distribution: Widely distributed. Crosses the placenta and enters breast milk in low concentrations. CSF penetration sufficient to treat meningitis.

Metabolism and Excretion: Partly metabolized, partly excreted in the urine.

Half-life: 5.4–10.9 hr.

CONTRAINDICATIONS AND PRECAUTIONS

Contraindicated in: ■ Hypersensitivity to cephalosporins ■ Serious hypersensitivity to penicillins.

Use Cautiously in: ■ Pregnancy or lactation (safety not established).

ADVERSE REACTIONS AND SIDE EFFECTS*

GI: nausea, vomiting, diarrhea, cramps, PSEUDOMEMBRANOUS COLITIS.

Derm: rashes, urticaria.

Hemat: blood dyscrasias, hemolytic anemia.

Local: phlebitis at IV site, pain at IM site.

Misc: superinfection, allergic reactions including ANAPHYLAXIS and serum sickness.

INTERACTIONS

Drug–Drug: None significant.

ROUTE AND DOSAGE

■ **IM, IV (Adults):** 1–2 g/day, single dose or divided doses q 12 hr (250 mg single dose for uncomplicated gonorrhea).

■ **IM, IV (Children):** 50–75 mg/kg/day single dose or divided doses q 12 hr (50 mg/kg q 12 hr for meningitis; may precede with 75 mg/kg loading dose or 80 mg/kg q 12 hr for 3 doses, then q 24 hr).

C

AVAILABILITY

- *Injection:* 500 mg, 1 g, 2 g, 10 g.

TIME/ACTION PROFILE (blood levels)

	ONSET	PEAK
IM	rapid	1–2 hr
IV	rapid	end of infusion

NURSING IMPLICATIONS

ASSESSMENT

- Assess patient for infection (vital signs; appearance of wound, sputum, urine, and stool; WBC) at beginning and throughout course of therapy.
- Obtain a history before initiating therapy to determine previous use of and reactions to penicillins or cephalosporins. Persons with a negative history of penicillin sensitivity may still have an allergic response.
- Obtain specimens for culture and sensitivity prior to initiating therapy. First dose may be given before receiving results.
- Observe patient for signs and symptoms of anaphylaxis (rash, pruritus, laryngeal edema, wheezing). Discontinue the drug and notify the physician immediately if these occur. Keep epinephrine, an antihistamine, and resuscitation equipment close by in the event of an anaphylactic reaction.
- **Lab Test Considerations:** May cause increased BUN, creatinine, AST (SGOT), ALT (SGPT), bilirubin, and alkaline phosphatase levels.
- May cause false-positive results for Coombs' test and urine glucose when copper sulfate method is used (Clinitest). Use glucose enzymatic tests (Clinistix, Tes-Tape) to test urine glucose.

POTENTIAL NURSING DIAGNOSES

- Infection, high risk for (indications, side effects).
- Diarrhea (adverse reactions).
- Knowledge deficit related to medication regimen (patient/family teaching).

IMPLEMENTATION

- **General Info:** Reconstituted solution may vary in color from light yellow to amber.
- **IM:** Reconstitute IM doses with 0.9 ml of Sterile or Bacteriostatic Water for Injection, D5W, or 0.9% NaCl for Injection in each 250-mg vial, 1.8 ml in each 500-mg vial, 3.6 ml in each 1-g vial or 7.2 ml in each 2-g vial. Physician may order dilution with 1% lidocaine HCl to minimize injection discomfort.
- Inject deep into a well-developed muscle mass; massage well.
- **IV:** Change IV sites every 48–72 hr to prevent phlebitis.
- **Intermittent Infusion:** For intermittent infusion reconstitute each 250-mg vial with 2.4 ml, each 500-mg vial with 4.8 ml, each 1-g vial with 9.6 ml, and each 2-g vial with 19.2 ml of Sterile Water for Injection, 0.9% NaCl, or D5W. Do not use preparations containing benzyl alcohol when used for neonates.
- Solution may be diluted further in 50–100 ml of 0.9% NaCl, D5W, D10W, D5/0.45% NaCl, or lactated Ringer's solution. Stable for 3 days at room temperature.
- *Rate:* Administer infusion over 30–60 min. Monitor for phlebitis.
- **Y-Site Compatibility:** ■ acyclovir ■ fludarabine ■ foscarnet ■ meperidine ■ morphine ■ sargramastim ■ zidovudine.
- **Y-Site Incompatibility:** ■ fluconazole ■ vancomycin.
- **Additive Incompatibility:** Do not admix with aminoglycosides; if administered concurrently, administer in separate sites.

PATIENT/FAMILY TEACHING

- Advise patient to report the signs of superinfection (furry overgrowth on the tongue, vaginal itching or discharge, loose or foul-smelling stools) and allergy.
- Instruct patient to notify physician if fever and diarrhea develop, especially if stool contains blood, pus, or mu-

cus. Advise patient not to treat diarrhea without consulting physician or pharmacist.

EVALUATION

Clinical response to therapy can be evaluated by: ▪ Resolution of the signs and symptoms of infection. Length of time for complete resolution depends on the organism and site of infection.

CEFUROXIME
(se-fyoor-**ox**-eem)
Ceftin, Kefurox, Zinacef

CLASSIFICATION(S):
Anti-infective (second generation cephalosporin)
Pregnancy Category B

INDICATIONS

▪ Treatment of the following infections: □ Respiratory tract infections □ Skin and skin structure infections □ Bone and joint infections □ Urinary tract and gynecologic infections including uncomplicated gonorrhea □ Septicemia and meningitis ▪ Oral form to treat pharyngitis, tonsillitis, and otitis ▪ Has been used as a perioperative prophylactic anti-infective.

ACTION

▪ Binds to bacterial cell wall membrane, causing cell death. **Therapeutic Effect:** ▪ Bactericidal action against susceptible bacteria. **Spectrum:** ▪ Many gram-positive cocci including: □ *Streptococcus pneumoniae* □ Group A beta-hemolytic streptococci □ Penicillinase-producing staphylococci ▪ Increased activity against several other important gram-negative pathogens including: □ *Haemophilus influenzae* □ Acinetobacter □ Enterobacter □ *Escherichia coli* □ *Klebsiella pneumoniae* □ *Neisseria gonorrhea* (including penicillinase-producing strains) □ Providencia □ Proteus □ Serratia ▪ Also active against *Bacteroides fragilis* ▪ Has no activity

against: □ Methicillin-resistant staphylococci □ Enterococcus.

PHARMACOKINETICS

Absorption: Well absorbed following IM administration. Oral absorption is enhanced by food (52% with food, 37% fasting).

Distribution: Widely distributed. Penetration into CSF sufficient to treat meningitis. Crosses the placenta and enters breast milk in low concentrations.

Metabolism and Excretion: Excreted primarily unchanged by the kidneys.

Half-life: 1.3 hr (increased in renal impairment).

CONTRAINDICATIONS AND PRECAUTIONS

Contraindicated in: ▪ Hypersensitivity to cephalosporins ▪ Serious hypersensitivity to penicillins.

Use Cautiously in: ▪ Renal impairment (dosage reduction required if creatinine clearance <20 ml/min) ▪ Pregnancy and lactation (safety not established, but has been used in obstetric surgery).

ADVERSE REACTIONS AND SIDE EFFECTS*

GI: <u>nausea</u>, <u>vomiting</u>, cramps, <u>diarrhea</u>, PSEUDOMEMBRANOUS COLITIS.

Derm: <u>rashes</u>, urticaria.

Hemat: blood dyscrasias, hemolytic anemia.

Local: <u>phlebitis</u> at IV site, <u>pain</u> at IM site.

Misc: superinfection, allergic reactions including ANAPHYLAXIS and serum sickness.

INTERACTIONS

Drug–Drug: ▪ Probenecid decreases excretion and increases blood levels.

ROUTE AND DOSAGE

▪ **PO (Adults and Children >12 yr):** 125–500 mg twice daily. For uncomplicated gonorrhea 1 g single dose.

▪ **PO (Children <12 yr):** 125 mg

---

*<u>Underlines</u> indicate most frequent; CAPITALS indicate life-threatening.

twice daily (250 mg twice daily for otitis media in children >2 yr).

- **IM, IV (Adults):** 2.25–9 g/day in divided doses q 6–8 hr. (For uncomplicated gonorrhea—1.5 g IM single dose with 1 g probenecid PO).
- **IM, IV (Children and Infants >3 mo):** 50–100 mg/kg/day in divided doses every 6–8 hr (for meningitis: 200–240 mg/kg/day in divided doses q 6–8 hr).

AVAILABILITY

- **Tablets:** 125 mg, 250 mg, 500 mg
- **Injection:** 150 mg, 1.5 g, 7.5 g.

TIME/ACTION PROFILE (blood levels)

	ONSET	PEAK
PO	rapid	2 hr
IM	rapid	15–60 min
IV	rapid	end of infusion

NURSING IMPLICATIONS

ASSESSMENT

- ▫ Assess patient for infection (vital signs; appearance of wound, sputum, urine, and stool; WBC) at beginning and throughout course of therapy.
- ▫ Obtain a history before initiating therapy to determine previous use of and reactions to penicillins or cephalosporins. Persons with a negative history of penicillin sensitivity may still have an allergic response.
- ▫ Obtain specimens for culture and sensitivity prior to initiating therapy. First dose may be given before receiving results.
- ▫ Observe patient for signs and symptoms of anaphylaxis (rash, pruritus, laryngeal edema, wheezing). Discontinue the drug and notify the physician immediately if these occur. Keep epinephrine, an antihistamine, and resuscitation equipment close by in the event of an anaphylactic reaction.
- **Lab Test Considerations:** May cause false-positive results for Coombs' test and urine glucose when tested with copper sulfate method (Clinitest). Use glucose enzymatic tests (Clinistix or Tes-Tape) to test urine glucose.

- ▫ May cause false-negative blood glucose test results with ferricyanide tests. Use glucose enzymatic or hexokinase tests to determine blood glucose concentrations.
- ▫ May cause increased AST (SGOT), ALT (SGPT), alkaline phosphatase and bilirubin levels and decreased hemoglobin and hematocrit levels.

POTENTIAL NURSING DIAGNOSES

- Infection, high risk for (indications, side effects).
- Diarrhea (adverse reactions).
- Knowledge deficit related to medication regimen (patient/family teaching).

IMPLEMENTATION

- **General Info:** Reconstituted solution is light yellow to amber in color. Do not use solution that is cloudy or contains a precipitate.
- **PO:** Tablets may be crushed and mixed with food; however, crushed tablets have a strong, persistent bitter taste. Alternative therapy should be considered for children that cannot swallow tablets.
- **IM:** Reconstitute IM doses with 3.6 ml of Sterile Water for Injection to each 750-mg vial.
- ▫ Inject deep into a well-developed muscle mass; massage well.
- **IV:** Change IV sites every 48–72 hr to prevent phlebitis.
- **Direct IV:** Add 8 ml of Sterile Water for Injection to each 750-mg vial or 16 ml to 1.5-g vial for a concentration of 90 mg/ml.
- **Rate:** Administer slowly over 3–5 min.
- **Intermittent Infusion:** Solution may be further diluted in 100 ml of 0.9% NaCl, D5W, D10W, D5/0.45% NaCl, or D5/0.9% NaCl. Stable for 24 hr at room temperature and 1 wk if refrigerated.
- **Rate:** Administer over 30 min. Monitor for phlebitis.
- **Continuous Infusion:** May also be diluted in 500–1000 ml for continuous infusion.
- **Y-Site Compatibility:** ■ acyclovir

- atracurium ■ cyclophosphamide
■ famotidine ■ fludarabine ■ foscarnet
■ hydromorphone ■ meperidine ■ morphine ■ ondansetron ■ pancuronium
■ perphenazine ■ sargramostim ■ vecuronium.
- **Y-Site Incompatibility:** ■ fluconazole.
- **Additive Incompatibility:** Do not admix with aminoglycosides; if administered concurrently, administer in separate sites.

PATIENT/FAMILY TEACHING

□ Instruct patient to take medication around the clock and to finish drug completely, even if feeling better. Caution patient that sharing of this medication may be dangerous.
□ Advise patient to report the signs of superinfection (furry overgrowth on the tongue, vaginal itching or discharge, loose or foul-smelling stools) and allergy.
□ Instruct patient to notify physician if fever and diarrhea develop, especially if stool contains blood, pus, or mucus. Advise patient not to treat diarrhea without consulting physician or pharmacist.

EVALUATION

Clinical response to therapy can be evaluated by: ■ Resolution of the signs and symptoms of infection. Length of time for complete resolution depends on the organism and site of infection.

CEPHALEXIN
(sef-a-**lex**-in)
Biocel, C-Lexin, Cefanex, {Ceporex}, Keflet, Keflex, Keftab, {Novolexin}, {Nu-Cephalex}, {Zartan}

CLASSIFICATION(S):
Anti-infective (first generation cephalosporin)
Pregnancy Category B

INDICATIONS

- Treatment of: □ Serious skin and skin structure infections □ Urinary tract in-

fections □ Bone and joint infections □ Septicemia □ Respiratory tract infections □ Otitis media.

ACTION

■ Binds to bacterial cell wall membrane, causing cell death. **Therapeutic Effect:** ■ Bactericidal action against susceptible bacteria. **Spectrum:** ■ Active against many gram-positive cocci including: □ *Streptococcus pneumoniae* □ Group A beta-hemolytic streptococci □ Penicillinase-producing staphylococci ■ Active against some gram-negative rods including: □ *Klebsiella pneumoniae* □ *Proteus mirabilis* □ *Escherichia coli* ■ Not active against: □ Methicillin-resistant staphylococci □ *Bacteroides fragilis* □ Enterococcus.

PHARMACOKINETICS

Absorption: Well absorbed following oral administration.
Distribution: Widely distributed. Crosses the placenta and enters breast milk in low concentrations. Minimal penetration into CSF.
Metabolism and Excretion: Excreted almost entirely unchanged by the kidneys.
Half-life: 0.5–1.2 hr; cephradine, 0.7–2 hr.

CONTRAINDICATIONS AND PRECAUTIONS

Contraindicated in: ■ Hypersensitivity to cephalosporins ■ Serious hypersensitivity to penicillins.
Use Cautiously in: ■ Renal impairment (dosage reduction required) ■ Patients >50 yr (increased risk of renal toxicity) ■ Pregnancy or lactation (safety not established).

ADVERSE REACTIONS AND SIDE EFFECTS*

GI: <u>nausea</u>, <u>vomiting</u>, cramps, <u>diarrhea</u>, PSEUDOMEMBRANOUS COLITIS.
GU: nephrotoxicity.
Derm: <u>rashes</u>, urticaria.
Hemat: blood dyscrasias, hemolytic anemia.

{} = Available in Canada only.
*<u>Underlines</u> indicate most frequent; CAPITALS indicate life-threatening.

Local: phlebitis at IV site, pain at IM site.
Misc: superinfection, allergic reactions including ANAPHYLAXIS and serum sickness.

INTERACTIONS

Drug–Drug: ▪ **Probenecid** decreases excretion and increases blood levels.

ROUTE AND DOSAGE

▪ **PO (Adults):** 250–500 mg q 6 hr (500 mg q 12 hr for cystitis).
▪ **PO (Children):** 25–50 mg/kg/day in divided doses q 6 hr.

AVAILABILITY

▪ *Tablets:* 250 mg, 500 mg, 1 g ▪ *Capsules:* 250 mg, 500 mg ▪ *Oral suspension:* 100 mg/ml, 125 mg/5 ml, 250 mg/5 ml.

TIME/ACTION PROFILE (blood levels)

	ONSET	PEAK
PO	rapid	1 hr

NURSING IMPLICATIONS

ASSESSMENT

▫ Assess patient for infection (vital signs; appearance of wound, sputum, urine, and stool; WBC; earache) at beginning and throughout therapy.
▫ Obtain a history before initiating therapy to determine previous use of and reactions to penicillins or cephalosporins. Persons with a negative history of penicillin sensitivity may still have an allergic response.
▫ Obtain specimens for culture and sensitivity prior to initiating therapy. First dose may be given before receiving results.
▫ Observe patient for signs and symptoms of anaphylaxis (rash, pruritus, laryngeal edema, wheezing). Discontinue the drug and notify the physician immediately if these occur. Keep epinephrine, an antihistamine, and resuscitation equipment close by in the event of an anaphylactic reaction.
▪ **Lab Test Considerations:** May cause false-positive results for Coombs' test and urine glucose when tested with copper sulfate method (Clinitest). Use glucose enzymatic tests (Clinistix or Tes-Tape) to test urine glucose.
▫ May cause elevated AST (SGOT), ALT (SGPT), and alkaline phosphatase levels.

POTENTIAL NURSING DIAGNOSES

▪ Infection, high risk for (indications, side effects).
▪ Knowledge deficit related to medication regimen (patient/family teaching).
▪ Noncompliance related to medication regimen (patient/family teaching).

IMPLEMENTATION

▪ **PO:** Administer with food or milk to minimize GI irritation. Food slows but does not decrease absorption.
▫ Refrigerate oral suspensions.

PATIENT/FAMILY TEACHING

▫ Instruct patients to finish the medication completely as directed, even if feeling better. Advise patients that sharing of this medication may be dangerous.
▫ Advise patient to report the signs of superinfection (furry overgrowth on the tongue, vaginal itching or discharge, loose or foul-smelling stools) and allergy.
▫ Instruct patient to notify physician if fever and diarrhea develop, especially if stool contains blood, mucus, or pus. Advise patient not to treat diarrhea without consulting physician or pharmacist.

EVALUATION

Clinical response to therapy can be evaluated by: ▪ Resolution of the signs and symptoms of infection. Length of time for complete resolution depends on the organism and site of infection.

CEPHALOTHIN
(sef-**a**-loe-thin)
{Ceporacin}, {Keflin}, Keflin Neutral, Seffin Neutral

CLASSIFICATION(S):
Anti-infective (first generation cephalosporin)
Pregnancy Category B

INDICATIONS

■ Treatment of: □ Serious skin and skin structure infections □ Urinary tract infections □ Bone and joint infections □ Endocarditis □ Septicemia ■ Also used as a perioperative prophylactic anti-infective.

ACTION

■ Binds to bacterial cell wall membrane, causing cell death. **Therapeutic Effect:** ■ Bactericidal action against susceptible bacteria. **Spectrum:** ■ Active against many gram-positive cocci including: □ *Streptococcus pneumoniae* □ Group A beta-hemolytic streptococci □ Penicillinase-producing staphylococci ■ Active against some gram-negative rods including: □ *Klebsiella pneumoniae* □ *Proteus mirabilis* □ *Escherichia coli* ■ Not active against: □ Methicillin-resistant staphylococci □ *Bacteroides fragilis* □ Enterococcus.

PHARMACOKINETICS

Absorption: Well absorbed following IM administration.
Distribution: Widely distributed. Crosses the placenta and enters breast milk in low concentrations. Minimal penetration into CSF.
Metabolism and Excretion: Excreted almost entirely unchanged by the kidneys.
Half-life: 0.5–1 hr.

CONTRAINDICATIONS AND PRECAUTIONS

Contraindicated in: ■ Hypersensitivity to cephalosporins ■ Serious hypersensitivity to penicillins.
Use Cautiously in: ■ Renal impairment (dosage reduction required if creatinine clearance <80 ml/min) ■ Patients >50 yr (increased risk of renal

toxicity) ■ Pregnancy or lactation (safety not established).

ADVERSE REACTIONS AND SIDE EFFECTS*

GI: nausea, vomiting, cramps, diarrhea, PSEUDOMEMBRANOUS COLITIS.
GU: nephrotoxicity.
Derm: rashes, urticaria.
Hemat: blood dyscrasias, hemolytic anemia.
Local: phlebitis at IV site, pain at IM site.
Misc: superinfection, allergic reactions including ANAPHYLAXIS and serum sickness.

INTERACTIONS

Drug–Drug: ■ **Probenecid** decreases excretion and increases blood levels ■ May potentiate nephrotoxicity from other **nephrotoxic agents (aminoglycosides)**.

ROUTE AND DOSAGE

■ **IM, IV (Adults):** 0.5–2 g q 4–6 hr (up to 2 g q 4 hr).
■ **IM, IV (Children):** 80–160 mg/kg/day in divided doses q 4–6 hr.

AVAILABILITY

■ *Injection:* 1 g, 2 g, 20 g.

TIME/ACTION PROFILE (blood levels)

	ONSET	PEAK
IM	rapid	0.5 hr
IV	rapid	end of infusion

NURSING IMPLICATIONS

ASSESSMENT

□ Assess patient for infection (vital signs; appearance of wound, sputum, urine, and stool; WBC) at beginning and throughout course of therapy.
□ Obtain a history before initiating therapy to determine previous use of and reactions to penicillins or cephalosporins. Persons with a negative history of penicillin sensitivity may still have an allergic response.

□ Obtain specimens for culture and sensitivity prior to initiating therapy. First dose may be given before receiving results.

□ Observe patient for signs and symptoms of anaphylaxis (rash, pruritus, laryngeal edema, wheezing). Discontinue the drug and notify the physician immediately if these occur. Keep epinephrine, an antihistamine, and resuscitation equipment close by in the event of an anaphylactic reaction.

□ Monitor intake and output ratios and daily weight. Patients with impaired renal function, over age 50, or receiving other nephrotoxic drugs are at risk for developing nephrotoxicity with high-dose therapy.

▪ **Lab Test Considerations:** May cause false-positive results for Coombs' test and urine glucose when tested with copper sulfate method (Clinitest). Use glucose enzymatic tests (Clinistix or Tes-Tape) to test urine glucose.

□ May cause increased BUN, AST (SGOT), ALT (SGPT), and alkaline phosphatase levels.

POTENTIAL NURSING DIAGNOSES

▪ Infection, high risk for (indications, side effects).

▪ Diarrhea (adverse reactions).

▪ Knowledge deficit related to medication regimen (patient/family teaching).

IMPLEMENTATION

▪ **General Info:** Darkened color of solution does not affect potency. Do not administer solution that is cloudy or contains a precipitate.

▪ **IM:** Reconstitute IM doses with 4 ml of Sterile Water for Injection to each 1-g vial. May use additional diluent (0.2–0.4 ml) and warm slightly to facilitate dissolution.

□ Inject deep into a well-developed muscle mass; massage well.

▪ **IV:** Change IV sites every 48–72 hr to prevent phlebitis.

□ Hydrocortisone 10–25 mg may be added to infusions containing 4–6 g or more of cephalothin to decrease the incidence of thrombophlebitis.

▪ **Direct IV:** Dilute in at least 1 g/10 ml of Sterile Water for Injection, D5W, or 0.9% NaCl.

▪ *Rate:* Administer slowly over 3–5 min.

▪ **Intermittent Infusion:** Reconstituted 1-g or 2-g solution may be further diluted in 50 ml of D5W, D10W, D5/0.9% NaCl, D5/LR, lactated Ringer's solution, or 0.9% NaCl. Stable for 24 hr at room temperature and 96 hr if refrigerated.

▪ *Rate:* Administer over 15–30 min. Monitor for phlebitis.

▪ **Continuous Infusion:** May also be diluted in 500–1000 ml for continuous infusion.

▪ **Syringe Compatibility:** ▪ cimetidine.

▪ **Syringe Incompatibility:** ▪ metoclopramide.

▪ **Y-Site Compatibility:** Discontinue other IV solutions during IV administration of cephalothin.

▪ **Additive Compatibility:** ▪ hydrocortisone sodium succinate.

▪ **Additive Incompatibility:** Do not admix with aminoglycosides; if administered concurrently, administer in separate sites.

PATIENT/FAMILY TEACHING

□ Advise patient to report the signs of superinfection (furry overgrowth on the tongue, vaginal itching or discharge, loose or foul-smelling stools) and allergy.

□ Instruct patient to notify physician if fever and diarrhea develop, especially if stool contains blood, mucus, or pus. Advise patient not to treat diarrhea without consulting physician or pharmacist.

EVALUATION

Clinical response to therapy can be evaluated by: ▪ Resolution of the signs and symptoms of infection. Length of time for complete resolution depends on the organism and site of infection.

CEPHAPIRIN
(sef-a-**pye**-rin)
Cefadyl

CLASSIFICATION(S):
Anti-infective (first generation cephalosporin)
Pregnancy Category B

INDICATIONS

■ Treatment of: □ Serious skin and skin structure infections □ Urinary tract infections □ Bone and joint infections □ Endocarditis □ Septicemia ■ Also used as a perioperative prophylactic anti-infective.

ACTION

■ Binds to bacterial cell wall membrane, causing cell death. **Therapeutic Effect:** ■ Bactericidal action against susceptible bacteria. **Spectrum:** ■ Active against many gram-positive bacteria including: □ *Streptococcus pneumoniae* □ Group A beta-hemolytic streptococci □ Penicillinase-producing staphylococci ■ Active against some gram-negative rods including: □ *Klebsiella pneumoniae* □ *Proteus mirabilis* □ *Escherichia coli* ■ Not active against: □ Methicillin-resistant staphylococci □ *Bacteroides fragilis* □ Enterococcus.

PHARMACOKINETICS

Absorption: Well absorbed following IM administration.
Distribution: Widely distributed. Crosses the placenta and enters breast milk in low concentrations. Minimal penetration into CSF.
Metabolism and Excretion: Excreted almost entirely unchanged by the kidneys.
Half-life: 0.4–0.8 hr.

CONTRAINDICATIONS AND PRECAUTIONS

Contraindicated in: ■ Hypersensitivity to cephalosporins ■ Serious hypersensitivity to penicillins.
Use Cautiously in: ■ Renal impair-

ment (dosage reduction required if serum creatinine >5 mg/dl) ■ Pregnancy or lactation (safety not established).

ADVERSE REACTIONS AND SIDE EFFECTS*

GI: nausea, vomiting, cramps, diarrhea.
Derm: rashes, urticaria.
Hemat: blood dyscrasias, hemolytic anemia, bleeding.
Local: phlebitis at IV site, pain at IM site.
Misc: superinfection, allergic reactions including ANAPHYLAXIS and serum sickness.

INTERACTIONS

Drug–Drug: ■ **Probenecid** decreases excretion and increases blood levels.

ROUTE AND DOSAGE

■ **IM, IV (Adults):** 0.5–1 g q 4–6 hr.
■ **IM, IV (Children > 3 mo):** 40–80 mg/kg/day in divided doses every 6 hr.

AVAILABILITY

■ *Injection:* 500 mg, 1 g, 2 g, 4 g, 20 g.

TIME/ACTION PROFILE (blood levels)

	ONSET	PEAK
IM	rapid	0.5
IV	rapid	end of infusion

NURSING IMPLICATIONS

ASSESSMENT

□ Assess patient for infection (vital signs; appearance of wound, sputum, urine, and stool; WBC) at beginning and throughout course of therapy.
□ Obtain a history before initiating therapy to determine previous use of and reactions to penicillins or cephalosporins. Persons with a negative history of penicillin sensitivity may still have an allergic response.
□ Obtain specimens for culture and sensitivity prior to initiating therapy. First dose may be given before receiving results.
□ Observe patient for signs and symp-

toms of anaphylaxis (rash, pruritus, laryngeal edema, wheezing). Discontinue the drug and notify the physician immediately if these occur. Keep epinephrine, an antihistamine, and resuscitation equipment close by in the event of an anaphylactic reaction.

■ **Lab Test Considerations:** May cause false-positive results for Coombs' test and urine glucose when tested with copper sulfate method (Clinitest). Use glucose enzymatic tests (Clinistix or Tes-Tape) to test urine glucose.

□ May cause transient increase in BUN, AST (SGOT), ALT (SGPT), alkaline phosphatase and bilirubin levels.

POTENTIAL NURSING DIAGNOSES
■ Infection, high risk for (indications, side effects).
■ Diarrhea (adverse reactions).
■ Knowledge deficit related to medication regimen (patient/family teaching).

IMPLEMENTATION
■ **General Info:** Solution color changes do not alter potency.
■ **IM:** Reconstitute IM doses with 1 or 2 ml of Sterile or Bacteriostatic Water for Injection to each 1- or 2-g vial, respectively.
□ Inject deep into a well-developed muscle mass; massage well.
■ **IV:** Change IV sites every 48–72 hr to prevent phlebitis.
■ **Direct IV:** Dilute in 10 ml or more of Bacteriostatic Water for Injection, D5W, or 0.9% NaCl.
■ *Rate:* Administer slowly over 3–5 min.
■ **Intermittent Infusion:** Reconstituted solution may be further diluted in 50–100 ml of 0.9% NaCl, D5W, D10W, D20W, D5/0.25% NaCl, D5/0.45% NaCl, D5/0.9% NaCl, or D5/LR. Stable for 24 hr at room temperature and 10 days if refrigerated.
■ *Rate:* Administer over 15–20 min. Monitor for phlebitis.
■ **Continuous Infusion:** Solution may also be diluted in 500–1000 ml for continuous infusion.
■ **Y-Site Compatibility:** ■ acyclovir ■ cyclophosphamide ■ famotidine ■ heparin ■ hydrocortisone sodium succinate ■ hydromorphone ■ magnesium sulfate ■ meperidine ■ morphine ■ multivitamins ■ perphenazine ■ potassium chloride.

■ **Additive Incompatibility:** Do not admix with aminoglycosides; if administered concurrently, administer in separate sites.

PATIENT/FAMILY TEACHING
□ Advise patient to report the signs of superinfection (furry overgrowth on the tongue, vaginal itching or discharge, loose or foul-smelling stools) and allergy.
□ Instruct patient to notify physician if fever and diarrhea develop, especially if stool contains blood, mucus, or pus. Advise patient not to treat diarrhea without consulting physician or pharmacist.

EVALUATION
Clinical response to therapy can be evaluated by: ■ Resolution of the signs and symptoms of infection. Length of time for complete resolution depends on the organism and site of infection.

CEPHRADINE
(**sef**-re-deen)
Velosef

CLASSIFICATION(S):
Anti-infective (first generation cephalosporin)
Pregnancy Category B

INDICATIONS
■ Treatment of: □ Serious skin and skin structure infections □ Urinary tract infections □ Bone and joint infection □ Respiratory tract infections □ Otitis media □ Septicemia ■ Has also been used as a perioperative prophylactic anti-infective.

ACTION
■ Binds to bacterial cell wall membrane, causing cell death. **Therapeutic Effect:**

- Bactericidal action against susceptible bacteria. **Spectrum:** • Active against many gram-positive cocci including: □ *Streptococcus pneumoniae* □ Group A beta-hemolytic streptococci □ Penicillinase-producing staphylococci • Active against some gram-negative rods including: □ *Klebsiella pneumoniae* □ *Proteus mirabilis* □ *Escherichia coli* • Not active against: □ Methicillin-resistant staphylococci □ *Bacteroides fragilis* □ Enterococcus.

PHARMACOKINETICS

Absorption: Well absorbed following oral and IM administration.
Distribution: Widely distributed. Crosses the placenta and enters breast milk in low concentrations. Minimal penetration into CSF.
Metabolism and Excretion: Excreted almost entirely unchanged by the kidneys.
Half-life: 0.7–2 hr.

CONTRAINDICATIONS AND PRECAUTIONS

Contraindicated in: • Hypersensitivity to cephalosporins • Serious hypersensitivity to penicillins.
Use Cautiously in: • Renal impairment (dosage reduction required if creatinine clearance <20 ml/min). • Pregnancy or lactation (safety not established).

ADVERSE REACTIONS AND SIDE EFFECTS*

GI: nausea, vomiting, cramps, diarrhea, PSEUDOMEMBRANOUS COLITIS.
Derm: rashes, urticaria.
Hemat: blood dyscrasias, hemolytic anemia.
Local: phlebitis at IV site, pain at IM site.
Misc: superinfection, allergic reactions including ANAPHYLAXIS and serum sickness.

INTERACTIONS

Drug–Drug: • Probenecid decreases excretion and increases blood levels.

ROUTE AND DOSAGE

- **PO (Adults):** 250–500 mg q 6 hr or 500–1000 mg q 12 hr.
- **PO (Children >9 mo):** 25–100 mg/kg/day in divided doses q 6–12 hr.
- **IM, IV (Adults):** 500–1000 mg q 6 hr.
- **IM, IV (Children >1 yr):** 50–100 mg/kg/day in divided doses q 6 hr.

AVAILABILITY

- **Capsules:** 250 mg, 500 mg • **Oral suspension:** 125 mg/5 ml, 250 mg/5 ml • **Injection:** 250 mg, 500 mg, 1 g, 2 g.

TIME/ACTION PROFILE (blood levels)

	ONSET	PEAK
PO, IM	rapid	1–2
IV	rapid	end of infusion

NURSING IMPLICATIONS

ASSESSMENT

□ Assess patient for infection (vital signs; appearance of wound, sputum, urine, and stool; WBC; earache) at beginning and throughout course of therapy.
□ Obtain a history before initiating therapy to determine previous use of and reactions to penicillins or cephalosporins. Persons with a negative history of penicillin sensitivity may still have an allergic response.
□ Obtain specimens for culture and sensitivity prior to initiating therapy. First dose may be given before receiving results.
□ Observe patient for signs and symptoms of anaphylaxis (rash, pruritus, laryngeal edema, wheezing). Discontinue the drug and notify the physician immediately if these occur. Keep epinephrine, an antihistamine, and resuscitation equipment close by in the event of an anaphylactic reaction.
- **Lab Test Considerations:** May cause false-positive results for Coombs' test and urine glucose when tested with copper sulfate method (Clinitest). Use glucose enzymatic tests (Clinistix or Tes-Tape) to test urine glucose.

*Underlines indicate most frequent; **CAPITALS** indicate life-threatening.

□ May cause transient increase in BUN, AST (SGOT), ALT (SGPT), LDH, alkaline phosphatase, and bilirubin levels.

POTENTIAL NURSING DIAGNOSES

- Infection, high risk for (indications, side effects).
- Knowledge deficit related to medication regimen (patient/family teaching).
- Noncompliance related to medication regimen (patient/family teaching).

IMPLEMENTATION

- **General Info:** Reconstituted parenteral doses may vary in color from light straw to yellow. Color changes do not alter potency.
- **PO:** Administer oral doses with food or milk to minimize GI irritation.
- □ Shake oral suspension well. Refrigerate.
- **IM:** Reconstitute IM doses with 1.2 ml of Sterile or Bacteriostatic Water for Injection in each 250-mg vial, 2 ml in each 500-mg vial, 4 ml in each 1-g vial.
- □ Inject deep into a well-developed muscle mass; massage well.
- **IV:** Change IV sites every 48–72 hr to prevent phlebitis.
- **Direct IV:** Add 5 ml of sterile water, D5W, or 0.9% NaCl to each 250- or 500-mg vial, 10 ml of diluent to each 1-g vial, and 20 ml to each 2-g vial.
- **Rate:** Administer slowly over 3–5 min.
- **Intermittent Infusion:** Dilute each g in at least 10 ml of D5W, D10W, 0.9% NaCl, or D5/0.9% NaCl. Stable for 10 hr at room temperature and 48 hr if refrigerated.
- **Rate:** Administer over 30–60 min. Monitor for phlebitis.
- **Additive Incompatibility:** ▪ Ringer's ▪ Lactated Ringer's solution ▪ calcium. Do not admix with aminoglycosides; if administered concurrently, administer in separate sites.

PATIENT/FAMILY TEACHING

- □ Instruct patients to finish the drug

completely as directed, even if feeling better. Advise patients that sharing of this medication may be dangerous.
- □ Advise patient to report the signs of superinfection (furry overgrowth on the tongue, vaginal itching or discharge, loose or foul-smelling stools) and allergy.
- □ Instruct patient to notify physician if fever and diarrhea develop, especially if stool contains blood, mucus, or pus. Advise patient not to treat diarrhea without consulting physician or pharmacist.

EVALUATION

Clinical response to therapy can be evaluated by: ▪ Resolution of the signs and symptoms of infection. Length of time for complete resolution depends on the organism and site of infection.

CHLORAL HYDRATE
(**klo**-ral **hye**-drate)
Aquachloral, Noctec, {Novachlorhydrate}

CLASSIFICATION(S):
Sedative/hypnotic
Schedule IV
Pregnancy Category C

INDICATIONS

- Short-term sedative and hypnotic (effectiveness decreases after 2 wk of use)
- Sedation or reduction of anxiety preoperatively (anesthetic adjunct).

ACTION

- Converted to trichloroethanol, which is the active drug. Has generalized CNS depressant properties. **Therapeutic Effect:** ▪ Sedation or induction of sleep.

PHARMACOKINETICS

Absorption: Well absorbed following oral or rectal administration.
Distribution: Widely distributed. Crosses the placenta and enters breast milk in low concentrations.

Metabolism and Excretion: Converted by liver to trichloroethanol, which is active. Trichloroethanol is, in turn, metabolized by the liver and kidneys to inactive compounds.
Half-life: 8–10 hr (trichloroethanol).

CONTRAINDICATIONS AND PRECAUTIONS

Contraindicated in: ▪ Hypersensitivity ▪ Coma or pre-existing CNS depression ▪ Uncontrolled severe pain ▪ Pregnancy and lactation ▪ Esophagitis, gastritis, or ulcer disease ▪ Proctitis (rectal use) ▪ Tartrazine hypersensitivity (some rectal products).

Use Cautiously in: ▪ Hepatic dysfunction ▪ Severe renal impairment ▪ Patients who may be suicidal or who may have been addicted to drugs previously ▪ Elderly patients (reduce dosage).

ADVERSE REACTIONS AND SIDE EFFECTS*

CNS: excess sedation, hangover, disorientation, headache, irritability, dizziness, incoordination.
Resp: respiratory depression.
Derm: rashes.
GI: nausea, vomiting, diarrhea, flatulence.
Misc: tolerance, psychological dependence, physical dependence.

INTERACTIONS

Drug–Drug: ▪ Additive CNS depression with other CNS **depressants** including **alcohol, antihistamines, antidepressants, sedative/hypnotics,** and **opioid analgesics** ▪ May potentiate **oral anticoagulants** ▪ When given within 24 hr of IV **furosemide** may cause diaphoresis, changes in blood pressure, and flushing.

ROUTE AND DOSAGE

Anxiety, Sedation
▪ **PO (Adults):** 250 mg 3 times daily.
▪ **Rect (Adults):** 325 mg 3 times daily.
▪ **PO, Rect (Children):** 8.3 mg/kg (up to 500 mg 3 times daily).

Hypnotic
▪ **PO, Rect (Adults):** 500–1000 mg at bedtime.
▪ **PO, Rect (Children):** 50 mg/kg (up to 1 g).

Preoperative
▪ **PO (Adults):** 500 mg–1 g 30 min before surgery.

Pre-EEG Sedation
▪ **PO (Children):** 25–50 mg/kg.

AVAILABILITY

▪ *Capsules:* 250 mg, 500 mg ▪ *Syrup:* 250 mg/5 ml, 500 mg/5 ml ▪ *Suppositories:* 324 mg, 500 mg, 648 mg.

TIME/ACTION PROFILE (sedation)

	ONSET	PEAK	DURATION
PO	30 min	UK	4–8 hr
Rect	0.5–1 hr	UK	4–8 hr

NURSING IMPLICATIONS

ASSESSMENT
▫ Assess mental status, sleep patterns, and potential for abuse prior to administering this medication. Prolonged use may lead to physical and psychological dependence. Limit amount of drug available to the patient.
▫ Assess alertness at time of peak effect. Notify physician if desired sedation does not occur or if paradoxical reaction occurs.
▪ **Lab Test Considerations:** Interferes with copper sulfate urine glucose test results (Clinitest). Test for urine glucose with glucose enzymatic tests (Clinistix or Tes-Tape).
▫ Interferes with tests for urinary 17-hydroxycorticosteroids and urinary catecholamines.

POTENTIAL NURSING DIAGNOSES
▪ Sleep pattern disturbance (indications).
▪ Anxiety (indications).
▪ Injury, high risk for (side effects).

IMPLEMENTATION
▪ **General Info:** Before administering, reduce external stimuli and provide

*Underlines indicate most frequent; **CAPITALS** indicate life-threatening.

comfort measures to increase effectiveness of medication.

□ Protect patient from injury. Place bed side rails up. Assist with ambulation. Remove cigarettes from patients receiving hypnotic dose.

□ When administered before outpatient procedures for sedation in children, dose should be administered at the facility where procedure is to be performed.

■ **PO:** Capsules should be swallowed whole with a full glass of water or juice to minimize gastric irritaton; do not chew. Dilute syrup in ½ glass of water or juice.

■ **Rect:** If suppository is too soft for insertion, chill in refrigerator for 30 min or run under cold water before removing foil wrapper.

PATIENT/FAMILY TEACHING

□ Instruct patient to take chloral hydrate exactly as directed. Missed doses should be omitted; do not double doses. If used for 2 wk or longer, abrupt withdrawal may result in CNS excitement, tremor, anxiety, hallucinations, and delirium.

□ Chloral hydrate causes drowsiness or dizziness. Caution patient to avoid driving or other activities requiring alertness until response to medication is known.

□ Caution patient that concurrent alcohol use may create an additive effect that results in tachycardia, vasodilation, flushing, headache, hypotension, and pronounced CNS depression. Alcohol and other CNS depressants should be avoided while taking chloral hydrate.

□ Advise patient to discontinue use and notify physician if skin rash, dizziness, irritability, impaired thought processes, headache, or motor incoordination occur.

EVALUATION

Effectiveness of therapy can be demonstrated by: ■ Sedation ■ Improvement in sleep pattern.

CHLORAMBUCIL
(klor-**am**-byoo-sill)
Leukeran

CLASSIFICATION(S):
Antineoplastic (alkylating agent)
Pregnancy Category D

INDICATIONS

■ Management of chronic lymphocytic leukemia, malignant lymphoma, and Hodgkin's disease (alone and in combination with other agents).

ACTION

■ An alkylating agent that interferes with cellular protein synthesis (cell cycle-phase nonspecific). **Therapeutic Effect:** ■ Death of rapidly replicating cells, particularly malignant cells.

PHARMACOKINETICS

Absorption: Rapidly and completely absorbed from the GI tract.
Distribution: Crosses the placenta.
Metabolism and Excretion: Extensively metabolized by the liver.
Half-life: 1.5 hr.

CONTRAINDICATIONS AND PRECAUTIONS

Contraindicated in: ■ Hypersensitivity ■ Previous resistance ■ Pregnancy or lactation.
Use Cautiously in: Patients with childbearing potential ■ Infection ■ Other chronic debilitating diseases.

ADVERSE REACTIONS AND SIDE EFFECTS*

Resp: pulmonary fibrosis.
GI: nausea, vomiting, stomatitis (rare).
GU: decreased sperm count, infertility.
Derm: rash, dermatitis, alopecia (rare).
Hemat: anemia, leukopenia, thrombocytopenia.
Metab: hyperuricemia.
Misc: allergic reactions, risk of second malignancy.

*Underlines indicate most frequent; **CAPITALS** indicate life-threatening.

INTERACTIONS

Drug–Drug: Additive bone marrow depression with other **bone marrow depressants (antineoplastics)** ▪ May decrease antibody response to **live vaccines** and increase the risk of adverse reactions.

ROUTE AND DOSAGE

▪ **PO (Adults):** 0.1–0.2 mg/kg/day (3–6 mg/m^2/day) for 3–6 wk, then adjust dose on basis of blood counts—other regimens are used.
▪ **PO (Children):** 0.1–0.2 mg/kg/day (4.5 mg/m^2/day) single dose or divided doses.

AVAILABILITY

▪ *Tablets:* 2 mg.

TIME/ACTION PROFILE (effects on white blood cell counts)

	ONSET	PEAK	DURATION
PO	7–14 days	7–14 days	14–28 days

NURSING IMPLICATIONS

ASSESSMENT

□ Assess for fever, sore throat, and signs of infection. If these symptoms occur, notify physician immediately.
□ Assess for bleeding (bleeding gums, bruising, petechiae; guaiac stools, urine, emesis). Avoid IM injections and rectal temperatures. Hold pressure on all venipuncture sites for at least 10 min.
□ Monitor intake and output ratios and daily weights. Notify physician if significant changes in totals occur.
□ Monitor for symptoms of gout (increased uric acid, joint pain, edema). Encourage patient to drink at least 2 liters of fluid/day. Allopurinol may be given to decrease uric acid levels. Alkalinization of urine may be ordered to increase excretion of uric acid.
□ Anemia may occur. Monitor for increased fatigue, dyspnea, and orthostatic hypotension.
▪ **Lab Test Considerations:** Monitor CBC and differential prior to and weekly during course of therapy. No-

tify physician of significant drops in granulocyte count. Leukopenia usually occurs around the third week of therapy and persists for 1–2 wk following a short course of therapy. The nadir of leukopenia occurs in 7–14 days after a single high dose, with recovery in 2–3 wk. The neutrophil count may decrease for 10 days after last dose. Monitor platelet count throughout therapy. Thrombocytopenia usually occurs around third week of therapy and persists for 1–2 wk following a short course of therapy. The nadir of thrombocytopenia occurs in 1–2 wk after a single dose, with recovery in 2–3 wk. Institute thrombocytopenia precautions if platelet count is <150,000/mm.^{3}
□ Monitor liver function tests, BUN, serum creatinine, and uric acid prior to and periodically during course of therapy. May cause elevated ALT (SGPT) and alkaline phosphatase, which may reflect hepatotoxicity.

POTENTIAL NURSING DIAGNOSES

▪ Injury, high risk for (side effects).
▪ Infection, high risk for (side effects).
▪ Knowledge deficit related to medication regimen (patient/family teaching).

IMPLEMENTATION

▪ **PO:** Administer oral medication either 1 hr before or 2 hr after meals. Can be compounded into a suspension by pharmacist for patients who have difficulty swallowing.

PATIENT/FAMILY TEACHING

□ Instruct patient to take medication exactly as directed, even if nausea or vomiting is a problem. Consult physician if vomiting occurs shortly after dose is taken. If a dose is missed and the medication is ordered daily, take when remembered that day. If ordered more frequently, take unless almost time for next dose. Do not double doses.
□ Instruct patient to report unusual bleeding. Advise patient of thrombocytopenia precautions (use soft toothbrush, electric razor, and avoid falls;

do not drink alcoholic beverages or take medication containing aspirin or ibuprofen, because these may precipitate gastric bleeding).

□ Caution patient to avoid crowds and persons with known infections. Physician should be informed immediately if symptoms of infection occur.

□ Instruct patient to inspect oral mucosa for redness and ulceration. If mouth sores occur, advise patient to use sponge brush and rinse mouth with water after eating and drinking. Consult physician if pain interferes with eating.

□ Advise patients on long-term therapy to notify physician immediately if cough, shortness of breath, and fever occur.

□ Instruct patient to inform physician if nausea and vomiting persist. Physician may order an antiemetic, although these side effects usually last less than 1 day and tend to decrease with continued therapy.

□ Discuss with patient the possibility of hair loss. Explore methods of coping.

□ This drug may cause irreversible gonadal suppression; however, patient should still use birth control. Instruct patient to inform physician if pregnancy is suspected.

□ Instruct patient not to receive any vaccinations without advice of physician.

EVALUATION
Effectiveness of therapy can be demonstrated by: ■ Improvement of hematopoietic values in leukemia ■ Decrease in size and spread of the tumor ■ Therapeutic effects of this drug are usually seen by the third week of therapy.

CHLORAMPHENICOL
(klor-am-**fen**-i-kole)
AK-Chlor, Chlorofair, Chloromycetin, Chloroptic, Econochlor, {Fenicol}, {Novochlorocap}, Ocu-Chlor, Ophthochlor, {Pentamy-

cetin}, {Sopamycetin}, Spectro-Chlor

CLASSIFICATION(S):
Anti-infective
Pregnancy Category UK

INDICATIONS
■ **PO, IV:** Management of the following serious infections when less toxic agents cannot be used: □ Skin and soft tissue infections □ Intra-abdominal infections □ CNS infections □ Meningitis □ Bacteremia ■ **Top, Otic, Ophth:** Local management of localized infections.

ACTION
■ Inhibits protein synthesis in susceptible bacteria at the level of the 50S bacterial ribosome. **Therapeutic Effect:** ■ Bacteriostatic action in susceptible organisms. **Spectrum:** ■ Wide variety of gram-positive aerobic organisms including: □ *Streptococcus pneumoniae* and other streptococci ■ Gram-negative pathogens: □ *Haemophilus influenzae* □ *Neisseria menigitidis* □ Salmonella □ Shigella ■ Anaerobes: □ *Bacteroides fragilis* □ *Bacteroides melaninogenicus* ■ Other organisms inhibited: □ Rickettsia □ Chlamydia □ Mycoplasma.

PHARMACOKINETICS
Absorption: Well absorbed following oral administration.
Distribution: Widely distributed. Crosses the blood–brain barrier with CSF levels 60% of serum values. Crosses the placenta; enters breast milk.
Metabolism and Excretion: Mostly metabolized by the liver. <10% excreted unchanged by the kidneys.
Half-life: 1.5–3.5 hr.

CONTRAINDICATIONS AND PRECAUTIONS
Contraindicated in: ■ Hypersensitivity ■ Previous toxic reaction to chloramphenicol.
Use Cautiously in: ■ Newborns ■ Se-

vere liver or renal disease (increased risk of adverse reactions) ▪ Elderly patients (increased risk of adverse reactions) ▪ Pregnancy or lactation (safety not established).

ADVERSE REACTIONS AND SIDE EFFECTS*

CNS: depression, confusion, headache.
EENT: optic neuritis, blurred vision.
GI: nausea, vomiting, diarrhea, bitter taste (IV only).
Derm: rashes.
Hemat: <u>bone marrow depression</u>, APLASTIC ANEMIA.
Neuro: peripheral neuritis.
Misc: GRAY SYNDROME in newborns, fever.

INTERACTIONS

Drug–Drug: ▪ May increase effects of the following drugs: **oral hypoglycemic agents, oral anticoagulants,** and **phenytoin** ▪ **Phenobarbital** or **rifampin** may decrease chloramphenicol blood levels ▪ May delay response to **vitamin B$_{12}$** or **folic acid** therapy ▪ Bone marrow depression may be additive with **bone-marrow-depressing agents (antineoplastics)** ▪ Chronic high-dose **acetaminophen** may increase toxicity.

ROUTE AND DOSAGE

- **PO, IV (Adults):** 12.5 mg/kg q 6 hr (up to 4 g/day).
- **PO, IV (Infants >2 wk and Children):** 12 mg/kg q 6 hr or 2.5 mg/kg q 12 hr.
- **PO, IV (Premature and Full-term Infants <2 wk):** 6.25 mg/kg q 6 hr.
- **Ophth (Adults and Children):** 1–2 drops of solution or small amount of ointment q 3–6 hr.
- **Otic (Adults and Children):** 2–3 drops 2–3 times/day.
- **Top (Adults and Children):** 1% cream applied 3–4 times daily.

AVAILABILITY

- *Capsules:* 250 mg ▪ *Oral suspension:* 150 mg/5 ml ▪ *Injection:* 100 mg/ml in 1 g-vials ▪ *Ophth ointment:* 10 mg/g ▪ *Ophth solution:* 25 mg/15 ml, 5 mg/ml ▪ *Cream:* 1% ▪ *Otic solution:* 0.5% ▪ *In combination with:* hydrocortisone (chloromycetin/hydrocortisone). See Appendix A.

TIME/ACTION PROFILE (blood levels)

	ONSET	PEAK
PO	rapid	1–3 hr
IV	rapid	end of infusion

NURSING IMPLICATIONS

ASSESSMENT

- **General Info:** Assess patient for infection (vital signs; wound appearance; sputum, urine, and stool; WBC) at beginning and throughout course of therapy.
- ▢ This drug should be administered systemically only to hospitalized patients or those under close medical supervision. Diagnosis should be confirmed with cultures prior to administration.
- ▢ Assess patients daily for signs of bone marrow depression (petechiae, sore throat, fatigue, unusual bleeding, bruising). Patients that have impaired liver or renal function, infants, children, and the elderly are at the greatest risk of developing adverse effects.
- **Premature Infants and Neonates:** Assess for gray syndrome (abdominal distension, drowsiness, low body temperature, cyanosis, hypotension, and respiratory distress).
- **Lab Test Considerations:** CBC and platelet count should be monitored every 2 days throughout therapy. The drug should be stopped if anemia, reticulocytopenia, leukopenia, or thrombocytopenia develops. Notify physician promptly.
- ▢ May cause false-positive copper sulfate urine glucose tests (Clinitest). Test urine glucose with glucose enzymatic tests (Clinistix or Tes-Tape).
- **Toxicity and Overdose:** Monitor se-

*Underlines indicate most frequent; **CAPITALS** indicate life-threatening.*

rum levels weekly. Therapeutic levels: peak, 5–25 mcg/ml.

POTENTIAL NURSING DIAGNOSES
- Infection, high risk for (indications, adverse effects).
- Knowledge deficit related to medication regimen (patient/family teaching).

IMPLEMENTATION
- **General Info:** Medication should be administered around the clock.
- **PO:** Give oral doses with a full glass of water 1 hr before or 2 hr after meals. Available as an oral suspension for patients with difficulty swallowing.
- **Direct IV:** Reconstitute to a 10% solution by adding 10 ml of Sterile Water for Injection or D5W to each 1 g. Do not use preparations containing benzyl alcohol in neonates.
- **Rate:** Inject slowly over at least 1 min.
- **Intermittent Infusion:** May be further diluted in 50–100 ml of D5W, D10W, D5/0.9% NaCl, D5/0.45% NaCl, D5/0.25% NaCl, D5/LR, 0.45% NaCl, 0.9% NaCl, or lactated Ringer's solution. Solution may form crystals at low temperatures. Shake well to dissolve crystals. Do not administer cloudy solutions.
- **Rate:** Administer over 30–60 min.
- **Syringe Compatibility:** ■ heparin.
- **Y-Site Compatibility:** ■ acyclovir ■ cyclophosphamide ■ enalaprilat ■ esmolol ■ foscarnet ■ hydromorphone ■ labetalol ■ magnesium sulfate ■ meperidine ■ morphine ■ perphenazine.
- **Y-Site Incompatibility:** ■ fluconazole.
- **Ophth:** See Appendix H for instillation of ophthalmic medications.
- **Top:** Cleanse area with soap and water prior to application.

PATIENT/FAMILY TEACHING
- **General Info:** Instruct patient to take medication exactly as directed and to finish prescription, even if feeling better. Missed doses should be taken as soon as remembered if not almost time for next dose. Do not double

doses. Caution patient that sharing of this medication may be dangerous.
- Advise patient to contact physician immediately if signs of unusual bleeding; bruising; fever; sore throat; nausea; vomiting; diarrhea; numbness, tingling, burning pain or weakness in hands or feet, occur. Medication should be discontinued with the onset of these symptoms.
- Instruct patient to report signs of superinfection (stomatitis, perianal itching, vaginal discharge, fever).
- Emphasize the importance of follow-up examinations. Bone marrow depression may develop weeks to months after drug therapy has been discontinued.
- **IV:** Reassure patient that bitter taste 15–20 sec following injection is limited to 2–3 min.
- **Ophth:** Inform patient solution may cause blurred vision for a few minutes after instillation.

EVALUATION
Clinical response to therapy may be determined by: ■ Resolution of the signs and symptoms of infection. Length of time for complete resolution depends on the organism and site of infection.

CHLORDIAZEPOXIDE
(klor-dye-az-e-**pox**-ide)
{Apo-Chlordiazepoxide}, Libritabs, Lipoxide, Librium, {Novopoxide}, {Solium}

CLASSIFICATION(S):
Sedative/hypnotic (benzodiazepine)
Schedule: IV
Pregnancy Category D

INDICATIONS

■ Adjunct in the management of anxiety and as a preoperative sedative ■ Treatment of symptoms of alcohol withdrawal.

ACTION

- Acts at many levels of the CNS to produce anxiolytic effect ▪ Depresses the CNS, probably by potentiating gamma aminobutyric acid (GABA), an inhibitory neurotransmitter. **Therapeutic Effects:** ▪ Sedation ▪ Relief of anxiety.

PHARMACOKINETICS

Absorption: Well absorbed from the GI tract. Absorption from IM sites may be slow and unpredictable.

Distribution: Widely distributed. Crosses the blood–brain barrier. Crosses the placenta and enters breast milk.

Metabolism and Excretion: Highly metabolized by the liver. Some products of metabolism are active as CNS depressants.

Half-life: 5–30 hr.

CONTRAINDICATIONS AND PRECAUTIONS

Contraindicated in: ▪ Hypersensitivity ▪ Cross-sensitivity with other benzodiazepines may occur ▪ Comatose patients or those with pre-existing CNS depression ▪ Uncontrolled severe pain ▪ Narrow-angle glaucoma ▪ Pregnancy and lactation ▪ Children ≤6 yr.

Use Cautiously in: ▪ Hepatic dysfunction ▪ Severe renal impairment ▪ Patients who may be suicidal or who may have been addicted to drugs previously ▪ Elderly or debilitated patients (initial dosage reduction required).

ADVERSE REACTIONS AND SIDE EFFECTS*

CNS: <u>dizziness</u>, <u>drowsiness</u>, hangover, paradoxical excitation, headache.
EENT: blurred vision.
GI: nausea, vomiting, diarrhea, constipation.
Derm: rashes.
Local: <u>pain</u> at IM site.
Misc: tolerance, psychological dependence, physical dependence.

INTERACTIONS

Drug–Drug: ▪ Alcohol, antidepres-

sants, antihistamines, and opioid analgesics—concurrent use results in additive CNS depression ▪ Cimetidine, oral contraceptives, disulfiram, fluoxetine, isoniazid, ketoconazole, metoprolol, propoxyphene, propranolol, or valproic acid may enhance its actions ▪ May decrease efficacy of levodopa ▪ Rifampin or barbiturates may decrease effectiveness of chlordiazepoxide ▪ Sedative effects may be decreased by theophylline.

ROUTE AND DOSAGE

Alcohol Withdrawal

- PO (Adults): 50–100 mg, repeated until agitation is controlled, up to 400 mg/day.
- IM, IV (Adults): 50–100 mg initially; may be repeated in 2–4 hr.

Anxiety

- PO (Adults): 5–25 mg 3–4 times daily.
- PO (Children >6 yr): 5 mg 2–4 times daily, up to 10 mg 2–3 times daily.
- IM, IV (Adults): 50–100 mg initially, then 25–50 mg 3–4 times daily as required (25–50 mg initially in elderly patients).

Preoperative Sedation

- PO (Adults): 5–10 mg 3–4 times daily for 24 hr preop.
- IM (Adults): 50–100 mg 1 hr preop.

AVAILABILITY

▪ *Capsules:* 5 mg, 10 mg, 25 mg ▪ *Tablets:* 5 mg, 10 mg, 25 mg ▪ *Injection:* 100 mg-ampule ▪ *In combination with:* amitriptyline, clindinium. See Appendix A.

TIME/ACTION PROFILE (sedation)

	ONSET	PEAK	DURATION
PO	1–2 hr	0.5–4 hr	up to 24 hr
IM	15–30 min	UK	UK
IV	1–5 min	UK	0.25–1 hr

NURSING IMPLICATIONS

ASSESSMENT

- **General Info:** Assess patient for anxiety and level of sedation (ataxia, diz-

*<u>Underlines</u> indicate most frequent; **CAPITALS** indicate life-threatening.

ziness, slurred speech) periodically throughout course of therapy.

□ Monitor blood pressure, heart rate, and respiratory rate frequently when administering parenterally. Contact physician immediately if significant changes occur.

□ Prolonged high-dose therapy may lead to psychological or physical dependence. Restrict the amount of drug available to patient.

▪ **Alcohol Withdrawal:** Assess patient for tremors, agitation, delirium, and hallucinations. Protect patient from injury.

▪ **Lab Test Considerations:** Patients on prolonged therapy should have CBC and liver function tests evaluated periodically. May cause an increase in serum bilirubin, AST (SGOT), and ALT (SGPT).

POTENTIAL NURSING DIAGNOSES

▪ Anxiety (indications).
▪ Injury, high risk for (side effects).
▪ Knowledge deficit related to medication regimen (patient/family teaching).

IMPLEMENTATION

▪ **General Info:** Use parenteral solution immediately after reconstitution and discard any unused portion.

□ Following parenteral administration have patient remain recumbent, and observe for 3 hr.

▪ **PO:** Administer after meals or with milk to minimize GI irritation. Tablets may be crushed and taken with food or fluids if patient has difficulty swallowing. Do not open capsules.

▪ **IM:** Reconstitute with 2 ml of diluent provided by manufacturer only. Do not use solution if opalescent or hazy. Agitate gently to minimize bubbling. Administer slowly, deep into a well-developed muscle mass to minimize pain at injection site. Solution reconstituted with IM diluent should not be given IV.

▪ **Direct IV:** Reconstitute 100 mg in 5 ml of 0.9% NaCl or Sterile Water for Injection. Do not use IM diluent.

▪ *Rate:* Administer prescribed dose slowly over at least 1 min. Rapid administration may cause apnea, hypotension, bradycardia, or cardiac arrest.

▪ **Syringe Incompatibility:** ▪ benzquinamide.

▪ **Y-Site Compatibility:** ▪ heparin ▪ hydrocortisone sodium succinate ▪ potassium chloride.

PATIENT/FAMILY TEACHING

□ Instruct patient to take chlordiazepoxide exactly as directed. If medication is less effective after a few weeks, check with physician, do not increase dose. Medication should be tapered at the completion of long-term therapy. Sudden cessation of medication may lead to withdrawal (insomnia, irritability, nervousness, tremors).

□ May cause drowsiness or dizziness. Caution patient to avoid driving or other activities requiring alertness until response to medication is known.

□ Advise patient to avoid the use of alcohol and other CNS depressants concurrently with this medication. Instruct patient to consult physician or pharmacist before taking over-the-counter medications.

□ Instruct patient to notify physician if pregnancy is suspected.

EVALUATION

Effectiveness of therapy can be demonstrated by: ▪ Decreased sense of anxiety □ Increased ability to cope ▪ Decreased tremulousness and more rational ideation when used for alcohol withdrawal.

CHLOROQUINE
(**klor**-oh-kwin)
Aralen

CLASSIFICATION(S):
Antimalarial
Pregnancy Category UK

INDICATIONS

▪ Suppression, prophylaxis, and treatment of malaria. **Unlabeled Use:**

- Treatment of severe rheumatoid arthritis.

ACTION

- Inhibits protein synthesis in susceptible organisms by inhibiting DNA and RNA polymerase. **Therapeutic Effects:**
- Death of plasmodia responsible for causing malaria ■ Improvement in inflammatory arthritis.

PHARMACOKINETICS

Absorption: Well absorbed following oral administration.
Distribution: Widely distributed; high tissue concentrations achieved. Crosses the placenta, enters breast milk.
Metabolism and Excretion: 30% metabolized by the liver. Metabolite also has antiplasmodial activity. 70% excreted unchanged by the kidneys.
Half-life: 72–120 hr.

CONTRAINDICATIONS AND PRECAUTIONS

Contraindicated in: ■ Hypersensitivity ■ Hypersensitivity to other 4-aminoquinolones (hydroxychloroquine) ■ Visual damage caused by chloroquine or other 4-aminoquinolones.
Use Cautiously in: ■ Liver disease ■ Alcoholism ■ Patients receiving hepatotoxic drugs ■ Psoriasis ■ G6-PD deficiency ■ Bone marrow depression ■ Pregnancy (although safety not established, has been used) ■ Children (extremely sensitive to chloroquine effects).

ADVERSE REACTIONS AND SIDE EFFECTS*

CNS: headache, fatigue, nervousness, anxiety, irritability, personality changes, confusion, SEIZURES, dizziness.
EENT: visual disturbances, keratopathy, retinopathy, ototoxicity.
CV: hypotension, ECG changes.
GI: epigastric discomfort, anorexia, nausea, vomiting, abdominal cramps, diarrhea.

GU: rusty yellow or brown discoloration of urine.
Derm: pigmentary changes, alopecia, pruritus, photosensitivity, skin erruptions, dermatoses.
Hemat: leukopenia, thrombocytopenia, agranulocytosis, APLASTIC ANEMIA.
Neuro: peripheral neuritis, neuromyopathy.

INTERACTIONS

Drug–Drug: ■ May increase the risk of hepatotoxicity when administered with other **hepatotoxic agents** ■ **Penicillamine** increases the risk of hematologic toxicity ■ Increased risk of dermatologic toxicity when given with other **agents having dermatologic toxicity** ■ May decrease rabies antibody titers when given concurrently with human diplod cell **rabies vaccine** ■ **Urinary acidifiers** may increase renal excretion and decrease effectiveness.
Drug–Food: ■ **Foods that acidify urine** (see Appendix K) may increase excretion and decrease effectiveness.

ROUTE AND DOSAGE

Doses expressed as chloroquine base: 1 mg of chloroquine base = 1.67 mg chloroquine phosphate or 1.25 mg chloroquine hydrochloride.

Malaria (Suppression or Chemoprophylaxis)

- **PO (Adults):** 300 mg once weekly, starting 1–2 wk prior to entering malarious areas and for 4 wk afterward.
- **PO (Children):** 5 mg/kg once weekly, starting 1–2 wk prior to entering malarious areas and for 4 wk afterward (not to exceed 300 mg/day).

Malaria (Uncomplicated Attacks)

- **PO (Adults):** 600 mg initially, then 300 mg at 6–8 hr, 24 hr, and 48 hr after initial dose (not to exceed 1 g/24 hr).
- **PO (Children):** 10 mg/kg initially, 5 mg/kg at 6 hr, 24 hr, and 48 hr after initial dose (not to exceed 12.5 mg/kg/24 hr).

C

*Underlines indicate most frequent; **CAPITALS** indicate life-threatening.

Malaria (Severe)
- **IM (Adults):** 160–200 mg may repeat in 6 hr (not to exceed 800 mg/24 hr).

Rheumatoid Arthritis
- **PO (Adults):** up to 2.4 mg/kg/day (based on ideal body weight).

AVAILABILITY

Chloroquine phosphate
- *Tablets:* 250 mg, 500 mg ▪ *In combination with:* primaquine.

Chloroquine hydrochloride
- *Injection:* 50 mg/ml.

TIME/ACTION PROFILE (onset of antimalarial activity is rapid, antiinflammatory activity may take up to 6 mo)

	ONSET	PEAK	DURATION
PO	rapid	1–2 hr	days–wks
IM	rapid	UK	days–wks

NURSING IMPLICATIONS

ASSESSMENT
- **General Info:** Determine baseline for future reference that includes current symptoms of disease prior to administration.
- □ Assess deep tendon reflexes periodically to determine muscle weakness. Therapy may be discontinued should this occur.
- **Malaria:** Assess patient for improvement in signs and symptoms of condition daily throughout course of therapy.
- **Rheumatoid Arthritis:** Assess degree of joint pain and limitation of motion monthly.
- **Lab Test Considerations:** Monitor CBC and platelet count periodically throughout therapy. May cause decreased WBC and platelet counts.

POTENTIAL NURSING DIAGNOSES
- Infection, high risk for (indications).
- Pain, chronic (indications).
- Knowledge deficit related to medication regimen (patient/family teaching).

IMPLEMENTATION
- **General Info:** For malaria prophylaxis, chloroquine therapy should be started 2 wk prior to potential exposures and continued for 6 wk after leaving the area.
- **PO:** Administer with milk or meals to minimize GI distress.
- □ Tablets may be crushed and placed inside empty capsules for patients with difficulty swallowing. Can be compounded into a suspension by pharmacist.
- **IM:** Parenteral administration may cause severe reaction (seizures, respiratory distress, shock, and cardiovascular collapse) or sudden death in children. Avoid if possible.
- □ Avoid intravenous injection; aspirate to ensure needle placement in muscle. Rotate sites. IM dose may be repeated in 6 hr if necessary. Change to oral route as soon as possible.

PATIENT/FAMILY TEACHING
- □ Instruct patient to take medication exactly as directed, and continue full course of therapy, even if feeling better. Missed doses should be taken as soon as remembered, except with regimens requiring doses more than once a day, for which missed doses should be taken within 1 hr or omitted. Do not double doses.
- □ Review methods of minimizing exposure to mosquitos with patients receiving chloroquine prophylactically (use repellant, wear long-sleeved shirt and long trousers, use screen or netting).
- □ Chloroquine may cause dizziness or lightheadedness. Caution patient to avoid driving or other activities requiring alertness until response to medication is known.
- □ Advise patients to avoid use of alcohol while taking chloroquine.
- □ Caution patient to keep chloroquine out of the reach of children; fatalities have occurred with ingestion of 3 or 4 tablets.
- □ Explain need for periodic ophthalmic examinations for patients on prolonged high-dose therapy. Advise patient that the risk of ocular damage

may be decreased by the use of dark glasses in bright light. Protective clothing and sunscreen should also be used to reduce risk of dermatoses.

▫ Inform patient that chloroquine may cause rusty yellow or brown discoloration of the urine.

▫ Advise patient to notify physician promptly if sore throat, fever, unusual bleeding or bruising, blurred vision, difficulty reading, visual changes, ringing in the ears, difficulty hearing, mental changes, or muscle weakness occur or if diarrhea, anorexia, nausea, stomach pain, vomiting or rash become pronounced or bothersome. Most adverse reactions are dose related.

■ **Rheumatoid Arthritis:** Instruct patient to contact physician if no improvement is noticed within a few days. Treatment may require up to 6 mo for full benefit.

EVALUATION
Effectiveness of therapy may be demonstrated by: ■ Prevention of or improvement in signs and symptoms of malaria ■ Management of rheumatoid arthritis.

CHLORPHENIRAMINE
(klor-fen-**eer**-a-meen)
Aller-Chlor, Chlo-Amine, Chlorate, Chlor-Niramine, Chlor-Pro, Chlor-Trimeton, {Chlor-Tripolon}, Chlorotab, Chlorspan, {Nonopheniram}, Telachlor, Teldrin, Pfeiffer's Allergy, Phenetron, Trimegen

CLASSIFICATION(S):
Antihistamine
Pregnancy Category B

INDICATIONS

■ Symptomatic relief of allergic symptoms caused by histamine release; most useful for nasal allergies and allergic dermatoses ■ Management of severe allergic or hypersensitivity reactions, including anaphylaxis and transfusion reactions.

ACTION

■ Blocks the following effects of histamine: ▫ Vasodilation ▫ Increased GI tract secretions ▫ Increased heart rate ▫ Hypotension. **Therapeutic Effect:** ■ Relief of symptoms associated with histamine excess usually seen in allergic conditions. Does not block the release of histamine.

PHARMACOKINETICS

Absorption: Well absorbed following oral and parenteral administration.
Distribution: Widely distributed. Minimal amounts excreted in breast milk. Crosses the blood-brain barrier.
Metabolism and Excretion: Extensively metabolized by the liver.
Half-life: 12–15 hr.

CONTRAINDICATIONS AND PRECAUTIONS

Contraindicated in: ■ Hypersensitivity ■ Acute attacks of asthma ■ Lactation (avoid use) ■ Known alcohol intolerance (some liquid forms).
Use Cautiously in: ■ Narrow-angle glaucoma ■ Liver disease ■ Elderly patients (more susceptible to adverse reactions) ■ Pregnancy (safety not established).

ADVERSE REACTIONS AND SIDE EFFECTS*

CNS: drowsiness, sedation, excitation (in children), dizziness.
CV: hypotension, hypertension, palpitations, arrhythmias.
EENT: blurred vision.
GI: dry mouth, obstruction, constipation.
GU: urinary hesitancy, retention.

INTERACTIONS

Drug–Drug: ■ Additive CNS depression with other **CNS depressants** including **alcohol, opioid analgesics,** and **sedative/hypnotics** ■ MAO inhibi-

---

{} = Available in Canada only.
*Underlines indicate most frequent; **CAPITALS** indicate life-threatening.

tors intensify and prolong anticholinergic effects of antihistamines ▪ Additive anticholinergic effects with other **drugs possessing anticholinergic properties** including **antidepressants, atropine, haloperidol, phenothiazines, quinidine,** and **disopyramide**.

ROUTE AND DOSAGE

- **PO (Adults):** 4 mg q 4–6 hr or 8–12 mg of extended-release formulation q 8–12 hr (not to exceed 24 mg/day).
- **PO (Children 6–12 yr):** 2 mg q 4–8 hr or 8 mg of extended-release formulation once daily (not to exceed 12 mg/day).
- **PO (Children 2–6 yr):** 1 mg q 4–6 hr.
- **SC, IM, IV (Adults):** 5–20 mg single dose (not to exceed 40 mg/day).
- **SC (Children):** 0.0875 mg/kg q 6 hr.

AVAILABILITY

- *Tablets:* 4 mg, 8 mg, 12 mg ▪ *Chewable tablets:* 2 mg ▪ *Timed-release tablets:* 8 mg, 12 mg ▪ *Timed-release capsules:* 8 mg, 12 mg ▪ *Syrup:* 2 mg/5 ml ▪ *Injection:* 10 mg/ml, 100 mg/ml ▪ *In combination with:* decongestants. See Appendix A.

TIME/ACTION PROFILE
(antihistaminic effects)

	ONSET	PEAK	DURATION
PO	15–30 min	6 hr	4–12 hr
SC	UK	UK	4–12 hr
IM	UK	UK	4–12 hr
IV	rapid	UK	4–12 hr
PO–ER	UK	UK	8–24 hr

NURSING IMPLICATIONS

ASSESSMENT

- ▫ Assess allergy symptoms (rhinitis, conjunctivitis, hives) prior to and periodically throughout course of therapy.
- ▫ Monitor pulse and blood pressure before initiating and throughout IV therapy.
- ▫ Assess lung sounds and character of bronchial secretions. Maintain fluid intake of 1500–2000 ml/day to decrease viscosity of secretions.
- **Lab Test Considerations:** May cause false-negative reactions on allergy skin tests; discontinue 4 days prior to testing.

POTENTIAL NURSING DIAGNOSES

- ▪ Airway clearance, ineffective (indications).
- ▪ Injury, high risk for (adverse reactions).
- ▪ Knowledge deficit related to medication regimen (patient/family teaching).

IMPLEMENTATION

- ▪ **PO:** Administer oral doses with food or milk to decrease GI irritation. Extended-release tablets and capsules should be swallowed whole, do not crush, break, or chew. Chewable tablets should not be swallowed whole; chew well before swallowing.
- ▪ **IM/SC:** The 20 mg/ml and 100 mg/ml solution are recommended for IM or SC route only.
- ▪ **Direct IV:** May be given undiluted. Use only the 10 mg/ml strength for IV administration.
- ▪ *Rate:* Administer each 10 mg dose over at least 1 min.

PATIENT/FAMILY TEACHING

- ▫ Instruct patient to take chlorpheniramine exactly as directed.
- ▫ Chlorpheniramine may cause drowsiness. Caution patient to avoid driving or other activities requiring alertness until response to drug is known.
- ▫ Caution patient to avoid using alcohol or other CNS depressants concurrently with this drug.
- ▫ Advise patient that good oral hygiene, frequent rinsing of mouth with water, and sugarless gum or candy may help relieve dryness of mouth.
- ▫ Instruct patient to contact physician if symptoms persist.

EVALUATION

Effectiveness of therapy can be demonstrated by: ▪ Decrease in allergic symptoms.

CHLORPROMAZINE
(klor-**proe**-ma-zeen)
{Chlorpromanyl}, {Largactil},
{Novo-Chlorpromazine}, Orma-
zine, Thorazine, Thor-prom

CLASSIFICATION(S):
Antipsychotic (phenothiazine),
Antiemetic
Pregnancy Category UK

C

INDICATIONS

▪ Acute and chronic psychoses, particularly when accompanied by increased psychomotor activity ▪ Nausea
and vomiting ▪ Intractable hiccups
▪ Preoperative sedation. **Unlabeled
Use:** ▪ Migraine headache.

ACTION

▪ Alters the effects of dopamine in the
CNS ▪ Possesses significant anticholinergic and alpha-adrenergic blocking
activity. **Therapeutic Effects:** ▪ Diminished signs and symptoms of psychosis
▪ Relief of nausea and vomiting ▪ Control of intractable hiccups.

PHARMACOKINETICS

Absorption: Absorption is variable following oral administration. Well absorbed following IM administration.
Distribution: Widely distributed, high
concentrations in the CNS. Crosses the
placenta and enters breast milk.
Metabolism and Excretion: Highly
metabolized by the liver and GI mucosa. Converted to some compounds
with antipsychotic activity.
Half-life: 30 hr.

CONTRAINDICATIONS AND PRECAUTIONS

Contraindicated in: ▪ Hypersensitivity ▪ Hypersensitivity to sulfites (injectable), povidone or benzyl alcohol (spansules) ▪ Cross-sensitivity with other
phenothiazines may occur ▪ Narrow-
angle glaucoma ▪ Bone marrow depression ▪ Severe liver disease ▪ Severe cardiovascular disease.
Use Cautiously in: ▪ Elderly or debilitated patients (initial dosage reduction
recommended) ▪ Pregnancy or lactation
(safety not established) ▪ Diabetes ▪ Respiratory disease ▪ Prostatic hypertrophy ▪ CNS tumors ▪ Epilepsy ▪ Intestinal obstruction.

ADVERSE REACTIONS AND SIDE EFFECTS*

CNS: sedation, extrapyramidal reac-
tions, tardive dyskinesia, NEUROLEPTIC
MALIGNANT SYNDROME.
EENT: dry eyes, blurred vision, lens
opacities.
CV: hypotension, tachycardia.
GI: constipation, dry mouth, ileus, an-
orexia, hepatitis.
GU: urinary retention.
Derm: rashes, photosensitivity, pig-
ment changes.
Endo: galactorrhea.
Hemat: AGRANULOCYTOSIS, leukope-
nia.
Metab: hyperthermia.
Misc: allergic reactions.

INTERACTIONS

Drug–Drug: ▪ Additive hypotension
with **antihypertensive agents** ▪ Additive
CNS depression with other **CNS depressants** including **alcohol, antidepressants, antihistamines, MAO inhibitors,
opioid analgesics, sedative/hypnotics,**
or **general anesthetics** ▪ **Phenobarbital** may decrease effectiveness ▪ Concurrent use with **lithium** may produce
acute encephalopathy, decreased chlorpromazine absorption, increased excretion of lithium, increased risk of extrapyramidal reactions, or masking of the
early signs of **lithium** toxicity ▪ **Antacids** or **adsorbent antidiarrheals** may
decrease adsorption ▪ Increased risk of
agranulocytosis with **antithyroid drugs**
▪ May decrease antiparkinson activity of **levodopa** and **bromocriptine**

- Decreases vasopressor response to **epinephrine** and **norepinephrine** - Decreases antihypertensive effect of **guanethidine** - Concurrent use with **beta blockers** may produce an increased response - Increased risk or anticholinergic effects with other **agents having anticholinergic properties** including antihistamines, tricyclic antidepressants, quinidine, or disopyramide.

ROUTE AND DOSAGE

Psychoses

- **PO (Adults):** 10–25 mg 2–4 times daily; increase by 20–50 mg/day every 3–4 days (usual dose is 200 mg/day; up to 1–2 g/day). Extended release capsules may be given 1–3 times daily.
- **PO (Children):** 0.55 mg/kg q 4–6 hr.
- **IM (Adults):** 25–50 mg initially, may be repeated in 1 hr, increase to maximum of 400 mg q 3–12 hr if needed (up to 1–2 g/day).
- **IM (Children >6 mo):** 0.55 mg/kg (15 mg/m^2) q 6–8 hr (not to exceed 40 mg/day in children 6 mo–5 yr, or 75 mg/day in children 5–12 yr).

Nausea and Vomiting

- **PO (Adults):** 10–25 mg q 4–6 hr.
- **PO (Children >6 mo):** 0.55 mg/kg or 15 mg/m^2 q 6–8 hr.
- **IM (Adults):** 25–50 mg q 3–4 hr.
- **IM (Children):** 0.55 mg/kg or 15 mg/m^2 q 6–8 hr.
- **Rect (Adults):** 50–100 mg q 6–8 hr.
- **Rect (Children):** 1 mg/kg q 6–8 hr.

Nausea and Vomiting During Surgery

- **IM (Adults):** 12.5 mg; may be repeated in 30 min.
- **IM (Children):** 0.275 mg/kg; may be repeated in 30 min.
- **IV (Adults):** Up to 25 mg slow infusion.
- **IV (Children):** 0.275 mg/kg slow infusion.

Preoperative Sedation

- **IM (Adults):** 12.5–25 mg 1–2 hr before surgery.
- **IM (Children):** 0.55 mg/kg 1–2 hr before surgery.

Intractable Hiccups

- **PO, IM (Adults):** 25–50 mg 3–4 times daily.
- **IV (Adults):** 25–50 mg slow infusion.

AVAILABILITY

- *Tablets:* 10 mg, 25 mg, 50 mg, 100 mg, 200 mg - *Sustained-release capsules:* 30 mg, 75 mg, 150 mg, 200 mg, 300 mg - *Syrup:* 10 mg/5 ml - *Concentrate:* 30 mg/ml, 100 mg/ml - *Suppositories:* 25 mg, 100 mg - *Injection:* 25 mg/ml.

TIME/ACTION PROFILE
(antipsychotic activity, antiemetic activity, sedation)

	ONSET	PEAK	DURATION
PO	30–60 min	UK	4–6 hr
PO–ER	30–60 min	UK	10–12 hr
Rect	1–2 hr	UK	3–4 hr
IM	UK	UK	4–8 hr
IV	rapid	UK	UK

NURSING IMPLICATIONS

ASSESSMENT

- **General Info:** Assess patient's mental status (orientation, mood, behavior) prior to and periodically throughout therapy.
- Monitor blood pressure (sitting, standing, lying), ECG, pulse, and respiratory rate prior to and frequently during the period of dosage adjustment. May cause Q-wave and T-wave changes in ECG.
- Observe patient carefully when administering medication to ensure medication is actually taken and not hoarded.
- Assess fluid intake and bowel function. Increased bulk and fluids in the diet may help minimize constipation.
- Monitor patient for onset of extrapyramidal side effects (akathisia—restless; dystonia—muscle spasms and twisting motions; pseudoparkinsonism—mask facies, rigidity, tremors, drooling, shuffling gait, dysphagia). Notify physician if these symptoms occur, as reduction in dosage or discontinuation of medication may be necessary. Physician may also order

trihexyphenidyl or diphenhydramine to control these symptoms.

□ Monitor for tardive dyskinesia (rhythmic movement of mouth, face, and extremities). Notify physician immediately if these symptoms occur, as these side effects may be irreversible.

□ Monitor for development of neuroleptic malignant syndrome (fever, respiratory distress, tachycardia, convulsions, diaphoresis, hypertension or hypotension, pallor, tiredness). Notify physician immediately if these symptoms occur.

■ **Preoperative Sedation:** Assess level of anxiety prior to and following administration.

■ **Migraine Headache:** Assess type, location, intensity, and duration of pain and accompanying symptoms.

■ **Lab Test Considerations:** CBC, liver function tests, and ocular examinations should be evaluated periodically throughout course of therapy. May cause decreased hematocrit, hemoglobin, leukocytes, granulocytes, platelets. May cause elevated bilirubin, AST (SGOT), ALT (SGPT), and alkaline phosphatase.

□ May cause false-positive or false-negative pregnancy tests and false-positive urine bilirubin test results.

POTENTIAL NURSING DIAGNOSES
■ Thought processes, altered (indications).
■ Knowledge deficit related to medication regimen (patient/family teaching).
■ Noncompliance (patient/family teaching).

IMPLEMENTATION
□ Keep patient recumbent for at least 30 min following parenteral administration to minimize hypotensive effects.
□ To prevent contact dermatitis, avoid getting solution on hands.
□ Phenothiazines should be discontinued 48 hr before and not resumed for 24 hr following metrizamide myelography, because they lower the seizure threshold.
■ **PO:** Administer oral doses with food,

milk, or a full glass of water to minimize gastric irritation. Tablets may be crushed. Do not open capsules; swallow whole. Spansules may be opened but contents should not be chewed. Dilute concentrate just prior to administration in 120 ml of coffee, tea, tomato or fruit juice, milk, water, soup, or carbonated beverages.

■ **Rect:** If suppository is too soft for insertion, chill in refrigerator for 30 min or run under cold water before removing foil wrapper.

■ **IM:** Do not inject SC. Inject slowly into deep, well-developed muscle. May be diluted with 0.9% NaCl or 2% procaine if ordered. Lemon-yellow color does not alter potency of solution. Do not administer solution that is markedly discolored or contains a precipitate.

■ **Direct IV:** For IV administration dilute with 0.9% NaCl in a 1 mg/ml concentration.

■ *Rate:* Inject slowly at a rate of 1 mg/1–2 min.

■ **Continuous Infusion:** May dilute 25–50 mg in 500–1000 ml of D5W, D10W, 0.45% NaCl, 0.9% NaCl, Ringer's or lactated Ringer's injection, dextrose/Ringer's or dextrose/lactated Ringer's combinations for intractable hiccups.

■ **Syringe Compatibility:** ■ atropine ■ butorphanol ■ diphenhydramine ■ doxapram ■ droperidol ■ fentanyl ■ glycopyrrolate ■ hydromorphone ■ hydroxyzine ■ meperidine ■ metoclopramide ■ midazolam ■ morphine ■ pentazocine ■ perphenazine ■ prochlorperazine ■ promazine ■ promethazine ■ scopolamine.

■ **Syringe Incompatibility:** ■ cimetidine ■ dimenhydrinate ■ heparin ■ pentobarbital ■ thiopental.

■ **Y-Site Compatibility:** ■ fluconazole ■ heparin ■ hydrocortisone sodium succinate ■ ondansetron ■ potassium chloride ■ vitamin B complex with C.

■ **Y-Site Incompatibility:** ■ fludarabine ■ sargamostim.

PATIENT/FAMILY TEACHING
□ Advise patient to take medication ex-

actly as directed and not to skip doses or double up on missed doses. Abrupt withdrawal may lead to gastritis, nausea, vomiting, dizziness, headache, tachycardia, and insomnia.

□ Inform patient of possibility of extrapyramidal symptoms and tardive dyskinesia. Instruct patient to report these symptoms immediately to physician.

□ Advise patients to make position changes slowly to minimize orthostatic hypotension.

□ Medication may cause drowsiness. Caution patient to avoid driving or other activities requiring alertness until response to the medication is known.

□ Caution patient to avoid taking alcohol or other CNS depressants concurrently with this medication.

□ Advise patient to use sunscreen and protective clothing when exposed to the sun. Exposed surfaces may develop a temporary pigment change (ranging from yellow-brown to grayish purple). Extremes of temperature (exercise, hot weather, hot baths or showers) should also be avoided, because this drug impairs body temperature regulation.

□ Instruct patient to use frequent mouth rinses, good oral hygiene, and sugarless gum or candy to minimize dry mouth. Consult physician or dentist if dry mouth continues for >2 wk.

□ Advise patient not to take chlorpromazine within 2 hr of antacids or antidiarrheal medication.

□ Inform patient that this medication may turn urine a pink-to-reddish-brown color.

□ Advise patient to notify physician or dentist of medication regimen prior to treatment or surgery.

□ Instruct patient to notify physician promptly if sore throat, fever, unusual bleeding or bruising, rash, weakness, tremors, visual disturbances, dark-colored urine, or clay-colored stools occur.

□ Emphasize the importance of routine follow-up examinations and continued participation in psychotherapy as indicated.

EVALUATION

Effectiveness of therapy can be demonstrated by: ▪ Decrease in excitable, paranoic, or withdrawn behavior. Therapeutic effects may not be seen for 7–8 wk ▪ Relief of nausea and vomiting ▪ Relief of hiccups ▪ Preoperative sedation ▪ Relief of migraine headache.

CHLORTHALIDONE
(klor-**thal**-i-doan)
{Apo-Chlorthalidone}, Hygroton, Thalitone, {Novothalidone}, {Uridon}

CLASSIFICATION(S):
Antihypertensive, Diuretic (thiazide-like)
Pregnancy Category B

INDICATIONS

▪ Alone or in combination with other agents in the management of mild to moderate hypertension ▪ Alone or in combination in the treatment of edema associated with congestive heart failure, the nephrotic syndrome, or pregnancy.

ACTION

▪ Increases excretion of sodium and water ▪ Promotes excretion of chloride, potassium, magnesium, and bicarbonate ▪ May produce arteriolar dilation. **Therapeutic Effects:** ▪ Lowering of blood pressure in hypertensive patients ▪ Diuresis with subsequent mobilization of edema.

PHARMACOKINETICS

Absorption: Well absorbed following oral administration.
Distribution: Distributed into extracellular space. Crosses the placenta and enters breast milk.

{} = Available in Canada only.

Metabolism and Excretion: 30–60% excreted unchanged by the kidneys.
Half-life: 54 hr.

CONTRAINDICATIONS AND PRECAUTIONS

Contraindicated in: ▪ Hypersensitivity ▪ Cross-sensitivity with sulfonamides may occur ▪ Anuria ▪ Lactation.

Use Cautiously in: ▪ Renal impairment ▪ Severe hepatic impairment ▪ Pregnancy (jaundice or thrombocytopenia may be seen in the newborn) ▪ Elderly patients (more sensitive to diuretic effects).

ADVERSE REACTIONS AND SIDE EFFECTS*

CNS: drowsiness, lethargy.
CV: hypotension.
GI: anorexia, nausea, vomiting, cramping, hepatitis.
Derm: rashes, photosensitivity.
Endo: hyperglycemia.
F and E: hypokalemia, hypochloremic alkalosis, hyponatremia, hypercalcemia, hypophosphatemia, hypomagnesemia, dehydration, hypovolemia.
Hemat: blood dyscrasias.
Metab: hyperuricemia, hyperlipidemia.
MS: muscle cramps.
Misc: pancreatitis.

INTERACTIONS

Drug–Drug: ▪ Additive hypotension with other **antihypertensives,** acute ingestion of **alcohol,** or **nitrates** ▪ Additive hypokalemia with **glucocorticoids, amphotericin B, mezlocillin, piperacillin,** or **ticarcillin** ▪ Decreases **lithium** excretion, may cause toxicity ▪ **Cholestyramine** or **colestipol** may decrease absorption.

Drug–Food: ▪ **Food** may increase extent of absorption.

ROUTE AND DOSAGE

▪ **PO (Adults):** 25–100 mg/day or 100 mg every other day or 3 times weekly.
▪ **PO (Children):** 2 mg/kg 3 times weekly.

AVAILABILITY

▪ **Tablets:** 25 mg, 50 mg, 100 mg ▪ **In combination with:** clonidine (Combipres), atenolol (Tenoretiz), or reserpine (Demi-Regroton, Regroton). See Appendix A.

TIME/ACTION PROFILE (diuretic effect)

	ONSET	PEAK	DURATION
PO	2 hr	2–6 hr	24–72 hr

NURSING IMPLICATIONS

ASSESSMENT

▪ **General Info:** Monitor blood pressure, intake and output, daily weight and assess feet, legs, and sacral area for edema daily.
▫ Assess patient, especially if taking cardiac glycosides, for anorexia, nausea, vomiting, muscle cramps, paresthesia, and confusion. Patients taking cardiac glycosides are at risk of digitalis toxicity due to the potassium-depleting effect of the diuretic.
▫ Assess patient for allergy to sulfonamides.
▪ **Lab Test Considerations:** Monitor electrolytes (especially potassium), blood glucose, BUN, and serum uric acid levels prior to and periodically throughout course of therapy.
▫ May cause increase in serum and urine glucose in diabetic patients.
▫ May cause an increase in serum bilirubin, calcium, and uric acid, and a decrease in serum magnesium, potassium, and sodium levels.
▫ May cause increased serum cholesterol, low-density lipoprotein, and triglyceride concentrations.

POTENTIAL NURSING DIAGNOSES

▪ Fluid volume excess (indications).
▪ Fluid volume deficit (side effects).
▪ Knowledge deficit related to medication regimen (patient/family teaching).

IMPLEMENTATION

▪ **General Info:** Administer in the morning to prevent disruption of sleep cycle.

- **PO:** May give with food or milk to minimize GI irritation. Tablets may be crushed and mixed with fluid to facilitate swallowing.

□ Intermittent dose schedule may be used for continued control of edema.

PATIENT/FAMILY TEACHING

□ Instruct patient to take this medication at the same time each day. If a dose is missed, take as soon as remembered, but not just before next dose is due. Do not double doses. Advise patients using chlorthalidone for hypertension to continue taking the medication even if feeling better.

□ Medication controls but does not cure hypertension.

□ Encourage patient to comply with additional interventions for hypertension (weight reduction, low-sodium diet, regular exercises, discontinuation of smoking, moderation of alcohol consumption, and stress management).

□ Instruct patient to monitor weight biweekly and notify physician of significant changes. Instruct patients with hypertension in correct technique for monitoring weekly blood pressure.

□ Caution patient to make position changes slowly to minimize orthostatic hypotension. This may be potentiated by alcohol.

□ Advise patient to use sunscreen (avoid those containing PABA) and protective clothing when in the sun to prevent photosensitivity reactions.

□ Instruct patient to follow a diet high in potassium (see Appendix K).

□ Advise patient to consult physician or pharmacist before taking over-the-counter medication concurrently with this therapy.

□ Advise patient to report muscle weakness, cramps, nausea, or dizziness to the physician.

□ Instruct patient to notify physician or dentist of medication regimen prior to treatment or surgery.

□ Emphasize the importance of routine follow-up examinations.

EVALUATION

Effectiveness of therapy can be demonstrated by: ■ Increase in urine output □ Decrease in edema ■ Decrease in blood pressure.

CHOLINE and MAGNESIUM SALICYLATES
(koe-leen mag-neez-ee-um sal-i-sil-ates)
Tricosal, Trilisate

CLASSIFICATION(S):
Nonopioid analgesic, Nonsteroidal anti-inflammatory agent, Antipyretic
Pregnancy Category C

INDICATIONS

■ Mild to moderate pain ■ Inflammatory disorders including: □ Rheumatoid arthritis □ Osteoarthritis ■ Fever.

ACTION

■ Produces analgesia and reduces inflammation by inhibiting the production of prostaglandins ■ Unlike aspirin, has no effect on platelet function. **Therapeutic Effects:** ■ Reduction of mild to moderate pain, inflammation, or fever.

PHARMACOKINETICS

Absorption: Well absorbed following oral administration.
Distribution: Rapidly and widely distributed. Crosses the placenta and enters breast milk.
Metabolism and Excretion: Extensively metabolized by the liver. Inactive metabolites excreted by the kidneys.
Half-life: 2–3 hr for low doses. For larger doses, half-life may increase up to 15–30 hr due to saturation of liver metabolism.

CONTRAINDICATIONS AND PRECAUTIONS

Contraindicated in: ■ Hypersensitivity to aspirin or other nonsteroidal anti-inflammatory agents (less cross-sensitivity than aspirin).

Use Cautiously in: ▪ Renal insufficiency (magnesium toxicity may occur) ▪ Severe liver impairment ▪ Pregnancy (may have adverse effects on fetus and mother) ▪ Lactation (safety not established) ▪ Children or adolescents with viral infections (may increase the risk of Reye's Syndrome).

ADVERSE REACTIONS AND SIDE EFFECTS*

EENT: tinnitus, hearing loss.

GI: dyspepsia, heartburn, epigastric distress, nausea, vomiting, anorexia, abdominal pain, GI BLEEDING, hepatotoxicity.

Misc: noncardiogenic pulmonary edema, allergic reactions including ANAPHYLAXIS or LARYNGEAL EDEMA.

INTERACTIONS

Drug–Drug: ▪ May increase toxicity of **penicillins, phenytoin, methotrexate, valproic acid, oral hypoglycemic agents,** and **sulfonamides** ▪ May antagonize the beneficial effects of **probenecid** or **sulfinpyrazone** ▪ May decrease effectiveness of concurrently administered **nonsteroidal anti-inflammatory agents** (except ketoprofen) ▪ **Glucocorticoids** may decrease serum salicylate levels ▪ **Urinary acidification** may increase serum salicylate levels ▪ **Alkalinization of the urine** or the ingestion of large amounts of **antacids** decreases serum salicylate levels ▪ May blunt the therapeutic response to **diuretics** or **antihypertensives** ▪ Increased risk of gastrointestinal irritation with **nonsteroidal anti-inflammatory agents** (effect less than aspirin) ▪ Increased risk of ototoxicity with **vancomycin.**

Drug–Food: ▪ **Foods capable of acidifying the urine** (see Appendix K) may enhance reabsorption and increase serum salicylate levels.

ROUTE AND DOSAGE

5 ml of liquid equivalent to 500 mg salicylate or 650 mg of aspirin. Tablet strength expressed in mg of salicylate: 500 mg tablet equivalent to 650 mg of aspirin, 750 mg tablet equivalent to 975 mg of aspirin, 1000 mg tablet equivalent to 1.3 g of aspirin.

▪ **PO (Adults):** 2–3 g of salicylate/day in 2–3 divided doses.
▪ **PO (Children >37 kg):** 2.2 g of salicylate/day in 2 divided doses.
▪ **PO (Children <37 kg):** 50 mg of salicylate/kg/day in 2 divided doses.

AVAILABILITY (listed as salicylate content)

▪ *Tablets:* 500 mg, 750 mg, 1000 mg
▪ *Liquid:* 500 mg/5 ml.

TIME/ACTION PROFILE (analgesia and fever reduction)*

	ONSET	PEAK	DURATION
PO	5–30 min	1–3 hr	3–6 hr

*Antirheumatic effect may take 2–3 wk of chronic dosing.

NURSING IMPLICATIONS

ASSESSMENT

▪ **General Info:** Patients who have asthma, allergies, and nasal polyps or who are allergic to tartrazine dyes are at an increased risk for developing hypersensitivity reactions.

▪ **Pain:** Assess pain and limitation of movement; note type, location, and intensity prior to and 1–3 hr following administration.

▪ **Fever:** Assess fever and note associated signs (diaphoresis, tachycardia, malaise, chills).

▪ **Toxicity and Overdose:** Observe patient for the onset of tinnitus, hyperventilation, agitation, mental confusion, lethargy, diarrhea, and sweating. If these symptoms appear, withhold medication and notify physician immediately.

POTENTIAL NURSING DIAGNOSES

▪ Pain (indications).
▪ Physical mobility, impaired (indications).
▪ Knowledge deficit related to medica-

---

*Underlines indicate most frequent; **CAPITALS** indicate life-threatening.

tion regimen (patient/family teaching).

IMPLEMENTATION

- **PO:** Administer after meals or with food or an antacid to minimize gastric irritation. Food slows but will not alter the total amount absorbed.

PATIENT/FAMILY TEACHING

- ☐ Instruct patient to take with a full glass of water and to remain in an upright position for 15–30 min after administration.
- ☐ Advise patient to report tinnitus, unusual bleeding of gums, bruising, or black, tarry stools, or fever lasting longer than 3 days.
- ☐ Caution patient to avoid concurrent use of alcohol with this medication to minimize possible gastric irritation.
- ☐ Advise patients on long-term therapy to inform physician or dentist of medication regimen prior to surgery.
- ☐ Centers for Disease Control warn against giving salicylates to children or adolescents with varicella (chickenpox) or influenza-like or viral illnesses because of a possible association with Reye's syndrome.

EVALUATION

Effectiveness of therapy can be demonstrated by: ■ Decrease in severity of mild to moderate discomfort ■ Increased ease of joint movement ■ Reduction of fever.

CHOLINE SALICYLATE
(**koe**-leen sal-i-sil-ate)
Arthropan

CLASSIFICATION(S):
Nonopioid analgesic, Nonsteroidal anti-inflammatory agent,
Antipyretic
Pregnancy Category UK

INDICATIONS

- ■ Treatment of mild to moderate pain
- ■ Management of inflammatory disorders including: ☐ Rheumatoid arthritis ☐ Osteoarthritis ■ Treatment of fever.

ACTION

- ■ Produces analgesia and reduces inflammation by inhibiting the production of prostaglandins ■ Unlike aspirin, has no effect on platelet function. **Therapeutic Effects:** ■ Analgesia resulting in reduction of mild to moderate pain ■ Reduction of inflammation ■ Reduction of fever.

PHARMACOKINETICS

Absorption: Well absorbed following oral administration.
Distribution: Rapidly and widely distributed. Crosses the placenta and enters breast milk.
Metabolism and Excretion: Extensively metabolized by the liver. Inactive metabolites excreted by the kidneys.
Half-life: 2–3 hr for low doses. For larger doses, half-life may increase up to 15–30 hr due to saturation of liver metabolism.

CONTRAINDICATIONS AND PRECAUTIONS

Contraindicated in: ■ Hypersensitivity to aspirin or other nonsteroidal anti-inflammatory agents (less cross-sensitivity than aspirin).
Use Cautiously in: ■ Renal insufficiency (magnesium toxicity may occur) ■ Severe liver impairment ■ Pregnancy (may have adverse effects on fetus and mother) ■ Lactation (safety not established) ■ Children or adolescents with viral infections (may increase the risk of Reye's Syndrome).

ADVERSE REACTIONS AND SIDE EFFECTS*

EENT: tinnitus, hearing loss.
GI: dyspepsia, heartburn, epigastric distress, nausea, vomiting, anorexia, abdominal pain, GI BLEEDING, hepatotoxicity.
Misc: noncardiogenic pulmonary edema, allergic reactions including ANAPHYLAXIS or LARYNGEAL EDEMA.

*Underlines indicate most frequent; **CAPITALS** indicate life-threatening.

INTERACTIONS

Drug–Drug: ▪ May increase toxicity of **penicillins, phenytoin, methotrexate, valproic acid, oral hypoglycemic agents,** and **sulfonamides** ▪ May antagonize the beneficial effects of **probenecid** or **sulfinpyrazone** ▪ May decrease effectiveness of concurrently administered **nonsteroidal anti-inflammatory agents** (except ketoprofen) ▪ **Glucocorticoids** may decrease serum salicylate levels ▪ **Urinary acidification** may increase serum salicylate levels ▪ **Alkalinization of the urine** or the ingestion of large amounts of **antacids** decreases serum salicylate levels ▪ May blunt the therapeutic response to **diuretics** or **antihypertensives** ▪ Increased risk of gastrointestinal irritation with **nonsteroidal anti-inflammatory agents** (effect less than aspirin) ▪ Increased risk of ototoxicity with **vancomycin**.

Drug–Food: ▪ **Foods capable of acidifying the urine** (see Appendix K) may enhance reabsorption and increase serum salicylate levels.

ROUTE AND DOSAGE

5 ml of liquid equivalent to 870 mg salicylate or 650 mg of aspirin.

Analgesic/Antipyretic

▪ **PO (Adults):** 435–669 mg ($\frac{1}{2}$–$\frac{3}{4}$ tsp) q 3 hr or 435–870 mg ($\frac{1}{2}$–1 tsp) q 4 hr or 870–1338 mg q 6 hr as needed.

▪ **PO (Children):** 2 g/m^2/day in 4–6 divided doses as needed.

Anti-Inflammatory

▪ **PO (Adults):** 4.8–7.2 g/day in divided doses.

▪ **PO (Children):** 107–133 mg/kg/day in divided doses.

AVAILABILITY

▪ *Solution:* 870 mg/5 ml.

TIME/ACTION PROFILE (analgesia and fever reduction)*

	ONSET	PEAK	DURATION
PO	5–30 min	1–3 hr	3–6 hr

*Antirheumatic effect may take 2–3 wk of chronic dosing.

NURSING IMPLICATIONS

ASSESSMENT

▪ **General Info:** Patients who have asthma, allergies, and nasal polyps or who are allergic to tartrazine dyes are at an increased risk for developing hypersensitivity reactions.

▪ **Pain:** Assess pain and limitation of movement; note type, location, and intensity prior to and 1–3 hr following administration.

▪ **Fever:** Assess fever and note associated signs (diaphoresis, tachycardia, malaise, chills).

▪ **Toxicity and Overdose:** Observe patient for the onset of tinnitus, hyperventilation, agitation, mental confusion, lethargy, diarrhea, and sweating. If these symptoms appear, withhold medication and notify physician immediately.

POTENTIAL NURSING DIAGNOSES

▪ Pain (indications).
▪ Physical mobility, impaired (indications).
▪ Knowledge deficit related to medication regimen (patient/family teaching).

IMPLEMENTATION

▪ **PO:** Administer after meals or with food or an antacid to minimize gastric irritation. Food slows but will not alter the total amount absorbed.

PATIENT/FAMILY TEACHING

▫ Instruct patient to take with a full glass of water and to remain in an upright position for 15–30 min after administration.

▫ Advise patient to report tinnitus, unusual bleeding of gums, bruising, or black, tarry stools, or fever lasting longer than 3 days.

▫ Caution patient to avoid concurrent use of alcohol with this medication to minimize possible gastric irritation.

▫ Advise patients on long-term therapy to inform physician or dentist of medication regimen prior to surgery.

▫ Centers for Disease Control warn against giving salicylates to children or adolescents with varicella (chickenpox) or influenza-like or viral illnesses because of a possible association with Reye's syndrome.

EVALUATION

Effectiveness of therapy can be demonstrated by: ▪ Decrease in severity of mild to moderate discomfort ▪ Increased ease of joint movement ▪ Reduction of fever.

CIMETIDINE
(sye-**met**-i-deen)
{Apo-Cimetidine}, {Novo-cimetine}, {Peptol}, Tagamet

CLASSIFICATION(S):
Antiulcer (histamine H_2 antagonist)
Pregnancy Category B

INDICATIONS

▪ Treatment of active duodenal ulcers and benign gastric ulcers ▪ Prophylaxis of duodenal ulcer ▪ Management of gastroesophageal reflux disease (GERD) ▪ Managment of gastric hypersecretory states (Zollinger–Ellison Syndrome). **Unlabeled Uses:** ▪ Prevention of upper GI bleeding ▪ Prevention of stress ulceration or aspiration pneumonitis.

ACTION

▪ Inhibits the action of histamine at the H_2-receptor site located primarily in gastric parietal cells, resulting in inhibition of gastric acid secretion. **Therapeutic Effects:** ▪ Healing and prevention of ulcers ▪ Decreased symptoms of gastroesophageal reflux ▪ Decreased secretion of gastric acid.

PHARMACOKINETICS

Absorption: Well absorbed following oral and IM administration.
Distribution: Widely distributed. Enters breast milk and probably crosses the placenta.
Metabolism and Excretion: 30% metabolized by the liver. Remainder is eliminated unchanged by the kidneys.
Half-life: 2 hr (increased in renal impairment).

CONTRAINDICATIONS AND PRECAUTIONS

Contraindicated in: ▪ Hypersensitivity.
Use Cautiously in: ▪ Elderly (more susceptible to adverse CNS reactions; dosage reduction recommended) ▪ Renal impairment (more susceptible to adverse CNS reactions; increased dosage interval recommended) ▪ Pregnancy or lactation.

ADVERSE REACTIONS AND SIDE EFFECTS*

CNS: <u>confusion</u>, dizziness, headache, drowsiness.
CV: bradycardia.
GI: nausea, diarrhea, constipation, hepatitis.
GU: nephritis, decreased sperm count.
Derm: rashes, exfoliative dermatitis, urticaria.
Endo: gynecomastia.
Hemat: AGRANULOCYTOSIS, APLASTIC ANEMIA, neutropenia, thrombocytopenia, anemia.
Local: pain at IM site.
MS: muscle pain.

INTERACTIONS

Drug–Drug: ▪ Cimetidine inhibits drug-metabolizing enzymes in the liver; may lead to increased blood levels and toxicity of the following—some **benzodiazepines** (not lorazepam, oxazepam, or temazepam), some **beta blockers** (labetalol, metoprolol, propranolol), **caffeine, calcium channel blockers, carbamazepine, chloroquine, lidocaine, metronidazole, moricizine, pentoxifylline, phenytoin, propafenone, quinidine, quinine, sulfonylureas, theophylline, triamterene, tricyclic antidepressants,** and **warfarin** ▪ Cimetidine decreases absorption of **ferrous (iron) salts, keto-**

conazole, fluconazole and tetracyclines ■ Anticholinergics and metoclopramide decrease absorption of cimetidine ■ The effects of succinlycholine, flecainide, procainamide, carmistine, and fluorouracil are increased by cimetidine ■ Effectiveness of cimetidine is decreased by cigarette smoking ■ Absorption of cimetidine is decreased by sucralfate (take cimetidine 2 hr before sucralfate).

ROUTE AND DOSAGE

Short-Term Treatment of Active Ulcers

- **PO (Adults):** 300 mg 4 times daily or 800 mg at bedtime or 400–600 mg twice daily (not to exceed 2.4 g/day).
- **PO (Children):** 20–40 mg/kg/day in 4 divided doses (10–15 mg/kg/day if renal function is impaired).
- **IM, IV (Adults):** 300 mg q 6 hr (not to exceed 2.4 g/day).
- **IM, IV (Children):** 5–10 mg/kg q 6–8 hr.
- **IV Infusion (Adults):** 900 mg infused over 24 hr (37.5 mg/hr); may be preceded by a 150 mg bolus dose.

Duodenal Ulcer Prophylaxis

- **PO (Adults):** 300 mg twice daily or 400 mg at bedtime.

Gastric Hypersecretory Conditions

- **PO, IM, IV (Adults):** 300–600 mg q 6 hr (up to 12 g/day has been used).

GERD

- **PO (Adults):** 800–1600 mg/day in divided doses.

Prevention of Upper-GI Bleeding

- **IV (Adults):** 50 mg/hr (25 mg/hr if creatinine clearance <30 ml/min).

Prophylaxis of Aspiration Pneumonitis

- **IM, IV (Adults):** 300 mg IM 1 hr before anesthesia, then 300 mg IV q 4 h until patient is conscious.

AVAILABILITY

- **Tablets:** 200 mg, 300 mg, 400 mg, 800 mg ■ **Oral liquid:** 300 mg/5 ml ■ **Injection:** 300 mg/2 ml-vials, 300 mg/50 ml 0.9% NaCl.

TIME/ACTION PROFILE (suppression of gastric acid secretion)

	ONSET	PEAK	DURATION
PO	30 min	45–90 min	4–5 hr
IM, IV	10 min	30 min	4–5 hr

NURSING IMPLICATIONS

C

ASSESSMENT

□ Assess patient for epigastric or abdominal pain and frank or occult blood in the stool, emesis, or gastric aspirate.

□ Assess elderly and debilitated patients routinely for confusion. Notify physician promptly should this occur.

■ **Lab Test Considerations:** CBC with differential should be monitored periodically throughout therapy.

□ May cause transient increase in serum transaminase and serum creatinine. Serum prolactin concentration may be increased following IV bolus. May also cause decreased parathyroid concentrations.

□ Antagonizes effects of pentagastrin and histamine during gastric acid secretion testing. Avoid administration for 24 hr preceding the test.

□ May cause false-negative results in skin tests using allergenic extracts. Cimetidine should be discontinued 24 hr prior to the test.

POTENTIAL NURSING DIAGNOSES

■ Pain (indications).

■ Knowledge deficit related to medication regimen (patient/family teaching).

IMPLEMENTATION

■ **PO:** Administer medication with meals or immediately afterward and at bedtime to prolong effect. If administering oral doses concurrently with antacids, give at least 1 hr apart.

□ Tablets have a characteristic odor.

■ **Direct IV:** Dilute each 300 mg in 20 ml of 0.9% NaCl for injection.

■ **Rate:** Administer over at least 2 min.

Rapid administration may cause hypotension and arrhythmias.

- **Intermittent Infusion:** Dilute each 300 mg in 50 ml of 0.9% NaCl, D5W, D10W, D5/LR, D5/0.9% NaCl, D5/0.45% NaCl, D5/0.25% NaCl, Ringer's or lactated Ringer's solution, or sodium bicarbonate. Diluted solution is stable for 48 hr at room temperature. Refrigeration may cause cloudiness but will not affect potency. Do not use solution that is discolored or contains precipitate.
- *Rate:* Administer over 15–20 min.
- **Continuous Infusion:** Dilute cimetidine 900 mg in 100–1000 ml of compatible solution (see Intermittent Infusion).
- *Rate:* Usually infused at a rate of 37.5 mg/hr, but should be individualized.
- **Y-Site Compatibility:** ■ acyclovir ■ aminophylline ■ amrinone ■ atracurium ■ enalaprilat ■ esmolol ■ fluconazole ■ fludarabine ■ foscarnet ■ heparin ■ hetastarch ■ labetalol ■ ondansetron ■ pancuronium ■ sargramostim ■ tolazoline ■ vecuronium ■ zidovudine.

PATIENT/FAMILY TEACHING

- **General Info:** Instruct patient to take medication as directed for the full course of therapy, even if feeling better. If a dose is missed, it should be taken as soon as remembered but not if almost time for next dose. Do not double doses.
- □ Inform patient that smoking interferes with the action of cimetidine. Encourage patient to quit smoking or at least not to smoke after last dose of the day.
- □ Cimetidine may cause drowsiness or dizziness. Caution patient to avoid driving or other activities requiring alertness until response to the drug is known.
- □ Advise patient to avoid alcohol, products containing aspirin or ibuprofen, and foods that may cause an increase in GI irritation.
- □ Advise patient to report onset of black, tarry stools, fever, sore throat,

diarrhea, dizziness, rash, confusion, or hallucinations to the physician promptly.

EVALUATION
Effectiveness of therapy can be demonstrated by: ■ Decrease in abdominal pain or prevention of gastric irritation and bleeding. Healing of duodenal ulcers can be seen by x-rays or endoscopy. Therapy is continued for at least 6 wk in treatment of ulcers ■ Decreased symptoms of esophageal reflux.

CIPROFLOXACIN
(sip-roe-**flox**-a-sin)
Ciloxan, Cipro

CLASSIFICATION(S):
Anti-infective (fluoroquinolone)
Pregnancy Category C

INDICATIONS

- **PO, IV:** Treatment of the following infections due to susceptible organisms:
  □ Lower respiratory tract infections
  □ Skin and skin structure infections
  □ Bone and joint infections □ Urinary tract infections ■ **PO:** Infectious diarrhea ■ **Ophth:** Management of corneal ulcers and conjunctivitis.

ACTION

- Inhibits bacterial DNA synthesis by inhibiting DNA gyrase. **Therapeutic Effect:** ■ Death of susceptible bacteria. **Spectrum:** ■ Broad activity includes many gram-positive pathogens: □ Staphylococci (including *Staphylococcus epidermidis* and methicillin-resistant strains of *Staphylococcus aureus*) □ *Streptococcus pyogenes* □ *Streptococcus pneumoniae* ■ Gram-negative spectrum notable for activity against: □ *E. coli* □ *Klebsiella* species □ Enterobacter □ *Salmonella* □ *Shigella* □ *Proteus vulgaris* □ *Providencia stuartii* □ *Providencia retgerii* □ *Morganella morganii* □ *Pseudomonas aeruginoa* □ *Serratia* □ *Haemophilus* species □ Acinetobacter □ *Neisseria gonorrhea* and *meningitidis* □ *Branhamella catarrhalis* □ Yersinia □ Vibrio □ Brucella □ Campylobacter □ Aeromonas species.

PHARMACOKINETICS

Absorption: Well absorbed (70%) following oral administration.

Distribution: Widely distributed. High tissue concentrations are achieved.

Metabolism and Excretion: 15% metabolized by the liver. 40–50% excreted unchanged by the kidneys.

Half-life: 4 hr (increased in renal disease).

CONTRAINDICATIONS AND PRECAUTIONS

Contraindicated in: ▪ Hypersensitivity ▪ Cross-sensitivity with other fluoroquinolones may exist ▪ Children <18 yr ▪ Pregnancy ▪ Hypersensitivity to benzalkonium chloride or EDTA (ophth only).

Use Cautiously in: ▪ Underlying CNS pathology ▪ Lactation (safety not established) ▪ ▪ Severe renal impairment (increased dosing interval required for oral ciprofloxacin if CCr <50 ml/min or for IV ciprofloxicin if CCr <30 ml/min).

ADVERSE REACTIONS AND SIDE EFFECTS*

CNS: tremors, <u>restlessness</u>, confusion, hallucination, SEIZURES, dizziness.

EENT: Ophth—lid margin crusting, crystals/scales, foreign body sensation, itching, conjuntival hyperemia.

GI: <u>nausea</u>, <u>diarrhea</u>, <u>vomiting</u>, <u>abdominal pain</u>; Ophth—bad taste in mouth.

GU: crystalluria, cylinduria, hematuria.

Derm: rash, photosensitivity.

Local: phlebitis at IV site (especially if infusion time is <30 min).

Misc: allergic reactions including ANAPHYLAXIS.

INTERACTIONS

Drug–Drug: ▪ Increases serum the-ophylline levels; may lead to toxicity ▪ Administration with **antacids, iron salts, sucralfate,** or **zinc sulfate** de-crease absorption of ciprofloxacin ▪ **Drugs that alkalinize the urine** increase the risk of crystalluria ▪ May increase nephrotoxicity of **cyclosporine** ▪ **Nitrofurantoin** may decrease effectiveness ▪ **Probenecid** increases blood levels ▪ May increase the effect of **warfarin** ▪ **Antineoplastics** may decrease ciprofloxacin blood levels ▪ **Caffeine** may decrease effectiveness of ciprofloxacin.

ROUTE AND DOSAGE

▪ **PO (Adults):** 250–750 mg q 12 hr (250-mg single dose for gonococcal urethritis).

▪ **IV (Adults):** 200–400 mg q 12 hr (administered as an infusion over 60 min).

▪ **Ophth (Adults):** 1–2 drops q 15–30 min until infection is controlled, then 1–2 drops 4–6 times daily.

AVAILABILITY

▪ *Tablets:* 250 mg, 500 mg, 750 mg
▪ *Injection:* 200-mg, 400-mg vials.

TIME/ACTION PROFILE (blood levels)

	ONSET	PEAK
PO	rapid	1–2 hr
IV	rapid	end of infusion

NURSING IMPLICATIONS

ASSESSMENT

□ Assess patient for infection (vital signs; appearance of wound, sputum, urine, and stool; WBC) at beginning and throughout course of therapy.

□ Obtain specimens for culture and sensitivity prior to initiating therapy. First dose may be given before receiving results.

□ Monitor intake and output. Intake should be at least 2000–3000 ml/day to prevent crystalluria.

▪ **Lab Test Considerations:** May cause elevated AST (SGOT), ALT (SGPT), alkaline phosphatase, bilirubin, BUN, creatinine, and LDH concentrations.

□ May cause elevated or decreased se-

*Underlines indicate most frequent; CAPITALS indicate life-threatening.

rum platelets and decreased RBCs and WBCs.

POTENTIAL NURSING DIAGNOSES
- Infection, high risk for (indications, side effects).
- Knowledge deficit related to medication regimen (patient/family teaching).
- Noncompliance related to medication regimen (patient/family teaching).

IMPLEMENTATION
- **PO:** Administer on an empty stomach, 2 hr after meals. If gastric irritation occurs, may be administered with meals. Food slows and may slightly decrease absorption.
- If antacids are prescribed concurrently, administer at least 2 hr before or after ciprofloxacin.
- Milk and yogurt decrease the absorption of ciprofloxacin. Do not take concurrently.
- **Intermittent Infusion:** Dilute ciprofloxacin to a concentration of 1–2 mg/ml with 0.9% NaCl or D5W. Stable for 14 days at refrigerated or room temperature.
- *Rate:* Administer over 60 min into a large vein to minimize venous irritation.
- **Y-Site Incompatibility:** ▪ Temporarily discontinue other solutions when administering ciprofloxacin ▪ heparin.
- **Ophth:** See Appendix H for instillation of ophthalmic medications.

PATIENT/FAMILY TEACHING
- Instruct patients to take medication completely as directed, even if feeling better. Advise patients that sharing of this medication may be dangerous.
- Ciprofloxacin may cause dizziness or lightheadedness. Caution patient to avoid driving or other activities requiring alertness until response to medication is known.
- Caution patient to use sunscreen and protective clothing to prevent photosensitivity reactions.
- Advise patient to report signs of superinfection (furry overgrowth on the tongue, vaginal itching or discharge, loose or foul-smelling stools).
- Instruct the patient to notify physician if symptoms do not improve.
- **Ophth:** Instruct patient in the proper technique for ophthalmic instillation. Emphasize the importance of not touching tip of applicator to any surface.

EVALUATION
Clinical response to therapy can be evaluated by: ▪ Resolution of the signs and symptoms of infection. Length of time for complete resolution depends on the organism and site of infection.

CISAPRIDE
(**siss**-a-pride)
Propulsid

CLASSIFICATION(S):
Gastrointestinal (antireflux)
Pregnancy Category C

INDICATIONS
▪ Management of nocturnal symptoms (heartburn) associated with gastroesophageal reflux disease (GERD).

ACTION
▪ Enhances the release of acetylcholine at the myenteric plexus. Increases the strength of esophageal peristalsis and increases lower esophageal sphincter pressure. Also acts as a serotonin-4 agonist. **Therapeutic Effect:** ▪ Reduced nocturnal symptoms of GERD.

PHARMACOKINETICS
Absorption: Rapidly absorbed following oral administration, although bioavailability is low (35–40%).
Distribution: Enters breast milk in low concentrations.
Metabolism and Excretion: Extensively metabolized by the liver (>90%).
Half-life: 8–10 hr.

CONTRAINDICATIONS AND PRECAUTIONS
Contraindicated in: ▪ Hypersensitivity ▪ Situations in which increased GI motility may be harmful (GI hemorrhage,

mechanical obstruction or perforation).
Use Cautiously in: ▪ Pregnancy, lactation, or children (safety not established).

ADVERSE REACTIONS AND SIDE EFFECTS*

CNS: headache, dizziness, fatigue, depression.
Resp: rhinitis, pharyngitis.
CV: chest pain.
GI: diarrhea, abdominal pain, dyspepsia, constipation, flatulence, vomiting.
F and E: dehydration.
MS: back pain, myalgia.

INTERACTIONS

Drug–Drug: ▪ **Anticholinergics** may decrease the effects of cisapride ▪ May accelerate the sedative effects of **benzodiazepines** or **alcohol** ▪ May increase the effects of **warfarin** ▪ May alter the effects of **drugs with narrow therapeutic margins** (digoxin, anticonvulsants; blood level monitoring recommended) ▪ **Cimetidine** increases plasma levels of cisapride ▪ GI absorption of **cimetidine** and **ranitidine** is accelerated.

ROUTE AND DOSAGE

▪ **PO (Adults):** 10–20 mg 4 times daily 15 min before meals and at bedtime.

AVAILABILITY

▪ *Tablets:* 10 mg.

TIME/ACTION PROFILE (effects on lower esophageal spincter pressure)

	ONSET	PEAK	DURATION
PO	30–60 min	70 min	UK

NURSING IMPLICATIONS

ASSESSMENT
▫ Assess patient for nocturnal symptoms (heartburn) associated with GERD.

POTENTIAL NURSING DIAGNOSES
▪ Pain (indications).
▪ Knowledge deficit related to medication regimen (patient/family teaching).

IMPLEMENTATION
▪ **PO:** Administer 15 min before each meal and at bedtime.

PATIENT/FAMILY TEACHING
▫ Instruct patient to take cisapride as directed, even if feeling better.
▫ Advise patient to avoid alcohol or other depressants while taking cisapride, as cisapride may enhance the sedative effects of these products.

EVALUATION
Effectiveness of therapy can be determined by: ▪ Decrease in nocturnal symptoms of GERD.

CISPLATIN
(sis-**pla**-tin)
CDDP, Platinol, Platinol-AQ

CLASSIFICATION(S):
Antineoplastic (alkylating agent)
Pregnancy Category UK

INDICATIONS

▪ Alone or in combination (with other antineoplastics, surgery, or radiation) in the management of: ▫ Metastatic testicular and ovarian carcinoma ▫ Advanced bladder cancer ▫ Head and neck cancer ▫ Cervical cancer ▫ Lung cancer ▫ Other tumors.

ACTION

▪ Inhibits DNA synthesis by producing cross-linking of parent DNA strands. (cell cycle-phase nonspecific). **Therapeutic Effect:** ▪ Death of rapidly replicating cells, particularly malignant cells.

PHARMACOKINETICS

Absorption: Following IV administration absorption is essentially complete.
Distribution: Widely distributed. Accumulates for months after administration.
Metabolism and Excretion: Excreted mainly by the kidneys.
Half-life: 30–100 hr.

*Underlines indicate most frequent; **CAPITALS** indicate life-threatening.

CONTRAINDICATIONS AND PRECAUTIONS

Contraindicated in: ▪ Hypersensitivity ▪ Pregnancy or lactation.

Use Cautiously in: ▪ Hearing loss ▪ Renal impairment (dosage reduction recommended) ▪ Electrolyte abnormalities ▪ Patients with childbearing potential ▪ Active infections ▪ Bone marrow depression ▪ Chronic debilitating illnesses.

ADVERSE REACTIONS AND SIDE EFFECTS*

CNS: SEIZURES.
EENT: ototoxicity, tinnitus.
GI: severe nausea, vomiting, diarrhea, hepatotoxicity.
GU: nephrotoxicity, infertility.
F and E: hypomagnesemia, hypokalemia, hypocalcemia.
Hemat: anemia, leukopenia, thrombocytopenia.
Local: phlebitis at IV site.
Metab: hyperuricemia.
Neuro: peripheral neuropathy.
Misc: anaphylactoid reactions.

INTERACTIONS

Drug–Drug: ▪ Additive nephrotoxicity and ototoxicity with other **nephro-** and **ototoxic drugs (aminoglycosides, loop diuretics)** ▪ Additive bone marrow depression with other **antineoplastic agents** or **radiation therapy**.

ROUTE AND DOSAGE

▪ **IV (Adults):** 20 mg/m^2 daily for 5 days or 50–70 mg/m^2, repeat q 3–4 wk in combination with other agents (up to 100 mg/m^2 q 4 wk if used as a single agent).

AVAILABILITY

▪ *Injection:* 10-mg, 50-mg, 100-mg vials.

TIME/ACTION PROFILE (effects on blood counts)

	ONSET	PEAK	DURATION
IV	UK	18–23 days	39 days

NURSING IMPLICATIONS

ASSESSMENT

▫ Monitor blood pressure, pulse, respiratory rate, and temperature frequently during administration. Notify physician of significant changes.

▫ Monitor intake and output and specific gravity frequently throughout therapy. Physician should be notified immediately if discrepancies occur. To reduce the risk of nephrotoxicity, a urinary output of at least 100 ml/hr should be maintained for 4 hr before initiating and for at least 24 hr after administration.

▫ Encourage patient to drink 2000–3000 ml/day to promote excretion of uric acid. Allopurinol and alkalinization of the urine may be ordered to help prevent uric acid nephropathy.

▫ Assess patency of IV site frequently during therapy. This medication may cause severe irritation and necrosis of tissue if extravasation occurs.

▫ Severe and protracted nausea and vomiting may occur as early as 1 hr after therapy and may last for 24 hr. Parenteral antiemetic agents should be administered 30–45 min prior to therapy and routinely around the clock for the next 24 hr as indicated. Monitor amount of emesis and notify physician if emesis exceeds guidelines to prevent dehydration.

▫ Assess for fever, chills, sore throat, and signs of infection. Notify physician if these symptoms occur.

▫ Monitor platelet count throughout therapy. Assess for bleeding (bleeding gums, bruising, petechiae; guaiac stools, urine, and emesis). Avoid IM injections and rectal temperatures. Apply pressure to venipuncture sites for 10 min.

▫ Anemia may occur. Monitor for increased fatigue, dyspnea, and orthostatic hypotension.

▫ Monitor for signs of anaphylaxis (facial edema, wheezing, tachycardia, hypotension). Discontinue medication immediately and notify physi-

*Underlines indicate most frequent; **CAPITALS** indicate life-threatening.

cian if these occur. Epinephrine and resuscitation equipment should be readily available.

▫ Medication may cause ototoxicity (especially in children) and neurotoxicity. Assess patient frequently for dizziness, tinnitus, hearing loss, loss of coordination, or numbness and tingling of extremities. These symptoms may be irreversible. Notify physician promptly if these occur.

▪ **Lab Test Considerations:** Monitor CBC prior to and routinely throughout course of therapy. The nadir of leukopenia, thrombocytopenia, and anemia occur within 18–23 days. Withhold further doses until WBC is >4000/mm^3 and platelet count is >100,000/mm^3.

▫ Monitor renal and hepatic function prior to and periodically throughout course of therapy. May cause nephrotoxicity (increased BUN and creatinine, and decreased calcium, magnesium, phosphate, and potassium levels). Do not administer additional doses until BUN is <25 mg/100 ml and serum creatinine is <1.5 mg/100 ml. May cause increased uric acid levels. Hepatotoxity may be manifested by increased AST (SGOT), ALT (SGPT), and bilirubin.

POTENTIAL NURSING DIAGNOSES
▪ Infection, high risk for (adverse reactions).
▪ Injury, high risk for (side effects).
▪ Knowledge deficit related to medication regimen (patient/family teaching).

IMPLEMENTATION
▪ **General Info:** Hydrate patient with at least 1–2 liters of IV fluid 8–12 hr before initiating therapy with cisplatin.
▫ Do not use aluminum needles or equipment during preparation or administration. Aluminum reacts with the drug, forms a black or brown precipitate, and renders it ineffective.
▫ Unopened vials of powder must be refrigerated.
▫ Solution should be prepared in a biologic cabinet. Wear gloves, gown, and

mask while handling medication. Discard equipment in specially designated containers (see Appendix I).

▪ **Intermittent Infusion:** Reconstitute 10-mg vials with 10 ml of Sterile Water for Injection and 50-mg vial with 50 ml. Stable for 2 hr if reconstituted with sterile water, for 72 hr with bacteriostatic water. Do not refrigerate, as crystals will form. Solution should be clear and colorless; discard if turbid or contains precipitates.

▫ Dilution in 2 liters of 5% dextrose in 0.3% or 0.45% NaCl containing 37.5 g of mannitol is recommended.

▪ *Rate:* Infuse over 6–8 hr.

▪ **Continuous Infusion:** Has been administered as continuous infusion over 24 hr to 5 days with resultant decrease in nausea and vomiting.

▪ **Syringe Compatibility:** ▪ bleomycin ▪ cyclophosphamide ▪ doxapram ▪ doxorubicin ▪ droperidol ▪ fluorouracil ▪ furosemide ▪ heparin ▪ leucovorin calcium ▪ methotrexate ▪ metoclopramide ▪ mitomycin ▪ vinblastine ▪ vincristine.

▪ **Y-Site Compatability:** ▪ bleomycin ▪ cyclophosphamide ▪ doxorubicin ▪ droperidol ▪ fludarabine ▪ fluorouracil ▪ furosemide ▪ heparin ▪ leucovorin calcium ▪ methotrexate ▪ metoclopromide ▪ mitomycin ▪ ondansetron ▪ sargramostim ▪ vinblastine ▪ vincristine.

▪ **Additive Compatability:** ▪ etoposide ▪ floxuridine ▪ hydroxyzine ▪ leucovorin calcium ▪ magnesium sulfate ▪ mannitol ▪ 0.9% NaCl ▪ D5/0.9% NaCl.

▪ **Additive Incompatability:** ▪ fluorouracil ▪ mesna ▪ sodium bicarbonate ▪ thiotepa.

PATIENT/FAMILY TEACHING
▫ Instruct patient to report pain at injection site immediately.
▫ Instruct patient to notify physician promptly if fever, sore throat, signs of infection, bleeding gums, bruising, petechiae; blood in stools, urine, or emesis; increased fatigue, dyspnea, or orthostatic hypotension occur.

Caution patient to avoid crowds and persons with known infections. Instruct patient to use soft toothbrush and electric razor, and to avoid falls. Caution patient not to drink alcoholic beverages or take medication containing aspirin or ibuprofen, as these may precipitate gastric bleeding.

□ Instruct patient to report promptly any numbness or tingling in extremities or face, difficulty with hearing or tinnitus, unusual swelling, or joint pain to physician.

□ Instruct patient not to receive any vaccinations without advice of physician.

□ Advise patient of the need for contraception although cisplatin may cause infertility.

□ Emphasize the need for periodic lab tests to monitor for side effects.

EVALUATION
Effectiveness of therapy may be determined by: ▪ Decrease in size or spread of malignancies ▪ Therapy should not be administered more frequently than every 3–4 wk, and only if lab values are within acceptable parameters and patient is not exhibiting signs of ototoxicity or other serious adverse effects.

CLARITHROMYCIN
(klare-**ith**-row-my-sin)
Biaxin

CLASSIFICATION(S):
Anti-infective (macrolide)
Pregnancy Category C

INDICATIONS
▪ Treatment of the following infections due to susceptible organisms: □ Upper respiratory tract infections including streptococcal pharyngitis and sinusitis □ Lower respiratory tract infections including bronchitis and pneumonia.

ACTION
▪ Inhibits protein synthesis at the level of the 50S bacterial ribosome. **Thera-**peutic Effect:** ▪ Bacteriostatic action against susceptible bacteria. **Spectrum:** ▪ Active against the following gram-positive aerobic bacteria: □ *Staphylococcus aureus* □ *Streptococcus pneumoniae* □ *Streptococcus pyogenes* (group A strep) ▪ Active against these gram-negative aerobic bacteria: □ *Haemophilus influenzae* □ *Moraxella catarrhalis* ▪ Also active against: □ *Mycoplasma* □ *Legionella* ▪ Not active against methicillin-resistant *Staphylococcus aureus*.

PHARMACOKINETICS
Absorption: Rapidly absorbed (50%) following oral administration.
Distribution: Widely distributed to body tissues and fluids. Tissue levels may exceed those in serum.
Metabolism and Excretion: 10–15% conversion by the liver to 14-hydroxyclarithromycin, which has anti-infective activity. 20–30% excreted unchanged in urine.
Half-life: 250-mg dose—3–4 hr; 500-mg dose—5–7 hr.

CONTRAINDICATIONS AND PRECAUTIONS
Contraindicated in: ▪ Hypersensitivity to clarithromycin, erythromycin, or other macrolide anti-infectives.
Use Cautiously in: ▪ Pregnancy (avoid use unless no alternatives available) ▪ Lactation and children <12 yr (safety not established) ▪ Severe liver and/or renal impairment (dosage adjustment required if creatinine clearance <30 ml/min).

ADVERSE REACTIONS AND SIDE EFFECTS*
CNS: headache.
GI: diarrhea, nausea, abnormal taste, dyspepsia, abdominal pain/discomfort.
Hemat: leukopenia, elevated prothrombin time.

INTERACTIONS
Drug–Drug: ▪ May increase serum levels and the risk of toxicity from **the-**

---

ophylline or **carbamazepine** ▪ May increase the effect of **oral anticoagulants** ▪ May decrease effects of **zidovudine** ▪ May increase risk of arrhythmias with **astemizole** or **terfenadine**.

ROUTE AND DOSAGE

▪ **PO (Adults):** 250–500 mg q 12 hr.

AVAILABILITY

▪ *Tablets:* 250 mg, 500 mg.

TIME/ACTION PROFILE (serum levels)

	ONSET	PEAK
PO	UK	2 hr

NURSING IMPLICATIONS

Assessment

□ Assess patient for infection (vital signs; appearance of wound, sputum, urine, and stool; WBC) at beginning and throughout course of therapy.

□ Obtain specimens for culture and sensitivity prior to initiating therapy. First dose may be given before receiving results.

▪ **Lab Test Considerations:** May cause increased serum bilirubin, AST (SGOT), ALT (SGPT), LDH, and alkaline phosphatase concentrations.

□ May rarely cause elevated prothrombin time, BUN, and serum creatinine. May occasionally cause decreased WBC.

Potential Nursing Diagnoses

▪ Infection, high risk for (indications, side effects).

▪ Knowledge deficit related to medication regimen (patient/family teaching).

▪ Noncompliance related to medication regimen (patient/family teaching).

Implementation

▪ **PO:** Administer around the clock, without regard to meals. Food slows but does not decrease the extent of absorption.

Patient/Family Teaching

□ Instruct patients to take medication around the clock and to finish the drug completely as directed, even if feeling better. Missed doses should be taken as soon as possible, with remaining doses evenly spaced throughout day. Advise patients that sharing of this medication may be dangerous.

□ Advise patient to report the signs of superinfection (black, furry overgrowth on the tongue, vaginal itching or discharge, loose or foul-smelling stools).

□ Instruct patient to notify the physician if fever and diarrhea develop, especially if stool contains blood, pus, or mucus. Advise patient not to treat diarrhea without consulting physician or pharmacist.

□ Advise patient to notify physician if pregnancy is planned or suspected.

□ Instruct the patient to notify the physician if symptoms do not improve.

Evaluation

Clinical response to therapy may be determined by: ▪ Resolution of the signs and symptoms of infection. Length of time for complete resolution depends on the organism and site of infection.

CLEMASTINE

(**klem**-as-teen)
Tavist

CLASSIFICATION(S):
Antihistamine
Pregnancy Category B

INDICATIONS

▪ Relief of allergic symptoms caused by histamine release.

ACTION

▪ Blocks the following effects of histamine: □ Vasodilation □ Increased GI tract secretions □ Increased heart rate □ Hypotension. **Therapeutic Effect:** ▪ Relief of symptoms associated with histamine excess usually seen in allergic conditions. Does not block the release of histamine.

PHARMACOKINETICS

Absorption: Well absorbed following oral administration.

Distribution: Enters breast milk in high concentrations.

Metabolism and Excretion: Extensively metabolized by the liver.

Half-life: UK.

CONTRAINDICATIONS AND PRECAUTIONS

Contraindicated in: ▪ Hypersensitivity ▪ Acute attacks of asthma ▪ Lactation (avoid use) ▪ Known alcohol intolerance (liquid form).

Use Cautiously in: ▪ Narrow-angle glaucoma ▪ Liver disease ▪ Elderly patients (more susceptible to adverse reactions) ▪ Pregnancy or children <6 yr (safety not established).

ADVERSE REACTIONS AND SIDE EFFECTS*

CNS: <u>drowsiness</u>, <u>sedation</u>, dizziness, confusion, paradoxical excitation (children).

CV: hypotension, <u>hypertension</u>, palpitations, arrhythmias.

EENT: <u>blurred vision</u>.

GI: <u>dry mouth</u>, obstruction, constipation.

GU: urinary hesitancy, retention.

Derm: sweating.

INTERACTIONS

Drug–Drug: ▪ Additive CNS depression with other **CNS depressants,** including **alcohol, opioid analgesics,** and **sedative/hypnotics** ▪ **MAO inhibitors** intensify and prolong the anticholinergic effects of antihistamines.

ROUTE AND DOSAGE

▪ **PO (Adults):** 1.34 mg twice daily or 2.68 mg 1–3 times daily.

▪ **PO (Children 6–12 yr):** 0.67–1.34 mg twice daily (not to exceed 4.02 mg/day).

AVAILABILITY

▪ *Tablets:* 1.34 mg, 2.68 mg ▪ *Syrup:* 0.67 mg/ml ▪ *In combination with:*

phenylpropanolamine (Tavist-D). See Appendix A.

TIME/ACTION PROFILE
(antihistaminic effects)

	ONSET	PEAK	DURATION
PO	15–60 min	1–2 hr	12 hr

NURSING IMPLICATIONS

ASSESSMENT

▫ Assess allergy symptoms (rhinitis, conjunctivitis, hives, urticaria) prior to and periodically throughout course of therapy.

▫ Assess lung sounds and character of bronchial secretions. Maintain fluid intake of 1500–2000 ml/day to decrease viscosity of secretions.

▪ **Lab Test Considerations:** May cause false-negative reactions on allergy skin tests; discontinue 3 days prior to testing.

▪ **Toxicity and Overdose:** Symptoms of toxicity in children include excitement, hyperreflexia, hallucinations, tremors, ataxia, fever, seizures, fixed dilated pupils, dry mouth, and facial flushing. The dose that causes seizures approximates the lethal dose. Adults are more likely to experience severe drowsiness.

POTENTIAL NURSING DIAGNOSES

▪ Airway clearance, ineffective (indications).

▪ Injury, high risk for (adverse reactions).

▪ Knowledge deficit related to medication regimen (patient/family teaching).

IMPLEMENTATION

▪ **PO:** Administer with food or milk to decrease GI irritation.

PATIENT/FAMILY TEACHING

▫ Instruct patient to take medication as directed. Do not take more than recommended amount. Missed doses should be taken as soon as remembered unless almost time for next dose. Do not double dose.

*<u>Underlines</u> indicate most frequent; **CAPITALS** indicate life-threatening.

□ Clemastine may cause drowsiness. Caution patient to avoid driving or other activities requiring alertness until response to drug is known.

□ Caution patient to avoid using alcohol or other CNS depressants concurrently with this drug.

□ Advise patient that good oral hygiene, frequent rinsing of mouth with water, and sugarless gum or candy may help relieve dry mouth. Patient should notify dentist if dry mouth persists for >2 wk.

□ Elderly patients are at risk for orthostatic hypotension. Advise patient to make position changes slowly.

□ Instruct patient to contact physician if symptoms persist or difficulty with urination, changes in vision, confusion, severe dry mouth, nose, and throat, or dizziness occur. Parents should notify physician if their child has difficulty sleeping, becomes unusually excited or irritable, or develops shortness of breath or facial flushing.

EVALUATION
Effectiveness of therapy can be demonstrated by: ■ Decrease in allergic symptoms.

CLINDAMYCIN
(klin-da-**mye**-sin)
Cleocin, {Dalacin C}

CLASSIFICATION(S):
Anti-infective (miscellaneous)
Pregnancy Category UK

INDICATIONS
■ **PO, IM, IV:** Treatment of the following serious infections due to susceptible organisms: □ Skin and skin structure infections □ Respiratory tract infections □ Septicemia □ Intra-abdominal infections □ Gynecologic infections □ Osteomyelitis ■ Endocarditis prophylaxis ■ **Top:** Treatment of severe acne ■ **Vag:** Treatment of bacterial vaginosis.

ACTION
■ Inhibits protein synthesis in susceptible bacteria at the level of the 50S ribosome. **Therapeutic Effect:** ■ Bactericidal or bacteriostatic, depending on susceptibility and concentration. **Spectrum:** ■ Active against most gram-positive aerobic cocci, including: □ Staphylococci □ *Streptococcus pneumoniae* □ Other streptococci, but not enterococcus ■ Has good activity against those anaerobic bacteria that cause bacterial vaginosis, including *Bacteroides fragilis* sp, *Gardinerella vaginalis, Mobiluncus* sp, *Mycoplasma hominus,* and *Corynebacterium.*

PHARMACOKINETICS
Absorption: Well absorbed following oral and IM administration. Minimal absorption following topical application.
Distribution: Widely distributed. Does not significantly cross blood–brain barrier. Crosses the placenta and enters breast milk.
Metabolism and Excretion: Mostly metabolized by the liver.
Half-life: 2–3 hr.

CONTRAINDICATIONS AND PRECAUTIONS
Contraindicated in: ■ Hypersensitivity ■ Previous pseudomembranous colitis ■ Severe liver impairment ■ Diarrhea ■ Known alcohol intolerance (topical solution, suspension).
Use Cautiously in: ■ Pregnancy or lactation (safety not established).

ADVERSE REACTIONS AND SIDE EFFECTS*
CNS: dizziness, vertigo, headache.
CV: hypotension, arrhythmias.
Derm: rashes.
GI: diarrhea, nausea, vomiting, PSEUDOMEMBRANOUS COLITIS, bitter taste (IV only).
Local: phlebitis at IV site.

{} = Available in Canada only.
*Underlines indicate most frequent; **CAPITALS** indicate life-threatening.

INTERACTIONS

Drug–Drug: ▪ **Kaolin** may decrease GI absorption ▪ May enhance the neuro-muscular blocking action of other **neuromuscular blocking agents** ▪ **Top:** Concurrent use with **irritants, abrasives,** or **desquamating agents** may result in additive irritation ▪ **Top:** Antagonizes the effects of topical **erythromycin.**

ROUTE AND DOSAGE

▪ **PO (Adults):** 150–450 mg q 6 hr.
▪ **PO (Children):** 8–25 mg/kg/day in divided doses q 6–8 hr. (Children ≤10 kg should receive at least 37.5 mg q 8 hr.)
▪ **IM, IV (Adults):** 600–1200 mg/day in 2–4 divided doses (up to 4.8 g/day IV has been used, single IM doses of >600 mg are not recommended).
▪ **IM, IV (Neonates):** 15–20 mg/kg/day in divided doses q 6–8 hr.
▪ **IM, IV (Neonates <1 mo):** 15–20 mg/kg/day in 3–4 divided doses.
▪ **IM, IV (Children >1 mo):** 20–40 mg/kg/day in 3–4 divided doses (350–450 mg/m²/day).
▪ **Vag:** 5 g applicatorful hs for 7 days.
▪ **Top:** 1% solution applied twice daily.

AVAILABILITY

▪ *Capsules:* 75 mg, 150 mg, 300 mg
▪ *Oral suspension:* 75 mg/5 ml ▪ *Injection:* 150 mg/ml ▪ *Topical:* 1% lotion, gel, solution, suspension ▪ *Vaginal:* 2% cream.

TIME/ACTION PROFILE (blood levels)

	ONSET	PEAK
PO	rapid	45 min
IM	rapid	1.3 hr
IV	rapid	end of infusion
Vag/Top	rapid	UK

NURSING IMPLICATIONS

ASSESSMENT

▫ Assess patient for infection (vital signs; appearance of wound, sputum, urine, and stool; WBC) at beginning and throughout course of therapy.
▫ Obtain specimens for culture and sensitivity prior to initiating therapy. First dose may be given before receiving results.
▫ Monitor bowel elimination. Diarrhea, abdominal cramping, fever, and bloody stools should be reported to physician promptly as a sign of drug-induced pseudomembranous colitis. This may begin up to several weeks following the cessation of therapy.
▫ Assess patient for hypersensitivity (skin rash, urticaria).
▪ **Lab Test Considerations:** Monitor CBC; may cause transient decrease in leukocytes, eosinophils, and platelets.
▫ May cause elevated alkaline phosphatase, bilirubin, CPK, AST (SGOT), and ALT (SGPT) concentrations.

POTENTIAL NURSING DIAGNOSES

▪ Infection, high risk for (indications, side effects).
▪ Diarrhea (side effects).
▪ Knowledge deficit related to medication regimen (patient/family teaching).

IMPLEMENTATION

▪ **PO:** Administer the oral form of the drug with a full glass of water. May be given with meals. Shake liquid preparations well. Do not refrigerate. Stable for 14 days at room temperature.
▪ **IM:** Do not administer >600 mg in a single IM injection.
▪ **Intermittent Infusion:** Do not administer as an undiluted IV bolus. Dilute each 300 mg for IV administration with at least 50 ml of D5W, D10W, D5/0.45% NaCl, D5/0.9% NaCl, D5/Ringer's injection, 0.9% NaCl, or lactated Ringer's solution for injection. Stable for 24 hr at room temperature. Crystals may occur if refrigerated but dissolve when warmed to room temperature. Do not administer solution with undissolved crystals.
▪ *Rate:* Administer each 300 mg over a minimum of 10 min. Do not give more than 1200 mg in a single 1-hr infusion.
▪ **Continuous Infusion:** May also be initially administered as a single rapid

infusion, followed by continuous IV infusion.
- **Syringe Compatibility:** - amikacin - aztreonam - gentamicin - heparin.
- **Syringe Incompatibility:** - tobramycin.
- **Y-Site Compatibility:** - cyclophosphamide - enalaprilat - esmolol - foscarnet - hydromorphone - labetolol - magnesium sulfate - meperidine - morphine - multivitamins - ondansetron - perphenazine - zidovudine.
- **Vag:** Applicators are supplied for vaginal administration.
- **Top:** Contact with eyes, mucous membranes, and open cuts should be avoided during topical application. If accidental contact occurs, rinse with copious amounts of cool water.
  □ Wash affected areas with warm water and soap, rinse, and pat dry prior to application. Apply to entire affected area.

Patient/Family Teaching
- **General Info:** Instruct patient to take medication around the clock and to finish the drug completely as directed, even if feeling better. If a dose is missed, take as soon as remembered. If almost time for next dose, space doses 2–4 hr apart. Advise patient that sharing of this medication may be dangerous.
  □ Instruct patient to notify physician immediately if diarrhea, abdominal cramping, fever, or bloody stools occur and not to treat with antidiarrheals without physician's approval.
  □ Advise patient to report signs of superinfection (furry overgrowth on the tongue, vaginal or anal itching or discharge).
  □ Notify physician if no improvement within a few days.
  □ Patients with a history of rheumatic heart disease or valve replacement need to be taught the importance of antimicrobial prophylaxis before invasive medical or dental procedures.
- **IV:** Inform patient that bitter taste occurring with IV administration is not significant.

- **Vaginal:** Instruct patient on proper use of vaginal applicator. Insert high into vagina at bedtime. Instruct patient to remain recumbent for at least 30 min following insertion. Advise patient to use sanitary napkin to prevent staining of clothing or bedding. Therapy should be continued during menstrual period.
  □ Advise patient to refrain from vaginal sexual intercourse during treatment.
  □ Caution patient that mineral oil in clindamycin cream may weaken latex or rubber condoms or diaphragms. Such products should not be used within 72 hr of vaginal cream.
- **Top:** Caution patient applying topical clindamycin that solution is flammable (vehicle is isopropyl alcohol). Avoid application while smoking or near heat or flame.
  □ Advise patient to notify physician if excessive drying of skin occurs.
  □ Advise patient to wait 30 min after washing or shaving area before applying.

Evaluation
Clinical response to therapy can be evaluated by: - Resolution of the signs and symptoms of infection. Length of time for complete resolution depends on the organism and site of infection - Endocarditis prophylaxis - Improvement in acne vulgaris lesions. Improvement should be seen in 6 wk but may take 8–12 wk for maximum benefit.

CLOFAZIMINE
(kloe-**fa**-zi-meen)
Lamprene

CLASSIFICATION(S):
Anti-infective (miscellaneous)
Pregnancy Category C

INDICATIONS
- In combination with other agents in the treatment of leprosy (Hansen's
  □ Draw the entire dose from below the froth line in the vial. Reconstituted

disease). **Unlabeled Use:** ▪ In combination with other agents in the treatment of atypical mycobacterial infections *(Mycobacterium avium-intracellulare)* in AIDS patients.

ACTION

▪ Binds to mycobacterial DNA, inhibiting mycobacterial protein synthesis and growth. **Therapeutic Effects:** ▪ Slow bactericidal action against susceptible mycobacteria ▪ Also has anti-inflammatory and immunosuppressive properties.

PHARMACOKINETICS

Absorption: Incompletely absorbed following oral administration. Degree of absorption depends on type of formulation and dose.
Distribution: Distributes to fatty and reticuloendothelial tissue concentrating as crystals. Does not enter CSF. Crosses the placenta and enters breast milk.
Metabolism and Excretion: 35–75% excreted unchanged in the feces. Small amounts eliminated in bile.
Half-life: 8 days (70 days in tissue).

CONTRAINDICATIONS AND PRECAUTIONS

Contraindicated in: ▪ Hypersensitivity.
Use Cautiously in: ▪ Has been used in pregnancy safely (skin discoloration of infants noted) ▪ Lactation (causes skin discoloration of nursing infant) ▪ Children <12 yr (safety not established) ▪ Abdominal pain or diarrhea ▪ Suicidal tendencies.

ADVERSE REACTIONS AND SIDE EFFECTS*

CNS: anxiety, depression, dizziness, drowsiness, fatigue.
EENT: red-brown discoloration of conjunctiva, cornea, and lacrimal fluid, dryness, burning, itching, irritation, lacrimation, visual loss.
GI: SPLENIC INFARCTION, BOWEL OBSTRUCTION, GI BLEEDING, abdominal

pain, epigastric pain, diarrhea, nausea, vomiting, anorexia, constipation.
Derm: dry skin, pinkish-brown discoloration of skin, rash, phototoxicity.
Misc: reddish-brown discoloration of sweat, sputum, urine, breast milk, feces, nasal secretions, and semen.

INTERACTIONS

Drug–Drug: ▪ **Dapsone** may negate the anti-inflammatory properties of clofazimine ▪ **Isoniazid** decreases skin concentrations and increases urinary excretion of clofazimine.

ROUTE AND DOSAGE

Leprosy
▪ **PO (Adults):** 50–100 mg/day (up to 300 mg/day).

Atypical Mycobacterium Infections
▪ **PO (Adults):** 100 mg q 8 hr.

AVAILABILITY

▪ *Capsules:* 50 mg, 100 mg.

TIME/ACTION PROFILE

	ONSET	PEAK	DURATION
PO	UK	UK	UK

NURSING IMPLICATIONS

ASSESSMENT

▪ **General Info:** Assess patient for mental depression and suicidal tendencies if skin discoloration occurs.
▪ **Leprosy:** Assess skin lesions periodically throughout treatment.
▪ **AIDS:** Assess vital signs, lung sounds, and respiratory status in patients with atypical mycobacterial infections.
▪ **Lab Test Considerations:** May cause increased erythrocyte sedimentation rate (ESR).
□ May cause elevated serum glucose, albumin, AST (SGOT), and bilirubin concentrations. May cause decreased serum potassium concentrations.

POTENTIAL NURSING DIAGNOSES

▪ Skin integrity, impaired (indications).

*Underlines indicate most frequent; **CAPITALS** indicate life-threatening.

- Body image disturbance (adverse reactions).
- Knowledge deficit related to medication regimen (patient/family teaching).

IMPLEMENTATION

- **PO:** Administer medication with meals or milk.

PATIENT/FAMILY TEACHING

- □ Instruct patient to take clofazimine as directed, at the same time every day; therapy may take years. Missed doses should be taken as soon as remembered if not almost time for next dose; do not double doses.
- □ May cause loss of vision, dizziness, or drowsiness. Caution patient to avoid driving or other activities requiring alertness until response to medication is known.
- □ Inform diabetic patients that clofazimine may cause elevated blood glucose test results.
- □ Advise patient to use sunscreen and protective clothing to prevent phototoxicity reactions.
- □ Instruct patient to use skin creams, lotions, or oils to treat rough, dry, or scaly skin.
- □ Inform patient that a reversible pink or red to brownish-black discoloration of the skin may occur within a few weeks of treatment. Several months or years after discontinuing clofazimine may be required for discoloration to disappear completely. May also cause discoloration of feces, lining of eyelids, sputum, sweat, tears, and urine.
- □ Instruct patient to notify physician promptly if abdominal pain, diarrhea, nausea or vomiting, jaundice, tarry stools, loss of vision, skin discoloration, or mental depression occurs.
- □ Advise patient to notify physician if no improvement is seen within 1–3 mo.

EVALUATION

Effectiveness of therapy may be determined by: ■ Improvement in skin lesions. Full therapeutic benefits may take up to 6 mo ■ Resolution of symptoms of atypical mycobacterial infection.

CLOMIPHENE
(**kloe**-mi-feen)
Clomid, Milophene, Serophene

CLASSIFICATION(S):
Hormone (ovulation inducer)
Pregnancy Category UK

INDICATIONS

■ Induces ovulation in anovulatory women who desire to become pregnant. Requires intact anterior pituitary, thyroid, and adrenal function. **Unlabeled Use:** ■ Male infertility caused by oligospermia.

ACTION

■ Stimulates release of pituitary gonadotropins, follicle-stimulating hormone, and luteinizing hormone, resulting in ovulation and the development of the corpus luteum. **Therapeutic Effect:** ■ Induction of ovulation.

PHARMACOKINETICS

Absorption: Well absorbed following oral administration.
Distribution: Not known.
Metabolism and Excretion: Apparently metabolized by the liver, with enterohepatic recirculation and biliary elimination. Excreted in feces.
Half-life: 5 days.

CONTRAINDICATIONS AND PRECAUTIONS

Contraindicated in: ■ Liver disease ■ Ovarian cysts ■ Pregnancy.
Use Cautiously in: ■ Known sensitivity to pituitary gonadotropins ■ Polycystic ovary syndrome.

ADVERSE REACTIONS AND SIDE EFFECTS*

CNS: nervousness, restlessness, headache, insomnia, lightheadedness, fatigue.

EENT: blurred vision, scotoma, photophobia, visual disturbances.
CV: flushing, hot flashes.
GI: distention, bloating, abdominal pain, nausea, vomiting, increased appetite.
GU: urinary frequency, increased urine volume.
Derm: rashes, urticaria, allergic dermatitis, reversible hair loss.
Endo: ovarian enlargement, cyst formation, breast discomfort, multiple births.
Metab: weight gain.

INTERACTIONS
Drug–Drug: None significant.

ROUTE AND DOSAGE
- **PO (Adults):** 25–50 mg/day for 5 days; if ovulation does not occur, a second course of 100 mg/day for 5 days may be given 30 days after the initial course. A maximum of 3 courses may be administered. Some patients require up to 250 mg/day.

AVAILABILITY
- *Tablets:* 50 mg.

TIME/ACTION PROFILE (ovulation)

	ONSET	PEAK	DURATION
PO	5–14 days	UK	UK

NURSING IMPLICATIONS
ASSESSMENT
- A pelvic examination to determine ovarian size should be completed prior to course of therapy.
- An endometrial biopsy is recommended in older patients prior to clomiphene therapy to rule out the presence of endometrial carcinoma.
- **Lab Test Considerations:** Estrogen excretion determinations, histological studies of the luteal phase endometrium, serum progesterone, and urinary excretion of pregnanediol may be used to determine whether ovulation has occurred following a course of clomiphene.
- Liver function tests should be performed prior to course of therapy.
- May cause increased serum thyroxine and thyroxine-binding globulin levels.

POTENTIAL NURSING DIAGNOSES
- Knowledge deficit related to medication regimen (patient/family teaching).

IMPLEMENTATION
- **General Info:** Clomiphene therapy is usually begun on the fifth day of the menstrual cycle.

PATIENT/FAMILY TEACHING
- Instruct patient to take clomiphene exactly as directed at the same time each day. Missed doses should be taken as soon as remembered and the dose doubled if not remembered until the time of the next dose. Notify physician if more than 1 dose is missed.
- Advise patient that conception should be attempted with intercourse every other day starting 48 hr prior to ovulation.
- Instruct patient in the correct method for measuring basal body temperature. A record of the daily basal body temperature should be maintained prior to and throughout course of therapy. Emphasize the importance of compliance with all aspects of therapy.
- Prior to therapy, patient should be informed of the potential for multiple births.
- Medication may cause visual disturbances or dizziness. Caution patient to avoid driving until the response to the medication is known.
- Instruct patient to notify physician immediately if pregnancy is suspected; clomiphene should not be taken during pregnancy.
- Advise patient that ophthalmologic examinations should be performed to evaluate the possibility of ocular toxicity if treatment is continued for more than 1 yr.
- Advise patient to notify physician promptly if bloating, stomach or pelvic pain, blurred vision, jaundice, persistent hot flashes, breast discomfort, headache, or nausea and vomiting occur.

▫ Emphasize the importance of close monitoring by the physician throughout course of therapy.

EVALUATION
Effectiveness of therapy can be demonstrated by: ▪ Occurrence of ovulation measured by estrogen excretion, biphasic body temperature curve, urinary excretion of pregnanediol at postovulatory levels, and endometrial histologic changes. If conception is not achieved after 3–4 courses of clomiphene, diagnosis should be re-evaluated.

CLOMIPRAMINE
(kloe-**mip**-ra-meen)
Anafranil

CLASSIFICATION(S):
Antipsychotic, Antiobsessive agent
Pregnancy Category UK

INDICATIONS
▪ Management of obsessive-compulsive disorder (OCD).

ACTION
▪ Potentiates the effect of serotonin (antiobsessional effect) and norepinephrine in the CNS. Also has moderate anticholinergic properties. **Therapeutic Effect:** ▪ Diminished obsessive-compulsive behavior.

PHARMACOKINETICS
Absorption: Well absorbed from the GI tract.
Distribution: Widely distributed.
Metabolism and Excretion: Extensively metabolized by the liver. Some conversion to a pharmacologically active metabolite (desmethylclomipramine). Undergoes enterohepatic recirculation and secretion into gastric juices. Appears to enter breast milk.
Half-life: 21–31 hr.

CONTRAINDICATIONS AND PRECAUTIONS
Contraindicated in: ▪ Hypersensitivity ▪ Pregnancy or lactation ▪ Narrow-angle glaucoma ▪ Recent myocardial infarction.
Use Cautiously in: ▪ History of seizures (threshold may be lowered) ▪ Children <10 yr (safety not established) ▪ Elderly patients ▪ Concurrent MAO inhibitor or clonidine use (avoid if possible) ▪ Patients with pre-existing cardiovascular disease ▪ Elderly men with prostatic hypertrophy (may be more susceptible to urinary retention) ▪ Hyperthyroidism (increased risk of arrhythmias).

ADVERSE REACTIONS AND SIDE EFFECTS*
CNS: SEIZURES, sedation, drowsiness, lethargy, weakness, aggressive behavior.
EENT: dry eyes, dry mouth, blurred vision, vestibular disorder.
CV: hypotension, ARRHYTHMIAS, ECG changes.
GI: orthostatic constipation, eructation.
GU: urinary retention, male sexual dysfunction.
Derm: photosensitivity, dry skin.
Endo: gynecomastia.
Hemat: anemia.
MS: muscle weakness.
Neuro: extrapyramidal reactions.
Misc: hyperthermia, weight gain.

INTERACTIONS
Drug–Drug: ▪ May cause hypotension and tachycardia when used with **MAO inhibitors** ▪ May prevent the therapeutic response to **antihypertensives** ▪ Use with **clonidine** may result in hypertensive crisis ▪ Additive CNS depression with other **CNS depressants** including **alcohol, antihistamines, opioid analgesics,** and **sedative/hypnotics** ▪ **Adrenergic** and **anticholinergic** side effects may be additive with other **agents having these properties** ▪ Effects and toxicity may be increased by concurrent **fluoxe-**

tine, **phenothazines, cimetidine,** or **oral contraceptives ▪ Nicotine** (cigarette smoke or nicotine gum) may increase metabolism and decrease effectiveness ▪ Transient delerium may occur with **disulfiram**.

ROUTE AND DOSAGE

▪ **PO (Adults):** 25 mg/day initially, increased over 2-wk period to 100 mg/day in divided doses. May be further increased over several weeks to maximum of 250 mg/day in divided doses. Once stabilizing dose is reached, entire daily dose may be given at bedtime.

▪ **PO (Children and Adolescents):** 25 mg/day initially, increased over 2-wk period to 3 mg/kg/day or 100 mg/day (whichever is smaller) in divided doses. May be further increased to 3 mg/kg/day or 200 mg/day (whichever is smaller) in divided doses. Once stabilizing dose is reached, entire daily dose may be given at bedtime.

AVAILABILITY

▪ *Capsules:* 25 mg, 50 mg, 75 mg.

TIME/ACTION PROFILE

	ONSET	PEAK	DURATION
PO	1–6 wk	UK	UK

NURSING IMPLICATIONS

ASSESSMENT

□ Monitor mental status and affect. Assess patient for frequency of obsessive-compulsive behaviors. Note degree to which these thoughts and behaviors interfere with daily functioning.

□ Observe for onset of extrapyramidal side effects (pill-rolling motions, drooling, tremors, rigidity, mask facies, shuffling gait, restlessness, muscle spasms, twisting motions). Notify physician immediately if these symptoms occur. Dosage reduction or discontinuation may be necessary. Physician may order antiparkinson agents to control extrapyramidal effects.

POTENTIAL NURSING DIAGNOSIS

▪ Coping, ineffective individual (obsessive-compulsive behaviors) related to repressed anxiety (indications).

▪ Injury, high risk for (side effects).

▪ Knowledge deficit related to medication regimen (patient/family teaching).

IMPLEMENTATION

▪ **PO:** Administer medication with or immediately following a meal to minimize gastric irritation. After titration of dosage, total daily dose may be given at bedtime.

PATIENT/FAMILY TEACHING

□ Instruct patient to take medication exactly as directed. Abrupt discontinuation may cause nausea, headache, and malaise.

□ May cause drowsiness and blurred vision. Caution patient to avoid driving and other activities requiring alertness until response to drug is known.

□ Advise patient to avoid alcohol or other CNS depressant drugs during course of therapy and for 3–7 days after cessation of therapy.

□ Instruct patient to notify physician if dry mouth or constipation persists or if urinary retention or uncontrolled movements or rigidity occur. Sugarless candy or gum may diminish dry mouth, and an increase in fluid intake or bulk may prevent constipation. If these symptoms persist, dosage reduction or discontinuation may be necessary.

□ Advise patient to inform physician if breast enlargement or sexual dysfunction occurs.

□ Caution patient to use sunscreen and protective clothing to prevent photosensitivity reactions.

□ Inform patient of need to monitor dietary intake as possible increase in appetite may lead to undesired weight gain.

□ Advise patient to notify physician or dentist of medication regimen prior to treatment or surgery.

□ Emphasize the importance of follow-up examinations to monitor effectiveness and side effects.

EVALUATION
Effectiveness of therapy can be demonstrated by: ▪ Diminished obsessive-compulsive behavior.

CLONAZEPAM
(kloe-**na**-ze-pam)
Klonopin, {Rivotril}

CLASSIFICATION(S):
Anticonvulsant (benzodiazepine)
Schedule IV
Pregnancy Category UK

INDICATIONS

▪ Prophylaxis of: □ Petit mal □ Petit mal variant □ Akinetic □ Myoclonic seizures **Unlabeled Uses:** ▪ Uncontrolled leg movements during sleep ▪ Neuralgias.

ACTION

▪ Produces anticonvulsant and sedative effects in the CNS. Mechanism is unknown but is probably similar to that of benzodiazepines (chlordiazepoxide, diazepam). **Therapeutic Effect:** ▪ Prevention of seizures.

PHARMACOKINETICS

Absorption: Well absorbed from the GI tract.
Distribution: Appears to cross the blood–brain barrier and the placenta.
Metabolism and Excretion: Mostly metabolized by the liver.
Half-life: 18–50 hr.

CONTRAINDICATIONS AND PRECAUTIONS

Contraindicated in: ▪ Hypersensitivity to clonazepam or other benzodiazepines ▪ Severe liver disease.
Use Cautiously in: ▪ Narrow-angle glaucoma ▪ Chronic respiratory disease ▪ Pregnancy or lactation (safety not established) ▪ Children (long-term effects on growth and maturation not known) ▪ Do not discontinue abruptly.

ADVERSE REACTIONS AND SIDE EFFECTS*

CNS: drowsiness, ataxia, hypotonia, behavioral changes.
EENT: abnormal eye movements, diplopia, nystagmus.
Resp: increased secretions.
CV: palpitations.
GI: constipation, diarrhea, hepatitis.
GU: dysuria, nocturia, urinary retention.
Hemat: anemia, leukopenia, thrombocytopenia, eosinophilia.
Misc: fever.

INTERACTIONS

Drug–Drug: ▪ **Alcohol, antidepressants, antihistamines,** and **opioid analgesics**—concurrent use results in additive CNS depression ▪ **Cimetidine, oral contraceptives, disulfiram, fluoxetine, isoniazid, ketoconazole, metoprolol, propoxyphene, propranolol,** or **valproic acid** may decrease the metabolism of clonazepam, enhancing its actions ▪ May decrease efficacy of **levodopa** ▪ **Rifampin** or **barbiturates** may increase the metabolism and decrease effectiveness of clonazepam ▪ Sedative effects may be decreased by **theophylline** ▪ May increase serum **phenytoin** levels ▪ **Phenytoin** may decrease serum clonazepam levels.

ROUTE AND DOSAGE

▪ **PO (Adults):** Initial daily dose not to exceed 1.5 mg given in 3 divided doses; may increase by 0.5–1 mg q 3rd day. Total daily maintenance dose not to exceed 20 mg.
▪ **PO (Children up to 10 yr or 30 kg):** Initial daily dose 0.01–0.03 mg/kg/day (not to exceed 0.05 mg/kg/day) given in 2–3 divided doses; increase by no more than 0.25–0.5 mg q 3rd day until therapeutic blood levels are reached. Daily dose not to exceed 0.2 mg/kg.

AVAILABILITY

▪ *Tablets:* 0.5 mg, 1 mg, 2 mg.

{} = Available in Canada only.
*Underlines indicate most frequent; **CAPITALS** indicate life-threatening.

TIME/ACTION PROFILE
(anticonvulsant activity)

	ONSET	PEAK	DURATION
PO	20–60 min	1–2 hr	6–12 hr

NURSING IMPLICATIONS

ASSESSMENT

□ Observe and record intensity, duration, and location of seizure activity.

□ Assess patient for drowsiness, unsteadiness, and clumsiness. These symptoms are dose-related and most severe during initial therapy; may decrease in severity or disappear with continued or long-term therapy.

▪ **Lab Test Considerations:** Evaluate liver function, CBC, and platelet counts periodically throughout course of prolonged therapy.

□ May cause decreased RBCs, WBCs, and platelets. May also cause increased AST (SGOT), ALT (SGPT), and alkaline phosphatase.

▪ **Toxicity and Overdose:** Therapeutic serum concentrations are 20–80 ng/ml.

POTENTIAL NURSING DIAGNOSES

▪ Injury, high risk for (indications, side effects).

▪ Knowledge deficit related to medication regimen (patient/family teaching).

IMPLEMENTATION

▪ **General Info:** Institute seizure precautions for patients on initial therapy or undergoing dosage manipulations.

▪ **PO:** Administer with food to minimize gastric irritation. Tablets may be crushed if patient has difficulty swallowing.

PATIENT/FAMILY TEACHING

□ Instruct patient to take medication exactly as directed. Missed doses should be taken within 1 hr or omitted; do not double doses. Abrupt withdrawal of clonazepam may cause status epilepticus, tremors, nausea, vomiting, and abdominal and muscle cramps.

□ Medication may cause drowsiness or dizziness. Advise patient to avoid driving or other activities requiring alertness until response to drug is known.

□ Caution patient to avoid taking alcohol or other CNS depressants concurrently with this medication.

□ Advise patient to notify physician or dentist of medication regimen prior to treatment or surgery.

□ Instruct patient and family to notify physician of unusual tiredness, bleeding, sore throat, fever, clay-colored stools, yellowing of skin, or behavioral changes.

□ Emphasize the importance of follow-up examinations to determine effectiveness of the medication.

□ Patient on anticonvulsant therapy should carry identification describing disease process and medication regimen at all times.

EVALUATION

Effectiveness of therapy can be demonstrated by: ▪ Decrease or cessation of seizure activity without undue sedation. Dosage adjustments may be required after several months of therapy ▪ Relief of leg movements during sleep ▪ Decrease in pain from neuralgia.

CLONIDINE
(**klon**-i-deen)
Catapres, Catapress-TTS,
{Dixarit}

CLASSIFICATION(S):
Antihypertensive (centrally acting adrenergic)
Pregnancy Category C

INDICATIONS

▪ Alone and in combination with other antihypertensives in the management of mild to moderate hypertension. **Unla-**

beled Uses: ▪ Management of opioid withdrawal, prophylaxis of vascular headaches, treatment of dysmenorrhea, treatment of menopausal syndrome.

ACTION

▪ Stimulates alpha-adrenergic receptors in the CNS. Result is inhibition of cardioacceleration and vasoconstriction center. **Therapeutic Effect:** ▪ Decrease in blood pressure.

PHARMACOKINETICS

Absorption: Well absorbed from the GI tract and through the skin.
Distribution: Widely distributed and crosses the blood–brain barrier. Enters breast milk.
Metabolism and Excretion: Mostly metabolized by the liver. 30% eliminated unchanged by the kidneys.
Half-life: 12–20 hr.

CONTRAINDICATIONS AND PRECAUTIONS

Contraindicated in: ▪ Hypersensitivity.
Use Cautiously in: ▪ Serious cardiac disease ▪ Cerebrovascular disease ▪ Renal insufficiency ▪ Pregnancy, lactation, or children (safety not established) ▪ Elderly patients (dosage reduction may be required) ▪ Do not discontinue abruptly.

ADVERSE REACTIONS AND SIDE EFFECTS*

CNS: <u>drowsiness</u>, nightmares, nervousness, depression.
CV: hypotension, bradycardia, palpitations.
GI: <u>dry mouth</u>, constipation.
GU: impotence.
Derm: rash.
F and E: sodium retention.
Metab: weight gain.
Misc: <u>withdrawal phenomenon</u>.

INTERACTIONS

Drug–Drug: ▪ Additive sedation with **CNS depressants** including **alcohol, antihistamines, opioid analgesics,** and **sedative/hypnotics** ▪ Additive hypoten-

sion with other **antihypertensive agents** and **nitrates** ▪ Additive bradycardia with **myocardial depressants,** including **beta-adrenergic blockers** ▪ **MAO inhibitors, amphetamines,** or **tricyclic antidepressants** may decrease antihypertensive effect ▪ Withdrawal phenomenon may be exaggerated by concurrent **tricyclic antidepressants** or discontinuation of **beta blockers** (discontinue beta blockers several days prior to discontinuing clonidine).

ROUTE AND DOSAGE

Hypertension
▪ **PO (Adults):** Initial dose 0.1 mg bid. Usual maintenance dose is 0.2–0.6 mg/day in 2–3 divided doses (up to 2.4 mg/day).
▪ **TD (Adults):** Transdermal system delivering 0.1–0.3 mg/24 hr system applied every 7 days.

Hypertensive Urgency
▪ **PO (Adults):** 0.1–0.2 mg initially, then 0.05–0.1 mg q h until BP controlled or total of 0.5–0.8 mg given, then start maintenance therapy.

Opioid Withdrawal
▪ **PO (Adults):** 0.3–1.2 mg/day, may be decreased by 50%/day for 3 days then discontinued or decreased by 0.1–0.2 mg/day.

Vascular Headache Prophylaxis
▪ **PO (Adults):** 0.025 mg 2–4 times daily (up to 0.15 mg/day in divided doses).

Dysmenorrhea
▪ **PO (Adults):** 0.025 mg twice daily for 14 days before and during menses.

Menopausal Syndrome
▪ **PO (Adults):** 0.025–0.075 mg twice daily.

AVAILABILITY

▪ *Tablets:* 0.1 mg, 0.2 mg, 0.3 mg
▪ *Transdermal systems:* Catapress-TTS 1 contains 2.5 mg total clonidine content, releases 0.1 mg/24 hr; Catapress-TTS 2 contains 5 mg total clonidine content, releases 0.2 mg/24 hr;

C

Catapress-TTS 3 contains 7.5 mg total clonidine content, releases 0.3 mg/24 hr
■ *In combination with:* chlorthalidone (Combipres). See Appendix A.

TIME/ACTION PROFILE
(antihypertensive effect)

	ONSET	PEAK	DURATION
PO	30–60 min	2–4 hr	8 hr
TD	2–3 days	UK	7 days*

*8 hr following removal of patch.

NURSING IMPLICATIONS

ASSESSMENT
■ **General Info:** Monitor intake and output ratios and daily weight, and assess for edema daily, especially at beginning of therapy.
■ **Hypertension:** Monitor blood pressure and pulse frequently during initial dosage adjustment and periodically throughout therapy. Notify physician of significant changes.
■ **Opioid Withdrawal:** Monitor patient for signs and symptoms of opioid withdrawal (tachycardia, fever, runny nose, diarrhea, sweating, nausea, vomiting, irritability, stomach cramps, shivering, unusually large pupils, weakness, difficulty sleeping, gooseflesh).
■ **Lab Test Considerations:** May cause transient increase in blood glucose levels.

POTENTIAL NURSING DIAGNOSES
■ Injury, high risk for (side effects).
■ Knowledge deficit related to medication regimen (patient/family teaching).
■ Noncompliance (patient/family teaching).

IMPLEMENTATION
■ **PO:** Administer last dose of the day at bedtime.
■ **Transdermal:** Transdermal system should be applied once every 7 days. May be applied to any hairless site; avoid cuts or callouses. Absorption is greater when placed on chest or upper arm, and decreased when placed on thigh. Rotate sites. Wash area with soap and water, dry thoroughly before application. Apply firm pressure over patch to ensure contact with skin, especially around edges. Remove old system and discard. System includes a protective adhesive overlay to be applied over medication patch to ensure adhesion should medication patch loosen.

PATIENT/FAMILY TEACHING
■ **General Info:** Instruct patient to take clonidine at the same time each day, even if feeling well. Clonidine controls but does not cure hypertension. If a dose is missed, take as soon as remembered. If more than 1 oral dose in a row is missed, or if transdermal system is late being changed by 3 or more days, consult physician. Oral clonidine should be gradually discontinued over 2–4 days to prevent rebound hypertension.
□ Encourage patient to comply with additional interventions for hypertension (weight reduction, low-sodium diet, discontinuation of smoking, moderation of alcohol consumption, regular exercise, and stress management). Patient should also avoid excessive amounts of tea, coffee, and cola.
□ Instruct patient and family on proper technique for blood pressure monitoring. Advise them to check blood pressure at least weekly and report significant changes to physician.
□ Clonidine may cause drowsiness. Advise patient to avoid driving or other activities requiring alertness until response to medication is known.
□ Caution patient to avoid sudden changes in position to decrease orthostatic hypotension. Use of alcohol, standing for long periods, exercising, and hot weather may increase orthostatic hypotension.
□ If dry mouth occurs, frequent mouth rinses, good oral hygiene, and sugarless gum or candy may decrease effect. If dry mouth continues for more than 2 wk, consult physician or dentist.

□ Caution patient to avoid concurrent use of alcohol or other CNS depressants with this medication.
□ Advise patient to consult physician or pharmacist before taking any cough, cold, or allergy remedies.
□ Advise patient to notify physician or dentist of medication regimen prior to treatment or surgery.
▪ **Transdermal:** Instruct patient on proper application of transdermal system. Do not cut or trim unit. Transdermal system can remain in place during bathing or swimming.

EVALUATION
Effectiveness of therapy can be demonstrated by: ▪ Decrease in blood pressure ▪ Decrease in the signs and symptoms of opioid withdrawal ▪ Prevention of vascular headaches ▪ Decrease in dysmenorrhea ▪ Decrease in symptoms of menopausal syndrome.

CLORAZEPATE
(klor-**az**-e-pate)
Gen-XENE, {Novoclopate},
Tranxene

CLASSIFICATION(S):
Antianxiety agent, Sedative/
hypnotic (benzodiazepine),
Anticonvulsant
Schedule IV
Pregnancy Category UK

INDICATIONS
▪ Treatment of anxiety ▪ Management of alcohol withdrawal ▪ Management of simple partial seizures.

ACTION
▪ Acts at many levels in the CNS to produce anxiolytic effect and CNS depression (by stimulating inhibitory GABA receptors) ▪ Produces skeletal muscle relaxation (by inhibiting spinal polysynaptic afferent pathways) ▪ Also has anticonvulsant effect (enhances presynaptic inhibition). **Therapeutic Effects:**
▪ Relief of anxiety ▪ Sedation ▪ Prevention of seizures.

PHARMACOKINETICS
Absorption: Well absorbed from the GI tract.
Distribution: Widely distributed. Crosses the placenta and enters breast milk.
Metabolism and Excretion: Metabolized by the liver. Some conversion to active compounds.
Half-life: 48 hr.

CONTRAINDICATIONS AND PRECAUTIONS
Contraindicated in: ▪ Hypersensitivity ▪ Cross-sensitivity with other benzodiazepines may exist ▪ Pre-existing CNS depression ▪ Severe uncontrolled pain ▪ Narrow-angle glaucoma ▪ Pregnancy or lactation.
Use Cautiously in: ▪ Pre-existing hepatic dysfunction ▪ Patients who may be suicidal or have been addicted to drugs in the past ▪ Elderly or debilitated patients (dosage reduction required) ▪ Severe pulmonary disease.

ADVERSE REACTIONS AND SIDE EFFECTS*
CNS: dizziness, drowsiness, lethargy, hangover, paradoxical excitation, mental depression, headache.
EENT: blurred vision.
Resp: respiratory depression.
GI: nausea, vomiting, diarrhea, constipation.
Derm: rashes.
Misc: tolerance, psychological dependence, physical dependence.

INTERACTIONS
Drug–Drug: ▪ **Alcohol, antidepressants, antihistamines,** and **opioid analgesics**—concurrent use results in additive CNS depression ▪ **Cimetidine, oral contraceptives, disulfram, fluoxetine, isoniazid, ketoconazole, metoprolol, propoxyphene, propranolol,** or **valproic acid** may decrease the

---

{} = Available in Canada only.
*Underlines indicate most frequent; CAPITALS indicate life-threatening.

metabolism of clorazepate, enhancing its actions ▪ May decrease efficacy of **levodopa** ▪ **Rifampin** or **barbiturates** may increase the metabolism and decrease effectiveness of clorazepate ▪ Sedative effects may be decreased by **theophylline**.

ROUTE AND DOSAGE
Anxiety
▪ **PO (Adults):** 15–60 mg/day in divided doses. May be given in a single dose of 11.25–22.5 mg at bedtime.
▪ **PO (Elderly/Debilitated Patients):** 7.5–15 mg/day.

Alcohol Withdrawal
▪ **PO (Adults):** 30 mg initially, then 15 mg 2–4 times daily on first day, then gradually decreased over subsequent days.

Anticonvulsant
▪ **PO (Adults):** 7.5 mg 3 times daily; can increase by no more than 7.5 mg/day at weekly intervals (daily dose not to exceed 90 mg).

AVAILABILITY
▪ **Tablets:** 3.75 mg, 7.5 mg, 11.25 mg, 15 mg, 22.5 mg ▪ **Capsules:** 3.75 mg, 7.5 mg, 15 mg.

TIME/ACTION PROFILE (sedation)

	ONSET	PEAK	DURATION
PO	1–2 hr	1–2 hr	up to 24 hr

NURSING IMPLICATIONS
ASSESSMENT
▪ **General Info:** Prolonged high-dose therapy may lead to psychological or physical dependence. Restrict amount of drug available to patient.
▪ **Anxiety:** Assess degree and manifestations of anxiety prior to and periodically throughout therapy.
▪ **Alcohol Withdrawal:** Assess patient experiencing alcohol withdrawal for tremors, agitation, delirium, and hallucinations. Protect from injury.
▪ **Seizures:** Observe and record intensity, duration, and location of seizure activity.

▪ **Lab Test Considerations:** Patients on high-dose therapy should receive routine evaluation of renal, hepatic, and hematologic function. May cause increased serum bilirubin, AST (SGOT), ALT (SGPT), and alkaline phosphatase concentrations.

POTENTIAL NURSING DIAGNOSES
▪ Anxiety (indications).
▪ Injury, high risk for (indications, side effects).
▪ Knowledge deficit related to medication regimen (patient/family teaching).

IMPLEMENTATION
▪ **PO:** If gastric irritation is a problem, may be administered with food or fluids. Capsule should be swallowed whole; do not open.
▫ Avoid administration of antacids within 1 hr of medication, as absorption of clorazepate may be delayed.

PATIENT/FAMILY TEACHING
▪ **General Info:** Instruct patient to take medication exactly as directed, not to skip or double up on missed doses. Abrupt withdrawal of clorazepate may cause status epilepticus, tremors, nausea, vomiting, and abdominal and muscle cramps.
▫ Medication may cause drowsiness or dizziness. Advise patient to avoid driving or other activities requiring alertness until response to drug is known.
▫ Caution patient to avoid taking alcohol or other CNS depressants concurrently with this medication.
▫ Instruct patient to contact physician immediately if pregnancy is suspected.
▫ Advise patient to notify physician or dentist of medication regimen prior to treatment or surgery.
▫ Emphasize the importance of follow-up examinations to determine effectiveness of the medication.
▪ **Seizures:** Patients on anticonvulsant therapy should carry identification describing disease process and medication regimen at all times.

EVALUATION

Effectiveness of therapy can be demonstrated by: ▪ Increase in sense of well-being □ Decrease in subjective feelings of anxiety ▪ Control of acute alcohol withdrawal ▪ Decrease or cessation of seizure activity without undue sedation.

CLOXACILLIN
(klox-a-**sill**-in)
{Apo-Cloxi}, Cloxapen, {No-vocloxin}, {Nu-Cloxi}, {Orbenin}, Tegopen

CLASSIFICATION(S):
Anti-infective (penicillinase-resistant penicillin)
Pregnancy Category B

INDICATIONS

▪ Treatment of the following infections due to penicillinase-producing staphylococci: □ Respiratory tract infections □ Sinusitis □ Skin and skin structure infections.

ACTION

▪ Binds to bacterial cell wall, leading to cell death. Resists the action of penicillinase, an enzyme capable of inactivating penicillin. **Therapeutic Effect:** ▪ Bactericidal action. **Spectrum:** ▪ Active against most gram-positive aerobic cocci, but less so than penicillin. ▪ Spectrum is notable for activity against: □ Penicillinase-producing strains of *Staphylococcus aureus* □ *Staphylococcus epidermidis* ▪ Not active against methicillin-resistant staphylococci.

PHARMACOKINETICS

Absorption: Moderately absorbed (37–60%) following oral administration.
Distribution: Widely distributed. Penetration into CSF is minimal. Crosses the placenta and enters breast milk.
Metabolism and Excretion: Some metabolism by the liver (9–22%) and some renal excretion of unchanged drug (30–45%).
Half-life: 0.5–1.1 hr (increased in severe hepatic and renal dysfunction).

CONTRAINDICATIONS AND PRECAUTIONS

Contraindicated in: ▪ Hypersensitivity to penicillins ▪ Should not be used as initial therapy in serious infections or in patients experiencing nausea or vomiting.
Use Cautiously in: ▪ Severe renal or hepatic impairment (dosage reduction required) ▪ Pregnancy or lactation (safety not established).

ADVERSE REACTIONS AND SIDE EFFECTS*

CNS: SEIZURES (high doses).
GI: <u>nausea</u>, <u>vomiting</u>, <u>diarrhea</u>, hepatitis.
GU: interstitial nephritis.
Derm: <u>rashes</u>, urticaria.
Hemat: blood dyscrasias.
Misc: superinfection, <u>allergic reactions</u>, including ANAPHYLAXIS and serum sickness.

INTERACTIONS

Drug–Drug: ▪ **Probenecid** decreases renal excretion and increases blood levels ▪ May alter the effect of **warfarin**.
Drug–Food: ▪ Food and acidic juices decrease absorption.

ROUTE AND DOSAGE

▪ **PO (Adults and Children >20 kg):** 250–500 mg q 6 hr.
▪ **PO (Children >1 mo and <20 kg):** 25–100 mg/kg/day in divided doses q 6 hr.

AVAILABILITY

▪ *Capsules:* 250 mg, 500 mg ▪ *Oral solution:* 125 mg/5 ml.

TIME/ACTION PROFILE (blood levels)

	ONSET	PEAK
PO	30 min	30–120 min

{} = Available in Canada only.
*<u>Underlines</u> indicate most frequent; **CAPITALS** indicate life-threatening.

NURSING IMPLICATIONS

ASSESSMENT

□ Assess patient for infection (vital signs; appearance of wound, sputum, urine, and stool; WBC) at beginning and throughout course of therapy.

□ Obtain a history before initiating therapy to determine previous use of and reactions to penicillins or cephalosporins. Persons with a negative history of penicillin sensitivity may still have an allergic response.

□ Obtain specimens for culture and sensitivity prior to initiating therapy. First dose may be given before receiving results.

□ Observe patient for signs and symptoms of anaphylaxis (rash, pruritus, laryngeal edema, wheezing, abdominal pain). Discontinue the drug and notify the physician immediately if these occur. Keep epinephrine, an antihistamine, and resuscitation equipment close by in the event of an anaphylactic reaction.

▪ **Lab Test Considerations:** CBC, BUN, creatinine, urinalysis, and liver function tests should be monitored periodically during therapy.

□ May cause an increased AST (SGOT) concentrations.

POTENTIAL NURSING DIAGNOSES

▪ Infection, high risk for (indications, side effects).

▪ Knowledge deficit related to medication regimen (patient/family teaching).

▪ Noncompliance related to medication regimen (patient/family teaching).

IMPLEMENTATION

▪ **PO:** Administer around the clock on an empty stomach at least 1 hr before or 2 hr after meals. Take with a full glass of water; acidic juices may decrease absorption of penicillins.

□ Use calibrated measuring device for liquid preparations. Shake well. Solution stable for 14 days if refrigerated.

PATIENT/FAMILY TEACHING

□ Instruct patient to take medication around the clock and to finish the drug completely as directed, even if feeling better. Missed doses should be taken as soon as remembered. Advise patient that sharing of this medication may be dangerous.

□ Advise patient to report signs of superinfection (black, furry overgrowth on the tongue, vaginal itching or discharge, loose or foul-smelling stools) and allergy.

□ Instruct patient to notify physician if fever and diarrhea develop, especially if stool contains blood, pus, or mucus. Advise patient not to treat diarrhea without consulting physician or pharmacist.

□ Instruct patient to notify physician if symptoms do not improve.

EVALUATION

Clinical response can be evaluated by:

▪ Resolution of the signs and symptoms of infection. Length of time for complete resolution depends on the organism and site of infection.

CLOZAPINE
(**cloz**-a-peen)
Clozaril

CLASSIFICATION(S):
Antipsychotic
Pregnancy Category B

INDICATIONS

▪ Treatment of schizophrenic patients who are unresponsive to or cannot tolerate standard therapy with other antipsychotic agents.

ACTION

▪ Binds to dopamine receptors in the CNS ▪ Also has anticholinergic and alpha-adrenergic blocking activity ▪ Produces less extrapyramidal reactions and tardive dyskinesia than standard antipsychotic therapy but carries high risk of hematologic abnormalities. **Therapeutic Effect:** ▪ Diminished schizophrenic behavior.

PHARMACOKINETICS

Absorption: Well absorbed following oral administration.

Distribution: Rapid and extensive distribution, crosses blood–brain barrier and placenta. 95% bound to plasma proteins.

Metabolism and Excretion: Mostly metabolized on first pass through the liver.

Half-life: 8–12 hr.

CONTRAINDICATIONS AND PRECAUTIONS

Contraindicated in: ▪ Hypersensitivity ▪ Bone marrow depression ▪ Lactation ▪ Severe CNS depression or coma.

Use Cautiously in: ▪ Prostatic enlargement ▪ Narrow-angle glaucoma ▪ Children <16 yr (safety not established) ▪ Malnourished patients or patients with cardiovascular, hepatic, or renal disease (use lower initial dose, titrate more slowly) ▪ Seizure disorder.

ADVERSE REACTIONS AND SIDE EFFECTS*

CNS: <u>sedation</u>, SEIZURES, <u>dizziness</u>, NEUROLEPTIC MALIGNANT SYNDROME.

EENT: visual disturbances, dry mouth, increased salivation.

CV: <u>hypotension</u>, <u>tachycardia</u>, ECG changes, hypertension.

GI: <u>constipation</u>, nausea, vomiting, abdominal discomfort.

Derm: sweating, rash.

Hemat: AGRANULOCYTOSIS, LEUKOPENIA.

Neuro: extrapyramidal reactions.

Misc: fever, weight gain.

INTERACTIONS

Drug–Drug: ▪ Additive anticholinergic effects with other **agents having anticholinergic properties** including **antihistamines, quinidine, disopyramide,** and **antidepressants** ▪ Additive CNS depression with **alcohol, antidepressants, antihistamines, opioid analgesics,** or **sedative/hypnotics** ▪ Additive hypotension with **nitrates,** acute ingestion of **alcohol,** or **antihypertensives** ▪ Increased risk of bone marrow suppression with **antineoplastic agents** or **radiation therapy** ▪ Use with **lithium** increases the risk of adverse CNS reactions, including seizures.

ROUTE AND DOSAGE

▪ **PO (Adults):** 25 mg 1–2 times daily initially, increase by 25–50 mg/day over a period of 2 wk up to target dose of 300–450 mg/day. May increase by up to 100 mg/day once or twice weekly (not to exceed 900 mg/day).

AVAILABILITY

▪ *Tablets:* 25 mg, 100 mg.

TIME/ACTION PROFILE
(antipsychotic effect)

	ONSET	PEAK	DURATION
PO	UK	wks	4–12 hr

NURSING IMPLICATIONS

ASSESSMENT

▫ Monitor patient's mental status (delusions, hallucinations, and behavior) prior to and periodically throughout therapy.

▫ Monitor blood pressure (sitting, standing, lying) and pulse rate prior to and frequently during initial dosage titration.

▫ Observe patient carefully when administering medication to ensure medication is actually taken and not hoarded.

▫ Monitor patient for onset of extrapyramidal side effects (akathesia—restlessness, dystonia—muscle spasms and twisting motions, or pseudoparkinsonism—mask facies, rigidity, tremors, drooling, shuffling gait, dysphagia). Notify physician if these symptoms occur, because reduction in dosage or discontinuation of medication may be necessary. Physician may also order trihexyphenidyl or diphenhydramine to control these symptoms.

▫ Although not yet reported for clozapine, monitor for possible tardive dyskinesia (rhythmic movement of mouth, face, and extremities). Notify physician immediately if these symptoms occur, as these side effects may be irreversible.

□ Monitor frequency and consistency of bowel movements. Increasing bulk and fluids in the diet may help minimize constipation.

□ Clozapine lowers the seizure threshold. Institute seizure precautions for patients with history of seizure disorder.

□ Transient fevers may occur, especially during first 3 wk of therapy. Fever is usually self-limiting, but may require discontinuation of medication. Also, monitor for development of neuroleptic malignant syndrome (fever, respiratory distress, tachycardia, convulsions, diaphoresis, hypertension or hypotension, pallor, tiredness). Notify physician immediately if these symptoms occur.

■ **Lab Test Considerations:** Monitor WBC and differential count prior to initiation of therapy, and WBC count weekly during therapy and for 4 wk after discontinuation of clozapine. Due to the risk of agranulocytosis, clozapine is only available in a 1-wk supply through the *Clozaril Patient Management System,* which combines WBC testing, patient monitoring, pharmacy, and drug distribution. If WBC is <3000 mm^3 or granulocyte count is <1500 mm^3, withhold clozapine and monitor patient for signs and symptoms of infection.

■ **Toxicity and Overdose:** Overdose is treated with activated charcoal and supportive therapy. Monitor patient for several days due to risk of delayed effects.

□ Avoid use of epinephrine and its derivatives when treating hypotension, and avoid quinidine and procainamide when treating arrhythmias.

POTENTIAL NURSING DIAGNOSES
■ Violence, high risk for: directed at others (indications).
■ Thought processes, altered: related to panic anxiety (indications).
■ Injury, high risk for (side effects).

IMPLEMENTATION
■ **PO:** Administer capsules with food or milk to decrease gastric irritation.

PATIENT/FAMILY TEACHING
□ Instruct patient to take medication exactly as directed. Patients on long-term therapy may need to discontinue gradually over 1–2 wk.

□ Inform patient of possibility of extrapyramidal symptoms. Instruct patient to report these symptoms immediately to physician.

□ Advise patients to make position changes slowly to minimize orthostatic hypotension.

□ May cause seizures and drowsiness. Caution patient to avoid driving or other activities requiring alertness while taking clozapine.

□ Caution patient to avoid concurrent use of alcohol, other CNS depressants, and over-the-counter medications without consulting physician.

□ Instruct patient to use frequent mouth rinses, good oral hygiene, and sugarless gum or candy to minimize dry mouth.

□ Advise patient to notify physician or dentist of medication regimen prior to treatment or surgery.

□ Instruct patient to notify physician promptly if sore throat, fever, lethargy, weakness, malaise, or flu-like symptoms occur. Patients should also notify physician if they become or intend to become pregnant.

□ Advise patient of need for continued medical follow-up for psychotherapy, eye examinations, and laboratory tests.

EVALUATION
Effectiveness of therapy can be demonstrated by: ■ Decreased psychotic ideation.

CODEINE
(koe-**deen**)
{Paveral}

INDICATIONS

- Alone and in combination with non-opioid analgesics in the management of mild to moderate pain ▪ Antitussive (in smaller doses). **Unlabeled Use:** ▪ Management of diarrhea.

ACTION

- Binds to opiate receptors in the CNS. Alters the perception of and response to painful stimuli, while producing generalized CNS depression. ▪ Decreases cough reflex ▪ Decreases GI motility. **Therapeutic Effects:** ▪ Decreased severity of pain ▪ Suppression of the cough reflex ▪ Decreased diarrhea.

PHARMACOKINETICS

Absorption: 50% absorbed from the GI tract. Completely absorbed from IM sites. Oral and parenteral doses are not equal.

Distribution: Widely distributed. Crosses the placenta and enters breast milk.

Metabolism and Excretion: Mostly metabolized by the liver. 10% converted to morphine. Minimal renal excretion (5–15%) of unchanged drug.

Half-life: 2.5–4 hr.

CONTRAINDICATIONS AND PRECAUTIONS

Contraindicated in: ▪ Hypersensitivity ▪ Pregnancy or lactation (avoid chronic use).

Use Cautiously in: ▪ Head trauma ▪ Increased intracranial pressure ▪ Severe renal, hepatic, or pulmonary disease ▪ Hypothyroidism ▪ Adrenal insufficiency ▪ Alcoholism ▪ Elderly or debilitated patients (dosage reduction required) ▪ Patients with undiagnosed abdominal pain ▪ Prostatic hypertrophy ▪ Has been used during labor; respiratory depression may occur in the newborn.

ADVERSE REACTIONS AND SIDE EFFECTS*

CNS: <u>sedation</u>, <u>confusion</u>, headache, euphoria, floating feeling, unusual dreams, hallucinations, dysphoria.

CV: <u>hypotension</u>, bradycardia.

EENT: miosis, diplopia, blurred vision.

Resp: respiratory depression.

GI: <u>nausea</u>, <u>vomiting</u>, <u>constipation</u>.

GU: urinary retention.

Derm: sweating, flushing.

Misc: tolerance, physical dependence, psychological dependence.

INTERACTIONS

Drug–Drug: ▪ Use with caution in patients receiving **MAO inhibitors** (reduce initial dosage to 25% of usual dose) ▪ Additive CNS depression with **alcohol, antidepressants, antihistamines,** and **sedative/hypnotics** ▪ Administration of **partial antagonists (buprenorphine, butorphanol, nalbuphine,** or **pentazocine)** may precipitate opioid withdrawal in physically dependent patients ▪ **Nalbuphine** or **pentazocine** may decrease analgesia.

ROUTE AND DOSAGE

Analgesia

- **PO, IM, SC (Adults):** 15–60 mg q 3–6 hr as needed.
- **PO, IM, SC (Children):** 0.5 mg/kg q 4–6 hr (up to 4 times daily) as needed.

Antitussive

- **PO, IM, SC (Adults):** 10–20 mg q 4–6 hr as needed (not to exceed 120 mg/day).
- **PO, IM, SC (Children 6–12 yr):** 5–10 mg q 4–6 hr as needed (not to exceed 60 mg/day).
- **PO, IM, SC (Children 2–5 yr):** 1 mg/kg/day in 4 divided doses (not to exceed 30 mg/day).

Antidiarrheal

- **PO (Adults):** 30 mg, may be repeated up to 4 times daily.

*<u>Underlines</u> indicate most frequent; **CAPITALS** indicate life-threatening.

AVAILABILITY

▪ *Tablets:* 15 mg, 30 mg, 60 mg ▪ *Oral solution:* {10 mg/5 ml}, 15 mg/5 ml ▪ *Injection:* 30 mg/ml, 60 mg/ml ▪ *In combination with:* antihistamines, decongestants, antipyretics, caffeine, and nonopioid analgesics. See Appendix A.

TIME/ACTION PROFILE (analgesia)

	ONSET	PEAK	DURATION
PO	30–45 min	60–120 min	4 hr
IM	10–30 min	30–60 min	4 hr
SC	10–30 min	UK	4 hr

NURSING IMPLICATIONS

Assessment

▪ **General Info:** Assess blood pressure, pulse, and respiratory rate before and periodically during administration.

□ Assess bowel function routinely. Increased intake of fluids and bulk, stool softeners, and laxatives may minimize constipating effects.

▪ **Pain:** Assess type, location, and intensity of pain prior to and 60 min following administration.

□ Prolonged use may lead to physical and psychological dependence and tolerance. This should not prevent patient from receiving adequate analgesia. Most patients who receive codeine for medical reasons do not develop psychological dependence. Progressively higher doses may be required to relieve pain with long-term therapy.

▪ **Cough:** Assess cough and lung sounds during antitussive use.

▪ **Lab Test Considerations:** May cause increased plasma amylase and lipase concentrations.

▪ **Toxicity and Overdose:** If overdose occurs, naloxone (Narcan) is the antidote.

Potential Nursing Diagnoses

▪ Pain (indications).
▪ Sensory-perceptual alteration: visual, auditory (side effects).
▪ Injury, high risk for (side effects).

Implementation

▪ **General Info:** Explain therapeutic value of medication prior to administration to enhance the analgesic effect.

□ Regularly administered doses may be more effective than prn administration. Analgesic is more effective if given before pain becomes severe.

□ Coadministration with nonopioid analgesics may have additive analgesic effects and permit lower doses.

□ Medications should be discontinued gradually after long-term use to prevent withdrawal symptoms.

□ When combined with nonopioid analgesics (aspirin, acetaminophen; #2 = 15 mg, #3 = 30 mg, #4 = 60 mg codeine). Codeine as an individual drug is a Schedule II substance. In combination with other drugs, tablet form is Schedule III, liquid is Schedule IV, and elixir or cough suppressant is Schedule V (see Appendix C).

▪ **PO:** Oral doses may be administered with food or milk to minimize GI irritation.

▪ **IM/SC:** Do not administer solution that is more than slightly discolored or contains a precipitate.

▪ **Syringe Compatibility:** ▪ glycopyrrolate ▪ hydroxyzine.

Patient/Family Teaching

□ Instruct patient on how and when to ask for pain medication.

□ Codeine may cause drowsiness or dizziness. Advise patient to call for assistance when ambulating or smoking. Caution ambulatory patient to avoid driving or other activities requiring alertness until response to medication is known.

□ Advise patient to make position changes slowly to minimize orthostatic hypotension.

□ Caution patient to avoid concurrent use of alcohol or other CNS depressants with this medication.

□ Encourage patient to turn, cough, and breathe deeply every 2 hr to prevent atelectasis.

Evaluation

Effectiveness of therapy can be demonstrated by: ▪ Decrease in severity of pain without a significant alteration in level of consciousness or respiratory status ▪ Suppression of cough ▪ Control of diarrhea.

COLCHICINE
(kol-chi-seen)

CLASSIFICATION(S):
Antigout agent
Pregnancy Category C

INDICATIONS

▪ Treatment of acute attacks of gouty arthritis (larger doses) ▪ Prevention of recurrences of gout (smaller doses). **Unlabeled Uses:** ▪ Treatment of hepatic cirrhosis and familial Mediterranean fever.

ACTION

▪ Interferes with the functions of white blood cells in initiating and perpetuating the inflammatory response to monosodium urate crystals. **Therapeutic Effects:** ▪ Decreased pain and inflammation in acute attacks of gout ▪ Prevention of recurrent attacks of gout.

PHARMACOKINETICS

Absorption: Absorbed from the GI tract, then re-enters GI tract from biliary secretions, when more absorption may occur.
Distribution: Concentrates in white blood cells.
Metabolism and Excretion: Partially metabolized by the liver. Secreted in bile back into GI tract. Eliminated in the feces. Small amount excreted in the urine.
Half-life: 20 min (plasma), 60 hr (white blood cells).

CONTRAINDICATIONS AND PRECAUTIONS

Contraindicated in: ▪ Hypersensitivity ▪ Pregnancy ▪ Severe renal or GI disease.
Use Cautiously in: ▪ Elderly or debilitated patients (toxicity may be cumula-

tive) ▪ Lactation or children (safety not established).

ADVERSE REACTIONS AND SIDE EFFECTS*

GI: <u>nausea</u>, <u>vomiting</u>, abdominal pain, <u>diarrhea</u>.
GU: anuria, hematuria, renal damage.
Derm: alopecia.
Hemat: AGRANULOCYTOSIS, APLASTIC ANEMIA, leukopenia, thrombocytopenia.
Local: phlebitis at IV site.
Neuro: peripheral neuritis.

INTERACTIONS

Drug–Drug: ▪ May cause reversible malabsorption of **vitamin B₁₂**.

ROUTE AND DOSAGE
Acute Gouty Arthritis

▪ **PO (Adults):** 0.5–1.3 mg, then 0.5–0.65 mg q 1–2 hr or 1–1.3 mg q 2 hr until relief or GI side effects occur (control of acute attack usually requires total cumulative dose of 4–10 mg).

Prophylaxis of Recurrence of Gouty Arthritis

▪ **PO (Adults):** 0.5–0.6 mg/day, 3–4 days/wk, up to 1–1.8 mg/day.

AVAILABILITY

▪ *Tablets:* 0.5 mg, 0.6 mg, {1 mg}.

TIME/ACTION PROFILE (anti-inflammatory activity)

	ONSET	PEAK	DURATION
PO	12 hr	24–72 hr	UK

NURSING IMPLICATIONS
ASSESSMENT

☐ Assess involved joints for pain, mobility, and edema throughout therapy. During initiation of therapy, monitor for drug response every 1–2 hr.
☐ Monitor intake and output ratios. Fluids should be encouraged to promote a urinary output of at least 2000 ml/day.
▪ **Lab Test Considerations:** In patients receiving prolonged therapy, monitor baseline and periodic CBC; notify physician if a significant decrease in values occurs.

*Underlines indicate most frequent; CAPITALS indicate life threatening.

- May cause an increase in AST (SGOT) and alkaline phosphatase.
- May cause false-positive results for urine hemoglobin.
- May interfere with results of urinary 17-hydroxycorticosteroid concentrations.
- **Toxicity and Overdose:** Assess patient for toxicity (weakness, abdominal discomfort, nausea, vomiting, diarrhea). If these symptoms occur, discontinue medication and notify physician. Opioids may be needed to treat diarrhea.

POTENTIAL NURSING DIAGNOSES
- Pain (indications).
- Physical mobility, impaired (indications).
- Knowledge deficit related to medication regimen (patient/family teaching).

IMPLEMENTATION
- **General Info:** Physician may order intermittent therapy with 3 days between courses to decrease risk of toxicity.
- **PO:** Administer oral doses with food to minimize gastric irritation.

PATIENT/FAMILY TEACHING
- Review medication administration schedule. Emphasize importance of taking medication at correct time: begin or increase dose when first symptoms of attack occur; stop or return to prophylactic dose when attack subsides. If dose is missed, take as soon as remembered unless almost time for next dose. Do not double doses.
- Advise patient to follow physician's recommendations regarding weight loss, diet, and alcohol consumption.
- Instruct patient to report nausea, vomiting, abdominal pain, diarrhea, unusual bleeding, or bruising, sore throat, fatigue, malaise, or rash to physician promptly. Medication should be withheld if gastric symptoms occur.
- Surgery may precipitate an acute attack of gout. Advise patient to confer with physician regarding dose 3 days before surgical or dental procedures.

EVALUATION
Therapeutic effects can be demonstrated by: ▪ Decrease in pain and swelling in affected joints within 12 hr ▫ Relief of symptoms within 24–48 hr ▪ Prevention of acute gout attacks.

COLFOSCERIL PALMITATE
(koll-**foss**-er-ill **pal**-mi-tate)
natural lung surfactant, Exosurf Neonatal

CLASSIFICATION(S):
Pulmonary surfactant
Pregnancy Category UK

INDICATIONS
▪ Treatment and prophylaxis of respiratory distress syndrome (RDS, hyaline membrane disease) in premature infants.

ACTION
▪ Replaces endogenous pulmonary surfactant in premature infants, allowing normal surface activity in alveoli. Cetyl alcohol in formulation spreads colfosceril on air-fluid surface, whereas Tyloxapal, a surfactant, disperses colfosceril and cetyl alcohol. **Therapeutic Effects:** ▪ Decreased incidence, mortality, and complications from RDS in premature infants.

PHARMACOKINETICS
Absorption: Administered directly to site of action. Systemic absorption not known.
Distribution: Rapidly distributes to lung tissue.
Metabolism and Excretion: Enters surfactant pathways where recycling and reutilization occur.
Half-life: UK.

CONTRAINDICATIONS AND PRECAUTIONS
Contraindications in: ▪ No known contraindications.
Use Cautiously in: ▪ No known cautions.

ADVERSE REACTIONS AND SIDE EFFECTS*

Resp: pulmonary hemorrhage, apnea.
CV: bradycardia, hypotension, vasoconstriction.
Misc: increased risk of sepsis following treatment.

INTERACTIONS

Drug–Drug: ▪ None known.

ROUTE AND DOSAGE

Prophylactic Treatment
▪ **Intratracheal (Premature Infants):** 5 ml/kg given as 2 half-doses of 2.5 ml/kg as soon as possible after birth, repeat 12 and 24 hr later if still mechanically ventilated.

Rescue Treatment
▪ **Intratracheal (Premature Infants):** 5 ml/kg given as 2 half-doses of 2.5 ml/kg as soon as diagnosis of RDS is made, give a second dose 12 hr later if still mechanically ventilated.

AVAILABILITY

▪ *Powder for intratracheal administration:* 108 mg/10-ml vial.

TIME/ACTION PROFILE (surfactant activity)

	ONSET	PEAK	DURATION
Intratracheal	rapid	UK	12 hr

NURSING IMPLICATIONS

ASSESSMENT

▢ Monitor ECG, heart rate, color, chest expansion, facial expression, transcutaneous oxygen saturation, and endotracheal tube patency continuously during dosing. Continuous bedside monitoring should continue for at least 30 min following dosing.
▪ **Lab Test Considerations:** Monitor arterial blood gases frequently to prevent hyperoxia or hypocarbia.
▪ **Toxicity and Overdose:** If chest expansion improves substantially after dosing, reduce peak inspiratory ventilator pressures immediately to pre-

vent lung overdistension and fatal pulmonary leak.
▢ If infant becomes pink and transcutaneous oxygen saturation is in excess of 95%, reduce FiO_2 in small but repeated steps immediately to prevent hyperoxia.
▢ If arterial or transcutaneous CO_2 measurements are less than 30 mmHg, ventilator rate should be reduced immediately to prevent hypocarbia.

POTENTIAL NURSING DIAGNOSES

▪ Impaired gas exchange (indications).

IMPLEMENTATION

▪ **General Info:** Only trained medical personnel with experience in airway and clinical management of unstable neonates should perform colfosceril instillation.
▢ Suction the infant endotracheally prior to instillation. Check position of endotracheal tube prior to instillation. Do not suction for 2 hr following instillation unless clinically necessary.
▢ If reflux occurs after instillation, stop drug administration and increase the peak inspiratory pressure on the ventilator by 4–5 cm H_2O until the endotracheal tube clears.
▢ If transcutaneous oxygen saturation drops more than 20% during instillation, stop administration and increase peak inspiratory pressure on the ventilator by 4–5 cm H_2O and increase the FiO_2 for 1–2 min, if necessary.
▪ **Inhalation:** Reconstitute *only* with diluent provided (preservative-free Sterile Water for Injection). Fill a 10- or 12-ml syringe with 8 ml of diluent using an 18- or 19-gauge needle. Allow the vacuum in the vial to draw the sterile water into the vial. Aspirate as much of the 8 ml as possible out of the vial and into the syringe while maintaining the vacuum, then suddenly release the syringe plunger. Repeat process 3–4 times to ensure mixing of contents. If vacuum is not present, do not use the vial.

*Underlines indicate most frequent; **CAPITALS** indicate life threatening.

drug is a milky white suspension. If suspension separates, gently shake or swirl to resuspend. Do not use if persistent large flakes or particles are present.

□ Instillation is accomplished through a special endotracheal tube adaptor.

■ *Rate:* Instill each half-dose slowly over 1–2 min in small bursts timed with inspiration. After the first 2.5 ml/kg half-dose is administered in the midline position, turn the infant's head and torso 45° to the right and continue mechanical ventilation for 30 sec. Once returned to the midline position, instill the second 2.5 ml/kg half-dose over 1–2 min and turn the infant's head and torso to the left for 30 sec while continuing mechanical ventilation. Then return infant to midline.

PATIENT/FAMILY TEACHING
□ Explain purpose of medication to parents.

EVALUATION
Effectiveness of therapy may be determined by: ■ Prevention of RDS ■ Improvement in lung compliance □ Improved oxygenation □ Normalization of arterial blood gases.

CONTRACEPTIVES, HORMONAL

MONOPHASIC ORAL CONTRACEPTIVES
mestranol/norethindrone
(**mes**-tre-nole)/(nor-eth-**in**-drone)
Genora 1/50, Nelova 1/50M, Norethin 1/50M, Norinyl 1 + 50, Ortho-Novum 1/50
ethinyl estradiol/norethindrone
(**eth**-in-il ess-tra-**dye**-ole)/(nor-eth-**in**-drone)
Brevicon, Genora 0.5/35, Genora 1/35, Loestrin 21 1.5/30, Loestrin 21 1/20, Modicon, N.E.E. 1/35, Nelova 0.5/35E, Nelova 1/35E, Norcept-E 1/35, Norethin 1/35E, Norinyl 1 + 35, Ortho-Novum 1/35, Ovcon 35, Ovcon-50, Norles-

trin 1/50, Norlestrin 2.5/50
ethinyl estradiol/ethynodiol
(**eth**-in-il ess-tra-**dye**-ole)/(e-thye-noe-**dye**-ole)
Demulen, Demulen 1/35
ethinyl estradiol/norgestrel
(**eth**-in-il ess-tra-**dye**-ole)/(nor-**jess**-trel)
Lo-Ovral, Ovral
ethinyl estradiol/levonorgestrel
(**eth**-in-il ess-tra-**dye**-ole)/(lee-voe-nor-**jess**-trel)
Levlen, Nordette
desogestrel/ethinyl estradiole
(dess-oh-**jess**-trel)/(**eth**-in-il ess-tra-**dye**-ole)
Desogen

BIPHASIC ORAL CONTRACEPTIVES
ethinyl estradiol/norethindrone
Nelova 10/11, Ortho Novum 10/11

TRIPHASIC ORAL CONTRACEPTIVES
ethinyl estradiol/norethindrone
Tri-Norinyl, Ortho Novum 7/7/7
ethinyl estradiol/norgestrel
Tri-Levlen, Triphasil

PROGESTIN-ONLY ORAL CONTRACEPTIVES
norethindrone
Micronor, Nor-Q.D.
norgestrel
Ovrette

CONTRACEPTIVE IMPLANT
levonorgestrel
Norplant

INJECTABLE CONTRACEPTIVE
medroxyprogesterone
(me-**drox**-ee-proe-jess-te-rone)
Depo-Provera

CLASSIFICATION(S):
Hormones (estrogens, progestins, contraceptives)
Pregnancy Category X

INDICATIONS
■ Prevention of pregnancy.

ACTION
■ **Monophasic Oral Contraceptives:** Provide a fixed dosage of estrogen/

progestin over a 21-day cycle. Ovulation is inhibited by suppression of follicle-stimulating hormone (FSH) and luteinizing hormone (LH). May alter cervical mucus and the endometrial environment, preventing penetration by sperm and implantation of the egg ▪ **Biphasic Oral Contraceptives:** Ovulation is inhibited by suppression of follicle-stimulating hormone (FSH) and luteinizing hormone (LH). May alter cervical mucus and the endometrial environment, preventing penetration by sperm and implantation of the egg. In addition, smaller dose of progestin in phase 1 allows for proliferation of endometrium. Larger amount in phase 2 allows for adequate secretory development ▪ **Triphasic Oral Contraceptives:** Ovulation is inhibited by suppression of follicle-stimulating hormone (FSH) and luteinizing hormone (LH). May alter cervical mucus and the endometrial environment, preventing penetration by sperm and implantation of the egg. Varying doses of estrogen/progestin may more closely mimic natural hormonal fluctuations ▪ **Progestin-Only Contraceptives and Contraceptive Implant:** Mechanism not clearly known. May alter cervical mucus and the endometrial environment, preventing penetration by sperm and implantation of the egg. Ovulation may also be suppressed ▪ **Medroxyprogesterone Injection:** Inhibits gonadotropin secretion, follicle maturation and ovulation. Also produces endometrial thinning. **Therapeutic Effect:** ▪ Prevention of pregnancy.

PHARMACOKINETICS

Absorption: Well absorbed following oral administration. Slowly absorbed from implant or IM injection.
Distribution: UK.
Metabolism and Excretion: Mostly metabolized by the liver.
Half-life: UK.

CONTRAINDICATIONS AND PRECAUTIONS

Contraindicated in: ▪ History of thromboembolic disorders, cardiovascular disease, cerebrovascular disease, liver tumors, or gallbladder disease ▪ Lactation (avoid use) ▪ Hypersensitivity to parabens (injectable only).
Use Cautiously in: ▪ Surgical procedures (discontinue 2–4 wk prior to surgery) ▪ History of cigarette smoking or age >30–35 yr (increased risk of cardiovascular or thromboembolic phenomenon ▪ Presence of other cardiovascular risk factors (obesity, hyperglycemia, elevated lipids, hypertension) ▪ History of diabetes mellitus, bleeding disorders, or headaches.

ADVERSE REACTIONS AND SIDE EFFECTS*

CNS: migraine headache, depression.
EENT: contact lens intolerance, retinal thrombosis, optic neuritis.
CV: PULMONARY EMBOLISM, CORONARY THROMBOSIS, CEREBRAL HEMORRHAGE, CEREBRAL THROMBOSIS, thrombophlebitis, thromboembolic phenomenon, Raynaud's disease, hypertension, edema.
GI: nausea, vomiting, abdominal cramps, bloating, gallbladder disease, cholestatic jaundice, liver tumors.
GU: breakthrough bleeding, spotting, dysmenorrhea, amenorrhea.
Derm: melasma, rash.
Endo: hyperglycemia.
Misc: weight change.

INTERACTIONS

Drug–Drug: ▪ Oral contraceptive efficacy may be decreased by **penicillins, chloramphenicol, dihydroergotamine, mineral oil, oral neomycin, sulfonamides, barbiturates** (except butalbital), **chronic alcohol use, carbamazepine, glucocorticoids** (systemic), **griseofulvin, phenylbutazone, phenytoin, primidone, rifampin,** or **tetracyclines** ▪ May increase the risk of toxicity from **tricyclic antidepressants** ▪ Increased risk of hepatic toxicity with **dantrolene** (estrogen only) ▪ **Carbamazepine** or **phenytoin** may decrease the efficacy of contraceptive implants ▪ **Cigarette smoking** increases the risk of thromboembolic phenomenon (estrogen only) ▪ May interfere with the effectiveness of **bromocriptine** ▪ May alter the effects of **warfarin** (increase or decrease).

ROUTE AND DOSAGE

Monophasic Oral Contraceptives

▪ **PO (Adults):** On 21-day regimen, take first tablet on first Sunday after menses begin (take on Sunday if menses begin on Sunday) for 21 days, then skip 7 days, then begin again. Regimen may also be started on first day of menses, continued for 21 days, then skip 7 days and begin again. Some regimens contain 7 placebo tablets, so that 1 tablet is taken every day for 28 days.

Biphasic Oral Contraceptives

▪ **PO (Adults):** Given in 2 phases. First phase is 10 days of smaller amount of progestin. Second phase is larger amount of progestin. Amount of estrogen remains constant for same length of time (total of 21 days), then skip 7 days, then begin again. Some regimens contain 7 placebo tablets for 28-day regimen.

Triphasic Oral Contraceptives

▪ **PO (Adults):** Progestin amount varies throughout a 21-day cycle. Estrogen component stays the same or may vary. Some regimens contain 7 placebo tablets for 28-day regimen.

Progestin Only Oral Contraceptives

▪ **PO (Adults):** Start on first day of menses. Taken daily and continuously.

Contraceptive Implant

▪ **Subdermal (Adults):** 6 capsules implanted subdermally during first 7 days of menses.

Injectable Contraceptive

▪ **IM (Adults):** 150 mg within first 5 days of menses or within 5 days postpartum, if not breast feeding. If breast feeding, give 6 wk postpartum.

AVAILABILITY

▪ **Tablets:** Usually in monthly packs with enough (21) active tablets to complete a 28-day cycle. Some contain 7 inert tablets to complete the cycle. ▪ **Implant:** package of 6 implantable capsules containing 36 mg of levonorgestrel each ▪ **Injectable:** 150 mg/ml.

TIME/ACTION PROFILE (prevention of pregnancy)

	ONSET	PEAK	DURATION
PO	1 mo	1 mo	1 mo*
Implant	1 mo	1 mo	5 yr
IM	1 mo	1 mo	3 mo

*Only during mo of taking contraceptive.

NURSING IMPLICATIONS

ASSESSMENT

□ Assess blood pressure prior to and periodically throughout therapy.

▪ **Lab Test Considerations:** Monitor hepatic function periodically throughout therapy.

□ *Estrogens-only*—May cause increased serum glucose, sodium, triglyceride, high-density lipoproteins (HDL), phospholipid, cortisol, prothrombin, and Factors VII, VIII, IX, and X levels. May cause decreased serum folate, pyridoxine, and antithrombin III levels.

□ May cause false interpretations of thyroid function tests, false increases in norepinephrine platelet-induced aggregability, and false decreases in metyrapone tests.

□ *Progestins-only*—May cause increased serum alkaline phosphatase, low-density lipoproteins (LDL), and urinary nitrogen concentrations. May cause decreased amino acids and high-density lipoprotein (HDL) concentrations.

□ *Estrogens and Progestins*—May cause decreased pregnanediol excretion concentrations. May cause increased serum proteins.

POTENTIAL NURSING DIAGNOSES

▪ Knowledge deficit related to medication regimen (patient/family teaching).

IMPLEMENTATION

▪ **PO:** Oral doses may be administered with or immediately after food to reduce nausea.

- **Levonorgestrel Implant:** 6-capsule implant is inserted subdermally in midportion of upper arm about 8–10 cm above the elbow crease.
- **IM:** Shake vial vigorously just before use to ensure uniform suspension. Administer deep IM into gluteal or deltoid muscle. If period between injections is >14 wk, determine that patient is not pregnant before administering the drug.

PATIENT/FAMILY TEACHING

□ Instruct patient to take oral medication as directed at the same time each day. Pills should be taken in proper sequence and kept in the original container.

□ *If single daily dose is missed:* take as soon as remembered; if not until next day, take 2 tablets and continue on regular dosing schedule. *If 2 days in a row are missed:* take 2 tablets a day for the next 2 days and continue on regular dosing schedule, using a second method of birth control for the remaining cycle. *If 3 days in a row are missed:* discontinue medication and use another form of birth control until period begins or pregnancy is ruled out; then begin a new cycle of tablets. *For 28-day dosing schedule:* if schedule is followed for first 21 days and 1 dose is missed of the last 7 tablets, it is important to take first tablet of next month's cycle on the regularly scheduled day.

□ Advise patient of the need to use another form of contraception for the first 3 wk when beginning to use oral contraceptives.

□ Advise patient that a second method of birth control should also be used during each cycle in which any of the following are used: *Oral Contraceptives*—alcohol (chronic use), barbiturates (except butalbital), carbamazepine, chloramphenicol, dihydroergotamine, glucocorticoids (systemic), griseofulvin, mineral oil, oral neomycin, penicillins, rifampin, sulfonamides, or tetracyclines. *Levonorgestrel Implant*—carbamazepine or phenytoin.

□ Explain dosage schedule and maintenance routine. Discontinuing medication suddenly may cause withdrawal bleeding.

□ If nausea becomes a problem, advise patient that eating solid food often provides relief.

□ Advise patient to report signs and symptoms of fluid retention (swelling of ankles and feet, weight gain), thromboembolic disorders (pain, swelling, tenderness in extremities, headache, chest pain, blurred vision), mental depression, or hepatic dysfunction (yellowed skin or eyes, pruritus, dark urine, light colored stools), or abnormal vaginal bleeding to physician.

□ Instruct patient to stop taking medication and notify physician if pregnancy is suspected.

□ Caution patient that cigarette smoking during estrogen therapy may increase risk of serious side effects, especially for women over age 35.

□ Caution patients to use sunscreen and protective clothing to prevent increased pigmentation.

□ Advise patient to notify physician or dentist of medication regimen prior to treatment or surgery.

□ Emphasize the importance of routine follow-up physical examinations including blood pressure; breast, abdomen, and pelvic examinations; and PAP smears every 6–12 mo.

EVALUATION

Effectiveness of therapy can be demonstrated by: ■ Prevention of pregnancy.

CORTICOTROPIN
(kor-ti-koe-**troe**-pin)
ACTH, Acthar, H.P. Acthar Gel

CLASSIFICATION(S):
Hormone (adrenocorticotrophic)
Pregnancy Category C

INDICATIONS

- Diagnosis of adrenocortical disorders
- Used as an anti-inflammatory or im-

munosuppressant when conventional glucocorticoid therapy has failed. **Unlabeled Use:** ▪ Myasthenia gravis.

ACTION

▪ Normally produced by the pituitary, stimulates the adrenal gland to produce both glucocorticoids (hydrocortisone) and mineralocorticoids (sodium retention). Action requires intact adrenal responsiveness ▪ Actions resemble those of glucocorticoid administration and include suppression of the normal immune response and inflammation ▪ Additional numerous intense metabolic effects ▪ Potent mineralocorticoid (soduim retention) ▪ Suppresses adrenal function with chronic use. **Therapeutic Effect:** ▪ Production of adrenal steroids following administration.

PHARMACOKINETICS

Absorption: ACTH is rapidly absorbed from IM and SC sites. Repository forms or zinc hydroxide are more slowly absorbed from IM and SC sites.
Distribution: Removed from plasma to many tissues. Does not cross the placenta.
Metabolism and Excretion: Metabolic fate not known.
Half-life: 15 min (plasma).

CONTRAINDICATIONS AND PRECAUTIONS

Contraindicated in: ▪ Hypersensitivity to pork proteins ▪ Serious infections, except for septic shock or tuberculous meningitis.
Use Cautiously in: ▪ Children (chronic use may lead to growth suppression) ▪ Chronic treatment may result in adrenal suppression ▪ Do not discontinue abruptly ▪ Additional doses may be needed during stress (infections, surgery) ▪ Use lowest possible dose for shortest period of time ▪ Pregnancy or lactation (safety not established).

ADVERSE REACTIONS AND SIDE EFFECTS* (with chronic use)

CNS: psychoses, depression, euphoria.

EENT: cataracts, increased intraocular pressure.
CV: edema, hypertension, congestive heart failure, thromboembolism.
GI: nausea, vomiting, increased appetite, weight gain, peptic ulceration.
Derm: petechiae, ecchymoses, fragility, decreased wound healing, hirsutism, acne.
Endo: menstrual irregularities, hyperglycemia, decreased growth in children, ADRENAL SUPPRESSION.
F and E: hypokalemia, sodium retention, metabolic alkalosis, hypocalcemia.
Local: atrophy at IM sites (repository dosage forms).
MS: weakness, myopathy, aseptic necrosis of joints, osteoporosis.
Misc: increases susceptibility to infections, pancreatitis, Cushingoid appearance (moon face, buffalo hump).

INTERACTIONS

Drug–Drug: ▪ Additive hypokalemia with **amphotericin B, mezlocillin, piperacillin, ticarcillin,** or **diuretics** ▪ Hypokalemia may increase the risk of **cardiac glycoside** toxicity ▪ May increase requirements for **insulin** or **oral hypoglycemic agents** ▪ **Phenytoin, phenobarbital,** and **rifampin** stimulate metabolism, may decrease effectiveness ▪ **Oral contraceptives** may block metabolism.

ROUTE AND DOSAGE

Anti-Inflammatory/Immunosuppressant

▪ **IM, SC (Adults):** 40–80 units/day (up to 120 units/day for multiple sclerosis) or 40–80 units q 24–48 hr of repository gelatin form.
▪ **IM, SC (Children):** 1.6 units/kg/day (50 units/m^2/day) in 3–4 divided doses or 0.8 units/kg/day or 25 units/m^2/day of repository form in 1–2 divided doses.

Diagnosis of Adrenal Disorders

▪ **IV (Adults):** 10–25 units infused over 8 hr.
▪ **IM (Adults):** 25 units.

*Underlines indicate most frequent; **CAPITALS** indicate life-threatening.

AVAILABILITY

■ *Powder for injection:* 40 units/vial, 80 units/vial ■ *Repository injection:* 40 units/vial, 80 units/ml.

TIME/ACTION PROFILE (effects on plasma cortisol levels)

	ONSET	PEAK	DURATION
IM (gelatin repository)	UK	3–12 hr	10–25 hr
IV	UK	1 hr	UK

NURSING IMPLICATIONS

ASSESSMENT

◻ In patients with a history of allergic reactions, monitor for hypersensitivity response (wheezing, rash or hives, bradycardia, irritability seizures, nausea, and vomiting). These reactions are more likely to occur with SC route or prolonged therapy. Patients allergic to porcine proteins should receive intradermal test dose prior to therapeutic or diagnostic dose.

◻ Monitor intake and output ratios and daily weights. Observe patient for peripheral edema, steady weight gain, rales/crackles, or dyspnea. Notify physician should these occur.

■ **Lab Test Considerations:** When used to diagnose adrenal insufficiency, plasma cortisol concentrations and urine 17-ketosteroids and 17-hydroxy-ketosteroids will be measured prior to and after administration of corticotropin. Therapeutic response is a rise in the plasma and urine steroid concentrations.

◻ Patients on prolonged courses of therapy should routinely have hematologic values, serum electrolytes, serum and urine glucose evaluated. May decrease WBC counts. May cause hyperglycemia, especially in persons with diabetes. May decrease serum potassium and calcium and increase serum sodium concentrations.

◻ Guaiac stools. Promptly report presence of guaiac-positive stools.

◻ May increase serum cholesterol and lipid values. May decrease serum protein-bound iodine and thyroxine concentrations.

◻ Suppresses reactions to allergy skin tests.

POTENTIAL NURSING DIAGNOSES

■ Infection, high risk for (side effects).

■ Knowledge deficit related to medication regimen (patient/family teaching).

IMPLEMENTATION

■ **General Info:** Reconstitute 25-unit vial with 1 ml of Sterile Water or 0.9% NaCl for Injection. Reconstitute 40-unit vial with 2 ml. Stable for 24 hr at room temperature, 7 days if refrigerated.

■ **IM, SC:** Shake suspension well before drawing up dose.

◻ Refrigerate repository form. Warm to room temperature before administering. Use 22-gauge needle. Administer deep IM; massage well. Rotate sites. Inform patient that injection is painful.

■ **IV:** Do not administer repository form IV. Ensure that label on vial states that it is for IV use.

■ **Direct IV:** Administer over 2 min.

■ **Intermittent Infusion:** Dilute 10–25 units in 500 ml of D5W, D5/0.9% NaCl, 0.9% NaCl, or lactated Ringer's solution.

■ *Rate:* Infuse over 8 hr. May also be ordered as 40 units to be infused over 12–48 hr.

PATIENT/FAMILY TEACHING

■ **General Info:** This drug causes immunosuppression and may mask symptoms of infection. Instruct patient to avoid people with known contagious illness and to report possible infections immediately.

◻ Review side effects with patient. Instruct patient to inform physician promptly if severe abdominal pain or tarry stools occur. Patient should also report unusual swelling, weight gain, tiredness, bone pain, bruising, non-healing sores, visual disturbances, or behavior changes.

◻ Encourage patients on long-term therapy to eat a diet high in protein, calcium, and potassium and low in sodium and carbohydrates (see Appendix K).

□ Instruct patient to inform physician if symptoms of underlying disease return or worsen.

□ Caution patient to avoid vaccinations without consulting physician.

▪ **Diagnostic Aid:** Explain purpose of corticotropin and need for lab tests.

EVALUATION
Effectiveness of therapy can be demonstrated by: ▪ Differentiation of primary from secondary adrenocortical insufficiency ▪ Decrease in presenting symptoms ▪ Induction of remission in multiple sclerosis.

CORTISONE
(**kor**-ti-sone)
Cortone

CLASSIFICATION(S):
Glucocorticoid (short-acting)
Pregnancy Category C

INDICATIONS
▪ Management of adrenocortical insufficiency. Use in other situations is limited due to mineralocorticoid activity.

ACTION
▪ Suppresses the normal immune response and inflammation ▪ Additional numerous intense metabolic effects ▪ Potent mineralocorticoid (sodium retention) ▪ Suppresses adrenal function with chronic use at doses >20 mg/day.
Therapeutic Effect: ▪ Replacement of cortisol in adrenal insufficiency.

PHARMACOKINETICS
Absorption: Absorption from the GI tract, but large amounts are rapidly inactivated. Converted to hydrocortisone following absorption. Slowly absorbed from IM sites.
Distribution: Widely distributed. Crosses the placenta and probably enters breast milk.

Metabolism and Excretion: Converted by the liver to hydrocortisone.
Half-life: 30 min.

CONTRAINDICATIONS AND PRECAUTIONS
Contraindications in: ▪ Serious infections.
Use Cautiously in: ▪ Children (chronic use may lead to growth suppression) ▪ Chronic treatment with doses >20 mg/day may also result in adrenal suppression ▪ Stress, including surgery or infection (additional doses may be required in patients receiving chronic therapy) ▪ Pregnancy or lactation (safety not established).

ADVERSE REACTIONS AND SIDE EFFECTS*
CNS: psychoses, depression, euphoria.
EENT: cataracts, increased intraocular pressure.
CV: edema, hypertension, congestive heart failure, thromboembolism.
GI: nausea, vomiting, increased appetite, weight gain, peptic ulceration.
Derm: petechiae, ecchymoses, fragility, decreased wound healing, hirsutism, acne.
Endo: menstrual irregularities, hyperglycemia, decreased growth in children, ADRENAL SUPPRESSION.
F and E: hypokalemia, sodium retention, metabolic alkalosis, hypocalcemia.
Local: atrophy at IM sites (repository dosage forms).
MS: weakness, myopathy, aseptic necrosis of joints, osteoporosis.
Misc: increases susceptibility to infections, pancreatitis, Cushingoid appearance (moon face, buffalo hump).

INTERACTIONS
Drug–Drug: ▪ Additive hypokalemia with **amphotericin B, mezlocillin, piperacillin, ticarcillin,** or **diuretics** ▪ Hypokalemia may increase the risk of **cardiac glycoside** toxicity ▪ May increase requirements for **insulin** or **oral hypoglycemic agents** ▪ **Phenytoin, pheno-**

barbital, and **rifampin** stimulate metabolism, may decrease effectiveness
- **Oral contraceptives** may block metabolism.

ROUTE AND DOSAGE
- **PO, IM (Adults):** 20–300 mg/day.

AVAILABILITY
- **Tablets:** 5 mg, 10 mg, 25 mg ■ **Injection:** 50 mg/ml.

TIME/ACTION PROFILE
(peak = blood levels;
duration = duration of adrenal
suppression or anti-inflammatory
activity)

	ONSET	PEAK	DURATION
PO	rapid	2 hr	1.25–1.5 days
IM	slow	20–48 hr	1.25–1.5 days

NURSING IMPLICATIONS
ASSESSMENT
- Assess patient for signs of adrenal insufficiency (hypotension, weight loss, weakness, nausea, vomiting, anorexia, lethargy confusion, restlessness) prior to and periodically throughout course of therapy.
- Monitor intake and output ratios and daily weights. Observe patient for peripheral edema, steady weight gain, rales/crackles, or dyspnea. Notify physician should these occur.
- Children should also have periodic evaluations of growth.
- **Lab Test Considerations:** Patients on prolonged courses of therapy should routinely have hematologic values, serum electrolytes, serum and urine glucose evaluated. May decrease WBC counts. May cause hyperglycemia, especially in persons with diabetes. May decrease serum potassium and calcium and increase serum sodium concentrations.
- Promptly report presence of guaiac-positive stools.
- May increase serum cholesterol and lipid values. May decrease serum protein-bound iodine and thyroxine concentrations.

- Suppresses reactions to allergy skin tests.
- Periodic adrenal function tests may be ordered to assess degree of hypothalamic-pituitary-adrenal axis suppression.

POTENTIAL NURSING DIAGNOSES
- Infection, high risk for (side effects).
- Knowledge deficit related to medication regimen (patient/family teaching).

IMPLEMENTATION
- **General Info:** If dose is ordered daily or every other day, administer in the morning to coincide with the body's normal secretion of cortisol.
- **PO:** Administer with meals to minimize gastric irritation.
- **IM/SC:** Shake suspension well before drawing up. IM doses should not be administered when rapid effect is desirable. Do not dilute with other solution or admix. Do not administer this preparation IV.

PATIENT/FAMILY TEACHING
- Instruct patient to take medication exactly as directed; do not skip or double up on missed doses. Stopping the medication suddenly may result in adrenal insufficiency (anorexia, nausea, fatigue, weakness, hypotension, dyspnea, and hypoglycemia). If these signs appear notify physician immediately. This can be life-threatening.
- Encourage patients on long-term therapy to eat a diet high in protein, calcium, and potassium and low in sodium and carbohydrates (see Appendix K).
- This drug causes immunosuppression and may mask symptoms of infection. Instruct patient to avoid people with known contagious illnesses and to report possible infections immediately.
- Review side effects with patient. Instruct patient to inform physician promptly if severe abdominal pain or tarry stools occur. Patient should also report unusual swelling, weight gain, tiredness, bone pain, bruising, non-

healing sores, visual disturbances, or behavior changes.

□ Advise patient to notify physician or dentist of medication regimen prior to treatment or surgery.

□ Instruct patient to inform physician if symptoms of underlying disease return or worsen.

□ Advise patient to carry identification in the event of an emergency in which patient cannot relate medical history.

□ Caution patient to avoid vaccinations without consulting physician.

□ Emphasize the importance of follow-up examinations to monitor progress and side effects.

EVALUATION
Effectiveness of therapy can be demonstrated by: ■ Decrease in presenting symptoms with minimal drug-related side effects.

COSYNTROPIN
(koe-sin-troe-pin)
Cortrosyn, Synacthen, Tetracosactrin

CLASSIFICATION(S):
Hormone (adrenocorticotrophic)
Pregnancy Category C

INDICATIONS
■ Diagnosis of adrenocortical disorders.

ACTION
■ A synthetic form of corticotropin (ACTH); stimulates the adrenal gland to produce both glucocorticoids (hydrocortisone) and mineralocorticoids (aldosterone). Action requires intact adrenal responsiveness ■ Actions resemble those of glucocorticoid administration and include suppression of the normal immune response and inflammation ■ Additional numerous intense metabolic effects ■ Potent mineralocorticoid (sodium retention). **Therapeutic Effect:** ■ Production of adrenal steroids following administration.

PHARMACOKINETICS
Absorption: ACTH is rapidly absorbed. Repository forms (gelatin or zinc hydroxide) are more slowly absorbed.
Distribution: Removed from plasma to many tissues. Does not cross the placenta.
Metabolism and Excretion: Metabolic fate not known.
Half-life: 15 min (plasma).

CONTRAINDICATIONS AND PRECAUTIONS
Contraindicated in: ■ Hypersensitivity ■ Serious infections.
Use Cautiously in: ■ Pregnancy or lactation (safety not established).

ADVERSE REACTIONS AND SIDE EFFECTS*
Misc: hypersensitivity reactions, including ANAPHYLAXIS.

INTERACTIONS
Drug–Drug: ■ **Estrogens** may block metabolism ■ **Glucocorticoids** will alter the results of testing.

ROUTE AND DOSAGE
■ **SC, IM, IV (Adults and Children >2 yr):** 0.25 mg.
■ **IM (Children <2 yr):** 0.125 mg.

AVAILABILITY
■ *Powder for injection:* 0.25 mg/vial.

TIME/ACTION PROFILE (effects on plasma cortisol levels)

	ONSET	PEAK	DURATION
IM, IV	UK	45–60 min	UK

NURSING IMPLICATIONS
ASSESSMENT
□ In patients with a history of allergic reactions, monitor for hypersensitivity response (wheezing, rash or hives, bradycardia, irritability seizures, nausea, and vomiting). Cosyntropin is less likely than ACTH to cause such a response.

- **Lab Test Considerations:** Plasma cortisol concentrations will be measured prior to and 30 or 60 min after administration of cosyntropin. Therapeutic response is a rise in the plasma cortisol of at least 7 mcg/100 ml above baseline or a final concentration of at least 18 mcg/100 ml. Administration of glucocorticoids on the day of the test will interfere with test results by causing elevated baseline plasma cortisol concentrations.

POTENTIAL NURSING DIAGNOSES
- Knowledge deficit related to medication regimen (patient/family teaching).

IMPLEMENTATION
- **General Info:** May be administered SC, IM, direct IV, and by IV infusion.
- Reconstitute 250-mcg vial with 1 ml of 0.9% NaCl for injection.
- Stable for 24 hr at room temperature, 21 days if refrigerated.
- **Direct IV:** Administer over 2 min.
- **Intermittent Infusion:** May be further diluted in D5W or 0.9% NaCl. Stable for 12 hr at room temperature.
- **Rate:** Infuse at a rate of 40 mcg/hr over 6 hr.

PATIENT/FAMILY TEACHING
- Explain purpose of cosyntropin and need for lab tests.

EVALUATION
Effectiveness of therapy can be demonstrated by: ▪ Differentiation of primary from secondary adrenocortical insufficiency.

CYCLOBENZAPRINE
(sye-kloe-**ben**-za-preen)
Cycloflex, Flexeril

CLASSIFICATION(S):
Skeletal muscle relaxant (centrally acting)
Pregnancy Category B

INDICATIONS
- In combination with other treatment modalities (physical therapy, bed rest) in the management of acute painful musculoskeletal conditions associated with muscle spasm.

ACTION
- Reduces tonic somatic muscle activity at the level of the brainstem. Structually similar to tricyclic antidepressants. **Therapeutic Effect:** ▪ Reduction in muscle spasm and hyperactivity without loss of function.

PHARMACOKINETICS
Absorption: Well absorbed from the GI tract.
Distribution: Distribution not known.
Metabolism and Excretion: Mostly metabolized by the liver.
Half-life: 1–3 days.

CONTRAINDICATIONS AND PRECAUTIONS
Contraindicated in: ▪ Hypersensitivity ▪ Should not be used within 14 days of MAO inhibitor therapy ▪ Immediate period after myocardial infarction ▪ Severe or symptomatic cardiovascular disease ▪ Cardiac conduction disturbances ▪ Hyperthyroidism.
Use Cautiously in: ▪ Cardiovascular disease ▪ Pregnancy, lactation, and children (safety not established) ▪ Therapy should be limited to 2–3 wk.

ADVERSE REACTIONS AND SIDE EFFECTS*
CNS: drowsiness, dizziness, fatigue, headache, nervousness, confusion.
EENT: dry mouth, blurred vision.
CV: arrhythmias.
GI: constipation, unpleasant taste, dyspepsia, nausea.
GU: urinary retention.

INTERACTIONS
Drug–Drug: ▪ Additive CNS depression with other **CNS depressants**, including **alcohol, antihistamines, opioid analgesics,** and **sedative/hypnotics** ▪ Additive anticholinergic effects with **drugs possessing anticholinergic properties,**

*Underlines indicate most frequent; **CAPITALS** indicate life-threatening.

including **antihistamines, antidepressants, atropine, disopyramide, haloperidol,** and **phenothiazines** ▪ Avoid use within 14 days of **MAO inhibitor** therapy (hyperpyretic crisis, convulsions, and death may occur) ▪ May blunt the response to **guanadrel** or **guanethidine.**

ROUTE AND DOSAGE
▪ **PO (Adults):** 10 mg 3 times daily (range 20–40 mg/day; not to exceed 60 mg/day).

AVAILABILITY
▪ *Tablets:* 10 mg.

TIME/ACTION PROFILE (skeletal muscle relaxation)

	ONSET	PEAK*	DURATION
PO	1 hr	4–6 hr	12–24 hr

*Full effects may not occur for 1–2 wk.

NURSING IMPLICATIONS

ASSESSMENT
▫ Assess patient for pain, muscle stiffness, and range of motion prior to and periodically throughout therapy.

POTENTIAL NURSING DIAGNOSES
▪ Pain (indications).
▪ Physical mobility, impaired (indications).
▪ Injury, high risk for (side effects).

IMPLEMENTATION
▪ PO: May be administered with meals to minimize gastric irritation.

PATIENT/FAMILY TEACHING
▫ Instruct patient to take medication exactly as directed; do not take more than the prescribed amount. Missed doses should be taken within 1 hr of time ordered, otherwise return to normal dosage schedule. Do not double doses.
▫ Medication may cause drowsiness, dizziness, and blurred vision. Caution patient to avoid driving or other activities requiring alertness until response to drug is known.
▫ Advise patient to avoid concurrent use of alcohol or other CNS depressants with this medication.
▫ If constipation becomes a problem, advise patient that increasing fluid intake and bulk in diet and stool softeners may alleviate this condition.
▫ Advise patient to notify physician if symptoms of urinary retention (distended abdomen, feeling of fullness, overflow incontinence, voiding small amounts) occur.
▫ Inform patient that good oral hygiene, frequent mouth rinses, and sugarless gum or candy may help relieve dry mouth.

EVALUATION
Effectiveness of therapy can be demonstrated by: ▪ Relief of muscular spasm in acute skeletal muscle conditions. Maximum effects may not be evident for 1–2 wk.

CYCLOPHOSPHAMIDE
(sye-kloe-**foss**-fa-mide)
Cytoxan, Neosar, {Procytox}

CLASSIFICATION(S):
Antineoplastic (alkylating agent), Immunosuppressant
Pregnancy Category C

INDICATIONS
▪ Alone or with other modalities (other chemotherapeutic agents, radiation therapy, surgery) in the management of: ▫ Hodgkin's disease ▫ Malignant lymphomas ▫ Multiple myeloma ▫ Leukemias ▫ Mycosis fungoides ▫ Neuroblastoma ▫ Ovarian carcinoma ▫ Breast carcinoma, and a variety of other tumors ▪ Treatment of minimal change nephrotic syndrome in children. **Unlabeled Uses:** ▪ Used as an immunosuppressant in the treatment of severe active rheumatoid arthritis or Wegener's granulomatosis.

ACTION
▪ Interferes with DNA replication and

{} = Available in Canada only.

RNA transcription, ultimately disrupting protein synthesis (cell cycle-phase nonspecific). **Therapeutic Effects:** ▪ Death of rapidly replicating cells, particularly malignant ones ▪ Also has immunosuppressant action in smaller doses.

PHARMACOKINETICS

Absorption: Inactive parent drug is well absorbed from the GI tract. Converted to active drug by the liver.

Distribution: Widely distributed. Limited penetration of the blood–brain barrier. Crosses the placenta and enters breast milk.

Metabolism and Excretion: Converted to active drug by the liver. 30% eliminated unchanged by the kidneys.

Half-life: 4–6.5 hr.

CONTRAINDICATIONS AND PRECAUTIONS

Contraindicated in: ▪ Hypersensitivity ▪ Pregnancy or lactation.

Use Cautiously in: ▪ Patients with childbearing potential ▪ Active infections ▪ Decreased bone marrow ▪ Other chronic debilitating illnesses.

ADVERSE REACTIONS AND SIDE EFFECTS*

CV: MYOCARDIAL FIBROSIS, hypotension.

Resp: pulmonary fibrosis.

GI: anorexia, nausea, vomiting.

GU: hemorrhagic cystitis, hematuria.

Derm: alopecia.

Endo: syndrome of inappropriate secretion of antidiuretic hormone (SIADH), gonadal suppression.

Hemat: anemia, thrombocytopenia, leukopenia.

Metab: hyperuricemia.

Misc: secondary neoplasms.

INTERACTIONS

Drug–Drug: ▪ **Phenobarbital** or **rifampin** may increase the toxicity of cyclophosphamide ▪ Concurrent **allopurinol** may exaggerate bone marrow depression ▪ May prolong neuromusclar block-ade from **succinylcholine** ▪ Cardiotoxicity may be additive with **other cardiotoxic agents (cytarabine, daunorubicin, doxorubicin)** ▪ Additive bone marrow depression with other **antineoplastics** or **radiation therapy** ▪ May potentiate the effects of **oral anticoagulants** ▪ May decrease antibody response to **live virus vaccines** and increase the risk of adverse reactions ▪ Prolongs the effects of **cocaine**.

ROUTE AND DOSAGE

Many regimens are used.

▪ **PO (Adults):** 1–5 mg/kg/day.

▪ **PO (Children):** *Induction*—2–8 mg/kg/day (60–250 mg/m²/day) in divided doses for 6 days or longer. *Maintenance*—2–5 mg/kg (50–150 mg/m²) twice weekly.

▪ **IV (Adults):** 40–50 mg/kg in divided doses over 2–5 days *or* 10–15 mg/kg q 7–10 days *or* 3–5 mg/kg twice weekly *or* 1.5–3 mg/kg/day. Other regimens may use larger doses.

▪ **IV (Children):** *Induction*—2–8 mg/kg/day (60–250 mg/m²/day) in divided doses for 6 days or longer. Total dose for 7 days may be given as a single dose. *Maintenance*—10–15 mg/kg every 7–10 days or 30 mg/kg q 3–4 wk.

AVAILABILITY

▪ *Tablets:* 25 mg, 50 mg ▪ *Injection:* 100 mg, 200 mg, 500 mg, 1-g and 2-g vials.

TIME/ACTION PROFILE (effects on blood counts)

	ONSET	PEAK	DURATION
PO	7 days	10–14 days	21 days
IV	7 days	10–14 days	21 days

NURSING IMPLICATIONS

Assessment

☐ Monitor blood pressure, pulse, respiratory rate, and temperature frequently during administration. Notify physician of significant changes.

*Underlines indicate most frequent; **CAPITALS** indicate life-threatening.

▫ Monitor urinary output frequently throughout therapy. To reduce the risk of hemorrhagic cystitis, fluid intake should be at least 3000 ml/day for adults and 1000–2000 ml/day for children.

▫ Assess for fever, chills, sore throat, and signs of infection. Notify physician if these symptoms occur.

▫ Monitor platelet count throughout therapy. Assess for bleeding (bleeding gums, bruising, petechiae; guaiac stools, urine, and emesis). Avoid IM injections and rectal temperatures. Apply pressure to venipuncture sites for 10 min.

▫ Assess nausea, vomiting, and appetite. Weigh weekly. Antiemetics may be given 30 min prior to administration of medication to minimize GI effects. Anorexia and weight loss can be minimized by feeding frequent light meals.

▫ Encourage patient to drink 2000–3000 ml/day to promote excretion of uric acid. Alkalinization of the urine may be ordered to help prevent uric acid nephropathy.

▫ Anemia may occur. Monitor for increased fatigue, dyspnea, and orthostatic hypotension.

▫ Assess cardiac and respiratory status for dyspnea, rales/crackles, weight gain, edema. Pulmonary toxicity may occur after prolonged therapy. Cardiotoxicity may occur early in therapy and is characterized by symptoms of congestive heart failure.

■ **Lab Test Considerations:** Monitor CBC and differential prior to and periodically throughout course of therapy. The nadir of leukopenia occurs in 7–12 days (recovery in 17–21 days). Leukocytes should be maintained between 2500–4000/mm³. May also cause thrombocytopenia (nadir 10–15 days), and rarely causes anemia.

▫ Monitor BUN, creatinine, and uric acid prior to and frequently during course of therapy to detect nephrotoxicity.

▫ Monitor ALT (SGPT), AST (SGOT), LDH, and serum bilirubin prior to and frequently during course of therapy to detect hepatotoxicity.

▫ Urinalysis should be evaluated before initiating therapy and frequently during course of therapy to detect hematuria or change in specific gravity indicative of SIADH.

▫ May suppress positive reactions to skin tests for candida, mumps, trichophyton, and tuberculin PPD. May also produce false-positive results in PAP smears.

POTENTIAL NURSING DIAGNOSES

■ Infection, high risk for (side effects).
■ Body image disturbance (side effects).
■ Knowledge deficit related to medication regimen (patient/family teaching).

IMPLEMENTATION

■ **PO:** Administer medication on an empty stomach. If severe gastric irritation develops, medication may be given with food.

▫ Oral preparations can be formed by diluting powder for injection in Aromatic Elixir to a concentration of 1–5 mg of cyclophosphamide/ml. Reconstituted preparations should be refrigerated and used within 2 wk.

■ **IV:** Solution for IV administration should be prepared in a biologic cabinet. Wear gloves, gown, and mask while handling IV medication. Discard IV equipment in specially designated containers (see Appendix I).

▫ Prepare IV solution by diluting each 100 mg with 5 ml of Sterile Water or Bacteriostatic Water for Injection containing parabens. Shake solution gently and allow to stand until clear. Use solution prepared without bacteriostatic water within 6 hr. Solution prepared with bacteriostatic water is stable for 24 hr at room temperature, 6 days if refrigerated.

■ **Direct IV:** Administer reconstituted solution directly at a rate of 100 mg over 1 min.

■ **Intermittent Infusion:** May be further diluted in up to 250 ml of D5W, 0.9% NaCl, D5/0.9% NaCl, 0.45% NaCl, lactated Ringer's solution, or dextrose/ Ringer's solution.

- **Syringe Compatibility:** ■ bleomycin ■ cisplatin ■ doxorubicin ■ droperidol ■ fentanyl ■ fluorouracil ■ heparin ■ leucovorin calcium ■ methotrexate ■ metoclopramide ■ mitomycin ■ vinblastine ■ vincristine.

- **Y-Site Compatibility:** Compatible via Y-site injection into port of free-flowing IV with ■ amikacin ■ ampicillin ■ bleomycin ■ cefamandole ■ cefazolin ■ cefoperazone ■ ceforanide ■ cefotaxime ■ cefoxitin ■ cefuroxime ■ cephalothin ■ cephapirin ■ chloramphenicol ■ cisplatin ■ clindamycin ■ doxorubicin ■ doxycycline ■ droperidol ■ erythromycin ■ fludarabine ■ fluorouracil ■ gentamicin ■ heparin ■ kanamycin ■ leucovorin calcium ■ methotrexate ■ metoclopramide ■ metronidazole ■ mezlocillin ■ minocycline ■ mitomycin ■ moxalactam ■ nafcillin ■ ondanestron ■ oxacillin ■ penicillin G potassium ■ piperacillin ■ ticarcillin ■ tobramycin ■ trimethoprim/sulfamethoxazole ■ vancomycin ■ vinblastine ■ vincristine.

PATIENT/FAMILY TEACHING

▫ Instruct patient to take dose in early morning. Emphasize need for adequate fluid intake for 72 hr after therapy. Patient should void frequently to decrease bladder irritation from metabolites excreted by the kidneys. Physician should be notified immediately if hematuria is noted. If a dose is missed physician should be contacted.

▫ Instruct patient to notify physician promptly if fever, sore throat, signs of infection, sores in the mouth or on the lips, yellow discoloration of skin or eyes, bleeding gums, bruising, petechiae, blood in urine, stool, or emesis or unusual swelling, joint pain, shortness of breath, or confusion occurs. Caution patient to avoid crowds and persons with known infections. Instruct patient to use soft toothbrush and electric razor and to avoid falls. Patient should also be cautioned not

to drink alcoholic beverages or to take products containing aspirin or ibuprofen, as these may precipitate GI hemorrhage.

▫ Advise patient that this medication may cause sterility and menstrual irregularities or cessation of menses. This drug is also teratogenic, and contraceptive measures should continue for at least 4 mo after completion of therapy.

▫ Discuss with patient the possibility of hair loss. Explore methods of coping. May also cause darkening of skin and fingernails.

▫ Instruct patient not to receive any vaccinations without advice of physician.

EVALUATION

Effectiveness of therapy can be demonstrated by: ■ Decrease in size or spread of malignant tumors ■ Improvement of hematologic status in patients with leukemia. Maintenance therapy is instituted if leukocyte count remains between 2500 and 4000/mm^3 and if patient does not demonstrate serious side effects.

CYCLOSPORINE
(sye-kloe-spor-een)
Ciclosporin, Cyclosporin A, Sandimmune

CLASSIFICATION(S):
Immunosuppressant
Pregnancy Category C

INDICATIONS

■ Prevention and treatment of rejection in renal, cardiac, and hepatic transplantation (with glucocorticoids).

ACTION

■ Inhibits normal immune responses (cellular and humoral) by inhibiting interleukin-2, a factor necessary for initiation of T-cell activity. **Therapeutic Effect:** ■ Prevention of rejection reactions.

PHARMACOKINETICS

Absorption: Erratically absorbed (range 10–60%) after oral administration, with significant first-pass metabolism by the liver.

Distribution: Widely distributed, mainly into extracellular fluid and blood cells. Crosses the placenta and enters breast milk.

Metabolism and Excretion: Extensively metabolized by the liver, excreted in bile, small amounts (6%) excreted unchanged by the kidneys.

Half-life: 19–27 hr.

CONTRAINDICATIONS AND PRECAUTIONS

Contraindicated in: ▪ Hypersensitivity to cyclosporine or polyoxethylated castor oil (vehicle for IV form) ▪ Should not be given to pregnant or lactating women unless benefits outweigh risks ▪ Disulfiram therapy or known alcohol intolerance ▪ (IV and oral liquid dosage forms contain alcohol).

Use Cautiously in: ▪ Severe hepatic impairment (dosage reduction recommended) ▪ Renal impairment (frequent dosage changes may be necessary) ▪ Active infection ▪ Children (larger or more frequent doses may be required).

ADVERSE REACTIONS AND SIDE EFFECTS*

CNS: tremor, SEIZURES, headache, flushing, confusion, psychiatric problems.

CV: hypertension.

Derm: hirsutism, gingival hyperplasia, acne.

GI: nausea, vomiting, diarrhea, anorexia, abdominal discomfort.

GU: nephrotoxicity.

F and E: hypomagnesemia, hyperkalemia.

Hemat: leukopenia, anemia, thrombocytopenia.

Metab: hyperuricemia, hyperlipidemia.

Neuro: paresthesia, hyperesthesia.

Misc: hepatotoxicity, infections, hypersensitivity reactions, hyperlipidemia.

INTERACTIONS

Drug–Drug: ▪ Increased risk of nephrotoxicity with **amphotericin B, aminoglycosides, fluoroquinolones, erythromycin, ketoconazole, NSAIDs, melphelan,** or **sulfonamides** ▪ Blood levels and risk of toxicity of cyclosporine are increased by **anabolic steroids, oral contraceptives, erythromycin, cimetidine, danazol, fluconazole, ketoconazole, miconazole,** and **calcium channel blockers** ▪ Additive immunosuppression with other **immunosuppressants** (**cyclophosphamide, azathioprine, glucocorticoids**) or **verapamil** ▪ **Barbiturates, phenytoin, rifampin, carbamazepine,** or **sulfonamides** may decrease the effect of cyclosporine ▪ Additive hyperkalemia may occur with **potassium-sparing diuretics, potassium supplements,** or **ACE inhibitors** ▪ Increases serum levels and the risk of toxicity from **digoxin** (decrease digoxin dose by 50%) ▪ Prolongs the action of **neuromuscular blocking agents** ▪ Increased risk of seizures with **imipenem/cilastatin** ▪ May decrease antibody response to **live virus vaccines** and increase the risk of adverse reactions ▪ Increased risk of rhabdomyolysis with **lovastatin**.

ROUTE AND DOSAGE

Many regimens are used.

- ▪ **PO (Adults and Children):** 15 mg/kg/day (first dose before transplant) for 1–2 wk, taper by 5% weekly to maintenance dose of 5–10 mg/kg/day.
- ▪ **IV (Adults and Children):** 5–6 mg/kg/day (⅓ PO dose) initially, change to PO as soon as possible.

AVAILABILITY

▪ *Soft gelatin capsules:* 25 mg, 100 mg ▪ *Oral solution:* 100 mg/ml ▪ *Injection:* 50 mg/ml in 5-ml ampules.

TIME/ACTION PROFILE (blood levels)

	ONSET	PEAK	DURATION
PO	UK	3.5 hr	UK
IV	UK	end of infusion	UK

*Underlines indicate most frequent; **CAPITALS** indicate life-threatening.

NURSING IMPLICATIONS

ASSESSMENT

- **General Info:** Assess for symptoms of organ rejection throughout therapy.
  - Monitor intake and output ratios, daily weight, and blood pressure throughout therapy. Notify physician of significant changes.
- **IV:** Monitor patient for signs and symptoms of hypersensitivity (wheezing, dyspnea, flushing of face or neck). Oxygen, epinephrine, and equipment for treatment of anaphylaxis should be available with each IV dose.
  - Nephrotoxicity may occur; monitor BUN and serum creatinine periodically. Notify physician if significant increases occur. May also cause decreased serum magnesium levels.
  - May cause hepatotoxicity; monitor for elevated AST (SGOT), ALT (SGPT), alkaline phoshatase, amylase, and bilirubin.
  - May cause increased serum potassium and uric acid levels.
  - Serum lipid levels may be elevated.
- **Toxicity and Overdose:** Serum cyclosporine levels should be evaluated periodically during therapy. Dose may be adjusted daily, in response to levels, during initiation of therapy. Trough levels of 250–800 ng/ml (blood) or 50–300 ng/ml (plasma) 24 hr after a dose is given have been shown to minimize side effects and rejection events.

POTENTIAL NURSING DIAGNOSES

- Infection, high risk for (side effects).
- Knowledge deficit related to medication regimen (patient/family teaching).

IMPLEMENTATION

- **General Info:** Given with other immunosuppressive agents. Protect transplant patients from staff and visitors who may carry infection. Maintain protective isolation as indicated.
- **PO:** Draw up oral solution in the pipette provided with the medication. Mix oral solution with milk, chocolate milk, or orange juice, preferably at room temperature. Stir well and drink at once. Use a glass container and rinse with more diluent to ensure that total dose is taken. Administer oral doses with meals. Wipe pipette dry; do not wash after use.
- **Intermittent Infusion:** Dilute each 1 ml (50 mg) of IV concentrate immediately before use with 20–100 ml of D5W or 0.9% NaCl for injection. Solution is stable for 24 hr in D5W. In 0.9% NaCl it is stable for 6 hr in a polyvinylchloride container and 12 hr in a glass container at room temperature.
- **Rate:** Infuse slowly over 2–6 hr via infusion pump.
- **Continuous Infusion:** May be administered over 24 hr.

PATIENT/FAMILY TEACHING

- Instruct patient to take medication at the same time each day, as directed. Do not skip doses or double up on missed doses. Take a missed dose as soon as remembered within 12 hr. Do not discontinue medication without physician's advice.
- Reinforce the need for lifelong therapy to prevent transplant rejection. Review symptoms of rejection for transplanted organ, and stress need to notify physician immediately if they occur.
- Advise patient of common side effects (nephrotoxicity, increased blood pressure, hand tremors, increased facial hair, gingival hyperplasia).
- Teach patient the correct method for monitoring blood pressure at home. Instruct patient to notify physician of significant changes in blood pressure or if hematuria, frequency, cloudy urine, or decreased urine output occur.
- Instruct patient on proper oral hygiene. Meticulous oral hygiene and regular dental care will help decrease gingival inflammation and hyperplasia.
- Instruct patient to consult with physician or pharmacist before taking any over-the-counter medications or re-

ceiving any vaccinations while taking this medication.

□ Advise patient to notify physician if pregnancy is planned or suspected.

□ Emphasize the importance of follow-up examinations and lab tests.

EVALUATION
Effectiveness of therapy may be determined by: ▪ Prevention of rejection of transplanted tissues.

CYPROHEPTADINE
(si-proe-**hep**-ta-deen)
Periactin

CLASSIFICATION(S):
Antihistamine
Pregnancy Category B

INDICATIONS

▪ Relief of allergic symptoms caused by histamine release. Most useful in conditions such as: □ Nasal allergies □ Allergic dermatoses □ Cold urticaria. **Unlabeled Uses:** ▪ Stimulation of appetite ▪ Suppression of vascular headaches.

ACTION

▪ Blocks the following effects of histamine: □ Vasodilation □ Increased GI tract secretions □ Increased heart rate □ Hypotension ▪ Also blocks the effects of serotonin, which may result in increased appetite and decreased vascular headaches. **Therapeutic Effects:** ▪ Relief of symptoms associated with histamine excess usually seen in allergic conditions, including cold urticaria ▪ Stimulation of appetite.

PHARMACOKINETICS

Absorption: Apparently well absorbed after oral dosing.
Distribution: Distribution not known.
Metabolism and Excretion: Almost completely metabolized by the liver.
Half-life: UK.

CONTRAINDICATIONS AND PRECAUTIONS

Contraindicated in: ▪ Hypersensitivity ▪ Acute attacks of asthma ▪ Lactation ▪ Known alcohol intolerance (syrup only).
Use Cautiously in: ▪ Elderly (more susceptible to adverse reactions) ▪ Pregnancy (safety not established) ▪ Narrow-angle glaucoma ▪ Liver disease.

ADVERSE REACTIONS AND SIDE EFFECTS*

CNS: drowsiness, sedation, excitation (in children).
CV: hypotension, palpitations, arrhythmias.
EENT: blurred vision.
GI: dry mouth, constipation.
GU: urinary hesitancy, retention.
Derm: rashes, photosensitivity.

INTERACTIONS

Drug–Drug: ▪ Additive CNS depression with other **CNS depressants,** including **alcohol, opioid analgesics,** and **sedative/hypnotics** ▪ **MAO inhibitors** may intensify and prolong the anticholinergic effects of antihistamines.

ROUTE AND DOSAGE

▪ **PO (Adults):** 4 mg q 8 hr (range 4–20 mg/day in 3 divided doses; up to 32 mg/day).
▪ **PO (Children 6–14 yr):** 2–4 mg q 6–8 hr (not to exceed 16 mg/day).
▪ **PO (Children 2–6 yr):** 2 mg q 8–12 hr (not to exceed 12 mg/day).

AVAILABILITY

▪ *Tablets:* 4 mg ▪ *Syrup:* 2 mg/5 ml.

TIME/ACTION PROFILE
(antihistaminic effects)

	ONSET	PEAK	DURATION
PO	15–60 min	1–2 hr	8 hr

NURSING IMPLICATIONS

ASSESSMENT
▪ **Allergy:** Assess symptoms (rhinitis,

---

*<u>Underlines</u> indicate most frequent; **CAPITALS** indicate life-threatening.

conjunctivitis, hives) prior to and periodically throughout therapy.

□ Assess lung sounds and respiratory function prior to and periodically throughout course of therapy. Medication may cause thickening of bronchial secretions. Maintain fluid intake of 1500–2000 ml/day to decrease viscosity of secretions.

■ **Appetite Stimulant:** Monitor food intake and weight routinely.

■ **Lab Test Considerations:** May cause false-negative reactions on allergy skin tests; discontinue 72 hr prior to testing.

□ Increased serum amylase and prolactin concentrations may occur when cyproheptadine is administered with a thyrotropin-releasing hormone.

POTENTIAL NURSING DIAGNOSES

■ Airway clearance, ineffective (indications).

■ Injury, high risk for (side effects).

■ Knowledge deficit related to medication regimen (patient/family teaching).

IMPLEMENTATION

■ **PO:** Administer with food, water, or milk to minimize gastric irritation.

PATIENT/FAMILY TEACHING

□ Instruct patient to take cyproheptadine exactly as directed. Missed dose should be taken as soon as remembered. Do not double doses. Syrup should be accurately measured using calibrated medication cup or measuring device.

□ Medication may cause drowsiness. Advise patient to avoid driving or other activities requiring alertness until response to the drug is known.

□ Advise patient to use sunscreen and protective clothing to prevent a photosensitivity reaction.

□ Caution patient to avoid concurrent use of alcohol and other CNS depressants.

□ Advise patient that frequent mouth rinses, good oral hygiene, and sugarless gum or candy may decrease dry mouth. Patient should notify dentist if dry mouth persists for >2 wk.

EVALUATION

Effectiveness of therapy can be demonstrated by: ■ Alleviation of allergic symptoms □ Alleviation of cold urticaria ■ Improvement of appetite.

CYTARABINE

(sye-**tare**-a-been)
Ara-C, cytosine arabinoside, Cytosar-U, {Cytosar}, Tarabine PFS

CLASSIFICATION(S):
Antineoplastic (antimetabolite)
Pregnancy Category C

INDICATIONS

■ **IV:** Used mainly in combination chemotherapeutic regimens for the treatment of leukemias and non-Hodgkin's lymphomas ■ **IT:** Treatment of meningeal leukemia.

ACTION

■ Inhibits DNA synthesis by inhibiting DNA polymerase (cell cycle-S phase specific). **Therapeutic Effect:** ■ Death of rapidly replicating cells, particularly malignant ones.

PHARMACOKINETICS

Absorption: Absorption occurs from SC sites, but blood levels are less than with IV administration.

Distribution: Widely distributed. Crosses the blood–brain barrier, but not in sufficient quantities. Crosses the placenta.

Metabolism and Excretion: Metabolized mostly by the liver; small amounts (<10%) excreted unchanged by the kidneys.

Half-life: 1–3 hr.

CONTRAINDICATIONS AND PRECAUTIONS

Contraindicated in: ■ Hypersensitivity ■ Pregnancy or lactation.

Use Cautiously in: ▪ Patients with childbearing potential ▪ Active infections ▪ Decreased bone marrow reserve ▪ Other chronic debilitating illnesses.

ADVERSE REACTIONS AND SIDE EFFECTS*

CNS: headache, CNS dysfunction (high dose).
EENT: high dose—hemorrhagic conjunctivitis, corneal toxicity.
Resp: high dose—pulmonary edema.
GI: nausea, vomiting, hepatitis; high dose—severe GI ulceration, hepatotoxicity, stomatitis.
Derm: rash, alopecia.
Endo: gonadal suppression.
Hemat: bone marrow depression.
Metab: hyperuricemia.
Misc: fever, cytarabine syndrome.

INTERACTIONS

Drug–Drug: Additive bone marrow depression with other **antineoplastics** or **radiation therapy** ▪ Increased risk of cardiomyopathy when used in high-dose regimens with **cyclophosphamide** ▪ May decrease antibody response to **live virus vaccines** and increase the risk of adverse reactions.

ROUTE AND DOSAGE

▪ **IV (Adults):** 100–200 mg/m²/day or 3 mg/kg/day as a continuous infusion over 24 hr or divided doses by rapid injection for 5–10 days; course may be repeated in 2 wk. High-dose regimen—2–3 g/m² over 1–3 hr every 12 hr for 2–6 days.
▪ **SC (Adults):** Maintenance dose—1 mg/kg 1–2 times weekly.
▪ **IT (Adults):** 30 mg/m² once every 4 days until CSF is normal, followed by an additional dose (range 5–75 mg/m² given every 1–4 days for 4 days).

AVAILABILITY

▪ *Injection:* 100 mg, 500 mg, 1-g and 2-g vials.

TIME/ACTION PROFILE (effects on white blood cell counts)

	ONSET	PEAK	DURATION
SC, IV (1st phase)	24 hr	7–9 days	12 days
SC, IV (2nd phase)	15–24 days	15–24 days	25–34 days

NURSING IMPLICATIONS

ASSESSMENT

▫ Assess for fever, sore throat, and signs of infection. If these symptoms occur notify physician immediately.
▫ Assess for bleeding (bleeding gums, bruising, petechiae; guaiac stools, urine, emesis). Avoid IM injections and rectal temperatures. Hold pressure on all venipuncture sites for at least 10 min.
▫ Monitor intake and output ratios and daily weights. Notify physician if significant changes in totals occur.
▫ Monitor for symptoms of gout (increased uric acid, joint pain, edema). Encourage patient to drink at least 2 liters of fluid each day. Allopurinol may decrease uric acid levels. Alkalinization of urine may increase excretion of uric acid.
▫ Assess nutritional status. Nausea and vomiting may occur within 1 hr of administration, especially if IV dose is administered rapidly. Administering an antiemetic prior to and periodically throughout therapy and adjusting diet as tolerated may help maintain fluid and electrolyte balance and nutritional status.
▫ Anemia may occur. Monitor for increased fatigue, dyspnea, and orthostatic hypotension.
▫ Monitor patient for developmnt of *cytarabine syndrome* (fever, myalgia, bone pain, chest pain, maculopapular rash, conjunctivitis, malaise) which usually occurs 6–12 hr following administration. Glucocorticoids may be used for treatment or preven-

*Underlines indicate most frequent; **CAPITALS** indicate life-threatening.

tion. If patient responds to glucocorticoids, continue cytarabine and glucocorticoids.

- **Lab Test Considerations:** Monitor CBC and differential prior to and frequently throughout therapy. Leukocyte counts begins to drop within 24 hr of administration. The initial nadir occurs in 7–9 days. After a small rise in the count, the second, deeper nadir occurs 15–24 days after administration. Leukocyte and thrombocyte counts usually begin to rise 10 days after the nadirs. Therapy is usually withdrawn if leukocyte count is $<1000/mm^3$ or platelet count is $<50,000/mm^3$. Frequent bone marrow examinations are also indicated.
  - ▫ Renal (BUN and creatinine) and hepatic function (AST [SGOT], ALT [SGPT], bilirubin, and LDH) should be monitored prior to and routinely throughout course of therapy.
  - ▫ May cause increase uric acid concentrations.

POTENTIAL NURSING DIAGNOSES

- Infection, high risk for (adverse reactions).
- Injury, high risk for (side effects).
- Knowledge deficit related to medication regimen (patient/family teaching).

IMPLEMENTATION

- **General Info:** Solution should be prepared in a biologic cabinet. Wear gloves, gown, and mask while handling IV medication. Discard IV equipment in specially designated containers (see Appendix I).
  - ▫ May be given SC, direct IV, intermittent IV, continuous IV, or IT.
- **SC/IV:** Reconstitute 100-mg vials with 5 ml of Bacteriostatic Water for Injection with benzyl alcohol 0.9%. Reconstitute 500-mg vials with 10 ml. Reconstituted solution is stable for 48 hr. Do not administer a cloudy solution.
- **Direct IV:** Administer each 100 mg direct IV push over 1–3 min.
- **Intermittent Infusion:** May be further diluted in 100 ml of 0.9% NaCl or

D5W. May also be diluted in D10W, D5/0.9% NaCl, Ringer's solution, lactated Ringer's solution, or D5/LR.
- *Rate:* Infuse over 30 min.
- **Continuous Infusion:** Rate and concentration for IV infusion are ordered individually by physician.
- **Syringe Compatibility:** ▪ metoclopramide.
- **Y-Site Compatibility:** ▪ fludarabine ▪ ondansetron ▪ sargramostim.
- **Additive Compatibility:** ▪ methotrexate ▪ potassium chloride ▪ prednisolone sodium phosphate ▪ vincristine.
- **Additive Incompatibility:** ▪ fluorouracil ▪ heparin ▪ regular insulin ▪ nafcillin ▪ oxacillin ▪ penicillin G sodium.
- **IT:** Reconstitute with preservative-free 0.9% NaCl or other suitable diluent. Use immediately to prevent bacterial contamination.

PATIENT/FAMILY TEACHING

- ▫ Caution patient to avoid crowds and persons with known infections. Physician should be informed immediately if symptoms of infection occur.
- ▫ Instruct patient to report unusual bleeding. Advise patient of thrombocytopenia precautions (use soft toothbrush and electric razor; avoid falls; do not drink alcoholic beverages or take medication containing aspirin or ibuprofen, as these may precipitate gastric bleeding).
- ▫ Instruct patient to inspect oral mucosa for redness and ulceration. If mouth sores occur advise patient to use sponge brush and rinse mouth with water after eating and drinking. Consult physician if pain interferes with eating.
- ▫ Advise patient that this medication may have teratogenic effects. Contraception should be practiced during therapy and for at least 4 mo after therapy is concluded.
- ▫ Instruct patient not to receive any vaccinations without advice of physician.
- ▫ Emphasize the need for periodic lab tests to monitor for side effects.

EVALUATION
Effectiveness of therapy can be demonstrated by: ▪ Improvement of hematopoietic values in leukemias ▪ Decrease in size and spread of the tumor in non-Hodgkin's lymphomas. Therapy is continued every 2 wk until patient is in complete remission or thrombocyte count or leukocyte count falls below acceptable levels.

CYTOMEGALOVIRUS IMMUNE GLOBULIN
(site-oh-**meg**-a-loe-vye-rus)
CMVIG

CLASSIFICATION(S):
Vaccine (immune globulin)
Pregnancy Category UK

INDICATIONS
▪ Suppression of cytomegalovirus (CMV) disease in CMV-negative recipients of transplanted CMV-positive kidneys.

ACTION
▪ Consists of IgG antibodies capable of providing passive immunity against CMV disease. **Therapeutic Effect:** ▪ Prevention of serious sequelae of CMV disease in renal transplant patients.

PHARMACOKINETICS
Absorption: Administered IV only, resulting in complete bioavailability.
Distribution: Distribution not known.
Metabolism and Excretion: UK.
Half-life: UK.

CONTRAINDICATIONS AND PRECAUTIONS
Contraindicated in: ▪ Hypersensitivity to immune globulins or albumin ▪ Selective IgA deficiency.
Use Cautiously in: ▪ Pregnancy or lactation (safety not established).

ADVERSE REACTIONS AND SIDE EFFECTS*
CV: hypotension.
Resp: wheezing.
GI: vomiting, nausea.
Derm: flushing.
MS: muscle cramps, back pain.
Misc: chills, fever, allergic reactions including ANAPHYLAXIS.

INTERACTIONS
Drug–Drug: ▪ May interfere with immune response to some **live virus vaccines** including **measles, mumps,** and **rubella virus vaccine** (do not administer within 3 mo of immune globulin).

ROUTE AND DOSAGE
▪ **IV (Adults):** 150 mg/kg within 72 hr of transplantation, followed by 100 mg/kg after 2, 4, 6, and 8 wk, then 50 mg/kg at 12 and 16 wk.

AVAILABILITY
▪ *Injection:* 2500-mg vial.

TIME/ACTION PROFILE (CMV antibody titers)

	ONSET	PEAK	DURATION
IV	rapid	UK	UK

NURSING IMPLICATIONS
ASSESSMENT
▫ Monitor vital signs prior to, during, and following infusion, and before any increases in infusion rate.
▫ Monitor patient for adverse reactions throughout therapy. If patient develops minor side effects (nausea, vomiting, muscle cramps, back pain, fever, flushing, chills) slow infusion rate or stop infusion temporarily. If hypotension or anaphylaxis occurs, stop infusion and administer treatment (epinephrine and diphenhydramine).

POTENTIAL NURSING DIAGNOSES
▪ Infection, high risk for (indications)
▪ Knowledge deficit related to medication regimen (patient/family teaching).

---

*Underlines indicate most frequent; CAPITALS indicate life-threatening.

IMPLEMENTATION

- **General Info:** Reconstitute with 50 ml of Sterile Water for Injection with a double-ended needle or large syringe. To avoid foaming, do not shake vial. If using a double-ended needle, insert into water first, as powder is supplied in an evacuated vial and water will transfer by suction. After water is transferred, release residual vacuum to speed dissolution. Rotate gently to wet undissolved powder. Allow 30 min for powder to dissolve. Solution should be clear, colorless, and free of particulate matter.
- **Intermittent Infusion:** Infusion should be started within 6 hr and completed within 12 hr of reconstitution.
- □ Administer via infusion pump through a separate IV line. If not possible, solution may be piggy-backed in an IV line containing 0.9% NaCl, D5W, D10W, D20W, or combinations of dextrose and saline, but do not dilute to more than 1:2. Do not use filters.
- **Rate:** Administer initial dose at 15 mg/kg/hr for first 30 min. If no adverse reactions occur, rate may be increased to 30 mg/kg/hr; if no adverse reactions occur in subsequent 30 min, rate may be increased to 60 mg/kg/hr. Do not exceed 75 ml/hr volume or 60 mg/kg/hr rate. Monitor patient closely during rate changes. May cause pain at injection site.
- □ During subsequent doses, rate may be increased in same increments every 15 min if no adverse reactions occur, until 60 mg/kg/hr maximum is reached.

PATIENT/FAMILY TEACHING

- □ Instruct patient to notify physician if any adverse reactions occur.
- □ May cause drowsiness. Caution patient to avoid driving or other activities requiring alertness after receiving medication until response to medication is known.

EVALUATION

Effectiveness of therapy can be demonstrated by: ▪ Prevention of serious sequelae of CMV disease, including blindness, in renal transplant patients.

DACARBAZINE
(da-**kar**-ba-zeen)
DTIC-Dome, {DTIC}

CLASSIFICATION(S):
Antineoplastic (alkylating agent)
Pregnancy Category C

D

INDICATIONS

▪ Used alone in the treatment of metastatic malignant melanoma ▪ Used in combination with other antineoplastic agents in the treatment of advanced Hodgkin's disease. **Unlabeled Use:** ▪ Treatment of metastatic sarcomas.

ACTION

▪ Disrupts DNA and RNA synthesis (cell cycle-phase nonspecific). **Therapeutic Effect:** ▪ Death of rapidly growing tissue cells, especially malignant cells.

PHARMACOKINETICS

Absorption: Poorly absorbed following oral administration. Must be given IV.
Distribution: Large volume of distribution; appears to concentrate in liver. Some penetration of CNS.
Metabolism and Excretion: 50% metabolized by the liver, 50% excreted unchanged by the kidneys.
Half-life: 5 hr (increased in renal disease).

CONTRAINDICATIONS AND PRECAUTIONS

Contraindicated in: ▪ Hypersensitivity ▪ Pregnancy or lactation.
Use Cautiously in: ▪ Patients with childbearing potential ▪ Active infections ▪ Decreased bone marrow reserve ▪ Other chronic debilitating diseases

- Children (safety not established)
- Renal disease.

ADVERSE REACTIONS AND SIDE EFFECTS*

GI: <u>nausea</u>, <u>vomiting</u>, <u>anorexia</u>, diarrhea, hepatic vein thrombosis, HEPATIC NECROSIS.

Derm: alopecia, photosensitivity, facial flushing.

Endo: gonadal suppression.

Hemat: <u>bone marrow depression</u>.

Local: <u>pain</u> at IV site, phlebitis at IV site, tissue necrosis.

MS: mylagia.

Neuro: facial paresthesia.

Misc: facial flushing, flu-like syndrome, malaise, fever, ANAPHYLAXIS.

INTERACTIONS

Drug–Drug: ▪ Additive bone marrow depression with other **antineoplastic agents** or **radiation therapy** ▪ Additive hepatotoxicity with other **hepatotoxic drugs** ▪ **Phenytoin** or **phenobarbital** may increase metabolism and decrease effectiveness ▪ May decrease antibody response to **live virus vaccines** and increase the risk of adverse reactions.

ROUTE AND DOSAGE

Other regimens are used.

Malignant Melanoma

- **IV (Adults):** 2–4.5 mg/kg/day for 10 days q 4 wk or 250 mg/m²/day for 5 days q 3 wk.

Hodgkin's Disease

- **IV (Adults):** 150 mg/m²/day for 5 days (in combination with other agents) q 4 wk or 375 mg/m² (with other agents) q 15 days.

AVAILABILITY

- *Injection:* 100-mg, 200-mg, 500-mg vials.

TIME/ACTION PROFILE (effects on blood counts)

	ONSET	PEAK	DURATION
IV (WBCs)	16–20 days	21–25 days	3–5 days
IV (platelets)	UK	16 days	3–5 days

NURSING IMPLICATIONS

ASSESSMENT

▫ Monitor vital signs prior to and frequently during therapy.

▫ Assess for fever, chills, sore throat, and signs of infection. Notify physician if these symptoms occur.

▫ Monitor platelet count throughout therapy. Assess for bleeding (bleeding gums, bruising, petechiae; guaiac stools, urine, and emesis). Avoid IM injections and rectal temperatures. Apply pressure to venipuncture sites for 10 min.

▫ Monitor IV site closely. Dacarbazine is an irritant. Instruct patient to notify nurse immediately if discomfort at IV site occurs. Discontinue IV immediately if infiltration occurs. Applications of hot packs may relieve pain, burning sensation, and irritation at injection site.

▫ Monitor intake and output, appetite, and nutritional intake. Assess for nausea and vomiting, which may be severe and last 1–12 hr. Administration of an antiemetic prior to and periodically during therapy and adjusting diet as tolerated may help maintain fluid and electrolyte balance and nutritional status. Nausea usually decreases on subsequent doses.

▪ **Lab Test Considerations:** Monitor CBC and differential prior to and periodically throughout therapy. The nadir of thrombocytopenia occurs in 16 days. The nadir of leukopenia occurs in 3–4 wk. Recovery begins in 5 days. Withhold dose and notify physician if platelet count is <100,000/mm³ or leukocyte count is <4000/mm³.

▫ Monitor for increased AST (SGOT), ALT (SGPT), uric acid, and BUN.

POTENTIAL NURSING DIAGNOSES

▪ Infection, high risk for (side effects).
▪ Injury, high risk for (side effects).
▪ Knowledge deficit related to medication regimen (patient/family teaching).

---

*<u>Underlines</u> indicate most frequent; **CAPITALS** indicate life-threatening.

IMPLEMENTATION

- **General Info:** Reconstitute each 100-mg vial with 9.9 ml of Sterile Water for Injection and each 200-mg vial with 19.7 ml to yield a concentration of 10 mg/ml. Solution is colorless or clear yellow. Do not use solution that has turned pink. Solution is stable for 8 hr at room temperature and for 72 hr if refrigerated.
- □ Solution should be prepared in a biologic cabinet. Wear gloves, gown, and mask while handling medication. Discard equipment in designated containers (see Appendix I).
- **Direct IV:** Administer over 1 min.
- **Intermittent Infusion:** Further dilute with 250 ml of D5W or 0.9% NaCl. Stable for 24 hr if refrigerated or 8 hr at room temperature.
- **Rate:** Administer over 15–30 min.
- **Y-Site Compatibility:** ▪ fludarabine ▪ ondansetron ▪ sargramostim.
- **Additive Compatibility:** ▪ bleomycin ▪ carmustine ▪ cyclophosphamide ▪ cytarabine ▪ dactinomycin ▪ doxorubicin ▪ fluorouracil ▪ mercaptopurine ▪ methotrexate ▪ vinblastine.
- **Additive Incompatibility:** ▪ hydrocortisone sodium succinate.

PATIENT/FAMILY TEACHING

- □ Instruct patient to notify physician if fever, chills, sore throat, signs of infection, bleeding gums, bruising, petechiae; or blood in urine, stool, or emesis occurs. Caution patient to avoid crowds and persons with known infections. Instruct patient to use soft toothbrush and electric razor. Patients should be cautioned not to drink alcoholic beverages or take products containing aspirin or ibuprofen.
- □ May cause photosensitivity. Instruct patient to avoid sunlight or wear protective clothing and use sunscreen for 2 days after therapy.
- □ Instruct patient to inform physician if flu-like syndrome occurs. Symptoms include fever, myalgia, and general malaise. May occur after several courses of therapy. Usually occurs 1 wk after administration. May persist for 1–3 wk. Physician may order acetaminophen for relief of symptoms.
- □ Discuss with patient the possibility of hair loss. Explore coping strategies.
- □ Advise patient of the need for contraception.
- □ Instruct patient not to receive any vaccinations without advice of physician.

EVALUATION

Effectiveness of therapy can be demonstrated by: ▪ Decrease in size and spread of malignant melanoma or Hodgkin's lymphoma.

D

DACTINOMYCIN
(dak-ti-noe-**mye**-sin)
actinomycin D, Cosmegen

CLASSIFICATION(S):
Antineoplastic (antibiotic)
Pregnancy Category C

INDICATIONS

▪ Used alone and in combination with other treatment modalities (other antineoplastic agents, radiation therapy, or surgery) in the management of: □ Wilms' tumor □ Rhabdomyosarcoma □ Ewing sarcoma □ Trophoblastic neoplasms □ Testicular carcinoma □ Other malignancies.

ACTION

▪ Inhibits RNA synthesis by forming a complex with DNA (cell cycle-phase nonspecific). **Therapeutic Effects:** ▪ Death of rapidly replicating cells, particularly malignant ones ▪ Also has immunosuppressive properties.

PHARMACOKINETICS

Absorption: Administered IV only.
Distribution: Widely distributed, but does not cross the blood–brain barrier. Crosses the placenta.
Metabolism and Excretion: Excreted in bile and subsequently in the feces as unchanged drug (50%); small amounts

(10%) excreted unchanged by the kidneys.

Half-life: 36 hr.

CONTRAINDICATIONS AND PRECAUTIONS

Contraindicated in: ▪ Hypersensitivity ▪ Pregnant or lactating women.

Use Cautiously in: ▪ Patients with childbearing potential ▪ Active infections ▪ Decreased bone marrow reserve ▪ Other chronic debilitating illnesses ▪ Obese or edematous patients (dose should be based on body surface area).

ADVERSE REACTIONS AND SIDE EFFECTS*

CNS: lethargy.
GI: nausea, vomiting, stomatitis, ulceration.
Derm: alopecia, rashes.
Endo: gonadal suppression.
Hemat: anemia, leukopenia, thrombocytopenia.
Local: phlebitis at IV site.
Misc: fever.

INTERACTIONS

Drug–Drug: ▪ Additive bone marrow depression with other **antineoplastics** or **radiation therapy** ▪ May decrease antibody response to **live virus vaccines** and increase risk of adverse reactions.

ROUTE AND DOSAGE

▪ **IV (Adults):** 10–15 mcg/kg/day for up to 5 days q 4–6 wk or 500 mcg/m² (up to 2 mo) weekly for 3 wk.
▪ **IV (Children >6 mo):** 15 mcg/kg (450 mcg/m²) daily for up to 5 days, 2.5 mg/m² divided into 7 daily doses, repeat q 4–6 wk.

AVAILABILITY

▪ *Injection:* 0.5-mg vials.

TIME/ACTION PROFILE (effects on blood counts)

	ONSET	PEAK	DURATION
IV	7 days	14 days	21–28 days

NURSING IMPLICATIONS

ASSESSMENT

▢ Monitor vital signs prior to and frequently during therapy.

▢ Assess for fever, chills, sore throat, and signs of infection. Notify physician if these symptoms occur.

▢ Monitor platelet count throughout therapy. Assess for bleeding (bleeding gums, bruising, petechiae; guaiac stools, urine, and emesis). Avoid IM injections and rectal temperatures. Apply pressure to venipuncture sites for 10 min.

▢ Assess IV site frequently for inflammation or infiltration. Patient should notify nurse if pain or irritation at injection site occurs. If extravasation occurs, infusion must be stopped and restarted in another vein to avoid damage to SC tissue. Notify physician immediately. Standard treatments include local injections of steroids and application of ice compresses. Saline may be infused through the line into infiltrated area to dilute the drug.

▢ Monitor intake and output, appetite, and nutritional intake. Assess for nausea and vomiting, which usually begin a few hours after administration and persist for up to 20 hr. Administration of an antiemetic prior to and periodically during therapy and adjusting diet as tolerated may help maintain fluid and electrolyte balance and nutritional status. IV fluids and allopurinol may be given to decrease uric acid levels in patients unable to maintain satisfactory oral intake.

▪ **Lab Test Considerations:** May cause increased uric acid levels.

▢ Monitor CBC and differential prior to and periodically throughout therapy. Platelets and leukocyte counts begin to drop 7–10 days after beginning therapy. The nadirs of thrombocytopenia and leukopenia occur in 3 wk. Recovery occurs 3 wk later.

▢ Monitor for hepatotoxicity (increased

---

*Underlines indicate most frequent; **CAPITALS** indicate life-threatening.

AST [SGOT], ALT [SGPT], LDH, and serum bilirubin).

POTENTIAL NURSING DIAGNOSES

- Infection, high risk for (adverse reactions).
- Oral mucous membranes, altered (side effects).
- Knowledge deficit related to medication regimen (patient/family teaching).

IMPLEMENTATION

- **General Info:** Avoid contact with skin. If spillage occurs, irrigate skin with copious amount of water for 15 min. If splashed into eye, irrigate with water and consult ophthalmologist.
- Solution for IV administration should be prepared in a biologic cabinet. Wear gloves, gown, and mask while handling IV medication. Discard IV equipment in specially designated containers (see Appendix I).
- **IV:** Reconstitute each 0.5 mg vial with 1.1 ml of Sterile Water for Injection without preservatives. Solution color is gold. Discard any unused solution.
- **Direct IV:** Change needle between reconstitution and direct IV administration.
- **Rate:** May be injected into Y-site or 3-way stopcock of free-flowing infusions of 0.9% NaCl or D5W at a rate of 500 mcg/min.
- **Intermittent Infusion:** May be further diluted in 50 ml of 0.9% NaCl or D5W.
- **Rate:** Infuse over 10–15 min.
- **Y-Site Compatibility:** ■ fludarabine ■ ondansetron ■ sargramostim.

PATIENT/FAMILY TEACHING

- Instruct patient to notify physician if fever, chills, sore throat, signs of infection, bleeding gums, bruising, petechiae, blood in urine, stool, or emesis occurs. Caution patient to avoid crowds and persons with known infections. Instruct patient to use soft toothbrush and electric razor. Patients should be cautioned not to drink alcoholic beverages or take products containing aspirin or ibuprofen.
- Instruct patient to inspect oral mucosa for erythema and ulceration. If ulceration occurs, advise patient to use sponge brush and rinse mouth with water after eating and drinking. Physician may order viscous lidocaine swishes if mouth pain interferes with eating.
- Inform patient that this medication may cause irreversible gonadal suppression. Advise patient that this medication may have teratogenic effects. Contraception should be used during therapy and for at least 4 mo after therapy is concluded.
- Discuss with patient the possibility of hair loss, which usually occurs 7–10 days after administration of dactinomycin. Explore coping strategies.
- Instruct patient not to receive any vaccinations without advice of physician.
- Emphasize the need for periodic lab tests to monitor for side effects.

EVALUATION

Effectiveness of therapy can be demonstrated by: ■ Decrease in size or spread of malignancy.

DANAZOL
(da-na-zole)
Danocrine, {Cyclomen}

CLASSIFICATION(S):
Hormone (androgen)
Pregnancy Category UK

INDICATIONS

■ Treatment of moderate endometriosis unresponsive to more conventional therapy ■ Palliative therapy of fibrocystic breast disease ■ Prophylaxis of hereditary angioedema.

ACTION

■ Inhibits pituitary output of gonadotropins, resulting in suppression of ovarian function. Has weak androgenic-anabolic activity. **Therapeutic Effects:** ■ Atrophy of ectopic endometrial tissue

{} = Available in Canada only.

in endometriosis ▪ Decreased pain and nodularity in fibrocystic breast disease ▪ Correction of biochemical abnormalities in hereditary angioedema.

PHARMACOKINETICS

Absorption: Absorbed from the GI tract.
Distribution: Distribution not known.
Metabolism and Excretion: Metabolized by the liver.
Half-life: 4.5 hr.

CONTRAINDICATIONS AND PRECAUTIONS

Contraindicated in: ▪ Hypersensitivity ▪ Male patients with breast or prostate cancer ▪ Hypercalcemia ▪ Severe hepatic, renal, or cardiac disease ▪ Pregnancy or lactation.
Use Cautiously in: ▪ Previous history of liver disease ▪ Coronary artery disease ▪ Prepubertal males.

ADVERSE REACTIONS AND SIDE EFFECTS*

CNS: <u>emotional lability</u>.
CV: <u>edema</u>.
Derm: <u>hirsutism</u>, <u>acne</u>, <u>oiliness</u>.
EENT: <u>deepening of voice</u>.
Endo: <u>decreased breast size</u> (females), <u>anovulation</u>, <u>amenorrhea</u>, decreased libido.
GU: testicular atrophy, clitoral enlargement, amenorrhea.
Metab: <u>weight gain</u>.
Misc: hepatitis (cholestatic jaundice).

INTERACTIONS

Drug–Drug: ▪ May potentiate **warfarin, oral hypoglycemic agents, insulin,** or **glucocorticoids** ▪ May increase **cyclosporine** levels and risk of toxicity.

ROUTE AND DOSAGE

Endometriosis
▪ **PO (Adults):** 200–800 mg/day in 2 divided doses for 3–6 mo (up to 9 mo).

Fibrocystic Breast Disease
▪ **PO (Adults):** 100–400 mg/day in 2 divided doses for 2–6 mo.

Hereditary Angioedema
▪ **PO (Adults):** 200 mg 2–3 times daily.

AVAILABILITY
▪ *Capsules:* 50 mg, 100 mg, 200 mg.

TIME/ACTION PROFILE (disease response)

	ONSET	PEAK	DURATION
PO (endometriosis)	UK	6–8 wk	60–90 days
PO (fibrocystic disease)	1 mo	2–6 mo	1 yr
PO (angioedema)	UK	1–3 mo	UK

NURSING IMPLICATIONS

ASSESSMENT
▪ **Endometriosis:** Assess patient for endometrial pain prior to and periodically throughout therapy.
▪ **Fibrocystic Breast Disease:** Assess patient for breast pain, tenderness, and nodules prior to and monthly throughout therapy.
▪ **Hereditary Angioedema:** Monitor patient for edematous attacks throughout therapy, especially during dosage adjustments.
▪ **Lab Test Considerations:** Liver function tests should be monitored periodically throughout therapy.
  □ Semen count and volume, viscosity, and motility determinations are recommended every 3–4 mo during treatment for hereditary angioedema, especially in adolescents.
  □ May alter results of glucose tolerance or thyroid function tests.

POTENTIAL NURSING DIAGNOSES
▪ Sexual dysfunction (side effects).
▪ Body image disturbance (side effects).
▪ Knowledge deficit related to medication regimen (patient/family teaching).

IMPLEMENTATION
▪ **General Info:** In patients with endometriosis or fibrocystic breast dis-

ease, therapy should be started during menstruation or preceded by a pregnancy test. Advise patient to notify physician immediately if pregnancy is suspected.

■ **PO:** Medication may be administered with meals to minimize GI irritation.

PATIENT/FAMILY TEACHING

■ **General Info:** Instruct patient to take medication exactly as prescribed. Missed doses should be taken as soon as remembered, if not almost time for next dose; do not double doses.

□ Advise patient to use a form of contraception other than oral contraceptives during therapy. Inform patient that amenorrhea is expected with higher doses. Instruct patient to notify physician if regular menstruation does not occur within 60–90 days after discontinuation of therapy.

□ Advise patient to notify physician if masculinizing effects occur (abnormal growth of facial hair or other body hair, deepening of the voice).

□ Emphasize the importance of routine visits to physician to check progress during therapy.

■ **Fibrocystic Breast Disease:** Teach patient the correct technique for monthly breast self-examination. Instruct patient to report increase in size of nodules to physician promptly.

EVALUATION

Effectiveness of therapy can be demonstrated by: ■ Decrease in symptoms of endometriosis. Therapy for endometriosis usually requires 3–6 mo and may extend to 9 mo to decrease symptoms. ■ Relief of pain and tenderness in fibrocystic breast disease, which is usually relieved by the first month and eliminated in 2–3 mo. Elimination of nodularity usually requires 4–6 mo. ■ Resolutions of signs and symptoms of hereditary angioedema. Initial response in hereditary angioedema may require 1–3 mo of therapy; efforts should be made to decrease dosage at 1–3-mo intervals.

DANTROLENE
(dan-troe-leen)
Dantrium

CLASSIFICATION(S):
Skeletal muscle relaxant (direct acting)
Pregnancy Category C (IV use)

INDICATIONS

■ **PO:** Treatment of spasticity associated with: □ Spinal cord injury □ Stroke □ Cerebral palsy □ Multiple sclerosis ■ **PO:** Prophylaxis of malignant hyperthermia ■ **IV:** Emergency treatment of malignant hyperthermia.

ACTION

■ Acts directly on skeletal muscle, causing relaxation by decreasing calcium release from sarcoplasmic reticulum in muscle cells ■ Prevents intense catabolic process associated with malignant hyperthermia. **Therapeutic Effects:** ■ Reduction of muscle spasticity ■ Prevention of malignant hyperthermia.

PHARMACOKINETICS

Absorption: 35% absorbed after oral administration.
Distribution: Distribution not known.
Metabolism and Excretion: Almost entirely metabolized by the liver.
Half-life: 8.7 hr.

CONTRAINDICATIONS AND PRECAUTIONS

Contraindicated in: ■ No contraindications to IV form in treatment of hyperthermia ■ Pregnancy and lactation ■ In situations where spasticity is used to maintain posture or balance.
Use Cautiously in: ■ Cardiac, pulmonary, or previous liver disease ■ Females, patients >35 yr (increased risk of hepatotoxicity).

ADVERSE REACTIONS AND SIDE EFFECTS*

CNS: <u>muscle weakness</u>, <u>drowsiness</u>, dizziness, malaise, headache, confu-

D

sion, nervousness, insomnia, light-headedness.
EENT: excessive lacrimation, visual disturbances.
Resp: pleural effusions.
CV: tachycardia, changes in blood pressure.
GI: diarrhea, anorexia, vomiting, GI bleeding, cramps, dysphagia, HEPATO-TOXICITY.
GU: frequency, incontinence, nocturia, dysuria, crytalluria, impotence.
Derm: pruritis, urticaria, photosensitivity, sweating.
Local: phlebitis, irritation at IV site.
Hemat: eosinophilia.
MS: myalgia.
Misc: drooling, chills, fever.

INTERACTIONS

Drug–Drug: ▪ Additive CNS depression with **CNS depressants,** including **alcohol, antihistamines, opioid analgesics, sedative/hypnotics,** and **parenteral magnesium sulfate** ▪ Increased risk of hepatotoxicity with other **hepatotoxic agents** or **estrogens** ▪ Increased risk of arrhythmias with **verapamil.**

ROUTE AND DOSAGE

Spasticity

▪ **PO (Adults):** 25 mg/day initially, increase to 25 mg 2–4 times daily, then by increments of 25 mg up to 100 mg 2–4 times daily if needed—dosage increments may be made q 4–7 days (not to exceed 400 mg/day).

▪ **PO (Children >5 yr):** 0.5 mg/kg twice daily; increase to 0.5 mg/kg 3–4 times daily, then by increments of 0.5 mg/kg up to 3 mg/kg 2–4 times daily (not to exceed 100 mg 4 times daily).

Hyperthermic Crisis

▪ **IV (Adults and Children):** 1 mg/kg; may repeat dose up to cumulative dose of 10 mg/kg, followed by 1–3 days of PO therapy (4–8 mg/kg/day in 4 divided doses).

Hyperthermia Prevention

▪ **PO (Adults and Children):** 4–8 mg/kg/day in 3–4 divided doses for 1–2 days prior to procedure, last dose 3–4 hr preop.

▪ **IV (Adults and Children):** 2.5 mg/kg prior to anesthesia.

AVAILABILITY

▪ *Capsules:* 25 mg, 50 mg, 100 mg ▪ *Injection:* 20 mg/vial.

TIME/ACTION PROFILE (effects on spasticity)

	ONSET	PEAK	DURATION
PO	1 wk	UK	6–12 hr
IV	rapid	rapid	UK

NURSING IMPLICATIONS

ASSESSMENT

▪ **General Info:** Assess bowel function periodically. Persistent diarrhea may warrant discontinuation of therapy.

▪ **Muscle Spasticity:** Assess neuromuscular status and muscle spasticity before initiating therapy and periodically during its course to determine response to therapy.

▪ **Malignant Hyperthermia:** Assess previous anesthesia history of all surgical patients. Also assess for family history of reactions to anesthesia (malignant hyperthermia or perioperative death).

□ Monitor ECG, vital signs, electrolytes, and urine output continuously when administering IV for malignant hyperthermia.

□ Monitor patient for difficulty swallowing and choking during meals on the day of administration.

▪ **Lab Test Considerations:** Hepatic and renal function and CBC should be evaluated prior to and periodically during therapy in patients receiving prolonged therapy. Liver function abnormalities (elevated AST [SGOT], ALT [SGPT], alkaline phosphatase, bilirubin) may require discontinuation of therapy.

POTENTIAL NURSING DIAGNOSES

▪ Physical mobility, impaired (indication).
▪ Pain (indications).
▪ Injury, high risk for (side effects).

IMPLEMENTATION

▪ **PO:** If gastric irritation becomes a

problem, may be administered with food. Oral suspensions may be made by opening capsules and adding them to fruit juices or other liquid. Drink immediately after mixing.

▪ **Direct IV:** Reconstitute each 20 mg with 60 ml of Sterile Water for Injection without a bacteriostatic agent for a concentration of 333 mcg/ml. Shake until solution is clear. Solution must be used within 6 hr. Protect diluted solution from direct light.

▪ *Rate:* Administer each single dose by rapid continuous IV push through Y tubing or 3-way stopcock. Follow immediately with subsequent doses as indicated. Medication is very irritating to tissues; observe infusion site frequently to avoid extravasation.

PATIENT/FAMILY TEACHING

▪ **General Info:** Advise patient not to take more medication than the amount prescribed, to minimize risk of hepatotoxicity and other side effects. If a dose is missed, do not take unless remembered within 1 hr. Do not double doses.

▢ May cause dizziness, drowsiness, lightheadedness, visual disturbances, and muscle weakness. Advise patient to avoid driving and other activities requiring alertness until response to drug is known.

▢ Caution patient to use sunscreen and protective clothing to prevent photosensitivity reactions.

▢ Advise patient to avoid taking alcohol or other CNS depressants concurrently with this medication.

▢ Instruct patient to notify physician if rash, itching, nausea, vomiting, abdominal discomfort, yellow eyes, dark urine, or clay-colored, bloody, or black tarry stools occur.

▢ Emphasize the importance of follow-up examinations to check progress in long-term therapy and blood tests to monitor for side effects.

▪ **Malignant Hyperthermia:** Patients with malignant hyperthemia should carry identification describing disease process at all times.

EVALUATION

Effectiveness of therapy can be demonstrated by: ▪ Relief of muscle spasm in musculoskeletal conditions. One wk or more may be required to see improvement; if there is no observed improvement in 45 days the medication is usually discontinued ▪ Prevention or decrease in temperature and skeletal rigidity in malignant hyperthermia.

DAUNORUBICIN   D
(daw-noe-**roo**-bi-sin)
Cerubidine

CLASSIFICATION(S):
Antineoplastic (antibiotic)
Pregnancy Category D

INDICATIONS

▪ Used in combination with other antineoplastic agents in the treatment of leukemias.

ACTION

▪ Forms a complex with DNA, which subsequently inhibits DNA and RNA synthesis (cell cycle-phase nonspecific). **Therapeutic Effect:** ▪ Death of rapidly replicating cells, particularly malignant ones. Also has immunosuppressive properties.

PHARMACOKINETICS

Absorption: Administered IV only, resulting in complete bioavailability.

Distribution: Widely distributed. Crosses the placenta.

Metabolism and Excretion: Extensively metabolized by the liver. Converted partially to a compound that also has antineoplastic activity. 40% eliminated by biliary excretion.

Half-life: 18.5 hr.

CONTRAINDICATIONS AND PRECAUTIONS

Contraindicated in: ▪ Hypersensitivity ▪ Congestive heart failure ▪ Arrhythmias ▪ Pregnant or lactating women.

Use Cautiously in: ▪ Patients with childbearing potential ▪ Active infections ▪ Decreased bone marrow reserve ▪ Other chronic debilitating illnesses ▪ May reactivate skin lesions produced by previous radiation therapy ▪ Hepatic or renal impairment (dosage reduction recommended if serum creatinine >3 mg/dl or serum bilirubin >1.2 mg/dl).

ADVERSE REACTIONS AND SIDE EFFECTS*

CV: CONGESTIVE HEART FAILURE, arrhythmias.
GI: nausea, vomiting, stomatitis, esophagitis.
GU: red urine.
Derm: alopecia.
Endo: gonadal suppression.
Hemat: bone marrow depression.
Local: phlebitis at IV site.
Metab: hyperuricemia.
Misc: fever, chills.

INTERACTIONS

Drug–Drug: ▪ Additive myelosuppression with other **antineoplastic agents** ▪ **Cyclophosphamide** increases the risk of cardiotoxicity ▪ May decrease antibody response to **live virus vaccines** and increase risk of adverse reactions.

ROUTE AND DOSAGE

Other dose regimens are used. In adults, cumulative dose should not exceed 550 mg/m² (450 mg/m² if previous chest radiation) or 300 mg/m² in children >2 yr.

▪ **IV (Adult <60 yr):** 45 mg/m²/day for 1–3 days, as part of combination regimen.
▪ **IV (Adults ≥60 yr):** 30 mg/m²/day for 1–3 days, as part of combination regimen.
▪ **IV (Children >2 yr):** 25 mg/m²/day as part of combination regimen.

AVAILABILITY

▪ *Injection:* 20 mg/vial.

TIME/ACTION PROFILE (effects on blood counts)

	ONSET	PEAK	DURATION
IV	7–10 days	10–14 days	21 days

NURSING IMPLICATIONS

ASSESSMENT

▢ Monitor vital signs prior to and frequently during therapy.
▢ Assess for fever, chills, sore throat, and signs of infection. Notify physician if these symptoms occur.
▢ Monitor platelet count throughout therapy. Assess for bleeding (bleeding gums, bruising, petechiae, guaiac stools, urine, and emesis). Avoid IM injections and rectal temperatures. Apply pressure to venipuncture sites for 10 min.
▢ Assess IV site frequently for inflammation or infiltration. Patient should notify nurse if pain or irritation at injection site occurs. If extravasation occurs, infusion must be stopped and restarted in another vein to avoid damage to SC tissue. Notify physician immediately. Standard treatments include local injections of steroids and application of ice compresses.
▢ Monitor intake and output, appetite, and nutritional intake. Assess for nausea and vomiting, which although mild, may persist for 24–48 hr. Administration of an antiemetic prior to and periodically during therapy and adjusting diet as tolerated may help maintain fluid and electrolyte balance and nutritional status. Encourage fluid intake of 2000–3000 ml/day. Physician may also order allopurinol and alkalinization of the urine to help prevent urate stone formation.
▢ Assess patient for evidence of congestive heart failure (peripheral edema, dyspnea, rales/crackles, weight gain, jugular venous distension); usually related to cumulative dose. Chest x-ray, echocardiography, and ECGs

may be ordered prior to and periodically throughout therapy. A 30% decrease in QRS voltage and decrease in systolic ejection fraction are early signs of cardiomyopathy.

- **Lab Test Considerations:** Monitor CBC and differential prior to and periodically throughout therapy. The leukocyte count nadir occurs 10–14 days after administration. Recovery usually occurs within 21 days after administration of daunorubicin.
- □ Monitor AST (SGOT), ALT (SGPT), LDH, and serum bilirubin. May cause transiently elevated serum phosphatase, bilirubin, and AST (SGOT) concentrations.
- □ Monitor uric acid levels.

POTENTIAL NURSING DIAGNOSES

- Infection, high risk for (adverse reactions).
- Cardiac output, decreased (side effects).
- Knowledge deficit related to medication regimen (patient/family teaching).

IMPLEMENTATION

- **General Info:** Solution should be prepared in a biologic cabinet. Wear gloves, gown, and mask while handling IV medication. Discard IV equipment in specially designated containers (see Appendix I).
- **IV:** Reconstitute each 20 mg with 4 ml of Sterile Water for Injection. Reconstituted medication is stable for 24 hr at room temperature, 48 hr if refrigerated. Protect from sunlight.
- □ Do not use aluminum needles when reconstituting or injecting daunorubicin, as aluminum darkens the solution.
- **Direct IV:** Dilute further in 10–15 ml of 0.9% NaCl. Administer direct IV push through Y-site or 3-way stopcock into free-flowing infusion of 0.9% NaCl or D5W.
- **Rate:** Administer over at least 3–5 min. Rapid administration rate may cause facial flushing or erythema along the vein.
- **Intermittent Infusion:** May be further

diluted in 50–100 ml of D5W, 0.9% NaCl, or lactated Ringer's solution.
- **Rate:** Infuse 50 ml over 10–15 min and 100 ml over 30–45 min.
- **Y-Site Compatibility:** ■ ondansetron.
- **Y-Site Incompatibility:** ■ fludarabine.
- **Additive Incompatibility:** Manufacturer does not recommend admixing daunorubicin.

PATIENT/FAMILY TEACHING

- □ Instruct patient to notify physician if fever, chills, sore throat, signs of infection, bleeding gums, bruising, petechiae, blood in urine, stool, or emesis occurs. Caution patient to avoid crowds and persons with known infections. Instruct patient to use soft toothbrush and electric razor. Patient should be cautioned not to drink alcoholic beverages or take products containing aspirin or ibuprofen.
- □ Instruct patient to inspect oral mucosa for erythema and ulceration. If ulceration occurs advise patient to use sponge brush and rinse mouth with water after eating and drinking. Consult physician if mouth pain interferes with eating. Period of highest risk is 3–7 days after administration of dose.
- □ Instruct patient to notify physician immediately if irregular heartbeat, shortness of breath, or swelling of lower extremities occurs.
- □ Discuss with patient possibility of hair loss. Explore methods of coping. Regrowth of hair usually begins within 5 wk after discontinuing therapy.
- □ Inform patient that medication may turn urine reddish color for 1–2 days following administration.
- □ Inform patient that this medication may cause irreversible gonadal suppression. Advise patient that this medication may have teratogenic effects. Contraception should be used during therapy and for at least 4 mo after therapy is concluded.
- □ Instruct patient not to receive any vaccinations without advice of physician.

▫ Emphasize the need for periodic lab tests to monitor for side effects.

EVALUATION

Effectiveness of therapy can be demonstrated by: ■ Improvement of hematologic status. Courses of therapy are usually administered no more frequently than every 21 days, to allow for bone marrow recovery.

DEFEROXAMINE
(de-fer-**ox**-a-meen)
Desferal

CLASSIFICATION(S):
Antidote (heavy metal antagonist)
Pregnancy Category C

INDICATIONS

■ Management of acute toxic iron ingestion ■ Management of secondary iron overload syndromes associated with multiple transfusion therapy.

ACTION

■ Chelates unbound iron, forming a water-soluble complex (ferrioxamine) in plasma that is easily excreted by the kidneys. **Therapeutic Effect:** ■ Removal of excess iron. Also chelates aluminum.

PHARMACOKINETICS

Absorption: Poorly absorbed following oral administration. Well absorbed following IM administration and SC administration.

Distribution: Appears to be widely distributed.

Metabolism and Excretion: Metabolized by tissues and plasma enzymes. Unchanged drug and chelated form excreted by the kidneys. 33% of iron removed is eliminated in the feces via the biliary excretion.

Half-life: 1 hr.

CONTRAINDICATIONS AND PRECAUTIONS

Contraindicated in: ■ Avoid use during pregnancy or in women who may become pregnant ■ Severe renal disease ■ Anuria.

Use Cautiously in: ■ Safe use in children <3 yr not established.

ADVERSE REACTIONS AND SIDE EFFECTS*

CV: tachycardia.

EENT: cataracts, blurred vision, ototoxicity.

GI: abdominal pain, diarrhea.

GU: red urine.

Local: pain at injection site, induration at injection site.

MS: leg cramps.

Misc: flushing, erythema, urticaria, hypotension, shock following rapid IV administration, allergic reactions, fever.

INTERACTIONS

Drug–Drug: ■ **Ascorbic acid** may increase the effectiveness of deferoxamine but may also increase cardiac iron toxicity.

ROUTE AND DOSAGE

IM route is preferred.

Acute Iron Intoxication

■ **IM (Adults and Children >3 yr):** 90 mg/kg (up to 1 g) q 8 hr (not to exceed 6 g/day).

■ **IV (Adults and Children):** 15 mg/kg/hr.

Chronic Iron Overload

■ **IM (Adults and Children >3 yr):** 0.5–1 g/day.

■ **IV (Adults and Children):** In addition to above IM dosage for chronic iron overload, 2-g doses may be given by slow IV infusion at the time each unit of blood is transfused.

■ **SC (Adults and Children >3 yr):** 1–2 g/day (20–40 mg/kg/day) by continuous SC infusion given over 8–24 hr.

■ **SC (Children <3 yr):** 10 mg/kg/day.

*Underlines indicate most frequent; **CAPITALS** indicate life-threatening.

AVAILABILITY

▪ *Injection:* 500 mg/vial.

TIME/ACTION PROFILE (effects on hematologic parameters)

	ONSET	PEAK	DURATION
IV	rapid	UK	UK
IM	UK	UK	UK
SC	UK	UK	UK

NURSING IMPLICATIONS

ASSESSMENT

□ In acute poisoning, assess time, amount, and type of iron preparation ingested.

□ Monitor signs of iron toxicity: early acute (abdominal pain, bloody diarrhea, emesis), late acute (decreased level of consciousness, shock, metabolic acidosis).

□ Monitor vital signs closely, especially during IV administration. Notify physician if hypotension, erythema, urticaria, or signs of allergic reaction occur. Keep epinephrine, an antihistamine, and resuscitation equipment close by in the event of an anaphylactic reaction.

□ May cause ocular or ototoxicity. Inform physician if decreased visual acuity or hearing loss occurs.

□ Monitor intake and output and urine color. Inform physician if patient is anuric. Chelated iron is excreted primarily by the kidneys; urine may turn red.

▪ **Lab Test Considerations:** Monitor serum iron, iron binding capacity, transferrin levels, and urinary iron excretion prior to and periodically throughout course of therapy.

□ Monitor liver function studies to assess damage from iron poisoning.

POTENTIAL NURSING DIAGNOSIS

▪ Injury, high risk for: poisoning (patient/family teaching).

▪ Knowledge deficit related to medication regimen (patient/family teaching).

IMPLEMENTATION

▪ **General Info:** Reconstitute contents of each vial with 2 ml of Sterile Water for Injection. Solution is stable for 1 wk after reconstitution if protected from light.

□ Used in conjunction with induction of emesis or gastric aspiration and lavage with sodium bicarbonate, and supportive measures for shock and metabolic acidosis in acute poisoning.

▪ **IM:** IM is the preferred route for acute poisoning unless accompanied by shock. Administer deep IM and massage well. Rotate sites. IM administration may cause transient severe pain.

▪ **SC:** SC route is used to treat chronically elevated iron levels.

□ Therapy is administered into abdominal subcutaneous tissue via infusion pump for 8–24 hr per treatment.

▪ **IV:** IV route is reserved for severe life-threatening poisoning. Reconstitute, then further dilute in D5W, 0.9% NaCl, or lactated Ringer's solution.

▪ **Rate:** Maximum infusion rate is 15 mg/kg/hr. Rapid infusion rate may cause hypotension, erythema, urticaria, wheezing, convulsions, tachycardia, or shock.

□ May be administered at the same time as blood transfusion in persons with chronically elevated serum iron levels. Use separate site for administration.

PATIENT/FAMILY TEACHING

□ Reinforce need to keep iron preparations, all medications, and hazardous substances out of the reach of children.

□ Reassure patient that red coloration of urine is expected and reflects excretion of excess iron.

□ Advise patient not to take vitamin C preparations without consulting physician, as tissue toxicity may increase.

□ Encourage patients requiring chronic therapy to keep follow-up appointments for lab tests. Physician may also order eye and hearing examinations every 3 mo.

EVALUATION
Effectiveness of therapy can be demonstrated by: ■ Return of serum iron concentrations to a normal level (50–150 mcg/100 ml).

DEMECLOCYCLINE
(dem-e-kloe-**sye**-kleen)
Declomycin

CLASSIFICATION(S):
Anti-infective (tetracycline)
Pregnancy Category UK

INDICATIONS

■ Treatment of various infections due to unusual organisms, including: □ *Mycoplasma* □ *Chlamydia* □ *Rickettsia* ■ Treatment of gonorrhea and syphillis in penicillin-allergic patients ■ Adjunctive treatment of severe acne and inclusion conjunctivitis and prevention of exacerbations of chronic bronchitis. **Unlabeled Use:** ■ Management of chronic syndrome of inappropriate secretion of antidiuretic hormone (SIADH).

ACTION

■ Inhibits bacterial protein synthesis at the level of the 30S ribosome. **Therapeutic Effect:** ■ Bacteriostatic action against susceptible bacteria. **Spectrum:** ■ Some gram-positive pathogens: □ *Bacillus anthracis* □ *Clostridium perfringens* □ *Clostridium tetani* □ *Listeria monocytogenes* □ *Nocardia* □ Propionibacterium acnes □ *Actinomyces isrealii* ■ Some gram-negative pathogens: □ *Haemophilus influenzae* □ *Legionella pneumophila* □ *Yersinia entercolitica* □ *Yersinia pestis* □ *Neisseria gonorrhea* □ *Neisseria meningitidis* ■ Also active against several unusual pathogens, including: □ *Mycoplasma* □ *Chlamydia* □ *Rickettsia*.

PHARMACOKINETICS

Absorption: Well absorbed (60–80%) following oral administration.

Distribution: Widely distributed throughout body fluids. Concentrates in bone, liver, spleen, tumors, and teeth. **Metabolism and Excretion:** Some biliary secretion, 40% excreted unchanged by the kidneys.
Half-life: 10–17 hr (increased in renal impairment).

CONTRAINDICATIONS AND PRECAUTIONS

Contraindicated in: ■ Hypersensitivity ■ Pregnancy (permanent staining of teeth in child) ■ Lactation and children <8 yr.
Use Cautiously in: ■ Cachectic or debilitated patients ■ Liver disease ■ Renal disease ■ Nephrogenic diabetes insipidus.

ADVERSE REACTIONS AND SIDE EFFECTS*

GI: <u>nausea</u>, <u>vomiting</u>, <u>diarrhea</u>, pancreatitis, esophagitis.
Derm: rashes, <u>photosensitivity</u>, urticaria.
Endo: nephrogenic diabetes insipidus (increased thirst, increased urination, weakness, fatigue).
Hemat: blood dyscrasias.
Misc: superinfection, hypersensitivity reactions.

INTERACTIONS

Drug–Drug: ■ May enhance the effect of **warfarin** ■ May decrease the effectiveness of **oral contraceptives** ■ **Calcium, iron,** and **magnesium** form insoluble compounds (chelates) and decrease absorption of demeclocycline ■ Decreases antidiuretic effect of **desmopressin**.
Drug–Food: ■ **Calcium** in foods or dairy products decreases absorption by forming insoluble compounds (chelates) ■ **Food** decreases absorption of demeclocycline.

ROUTE AND DOSAGE

Anti-infective
■ **PO (Adults):** 150 mg q 6 hr or 300 mg q 12 hr (up to 2.4 g/day).

---

*<u>Underlines</u> indicate most frequent; **CAPITALS** indicate life-threatening.

SIADH

- **PO (Adults):** 3.25–3.75 mg/kg q 6 hr.

AVAILABILITY

- **Capsules:** 150 mg ▪ **Tablets:** 150 mg, 300 mg.

TIME/ACTION PROFILE

	ONSET	PEAK	DURATION
PO (anti-infective)	UK	3–4 hr	
PO (SIADH)	5 days	UK	2–6 days

NURSING IMPLICATIONS

ASSESSMENT

- **Infection:** Assess patient for infection (vital signs; appearance of wound, sputum, urine, and stool; WBC) at beginning and throughout therapy.
- □ Obtain specimens for culture and sensitivity prior to initiating therapy. First dose may be given before receiving results.
- **SIADH:** Monitor intake and output ratios and assess edema in patients treated for syndrome of inappropriate antidiuretic hormone.
- **Lab Test Considerations:** Renal, hepatic, and hematopoietic functions should be monitored periodically during long-term therapy.
- □ May cause AST (SGOT), ALT (SGPT), serum alkaline phosphatase, bilirubin, and amylase concentrations. May interfere with urine glucose testing with copper sulfate method (Clinitest); use glucose enzymatic tests (Tes-Tape, Ketodiastix).

POTENTIAL NURSING DIAGNOSES

- Infections, high risk for (indications, side effects).
- Knowledge deficit related to medication regimen (patient/family teaching).
- Noncompliance related to medication regimen (patient/family teaching).

IMPLEMENTATION

- **General Info:** May cause yellow-brown discoloration and softening of teeth and bones if administered prenatally or during early childhood. Not recommended for children under 8 yr of age or during pregnancy or lactation.
- **PO:** Administer around the clock. May be taken with food if GI irritation occurs. Take with a full glass of liquid and at least 1 hr before going to bed to avoid esophageal irritation. Do not administer within 1–3 hr of other medications.
- □ Avoid administration of milk, calcium, antacids, magnesium-containing medications, or iron supplements within 1–3 hr of demeclocycline.

PATIENT/FAMILY TEACHING

- □ Instruct patient to take medication around the clock and to finish the drug completely as directed, even if feeling well. Advise patient that sharing of this medication may be dangerous.
- □ Advise patient to avoid taking milk or other dairy products or antacids concurrently with this medication.
- □ Caution patient to use sunscreen and protective clothing to prevent phototoxicity reactions.
- □ Advise patient to report signs of superinfection (black, furry overgrowth on the tongue, vaginal itching or discharge, loose or foul-smelling stools). Skin rash, pruritus, and urticaria should also be reported.
- □ Instruct patient to notify physician if symptoms do not improve.
- □ Caution patient to discard outdated or decomposed products, as they may be toxic.

EVALUATION

Clinical response can be evaluated by:
- Resolution of the signs and symptoms of infection. Length of time for complete resolution depends on the organism and site of infection ▪ Resolution of the signs and symptoms of SIADH.

DESMOPRESSIN
(des-moe-**press**-in)
Concentraid, DDAVP

INDICATIONS

■ **Intranasal:** Management of primary nocturnal enuresis unresponsive to other treatment modalities ■ **Intranasal, SC, IV:** Treatment of diabetes insipidus caused by a deficiency of vasopressin ■ **SC, IV:** Control bleeding in certain types of hemophilia and von Willebrand's disease ■ **Intranasal:** Concentraid product only used for testing of renal concentrating ability.

ACTION

■ An analogue of naturally occurring vasopressin (antidiuretic hormone). Primary action is enhanced reabsorption of water in the kidneys. **Therapeutic Effects:** ■ Prevention of nocturnal enuresis ■ Maintenance of appropriate body water content in diabetes insipidus ■ Control of bleeding in certain types of hemophilia or von Willebrand's disease.

PHARMACOKINETICS

Absorption: Some absorption (10–20%) from nasal mucosa.
Distribution: Distribution not fully known. Enters breast milk.
Metabolism and Excretion: Metabolism and excretion not known.
Half-life: 75 min.

CONTRAINDICATIONS AND PRECAUTIONS

Contraindicated in: ■ Hypersensitivity ■ Hypersensitivity to chlorobutanol ■ Patients with type IIB or platelet-type (pseudo) von Willebrand's disease.
Use Cautiously in: ■ Angina pectoris ■ Hypertension ■ Pregnancy or lactation (safety not established).

ADVERSE REACTIONS AND SIDE EFFECTS*

CNS: headache, drowsiness, listlessness.

EENT: *Intranasal*—rhinitis, nasal congestion.
Resp: dyspnea.
CV: hypertension, hypotension, and tachycardia (large IV doses only).
GI: nausea, mild abdominal cramps.
GU: vulval pain.
Derm: flushing.
F and E: water intoxication and hyponatremia.
Local: phlebitis at IV site.

INTERACTIONS

Drug–Drug: ■ **Chlorpropamide, clofibrate,** or **carbamazepine** may enhance the antidiuretic response to desmopressin ■ **Demeclocycline, lithium,** or **norepinephrine** may diminish the antidiuretic response to desmopressin.

ROUTE AND DOSAGE

Primary Nocturnal Enuresis

■ **Intranasal (Children ≥6 yr):** 20 mcg (10 mcg in each nostril) at bedtime (range 10–40 mcg).

Diabetes Insipidus

■ **Intranasal (Adults):** 10–40 mcg as single dose or in divided doses 1–3 times daily.
■ **Intranasal (Children 3 mo–12 yr):** 5–30 mcg as a single dose or in divided doses 2 times daily.
■ **SC, IV (Adults):** 2–4 mcg/day in 2 divided doses.

Antihemorrhage

■ **IV (Adults and Children >3 mo):** 0.3 mcg/kg repeated as needed.

Renal Concentrating Test

■ **Intranasal (Adults):** 40 mcg (20 mcg in each nostril—contents of 2 pipets).
■ **Intranasal (Children 1–12 yr):** 20 mcg (1 pipet).

AVAILABILITY

■ *Intranasal pipets:* 20 mcg/2 ml nasal solution (Concentraid) ■ *Nasal spray:* 10 mcg/spray—5-ml bottle = 50 doses (DDAVP) ■ *Rhinal tube delivery system:* 2.5-ml vials with applicator tubes (DDAVP) ■ *Injection:* 4-mcg/ml.

---

*Underlines indicate most frequent; **CAPITALS** indicate life-threatening.

TIME/ACTION PROFILE
(intranasal = antidiuretic effect;
IV = effect on factor VIII activity)

	ONSET	PEAK	DURATION
Intranasal	1 hr	1–5 hr	8–20 hr
IV	within min	15–30 min	3 hr (4–24 hr in mild hemophilia A)

NURSING IMPLICATIONS
ASSESSMENT
- **General Info:** Chronic intranasal use may cause tolerance or if administered more frequently than every 24–48 hr IV tachyphylaxis (short-term tolerance) may develop.
- **Nocturnal Enuresis:** Monitor frequency of enuresis throughout therapy.
- **Diabetes Insipidus:** Monitor urine osmolality and urine volume frequently to determine effects of medication. Assess patient for symptoms of dehydration (excessive thirst, dry skin and mucous membranes, tachycardia, poor skin turgor). Weigh patient daily and assess for edema.
- **Hemophilia:** When used in hemophilia A and von Willebrand's disease, monitor plasma factor VIII concentrations and bleeding time. Assess patient for signs of bleeding. Monitor ristocetin cofactor and Willebrand factor when used for von Willebrand's disease.
  □ Monitor blood pressure and pulse during IV infusion.
  □ Monitor intake and output and adjust fluid intake (especially in children and elderly) to avoid overhydration in patients receiving desmopressin for hemophilia.
- **Toxicity and Overdose:** Signs and symptoms of water intoxication include confusion, drowsiness, headache, weight gain, difficulty urinating, seizures, and coma.
  □ Treatment of overdose includes decreasing dosage and, if symptoms are severe, administration of furosemide.

POTENTIAL NURSING DIAGNOSES
- Fluid volume deficit (indications).

- Fluid volume excess (adverse reactions).
- Knowledge deficit related to medication regimen (patient/family teaching).

IMPLEMENTATION
- **General Info:** IV desmopressin has 10 times the antidiuretic effect of intranasal desmopressin.
- **Diabetes Insipidus:** Parenteral dose for antidiuretic effect is administered direct IV or SC.
- **Hemophilia:** Parenteral for antihemorrhage is administered via IV infusion.
- **Direct IV:** Administer each dose over 1 min for diabetes insipidus.
- **Intermittent Infusion:** Dilute each dose in 50 ml of 0.9% NaCl.
- *Rate:* Infuse slowly over 15–30 min for hemophilia.

PATIENT/FAMILY TEACHING
- **General Info:** Advise patient to notify physician if drowsiness, listlessness, headache, dyspnea, heartburn, nausea, abdominal cramps, vulval pain, or severe nasal congestion or irritation occurs.
  □ Caution patient to avoid concurrent use of alcohol with this medication.
- **Diabetes Insipidus:** Instruct patient on intranasal administration. Medication is supplied with a flexible calibrated catheter (rhinyle). Draw solution into rhinyle. Insert one end of tube into nostril, blow on the other end to deposit solution deep into nasal cavity. An air-filled syringe may be attached to the plastic catheter for children, infants, or obtunded patients. Tube should be rinsed under water after each use.
  □ If a dose is missed, instruct patient to take it as soon as remembered, not using if it is almost time for the next dose. Do not double doses.
  □ Advise patient that rhinitis or upper respiratory infection may decrease effectiveness of this therapy. If increased urine output occurs, patient should contact physician for dosage adjustment.

D

□ Patients with diabetes insipidus should carry identification describing disease process and medication regimen at all times.

EVALUATION
Effectiveness of therapy can be demonstrated by: ■ Decreased frequency of nocturnal enuresis ■ Decrease in urine volume □ Relief of polydipsia □ Increased urine osmolality ■ Control of bleeding in hemophilia.

DEXAMETHASONE
(dex-a-**meth**-a-sone)
Ak-Dex, Dalalone, Decadrol, Decadron, Decaject, {Deronil}, Dexacen, Dexasone, Dexon, Hexadrol, Mymethasone, Solurex

CLASSIFICATION(S):
Glucocorticoid (long-acting),
Anti-inflammatory agent
Pregnancy Category UK

INDICATIONS
■ Used systemically and locally in a wide variety of disorders including: □ Chronic inflammatory disorders □ Allergies □ Hematologic diseases □ Neoplasms □ Autoimmune problems □ Management of cerebral edema and septic shock □ Diagnostic agent in adrenal disorders. **Unlabeled Use:** ■ Short-term administration to high-risk mothers before delivery to prevent respiratory distress syndrome in the newborn.

ACTION
■ Suppresses inflammation and the normal immune response. Has numerous intense metabolic effects ■ Suppresses adrenal function at chronic doses of 0.75 mg/day. Practically devoid of mineralocorticoid (sodium-retaining) activity. **Therapeutic Effects:** ■ Suppression of inflammation and modification of the normal immune response.

PHARMACOKINETICS
Absorption: Well absorbed following oral and IM administration. Chronic high-dose topical or inhalation use may also lead to systemic absorption. IM acetate salt is long-acting.
Distribution: Widely distributed. Crosses the placenta and probably enters breast milk.
Metabolism and Excretion: Mostly metabolized by the liver; small amounts excreted unchanged by the kidneys.
Half-life: 110–210 min; Adrenal suppression lasts 2.75 days.

CONTRAINDICATIONS AND PRECAUTIONS
Contraindicated in: ■ Active untreated infections (except for certain forms of meningitis) ■ Avoid chronic use during lactation ■ Bisulfite, paraben, or alcohol hypersensitivity—some products contain bisulfites, parabens, or alcohol.
Use Cautiously in: ■ Chronic treatment (will lead to adrenal suppression) ■ Should never be abruptly discontinued ■ Supplemental doses may be needed during stress (surgery, infection) ■ Pregnancy (safety not established) ■ Children (chronic use will result in decreased growth) ■ Use lowest possible dose for shortest period of time.

ADVERSE REACTIONS AND SIDE EFFECTS*
CNS: headache, restlessness, psychoses, depression, euphoria, personality changes, increased intracranial pressure (children only).
EENT: cataracts, increased intraocular pressure.
CV: hypertension.
GI: nausea, vomiting, anorexia, peptic ulceration.
Derm: decreased wound healing, petechiae, ecchymoses, fragility, hirsutism, acne.
Endo: adrenal suppression, hyperglycemia.

{} = Available in Canada only.
*Underlines indicate most frequent; **CAPITALS** indicate life-threatening.

F and E: hypokalemia, hypokalemic alkalosis, fluid retention (long-term high doses).
Hemat: thromboembolism, thrombophlebitis.
Metab: weight loss, weight gain.
MS: muscle wasting, muscle pain, aseptic necrosis of joints, osteoporosis.
Misc: increased susceptibility to infection, cushingoid appearance (moon face, buffalo hump).

INTERACTIONS

Drug–Drug: ▪ Additive hypokalemia with diuretics, amphotericin B, mezlocillin, piperacillin, or ticarcillin ▪ Hypokalemia may increase the risk of cardiac glycoside toxicity ▪ May increase requirement for insulin or hypoglycemic agents.

ROUTE AND DOSAGE
Adrenal Insufficiency
▪ **PO (Children):** 23.3 mcg/kg or 670 mcg/m²/day in 3 divided doses.

Anti-Inflammatory and Most Other Uses (Dose is determined by response.)
▪ **PO (Adults):** 0.5–9 mg daily in single or 3–4 divided doses.
▪ **PO (Children):** 83.3–333.3 mcg/kg or 2.5–10 mg/m²/day in 3–4 divided doses.
▪ **IM, IV (Adults):** 0.5–24 mg/day (phosphate).
▪ **IM (Adults):** 8–16 mg/day (acetate).
▪ **Intra-Articular (Adults):** 4–16 mg (acetate) single dose, may be repeated q 1–3 wk.
▪ **Top (Adults):** Apply 3–4 times daily.
▪ **Top (Children):** Apply 1–2 times daily.
▪ **Inhalation (Adults):** 3 sprays 2–4 times daily (up to 12 sprays/day).
▪ **Inhalation (Children):** 2 sprays 2–4 times daily.
▪ **Ophth (Adults and Children):** 1–2 drops of solution or suspension q 1 hr during the day and q 2 hr at night or 1.25–2.5 cm of ointment 3–4 times daily initially, then 1–2 times daily, or use solution during day and ointment at night.

▪ **Nasal (Adults):** 2 sprays in each nostril 2–3 times daily.
▪ **Nasal (Children 6–12 yr):** 1–2 sprays in each nostril bid.

Cerebral Edema
▪ **IM, IV (Adults):** 10 mg initially, 4–6 mg q 6 hr (phosphate), may be decreased to 2 mg q 8–12 hr, then change to PO.
▪ **PO (Adults):** 2 mg q 8–12 hr.

Dexamethasone Suppression Test
▪ **PO (Adults):** 1 mg at 11 p.m. or 0.5 mg q 6 hr for 48 hr.

AVAILABILITY
▪ *Tablets:* 4 mg, 6 mg ▪ *Elixir:* 0.5 mg/5 ml ▪ *Oral solution:* 0.5 mg/5 ml, 1 mg/ml ▪ *Dexamethasone sodium phosphate injection:* 4 mg/ml, 10 mg/ml, 20 mg/ml, 24 mg/ml ▪ *Dexamethasone acetate injection (not for IV use):* 8 mg/ml, 16 mg/ml ▪ *Ophthalmic:* 0.1% solution, 0.1% suspension, 0.05% ointment ▪ *Topical:* 0.01%, 0.04% aerosol, 0.1% cream ▪ *Respiratory and intranasal inhaler:* 84 mcg/actuation—170 actuations/12.6 container.

TIME/ACTION PROFILE (peak = peak blood levels; duration = duration of adrenal suppression or anti-inflammatory activity)

	ONSET	PEAK	DURATION
PO	UK	1–2 hr	2.75 days
IM (phosphate)	rapid	UK	2.75 days
IV (phosphate)	rapid	UK	2.75 days
IM (acetate)	UK	8 hr	6 days
IA (acetate)	UK	UK	1–3 wk

NURSING IMPLICATIONS
ASSESSMENT
▪ **General Info:** This drug is indicated for many conditions. Assess involved systems prior to and periodically throughout course of therapy.
▫ Monitor intake and output ratios and daily weights. Observe patient for the appearance of peripheral edema, steady weight gain, rales/crackles, or dyspnea. Notify physician should these occur.

- Children should have periodic evaluations of growth.
- **Cerebral Edema:** Assess patient for changes in level of consciousness and headache throughout therapy.
- **Intra-articular:** Monitor pain, edema, and range of motion of affected joints.
- **Top:** Assess affected skin prior to and daily during therapy. Note degree of inflammation and pruritis.
- **Inhalation:** Monitor respiratory status and lung sounds.
- **Lab Test Considerations:** *Systemic—* Monitor serum electrolytes and glucose. May cause hyperglycemia, especially in persons with diabetes. May cause hypokalemia.
- Guaiac stools. Promptly report presence of guaiac-positive stools.
- Periodic adrenal function tests may be ordered to assess degree of hypothalamic-pituitary-adrenal axis suppression in systemic and chronic topical therapy.
- **Dexamethasone Suppression Test:** To diagnose Cushing's syndrome: obtain baseline cortisol level; administer dexamethasone at 11 p.m. and obtain cortisol levels at 8 a.m. the next day. Normal response is a decreased cortisol level.
- Alternative method: Obtain baseline 24-hr urine for 17-hydroxycorticosteroid (OHCS) concentrations, then begin 48-hr administration of dexamethasone. Second 24-hr urine for 17-OHCS is obtained after 24 hr of dexamethasone.

POTENTIAL NURSING DIAGNOSES

- Infection, high risk for (side effects).
- Knowledge deficit related to medication regimen (patient/family teaching).

IMPLEMENTATION

- **General Info:** If dose is ordered daily, administer in the morning to coincide with the body's normal secretion of cortisol.
- **PO:** Administer with meals to minimize gastric irritation.
- **Direct IV:** May be given undiluted. Do not administer suspension IV.

- *Rate:* Administer over 1 min.
- **Intermittent IV:** May be added to D5W or 0.9% NaCl solution. Administer infusions at prescribed rate. Diluted solution should be used within 24 hr.

DEXAMETHASONE SODIUM PHOSPHATE

- **Syringe Compatibility:** ▪ metoclopramide ▪ ranitadine.
- **Syringe Incompatibility:** ▪ doxapram ▪ glycopyrrolate.
- **Y-Site Compatibility:** ▪ acyclovir ▪ famotidine ▪ fluconazole ▪ fludarabine ▪ foscarnet ▪ heparin ▪ hydrocortisone ▪ meperidine ▪ morphine ▪ ondansetron ▪ potassium ▪ sargramostim ▪ vitamin B complex with C ▪ zidovudine.
- **Top:** Apply to clean, slightly moist skin. Wear gloves.
- Apply occlusive dressing only with physician's order. Apply aerosol form from a distance of 15 cm for 1–2 sec.
- **Inhalation:** Allow at least 1 min between inhalations of aerosol medication.
- **Ophth:** See Appendix H for instillation of ophthalmic medications.

PATIENT/FAMILY TEACHING

- **General Info:** Instruct patient to take medication exactly as directed, not to skip doses or double up on missed doses. Stopping the medication suddenly may result in adrenal insufficiency (anorexia, nausea, fatigue, weakness, hypotension, dyspnea, and hypoglycemia). If these signs appear, notify physician immediately. This can be life-threatening.
- Instruct patient on correct technique of medication administration. Emphasize importance of avoiding the eyes unless ophthalmic form is specified.
- Encourage patient on long-term therapy to eat diet high in protein, calcium, and potassium and low in sodium and carbohydrates (see Appendix K for foods included).
- This drug causes immunosuppression and may mask symptoms of infection. Instruct patient to avoid people with known contagious illnesses

and to report possible infections immediately.

□ Review side effects with patient. Instruct patient to inform physician promptly if severe abdominal pain or tarry stools occur. Patient should also report unusual swelling, weight gain, tiredness, bone pain, bruising, non-healing sores, visual disturbances, or behavior changes.

□ Instruct patient to inform physician if symptoms of underlying disease return or worsen.

□ Advise patient to carry identification describing medication regimen in the event of an emergency in which patient cannot relate medical history.

□ Caution patient to avoid vaccinations without consulting physician.

□ Explain need for continued medical follow-up to assess effectiveness and possible side effects of medication. Physician may order periodic lab tests and eye examinations.

□ Emphasize the importance of follow-up examinations to monitor progress and side effects.

▪ **Inhalation:** Advise patients using inhalation glucocorticoids and bronchodilator to use bronchodilator first and to allow 5 min to elapse before administering the glucocorticoid, unless otherwise directed by physician.

□ Instruct patient in the proper use of the metered-dose inhaler. See Appendix H for instructions.

EVALUATION

Effectiveness of therapy can be demonstrated by: ▪ Suppression of the inflammatory and immune responses in autoimmune disorders and allergic reactions ▪ Decrease in intracranial pressure.

DEXTROAMPHETAMINE
(dex-troe-am-**fet**-a-meen)
Dexedrine, Ferndex, Oxydess II,
Spancap #1

CLASSIFICATION(S):
CNS Stimulant
Schedule II
Pregnancy Category C

INDICATIONS

▪ Treatment of narcolepsy ▪ Adjunct in the management of attention deficit disorder (ADD).

ACTION

▪ Produces CNS stimulation by releasing norepinephrine from nerve endings. Pharmacologic effects: □ CNS and respiratory stimulation □ Vasoconstriction □ Mydriasis (pupillary dilation) □ Contraction of the urinary bladder sphincter. **Therapeutic Effects:** ▪ Increased motor activity and mental alertness and decreased fatigue in narcoleptic patients ▪ Increased attention span in attention deficit disorder.

PHARMACOKINETICS

Absorption: Well absorbed following oral administration.

Distribution: Widely distributed throughout body tissues with high concentrations in the brain and CSF. Crosses the placenta and enters breast milk. Potentially embryotoxic.

Metabolism and Excretion: Some metabolism by the liver. Urinary excretion is pH-dependent. Alkaline urine promotes reabsorption and prolongs action.

Half-life: 10–12 hr (6.8 hr in children).

CONTRAINDICATIONS AND PRECAUTIONS

Contraindicated in: ▪ Pregnancy or lactation ▪ Hyperexcitable states, including hyperthyroidism ▪ Psychotic personalities ▪ Suicidal or homicidal tendencies ▪ Chemical dependence ▪ Glaucoma ▪ Hypersensitivity to tartrazine (FDC yellow dye #5).

Use Cautiously in: ▪ Cardiovascular disease ▪ Hypertension ▪ Diabetes mellitus ▪ Elderly or debilitated patients ▪ Continual use (may result in psychological dependence or physical addiction).

ADVERSE REACTIONS AND SIDE EFFECTS*

CNS: <u>restlessness</u>, <u>tremor</u>, <u>hyperactivity</u>, <u>insomnia</u>, irritability, dizziness, headache.
CV: <u>tachycardia</u>, <u>palpitations</u>, hypertension, hypotension.
GI: nausea, vomiting, <u>anorexia</u>, dry mouth, cramps, diarrhea, constipation, metallic taste.
GU: impotence, increased libido.
Derm: urticaria.
Misc: psychological dependence, physical dependence.

INTERACTIONS

Drug–Drug: ▪ Additive adrenergic effects with other **adrenergic agents** ▪ Use with **monoamine oxidase inhibitors** can result in hypertensive crisis ▪ Alkalinizing the urine (**sodium bicarbonate, acetazolamide**), prolongs effect ▪ Acidification of urine (**ammonium chloride,** large doses of **ascorbic acid**) decreases effect ▪ **Phenothiazines** may decrease effect of dextroamphetamine ▪ May antagonize the response to **antihypertensives** ▪ Increased risk of cardiovascular side effects with **beta blockers** or **tricyclic antidepressants**.

ROUTE AND DOSAGE

Attention Deficit Disorder
▪ **PO (Children >6 yr):** 5–10 mg/day in 1–2 doses, increase by 5 mg at weekly intervals. Sustained-release capsules may be given once daily.
▪ **PO (Children 3–5 yr):** 2.5 mg/day, increase by 2.5 mg at weekly intervals.

Narcolepsy
▪ **PO (Adults):** 5–60 mg/day single dose or in divided doses.

AVAILABILITY

▪ *Tablets:* 5 mg, 10 mg ▪ *Sustained-release capsules:* 5 mg, 10 mg, 15 mg.

TIME/ACTION PROFILE (CNS stimulation)

	ONSET	PEAK	DURATION
PO	1–2 hr	UK	2–10 hr
PO-ER	UK	UK	up to 24 hr

NURSING IMPLICATIONS

ASSESSMENT
▪ **General Info:** Monitor blood pressure, pulse, and respiration before administering and periodically throughout course of therapy.
▫ May produce a false sense of euphoria and well-being. Provide frequent rest periods and observe patient for rebound depression after the effects of the medication have worn off.
▫ Has high dependence and abuse potential. Tolerance to medication occurs rapidly; do not increase dose.
▪ **Attention Deficit Disorders:** Assess attention span, impulse control, and interactions with others in children.
▪ **Narcolepsy:** Observe and document frequency of episodes.

POTENTIAL NURSING DIAGNOSES
▪ Thought processes, altered (side effects).
▪ Knowledge deficit related to medication regimen (patient/family teaching).

IMPLEMENTATION
▪ **General Info:** Therapy should utilize the lowest effective dose.
▪ **PO:** Sustained-release capsules should be swallowed whole; do not break, crush, or chew.

PATIENT/FAMILY TEACHING
▪ **General Info:** Instruct patient to take medication at least 6 hr before bedtime to avoid sleep disturbances. Missed doses should be taken as soon as remembered up to 6 hr before bedtime. Do not double doses. Instruct patient not to alter dosage without consulting physician. Abrupt cessation with high doses may cause

---

*<u>Underlines</u> indicate most frequent; **CAPITALS** indicate life-threatening.

extreme fatigue and mental depression.

- ☐ Inform patient that the effects of drug-induced dry mouth can be minimized by rinsing frequently with water or chewing sugarless gum or candies.
- ☐ Advise patient to avoid the intake of large amounts of caffeine.
- ☐ Medication may impair judgment. Advise patients to use caution when driving or during other activities requiring alertness.
- ☐ Advise patient to notify physician if nervousness, restlessness, insomnia, dizziness, anorexia, or dry mouth becomes severe.
- ☐ Inform patient that physician may order periodic holiday from the drug to assess progress and decrease dependence.

EVALUATION
Effectiveness of therapy can be demonstrated by: ▪ Decreased incidence of narcolepsy ▪ Improved attention span and social interactions.

DEXTROMETHORPHAN
(dex-troe-meth-**or**-fan)
{Balminil DM}, Benylin DM, {Broncho-Grippol-DM}, Children's Hold, {DM Syrup}, Hold DM, {Koffex}, {Neo-DM}, {Ornex-DM}, Pertussin CS, Pertussin ES, {Robidex}, Robitussin Cough Calmers, Robitussin Pediatric, Scot-Tussin DM Cough Chasers, {Sedatuss}, Sucrets Cough Control, St. Joseph Cough Suppressant, Suppress, Trocal, Vicks Formula 44, Vicks Formula 44 Pediatric Formula

CLASSIFICATION(S):
Antitussive
Pregnancy Category UK

INDICATIONS
▪ Symptomatic relief of coughs caused by minor viral upper respiratory tract infections or inhaled irritants ▪ Most effective for chronic nonproductive cough ▪ A common ingredient in nonprescription cough and cold preparations.

ACTION
▪ Suppresses the cough reflex by a direct effect on the cough center in the medulla. Related to opioids structurally but has no analgesic properties. **Therapeutic Effect:** ▪ Relief of irritating nonproductive cough.

PHARMACOKINETICS
Absorption: Rapidly absorbed from the GI tract. Extended-release product is slowly absorbed.

Distribution: Distribution not known. Probably crosses the placenta and enters breast milk.

Metabolism and Excretion: Probably metabolized by the liver.

Half-life: UK.

CONTRAINDICATIONS AND PRECAUTIONS
Contraindicated in: ▪ Hypersensitivity ▪ Patients taking monoamine oxidase inhibitors ▪ Should not be used for chronic productive coughs ▪ Some products contain alcohol and should be avoided in patients with known intolerance.

Use Cautiously in: ▪ Cough that lasts more than 1 wk or is accompanied by fever, rash, or headache—physician should be consulted ▪ Pregnancy, lactation, or children <2 yr (safety not established).

ADVERSE REACTIONS AND SIDE EFFECTS*
CNS: high dose—dizziness, sedation.
GI: nausea.

INTERACTIONS
Drug–Drug: ▪ Use with **MAO inhibitors** may result in excitation, hypotension, and hyperpyrexia ▪ Additive CNS depression with **antihistamines, alcohol, antidepressants, sedative/hypnotics,** or **opioid analgesics.**

ROUTE AND DOSAGE

- **PO (Adults and Children >12 yr):** 10–20 mg q 4 hr or 30 mg q 6–8 hr or 60 mg of extended-release preparation bid (not to exceed 120 mg/day).
- **PO (Children 6–12 yr):** 5–10 mg q 4 hr or 15 mg q 6–8 hr or 30 mg of extended-release preparation q 12 hr (not to exceed 60 mg/day).
- **PO (Children 2–6 yr):** 2.5–7.5 mg q 4–8 hr or 15 mg of extended-release preparation q 12 hr (not to exceed 30 mg/day).

AVAILABILITY

- *Lozenges:* 2.5 mg, 5 mg ▪ *Liquid:* 3.5 mg/5 ml, 7.5 mg/5 ml, 15 mg/5 ml ▪ *Syrup:* 15 mg/15 ml, 10 mg/5 ml ▪ *Sustained-action liquid:* 30 mg/5 ml ▪ *In combination with:* antihistamines, decongestants, and expectorants in cough and cold preparations. See Appendix A.

TIME/ACTION PROFILE (cough suppression)

	ONSET	PEAK	DURATION
PO	15–30 min	UK	3–6 hr
PO-ER	UK	UK	9–12 hr

NURSING IMPLICATIONS

ASSESSMENT

- **General Info:** Assess frequency and nature of cough, lung sounds, and amount and type of sputum produced. Unless contraindicated, maintain fluid intake of 1500–2000 ml to decrease viscosity of bronchial secretions.

POTENTIAL NURSING DIAGNOSES

- Airway clearance, ineffective (indications).
- Knowledge deficit related to medication regimen (patient/family teaching).

IMPLEMENTATION

- **PO:** Do not give fluids immediately after administering to prevent dilution of vehicle. Shake oral suspension well before administration.

PATIENT/FAMILY TEACHING

- ◻ Instruct patient to cough effectively: sit upright and take several deep breaths before attempting to cough.
- ◻ Advise patient to minimize cough by avoiding irritants, such as cigarette smoke, fumes, and dust. Humidification of environmental air, frequent sips of water, and sugarless hard candy may also decrease the frequency of dry, irritating cough.
- ◻ Caution patient to avoid taking alcohol or other CNS depressants concurrently with this medication.
- ◻ May occasionally cause dizziness or drowsiness. Caution patient to avoid driving or other activities requiring alertness until response to the medication is known.
- ◻ Advise patient that any cough lasting over 1 wk or accompanied by fever, chest pain, persistent headache, or skin rash warrants medical attention.

EVALUATION

Effectiveness of therapy can be demonstrated by: ▪ Decrease in frequency and intensity of cough without eliminating patient's cough reflex.

DEXTROSE
Glucose, Glutose, Insta-glucose, Insulin Reaction

CLASSIFICATION(S):
Caloric agent (carbohydrate)
Pregnancy Category C

INDICATIONS

- Lower-concentration (2.5–11.5%) injection is used to provide hydration and calories ▪ Higher concentrations (up to 70%) are used IV to treat hypoglycemia and in combination with amino acids to provide calories for parenteral nutrition ▪ Oral forms are used to correct hypoglycemia in conscious patients.

ACTION

- Provides calories. **Therapeutic Effects:** ▪ Provision of calories ▪ Prevention and treatment of hypoglycemia.

PHARMACOKINETICS

Absorption: Well absorbed following oral administration.

Distribution: Widely distributed and rapidly utilized.

Metabolism and Excretion: Metabolized to carbon dioxide and water. When renal threshold is exceeded, dextrose is excreted unchanged by the kidneys.

Half–life: UK.

CONTRAINDICATIONS AND PRECAUTIONS

Contraindicated in: ▪ Allergy to corn or corn products ▪ Hypertonic solution (>5%) should not be given to patients with CNS bleeding or anuria or who are at risk of dehydration.

Use Cautiously in: ▪ Known diabetic patients (frequent lab assessment necessary to quantitate appropriate doses) ▪ Chronic alcoholics or severely malnourished patients (administration requires initial pretreatment with thiamine).

ADVERSE REACTIONS AND SIDE EFFECTS*

Endo: inappropriate insulin secretion (long-term use).

F and E: hypokalemia, hypophosphatemia, hypomagnesemia, fluid overload.

Local: local pain and irritation at IV site (hypertonic solution).

Metab: hyperglycemia, glycosuria.

INTERACTIONS

Drug–Drug: ▪ Will alter requirements for **insulin** or **oral hypoglycemic agents** in diabetic patients.

ROUTE AND DOSAGE

Hydration (as 5% solution)
▪ **IV (Adults and Children):** 0.5–0.8 g/kg/hr.

Hypoglycemia
▪ **PO (Conscious Adults and Children):** 10–20 g, may repeat in 10–20 min.
▪ **IV (Adults):** 20–50 ml of 50% solution infused slowly (3 ml/min).

▪ **IV (Infants and Neonates):** 250–500 mg/kg/dose (as 25% dextrose) repeated doses of 10–12 ml of 25% dextrose may be required.

AVAILABILITY

▪ *Oral gel:* 40% ▪ *Chewable tablets:* 5 g ▪ *Solution for injection:* 2.5%, 5%, 10%, 20%, 25%, 30%, 40%, 50%, 60%, 70% ▪ *In combination with:* sodium chloride, other electrolytes, and amino acids.

TIME/ACTION PROFILE (effects on blood sugar in diabetic patients)

	ONSET	PEAK	DURATION
PO	rapid	rapid	brief
IV	rapid	rapid	brief

NURSING IMPLICATIONS

ASSESSMENT

▫ Assess the hydration status of patients receiving IV dextrose. Monitor intake and output and electrolyte concentrations. Assess patient for dehydration or edema.

▫ Assess nutritional status, function of gastrointestinal tract, and caloric needs of patient.

▫ Diabetics and patients receiving hypertonic dextrose solution (>5%) should have serum glucose monitored regularly.

▫ Monitor IV site frequently for phlebitis and infection.

▪ **Lab Test Considerations:** May cause an elevated serum glucose.

POTENTIAL NURSING DIAGNOSES

▪ Fluid volume deficit (indications).
▪ Nutrition, altered: less than body requirements (indications).
▪ Fluid volume excess (adverse reactions).

IMPLEMENTATION

▪ **General Info:** Dextrose solution alone does not contain enough calories to sustain an individual for a prolonged period. Dextrose contains 3.4 kcal/g. D5W contains 170 cal/liter and D10W contains 340 cal/liter.

---

*Underlines indicate most frequent; **CAPITALS** indicate life-threatening.

- **PO:** Concentrated dextrose gels and chewable tablets may be used in the treatment of hypoglycemia in conscious patients. The dose should be repeated if symptoms persist and serum glucose has not increased by at least 20 mg/100 ml within 20 min.
- **IV:** Hypertonic dextrose solution (>5%) should be administered IV into a central vein. For emergency treatment of hypoglycemia administer slowly into a large peripheral vein to prevent phlebitis or sclerosis of the vein. Assess IV site frequently. Rapid infusions may cause hyperglycemia or fluid shifts. When hypertonic solution is discontinued, taper solution and administer D5W or D10W to prevent rebound hypoglycemia.
- Patients requiring prolonged infusions of dextrose should have electrolytes added to the dextrose solution to prevent water intoxication and maintain fluid and electrolyte balance.
- **Additive Incompatibility:** ▪ whole blood.

PATIENT/FAMILY TEACHING
- Explain the purpose of dextrose administration to patient.
- Instruct diabetic patient on the correct method for self-blood glucose monitoring.
- Advise patient on when and how to administer dextrose products for hypoglycemia.

EVALUATION
Effectiveness of therapy can be demonstrated by: ▪ Correction and maintenance of adequate hydration status and normal serum glucose levels ▪ Maintenance of adequate caloric intake.

DEZOCINE
(dez-oh-seen)
Dalgan

CLASSIFICATION(S):
Opioid analgesic (agonist/ antagonist)
Pregnancy Category C

INDICATIONS
- Short-term management of moderate to severe pain.

ACTION
- Binds to opiate receptors in the CNS
- Alters the perception of and the response to painful stimuli, while causing generalized CNS depression ▪ Has partial antagonist properties, which may result in opioid withdrawal in physically dependent patients. **Therapeutic Effect:** ▪ Relief of moderate to severe pain.

PHARMACOKINETICS
Absorption: Rapidly and completely absorbed following IM administration.
Distribution: Distribution not known.
Metabolism and Excretion: Mostly metabolized by the liver. <1% excreted unchanged by the kidneys.
Half-life: 2.4 hr (range 1.2–7.4 hr).

CONTRAINDICATIONS AND PRECAUTIONS
Contraindicated in: ▪ Hypersensitivity to dezocine or bisulfites.
Use Cautiously in: ▪ Head trauma ▪ Increased intracranial pressure ▪ Severe renal, hepatic, or pulmonary disease (dosage reduction recommended) ▪ Undiagnosed abdominal pain ▪ Geriatric, debilitated, or very ill patients (initial dosage reduction recommended) ▪ Pregnancy, labor, lactation, or children <18 yr (safety not established) ▪ Patients who are physically dependent on agonist opiod analgesics (may precipitate withdrawal).

ADVERSE REACTIONS AND SIDE EFFECTS*
CNS: <u>drowsiness</u>, anxiety, confusion, crying, dizziness, lightheadedness, slurred speech.
EENT: miosis, blurred vision, double vision.
CV: orthostatic hypotension.
Resp: respiratory depression.
GI: nausea, vomiting, abdominal pain, constipation, dry mouth.

*<u>Underlines</u> indicate most frequent; **CAPITALS** indicate life-threatening.

GU: urinary frequency, hesitancy, retention.

Derm: flushing or redness of skin.

Misc: tolerance, physical dependence, psychological dependence.

INTERACTIONS

Drug–Drug: ▪ Use with caution in patients receiving **MAO inhibitors** (may result in unpredictable reactions) ▪ Additive CNS depression with **alcohol, antihistamines,** and **sedative/hypnotics** ▪ May precipitate withdrawal in patients who are dependent on **opioid analgesic agonists** ▪ May diminish the analgesic effects of other **opioid analgesics.**

ROUTE AND DOSAGE

▪ **IM (Adults):** 10 mg (range: 5–20 mg) every 3–6 hr as needed.

▪ **IV (Adults):** 5 mg initially (range: 2.5–10 mg) every 2–4 hr as needed.

AVAILABILITY

▪ *Injection:* 5 mg/ml, 10 mg/ml, 15 mg/ml.

TIME/ACTION PROFILE (analgesic)

	ONSET	PEAK	DURATION
IM	within 30 min	1–2 hr	3–6 hr
IV	within 15 min	UK	2–4 hr

NURSING IMPLICATIONS

ASSESSMENT

□ Assess type, location, and intensity of pain prior to and 60 min following IM and 30 min following IV administration.

□ Assess blood pressure, pulse, and respirations before and periodically during administration. Dezocine does produce respiratory depression, but this does not markedly increase with increased doses.

□ While this drug has a low potential for dependence, prolonged use may lead to physical and psychological dependence and tolerance. This should not prevent patient from receiving adequate analgesia. Most patients who receive dezocine for medical reasons do not develop psychological dependence. If tolerance develops, changing to an opioid agonist may be required to relieve pain.

□ Assess prior analgesic history. Antagonistic properties may induce withdrawal symptoms (vomiting, restlessness, abdominal cramps, and increased blood pressure and temperature) in patients physically dependent on opioids.

▪ **Toxicity and Overdose:** If overdose occurs, naloxone (Narcan) is the antidote.

POTENTIAL NURSING DIAGNOSES

▪ Pain (indications).

▪ Injury, high risk for (side effects).

▪ Sensory-perceptual alteration: visual, auditory (side effects).

IMPLEMENTATION

▪ **General Info:** Explain therapeutic value of medication prior to administration to enhance the analgesic effect.

□ Regularly administered doses may be more effective than prn administration. Analgesic is more effective if given before pain becomes severe.

□ Coadministration with nonopioid analgesics may have additive effects and permit lower opioid doses.

▪ **IM:** Administer IM injections deep into well-developed muscle. Rotate sites of injections. Avoid SC injections.

▪ **Direct IV:** May give IV undiluted.

▪ *Rate:* Administer slowly, each 5 mg over 3–5 min.

PATIENT/FAMILY TEACHING

□ Instruct patient on how and when to ask for pain medication.

□ Dezocine may cause drowsiness or dizziness. Advise patient to call for assistance when ambulating and to avoid driving or other activities requiring alertness until response to the medication is known.

□ Caution patient to make position changes slowly to minimize orthostatic hypotension.

□ Advise patient that frequent mouth

rinses, good oral hygiene, and sugar-less gum or candy may decrease dry mouth.
- Encourage patient to turn, cough, and breathe deeply every 2 hr to prevent atelectasis.
- Advise patient to avoid concurrent use of alcohol or other CNS depres-sants with this medication.

EVALUATION
Effectiveness of therapy can be demon-strated by: ▪ Decrease in severity of pain without a significant alteration in level of consciousness or respiratory status.

DIAZEPAM
(dye-**az**-e-pam)
{Apo-Diazepam}, {Diazemuls}, {Novodipam}, T-Quil, Valium, Valrelease, Vazepam, {Vivol}, Zetran

CLASSIFICATION(S):
Sedative/hypnotic (benzodiaze-pine), Anticonvulsant (benzodi-azepine), Skeletal muscle relax-ant (centrally acting)
Schedule IV
Pregnancy Category D

INDICATIONS
▪ Management of anxiety ▪ Preoperative sedation ▪ Light anesthesia ▪ Amnesia ▪ Treatment of status epilepticus ▪ Skel-etal muscle relaxant ▪ Management of the symptoms of alcohol withdrawal **Unlabeled Use:** ▪ **Rectal:** Control of seizures.

ACTION
▪ Depresses the CNS, probably by po-tentiating gamma-aminobutyric acid (GABA), an inhibitory neurotransmitter ▪ Produces skeletal muscle relaxation by inhibiting spinal polysynaptic af-ferent pathways ▪ Has anticonvulsant properties due to enhanced presynaptic

inhibition. **Therapeutic Effects:** ▪ Relief of anxiety ▪ Sedation ▪ Amnesia ▪ Skele-tal muscle relaxation ▪ Cessation of sei-zure activity.

PHARMACOKINETICS
Absorption: Rapidly absorbed from the GI tract. Absorption from IM sites may be slow and unpredictable. Also absorbed from rectal mucosa.
Distribution: Widely distributed. Crosses the blood–brain barrier. Crosses the placenta and enters breast milk.
Metabolism and Excretion: Highly metabolized by the liver. Some products of metabolism are active as CNS de-pressants.
Half-life: 20–70 hr.

CONTRAINDICATIONS AND PRECAUTIONS
Contraindicated in: ▪ Hypersensitivity ▪ Cross-sensitivity with other benzo-diazepines may exist ▪ Comatose pa-tients ▪ Pre-existing CNS depression ▪ Uncontrolled severe pain ▪ Narrow-angle glaucoma ▪ Pregnancy or lacta-tion ▪ Known alcohol or propylene gly-col intolerance (injection only).
Use Cautiously in: ▪ Hepatic dysfunc-tion ▪ Severe renal impairment ▪ Pa-tients who may be suicidal or who may have been addicted to drugs previously ▪ Elderly or debilitated patients (dosage reduction required) ▪ Children (dosage should not exceed 0.25 mg/kg).

ADVERSE REACTIONS AND SIDE EFFECTS*
CNS: dizziness, drowsiness, lethargy, hangover, paradoxical excitation, men-tal depression, headache.
CV: hypotension (IV only).
Derm: rashes.
EENT: blurred vision.
GI: nausea, vomiting, diarrhea, consti-pation.
Local: venous thrombosis, phlebitis (IV).

{} = Available in Canada only.
*Underlines indicate most frequent; **CAPITALS** indicate life-threatening.

Resp: respiratory depression.
Misc: tolerance, psychological dependence, physical dependence.

INTERACTIONS

Drug–Drug: ▪ **Alcohol, antidepressants, antihistamines,** and **opioid analgesics**—concurrent use results in additive CNS depression ▪ **Cimetidine, oral contraceptives, disulfiram, fluoxetine, isoniazid, ketoconazole, metoprolol, propoxyphene, propranolol,** or **valproic acid** may decrease the metabolism of diazepam, enhancing its actions ▪ May decrease the efficacy of **levodopa** ▪ **Rifampin** or **barbiturates** may increase the metabolism and decrease effectiveness of diazepam ▪ Sedative effects may be decreased by **theophylline.**

ROUTE AND DOSAGE

Antianxiety, Anticonvulsant

- ▪ **PO (Adults):** 2–10 mg 2–4 times daily or 15–30 mg of extended-release form once daily.
- ▪ **PO (Children >6 mo):** 1–2.5 mg 3–4 times daily.
- ▪ **IM, IV (Adults):** 2–10 mg, may repeat in 3–4 hr if needed.

Precardioversion

- ▪ **IV (Adults):** 5–15 mg 5–10 min precardioversion.

Pre-Endoscopy

- ▪ **IV (Adults):** up to 20 mg
- ▪ **IM (Adults):** 5–10 mg 30 min pre-endoscopy.

Status Epilepticus

- ▪ **IV (Adults):** 5–10 mg, may repeat q 10–15 min total of 30 mg, may repeat regimen again in 2–4 hr (IM route may be used if IV route unavailable).
- ▪ **IM, IV (Children >5 yr):** 1 mg q 2–5 min total of 10 mg, repeat q 2–4 hr.
- ▪ **IM, IV (Children 1 mo–5 yr):** 0.2–0.5 mg q 2–5 min to maximum of 5 mg, may repeat q 2–4 hr.
- ▪ **Rectal (Adults):** 0.15–0.5 mg/kg (up to 20 mg/dose).
- ▪ **Rectal (Geriatrics):** 0.2–0.3 mg/kg.
- ▪ **Rectal (Children):** 0.2–0.5 mg/kg.

Skeletal Muscle Relaxation

- ▪ **PO (Adults):** 2–10 mg 3–4 times daily or 15–30 mg of extended-release form once daily. 2–2.5 mg 1–2 times daily initially in elderly or debilitated patients.
- ▪ **IM, IV (Adults):** 5–10 mg (2–5 mg in debilitated patients) may repeat in 2–4 hr.

Alcohol Withdrawal

- ▪ **PO (Adults):** 10 mg 3–4 times in first 24 hr, decrease to 5 mg 3–4 times daily.
- ▪ **IM, IV (Adults):** 10 mg initially, then 5–10 mg in 3–4 hr as needed.

AVAILABILITY

▪ *Tablets:* 2 mg, 5 mg, 10 mg ▪ *Sustained release capsules:* 15 mg ▪ *Oral solution:* 5 mg/5 ml, 5 mg/ml ▪ *Injection:* 5 mg/ml (contains 10% alcohol and 40% propylene glycol) ▪ {*Sterile emulsion for injection:* 5 mg/ml [contains egg phospholipids and soybean oil]}.

TIME/ACTION PROFILE (sedation)

	ONSET	PEAK	DURATION
PO	30–60 min	1–2 hr	up to 24 hr
PO-ER	UK	UK	24 hr
IM	within 20 min	0.5–1.5 hr	UK
IV	1–5 min	15–30 min	15–60 min*

*In status epilepticus anticonvulsant duration is 15–20 min.

NURSING IMPLICATIONS

ASSESSMENT

- ▪ **General Info:** Monitor blood pressure, pulse, and respiratory rate prior to and periodically throughout therapy and frequently during IV therapy.
- ▫ Assess IV site frequently during administration; diazepam may cause phlebitis and venous thrombosis.
- ▫ Prolonged high-dose therapy may lead to psychological or physical dependence. Restrict amount of drug available to patient. Observe depressed patients closely for suicidal tendencies.
- ▪ **Anxiety:** Assess degree of anxiety and level of sedation (ataxia, dizziness, slurred speech) prior to and periodically throughout therapy.

D

- **Seizures:** Observe and record intensity, duration, and location of seizure activity. The initial dose of diazepam offers seizure control for 15–20 min after administration. Institute seizure precautions.
- **Muscle Spasms:** Assess muscle spasm, associated pain, and limitation of movement prior to and throughout course of therapy.
- **Alcohol Withdrawal:** Assess patient experiencing alcohol withdrawal for tremors, agitation, delirium, and hallucinations. Protect patient from injury.
- **Lab Test Considerations:** Hepatic and renal function, and CBC should be evaluated periodically throughout course of prolonged therapy.

POTENTIAL NURSING DIAGNOSES
- Anxiety (indications).
- Physical mobility, impaired (indications).
- Injury, high risk for (side effects).

IMPLEMENTATION
- **General Info:** Patient should be kept on bedrest and observed for at least 3 hr following parenteral administration.
- **PO:** Administer with food to minimize gastric irritation. Tablets may be crushed and taken with food or water if patient has difficulty swallowing. Swallow sustained-release capsules whole; do not crush, break, or chew.
  □ Mix Intensol preparation with liquid or semisolid food such as water, juices, soda, applesauce, or pudding. Administer entire amount immediately. Do not store.
- **IM:** IM injections are painful and erratically absorbed. If IM route is used, inject deeply into deltoid muscle for maximum absorption.
- **IV:** Resuscitation equipment should be available when diazepam is administered IV.
- **Direct IV:** For IV administration do not dilute or mix with any other drug. If direct IV push is not feasible, administer IV push into tubing as close to insertion site as possible. Continu-

ous infusion is not recommended because of precipitation in IV fluids and absorption of diazepam into infusion bags and tubing. Injection may cause burning and venous irritation; avoid small veins.
- *Rate:* Administer slowly at a rate of 5 mg over at least 1 min. Infants and children should receive total dose over a minimum of 3–5 min. Rapid injection may cause apnea, hypotension, bradycardia, or cardiac arrest.
- **Syringe Compatibility:** ▪ cimetidine.
- **Syringe Incompatibility:** ▪ heparin.
- **Y-Site Incompatibility:** ▪ atracurium ▪ heparin ▪ pancuronium ▪ potassium chloride ▪ vecuronium.
- **Rectal:** Diazepam Injection has been used for rectal administration. Instill via catheter or cannula fitted to the syringe or directly from a 1-ml syringe inserted 4–5 cm into the rectum. A dilution of Diazepam Injection with propylene glycol containing 1 mg/ml has also been used.
  □ Do not dilute with other solutions, IV fluids, or medications.

PATIENT/FAMILY TEACHING
- **General Info:** Instruct patient to take medication exactly as directed; not to take more than prescribed, or to increase dose if less effective after a few weeks without checking with physician. Abrupt withdrawal of diazepam may cause insomnia, unusual irritability or nervousness, and seizures. Advise patient that sharing of this medication may be dangerous.
  □ Medication may cause drowsiness, clumsiness, or unsteadiness. Advise patient to avoid driving or other activities requiring alertness until response to medication is known.
  □ Caution patient to avoid taking alcohol or other CNS depressants concurrently with this medication.
  □ Advise patient to notify physician if pregnancy is suspected or planned.
  □ Emphasize the importance of follow-up examinations to determine effectiveness of the medication.
- **Seizures:** Patients on anticonvulsant

therapy should carry identification describing disease process and medication regimen at all times.

EVALUATION

Effectiveness of therapy can be demonstrated by: ▪ Decrease in anxiety level. Full therapeutic antianxiety effects occur after 1–2 wk of therapy ▪ Control of seizures ▪ Decrease in muscle spasms ▪ Decreased tremulousness and more rational ideation when used for alcohol withdrawal.

DIAZOXIDE
(dye-az-**ox**-ide)
Hyperstat, Proglycem

CLASSIFICATION(S):
Antihypertensive (vasodilator),
Hyperglycemic
Pregnancy Category C (PO)

INDICATIONS

▪ **IV:** Emergency treatment of hypertension ▪ **PO:** Treatment of hypoglycemia associated with hyperinsulinism or other causes.

ACTION

▪ Directly relaxes vascular smooth muscle in peripheral arterioles. Produces reflex tachycardia and increased cardiac output ▪ Inhibits insulin release from the pancreas and decreases peripheral utilization of glucose. **Therapeutic Effects:** ▪ Lowering of blood pressure ▪ Increased blood glucose.

PHARMACOKINETICS

Absorption: Well absorbed following oral administration.
Distribution: Crosses the blood–brain barrier and placenta.
Metabolism and Excretion: 50% metabolized by the liver. 50% excreted unchanged by the kidneys.
Half-life: 21–45 hr.

CONTRAINDICATIONS AND PRECAUTIONS

Contraindicated in: ▪ Hypersensitivity ▪ Hypersensitivity to bisulfites (IV only). Cross sensitivity with sulfonamides may occur.
Use Cautiously in: ▪ Diabetics (hyperglycemia accompanies use) ▪ Pregnancy and lactation (safety not established—may inhibit labor) ▪ Cardiovascular disease ▪ Uremia.

ADVERSE REACTIONS AND SIDE EFFECTS*

CV: edema, <u>tachycardia</u>, angina, arrhythmias, <u>hypotension</u>, flushing, congestive heart failure.
Derm: hirsutism.
Endo: <u>hyperglycemia</u>.
F and E: <u>sodium and water retention</u>.
Local: phlebitis at IV site.

INTERACTIONS

Drug–Drug: ▪ Concurrent **diuretic** therapy may potentiate hyperglycemic, hyperuricemic, and hypotensive effects ▪ May increase the metabolism and decrease the effectiveness of **phenytoin** ▪ **Phenytoin, corticosteroids,** and **estrogen/progesterone** may increase hyperglycemia ▪ May increase the effects of **warfarin** ▪ May alter the effects of **insulin** or **oral hypoglycemic agents**.

ROUTE AND DOSAGE

Hypertension

▪ **IV (Adults and Children):** 1–3 mg/kg every 5–15 min (not to exceed 150 mg/dose).

Hypoglycemia

▪ **PO (Adults and Children):** 3–8 mg/kg/day given in divided doses every 8–12 hr.
▪ **PO (Infants and Newborns):** 8–15 mg/kg/day in divided doses every 8–12 hr.

AVAILABILITY

▪ *Capsules:* 50 mg ▪ *Oral suspension:* 50 mg/ml ▪ *Injection:* 15 mg/ml, 300 mg/20 ml.

D

---

*<u>Underlines</u> indicate most frequent; **CAPITALS** indicate life-threatening.

TIME/ACTION PROFILE

	ONSET	PEAK	DURATION
PO*	1 hr	8–12 hr	8 hr
IV†	immediate	5 min	3–12 hr

*Blood sugar.
†Blood pressure.

NURSING IMPLICATIONS

ASSESSMENT

■ **General Info:** Assess for allergy to sulfonamide drugs.

□ Assess patient routinely for signs and symptoms of congestive heart failure (peripheral edema, dyspnea, rales/crackles, fatigue, weight gain, jugular venous distension). Notify physician if these occur.

■ **Hypertension:** Monitor blood pressure and pulse every 5 min until stable and then hourly. Report significant changes to physician immediately.

■ **Hypoglycemia:** Assess patient for signs of hyperglycemia (drowsiness, fruity breath, increased urination, unusual thirst). Monitor blood glucose on diabetic patients requiring frequent doses.

■ **Lab Test Considerations:** May cause increased serum glucose, BUN, alkaline phosphatase, AST (SGOT), sodium and uric acid levels.

□ Monitor blood glucose in diabetic patients requiring frequent parenteral doses.

□ May cause decreased creatinine clearance, hematocrit, and hemoglobin.

■ **Toxicity and Overdose:** If severe hypotension occurs, treatment includes Trendelenburg position, volume infusion, and sympathomimetics (norepinephrine).

□ Patients who develop marked hyperglycemia must be monitored for 7 days while blood glucose concentrations stabilize.

POTENTIAL NURSING DIAGNOSES

■ Cardiac output, decreased (side effects).

■ Knowledge deficit related to medication regimen (patient/family teaching).

IMPLEMENTATION

■ **General Info:** Loop diuretics are commonly given concurrently with this medication to prevent sodium and water retention.

□ Oral and injectable solution must be protected from light. Do not administer darkened solution.

■ **PO:** Shake oral suspension well before use.

■ **Direct IV:** Do not administer SC or IM. Injection may cause warmth and pain along injected vein. Monitor IV site closely; extravasation causes cellulitis and pain. Cold packs may be applied if extravasation occurs.

■ *Rate:* Administer undiluted over 30 sec or less only into a peripheral vein to prevent cardiac arrhythmias. May be repeated every 5–15 min as indicated.

□ Have patient remain recumbent for at least 1 hr following IV administration. Take blood pressure standing prior to ambulation.

■ **Syringe Compatibility:** ■ heparin.

■ **Y-Site Incompatibility:** ■ hydralazine ■ propranolol.

PATIENT/FAMILY TEACHING

■ **Hypoglycemia:** Instruct patient to take medication as directed, at the same time each day.

□ Encourage patient to follow prescribed diet, medication, and exercise regimen to prevent hypoglycemic or hyperglycemic episodes.

□ Review signs of hypoglycemia and hyperglycemia with patient.

□ Advise patient not to switch from capsule to oral suspension form without consulting physician, as oral suspension produces higher blood concentrations.

■ **Hypertension:** Instruct patient to make position changes slowly to minimize orthostatic hypotension.

□ Caution patient to avoid taking other medications, especially over-the-counter cold medicine, without consulting physician or pharmacist.

□ Emphasize the importance of routine follow-up examinations, especially during the first few weeks of therapy.

EVALUATION

Effectiveness of therapy can be demonstrated by: ▪ Decrease in blood pressure without the appearance of side effects. This drug is utilized in short-term treatment of hypertension. Oral antihypertensives should be introduced as soon as the hypertensive crisis is controlled ▪ Management of hypoglycemia and return to normal serum glucose concentrations. If diazoxide is not effective within 2–3 wk, therapy should be re-evaluated.

DICLOFENAC
(dye-**kloe**-fen-ak)
Voltaren, {Voltaren SR}

CLASSIFICATION(S):
Nonsteroidal anti-inflammatory agent
Pregnancy Category B

INDICATIONS

▪ **PO:** Management of inflammatory disorders including: ▫ Rheumatoid arthritis ▫ Osteoarthritis ▫ Ankylosing spondylitis ▪ **Ophth:** Management of inflammation following cataract extraction.

ACTION

▪ Inhibits prostaglandin synthesis. **Therapeutic Effects:** ▪ Suppression of pain and inflammation.

PHARMACOKINETICS

Absorption: Well absorbed following oral administration. Tablets are delayed-release dosage form. Absorption also occurs following ophthalmic administration.
Distribution: Crosses the placenta and enters breast milk.
Metabolism and Excretion: At least 50% metabolized on first pass through the liver.
Half-life: 1.2–2 hr.

CONTRAINDICATIONS AND PRECAUTIONS

Contraindicated in: ▪ Hypersensitivity ▪ Cross-sensitivity may exist with other nonsteroidal anti-inflammatory agents, including aspirin ▪ Active GI bleeding or ulcer disease ▪ Patients who wear soft contact lenses (ophthalmic product only) ▪ Hypersensitivity to castor oil (ophth only).
Use Cautiously in: ▪ Severe cardiovascular, renal, or hepatic disease ▪ Past history of ulcer disease ▪ Pregnancy, lactation, and children (safety not established) ▪ Elderly patients (dosage reduction recommended; may be more susceptible to adverse reactions) ▪ History of bleeding tendency.

ADVERSE REACTIONS AND SIDE EFFECTS*

Listed as occurring with oral use of diclofenac, except for **EENT.**

CV: hypertension, drowsiness, dizziness, headache.
EENT: Ophth—stinging, anterior chamber reactions, ocular allergy.
GI: abdominal pain, dyspepsia, heartburn, diarrhea, GI BLEEDING, elevated liver enzymes.
GU: frequency, dysuria, hematuria, nephritis, proteinuria, acute renal failure.
Derm: rashes, eczema, photosensitivity.
F and E: edema.
Hemat: prolonged bleeding time.
Misc: allergic reactions, including ANAPHYLAXIS.

INTERACTIONS (Listed as occurring with oral use of diclofenac)

Drug–Drug: ▪ Concurrent use with **aspirin** may decrease effectiveness ▪ Additive adverse GI effects with **aspirin, other nonsteroidal anti-inflammatory agents, potassium supplements, colchicine, glucocorticoids, or alcohol** ▪ Chronic use with **acetaminophen** may increase the risk of adverse renal reactions ▪ May decrease the effectiveness of

D

diuretics, **antihypertensive** therapy, **insulin**, or **hypoglycemic agents** ▪ Increases serum **digoxin** levels (dosage adjustment may be necessary) ▪ May increase serum **lithium** levels and increase the risk of toxicity ▪ Increases the risk of toxicity from **methotrexate** ▪ **Probenecid** increases risk of toxicity from diclofenac ▪ Increased risk of bleeding with **cefamandole, cefotetan, cefoperazone, plicamycin, thrombolytic agents,** or **anticoagulants** ▪ Increased risk of adverse hematologic reactions with **antineoplastic agents** or **radiation therapy** ▪ Concurrent use with **potassium-sparing diuretics** increases the risk of hyperkalemia ▪ Concurrent use with **gold compounds** may increase the risk of adverse renal reactions.

ROUTE AND DOSAGE

Rheumatoid Arthritis
▪ **PO (Adults):** 150–200 mg/day in 2–4 divided doses initially; when response is obtained, decrease to minimum required to control symptoms (range 75–100 mg/day in 3 divided doses). Extended-release product may be given once daily.

Osteoarthritis
▪ **PO (Adults):** 100–150 mg/day in 2–3 divided doses initially; when response is obtained, decrease to minimum required to control symptoms.

Ankylosing Spondylitis
▪ **PO (Adults):** 100–125 mg/day in 4–5 divided doses initially; when response is obtained, decrease to minimum required to control symptoms.

Postcataract Surgery
▪ **Ophth (Adults):** 1 drop of 0.1% solution 4 times daily for 2 wk starting 24 hr after procedure.

AVAILABILITY

▪ *Enteric-coated tablets:* 25 mg, 50 mg, 75 mg ▪ {*Extended-release tablets:* 75 mg, 100 mg} ▪ *Ophth solution:* 1%.

TIME/ACTION PROFILE (anti-inflammatory effects)

	ONSET	PEAK	DURATION
PO	few days–1 wk	2 wk or more	UK
Ophth	rapid	UK	UK

NURSING IMPLICATIONS

ASSESSMENT
▪ **PO:** Assess arthritic pain (note type, location, intensity) and limitation of movement prior to and periodically during therapy.
▫ Patients who have asthma, aspirin-induced allergy, and nasal polyps are at increased risk for developing hypersensitivity reactions.
▪ **Ophth:** Assess patient for eye inflammation throughout therapy.

POTENTIAL NURSING DIAGNOSES
▪ Pain (indications).
▪ Physical mobility, impaired (indications).
▪ Knowledge deficit related to medication regimen (patient/family teaching).

IMPLEMENTATION
▪ **PO:** Administer after meals or with food to minimize gastric irritation. Do not crush or chew enteric-coated or sustained-release tablets.
▪ **Ophth:** See Appendix H for instillation of ophthalmic medications.

PATIENT/FAMILY TEACHING
▪ **PO:** Instruct patient to take diclofenac with a full glass of water and to remain in an upright position for 15–30 min after administration.
▫ Caution patient to avoid concurrent use of alcohol, aspirin, ibuprofen, acetaminophen, or other OTC medications without consulting physician or pharmacist.
▫ May cause drowsiness or dizziness. Caution patient to avoid driving or other activities requiring alertness until response to medication is known.

□ Caution patient to wear sunscreen and protective clothing to prevent photosensitivity reactions.

□ Advise patient to consult physician if rash, itching, visual disturbances, tinnitus, weight gain, edema, black stools, or persistent headache occurs.

■ Ophth: Instruct patient on correct technique for instillation of drops.

□ Inform patient that concurrent use of hydrogel soft contact lenses may cause ocular irritation.

EVALUATION

Effectiveness of therapy can be demonstrated by: ■ Decrease in severity of mild to moderate discomfort □ Increased ease of joint movement. Patients who do not respond to one nonsteroidal anti-inflammatory agent may respond to another ■ Decrease in ocular irritation following cataract surgery.

DICLOXACILLIN
(dye-**klox**-a-sill-in)
Dycill, Dynapen, Pathocil

CLASSIFICATION(S):
Anti-infective (penicillinase-resistant penicillin)
Pregnancy Category B

INDICATIONS

■ Treatment of infections due to susceptible strains of penicillinase-producing staphylococci: □ Respiratory tract infections □ Sinusitis □ Skin and skin structure infections.

ACTION

■ Binds to bacterial cell wall, leading to cell death. Resists the action of penicillinase, an enzyme capable of inactivating penicillin. **Therapeutic Effect:** ■ Bactericidal action against susceptible bacteria. **Spectrum:** ■ Active against most gram-positive aerobic cocci, but less so than penicillin. Spectrum is notable for activity against penicillinase-producing strains of: □ *Staph-*

ylococcus aureus □ *Staphylococcus epidermidis* ■ Not active against methicillin-resistant staphylococci.

PHARMACOKINETICS

Absorption: Rapidly but incompletely (35–76%) absorbed from the GI tract.
Distribution: Widely distributed. Penetration into CSF is minimal. Crosses the placenta and enters breast milk.
Metabolism and Excretion: Some metabolism by the liver (6–10%) and some renal excretion of unchanged drug (60%). Small amounts eliminated in the feces via the bile.
Half-life: 0.5–1 hr (increased in severe hepatic and renal dysfunction).

CONTRAINDICATIONS AND PRECAUTIONS

Contraindicated in: ■ Hypersensitivity ■ Should not be used as initial therapy in serious infections or in patients experiencing nausea or vomiting ■ Newborns.
Use Cautiously in: ■ Severe renal or hepatic impairment (dosage reduction required) ■ Pregnancy or lactation (safety not established).

ADVERSE REACTIONS AND SIDE EFFECTS*

CNS: SEIZURES (high doses).
GI: <u>nausea</u>, <u>vomiting</u>, <u>diarrhea</u>, hepatitis.
GU: interstitial nephritis.
Derm: <u>rashes</u>, urticaria.
Hemat: blood dyscrasias.
Misc: superinfection, <u>allergic reactions</u>, including ANAPHYLAXIS and serum sickness.

INTERACTIONS

Drug–Drug: ■ **Probenecid** decreases renal excretion and increases blood levels ■ May alter the effect of **warfarin**.
Drug–Food: ■ **Food** or **acidic beverages** decrease absorption.

ROUTE AND DOSAGE

■ **PO (Adults and Children ≥40 kg):** 125–250 mg q 6 hr (up to 6 g/day).

---

*<u>Underlines</u> indicate most frequent; **CAPITALS** indicate life-threatening.

- **PO (Children <40 kg):** 12.5–25 mg/kg/day in divided doses q 6 hr.

AVAILABILITY

- *Capsules:* 125 mg, 250 mg, 500 mg
- *Oral Solution:* 62.5 mg/5 ml.

TIME/ACTION PROFILE (blood levels)

	ONSET	PEAK
PO	30 min	0.5–2 hr

NURSING IMPLICATIONS

ASSESSMENT

- Assess patient for infection (vital signs; appearance of wound, sputum, urine, and stool; WBC) at beginning and throughout course of therapy.
- Obtain a history before initiating therapy to determine previous use of and reactions to penicillins or cephalosporins. Persons with a negative history of penicillin sensitivity may still have an allergic response.
- Obtain specimens for culture and sensitivity prior to initiating therapy. First dose may be given before receiving results.
- Observe patient for signs and symptoms of anaphylaxis (rash, pruritus, laryngeal edema, wheezing, abdominal pain). Discontinue drug and notify physician immediately if these occur. Keep epinephrine, an antihistamine, and resuscitation equipment close by in the event of an anaphylactic reaction.
- **Lab Test Considerations:** CBC, BUN, creatinine, urinalysis, and liver function tests should be monitored periodically during therapy. May cause an increased AST (SGOT) concentrations.

POTENTIAL NURSING DIAGNOSES

- Infection, high risk for (indications, side effects).
- Knowledge deficit related to medications regimen (patient/family teaching).
- Noncompliance related to medication regimen (patient/family teaching).

IMPLEMENTATION

- **PO:** Administer around the clock on an empty stomach at least 1 hr before or 2 hr after meals. Take with a full glass of water; acidic juices may decrease absorption of penicillins.
- Use calibrated measuring device for liquid preparations. Shake well. Solution is stable for 14 days if refrigerated.

PATIENT/FAMILY TEACHING

- Instruct patient to take medication around the clock and to finish the drug completely as directed, even if feeling better. Missed doses should be taken as soon as remembered. Advise patient that sharing of this medication may be dangerous.
- Advise patient to report signs of superinfection (black, furry overgrowth on the tongue, vaginal itching or discharge, loose or foul-smelling stools) and allergy.
- Instruct patient to notify physician if fever and diarrhea develop, especially if stool contains blood, pus, or mucus. Advise patient not to treat diarrhea without consulting physician or pharmacist.
- Instruct patient to notify physician if symptoms do not improve.

EVALUATION

Clinical response to therapy can be evaluated by: ■ Resolution of the signs and symptoms of infection. Length of time for complete resolution depends on the organism and site of infection.

DIDANOSINE
(dye-**dan**-oh-seen)
dideoxyinosine, Videx

CLASSIFICATION(S):
Antiviral
Pregnancy Category B

INDICATIONS

- Treatment of advanced human immunodeficiency virus (HIV) infection (acquired immunodeficiency syndrome [AIDS]).

ACTION

- Inhibits viral replication by interfering with viral RNA-directed DNA polymerase (reverse transcriptase). Must be converted intracellularly by the phosphorylation process to its active form. **Therapeutic Effects:** - Virustatic action against susceptible viruses - Increase in CD4 cell counts that may result in slowed progression and decreased incidence of opportunistic infections in HIV-infected patients. **Spectrum:** - Active against retroviruses, including the human immunodeficiency virus.

PHARMACOKINETICS

Absorption: Rapidly degrades at gastric pH. Buffers in formulation neutralize gastric acid and allow for maximal absorption (33–37%).
Distribution: CSF levels are 21% of plasma levels in adults.
Metabolism and Excretion: 55% eliminated by the kidneys (urinary excretion appears to be less in children).
Half-life: 1.6 hr (0.8 hr in children).

CONTRAINDICATIONS AND PRECAUTIONS

Contraindicated in: - Hypersensitivity - Lactation - Phenylketonuria (tablets contain phenylalanine).
Use Cautiously in: - History of gout - Patients on sodium-restricted diets (tablets contain 264.5 mg sodium) - Renal impairment (dosage modification required if CCr <60 ml/min) - History of seizures.

ADVERSE REACTIONS AND SIDE EFFECTS*

CNS: <u>headache</u>, weakness, insomnia, pain, dizziness, SEIZURES, lethargy.
EENT: <u>rhinitis</u>, ear pain, photophobia, epistaxis.
Resp: <u>cough</u>, asthma.
CV: hypertension, edema, vasodilation, arrhythmias.

GI: PANCREATITIS, <u>diarrhea</u>, <u>nausea</u>, vomiting, abdominal pain, dry mouth, <u>anorexia</u>, weight loss, constipation, stomatitis, <u>liver function abnormalities</u>, LIVER FAILURE.
GU: urinary frequency.
Derm: rash, alopecia, ecchymoses.
Hemat: leukopenia, <u>granulocytopenia</u>, anemia, bleeding.
Metab: hyperlipidemia, hyperuricemia.
MS: myalgia, arthritis.
Neuro: <u>peripheral neuropathy</u>, poor coordination.
Misc: <u>chills</u>, <u>fever</u>.

D

INTERACTIONS

Drug–Drug: - Presence of buffers in didanosine will decrease absorption of **ketoconazole, dapsone, tetracyclines, fluoroquinolones** - Increased risk of peripheral neuropathy with other **drugs causing peripheral neuropathy** - Increased risk of pancreatitis with other **drugs causing pancreatitis**.
Drug–Food: - Administration of didanosine with **food** decreases absorption by 50%.

ROUTE AND DOSAGE

When tablets are used, adults and children >1 yr should receive 2 tablets/dose to ensure adequate buffering. Children <1 yr may receive 1 tablet.

- **PO (Adults ≥60 kg):** *Tablets*—200 mg bid; *buffered powder packets*—250 mg bid.
- **PO (Adults <60 kg):** *Tablets*—125 mg bid; *buffered powder packets*—167 mg bid.
- **PO (Children with BSA 1.1–1.4 m²):** *Tablets*—100 mg bid; *reconstituted pediatric powder*—125 mg bid.
- **PO (Children with BSA 0.8–1 m²):** *Tablets*—75 mg bid; *reconstituted pediatric powder*—94 mg bid.
- **PO (Children with BSA 0.5–0.7 m²):** *Tablets*—50 mg bid; *reconstituted pediatric powder*—62 mg bid.
- **PO (Children with BSA <0.4 m²):** *Tablets*—25 mg bid; *reconstituted pediatric powder*—31 mg bid.

AVAILABILITY

■ *Chewable/dispersable buffered tablets:* 25 mg, 50 mg, 100 mg, 150 mg
■ *Buffered powder packets for oral solution:* 100 mg, 167 mg, 250 mg, 375 mg ■ *Pediatric powder for oral solution:* 10 mg/ml, 20 mg/ml.

TIME/ACTION PROFILE (antiviral plasma levels)

	ONSET	PEAK
PO	UK	0.5–1 hr

NURSING IMPLICATIONS

ASSESSMENT

□ Monitor patient for symptoms of opportunistic infection prior to and throughout therapy.
□ Monitor patient for peripheral neuropathy (distal numbness, tingling, or pain in feet or hands) throughout therapy. Dose may need to be decreased.
□ Monitor patient for symptoms of pancreatitis (abdominal pain, nausea, vomiting, increased amylase concentrations). May require discontinuation of therapy. Pancreatitis may be fatal.
■ **Lab Test Considerations:** Monitor CBC and hepatic function throughout therapy. May cause leukopenia, granulocytopenia, thrombocytopenia, and anemia. May cause elevated AST (SGOT), ALT (SGPT), alkaline phosphatase, bilirubin, uric acid, and amylase concentrations.

POTENTIAL NURSING DIAGNOSES

■ Infection, high risk for (indications, side effects).
■ Injury, high risk for (side effects).
■ Knowledge deficit related to medication regimen (patient/family teaching).

IMPLEMENTATION

■ **General Info:** If diarrhea develops in patients taking buffered powder for oral solution, chewable/dispersible buffered tablets may cause less diarrhea.
□ If solution or powder spills or leaks, a wet mop or damp sponge should be used for cleaning to avoid generation of dust. Clean surface with soap and water as needed.
■ **PO:** Administer every 12 hr on an empty stomach, 1 hr before or 2 hr after meals. Food may decrease the absorption of didanosine by 50%. Do not administer ketoconazole, dapsone, tetracyclines, or fluoroquinolones within 2 hr of didanosine.
□ Tablets should be chewed thoroughly, manually crushed or dispersed in at least 1 oz of water prior to administration. To disperse, add 1 or 2 tablets to at least 1 oz of water and stir until a uniform dispersion forms. Dispersion should be taken immediately.
□ Buffered powder for oral solution should be mixed in at least 4 oz of water; do not mix with fruit juice or other acid-containing liquid. Stir 2–3 min until the powder dissolves completely. Solution should be taken immediately.
□ Solution for pediatric use is mixed by pharmacist and is stable for 30 days if refrigerated. Shake admixture immediately before administering.

PATIENT/FAMILY TEACHING

□ Instruct patient on the importance of taking didanosine exactly as directed, even if feeling better. Caution patient not to share or trade this medication with others.
□ May cause dizziness. Caution patient to avoid driving or other activities requiring alertness until response to medication is known.
□ Advise patient to consult physician or pharmacist before taking other medications concurrently with didanosine.
□ Caution patient to avoid crowds and persons with known infections.
□ Advise patient to notify physician immediately if numbness or tingling of the hands or feet, stomach pain, nausea, or vomiting occur.
□ Caution patient to avoid sexual contact, to use a condom to prevent transmission of HIV, and not to share needles with anyone.

□ Children should have dilated retinal examinations every 6 mo during therapy.
□ Emphasize the importance of regular examinations to monitor for side effects.

EVALUATION
Effectiveness of therapy may be determined by: ■ Slowed progression or decreased incidence of opportunistic infection.

DIENESTROL
(dye-en-**ess**-trole)
DV, Ortho Dienestrol

CLASSIFICATION(S):
Hormone (estrogen)
Pregnancy Category X

INDICATIONS
■ Symptomatic management of atrophic vaginitis in postmenopausal women.

ACTION
■ Estrogens promote the growth and development of female sex organs and the maintenance of secondary sex characteristics in women. Metabolic effects include: □ Reduced blood cholesterol □ Protein synthesis □ Sodium and water retention. **Therapeutic Effect:** ■ Restoration of integrity of the vaginal mucosa in postmenopausal women.

PHARMACOKINETICS
Absorption: Readily absorbed through skin and mucous membranes.
Distribution: Amounts absorbed are widely distributed.
Metabolism and Excretion: Amounts absorbed are metabolized by the liver.
Half-life: UK.

CONTRAINDICATIONS AND PRECAUTIONS
Contraindicated in: ■ Thromboembolic disease ■ Undiagnosed vaginal bleeding ■ Pregnancy (use may result in harm to the fetus) ■ Lactation.

Use Cautiously in: ■ Patients with serious cardiac, hepatic, or renal disease ■ May increase the risk of endometrial carcinoma.

ADVERSE REACTIONS AND SIDE EFFECTS*
CNS: headache, dizziness, depression.
CV: edema, hypertension.
GI: nausea, vomiting, abdominal cramps, bloating, jaundice.
GU: breakthrough bleeding, dysmenorrhea, vaginal candidiasis, cystitis.
Derm: pigmentation, rashes.
Endo: hyperglycemia.
F and E: hypercalcemia, sodium and water retention.
Hemat: thromboembolism.
Misc: breast tenderness, enlargement, change in libido.

INTERACTIONS
Drug–Drug: ■ May alter requirements for **oral anticoagulants, oral hypoglycemic agents,** or **insulin.**

ROUTE AND DOSAGE
■ **Vag (Adults):** 1 applicatorful 1–2 times daily for 1–2 wk, then ½ dose for 1–2 wk. Maintenance dose of 1 applicator 1–3 times/wk.

AVAILABILITY
■ *Vaginal cream:* 0.01%.

TIME/ACTION PROFILE (symptomatic relief of atrophic vaginitis)*

	ONSET	PEAK	DURATION
Vag	days	UK	UK

*Response is highly variable.

NURSING IMPLICATIONS
ASSESSMENT
□ Blood pressure should be monitored periodically throughout therapy.
□ Monitor intake and output ratios and weekly weight. Report significant discrepancies or steady weight gain to physician.
■ **Lab Test Considerations:** May cause

increased serum glucose and triglycerides.

□ May alter prothrombin levels.

POTENTIAL NURSING DIAGNOSES

■ Sexual dysfunction (indications).

■ Knowledge deficit related to medication regimen (patient/family teaching).

IMPLEMENTATION

■ **Vag:** Manufacturer provides applicator with cream.

PATIENT/FAMILY TEACHING

□ Instruct patient in the correct use of vaginal applicator. Patient should remain recumbent for at least 30 min after administration. May use sanitary napkin to protect clothing, but do not use tampons.

□ Explain dosage schedule and maintenance routine. Discontinuing medication suddenly may cause withdrawal bleeding.

□ Advise patient to report signs and symptoms of fluid retention (swelling of ankles and feet, weight gain), thromboembolic disorders (pain, swelling, tenderness in extremities, headache, chest pain, blurrred vision), mental depression, unusual vaginal bleeding, or hepatic dysfunction (yellowed skin or eyes, pruritus, dark urine, light-colored stools) to physician.

□ Instruct patient to stop taking medication and notify physician if pregnancy is suspected.

□ Caution patient that cigarette smoking during estrogen therapy may increase risk of serious side effects, especially for women over age 35.

□ Emphasize the importance of routine follow-up physical examinations, including blood pressure; breast, abdomen, and pelvic examinations; and PAP smears every 6–12 mo.

EVALUATION

Effectiveness of therapy can be demonstrated by: ■ Decrease in vaginal and vulval itching, inflammation, and dryness.

DIETHYLSTILBESTROL

(dye-eth-il-stil-**bess**-trole)
DES, {Honvol}, Stilphostrol

CLASSIFICATION(S):
Hormone (estrogen), Antineoplastic (hormone)
Pregnancy Category X

INDICATIONS

■ Palliatively in advanced, inoperable metastatic prostate carcinoma and postmenopausal breast carcinoma (Stilphostrol used for prostate carcinoma only).

ACTION

■ Promotes the growth and development of female sex organs and the maintenance of secondary sex characteristics in women ■ Metabolic effects include reduced blood cholesterol, protein synthesis, and sodium and water retention. **Therapeutic Effects:** ■ Decreased tumor spread in androgen-sensitive tumors.

PHARMACOKINETICS

Absorption: Well absorbed from the GI tract.
Distribution: Widely distributed. Crosses the placenta and probably enters breast milk.
Metabolism and Excretion: Metabolized by the liver.
Half-life: UK.

CONTRAINDICATIONS AND PRECAUTIONS

Contraindicated in: ■ Thromboembolic disease ■ Undiagnosed vaginal bleeding ■ Pregnancy (use may result in harm to the fetus) ■ Lactation.
Use Cautiously in: ■ Underlying cardiovascular disease ■ Severe hepatic or renal disease ■ May increase the risk of endometrial carcinoma.

ADVERSE REACTIONS AND SIDE EFFECTS*

CNS: headache, dizziness, lethargy.

{} = Available in Canada only.
*Underlines indicate most frequent; CAPITALS indicate life-threatening.

CV: <u>edema</u>, THROMBOEMBOLISM, <u>hypertension</u>, MYOCARDIAL INFARCTION.

EENT: worsening of myopia or astigmatism, <u>intolerance to contact lenses</u>.

GI: <u>nausea</u>, vomiting, anorexia, increased appetite, <u>weight changes</u>, jaundice.

GU: females—<u>breakthrough bleeding</u>, <u>dysmenorrhea</u>, <u>amenorrhea</u>, cervical erosions, vaginal candidiasis, loss of libido; males—<u>testicular atrophy</u>, <u>impotence</u>.

Derm: <u>acne</u>, urticaria, <u>oily skin</u>, pigmentation, photosensitivity.

Endo: hyperglycemia, <u>gynecomastia</u>, (males).

F and E: sodium and water retention, hypercalcemia.

MS: leg cramps.

Misc: <u>breast tenderness</u>.

INTERACTIONS

Drug–Drug: ▪ May alter requirement for **oral anticoagulants, oral hypoglycemic agents,** or **insulin** ▪ **Barbiturates** or **rifampin** may decrease effectiveness.

ROUTE AND DOSAGE

Postmenopausal Breast Carcinoma
▪ **PO (Adults):** 15 mg/day.

Prostate Carcinoma
▪ **PO (Adults):** 1–3 mg/day of diethylstilbestrol or 50–200 mg 3 times daily as diethylstilbestrol diphosphate (Stilphostrol).

▪ **IV (Adults):** 500 mg–1 g/day initially until response is obtained (5 or more days), then 250–500 mg 1–2 times weekly.

AVAILABILITY

Diethylstilbestrol
▪ *Tablets:* 1 mg, 5 mg.

Diethylstilbestrol diphosphate
▪ *Tablets:* 50 mg ▪ *Injection:* 0.25 g.

TIME/ACTION PROFILE (estrogen replacement effect)

	ONSET	PEAK	DURATION
PO	rapid*	UK	UK

*Onset of response for carcinomas may take 4–8 wk.

NURSING IMPLICATIONS

ASSESSMENT
□ Assess blood pressure prior to and periodically throughout therapy.
□ Monitor intake and output ratios and weekly weight. Report significant discrepancies or steady weight gain to physician.
▪ **Lab Test Considerations:** May cause increased serum glucose, sodium, triglyceride, phospholipid, cortisol, prolactin, prothrombin, and factors VII, VIII, IX, and X levels. May decrease serum folate, pyridoxine, antithrombin III, and pregnanediol excretion concentrations.
□ May alter thyroid hormone assays.
□ May cause hypercalcemia in patients with metastatic bone lesions.

POTENTIAL NURSING DIAGNOSES
▪ Knowledge deficit related to medication regimen (patient/family teaching).

IMPLEMENTATION
▪ **PO:** Administer oral doses with or immediately after food to reduce nausea.
□ Do not crush or chew enteric-coated tablets.
▪ **IV:** Dilute solution in 250–500 ml of D5W or 0.9% NaCl.
▪ *Rate:* Infuse at a rate of 1–2 ml/min for the first 10–15 min. If infusion is tolerated, adjust the rate so that the entire dose has infused within 1 hr.

PATIENT/FAMILY TEACHING
□ Instruct patient to take oral medication as directed. If a dose is missed, take as soon as remembered as long as it is not just before next dose. Do not double doses.
□ If nausea becomes a problem, advise patient that eating solid food often provides relief.
□ Advise patient to report signs and symptoms of fluid retention (swelling of ankles and feet, weight gain), thromboembolic disorders (pain, swelling, tenderness in extremities, headache, chest pain, blurred vision), mental depression, or hepatic dysfunction (yellowed skin or eyes, pruri-

D

tus, dark urine, light-colored stools) to physician.

□ Instruct patient to stop taking medication and notify physician if pregnancy is suspected. Caution patient of the increase in cervical and vaginal carcinoma in female offspring and in testicular tumors in male offspring if this drug is taken during pregnancy.

□ Caution patient that cigarette smoking during estrogen therapy may increase risk of serious side effects, especially for women over age 35.

□ Advise patient to notify physician or dentist of medication regimen prior to treatment or surgery.

□ Caution patient to use sunscreen and protective clothing to prevent photosensitivity reactions.

□ Emphasize the importance of routine follow-up physical examinations including blood pressure; breast, abdomen, and pelvic examinations; and PAP smears every 6–12 mo.

EVALUATION

Effectiveness of therapy can be demonstrated by: ▪ Control of the spread of advanced metastatic breast or prostatic cancer.

DIFLUNISAL
(dye-**floo**-ni-sal)
Dolobid

CLASSIFICATION(S):
Nonopioid analgesic, Nonsteroidal inflammatory agent
Pregnancy Category C

INDICATIONS

▪ Management of inflammatory disorders including: □ Rheumatoid arthritis □ Osteoarthritis ▪ Analgesic in the treatment of mild to moderate pain.

ACTION

▪ Inhibits prostaglandin synthesis ▪ Diflunisal is a salicylate similar to as-

pirin. **Therapeutic Effects:** ▪ Suppression of pain and inflammation.

PHARMACOKINETICS

Absorption: Well absorbed from the GI tract.
Distribution: Crosses the placenta and enters breast milk.
Metabolism and Excretion: Metabolized by the liver.
Half-life: 8–12 hr.

CONTRAINDICATIONS AND PRECAUTIONS

Contraindicated in: ▪ Hypersensitivity ▪ Cross-sensitivity may exist with other NSAIAs, including aspirin ▪ Active GI bleeding or ulcer disease.
Use Cautiously in: ▪ Severe cardiovascular, renal, or hepatic disease ▪ History of ulcer disease ▪ Pregnancy, lactation, or children (safety not established) ▪ Adolescents (may increase the risk of Reye's syndrome if used during viral illness).

ADVERSE REACTIONS AND SIDE EFFECTS*

CNS: headache, drowsiness, psychic disturbances, dizziness.
EENT: blurred vision, tinnitus, rhinitis.
CV: edema, changes in blood pressure, arrhythmias.
GI: nausea, vomiting, diarrhea, constipation, GI bleeding, discomfort.
GU: renal failure.
Derm: rashes.
Hemat: blood dyscrasias, prolonged bleeding time.
MS: muscle aches.
Misc: allergic reactions, including ANAPHYLAXIS, chills.

INTERACTIONS

Drug–Drug: ▪ Concurrent use with **aspirin** may decrease effectiveness ▪ Additive adverse GI effects with **aspirin,** other **nonsteroidal anti-inflammatory agents, potassium supplements, colchicine, glucocorticoids,** or **alcohol** ▪ Chronic use with **acetaminophen** may increase the risk of adverse renal and

---

*Underlines indicate most frequent; **CAPITALS** indicate life-threatening.

hepatic reactions ▪ May decrease the effectiveness of **diuretics or antihypertensive** therapy ▪ May increase the hypoglycemic effects of **insulin** or **oral hypoglycemic agents** ▪ May increase serum **lithium** levels and increase the risk of toxicity ▪ Increases the risk of toxicity from **methotrexate** ▪ **Probenecid** increases risk of toxicity from diflunisal ▪ Increased risk of bleeding with **cefamandole, cefotetan, cefoperazone, moxalactam** or **plicamycin, thrombolytic agents,** or **anticoagulants** ▪ Increased risk of adverse hematologic reactions with **antineoplastic agents** or **radiation therapy** ▪ Administration with **antacids** decrease absorption of diflunisal ▪ May increase the risk of adverse renal reactions when used with **gold compounds**.

ROUTE AND DOSAGE

Analgesia
▪ **PO (Adults):** 500–1000 mg initally, then 250–500 mg q 8–12 hr.

Anti-inflammatory
▪ **PO (Adults):** 500–1000 mg/day in 2 divided doses.

AVAILABILITY
▪ *Tablets:* 250 mg, 500 mg.

TIME/ACTION PROFILE

	ONSET	PEAK	DURATION
analagesic	60 min	2–3 hr	8–12 hr
anti-inflammatory	few days–1 wk	2 wk	UK

NURSING IMPLICATIONS

Assessment
▪ **General Info:** Patients who have asthma, aspirin-induced allergy, and nasal polyps are at increased risk for developing hypersensitivity reactions.
▪ **Arthritis:** Assess pain and range of motion prior to and periodically during therapy.
▪ **Pain:** Assess pain (type, location, and intensity) prior to and 1–2 hr following administration.
▪ **Lab Test Considerations:** BUN, serum creatinine, CBC, and liver func-

tion tests should be evaluated periodically in patients receiving prolonged course of therapy.
□ Serum potassium, creatinine, AST (SGOT), ALT (SGPT), and LDH may show increased levels. Serum uric acid levels may be decreased.
□ May cause minimally prolonged bleeding time, which may persist for less than 1 day following discontinuation of therapy.

Potential Nursing Diagnoses
▪ Pain (indications).
▪ Physical mobility, impaired (indications).
▪ Knowledge deficit related to medication regimen (patient/family teaching).

Implementation
▪ **General Info:** Coadministration with opioid analgesics may have additive analgesic effects and may permit lower opioid doses.
▪ **PO:** For rapid initial effect, administer 30 min before or 2 hr after meals. May be administered with food, milk, or antacids to decrease GI irritation. Food slows but does not reduce the extent of absorption. Capsules should be swallowed whole; do not crush or chew.

Patient/Family Teaching
□ Advise patient to take this medication with a full glass of water and to remain in an upright position for 15–30 min after administration.
□ Instruct patient to take medication exactly as directed. If a dose is missed, it should be taken as soon as remembered but not if almost time for the next dose. Do not double doses.
□ This medication may cause drowsiness or dizziness. Advise patient to avoid driving or other activities requiring alertness until response to the medication is known.
□ Caution patient to avoid concurrent use of alcohol, aspirin, ibuprofen, acetaminophen, or other over-the-counter medications without consulting physician or pharmacist.
□ Instruct patient to notify physician if

rash, itching, chills, rhinitis, fever, muscle aches, visual disturbances, weight gain, edema, black stools, or persistent headache occur.
□ Centers for Disease Control warn against giving aspirin or salicylates to children or adolescents with varicella (chicken pox) or influenza-like or viral illnesses because of a possible association with Reye's syndrome.

EVALUATION
Effectiveness of therapy can be demonstrated by: ▪ Decrease in severity of mild to moderate pain ▪ Improved joint mobility. Partial arthritic relief is usually seen within 1–2 wk with maximum effectiveness seen in several weeks. Patients who do not respond to one nonsteroidal anti-inflammatory agent may respond to another.

DIGITOXIN
(di-ji-**tox**-in)
Crystodigin

CLASSIFICATION(S):
Cardiac glycoside, Inotropic agent, Antiarrhythmic
Pregnancy Category C

INDICATIONS
▪ Alone or in combination with other agents (diuretics, vasodilators) in the treatment of congestive heart failure ▪ Used to slow the ventricular rate in tachyarrhythmias, such as atrial fibrillation and atrial flutter ▪ Used to terminate paroxysmal atrial tachycardia.

ACTION
▪ Increases the force of myocardial contraction ▪ Prolongs refractory period of the AV node ▪ Decreases conduction through the SA and AV node. **Therapeutic Effects:** ▪ Increased cardiac output (positive inotropic effect) and slowing of the heart rate (negative chronotropic effect).

PHARMACOKINETICS
Absorption: Completely absorbed following oral administration.
Distribution: Widely distributed.
Metabolism and Excretion: Primarily metabolized by the liver. Some metabolites have cardiac activity.
Half-life: 5–7 days.

CONTRAINDICATIONS AND PRECAUTIONS
Contraindicated in: ▪ Hypersensitivity ▪ Uncontrolled ventricular arrhythmias ▪ AV block ▪ Idiopathic hypertrophic subaortic stenosis ▪ Constrictive pericarditis.
Use Cautiously in: ▪ Electrolyte abnormalities (hypokalemia, hypercalcemia, and hypomagnesemia may predispose to cardiac glycoside toxicity) ▪ Pregnancy and lactation (safety has not been established) ▪ Elderly (particularly sensitive to toxic effects) ▪ Myocardial infarction.

ADVERSE REACTIONS AND SIDE EFFECTS*
CNS: <u>fatigue</u>, weakness, headache.
EENT: blurred vision, yellow vision.
CV: ARRHYTHMIAS, <u>bradycardia</u>, ECG changes.
Endo: gynecomastia.
GI: <u>nausea</u>, <u>vomiting</u>, <u>anorexia</u>, diarrhea.
Hemat: thrombocytopenia.

INTERACTIONS
Drug–Drug: ▪ Thiazide diuretics, mezlocillin, piperacillin, ticarcillin, amphotericin B, and glucocorticoids, which cause hypokalemia, may increase the risk of toxicity ▪ Use with quinidine, verapamil, amiodarone, or diltiazem increases serum levels of digitoxin ▪ Additive bradycardia may occur with beta-adrenergic blocking agents and other antiarrhythmic agents (quinidine, disopyramide) ▪ Absorption is decreased by concurrent antacids, kaolin-pectin, cholestyramine, or colestipol ▪ Concurrent use with pheno-

---

*<u>Underlines</u> indicate most frequent; **CAPITALS** indicate life-threatening.

barbital, phenytoin, or **rifampin** may result in decreased effectiveness of digitoxin ▪ Use with **succinylcholine** may increase cardiac irritability.

ROUTE AND DOSAGE
▪ **PO (Adults and Children >12 yr):** 1.2–1.6 mg (digitalizing dose) initially given in divided doses over 24 hr, followed by 150 mcg daily (range 50–300 mcg).

AVAILABILITY
▪ *Tablets:* 50 mcg, 100 mcg, 150 mcg, 200 mcg.

TIME/ACTION PROFILE (antiarrhythmic or inotropic effects, provided that a loading dose has been given)

	ONSET	PEAK	DURATION
PO	30 min–2 hr	4–12 hr	2–3 wk

NURSING IMPLICATIONS

ASSESSMENT
□ Monitor apical pulse for 1 full min prior to administering. Withhold dose and notify physician if pulse rate is <60 bpm. Also notify physician promptly of any significant changes in rate, rhythm, or quality of pulse.
□ Monitor intake and output ratios and daily weights. Assess for peripheral edema and auscultate lungs for rales/crackles throughout therapy.
□ Before administering initial loading dose, determine if patient has taken any digitalis preparations in the preceding 2–3 wk, to prevent toxicity.
□ Monitor ECG periodically throughout therapy.
▪ **Lab Test Considerations:** Serum electrolyte levels, especially potassium, magnesium, and calcium, and renal and hepatic functions should be evaluated periodically during course of therapy. Notify physician prior to giving dose if patient is hypokalemic. Hypokalemia, hypomagnesemia, or hypercalcemia may make the patient more susceptible to digitalis toxicity.

▪ **Toxicity and Overdose:** Therapeutic serum digitoxin levels range from 20 to 35 ng/ml. Serum digitoxin levels may be drawn 4–10 hr after a dose, although levels are usually drawn immediately prior to the next dose.
□ Observe patient for signs and symptoms of toxicity (anorexia, nausea, vomiting, abdominal pain, visual disturbances, headache, confusion, unusually slow or irregular pulse). If these appear, withhold drug and notify physician immediately.
□ If signs of life-threatening digitoxin toxicity occur, potassium, phenytoin, and digoxin immune Fab (Digibind) may be used for treatment.

POTENTIAL NURSING DIAGNOSES
▪ Cardiac output, decreased (indications).
▪ Knowledge deficit related to medication regimen (patient/family teaching).

IMPLEMENTATION
▪ **General Info:** For rapid digitalization the initial dose is higher than the maintenance dose. ¼–½ the total digitalizing dose may be given initially. The remainder of the dose will be given in ¼ increments in 4–8 hr intervals.
▪ **PO:** Oral preparations can be administered without regard to meals. Tablets can be crushed and administered with food or fluids if patient has difficulty swallowing.

PATIENT/FAMILY TEACHING
□ Instruct patient to take medication exactly as directed, at the same time each day. If a dose is missed, take within 12 hr. Do not double doses. Consult physician if doses for 2 or more days are missed.
□ Teach patient to take own pulse and to contact physician before taking medication if pulse rate is <60 or >100.
□ Review signs and symptoms of digitalis toxicity with patient and family. Advise patient to notify physician immediately if symptoms of toxicity or congestive heart failure occur. Inform

patient that these symptoms may be mistaken for those of colds and flu.

□ Instruct patient to keep digitoxin tablets in their original container and not to mix in pill boxes with other medications, as they may look similar and be mistaken for other medications.

□ Advise patient that sharing of this medication can be dangerous.

□ Caution patient to avoid concurrent use of over-the-counter medications, especially antacids and cold preparations, without consulting physician.

□ Advise patient to notify physician or dentist of this medication regimen prior to treatment.

□ Advise patient to carry identification describing condition and medication regimen at all times.

□ Emphasize the importance of routine follow-up examinations to determine effectiveness and to monitor for toxicity.

EVALUATION

Effectiveness of therapy can be demonstrated by: ▪ Decrease in severity of congestive heart failure □ Increase in cardiac output ▪ Decrease in ventricular response in atrial tachyarrhythmias ▪ Resolution of paroxysmal atrial tachycardia.

DIGOXIN
(di-**jox**-in)
Lanoxicaps, Lanoxin, {Novo-digoxin}

CLASSIFICATION(S):
Cardiac glycoside, Inotropic agent, Antiarrhythmic
Pregnancy Category C

INDICATIONS

▪ Alone or in combination with other agents (diuretics, vasodilators) in the treatment of congestive heart failure ▪ Used to slow the ventricular rate in tachyarrhythmias, such as atrial fibril-

lation and atrial flutter ▪ Used to terminate paroxysmal atrial tachycardia.

ACTION

▪ Increases the force of myocardial contraction ▪ Prolongs refractory period of the AV node ▪ Decreases conduction through the SA and AV node. **Therapeutic Effects:** ▪ Increased cardiac output and slowing of the heart rate.

PHARMACOKINETICS

Absorption: 60–85% absorbed following oral administration of tablets. 75–80% absorbed following administration of elixir. Absorption from liquid-filled capsules is 90–100%. 80% absorbed from IM sites, but this route is not recommended due to extreme pain and irritation.

Distribution: Widely distributed. Crosses the placenta and enters breast milk.

Metabolism and Excretion: Excreted almost entirely unchanged by the kidneys.

Half-life: 34–44 hr (increased in renal impairment).

CONTRAINDICATIONS AND PRECAUTIONS

Contraindicated in: ▪ Hypersensitivity ▪ Uncontrolled ventricular arrhythmias ▪ AV block ▪ Idiopathic hypertrophic subaortic stenosis ▪ Constrictive pericarditis ▪ Known alcohol intolerance (elixir only).

Use Cautiously in: ▪ Electrolyte abnormalities (hypokalemia, hypercalcemia, and hypomagnesemia may predispose to cardiac glycoside toxicity) ▪ Pregnancy and lactation (although safety has not been established, digoxin has been used during pregnancy without adverse effects on the fetus) ▪ Elderly patients (particularly sensitive to toxic effects) ▪ Myocardial infarction ▪ Renal impairment (dosage reduction required) ▪ Obese patients (dose should be based on ideal body weight).

ADVERSE REACTIONS AND SIDE EFFECTS*

CNS: <u>fatigue</u>, weakness, headache, blurred vision, yellow vision.

CV: ARRHYTHMIAS, <u>bradycardia</u>, ECG changes.

GI: <u>nausea</u>, <u>vomiting</u>, <u>anorexia</u>, diarrhea.

Endo: gynecomastia.

Hemat: thrombocytopenia.

INTERACTIONS

Drug–Drug: ▪ **Thiazide** and **loop diuretics, mezlocillin, piperacillin, ticarcillin, amphotericin B,** and **glucocorticoids** which cause hypokalemia may increase the risk of toxicity ▪ **Quinidine, cyclosporine, amiodarone, verapamil, diltiazem, propofenone,** and **diflunisal** increase serum levels of digoxin and may lead to toxicity (dosage reduction recommended) ▪ **Spironolactone** increases digoxin half-life (reduced dosage or increased dosing interval may be required) ▪ Additive bradycardia may occur with **beta-adrenergic blocking agents** and other **antiarrhythmic agents (quinidine, disopyramide)** ▪ Absorption is decreased by concurrent **antacids, kaolin-pectin, cholestyramine,** or **colestipol** ▪ **Thyroid hormones** may decrease therapeutic effects.

Drug–Food: Concurrent ingestion of a **high-fiber meal** may decrease the absorption of digoxin.

ROUTE AND DOSAGE

For rapid effect, a larger initial loading or "digitalizing" dose should be administered in several divided doses over 12–24 hr. Maintenance doses must be determined by renal function. All dosing must be evaluated by individual response. In general, doses required for atrial arrhythmias are higher than those for inotropic effect. Digoxin 0.25 mg tablets = 0.2 mg liquid-filled capsules.

Oral Digoxin Tablets or Elixir

▪ **PO (Adults):** 8–12 mcg/kg (6–10 mcg/kg for inotropic effect, 10–15 mcg/kg for atrial arrhythmias). Give half of this initially, remainder at 4–8 hr intervals based on response. Maintenance dose: 15–25% of loading dose. Usual adult oral dose 0.1–0.25 mg/day.

▪ **PO (Children >10 yr):** 10–15 mcg/kg. Give half of this initially, remainder at 6–8 hr intervals based on response. Maintenance dose: 25–35% of loading dose given as a single daily dose.

▪ **PO (Children 5–10 yr):** 20–35 mcg/kg initially in several divided doses given every 6–8 hr. Maintenance dose: 25–35% of initial dose given as a single daily dose.

▪ **PO (Children 2–5 yr):** 30–40 mcg/kg initially in several divided doses given every 6–8 hr. Maintenance dose: 25–35% of loading dose given as a single daily dose.

▪ **PO (Children 1–24 mo):** 35–60 mcg/kg initially in several divided doses given every 6–8 hr. Maintenance dose: 25–35% of loading dose given as a single daily dose.

▪ **PO (Neonates <1 mo):** 25–35 mcg/kg initially in several divided doses given every 6–8 hr. Maintenance dose: 25–35% of loading dose given as a single daily dose.

Digoxin Liquid-Filled Capsules

▪ **PO (Adults and Children >10 yr):** 8–12 mcg/kg initially in several divided doses given every 6–8 hr. Maintenance dose: 15–35% of initial dose given as a single daily dose or 2 divided doses (if dose >300 mcg give as 2 divided doses).

▪ **PO (Children 5–10 yr):** 15–30 mcg/kg initially in several divided doses given every 6–8 hr. Maintenance dose: 25–35% of initial dose given in 2–3 divided doses/day.

▪ **PO (Children 2–5 yr):** 25–35 mcg/kg initially in several divided doses given every 6–8 hr. Maintenance dose: 25–35% of initial dose given in 2–3 divided doses/day.

IV Digoxin

▪ **IV (Adults and Children >10 yr):** 8–

12 mcg/kg initially in several divided doses given every 4–8 hr (every 6–8 hr in children). Maintenance dose: 25–35% of initial dose given as a single daily dose.

- **IV (Children 5–10 yr):** 15–30 mcg/kg initially in several divided doses given every 6–8 hr. Maintenance dose: 25–35% of initial dose given in 2–3 divided doses/day.
- **IV (Children 2–5 yr):** 25–35 mcg/kg initially in several divided doses given every 6–8 hr. Maintenance dose: 25–35% of initial dose given in 2–3 divided doses/day.
- **IV (Children 1–24 mo):** 30–50 mcg/kg initially in several divided doses given every 6–8 hr. Maintenance dose: 25–35% of initial dose given in 2–3 divided doses/day.
- **IV (Neonates):** 20–30 mcg/kg initially in several divided doses given every 6–8 hr. Maintenance dose: 25–35% of initial dose given in 2 divided doses/day.

AVAILABILITY

- **Tablets:** 0.125 mg, 0.25 mg, 0.5 mg
- **Capsules:** 0.05 mg, 0.1 mg, 0.2 mg
- **Pediatric elixir:** 0.05 mg/ml ▪ **Injection:** 0.25 mg/ml ▪ **Pediatric injection:** 0.1 mg/ml.

TIME/ACTION PROFILE (antiarrhythmic or inotropic effects, provided that a loading dose has been given. Duration listed is that for normal renal function; in impaired renal function, duration will be longer.)

	ONSET	PEAK	DURATION
PO	0.5–2 hr	6–8 hr	2–4 days
IM	30 min	4–6 hr	2–4 days
IV	5–30 min	1–5 hr	2–4 days

NURSING IMPLICATIONS

Assessment

▫ Monitor apical pulse for 1 full min prior to administering. Withhold dose and notify physician if pulse rate is <60 bpm in an adult or <70 bpm in a child, or <90 bpm in an infant.

Also notify physician promptly of any significant changes in rate, rhythm, or quality of pulse.

▫ Blood pressure should be monitored periodically in patients receiving IV digoxin.

▫ Monitor ECG throughout IV administration and periodically throughout therapy. Notify physician if bradycardia or new arrhythmias occur.

▫ Observe IV site for redness or infiltration; extravasation can lead to tissue irritation and sloughing.

▫ Monitor intake and output ratios and daily weights. Assess for peripheral edema, and auscultate lungs for rales/crackles at least every 8 hr.

▫ Before administering initial loading dose, determine if patient has taken any digitalis preparations in the preceding 2–3 wk.

- **Lab Test Considerations:** Serum electrolyte levels, especially potassium, magnesium, and calcium, renal, and hepatic functions should be evaluated periodically during course of therapy. Notify physician prior to giving dose if patient is hypokalemic. Hypokalemia, hypomagnesemia, or hypercalcemia may make the patient more susceptible to digitalis toxicity.

- **Toxicity and Overdose:** Therapeutic serum digoxin levels range from 0.5 to 2 ng/ml. Serum digoxin levels may be drawn 4–10 hr after a dose is administered, although they are usually drawn immediately prior to the next dose.

▫ Observe patient for signs and symptoms of toxicity. In adults and older children the first signs of toxicity usually include abdominal pain, anorexia, nausea, vomiting, visual disturbances, bradycardia, and other arrhythmias. In infants and small children the first symptoms of overdose are usually cardiac arrhythmias. If these appear, withhold drug and notify physician immediately.

▫ If signs of toxicity occur and are not severe, discontinuation of digoxin may be all that is required.

▫ If hypokalemia is present and renal

function is adequate, potassium salts may be administered. Do not administer if hyperkalemia or heart block exists.

□ Correction of arrhythmias due to digitalis toxicity may be attempted with lidocaine, procainamide, quinidine, propranolol, or phenytoin. Temporary ventricular pacing may be useful in advanced heart block.

□ Treatment of life-threatening arrhythmias may include administration of digoxin immune Fab (Digibind), which binds to the digoxin molecule in the blood and is excreted by the kidneys.

POTENTIAL NURSING DIAGNOSES

■ Cardiac output, decreased (indications).

■ Knowledge deficit related to medication regimen (patient/family teaching).

IMPLEMENTATION

■ **General Info:** For rapid digitalization the initial dose is higher than the maintenance dose. ¼–½ of the total digitalizing dose is given initially. The remainder of the dose will be administered in ¼ increments at 4–6-hr intervals.

□ When changing from parenteral to oral dosage forms, dosage adjustments may be necessary because of pharmacokinetic variations in percent of digoxin absorbed, except when changing from parenteral to liquid-filled soft capsules.

■ **PO:** Oral preparations can be administered without regard to meals. Tablets can be crushed and administered with food or fluids if patient has difficulty swallowing. Use calibrated measuring device for liquid preparations. Do not alternate between dosage forms; bioavailability of capsules is not equal to tablets or elixir.

■ **IM:** Administer deep into gluteal muscle and massage well to reduce painful local reactions. Do not administer more than 2 ml of digoxin in each IM site. IM administration is not generally recommended.

■ **Direct IV:** IV doses may be given undiluted or each 1 ml may be diluted in 4 ml of Sterile Water, 0.9% NaCl, D5W, or lactated Ringer's solution for Injection. Less diluent will cause precipitation. Use diluted solution immediately. Do not use solution that is discolored or contains precipitate.

■ *Rate:* Administer each dose through Y-site injection or 3-way stopcock over a minimum of 5 min.

■ **Syringe Compatibility:** ■ heparin.

■ **Y-Site Compatibility:** ■ famotidine ■ meperidine ■ milrinone ■ morphine ■ potassium chloride.

■ **Y-Site Incompatibility:** ■ fluconazole ■ foscarnet.

■ **Additive Incompatibility:** Manufacturer recommends that digoxin not be admixed with other drugs.

PATIENT/FAMILY TEACHING

□ Instruct patient to take medication exactly as directed, at the same time each day. Missed doses should be taken within 12 hr of scheduled dose or not taken at all. Do not double doses. Consult physician if doses for 2 or more days are missed. Do not discontinue medication without consulting physician.

□ Teach patient to take pulse and to contact physician before taking medication if pulse rate is <60 or >100.

□ Review signs and symptoms of digitalis toxicity with patient and family. Advise patient to notify physician immediately if these or symptoms of congestive heart failure occur. Inform patient that these symptoms may be mistaken for those of colds or flu.

□ Instruct patient to keep digoxin tablets in their original container and not to mix in pill boxes with other medications, as they may look similar and may be mistaken for other medications.

□ Advise patient that sharing of this medication can be dangerous.

□ Caution patient to avoid concurrent use of over-the-counter medications without consulting physician. Advise patient to avoid taking antacids or antidiarrheals within 2 hr of digoxin.

□ Advise patient to notify physician or dentist of this medication regimen prior to treatment.
□ Patients taking digoxin should carry identification describing disease process and medication regimen at all times.
□ Emphasize the importance of routine follow-up examinations to determine effectiveness and to monitor for toxicity.

EVALUATION
Effectiveness of therapy can be demonstrated by: ▪ Decrease in severity of congestive heart failure ▪ Increase in cardiac output ▪ Decrease in ventricular response in tachyarrhythmias ▪ Termination of paroxysmal atrial tachycardia.

DIGOXIN IMMUNE FAB
(di-**jox**-in im-**myoon** FAB)
Digibind

CLASSIFICATION(S):
Antidote (for digoxin, digitoxin)
Pregnancy Category C

INDICATIONS
▪ Management of serious life-threatening overdosage with digoxin or digitoxin.

ACTION
▪ An antibody produced in sheep that binds antigenically to unbound digoxin or digitoxin in serum. **Therapeutic Effect:** ▪ Binding and subsequent removal of digoxin or digitoxin, preventing toxic effects in overdose.

PHARMACOKINETICS
Absorption: Administered IV only, resulting in complete bioavailability.
Distribution: Widely distributed throughout extracellular space.
Metabolism and Excretion: Excreted by the kidneys as the bound complex (digoxin immune Fab plus digoxin or digitoxin).
Half-life: 14–20 hr.

CONTRAINDICATIONS AND PRECAUTIONS
Contraindicated in: ▪ No known contraindications.
Use Cautiously in: ▪ Known hypersensitivity to sheep proteins or products ▪ Children, pregnancy, or lactation (safety not established).

ADVERSE REACTIONS AND SIDE EFFECTS*
CV: re-emergence of atrial fibrillation, re-emergence of congestive heart failure.
F and E: HYPOKALEMIA.

INTERACTIONS
Drug–Drug: ▪ Prevents response to digoxin or digitoxin.

ROUTE AND DOSAGE
When Digoxin or Digitoxin Dose is *Not* Known
▪ IV (Adults and Children): 800 mg.

When Digoxin or Digitoxin Dose or Serum Digoxin Level (SDL) is Known
Calculate total dose or body load (TBL) in mg of digoxin or digitoxin. If digoxin was ingested orally as tablets or elixir multiply by 0.8. TBL may also be calculated from serum digoxin level (SDL) as follows: TBL = SDL (5.6) (patient's weight in kg) ÷ 1000.
▪ IV (Adults and Children): Total body load (TBL) × 66.7 = dose of digoxin immune Fab (mg).

Skin Test
▪ Intradermal (Adults): 10 mcg.

AVAILABILITY
▪ *Injection:* 40 mg/vial. Each vial will bind 0.6 mg of digoxin or digitoxin.

TIME/ACTION PROFILE (reversal of arrhythmias and hyperkalemia; reversal of inotropic effect may take several hr)

	ONSET	PEAK	DURATION
IV	30 min (variable)	UK	2–6 hr

---

*Underlines indicate most frequent; **CAPITALS** indicate life-threatening.

NURSING IMPLICATIONS

ASSESSMENT

- □ Monitor ECG, pulse, blood pressure, and body temperature prior to and throughout treatment. Patients with atrial fibrillation may develop a rapid ventricular response as a result of decreased digoxin or digitoxin levels.
- □ Assess patient for increase in signs of congestive heart failure (peripheral edema, dyspnea, rales/crackles, weight gain).
- ▪ **Lab Test Considerations:** Monitor serum digoxin or digitoxin levels prior to administration.
- □ Monitor serum potassium levels frequently during treatment. Prior to treatment hyperkalemia usually coexists with toxicity. Levels may decrease rapidly; hypokalemia should be treated promptly.
- □ Free serum digoxin or digitoxin levels fall rapidly following administration. Total body concentrations rise suddenly after administration but are bound to the Fab molecule and are inactive. Total body concentrations will decrease to undetectable levels within several days. Serum digoxin or digitoxin levels are not valid for 5–7 days following administration.

POTENTIAL NURSING DIAGNOSES

- ▪ Knowledge deficit related to medication regimen (patient/family teaching).

IMPLEMENTATION

- ▪ **General Info:** Cardiopulmonary resuscitation equipment and medications should be available during administration.
- □ Delay redigitalization for several days until the elimination of digoxin immune Fab from the body is complete.
- □ *Test Dose:* Patients with a high risk for allergy to digoxin immune Fab or sheep proteins should have skin testing for allergy prior to administration. Prepare skin test solution by diluting 0.1 ml of the reconstituted solution (10 mg/ml) in 9.9 ml of 0.9% NaCl to produce a 10 ml solution (100 mcg/ml). Testing may be administered by intradermal injection or scratch test. For intradermal use, inject 0.1 ml intradermally. For scratch test place 1 drop of solution on the skin and make a ¼-in scratch through the drop with a sterile needle. Following either method, inspect for urticarial wheal surrounded by erythema after 20 min. If a positive skin test occurs, use of digoxin immune Fab should be avoided unless absolutely necessary.
- ▪ **Intermittent Infusion:** Reconstitute each 40 mg for IV administration in 4 ml of Sterile Water for Injection and mix gently. Solution will contain a concentration of 10 mg/ml. May be further diluted with 0.9% NaCl for IV infusion. Reconstituted solution should be used immediately but is stable for 4 hr if refrigerated.
- □ In infants and small children, monitor for fluid overload. For small doses, a reconstituted 40-mg vial can be diluted with 36 ml of 0.9% NaCl for a concentration of 1 mg/ml. Administer with a tuberculin syringe.
- ▪ *Rate:* Administer reconstituted solution by IV infusion through a 0.22-micron membrane filter over 30 min. If cardiac arrest is imminent, rapid direct IV injection may be used.

PATIENT/FAMILY TEACHING

- □ Explain the procedure and purpose of the treatment to the patient.

EVALUATION

Effectiveness of therapy can be demonstrated by: ▪ Resolution of signs and symptoms of digoxin or digitoxin toxicity □ Decreased digoxin or digitoxin level without major side effects.

D

DIHYDROTACHYSTEROL
(dye-hye-droh-tak-**iss**-ter-ole)
DHT, Hytakerol, vitamin D analogue

CLASSIFICATION(S):
Vitamin (fat-soluble)
Pregnancy Category C

INDICATIONS

- Treatment of hypophosphatemia
- Treatment of hypocalcemia ▪ Prevention and treatment of rickets ▪ Prevention and treatment of vitamin D deficiency ▪ Prevention and treatment of postoperative and idiopathic tetany. **Unlabeled Use:** ▪ Renal osteodystrophy.

ACTION

- Promotes the absorption of calcium and phosphorous ▪ Regulates calcium homeostasis in conjunction with parathyroid hormone and calcitonin. **Therapeutic Effect:** ▪ Treatment and prevention of deficiency states, particularly bone manifestations.

PHARMACOKINETICS

Absorption: Well absorbed in an inactive form.
Distribution: Stored in the liver and other fatty tissues.
Metabolism and Excretion: Converted to active form by sunlight and the liver. Metabolized and excreted by the kidneys.
Half-life: UK.

CONTRAINDICATIONS AND PRECAUTIONS

Contraindicated in: ▪ Hypersensitivity ▪ Hypercalcemia ▪ Vitamin D toxicity ▪ Lactation (large doses).
Use Cautiously in: ▪ Patients receiving cardiac glycosides ▪ Pregnancy (larger doses; safety not established).

ADVERSE REACTIONS AND SIDE EFFECTS*

- Do not occur at dose within the range of daily requirements.

INTERACTIONS

Drug–Drug: ▪ **Cholestyramine, colestipol,** or **mineral oil** decrease absorption of vitamin D analogues ▪ Use with **thiazide diuretics** in patients with hypoparathyroidism may result in hypercalcemia ▪ **Glucocorticoids** decrease the effectiveness of vitamin D analogues ▪ Use with **cardiac glycosides** increases

the risk of arrhythmias ▪ Vitamin D requirements are increased by **phenytoin** and other **hydantoin anticonvulsants, sucralfate, barbiturates,** and **primidone.**

ROUTE AND DOSAGE

Hypocalcemic Tetany
- **PO (Adults):** 0.75–2.5 mg/day for 3 days, then 0.25–1 mg daily.

Hypoparathyroidism or Pseudohypoparathyroidism
- **PO (Adults):** 0.75–2.5 mg/day initially for several days, then 0.2–1 mg/day (up to 1.5 mg/day).
- **PO (Children):** 1–5 mg/day for 4 days, then 0.5–1.5 mg/day.

Renal Osteodystrophy
- **PO (Adults):** 0.1–0.25 mg/day initially, then 0.2–1 mg/day.

AVAILABILITY

- *Tablets:* 0.125 mg, 0.2 mg, 0.4 mg
- *Capsules:* 0.125 mg ▪ *Oral solution:* 0.2 mg/ml, 0.25 mg/ml.

TIME/ACTION PROFILE (effects on serum calcium)

	ONSET	PEAK	DURATION
PO	several hr	1–2 wk	2 wk

NURSING IMPLICATIONS

ASSESSMENT

- ☐ Observe patient for evidence of hypocalcemia (paresthesia, muscle twitching, laryngospasm, colic, cardiac arrhythmias, and Chvostek's or Trousseau's signs). Protect symptomatic patient by raising and padding side rails; keep bed in low position.
- ☐ Assess patient for bone pain and weakness prior to and throughout course of therapy.
- ▪ **Lab Test Considerations:** Serum calcium levels should be drawn weekly during initial therapy. Monitor BUN, serum creatinine, alkaline phosphatase parathyroid hormone levels, creatinine clearance, and 24-hr uri-

*Underlines indicate most frequent; **CAPITALS** indicate life-threatening.

nary calcium periodically. Monitor serum phosphorous levels prior to and periodically throughout course of therapy.

- **Toxicity and Overdose:** Toxicity is manifested as hypercalcemia. Assess for nausea, vomiting, anorexia, weakness, constipation, headache, bone pain, and metallic taste. Later symptoms include polyuria, polydipsia, photophobia, rhinorrhea, pruritis, and cardiac arrhythmias.
- □ Treatment includes discontinuing dihydrotachysterol, instituting a low-calcium diet, and administering a laxative. IV hydration and loop diuretics may be ordered to increase urinary excretion of calcium. Hemodialysis may also be used.

POTENTIAL NURSING DIAGNOSES
- Nutrition, altered: less than body requirements (indications).
- Knowledge deficit related to medication regimen (patient/family teaching).

IMPLEMENTATION
- **PO:** May be administered without regard to meals. Measure solution accurately with calibrated dropper provided by manufacturer.

PATIENT/FAMILY TEACHING
- □ Advise patient to take as directed. Take missed doses as soon as remembered; do not double up on doses.
- □ Encourage patient to comply with diet recommendations of physician. Explain that the best source of vitamins is a well-balanced diet with foods from the 4 basic food groups. See Appendix K for foods high in vitamin D.
- □ See Appendix K for foods high in calcium. Renal patients must still consider renal failure diet in food selection. Physician may order concurrent calcium supplement.
- □ Review symptoms of overdosage and instruct patient to report these promptly to physician.
- □ Emphasize the importance of follow-up examinations to evaluate progress.

EVALUATION
Effectiveness of therapy can be demonstrated by: ■ Normalization of serum calcium levels in hypocalcemic tetany and hypoparathyroidism.

DILTIAZEM
(dil-**tye**-a-zem)
{Apo-Diltiaz}, Cardizem, Cardizem SR, Cardizem CD, Dilacor XR

CLASSIFICATION(S):
Calcium channel blocker, Antianginal, Coronary vasodilator
Pregnancy Category C

INDICATIONS
- **PO:** Management of angina pectoris due to coronary insufficiency or vasospasm (Prinzmetal's angina) ■ **PO:** Alone or in combination with other agents in the management of hypertension (SR, CD, XR product only) ■ **IV:** Conversion of atrial arrhythmias including atrial fibrillation, atrial flutter, and paroxysmal supraventricular tachycardia (PSVT).

ACTION
- Inhibits the transport of calcium into myocardial and vascular smooth muscle cells, resulting in inhibition of excitation-contraction coupling and subsequent contraction ■ May decrease SA and AV node conduction. **Therapeutic Effect:** ■ **PO:** Coronary vasodilation and subsequent decrease in frequency and severity of attacks of angina pectoris ■ **PO:** Lowering of blood pressure ■ **IV:** Suppression of atrial tachyarrhythmias.

PHARMACOKINETICS
Absorption: Well absorbed after oral administration, but large amounts are rapidly metabolized.
Distribution: Distribution not known.

Metabolism and Excretion: Mostly metabolized by the liver.
Half-life: 3.5–9 hr.

CONTRAINDICATIONS AND PRECAUTIONS

Contraindicated in: ▪ Hypersensitivity ▪ Sick sinus syndrome (without a pacemaker) ▪ 2nd- and 3rd-degree heart block ▪ Severe hypotension.
Use Cautiously in: ▪ Severe hepatic disease (dosage reduction may be required) ▪ Congestive heart failure ▪ Pregnancy, lactation, or children (safety not established).

ADVERSE REACTIONS AND SIDE EFFECTS*

CNS: dizziness, headache, tremors, mood changes, fatigue, drowsiness.
CV: arrhythmias, edema, hypotension, syncope, palpitations, congestive heart failure, 2nd- and 3rd-degree heart block.
GI: anorexia, constipation, nausea, abdominal discomfort, hepatitis, gingival hyperplasia.
Derm: rash, petechiae, photosensitivity, pruritus, sweating, flushing.
Local: itching and burning at IV site.

INTERACTIONS

Drug–Drug: ▪ May increase serum **digoxin** levels (dosage reduction may be required) ▪ Increased risk of bradycardia, conduction defects, or congestive heart failure when used with **beta-adrenergic blockers, digoxin** or **disopyramide** ▪ **Phenytoin** and **phenobarbital** may hasten metabolism and decrease effectiveness ▪ **Cimetidine** and **propranolol** may slow metabolism and lead to toxicity ▪ May decrease metabolism and increase risk of toxicity from **cyclosporine** or **carbamazepine** ▪ Additive hypotension with other **antihypertensives,** acute ingestion of **alcohol,** or **nitrates.**

ROUTE AND DOSAGE

▪ **PO (Adults):** 30–120 mg 3–4 times daily or 60–120 mg twice daily as SR

capsules or 180–240 mg day once daily as CD or XR capsules (up to 360 mg/day).
▪ **IV (Adults):** 0.25 mg/kg may repeat in 15 min with a dose of 0.35 mg/kg. May follow with continuous infusion at 10 mg/hr (range 5–15 mg/hr) for up to 24 hr.

AVAILABILITY

▪ *Tablets:* 30 mg, 60 mg, 90 mg, 120 mg ▪ *Sustained-release capsules SR:* 60 mg, 90 mg, 120 mg ▪ *CD:* 120 mg, 180 mg, 240 mg, 300 mg ▪ *XR:* 180 mg, 240 mg ▪ *Injection:* 5 mg/ml.

TIME/ACTION PROFILE
(cardiovascular effects)

	ONSET	PEAK	DURATION
PO	30 min	2–3 hr	6–8 hr
PO-SR	UK	UK	12 hr
PO-CD	UK	14 days*	UK
PO-XR	UK	14 days*	UK
IV	2–5 min	UK	UK

*Maximum antihypertensive effect with chronic therapy.

NURSING IMPLICATIONS

Assessment

▪ **General Info:** Monitor blood pressure and pulse before and periodically during therapy.
▫ Monitor intake and output ratios and daily weight. Assess patient for signs of congestive heart failure (peripheral edema, rales/crackles, dyspnea, weight gain).
▫ Patients receiving cardiac glycosides concurrently with diltiazem should have routine serum digoxin levels and be monitored for signs and symptoms of digitalis toxicity.
▫ Monitor ECG frequently during dosage titration and periodically in patients receiving long-term therapy. May cause prolonged PR interval.
▪ **Angina:** Assess location, duration, intensity, and precipitating factors of patient's anginal pain.
▪ **Arrhythmias:** Monitor ECG continuously during administration. Notify

*Underlines indicate most frequent; **CAPITALS** indicate life-threatening.

physician promptly if bradycardia or prolonged hypotension occur. Emergency equipment and medication should be available. Monitor blood pressure and pulse before and frequently during administration.

- **Lab Test Considerations:** Monitor renal and hepatic functions periodically during long-term therapy. May cause increase in hepatic enzymes after several days of therapy, which return to normal upon discontinuation of therapy.
- □ Total serum calcium concentrations are not affected by calcium channel blockers.

POTENTIAL NURSING DIAGNOSES

- Cardiac output, decreased (indications).
- Pain (indications).
- Knowledge deficit related to medication regimen (patient/family teaching).

IMPLEMENTATION

- **PO:** May be administered with meals if gastric irritation becomes a problem. Crush and mix with food or fluids for patients having difficulty swallowing. Do not open, crush, or chew sustained-release capsules.
- **Direct IV:** May be administered undiluted.
- *Rate:* Administer each dose as a bolus over 2 min.
- **Continuous Infusion:** Dilute 125 mg in 100 ml, 250 mg in 250 ml, or 250 mg in 500 ml of 0.9% NaCl, D5W, or D5/0.45% NaCl for concentrations of 1 mg/ml, 0.83 mg/ml, or 0.45 mg/ml, respectively.
- *Rate:* Initial infusion should be administered at a rate of 10 mg/hr. May increase in increments of 5 mg/hr, up to 15 mg/hr if further reduction in heart rate is required. Some patients may respond to a rate of 5 mg/hr. Infusion may be continued up to 24 hr.

PATIENT/FAMILY TEACHING

- **General Info:** Advise patient to take medication exactly as directed, not to skip or double up on missed doses. Consult physician prior to discontin-

uation of therapy; gradual discontinuation may be necessary.

- □ Instruct patient to take pulse prior to taking diltiazem. Patients should hold medication and consult physician if pulse is <50 bpm.
- □ Caution patient to make position changes slowly to minimize orthostatic hypotension.
- □ Medication may cause dizziness. Advise patient to avoid driving or other activities requiring alertness until response to medication is known.
- □ Instruct patient to avoid concurrent use of alcohol or over-the-counter medications without consulting physician or pharmacist.
- □ Diltiazem may occasionally cause gingival hyperplasia. Advise patient to maintain good oral hygiene and have regular dental examinations and cleaning to prevent gingival tenderness, bleeding, and enlargement.
- □ Caution patient to wear protective clothing and use sunscreen to prevent photosensitivity reactions.
- **Angina:** Advise patient to contact physician if chest pain does not improve or worsens after therapy, or if it is accompanied by diaphoresis or shortness of breath.
- □ Caution patient to discuss exercise restrictions with physician prior to exertion.
- □ Advise patient that nitroglycerin SL may be used concurrently as directed for acute anginal attacks.
- **Hypertension:** Encourage patient to comply with additional methods for controlling hypertension (weight reduction, low-sodium diet, discontinuation of smoking, moderation of alcohol consumption, regular exercise, stress management). Diltiazem controls but does not cure hypotension.
- □ Instruct patient and family in proper technique for monitoring blood pressure. Advise patient to take blood pressure weekly and to report significant changes to physician.

EVALUATION

Effectiveness of therapy can be demonstrated by: ■ Decrease in frequency and severity of anginal attacks □ Decreased need for nitrate therapy □ Increase in activity tolerance and sense of well-being ▪ Decrease in blood pressure ▪ Suppression of atrial tachyar-rhythmias.

DIMENHYDRINATE
(dye-men-**hye**-dri-nate)
Calm X, Dimetabs, Dinate, Dommanate, Dramamine, Dramanate, Dramilin, Dramocen, Dramoject, {Gravol}, Hydrate, Marmine, {Nauseatol}, Nico-Vert, {Novodimenate}, {PMS-Dimenhydrinate}, Tega-Vert, {Travamine}, Triptone, Wehamine

CLASSIFICATION(S):
Antihistamine, Antiemetic
Pregnancy Category B

INDICATIONS

▪ Treatment and prevention of nausea, vomiting, dizziness, and vertigo accompanying motion sickness.

ACTION

▪ Inhibits vestibular stimulation ▪ Has significant CNS depressant, anticholinergic, antihistaminic, and antiemetic properties. **Therapeutic Effect:** ▪ Decreased vestibular stimulation, which may prevent motion sickness.

PHARMACOKINETICS

Absorption: ▪ Well absorbed following oral or IM administration ▪ Alcohol intolerance (some liquid products).
Distribution: Distribution not known. Probably crosses the placenta and enters breast milk.
Metabolism and Excretion: Metabolized by the liver.
Half-life: UK.

CONTRAINDICATIONS AND PRECAUTIONS

Contraindicated in: ▪ Hypersensitivity.
Use Cautiously in: ▪ Narrow-angle glaucoma ▪ Seizure disorders ▪ Prostatic hypertrophy.

ADVERSE REACTIONS AND SIDE EFFECTS*

CNS: <u>drowsiness</u>, paradoxical excitation (children), dizziness, headache.
EENT: blurred vision, tinnitus.
CV: palpitations, hypotension.
GI: dry mouth, <u>anorexia</u>, constipation, diarrhea.
GU: frequency, dysuria.
Local: pain at IM site.

INTERACTIONS

Drug–Drug: ▪ Additive CNS depression with other **antihistamines, alcohol, narcotic analgesics,** and **sedative/hypnotics** ▪ May mask signs or symptoms of ototoxicity in patients receiving **ototoxic drugs (aminoglycosides, ethacrynic acid)** ▪ Additive anticholinergic properties with **tricyclic antidepressants, quinidine,** or **disopyramide** ▪ **MAO inhibitors** intensify and prolong the anticholinergic effects of antihistamines.

ROUTE AND DOSAGE

▪ **PO, Rectal (Adults):** 50–100 mg q 4–6 hr (not to exceed 400 mg/day).
▪ **IM, IV (Adults):** 50 mg q 4 hr.
▪ **PO, Rectal (Children 6–12 yr):** 25–50 mg q 6–8 hr (not to exceed 150 mg/day).
▪ **PO, Rectal (Children 2–5 yr):** 12.5–25 mg q 6–8 hr (not to exceed 75 mg/day).
▪ **IM, IV (Children):** 1.25 mg/kg q 6–8 hr.

AVAILABILITY

▪ *Tablets:* 50 mg ▪ *Chewable tablets:* 50 mg ▪ *Capsules:* 50 mg ▪ *Liquid:* 12.5

mg/4 ml ▪ {*Suppositories:* 50 mg, 100 mg} ▪ *Injection:* 50 mg/ml.

TIME/ACTION PROFILE (antimotion sickness, antiemetic activity)

	ONSET	PEAK	DURATION
PO	15–60 min	1–2 hr	3–6 hr
IM	20–30 min	1–2 hr	3–6 hr
IV	rapid	UK	3–6 hr

NURSING IMPLICATIONS

ASSESSMENT

□ Assess nausea, vomiting, bowel sounds, and abdominal pain prior to and after the administration of this drug. Dimenhydrinate may mask the signs of an acute abdomen.
□ Monitor intake and output, including emesis. Assess patient for signs of dehydration (excessive thirst, dry skin and mucous membranes, tachycardia, increased urine specific gravity, poor skin turgor).
▪ **Lab Test Considerations:** Will cause false-negative allergy skin tests; discontinue 72 hr prior to testing.

POTENTIAL NURSING DIAGNOSES

▪ Fluid volume deficit (indications).
▪ Nutrition, altered: less than body requirements (indications).
▪ Injury, high risk for (side effects).

IMPLEMENTATION

▪ **General Info:** When used for prophylaxis of motion sickness, administer at least 30 min and preferably 1–2 hr before exposure to conditions that may precipitate motion sickness.
▪ **PO:** Use calibrated measuring device when administering liquid dose.
▪ **IM:** Administer into well-developed muscle; massage well.
▪ **Direct IV:** Dilute 50 mg in 10 ml of 0.9% NaCl for injection.
▪ **Rate:** Inject over 2 min.
▪ **Syringe Compatibility:** ▪ atropine ▪ diphenhydramine ▪ droperidol ▪ fentanyl ▪ heparin ▪ meperidine ▪ metoclopramide ▪ morphine ▪ pentazocine ▪ perphenazine ▪ ranitidine ▪ scopolamine. Mix immediately before use.
▪ **Syringe Incompatibility:** ▪ butorpha-

nol ▪ chlorpromazine ▪ glycopyrrolate ▪ hydroxyzine ▪ midazolam ▪ pentobarbital ▪ prochlorperazine ▪ promazine ▪ promethazine ▪ thiopental.
▪ **Y-Site Compatibility:** ▪ acyclovir.
▪ **Solution Compatibility:** D5W, 0.45% NaCl, 0.9% NaCl, Ringer's solution, lactated Ringer's solution, dextrose/saline combinations, or dextrose/Ringer's combinations.

PATIENT/FAMILY TEACHING

□ Medication may cause drowsiness and sedation. Advise patient to avoid driving or other activities requiring alertness until response to the drug is known.
□ Inform patient that this medication may cause dry mouth. Frequent oral rinses, good oral hygiene, and sugarless gum or candy may minimize this effect.
□ Caution patient to avoid alcohol and other CNS depressants concurrently with this medication.

EVALUATION

Effectiveness of therapy can be demonstrated by: ▪ Prevention or decreased severity of nausea and vomiting.

DIMERCAPROL
(dye-mer-**cap**-role)
British anti-lewisite, BAL in Oil, dimercaptopropanol

CLASSIFICATION(S):
Antidote (heavy metal antagonist)
Pregnancy Category C

INDICATIONS

▪ Treatment of acute: □ Mercury □ Gold □ Arsenic poisoning ▪ Adjunct (with edetate calcium disodium) in the treatment of severe lead poisoning accompanied by encephalopathy.

ACTION

▪ Binds up heavy metals in a reversible complex so that they cannot bind to tissues and cause organ damage. **Therapeutic Effect:** ▪ Prevention of organ damage from mercury, gold, arsenic, or lead poisoning.

PHARMACOKINETICS

Absorption: Well absorbed following IM administration.

Distribution: Widely distributed with high concentrations in liver and kidneys. Also penetrates brain.

Metabolism and Excretion: 50% excreted as complex with heavy metal by kidneys and in bile. 50% rapidly metabolized by the liver.

Half-life: UK (metabolism and excretion are complete within 6–24 hr).

CONTRAINDICATIONS AND PRECAUTIONS

Contraindicated in: ▪ Hypersensitivity ▪ Hypersensitivity to peanut products (vehicle is peanut oil) ▪ Impaired liver function (except postarsenical jaundice).

Use Cautiously in: ▪ Renal impairment (dosage reduction required) ▪ Hypertension ▪ Pregnancy or lactation (safety not established).

ADVERSE REACTIONS AND SIDE EFFECTS*

CNS: SEIZURES, coma, stupor, anxiety, nervousness, restlessness, weakness.

EENT: blepheral spasm, lacrimation, rhinorrhea.

Resp: unpleasant breath odor.

CV: increased blood pressure.

GI: nausea, vomiting, pain in teeth, abdominal pain.

GU: nephrotoxicity.

Derm: sweating.

Hemat: hemolysis (in G6-PD-deficient patients), transient leukopenia (children).

Local: pain at IM site, sterile abscesses at IM sites.

MS: muscle ache, muscle spasm, painful extremities.

Misc: feeling of constriction in throat, chest, or hands; burning sensation in lips, mouth, throat, eyes, or penis; fever (children).

INTERACTIONS

Drug–Drug: ▪ Forms a toxic complex with **iron** ▪ Nephrotoxicity decreased by agents that alkalinize the urine.

Drug–Food: ▪ Nephrotoxicity decreased by foods that alkalinize the urine.

ROUTE AND DOSAGE

Severe Lead Poisoning (with edetate Ca disodium)

▪ **IM (Adults):** 4 mg/kg q 4 hr for 2–7 days. Regimen may be repeated after 2-day rest.

▪ **IM (Children):** 75 mg/m^2 q 4 hr for 5 days. Regimen may be repeated after 2-day rest.

Severe Arsenic or Gold Poisoning

▪ **IM (Adults):** 3 mg/kg q 4 hr for 2 days, then qid on the third day, then bid for 10 days or until complete recovery.

Mild Arsenic or Gold Poisoning

▪ **IM (Adults):** 2.5 mg/kg q 4 hr for 2 days, then bid on the third day, then qid for 10 days or until complete recovery.

Gold-induced Dermatitis

▪ **IM (Adults):** 2.5 mg/kg q 4 hr for 2 days, then bid for 7 days.

AVAILABILITY

▪ *Injection:* 100 mg/ml.

TIME/ACTION PROFILE (blood levels of heavy metals)

	ONSET	PEAK	DURATION
IM	UK	UK	4 hr

NURSING IMPLICATIONS

ASSESSMENT

▢ Determine time and amount of ingestion of heavy metal (arsenic, lead) or time and amount of administration of gold.

▢ Assess patient for symptoms of toxicity from ingested substance.

▢ Monitor blood pressure and pulse throughout therapy. Systolic blood pressure may rise, and tachycardia may occur 15–30 min after adminis-

---

*Underlines indicate most frequent; **CAPITALS** indicate life-threatening.

tration. Blood pressure usually returns to normal within 2 hr.

- Monitor intake and output and notify physician if significant discrepancies occur or if urine output decreases. Physician may order alkalinization of urine to prevent nephrotoxicity.
- Monitor temperature throughout therapy. May cause fever in children after second or third dose, which persists until discontinuation of therapy.
- **Lab Test Considerations:** May cause decreased values of I^{131} thyroid uptake if test is performed during or immediately following dimercaprol therapy.

POTENTIAL NURSING DIAGNOSES
- Poisoning, high risk for (indications).
- Home maintenance management, impaired (indications).
- Knowledge deficit related to ingestion and medication regimen (patient/family teaching).

IMPLEMENTATION
- **General Info:** Dimercaprol is most effective when administered within 1–2 hr after ingestion.
- Administration of ephedrine or an antihistamine may prevent or treat histamine-like side effects.
- Commonly used concurrently with edetate calcium disodium when used to treat lead poisoning.
- Contact of the solution with the skin may cause dermatitis. Wash hands immediately.
- **IM:** Administer only deep IM. Injection is painful and may cause sterile abscess.
- Solution is yellow and viscous, with a pungent odor. May be turbid and contain sediment. This does not indicate deterioration of solution.
- If administered concurrently with edetate calcium disodium, use different sites for injections.

PATIENT/FAMILY TEACHING
- Explain purpose of therapy to patient or parents.
- Inform patient that injection is painful and may cause an unpleasant garlic-like breath odor.
- Instruct patient to notify physician if headache, burning of lips, sweating, or tearing occurs.

EVALUATION
Effectiveness of therapy can be demonstrated by: ■ Resolution of the symptoms of lead, arsenic, or gold toxicity.

DINOPROSTONE
(dye-noe-**prost**-one)
Prostin E₂

CLASSIFICATION(S):
Abortifacient (prostaglandin),
Oxytocic
Pregnancy Category UK

INDICATIONS
- **Endocervical Gel:** □ Used to "ripen" the unfavorable cervix in pregnancy at or near term, when induction of labor is indicated. ■ **Vaginal Suppository:** □ Induction of midtrimester abortion □ Management of missed abortion up to 28 wk □ Management of nonmetastatic gestational trophoblastic disease (benign hydatidiform mole).

ACTION
- Produces contractions similar to those occurring during labor at term by stimulating the myometrium (oxytocic effect) ■ Initiates softening, effacement, and dilation of the cervix ("ripening") ■ Also stimulates GI smooth muscle.
Therapeutic Effects: ■ Initiation of labor ■ Expulsion of fetus.

PHARMACOKINETICS
Absorption: Rapidly absorbed.
Distribution: Distribution not known. Action is mostly local.
Metabolism and Excretion: Metabolized by enzymes in lung, kidneys, spleen, and liver tissue.
Half-life: UK.

CONTRAINDICATIONS AND PRECAUTIONS
Contraindicated in: ■ Hypersensitivity

to prostaglandins or additives in the gel or suppository ■ The gel should be avoided in situations where prolonged uterine contractions should be avoided including □ Previous Cesarean section or uterine surgery □ Cephalopelvic disproportion □ Traumatic delivery or difficult labor □ Multiparity □ Hyperactive or hypertonic uterus □ Fetus distress (if delivery is not imminent) □ Unexplained vaginal bleeding □ Placenta previa □ Vasa previa □ Active herpes genitalis □ Obstetric emergency requiring surgical intervention □ Situations where vaginal delivery is contraindicated ■ Neither product should be used in the presence of acute pelvic inflammatory disease or ruptured membranes.

Use Cautiously in: ■ Uterine scarring ■ Asthma ■ Hypotension ■ Cardiac disease ■ Adrenal disorders ■ Anemia ■ Jaundice ■ Diabetes mellitus ■ Epilepsy ■ Glaucoma ■ Pulmonary, renal, or hepatic disease.

ADVERSE REACTIONS AND SIDE EFFECTS*

Endocervical Gel
GU: uterine contractile abnormalities, warm feeling in vagina.
MS: back pain.
Misc: fever.

Suppository
CNS: <u>headache</u>, drowsiness, syncope.
Resp: coughing, dyspnea, wheezing.
CV: <u>hypotension</u>, hypertension.
GI: <u>nausea</u>, <u>vomiting</u>, <u>diarrhea</u>.
GU: uterine rupture, urinary tract infection, vaginal/uterine pain.
Misc: chills, fever, allergic reactions, including ANAPHYLAXIS.

INTERACTIONS
Drug–Drug: ■ Augments the effects of other **oxytocics**.

ROUTE AND DOSAGE
Cervical Ripening
■ **Cervical (Adults):** 0.5 mg, if response is unfavorable, may repeat in 6 hr (not to exceed 1.5 mg/24 hr).

Abortifacient
■ **Vaginal Suppository (Adults):** 20 mg, repeat q 3–5 hr (not to exceed 240 mg total).

AVAILABILITY
■ **Endocervical gel:** 0.5 mg dinoprostone in 3 g of gel vehicle in a prefilled syringe with catheters ■ **Vaginal suppository:** 20 mg.

TIME/ACTION PROFILE

	ONSET	PEAK	DURATION
cervical ripening (gel)	rapid	30–45 min	UK
abortion time (suppository)	10 min	12–24 hr	2–3 hr

NURSING IMPLICATIONS
ASSESSMENT
■ **Abortifacient:** Monitor frequency, duration, and force of contractions and uterine resting tone.
□ Monitor temperature, pulse, and blood pressure periodically throughout course of therapy. Dinoprostone-induced fever (elevation >1.1°C or 2°F) usually occurs within 15–45 min following insertion of suppository. This returns to normal 2–6 hr after discontinuation or removal of suppository from vagina.
□ Auscultate breath sounds. Wheezing and sensation of chest tightness may indicate hypersensitivity reaction.
□ Assess for nausea, vomiting, and diarrhea. Vomiting occurs in about 67% of patients and diarrhea in about 40% of patients. Premedication with antiemetic and an antidiarrheal may be ordered.
□ Monitor amount and type of vaginal discharge. Notify physician immediately if symptoms of hemorrhage (increased bleeding, hypotension, pallor, tachycardia) occur.
■ **Cervical Ripening:** Monitor uterine activity, fetal status, and dilation and effacement of cervix continuously throughout therapy. Assess for hyper-

tonus, sustained uterine contractility, and fetal distress.

POTENTIAL NURSING DIAGNOSES
- Knowledge deficit related to medication regimen (patient/family teaching).

IMPLEMENTATION
- **Abortifacient:** Warm the suppository to room temperature just prior to use. Can be made into a gel by pharmacist.
- Wear gloves when handling unwrapped suppository to prevent absorption through skin.
- Patient should remain supine for 10 min following insertion of suppository, then she may be ambulatory.
- **Cervical Ripening:** Determine degree of effacement prior to insertion of the endocervical catheter. Do not administer above the level of the internal os. Use the 20-mm endocervical catheter if no effacement is present and the 10-mm catheter if the cervix is 50% effaced.
- Use caution to prevent contact of dinoprostone gel with skin. Wash hands thoroughly with soap and water after administration.
- Bring gel to room temperature just prior to administration. Do not force warming with external sources (water bath, microwave). Remove peel-off seal from end of syringe, then remove the protective end cap and insert end cap into plunger stopper assembly in barrel of syringe. Aseptically remove catheter from package. Firmly attach catheter hub to syringe tip; click is evidence of attachment. Fill catheter with sterile gel by pushing plunger to expel air from catheter prior to administration to patient. Gel is stable for 24 mo if refrigerated.
- Patient should be in dorsal position with cervix visualized using a speculum. Introduce gel with catheter into cervical canal using sterile technique. Administer gel by gentle expulsion of syringe and then remove catheter. Do not attempt to administer small amount of gel remaining in syringe. Use syringe for only 1 patient; discard syringe, catheter, and unused package contents after using.
- Patient should remain supine for 15–30 min following administration to minimize leakage from cervical canal.
- Oxytocin may be administered 6–12 hr following desired response from dinoprostone gel. If no cervical/uterine response to initial dose of dinoprostone is obtained, repeat dose may be administered in 6 hr.

PATIENT/FAMILY TEACHING
- **General Info:** Explain purpose of medication and vaginal examinations.
- **Abortifacient:** Instruct patient to notify physician immediately if fever and chills, foul-smelling vaginal discharge, lower abdominal pain, or increased bleeding occurs.
- Provide emotional support throughout therapy.
- **Cervical Ripening:** Inform patient that she may experience a warm feeling in her vagina during administration.
- Advise patient to notify physician or nurse if contractions become prolonged.

EVALUATION
Effectiveness of therapy can be demonstrated by: ▪ Complete abortion. Continuous administration for more than 2 days is not usually recommended ▪ Cervical ripening and induction of labor.

DIPHENHYDRAMINE
(dye-fen-**hye**-dra-meen)
{Allerdryl}, AllerMax, Belix, Bena-D, Benadryl, Benahist, Ben-Allergin, Benaphen, Benoject, Benylin, Bydramine, Dihydrex, Diphen, Diphenacen, Diphenadryl, Dormarex 2, Genahist, Gen-D-phen, Hydramine, Hydramyn, Hyrexin, {Insomnal}, Maximum Strength Nytol, Nervine Night-

time Sleep-Aid, Nidryl, Nordryl, Phendry, Sleep-Eze 3, Sominex, Tusstat, Twilite, Valdrene, Wehdryl

CLASSIFICATION(S):
Antihistamine, Antitussive
Pregnancy Category B

INDICATIONS

■ Relief of allergic symptoms caused by histamine release including: □ Anaphylaxis □ Nasal allergies □ Allergic dermatoses ■ Parkinson's disease and dystonic reactions from medications ■ Mild night-time sedation ■ Prevention of motion sickness ■ Antitussive.

ACTION

■ Blocks the following effects of histamine: □ Vasodilation □ Increased GI tract secretions □ Increased heart rate □ Hypotension ■ Significant CNS depressant and anticholinergic properties. **Therapeutic Effects:** ■ Relief of symptoms associated with histamine excess ■ Relief of acute dystonic reactions ■ Prevention of motion sickness ■ Suppression of cough.

PHARMACOKINETICS

Absorption: Well absorbed following oral and IM administration. Minimal systemic absorption may follow topical administration.
Distribution: Widely distributed. Crosses the placenta and enters breast milk.
Metabolism and Excretion: Metabolized by the liver (95%).
Half-life: 2.4–7 hr.

CONTRAINDICATIONS AND PRECAUTIONS

Contraindicated in: ■ Hypersensitivity ■ Acute attacks of asthma ■ Lactation ■ Known alcohol intolerance (some liquid products).
Use Cautiously in: ■ Elderly patients (more susceptible to adverse drug reactions; dosage reduction recommended)

■ Severe liver disease ■ Narrow-angle glaucoma ■ Seizure disorders ■ Prostatic hypertrophy ■ Pregnancy (safety not established).

ADVERSE REACTIONS AND SIDE EFFECTS*

CNS: <u>drowsiness</u>, paradoxical excitation (children), dizziness, headache.
EENT: blurred vision, tinnitus.
CV: palpitations, hypotension.
GI: <u>dry mouth</u>, <u>anorexia</u>, constipation, diarrhea.
GU: frequency, dysuria, urinary retention.
Derm: photosensitivity.
Local: pain at IM site.

INTERACTIONS

Drug–Drug: ■ Additive CNS depression with other **antihistamines, alcohol, opioid analgesics,** and **sedative/hypnotics** ■ Additive anticholinergic properties with **tricyclic antidepressants, quinidine,** or **disopyramide** ■ **MAO inhibitors** intensify and prolong the anticholinergic effects of antihistamines.

ROUTE AND DOSAGE

■ **PO (Adults):** 25–50 mg q 4–6 hr.
■ **PO (Children >9.1 kg):** 12.5–25 mg q 4–6 hr.
■ **PO (Children <9.1 kg):** 6.25–12.5 mg q 4–6 hr.
■ **IM, IV (Adults):** 10–50 mg single dose (may need up to 100 mg dose, not to exceed 400 mg/day).
■ **IM, IV (Children):** 1.25 mg/kg 4 times daily (not to exceed 300 mg/day).
■ **Top (Adults and Children >2 yr):** 1–2% cream, lotion, or spray 3–4 times daily.

AVAILABILITY

■ *Capsules:* 25 mg, 50 mg ■ *Tablets:* 25 mg, 50 mg ■ *Elixir:* 12.5 mg/5 ml ■ *Syrup:* 12.5 mg/5 ml ■ *Injection:* 50 mg/ml ■ *Cream:* 1%, 2% ■ *Spray:* 1%, 2% ■ *Lotion:* 1% ■ *In combination with:* analgesics, decongestants, and

---

*Underlines indicate most frequent; **CAPITALS** indicate life-threatening.

expectorants, in over-the-counter pain, sleep, cough, and cold preparations; and with camphor and calamine in topical preparations. See Appendix A.

TIME/ACTION PROFILE
(antihistaminic effects)

	ONSET	PEAK	DURATION
PO	15–60 min	1–4 hr	4–8 hr
IM	20–30 min	1–4 hr	4–8 hr
IV	rapid	UK	4–8 hr

NURSING IMPLICATIONS

ASSESSMENT

- **General Info:** Diphenhydramine has multiple uses. Determine why the medication was ordered and assess symptoms that apply to the individual patient.
- **Prevention and Treatment of Anaphylaxis:** Assess for urticaria and for patency of airway.
- **Allergic Rhinitis:** Assess degree of nasal stuffiness, rhinorrhea, and sneezing.
- **Parkinsonism and Extrapyramidal Reactions:** Assess movement disorder prior to and following administration.
- **Insomnia:** Assess sleep patterns.
- **Motion Sickness and Nausea Associated with Chemotherapy:** Assess nausea, vomiting, bowel sounds, and abdominal pain.
- **Cough Suppressant:** Assess frequency and nature of cough, lung sounds, and amount and type of sputum produced. Unless contraindicated, maintain fluid intake of 1500–2000 ml daily to decrease viscosity of bronchial secretions.
- **Pruritis:** Assess degree of itching and skin rash and inflammation.
- **Lab Test Considerations:** Diphenhydramine may decrease skin response to allergy tests. Discontinue 4 days prior to skin testing.

POTENTIAL NURSING DIAGNOSES

- Sleep pattern disturbance (indications).
- Fluid volume deficit, high risk for (indications).
- Injury, high risk for (side effects).

IMPLEMENTATION

- **General Info:** When used for insomnia, administer 20 min before bedtime and schedule nursing activities to minimize interruption of sleep.
  - When used for prophylaxis of motion sickness administer at least 30 min and preferably 1–2 hr before exposure to conditions that may precipitate motion sickness.
- **PO:** Administer with meals or milk to minimize GI irritation. Capsule may be emptied and contents taken with water or food.
- **IM:** Administer into well-developed muscle. Avoid SC injections.
- **Direct IV:** May give undiluted. May be further diluted in 0.9% NaCl, 0.45% NaCl, D5W, D10W, D5/0.9% NaCl, D5/0.45% NaCl, D5/0.25% NaCl, Ringer's solution, lactated Ringer's solution, and dextrose/Ringer's combinations.
- **Rate:** Inject 25 mg over at least 1 min.
- **Syringe Compatibility:** ■ atropine ■ butorphanol ■ chlorpromazine ■ cimetidine ■ dimenhydrinate ■ droperidol ■ fentanyl ■ glycopyrrolate ■ hydromorphone ■ hydroxyzine ■ meperidine ■ metoclopramide ■ midazolam ■ morphine ■ nalbuphine ■ pentazocine ■ perphenazine ■ prochlorperazine ■ promazine ■ promethazine ■ ranitidine ■ scopolamine. Compatible only for brief periods; prepare immediately before injection.
- **Syringe Incompatibility:** ■ pentobarbital ■ phenobarbital ■ phenytoin ■ thiopental.
- **Y-Site Compatibility:** ■ acyclovir ■ fluconazole ■ fludarabine ■ heparin ■ hydrocortisone ■ meperidine ■ ondansetron ■ potassium chloride.
- **Y-Site Incompatibility:** ■ foscarnet.

PATIENT/FAMILY TEACHING

- **General Info:** Instruct patient to take medication exactly as directed; do not exceed recommended amount.
  - May cause drowsiness and sedation. Advise patient to avoid driving or other activities requiring alertness until response to drug is known.

▫ Inform patient that this drug may cause dry mouth. Frequent oral rinses, good oral hygiene, and sugarless gum or candy may minimize this effect. Notify dentist if dry mouth persists for more than 2 wk.

▫ Advise patient to use sunscreen and protective clothing to prevent photosensitivity reactions.

▫ Caution patient to avoid use of alcohol and other CNS depressants concurrently with this medication.

▫ Advise patients taking diphenhydramine in OTC preparations to notify the physician if symptoms worsen or persist for more than 7 days.

▪ Top: Instruct patient to cleanse affected skin prior to application, to avoid application to raw or blistered skin, and to discontinue use and contact physician if irritation occurs.

EVALUATION

Effectiveness of therapy can be demonstrated by: ▪ Prevention of or decreased urticaria in anaphylaxis or other allergic reactions ▪ Decreased dyskinesia in parkinsonism and extrapyramidal reactions ▪ Sedation when used as a sedative/hypnotic ▪ Prevention of or decreased nausea and vomiting caused by motion sickness ▪ Decrease in frequency and intensity of cough without eliminating cough reflex.

DIFENOXIN/ATROPINE
(dye-fen-**ox**-in/**a**-troe-peen)
Motofen

DIPHENOXYLATE/ATROPINE
(dye-fen-**ox**-i-late/**a**-troe-peen)
Diphenatol, Lofene, Logen, Lomanate, Lomotil, Lonox, Lo-Trol, Nor-mil

CLASSIFICATION(S):
Antidiarrheal
Schedule IV (difenoxin/atropine),
V (diphenoxylate/atropine)
Pregnancy Category C

INDICATIONS

▪ Adjunctive therapy in the treatment of diarrhea.

ACTION

▪ Inhibits excess GI motility ▪ Structurally related to narcotic analgesics but has no analgesic properties ▪ Atropine added to discourage abuse. **Therapeutic Effect:** ▪ Decreased GI motility with subsequent decrease in diarrhea.

PHARMACOKINETICS

Absorption: Well absorbed from the GI tract.
Distribution: Distribution not known. Enters breast milk.
Metabolism and Excretion: Diphenoxylate is mostly metabolized by the liver with some conversion to an active antidiarrheal compound (difenoxin). Difenoxin is metabolized by the liver to inactive compounds. Minimal excretion in the urine.
Half-life: 2.5 hr (diphenoxylate).

CONTRAINDICATIONS AND PRECAUTIONS

Contraindicated in: ▪ Hypersensitivity ▪ Severe liver disease ▪ Infectious diarrhea (due to *E. Coli, Salmonella,* or *Shigella*) ▪ Diarrhea associated with Pseudomembranous colitis ▪ Dehydrated patients ▪ Narrow-angle glaucoma ▪ Children <2 yr ▪ Known alcohol intolerance (some liquid diphenoxylate products only).

Use Cautiously in: ▪ Patients physically addicted to opioid analgesics ▪ Inflammatory bowel disease ▪ Prostatic hypertrophy ▪ Pregnancy and lactation (safety not established) ▪ Children (especially children with Down's syndrome—increased sensitivity to atropine) ▪ Difenoxin not recommended for use in children <12 yr.

ADVERSE REACTIONS AND SIDE EFFECTS*

CNS: *difenoxin*—dizziness, lightheadedness, drowsiness, headache, tired-

---

*Underlines indicate most frequent; CAPITALS indicate life-threatening.

ness, nervousness, insomnia, confusion; *diphenoxylate*—<u>drowsiness</u>, dizziness.
EENT: *difenoxin*—blurred vision, burning eyes; *diphenoxylate*—blurred vision, dry eyes.
CV: *diphenoxylate*—tachycardia.
GI: *diphenoxylate*—<u>constipation</u>, ileus, dry mouth; *difenoxin*—nausea, vomiting, constipation, dry mouth, epigastric distress.
GU: *diphenoxylate*—urinary retention.
Derm: *diphenoxylate*—flushing.

INTERACTIONS
Drug–Drug: ▪ Additive CNS depression with other **CNS depressants** including **alcohol, antihistamines, opioid analgesics,** and **sedative/hypnotics** ▪ Additive anticholinergic properties with other **drugs having anticholinergic properties** including **tricyclic antidepressants** and **disopyramide** ▪ Use with **MAO inhibitors** may result in hypertensive crisis.

ROUTE AND DOSAGE
Diphenoxylate/Atropine
Doses given are in terms of diphenoxylate—each tablet contains 2.5 mg diphenoxylate with 0.025 mg of atropine; each 5 ml of liquid contains 2.5 mg diphenoxylate with 0.025 mg of atropine.
▪ **PO (Adults):** 2.5–5 mg 3–4 times daily initially then 2.5 mg 2–3 times daily (not to exceed 20 mg/day).
▪ **PO (Children 9–12 yr):** 1.75–2.5 mg 4 times daily.
▪ **PO (Children 6–9 yr):** 1.25–2.5 mg 4 times daily.
▪ **PO (Children 5–6 yr):** 1.25–2.25 mg 4 times daily.
▪ **PO (Children 4–5 yr):** 1–2 mg 4 times daily.
▪ **PO (Children 3–4 yr):** 1–1.5 mg 4 times daily.
▪ **PO (Children 2–3 yr):** 0.75–1.5 mg 4 times daily.

Difenoxin/Atropine
Doses given are in terms of difenoxin—each tablet contains 1 mg difenoxin with 0.025 mg of atropine.
▪ **PO (Adults):** 2 tablets initially then

1 tablet after each loose stool or every 3–4 hr as needed (not to exceed 8 tablets/day).

AVAILABILITY
Diphenoxylate/Atropine
▪ *Tablets:* 2.5 mg diphenoxylate/0.025 mg atropine ▪ *Liquid:* (some products contain alcohol) 2.5 mg diphenoxylate/0.025 mg atropine per 5 ml.
Difenoxin/Atropine
▪ *Tablets:* 1 mg difenoxin/0.025 mg atropine.

TIME/ACTION PROFILE (antidiarrheal action)

	ONSET	PEAK	DURATION
PO (difenoxin)	45–60 min	2 hr	3–4 hr
PO (diphenoxylate)	45–60 min	2 hr	3–4 hr

NURSING IMPLICATIONS
ASSESSMENT
▫ Assess the frequency and consistency of stools and bowel sounds prior to and throughout course of therapy.
▫ Assess patient's fluid and electrolyte balance and skin turgor for dehydration.
▪ **Lab Test Considerations:** Liver function tests should be evaluated periodically during prolonged therapy.
▫ Diphenoxylate/atropine may cause increased serum amylase concentrations.

POTENTIAL NURSING DIAGNOSES
▪ Diarrhea (indications).
▪ Constipation (side effects).
▪ Knowledge deficit related to medication regimen (patient/family teaching).

IMPLEMENTATION
▪ **General Info:** Risk of dependence increases with high-dose, long-term use. Atropine has been added to discourage abuse.
▪ **PO:** Diphenoxylate/atropine tablets may be administered with food if GI irritation occurs. Tablets may be crushed and administered with patient's fluid of choice. Use calibrated

measuring device for liquid preparations.

PATIENT/FAMILY TEACHING

☐ Instruct patient to take medication exactly as directed. Do not take more than the prescribed amount because of the habit-forming potential and risk of overdose in children.

☐ Medication may cause drowsiness. Advise patient to avoid driving or other activities requiring alertness until response to drug is known.

☐ Advise patient that frequent mouth rinses, good oral hygiene, and sugarless gum or candy may relieve dry mouth.

☐ Caution patient to avoid alcohol and other CNS depressants concurrently with this medication.

☐ Instruct patient to notify physician if diarrhea persists or if fever, abdominal pain, or palpitations occur.

EVALUATION

Effectiveness of therapy can be demonstrated by: ■ Decrease in diarrhea. Treatment should be continued for 24–36 hr before it is considered ineffective in treatment of acute diarrhea.

DIPYRIDAMOLE

(dye-peer-**id**-a-mole)

{Apo-Dipyridamole}, Persantine, Persantine IV

CLASSIFICATION(S):
Antiplatelet agent, Diagnostic agent (coronary vasodilator)
Pregnancy Category B

INDICATIONS

■ **PO:** Prevention of thromboembolism in patients with prosthetic heart valves (with warfarin) ■ **PO:** Maintains patency after surgical grafting procedures, including coronary artery bypass (with aspirin) ■ **IV:** Diagnostic agent in lieu of exercise during thallium myocardial perfusion imaging.

ACTION

■ **PO:** Decreases platelet aggregation by inhibiting the enzyme phosphodiesterase ■ **IV:** Produces coronary vasodilation by inhibiting adenosine uptake. **Therapeutic Effects:** ☐ *PO:* Inhibition of platelet aggregation and subsequent thromboembolic events ☐ *IV:* In diagnostic thallium imaging dipyridamole dilates normal coronary arteries, reducing flow to vessels that are narrowed and causing abnormal thallium distribution.

PHARMACOKINETICS

Absorption: Moderately absorbed (30–60%) after oral administration.
Distribution: Widely distributed. Crosses the placenta. Enters breast milk.
Metabolism and Excretion: Metabolized by the liver, excreted in the bile.
Half-life: 10 hr.

CONTRAINDICATIONS AND PRECAUTIONS

Contraindicated in: ■ Hypersensitivity.
Use Cautiously in: ■ Hypotensive patients ■ Patients with platelet defects ■ Pregnancy (although safety not established, has been used without harm during pregnancy) ■ Lactation or children <12 yr (safety not established).

ADVERSE REACTIONS AND SIDE EFFECTS*

CNS: <u>headache</u>, <u>dizziness</u>, weakness, syncope; IV only—transient cerebral ischemia.
CV: flushing, <u>hypotension</u>; IV only—MYOCARDIAL INFARCTION, arrhythmias.
Resp: IV only—bronchospasm.
GI: GI upset, <u>nausea</u>, vomiting, diarrhea.
Derm: rash.

INTERACTIONS

Drug–Drug: ■ Additive effects with **aspirin** on platelet aggregation ■ Risk of

---

bleeding may be increased when used with **anticoagulants, thrombolytics, non-steroidal anti-inflammatory agents,** or **sulfinpyrazone** ▪ Increased risk of hypotension with **alcohol** ▪ **Theophylline** may negate the effects of dipyridamole during diagnostic thallium imaging.

ROUTE AND DOSAGE

▪ **PO (Adults):** 75–100 mg 4 times daily in divided doses.
▪ **IV (Adults):** 570 mcg/kg.

AVAILABILITY

▪ *Tablets:* 25 mg, 50 mg, 75 mg ▪ *Injection:* 10 mg/2 ml.

TIME/ACTION PROFILE
(PO = antiplatelet activity,
IV = coronary vasodilation)

	ONSET	PEAK	DURATION
PO	UK	UK	UK
IV	UK	6.5 min*	30 min

*From start of infusion.

NURSING IMPLICATIONS

ASSESSMENT

▪ **PO:** Monitor blood pressure and pulse before instituting therapy and regularly during period of dosage adjustment.
▪ **IV:** Monitor vital signs during and for 10–15 min following infusion. Obtain ECG in at least 1 lead. If severe chest pain or bronchospasm occurs, administer IV aminophylline 50–250 mg at a rate of 50–100 mg over 30–60 sec. If hypotension is severe, place patient in a supine position with head tilting down. If chest pain is unrelieved with aminophylline 250 mg, administer nitroglycerin SL. If chest pain is still unrelieved, treat as myocardial infarction.
▪ **Lab Test Considerations:** Bleeding time should be monitored periodically throughout course of therapy.

POTENTIAL NURSING DIAGNOSES

▪ Cardiac output, decreased (indications).
▪ Pain (indications).

▪ Knowledge deficit related to medication regimen (patient/family teaching).

IMPLEMENTATION

▪ **PO:** Administer with a full glass of water at least 1 hr before or 2 hr after meals for faster absorption. If GI irritation occurs, may be administered with or immediately after meals. Tablets may be crushed and mixed with food if patient has difficulty swallowing. Pharmacist may make a suspension.
▪ **Intermittent Infusion:** Dilute in at least a 1:2 ratio of 0.45% NaCl, 0.9% NaCl, or D5W for a total volume of 20–50 ml. Undiluted dipyridamole may cause venous irritation.
▪ *Rate:* Infuse dose over 4 min.

PATIENT/FAMILY TEACHING

▪ **PO:** Instruct patient to take medication at evenly spaced intervals as prescribed. If a dose is missed, take as soon as remembered unless the next scheduled dose is within 4 hr. Do not double doses. Benefit of medication may not be apparent to patient; encourage patient to continue taking medication as directed.
▫ Caution patient to make position changes slowly to minimize orthostatic hypotension.
▫ Advise patient to avoid the use of alcohol, as it may potentiate the hypotensive effects. Tobacco products should also be avoided because nicotine causes vasoconstriction.
▫ Advise patient to consult physician or pharmacist before taking over-the-counter medications concurrently with this medication.
▫ Instruct patient to notify physician if unusual bleeding or bruising occurs.
▪ **IV:** Instruct patient to notify physician immediately if dyspnea or chest pain occurs.

EVALUATION

Effectiveness of therapy can be demonstrated by: ▪ Prevention of postoperative thromboembolic complications associated with prosthetic heart valves ▪ Maintenance of patency after

D

surgical graft procedures ▪ Coronary vasodilation in thallium myocardial perfusion imaging.

DISOPYRAMIDE
(dye-soe-**peer**-a-mide)
Norpace, Norpace CR, {Rythmodan}, {Rythmodan-LA}

CLASSIFICATION(S):
Antiarrhythmic (group I)
Pregnancy Category C

INDICATIONS

▪ Suppression and prevention of unifocal and multifocal PVCs, paired PVCs, and ventricular tachycardia. **Unlabeled Use:** ▪ Treatment and prevention of supraventricular tachyarrhythmias.

ACTION

▪ Decreases myocardial excitability and conduction velocity ▪ May depress myocardial contractility ▪ Also has anticholinergic properties ▪ Little effect on heart rate, but has a direct negative inotropic effect. **Therapeutic Effect:** ▪ Suppression of ventricular arrhythmias.

PHARMACOKINETICS

Absorption: Well absorbed from the GI tract.
Distribution: Widely distributed throughout extracellular fluid. Enters breast milk.
Metabolism and Excretion: Metabolized by the liver. 10% excreted unchanged in the feces, 50% excreted unchanged by the kidneys.
Half-life: 8–18 hr (increased in hepatic or renal impairment).

CONTRAINDICATIONS AND PRECAUTIONS

Contraindicated in: ▪ Hypersensitivity ▪ Cardiogenic shock ▪ 2nd-degree and 3rd-degree heart block ▪ Sick sinus syndrome (without a pacemaker).

Use Cautiously in: ▪ Left ventricular dysfunction (use lower doses) ▪ Possible cardiac decompensation (dosage reduction recommended) ▪ Hepatic or renal insufficiency (dosage reduction recommended if CCr ≤40 ml/min) ▪ Elderly men with prostatic enlargement ▪ Myasthenia gravis ▪ Glaucoma ▪ Pregnancy or lactation (safety not established).

ADVERSE REACTIONS AND SIDE EFFECTS*

CNS: blurred vision, dizziness, headache, fatigue.
CV: CONGESTIVE HEART FAILURE, edema, dyspnea, AV block, hypotension.
EENT: dry eyes, dry throat.
GI: <u>dry mouth</u>, <u>constipation</u>, nausea, abdominal pain, flatulence.
GU: <u>urinary hesitancy</u>, <u>retention</u>.
Endo: hypoglycemia.
Misc: impaired temperature regulation.

INTERACTIONS

Drug–Drug: ▪ May potentiate anticoagulant effect of **warfarin** ▪ **Rifampin, phenobarbital,** and **phenytoin** may decrease blood levels and effectiveness ▪ **Cimetidine** may decrease metabolism and increase blood levels ▪ May have additive toxic cardiac effects when used with other **antiarrhythmics** (prolonged conduction and decreased cardiac output), especially **verapamil**—avoid using disopyramide for 48 hr before or 24 hr after ▪ Anticholinergic side effects may be additive with other **drugs having anticholinergic properties** including **antihistamines** and **tricyclic antidepressants** ▪ Increased risk of arrhythmias with **pimozide**.

ROUTE AND DOSAGE

▪ **PO (Adults >50 kg):** 300 mg initially as immediate-release capsules followed by 150 mg q 6 hr (as immediate-release capsules) or 300 mg q 12 hr as CR or LA dosage form (up to 800 mg/day).

{} = Available in Canada only.

*<u>Underlines</u> indicate most frequent; **CAPITALS** indicate life-threatening.

- **PO (Adults <50 kg or patients with left ventricular dysfunction):** 200 mg initially as immediate-release capsules followed by 400 mg/day— 100 mg q 6 hr (as immediate-release capsules) or 200 mg q 12 hr as CR or LA dosage form.
- **PO (Children 12–18 yr):** 6–15 mg/kg daily, in divided doses q 6 hr.
- **PO (Children 4–12 yr):** 10–15 mg/kg daily in divided doses q 6 hr.
- **PO (Children 1–4 yr):** 10–20 mg/kg daily in divided doses q 6 hr.
- **PO (Children <1 yr):** 10–30 mg/kg daily in divided doses q 6 hr.

AVAILABILITY

- *Capsules:* 100 mg, 150 mg ▪ *Extended-release capsules:* 100 mg, 150 mg ▪ {*Extended-release tablets:* 250 mg}.

TIME/ACTION PROFILE
(antiarrhythmic effects)

	ONSET	PEAK	DURATION
PO	0.5–3.5 hr	2.5 hr	1.5–8.5 hr
PO-CR	0.5–3.5 hr	4.9 hr	12 hr

NURSING IMPLICATIONS

ASSESSMENT

- Monitor blood pressure, pulse, and ECG prior to and routinely throughout therapy. Check pulse prior to administering medication; withhold and notify physician if <60 or >120 bpm, or if changes in rhythm occur.
- Monitor intake and output ratios and daily weight; assess for edema and urinary retention daily.
- Assess patient for signs of congestive heart failure (peripheral edema, rales/crackles, dyspnea, weight gain, jugular venous distention). Notify physician if these occur.
- **Lab Test Considerations:** Renal and hepatic functions and serum potassium levels should be evaluated periodically throughout therapy.
- May cause elevated serum BUN, cholesterol, and triglyceride levels.
- May cause decreased blood glucose concentrations.

POTENTIAL NURSING DIAGNOSES

- Cardiac output, decreased (indications).
- Oral mucous membranes, altered: (side effects).
- Knowledge deficit related to medication regimen (patient/family teaching).

IMPLEMENTATION

- **General Info:** When changing from quinidine sulfate or procainamide to disopyramide, regular maintenance dose of disopyramide may be given 6–12 hr after last dose of quinidine sulfate or 3–6 hr after last dose of procainamide.
- Extended-release form (CR capsules or LA tablets) is indicated for maintenance therapy only. When changing from regular form to extended-release forms, give the first dose of extended-release form 6 hr after the last regular dose.
- **PO:** Administer medication on an empty stomach, 1 hr before or 2 hr after meals. Controlled-release capsules (CR) and long-acting tablets (LA) must be swallowed whole; do not break open, crush, or chew.
- Pharmacist may prepare a suspension with 100 mg capsules and cherry syrup.

PATIENT/FAMILY TEACHING

- Advise patient to take medication around the clock, exactly as directed. Do not discontinue medication without consulting physician. If a dose is missed, take as soon as remembered unless within 4 hr of next dose. Do not double doses.
- Medication may cause dizziness. Caution patients to avoid driving or other activities requiring alertness until response to medication is known.
- Instruct patient to make position changes slowly to minimize orthostatic hypotension.
- Advise patient that frequent mouth rinses, good oral hygiene, and sugarless gum or candy may help relieve dry mouth.
- Caution patient to avoid extremes of

temperature, as this medication may cause impairment of body temperature regulation. Patient should use sunscreen and protective clothing to prevent photosensitivity reactions.

□ Advise patient to consult physician or pharmacist prior to taking over-the-counter medications or alcohol concurrently with this medication.

□ If constipation becomes a problem, advise patient that increasing bulk and fluids in the diet and exercise may minimize constipation.

□ Instruct patient to notify physician if dry mouth, difficult urination, constipation, or blurred vision persist.

EVALUATION

Effectiveness of therapy can be demonstrated by: ▪ Suppression of PVCs and ventricular tachycardia ▪ Prevention of further arrhythmias.

DISULFIRAM
(dye-**sul**-fi-ram)
Antabuse

CLASSIFICATION(S):
Alcohol abuse deterrent
Pregnancy Category UK

INDICATIONS

▪ Management of alcohol dependence
▪ Discourages further abuse of alcohol in programs combining support and psychotherapy.

ACTION

▪ Inhibits the enzyme aldehyde dehydrogenase, resulting in accumulation of toxic concentrations of acetaldehyde following ingestion of alcohol. **Therapeutic Effect:** ▪ Production of uncomfortable hypersensitivity reaction following alcohol ingestion (disulfiram reaction or acetaldehyde syndrome).

PHARMACOKINETICS

Absorption: Rapidly absorbed following oral administration, but effect is delayed.

Distribution: Initially distributes to fat.

Metabolism and Excretion: Metabolized by the liver. 5–20% excreted unchanged in feces.

Half-life: UK. Up to 20% remains in the body for 7 days.

CONTRAINDICATIONS AND PRECAUTIONS

Contraindicated in: ▪ Previous allergic reactions to disulfiram or rubber contact dermatitis (thiuram derivatives) ▪ Alcohol intoxication ▪ Cardiovascular disease ▪ Psychoses.

Use Cautiously in: ▪ Diabetes mellitus ▪ Hypothyroidism ▪ Seizures or abnormal EEG ▪ Cerebral hemorrhage ▪ Nephritis ▪ History of liver disease ▪ History of drug dependence ▪ Pregnancy, lactation, or children (safety not established).

ADVERSE REACTIONS AND SIDE EFFECTS*

CNS: drowsiness, fatigue, impotence, headache, vertigo, insomnia, abnormal gait, slurred speech, disorientation, confusion, personality changes, seizures, delirium, psychoses, bizarre behavior, encephalopathy.

EENT: optic neuritis.

GI: hepatitis.

GU: impotence.

Derm: acneform rash, allergic dermatitis.

Hemat: blood dyscrasias.

Neuro: peripheral neuropathy, polyneuritis.

Misc: ingestion or application of alcohol results in disulfiram reaction (see Drug–Drug Interactions).

INTERACTIONS

Drug–Drug: ▪ Concurrent use with **alcohol** in any form (cough and cold preparations, skin liniments, aftershaves) will produce the disulfiram reaction ▪ Disulfiram increases blood levels and the risk of toxicity of **phenytoin, isoniazid, metronidazole, diazepam, chlordiazepoxide,** and **paraldehyde.**

---

*Underlines indicate most frequent; **CAPITALS** indicate life-threatening.

Drug–Food: ▪ Concurrent use with any food containing **alcohol** will result in disulfiram reaction.

ROUTE AND DOSAGE

▪ **PO (Adults):** 500 mg/day for 1–2 wk, then 250 mg/day (range 125–500 mg/day).

AVAILABILITY

▪ *Tablets:* 250 mg, 500 mg.

TIME/ACTION PROFILE (ability to produce disulfiram reaction following exposure to alcohol)

	ONSET	PEAK	DURATION
PO	5–10 min (3–12 hr)*	UK	1–2 wk

*Onset of reaction is 5–10 min following alcohol ingestion during chronic dosing. After initial dose, reaction may be delayed up to 12 hr.

NURSING IMPLICATIONS

ASSESSMENT

▢ Assess patient for use of alcohol in any form within the 12 hr prior to administration of disulfiram. Patients should be free of alcohol intake for at least 12 hr prior to initiation of therapy.

▪ **Lab Test Considerations:** Monitor CBC periodically and SMA-12 levels every 6 mo throughout therapy.

▢ Doses of 500 mg/day may cause an increase in serum cholesterol concentrations.

▢ Monitor hepatic function tests prior to and at periodic intervals during therapy. May cause elevated AST (SGOT) and ALT (SGPT) levels.

POTENTIAL NURSING DIAGNOSES

▪ Coping, ineffective individual (indications).

▪ Knowledge deficit related to medication regimen (patient/family teaching).

IMPLEMENTATION

▪ **General Info:** Disulfiram should *never* be administered without the patient's knowledge.

▢ Check alcohol content of other medications patient is taking prior to administration. Do not administer within 12 hr of alcohol-containing preparations.

▢ The alcohol-disulfiram test is considered unnecessary by most clinicians and may be associated with increased drug toxicity. Explicit descriptions of the reaction following ingestion of alcohol are considered sufficient to deter the patient from ingesting alcohol during treatment. If the test is considered necessary, it should be performed under careful medical supervision with adequate facilities, including oxygen, in the event of a severe reaction. This test should not be performed on patients over 50 yr. The test consists of slowly administering 15 ml of 100-proof alcohol after 1–2 wk of disulfiram therapy. The dose may be repeated once but should not exceed 30 ml of alcohol. Discontinue alcohol at the first sign of symptoms.

▪ **PO:** Tablets may be crushed and mixed with beverages.

▢ If daytime drowsiness occurs, dose may be given at bedtime.

PATIENT/FAMILY TEACHING

▢ Inform patient and family of the nature of the medication, the disulfiram-alcohol reaction, and its consequences. Instruct patient in the importance of compliance with disulfiram therapy. Alcohol in all forms, including beer, wine, liquor, vinegars, cough mixtures, sauces, aftershave lotions, liniments, and colognes, should be avoided. Advise patient that alcohol intake within 12 hr prior to or 14 days following administration may cause the disulfiram-alcohol reaction (blurred vision, chest pain, confusion, dizziness or fainting, fast or pounding heartbeat, flushing or redness of face, nausea, vomiting, dyspnea, unusual sweating, severe weakness, seizures, myocardial infarction, unconsciousness, death). Effects of this reaction may last 30 min to several hours.

▢ Advise patient to check all medications for alcohol content.

▢ Medication may cause drowsiness.

Caution patient to avoid driving or other activities requiring alertness until response to drug is known.
□ Caution patient to avoid taking CNS depressants during disulfiram therapy.
□ Instruct patient to carry identification describing medication regimen at all times. Physician should be notified if visual changes or rash occur.
□ Emphasize the importance of follow-up visits to the physician to monitor progress in long-term therapy and participation in alcohol-abuse therapy.

EVALUATION

Effectiveness of therapy can be demonstrated by: ▪ Maintenance of sobriety in the treatment of chronic alcoholism or avoidance of alcohol intake.

DOBUTAMINE
(doe-**byoo**-ta-meen)
Dobutrex

CLASSIFICATION(S):
Inotropic agent
Pregnancy Category UK

INDICATIONS

▪ Short-term management of heart failure due to depressed contractility from organic heart disease or surgical procedures.

ACTION

▪ Stimulates beta$_1$ (myocardial) adrenergic receptors with relatively minor effect on heart rate or peripheral blood vessels. **Therapeutic Effect:** ▪ Increased cardiac output without significantly increasing heart rate.

PHARMACOKINETICS

Absorption: Administered by IV infusion only, resulting in complete bioavailability.
Distribution: Distribution not known.
Metabolism and Excretion: Metabolized by the liver and other tissues.

Half-life: 2 min.

CONTRAINDICATIONS AND PRECAUTIONS

Contraindicated in: ▪ Hypersensitivity ▪ Hypersensitivity to bisulfites (contains bisulfite) ▪ Idiopathic hypertropic subaortic stenosis.
Use Cautiously in: ▪ Myocardial infarction ▪ Atrial fibrillation (pretreatment with cardiac glycosides recommended) ▪ Pregnancy, lactation, and children (safety not established).

ADVERSE REACTIONS AND SIDE EFFECTS*

CNS: headache.
Resp: shortness of breath.
CV: <u>tachycardia</u>, <u>hypertension</u>, <u>premature ventricular contractions</u>, angina pectoris.
GI: nausea, vomiting.
Misc: nonanginal chest pain.

INTERACTIONS

Drug–Drug: ▪ Use with **nitroprusside** may have a synergistic effect on increasing cardiac output ▪ **Beta-adrenergic blocking agents** may negate the effect of dobutamine ▪ Increased risk of arrhythmias or hypertension with some **anesthetics (cyclopropane, halothane), MAO inhibitors, oxytocics,** or **tricyclic antidepressants**.

ROUTE AND DOSAGE

See infusion rate chart in Appendix D.
▪ **IV (Adults):** 2.5–15 mcg/kg/min.

AVAILABILITY

▪ *Injection:* 250 mg/20-ml vial.

TIME/ACTION PROFILE (inotropic effects)

	ONSET	PEAK	DURATION
IV	1–2 min	10 min	brief (min)

NURSING IMPLICATIONS

ASSESSMENT

□ Monitor blood pressure, heart rate, ECG, pulmonary capillary wedge pressure (PCWP), cardiac output, central venous pressure (CVP), and urinary output continuously during the administration of this medication.

□ An increase in systolic blood pressure of 10–20 mmHg and an increase in heart rate of 5–15 bpm occurs in most patients. Observe patient closely for extreme increases in blood pressure, heart rate, or ectopy. This may indicate a need for dosage reduction. Notify physician.

□ Diabetic patients may require an increase in insulin. Monitor blood glucose levels closely.

■ **Toxicity and Overdose:** If overdose occurs, reduction or discontinuation of therapy is the only treatment necessary due to the short duration of dobutamine.

POTENTIAL NURSING DIAGNOSES

■ Cardiac output, decreased (indications).
■ Tissue perfusion, altered: (indications).

IMPLEMENTATION

■ **General Info:** Correct hypovolemia with volume expanders prior to initiating dobutamine therapy.

■ **IV:** Reconstitute 250-mg vial with 10 ml of Sterile Water or D5W for Injection. If not completely dissolved, add another 10 ml of diluent. Dilute in at least 50 ml of D5W, 0.9% NaCl, sodium lactate, 0.45% NaCl, D5/0.45% NaCl, D5/0.9% NaCl, D5/LR, or lactated Ringer's solution. Standard concentrations range from 250 mcg/ml to 1000 mcg/ml. Concentrations should not exceed 5 mg of dobutamine per ml. Slight pink color of solution does not alter potency. Solution is stable for 24 hr at room temperature.

■ **Continuous Infusion:** Administer via infusion pump. Rate of administration is titrated according to patient response (heart rate, presence of ectopic activity, blood pressure, urine output, CVP, PCWP, cardiac output); see Appendix D.

■ **Y-Site Compatibility:** ■ amrinone ■ atracurium ■ bretylium ■ calcium chloride ■ calcium gluconate ■ diazepam ■ dopamine ■ enalaprilat ■ famotidine ■ insulin ■ lidocaine ■ magnesium sulfate ■ meperidine ■ nitroglycerin ■ pancuronium ■ potassium chloride ■ protamine ■ ranitidine ■ sodium nitroprusside ■ streptokinase ■ tobramycin ■ tolazoline ■ vecuronium ■ verapamil ■ zidovudine.

■ **Y-Site Incompatibility:** ■ acyclovir ■ alteplase ■ aminophylline ■ foscarnet ■ phytonadione.

PATIENT/FAMILY TEACHING

□ Explain to patient the rationale for instituting this medication and the need for frequent monitoring.

□ Instruct patient to notify nurse immediately of pain or discomfort at the site of administration.

EVALUATION

Effectiveness of therapy can be demonstrated by: ■ Increase in cardiac output
□ Improved hemodynamic parameters
□ Increased urine output.

DOCUSATE
(dok-yoo-sate)

DOCUSATE CALCIUM
DC Softgels, Pro-Cal-Sof, Sulfalax, Surfak

DOCUSATE POTASSIUM
Dialose, Diocto-K, Kasof

DOCUSATE SODIUM
Colace, Dioeze, Diocto, Diosul, Disonate, DOK, DOS Softgels, DOSS, Doxinate, DSS, Laxinate 100, Modane Soft, Regulax SS, {Regulex}, Regutol, Therevac, Therevac SB

CLASSIFICATION(S):
Laxative (stool softener)
Pregnancy Category C

INDICATIONS

■ **PO:** Prevention of constipation (in patients who should avoid straining, such as after myocardial infarction or rectal surgery) ▪ **Rectal:** Used by enema to soften fecal impaction.

ACTION

▪ Promotes incorporation of water into stool, resulting in softer fecal mass ▪ May also promote electrolyte and water secretion into the colon. **Therapeutic Effect:** ▪ Softening and passage of stool.

PHARMACOKINETICS

Absorption: Small amounts may be absorbed from the small intestine after oral administration. Absorption from the rectum is not known.
Distribution: Distribution not known.
Metabolism and Excretion: Amounts absorbed after oral administration are eliminated in bile.
Half-life: UK.

CONTRAINDICATIONS AND PRECAUTIONS

Contraindicated in: ▪ Hypersensitivity ▪ Abdominal pain, nausea, or vomiting especially when associated with fever or other signs of an acute abdomen.
Use Cautiously in: ▪ Excessive or prolonged use may lead to dependence ▪ Has been used during pregnancy and lactation ▪ Should not be used if prompt results are desired.

ADVERSE REACTIONS AND SIDE EFFECTS*

EENT: throat irritation.
GI: mild cramps.
Derm: rashes.

INTERACTIONS

Drug–Drug: None significant.

ROUTE AND DOSAGE

Docusate Calcium
▪ **PO (Adults):** 240 mg once daily.
▪ **PO (Children ≥6 yr and Adults With Minimal Requirements):** 50–150 mg once daily.

Docusate Potassium
▪ **PO (Adults):** 100–300 mg once daily.

▪ **PO (Children ≥6 yr):** 100 mg once daily at bedtime.

Docusate Sodium
▪ **PO (Adults and Older Children):** 50–500 mg once daily.
▪ **PO (Children 6–12 yr):** 40–120 mg once daily.
▪ **PO (Children 3–6 yr):** 20–60 mg once daily.
▪ **PO (Children <3 yr):** 10–40 mg.
▪ **Rect—Enema (Adults):** 50–100 mg or 1 unit containing 283 mg docusate sodium, soft soap, and glycerin.

AVAILABILITY

Docusate Calcium
▪ *Capsules:* 50 mg, 240 mg.
Docusate Potassium
▪ *Capsules:* 100 mg, 240 mg.
Docusate Sodium
▪ *Tablets:* 100 mg ▪ *Capsules:* 50 mg, 100 mg, 240 mg, 250 mg ▪ *Syrup:* 50 mg/15 ml, 60 mg/15 ml ▪ *Liquid:* 150 mg/15 ml ▪ *Solution:* 50 mg/ml ▪ *Enema:* 283 mg/3.9-g capsule ▪ *In combination with:* Stimulant laxatives. See Appendix A.

TIME/ACTION PROFILE (softening of stool)

	ONSET	PEAK	DURATION
PO	1–3 days	UK	UK
Rectal	min–hr	UK	UK

NURSING IMPLICATIONS

ASSESSMENT
▫ Assess patient for abdominal distention, presence of bowel sounds, and usual pattern of bowel function.
▫ Assess color, consistency, and amount of stool produced.

POTENTIAL NURSING DIAGNOSES
▪ Constipation (indications).
▪ Knowledge deficit related to medication regimen (patient/family teaching).

IMPLEMENTATION
▪ **General Info:** This medication does not stimulate intestinal peristalsis.

*Underlines indicate most frequent; **CAPITALS** indicate life-threatening.

- **PO:** Administer with a full glass of water or juice. May be administered on an empty stomach for more rapid results.
- Oral solution may be diluted in milk or fruit juice to decrease bitter taste.

PATIENT/FAMILY TEACHING
- Advise patients that laxatives should be used only for short-term therapy. Long-term therapy may cause electrolyte imbalance and dependence.
- Encourage patients to use other forms of bowel regulation, such as increasing bulk in the diet, increasing fluid intake, increasing mobility. Normal bowel habits are variable and may vary from 3 times/day to 3 times/wk.
- Instruct patients with cardiac disease to avoid straining during bowel movements (Valsalva maneuver).
- Advise patient not to use laxatives when abdominal pain, nausea, vomiting, or fever is present.

EVALUATION
Effectiveness of therapy can be demonstrated by: ▪ A soft, formed bowel movement, usually within 24–48 hr. May require 3–5 days of therapy for results.

DOPAMINE
(dope-a-meen)
Dopastat, Intropin, {Revimine}

CLASSIFICATION(S):
Vasopressor, Inotropic agent
Pregnancy Category C

INDICATIONS
▪ Adjunct to standard measures to improve: □ Blood pressure □ Cardiac output □ Urine output in treatment of shock unresponsive to fluid replacement.

ACTION
▪ Small doses (0.5–2 mcg/kg/min) stimulate dopaminergic receptors, producing renal vasodilation ▪ Larger doses (2–10 mcg/kg/min) stimulate dopaminergic and beta$_1$-adrenergic recep-

tors, producing cardiac stimulation and renal vasodilation ▪ Doses greater than 10 mcg/kg/min stimulate alpha-adrenergic receptors and may cause renal vasoconstriction. **Therapeutic Effects:** ▪ Increased cardiac output, increased blood pressure, and improved renal blood flow.

PHARMACOKINETICS
Absorption: Administered IV only, resulting in complete bioavailability.
Distribution: Widely distributed after IV administration, but does not cross the blood–brain barrier.
Metabolism and Excretion: Metabolized in liver, kidneys, and plasma.
Half-life: 2 min.

CONTRAINDICATIONS AND PRECAUTIONS
Contraindicated in: ▪ Tachyarrhythmias ▪ Pheochromocytoma ▪ Hypersensitivity to bisulfites (some products).
Use Cautiously in: ▪ Occlusive vascular diseases ▪ Pregnancy, lactation, and children (safety not established).

ADVERSE REACTIONS AND SIDE EFFECTS*
CNS: headache.
EENT: mydriasis (high dose).
Resp: dyspnea.
CV: arrhythmias, hypotension, palpitations, angina, ECG change, vasoconstriction.
GI: nausea, vomiting.
Derm: piloerection.
Local: irritation at IV site.

INTERACTIONS
Drug–Drug: ▪ Use with **MAO inhibitors** or **ergot alkaloids (ergotamine)** results in severe hypertension ▪ Use with **IV phenytoin** may cause hypotension and bradycardia ▪ Use with **general anesthetics** may result in arrhythmias ▪ **Beta-adrenergic blockers** may antagonize cardiac effects.

ROUTE AND DOSAGE
See infusion rate table in Appendix D.

- **IV (Adults):** 0.5–5 mcg/kg/min initially, increase at 10–30 min intervals up to 50 mcg/kg/min.

AVAILABILITY

- *Injection:* 40 mg/ml, 80 mg/ml, 160 mg/ml.

TIME/ACTION PROFILE
(hemodynamic effects)

	ONSET	PEAK	DURATION
IV	5 min	rapid	<10 min

NURSING IMPLICATIONS

ASSESSMENT

- Monitor blood pressure, pulse, respiration, ECG, and hemodynamic parameters every 5–15 min during and after administration. Notify physician if significant changes in vital signs or arrhythmias occur. Consult physician for parameters for pulse, blood pressure, or ECG changes for adjusting dosage or discontinuing medication.
- Monitor urine output frequently throughout administration. Notify physician promptly if urine output decreases.
- Palpate peripheral pulses and assess appearance of extremities routinely throughout dopamine administration. Notify physician if quality of pulse deteriorates or if extremities become cold or mottled.
- If hypotension occurs, administration rate should be increased. If hypotension continues, more potent vasoconstrictors (norepinephrine) may be administered.
- **Toxicity and Overdose:** If excessive hypertension occurs, rate of infusion should be decreased or temporarily discontinued until blood pressure is decreased. Although additional measures are usually not necessary due to short duration of dopamine, phentolamine may be administered if hypertension continues.

POTENTIAL NURSING DIAGNOSES

- Cardiac output, decreased (indications).

- Tissue perfusion, altered (indications).

IMPLEMENTATION

- **General Info:** Hypovolemia should be corrected prior to administration of dopamine.
- Administer into a large vein, and assess administration site frequently. Extravasation may cause severe irritation, necrosis, and sloughing of tissue. If extravasation occurs, affected area should be infiltrated with 10–15 ml of 0.9% NaCl containing 5–10 mg of phentolamine.
- **Continuous Infusion:** Dilute 200–400 mg in 250–500 ml of 0.9% NaCl, D5W, D5/LR, D5/0.45% NaCl, D5/ 0.9% NaCl, or in lactated Ringer's solution for IV infusion. Concentrations commonly used are 800 mcg/ml or 0.8 mg/ml (200 mg/250 ml) and 1.6 mg/ml (400 mg/250 ml). Dilute immediately prior to administration. Yellow or brown discoloration indicates decomposition. Discard solution that is cloudy, discolored, or contains a precipitate. Solution is stable for 24 hr.
- *Rate:* Administer at a rate of 0.5–5 mcg/kg/min, and increase by 1–4 mcg/kg/min at 10–30 min intervals until desired dosage is obtained. Infusion must be administered via infusion pump to ensure precise amount delivered. Rate of administration is titrated according to patient response (blood pressure, heart rate, urine flow, peripheral perfusion, presence of ectopic activity, cardiac output); see Appendix D.
- **Y-Site Compatibility:** ▪ amrinone ▪ atracurium ▪ dobutamine ▪ esmolol ▪ famotidine ▪ foscarnet ▪ heparin ▪ hydrocortisone sodium succinate ▪ labetalol ▪ lidocaine ▪ meperidine ▪ morphine ▪ nitroglycerin ▪ pancuronium ▪ potassium chloride ▪ ranitidine ▪ sodium nitroprusside ▪ streptokinase ▪ tolazoline ▪ vecuronium ▪ verapamil ▪ vitamin B complex with C ▪ zidovudine.
- **Y-Site Incompatibility:** ▪ acyclovir ▪ alteplase.

D

PATIENT/FAMILY TEACHING

□ Advise patient to inform nurse immediately if chest pain, dyspnea, numbness, tingling, or burning of extremities occurs.

□ Instruct patient to inform nurse immediately of pain or discomfort at the site of administration.

EVALUATION

Effectiveness of therapy can be demonstrated by: ▪ Increase in blood pressure □ Increase in peripheral circulation □ Increase in urine output.

DOXACURIUM

(dox-a-**cure**-ee-yum)
Nuromax

CLASSIFICATION(S):
Neuromuscular blocking agent
(nondepolarizing)
Pregnancy Category C

INDICATIONS

▪ Induction of skeletal muscle paralysis and facilitation of intubation after induction of anesthesia in surgical procedures.

ACTION

▪ Prevents neuromuscular transmission by blocking the effect of acetylcholine at the myoneural junction. Has no analgesic or anxioytic properties. **Therapeutic Effect:** ▪ Skeletal muscle paralysis.

PHARMACOKINETICS

Absorption: Administered IV only, resulting in complete bioavailability.
Distribution: Distribution not known.
Metabolism and Excretion: Excreted primarily unchanged in urine and bile.
Half-life: 90–120 min (increased in kidney transplant patients).

CONTRAINDICATIONS AND PRECAUTIONS

Contraindicated in: ▪ Hypersensitivity to doxacurium or benzyl alcohol ▪ New-

born infants (benzyl alcohol may produce fatal reactions).
Use Cautiously in: ▪ Pregnancy, lactation, or children <2 yr (safety not established) ▪ Elderly patients (slower onset of neuromuscular blockade) ▪ Electrolyte or acid base abnormalities (unpredictable response) ▪ Burn patients (may have resistance) ▪ Neuromuscular diseases (exaggerated response).

ADVERSE REACTIONS AND SIDE EFFECTS*

Almost all adverse reactions to doxacurium are extensions of pharmacologic effects.
Resp: APNEA, respiratory insufficiency.
CV: hypotension.
Derm: flushing.
MS: muscle weakness.

INTERACTIONS

Drug–Drug: ▪ **Carbamazepine** and **phenytoin** decrease duration of block and increase time of onset ▪ Intensity and duration of paralysis may be prolonged by **aminoglycoside antibiotics, polymyxin B, colistin, clindamycin, lidocaine, quinidine, procainamide, beta-adrenergic blocking agents, potassium-losing diuretics,** and **magnesium** ▪ **Isoflurane, enflurane, halothane,** or **succinylcholine** potentiate effects (decrease doxacurium dosage).

ROUTE AND DOSAGE

▪ **IV (Adults):** 50 mcg/kg (may need up to 80 mcg/kg for prolonged effect; 25 mcg/kg for succinylcholine-assisted intubation) initially, followed 60–100 min later by 5–10 mcg/kg, repeated as required.

▪ **IV (Children 2–12 yr):** 30–50 mcg/kg initially, maintenance doses may be required more frequently than in adults.

AVAILABILITY

▪ *Injection:* 1 mg/ml.

---

*Underlines indicate most frequent; **CAPITALS** indicate life-threatening.

TIME/ACTION PROFILE (skeletal muscle paralysis)

	ONSET	PEAK	DURATION
IV*	5 min	UK	100 min

*For a 0.05 mg/kg dose in an adult.

NURSING IMPLICATIONS

ASSESSMENT

□ Assess respiratory status continuously throughout doxacurium therapy. Doxacurium should be used only by individuals experienced in endotracheal intubation, and equipment for this procedure should be readily available.

□ Neuromuscular response to doxacurium should be monitored with a peripheral nerve stimulator. Paralysis is initially selective and usually occurs sequentially in the following muscles: levator muscles of eyelids, muscles of mastication, limb muscles, abdominal muscles, muscles of the glottis, intercostal muscles, and the diaphragm. Recovery of muscle function usually occurs in reverse order.

□ Observe the patient for residual muscle weakness and respiratory distress during the recovery period.

▪ **Toxicity and Overdose:** If overdose occurs, use peripheral nerve stimulator to determine the degree of neuromuscular blockade. Maintain airway patency and ventilation until recovery of normal respirations occurs.

□ Administration of anticholinesterase agents (neostigmine, pyridostigmine) may be used to antagonize the action of doxacurium once the patient has demonstrated some spontaneous recovery from neuromuscular block. Atropine is usually administered prior to or concurrently with anticholinesterase agents to counteract the muscarinic effects.

□ Administration of fluids and vasopressors may be necessary to treat severe hypotension or shock.

POTENTIAL NURSING DIAGNOSES

▪ Breathing pattern, ineffective (indications).

▪ Communication, impaired: verbal (side effects).

▪ Fear (side effects).

IMPLEMENTATION

▪ **General Info:** Dose is titrated to patient response.

□ Doxacurium has no effect on consciousness or the pain threshold. Adequate anesthesia should *always* be used when doxacurium is used as an adjunct to surgical procedures.

□ Store at room temperature.

▪ **Direct IV:** Administer initial IV dose as a bolus over 1 min. Maintenance dose is usually required 60 min following initial dose of 0.025 mg/kg or 100 min following initial dose of 0.05 mg/kg. May be diluted further in D5W or 0.9% NaCl. Use diluted doxacurium within 8 hr. Discard unused diluted doxacurium after 8 hr.

▪ *Rate:* Administer every 30–45 min.

▪ **Y-Site Compatibility:** ▪ D5/0.9% NaCl ▪ LR ▪ D5/LR ▪ alfentanil ▪ fentanyl ▪ sufentanil.

▪ **Additive Incompatibility:** Incompatible with most barbiturates or sodium bicarbonate; do not administer in the same syringe or through the same needle during infusion.

PATIENT/FAMILY TEACHING

□ Explain all procedures to patient receiving doxacurium therapy without anesthesia, as consciousness is not affected by atracurium alone.

□ Reassure patient that communication abilities will return as the medication wears off.

EVALUATION

Effectiveness of therapy can be demonstrated by: ▪ Adequate suppression of the twitch response when tested with peripheral nerve stimulation and subsequent muscle paralysis.

DOXAPRAM
(dox-a-pram)
Dopram

INDICATIONS

- Used in carefully selected short-term situations with other supportive measures to treat postoperative CNS and respiratory depression due to CNS depressants ▪ Short-term postoperative stimulation of deep breathing with other supportive measures ▪ Prevention of acute hypercapnea during administration of oxygen to patients with acute respiratory insufficiency due to COPD (short-term only—less than 2 hr).

ACTION

- In low doses, stimulates breathing by activating carotid receptors ▪ Larger doses directly stimulate the respiratory center in medulla as well as produce generalized CNS stimulation. **Therapeutic Effect:** ▪ Transient increase in tidal volume, small increase in respiratory rate. Oxygenation is not increased.

PHARMACOKINETICS

Absorption: Administered IV only, results in complete bioavailability.
Distribution: Distribution in humans not known.
Metabolism and Excretion: Rapidly metabolized. Metabolites mostly excreted by the kidneys.
Half-life: 2.4–4 hr.

CONTRAINDICATIONS AND PRECAUTIONS

Contraindicated in: ▪ Hypersensitivity ▪ Patients on ventilators ▪ Head trauma ▪ Seizures ▪ Flail chest ▪ Pulmonary embolism ▪ Pneumothorax ▪ Pulmonary fibrosis ▪ Acute asthma ▪ Extreme dyspnea ▪ Cardiovascular or cerebrovascular disease ▪ Newborns (contains benzyl alcohol).
Use Cautiously in: ▪ Patients with a history of asthma or arrhythmias ▪ Increased intracranial pressure ▪ Hyperthyroidism ▪ Pheochromocytoma ▪ Serious uncorrected metabolic disorders ▪ Pregnancy, lactation, or children <12 yr (safety not established) ▪ Should not be used routinely as a respiratory stimulant.

ADVERSE REACTIONS AND SIDE EFFECTS*

CNS: SEIZURES†, headache, dizziness, apprehension, disorientation.
EENT: miosis, sneezing, gagging.
Resp: dyspnea†, bronchospasm, laryngospasm, coughing, rebound hypoventilation.
CV: elevated blood pressure†, tachycardia†, arrhythmias†, hypotension, chest pain, changes in heart rate, T-wave inversion.
GI: nausea, vomiting, diarrhea, desire to defecate.
GU: perineal or genital burning sensation, urinary retention, spontaneous voiding.
Derm: flushing, sweating, pruritus.
Hemat: hemolysis.
Local: irritation at IV site.
Metab: hyperpyrexia.
MS: skeletal muscle hyperactivity†, muscle spasticity†, involuntary movement†.
Neuro: paresthesia, positive bilateral Babinski's sign, generalized clonus.

INTERACTIONS

Drug–Drug: ▪ Pressor effects may be increased by concurrent use of **sympathomimetic amines** or **MAO inhibitors** ▪ May mask effects of **skeletal muscle relaxants**.

ROUTE AND DOSAGE

Respiratory Depression Following Anesthesia

- **IV (Adults):** 0.5–1 mg/kg (not to exceed 1.5 mg/kg) initially, may repeat every 5 min to a total of 2 mg/kg or as an infusion at 5 mg/min until response is obtained, then decrease infusion rate to 1–3 mg/min (total dose

†Early signs of toxicity.
*Underlines indicate most frequent; **CAPITALS** indicate life-threatening.

by infusion method should not exceed 4 mg/kg).

Drug-Induced CNS Depression

■ **IV (Adults):** 2 doses of 1–2 mg/kg may be repeated at 5-min intervals. Can repeat in 1–2 hr until spontaneous breathing or total of 3 g/24 hr given. If response occurs in 1–2 hr, can infuse at rate of 1–3 mg/min for up to 2 hr. Total dose not to exceed 3 g/24 hr.

Acute Hypercapnea

■ **IV (Adults):** 1–2 mg/min (up to 3 mg/min). Should not be used for more than 2 hr.

AVAILABILITY

■ *Injection:* 20 mg/ml.

TIME/ACTION PROFILE (increases in minute volume)

	ONSET	PEAK	DURATION
IV	20–40 sec	1–2 min	5–12 min

NURSING IMPLICATIONS

ASSESSMENT

□ Because of narrow margin of safety and indications for use, patient must be monitored constantly when receiving doxapram and for 1 hr after medication is discontinued and patient is fully alert.

□ Monitor respiratory status (rate, rhythm, and depth of respirations) and ABGs. Ensure that patient has patent airway and is adequately oxygenated. Relapse of respiratory depression may occur if CNS depressant has long duration of action. To encourage maximal chest expansion and to prevent aspiration, position patient on side; elevate head of bed.

□ Monitor neurologic status (level of consciousness and deep tendon reflexes). Notify physician if reflexes become hyperactive or if spasticity occurs.

□ Monitor vital signs, ECG, and hemodynamic parameters. May cause tachycardia, hypertension, increased cardiac output, increased pulmonary artery pressure. Notify physician if there is significant change in hemo-

dynamic parameters, arrhythmias, or chest pain. Patients with COPD may be at increased risk for arrhythmias because of hypoxia.

□ Obtain baseline weight to ensure correct dosage.

□ Inspect infusion site. May cause thrombophlebitis (erythema, swelling, and pain or skin irritation).

■ **Lab Test Considerations:** Monitor ABGs prior to and every 30 min during therapy. Notify physician immediately if ABGs deteriorate. Physician may order cessation of drug, intubation, and mechanical ventilation.

□ Monitor hemoglobin, hematocrit, erythrocyte, and leukocyte count. Rapid infusion may cause hemolysis.

□ May cause elevated BUN and proteinuria.

■ **Toxicity and Overdose:** Toxicity is manifested by severe hypertension, tachycardia, and hyperactive reflexes or seizures. Infusion should be stopped immediately. Seizures may be controlled with diazepam or a short-acting barbiturate. Resuscitative equipment should be available at all times.

POTENTIAL NURSING DIAGNOSES

■ Breathing pattern, ineffective (indications).

■ Knowledge deficit related to medication regimen (patient/family teaching).

IMPLEMENTATION

■ **Direct IV:** Administer over 5 min.

■ **Intermittent Infusion:** Dilute 250 mg in 250 ml of D5W, D10W, or 0.9% NaCl to yield a concentration of 1 mg/ml. Dilute 400 mg (20-mg vial) in 180 ml of IV fluid to yield a 2 mg/ml concentration. Dosages vary with patient's condition. Infusion is limited to 2 hr. Administer via infusion pump to ensure accurate dosage.

■ **Syringe Compatibility:** ■ bumetanide ■ chlorpromazine ■ cimetidine ■ hydroxyzine ■ imipramine ■ isoniazid ■ phytonadione ■ pyridoxine ■ terbutaline ■ thiamine.

■ **Syringe Incompatibility:** ■ aminophylline ■ ascorbic acid ■ dexamethasone ▪ folic acid ▪ furosemide ▪ hydrocortisone ▪ methylprednisolone.

PATIENT/FAMILY TEACHING

□ Instruct patient to notify nurse immediately if shortness of breath worsens.

EVALUATION

Effectiveness of therapy can be demonstrated by: ▪ Reversal of respiratory and nervous system depression associated with CNS depressants ▪ Postoperative respiratory depression not associated with skeletal muscle relaxants ▪ Prevention of acute respiratory insufficiency in patients with COPD. Doxapram is not used often because of its narrow margin of safety.

DOXAZOSIN
(dox-**ay**-zoe-sin)
Cardura

CLASSIFICATION(S):
Antihypertensive (peripherally acting antiadrenergic)
Pregnancy Category B

INDICATIONS

▪ Treatment of hypertension, alone or in combination with other agents.

ACTION

▪ Dilates both arteries and veins by blocking postsynaptic alpha$_1$-adrenergic receptors. **Therapeutic Effect:** ▪ Lowering of blood pressure.

PHARMACOKINETICS

Absorption: Well absorbed following oral administration.
Distribution: Distribution not known. Appears to enter breast milk. 98% bound to plasma proteins.
Metabolism and Excretion: Extensively metabolized by the liver.
Half-life: 22 hr.

CONTRAINDICATIONS AND PRECAUTIONS

Contraindicated in: ▪ Hypersensitivity.
Use Cautiously in: ▪ Pregnancy, lacta-
tion, or children (safety not established) ▪ Hepatic dysfunction.

ADVERSE REACTIONS AND SIDE EFFECTS*

CNS: <u>dizziness</u>, <u>headache</u>, depression, somnolence, nervousness, weakness, fatigue.
EENT: epistaxis, blurred vision, abnormal vision, conjunctivitis, vertigo.
Resp: dyspnea.
CV: <u>first dose orthostatic hypotension</u>, palpitations, arrhythmias, chest pain, edema.
GI: nausea, vomiting, dry mouth, diarrhea, constipation, abdominal discomfort, flatulence.
GU: decreased libido, sexual dysfunction.
Derm: flushing, rash.
MS: arthritis, arthralgia, myalgia, gout.

INTERACTIONS

Drug–Drug: ▪ Additive hypotension with acute ingestion of **alcohol,** other **antihypertensive agents,** or **nitrates** ▪ **Nonsteroidal anti-inflammatory agents** may decrease antihypertensive effects ▪ May decrease antihypertensive effect of **clonidine.**

ROUTE AND DOSAGE

▪ **PO (Adults):** 1 mg once daily at bedtime, may be gradually increased at 2-wk intervals to 2–16 mg/day, incidence of postural hypotension greatly increased at doses >4 mg/day.

AVAILABILITY

▪ *Tablets:* 1 mg, 2 mg, 4 mg, 8 mg.

TIME/ACTION PROFILE

	ONSET	PEAK	DURATION
PO	1–2 hr	2–6 hr	24 hr

NURSING IMPLICATIONS

ASSESSMENT

□ Monitor blood pressure and pulse frequently between 2–6 hr after a dose during initial dosage adjustment and with each increase in dose, and peri-

---

*<u>Underlines</u> indicate most frequent; **CAPITALS** indicate life-threatening.

odically throughout course of therapy. Notify physician of significant changes.

□ Assess patient for first dose orthostatic hypotension and syncope. Incidence may be dose related. Observe patient closely during this period and take precautions to prevent injury.

□ Monitor intake and output ratios and daily weight, and assess for edema daily, especially at beginning of therapy. Notify physician of weight gain or edema.

▪ **Lab Test Considerations:** May cause elevated serum sodium levels.

POTENTIAL NURSING DIAGNOSES

▪ Injury, high risk for (side effects).
▪ Knowledge deficit related to medication regimen (patient/family teaching).
▪ Noncompliance (patient/family teaching).

IMPLEMENTATION

□ May be administered concurrently with a diuretic or other antihypertensive.

PATIENT/FAMILY TEACHING

□ Emphasize the importance of continuing to take this medication, even if feeling well. Instruct patient to take medication at the same time each day. If a dose is missed, take as soon as remembered unless almost time for next dose. Do not double doses.

□ Encourage patient to comply with additional interventions for hypertension (weight reduction, low sodium diet, discontinuation of smoking, moderation of alcohol consumption, regular exercise, and stress management).

□ Instruct patient and family on proper technique for blood pressure monitoring. Advise them to check blood pressure at least weekly and report significant changes to physician.

□ Doxazosin may cause drowsiness or dizziness. Advise patient to avoid driving or other activities requiring alertness until response to medication is known.

□ Caution patient to avoid sudden changes in position to decrease orthostatic hypotension.

□ Advise patient to consult physician or pharmacist before taking any cough, cold, or allergy remedies. Patients should also avoid excessive amounts of coffee, tea, or cola.

□ Emphasize the importance of follow-up visits to determine effectiveness of therapy.

EVALUATION

Effectiveness of therapy can be measured by: ▪ Decrease in blood pressure without appearance of side effects.

DOXEPIN
(**dox**-e-pin)
Sinequan, {Triadapin}

CLASSIFICATION(S):
Antidepressant (tricyclic), Antianxiety agent
Pregnancy Category C

INDICATIONS

▪ Used in conjunction with psychotherapy in the management of various forms of endogenous depression ▪ Also used in the treatment of anxiety. **Unlabeled Use:** ▪ Management of chronic pain syndromes.

ACTION

▪ Prevents the reuptake of norepinephrine and serotonin by presynaptic neurons; resultant accumulation of neurotransmitters potentiates their activity ▪ Also possesses significant anticholinergic properties. **Therapeutic Effects:** ▪ Relief of depression ▪ Decreased anxiety.

PHARMACOKINETICS

Absorption: Well absorbed from the GI tract, although much is metabolized on first pass through the liver.
Distribution: Widely distributed. Enters breast milk. Probably crosses the placenta.

{} = Available in Canada only.

Metabolism and Excretion: Metabolized by the liver. Some conversion to active antidepressant compound. May re-enter gastric juice via secretion from enterohepatic circulation, where more absorption may occur.

Half-life: 8–25 hr.

CONTRAINDICATIONS AND PRECAUTIONS

Contraindicated in: ▪ Hypersensitivity ▪ Narrow-angle glaucoma ▪ Pregnancy or lactation ▪ Period immediately after myocardial infarction.

Use Cautiously in: ▪ Elderly patients (initial dosage reduction recommended) ▪ Pre-existing cardiovascular disease (increased risk of adverse reactions) ▪ Prostatic enlargement (more susceptible to urinary retention) ▪ Seizures ▪ Anticholinergic side effects (may require dosage modification or drug discontinuation) ▪ Dosage requires slow titration, therapeutic response may take up to 6 wk.

ADVERSE REACTIONS AND SIDE EFFECTS*

CNS: drowsiness, sedation, lethargy, fatigue, confusion, agitation, hallucinations.

EENT: blurred vision, increased intraocular pressure.

CV: hypotension, ECG abnormalities, arrhythmias.

GI: dry mouth, constipation, paralytic ileus, hepatitis, nausea, increased appetite.

GU: urinary retention.

Derm: rashes, photosensitivity.

Hemat: blood dyscrasias.

Misc: hypersensitivity reactions.

INTERACTIONS

Drug–Drug: ▪ May cause hypotension, tachycardia, and potentially fatal reactions when used with **MAO inhibitors** (avoid concurrent use—discontinue 2 wk prior to doxepin) ▪ May prevent the therapeutic response to most **antihypertensives** ▪ May cause severe hypertension when used with **clonidine** (avoid

concurrent use) ▪ Additive CNS depression with other **CNS depressants** including **alcohol, antihistamines, opioid analgesics,** and **sedative/hypnotics** ▪ **Adrenergic** and **anticholinergic** side effects may be additive with other agents having these properties ▪ **Cimetidine, fluoxetine, phenothiazines,** or **oral contraceptives** increase levels and may cause toxicity ▪ May produce transient delirium with **disulfiram** ▪ **Smoking** may increase metabolism and decrease effectiveness.

ROUTE AND DOSAGE

▪ **PO (Adults):** 25–150 mg/day single bedtime dose or 2–3 divided doses, increase gradually (up to 300 mg/day, single dose should not exceed 150 mg).

AVAILABILITY

▪ *Capsules:* 10 mg, 25 mg, 50 mg, 75 mg, 100 mg, 150 mg ▪ *Oral concentrate:* 10 mg/ml.

TIME/ACTION PROFILE
(antidepressant activity)

	ONSET	PEAK	DURATION
PO	2–3 wk	up to 6 wk	days–wks

NURSING IMPLICATIONS

ASSESSMENT

▪ **General Info:** Monitor blood pressure and pulse rate prior to and during initial therapy.

▪ **Depression:** Assess mental status frequently. Confusion, agitation, and hallucinations may occur during initiation of therapy and may require dosage reduction. Monitor mood changes. Assess for suicidal tendencies, especially during early therapy. Restrict amount of drug available to patient.

▪ **Anxiety:** Assess degree and manifestations of anxiety prior to and throughout therapy.

▪ **Pain:** Assess the type, location, and severity of pain prior to and periodically throughout therapy.

*Underlines indicate most frequent; **CAPITALS** indicate life-threatening.

- **Lab Test Considerations:** Assess leukocyte and differential blood counts, hepatic function, and serum glucose periodically. May cause elevated serum bilirubin and alkaline phosphatase levels. May cause bone marrow depression. Serum glucose may be increased or decreased.

POTENTIAL NURSING DIAGNOSES

- Coping, ineffective individual (indications).
- Injury, high risk for (side effects).
- Knowledge deficit related to medication regimen (patient/family teaching).

IMPLEMENTATION

- **General Info:** May be given as a single dose at bedtime to minimize sedation during the day. Dose increases should be made at bedtime because of sedation. Dose titration is a slow process; may take weeks to months.
- **PO:** Administer medication with or immediately following a meal to minimize gastric irritation. Capsules may be opened and mixed with foods or fluids if patient has difficulty swallowing.
- Oral concentrates must be diluted in at least 120 ml of water, milk, or juice. Do not mix with carbonated beverages or grape juice. Use calibrated measuring device to ensure accurate amount.

Patient/Family Teaching

- Instruct patient to take medication exactly as directed. Do not skip or double up on missed doses. Inform patient that at least 2 wk are needed before drug effects may be noticed. Abrupt discontinuation may cause nausea, headache, and malaise.
- Doxepin may cause drowsiness and blurred vision. Caution patient to avoid driving and other activities requiring alertness until response to the medication is known.
- Orthostatic hypotension, sedation, and confusion are common during early therapy, especially in the elderly. Protect patient from falls and advise patient to make position changes slowly.
- Advise patient to avoid alcohol or other CNS depressant drugs during and for at least 3–7 days after therapy has been discontinued.
- Advise patient to notify physician if urinary retention occurs or if dry mouth or constipation persists. Frequent rinses, good oral hygiene, and sugarless hard candy or gum may diminish dry mouth. An increase in fluid intake, fiber, and exercise may prevent constipation. If these symptoms persist, dosage reduction or discontinuation may be necessary.
- Caution patient to use sunscreen and protective clothing to prevent photosensitivity reactions.
- Inform patient of need to monitor dietary intake. Increase in appetite is possible and may lead to undesired weight gain.
- Advise patient to notify physician or dentist of medication regimen prior to treatment or surgery.
- Therapy for depression is usually prolonged. Emphasize the importance of follow-up examinations to monitor effectiveness and side effects.

EVALUATION

Effectiveness of therapy can be demonstrated by: ▪ Increased sense of well-being □ Renewed interest in surroundings □ Increased appetite □ Improved energy level □ Improved sleep ▪ Decrease in anxiety ▪ Decrease in chronic pain. Patients may require 2–6 wk of therapy before full therapeutic effects of medication are evident.

DOXORUBICIN
(dox-oh-**roo**-bi-sin)
Adriamycin PFS, Adriamycin RDF, Rubex

CLASSIFICATION(S):
Antineoplastic (anthracycline)
Pregnancy Category UK

INDICATIONS
■ Alone and in combination with other treatment modalities (surgery, radiation therapy) in the treatment of various solid tumors including: ▫ Breast ▫ Ovarian ▫ Bladder ▫ Bronchogenic carcinoma ■ Also useful in malignant lymphomas and leukemias.

ACTION
■ Inhibits DNA and RNA synthesis by forming a complex with DNA; (action is cell cycle-S phase specific) ■ Also has immunosuppressive properties. **Therapeutic Effect:** ■ Death of rapidly replicating cells, particularly malignant ones.

PHARMACOKINETICS
Absorption: Administered IV only, resulting in complete bioavailability.
Distribution: Widely distributed. Does not cross the blood–brain barrier.
Metabolism and Excretion: Mostly metabolized by the liver. Converted by liver to compound, which also has antineoplastic activity. Excreted predominantly in the bile, 50% as unchanged drug. Less than 5% eliminated unchanged in the urine.
Half-life: 16.7 hr.

CONTRAINDICATIONS AND PRECAUTIONS
Contraindicated in: ■ Hypersensitivity ■ Pregnancy or lactation.
Use Cautiously in: ■ Previous congestive heart failure or arrhythmias ■ Patients with childbearing potential ■ Infections ■ Depressed bone marrow reserve ■ Other chronic debilitating illnesses ■ Liver impairment (dosage reduction required if serum bilirubin >1.2 mg/dl).

ADVERSE REACTIONS AND SIDE EFFECTS*
CV: CARDIOMYOPATHY, ECG changes.
Derm: alopecia.
Endo: gonadal suppression.
GI: stomatitis, esophagitis, nausea, vomiting, diarrhea.

GU: red urine.
Hemat: anemia, leukopenia, thrombocytopenia.
Local: phlebitis at IV site, tissue necrosis.
Metab: hyperuricemia.
Misc: hypersensitivity reactions.

INTERACTIONS
Drug–Drug: ■ Additive bone marrow depression with other **antineoplastics** or **radiation therapy** ■ May aggravate skin reactions at previous **radiation therapy** sites ■ May increase risk of hemorrhagic cystitis from **cyclophosphamide** or hepatitis from **mercaptopurine** ■ Cardiac toxicity may be enhanced by **radiation therapy** or **cyclophosphamide** ■ May decrease antibody response to **live virus vaccines** and increase the risk of adverse reactions.

ROUTE AND DOSAGE
■ **IV (Adults):** 60–75 mg/m^2 daily repeat q 21 days or 25–30 mg/m^2 daily for 2–3 days, repeat q 3–4 wk or 20 mg/m^2/wk. Total cumulative dose should not exceed 550 mg/m^2 without monitoring of cardiac function.

AVAILABILITY
■ *Injection:* 10-mg, 20-mg, 50-mg, 100-mg, 150-mg vials.

TIME/ACTION PROFILE (effect on blood counts)

	ONSET	PEAK	DURATION
IV	10 days	14 days	21–24 days

NURSING IMPLICATIONS
ASSESSMENT
▫ Monitor blood pressure, pulse, respiratory rate, and temperature frequently during administration. Notify physician of significant changes.
▫ Assess for fever, chills, sore throat, and signs of infection. Notify physician if these symptoms occur.
▫ Monitor platelet count throughout therapy. Assess for bleeding (bleeding gums, bruising, petechiae, guaiac

*Underlines indicate most frequent; CAPITALS indicate life-threatening

stools, urine, and emesis). Avoid IM injections and rectal temperatures. Apply pressure to venipuncture sites for 10 min.
□ Anemia may occur. Monitor for increased fatigue, dyspnea, and orthostatic hypotension.
□ Monitor intake and output ratios, and inform physician if significant discrepancies occur. Encourage fluid intake of 2000–3000 ml/day. Physician may also order allopurinol and alkalinization of the urine to decrease serum uric acid levels and to help prevent urate stone formation.
□ Severe and protracted nausea and vomiting may occur as early as 1 hr after therapy and may last 24 hr. Parenteral antiemetic agents should be administered 30–45 min prior to therapy and routinely around the clock for the next 24 hr as indicated. Monitor amount of emesis and notify physician if emesis exceeds guidelines to prevent dehydration.
□ Monitor for development of signs of myocardial toxicity, which may be either acute and transient (ST segment depression, flattened T wave, sinus tachycardia, and extrasystoles) or of late onset and characterized by congestive heart failure (peripheral edema, dyspnea, rales/crackles, weight gain). Chest x-ray, echocardiography, ECGs and radionuclide angiography may be ordered prior to and periodically throughout therapy.
□ Assess injection site frequently for redness, irritation, or inflammation. Medication may infiltrate painlessly. If extravasation occurs, infusion must be stopped and restarted elsewhere to avoid damage to SC tissue. Standard treatments include leaving original needle in place, injecting the area with glucocorticoids, and applying ice compresses.
■ **Lab Test Considerations:** Monitor CBC and differential prior to and periodically throughout therapy. The leukocyte count nadir occurs 10–14 days after administration and recovery usually occurs by the 21st day.

Thrombocytopenia and anemia may also occur.
□ Monitor renal (BUN and creatinine) and hepatic (AST [SGOT], ALT [SGPT], LDH, and serum bilirubin) function prior to and periodically throughout course of therapy. May cause increased serum and urine uric acid concentrations.

POTENTIAL NURSING DIAGNOSES
■ Infection, high risk for (adverse reactions).
■ Nutrition, altered: less than body requirements (adverse reactions).
■ Knowledge deficit related to medication regimen (patient/family teaching).

IMPLEMENTATION
■ **General Info:** Solution should be prepared in a biologic cabinet. Wear gloves, gown, and mask while handling medication. Discard IV equipment in specially designated containers (see Appendix I).
□ Aluminum needles may be used to administer doxorubicin but should not be used during storage, as prolonged contact results in discoloration of solution and formation of a dark precipitate. Solution is red.
■ **Direct IV:** Dilute each 10 mg with 5 ml of 0.9% NaCl (nonbacteriostatic) for injection. Shake to dissolve completely. Do not add to IV solution. Reconstituted medication is stable for 24 hr at room temperature and 48 hr if refrigerated. Protect from sunlight.
■ *Rate:* Administer each dose over 3–5 minutes through Y-site or 3-way stopcock of a free-flowing infusion of 0.9% NaCl or D5W. Facial flushing and erythema along vein involved frequently occur when administration is too rapid.
■ **Syringe Compatibility:** ■ bleomycin ■ cisplatin ■ cyclophosphamide ■ droperidol ■ fluorouracil ■ leucovorin calcium ■ methotrexate ■ metoclopromide ■ mitomycin ■ vincristine.
■ **Syringe Incompatibility:** ■ furosemide ■ heparin.
■ **Y-Site Compatibility:** ■ bleomycin

▪ cisplatin ▪ cyclophosphamide ▪ droperidol ▪ fludarabine ▪ fluorouracil ▪ leucovorin calcium ▪ methotrexate ▪ metoclopromide ▪ mitomycin ▪ ondansetron ▪ sargramostim ▪ vinblastine ▪ vincristine.

▪ **Y-Site Incompatibility:** ▪ aminophylline ▪ cephalothin ▪ dexamethasone ▪ furosemide ▪ heparin.

PATIENT/FAMILY TEACHING

□ Instruct patient to notify physician promptly if fever, sore throat, signs of infection, bleeding gums, bruising, petechiae, blood in stools or urine, emesis, increased fatigue, dyspnea, or orthostatic hypotension occur. Caution patient to avoid crowds and persons with known infections. Instruct patient to use soft toothbrush and electric razor and to avoid falls. Patients should be cautioned not to drink alcoholic beverages or take medication containing aspirin or ibuprofen, as these may precipitate gastric bleeding.

□ Instruct patient to report pain at injection site immediately.

□ Instruct patient to inspect oral mucosa for erythema and ulceration. If ulceration occurs advise patient to use sponge brush, rinse mouth with water after eating and drinking, and confer with physician if mouth pain interferes with eating. The risk of developing stomatitis is greatest 5–10 days after a dose; the usual duration is 3–7 days.

□ Advise patient that this medication may have teratogenic effects. Contraception should be used during and for at least 4 mo after therapy is concluded. Inform patient before initiating therapy that this medication may cause irreversible gonadal suppression.

□ Instruct patient to notify physician immediately if irregular heartbeat, shortness of breath, or swelling of lower extremities occurs.

□ Discuss the possibility of hair loss with patient. Explore methods of coping. Regrowth usually occurs 2–3 mo after discontinuation of therapy.

□ Instruct patient not to receive any vaccinations without advice of physician.

□ Inform patient that medication may cause urine to appear red for 1–2 days.

□ Instruct patient to notify physician if skin irritation occurs at site of previous radiation therapy.

□ Emphasize the need for periodic lab tests to monitor for side effects.

EVALUATION

Effectiveness of therapy can be demonstrated by: ▪ Decrease in size or spread of malignancies in solid tumors ▪ Improvement of hematologic status in leukemias.

D

DOXYCYCLINE
(dox-i-**sye**-kleen)
{Apo-Doxy}, Doryx, Doxy, Doxy-Caps, Doxychel, {Doxycin}, Monodox, {Novodoxyclin}, Vibramycin, Vibra-Tabs, Vovox

CLASSIFICATION(S):
Anti-infective (tetracycline)
Pregnancy Category UK

INDICATIONS

▪ Used most commonly in the treatment of infections due to unusual organisms including: □ *Mycoplasma* □ *Chlamydia* □ *Rickettsia* ▪ Also useful in the treatment of gonorrhea and syphilis in penicillin-allergic patients. **Unlabeled Uses:** ▪ Treatment of "traveler's diarrhea" ▪ Prevention of exacerbations of chronic bronchitis □ Treatment of Lyme disease.

ACTION

▪ Inhibits bacterial protein synthesis at the level of the 30S ribosome. **Therapeutic Effect:** ▪ Bacteriostatic action against susceptible bacteria. **Spectrum:** ▪ Some gram-positive pathogens:

□ *Bacillus anthracis* □ *Clostridium perfringens* □ *Clostridium tetani* □ *Listeria monocytogenes* □ *Nocardia* □ *Propionbacterium acnes* □ *Actinomyces isrealii* ■ Some gram-negative pathogens: □ *Haemophilus influenzae* □ *Legionella pneumophila* □ *Versinia entercolitica* □ *Versinia pestis* □ *Neisseria gonorrhea* □ *Neisseria meningitidis* ■ Also active against several other pathogens, including: □ *Mycoplasma* □ *Treponema pallidum* □ *Chlamydia* □ *Rickettsia* □ *Borrelia burgdorferi.*

PHARMACOKINETICS

Absorption: Well absorbed from the GI tract.
Distribution: Widely distributed, some penetration into CSF. Crosses the placenta and enters breast milk.
Metabolism and Excretion: 20–40% excreted unchanged by the urine. Some inactivation in the intestine and some enterohepatic circulation with excretion in bile and feces.
Half-life: 14–17 hr (increased in severe renal impairment).

CONTRAINDICATIONS AND PRECAUTIONS

Contraindicated in: ■ Hypersensitivity ■ Children <8 yr (permanent staining of teeth) ■ Pregnancy or lactation.
Use Cautiously in: ■ Cachectic or debilitated patients ■ Hepatic or renal disease.

ADVERSE REACTIONS AND SIDE EFFECTS*

GI: nausea, vomiting, diarrhea, pancreatitis, esophagitis, hepatotoxicity.
Hemat: blood dyscrasias.
Derm: rashes, photosensitivity.
Local: phlebitis at IV site.
Misc: superinfection, hypersensitivity reactions.

INTERACTIONS

Drug–Drug: ■ May enhance the effect of **oral anticoagulants** ■ **Barbiturates, phenytoin,** or **carbamazepine** may decrease the activity of doxycycline ■ May

decrease the effectiveness of **oral contraceptives** ■ **Calcium, iron,** or **magnesium** form chelates and decrease absorption (effect is less with doxycycline than with other tetracyclines).
Drug–Food: ■ **Calcium** in foods or dairy products decreases absorption by forming an insoluble chelate (effect is less with doxycycline than with other tetracyclines).

ROUTE AND DOSAGE

■ **PO, IV (Adults):** 100–200 mg/day given once daily or in divided doses q 12 hr.
■ **PO, IV (Children >8 yr):** 2.2–4.4 mg/kg/day given once daily or in divided doses q 12 hr.

AVAILABILITY

■ *Tablets:* 50 mg ■ *Capsules:* 50 mg, 100 mg ■ *Delayed-release capsules:* 100 mg ■ *Oral suspension:* 25 mg/5 ml ■ *Syrup:* 50 mg/5 ml ■ *Injection:* 100-mg, 200-mg vials.

TIME/ACTION PROFILE (blood levels)

	ONSET	PEAK
PO	1–2 hr	1.5–4 hr
IV	rapid	end of infusion

NURSING IMPLICATIONS

ASSESSMENT

□ Assess patient for infection (vital signs; appearance of wound, sputum, urine, and stool; WBC) at beginning and throughout course of therapy.
□ Obtain specimens for culture and sensitivity prior to initiating therapy. First dose may be given before receiving results.
□ Assess IV site frequently; may cause thrombophlebitis.
■ **Lab Test Considerations:** Renal, hepatic, and hematopoietic functions should be monitored periodically during long-term therapy.
□ May cause increased AST (SGOT), ALT (SGPT), serum alkaline phosphatase, bilirubin, and amylase concentrations. May interfere with urine

glucose testing with copper sulfate method (Clinitest); use glucose enzymatic tests (Tes-Tape, Ketodiastix).

POTENTIAL NURSING DIAGNOSES

- Infection, high risk for (indications, side effects).
- Knowledge deficit related to medication regimen (patient/family teaching).
- Noncompliance related to medication regimen (patient/family teaching).

IMPLEMENTATION

- **General Info:** May cause yellow-brown discoloration and softening of teeth and bones if administered prenatally or during early childhood. Not recommended for children under 8 yr or during pregnancy or lactation.
- **PO:** Administer the oral form of the drug around the clock. May be taken with food. Take with a full glass of liquid and at least 1 hr before going to bed to avoid esophageal ulceration. Use calibrated measuring for liquid preparations. Shake liquid preparations well. Do not administer within 1–3 hr of other medications.
- Avoid administration of calcium, antacids, magnesium-containing medications, or iron supplements within 1–3 hr of oral doxycycline.
- **Intermittent Infusion:** Dilute each 100 mg with 10 ml of Sterile Water or 0.9% NaCl for Injection. Dilute further in 100–1000 ml of 0.9% NaCl, D5W, D5/LR, Ringer's, or lactated Ringer's solution. Solution is stable for 12 hr at room temperature and 72 hr if refrigerated. If diluted with D5/LR or lactated Ringer's solution, administer within 6 hr. Protect solution from direct sunlight. Concentrations of less than 1 mcg/ml or greater than 1 mg/ml are not recommended.
- *Rate:* Administer over a minimum of 1–4 hr. Avoid rapid administration. Avoid extravasation.
- **Y-Site Compatibility:** ▪ acyclovir ▪ cyclophosphamide ▪ fludarabine ▪ hydromorphone ▪ magnesium sulfate ▪ meperidine ▪ morphine ▪ ondansetron ▪ perphenazine ▪ sargramostim.

PATIENT/FAMILY TEACHING

- Instruct patient to take medication around the clock and to finish the drug completely as directed, even if feeling better. Advise patient that sharing of this medication may be dangerous.
- Caution patient to use sunscreen and protective clothing to prevent photosensitivity reactions.
- Advise patient to report the signs of superinfection (black, furry overgrowth on the tongue, vaginal itching or discharge, loose or foul-smelling stools). Skin rash, pruritus, and urticaria should also be reported.
- Instruct patient to notify physician if symptoms do not improve.
- Caution patient to discard outdated or decomposed products, as they may be toxic.

EVALUATION

Clinical response to therapy can be evaluated by: ▪ Resolution of the signs and symptoms of infection. Length of time for complete resolution depends on the organism and site of infection.

DRONABINOL

(droe-**nab**-i-nol)
delta-9-tetrahydrocannabinol, THC, Marinol

CLASSIFICATION(S):
Antiemetic (cannabinoid)
Schedule II
Pregnancy Category B

INDICATIONS

▪ Prevention of serious nausea and vomiting from cancer chemotherapy when other more conventional agents have failed ▪ Management of anorexia, which may accompany the acquired immunodeficiency syndrome (AIDS).

ACTION

▪ Active ingredient in marijuana ▪ Has a wide variety of CNS effects, including inhibition of the vomiting control mechanism in the medulla oblongata. **Thera-**

peutic Effects: ▪ Suppression of nausea and vomiting ▪ Stimulates appetite in patients with AIDS.

PHARMACOKINETICS

Absorption: Extensively metabolized following absorption, resulting in poor bioavailability (10–20%).

Distribution: Enters breast milk in high concentrations. Highly lipid-soluble. Persists in tissues for prolonged period of time.

Metabolism and Excretion: Extensively metabolized. 50% excreted via biliary elimination. At least 1 metabolite is psychoactive.

Half-life: 25–36 hr.

CONTRAINDICATIONS AND PRECAUTIONS

Contraindicated in: ▪ Hypersensitivity to dronabinol, marijuana, or sesame oil ▪ Nausea and vomiting due to any other causes ▪ Should be used only in supervised patients ▪ Lactation.

Use Cautiously in: ▪ Patients who have abused drugs or been drug-dependent in the past ▪ Chronic use may lead to withdrawal syndrome on discontinuation ▪ Pregnancy (do not use unless clearly indicated) ▪ Safety in children <18 not established.

ADVERSE REACTIONS AND SIDE EFFECTS*

CNS: drowsiness, heightened awareness, dizziness, concentration difficulty, perceptual difficulty, coordination impairment, headache, irritability, depression, weakness, hallucinations, memory loss, ataxia, paranoia, disorientation, tinnitus, nightmares, speech difficulty, impaired judgment.

EENT: dry mouth, visual distortion.

CV: tachycardia, syncope.

GI: diarrhea.

Derm: facial flushing, perspiring.

MS: muscular pain.

Neuro: paresthesia.

Misc: physical dependence, psychological dependence (high doses or prolonged therapy).

INTERACTIONS

Drug–Drug: ▪ Additive CNS depression with **alcohol, antihistamines, opioid analgesics, tricyclic antidepressants,** and **sedative/hypnotics** ▪ Increased risk of tachycardia with **amphetamines, cocaine, sympathomimetics, anticholinergics, antihistamines,** and **tricyclic antidepressants.**

ROUTE AND DOSAGE

Antiemetic

▪ **PO (Adults):** 5 mg/m^2 1–3 hr prior to chemotherapy; may repeat every 2–4 hr after chemotherapy to a total of 4–6 doses/day. If initial dose is ineffective and no significant adverse reactions have occurred, dosage may be increased by 2.5 mg/m^2 to a maximum of 15 mg/m^2.

Appetite Stimulant

▪ **PO (Adults):** 2.5–10 mg/day in 1–2 divided doses (up to 20 mg/day).

AVAILABILITY

▪ *Gelatin capsules:* 2.5 mg, 5 mg, 10 mg.

TIME/ACTION PROFILE (antiemetic effect)

	ONSET	PEAK	DURATION
PO	UK	2 hr	6 hr

NURSING IMPLICATIONS

ASSESSMENT

▢ Assess nausea, vomiting, appetite, bowel sounds, and abdominal pain prior to and following the administration of this drug.

▢ Monitor hydration and nutritional status and intake and output. Patients with severe nausea and vomiting may require IV fluids in addition to antiemetics.

▢ Monitor blood pressure and heart rate periodically throughout therapy.

▢ Patients on dronabinol therapy should be monitored closely for side effects because the effects of dronabinol vary with each patient.

*Underlines indicate most frequent; **CAPITALS** indicate life-threatening.

POTENTIAL NURSING DIAGNOSES
- Fluid volume deficit, high risk for (indications).
- Nutrition, altered: less than body requirements (indications).
- Injury, high risk for (side effects).

IMPLEMENTATION
- **General Info:** Dronabinol capsules should be refrigerated but not frozen.
- Physical or psychological dependence may occur with high doses or prolonged therapy, causing a withdrawal syndrome (irritability, restlessness, insomnia, hot flashes, sweating, rhinorrhea, loose stools, hiccups, anorexia) when discontinued. This is unlikely to occur with therapeutic doses and short-term use of dronabinol.
- **Antiemetic:** This drug may be administered prophylactically 1–3 hr prior to chemotherapy and repeated every 2–4 hr after chemotherapy up to 4–6 doses daily.
- **Anorexia:** Give 2.5 mg bid before lunch and supper initially. Reduce dose to 2.5 mg/day in the evening or at bedtime for patients unable to tolerate 5 mg/day dose. May increase dose to 2.5 mg at lunch and 5 mg before supper or 5 mg at lunch and 5 mg after supper if further therapeutic effect is desired, and adverse effects are minimal. Most patients respond to 2.5 mg bid dose, but up to 10 mg bid has been tolerated in about 50% of patients. Adverse effects are usually dose related.

PATIENT/FAMILY TEACHING
- Instruct patient to take dronabinol exactly as directed. Take missed doses as soon as remembered but not if almost time for next dose; do not double doses. Signs of overdose (mood changes, confusion, hallucinations, depression, nervousness, fast or pounding heartbeat) may occur with increased doses.
- Advise patient to call for assistance when ambulating, as this drug may cause dizziness, drowsiness, and impaired judgment and coordination. Avoid driving or other activities requiring alertness until response to the drug is known.
- Instruct patient to make position changes slowly to minimize orthostatic hypotension.
- Caution patient to avoid taking alcohol or other CNS depressants during dronabinol therapy.
- Advise patient and family to use general measures to decrease nausea (begin with sips of liquids and small nongreasy meals, provide oral hygiene, remove noxious stimuli from environment).

EVALUATION
Effectiveness of therapy can be demonstrated by: ■ Prevention of and decrease in nausea and vomiting associated with chemotherapy ■ Decrease in anorexia in patients with AIDS.

DROPERIDOL
(droe-**per**-i-dole)
Inapsine

CLASSIFICATION(S):
Tranquilizer (butyrophenone),
Antiemetic (butyrophenone)
Pregnancy Category C

INDICATIONS
■ Used to produce tranquilization and as an adjunct to general and regional anesthesia ■ Also useful in decreasing postoperative or postprocedure nausea and vomiting ■ May be used in combination with fentanyl (see **Droperidol/Fentanyl**).

ACTION
■ Similar to haloperidol, alters the action of dopamine in the CNS. **Therapeutic Effects:** ■ Tranquilization ■ Suppression of nausea and vomiting in selected situations.

PHARMACOKINETICS
Absorption: Well absorbed following IM administration.

Distribution: Appears to cross the blood–brain barrier and placenta.

Metabolism and Excretion: Mainly metabolized by the liver. Only 10% excreted unchanged by the kidneys.

Half-life: UK.

CONTRAINDICATIONS AND PRECAUTIONS

Contraindicated in: ▪ Hypersensitivity ▪ Known intolerance ▪ Narrow-angle glaucoma ▪ Bone marrow depression ▪ CNS depression ▪ Severe liver or cardiac disease.

Use Cautiously in: ▪ Elderly, debilitated, or severely ill patients (smaller doses should be used) ▪ Diabetics ▪ Respiratory insufficiency ▪ Prostatic hypertrophy ▪ CNS tumors ▪ Intestinal obstruction ▪ Cardiac disease ▪ Seizures (may lower seizure threshold) ▪ Severe liver disease ▪ Pregnancy, lactation, and children <2 yr (although safety not established, droperidol has been used during cesarean section without respiratory depression in the newborn).

ADVERSE REACTIONS AND SIDE EFFECTS*

CNS: excessive sedation, extrapyramidal reactions, tardive dyskinesia, restlessness, confusion, hyperactivity, dizziness, nightmares, mental depression, hallucinations, SEIZURES, anxiety, abnormal EEG.

EENT: dry eyes, blurred vision.

Resp: bronchospasm, laryngospasm.

CV: hypotension, tachycardia.

GI: dry mouth, constipation.

Misc: chills, shivering, facial sweating.

INTERACTIONS

Drug–Drug: ▪ Additive hypotension with **antihypertensives** or **nitrates** ▪ Additive CNS depression with other **CNS depressants,** including **alcohol, antihistamines, antidepressants, opioid analgesics,** and other **sedatives.**

ROUTE AND DOSAGE

Premedication

▪ **IV, IM (Adults):** 2.5–10 mg 30–60 min prior to induction of anesthesia. Additional doses of 1.25–2.5 mg IV may be needed.

▪ **IM, IV (Children 2–12 yr):** 88–165 mcg/kg.

Adjunct for Induction of General Anesthesia (IV route preferred)

▪ **IM, IV (Adults):** 0.22–0.275 mg/kg with anesthetic or analgesic. Additional doses of 1.25–2.5 mg IV may be needed.

▪ **IM, IV (Children 2–12 yr):** 88–165 mcg/kg.

Adjunct for Maintenance of General Anesthesia

▪ **IV (Adults):** 1.25–2.5 mg.

Used without General Anesthesia During Diagnostic Procedures

▪ **IM (Adults):** 2.5–10 mg 30–60 min prior to procedure. Additional doses of 1.25–2.5 mg may be needed.

Adjunct in Regional Anesthesia

▪ **IM, IV (Adults):** 2.5–5 mg.

AVAILABILITY

▪ *Injection:* 2.5 mg/ml.

TIME/ACTION PROFILE (sedation)

	ONSET	PEAK	DURATION*
IM	3–10 min	30 min	2–4 hr
IV	3–10 min	30 min	2–4 hr

*Listed as duration of tranquilization; alterations in consciousness may last up to 12 hr.

NURSING IMPLICATIONS

ASSESSMENT

▪ **General Info:** Monitor blood pressure and heart rate frequently throughout course of therapy. Notify physician of significant changes immediately. Hypotension may be treated with parenteral fluids if hypovolemia is a causal factor. Vasopressors (norepinephrine, phenylephrine) may be needed. Avoid use of epinephrine, as droperidol reverses its pressor effects and may cause paradoxical hypotension.

□ Assess patient for level of sedation following administration.

□ Observe patient for extrapyramidal

---

*Underlines indicate most frequent; **CAPITALS** indicate life-threatening.

symptoms (dystonia, oculogyric crisis, extended neck, flexed arms, tremor, restlessness, hyperactivity, anxiety) throughout therapy. Notify physician should these occur. An anticholinergic antiparkinsonian agent may be used to treat these symptoms.
- **Nausea and Vomiting:** Assess nausea, vomiting, bowel sounds, and abdominal pain prior to and following administration.

POTENTIAL NURSING DIAGNOSES
- Injury, high risk for (side effects).
- Knowledge deficit related to medication regimen (patient/family teaching).

IMPLEMENTATION
- **IM/IV:** May be administered IM or IV.
- **Direct IV:** Administer each dose slowly over at least 1 min.
- **Intermittent Infusion:** May be added to 250 ml of D5W, 0.9% NaCl, or lactated Ringer's solution and administered by slow IV infusion.
- **Syringe Compatibility:** ▪ atropine ▪ bleomycin ▪ butorphanol ▪ chlorpromazine ▪ cimetidine ▪ cisplatin ▪ cyclophosphamide ▪ dimenhydrinate ▪ diphenhydramine ▪ doxorubicin ▪ fentanyl ▪ glycopyrrolate ▪ hydroxyzine ▪ meperidine ▪ metoclopramide ▪ midazolam ▪ mitomycin ▪ morphine ▪ nalbuphine ▪ pentazocine ▪ perphenazine ▪ prochlorperazine ▪ promazine ▪ promethazine ▪ scopolamine ▪ vinblastine ▪ vincristine.
- **Syringe Incompatibility:** ▪ fluorouracil ▪ furosemide ▪ heparin ▪ leucovorin calcium ▪ methotrexate ▪ pentobarbital.
- **Y-Site Compatibility:** ▪ bleomycin ▪ buprenorphine ▪ cisplatin ▪ cyclophosphamide ▪ doxorubicin ▪ fluconazole ▪ hydrocortisone sodium succinate ▪ meperidine ▪ metoclopramide ▪ mitomycin ▪ ondansetron ▪ potassium chloride ▪ sargramostim ▪ vinblastine ▪ vincristine ▪ vitamin B complex with C.
- **Y-Site Incompatibility:** ▪ fluorouracil

▪ foscarnet ▪ furosemide ▪ leucovorin calcium ▪ methotrexate ▪ nafcillin.
- **Additive Incompatibility:** ▪ barbiturates.

PATIENT/FAMILY TEACHING
□ Caution patient to make position changes slowly to minimize orthostatic hypotension.
□ Medication causes drowsiness. Advise patient to call for assistance during ambulation and transfer.

EVALUATION
Effectiveness of therapy can be demonstrated by: ▪ General quiescence and reduced motor activity ▪ Decreased nausea and vomiting.

D

DROPERIDOL/FENTANYL
(droe-**per**-i-dole/**fen**-ta-nil)
Innovar

CLASSIFICATION(S):
Combination butyrophenone (droperidol) plus opioid analgesic (fentanyl)
Schedule II
Pregnancy Category C

INDICATIONS
- Used to produce tranquilization and analgesia during diagnostic or surgical procedures ▪ Adjunct in various types of anesthesia.

ACTION
- *Droperidol* alters the action of dopamine in the CNS ▪ *Fentanyl* is an opioid analgesic that binds to opiate receptors in the CNS, altering the response to and perception of pain. **Therapeutic Effect of Combination:** ▪ Neuroleptanalgesia (quiescence, decreased motor activity, and analgesia without loss of consciousness).

PHARMACOKINETICS
Distribution: Droperidol appears to cross the blood–brain barrier and placenta.

Metabolism and Excretion: Both droperidol and fentanyl are mainly metabolized by the liver with small amounts (10–20%) excreted unchanged by the kidneys.
Half-life: UK for both drugs.

CONTRAINDICATIONS AND PRECAUTIONS

Contraindicated in: ▪ Hypersensitivity ▪ Known intolerance ▪ Narrow-angle glaucoma ▪ Bone marrow depression ▪ CNS depression ▪ Severe liver or cardiac disease.

Use Cautiously in: ▪ Elderly, debilitated, or severely ill patients (lower doses should be used) ▪ Diabetics ▪ Patients with severe pulmonary or hepatic disease ▪ Prostatic hypertrophy ▪ CNS tumors ▪ Increased intracranial pressure ▪ Head trauma ▪ Intestinal obstruction ▪ Undiagnosed abdominal pain ▪ Adrenal insufficiency ▪ Hypothyroidism ▪ Alcoholism ▪ Cardiac disease ▪ Seizures (may lower seizure threshold) ▪ Pregnancy, lactation, and children <2 yr (safety not established).

ADVERSE REACTIONS AND SIDE EFFECTS*

CNS: excessive sedation, extrapyramidal reactions, tardive dyskinesia, restlessness, confusion, hyperactivity, dizziness, nightmares, mental depression, hallucinations, euphoria, floating feeling, dysphoria.
EENT: dry eyes, blurred vision, miosis, diplopia.
Resp: bronchospasm, laryngospasm, apnea, respiratory depression.
CV: hypotension, tachycardia, bradycardia.
GI: dry mouth, constipation, nausea, vomiting.
GU: urinary retention.
Derm: sweating, flushing.
MS: skeletal and thoracic muscle rigidity.
Misc: chills, shivering, facial sweating.

INTERACTIONS

Drug–Drug: ▪ Additive hypotension with **antihypertensives** or **nitrates** ▪ Additive CNS depression with other **CNS depressants,** including **alcohol, antihistamines, antidepressants,** and other **sedative/hypnotics** or **opioid analgesics** (decrease dose of opioids if given within 8 hr of droperidol/fentanyl) ▪ Avoid using in patients who have received **MAO inhibitors** within 14 days.

ROUTE AND DOSAGE

Each ml contains 2.5 mg droperidol and 0.05 mg fentanyl. Because droperidol is much longer acting than fentanyl, additional doses of fentanyl alone may be given to prevent accumulation of droperidol.

Premedication
▪ **IM (Adults):** 0.5–2 ml 45–60 min prior to surgery.
▪ **IM (Children):** 0.25 ml/20 lb body weight 45–60 min prior to surgery.

Adjunct to General Anesthesia
▪ **IV (Adults):** 1 ml/20–25 lb body weight administered in small increments or as an infusion until somnolence occurs. Additional fentanyl may be used to maintain analgesia. In prolonged procedures, additional doses of 0.5–1 ml of droperidol/fentanyl **IV** may be required if lightening of tranquilization and analgesia occurs.
▪ **IV (Children >2 yr):** 0.5 ml/20 lb body weight administered in small increments or as an infusion until somnolence occurs. Additional fentanyl may be used to maintain analgesia.

Used without a General Anesthetic in Diagnostic Procedures
▪ **IM (Adults):** 0.5–2 ml 45–60 min prior to procedure. Additional fentanyl used to maintain analgesia. In prolonged procedures, additional doses of 0.5–1 ml of droperidol/fenta-

nyl **IV** may be required if lightening of tranquilization and analgesia occurs.

Adjunct to Regional Anesthesia
- **IM, IV (Adults):** 1–2 ml.

AVAILABILITY
- **Injection:** 2.5 mg droperidol and 0.05 mg fentanyl/ml.

TIME/ACTION PROFILE (noted as tranquilizing effects of droperidol, analgesic effects of fentanyl)

	ONSET	PEAK	DURATION*
IM droperidol	3–10 min	30 min	up to 12 hr
IM fentanyl	7–15 min	20–30 min	1–2 hr
IV droperidol	3–10 min	30 min	up to 12 hr
IV fentanyl	1–2 min	3–5 min	0.5–1 hr

*Listed as duration of tranquilization; alterations in consciousness may last up to 12 hr. Effects on respiratory depression outlast analgesic effects.

NURSING IMPLICATIONS

ASSESSMENT
- May cause pronounced respiratory depression. Monitor respiratory rate, ECG, and blood pressure frequently throughout course of therapy. Notify physician of significant changes immediately. Hypotension may be treated with parenteral fluids if hypovolemia is a causal factor. Vasopressors (norepinephrine, phenylephrine) may be needed. Avoid use of epinephrine, as droperidol reverses its pressor effects and may cause paradoxical hypotension.
- Doses of opioid analgesics administered following administration of droperidol/fentanyl should be decreased to ¼–⅓ the normal dose for 8 hr following the administration of droperidol/fentanyl.
- Observe patient for extrapyramidal symptoms (dystonia, oculogyric crisis, extended neck, flexed arms,

tremor, restlessness, hyperactivity, anxiety) throughout therapy. Notify physician should these occur. An anticholinergic antiparkinsonian agent may be used to treat these symptoms.
- **Lab Test Considerations:** May cause elevated serum amylase and lipase concentrations.
- **Toxicity and Overdose:** Naloxone (Narcan) may reverse respiratory depression. Dose may need to be repeated, as fentanyl has a longer duration than naloxone.
- Bradycardia may be treated with atropine.

POTENTIAL NURSING DIAGNOSES
- Pain (indications).
- Injury, high risk for (side effects).

IMPLEMENTATION
- **Direct IV:** Administer slowly over at least 1 min.
- **Intermittent Infusion:** Droperidol/fentanyl 10 ml may be added to 250 ml of D5W and infused until the onset of somnolence as an adjunct to general anesthesia.
- **Syringe Compatibility:** ■ benzquinamide ■ glycopyrrolate.
- **Syringe Incompatibility:** ■ heparin.
- **Y-Site Compatibility:** ■ hydrocortisone sodium succinate ■ potassium chloride.
- **Y-Site Incompatibility:** ■ nafcillin.
- **Additive Incompatibility:** ■ barbiturates.

PATIENT/FAMILY TEACHING
- Caution patient to make position changes slowly to minimize orthostatic hypotension.
- Medication causes drowsiness. Advise patient to call for assistance during ambulation and transfer and to avoid driving or other activities requiring alertness for 24 hr after last dose.

EVALUATION
Effectiveness of therapy can be demonstrated by: ■ General quiescence, reduced motor activity, and pronounced analgesia.

D

DYPHYLLINE
(dye-fi-lin)
Dilor, Dyflex, Lufyllin, Neothylline, {Protophylline}

CLASSIFICATION(S):
Bronchodilator (phosphodiesterase inhibitor)
Pregnancy Category C

INDICATIONS

- Bronchodilator in reversible airway obstruction due to asthma or COPD.

ACTION

- Inhibits phosphodiesterase, producing increases in tissue concentrations of cyclic adenosine monophosphate (cAMP). Increased levels of cAMP result in: □ Bronchodilation □ CNS stimulation □ Positive inotropic and chronotropic effects □ Diuresis □ Gastric acid secretion. Dyphylline is a chemical derivative of theophylline. **Therapeutic Effect:** ▪ Bronchodilation.

PHARMACOKINETICS

Absorption: Well absorbed (75%) following oral administration.
Distribution: Achieves high concentrations in breast milk.
Metabolism and Excretion: 85% excreted unchanged by the kidneys.
Half-life: 1.8–2.1 hr (increased in renal impairment).

CONTRAINDICATIONS AND PRECAUTIONS

Contraindicated in: ▪ Hypersensitivity ▪ Some products contain benzyl alcohol and/or bisulfites—avoid use in patients with hypersensitivities to these compounds ▪ Known alcohol intolerance (elixir only) ▪ Lactation ▪ Uncontrolled arrhythmias ▪ Hyperthyroidism.
Use Cautiously in: ▪ Pregnancy or children (safety not established) ▪ Severe cardiovascular disease ▪ Peptic ulcer disease.

ADVERSE REACTIONS AND SIDE EFFECTS*

CNS: <u>nervousness</u>, <u>anxiety</u>, headache, insomnia, SEIZURES.
Resp: tachypnea.
CV: <u>tachycardia</u>, palpitations, arrhythmias, angina pectoris.
GI: <u>nausea</u>, <u>vomiting</u>, anorexia, cramps.
GU: albuminuria, hematuria, diuresis.
Neuro: tremor.
Misc: hyperglycemia, syndrome of inappropriate secretion of antidiuretic hormone (SIADH).

INTERACTIONS

Drug–Drug: ▪ Additive CV and CNS side effects with **adrenergic (sympathomimetic) agents** ▪ Additive bronchodilation with other **bronchodilators** ▪ **Probenecid** decreases renal excretion and increases blood levels ▪ **Beta-adrenergic blockers** may decrease therapeutic effects of dyphylline ▪ May decrease sedation from **benzodiazepines**.

ROUTE AND DOSAGE

Chronic Therapy
- PO (Adults): 15 mg/kg q 6 hr.
- IM (Adults): 250–500 mg q 6 hr.

AVAILABILITY

▪ *Tablets:* 200 mg, 400 mg ▪ *Elixir:* 100 mg/15 ml, 160 mg/15 ml ▪ *Injection:* 250 mg/ml.

TIME/ACTION PROFILE
(bronchodilation)

	ONSET	PEAK	DURATION
PO	UK	1 hr	6 hr

NURSING IMPLICATIONS

ASSESSMENT
□ Assess blood pressure, pulse, respiration, and lung sounds before administering medication and throughout therapy.
□ Patients with a history of cardiovas-

{} = Available in Canada only.
*<u>Underlines</u> indicate most frequent; **CAPITALS** indicate life-threatening.

cular problems should be monitored for ECG changes.

□ Monitor intake and output ratios for an increase in diuresis.

▪ **Toxicity and Overdose:** Standard theophylline assays do not measure dyphylline concentrations.

POTENTIAL NURSING DIAGNOSES

▪ Airway clearance, ineffective (indications).

▪ Activity intolerance (indications).

▪ Knowledge deficit related to medication regimen (patient/family teaching).

IMPLEMENTATION

▪ **General Info:** Administer around the clock to maintain therapeutic plasma levels.

□ Determine if patient has had another form of theophylline prior to administering initial dose.

▪ **PO:** Administer 1 hr before or 2 hr after meals for rapid absorption. May be administered after meals to minimize GI irritation. Food slows but does not reduce the extent of absorption. Measure dose of liquid forms, using calibrated medication cup.

▪ **IM:** Do not use if precipitate is present. May be caused by exposure to cold.

□ Inject slowly; avoid IV administration.

PATIENT/FAMILY TEACHING

□ Emphasize the importance of taking only the prescribed dose at the prescribed time intervals. Missed doses should be taken as soon as remembered or omitted if close to next dose.

□ Encourage patient to drink adequate liquids (2000 ml/day minimum) to decrease the viscosity of the airway secretions.

□ Advise patient to avoid over-the-counter cough, cold, or breathing preparations without consulting physician or pharmacist. These medications may increase side effects and cause arrhythmias.

□ Advise patient to minimize intake of xanthine-containing foods or beverages (colas, coffee, chocolate).

□ Encourage patients not to smoke, as smoking may irritate respiratory tract.

□ Advise patient to contact physician promptly if the usual dose of medication fails to produce the desired results, symptoms worsen after treatment, or toxic effects (anorexia, nausea, vomiting, restlessness, insomnia, tachycardia, arrhythmias, seizures) occur.

EVALUATION

Effectiveness of therapy can be demonstrated by: ▪ Increased ease in breathing and clearing of lung fields on auscultation.

E

EDETATE CALCIUM DISODIUM
(**ee**-de-tate **kal**-see-yum dye-**sode**-ee-yum)
calcium disodium vernesate, calcium EDTA, edathamil calcium disodium, sodium calcium edetate

CLASSIFICATION(S):
Antidote (lead chelator)
Pregnancy Category UK

INDICATIONS

▪ Management of acute and chronic lead poisoning, including encephalopathy and nephropathy.

ACTION

▪ Removes toxic amounts of lead or other divalent or trivalent cations by their displacement of calcium in edetate calcium disodium. Result is a soluble complex that is excreted by the kidneys. **Therapeutic Effect:** ▪ Removal of toxic amounts of lead from the blood and other tissues.

PHARMACOKINETICS

Absorption: Well absorbed following IM administration.

Distribution: Distributed to extracellular fluid. Does not cross the blood–brain barrier.

Metabolism and Excretion: Rapidly

excreted by the kidneys as unchanged drug or lead complex.

Half-life: IM—20–60 min; IV—1.5 hr.

CONTRAINDICATIONS AND PRECAUTIONS

Contraindicated in: ▪ Anuria.

Use Cautiously in: ▪ Underlying renal disease (dosage reduction required if serum creatinine >2 mg/dl) ▪ Cardiac arrhythmias ▪ Pregnancy or lactation (safety not established) ▪ Lead encephalopathy (should be used with concurrent dimercaprol).

ADVERSE REACTIONS AND SIDE EFFECTS*

CNS: headache, malaise, fatigue.

EENT: sneezing, lacrimation, nasal, congestion.

CV: ECG changes (inverted T waves), hypotension.

GI: nausea, vomiting.

GU: nephrotoxicity, glycosuria.

F and E: hypercalcemia.

Local: pain at IM site, phlebitis at IV site.

MS: mylagia, arthralgia, leg cramps.

Neuro: numbness, tingling.

Misc: excessive thirst, fever, chills, histamine-like reaction.

INTERACTIONS

Drug–Drug: ▪ May increase the risk of **cardiac glycoside** toxicity ▪ **Glucocorticoids** increase nephrotoxicity ▪ Decrease the duration of action of **zinc insulin** preparations.

ROUTE AND DOSAGE

Lead Mobilization Test
▪ **IM, IV (Adults):** 1 g.
▪ **IM, IV (Children):** 15 mg/kg (500 mg/ m^2, not to exceed 1 g).

Lead Poisoning
▪ **IM, IV (Adults):** 15–25 mg/kg (0.5–0.75 g/m^2) q 12 hr for 3–5 days (not to exceed 2 g/day). May be repeated after 2-day rest period.
▪ **IM, IV (Children):** 1–1.5 g/m^2/day in 4 divided doses for 5 days. May be repeated after 2-day rest period.

AVAILABILITY

▪ *Injection:* 200 mg/ml, 5-ml ampules.

TIME/ACTION PROFILE (urinary lead excretion)

	ONSET	PEAK	DURATION
IM	UK	UK	UK
IV	1 hr	24–48 hr	UK

NURSING IMPLICATIONS

ASSESSMENT

▫ Assess patient and family members for evidence of lead poisoning prior to and periodically throughout course of therapy. Acute lead poisoning is characterized by a metallic taste, colicky abdominal pain, vomiting, diarrhea, oliguria, and coma. Symptoms of chronic poisoning vary with severity and include anorexia, a blue-black line along the gums, intermittent vomiting, paresthesia, encephalopathy, seizures, and coma.

▫ Monitor intake and output and daily weight. Notify physician of any discrepancies. If patient is anuric, edetate calcium disodium should be held until urine flow is established by IV hydration.

▫ Monitor neurologic status closely (level of consciousness, pupil response, movement). Notify physician immediately of any changes. Infuse slowly; rapid infusion rate may increase intracranial pressure. Physician may also order fluid restriction to prevent increased intracranial pressure.

▫ Monitor vital signs and ECG frequently. Notify physician if hypotension or T wave inversion occur. Physician should also be notified if fever, chills, malaise, or nasal congestion occur. This histamine-like response reaction usually resolves in 48 hr.

▪ **Lab Test Considerations:** Monitor serum and urine lead levels prior to and periodically throughout therapy. Wait at least 1 hr after infusing edetate cal-

---

*Underlines indicate most frequent; **CAPITALS** indicate life-threatening.

cium disodium before drawing serum lead level.

□ Monitor urinalysis daily and serum creatinine, BUN, alkaline phosphatase, calcium, and phosphorous levels. Both lead and edetate calcium disodium are nephrotoxic. Notify physician if hematuria, proteinuria, or large renal epithelial cells are present.

□ May cause an increase in urine glucose.

POTENTIAL NURSING DIAGNOSES

- Poisoning, high risk for (indications, patient/family teaching).
- Home maintenance management, impaired (indications).
- Knowledge deficit related to medication and dietary regimens (patient/family teaching).

IMPLEMENTATION

- **General Info:** Administer IM or IV; oral administration may increase absorption of lead.
- □ Patients with serum lead levels of 100 mcg/dl or more, or those with lead encephalopathy may also be treated with dimercaprol (BAL). Administer these medications at separate sites.
- **IM:** IM is the preferred route for children and patients with lead encephalopathy. Procaine hydrochloride 1% (1 ml procaine to 1 ml edetate calcium disodium ratio, for a final concentration of 0.5% procaine) is usually ordered to minimize pain at the injection site. Administer deep IM into well-developed muscle; massage well. Rotate sites.
- **Intermittent Infusion:** Dilute 5 ml with 250–500 ml of D5W or 0.9% NaCl for a final concentration of 2–4 mg/ml.
- **Rate:** Administer over 1 hr in asymptomatic adults and over 2 hr in symptomatic patients. Use infusion pump to control rate accurately.
- **Continuous Infusion:** May also be administered as a single daily infusion over 8–24 hr.
- **Additive Compatibility:** ▪ netilmicin.
- **Additive Incompatibility:** ▪ D10W,

lactated Ringer's solution, amphotericin B, or hydralazine.

PATIENT/FAMILY TEACHING

- **Home Care Issues:** Discuss need for follow-up appointments to monitor lead levels. Additional treatments may be necessary.
- □ Consult public health department regarding potential sources of lead poisoning in the home, workplace, and recreational areas.

EVALUATION

Effectiveness of therapy can be demonstrated by: ▪ Decrease in symptoms of lead poisoning □ Decrease in serum lead levels to below 50 mcg/dl, although the normal upper limit is 29 mcg/dl.

E

EDROPHONIUM

(ed-roe-**fone**-ee-yum)
Enlon, Reversol, Tensilon

CLASSIFICATION(S):
Cholinergic (anticholinesterase)
Pregnancy Category C

INDICATIONS

▪ Diagnosis of myasthenia gravis ▪ Assessment of adequacy of anticholinesterase therapy in myasthenia gravis ▪ Differentiating myasthenic from cholinergic crisis ▪ Reversal of nondepolarizing neuromuscular blockers.

ACTION

▪ Inhibits the breakdown of acetylcholine so that it accumulates and has a prolonged effect. Effects include miosis, increased intestinal and skeletal muscle tone, bronchial and ureteral constriction, bradycardia, increased salivation, lacrimation, and sweating. **Therapeutic Effects:** ▪ Improved but short-lived cranial muscular function in patients with myasthenia gravis ▪ Reversal of nondepolarizing neuromuscular blockers.

PHARMACOKINETICS

Absorption: Absorption following IM and SC administration not known.

Distribution: Distribution not known.
Metabolism and Excretion: Metabolic fate not known.
Half-life: UK.

CONTRAINDICATIONS AND PRECAUTIONS

Contraindicated in: ▪ Hypersensitivity ▪ Mechanical obstruction of the GI or GU tract ▪ Pregnancy (may cause uterine irritability after IV administration near term; newborns may display muscle weakness) ▪ Lactation ▪ Hypersensitivity to bisulfites.

Use Cautiously in: ▪ History of asthma ▪ Ulcer disease ▪ Cardiovascular disease ▪ Epilepsy ▪ Hyperthyroidism ▪ Because some patients may be extremely sensitive to the effects of anticholinesterases, atropine should be available in case of excessive dosage.

ADVERSE REACTIONS AND SIDE EFFECTS*

CNS: dizziness, weakness, SEIZURES.
EENT: miosis, lacrimation.
Resp: excess secretions, bronchospasm.
CV: bradycardia, hypotension.
GI: abdominal cramps, nausea, vomiting, diarrhea, excess salivation.
Derm: rashes, sweating.
MS: fasciculation.

INTERACTIONS

Drug–Drug: ▪ Action may be antagonized by **drugs possessing anticholinergic properties,** including **antihistamines, antidepressants, atropine, haloperidol, phenothiazines, quinidine,** and **disopyramide** ▪ Prolongs action of depolarizing **muscle-relaxing agents (succinylcholine, decamethonium)** ▪ May lead to excessive bradycardia in patients receiving **cardiac glycosides.**

ROUTE AND DOSAGE

Diagnosis of Myasthenia Gravis

▪ **IV (Adults):** 2 mg, if no response administer 8 more mg; may repeat test in 30 min. If cholinergic response occurs, administer atropine 0.4–0.5 mg IV.

▪ **IV (Children >34 kg):** 2 mg, if no response may administer 1 mg q 30–45 sec to a total of 10 mg. If cholinergic response occurs, administer atropine IV.

▪ **IV (Children <34 kg):** 1 mg, if no response may administer 1 mg q 45 sec to a total of 5 mg. If cholinergic response occurs, administer atropine IV.

▪ **IV (Infants):** 0.5 mg.

▪ **IM (Adults):** 10 mg. If cholinergic response occurs, may repeat 2 mg dose in 30 min to rule out false negative reaction.

▪ **IM (Children <34 kg):** 2 mg.

▪ **IM (Children >34 kg):** 5 mg.

Assessment of Anticholinesterase Therapy

▪ **IV (Adults):** 1–2 mg 1 hr after oral anticholinesterase dose.

Differentiation of Cholinergic from Myasthenic Crisis

▪ **IV (Adults):** 1 mg, may give additional 1 mg 1 min later.

Reversal of Nondepolarizing Neuromuscular Blocking Agents

▪ **IV (Adults):** 10 mg, may repeat q 5–10 min (not to exceed 40 mg).

AVAILABILITY

▪ *Injection:* 10 mg/ml ▪ *In combination with:* atropine (Enlon-Plus). See Appendix A.

TIME/ACTION PROFILE (cholinergic activity)

	ONSET	PEAK	DURATION
IM	2–10 min	UK	5–30 min
IV	30–60 sec	UK	5–10 min

NURSING IMPLICATIONS

ASSESSMENT

▪ **General Info:** Assess neuromuscular status (ptosis, diplopia, vital capacity, ability to swallow, extremity strength) prior to and immediately after administration of medication.

---

*Underlines indicate most frequent; **CAPITALS** indicate life-threatening.

□ To differentiate myasthenic from cholinergic crisis, assess for increased weakness, diaphoresis, increased saliva and bronchial secretions, dyspnea, nausea, vomiting, diarrhea, and bradycardia. If these symptoms occur, patient is in cholinergic crisis. If strength improves, patient is in a myasthenic crisis.

■ **Toxicity and Overdose:** Atropine may be used for treatment of cholinergic symptoms. Oxygen and resuscitation equipment should be available.

POTENTIAL NURSING DIAGNOSES

■ Breathing pattern, ineffective (indications).
■ Knowledge deficit related to medication regimen (patient/family teaching).

IMPLEMENTATION

■ **General Info:** For myasthenia gravis patients, diagnostic IV dose and dose to differentiate myasthenic from cholinergic crisis is administered by a physician.
■ **IV:** IV doses are administered undiluted with a tuberculin syringe.
■ **Y-Site Compatibility:** ■ heparin ■ hydrocortisone ■ potassium chloride ■ vitamin B complex with C.

PATIENT/FAMILY TEACHING

□ Inform patient that the effects of this medication last up to 30 min.

EVALUATION

Effectiveness of medication can be demonstrated by: ■ Relief of myasthenic symptoms ■ Differentiation of myasthenic from cholinergic crisis ■ Reversal of paralysis after anesthesia.

ENALAPRIL
(e-**nal**-a-pril)
Vasotec

ENALAPRILAT
(e-**nal**-a-pril-at)
Vasotec

CLASSIFICATION(S):
Antihypertensive, Angiotensin converting enzyme (ACE) inhibitor
Pregnancy Category C (first trimester), Category D (second trimester)

INDICATIONS

■ Alone or in combination with other antihypertensives in the management of hypertension ■ Used in combination with other drugs (diuretics, cardiac glycosides) in the management of congestive heart failure.

ACTION

■ Prevents the production of angiotensin II, a potent vasoconstrictor that stimulates the production of aldosterone by blocking its conversion to the active form. Result is systemic vasodilation. **Therapeutic Effects:** ■ Lowering of blood pressure in hypertensive patients ■ Decreased preload and afterload in patients with congestive heart failure.

PHARMACOKINETICS

Absorption: Well absorbed following oral administration.
Distribution: Minimal crossing of the blood–brain barrier. Rest of distribution not known.
Metabolism and Excretion: Following absorption, enalapril is converted to enalaprilat, the active metabolite. 60% excreted by the kidneys (40% as enalaprilat, 20% as enalapril).
Half-life: 11 hr (increased in renal impairment).

CONTRAINDICATIONS AND PRECAUTIONS

Contraindicated in: ■ Hypersensitivity ■ Cross-sensitivity with other ACE inhibitors may exist ■ Pregnancy (may cause fetal malformation or death; hypotension, oliguria, or hypokalemia may occur in newborn).
Use Cautiously in: ■ Renal impairment (dosage reduction required if serum creatinine >3 mg/dl) ■ Second or

E

third trimester of pregnancy ▪ Lactation and children (safety not established) ▪ Hypotension may be exaggerated during surgery/anesthesia ▪ Aortic stenosis ▪ Cerebrovascular disease ▪ Cardiac insufficiency ▪ Hyponatremia or concurrent diuretic therapy (initial dosage reduction recommended).

Extreme Caution in: ▪ Patients with a family history of hereditary angioedema.

ADVERSE REACTIONS AND SIDE EFFECTS*

CNS: headache, dizziness, fatigue.
Resp: cough.
CV: hypotension, tachycardia, angina pectoris.
GI: anorexia, diarrhea, nausea, impaired taste.
GU: impotence.
Derm: rashes.
F and E: hyperkalemia.
Misc: fever, ANGIOEDEMA with laryngospasm.

INTERACTIONS

Drug–Drug: ▪ Additive hypotension with other **antihypertensives, phenothiazines,** acute ingestion of **alcohol,** and **vasodilators** ▪ Hyperkalemia may result with concurrent **potassium supplements, cyclosporine,** or **potassium-sparing diuretics** ▪ Antihypertensive response may be blunted by **nonsteroidal anti-inflammatory agents** ▪ Absorption may be decreased by **antacids** ▪ Increases levels and may increase the risk of **lithium** or **digoxin** toxicity ▪ Risk of hypersensitivity reactions increased by concurrent **allopurinol** ▪ **Capsaicin** may increase the incidence of cough ▪ Effectiveness may be decreased by **rifampin.**
Drug–Food: ▪ Hyperkalemia may result from a **high-potassium diet.**

ROUTE AND DOSAGE

Enalapril/Enalaprilat

▪ **PO (Adults):** *Hypertension*—Initial dose 5 mg/day, increased as required by response (usual range 10–40 mg/day in 1–2 divided doses). *Conges-*

tive heart failure—Initial dose 2.5 mg 1–2 times daily, increased as required by response (usual range 5–20 mg/day in 1–2 divided doses).
▪ **IV (Adults):** 0.625–1.25 mg (0.625 mg if receiving diuretics) q 6 hr.

AVAILABILITY

▪ **Tablets:** 2.5 mg, 5 mg, 10 mg, 20 mg
▪ **Injection:** 1.25 mg/ml ▪ **In combination with:** hydrochlorothiazide (Vaserectic). See Appendix A.

TIME/ACTION PROFILE (effect on blood pressure)

	ONSET	PEAK	DURATION
PO	1 hr	4–6 hr	24 hr
IV	15 min	1–4 hr	6 hr

NURSING IMPLICATIONS

ASSESSMENT

▢ Monitor blood pressure and pulse frequently during initial dosage adjustment and periodically throughout course of therapy. Notify physician of significant changes.

▢ Monitor weight and assess patient routinely for resolution of fluid overload (peripheral edema, rales/crackles, dyspnea, weight gain, jugular venous distension).

▪ **Lab Test Considerations:** Monitor BUN, creatinine, and electrolyte levels periodically. Serum potassium may be increased and BUN and creatinine transiently increased, while sodium levels may be decreased.

POTENTIAL NURSING DIAGNOSES

▪ Cardiac output, decreased (indications, side effects).
▪ Knowledge deficit related to medication regimen (patient/family teaching).
▪ Noncompliance (patient/family teaching).

IMPLEMENTATION

▪ **PO:** Precipitous drop in blood pressure during first 1–3 hr following first dose may require volume expansion with normal saline but is not nor-

mally considered an indication for stopping therapy. Monitor closely for at least 1 hr after blood pressure has stabilized.
- **Direct IV:** May be administered undiluted.
- *Rate:* Administer over 5 min.
- **Intermittent Infusion:** Dilute in 50 ml of D5W, 0.9% NaCl, D5/0.9% NaCl, or D5/LR. Diluted solution is stable for 24 hr.
- *Rate:* Administer as a slow infusion.
- **Y-Site Compatibility:** ■ amikacin ■ aminophylline ■ ampicillin ■ ampicillin/sulbactam ■ aztreonam ■ butorphanol ■ calcium gluconate ■ cefazolin ■ cefoperazone ■ ceftazidime ■ ceftizoxime ■ chloramphenicol ■ cimetidine ■ clindamycin ■ erythromycin lactobionate ■ esmolol ■ famotidine ■ fentanyl ■ ganciclovir ■ gentamicin ■ heparin ■ hetastarch ■ hydrocortisone sodium succinate ■ labetalol ■ lidocaine ■ magnesium sulfate ■ methylprednisolone sodium succinate ■ metronidazole ■ morphine ■ nafcillin ■ penicillin G potassium ■ phenobarbital ■ piperacillin ■ potassium chloride ■ potassium phosphate ■ ranitidine ■ sodium acetate ■ tobramycin ■ trimethoprim/sulfamethoxazole ■ vancomycin.
- **Y-Site Incompatibility:** ■ amphotericin B ■ phenytoin.

PATIENT/FAMILY TEACHING
- □ Instruct patient to take enalapril exactly as directed, even if feeling well. Missed doses should be taken as soon as remembered but not if almost time for next dose. Do not double doses. Medication controls but does not cure hypertension. Caution patient not to discontinue enalapril therapy unless directed by physician.
- □ Encourage patient to comply with additional interventions for hypertension (weight reduction, discontinuation of smoking, moderation of alcohol consumption, regular exercise, and stress management).
- □ Instruct patient and family on proper technique for blood pressure monitoring. Advise them to check blood pres-

sure at least weekly and report significant changes to physician.
- □ Caution patient to avoid salt substitutes or foods containing high levels of potassium or sodium, unless directed by physician (see Appendix K).
- □ Advise patient that enalapril may cause an impairment of taste that generally reverses itself within 8–12 wk, even with continued therapy.
- □ Caution patient to change positions slowly to minimize orthostatic hypotension, particularly after initial dose. Also advise patient that exercise or hot weather may increase hypotensive effects.
- □ Advise patient to consult physician or pharmacist before taking any over-the-counter medications, especially cold remedies. Patient should also avoid excessive amounts of tea, coffee, or cola.
- □ Enalapril may cause dizziness. Caution patient to avoid driving and other activities requiring alertness until response to medication is known.
- □ Advise patient to inform physician or dentist of medication regimen prior to treatment or surgery.
- □ Instruct patient to notify physician if rash, mouth sores, sore throat, fever, swelling of hands or feet, irregular heartbeat, chest pain, dry cough, swelling of face, eyes, lips, or tongue, or difficulty breathing occurs.
- □ Advise patient to notify physician if pregnancy is planned or suspected.
- □ Emphasize the importance of follow-up examinations to monitor progress.

EVALUATION
Effectiveness of therapy can be demonstrated by: ■ Decrease in blood pressure without appearance of side effects ■ Decrease in signs and symptoms of congestive heart failure.

ENOXACIN
(e-**nox**-a-sin)
Penetrex

INDICATIONS

■ Treatment of the following infections due to susceptible organisms □ Sexually transmitted disease, including uncomplicated urethral or cervical gonorrhea □ Uncomplicated urinary tract infections.

ACTION

■ Inhibits bacterial DNA synthesis by inhibiting DNA gyrase. **Therapeutic Effect:** ■ Death of susceptible bacteria. **Spectrum:** ■ Includes activity against staphylococci, *Aeromonas* sp, *Citrobacter* sp, *Enterobacter* sp, *Escherichia coli, Hemophilus ducreyi, Klebsiella pneumoniae, Klebsiella* sp, *Moranella morganii, Neisseria gonorrhea, Proteus vulgaris, Proteus mirabilis, Providencia alcalifaciens, Providencia stuartii, Pseudomonas aeruginosa,* and Serratia.

PHARMACOKINETICS

Absorption: Well absorbed following oral administration (90% bioavailability).

Distribution: Widely distributed to body tissues and fluids.

Metabolism and Excretion: >40% excreted unchanged by the kidneys. 20% metabolized by the liver.

Half-life: 3–6 hr (increased in renal disease).

CONTRAINDICATIONS AND PRECAUTIONS

Contraindicated in: ■ Hypersensitivity to enoxacin or other quinolones ■ Children <18 yr ■ Pregnancy.

Use Cautiously in: ■ Underlying CNS pathology ■ Lactation (high milk concentrations achieved, safety not established) ■ Severe renal impairment (dosage reduction required if CCr ≤30 ml/min/1.73 m^2).

ADVERSE REACTIONS AND SIDE EFFECTS*

CNS: headache, dizziness, insomnia, SEIZURES, somnolence.

GI: <u>nausea</u>, diarrhea, vomiting, abdominal pain, unusual taste, dry mouth, dyspepsia, PSEUDOMEMBRANOUS COLITIS.

Derm: pruritis, rash, photosensitivity.

INTERACTIONS

Drug–Drug: ■ Increases serum **theophylline** levels and may lead to toxicity ■ Administration with **antacids, iron salts, bismuth subsalicylate, sucralfate,** or **zinc salts** decrease absorption of enoxacin ■ May increase the effects of **warfarin** ■ Enoxacin may increase serum **digoxin** levels resulting in toxicity ■ Clearance of **caffeine** is reduced, and toxicity may occur ■ **Cimetidine** decreases metabolism ■ Concurrent use with **antineoplastic agents** may decrease levels.

ROUTE AND DOSAGE

Urinary Tract Infections
■ PO (Adults): 400–800 mg/day in divided doses q 12 hr.

Sexually Transmitted Diseases
■ PO (Adults): 400-mg, single dose.

AVAILABILITY

■ *Tablets:* 200 mg, 400 mg.

TIME/ACTION PROFILE (blood levels)

	ONSET	PEAK
PO	Rapid	UK

NURSING IMPLICATIONS

ASSESSMENT

□ Assess patient for infection (vital signs, urinalysis, frequency and urgency of urination, WBC, fever, cloudy or foul-smelling urine) at beginning and throughout therapy.

□ Obtain specimens for culture and sensitivity prior to initiating therapy. First dose may be given before receiving results.

---

*<u>Underlines</u> indicate most frequent; **CAPITALS** indicate life-threatening.

- **Lab Test Considerations:** May cause increased AST (SGOT), ALT (SGPT), and serum alkaline phosphatase.
- □ May cause decreased hemoglobin and hematocrit concentrations.

POTENTIAL NURSING DIAGNOSES
- Infection, high risk for (indications), side effects).
- Knowledge deficit related to medication regimen (patient/family teaching).
- Noncompliance related to medication regimen (patient/family teaching).

IMPLEMENTATION
- **PO:** Administer around the clock on an empty stomach, at least 1 hr before or 2 hr after meals, with a full glass of water.

PATIENT/FAMILY TEACHING
- □ Instruct patient to take medication around the clock and to finish the drug completely as directed, even if feeling better. If a dose is missed, take as soon as remembered unless almost time for next dose; do not double doses. Advise patient that sharing of this medication may be dangerous.
- □ Encourage patient to maintain a fluid intake of at least 1200–1500 ml/day.
- □ Advise patient that antacids or medications containing iron or zinc will decrease absorption and should not be taken within 4 hr before or 2 hr after taking this medication.
- □ May cause dizziness and drowsiness. Caution patient to avoid driving or other activities requiring alertness until response to medication is known.
- □ Caution patient to use sunscreen and protective clothing to prevent photosensitivity reactions.
- □ Instruct patient to notify physician immediately if rash occurs or if symptoms do not improve within a few days of therapy.

EVALUATION
Clinical response can be evaluated by:
- Resolution of the signs and symptoms of infection. Length of time for complete resolution depends on organism and site of infection.

ENOXAPARIN
(ee-**nox**-a-par-in)
Lovenox

CLASSIFICATION(S):
Antithrombotic (low molecular weight heparin)
Pregnancy Category B

INDICATIONS
- Prevention of deep vein thrombosis (a cause of pulmonary embolism) following hip replacement surgery.

ACTION
- Prevents the conversion of prothrombin to thrombin via its effects on factor X_a. Enoxaparin is low molecular weight heparin. **Therapeutic Effect:** - Prevention of thrombus formation.

PHARMACOKINETICS
Absorption: Well absorbed following SC administration (92%).
Distribution: Distribution not known.
Metabolism and Excretion: Metabolism and excretion not known.
Half-life: 4.5 hr.

CONTRAINDICATIONS AND PRECAUTIONS
Contraindicated in: - Patients with active bleeding, thrombocytopenia associated with antiplatelet antibodies in the presence of enoxaparin - Hypersensitivity to enoxaparin or pork proteins.
Use Cautiously in: - Patients with bleeding disorders, uncontrolled arterial hypertension, history or recent GI bleed or ulceration - Elderly patients and patients with renal impairment (more sensitive to the effects of enoxaparin).
Extreme Caution: - Patients with a history of heparin-induced thrombocytopenia - Recent brain, spinal or ophthalmologic surgery - Bacterial endocarditis - Congenital or acquired bleeding problems - Active GI bleeding or ulceration.

E

ADVERSE REACTIONS AND SIDE EFFECTS*

CNS: edema.
Hemat: BLEEDING, thrombocytopenia, anemia.
Local: irritation, pain, hematoma, and erythema at injection site.

INTERACTIONS

Drug–Drug: ▪ Risk of bleeding may be increased by concurrent use of other **anticoagulants** or **antiplatelet drugs** (including **nonsteroidal anti-inflammatory agents**).

ROUTE AND DOSAGE

▪ **SC (Adults):** 30 mg twice daily started within 24 hr following surgery.

AVAILABILITY

▪ *Prefilled syringes:* 30 mg/0.3 ml.

TIME/ACTION PROFILE
(antithrombotic effect)

	ONSET	PEAK	DURATION
SC	UK	UK	12 hr

NURSING IMPLICATIONS

ASSESSMENT

▪ **General Info:** Assess patient for signs of bleeding and hemorrhage (bleeding gums, nose bleed, unusual bruising, black tarry stools, hematuria, fall in hematocrit or blood pressure, guaiac-positive stools). Notify physician if these occur.
▪ **SC:** Observe injection sites for hematomas or ecchymosis or inflammation.
▪ **Lab Test Considerations:** Monitor CBC and platelet count periodically throughout therapy.

POTENTIAL NURSING DIAGNOSES

▪ Tissue perfusion, altered (indications).
▪ Injury, high risk for (side effects).
▪ Knowledge deficit related to medication regimen (patient/family teaching).

IMPLEMENTATION

▪ **General Info:** Administration should begin as soon as possible after surgery, but not more than 24 hr postoperatively and should be continued throughout period of postoperative care until risk of deep vein thrombosis has lessened, usually 7–10 days.
▪ **SC:** Administer deep into SC tissue. Alternate injection sites between the left and right anterolateral and left and right posterolateral abdominal wall. Inject whole length of needle into a skin fold held between thumb and forefinger; hold skin fold throughout injection. Do not administer IM because of the danger of hematoma formation. Solution should be clear colorless to pale yellow; do not inject solution containing particulate matter.

PATIENT/FAMILY TEACHING

□ Advise patient to report any symptoms of unusual bleeding or bruising to nurse or physician immediately.
□ Instruct patient not to take aspirin, medications containing aspirin, or ibuprofen while on enoxaparin therapy.

EVALUATION

Clinical response to therapy is indicated by: ▪ Prevention of deep vein thrombosis.

EPHEDRINE
(e-**fed**-drin)
Kondon's Nasal Jelly, Pretz-D

CLASSIFICATION(S):
Bronchodilator (alpha- and beta-adrenergic), Nasal decongestant, Vasopressor
Pregnancy Category C

INDICATIONS

▪ **PO, IM, IV, SC:** Used as a bronchodilator in the management of reversible airway obstruction due to asthma or COPD ▪ **PO, Nasal:** Relief of nasal congestion in viral upper respiratory tract infections or allergic rhinitis ▪ **PO:** Management of orthostatic hypotension ▪ Management of acute hypotension associated with overdosage of antihypertensive agents ▪ **PO:** Management of mental depression or narcolepsy.

ACTION
▪ An alpha- and beta-adrenergic agonist. Beta-adrenergic agonist effects result in accumulation of cyclic AMP at beta-adrenergic receptors, producing bronchodilation, CNS and cardiac stimulation, diuresis, and gastric acid secretion. Primary alpha-adrenergic effect is peripheral vasoconstriction. **Therapeutic Effects:** ▪ Bronchodilation ▪ Vasoconstriction with decreased congestion ▪ Restoration of blood pressure ▪ CNS stimulation.

PHARMACOKINETICS
Absorption: Well absorbed following oral, IM, or SC administration.
Distribution: Probably crosses the placenta and enters breast milk.
Metabolism and Excretion: Small amounts slowly metabolized by the liver. Mostly excreted unchanged by the kidneys.
Half-life: 3–6 hr (depends on urine pH).

CONTRAINDICATIONS AND PRECAUTIONS
Contraindicated in: ▪ Hypersensitivity ▪ Known intolerance ▪ Angle-closure glaucoma ▪ Cyclopropane or halothane anesthesia ▪ Thyrotoxicosis ▪ Diabetes mellitus ▪ Pregnancy ▪ Hypertension ▪ Severe cardiovascular disease.
Use Cautiously in: ▪ Cardiovascular disease ▪ Lactation ▪ Prostatic hypertrophy.

ADVERSE REACTIONS AND SIDE EFFECTS*
CNS: CNS stimulation, nervousness, anxiety paranoid state (long-term use), dizziness, lightheadedness, vertigo.

EENT: rebound congestion (nasal use), local irritation.
Resp: breathing difficulties.
CV: angina pectoris, palpitations, tachycardia, ARRHYTHMIAS.
GU: urinary retention, decreased urine output.
Misc: rapid development of tolerance (tachyphylaxis), diaphoresis.

INTERACTIONS
Drug–Drug: Cyclopropane, cardiac glycosides, or halothane increases risk of arrhythmias ▪ Additive effects with other adrenergic (sympathomimetic) agents ▪ Use with MAO inhibitors may result in hypertensive crisis ▪ Pressor response may be reduced by reserpine, methyldopa, or furosemide ▪ Theophylline increases the risk of adverse effects ▪ Reflex bradycardia and pressor effects are decreased by atropine ▪ Acidifying the urine (ammonium chloride) decreases half-life ▪ Alkalinizing the urine (sodium bicarbonate) increases the half-life.

ROUTE AND DOSAGE
Bronchodilator, Nasal Decongestant
▪ **PO (Adults):** 25–50 mg q 3–4 hr as needed.
▪ **PO (Children):** 2–3 mg/kg/day or 100 mg/m^2/day in 4–6 divided doses.
▪ **IV, IM, SC (Adults):** 12.5–25 mg.
▪ **Top (Adults and Children >6 yr):** Nasal/Solution, spray, or jelly should not be used more frequently than q 4 hr or for more than 3–4 days.

Vasopressor
▪ **IV (Adults):** 10–25 mg as a slow injection; additional doses may be given in 5–10 min (not to exceed 150 mg/24 hr).
▪ **SC, IM (Adults):** 25–50 mg (range 10–50 mg), may be followed by second IM dose of 50 mg or an IV dose of 25 mg (not to exceed 150 mg/24 hr).
▪ **IV, SC (Children):** 3 mg/kg/day or 25–100 mg/m^2/day in 4–6 divided doses.

Orthostatic Hypotension
- **PO (Adults):** 25 mg 1–4 times daily.
- **PO (Children):** 3 mg/kg/day in 4–6 divided doses.

CNS Stimulant
- **PO (Adults):** 25–50 mg q 3–4 hr as needed.
- **PO (Children):** 3 mg/kg/day or 100 mg/m²/day in 4–6 divided doses.

AVAILABILITY
- *Capsules:* 25 mg, 50 mg ▪ *Syrup:* 20 mg/5 ml ▪ *Nasal spray:* 0.25% ▪ *Nasal drops:* 0.5% ▪ *Nasal jelly:* 1% ▪ *Injection:* 25 mg/ml, 50 mg/ml ▪ *In combination with:* antihistamines, decongestants, antitussives in cough and cold preparation.

TIME/ACTION PROFILE (PO, SC, IM = bronchodilation, IV = pressor response, Top = nasal decongestion)

	ONSET	PEAK	DURATION
PO	15–60 min	UK	3–5 hr
SC	UK	UK	1 hr
IM	10–20 min	UK	1 hr
IV	UK	UK	1 hr
Top	UK	UK	6 hr

NURSING IMPLICATIONS

ASSESSMENT
- **Bronchodilator:** Assess lung sounds, pulse, and blood pressure before administration and during peak of medication.
- **Vasopressor:** Monitor blood pressure, pulse, ECG, and respiratory rate frequently during IV administration.
- **Nasal Decongestant:** Assess patient for nasal and sinus congestion prior to and periodically during therapy.
- **CNS Stimulant:** Assess sleep patterns and mental status of patients treated for narcolepsy or mental depression.

POTENTIAL NURSING DIAGNOSES
- Tissue perfusion, altered (indications).
- Airway clearance, ineffective (indications).
- Knowledge deficit related to medication regimen (patient/family teaching).

IMPLEMENTATION
- **General Info:** Tolerance to ephedrine may develop with prolonged or excessive use. Effectiveness may be restored by discontinuing for a few days and then readministering.
- **PO:** Administer last dose each day a few hours before bedtime to minimize insomnia.
- **IV:** Use only clear solutions. Discard any unused solution.
- **Direct IV:** Inject undiluted through Y-site or 3-way stopcock.
- *Rate:* Administer slowly, each 10 mg over at least 1 min.
- **Solution Compatibility:** ▪ D5W ▪ D10W ▪ 0.45% NaCl ▪ 0.9% NaCl ▪ Ringer's and lactated Ringer's solution ▪ dextrose/saline combinations ▪ dextrose/Ringer's or lactated Ringer's combinations.

PATIENT/FAMILY TEACHING
- Instruct patient to take ephedrine exactly as directed. If on a scheduled dosing regimen, take a missed dose as soon as remembered, spacing remaining doses at regular intervals. Do not double doses. Caution patient not to exceed recommended dose.
- Instruct patient to contact physician immediately if shortness of breath is not relieved by medication or is accompanied by diaphoresis, dizziness, palpitations, or chest pain.
- Advise patient to consult physician or pharmacist before taking any over-the-counter medications or alcoholic beverages concurrently with this therapy.

EVALUATION
Effectiveness of therapy can be demonstrated by: ▪ Prevention or relief of bronchospasm ▪ Increase in blood pressure, when used as a vasopressor ▪ Decrease in sinus and nasal congestion ▪ Improvement in mental status and increase in alertness, when used as a CNS stimulant.

EPINEPHRINE (inhalation)
(ep-i-**nef**-rin)
Adrenalin, AsthmaHaler, Bronk-aid, Dysne-Inhal, Medihaler-Epi, Primatene

RACEMIC EPINEPHRINE (inhalation)
AsthmaNefrin, microNEFRIN, S-2 Inhalant, Vaponefrin

EPINEPHRINE (parenteral)
EpiPen, EpiPen Jr

EPINEPHRINE (parenteral suspension)
Sus-Phrine

EPINEPHRINE (ophthalmic)
Epifrin, Epinal, Epitrate, Eppy/N, Glaucon

CLASSIFICATION(S):
Bronchodilator (adrenergic),
Cardiac stimulant, Ophthalmic
(antiglaucoma)
Pregnancy Category C

INDICATIONS

▪ **IV, SC, Inhalation:** Bronchodilator in the symptomatic treatment of asthma and other forms of reversible airway disease, which may occur in association with chronic bronchitis and emphysema ▪ **IV, SC:** Treatment of anaphylaxis ▪ **IV, Intracardiac:** Cardiac arrest ▪ **Ophth:** Treatment of open-angle glaucoma ▪ **Local:** As an adjunct in the localization of anesthesia.

ACTION

▪ Beta$_1$- and beta$_2$-adrenergic agonist, which produces an accumulation of cyclic adenosine monophosphate (cAMP). Increased levels of cAMP at beta-adrenergic receptors produce bronchodilation, CNS and cardiac stimulation, diuresis, and gastric acid secretion ▪ When injected locally, stimulates alpha-adrenergic receptors in blood vessels of the skin, producing vasoconstriction. **Therapeutic Effects:** ▪ Bronchodilation ▪ Cardiac stimulation ▪ Vasoconstriction ▪ The following oph-

thalmic effects: □ Decreased formation of aqueous humor □ Increased aqueous outflow □ Conjunctival vasoconstriction □ Mydriasis ▪ Localization of anesthetics.

PHARMACOKINETICS

Absorption: Absorbed but rapidly metabolized following oral administration. Systemic absorption may follow ophthalmic administration or large and repeated inhalation doses.
Distribution: Does not cross the blood–brain barrier. Crosses the placenta and enters breast milk.
Metabolism and Excretion: Action is rapidly terminated by metabolism and uptake by nerve endings.
Half-life: UK.

CONTRAINDICATIONS AND PRECAUTIONS

Contraindicated in: ▪ Hypersensitivity to sympathomimetics ▪ May contain bisulfites—avoid use in patients with bisulfite hypersensitivity.
Use Cautiously in: ▪ Elderly (more susceptible to adverse reactions—dosage reduction may be required) ▪ Pregnancy and lactation (safety not established) ▪ Cardiovascular disease ▪ Arrhythmias ▪ Hypertension ▪ Hyperthyroidism ▪ Glaucoma (except for ophthalmic use in open-angle glaucoma) ▪ Diabetes mellitus (may increase the need for insulin or oral hypoglycemic agents) ▪ Excessive use of inhaler may lead to tolerance, paradoxical bronchospasm, systemic absorption, and side effects.

ADVERSE REACTIONS AND SIDE EFFECTS*

CNS: nervousness, restlessness, insomnia, tremor, headache.
CV: hypertension, arrhythmias, angina.
Endo: hyperglycemia.
GI: nausea, vomiting.
GU: urinary retention, hesitancy.

INTERACTIONS

Drug–Drug: ▪ Additive effect with

other **adrenergic (sympathomimetic) agents,** including **decongestants** ▪ Use with **MAO inhibitors** may lead to hypertensive crisis ▪ Increased risk of arrhythmias with **general anesthetics** or **cardiac glycosides** ▪ **Beta-adrenergic blockers** may block therapeutic response (however, **ophthalmic beta blockers** may be used with **ophthalmic epinephrine,** resulting in additive lowering of intraocular pressure).

ROUTE AND DOSAGE
See infusion rate table in Appendix D.

Epinephrine Solution—Parenteral Bronchodilator
▪ **SC (Adults):** 0.2–0.5 mg q 20 min–4 hr (up to 1 mg/dose).

Anaphylactic Reactions
▪ **IM, SC (Adults):** 0.2–0.5 mg, may repeat q 10–15 min (up to 1 mg/dose).
▪ **SC (Children):** 0.01 mg/kg repeat q 15 min for 2 doses, then q 4 hr as needed (not to exceed 0.5 mg/dose).

Vasopressor, Anaphylactic Shock
▪ **IM, SC (Adults):** 0.5 mg, may repeat in 5 min, may be followed by IV administration.
▪ **IV (Adults):** 0.1–0.25 mg (up to 0.5 mg) may repeat q 5–15 min or followed by infusion at 1 mcg/min; may be increased to a maximum of 4 mcg/min.
▪ **IM, IV, SC (Children):** 10 mcg/kg (up to 0.3 mg) may repeat q 5–15 min.

Cardiac Arrest
▪ **IV, Intracardiac, Endotracheal (Adults):** 0.1–1 mg, repeat q 5 min as needed.
▪ **IV, Intracardiac, Endotracheal (Children):** 5–10 mcg/kg q 5 min, may be followed by IV infusion at an initial rate of 0.1 mcg/kg/min, not to exceed 1.5 mcg/kg/min.

Epinephrine Suspension—Parenteral Bronchodilator
▪ **SC (Adults):** 0.5 mg initially, then 0.5–1.5 mg no more often than q 6 hr as needed.
▪ **SC (Children):** 25 mcg/kg no more often than q 6 hr as needed.

Epinephrine Inhalation
▪ **Inhalation (Adults and Children):** 1–2 inhalations of 1:100 or 2.25% racepinephrine (0.2 mg/dose). May repeat q 3 hr.

Epinephrine Ophthalmic
▪ **Ophth (Adults):** 1 drop 1–2 times daily.

AVAILABILITY
▪ *Solution for injection:* 1:1000 (1 mg/ml), 1:10,000 (0.1 mg/ml) ▪ *Pediatric solution for injection:* 1:100,000 (0.01 mg/ml) ▪ *Suspension for injection:* 1:200 (5 mg/ml) ▪ *Auto-injector:* 0.5 mg/ml, 1 mg/ml ▪ *Solution for inhalation:* 1:100, 2.25% (racepinephrine), 2% (racepinephrine) ▪ *Aerosol:* 0.16 mg/spray, 0.25 mg/spray, 0.2 mg/spray ▪ *Ophth solution:* 0.25%, 0.5%, 1%, 2%.

TIME/ACTION PROFILE (SC, IM, IV, Inhaln = bronchodilation, Ophth = lowering of intraocular pressure)

	ONSET	PEAK	DURATION
SC	5–10 min	20 min	20–30 min*
IM	5–10 min	20 min	20–30 min
IV	rapid	20 min	20–30 min
Inhaln	3–5 min	20 min	1–3 hr
Ophth	within 1 hr	4–8 hr	24 hr

*Epinephrine suspension has a duration of 6–12 hr.

NURSING IMPLICATIONS
ASSESSMENT
▪ **IV:** Monitor blood pressure, pulse, and respiratory rate prior to and every 5 min during IV administration. Patients receiving IV epinephrine should have continuous ECG monitoring.
▪ **Bronchodilator:** Assess lung sounds before and after treatment. Note amount, color, and character of sputum produced, and notify physician of abnormal findings.
▫ Observe patient closely for symptoms of relief. If no relief occurs within 20 min of treatment, or if symptoms worsen, notify physician immediately.

□ Observe patient for drug tolerance and rebound bronchospasm. Patients requiring more than 3 inhalation treatments in 24 hr should be under close supervision. If minimal or no relief is seen after 3–5 inhalation treatments within 6–12 hr, further treatment with aerosol alone is not recommended.

▪ **Lab Test Considerations:** May cause an increase in blood glucose and serum lactic acid concentrations.

POTENTIAL NURSING DIAGNOSES

▪ Airway clearance, ineffective (indications).
▪ Cardiac output, decreased (indications).
▪ Knowledge deficit related to medication regimen (patient/family teaching).

IMPLEMENTATION

▪ **General Info:** Medication should be administered promptly at the onset of bronchospasm.

□ Check dose, concentration, and route of administration carefully prior to administration. Fatalities have occurred from medication errors. Use a tuberculin syringe for SC injection to ensure that correct amount of medication is administered. Suspension is for SC use *only*.

□ Do not use solutions that are pinkish or brownish or that contain a precipitate.

□ For anaphylactic shock, volume replacement should be administered concurrently with epinephrine. Antihistamines and glucocorticoids may be used in conjunction with epinephrine.

▪ **SC/IM:** Medication can cause irritation of tissue. Rotate injection sites to prevent tissue necrosis. Massage injection sites well after administration to enhance absorption and to decrease local vasoconstriction. Avoid IM administration in gluteal muscle. Shake suspension well before administering; inject promptly to prevent settling.

▪ **IV:** Dilute 1 mg (1 ml) of 1:1000 solution in at least 10 ml of 0.9% NaCl for injection to prepare a 1:10,000 solution. Discard any solution not used within 24 hr of preparation.

▪ **Direct IV:** Administer each 1 mg over at least 1 min; more rapid administration may be used during cardiac resuscitation.

▪ **Continuous Infusion:** For maintenance, solution may be further diluted in 500 ml of D5W, D10W, 0.9% NaCl, D5/LR, D5/Ringer's solution, dextrose/saline combinations, or Ringer's or lactated Ringer's solution. Administer through Y-site or 3–way stopcock via infusion pump to ensure accurate dosage.

▪ **Syringe Compatibility:** ▪ doxapram ▪ heparin ▪ milrinone.

▪ **Y-Site Compatibility:** ▪ amrinone ▪ atracurium ▪ calcium chloride ▪ calcium gluconate ▪ famotidine ▪ heparin ▪ hydrocortisone sodium succinate ▪ pancuronium ▪ phytonadione ▪ potassium chloride ▪ vecuronium.

▪ **Y-Site Incompatibility:** ▪ ampicillin.

▪ **Additive Incompatibility:** ▪ aminophylline ▪ sodium bicarbonate.

▪ **Inhalation:** When using epinephrine inhalation solution, 10 drops of 1% base solution should be placed in the reservoir of the nebulizer.

□ The 2.25% inhalation solution of racepinephrine must be diluted for use in the combination nebulizer/respirator.

□ Allow 1–2 min to elapse between inhalations of epinephrine inhalation solution, epinephrine inhalation aerosol, or epinephrine bitartrate inhalation aerosol to make certain the second inhalation is necessary.

□ When epinephrine is used concurrently with glucocorticoid or ipratropium inhalations, administer bronchodilator first and other medications 5 min apart to prevent toxicity from inhaled fluorocarbon propellants.

▪ **Endotracheal:** Epinephrine can be injected directly into the bronchial tree via the endotracheal tube if the patient has been intubated. Use the same dose as for IV injection.

E

- **Ophth:** See Appendix H for administration of ophthalmic medications. If used with miotics, instill miotics first.

PATIENT/FAMILY TEACHING

- **General Info:** Advise patient taking epinephrine for asthma, bronchitis, emphysema, or other obstructive pulmonary diseases to contact physician immediately if there is no response to the usual dose of epinephrine or if angina develops. This may signify worsening of condition and requires evaluation of therapy.
- **Inhalation:** Instruct patient to rinse mouth after each inhalation to prevent dryness.
□ Advise patient to consult physician or pharmacist prior to taking any over-the-counter medications concurrently with epinephrine.
□ Advise patient to report bronchial irritation, restlessness, or insomnia to physician promptly. A decrease in medication dose may be necessary.
- **Auto-injector:** Instruct patients using auto-injector for anaphylactic reactions to remove gray safety cap, placing black tip on thigh at right angle to leg. Press hard into thigh until auto-injector functions, hold in place several seconds, remove, and discard properly. Massage injected area for 10 sec.
- **Ophth:** Emphasize the importance of not touching the applicator tip to any surface.
□ Instruct patient to report immediately any decrease in visual acuity.
□ Advise patient not to use solution if it is brown or contains particulate matter. Solution should be discarded 3 mo after dropper is placed in solution.
□ Instruct patients not to use while wearing soft contact lenses.

EVALUATION

Effectiveness of therapy can be demonstrated by: ▪ Decrease in wheezing and respiratory distress ▪ Reversal of signs and symptoms of anaphylaxis ▪ Increase in cardiac rate and output, when used in cardiac resuscitation ▪ Decrease in intraocular pressure ▪ Localization of local anesthetic.

EPOETIN ALFA
(ee-**poe**-e-tin al-fa)
Epogen, EPO, erythropoietin, Procrit

CLASSIFICATION(S):
Hormone (erythropoietin, recombinant)
Pregnancy Category C

INDICATIONS

- Treatment of anemia associated with chronic renal failure ▪ Management of anemia secondary to zidovudine (AZT) therapy in HIV-infected patients ▪ Management of anemia from chemotherapy in patients with nonmyeloid malignancies (Procrit only).

ACTION

- Stimulates erythropoiesis (production of red blood cells). **Therapeutic Effect:** ▪ Maintains and may elevate red blood cell counts, decreasing the need for transfusions.

PHARMACOKINETICS

Absorption: Well absorbed following SC administration.
Distribution: Distribution not known.
Metabolism and Excretion: Metabolism and excretion not known.
Half-life: 4–13 hr.

CONTRAINDICATIONS AND PRECAUTIONS

Contraindicated in: ▪ Hypersensitivity to albumin or mammalian cell-derived products ▪ Uncontrolled hypertension ▪ Patients with erythropoietin levels >200 mU/ml.
Use Cautiously in: ▪ History of seizures ▪ Pregnancy, lactation, or children (safety not established).

ADVERSE REACTIONS AND SIDE EFFECTS*

CNS: SEIZURES, headache.
CV: thrombotic events (hemodialysis patients), <u>hypertension</u>.
Derm: transient rashes.
Endo: resumption of menses, restored fertility.

INTERACTIONS

Drug–Drug: ▪ May increase the requirement for **heparin** anticoagulation during hemodialysis.

ROUTE AND DOSAGE

Anemia of Chronic Renal Failure

▪ **SC, IV (Adults):** 50–100 units/kg 3 times weekly initially, then adjust dosage by changes of 25 units/kg/dose to maintain target range of Hct. Usual maintenance dose 25 units/kg 3 times weekly.

Anemia Secondary to Zidovudine (AZT) Therapy

▪ **IV, SC (Adults):** 100 units/kg 3 times weekly for 8 wk, if inadequate response, may increase by 50–100 units/kg every 4–8 wk, up to 300 units/kg 3 times weekly.

Anemia from Chemotherapy

▪ **SC (Adults):** 150 units/kg 3 times weekly; may increase after 8 wk up to 300 units/kg 3 times weekly.

AVAILABILITY

▪ *Injection:* 2000 units/ml, 3000 units/ml, 4000 units/ml, 10,000 units/ml.

TIME/ACTION PROFILE (increase in RBCs)

	ONSET*	PEAK	DURATION
IV, SC	10 days	2–6 wk	UK

*Increase in reticulocytes.

NURSING IMPLICATIONS

ASSESSMENT

▫ Monitor blood pressure prior to and throughout course of therapy. Inform physician if severe hypertension is present or if blood pressure begins to increase. Uncontrolled hypertension is a contraindication for epoetin alfa therapy. Additional antihypertensive therapy may be required during initiation of therapy.
▫ Monitor response for symptoms of anemia (fatigue, dyspnea, pallor).
▫ Monitor dialysis shunts (thrill and bruit) and status of artificial kidney during hemodialysis. Heparin dose may need to be increased to prevent clotting. Patients with underlying vascular disease should be monitored for impaired circulation.
▪ **Lab Test Considerations:** Serum ferritin, transferrin, and iron levels should also be monitored to assess need for concurrent iron therapy. Transferrin saturation should be at least 20% and ferritin should be at least 100 ng/ml.
▫ Monitor renal function studies and electrolytes closely, as resulting increased sense of well-being may lead to decreased compliance with other therapies for renal failure. Increases in BUN, creatinine, uric acid, phosphorous, and potassium may occur.
▫ May cause increase in WBCs and platelets. May decrease bleeding times.
▫ *Anemia of Chronic Renal Failure:* Hematocrit should be monitored prior to and twice weekly during initial therapy, and regularly after target range (30–33%) has been reached and maintenance dose is determined. Other hemopoietic parameters (hemoglobin, reticulocyte count, and RBC count) also should be monitored prior to and periodically throughout therapy. Reticulocyte count usually begins to rise 10 days after initiation of therapy. Hemoglobin, hematocrit, and RBC levels begin to increase after 2–6 wk of therapy. Notify physician if hematocrit increases more than 4 points in a 2-wk period, as this increases the likelihood of a hypertensive reaction and seizures. If hematocrit exceeds 36%, dose should be withheld until hematocrit is 33%.

E

*<u>Underlines</u> indicate most frequent; **CAPITALS** indicate life-threatening.

Dose should be reduced by 25 units/kg upon resumption.

□ *Anemia Secondary to Zidovudine Therapy:* Before initiating therapy, determine endogenous serum erythropoietin level prior to transfusion. Patients receiving zidovudine with endogenous serum erythropoietin levels >500 mU/ml may not respond to therapy.

□ Monitor hematocrit weekly during dosage adjustment. If hematocrit exceeds 40%, discontinue dose until hematocrit drops to 36%, then decrease dose by 25%.

□ *Anemia from Chemotherapy:* Monitor hematocrit weekly until stable. Patients with lower baseline serum erythropoietin levels may respond more rapidly; not recommended if levels >200 mU/ml. If hematocrit exceeds 40%, hold dose until it falls to 36%, then decrease dose by 25%. If initial dose response is >4 percentage points in any 2-wk period, reduce dose.

POTENTIAL NURSING DIAGNOSES

- Activity intolerance (indications).
- Knowledge deficit related to medication and dietary regimen (patient/family teaching).
- Noncompliance (patient/family teaching).

IMPLEMENTATION

- **General Info:** Transfusions are still required for severe symptomatic anemia, as several weeks are required before therapeutic response occurs.
- □ Institute seizure precautions in patients who experience greater than a 4-point increase in hematocrit in a 2-wk period or exhibit any change in neurologic status. Risk of seizures is greatest during the first 90 days of therapy.
- □ Do not shake vial, as inactivation of medication may occur. Discard vial immediately after withdrawing dose.
- **SC:** This route is often used for patients not requiring dialysis.

- **IV:** May be administered as direct injection or bolus via venous line at end of dialysis session.

PATIENT/FAMILY TEACHING

- □ Stress importance of compliance with dietary restrictions, medications, and dialysis. Foods high in iron and low in potassium include liver, pork, veal, beef, mustard and turnip greens, peas, eggs, broccoli, kale, blackberries, strawberries, apple juice, watermelon, oatmeal, and enriched bread. Epoetin alfa will result in increased sense of well-being, but it does not cure underlying renal disease.
- □ Explain rationale for concurrent iron therapy (increased red blood cell production requires iron).
- □ Discuss possible return of menses and fertility in females of childbearing age. Patient should discuss contraceptive options with physician.
- □ Discuss ways of preventing self-injury in patients at risk for seizures. Driving and activities requiring continuous alertness should be avoided.

EVALUATION

Clinical response is indicated by: ▪ Increase in hematocrit to 30–33% and subsequent improvement in symptoms of anemia in patients with chronic renal failure ▪ Increase in hematocrit to >40% in anemia secondary to zidovudine therapy ▪ Increase in hematocrit in patients with anemia due to chemotherapy.

ERGOCALCIFEROL
(er-goe-kal-**sif**-e-role)
Calciferol, Deltalin, Drisdol, {Ostoforte}, {Radiostol}, vitamin D₂

CLASSIFICATION(S):
Vitamin (fat-soluble)
Pregnancy Category C

INDICATIONS

- Prophylaxis and treatment of vitamin D deficiency ▪ Treatment of hypophosphatemia or hypocalcemia ▪ Treatment of osteodystrophy ▪ Treatment of osteomalacia secondary to chronic anticonvulsant therapy ▪ Treatment of rickets. **Unlabeled Uses:** ▪ Renal osteodystrophy ▪ Treatment and prophylaxis of postoperative and idiopathic tetany.

ACTION

- Promotes the absorption of calcium and phosphorous ▪ Regulates calcium homeostasis in conjunction with parathyroid hormone and calcitonin. **Therapeutic Effect:** ▪ Treatment and prevention of deficiency states, particularly bone manifestations.

PHARMACOKINETICS

Absorption: Well absorbed in an inactive form.
Distribution: Stored in the liver and other fatty tissues.
Metabolism and Excretion: Converted to active form by sunlight and the liver. Metabolized and excreted by the kidney.
Half-life: UK.

CONTRAINDICATIONS AND PRECAUTIONS

Contraindicated in: ▪ Hypersensitivity ▪ Hypercalcemia ▪ Vitamin D toxicity ▪ Lactation (large doses).
Use Cautiously in: ▪ Patients receiving cardiac glycosides ▪ Pregnancy (larger doses; safety not established).

ADVERSE REACTIONS AND SIDE EFFECTS*

- Do not occur at doses within the range of daily requirements.

INTERACTIONS

Drug–Drug: ▪ **Cholestyramine, colestipol,** or **mineral oil** decreases absorption of vitamin D analogs ▪ Use with **thiazide diuretics** in patients with hypoparathyroidism may result in hypercalcemia ▪ **Glucocorticoids** decrease the effectiveness of vitamin D analogs ▪ Use with **cardiac glycosides** increases the risk of arrhythmias ▪ Vitamin D requirements are increased by **phenytoin** and other **hydantoin anticonvulsants, sucralfate, barbiturates,** and **primidone.**

ROUTE AND DOSAGE

Vitamin D Deficiency
- PO (Adults): 1000–2000 units/day initially, then 400 units/day maintenance.
- PO (Children): 1000–4000 units/day initially, then 400 units/day maintenance.

Vitamin D-Resistant Rickets
- PO (Adults): 12,000–500,000 units/day.

Vitamin D-Dependent Rickets
- PO (Adults): 10,000–60,000 units/day (up to 150,000 units/day).
- PO (Children): 3000–10,000 units/day, up to 50,000 units/day.

Familial Hypophosphatemia
- PO (Adults): 50,000–100,000 units/day.

Osteomalacia from Anticonvulsants
- PO (Adults): 1000–4000 units/day.
- PO (Children): 1000 units/day.

Hypoparathyroidism
- PO (Adults): 50,000–150,000 units/day.
- PO (Children): 50,000–200,000 units/day.

Renal Osteodystrophy
- PO (Adults): 10,000–300,000 units/day.
- PO (Children): 4000–40,000 units/day.

Malabsorption
- IM (Adults and Children): 10,000 units/day.

AVAILABILITY

- *Liquid:* 8000 units/ml ▪ *Capsules:* 50,000 units ▪ *Tablets:* 50,000 units ▪ *Injection:* 500,000 units/ml.

TIME/ACTION PROFILE (effects on serum calcium levels)

	ONSET	PEAK	DURATION
PO	12–24 hr*	UK	up to 6 mo*

*Therapeutic effect may take 10–14 days.

NURSING IMPLICATIONS

ASSESSMENT

- **General Info:** Assess for symptoms of vitamin deficiency prior to and periodically throughout therapy.
- □ Observe patient for evidence of hypocalcemia (paresthesias, muscle twitching, laryngospasm, colic, cardiac arrhythmias, and Chvostek's or Trousseau's sign). Protect symptomatic patient by raising and padding side rails; keep bed in low position.
- **Children:** Monitor height and weight; growth arrest may occur in prolonged high-dose therapy.
- **Ricketts/Osteomalacia:** Assess patient for bone pain and weakness prior to and throughout course of therapy.
- **Lab Test Considerations:** Monitor serum phosphorous levels prior to and periodically throughout course of therapy. Serum phosphorous must be controlled prior to initiating therapy. Aluminum carbonate or aluminum hydroxide is used for this purpose in dialysis patients.
- □ Serum calcium levels should be drawn weekly during initial therapy. Monitor BUN, serum creatinine, alkaline phosphatase, parathyroid hormone levels, creatine clearance, and 24-hr urinary calcium periodically. A fall in alkaline phosphatase levels may signal onset of hypercalcemia.
- **Toxicity and Overdose:** Toxicity is manifested as hypercalcemia. Assess for nausea, vomiting, anorexia, weakness, constipation, headache, bone pain, and metallic taste. Later symptoms include polyuria, polydipsia, photophobia, rhinorrhea, pruritis, and cardiac arrhythmias. Treatment includes discontinuing ergocalciferol and instituting a low-calcium diet. IV

hydration, loop diuretics, and urinary acidification may be ordered to increase urinary excretion of calcium. Dialysis may also be used.

POTENTIAL NURSING DIAGNOSES

- Nutrition, altered: less than body requirements (indications).
- Knowledge deficit related to medication regimen (patient/family teaching).

IMPLEMENTATION

- **General Info:** Because solitary vitamin deficiencies are rare, combinations are commonly administered.
- **PO:** May be administered without regard to meals. Measure solution accurately with calibrated dropper provided by manufacturer. May be mixed with juice, cereal, or food.
- **IM:** Injection is oil-based; avoid IV administration.

PATIENT/FAMILY TEACHING

- □ Advise patient to take as directed. If dose is missed, take as soon as remembered; do not double up on doses.
- □ Encourage patients to comply with diet recommendations of physician. Explain that the best source of vitamins is a well-balanced diet with foods from the 4 basic food groups.
- □ See Appendix K for foods high in calcium and vitamin D. Renal patients must still consider renal failure diet in food selection. Physician may order concurrent calcium supplement.
- □ Patients self-medicating with vitamin supplements should be cautioned not to exceed RDA (see Appendix L). The effectiveness of megadoses for treatment of various medical conditions is unproven and may cause side effects.
- □ Review symptoms of overdosage and instruct patient to report these promptly to physician.
- □ Emphasize the importance of follow-up examinations to evaluate progress.

EVALUATION

Effectiveness of therapy can be demonstrated by: ■ Decrease in the symptoms of vitamin D deficiency ■ Normalization of serum calcium levels in hypoparathyroidism ▪ Improvement in symptoms of vitamin D-resistant rickets.

ERGONOVINE
(er-goe-**noe**-veen)
Ergometrine, Ergotrate

CLASSIFICATION(S):
Oxytocic
Pregnancy Category UK

INDICATIONS

▪ Prevention and treatment of postpartum or postabortion hemorrhage caused by uterine atony or involution. **Unlabeled Use:** ▪ As a diagnostic agent to provoke coronary artery spasm.

ACTION

▪ Directly stimulates uterine and vascular smooth muscle. **Therapeutic Effect:** ▪ Uterine contraction.

PHARMACOKINETICS

Absorption: Well absorbed following oral or IM administration.
Distribution: Distribution not known.
Metabolism and Excretion: UK. Probably metabolized by the liver.
Half-life: UK.

CONTRAINDICATIONS AND PRECAUTIONS

Contraindicated in: ▪ Hypersensitivity ▪ Avoid chronic use ▪ Should not be used to induce labor.
Use Cautiously in: ▪ Hypertensive or eclamptic patients (increased susceptibility to hypertensive and arrhythmogenic side effects) ▪ Severe hepatic or renal disease ▪ Sepsis ▪ Third stage of labor.

ADVERSE REACTIONS AND SIDE EFFECTS*

CNS: dizziness, headache.
CV: palpitations, chest pain, hypertension, arrhythmias.
Derm: sweating.

EENT: tinnitus.
GI: nausea, vomiting.
Resp: dyspnea.
Misc: allergic reactions.

INTERACTIONS

Drug–Drug: ▪ Excessive vasoconstriction may result when used with other **vasopressors,** such as **dopamine** or **nicotine**.

ROUTE AND DOSAGE

Oxytocic
▪ **PO, SL (Adults):** 0.2–0.4 mg q 6–12 hr (usual course is 48 hr).
▪ **IM, IV (Adults):** 0.2 mg q 2–4 hr for up to 5 doses; then change to PO.

Provocative Agent for Coronary Artery Spasm
▪ **IV (Adults):** 50 mcg q 5 min until chest pain occurs or a total dose of 400 mcg has been given.

AVAILABILITY

▪ *Tablets:* 0.2 mg ▪ *Injection:* 0.2 mg/ml, {0.2 mg/ml}.

TIME/ACTION PROFILE (uterine contractions)

	ONSET	PEAK	DURATION
PO	5–15 min	UK	3 hr or longer
IM	2–5 min	UK	3 hr or longer
IV	immediate	UK	45 min

NURSING IMPLICATIONS

ASSESSMENT
▫ Monitor blood pressure, pulse, and respirations every 15–30 min until transfer to the postpartum unit, then every 1–2 hr. Inform physician if hypertension, chest pain, arrhythmias, headache, or change in neurologic status occurs.
▫ Monitor amount and type of vaginal discharge. Notify physician immediately if symptoms of hemorrhage (increased bleeding, hypotension, pallor, tachycardia) occur.
▫ Palpate uterine fundus, note position and consistency. Notify physician if

{} = Available in Canada only.
*Underlines indicate most frequent; **CAPITALS** indicate life-threatening.

fundus fails to contract in response to ergonovine. Assess patient for severe cramping; physician may reduce the dose.

□ Assess for signs of ergotism (cold, numb fingers and toes, nausea, vomiting, diarrhea, headache, muscle pain, weakness).

□ If patient fails to respond to ergonovine, check serum calcium level. Correction of hypocalcemia may restore responsiveness.

■ **Lab Test Considerations:** May cause decreased serum prolactin level, which inhibits synthesis of breast milk.

■ **Toxicity and Overdose:** Toxicity, initially manifested as ergotism, may cause seizures and gangrene. Seizures are treated with anticonvulsants. Vasodilators and heparin may be ordered to improve circulation to extremities. Amputation is required for gangrene.

POTENTIAL NURSING DIAGNOSES

■ Tissue perfusion, altered (indications).

■ Injury, high risk for (side effects).

■ Knowledge deficit related to medication regimen (patient/family teaching).

IMPLEMENTATION

■ **General Info:** Do not administer solution that is discolored or contains a precipitate.

■ **PO:** Administration is usually limited to 48 hr postpartum, by which time the danger of hemorrhage from uterine atony has passed.

□ Tablets may be administered SL.

■ **IM:** The preferred route is IM. Firm uterine contractions are produced within a few minutes. Dose may need to be repeated every 2–4 hr for full therapeutic effect.

■ **Direct IV:** The IV route is reserved for severe uterine bleeding. Dilute with 5 ml of 0.9 % NaCl.

■ *Rate:* Administer slow IV push over at least 1 min through Y-site injection of an IV of D5W or 0.9% NaCl.

PATIENT/FAMILY TEACHING

□ Review symptoms of toxicity with patient. Instruct her to report occurrence of these immediately.

□ Inform patient that uterine cramping demonstrates effectiveness of therapy.

□ Explain need for pad count to determine degree of bleeding. Instruct patient to report immediately an increase in degree of bleeding or passage of clots.

□ Instruct patient to report breastfeeding difficulties.

□ Caution patient not to smoke while receiving ergonovine, as nicotine is also a vasoconstrictor.

EVALUATION

Effectiveness of therapy is demonstrated by: ■ Uterine contraction and cramping in the prevention or cessation of uterine hemorrhage after delivery or abortion.

ERGOTAMINE
(er-**got**-a-meen)
{Ergomar}, Ergostat, {Gynergen}, {Medihaler Ergotamine}

DIHYDROERGOTAMINE
(dye-hye-droe-er-**got**-a-meen)
D.H.E. 45

CLASSIFICATION(S):
Vascular headache suppressant (alpha-adrenergic blocking agent)
Pregnancy Category X

INDICATIONS

■ Treatment of vascular headaches including □ Migraine □ Cluster headaches.

ACTION

■ In therapeutic doses produces vasoconstriction of dilated blood vessels by

---

stimulating alpha-adrenergic receptors
■ Larger doses may produce alpha-adrenergic blockade and vasodilation
■ Also has antiserotonin activity. **Therapeutic Effect:** ■ Constriction of dilated carotid artery bed with resolution of vascular headache.

PHARMACOKINETICS

Absorption: Unpredictably absorbed (60%) from the GI tract. Oral absorption may be enhanced by caffeine. Sublingual absorption is poor. Dihydroergotamine is rapidly absorbed following IM and SC administration.
Distribution: Ergotamine crosses the blood–brain barrier and enters breast milk.
Metabolism and Excretion: Both ergotamine and dihydroergotamine are highly metabolized (90%) by the liver. Some metabolites are active.
Half-life: Ergotamine (2 phases):—2.7 hr first phase; 21 hr second phase. Dihydroergotamine (2 phases)—2.3 min–1.45 hr first phase; 18–32 hr second phase.

CONTRAINDICATIONS AND PRECAUTIONS

Contraindicated in: ■ Serious infections ■ Peripheral vascular disease ■ Cardiovascular disease ■ Hypertension ■ Severe renal or liver disease ■ Malnutrition ■ Pregnancy ■ Lactation ■ Hypersensitivity to fluorocarbon propellants (inhalation only) ■ Known alcohol intolerance (dihydroergotamine injection only).
Use Cautiously in: ■ Illnesses associated with peripheral vascular pathology such as diabetes mellitus ■ Children <6 yr (safety not established).

ADVERSE REACTIONS AND SIDE EFFECTS*

CV: sinus tachycardia, sinus bradycardia, intermittent claudication, arterial spasm, angina pectoris, MYOCARDIAL INFARCTION.

GI: nausea, vomiting, abdominal pain, diarrhea, polydypsia.
MS: muscle pain, extremity stiffness, stiff neck, stiff shoulders.
Neuro: leg weakness, numbness or tingling in fingers or toes.
Misc: fatigue.

INTERACTIONS

Drug–Drug: ■ Concurrent use with **beta-adrenergic blockers, oral contraceptives, vasoconstrictors, macrolide anti-infectives** or **heavy cigarette smoking (nicotine)** may increase the risk of peripheral vasoconstriction ■ When used concurrently with prophylactic **methysergide** (another ergot alkaloid) dosage of ergotamine should be decreased by 50% ■ Dihydrotamine antagonizes the antianginal effects of **nitrates** ■ Concurrent use with **sumatriptan** may result in prolonged vasoconstriction (allow 24 hr between use).

ROUTE AND DOSAGE

Ergotamine
■ **PO, SL (Adults):** 2 mg initially, then 1–2 mg q 30 min until attack subsides or a total of 6 mg has been given. Should not be used more than twice weekly, with at least 5 days between courses. 1–2 mg PO at bedtime daily for 10–14 days has been used to terminate series of cluster headaches.

Dihydroergotamine
■ **IM, SC (Adults):** 1 mg, may repeat in 1 hr to a total of 3 mg (not to exceed 3 mg/day or 6 mg/wk).
■ **IM, SC (Children ≥6 yr):** 0.5 mg may be repeated in 1 hr.
■ **IV (Adults):** 0.5 mg, may repeat in 1 hr (not to exceed 2 mg/day or 6 mg/wk). For chronic intractable headache, 0.5–1 mg q 8 hr may be given until relief (not to exceed 6 mg/wk).
■ **IV (Children ≥6 yr):** 0.25 mg may be repeated in 1 hr.

AVAILABILITY

Ergotamine

- **Sublingual tablets:** 0.2 mg ▪ {**Tablets:** 1 mg} ▪ **In combination with:** caffeine, barbiturates, and belladonna alkaloids in preparations for vascular headaches. See Appendix A.

Dihydroergotamine

- **Injection:** 1 mg/ml (contains alcohol).

TIME/ACTION PROFILE (relief of headache)

	ONSET	PEAK	DURATION
PO (ergotamine)	1–2 hr (variable)	1–5 hr	UK
SL (ergotamine)	UK	UK	UK
IM, IV, SC (dihydroergotamine)	15–30 min	15 min–2 hr	8 hr

NURSING IMPLICATIONS

ASSESSMENT

- ▢ Assess frequency, location, duration, and characteristics (pain, nausea, vomiting, visual disturbances) of chronic headaches. During acute attack assess type, location, and intensity of pain prior to and 60 min after administration.
- ▢ Monitor blood pressure and peripheral pulses periodically during therapy. Inform physician if significant hypertension occurs.
- ▢ Assess for signs of ergotism (cold, numb fingers and toes, nausea, vomiting, headache, muscle pain, weakness).
- ▢ Assess for nausea and vomiting. Ergotamine stimulates the chemoreceptor trigger zone. Metoclopramide 10 mg IV may be given as an antiemetic 3–5 min prior to administration of dihydroergotamine IV.
- ▪ **Toxicity and Overdose:** Toxicity is manifested by severe ergotism (chest pain, abdominal pain, persistent paresthesia in the extremities) and gan-

grene. Vasodilators, dextran, or heparin may be ordered to improve circulation.

POTENTIAL NURSING DIAGNOSES

- ▪ Pain, acute (indications).
- ▪ Injury, high risk for (side effects).
- ▪ Knowledge deficit related to medication regimen (patient/family teaching).

IMPLEMENTATION

- ▪ **General Info:** Administer as soon as patient reports prodromal symptoms or headache.
- ▪ **SL:** Allow tablet to dissolve under tongue. Do not allow patient to eat, drink, or smoke while tablet is dissolving.
- ▪ **Direct IV:** Dihydroergotamine may be administered undiluted.
- ▪ **Rate:** Administer over 1 min.

PATIENT/FAMILY TEACHING

- ▪ **General Info:** Instruct patient to take ergotamine at the first sign of an impending headache and not to exceed the maximum dose prescribed by the physician.
- ▢ Encourage patient to rest in a quiet, dark room after taking ergotamine.
- ▢ Review symptoms of toxicity. Instruct patient to report these to physician promptly.
- ▢ Caution patient not to smoke and to avoid exposure to cold, as these vasoconstrictors may further impair peripheral circulation.
- ▢ Advise patient to avoid alcohol, as it may precipitate vascular headaches.
- ▢ Instruct female patients to inform physician if they plan or suspect pregnancy. Ergotamine should not be taken during pregnancy.
- ▪ **IM/SC:** Inject at the first sign of a headache and repeat at 1-hr intervals up to 3 doses. Once minimal effective dose is determined, adjust dose for subsequent attacks.

EVALUATION

Effectiveness of therapy can be demonstrated by: ▪ Prevention or relief of pain from vascular headaches.

ERYTHROMYCIN
(eh-rith-roe-**mye**-sin)

ERYTHROMYCIN BASE
{Apo-Erythro-EC}, E-base, E-mycin, {Erybid}, Eryc, Eryc-Sprinkle, Ery-tab, {Erythromid}, PCE Dispersatabs, Robimycin

ERYTHROMYCIN ESTOLATE
Erythrozone, Ilosone, {Novorythro}

ERYTHROMYCIN ETHYL-SUCCINATE
{Apo-Erythro-ES}, E.E.S., EryPed, Erythro

ERYTHROMYCIN GLUCEPTATE

ERYTHROMYCIN LACTO-BIONATE
Erythrocin

ERTHROMYCIN STEARATE
Eramycin, Erythrocin, {Novorythro}, Erythrocot, My-E, Wintrocin, Wyamycin S

ERYTHROMYCIN (OPHTHALMIC)
Ilotycin

ERYTHROMYCIN (TOPICAL)
Akne-Mycin, Erycette, Erygel, Erymax, ETS, Mythromycin, Staticin, T-stat

CLASSIFICATION(S):
Anti-infective (macrolide)
Pregnancy Category B

INDICATIONS

■ **PO, IV:** Treatment of the following infections due to susceptible organisms: □ Upper and lower respiratory tract infections □ Otitis media (with sulfonamides) □ Skin and skin structure infections □ Pertussis □ Diphtheria □ Erythrasma □ Intestinal amebiasis □ Pelvic inflammatory disease □ Nongonococcal urethritis □ Syphilis □ Legionnaire's disease □ Rheumatic fever ■ **Top:** Treatment of acne ■ **Ophth:** ■ Treatment of superficial ocular infections ■ Useful in situations in which penicillin is the most appropriate drug but cannot be used because of previous hypersensitivity reactions, including: □ Streptococcal infections □ Treatment of syphilis or gonorrhea □ Endocarditis prophylaxis.

ACTION

■ Suppresses protein synthesis at the level of the 50S bacterial ribosome. **Therapeutic Effect:** ■ Bacteriostatic action against susceptible bacteria. **Spectrum:** ■ Active against many gram-positive cocci, including: □ Streptococci □ Staphylococci ■ Gram-positive bacilli, including: □ *Clostridium* □ *Corynebacterium* ■ Several gram-negative pathogens, notably: □ *Neisseria* □ *Haemophilus influenzae* □ *Legionella pneumophila* ■ *Mycoplasma* and *Chlamydia* are also usually susceptible.

PHARMACOKINETICS

Absorption: Well absorbed from the duodenum following oral administration. Minimal absorption may follow topical or ophthalmic use.

Distribution: Widely distributed. Minimal penetration into CSF. Crosses the placenta and enters breast milk.

Metabolism and Excretion: Partially metabolized by the liver, excreted mainly unchanged in the bile. Small amounts excreted unchanged in the urine.

Half-life: 1.4–2 hr.

CONTRAINDICATIONS AND PRECAUTIONS

Contraindicated in: ■ Hypersensitivity ■ Hepatic dysfunction (estolate salt) ■ Pregnancy (estolate salt) ■ Known alcohol intolerance (most topicals). Products containing benzyl alcohol should be avoided in neonates.

Use Cautiously in: ■ Liver disease ■ Salts other than the estolate salt may be used in pregnancy to treat *Chlamydia* infections or syphilis ■ Tartrazine sensitivity (some products contain tartrazine—FDC yellow dye #5).

ADVERSE REACTIONS AND SIDE EFFECTS*

GI: <u>nausea</u>, <u>vomiting</u>, diarrhea, abdominal pain, cramping, hepatitis.
EENT: ototoxicity.
Derm: rashes.
Local: <u>phlebitis</u> at IV site.
Misc: allergic reactions, superinfection.

INTERACTIONS

Drug–Drug: ▪ Increases activity and may increase the risk of toxicity from **alfentanil, astemizole, bromocriptine, theophylline, carbamazepine, cyclosporine, disopyramide, ergot alkaloids, oral anticoagulants, methylprednisolone, terfenadine,** or **triazolam** ▪ May increase serum **digoxin** levels in a small percentage of patients ▪ **Top:** Concurrent use with **irritants, abrasives,** or **desquamating agents** may result in increased irritation ▪ **Top: Topical clindamycin** may antagonize beneficial effects.

ROUTE AND DOSAGE

250 mg of erythromycin base, estolate, or stearate = 400 mg of erythromycin ethylsuccinate.

▪ **PO (Adults):** Base, estolate, stearate—250–500 mg q 6–12 hr, ethylsuccinate—400–800 mg q 6–8 hr.
▪ **PO (Children):** 30–50 mg/kg/day in divided doses q 6–12 hr (up to 100 mg/kg/day).
▪ **IV (Adults):** Gluceptate and lactobionate only—1–4 g/day in divided doses q 6 hr, or as a continuous infusion.
▪ **IV (Children):** Gluceptate and lactobionate only—15–20 mg/kg/day in divided doses q 6 hr or as a continuous infusion.
▪ **Top (Adults and Children >12 yr):** 2% ointment, gel, or solution bid.
▪ **Ophth (Adults):** 0.5% ointment to conjunctiva 1 or more times daily.

AVAILABILITY

Erythromycin Base

▪ *Enteric-coated tablets:* 250 mg, 333 mg ▪ *Tablets with polymer-coated particles* 333 mg, 500 mg ▪ *Film-coated tablets:* 500 mg ▪ *Delayed-release capsules:* {125 mg}, 250 mg ▪ *Topical ointment:* 2% ▪ *Topical gel:* 2% ▪ *Ophthalmic ointment:* 5 mg/g.

Erythromycin Estolate

▪ *Tablets:* 500 mg ▪ *Capsules:* 250 mg ▪ *Oral suspension:* 125 mg/5 ml, 250 mg/5 ml.

Erythromycin Stearate

▪ *Film-coated tablets:* 250 mg, 500 mg.

Erythromycin Ethylsuccinate

▪ *Chewable tablets:* 200 mg ▪ *Tablets:* 400 mg ▪ *Oral suspension:* 200 mg/5 ml, 400 mg/5 ml ▪ *Drops:* 100 mg/2.5 ml ▪ *In combination with:* sulfisoxazole (Eryzole, Pediazole). See Appendix A.

Erythromycin Lactobionate

▪ *Injection:* 500 mg, 1 g.

TIME/ACTION PROFILE (blood levels)

	ONSET	PEAK
PO	1 hr	1–4 hr
IV	rapid	end of infusion

NURSING IMPLICATIONS

ASSESSMENT

□ Assess patient for infection (vital signs; appearance of wound, sputum, urine, and stool; WBC) at beginning and throughout course of therapy.
□ Obtain specimens for culture and sensitivity prior to initiating therapy. First dose may be given before receiving results.
▪ **Lab Test Considerations:** Liver function tests should be performed periodically on patients receiving high-dose, long-term therapy.
□ May cause increased serum bilirubin, AST (SGOT), ALT (SGPT), and alkaline phosphatase concentrations.
□ May cause false elevations of urinary catecholamines.

---

*Underlines indicate most frequent; **CAPITALS** indicate life-threatening.

POTENTIAL NURSING DIAGNOSES

- Infection, high risk for (indications, side effects).
- Knowledge deficit related to medication regimen (patient/family teaching).
- Noncompliance related to medication regimen (patient/family teaching).

IMPLEMENTATION

- **PO:** Administer around the clock on an empty stomach, at least 1 hr before or 2 hr after meals. May be taken with food if GI irritation occurs. Should not be taken with fruit juices. Take each dose with a full glass of water.
- Use calibrated measuring device for liquid preparations. Shake well before using.
- Chewable tablets should be crushed or chewed and not swallowed whole.
- Do not open, crush, or chew delayed-release capsules or tablets; swallow whole. Enteric-coated tablets may be administered regardless of meals.
- **IV:** Add 10 ml of Sterile Water for Injection without preservatives to 250- or 500-mg vials and 20 ml to 1-g vial. Solution is stable for 7 days after reconstitution if refrigerated.
- **Intermittent Infusion:** Dilute further in 100–250 ml of 0.9% NaCl or D5W.
- **Rate:** Administer slowly over 20–60 min to avoid phlebitis. Assess for pain along vein; slow rate if pain occurs; apply ice and notify physician if unable to relieve pain.
- **Continuous Infusion:** May also be administered as an infusion in a dilution of 1 g/liter of 0.9% NaCl, D5W, or lactated Ringer's solution over 4 hr.

ERYTHROMYCIN GLUCEPTATE

- **Syringe Incompatibility:** ■ heparin.
- **Additive Compatibility:** ■ calcium gluconate ■ dimenhydrinate ■ heparin ■ hydrocortisone sodium succinate ■ potassium chloride ■ sodium bicarbonate.
- **Additive Incompatibility:** ■ aminophylline ■ pentobarbital ■ secobarbital.

ERTHROMYCIN LACTOBIONATE

- **Syringe Incompatibility:** ■ heparin.

- **Y-Site Compatibility:** ■ acyclovir ■ cyclophosphamide ■ enalaprilat ■ esmolol ■ famotidine ■ foscarnet ■ hydromorphone ■ labetalol ■ magnesium sulfate ■ meperidine ■ morphine ■ multivitamins ■ perphenazine ■ vitamin B complex with C ■ zidovudine.
- **Y-Site Incompatibility:** ■ fluconazole.
- **Additive Compatibility:** cimetidine ■ hydrocortisone sodium succinate ■ pentobarbital ■ potassium chloride ■ prednisolone ■ sodium bicarbonate.
- **Additive Incompatibility:** ■ heparin ■ metoclopramide ■ vitamin B complex with C.
- **Ophth:** See Appendix H for administration of ophthalmic preparations.
- **Top:** Cleanse area prior to application. Wear gloves during application.

E

PATIENT/FAMILY TEACHING

- Instruct patient to take medication around the clock and to finish the drug completely as directed, even if feeling better. Missed doses should be taken as soon as remembered, with remaining doses evenly spaced throughout day. Advise patient that sharing of this medication may be dangerous.
- May cause nausea, vomiting, diarrhea, or stomach cramps; notify physician if these effects persist or if severe abdominal pain, yellow discoloration of the skin or eyes, darkened urine, pale stool, or unusual tiredness develops.
- Advise patient to report signs of superinfection (black, furry overgrowth on the tongue, vaginal itching or discharge, loose or foul-smelling stools).
- Instruct patient to notify the physician if symptoms do not improve.
- Patients with a history of rheumatic heart disease or valve replacement need to be taught the importance of using antimicrobial endocarditis prophylaxis before invasive medical or dental procedures.

EVALUATION

Clinical response can be determined by: ■ Resolution of the signs and symptoms of infection. Length of time for complete resolution depends on the organism and site of infection ▪ Improvement of acne lesions ▪ Endocarditis prophylaxis.

ESMOLOL
(ez-moe-lole)
Brevibloc

CLASSIFICATION(S):
Beta-adrenergic blocker (selective), Antiarrhythmic (group II)
Pregnancy Category C

INDICATIONS

▪ Short-term management of supraventricular tachyarrhythmias. **Unlabeled Use:** ▪ Lowering of blood pressure during surgical procedures.

ACTION

▪ Blocks stimulation of beta$_1$ (myocardial) receptor sites, with less effect on beta$_2$ (pulmonary and vascular) receptor sites. Results in decreased heart rate, decreased contractility, lowering of blood pressure, and decreased AV conduction. **Therapeutic Effect:** ▪ Slowing of the ventricular response in supraventricular tachyarrhythmias.

PHARMACOKINETICS

Absorption: Administered by IV route, resulting in complete bioavailability.
Distribution: Rapidly and widely distributed.
Metabolism and Excretion: Metabolized by enzymes in red blood cells and the liver.
Half-life: 9 min.

CONTRAINDICATIONS AND PRECAUTIONS

Contraindicated in: ▪ Uncompensated congestive heart failure ▪ Pulmonary edema ▪ Cardiogenic shock ▪ Bradycardia ▪ 2nd- or 3rd-degree heart block.
Use Cautiously in: ▪ Thyrotoxicosis

▪ Hypoglycemia (symptoms may be masked) ▪ Pregnancy, lactation, or children <18 yr (safety not established).

ADVERSE REACTIONS AND SIDE EFFECTS*

CNS: dizziness, headache, confusion, agitation, somnolence, weakness.
EENT: visual disturbances.
Resp: bronchospasm, wheezing.
CV: hypotension, chest pain, pulmonary edema, PVCs, ECG changes, bradycardia.
GI: nausea, vomiting, constipation, abdominal pain, dyspepsia.
GU: urinary retention.
Derm: rash.
Local: phlebitis at IV site.
Misc: peripheral ischemia, fever, chills.

INTERACTIONS

Drug–Drug: ▪ **General anesthesia, IV phenytoin,** and **verapamil** may cause additive myocardial depression ▪ Additive bradycardia may occur with **cardiac glycosides** ▪ Additive hypotension may occur with other **antihypertensive agents,** acute ingestion of **alcohol,** or **nitrates** ▪ Concurrent use with **amphetamines, cocaine, ephedrine, epinephrine, norepinephrine, phenylephrine,** or **pseudoephedrine** may result in excess alpha-adrenergic stimulation, hypertension, and bradycardia ▪ May negate the beneficial beta$_1$ cardiac effects of **dopamine** or **dobutamine** ▪ Concurrent **thyroid** administration may decrease effectiveness ▪ Use with **insulin** may result in prolonged hypoglycemia ▪ May prolong the effects of **succinylcholine** ▪ May decrease effectiveness of **theophylline.**

ROUTE AND DOSAGE

See infusion rate table in Appendix D.

▪ **IV (Adults):** 500-mcg/kg loading dose over 1 min initially, followed by 50-mcg/kg/min infusion for 4 min; if no response within 5 min, give second loading dose of 500 mcg/kg over 1 min and increase infusion to 100 mcg/

---

*Underlines indicate most frequent; **CAPITALS** indicate life-threatening.

kg/min for 4 min. If no response, repeat loading dose of 500 mcg/kg over 1 min and increase infusion rate by 50 mcg/kg/min increments (not to exceed 200 mcg/kg/min). As therapeutic end point is achieved, eliminate loading doses and decrease dosage increments to 25 mcg/kg/min.

AVAILABILITY

- **Injection:** 10 mg/ml, 250 mg/ml.

TIME/ACTION PROFILE
(cardiovascular effects)

	ONSET	PEAK	DURATION
IV	min	UK	1–20 min

NURSING IMPLICATIONS

ASSESSMENT

- Monitor blood pressure, heart rate, and ECG frequently throughout course of therapy. The risk of hypotension is greatest within the first 30 min of initiating esmolol infusion.
- Assess infusion site frequently throughout therapy. Concentrations of greater than 10 mg/ml may cause redness, swelling, skin discoloration, and burning at the injection site. Do not use butterfly needles for administration. If venous irritation occurs, stop the infusion and resume at another site.
- Monitor intake and output ratios and daily weight. Assess patient for signs and symptoms of congestive heart failure (peripheral edema, dyspnea, rales/crackles, weight gain, jugular venous distension).
- **Lab Test Considerations:** Monitor blood sugar closely in diabetic patients, because esmolol may mask signs and symptoms of hypoglycemia and may potentiate insulin-induced hypoglycemia.
- **Toxicity and Overdose:** Monitor patient for signs of overdose (bradycardia, severe dizziness or fainting, severe drowsiness, dyspnea, bluish fingernails or palms, seizures). Notify physician immediately if these signs occur.

- Treatment of esmolol overdose is symptomatic and supportive. Due to the short action of esmolol, discontinuation of therapy may relieve acute toxicity.
- Symptomatic bradycardia may be treated with atropine, isoproterenol, dobutamine, epinephrine, or a transvenous pacemaker.
- Premature ventricular contractions may be treated with lidocaine or phenytoin. Avoid the use of quinidine, procainamide, or disopyramide, as they may further depress myocardial function.
- Congestive heart failure may be treated with oxygen, cardiac glycosides, and/or diuretics.
- Hypotension may be treated with Trendelenberg position and IV fluids unless contraindicated. Vasopressors (epinephrine, norepinephrine, dopamine, dobutamine) may also be used. Hypotension does not respond to beta$_2$ agonists.
- Glucagon has been used to treat bradycardia and hypotension.
- A beta$_2$-adrenergic agonist (isoproterenol) and/or theophylline may be used to treat bronchospasm.

POTENTIAL NURSING DIAGNOSES

- Cardiac output, decreased (indications).
- Injury, high risk for (side effects).
- Knowledge deficit related to medication regimen (patient/family teaching).

IMPLEMENTATION

- **General Info:** To convert to other antiarrhythmic agents following esmolol administration, administer the first dose of the antiarrhythmic agent and decrease the esmolol dose by 50% after 30 min. If an adequate response is maintained for 1 hr following the second dose of the antiarrhythmic agent, discontinue the esmolol.
- **Intermittent Infusion:** Esmolol must be diluted and administered via IV infusion. To dilute for infusion, remove 20 ml from a 500-ml bottle of D5W, D5/LR, D5/0.45% NaCl, D5/

E

0.9% NaCl, 0.45% NaCl, 0.9% NaCl, or lactated Ringer's solution. Add 5 g of esmolol to the bottle, for a concentration of 10 mg/ml. Solution is stable for 24 hr at room temperature.

- **Rate:** The loading dose of esmolol is administered over 1 min, followed by a maintenance dose via IV infusion over 5 min. If the response is not adequate, procedure is repeated every 5 min with an increase in the maintenance dose. Titration of dose is based on desired heart rate or undesired decrease in blood pressure. The maintenance dose should not be >200 mcg/kg/min and can be administered for up to 48 hr. Esmolol infusions should not be abruptly discontinued; eliminate loading doses and decrease dosage by 25 mcg/kg/min (see Appendix D).
- **Y-Site Compatibility:** ▪ amikacin ▪ aminophylline ▪ ampicillin ▪ atracurium ▪ butorphanol ▪ calcium chloride ▪ cefazolin ▪ cefoperazone ▪ ceftazidime ▪ ceftizoxime ▪ chloramphenicol ▪ cimetidine ▪ clindamycin ▪ dopamine ▪ enalaprilat ▪ erythromycin lactobionate ▪ famotidine ▪ fentanyl ▪ gentamicin ▪ heparin ▪ hydrocortisone sodium succinate ▪ magnesium sulfate ▪ methyldopa ▪ metronidazole ▪ morphine ▪ nafcillin ▪ pancuronium ▪ penicillin G potassium ▪ phenytoin ▪ piperacillin ▪ polymyxin B ▪ potassium chloride ▪ potassium phosphate ▪ ranitidine ▪ sodium acetate ▪ streptomycin ▪ tobramycin ▪ trimethoprim/sulfamethoxazole ▪ vancomycin ▪ vecuronium.
- **Y-Site Compatibility:** ▪ furosemide.

PATIENT/FAMILY TEACHING
▫ Caution patient to make position changes slowly to minimize orthostatic hypotension.
▫ May cause drowsiness and dizziness. Caution patient to call for assistance during ambulation or transfer.

EVALUATION
Effectiveness of therapy can be demonstrated by: ▪ Decrease in or control of supraventricular tachyarrhythmias with-

out the appearance of detrimental side effects.

ESTAZOLAM
(ess-**taz**-oh-lam)
ProSom

CLASSIFICATION(S):
Sedative/hypnotic (benzodiazepine)
Schedule IV
Pregnancy Category X

INDICATIONS
▪ Short-term management of insomnia.

ACTION
▪ Depresses the CNS, probably by potentiating gamma-aminobutyric acid (GABA), an inhibitory neurotransmitter. **Therapeutic Effect:** ▪ Relief of insomnia.

PHARMACOKINETICS
Absorption: Well absorbed following oral administration.
Distribution: Highly lipid-soluble. Crosses the blood–brain barrier and placenta. Enters breast milk.
Metabolism and Excretion: Mostly metabolized by the liver. Metabolites do not have CNS depressant activity.
Half-life: 10–24 hr.

CONTRAINDICATIONS AND PRECAUTIONS
Contraindicated in: ▪ Hypersensitivity ▪ Cross-sensitivity with other benzodiazepines may exist ▪ Pre-existing CNS depression ▪ Severe uncontrolled pain ▪ Narrow-angle glaucoma ▪ Pregnancy or lactation.
Use Cautiously in: ▪ Hepatic dysfunction, elderly, very small or debilitated patients (initial dosage reduction may be necessary) ▪ Patients who are suicidal or who may have been addicted to drugs previously.

ADVERSE REACTIONS AND SIDE EFFECTS*

CNS: somnolence, weakness, hypokinesia, hangover, abnormal thinking, anxiety, agitation, amnesia, apathy, hostility, seizures, sleep disorders, stupor, twitch.
EENT: ear pain, eye irritation, photophobia.
Resp: RESPIRATORY DEPRESSION, cold symptoms, pharyngitis, asthma, dyspnea, sinusitis, rhinitus.
GI: dyspepsia, changes in appetite, flatulence, gastritis, abdominal pain.
GU: urinary frequency, urinary hesitancy, menstrual cramps, vaginal discharge, vaginal itching.
Derm: urticaria.
MS: lower extremity pain, back pain, stiffness, neck pain, myalgia, muscle spasm, arthritis.
Misc: allergic reactions, chills, thirst, psychological dependence, physical dependence.

INTERACTIONS

Drug–Drug: ■ Additive CNS depression with **alcohol, antihistamines, antidepressants, MAO inhibitors,** other **sedative/hypnotics,** or **opioid analgesics** ■ **Cimetidine** or **oral contraceptives** may decrease metabolism and increase effects of estazolam ■ May decrease efficacy of **levodopa** ■ **Rifampin** or **cigarette smoking** increase metabolism and decrease effectiveness ■ **Theopylline** may antagonize the effectiveness of estazolam.

ROUTE AND DOSAGE

■ **PO (Adults):** 1 mg at bedtime (range 0.5–2 mg).

AVAILABILITY

■ *Tablets:* 1 mg, 2 mg.

TIME/ACTION PROFILE (hypnotic activity)

	ONSET	PEAK*	DURATION
PO	15–30 min	2 hr	6–8 hr

*Plasma level.

NURSING IMPLICATIONS

ASSESSMENT

□ Assess sleep patterns prior to and periodically throughout course of therapy.
□ Prolonged therapy may lead to psychological or physical dependence. Restrict amount of drug available to patient, especially if patient is depressed, suicidal, or has a history of addiction.
■ **Lab Test Considerations:** Monitor CBC, urinalysis, and serum chemistries periodically during prolonged therapy.

POTENTIAL NURSING DIAGNOSES

■ Sleep pattern disturbance (indications).
■ Injury, high risk for (side effects).
■ Knowledge deficit related to medication regimen (patient/family teaching).

IMPLEMENTATION

■ **General Info:** Supervise ambulation and transfer of patients following administration. Remove cigarettes. Side rails should be raised and call bell within reach at all times.

PATIENT/FAMILY TEACHING

□ Advise patient to take medication exactly as directed. Discuss the importance of preparing environment for sleep (dark room, quiet, avoidance of nicotine and caffeine). Gradual discontinuation may be required following prolonged therapy. May cause disturbed sleep for the first 2 nights following discontinuation of estazolam.
□ Medication may cause daytime drowsiness. Caution patient to avoid driving and other activities requiring alertness until response to medication is known.
□ Caution patients to avoid taking alcohol or other CNS depressants concurrently with this medication.
□ Instruct patient to contact physician immediately if pregnancy is planned or suspected.

E

*Underlines indicate most frequent; **CAPITALS** indicate life-threatening.

EVALUATION
Effectiveness of therapy can be demonstrated by: ▪ Improvement in sleep pattern.

ESTRADIOL
(ess-tra-**dye**-ole)
Estrace

ESTRADIOL CYPIONATE
dep Gynogen, Depo-Estradiol, Depogen, Dura-Estrin, E-Cypionate, Estra-D, Estro-Cyp, Estrofem, Estroject-LA, Estronol-LA, Hormogen Depot

ESTRADIOL VALERATE
Deladiol, Delestrogen, Dioval XX, Duragen, Estradiol L.A., Estra-L, Estraval, Estravel, {Femogex}, Gynogen L.A., L.A.E., Valergen

ESTRADIOL TRANSDERMAL SYSTEM
Estrace, Estraderm TTS

CLASSIFICATION(S):
Hormone (estrogen)
Pregnancy Category X

INDICATIONS
▪ **PO, IM, Transdermal:** Treatment of moderate to severe vasomotor symptoms of menopause and of various estrogen-deficiency states including: □ Female hypogonadism □ Ovariectomy □ Primary ovarian failure ▪ **PO:** Inoperable metastatic postmenopausal breast or prostate carcinoma ▪ **Transdermal:** Treatment and prevention of postmenopausal osteoporosis. ▪ **Vaginal:** Management of atrophic vaginitis which may occur with menopause.

ACTION
▪ Estrogens promote the growth and development of female sex organs and the maintenance of secondary sex characteristics in women ▪ Metabolic effects include reduced blood cholesterol, protein synthesis, and sodium and water retention. **Therapeutic Effects:** ▪ Restoration of hormonal balance in various deficiency states ▪ Treatment of hormone-sensitive tumors.

PHARMACOKINETICS
Absorption: Well absorbed following oral administration. Readily absorbed through skin and mucous membranes.
Distribution: Widely distributed. Crosses the placenta and enters breast milk.
Metabolism and Excretion: Mostly metabolized by the liver and other tissues. Enterohepatic recirculation occurs, and more absorption may occur from the GI tract.
Half-life: UK.

CONTRAINDICATIONS AND PRECAUTIONS
Contraindicated in: ▪ Thromboembolic disease ▪ Undiagnosed vaginal bleeding ▪ Pregnancy (may result in harm to the fetus) ▪ Lactation.
Use Cautiously in: ▪ Underlying cardiovascular disease ▪ Severe hepatic or renal disease ▪ May increase the risk of endometrial carcinoma.

ADVERSE REACTIONS AND SIDE EFFECTS*
CNS: headache, dizziness, lethargy.
EENT: worsening of myopia or astigmatism, intolerance to contact lenses.
CV: edema, thromboembolism, hypertension, myocardial infarction.
GI: nausea, vomiting, anorexia, increased appetite, weight changes, jaundice.
GU: females—breakthrough bleeding, dysmenorrhea, amenorrhea, cervical erosions, vaginal candidiasis, loss of libido; males—testicular atrophy, impotence.
Derm: acne, urticaria, oily skin, pigmentation.
Endo: hyperglycemia, gynecomastia (males).
F and E: sodium and water retention, hypercalcemia.

{} = Available in Canada only.
*Underlines indicate most frequent; **CAPITALS** indicate life-threatening.

MS: leg cramps.
Misc: breast tenderness.

INTERACTIONS

Drug–Drug: ▪ May alter requirement for **oral anticoagulants, oral hypoglycemic agents,** or **insulin** ▪ **Barbiturates** or **rifampin** may decrease effectiveness.

ROUTE AND DOSAGE

Vasomotor Symptoms of Menopause, Atrophic Vaginitis, Female Hypogonadism, Ovarian Failure (Estrogen Replacement)

▪ **PO (Adults):** 0.5–2 mg daily or in a cycle.
▪ **IM (Adults):** 1–5 mg monthly (estradiol cypionate) or 10–20 mg (estradiol valerate) monthly.
▪ **Transdermal: (Adults):** 50- or 100-mcg/24 hr transdermal patch applied twice weekly.
▪ **Vag (Adults):** 2–4 g cream (0.2–0.4 mg estradiol) daily for 1–2 wk, then decrease to 1–2 g for 1–2 wk, then maintenance dose of 1 g 1–3 times weekly for 3 wk, then off for 1 wk, then repeat cycle once vaginal mucosa has been restored.

Postmenopausal Breast Carcinoma
▪ **PO (Adults):** 10 mg 3 times daily.

Prostate Carcinoma
▪ **PO (Adults):** 1–2 mg 3 times daily.
▪ **IM (Adults):** 30 mg q 1–2 wk (estradiol valerate).

AVAILABILITY

▪ *Tablets:* 1 mg, 2 mg ▪ *Injection (valerate in oil):* 10 mg/ml, 20 mg/ml, 40 mg/ml ▪ *Injection (cypionate in oil):* 5 mg/ml ▪ *Transdermal systems:* 0.05 mg/24 hr release rate (4 mg estradiol content), 0.1 mg/24 hr release rate (8 mg estradiol content) ▪ *Vaginal cream:* 100 mcg/g.

TIME/ACTION PROFILE (estrogenic effects)

	ONSET	PEAK	DURATION
PO	UK	UK	UK
IM	UK	UK	UK
TD	UK	UK	3–4 days

NURSING IMPLICATIONS

ASSESSMENT

☐ Assess blood pressure prior to and periodically throughout therapy.
☐ Monitor intake and output ratios and weekly weight. Report significant discrepancies or steady weight gain to physician.
▪ **Lab Test Considerations:** Monitor hepatic function prior to and periodically throughout therapy.
☐ May cause increased serum glucose, sodium, triglyceride, phospholipid, cortisol, prolactin, prothrombin and factors VII, VIII, IX, and X levels. May decrease serum folate, pyridoxine, antithrombin III, and pregnanediol excretion concentrations.
☐ May alter thyroid hormone assays.
☐ May cause hypercalcemia in patients with metastatic bone lesions.

POTENTIAL NURSING DIAGNOSES
▪ Sexual dysfunction (indications).
▪ Knowledge deficit related to medication regimen (patient/family teaching).

IMPLEMENTATION
▪ **PO:** Administer with or immediately after food to reduce nausea.
▪ **Vag:** Manufacturer provides applicator with cream. Dosage is marked on the applicator.
▪ **Transdermal:** When switching from PO form, begin transdermal therapy 1 wk after the last dose or when symptoms reappear.
▪ **IM:** Injection has oil base. Roll syringe to ensure even dispersion. Administer deep IM. Avoid IV administration.

PATIENT/FAMILY TEACHING
▪ **General Info:** Instruct patient to take medication as directed. If a dose is missed, take as soon as remembered as long as it is not just before next dose. Do not double doses.
☐ If nausea becomes a problem, advise patient that eating solid food often provides relief.
☐ Advise patient to report signs and symptoms of fluid retention (swelling of ankles and feet, weight gain),

thromboembolic disorders (pain, swelling, tenderness in extremities, headache, chest pain, blurred vision), mental depression, or hepatic dysfunction (yellowed skin or eyes, pruritus, dark urine, light-colored stools) to physician.

□ Instruct patient to stop taking medication and notify physician if pregnancy is suspected.

□ Advise patient to notify physician or dentist of medication regimen prior to treatment or surgery.

□ Explain dosage schedule and maintenance routine. Discontinuing medication suddenly may cause withdrawal bleeding.

□ Caution patient that cigarette smoking during estrogen therapy may cause increased risk of serious side effects, especially for women over age 35.

□ Caution patient to use sunscreen and protective clothing to prevent increased pigmentation.

□ Advise patient treated for osteoporosis that exercise has been found to arrest and reverse bone loss. The patient should discuss any exercise limitations with physician before beginning program.

□ Emphasize the importance of routine follow-up physical examinations, including blood presssure; breast, abdomen, and pelvic examinations; and PAP smears, every 6–12 mo.

▪ **Vag:** Instruct patient in the correct use of applicator. Patient should remain recumbent for at least 30 min after administration. May use sanitary napkin to protect clothing, but do not use tampon.

▪ **Transdermal Patch:** Instruct patient to wash and dry hands first. Apply disk to intact skin on hairless portion of abdomen. Press disk for 10 sec to ensure contact with skin (especially around edges). Avoid areas where clothing may rub disk loose. Change site with each administration to prevent skin irritation. Do not reuse site for 1 wk. Disk may be reapplied if it falls off.

EVALUATION

Effectiveness of therapy can be demonstrated by: ▪ Resolution of menopausal vasomotor symptoms ▪ Decreased vaginal and vulval itching, inflammation, or dryness associated with menopause ▪ Normalization of estrogen levels in patients with ovariectomy or hypogonadism ▪ Control of the spread of advanced metastatic breast or prostate cancer.

ESTRAMUSTINE
(ess-tra-**muss**-teen)
Emcyt

CLASSIFICATION(S):
Antineoplastic agent
(hormone/alkylating agent)
Pregnancy Category UK

INDICATIONS

▪ Palliative treatment of advanced metastatic prostate cancer.

ACTION

▪ Consists of combination of mechlorethamine, an alkylating agent, and estradiol, an estrogenic compound. Antineoplastic activity may be due to either component or the combination ▪ Also decreases serum testosterone levels.
Therapeutic Effect: ▪ Decreased spread of prostate cancer.

PHARMACOKINETICS

Absorption: Well absorbed (75%) following oral administration. During absorption, converted to estromustine and then to estrogenic compounds and mechlorethamine.
Distribution: Presence of estrogen enhances delivery to tissues with estrogen receptors. Concentrates in prostatic tissue.
Metabolism and Excretion: Eliminated primarily by biliary and fecal excretion. Small amounts excreted by kidneys.
Half-life: 20 hr.

CONTRAINDICATIONS AND PRECAUTIONS

Contraindicated in: ▪ Thromboembolism, recent stroke, or myocardial infarction ▪ Cross-sensitivity or tolerance to estradiol or mechlorethamine may exist.

Use Cautiously in: ▪ History of thromboembolic disorders ▪ Hypercalcemia ▪ Peptic ulcer ▪ Active infection including recent chickenpox or herpes zoster ▪ Renal or hepatic impairment ▪ Gallbladder disease ▪ Cardiovascular disease ▪ Cerebrovascular disease ▪ Migraine headaches ▪ Metabolic bone disease ▪ Epilepsy ▪ Asthma ▪ Bone marrow depression ▪ Patients with childbearing potential.

ADVERSE REACTIONS AND SIDE EFFECTS*

CNS: insomnia.
CV: edema, thromboembolism, hypertension.
GI: nausea, diarrhea, vomiting.
Endo: gynecomastia, decreased libido, gonadal suppression (azoospermia), hyperglycemia.
Derm: rashes.
F and E: sodium and water retention.
Hemat: anemia, leukopenia, thrombocytopenia.
Misc: allergic reactions, fever.

INTERACTIONS

Drug–Drug: ▪ **Cigarette smoking** increases the risk of adverse vascular effects ▪ **Calcium supplements** form an insoluble complex with estramustine that cannot be absorbed ▪ Increases effects and risk of toxicity with **glucocorticoids** (dosage reduction may be necessary) ▪ May decrease appropriate immune response to **live virus vaccines** and increase risk of adverse reactions.

Drug–Food: ▪ **Calcium** in dairy foods forms an insoluble complex with estramustine that cannot be absorbed.

ROUTE AND DOSAGE

▪ **PO (Adults):** 600 mg/m²/day in 3 divided doses or 14 mg/kg/day (range 10–16 mg/kg) in 3–4 divided doses.

AVAILABILITY

▪ *Capsules:* 140 mg.

TIME/ACTION PROFILE (effect on tumor spread)

	ONSET	PEAK	DURATION
PO	30–90 days	UK	6 wk*

*Persistence of hematologic effects.

NURSING IMPLICATIONS

ASSESSMENT

▫ Monitor blood pressure periodically throughout therapy.
▫ Monitor intake and output ratios and weekly weight. Report significant discrepancies or steady weight gain to physician.
▫ Monitor blood glucose closely in diabetic patients. May decrease glucose tolerance.
▪ **Lab Test Considerations:** Monitor hematologic and hepatic functions periodically throughout therapy. May cause leukopenia and thrombocytopenia. May also cause elevated LDH, AST (SGOT), and bilirubin levels.

POTENTIAL NURSING DIAGNOSES

▪ Knowledge deficit related to medication regimen (patient/family teaching).

IMPLEMENTATION

▪ **PO:** Administer with water 1 hr before or 2 hr after meals. Milk, milk products, and calcium-rich foods or calcium-containing antacids impair the absorption of estramustine and must not be taken simultaneously.

PATIENT/FAMILY TEACHING

▫ Instruct patient to take estramustine exactly as directed.
▫ Instruct patient to store capsules in the refrigerator, but may be kept at room temperature for 24–48 hr without losing potency.
▫ Advise patient of the need for contraception throughout therapy.

E

□ Advise patient to report signs and symptoms of fluid retention (swelling of ankles and feet, weight gain) and thromboembolic disorders (pain, swelling, tenderness in extremities, headache, chest pain, blurred vision) to physician.

EVALUATION
Effectiveness of therapy may be demonstrated by: ▪ Decrease in spread of prostate cancer. May require 30–90 days to determine maximum effects of therapy.

ESTROGENS, CONJUGATED
(**ess**-troe-jenz)
{C.E.S.}, conjugated estrogens, {Conjugated Estrogens C.S.D.}, Premarin

CLASSIFICATION(S):
Hormone (estrogen)
Pregnancy Category X

INDICATIONS

▪ **PO:** Treatment of moderate to severe vasomotor symptoms of menopause ▪ **PO:** Various estrogen-deficiency states, including: □ Female hypogonadism □ Ovariectomy □ Primary ovarian failure ▪ **PO:** Adjunctive therapy of postmenopausal osteoporosis ▪ **PO:** Adjunctive therapy of advanced inoperable metastatic breast and prostatic carcinoma ▪ **IM, IV:** Uterine bleeding due to hormonal imbalance ▪ **Vag:** Management of atrophic vaginitis.

ACTION

▪ Estrogens promote the growth and development of female sex organs and the maintenance of secondary sex characteristics in women ▪ Metabolic effects include reduced blood cholesterol, protein synthesis, and sodium and water retention. **Therapeutic Effects:** ▪ Restoration of hormonal balance in various deficiency states and treatment of hormone-sensitive tumors.

PHARMACOKINETICS

Absorption: Well absorbed following oral administration. Readily absorbed through skin and mucous membranes.
Distribution: Widely distributed. Crosses the placenta and enters breast milk.
Metabolism and Excretion: Mostly metabolized by the liver and other tissues. Enterohepatic recirculation occurs, and more absorption may occur from the GI tract.
Half-life: UK.

CONTRAINDICATIONS AND PRECAUTIONS

Contraindicated in: ▪ Thromboembolic disease ▪ Undiagnosed vaginal bleeding ▪ Pregnancy (may result in harm to the fetus) ▪ Lactation.
Use Cautiously in: ▪ Underlying cardiovascular disease ▪ Severe hepatic or renal disease ▪ May increase the risk of endometrial carcinoma.

ADVERSE REACTIONS AND SIDE EFFECTS (systemic use)*

CNS: headache, dizziness, lethargy, mental depression.
EENT: worsening of myopia or astigmatism, intolerance to contact lenses.
CV: edema, thromboembolism, hypertension, myocardial infarction.
GI: nausea, vomiting, anorexia, increased appetite, weight changes, jaundice.
GU: females—breakthrough bleeding, dysmenorrhea, amenorrhea, cervical erosions, vaginal candidiasis, loss of libido; males—testicular atrophy, impotence.
Derm: acne, urticaria, oily skin, pigmentation.
Endo: hyperglycemia, gynecomastia (males).
F and E: sodium and water retention, hypercalcemia.
MS: leg cramps.
Misc: breast tenderness.

{} = Available in Canada only.
*Underlines indicate most frequent; **CAPITALS** indicate life-threatening.

INTERACTIONS

Drug–Drug: ▪ May alter requirement for **oral anticoagulants, oral hypoglycemic agents,** or **insulin** ▪ **Barbiturates** or **rifampin** may decrease effectiveness ▪ **Cigarette smoking** increases the risk of adverse cardiovascular reactions.

ROUTE AND DOSAGE

Ovariectomy, Primary Ovarian Failure

▪ **PO (Adults):** 1.25 mg daily or in a cycle.

Menopausal Symptoms

▪ **PO (Adults):** 0.3–1.25 mg daily or in a cycle.

Osteoporosis

▪ **PO (Adults):** 0.625 mg daily or in a cycle.

Hypogonadism

▪ **PO (Adults):** 2.5–7.5 mg daily or in a cycle.

Inoperable Breast Carcinoma— Males and Postmenopausal Females

▪ **PO (Adults):** 10 mg tid.

Inoperable Prostate Carcinoma

▪ **PO (Adults):** 1.25–2.5 mg tid.

Uterine Bleeding

▪ **IM, IV (Adults):** 25 mg, may repeat in 6–12 hr if necessary.

Atrophic Vaginitis

▪ **Vag (Adults):** 2–4 g of cream daily for 21 days, off for 7 days, then repeat.

AVAILABILITY

▪ *Tablets:* 0.3 mg, 0.625 mg, 0.9 mg, 1.25 mg, 2.5 mg ▪ *Injection:* 25 mg/vial ▪ *Vaginal cream:* 0.625 mg/g.

TIME/ACTION PROFILE (estrogenic effects)*

	ONSET	PEAK	DURATION
PO	rapid	UK	UK
IM	delayed	UK	UK
IV	rapid	UK	UK

*Tumor response may take several wks.

NURSING IMPLICATIONS

ASSESSMENT

▪ **General Info:** Assess blood pressure prior to and periodically throughout therapy.

▫ Monitor intake and output ratios and weekly weight. Report significant discrepancies or steady weight gain to physician.

▪ **Menopause:** Assess frequency and severity of vasomotor symptoms.

▪ **Lab Test Considerations:** Monitor hepatic function periodically during long-term therapy.

▫ May cause increased serum glucose, sodium, triglyceride, phospholipid, cortisol, prolactin, prothrombin and factors VII, VIII, IX, and X levels. May decrease serum folate, pyridoxine, antithrombin III, and pregnanediol excretion concentrations.

▫ May cause hypercalcemia in patients with metastatic bone lesions.

▫ May cause false interpretations of thyroid function tests, false increases in sulfobromophthalein (BSP) and norepinephrine platelet-induced aggregability, and false decreases in metyrapone tests.

POTENTIAL NURSING DIAGNOSES

▪ Sexual dysfunction (indications).

▪ Knowledge deficit related to medication regimen (patient/family teaching).

IMPLEMENTATION

▪ **PO:** Administer with or immediately after food to reduce nausea.

▪ **Vag:** Manufacturer provides applicator with cream. Dose is marked on the applicator. Wash applicator with mild soap and warm water after each use.

▪ **IM:** To reconstitute, withdraw at least 5 ml of air from dry container and then slowly introduce the sterile diluent against the container side. Gently agitate container to dissolve; do not shake vigorously. Solution is stable for 60 days if refrigerated. Do not use if precipitate is present or if solution is darkened.

▪ **Direct IV:** Reconstitute as for IM. Inject into distal port tubing of free-flowing IV of 0.9% NaCl, D5W, or lactated Ringer's solution.

E

- **Rate:** Administer slowly (no faster than 5 mg/min) to prevent flushing.
- **Y-Site Compatibility:** ■ heparin ■ potassium chloride ■ vitamin B complex with C.
- **Additive Incompatibility:** ■ ascorbic acid or acidic solutions.

PATIENT/FAMILY TEACHING

- **General Info:** Instruct patient to take oral medication as directed. If a dose is missed, take as soon as remembered, but not just before next dose. Do not double doses.
- □ Explain dosage schedule and maintenance routine. Discontinuing medication suddenly may cause withdrawal bleeding. Bleeding is anticipated during the week conjugated estrogens are withheld.
- □ If nausea becomes a problem, advise patient that eating solid food often provides relief.
- □ Advise patient to report signs and symptoms of fluid retention (swelling of ankles and feet, weight gain), thromboembolic disorders (pain, swelling, tenderness in extremities; headache; chest pain; blurred vision), depression, hepatic dysfunction (yellowed skin or eyes, pruritus, dark urine, light-colored stools), or abnormal vaginal bleeding to physician.
- □ Instruct patient to stop taking medication and notify physician if pregnancy is suspected.
- □ Caution patient that cigarette smoking during estrogen therapy may increase risk of serious side effects, especially for women over age 35.
- □ Caution patients to use sunscreen and protective clothing to prevent increased pigmentation.
- □ Advise patient to notify physician or dentist of medication regimen prior to treatment or surgery.
- □ Advise patient treated for osteoporosis that exercise has been found to arrest and reverse bone loss. The patient should discuss any exercise limitations with physician before beginning program.
- □ Emphasize the importance of routine follow-up physical examinations, including blood pressure; breast, abdomen, and pelvic examinations; and PAP smears every 6–12 mo. Physician will evaluate possibility of discontinuing medication every 3–6 mo.
- **Vag:** Instruct patient in the correct use of applicator. Patient should remain recumbent for at least 30 min after administration. May use sanitary napkin to protect clothing, but do not use tampon. If a dose is missed, do not use the missed dose, but return to regular dosing schedule.

EVALUATION

Effectiveness of therapy can be demonstrated by: ■ Resolution of menopausal vasomotor symptoms □ Decreased vaginal and vulval itching, inflammation, or dryness associated with menopause ■ Normalization of estrogen levels in patients with ovariectomy or hypogonadism ■ Control of the spread of advanced metastatic breast or prostate cancer ■ Prevention of osteoporosis.

ESTROPIPATE
(ess-troe-**pi**-pate)
Ogen, Ortho-Est, piperazine estrone sulfate

CLASSIFICATION(S):
Hormone (estrogen)
Pregnancy Category X

INDICATIONS

■ **PO:** Treatment of vasomotor symptoms of menopause ■ **PO:** Treatment of various estrogen-deficiency states, including: □ Female hypogonadism □ Ovariectomy □ Primary ovarian failure ■ Adjunctive therapy of postmenopausal osteoporosis ■ **Vag:** Management of atrophic vaginitis.

ACTION

■ Estrogens promote the growth and development of female sex organs and the maintenance of secondary sex characteristics in women ▪ Metabolic effects include reduced blood cholesterol, protein synthesis, and sodium and water retention. **Therapeutic Effect:** ▪ Restoration of hormonal balance in various deficiency states.

PHARMACOKINETICS

Absorption: Well absorbed following oral administration. Readily absorbed through skin and mucous membranes.

Distribution: Widely distributed. Crosses the placenta and enters breast milk.

Metabolism and Excretion: Mostly metabolized by the liver and other tissues. Enterohepatic recirculation occurs, and more absorption may occur from the GI tract.

Half-life: UK.

CONTRAINDICATIONS AND PRECAUTIONS

Contraindicated in: ▪ Thromboembolic disease ▪ Undiagnosed vaginal bleeding ▪ Pregnancy (may result in harm to the fetus) ▪ Lactation.

Use Cautiously in: ▪ Underlying cardiovascular disease ▪ Severe hepatic or renal disease ▪ May increase the risk of endometrial carcinoma.

ADVERSE REACTIONS AND SIDE EFFECTS (systemic use)*

CNS: headache, dizziness, lethargy.

EENT: worsening of myopia or astigmatism, intolerance to contact lenses.

CV: edema, thromboembolism, hypertension, myocardial infarction.

GI: nausea, vomiting, anorexia, increased appetite, weight changes, jaundice.

GU: females—breakthrough bleeding, dysmenorrhea, amenorrhea, cervical erosions, vaginal candidiasis, loss of libido; males—testicular atrophy, impotence.

Derm: acne, urticaria, oily skin, pigmentation.

Endo: hyperglycemia, gynecomastia (males).

F and E: sodium and water retention, hypercalcemia.

MS: leg cramps.

Misc: breast tenderness.

INTERACTIONS

Drug–Drug: ▪ May alter requirement for **oral anticoagulants, oral hypoglycemic agents,** or **insulin** ▪ **Barbiturates** or **rifampin** may decrease effectiveness ▪ **Cigarette smoking** increases the risk of adverse cardiovascular reactions.

ROUTE AND DOSAGE

Vasomotor Symptoms of Menopause, Atrophic Vaginitis, Osteoporosis

▪ **PO (Adults):** 0.75–6 mg daily or in a cycle.

▪ **Vag (Adults):** 2–4 g of 0.15% cream daily for 3 wk, then off for 1 wk, then repeat cycle.

Female Hypogonadism, Ovarian Failure

▪ **PO (Adults):** 1.5–9 mg daily or in a cycle.

AVAILABILITY

▪ *Tablets:* 0.625 mg (0.75 mg estropipate), 1.25 mg (1.5 mg estropipate), 2.5 mg (3 mg estropipate), 5 mg (6 mg estropipate) ▪ *Vaginal cream:* 1.5 mg/g.

TIME/ACTION PROFILE (estrogenic effects)

	ONSET	PEAK	DURATION
PO	UK	UK	UK

NURSING IMPLICATIONS

ASSESSMENT

▪ **General Info:** Assess blood pressure prior to and periodically throughout therapy.

▫ Monitor intake and output ratios and weekly weight. Report significant discrepancies or steady weight gain to physician.

▪ **Menopause:** Assess frequency and severity of vasomotor symptoms.

---

*Underlines indicate most frequent; **CAPITALS** indicate life-threatening.

- **Lab Test Considerations:** Monitor hepatic function periodically during long-term therapy.
- May cause increased serum glucose, sodium, triglyceride, phospholipid, cortisol, prolactin, prothrombin and factors VII, VIII, IX, and X levels. May decrease serum folate, pyridoxine, antithrombin III, and pregnanediol excretion concentrations.
- May cause false interpretations of thyroid function tests, false increases in sulfobromophthalein (BSP) and norepinephrine platelet-induced aggregability, and false decreases in metyrapone tests.

POTENTIAL NURSING DIAGNOSES

- Sexual dysfunction (indications).
- Knowledge deficit related to medication regimen (patient/family teaching).

IMPLEMENTATION

- **PO:** Administer PO doses with or immediately after food to reduce nausea.
- **Vag:** Manufacturer provides applicator with cream. Dose is marked on the applicator. Wash applicator with mild soap and warm water after each use.

PATIENT/FAMILY TEACHING

- **General Info:** Instruct patient to take oral medication as directed. If a dose is missed, take as soon as remembered as long as it is not just before next dose. Do not double doses.
- Explain medication schedule to women on 21-day cycle followed by 7 days of not taking medication. Encourage patient to take medication at the same time each day.
- If nausea becomes a problem, advise patient that eating solid food often provides relief.
- Advise patient to report signs and symptoms of fluid retention (swelling of ankles and feet, weight gain), thromboembolic disorders (pain, swelling, tenderness in extremities; headache; chest pain; blurred vision), mental depression, hepatic dysfunction (yellowed skin or eyes, pruri-

tus, dark urine, light-colored stools), or abnormal vaginal bleeding to physician.
- Instruct patient to stop taking medication and notify physician if pregnancy is suspected.
- Caution patient that cigarette smoking during estrogen therapy may increase risk of serious side effects, especially for women over age 35.
- Caution patient to use sunscreen and protective clothing to prevent increased pigmentation.
- Advise patient to notify physician or dentist of medication regimen prior to treatment or surgery.
- Advise patient treated for osteoporosis that exercise has been found to arrest and reverse bone loss. The patient should discuss any exercise limitations with physician before beginning program.
- Emphasize the importance of routine follow-up physical examinations, including blood pressure; breast, abdomen, and pelvic examinations; and PAP smears, every 6–12 mo. Physician will evaluate possibility of discontinuing medication every 3–6 mo.
- **Vag:** Instruct patient in the correct use of applicator. Patient should remain recumbent for at least 30 min after administration. May use sanitary napkin to protect clothing, but do not use tampon. If a dose is missed, do not use the missed dose, but return to regular dosing schedule.

EVALUATION

Effectiveness of therapy can be demonstrated by: ■ Resolution of menopausal vasomotor symptoms □ Decreased vaginal and vulval itching, inflammation, or dryness associated with menopause ■ Normalization of estrogen levels in patients with ovariectomy or hypogonadism ■ Prevention of osteoporosis.

ETHAMBUTOL
(e-**tham**-byoo-tole)
{Etibi}, Myambutol

{} = Available in Canada only.

CLASSIFICATION(S):
Antitubercular
Pregnancy Category UK

INDICATIONS

▪ Used in combination with at least one other drug in the treatment of active tuberculosis or other mycobacterial diseases.

ACTION

▪ Inhibits the growth of mycobacteria. **Therapeutic Effect:** ▪ Tuberculostatic effect against susceptible organisms.

PHARMACOKINETICS

Absorption: Rapidly and well (80%) absorbed from the GI tract.

Distribution: Widely distributed into many body tissues and fluids. Crosses the blood–brain barrier, but only in small amounts. Crosses the placenta and enters breast milk.

Metabolism and Excretion: 50% metabolized by the liver, 50% eliminated unchanged by the kidneys.

Half-life: 3.3 hr (increased in renal or hepatic impairment).

CONTRAINDICATIONS AND PRECAUTIONS

Contraindicated in: ▪ Hypersensitivity ▪ Optic neuritis.

Use Cautiously in: ▪ Renal and severe hepatic impairment (dosage reduction required) ▪ Children <13 yr (safety not established) ▪ Pregnancy (although safety not established, ethambutol has been used with isoniazid to treat tuberculosis in pregnant women without adverse effects on the fetus) ▪ Lactation.

ADVERSE REACTIONS AND SIDE EFFECTS*

CNS: headache, malaise, dizziness, confusion, hallucinations.
EENT: <u>optic neuritis</u>.
GI: nausea, vomiting, anorexia, abdominal pain, hepatitis.
Metab: hyperuricemia.
MS: joint pain.

Neuro: peripheral neuritis.
Misc: fever, anaphylactoid reactions.

INTERACTIONS

Drug–Drug: ▪ Neurotoxicity may be additive with other **neurotoxic agents**.

ROUTE AND DOSAGE

▪ **PO (Adults and Children >13 yr):** 15–25 mg/kg/day.

AVAILABILITY

▪ *Tablets:* 100 mg, 400 mg.

TIME/ACTION PROFILE (blood levels)

	ONSET	PEAK
PO	rapid	2–4 hr

E

NURSING IMPLICATIONS

ASSESSMENT

▫ Mycobacterial studies and susceptibility tests should be performed prior to and periodically throughout therapy to detect possible resistance.
▫ Assess lung sounds and character and amount of sputum periodically throughout therapy.
▫ Assessments of visual function should be done frequently during course of therapy. Advise patient to report blurring of vision, constriction of visual fields, or changes in color perception immediately. Visual impairment, if not identified early, may lead to permanent sight impairment.
▪ **Lab Test Considerations:** Renal and hepatic functions, CBC, and uric acid levels should be monitored routinely throughout therapy.

POTENTIAL NURSING DIAGNOSES

▪ Infection, high risk for (indications).
▪ Sensory-perceptual alteration (side effects).
▪ Knowledge deficit related to medication regimen (patient/family teaching).

IMPLEMENTATION

▪ **General Info:** Ethambutol is given as a single daily dose and should be taken at the same time each day.

---

*<u>Underlines</u> indicate most frequent; **CAPITALS** indicate life-threatening.

Some regimens require dosing 2–3 times/week.
- **PO:** Administer with food or milk to minimize GI irritation.

PATIENT/FAMILY TEACHING
- ▢ Instruct patient to take medication exactly as prescribed by physician. Do not skip or double up on missed doses. A full course of therapy may take months to years. Do not discontinue without consulting physician, even though symptoms may disappear.
- ▢ Advise patient to notify physician if pregnancy is suspected.
- ▢ Instruct patient to notify physician if no improvement is seen in 2–3 wk. Physician should also be notified if unexpected weight gain or decreased urine output occurs.
- ▢ Emphasize the importance of routine examinations to evaluate progress and ophthalmic examinations if signs of optic neuritis occur.

EVALUATION
Effectiveness of therapy can be demonstrated by: ▪ Resolution of clinical symptoms of tuberculosis ▢ Decrease in acid-fast bacteria in sputum samples ▢ Improvement in chest x-rays. Therapy for tuberculosis is usually continued for at least 1–2 yr.

ETHOSUXIMIDE
(eth-oh-**sux**-i-mide)
Zarontin

CLASSIFICATION(S):
Anticonvulsant
Pregnancy Category UK

INDICATIONS

▪ Management of absence seizures (petit mal). **Unlabeled Use:** ▪ Management of myoclonic (partial) seizures.

ACTION

▪ Elevates the seizure threshold ▪ Suppresses abnormal wave and spike activity associated with absence (petit mal) seizures. **Therapeutic Effect:** ▪ Prevention of absence (petit mal) seizures.

PHARMACOKINETICS

Absorption: Rapidly and completely absorbed from the GI tract following oral administration.
Distribution: Freely distributed throughout body water.
Metabolism and Excretion: Mostly metabolized by the liver. 10% excreted unchanged by the kidneys.
Half-life: 60 hr (adults); 30 hr (children).

CONTRAINDICATIONS AND PRECAUTIONS

Contraindicated in: ▪ Hypersensitivity.
Use Cautiously in: ▪ Hepatic or renal disease ▪ Pregnancy or lactation (safety not established) ▪ Do not discontinue abruptly.

ADVERSE REACTIONS AND SIDE EFFECTS*

CNS: drowsiness, headaches, euphoria, irritability, hyperactivity, psychiatric disturbances, dizziness, ataxia, increased frequency of grand mal SEIZURES.
Derm: urticaria, rashes, hirsutism.
EENT: blurred vision.
GI: <u>anorexia</u>, <u>gastric upset</u>, <u>nausea</u>, <u>vomiting</u>, <u>cramping</u>, <u>weight loss</u>, <u>diarrhea</u>, hiccups.
GU: vaginal bleeding, pink or brown discoloration of urine.
Hemat: APLASTIC ANEMIA, AGRANULOCYTOSIS, leukopenia, eosinophilia.
Misc: allergic reactions, including STEVENS-JOHNSON SYNDROME.

INTERACTIONS

Drug–Drug: ▪ Seizure threshold may be lowered by **phenothiazines, antidepressants,** or **MAO inhibitors** ▪ Additive CNS depression with other **CNS depressants,** including **alcohol, antihistamines, antidepressants, opioid analgesics,** and **sedative/hypnotics** ▪ **Phenytoin** may increase metabolism and decrease effectiveness.

*<u>Underlines</u> indicate most frequent; **CAPITALS** indicate life-threatening.

ROUTE AND DOSAGE

- **PO (Adults and Children >6 yr):**
250 mg bid initially, may increase by
250 mg/day q 4–7 days up to 1.5 g/
day given in divided doses bid (usual
maintenance dose 20 mg/kg/day).
- **PO (Children 3–6 yr):** 250 mg/day
as a single dose initially, increase by
250 mg/day q 4–7 days up to 1 g/day.

AVAILABILITY

- *Capsules:* 250 mg • *Syrup:* 250 mg/5
ml.

TIME/ACTION PROFILE
(anticonvulsant activity)

	ONSET	PEAK	DURATION
PO	hr–days	days	days

NURSING IMPLICATIONS

ASSESSMENT

- Assess location, duration, and characteristics of seizure activity.
- Assess patient's mood, behavioral patterns, and facial expressions. Patients with a history of psychiatric disorders have an increased risk of developing behavioral changes. These symptoms may necessitate withdrawal of the medication.
- **Lab Test Considerations:** CBC, hepatic function tests, and urinalysis should be monitored routinely throughout the course of prolonged therapy.
- May cause false-positive results of direct Coombs' test.
- **Toxicity and Overdose:** Therapeutic serum ethosuximide levels range from 40–100 mcg/ml.

POTENTIAL NURSING DIAGNOSES

- Injury, high risk for (indications, side effects).
- Knowledge deficit related to medication regimen (patient/family teaching).

IMPLEMENTATION

- **PO:** Measure liquid preparations with calibrated measuring device.
- Administer with food or fluids to minimize GI irritation.

PATIENT/FAMILY TEACHING

- Instruct patient to take medication exactly as directed. If a dose is missed, take as soon as remembered within 4 hr, then continue on dosage schedule. Do not double doses. Do not discontinue medication without advice of physician. Sudden withdrawal may precipitate seizures.
- Medication may cause dizziness, drowsiness, or blurred vision. Caution patient to avoid driving or other activities requiring alertness until response to medication is known. Do not resume driving until physician gives clearance based on control of seizure disorder.
- Inform patient that medication may turn urine pink or brown.
- Advise patient to avoid alcohol while taking this medication.
- Advise patient to consult physician or pharmacist before taking any over-the-counter medications concurrently with this drug.
- Instruct patient to notify physician if skin rash, joint pain, sore throat, fever, unusual bleeding or bruising, swollen glands, or pregnancy occurs.
- Advise patient to carry identification describing disease process and medication regimen at all times.
- Emphasize the importance of follow-up examinations to monitor progress and side effects.

EVALUATION

Effectiveness of therapy can be demonstrated by: • Decrease or cessation of seizure activity without excessive sedation.

ETIDRONATE
(eh-tih-**droe**-nate)
Didronel

CLASSIFICATION(S):
Electrolyte modifier (hypo-calcemic)
**Pregnancy Category B (oral),
C (IV)**

INDICATIONS

- Treatment of Paget's disease of bone
- Treatment and prophylaxis of heterotopic calcification associated with total hip replacement or spinal cord injury
- Used with other agents (saline diuresis) in the management of hypercalcemia associated with malignancies.

ACTION

- Blocks the growth of calcium hydroxyapatite crystals by binding to calcium phosphate. **Therapeutic Effects:** • Decreased bone resorption and turnover.

PHARMACOKINETICS

Absorption: Absorption is generally poor (1–6%) following oral administration.

Distribution: Half of the absorbed dose is bound to hydroxyapatite crystals in areas of increased osteogenesis.

Metabolism and Excretion: Unabsorbed drug is eliminated in the feces. 50% of the absorbed dose is excreted unchanged by the kidneys.

Half-life: 5–7 hr.

CONTRAINDICATIONS AND PRECAUTIONS

Contraindicated in: • Hypersensitivity • Severe renal impairment (serum creatinine >5 mg/dl) • Hypercalcemia due to hyperparathyroidism.

Use Cautiously in: • Long bone fractures • Congestive heart failure • Hypocalcemia • Hypovitaminosis D • Moderate renal impairment (dosage reduction recommended if serum creatinine 2.5–4.9 mg/dl) • Pregnancy, lactation, or children (safety not established).

ADVERSE REACTIONS AND SIDE EFFECTS*

GI: diarrhea, nausea; IV—loss of taste, metallic taste.
GU: nephrotoxicity.
Derm: rash.
MS: bone pain, bone tenderness, microfractures.

INTERACTIONS

Drug–Drug: • Antacids or mineral supplements or buffers (as in didanosine) containing calcium, aluminum, iron, or magnesium may decrease the absorption of etidronate • Hypocalcemic effect may be additive with calcitonin.

Drug–Food: • Foods containing large amounts of calcium, aluminum, iron, or magnesium may decrease the absorption of etidronate.

ROUTE AND DOSAGE

Paget's Disease

- PO (Adults): 5–10 mg/kg/day single dose for up to 6 mo or 11–20 mg/kg/day for not more than 3 mo.

Heterotopic Ossification, Hip Replacement

- PO (Adults): 20 mg/kg/day for 1 mo prior to and 3 mo following surgery.

Heterotopic Ossification, Spinal Cord Injury

- PO (Adults): 20 mg/kg/day for 2 wk, then decreased to 10 mg/kg/day for 10 wk.

Hypercalcemia

- IV (Adults): 7.5 mg/kg/day for 3 days, then change to 20 mg/kg/day PO.

AVAILABILITY

- *Tablets:* 200 mg, 400 mg • *Injection:* 300 mg/6 ml.

TIME/ACTION PROFILE

	ONSET	PEAK	DURATION
PO (Paget's disease)	1 mo*	UK	1 yr
PO (heterotopic calcification)	UK	UK	several mons
IV (hypercalcemia)	24 hr†	3 days	11 days

*As measured by decreased urinary hydroxyproline.
†As measured by decreased urinary calcium excretion.

NURSING IMPLICATIONS

ASSESSMENT

- **General Info:** Assess patient for bone

pain, weakness, or loss of function prior to and throughout course of therapy. Bone pain may persist or increase in patients with Paget's disease; it usually subsides days to months after therapy is discontinued. Confer with physician regarding analgesic to control pain.

- **Heterotopic Ossification:** Monitor for inflammation and pain at the site and loss of function if ossification occurs near a joint.
- **Hypercalcemia:** Monitor symptoms of hypercalcemia (nausea, vomiting, anorexia, weakness, constipation, thirst, and cardiac arrhythmias).
- Observe patient carefully for evidence of hypocalcemia (paresthesia, muscle twitching, laryngospasm, colic, cardiac arrhythmias, and Chvostek's or Trousseau's sign). Protect symptomatic patients by elevating and padding side rails; keep bed in low position. Risk of hypocalcemia is greatest after 3 days of continuous IV therapy.
- **Lab Test Considerations:** Etidronate interferes with bone uptake of Technetium[99] in diagnostic scans.
- *Paget's Disease:* Decreased urinary excretion of hydroxyproline and serum alkaline phosphatase are often the first clinical signs of effectiveness. These values are monitored every 3 mo. Treatment is restarted when levels return to 75% of pretreatment values. Serum phosphate levels are also monitored prior to and 4 wk after beginning therapy. Dosage may be reduced if serum phosphate is elevated without corresponding decrease in urinary excretion of hydroxyproline or serum alkaline phosphatase.
- *Hypercalcemia:* Monitor serum calcium and albumin levels to determine effectiveness of therapy.
- Monitor BUN and creatine prior to and periodically throughout course of therapy. Stable or reversible increases in BUN and creatinine may occur in patients with hypercalcemia.

POTENTIAL NURSING DIAGNOSES

- Pain (indications, side effects).
- Injury, high risk for (indications).
- Knowledge deficit related to medication regimen (patient/family teaching).

IMPLEMENTATION

- **Hypercalcemia:** Used as adjunctive treatment after IV hydration and loop diuretics have restored urine output.
- **PO:** Administer on empty stomach, as food decreases absorption.
- **Intermittent Infusion:** Dilute in at least 250 ml of 0.9% NaCl. Solution is stable for 48 hr. Oral etidronate may be started on the day after last infusion.
- *Rate:* Infuse over at least 2 hr.

PATIENT/FAMILY TEACHING

- Advise patient to take as directed. If dose is missed, take as soon as remembered unless almost time for next dose. Do not double up on doses. Dose should not be taken within 2 hr of eating (especially products high in calcium) or taking vitamins or antacids, as absorption will be impaired.
- Instruct patient to notify physician if diarrhea occurs. Physician may divide the dose throughout the day to control diarrhea.
- Encourage patients to comply with physician's diet recommendations. Diet should contain adequate amounts of calcium and vitamin D (see Appendix K).
- Explain to patient receiving IV dose that metallic taste is not uncommon and usually disappears in a few hours.
- Advise patient to report signs of hypercalcemic relapse (bone pain, anorexia, nausea, vomiting, thirst, lethargy) to physician promptly.
- Emphasize need for keeping follow-up appointments to monitor progress, even after medication is discontinued, in order to detect relapse.

EVALUATION

Effectiveness of therapy can be demonstrated by: ▪ Lowered serum calcium levels ▪ Decreased bone pain and fractures in Paget's disease ▪ Prevention or treatment of heterotopic ossification.

Normal serum calcium levels are usually attained in 2–8 days in hypercalcemia associated with boney metastasis. Therapy may be repeated once after 1 wk.

ETODOLAC
(ee-**toe**-doe-lak)
Lodine

CLASSIFICATION(S):
Nonsteroidal anti-inflammatory agent, *Nonopioid analgesic*
Pregnancy Category C

INDICATIONS
▪ Management of osteoarthritis ▪ Treatment of mild to moderate pain.

ACTION
▪ Inhibits prostaglandin synthesis. **Therapeutic Effect:** ▪ Suppression of inflammation and pain.

PHARMACOKINETICS
Absorption: Well absorbed following oral administration.
Distribution: Highly bound to plasma proteins. Remainder of distribution not known.
Metabolism and Excretion: Not known.
Half-life: UK.

CONTRAINDICATIONS AND PRECAUTIONS
Contraindicated in: ▪ Hypersensitivity ▪ Active GI bleeding or ulcer disease ▪ Cross-sensitivity may exist with other nonsteroidal anti-inflammatory agents, including aspirin.
Use Cautiously in: ▪ Severe cardiovascular, renal, or hepatic disease ▪ History of ulcer disease ▪ Pregnancy, lactation, or children (safety not established).

ADVERSE REACTIONS AND SIDE EFFECTS*
CNS: weakness, malaise, dizziness, depression, nervousness, somnolence, insomnia, syncope.

EENT: blurred vision, tinnitus, photophobia.
Resp: asthma.
CV: fluid retention, edema, hypertension, congestive heart failure, palpitations.
GI: dyspepsia, abdominal pain, diarrhea, flatulence, nausea, constipation, gastritis, GI BLEEDING, melena, vomiting, thirst, dry mouth, drug-induced hepatitis, stomatitis.
GU: renal failure, dysuria, urinary frequency.
Derm: pruritus, rashes, flushing, ecchymoses, hyperpigmentation, sweating.
Hemat: anemia, prolonged bleeding time, thrombocytopenia.
Misc: chills, fever, allergic reactions including ANAPHYLAXIS, ANGIOEDEMA, STEVENS-JOHNSON SYNDROME.

INTERACTIONS
Drug–Drug: ▪ Concurrent use with aspirin may decrease effectiveness ▪ Additive adverse GI effects with aspirin, other **nonsteroidal anti-inflammatory agents, potassium supplements, glucocorticoids,** or **alcohol** ▪ Chronic use with **acetaminophen** may increase the risk of adverse renal reactions ▪ May decrease the effectiveness of **diuretics** or **antihypertensive** therapy ▪ May increase serum **lithium** levels and increase the risk of toxicity ▪ Increases the risk of toxicity from **methotrexate** ▪ Increased risk of bleeding with **cefamandole, cefotetan, cefoperazone, valproic acid** or **plicamycin, thrombolytic agents,** or **anticoagulants** ▪ Increased risk of adverse hematologic reactions with **antineoplastic agents** or **radiation therapy** ▪ May increase the risk of nephrotoxicity from **cyclosporine.**

ROUTE AND DOSAGE
Osteoarthritis
▪ **PO (Adults):** 600–1200 mg/day in divided doses given q 6–8 hr initially, followed by adjustment to maintenance dose of 200–1200 mg/day in divided doses given 2–4 times daily

---

*Underlines indicate most frequent; **CAPITALS** indicate life-threatening.

(200 mg 3–4 times daily, 300 mg 2–4 times daily, or 400 mg 2–4 times daily; not to exceed 1200 mg/day in patients >60 kg or 20 mg/kg in patients ≤60 kg).

Analgesia
- **PO (Adults):** 400 mg initially, then 200–400 mg q 6–8 hr (not to exceed 1200 mg/day in patients >60 kg or 20 mg/kg in patients ≤60 kg).

AVAILABILITY
- *Capsules:* 200 mg, 300 mg.

TIME/ACTION PROFILE (analgesic effect)

	ONSET	PEAK	DURATION
PO (analgesic)	0.5 hr	1–2 hr	4–12 hr
PO (anti-inflammatory)	days–wks	UK	UK

NURSING IMPLICATIONS

ASSESSMENT
- **General Info:** Patients who have asthma, aspirin-induced allergy, and nasal polyps are at increased risk for developing hypersensitivity reactions. Monitor for rhinitis, asthma, and urticaria.
- **Osteoarthritis:** Assess pain and range of movement prior to and 1–2 hr following administration.
- **Pain:** Assess location, duration, and intensity of the pain prior to and 60 min following administration.

POTENTIAL NURSING DIAGNOSES
- Pain (indications).
- Physical mobility, impaired (indications).
- Knowledge deficit related to medication regimen (patient/family teaching).

IMPLEMENTATION
- **General Info:** Coadministration with opioid analgesics may have additive analgesic effects and may permit lower opioid doses.
- **PO:** For rapid initial effect, administer 30 min before or 2 hr after meals. May be administered with food, milk, or antacids to decrease GI irritation.

Food slows but does not reduce the extent of absorption.

PATIENT/FAMILY TEACHING
- Advise patients to take this medication with a full glass of water and to remain in an upright position for 15–30 min after administration.
- Instruct patient to take medication exactly as directed. If a dose is missed, take as soon as remembered but not if almost time for next dose. Do not double doses.
- This medication may occasionally cause drowsiness or dizziness. Advise patient to avoid driving or other activities requiring alertness until response to the medication is known.
- Caution patient to avoid the concurrent use of alcohol, aspirin, ibuprofen, acetaminophen, or other over-the-counter medications without consultation with physician or pharmacist.
- Instruct patient to notify physician if rash, itching, chills, fever, visual disturbances, tinnitus, weight gain, edema, black stools, persistent or severe diarrhea, or persistent headache occur.
- Advise patient to inform physician or dentist of medication regimen prior to treatment or surgery.

EVALUATION
Effectiveness of therapy can be demonstrated by: ■ Decreased severity of pain ■ Improved joint mobility. Patients who do not respond to one nonsteroidal anti-inflammatory agent may respond to another.

ETOPOSIDE
(e-**toe**-poe-side)
VePesid

CLASSIFICATION(S):
Antineoplastic (podophyllotoxin derivative)
Pregnancy Category D

INDICATIONS
- Alone and in combination with other treatment modalities (other antineo-

plastic agents, radiation therapy, surgery) in the management of refractory testicular neoplasms and small cell carcinoma of the lung. **Unlabeled Uses:** ▪ Lymphomas and some leukemias.

ACTION

▪ Damages DNA prior to mitosis (cycle-dependent and phase-specific). **Therapeutic Effect:** ▪ Death of rapidly replicating cells, particularly malignant ones.

PHARMACOKINETICS

Absorption: Variably absorbed following oral administration.
Distribution: Rapidly distributed, does not appear to enter the CSF significantly but does appear to cross the placenta. Enters breast milk.
Metabolism and Excretion: Some metabolism by the liver, 45% excreted unchanged by the kidneys.
Half-life: 7 hr (range 3–12 hr).

CONTRAINDICATIONS AND PRECAUTIONS

Contraindicated in: ▪ Hypersensitivity ▪ Pregnancy ▪ Lactation ▪ Patients with known intolerance to benzyl alcohol, ethyl alcohol, or polyethylene glycol.
Use Cautiously in: ▪ Patients with childbearing potential ▪ Active infections ▪ Decreased bone marrow reserve ▪ Other chronic debilitating illnesses.

ADVERSE REACTIONS AND SIDE EFFECTS*

CNS: somnolence, fatigue, headache, vertigo.
Resp: bronchospasm, pulmonary edema.
CV: hypotension (IV), myocardial infarction, congestive heart failure.
GI: nausea, vomiting.
Hemat: leukopenia, thrombocytopenia.
Local: phlebitis at IV site.
Derm: alopecia.
Endo: gonadal suppression.
MS: muscle cramps.
Neuro: peripheral neuropathy.

Misc: allergic reactions, including ANAPHYLAXIS, fever.

INTERACTIONS

Drug–Drug: ▪ Additive bone marrow depression with other **antineoplastics** or **radiation therapy** ▪ May impair normal immune response to **live virus vaccines** and increase the risk of adverse reactions.

ROUTE AND DOSAGE

Testicular Neoplasms

▪ **IV (Adults):** 50–100 mg/m^2 daily for 5 days, repeat every 3–4 wk, or 100 mg/m^2 on days 1, 3, and 5 every 3–4 wk.

Small Cell Carcinoma of the Lung

▪ **PO (Adults):** 70 mg/m^2 (rounded to the nearest 50 mg)/day for 4 days, repeated every 3–4 wk up to 100 mg/m^2 (rounded to the nearest 50 mg)/day for 5 days every 3–4 wk.
▪ **IV (Adults):** 35 mg/m^2 daily for 4 days up to 50 mg/m^2 daily for 5 days every 3–4 wk.

AVAILABILITY

▪ *Capsules:* 50 mg ▪ *Injection:* 20 mg/ml.

TIME/ACTION PROFILE (noted as effects on blood counts)

	ONSET	PEAK	DURATION
PO	7–14 days	9–16 days	20 days
IV	7–14 days	9–16 days	20 days

NURSING IMPLICATIONS

ASSESSMENT

□ Monitor blood pressure prior to and every 15 min during infusion. If hypotension occurs, stop infusion and notify physician. After stabilizing blood pressure with IV fluids and supportive measures, infusion may be resumed at slower rate.
□ Monitor for hypersensitivity reaction (fever, chills, pruritus, urticaria, bronchospasm, tachycardia, hypotension). If these occur, stop infusion and notify physician. Keep epineph-

*Underlines indicate most frequent; **CAPITALS** indicate life-threatening.

rine, an antihistamine, and resuscitative equipment close by in the event of an anaphylactic reaction.

□ Assess for fever, chills, sore throat, and signs of infection. Notify physician if these symptoms occur.

□ Assess for bleeding (bleeding gums, bruising, petechiae; guaiac stools, urine, and emesis). Avoid IM injections and rectal temperatures. Apply pressure to venipuncture sites for 10 min.

□ Monitor intake and output, appetite, and nutritional intake. Etoposide causes nausea and vomiting in 30% of patients. Confer with physician regarding prophylactic use of an antiemetic.

□ Adjust diet as tolerated to help maintain fluid and electrolyte balance and nutritional status.

▪ **Lab Test Considerations:** Monitor CBC and differential prior to and periodically throughout therapy. The nadir of leukopenia occurs in 7–14 days. Notify physician if leukocyte count is <1000/mm^3. The nadir of thrombocytopenia occurs in 9–16 days. Notify physician if the platelet count is <75,000/mm^3. Recovery of leukopenia and thrombocytopenia occurs in 20 days.

□ Monitor liver function studies (AST [SGOT], ALT [SGPT], LDH, bilirubin) and renal function studies (BUN, creatinine) prior to and periodically throughout therapy to detect hepatotoxicity and nephrotoxicity.

□ May cause increased uric acid. Monitor levels periodically during therapy.

POTENTIAL NURSING DIAGNOSES

▪ Injury, high risk for (side effects).
▪ Infection, high risk for (side effects).
▪ Knowledge deficit related to medication regimen (patient/family teaching).

IMPLEMENTATION

▪ **General Info:** Avoid contact with skin. Use Luer-Lok tubing to prevent accidental leakage. If contact with skin occurs, immediately wash skin with soap and water.

□ Solution should be prepared in a biologic cabinet. Wear gloves, gown, and mask while handling medication. Discard equipment in designated containers (see Appendix I).

▪ **PO:** Capsules should be refrigerated.

▪ **Intermittent Infusion:** Dilute 5-ml vial with 250–500 ml of D5W or 0.9% NaCl for a concentration of 0.4–0.2 mg/ml. The 0.2-mg/ml solution is stable for 96 hr. The 0.4-mg/ml solution is stable for 48 hr. Concentrations >0.4 mg/ml are not recommended, as crystallization is likely. Discard solution if crystals are present.

▪ *Rate:* Infuse slowly over 30–60 min.

▪ **Y-Site Compatibility:** ▪ fludarabine ▪ ondansetron ▪ sargramostim.

▪ **Additive Compatibility:** ▪ cisplatin ▪ floxuridine ▪ fluorouracil ▪ ifosfamide.

E

PATIENT/FAMILY TEACHING

□ Instruct patient to take etoposide exactly as directed, even if nausea or vomiting occurs. If vomiting occurs shortly after dose is taken, consult physician. If a dose is missed, do not take at all.

□ Advise patient to notify physician if fever, chills, sore throat, signs of infection, bleeding gums, bruising, petechiae, or blood in urine, stool, or emesis occurs. Caution patient to avoid crowds and persons with known infections. Instruct patient to use soft toothbrush and electric razor. Patient should be cautioned not to drink alcoholic beverages or take products containing aspirin or ibuprofen.

□ Instruct patient to notify physician if rapid heartbeat, difficulty breathing, abdominal pain, yellow skin, weakness, paresthesia, or gait disturbances occur.

□ Instruct patient to inspect oral mucosa for redness and ulceration. If mouth sores occur, advise patient to use sponge brush and rinse mouth with water after eating and drinking. Viscous lidocaine swishes may be used if pain interferes with eating.

□ Discuss with patient the possibility of hair loss. Explore coping strategies.
□ Advise patient to use contraception.
□ Instruct patient not to receive any vaccinations without advice of physician.
□ Emphasize the need for periodic lab tests to monitor for side effects.

EVALUATION
Effectiveness of therapy can be demonstrated by: ▪ Decrease in size or spread of malignancies in solid tumors ▪ Improvement of hematologic status in leukemias.

ETRETINATE
(e-**tret**-i-nate)
Tegison

CLASSIFICATION(S):
Antipsoriatic (retinoid)
Pregnancy Category X

INDICATIONS

▪ Alone or as adjunct therapy in the management of severe recalcitrant psoriasis resistant to more conventional methods of treatment (topical tars, psoralens, UVB light, or methotrexate).

ACTION

▪ Structurally resembles vitamin A, though mechanism of action is not known. **Therapeutic Effect:** ▪ Improvement in psoriatic lesions.

PHARMACOKINETICS

Absorption: Inactive form is well absorbed following oral administration.
Distribution: Concentrates in dermal tissues and liver; stored in adipose tissue. Crosses the placenta.
Metabolism and Excretion: Highly metabolized by the liver, mostly on first pass through, where conversion to an active metabolite occurs.
Half-life: 120 days.

CONTRAINDICATIONS AND PRECAUTIONS

Contraindicated in: ▪ Hypersensitivity to retinoids ▪ Pregnancy ▪ Lactation ▪ Patients who are trying to conceive, who use unreliable methods of contraception, or who are planning to become pregnant in the future.
Use Cautiously in: ▪ Patients with a history of liver disease ▪ Children (safety not established).

ADVERSE REACTIONS AND SIDE EFFECTS*

CNS: fatigue, headache, fever, dizziness, pseudotumor cerebrii, anxiety, depression, abnormal thinking.
EENT: dry nose, chapped lips, sore throat, nose bleeds, cheilitis, sore tongue, rhinorrhea, eye irritation, eye pain, decreased visual acuity, abnormal lacrimation, visual defects, otitis, hearing changes, photophobia.
Resp: dyspnea, coughing, increased sputum, pharyngitis.
CV: thrombotic events, edema, arrhythmias, chest pain, syncope.
GI: dry mouth, gingival bleeding, abdominal pain, appetite changes, nausea, hepatitis, constipation, weight loss, abnormal taste, melana, mouth ulcers, flatulence.
GU: proteinuria, hemoglobinuria, WBCs in urine, polyuria, urinary retention, atropic vaginitis.
Derm: hair loss, peeling of skin, itching, redness, skin fragility, photosensitivity, abnormal fingernails, clamminess, granuloma, skin odor, increased pore size, sensory impairment, atropy, fissures, impaired healing, herpes simplex, hirsutism, infections, ulceration.
Endo: irregular menses.
F and E: abnormal calcium, abnormal potassium, abnormal phosphorus, abnormal CO_2, abnormal sodium, abnormal chloride.
Metab: hyperglycemia, hypoglycemia, hypertriglyceridemia, hypercholesterolemia, elevated HDL.

---

*Underlines indicate most frequent; **CAPITALS** indicate life-threatening.

MS: hyperostosis, bone and joint pain, myalgia, gout, hyperkinesia, hypotonia. **Misc:** increased risk of neoplasm.

INTERACTIONS

Drug–Drug: ▪ Electrolyte abnormalities may increase the risk of **cardiac glycoside** toxicity ▪ Additive toxicity with **vitamin A compounds** ▪ Increased risk of pseudotumor cerebrii with **tetracycline** ▪ Use with **alcohol** has an additive effect on increasing serum triglycerides ▪ Additive risk of hepatotoxicity with other **hepatotoxic agents** ▪ Additive risk of photosensitivity with other **photosensitizing agents** ▪ Concurrent use with **topical irritants, abrasives, or desquamating agents** may result in additive irritation.

Drug–Food: ▪ Absorption is enhanced by concurrent administration of **high-fat foods** or **milk**.

ROUTE AND DOSAGE

▪ **PO (Adults):** 0.75–1 mg/kg/day initially in divided doses for 8–16 wk, then lower to maintenance dose of 0.5–0.75 mg/kg/day. Erythrodermic psoriasis may respond to lower doses.

AVAILABILITY

▪ *Capsules:* 10 mg, 25 mg.

TIME/ACTION PROFILE (improvement in skin lesions)

	ONSET	PEAK	DURATION
PO	wks	wks–mos	yrs

NURSING IMPLICATIONS

Assessment

□ Assess skin prior to and periodically during therapy. Transient worsening of psoriasis may occur at initiation of therapy.

▪ **Lab Test Considerations:** Monitor liver function (AST [SGOT], ALT [SGPT], and LDH) every 1–2 wk during the first 1–3 mo of therapy and every 1–3 mo for the rest of the course of therapy. Inform physician if these values become elevated; therapy may be discontinued.

□ Monitor blood lipids (cholesterol, HDL, triglycerides) every 1–2 wk in the beginning of therapy and periodically thereafter. Inform physician of increased cholesterol and triglyceride levels or decrease in HDL.

□ Obtain periodic CBC, urinalysis, and serum electrolytes. Etretinate may alter (increase or decrease) hematocrit, hemoglobin, platelets, and WBC. May cause proteinuria, hematuria, glucose, and acetone in the urine. May increase or decrease sodium, potassium, calcium, and phosphate levels. May cause increased BUN and creatinine.

Potential Nursing Diagnoses

▪ Body image disturbance (indications).
▪ Knowledge deficit related to medication regimen (patient/family teaching).

Implementation

▪ **PO:** Absorption is enhanced by taking with milk or fatty foods.

Patient/Family Teaching

□ Instruct patient to take etretinate exactly as directed. If a dose is missed, take as soon as remembered with milk or fatty food; do not take if almost time for next dose. Do not double doses. Inform patient that condition may appear to worsen during initial therapy.

□ Caution patient not to take vitamin A supplements while taking etretinate. Hypervitaminosis A may result. Excessive alcohol and excessive ingestion of foods high in fat should be avoided to reduce the risk of hypertriglyceridemia and cardiovascular problems.

□ May cause dizziness or blurred vision. Caution patient to avoid driving or other activities requiring alertness until response to the medication is known. May impair night vision. Driving after dark should be avoided.

□ Inform patient that dry skin and chapped lips will occur. Applying lubricant to lips will help cheilitis. Physician should be notified if these symptoms become bothersome.

- Advise patient that oral rinses, sugarless gum or candy, or frequent oral hygiene may help relieve dry mouth.
- Discuss possibility of excessively dry eyes with patient who wears contact lenses. Patient may need to wear glasses during course of therapy.
- Advise female patients to use contraception throughout therapy. This drug is contraindicated during pregnancy. Physician may order pregnancy test 2 wk prior to initiation of therapy and start therapy on day 2 or 3 of the menstrual cycle. Teratogenic effects may persist for years. Patient should discuss this with the physician before attempting pregnancy.
- Caution patient not to donate blood while taking etretinate. After discontinuation, patient should have physician's approval prior to donating blood to prevent the possibility of a pregnant patient receiving the blood.
- Caution patient to minimize exposure to sunlight and to avoid sunlamps to prevent photosensitivity reactions.
- Instruct patient to report bone or joint pain, eye irritation, visual changes, abdominal pain, yellow skin, or unusual bruising.
- Inform patient of need for medical follow-up. Physician may order periodic ophthalmic examinations and bone x-rays.

EVALUATION

Effectiveness of therapy can be demonstrated by: ■ Improvement or resolution of skin lesions in psoriasis. Therapy may take 2–3 mo before full effects are seen. Therapy is discontinued in 1 mo if no effect is seen, when lesions resolve, or after 4–9 mo. Relapse may occur after discontinuation of therapy.

FACTOR IX COMPLEX (human)
Konyne 80, Profilnine Heat-Treated, Proplex T, Proplex SX-T

FACTOR IX (human)
AlphaNine, AlphaNine SD, Mononine

CLASSIFICATION(S):
Blood derivative (clotting factor)
Pregnancy Category C

INDICATIONS

■ Treatment of active or impending bleeding due to Factor IX deficiency (Hemophilia B, Christmas disease) ■ Treatment of bleeding in patients with Factor VIII inhibitors ■ Prevention and treatment of bleeding in patients with Factor VII deficiency (Proplex T only) ■ Rapid reversal of the effect of oral anticoagulants in emergency situations (Factor IX complex only).

ACTION

■ Factor IX complex (human) contains blood coagulation factors II, VII, IX, and X (Proplex SX-T has less factor VII). Factor IX complex (human) contains factor IX activity only. **Therapeutic Effects:** ■ Replacement of deficient factor IX in Hemophilia B ■ Restoration of hemostasis.

PHARMACOKINETICS

Absorption: Administered IV only, resulting in complete bioavailability.
Distribution: Distribution not known.
Metabolism and Excretion: Rapidly cleared from plasma by utilization in clotting process.
Half-life: *Factor IX*—24–32 hr; *Factor VII*—3–6 hr.

CONTRAINDICATIONS AND PRECAUTIONS

Contraindicated in: ■ Factor VII deficiency (except Proplex T) ■ Intravascular coagulation or fibrinolysis associated with liver disease.
Use Cautiously in: ■ Postoperative period (increased risk of thrombosis) ■ Blood groups A, B, or AB.

ADVERSE REACTIONS AND SIDE EFFECTS*

CNS: headache, somnolence, lethargy.
CV: changes in heart rate, changes in blood pressure.
GI: nausea, vomiting.
Derm: flushing, urticaria.
Hemat: thrombosis, disseminated intravascular coagulation.
Neuro: tingling.
Misc: fever, chills, risk of transmission of viral hepatitis, risk of transmission of HIV virus, hypersensitivity reactions.

INTERACTIONS

Drug–Drug: ▪ Use with **aminocaproic acid** may increase the risk of thrombosis.

ROUTE AND DOSAGE

The following general formula may be used: Dose (units) = body weight (kg) $\times (0.8 - 1) \times$ desired factor IX increase (in % of normal).

Factor IX Complex (Human)

Treatment of Bleeding in Patients with Hemophilia B
▪ **Adults and Children:** Amount necessary to establish 25% of normal Factor IX activity or 60–75 units/kg initially, followed by 10–20 units/kg/day for 1 wk.

Prophylaxis of Bleeding in Patients with Hemophilia B
▪ **Adults and Children:** 10–20 units/kg 1–2 times weekly.

Treatment of Bleeding in Patients with Hemophilia A and Inhibitors of Factor VIII
▪ **Adults and Children:** 75 units/kg, repeat dose 12 hr later.

Reversal of Oral Anticoagulant Activity
▪ **Adults and Children:** 15 units/kg.

Factor VII Deficiency (Proplex T only)
▪ **Adults and Children:** 0.5 units/kg × body weight (kg) × desired factor IX increase (in % of normal). Repeat every 4–6 hr as needed. For surgical procedures, raise level above 25% (40–60% of normal).

Factor IX (Human)

AlphaNine, AlphaNine SD
minor to moderate hemorrhage:
▪ **Adults and Children:** Dose sufficient to increase plasma Factor IX level to 20–30% as a single dose.

more serious hemorrhage or surgery:
▪ **Adults and Children:** Dose sufficient to increase plasma Factor IX level to 30–50% given as daily infusions.

dental extractions:
▪ **Adults and Children:** Dose sufficient to increase plasma Factor IX level to 50%. Repeat as needed.

Mononine
minor hemorrhage:
▪ **Adults and Children:** Dose sufficient to increase plasma Factor IX level to 15–25% (20–30 units/kg), may repeat in 24 hr.

major trauma or surgery:
▪ **Adults and Children:** Dose sufficient to increase plasma Factor IX level to 25–50% (75 units/kg) every 18–30 hr for up to 10 days.

AVAILABILITY

▪ *Injection:* Vials labeled with number of units.

TIME/ACTION PROFILE (hemostasis)

	ONSET	PEAK	DURATION
IV	immediate	UK	1–2 days

NURSING IMPLICATIONS

Assessment

☐ Monitor blood pressure, pulse, and respirations frequently.
☐ Obtain history of current trauma; estimate amount of blood loss.
☐ Monitor for renewed or increased bleeding every 15–30 min. Immobilize and apply ice to affected joints.
☐ Monitor intake and output ratios; note urine color. Notify physician if

*Underlines indicate most frequent; CAPITALS indicate life-threatening.

significant discrepancy occurs or urine becomes red or orange. Patients with type A, B, and AB blood are especially at risk for hemolytic reaction.

□ If hypersensitivity reaction (fever, chills, tingling, headache, urticaria, changes in blood pressure or pulse, nausea and vomiting, lethargy) occurs, slow infusion and notify physician.

□ Monitor coagulation studies before, during, and after therapy to assess effectiveness of therapy.

POTENTIAL NURSING DIAGNOSES

■ Tissue perfusion, altered (indications).

■ Injury, high risk for (indications).

■ Knowledge deficit related to medication regimen (patient/family teaching).

IMPLEMENTATION

■ **General Info:** Dosage varies with degree of clotting factor deficit, desired level of clotting factors, and weight.

□ Obtain type and cross-match of blood in case a transfusion is necessary.

□ To control bleeding after major trauma or surgery, factor IX levels should be maintained at 25% of normal for at least 1 wk. At 50% or greater of normal there is a risk of a thromboembolic reaction or disseminated intravascular coagulopathy.

□ Hepatitis B vaccine may be given prior to therapy to prevent hepatitis.

□ Inform all personnel of patient's bleeding tendency, to prevent further trauma. Apply pressure to all venipuncture sites for at least 5 min; avoid all IM injections.

■ **Direct IV:** Refrigerate concentrate until just prior to reconstitution. Warm diluent (Sterile Water for Injection) to room temperature before reconstituting. Use plastic syringe for preparation and administration. Use the filter needle provided by the manufacturer as an air vent to the vial when reconstituting. After adding diluent rotate vial gently until completely dissolved. Do not refrigerate after reconstitution. Begin administration within 3 hr. Reconstituted solution is stable for 12 hr at room temperature.

■ *Rate:* Administer IV no faster than 3 ml/min (100 units/min). Do not admix. Temporarily stop infusion and resume at slower rate if facial flushing or tingling occurs.

PATIENT/FAMILY TEACHING

□ Instruct patient to notify nurse immediately if bleeding recurs.

□ Advise patient to carry identification describing disease process at all times.

□ Caution patient to avoid products containing aspirin or ibuprofen, as they may further impair clotting.

□ Review with patient methods of preventing bleeding (use of soft toothbrush, avoid IM and SC injections, avoid potentially traumatic activities).

□ Advise patient that the risk of hepatitis or AIDS transmission may be decreased by use of heat-treated preparations. Current screening programs and vaccination with hepatitis B vaccine should help decrease the risk.

□ Reinforce need for patients with hemophilia to receive close medical supervision. Physician may order factor IX therapy 2–3 times per week for prophylaxis against spontaneous bleeding.

EVALUATION

Effectiveness of therapy can be demonstrated by: ■ Prevention of spontaneous bleeding or cessation of bleeding in patients with factor IX deficiency (hemophilia B, Christmas disease), factor VIII inhibitors, factor VII deficiency, or anticoagulant overdose.

FAMOTIDINE
(fa-**moe**-ti-deen)
Pepcid

CLASSIFICATION(S):
Histamine H_2 receptor antagonist, Antiulcer
Pregnancy Category B

INDICATIONS

- Short-term and maintenance treatment of active duodenal ulcers
- Management of gastric hypersecretory states (Zollinger-Ellison syndrome)
- Short-term treatment of benign gastric ulcers
- Treatment of gastroesophageal reflux disease (GERD).

ACTION

- Inhibits the action of histamine at the H_2 receptor site located primarily in gastric parietal cells, thereby inhibiting gastric acid secretion. **Therapeutic Effect:** ▪ Healing and prevention of ulcers.

PHARMACOKINETICS

Absorption: 40–45% absorbed following oral administration.

Distribution: Distribution not known. Probably does not cross the placenta or enter CSF.

Metabolism and Excretion: Up to 65–70% eliminated unchanged by the kidneys. 30–35% metabolized by the liver.

Half-life: 2.5–3.5 hr (increased in renal impairment).

CONTRAINDICATIONS AND PRECAUTIONS

Contraindicated in: ▪ Hypersensitivity ▪ Hypersensitivity to benzyl alcohol (IV only).

Use Cautiously in: ▪ Severe renal impairment (dosage reduction recommended if creatinine clearance <10 ml/min) ▪ Pregnancy, lactation, or children (safety not established).

ADVERSE REACTIONS AND SIDE EFFECTS*

CNS: <u>dizziness</u>, <u>headache</u>, drowsiness.
EENT: swelling of eyelids, tinnitus.
Resp: bronchospasm.
CV: palpitations, bradycardia, hypotension (IV).
GI: diarrhea, nausea, <u>constipation</u>, dry mouth.
Derm: facial edema, loss of hair, rash.
MS: joint pain, muscle pain.
Misc: fever.

INTERACTIONS

Drug–Drug: ▪ **Antacids** may slightly decrease the absorption of famotidine ▪ Decreases the absorption of **ketoconazole**.

ROUTE AND DOSAGE

Duodenal Ulcers

- **PO (Adults):** 40 mg at bedtime or 20 mg bid initially for 2–8 wk, followed by maintenance therapy of 20 mg daily at bedtime.
- **IV (Adults):** 20 mg q 12 hr.

Gastroesophageal Reflux Disease (GERD)

- **PO (Adults):** 20–40 mg twice daily.

Gastric Hypersecretory Conditions

- **PO (Adults):** 20 mg q 6 hr (range 20–160 mg q 6 hr).
- **IV (Adults):** 20 mg q 12 hr, higher doses may be necessary.

Benign Gastric Ulcer

- **PO (Adults):** 40 mg once daily at bedtime.

AVAILABILITY

- *Tablets:* 20 mg, 40 mg ▪ *Oral suspension:* 40 mg/5 ml ▪ *Injection:* 10 mg/ml.

TIME/ACTION PROFILE (inhibition of gastric acid secretion)

	ONSET	PEAK	DURATION
PO	within 1 hr	1–4 hr	6–12 hr
IV	within 1 hr	0.5–3 hr	8–15 hr

NURSING IMPLICATIONS

ASSESSMENT

- ▫ Assess patient routinely for epigastric or abdominal pain and frank or occult blood in the stool, emesis, or gastric aspirate.
- ▪ **Lab Test Considerations:** CBC with differential should be monitored periodically throughout therapy.
- ▫ Antagonizes effects of pentagastrin and histamine during gastric acid secretion tests. Avoid administration during the 24 hr preceding the test.
- ▫ May cause false-negative results in

---

*<u>Underlines</u> indicate most frequent; **CAPITALS** indicate life-threatening.

skin tests using allergen extracts. Famotidine should be discontinued prior to the test.

POTENTIAL NURSING DIAGNOSES
- Pain (indications).
- Knowledge deficit related to medication regimen (patient/family teaching).

IMPLEMENTATION
- **PO:** May be administered with food or liquids. Antacids may be administered concurrently for relief of gastric pain.
- Shake oral suspension prior to administration. Discard unused suspension after 30 days.
- **Direct IV:** Dilute 2 ml (10 mg/ml solution) in 5 or 10 ml of 0.9% NaCl for injection.
- *Rate:* Administer over at least 2 min. Rapid administration may cause hypotension.
- **Intermittent Infusion:** Dilute each 20 mg in 100 ml of 0.9% NaCl, D5W, D10W, lactated Ringer's solution, or sodium bicarbonate. Diluted solution is stable for 48 hr at room temperature. Do not use solution that is discolored or contains a precipitate.
- *Rate:* Administer over 15–30 min.
- **Y-Site Compatibility:** ■ aminophylline ■ ampicillin ■ ampicillin/sulbactam ■ amrinone ■ atropine ■ bretylium ■ calcium gluconate ■ cefazolin ■ cefoperazone ■ cefotaxime ■ cefotetan ■ cefoxitin ■ ceftazidime ■ ceftizoxime ■ cefuroxime ■ cephalothin ■ cephapirin ■ dexamethasone ■ digoxin ■ dobutamine ■ dopamine ■ enalaprilat ■ epinephrine ■ erythromycin lactobionate ■ esmolol ■ fluconazole ■ fludarabine ■ furosemide ■ gentamicin ■ heparin ■ hydrocortisone sodium succinate ■ imipenem/cilastatin ■ insulin ■ isoproterenol ■ labetalol ■ lidocaine ■ magnesium sulfate ■ meperidine ■ methylprednisolone ■ metoclopramide ■ mezlocillin ■ midazolam ■ morphine ■ nafcillin ■ nitroglycerin ■ norepinephrine ■ ondansetron ■ oxacillin ■ phenylephrine ■ phenytoin ■ piperacillin ■ potassium chloride ■ potassium phosphate ■ procainamide ■ sargramostim ■ sodium bicarbonate ■ sodium nitroprusside ■ theophylline ■ thiamine ■ ticarcillin ■ ticarcillin/clavulanate ■ verapamil.

PATIENT/FAMILY TEACHING
- Instruct patient to take medication as directed for the full course of therapy, even if feeling better. If a dose is missed it should be taken as soon as remembered, but not if almost time for next dose. Do not double doses.
- Inform patient that smoking interferes with the action of famotidine. Encourage patient to quit smoking or at least not to smoke after last dose of the day.
- May cause drowsiness or dizziness. Caution patient to avoid driving or other activities requiring alertness until response to the drug is known.
- Advise patient to avoid alcohol, products containing aspirin or ibuprofen, and foods that may cause an increase in GI irritation.
- Inform patient that increased fluid and fiber intake and exercise may minimize constipation.
- Advise patient to report onset of black, tarry stools; fever; diarrhea; dizziness; or rash to the physician promptly.

EVALUATION
Effectiveness of therapy can be demonstrated by: ■ Decrease in abdominal pain □ Prevention of gastric irritation and bleeding. Healing of duodenal ulcers can be seen by x-rays or endoscopy ■ Decrease in the signs and symptoms of gastroesophageal reflux disease.

FAT EMULSION
(fat ee-**mul**-shun)
Intralipid, Liposyn

CLASSIFICATION(S):
Caloric agent (nonprotein)
Pregnancy Category C

INDICATIONS

- Provision of nonprotein calories to patients whose total caloric needs cannot be met by carbohydrate (glucose) alone, usually as part of parenteral nutrition
- Treatment and prevention of essential fatty acid deficiency in patients receiving long-term parenteral nutrition.

ACTION

- Acts as a nonprotein calorie source. **Therapeutic Effect:** ■ Provision of essential fatty acids and nonprotein calories.

PHARMACOKINETICS

Absorption: Administered IV only, resulting in complete bioavailability.
Distribution: Distributes into intravascular space.
Metabolism and Excretion: Cleared by conversion to triglycerides, then to free fatty acids and glycerol by lipoprotein lipase. Free fatty acids are transported to tissues where they may be oxidized as an energy source or re-stored as triglycerides.
Half-life: UK.

CONTRAINDICATIONS AND PRECAUTIONS

Contraindicated in: ■ Hyperlipidemias ■ Lipoid nephrosis ■ Pancreatitis accompanied by lipemia ■ Hypersensitivity to egg products (emulsifier is egg yolk phospholipid).
Use Cautiously in: ■ Thromboembolic disorders ■ Severe liver or pulmonary disease ■ Anemia or bleeding disorders ■ Patients who are at risk for fat embolism ■ Preterm infants.

ADVERSE REACTIONS AND SIDE EFFECTS*

CV: chest pain.
GI: vomiting, hepatomegaly,† splenomegaly.†
Derm: jaundice.†
Local: phlebitis at IV site.
Misc: fever, chills, shivering, overloading syndrome,† infection, hypersensitivity reactions.

INTERACTIONS

Drug–Drug: ■ None significant.

ROUTE AND DOSAGE

Fat calories should not make up more than 60% of total calories.

Total Parenteral Nutrition

- **IV (Adults):** 10% emulsion—1 ml/min for initial 15–30 min, then increase to 83–125 ml/hr, not to exceed 500 ml on first day. Dosage may be increased on second day. Not to exceed 2.5 g/kg/day. 20% emulsion—0.5 ml for initial 15–30 min, then increase to 62.5 ml/hr, not to exceed 250 ml of Liposyn or 500 ml of Intralipid. Dosage may be increased on second day. Not to exceed 3 g/kg/day.
- **IV (Children):** 10% emulsion—0.1 ml/min for initial 10–15 min, then increase to 1 g/kg over 4 hr; rate should not exceed 100 ml/hr. 20% emulsion—0.05 ml/min for initial 10–15 min, then increase to 1 g/kg over 4 hr, rate should not exceed 50 ml/hr. Total should not exceed 3 g/kg/day.

Essential Fatty Acid Deficiency

- **IV (Adults and Children):** Provide 8–10% of caloric intake as fat.

AVAILABILITY

■ *Emulsion for IV Use 10%:* 50 ml, 100 ml, 200 ml, 250 ml, 500 ml ■ *Emulsion for IV Use 20%:* 50 ml, 100 ml, 200 ml, 250 ml, 500 ml.

TIME/ACTION PROFILE

	ONSET	PEAK	DURATION
IV	UK	UK	UK

NURSING IMPLICATIONS

ASSESSMENT

- Monitor weight every other day in adults and daily in infants and children receiving fat emulsion to assist in meeting caloric requirements.
- Assess patient for allergy to eggs prior to therapy. Acute hypersensitivity reaction with pruritic urticaria

†Seen only with long-term use.
*Underlines indicate most frequent; **CAPITALS** indicate life-threatening.

may occur in patients allergic to eggs.

- **Lab Test Considerations:** Monitor triglyceride and fatty acid levels routinely to determine patient's capacity to eliminate infused fat from the circulation.
- □ Monitor hemoglobin, hematocrit, liver function, blood coagulation, and platelet count (especially in neonates). Notify physician promptly for abnormalities. Therapy may be discontinued.
- **Toxicity and Overdose:** If signs of overloading syndrome (focal seizures, fever, leukocytosis, splenomegaly, shock) or elevated triglyceride or free fatty acid levels occur, infusion should be stopped and the patient reevaluated prior to reinstituting therapy.

POTENTIAL NURSING DIAGNOSES

- Nutrition, altered: less than body requirements (indications).
- Knowledge deficit related to medication regimen (patient/family teaching).

IMPLEMENTATION

- **General Info:** Fat emulsion should compose no more than 60% of patient's total caloric intake. The remaining 40% should be composed of carbohydrates and amino acids.
- □ Fat emulsion may be administered via peripheral or central venous catheter. Administer via infusion pump to ensure accurate rate. Monitor peripheral sites for phlebitis.
- □ Fat emulsion may be admixed ("3-in-1") or administered simultaneously with amino acid and dextrose solutions. Infuse fat emulsion via Y-site near the infusion site. Due to the lower specific gravity, the fat emulsion solution must be hung higher than the amino acid and dextrose solutions to prevent the fat emulsion from backing up into the amino acid and dextrose line.
- □ Do not use filters during administration.

- □ Use tubing provided by the manufacturer. Change IV tubing after each dose of fat emulsion.
- □ Do not use solutions in which the emulsion has separated or appears oily.
- □ Discard all unused portions.
- **Intermittent Infusion:** For adults the initial infusion rate should be 1 ml/min for the 10% solution and 0.5 ml/min for the 20% solution for the first 15–30 min. If no adverse reactions occur, the rate may be increased to 120 ml/hr for the 10% solution and 62.5 ml/hr for the 20% solution.
- □ No more than 500 ml of the 10% solution should be infused the first day. Dose may be increased on subsequent days.
- □ No more than 500 ml of the 20% solution of Intralipid should be infused the first day. Dose may be increased the following day.
- □ For children the initial infusion rate should be 0.1 ml/min of the 10% solution and 0.05 ml/min for the 20% solution for the first 10–15 min. If no adverse reactions occur, the rate may be increased to 1 g/kg over 4 hr. Do not exceed a rate of 100 ml/hr for the 10% solution or 50 ml/hr for the 20% solution.
- **Y-Site Compatibility:** ampicillin cefamandole cefazolin cefoxitin cephapirin clindamycin digoxin dopamine erythromycin lactobionate furosemide gentamicin isoproterenol kanamycin lidocaine norepinephrine oxacillin penicillin G potassium ticarcillin tobramycin.
- **Y-Site Incompatibility:** amikacin.
- **Additive Incompatibility:** Although compatibility studies have been done, manufacturer recommends that fat emulsion not be admixed with any other medication.

PATIENT/FAMILY TEACHING

- □ Explain the purpose of fat emulsion to the patient prior to administration.

EVALUATION
Effectiveness of therapy may be determined by: ▪ Weight gain □ Maintenance of normal serum triglyceride and fatty acid levels.

FELBAMATE
(fell-ba-mate)
Felbatol

CLASSIFICATION(S):
Anticonvulsant
Pregnancy Category C

INDICATIONS

▪ Used as initial therapy alone (monotherapy) or as adjunctive therapy with other anticonvulsants to control a variety of seizures in adults ▪ Adjunctive therapy with other anticonvulsants in children (2–14 yr) who have seizures associated with Lennox-Gastaut Syndrome.

ACTION

▪ Probably acts by raising seizure threshold and preventing seizure spread. Therapeutic Effect: ▪ Decreased incidence of seizures.

PHARMACOKINETICS

Absorption: Well absorbed following oral administration.
Distribution: Distribution not known.
Metabolism and Excretion: 40–50% excreted unchanged in urine. 40% metabolized by the liver.
Half-life: 20–23 hr.

CONTRAINDICATIONS AND PRECAUTIONS

Contraindicated in: ▪ Hypersensitivity.
Use Cautiously in: ▪ Patients with a history of hypersensitivity to other carbamates (meprobamate).

ADVERSE REACTIONS AND SIDE EFFECTS*

CNS: insomnia, headache, fatigue, somnolence, agitation, psychological disturbances, dizziness, weakness, malaise, agressive behavior.
EENT: diplopia, blurred vision.
CV: palpitations, tachycardia.
GI: anorexia, vomiting, nausea, dyspepsia, constipation, abnormal taste.
Derm: pruritis.
Neuro: ataxia.
Misc: weight increase, flu-like syndrome.

INTERACTIONS

Drug–Drug: ▪ Increases blood levels and risk of toxicity from phenytoin (decreases phenytoin dosage by 20%) ▪ Decreases carbamazepine blood levels, but increases levels of carbamazepine epoxide, an active metabolite ▪ Due to potential interactions, doses of carbamazepine, penytoin, and valproic acid should be decreased by 20–33% when initiating felbamate therapy. Further reductions may be required.

ROUTE AND DOSAGE

▪ PO (Adults and Children >14 yr):
If used alone, start with 1200 mg/day in 3–4 divided doses. May be increased by 600 mg/day at 2-wk intervals up to a total of 3600 mg. If converting from other agents, start with 1200 mg/day in 3–4 divided doses, and decrease other anticonvulsants by ⅓. After 1 wk increase to 2400 mg/day in 3–4 divided doses and decrease other anticonvulsants by up to ⅓. After another week, increase felbamate to 3600 mg/day in divided doses, while continuing to decrease doses of other anticonvulsants. If using as adjunctive therapy (with other agents), start with 1200 mg/day in 3–4 divided doses, decreasing doses of other anticonvulsants by 20%. Increase dose at weekly intervals by 1200 mg/day to 3600 mg/day. Decrease doses of other anticonvulsants as necessary.
▪ PO (Children): As adjunctive therapy, start at 15 mg/kg/day in 3–4 divided doses, decreasing the dose of other anticonvulsants by 20%. In-

F

*Underlines indicate most frequent; CAPITALS indicate life-threatening.

crease dosage by 15 mg/kg/day at 1-wk intervals to 45 mg/kg/day. Decrease doses of other anticonvulsants as necessary.

AVAILABILITY

▪ *Tablets:* 400 mg, 600 mg ▪ *Oral suspension:* 400 mg/5 ml.

TIME/ACTION PROFILE
(anticonvulsant activity)

	ONSET	PEAK	DURATION
PO	UK	UK	UK

NURSING IMPLICATIONS

ASSESSMENT

□ Assess location, duration, and characteristics of seizure activity.
▪ **Lab Test Considerations:** Monitor CBC with differential periodically during therapy.
□ May cause elevated AST (SGOT) and ALT (SGPT) levels.
▪ **Toxicity and Overdose:** When used as adjunctive therapy with other anticonvulsants, monitor serum blood levels of other anticonvulsants throughout therapy.

POTENTIAL NURSING DIAGNOSES

▪ Injury, high risk for (indications, side effects).
▪ Knowledge deficit related to medication regimen (patient/family teaching).

IMPLEMENTATION

▪ **General Info:** Implement seizure precautions.
▪ **PO:** May be administered with food or antacids to minimize gastric irritation.

PATIENT/FAMILY TEACHING

□ Instruct patient to take felbamate exactly as directed. If a dose is missed, take as soon as remembered but not just before next dose; do not double doses. Notify physician if more than 1 dose is missed. Medication should be gradually discontinued to prevent seizures and status epilepticus.
□ May cause dizziness and drowsiness. Advise patients to avoid driving or other activities requiring alertness until response to medication is known.
□ Instruct patient that fever, sore throat, mouth ulcers, petechiae, unusual bleeding or bruising, abdominal pain, chills, pale stools, dark urine, or jaundice should be reported to the physician immediately.
□ Advise patient not to take alcohol or other CNS depressants concurrently with this medication.
□ Advise patient to use a nonhormonal form of contraception while taking felbamate.
□ Instruct patient to notify physician or dentist of medication regimen prior to treatment or surgery.
□ Advise patient to carry identification describing disease and medication regimen at all times.

EVALUATION

Clinical response to therapy can be indicated by: ▪ Absense or reduction of seizure activity.

FELODIPINE
(fell-**oh**-di-peen)
Plendil

CLASSIFICATION(S):
Calcium channel blocker, Antihypertensive
Pregnancy Category C

INDICATIONS

▪ Alone or with other agents in the management of hypertension.

ACTION

▪ Inhibits the transport of calcium into myocardial and vascular smooth muscle cells, resulting in inhibition of excitation-contraction coupling and subsequent contraction. Result is systemic vasodilation. **Therapeutic Effect:** ▪ Reduction of blood pressure in hypertensive patients.

PHARMACOKINETICS

Absorption: Although well absorbed following oral administration, extensive metabolism leads to decreased bioavailability (20%).

Distribution: Distribution not known.

Metabolism and Excretion: Extensively metabolized. <0.5% excreted unchanged in urine.

Half-life: 11–16 hr.

CONTRAINDICATIONS AND PRECAUTIONS

Contraindicated in: ▪ Hypersensitivity.

Use Cautiously in: ▪ Hypotensive patients ▪ Congestive heart failure or compromised left ventricular function (especially in combination with beta-blocker therapy) ▪ Patients >65 yr or patients with impaired liver function (daily dosage should not exceed 10 mg) ▪ Pregnancy, lactation, or children (safety not established) ▪ Cardiac conduction defects.

ADVERSE REACTIONS AND SIDE EFFECTS*

CNS: <u>headache</u>, <u>dizziness</u>, weakness, syncope, anxiety, insomnia, psychiatric disturbances.

EENT: nasal congestion, pharyngitis, epistaxis.

Resp: cough, dyspnea, wheezing.

CV: <u>peripheral edema</u>, MYOCARDIAL INFARCTION, hypotension, chest pain, AV block, tachycardia.

GI: nausea, diarrhea, constipation, vomiting, dry mouth, flatulence, gingival hyperplasia.

GU: sexual difficulties.

Derm: flushing, rash, pruritus.

Hemat: anemia.

MS: muscle cramps, back pain.

Neuro: paresthesia.

INTERACTIONS

Drug–Drug: ▪ Additive hypotension with other **antihypertensives, nitrates,** or acute ingestion of **alcohol** ▪ **Cimetidine** or **ranitidine** decrease metabolism and may increase the effects of felodipine ▪ Combination with **beta blockers** may result in myocardial depression.

ROUTE AND DOSAGE

▪ **PO (Adults):** 5 mg once daily initially. May increase at 2-wk intervals. Usual daily dose is 5–10 mg (not to exceed 20 mg/day).

AVAILABILITY

▪ *Extended-release tablets:* 5 mg, 10 mg.

TIME/ACTION PROFILE (antihypertensive effect)

	ONSET	PEAK	DURATION
PO	2–5 hr	UK	up to 24 hr

NURSING IMPLICATIONS

ASSESSMENT

▫ Monitor blood pressure and pulse prior to and periodically throughout therapy. Monitor ECG periodically in patients receiving prolonged therapy.

▫ Monitor intake and output ratios and daily weight. Assess patient for signs of congestive heart failure (peripheral edema, rales/crackles, dyspnea, weight gain, jugular venous distention).

▪ **Lab Test Considerations:** Monitor hepatic function periodically in patients receiving long-term therapy. May cause elevated liver function tests.

POTENTIAL NURSING DIAGNOSES

▪ Cardiac output, decreased (indications).

▪ Knowledge deficit related to medication regimen (patient/family teaching).

IMPLEMENTATION

▪ **PO:** Administer once daily. Tablets should be swallowed whole; do not crush or chew.

PATIENT/FAMILY TEACHING

▫ Advise patient to take medication exactly as directed, not to skip or double up on missed doses. Felodipine may need to be discontinued gradually.

▫ Encourage patient to comply with additional interventions for hyperten-

---

*<u>Underlines</u> indicate most frequent; **CAPITALS** indicate life-threatening.

sion (weight reduction, smoking cessation, moderation of alcohol consumption, regular exercise, stress management). Felodipine controls but does not cure hypertension.

□ Caution patients to make position changes slowly to minimize orthostatic hypotension.

□ Felodipine may cause dizziness. Advise patient to avoid driving or other activities requiring alertness until response to the medication is known.

□ Instruct patient to avoid concurrent use of alcohol or over-the-counter medications without consulting physician or pharmacist.

□ Advise patient to notify the physician if irregular heart beats, dyspnea, swelling of hands and feet, pronounced dizziness, nausea, constipation or hypotension occur.

EVALUATION
Effectiveness of therapy can be demonstrated by: ▪ Decrease in blood pressure.

FENOPROFEN
(fen-oh-**proe**-fen)
Nalfon

CLASSIFICATION(S):
Nonsteroidal anti-inflammatory
agent, Nonopioid analgesic
Pregnancy Category B

INDICATIONS

▪ Management of inflammatory disorders, including: □ Rheumatoid arthritis □ Osteoarthritis ▪ Analgesic in the treatment of mild to moderate pain, including dysmenorrhea.

ACTION

▪ Inhibits prostaglandin synthesis. **Therapeutic Effects:** ▪ Suppression of pain and inflammation.

PHARMACOKINETICS

Absorption: Well absorbed from the GI tract.

Distribution: Does not cross the placenta. Enters breast milk in low concentrations.

Metabolism and Excretion: Mostly metabolized by the liver. Small amounts (2–5%) excreted unchanged by the kidneys.

Half-life: 3 hr.

CONTRAINDICATIONS AND PRECAUTIONS

Contraindicated in: ▪ Hypersensitivity ▪ Cross-sensitivity may exist with other NSAIAs, including aspirin ▪ Active GI bleeding or ulcer disease.

Use Cautiously in: ▪ Severe cardiovascular, renal, or hepatic disease ▪ Patients with a history of ulcer disease ▪ Pregnancy, lactation, or children (safety not established).

ADVERSE REACTIONS AND SIDE EFFECTS*

CNS: headache, drowsiness, psychic disturbances, dizziness.

EENT: blurred vision, tinnitus.

CV: edema, arrhythmias.

GI: nausea, dyspepsia, vomiting, constipation, GI BLEEDING, discomfort, HEPATITIS.

GU: renal failure, hematuria, cystitis.

Derm: rashes.

Hemat: blood dyscrasias, prolonged bleeding time.

Misc: allergic reactions, including ANAPHYLAXIS.

INTERACTIONS

Drug–Drug: ▪ Concurrent use with **aspirin** or **antacids** may decrease effectiveness ▪ Additive adverse GI effects with **aspirin**, other **nonsteroidal anti-inflammatory agents, potassium supplements, glucocorticoids,** or **alcohol** ▪ Chronic use with **acetaminophen** may increase the risk of adverse renal reactions ▪ May increase the risk of hypo-

---

*Underlines indicate most frequent; **CAPITALS** indicate life-threatening.

glycemia with **insulin** or **oral hypoglycemic agents** ▪ May decrease the effectiveness of **diuretics** or **antihypertensive** therapy ▪ May increase serum **lithium** levels and increase the risk of toxicity ▪ Increases the risk of toxicity from **methotrexate** ▪ Increased risk of bleeding with **cefamandole, cefotetan, cefoperazone, valproic acid** or **plicamycin, heparin, thrombolytic agents,** or **oral anticoagulants** ▪ Increased risk of adverse hematologic reactions with **antineoplastic agents** or **radiation therapy** ▪ **Phenobarbital** may increase metabolism and decrease effectiveness of fenoprofen ▪ May increase the risk of nephrotoxicity with **cyclosporine.**

ROUTE AND DOSAGE

Analgesia
▪ **PO (Adults):** 200 mg q 4–6 hr.

Anti-inflammatory
▪ **PO (Adults):** 300–600 mg 3–4 times daily (not to exceed 3.2 g/day).

AVAILABILITY
▪ *Capsules:* 200 mg, 300 mg ▪ *Tablets:* 600 mg.

TIME/ACTION PROFILE

	ONSET	PEAK	DURATION
PO (analgesic activity)	15–30 min	1–2 hr	4–6 hr
PO (anti-inflammatory activity)	several days	2–3 wk	UK

NURSING IMPLICATIONS

ASSESSMENT
▪ **General Info:** Patients who have asthma, aspirin-induced allergy, and nasal polyps are at increased risk for developing hypersensitivity reactions. Monitor for rhinitis, asthma, and urticaria.
▪ **Arthritis:** Assess pain and range of movement prior to and 1–2 hr following administration.
▪ **Pain:** Assess pain (type, location, and intensity) prior to and 1–2 hr following administration.

▪ **Lab Test Considerations:** BUN, serum creatinine, CBC, and liver function tests should be evaluated periodically in patients receiving prolonged course of therapy.
▫ Serum potassium, alkaline phosphatase, LDH, AST (SGOT) and ALT (SGPT) may show increased levels. Bleeding time may also be prolonged.

POTENTIAL NURSING DIAGNOSES
▪ Pain (indications).
▪ Physical mobility, impaired (indications).
▪ Knowledge deficit related to medication regimen (patient/family teaching).

IMPLEMENTATION
▪ **General Info:** Coadministration with opioid analgesics may have additive analgesic effects and may permit lower opioid doses.
▪ **PO:** For rapid initial effect, administer 30 min before or 2 hr after meals.
▪ **Dysmenorrhea:** Administer as soon as possible after the onset of menses. Prophylactic use has not been proven effective.

PATIENT/FAMILY TEACHING
▫ Advise patient to take this medication with a full glass of water and to remain in an upright position for 15–30 min after administration.
▫ Instruct patient to take medication exactly as directed. If a dose is missed, take as soon as remembered, but not if almost time for next dose. Do not double doses.
▫ May cause drowsiness or dizziness. Advise patient to avoid driving or other activities requiring alertness until response to the medication is known.
▫ Caution patient to avoid the concurrent use of alcohol, aspirin, ibuprofen, acetaminophen, or other over-the-counter medications without consulting physician or pharmacist.
▫ Instruct patient to notify physician if rash, itching, chills, fever, muscle aches, visual disturbances, tinnitus, weight gain, edema, black stools, or persistent headache occur.

F

□ Advise patient to inform physician or dentist of medication regimen prior to treatment or surgery.

EVALUATION

Effectiveness of therapy can be demonstrated by: ■ Decrease in severity of pain ■ Improved joint mobility. Partial arthritic relief is usually seen within a few days, but maximum effects may require 2–3 wk of continuous therapy. Patients who do not respond to one nonsteroidal anti-inflammatory agent may respond to another.

FENTANYL (Parenteral)
(**fen**-ta-nil)
Sublimaze

CLASSIFICATION(S):
Opioid analgesic (agonist)
Schedule II
Pregnancy Category C

INDICATIONS

■ Management of: □ Perioperative pain □ Intraoperative pain □ Postoperative pain ■ Treatment and prevention of perioperative tachypnea and emergence delirium ■ Supplement to general or regional analgesia—combination with droperidol produces neuroleptanalgesia (quiescence, decreased motor activity, and analgesia without loss of consciousness).

ACTION

■ Binds to opiate receptors in the CNS, altering the response to and perception of pain ■ Produces CNS depression. **Therapeutic Effect:** ■ Relief of moderate to severe pain.

PHARMACOKINETICS

Absorption: Well absorbed following IM administration.
Distribution: Distribution not known.
Metabolism and Excretion: Mostly metabolized by the liver. 10–25% excreted unchanged by the kidneys.

Half-life: 3.6 hr (increased after cardiopulmonary bypass and in elderly patients).

CONTRAINDICATIONS AND PRECAUTIONS

Contraindicated in: ■ Hypersensitivity ■ Known intolerance.
Use Cautiously in: ■ Elderly or debilitated patients ■ Severely ill patients ■ Diabetics ■ Patients with severe pulmonary or hepatic disease ■ CNS tumors ■ Increased intracranial pressure ■ Head trauma ■ Adrenal insufficiency ■ Undiagnosed abdominal pain ■ Hypothyroidism ■ Alcoholism ■ Cardiac disease, particularly arrhythmias ■ Pregnancy, lactation, and children <2 yr (safety not established).

ADVERSE REACTIONS AND SIDE EFFECTS*

CNS: euphoria, floating feeling, dysphoria, hallucinations, depression, excessive sedation.
Resp: respiratory depression, APNEA, laryngospasm, bronchoconstriction.
CV: bradycardia.
GI: constipation, nausea, vomiting.
MS: skeletal and thoracic muscle rigidity.

INTERACTIONS

Drug–Drug: ■ Avoid use in patients who have received **MAO inhibitors** within the previous 14 days (may produce unpredictable, potentially fatal reactions) ■ Additive CNS and respiratory depression with other **CNS depressants,** including **alcohol, antihistamines, antidepressants,** and other **sedative/hypnotics** ■ Increased risk of hypotension with **benzodiazepines.**

ROUTE AND DOSAGE

Preoperative Use
■ **IM (Adults):** 50–100 mcg 30–60 min before surgery.

Adjunct to General Anesthesia
■ **IV (Adults):** Low dose—2 mcg/kg. Moderate dose—2–20 mcg/kg, addi-

---

tional doses of 25–100 mcg may be given IV or IM as necessary. High dose—20–50 mcg/kg; additional doses ranging from 25 mcg to 50% of original dose may be repeated as necessary.

Adjunct to Regional Anesthesia
■ IM, IV (Adults): 50–100 mcg.

Postoperative Use (Recovery Room)
■ IM (Adults): 50–100 mcg, may repeat in 1–2 hr.

To Provide General Anesthesia
■ IV (Adults): 50–100 mcg/kg (up to 150 mcg/kg) with oxygen and a skeletal muscle relaxant.
■ IV (Children 2–12 yr): 2–3 mcg/kg.

AVAILABILITY

■ *Injection:* 0.05 mg/ml ■ *In combination with:* droperidol.

TIME/ACTION PROFILE (analgesia; respiratory depression may last longer than analgesia)

	ONSET	PEAK	DURATION
IM	7–15 min	20–30 min	1–2 hr
IV	1–2 min	3–5 min	0.5–1 hr

NURSING IMPLICATIONS

ASSESSMENT

▫ Monitor respiratory rate and blood pressure frequently throughout course of therapy. Notify physician of significant changes immediately. The respiratory depressant effects of fentanyl last longer than the analgesic effects. Subsequent opioid doses should be reduced by ¼–⅓ of the usually recommended dose. Monitor closely.

▫ Assess type, location, and intensity of pain prior to and 10 min following IM administration or 1–2 min following IV administration when fentanyl is used to treat pain.

■ **Lab Test Considerations:** May cause elevated serum amylase and lipase concentrations.

■ **Toxicity and Overdose:** If overdose

occurs, naloxone (Narcan) is the antidote.

POTENTIAL NURSING DIAGNOSES
■ Pain (indications).
■ Breathing pattern, ineffective (adverse reactions).
■ Injury, high risk for (side effects).

IMPLEMENTATION

■ **General Info:** Benzodiazepines may be administered prior to administration of fentanyl to reduce the induction dose requirements and decrease the time to loss of consciousness. This combination may also increase the risk of hypotension.

▫ Opioid antagonist, oxygen, and resuscitative equipment should be readily available during the administration of fentanyl.

■ **Direct IV:** Administer slowly over at least 1–2 min. Slow IV administration may reduce the incidence or severity of muscle rigidity, bradycardia, or hypotension.

■ **Intermittent Infusion:** Fentanyl may also be diluted with D5W, 0.9% NaCl, D5/LR, or lactated Ringer's solution for infusion and administered until the onset of somnolence as an adjunct to general anesthesia.

■ **Syringe Compatibility:** ■ atropine ■ butorphanol ■ chlorpromazine ■ cimetidine ■ dimenhydrinate ■ diphenhydramine ■ droperidol ■ heparin ■ hydromorphone ■ hydroxyzine ■ meperidine ■ metoclopramide ■ midazolam ■ morphine ■ pentazocine ■ perphenazine ■ prochlorperazine edisylate ■ promazine ■ promethazine ■ ranitidine ■ scopolamine.

■ **Syringe Incompatibility:** ■ pentobarbital.

■ **Y-Site Compatibility:** ■ atracurium ■ enalaprilat ■ esmolol ■ heparin ■ hydrocortisone sodium succinate ■ labetalol ■ nafcillin ■ pancuronium ■ potassium chloride ■ vecuronium ■ vitamin B complex with C.

■ **Additive Compatibility:** ■ bupivacaine.

■ **Additive Incompatibility:** ■ methohexital ■ pentobarbital ■ thiopental.

F

PATIENT/FAMILY TEACHING

□ Caution patient to make position changes slowly to minimize orthostatic hypotension.

□ Medication causes dizziness and drowsiness. Advise patient to call for assistance during ambulation and transfer, and to avoid driving or other activities requiring alertness for 24 hr after administration of fentanyl during outpatient surgery.

□ Instruct patient to avoid alcohol or other CNS depressants for 24 hr after administration of fentanyl for outpatient surgery.

EVALUATION

Effectiveness of therapy can be demonstrated by: ■ General quiescence □ Reduced motor activity ■ Pronounced analgesia.

FENTANYL TRANSDERMAL
(fen-ta-nil)
Duragesic

CLASSIFICATION(S):
Opioid analgesic (agonist)
Controlled Substance Schedule II
Pregnancy Category C

INDICATIONS

■ Management of chronic pain in patients requiring opioid analgesic therapy ■ Transdermal fentanyl is not recommended for the control of postoperative pain.

ACTION

■ Binds to opiate receptors in the CNS, altering the response to and perception of pain. **Therapeutic Effect:** ■ Decrease in severity of chronic pain.

PHARMACOKINETICS

Absorption: Well absorbed (92% of dose) through skin surface under transdermal patch, creating a depot in the upper skin layers. Release from transdermal system into systemic circulation increases gradually to a constant rate providing continuous delivery for 72 hr.

Distribution: Crosses the placenta and enters breast milk.

Metabolism and Excretion: Mostly metabolized by the liver. 10–25% excreted unchanged by the kidneys.

Half-life: 17 hr following removal of patch (due to continued release from deposition of drug in skin layers).

CONTRAINDICATIONS AND PRECAUTIONS

Contraindicated in: ■ Hypersensitivity to fentanyl or adhesives ■ Known intolerance ■ Acute pain (onset not rapid enough) ■ Alcohol intolerance (small amounts of alcohol released into skin).

Use Cautiously in: ■ Patients >60 yr, cachectic or debilitated patients (dosage reduction suggested due to altered drug disposition) ■ Severely ill patients ■ Diabetics ■ Patients with severe pulmonary or hepatic disease ■ CNS tumors ■ Increased intracranial pressure ■ Head trauma ■ Adrenal insufficiency ■ Undiagnosed abdominal pain ■ Hypothyroidism ■ Alcoholism ■ Cardiac disease, particularly bradyarrhythmias ■ Pregnancy, lactation, and children <2 yr (safety not established) ■ Fever (increases release of fentanyl from delivery system) ■ Titration period (additional analgesics may be required).

ADVERSE REACTIONS AND SIDE EFFECTS*

CNS: drowsiness, confusion, weakness, dizziness, restlessness.

Resp: respiratory depression, APNEA, laryngospasm, bronchoconstriction.

CV: bradycardia.

GI: constipation, dry mouth, nausea, vomiting, anorexia.

Derm: sweating, erythema.

Local: application site reactions.

MS: skeletal and thoracic muscle rigidity.

Misc: physical dependence, psychological dependence.

---

*Underlines indicate most frequent; **CAPITALS** indicate life-threatening.

INTERACTIONS

Drug–Drug: ▪ Avoid use in patients who have received **MAO inhibitors** within the previous 14 days (may produce unpredictable, potentially fatal reactions) ▪ Additive CNS and respiratory depression with other **CNS depressants** including **alcohol, antihistamines, antidepressants,** and **sedative/hypnotics** ▪ **Disulfiram, cefoperazone, cefotetan, cefamandole,** and **metronidazole** may produce adverse reactions due to release of small amounts of alcohol from transdermal system.

ROUTE AND DOSAGE

▪ **Transdermal (Adults):** 25 mcg/hr is the initial dose in patients who have not been receiving opioids prior to institution of transdermal fentanyl. To calculate the dosage of transdermal fentanyl required in patients who are already receiving opioid analgesics, assess the 24-hr requirement of currently used opioid. Using the equianalgesic table in Appendix B, convert this to an equivalent amount of morphine/24 hr. Conversion to fentanyl transdermal may be accomplished by using the fentanyl conversion table, which also appears in Appendix B. During dosage titration, additional short-acting opioids should be available for any breakthrough pain that may occur. Morphine 10 mg IM or 60 mg PO q 4 hr (60 mg/24 hr IM or 360 mg/24 hr PO) is considered to be approximately equivalent to transdermal fentanyl 100 mcg/hr. Transdermal patch lasts 72 hr in most patients. Some patients require a new patch every 48 hr.
▪ **Transdermal (Adults >60 yr, Debilitated or Cachectic Patients):** Initial dose should be 25 mcg/hr unless previous opioid use was >135 mg morphine PO/day (or other opioid equivalent).

AVAILABILITY

▪ *Transdermal systems:* 25 mcg/hr (contains 2.5 mg fentanyl in a 10-cm^2 patch), 50 mcg/hr (contains 5 mg fentanyl in a 20-cm^2 patch), 75 mcg/hr (contains 7.5 mg fentanyl in a 30-cm^2 patch), 100 mcg/hr (contains 10 mg fentanyl in a 40-cm^2 patch).

TIME/ACTION PROFILE (decreased pain)

	ONSET	PEAK	DURATION
TD	6 hr*	12–24 hr	72 hr†

*Achievement of blood levels associated with analgesia. Maximal response and dose titration may take up to 6 days.
†While patch is worn.

NURSING IMPLICATIONS

ASSESSMENT

□ Assess type, location, and intensity of pain prior to and 24 hr after application and periodically throughout therapy. Pain should be monitored frequently during initiation of therapy as should dosage changes to assess need for supplementary analgesics.
□ Assess blood pressure, pulse, and respiratory rate before and periodically during administration.
□ Prolonged use may lead to physical and psychological dependence and tolerance. This should not prevent patient from receiving adequate analgesia. Most patients who receive opioid analgesics for medical reasons do not develop psychological dependence.
□ Progressively higher doses may be required to relieve pain with long-term therapy. It may take up to 6 days after increasing doses to reach equilibrium, so patients should wear higher dose through 2 applications before increasing dose again.
□ Assess bowel function routinely. Increased intake of fluids and bulk, stool softeners, and laxatives may minimize constipating effects.
▪ **Lab Test Considerations:** May increase plasma amylase and lipase levels.
▪ **Toxicity and Overdose:** If overdosage occurs, naloxone (Narcan) is the antidote. Monitor patient closely, dose may need to be repeated or may need to be administered as an infusion be-

cause of long duration of action despite removal of patch.

POTENTIAL NURSING DIAGNOSES

- Pain (indications).
- Sensory-perceptual alteration: visual, auditory (side effects).
- Injury, high risk for (side effects).
- Knowledge deficit related to medication regimen (patient/family teaching).

IMPLEMENTATION

- **General Info:** Supplemental doses of short-acting opioid analgesics should be used to manage pain until relief is obtained with the transdermal system. Patients may continue to require supplemental narcotics for breakthrough pain. If >100 mcg/hr is required, use multiple systems.
- Dosage is titrated based on the patient's report of pain until adequate analgesia is attained. Dose is determined by calculating the previous 24-hr analgesic requirement and converting to the equianalgesic morphine dose using Appendix B. The conversion ratio from morphine to transdermal fentanyl is conservative; 50% of patients may require a dose increase after initial application. Increase after 3 days based on required daily doses of supplemental analgesics. Increases should be based on ratio of 90 mg/24 hr of oral morphine to 25 mcg/hr increase in transdermal fentanyl dose. Patients requiring >300 mcg/hr may need other methods of opioid analgesic administration.
- Coadministration with nonopioid analgesics may have additive analgesic effects and permit lower opioid doses.
- To convert to another opioid analgesic, remove transdermal fentanyl system and begin treatment with half the equianalgesic dose of the new analgesic in 12–18 hr.
- Medication should be discontinued gradually after long-term use to prevent withdrawal symptoms.
- **Transdermal:** Apply system to upper torso on a flat, nonirritated, and non-

irradiated site. If skin preparation is necessary, use clear water and clip, do not shave, hair. Allow skin to dry completely before application. Apply immediately after removing from package and press firmly in place with palm of hand for 10–20 sec, especially around the edges, to make sure contact is complete. For continued use, remove used system and fold so that adhesive edges are together. Flush system down toilet immediately upon removal. Apply new system to a different site. Discard unused systems by removing from pouch and flushing down the toilet.

PATIENT/FAMILY TEACHING

- Instruct patient how and when to ask for pain medication.
- Instruct patient in correct method for application and disposal of transdermal system.
- Medication may cause drowsiness or dizziness. Caution patient to call for assistance when ambulating or smoking and to avoid driving or other activities requiring alertness until response to medication is known.
- Advise patient to make position changes slowly to minimize dizziness.
- Caution patient to avoid concurrent use of alcohol or other CNS depressants with this medication.

EVALUATION

Effectiveness of therapy can be demonstrated by: ■ Decrease in severity of pain without a significant alteration in level of consciousness, respiratory status, or blood pressure.

FERROUS SALTS

ferrous fumarate
(**fer**-us **fyoo**-ma-rate)
Femiron, Feostat, Fumasorb, Fumerin, Hemocyte, Ircon, {Neo-Fer}, {Novofumar}, {Palafer}, Palmiron, Span-FF

{} = Available in Canada only.

ferrous gluconate
(**fer**-us **gloo**-koe-nate)
{Apo-Ferrous Gluconate}, Fergon,
Ferralet, {Fertinic}, {Novoferro-
gluc}, Simron

ferrous sulfate
(**fer**-us **sul**-fate)
{Apo-Ferrous Sulfate}, Feosol,
Fer-In-Sol, Fer-Iron, {Fero-Grad},
Fero-Gradumet, Ferralyn, Ferra-
TD, Mol-Iron, {Novoferrosulfa},
{PMS Ferrous Sulfate}, Slow Fe

CLASSIFICATION(S):
Antianemic, Iron supplement
Pregnancy Category UK

INDICATIONS
▪ Prevention and treatment of iron deficiency anemias.

ACTION
▪ An essential mineral found in hemoglobin, myoglobin, and a number of enzymes ▪ Allows oxygen transport from
lungs to tissues via hemoglobin. **Therapeutic Effect:** ▪ Correction of iron deficiency states ▪ Iron supplementation.

PHARMACOKINETICS
Absorption: 5–10% of dietary iron is
absorbed. In deficiency states this may
increase up to 30%. Therapeutically administered iron may be 60% absorbed.
Absorbed by active and passive transport processes.
Distribution: Crosses the placenta.
Metabolism and Excretion: Mostly re-
cycled, small daily losses occurring
through desquamation, sweat, urine,
and bile.
Half-life: UK.

CONTRAINDICATIONS AND PRECAUTIONS
Contraindicated in: ▪ Primary he-
mochromatosis ▪ Hemolytic anemias
▪ Some products contain tartrazine
(FDC #5)—use cautiously in patients
with tartrazine sensitivity.
Use Cautiously in: ▪ Peptic ulcer
▪ Ulcerative colitis or regional enteritis

(condition may be aggravated) ▪ Indis-
criminate chronic use (may lead to iron
overload).

ADVERSE REACTIONS AND SIDE EFFECTS*
GI: constipation, diarrhea, nausea,
dark stools, epigastric pain, GI
bleeding.
Misc: staining of teeth (liquid preparations).

INTERACTIONS
Drug–Drug: ▪ **Tetracycline** and **antacids** inhibit the absorption of iron by
forming insoluble compounds ▪ **Tetracycline** absorption is also decreased by
concurrent iron administration ▪ Iron
decreases the absorption of **fluoroquinolones** or **penicillamine** ▪ **Chloramphenicol** and **vitamin E** may impair the
hematologic response to iron therapy
▪ **Vitamin C** may slightly increase the
absorption of iron.
Drug–Food: ▪ Iron absorption is decreased by ⅓–½ by concurrent administration of food.

ROUTE AND DOSAGE
**Dosage Expressed in mg
Individual Salts**

Ferrous Fumarate—Prophylactic
▪ **PO (Adults):** 200 mg/day.
▪ **PO (Children):** 3 mg/kg/day.

Ferrous Fumarate—Therapeutic
▪ **PO (Adults):** 200 mg 3–4 times daily.
Controlled-release capsules may be
given twice daily.
▪ **PO (Children):** 3–6 mg/kg 3 times
daily.

Ferrous Gluconate—Prophylactic
▪ **PO (Adults):** 325/day.
▪ **PO (Children >2 yr):** 8 mg/kg/day.

Ferrous Gluconate—Therapeutic
▪ **PO (Adults):** 325–650 mg qid. Sustained-release capsules may be given
twice daily.
▪ **PO (Children >2 yr):** 16 mg/kg tid.

Ferrous Sulfate—Prophylactic
▪ **PO (Adults):** 300–325 mg/day.
▪ **PO (Children):** 5 mg/kg/day.

F

Ferrous Sulfate—Therapeutic

- **PO (Adults):** 300 mg 2–4 times daily. Timed-release tablets may be given twice daily.
- **PO (Children):** 10 mg/kg tid.

Dosage Expressed in mg Elemental Iron

- **PO (Adults):** 50–100 mg 3 times daily.
- **PO (Children):** 4–6 mg/kg/day in 3 divided doses.
- **PO (Infants):** 1–2 mg/kg/day.
- **PO (Pregnant Women):** 30–60 mg/day.

AVAILABILITY

Ferrous Fumarate (33% elemental iron)

- *Tablets:* 63 mg, 195 mg, 200 mg, 324 mg, 325 mg, 35 mg ▪ *Chewable tablets:* 100 mg ▪ *Controlled-release capsules:* 325 mg ▪ *Suspension:* 100 mg/5 ml ▪ *Drops:* 45 mg/0.6 ml ▪ *In combination with:* vitamin C, docusate. See Appendix A.

Ferrous Gluconate (11.6% elemental iron)

- *Tablets:* 300 mg, 320 mg, 325 mg ▪ *Sustained-release tablets:* 320 mg ▪ *Soft gelatin capsules:* 86 mg ▪ *Elixir:* 300 mg/5 ml.

Ferrous Sulfate (20–30% elemental iron)

- *Tablets:* 195 mg, 300 mg, 324 mg ▪ *Capsules:* 250 mg ▪ *Timed-release tablets:* 525 mg ▪ *Syrup:* 90 mg/5 ml ▪ *Elixir:* 220 mg/5 ml ▪ *Drops:* 125 mg/1 ml ▪ *In combination with:* ascorbic acid, antacids. See Appendix A.

TIME/ACTION PROFILE (effects on erythropoiesis)

	ONSET	PEAK	DURATION
PO	4 days	7–10 days	2–4 mo

NURSING IMPLICATIONS

ASSESSMENT

- Assess patient's nutritional status and dietary history to determine possible cause of anemia and need for patient teaching.
- Assess bowel function for constipation or diarrhea. Notify physician and use appropriate nursing measures should these occur.
- **Lab Test Considerations:** Hemoglobin, hematocrit, and reticulocyte values should be monitored prior to and every 3 wk during the first 2 mo of therapy and periodically thereafter. Serum ferritin and iron levels may also be monitored to assess effectiveness of therapy.
- Occult blood in stools may be obscured by black coloration of iron in stool. Guaiac test results may occasionally be false-positive. Benzidine test results are not affected by iron preparations.
- **Toxicity and Overdose:** Early symptoms of overdose include stomach pain, fever, nausea, vomiting (may contain blood), and diarrhea. Late symptoms include bluish lips, fingernails, and palms; drowsiness; weakness; tachycardia; seizures; metabolic acidosis; hepatic injury; and cardiovascular collapse. The patient may appear to recover prior to the onset of late symptoms. Therefore, hospitalization continues for 24 hr after patient becomes asymptomatic to monitor for delayed onset of shock or GI bleeding. Late complications of overdose include intestinal obstruction, pyloric stenosis, and gastric scarring.
- Treatment includes inducing emesis with syrup of ipecac. If patient is comatose or seizing, gastric lavage with sodium bicarbonate is performed. Deferoxamine is the antidote. Additional supportive treatments to maintain fluid and electrolyte balance and correction of metabolic acidosis are also indicated.

POTENTIAL NURSING DIAGNOSES

- Activity intolerance (indications).
- Knowledge deficit related to medication and dietary regimen (patient/family teaching).

IMPLEMENTATION

- **PO:** Oral preparations are most effectively absorbed if administered 1 hr before or 2 hr after meals. If gastric irritation occurs, administer with meals. Tablets and capsules should be taken with a full glass of water or juice. Do not crush or chew enteric-coated tablets and do not open capsules.
- □ Liquid preparations may stain teeth. Dilute well and administer with a straw or place drops at back of throat. Feosol elixir should be diluted in water only. Fer-in-Sol liquid or syrup may be diluted in water or fruit juice.
- □ Avoid using antacids, coffee, tea, dairy products, eggs, or whole grain breads within 1 hr before and 2 hr after administration of ferrous salts.

PATIENT/FAMILY TEACHING

- □ Encourage patient to comply with medication regimen. If a dose is missed, take as soon as remembered within 12 hr, otherwise return to regular dosing schedule. Do not double doses.
- □ Advise patient that stools may become dark green or black and that this change is harmless.
- □ Instruct patient to follow a diet high in iron (see Appendix K).
- □ Discuss with parents the risk of children overdosing on iron. Medication should be stored in the original childproof container and kept out of reach of children. Do not refer to vitamins as candy. Medical help should be sought immediately if overdose is suspected, as death may occur. Parents should have syrup of ipecac at home and call pediatrician, emergency department, or poison control center for instructions before administering.

EVALUATION

Clinical response to therapy is indicated by: ▪ Increase in hemoglobin, which may reach normal parameters after 1–2 mo of therapy. May require 3–6 mo for normalization of body iron stores.

FIBRINOLYSIN AND DESOXYRIBONUCLEASE
(fye-brin-oh-**lye**-sin/dez-ox-ee-rye-boe-**nuke**-lee-ase)
Elase

CLASSIFICATION(S):
Topical (enzyme)
Pregnancy Category UK

INDICATIONS

- ▪ Used as a topical debriding agent in the management of surgical wounds and other lesions including: □ Burns □ Ulcers ▪ Vaginitis □ Cervicitis ▪ As a debriding irrigant in: □ Infected wounds □ Sinus tracts □ Fistulae □ Lesions (with concurrent systemic anti-infective therapy).

ACTION

- ▪ Fibrinolysin breaks down fibrin in clots and fibrinous exudates ▪ Desoxyribonuclease degrades proteins present in devitalized tissues found in areas of purulent exudate. **Therapeutic Effect:** ▪ Removal of necrotic material (fibrin, purulent exudates), which may result in improved healing and response to other treatment modalities.

PHARMACOKINETICS

Absorption: Negligible systemic absorption.
Distribution: Distribution not known.
Metabolism and Excretion: Metabolism and excretion not known.
Half-life: UK (no activity left after 24 hr).

CONTRAINDICATIONS AND PRECAUTIONS

Contraindicated in: ▪ Hypersensitivity ▪ Hypersensitivity to bovine products or mercury compounds (contains thimerisol).
Use Cautiously in: ▪ Presence of infection (systemic anti-infectives may be required).

F

ADVERSE REACTIONS AND SIDE EFFECTS*

Local: hyperemia (large doses only).
Misc: hypersensitivity reactions, including ANAPHYLAXIS.

INTERACTIONS

Drug–Drug: ▪ None significant.

ROUTE AND DOSAGE

▪ **Top (Adults and Children):** Pack wound with gauze strips soaked in freshly prepared solution (wet to dry method) q 6–8 hr for 2–4 days or instill and irrigate with solution q 6–10 hr.
▪ **Vag (Adults):** 5 ml of ointment deep into vagina at bedtime nightly for 5 nights or instill 10 ml of solution into vagina, wait 2–3 min, and insert cotton tampon; follow next day with instillation of ointment.

AVAILABILITY

▪ **Powder:** 25 units fibrinolysin and 15,000 units desoxyribonuclease/vial in 30-ml vials ▪ **Oint:** 1 unit fibrinolysin and 666.6 units desoxyribonuclease/g in 10- and 30-g tubes ▪ **In combination with:** chloramphenicol (Elase-Chloromycetin). See Appendix A.

TIME/ACTION PROFILE (formation of granulation tissue)

	ONSET	PEAK	DURATION
Top	2–4 days	UK	UK

NURSING IMPLICATIONS

ASSESSMENT

▪ **General Info:** Assess wound dimensions, depth, exudate, and tissue characteristics prior to and periodically throughout course of therapy.
▫ Monitor skin surrounding wound. Notify physician if severe irritation and inflammation occur.
▫ Assess for pain associated with dressing changes. Confer with physician regarding analgesics for premedication prior to dressing changes.
▪ **Vag:** Assess for irritation, bleeding, or discharge.

POTENTIAL NURSING DIAGNOSES

▪ Tissue integrity, altered (indications).
▪ Knowledge deficit related to medication regimen (patient/family teaching).

IMPLEMENTATION

▪ **Top Oint:** Flush wound with water, saline irrigation, or hydrogen peroxide. Pat dry. Apply thin layer of ointment to wound and cover with nonadherent dressing. Change at least daily.
▪ **Top Solution:** Prepare solution by mixing 1 vial of powder with 10–50 ml of 0.9% NaCl. Solution is stable for 24 hr.
▫ Saturate gauze in solution and apply as wet to dry dressing every 6–8 hr. May be used to irrigate infected cavities or tracts (abscesses, empyemas, subcutaneous hematomas, or fistulae). Drain and replace solution every 6–10 hr to ensure enzyme activity and remove debrided tissue and exudate. Blood-tinged drainage may indicate growth of healthy tissue.
▫ In severe cases, 10 ml should be instilled vaginally by physician. Tampon is then inserted 1–2 min later and kept in place until the next day.
▪ **Vag Oint:** Administer 5 ml with applicator. Do not use tampons.

PATIENT/FAMILY TEACHING

▪ **Vag:** Instruct patient in the correct use of applicator. Patient should remain recumbent for at least 30 min after administration. May use sanitary napkin to protect clothing, but do not use tampon. Emphasize importance of follow-up appointment to evaluate effectiveness of treatment.

EVALUATION

Effectiveness of therapy can be demonstrated by: ▪ Debridement of necrotic tissue ▫ Formulation of granulation tissue ▪ Resolution of symptoms of vaginitis and cervicitis.

---

*Underlines indicate most frequent; **CAPITALS** indicate life-threatening.

FILGRASTIM

(fill-**grass**-stim)
Neupogen, G-CSF, granulocyte-colony stimulating factor

CLASSIFICATION(S):
Colony stimulating factor
Pregnancy Category C

INDICATIONS

- Prevention of febrile neutropenia and associated infection in patients who have received bone-marrow-depressing antineoplastic agents for the treatment of nonmyeloid malignancies.

ACTION

- A glycoprotein that binds to and stimulates immature neutrophils to divide and differentiate. Also activates mature neutrophils. **Therapeutic Effect:**
- Decreased incidence of infection in patients who received bone-marrow-depressing antineoplastic agents.

PHARMACOKINETICS

Absorption: Well absorbed following subcutaneous administration.
Distribution: Distribution not known.
Metabolism and Excretion: Metabolism and excretion not known.
Half-life: UK.

CONTRAINDICATIONS AND PRECAUTIONS

Contraindicated in: ▪ Hypersensitivity to E. *Coli*-derived proteins.
Use Cautiously in: ▪ Pregnancy, lactation, or children (safety not established) ▪ Malignancy with myeloid characteristics ▪ Pre-existing cardiac disease.

ADVERSE REACTIONS AND SIDE EFFECTS*

Resp: respiratory distress syndrome.
CV: hypotension, myocardial, infarction, arrhythmias.
MS: medullary bone pain.

INTERACTIONS

Drug–Drug: ▪ Simultaneous use with **antineoplastic agents** may have adverse effects on rapidly proliferating neutrophils—avoid use for 24 hr before and 24 hr following chemotherapy.

ROUTE AND DOSAGE

- **IV, SC (Adults):** 5 mcg/kg/day as a single injection daily for up to 2 wk. Dosage may be increased by 5 mcg/kg during each cycle of chemotherapy depending on blood counts.

AVAILABILITY

- *Injection:* 300 mcg/ml in 1- and 1.6-ml vials.

TIME/ACTION PROFILE

	ONSET	PEAK	DURATION
IV, SC	UK	UK	4 days*

*Return of neutrophil count to baseline.

NURSING IMPLICATIONS

ASSESSMENT

- ▫ Monitor heart rate, blood pressure, and respiratory status prior to and periodically during therapy.
- ▫ Assess bone pain throughout therapy. Pain is usually mild to moderate and controllable with nonopioid analgesics.
- ▪ **Lab Test Considerations:** Obtain a CBC and platelet count prior to chemotherapy and twice weekly during therapy to avoid leukocytosis. Monitor absolute neutrophil count (ANC). A transient rise is seen 1–2 days after initiation of therapy, but therapy should not be discontinued until ANC $>10,000/mm^3$.
- ▫ May cause transient increases in uric acid, LDH, and alkaline phosphatase concentrations.

POTENTIAL NURSING DIAGNOSES

- ▪ Infection, high risk for (indications).
- ▪ Pain (side effects).
- ▪ Knowledge deficit related to medica-

F

*Underlines indicate most frequent; **CAPITALS** indicate life-threatening.

tion regimen (patient/family teaching).

IMPLEMENTATION

▫ Administer no earlier than 24 hr following cytotoxic chemotherapy and not during the 24 hr before administration of chemotherapy.

▫ Refrigerate, do not freeze. Do not shake. May warm to room temperature for up to 6 hr prior to injection. Discard if left at room temperature for >6 hr. Vial is for 1 time use only.

▪ SC: If dose requires >1 ml of solution, may be divided into 2 injection sites.

PATIENT/FAMILY TEACHING

▪ Home Care Issues: Instruct patient on correct technique and proper disposal for home administration. Caution patient not to reuse needle, vial, or syringe. Provide patient with a puncture-proof container for needle and syringe disposal.

EVALUATION

Effectiveness of therapy can be demonstrated by: ▪ Decreased incidence of infection in patients who receive bone-marrow-depressing antineoplastic agents.

FINASTERIDE
(fin-**ass**-te-ride)
Proscar

CLASSIFICATION(S):
Androgen inhibitor
Pregnancy Category X

INDICATIONS

▪ Used in the treatment of benign prostatic hyperplasia (BPH).

ACTION

▪ Inhibits the enzyme 5a-reductase, which is responsible for converting testosterone to its potent metabolite 5a-dihydrotestosterone in prostate, liver, and skin. 5a-dihydrotestosterone is partially responsible for prostatic hyper-

plasia. **Therapeutic Effect:** Reduced prostate size with associated decrease in urinary symptoms.

PHARMACOKINETICS

Absorption: Well absorbed following oral administration (63%).

Distribution: Enters prostatic tissue and crosses the blood–brain barrier. Remainder of distribution not known.

Metabolism and Excretion: Mostly metabolized. 39% excreted in urine as metabolites. 57% excreted in feces.

Half-life: 6 hr (range 6–15 hr; slightly increased in patients >70 yr).

CONTRAINDICATIONS AND PRECAUTIONS

Contraindicated in: ▪ Hypersensitivity. Finasteride is not intended for use in children or during pregnancy or lactation.

Use Cautiously in: ▪ Patients with hepatic impairment or obstructive uropathy.

ADVERSE REACTIONS AND SIDE EFFECTS*

GU: impotence, decreased libido, decreased volume of ejaculate.

INTERACTIONS

Drug–Drug: ▪ Anticholinergics, adrenergic bronchodilators, and theophylline may decrease the beneficial effects of finasteride.

ROUTE AND DOSAGE

▪ PO (Adult Males): 5 mg once daily.

AVAILABILITY

▪ *Tablets:* 5 mg.

TIME/ACTION PROFILE (reduction in dihydrotestosterone levels)

	ONSET	PEAK	DURATION
PO	Rapid	8 hr	2 wk

NURSING IMPLICATIONS

ASSESSMENT

▫ Assess patient for symptoms of prostatic hypertrophy (urinary hesitancy, feeling of incomplete bladder empty-

---

*Underlines indicate most frequent; **CAPITALS** indicate life-threatening.

ing, interruption of urinary stream, impairment of size and force of urinary stream, terminal urinary dribbling, straining to start flow, dysuria, urgency) prior to and periodically throughout therapy.

□ Digital rectal examinations should be performed prior to and periodically throughout therapy.

■ **Lab Test Considerations:** Serum prostate specific antigen (PSA) concentrations, which are used to screen for prostate cancer, may be evaluated prior to and periodically throughout therapy. Finasteride may cause a decrease in serum PSA levels.

POTENTIAL NURSING DIAGNOSES
■ Urinary elimination, altered (indications).
■ Knowledge deficit related to medication regimen (patient/family teaching).

IMPLEMENTATION
■ **PO:** Administer once daily with or without meals.

PATIENT/FAMILY TEACHING
□ Instruct patient to take finasteride as directed, even if symptoms improve or are unchanged. At least 6–12 mo of therapy may be necessary to determine whether or not an individual will respond to finasteride.
□ Inform patient that the volume of ejaculate may be decreased during therapy, but that this will not interfere with normal sexual function.
□ Caution patient that finasteride poses a potential risk to a male fetus. Women who are pregnant or may become pregnant should avoid exposure to semen of a partner taking finasteride and should not handle crushed finasteride because of the potential for absorption.
□ Emphasize the importance of periodic follow-up examinations to determine whether a clinical response has occurred.

EVALUATION
Clinical response to therapy can be determined by: ■ Decrease in urinary symptoms of benign prostatic hypertrophy.

FLECAINIDE
(flek-a-nide)
Tambocor

CLASSIFICATION(S):
Antiarrhythmic (group IC)
Pregnancy Category C

INDICATIONS
■ Treatment of life-threatening ventricular arrhythmias, including ventricular tachycardia ■ Treatment of supraventricular tachyarrhythmias.

ACTION
■ Slows conduction in cardiac tissue by altering transport of ions across cell membranes. **Therapeutic Effect:** ■ Suppression of arrhythmias.

PHARMACOKINETICS
Absorption: Well absorbed from the GI tract following oral administration.
Distribution: Widely distributed.
Metabolism and Excretion: Mostly metabolized by the liver. 30% excreted unchanged by the kidneys.
Half-life: 11–14 hr.

CONTRAINDICATIONS AND PRECAUTIONS
Contraindicated in: ■ Hypersensitivity ■ Cardiogenic shock.
Use Cautiously in: ■ Congestive heart failure (dosage reduction may be required) ■ Pre-existing sinus node dysfunction or 2nd- or 3rd-degree heart block (without a pacemaker) ■ Renal impairment (dosage reduction required if creatinine clearance <35 ml/min) ■ Pregnancy, lactation, or children (safety not established).

ADVERSE REACTIONS AND SIDE EFFECTS*
CNS: dizziness, nervousness, headache, fatigue, tremor.
EENT: blurred vision, visual disturbances, diplopia.

*Underlines indicate most frequent, CAPITALS indicate life-threatening.

Resp: dyspnea, bronchospasm.
CV: ARRHYTHMIAS, congestive heart failure, palpitations, chest pain, edema, ECG changes.
GI: <u>nausea</u>, dyspepsia, vomiting, anorexia.
GU: impotence, urinary retention, polyuria.
Derm: rashes, increased sweating.
MS: myalgia, arthralgia.
Neuro: perioral numbness and paresthesia.
Misc: malaise, fever, swelling of tongue and lips.

INTERACTIONS

Drug–Drug: ▪ Additive cardiac effects with other **antiarrhythmics**, including **calcium channel blockers** ▪ **Disopyramide** or **verapamil** may have additive myocardial depressant effects; combination use should be undertaken cautiously ▪ Increases serum **digoxin** levels by a small amount (15–25%) ▪ Concurrent **beta-adrenergic blocker** therapy may result in increased levels of beta-adrenergic blocker and flecainide ▪ **Alkalinizing agents** promote reabsorption, increase blood levels, and may cause toxicity ▪ **Acidifying agents** increase renal elimination and may decrease effectiveness of flecainide (if urine pH <5) ▪ **Amiodarone** increases flecainide levels and may result in toxicity (flecainide dosage reduction recommended).
Drug–Food: ▪ **Foods that increase urine pH** to >7 result in increased blood levels (strict **vegetarian diet**). ▪ **Foods or beverages that decrease urine pH** to <5 increase renal elimination and may decrease effectiveness of flecainide (**acidic juices**).

ROUTE AND DOSAGE

▪ **PO (Adults):** 50–100 mg q 12 hr initially, increased by 50 mg bid until response is obtained or maximum total daily dose of 400 mg is reached. Some patients may require q 8 hr dosing.

AVAILABILITY

▪ *Tablets:* 50 mg, 100 mg, 150 mg.

TIME/ACTION PROFILE (antiarrhythmic effects)

	ONSET	PEAK	DURATION
PO	days	days–wks	12 hr

NURSING IMPLICATIONS

ASSESSMENT

▫ Monitor ECG or Holter monitor prior to and periodically throughout therapy. May cause QRS widening, PR prolongation, and QT prolongation.
▫ Monitor blood pressure and pulse periodically throughout course of therapy.
▫ Monitor intake and output ratios and daily weight. Assess patient for signs of congestive heart failure (peripheral edema, rales/crackles, dyspnea, weight gain, jugular venous distension).
▪ **Lab Test Considerations:** Renal, pulmonary, and hepatic functions and CBC should be evaluated periodically on patients receiving long-term therapy.
▫ May cause elevations in serum alkaline phosphatase during prolonged therapy.
▪ **Toxicity and Overdose:** Therapeutic blood levels range from 0.2 to 1.0 mcg/ml.

POTENTIAL NURSING DIAGNOSES

▪ Cardiac output, decreased (indications).
▪ Knowledge deficit related to medication regimen (patient/family teaching).

IMPLEMENTATION

▪ **General Info:** Previous antiarrhythmic therapy (except lidocaine) should be withdrawn 2–4 half-lives before starting flecainide.
▫ Dosage adjustments should be at least 4 days apart due to the long half-life of flecainide.
▪ **PO:** May be administered with meals if GI irritation becomes a problem.

PATIENT/FAMILY TEACHING

▫ Instruct patient to take medication around the clock exactly as directed, even if feeling better. Missed doses should be taken as soon as remembered if within 6 hr; omit if remembered later. Gradual dosage reduction may be necessary.

□ Medication may cause dizziness or visual disturbances. Caution patient to avoid driving and other activities requiring alertness until response to medication is known.

□ Advise patient to notify physician or dentist of medication regimen prior to treatment or surgery.

□ Instruct patient to notify physician if chest pain, shortness of breath, or diaphoresis occurs.

□ Advise patient to carry identification describing disease process and medication regimen at all times.

□ Emphasize the importance of follow-up examinations to monitor progress.

EVALUATION
Effectiveness of therapy can be demonstrated by: ▪ Decrease in frequency of life-threatening ventricular arrhythmias ▪ Decrease in supraventricular tachyarrhythmias.

FLOXURIDINE
(flox-**yoor**-i-deen)
FUDR

CLASSIFICATION(S):
Antineoplastic (antimetabolite)
Pregnancy Category D

INDICATIONS
▪ Treatment of hepatic and gastrointestinal carcinoma. **Unlabeled Uses:** ▪ Carcinoma of: □ Breast □ Ovary □ Cervix □ Bladder □ Kidney.

ACTION
▪ Inhibits DNA and RNA synthesis by preventing thymidine production (cell cycle-S phase specific). **Therapeutic Effect:** ▪ Death of rapidly replicating cells, particularly malignant ones.

PHARMACOKINETICS
Absorption: Administered intra-arterially only, resulting in direct delivery to tumor sites. Rapidly converted to floxuridine monophosphate (an active metabolite) and fluorouracil.
Distribution: Distributes mostly to tumor site as a result of elective intra-arterial administration.
Metabolism and Excretion: Fluorouracil undergoes cellular inactivation and metabolism by the liver. 60–80% excreted by the lungs as respiratory CO_2. Small amounts of fluorouracil (<10–15%) excreted unchanged by the kidneys.
Half-life: Fluorouracil—20 hr.

CONTRAINDICATIONS AND PRECAUTIONS
Contraindicated in: ▪ Hypersensitivity ▪ Pregnancy or lactation.
Use Cautiously in: ▪ Patients with childbearing potential ▪ Infections ▪ Depressed bone marrow reserve ▪ Other chronic debilitating illnesses.

ADVERSE REACTIONS AND SIDE EFFECTS*
CNS: acute cerebellar dysfunction.
GI: nausea, vomiting, stomatitis, diarrhea.
Derm: alopecia, maculopapular rash, nail loss, melanosis of nails, phototoxicity.
Endo: gonadal suppression.
Hemat: anemia, leukopenia, thrombocytopenia.
Misc: fever.

INTERACTIONS
Drug–Drug: ▪ Additive bone marrow depression with other **bone marrow depressants** (other **antineoplastics** and **radiation therapy**) ▪ May decrease antibody response to **live virus vaccines** and increase risk of adverse reactions.

ROUTE AND DOSAGE
▪ **Intra-Arterial (Adults):** 100–600 mcg/kg/day as a continuous infusion

for 14–21 days, followed by a 2-wk rest.

AVAILABILITY

▪ *Injection:* 500 mg in 5- or 10-mg vials.

TIME/ACTION PROFILE (effects on blood counts)

	ONSET	PEAK	DURATION
Intra-arterial	1–9 days	9–21 days	30 days

NURSING IMPLICATIONS

ASSESSMENT

☐ Monitor vital signs prior to and frequently during therapy.

☐ Assess mucous membranes, number and consistency of stools, and frequency of vomiting. Assess for fever, chills, sore throat, and signs of infection. Assess for bleeding (bleeding gums, bruising, petechiae; guaiac stools, urine, and emesis). Avoid IM injections and rectal temperatures. Apply pressure to venipuncture sites for 10 min. Notify physician if symptoms of toxicity (stomatitis or esophagopharyngitis, uncontrollable vomiting, diarrhea, GI bleeding, leukocyte count <3500/mm³, platelet count <100,000/mm³, hemorrhage from any site, or erythema at catheter insertion site) occur, as drug will need to be discontinued.

☐ Monitor intake and output, appetite, and nutritional intake. Adjusting diet as tolerated may help maintain fluid and electrolyte balance and nutritional status.

☐ Assess for abdominal pain, cramping, anorexia, or jaundice with hepatic artery infusion. These symptoms may indicate hepatotoxicity. Heartburn or black tarry stools may indicate dislodgement of catheter.

☐ Monitor site of intra-arterial infusion for bleeding, localized skin reaction, or impaired circulation, which may indicate catheter displacement.

▪ **Lab Test Considerations:** Hepatic, renal, and hematologic functions should be monitored prior to and periodically throughout therapy. Notify physician immediately if WBC <3500/mm³ or platelets <100,000/mm³. These are criteria for discontinuation of the medication. Increased serum alkaline phosphatase, AST (SGOT), ALT (SGPT), LDH, and bilirubin may indicate drug-induced hepatotoxicity or biliary sclerosis.

☐ Interferes with BSP, prothrombin, and sedimentation rate assays.

POTENTIAL NURSING DIAGNOSES

▪ Infection, high risk for (side effects).

▪ Nutrition, altered: less than body requirements (side effects).

▪ Knowledge deficit related to medication regimen (patient/family teaching).

IMPLEMENTATION

▪ **General Info:** Solution should be prepared in a biologic cabinet. Wear gloves, gown, and mask while handling medication. Discard equipment in specially designated containers (see Appendix I).

▪ **Intra-arterial Infusion Pump:** Reconstitute 5-ml vial with 5 ml of Sterile Water for Injection, to yield a concentration of 100 mg/ml. Further dilute in D5W or 0.9% NaCl to volume required by arterial infusion pump. Stable for 2 wk if refrigerated.

▪ **Y-Site Compatibility:** ▪ fludarabine ▪ ondansetron ▪ sargramostim.

▪ **Additive Compatibility:** ▪ carboplatin ▪ cisplatin ▪ etoposide ▪ fluorouracil ▪ heparin ▪ leucovorin.

PATIENT/FAMILY TEACHING

☐ Instruct patient to notify physician if fever, chills, sore throat, signs of infection, bleeding gums, bruising, petechiae, blood in urine or stool, jaundice, abdominal pain, local irritation at the site of arterial cannulization, or emesis occurs. Caution patient to avoid crowds and persons with known infections. Instruct patient to use soft toothbrush and electric razor. Patient should be cautioned not to drink alcoholic beverages or take products containing aspirin or ibuprofen.

- Advise patient to rinse mouth with clear water after eating and drinking and to avoid flossing to minimize stomatitis. Physician may order viscous lidocaine if mouth pain interferes with eating.
- Discuss with patient the possibility of hair loss. Explore methods of coping.
- Caution patient to use sunscreen and protective clothing to prevent phototoxicity reactions.
- Instruct patient not to receive any vaccinations without advice of physician.
- Emphasize the importance of routine follow-up lab tests to monitor progress and to check for side effects.
- Review with patient the need for contraception during therapy.

EVALUATION
Effectiveness of therapy can be demonstrated by: ■ Tumor size regression.

FLUCONAZOLE
(floo-**kon**-a-zole)
Diflucan

CLASSIFICATION(S):
Antifungal
Pregnancy Category C

INDICATIONS

■ Treatment of fungal infections due to susceptible organisms, including: □ Oropharyngeal or esophageal candidiasis □ Serious systemic candidal infections □ Urinary tract infections □ Peritonitis □ Cryptococcal meningitis.

ACTION

■ Inhibits synthesis of fungal sterols, a necessary component of the cell wall. **Therapeutic Effects:** ■ Fungistatic action against susceptible organisms ■ May be fungicidal in higher concentrations. **Spectrum:** ■ *Cryptococcus* neoforms ■ *Candida* sp.

PHARMACOKINETICS

Absorption: Well absorbed following oral administration.

Distribution: Widely distributed, good penetration into cerebrospinal fluid, eye, and peritoneum.
Metabolism and Excretion: >80% excreted unchanged by the kidneys. <10% metabolized by the liver.
Half-life: 30 hr (increased in renal impairment).

CONTRAINDICATIONS AND PRECAUTIONS

Contraindicated in: ■ Hypersensitivity to fluconazole or other azole antifungals.
Use Cautiously in: ■ Renal impairment (dosage reduction required if creatinine clearance <50 ml/min) ■ Underlying liver disease ■ Pregnancy, lactation, or children (safety not established).

ADVERSE REACTIONS AND SIDE EFFECTS*

Incidence of adverse reactions is increased in AIDS patients.
CNS: headache.
GI: nausea, vomiting, abdominal discomfort, diarrhea, HEPATOTOXICITY.
Derm: exfoliative skin disorders including STEVENS-JOHNSON SYNDROME.

INTERACTIONS

Drug–Drug: ■ Increases the activity of **warfarin** ■ **Rifampin** decreases blood levels ■ Increases the hypoglycemic effects of **tolbutamide, glyburide,** or **glipizide** ■ Increases blood levels of **cyclosporine** and **phenytoin.**

ROUTE AND DOSAGE

■ **PO, IV (Adults):** 100–400 mg/day.

AVAILABILITY

■ *Tablets:* 50 mg, 100 mg, 200 mg ■ *Injection:* 200 mg, 400 mg.

TIME/ACTION PROFILE (blood levels)

	ONSET	PEAK
PO	UK	1–2 hr
IV	rapid	end of infusion

F

NURSING IMPLICATIONS

ASSESSMENT

□ Assess infected area and monitor cerebrospinal fluid cultures prior to and periodically throughout therapy.

□ Specimens for culture should be taken prior to instituting therapy. Therapy may be started before results are obtained.

■ **Lab Test Considerations:** BUN and serum creatinine should be monitored prior to and periodically during therapy as patients with renal dysfunction will require dosage adjustment.

□ Liver function tests should be monitored prior to and periodically throughout course of therapy. May cause increased AST (SGOT), ALT (SGPT), serum alkaline phosphate, and bilirubin concentrations.

POTENTIAL NURSING DIAGNOSES

■ Infection, high risk for (indications).

■ Knowledge deficit related to medication regimen (patient/family teaching).

IMPLEMENTATION

■ **General Info:** Since bioavailability is similar, oral and IV doses are equal.

■ **Intermittent Infusion:** Open overwrap immediately before infusion. Inner bag may have slight opacity that will diminish gradually. Do not administer solution that is cloudy or has a precipitate. Check for leaks by squeezing inner bag. If found, discard container as unsterile.

□ Do not set tubing as part of a series of connections as this may cause air embolism.

■ *Rate:* Infuse at a maximum rate of 200 mg/hr.

■ **Y-Site Compatibility:** ■ acyclovir ■ amikacin ■ aminophylline ■ ampicillin/sulbactam ■ aztreonam ■ benztropine ■ cefazolin ■ cefotetan ■ cefoxitin ■ chlorpromazine ■ cimetidine ■ dexamethasone sodium phosphate ■ diphenhydramine ■ droperidol ■ famotidine ■ fludarabine ■ foscarnet ■ ganciclovir ■ gentamicin ■ heparin ■ hydrocortisone ■ immune globulin ■ leucovorin ■ meperidine ■ metoclopramide ■ metronidazole ■ midazolam ■ morphine ■ nafcillin ■ ondansetron ■ oxacillin ■ penicillin G potassium ■ phenytoin ■ prochlorperazine ■ promethazine ■ sargramostim ■ ticarcillin/clavulanate ■ tobramycin ■ vancomycin ■ zidovudine.

■ **Y-Site Incompatibility:** ■ amphotericin B ■ ampicillin ■ calcium gluconate ■ cefotaxime ■ ceftriaxone ■ ceftazidime ■ cefuroxime ■ chloramphenicol ■ clindamycin ■ diazepam ■ digoxin ■ erythromycin lactobionate ■ furosemide ■ haloperidol ■ hydroxyzine ■ imipenem/cilastatin ■ pentamidine ■ ticarcillin ■ trimethoprim/sulfamethoxazole.

■ **Additive Incompatibility:** Manufacturer does not recommend admixing.

PATIENT/FAMILY TEACHING

□ Instruct patient to take medication exactly as directed, even if feeling better. Doses should be taken at the same time each day. If a dose is missed, take as soon as remembered, but not if almost time for next dose. Do not double doses.

□ Instruct patient to notify physician if abdominal pain, fever, or diarrhea become pronounced or if signs and symptoms of liver dysfunction (unusual fatigue, anorexia, nausea, vomiting, jaundice, dark urine, or pale stools) occur.

EVALUATION

Effectiveness of therapy can be demonstrated by: ■ Resolution of clinical and laboratory indications of fungal infections. Full course of therapy may require weeks or months of treatment following resolution of symptoms.

FLUCYTOSINE
(floo-**sye**-toe-seen)
Ancobon, {Ancotil}, 5-FC

INDICATIONS

- Used in the treatment of serious fungal infections including: □ Endocarditis □ Meningitis □ Septicemia □ Urinary tract infections □ Pulmonary infections.

ACTION

- Following penetration into fungi, converted to fluorouracil, which interferes with fungal DNA and RNA synthesis
- Synergistic action with amphotericin B against some fungi. **Therapeutic Effect:** - Fungicidal action against susceptible organisms. **Spectrum:** - Active against only a small number of fungi, mainly □ Candida □ Cryptococcus.

PHARMACOKINETICS

Absorption: Well absorbed from the GI tract following oral administration.
Distribution: Widely distributed. Crosses the blood–brain barrier. Crosses the placenta.
Metabolism and Excretion: 80–90% excreted unchanged by the kidneys.
Half-life: 2.5–8 hr (increased in renal impairment).

CONTRAINDICATIONS AND PRECAUTIONS

Contraindicated in: - Hypersensitivity - Pregnancy or lactation.
Use Cautiously in: - Renal impairment (blood level monitoring and increased dosage interval recommended if creatinine clearance <40 ml/min) - Bone marrow depression (especially following radiation therapy or antineoplastic drugs).

ADVERSE REACTIONS AND SIDE EFFECTS*

CNS: dizziness, lightheadedness, drowsiness, confusion.
GI: nausea, vomiting, diarrhea, bloating.

Hemat: leukopenia, anemia, pancytopenia, thrombocytopenia.

INTERACTIONS

Drug–Drug: - Additive bone marrow depression with other bone marrow depressant drugs, including **antineoplastic agents** and **radiation therapy** - **Amphotericin B** may increase toxicity of flucytosine but may also increase antifungal activity - **Cytarabine** may decrease antifungal activity.

ROUTE AND DOSAGE

- **PO (Adults):** 12.5–37.5 mg/kg q 6 hr.
- **PO (Children):** 12.5–37.5 mg/kg q 6 hr or 375–562.5 mg/m² q 6 hr.

AVAILABILITY

- *Capsules:* 250 mg, 500 mg.

TIME/ACTION PROFILE (antifungal blood levels)

	ONSET	PEAK
PO	rapid	4–6 hr

F

NURSING IMPLICATIONS

ASSESSMENT

- □ Assess patient for signs and symptoms of systemic fungal infection prior to and periodically throughout therapy.
- □ Obtain specimens for culture prior to initiating therapy. First dose may be given before receiving results.
- **Lab Test Considerations:** Renal, hepatic, and hematologic functions should be monitored prior to and periodically throughout course of therapy.

POTENTIAL NURSING DIAGNOSES

- Infection, high risk for (indications).
- Fluid volume deficit, potential (adverse reactions).
- Knowledge deficit related to medication regimen (patient/family teaching).

IMPLEMENTATION

- **General Info:** The number 5 in 5-

*Underlines indicate most frequent; **CAPITALS** indicate life-threatening.

flourouracil is part of the drug name and not the dose.

- **PO:** To reduce nausea and vomiting, administer capsules a few at a time over 15 min.

PATIENT/FAMILY TEACHING

☐ Advise patient to take medication exactly as directed, even if feeling better. Missed doses should be taken as soon as remembered, if not almost time for next dose; do not double doses.

☐ May cause dizziness, lightheadedness, or drowsiness. Caution patient to avoid driving and other activities requiring alertness until response to medication is known.

☐ Instruct patient to notify physician promptly if rash, fever, sore throat, diarrhea, unusual bleeding or bruising, unusual tiredness, or weakness occur.

☐ Emphasize the importance of follow-up examinations to determine effectiveness of treatment.

EVALUATION

Effectiveness of therapy can be demonstrated by: ■ Resolution of the signs and symptoms of fungal infection. Duration of therapy is generally 4–6 wk but may continue for several months.

FLUDARABINE
(floo-**dar**-a-been)
Fludara

CLASSIFICATION(S):
Antineoplastic (antimetabolite)
Pregnancy Category D

INDICATIONS

■ Treatment of B-cell chronic lymphocytic leukemia unresponsive to standard therapy ■ Treatment of non-Hodgkin's lymphoma.

ACTION

■ Converted intracellularly to an active phosphorylated metabolite that inhibits DNA synthesis. **Therapeutic Effect:** ■ Death of rapidly replicating cells, particularly malignant ones.

PHARMACOKINETICS

Absorption: Administered IV only, resulting in complete bioavailability.
Distribution: Distribution not known.
Metabolism and Excretion: Following administration, rapidly converted to an active metabolite, which when phosphorylated intracellularly exerts antineoplastic activity. 23% of initial active metabolite excreted unchanged by the kidneys.
Half-life: 10 hr (for initial active metabolite).

CONTRAINDICATIONS AND PRECAUTIONS

Contraindicated in: ■ Hypersensitivity to fludarabine, mannitol, or sodium hydroxide ■ Pregnancy or lactation.
Use Cautiously in: ■ Renal impairment (dosage reduction may be necessary) ■ Patients with childbearing potential ■ Bone marrow depression ■ Chronic debilitating illness ■ Children (safety not established).

ADVERSE REACTIONS AND SIDE EFFECTS*

CNS: NEUROTOXICITY, malaise, <u>fatigue</u>, <u>weakness</u>, agitation, confusion, visual disturbances, coma.
Resp: pulmonary hypersensitivity, cough, dyspnea.
CV: <u>edema</u>.
GI: <u>nausea</u>, <u>vomiting</u>, anorexia, <u>diarrhea</u>, GI bleeding, stomatitis.
Derm: rashes.
Endo: gonadal suppression.
Hemat: <u>anemia</u>, <u>leukopenia</u>, <u>thrombocytopenia</u>.
MS: <u>myalgia</u>.
Neuro: peripheral neuropathy.
Misc: tumor lysis syndrome.

INTERACTIONS

Drug–Drug: ■ Additive bone marrow suppression with other **antineoplastic agents** or **radiation therapy** ■ May de-

*Underlines indicate most frequent; CAPITALS indicate life-threatening.

crease antibody response to **live virus vaccines** and increase the risk of adverse reactions.

ROUTE AND DOSAGE

- **IV (Adults):** 25 mg/m^2 daily for 5 days, repeat course every 28 days.

AVAILABILITY

- *Injection:* 50 mg/vial.

TIME/ACTION PROFILE (effects on blood counts)

	ONSET	PEAK	DURATION
IV	UK	13–16 days	UK

NURSING IMPLICATIONS

ASSESSMENT

- Assess patient for visual changes, weakness, confusion, and changes in level of consciousness throughout and for 60 days following therapy, as neurologic effects resulting in blindness, coma, and death have been reported.
- Assess for fever, sore throat, and signs of infection. If these symptoms occur, notify physician immediately.
- Assess for bleeding (bleeding gums, bruising, petechiae, guaiac stools, urine, emesis). Avoid IM injections and rectal temperatures. Hold pressure on all venipuncture sites for at least 10 min.
- Monitor respiratory status, intake and output ratios, and daily weights. Notify physician if significant changes occur.
- Assess nutritional status. Administering an antiemetic prior to and periodically throughout therapy and adjusting diet as tolerated may help maintain fluid and electrolyte balance and nutritional status.
- Anemia may occur. Monitor for increased fatigue, dyspnea, and orthostatic hypotension.
- May cause tumor lysis syndrome resulting in hyperuricemia, hyperphosphatemia, hypocalcemia, metabolic acidosis, hyperkalemia, hematuria, urate crystalluria, and renal failure. Monitor for flank pain and hematuria.
- **Lab Test Considerations:** Monitor CBC, differential, and platelet counts prior to and frequently throughout therapy. The nadir for granulocytes occurs in 13 days (range 3–25 days) and for platelets in 16 days (range 2–32 days) after administration.

POTENTIAL NURSING DIAGNOSES

- Infection, high risk for (adverse reactions).
- Injury, high risk for (side effects).
- Knowledge deficit related to medication regimen (patient/family teaching).

IMPLEMENTATION

- **General Info:** Solution should be prepared in a biologic cabinet. Wear gloves, gown, and mask while handling IV medication. Discard IV equipment in specially designated containers (see Appendix I).
- **IV:** Reconstitute with 2 ml of Sterile Water for Injection; solid cake should dissolve in <15 sec. Reconstituted solution is stable for 8 hr.
- **Intermittent Infusion:** Dilute further in 100–125 ml of 0.9% NaCl or D5W.
- *Rate:* Infuse over 30 min.
- **Y-Site Compatibility:** ■ amikacin ■ aminophylline ■ ampicillin ■ ampicillin/sulbactam ■ aztreonam ■ bleomycin ■ butorphanol ■ carboplatin ■ carmustine ■ cefazolin ■ cefoperazone ■ ceforanide ■ cefotaxime ■ cefotetan ■ ceftazidime ■ ceftizoxime ■ ceftriaxone ■ cefuroxime ■ cimetidine ■ cisplatin ■ clindamycin ■ cyclophosphamide ■ cytarabine ■ dacarbazine ■ dactinomycin ■ dexamethasone sodium phosphate ■ diphenhydramine ■ doxorubicin ■ doxycycline ■ droperidol ■ etoposide ■ famotidine ■ floxuridine ■ fluconazole ■ fluorouracil ■ furosemide ■ gentamicin ■ haloperidol ■ heparin ■ hydrocortisone ■ hydromorphone ■ ifosfamide ■ imipenem/cilastatin ■ lorazepam ■ magnesium sulfate ■ mannitol ■ mechlorethamine ■ meperidine ■ mesna ■ methotrexate ■ methylprednisolone sodium succi-

F

nate ▪ metoclopramide ▪ mezlocillin ▪ minocycline ▪ mitoxantrone ▪ morphine ▪ multivitamins ▪ nalbuphine ▪ netilmicin ▪ ondansetron ▪ pentostatin ▪ potassium chloride ▪ promethazine ▪ ranitidine ▪ sodium bicarbonate ▪ ticarcillin ▪ ticarcillin/clavulanate ▪ tobramycin ▪ trimethoprim/sulfamethoxazole ▪ vanomycin ▪ vinblastine ▪ vincristine ▪ zidovudine.

▪ **Y-Site Incompatibility:** ▪ acyclovir ▪ amphotericin B ▪ chlorpromazine ▪ daunorubicin ▪ ganciclovir ▪ hydroxyzine ▪ miconazole ▪ prochlorperazine.

PATIENT/FAMILY TEACHING

☐ Caution patient to avoid crowds and persons with known infections. Physician should be informed immediately if symptoms of infection occur.

☐ Instruct patient to report unusual bleeding. Advise patient of thrombocytopenia precautions (use soft toothbrush, electric razor, and avoid falls.) Do not drink alcoholic beverages or take medication containing aspirin or ibuprofen, as these may precipitate gastric bleeding.

☐ Instruct patient to inspect oral mucosa for redness and ulceration. If mouth sores occur, advise patient to use sponge brush and rinse mouth with water after eating and drinking. Consult physician if pain interferes with eating.

☐ Advise patient that this medication may have teratogenic effects. Contraception should be used during therapy and for at least 4 mo after therapy is concluded.

☐ Instruct patient not to receive any vaccinations without advice of physician.

☐ Emphasize the need for periodic lab tests to monitor for side effects.

EVALUATION

Effectiveness of therapy can be demonstrated by: ▪ Improvement of hematopoietic values in leukemias ▪ Decrease in size and spread of the tumor in non-Hodgkin's lymphomas. The 5-day course of therapy is continued every 28 days until patient is in complete remission, or neurotoxicity occurs.

FLUDROCORTISONE
(floo-droe-**kor**-ti-sone)
Florinef

CLASSIFICATION(S):
Mineralocorticoid
Pregnancy Category C

INDICATIONS

▪ Management of sodium loss and hypotension associated with adrenocortical insufficiency in conjunction with hydrocortisone or cortisone ▪ Management of sodium loss due to congenital adrenogenital syndrome (congenital adrenal hyperplasia).

ACTION

▪ Causes sodium reabsorption, hydrogen and potassium excretion, and water retention by its effects on the distal renal tubule. **Therapeutic Effects:** ▪ Maintenance of sodium balance and blood pressure in patients with adrenocortical insufficiency.

PHARMACOKINETICS

Absorption: Well absorbed following oral administration.
Distribution: Appears to be widely distributed; probably enters breast milk.
Metabolism and Excretion: Mostly metabolized by the liver.
Half-life: 3.5 hr.

CONTRAINDICATIONS AND PRECAUTIONS

Contraindicated in: ▪ Hypersensitivity.
Use Cautiously in: ▪ Congestive heart failure ▪ Addison's disease (patients may have exaggerated response) ▪ Pregnancy, lactation, or children (safety not established).

ADVERSE REACTIONS AND SIDE EFFECTS*

CNS: headaches, dizziness.
CV: edema, congestive heart failure, hypertension, arrhythmias.
GI: nausea, anorexia.
Endo: weight gain, adrenal suppression.
F and E: hypokalemia, hypokalemic alkalosis.
MS: arthralgia, tendon contractures, muscular weakness.
Neuro: ascending paralysis.
Misc: hypersensitivity reactions.

INTERACTIONS

Drug–Drug: ▪ Use with **diuretics, mezlocillin, piperacillin,** or **amphotericin B** may result in exaggerated hypokalemia ▪ Hypokalemia may increase the risk of **cardiac glycoside** toxicity ▪ May produce prolonged neuromuscular blockade following the use of **nondepolarizing neuromuscular blocking agents** ▪ **Phenobarbital** or **rifampin** may increase the metabolism and may decrease the effectiveness of fludrocortisone.

Drug–Food: ▪ Ingestion of large amounts of **salt** or **sodium-containing foods** may cause excessive sodium retention and potassium loss.

ROUTE AND DOSAGE

▪ **PO (Adults):** 100 mcg/day (range 100 mcg 3 times weekly–200 mcg daily). Doses as small as 0.05 mg daily may be required by some patients. Use with 10–37.5 mg cortisone daily or 10–30 mg hydrocortisone daily.
▪ **PO (Children):** 50–100 mcg/day.
▪ **PO (Infants):** 0.1–0.2 mg/24 hr.

AVAILABILITY

▪ *Tablets:* 0.1 mg.

TIME/ACTION PROFILE
(mineralocorticoid activity)

	ONSET	PEAK	DURATION
PO	UK	UK	1–2 days

NURSING IMPLICATIONS

ASSESSMENT

▫ Monitor blood pressure periodically throughout course of therapy. Inform physician of significant changes. Hypotension may indicate insufficient dosage.
▫ Monitor for fluid retention (weigh daily, assess for edema, and auscultate lungs for rales/crackles).
▪ **Lab Test Considerations:** Monitor serum electrolytes periodically throughout therapy. Fludrocortisone causes decreased serum potassium levels.

POTENTIAL NURSING DIAGNOSES

▪ Fluid volume deficit (indications).
▪ Fluid volume excess (side effects).
▪ Knowledge deficit related to medication regimen (patient/family teaching).

IMPLEMENTATION

▪ **PO:** Tablets are scored and may be broken if dosage adjustment is necessary.

PATIENT/FAMILY TEACHING

▫ Instruct patient to take medication exactly as directed. If a dose is missed, take as soon as remembered but not just before next dose is due. Explain that lifelong therapy is necessary and that abrupt discontinuation may lead to Addisonian crisis. Patient should keep an adequate supply available at all times.
▫ Advise patient to follow dietary modification prescribed by physician. Instruct patient to follow a diet high in potassium (see Appendix K). Amount of sodium allowed in diet varies with pathophysiology.
▫ Instruct patient to inform physician if weight gain or edema, muscle weakness, cramps, nausea, anorexia, or dizziness occurs.
▫ Advise patient to carry identification describing disease process and medication regimen at all times.

EVALUATION

Effectiveness of therapy can be demonstrated by: ▪ Normalization of fluid and

F

electrolyte balance without the development of hypokalemia or hypertension.

FLUMAZENIL
(flu-**maz**-e-nil)
Mazicon

CLASSIFICATION(S):
Antidote (benzodiazepine antagonist)
Pregnancy Category C

INDICATIONS

- Used to completely or partially reverse the effects of benzodiazepines when they are used as general anesthetics, or during diagnostic or therapeutic procedures. Also used in the management of intentional or accidental overdose of benzodiazepines.

ACTION

- Flumazenil is a benzodiazepine derivative that antagonizes the CNS depressant effects of benzodiazepine compounds. It has no effect on CNS depression of other causes including opioid analgesics, alcohol, barbiturates, or general anesthetics. **Therapeutic Effect:** ■ Reversal of benzodiazepine effects.

PHARMACOKINETICS

Absorption: IV administration results in complete bioavailability.
Distribution: Distribution not known.
Metabolism and Excretion: Metabolism of flumazenil occurs primarily in the liver.
Half-life: 41–79 min.

CONTRAINDICATIONS AND PRECAUTIONS

Contraindicated in: ■ Hypersensitivity to flumazenil or benzodiazepines ■ Patients receiving benzodiazepines for life-threatening medical problems including status epilepticus or increased intracranial pressure should not be given flumazenil ■ Serious cyclic antidepressant overdosage should not be managed with flumazenil.
Use Cautiously in: ■ Pregnancy, lactation, or children (safety not established) ■ Mixed CNS depressant overdosage (effects of other agents may emerge when benzodiazepine effect is removed) ■ History of seizures (seizures are more likely to occur in patients who are experiencing sedative/hypnotic withdrawal, patients who have recently received repeated doses of benzodiazepines or those who have a prior history of seizure activity).

ADVERSE REACTIONS AND SIDE EFFECTS*

CNS: <u>dizziness</u>, agitation, emotional lability, headache, fatigue, SEIZURES, confusion, somnolence, sleep disorders.
EENT: Abnormal vision, blurred vision, abnormal hearing.
CV: arrhythmias, chest pain, hypertension.
GI: <u>nausea</u>, <u>vomiting</u>, hiccups.
Derm: sweating, flushing.
Local: pain at injection site, injection-site reactions, phlebitis.
Neuro: paresthesia.
Misc: rigors, shivering.

INTERACTIONS

Drug–Drug: ■ None significant.
Drug–Food: ■ Administration of food during flumazenil infusion increases the clearance and may decrease the effect of flumazenil.

ROUTE AND DOSAGE

Reversal of Consciousness Sedation or General Anesthesia
- IV (Adults): 0.2 mg. Additional doses may be given at 1-min intervals until desired results are obtained, up to a total dose of 1 mg. If resedation occurs, additional doses may be given at 20-min intervals, given no more than 1 mg at a time, not to exceed 3 mg per hour.

Suspected Benzodiazepine Overdose
- IV (Adults): 0.2 mg. A second dose of 0.3 mg may be given 30 sec later. Ad-

---

*<u>Underlines</u> indicate most frequent; **CAPITALS** indicate life-threatening.

ditional doses of 0.5 mg may be given at 1-min intervals if necessary, to a total dose of 3 mg. Usual dose required is 1–3 mg. If resedation occurs, additional doses may be given at 20-min intervals, given no more than 1 mg at a time, not to exceed 3 mg per hour.

AVAILABILITY

- **Injection:** 0.1 mg/ml in 5- and 10-mg vials.

TIME/ACTION PROFILE (reversal of benzodiazepine effects)

ONSET	PEAK	DURATION
IV	1–2 min	6–10 min	UK

NURSING IMPLICATIONS

ASSESSMENT

- **General Info:** Assess level of consciousness and respiratory status prior to and throughout therapy. Observe patient for at least 2 hr following administration for the appearance of resedation. Hypoventilation may occur.
- **Overdose:** Attempt to assess time of ingestion and amount and type of benzodiazepine taken. Knowledge of agent ingested allows an estimate of duration of CNS depression.

POTENTIAL NURSING DIAGNOSES

- Injury, high risk for (indications).
- Poisoning, high risk for (indications).

IMPLEMENTATION

- **General Info:** Assure that patient has a patent airway before administration of flumazenil.
- Observe IV site frequently for redness or irritation. Administer through a free-flowing IV infusion into a large vein to minimize pain at the injection site.
- Optimal emergence should be undertaken slowly to decrease undesirable effects including confusion, agitation, emotional lability, and perceptual distortion.
- Institute seizure precautions. Seizures are more likely to occur in patients who are experiencing seda-

tive/hypnotic withdrawal, patients who have recently received repeated doses of benzodiazepines, or those who have a prior history of seizure activity. Seizures may be treated with benzodiazepines, barbiturates, or phenytoin. Larger than normal doses of benzodiazepines may be required.

- **Overdose:** If no effects are seen following administration of flumazenil, consider other causes of decreased level of consciousness (alcohol, barbiturates, opioid analgesics).
- **Direct IV:** May be administered undiluted or diluted in syringe with D5W, 0.9% NaCl, or lactated Ringer's solution. Diluted solution should be discarded after 24 hr.
- **Rate:** Administer each dose over 15 sec.

PATIENT/FAMILY TEACHING

- Flumazenil does not consistently reverse the amnestic effects of benzodiazepines. Provide patient and family with written instructions for postprocedure care. Inform family that patient may appear alert at the time of discharge, but the sedative effects of the benzodiazepine may recur. Instruct patient to avoid driving or other activities requiring alertness for at least 24 hr after discharge.
- Instruct patient not to take any alcohol or nonprescription drugs for at least 18–24 hr after discharge.
- Resumption of usual activities should occur only when no residual effects of the benzodiazepine remain.

EVALUATION

Clinical response to therapy can be determined by: ▪ Improved level of consciousness ◻ Decrease in respiratory depression caused by benzodiazepines.

FLUNISOLIDE
(floo-**nis**-oh-lide)
AeroBid, AeroBib-M, Nasalide, {Rhinalar}

CLASSIFICATION(S):
Glucocorticoid (long-acting),
Anti-inflammatory
Pregnancy Category C

INDICATIONS

- **Inhalation:** Anti-inflammatory and immunosuppressant in the treatment of chronic steroid-dependent asthma. May decrease requirement for or avoid use of systemic glucocorticoids ▪ **Intranasal:** Used in the management of allergic rhinitis and other chronic nasal inflammatory conditions, including nasal polyps.

ACTION

- Potent, locally acting anti-inflammatory and immune modifier. **Therapeutic Effects:** ▪ Decrease in symptoms of chronic asthma and allergic rhinitis.

PHARMACOKINETICS

Absorption: Action following inhalant is mostly local. Additional drug may be swallowed, but systemic bioavailability is minimal at recommended doses. Readily absorbed following nasal inhalant.

Distribution: Distribution not known.

Metabolism and Excretion: Mostly metabolized by the liver.

Half-life: 1–2 hr.

CONTRAINDICATIONS AND PRECAUTIONS

Contraindicated in: ▪ Hypersensitivity ▪ Hypersensitivity to fluorocarbon propellants (inhaler only) ▪ Acute attacks of asthma or allergic rhinitis.

Use Cautiously in: ▪ Nasal ulcers (intranasal form) ▪ Untreated bacterial, viral, or fungal infections ▪ Chronic treatment at higher-than-recommended doses may lead to adrenal suppression ▪ Systemic glucocorticoid therapy should not be abruptly discontinued when inhalation or intranasal therapy is started ▪ Pregnancy, lactation, or children <6 yr (safety not established).

ADVERSE REACTIONS AND SIDE EFFECTS*

CNS: headache, dizziness.

EENT: Nasal—<u>nasal burning</u>, <u>nasal irritation</u>, nasal bleeding, <u>sneezing attacks</u>; Inhalation—oropharyngeal fungal infections.

Resp: Inhalation—wheezing, bronchospasm.

GI: Nasal—nausea, vomiting, abdominal bloating.

Misc: ADRENAL SUPPRESSION at greater than recommended doses.

INTERACTIONS

Drug–Drug: ▪ None significant at recommended doses.

ROUTE AND DOSAGE

- **Inhalation (Adults):** 2 inhalations bid (not to exceed 4 sprays bid).
- **Inhalation (Children 6–15 yr):** 2 inhalations bid.
- **Nasal (Adults):** 2 sprays in each nostril bid, may be increased to 3 sprays in each nostril bid (not to exceed 8 sprays in each nostril daily).
- **Nasal (Children 6–14 yr):** 1 spray in each nostril tid, or 2 sprays in each nostril bid (not to exceed 4 sprays in each nostril daily).

AVAILABILITY

- *Aerosol for inhalation:* 250 mcg/actuation in 7-g cannister (100 metered doses) ▪ *Nasal spray:* 25 mcg/actuation in 25-ml bottle (≥200 sprays/bottle).

TIME/ACTION PROFILE

	ONSET	PEAK	DURATION
Inhaln	UK	1–4 wk	UK
Nasal	2–3 days	2–3 wk	UK

NURSING IMPLICATIONS

ASSESSMENT

- **General Info:** Assess patients changing from systemic glucocorticoids to flunisolide for signs of adrenal insufficiency (anorexia, nausea, weakness, fatigue, hypotension, hypoglycemia) during initial therapy. If these signs appear, notify physician immediately. This can be life-threatening.

- **Asthma:** Assess breathing pattern and lung sounds periodically throughout therapy. Alternative therapy is indicated for relief of an acute asthmatic attack.
- **Rhinitis:** Monitor degree of nasal stuffiness, amount and color of nasal discharge, and frequency of sneezing.
- **Lab Test Considerations:** Periodic adrenal function tests may be ordered in chronic therapy to assess degree of hypothalamic-pituitary-adrenal (HPA) axis suppression.

POTENTIAL NURSING DIAGNOSES

- Airway clearance, ineffective (indications).
- Infection, high risk for (side effects).
- Knowledge deficit related to medication regimen (patient/family teaching).

IMPLEMENTATION

- **General Info:** Attempts should be made to decrease dose to lowest amount required to control symptoms.
- **Nasal Spray:** Patient also using topical decongestant should be given decongestant 5–15 min before flunisolide. Instruct patient to blow nose gently, if unable to breathe freely through nasal passages, in advance of medication administration.
- **Inhalation:** Patients also using inhalation bronchodilators should be given bronchodilator 5 min before administering flunisolide.
- ☐ Allow at least 1-2 min between inhalations of aerosol medication.

PATIENT/FAMILY TEACHING

- **General Info:** Advise patient to take medication exactly as directed. If a dose is missed, take as soon as remembered unless almost time for next dose.
- ☐ Advise patient to carry identification in the event of an emergency in which patient cannot relate medical history.

- ☐ Caution patient to avoid smoking, known allergens, and other respiratory irritants.
- **Metered-Dose Inhaler:** Caution patient not to exceed recommended dose. Maximum dosage for adults is 4 per day.
- ☐ Instruct patient in proper use of metered-dose inhaler. See Appendix H for instructions.
- ☐ Advise patient to rinse mouth and gargle with water after each dose of inhaler to minimize throat irritation and *Candida* infection.
- ☐ Explain need for continued medical follow-up to assess effectiveness and possible side effects of medication. Physician may order periodic pulmonary function tests.
- ☐ Instruct patient to inform physician if symptoms of asthma attack or oral infection occur.
- **Nasal Spray:** Caution patient not to exceed maximal daily dose of 8 sprays per nostril for adults or 4 sprays for children <14 yr.
- ☐ Instruct patient in correct technique for administering nasal spray (see Appendix H). Warn patient that temporary nasal stinging may occur.
- ☐ Instruct patient to notify physician if symptoms do not improve within 1 mo or if nasal discharge becomes purulent.

EVALUATION

Effectiveness of therapy can be demonstrated by: ■ Prevention of bronchospasm in asthma ■ Resolution of nasal stuffiness, discharge, and sneezing in seasonal or perennial rhinitis.

FLUORIDE SUPPLEMENTS
(floor-ide)

oral fluoride
{Fluor-A-Day}, Fluoritab, {Fluotic}, Flura, Flura-Drops, Flura-Loz, Karidium, Luride, Pediaflor, Pedi-Dent, Pharmaflur, Phos-Flur, {Solu-Flur}

F

topical fluoride
ACT, Fluorigard, Fluorinse, Gel
Kam, Gel-Tin, Karigel, Listermint
with Fluoride, Minute-Gel, Point
Two, Stop, Thera-Flur

CLASSIFICATION(S):
Mineral supplement
Pregnancy Category UK

INDICATIONS

▪ Prevention of dental caries in children in areas where there is insufficient fluoride in drinking water.

ACTION

▪ Fluoride becomes incorporated into bone and teeth, where it serves to stabilize crystalline matrix. It promotes remineralization and may retard the growth of dental plaque. The presence of fluoride on the enamel surface of teeth promotes resistance to acid and prevents caries. **Therapeutic Effect:** ▪ Decreased incidence of dental caries in children.

PHARMACOKINETICS

Absorption: Well absorbed following oral administration.
Distribution: Stored in bone and developing teeth. Readily crosses the placenta, small amounts enter breast milk.
Metabolism and Excretion: 50% excreted unchanged by the kidneys. Small amounts excreted in feces and sweat.
Half-life: UK.

CONTRAINDICATIONS AND PRECAUTIONS

Contraindicated in: ▪ Hypersensitivity ▪ Dietary sodium restriction ▪ Where fluoride in drinking water exceeds 0.7 parts per million (ppm) ▪ Some products contain tartrazine and other additives; avoid use in patients with known intolerance ▪ Severe renal impairment.
Use Cautiously in: ▪ Situations where fluoride content of water is not known.

ADVERSE REACTIONS AND SIDE EFFECTS*

CNS: headache, weakness.
GI: gastric distress.
Derm: eczema, atopic dermatitis, urticaria.
Misc: mottling of teeth (toxicity).

INTERACTIONS

Drug–Drug: ▪ If taken concurrently with **calcium supplements,** calcium fluoride forms, and fluoride will not be absorbed. **Aluminum hydroxide** decreases absorption of fluoride.
Drug–Food: ▪ If taken concurrently with **dairy foods,** calcium fluoride forms and fluoride will not be absorbed.

ROUTE AND DOSAGE

Children <3 yr should not receive 1-mg tablets. 1-mg tablets should not be used if fluoride content of drinking water is >0.3 ppm.

Oral Fluoride—Fluoride Content of Drinking Water <0.3 ppm
▪ **PO (Children <2 yr):** 0.25 mg/day.
▪ **PO (Children 2–3 yr):** 0.5 mg/day.
▪ **PO (Children 3–12 yr):** 1 mg/day.

Oral Fluoride—Fluoride Content of Drinking Water 0.3–0.7 ppm
▪ **PO (Children <2 yr):** 0.125 mg/day.
▪ **PO (Children 2–3 yr):** 0.25 mg/day.
▪ **PO (Children 3–14 yr):** 0.25–0.75 mg/day.

Topical Fluoride
▪ **Topical (Adults and Children >12 yr):** 10 ml/day. (Point-Two is used once weekly.)
▪ **Topical (Children 6–12 yr):** 5–10 ml/day. (Point-Two is used once weekly.)

AVAILABILITY (listed as fluoride content)

▪ *Tablets:* 1 mg ▪ *Chewable tablets:* 0.5 mg, 1 mg ▪ *Drops:* 0.125 mg/drop, 0.25 mg/drop, 0.5 mg/drop ▪ *Lozenges:* 1 mg ▪ *Solution:* 0.2 mg/ml ▪ *Rinse:* 0.01%, 0.02%, 0.09% ▪ *Gel:* 0.5%, 1%, 1.23%.

---

*Underlines indicate most frequent; **CAPITALS** indicate life-threatening.

TIME/ACTION PROFILE (blood levels)

	ONSET	PEAK	DURATION
PO	UK	30–60 min	UK

NURSING IMPLICATIONS

ASSESSMENT
□ Examine teeth for staining or mottling periodically. Notify dentist if this occurs.

POTENTIAL NURSING DIAGNOSES
▪ Knowledge deficit related to medication regimen.

IMPLEMENTATION
□ Drops may be administered undiluted orally or mixed with food or fluids.
□ Do not administer sodium fluoride within 2 hr of milk or other dairy products; will cause decreased absorption of sodium fluoride.

PATIENT/FAMILY TEACHING
□ Instruct patient to take fluoride supplement as directed, according to directions included with each preparation.
□ Rinses and gel are most effective if used immediately after brushing or flossing and just before sleep. Instruct patient to expectorate any excess; *do not swallow.* Patient should not eat, drink, or rinse mouth for 30 min after application.
□ Encourage patient to have routine dental examinations to monitor dental hygiene.

EVALUATION
Effectiveness of therapy is determined by: ▪ Prevention of dental caries.

FLUOROURACIL
(flure-oh-**yoor**-a-sill)
Adrucil, Efudex, Fluoroplex, 5-FU

CLASSIFICATION(S):
Antineoplastic (antimetabolite)
Pregnancy Category UK

INDICATIONS
▪ **IV:** Used alone and in combination with other modalities (surgery, radiation therapy, other antineoplastic agents) in the treatment of: □ Colon □ Breast □ Rectal □ Gastric □ Pancreatic carcinoma ▪ **Topical:** Management of multiple actinic (solar) keratoses and superficial basal cell carcinoma.

ACTION
▪ Inhibits DNA and RNA synthesis by preventing thymidine production (cell cycle-S phase specific). **Therapeutic Effect:** ▪ Death of rapidly replicating cells, particularly malignant ones.

PHARMACOKINETICS
Absorption: Minimal absorption (5–10%) following topical application.
Distribution: Widely distributed. Concentrates and persists in tumors.
Metabolism and Excretion: Converted to floxuridine monophosphate (an active metabolite). Undergoes cellular inactivation and metabolism by the liver. 60–80% excreted by lungs as respiratory CO_2. Small amounts (<10–15%) excreted unchanged by the kidneys.
Half-life: 20 hr.

CONTRAINDICATIONS AND PRECAUTIONS
Contraindicated in: ▪ Hypersensitivity ▪ Pregnancy or lactation.
Use Cautiously in: ▪ Patients with childbearing potential ▪ Infections ▪ Depressed bone marrow reserve ▪ Other chronic debilitating illnesses ▪ Obese patients, patients with edema or ascites (dose should be based on ideal body weight).

ADVERSE REACTIONS AND SIDE EFFECTS*
CNS: acute cerebellar dysfunction.
GI: nausea, vomiting, stomatitis, diarrhea.
Derm: alopecia, maculopapular rash, nail loss, melanosis of nails, phototoxicity.
Endo: gonadal suppression.

*Underlines indicate most frequent; **CAPITALS** indicate life-threatening.

Hemat: anemia, leukopenia, thrombocytopenia.
Local: thrombophlebitis.
Misc: fever.

INTERACTIONS

Drug–Drug: ▪ Additive bone marrow depression with other **bone marrow depressants** (other **antineoplastics** and **radiation therapy**) ▪ May decrease antibody response to **live virus vaccines** and increase risk of adverse reactions.

ROUTE AND DOSAGE

Doses may vary greatly, depending on tumor, patient condition, and protocol use.

▪ **IV (Adults):** _Initial dose_—12 mg/kg/day for days 1–4, then 6 mg/kg on days 6, 8, 10, and 12; or 7–12 mg/kg/day for 4 days followed by 3-day rest, then 7–10 mg/kg q 3–4 days for 3 doses. _Maintenance_—7–12 mg/kg q 7–10 days or 300–500 mg/m²/day for 4–5 days (no single daily dose should exceed 800 mg). ▪ **Poor-Risk Patients:** 3–6 mg/kg/day on days 1–3, 3 mg/kg/day on days 5, 7, 9 (not to exceed 400 mg/dose). Doses of 370–425 mg/m²/day for 5 days have been used in combination with leucovorin.

▪ **Top (Adults):** 1% or 2% solution or cream bid to lesion on head or neck, 5% solution or cream bid to other areas.

AVAILABILITY

▪ _Injection:_ 50 mg/ml ▪ _Cream:_ 1%, 5% ▪ _Solution:_ 1%, 2%, 5%.

TIME/ACTION PROFILE (IV = effects on blood counts, Top = dermatologic effects)

	ONSET	PEAK	DURATION
IV	1–9 days	9–21 days (nadir)	30 days
Top	2–3 days	2–6 wk	1–2 mo

NURSING IMPLICATIONS

Assessment

▪ **General Info:** Monitor vital signs prior to and frequently during therapy.
□ Assess mucous membranes, number and consistency of stools, and frequency of vomiting. Assess for fever, chills, sore throat, and signs of infection. Assess for bleeding (bleeding gums, bruising, petechiae; guaiac stools, urine, and emesis). Avoid IM injections and rectal temperatures. Apply pressure to venipuncture sites for 10 min. Notify physician if symptoms of toxicity (stomatitis or esophagopharyngitis, uncontrollable vomiting, diarrhea, GI bleeding, leukocyte count <3500/mm³, platelet count <100,000/mm³, or hemorrhage from any site) occur, as drug will need to be discontinued.

□ Assess IV site frequently for inflammation or infiltration. Patient should notify nurse if pain or irritation at injection site occurs. May cause thrombophlebitis. If extravasation occurs, infusion must be stopped and restarted in another vein to avoid damage to SC tissue. Notify physician immediately. Standard treatment includes application of ice compresses.

□ Monitor intake and output, appetite, and nutritional intake. GI effects usually occur on fourth day of therapy. Adjusting diet as tolerated may help maintain fluid and electrolyte balance and nutritional status.

□ Monitor patient for cerebellar dysfunction (weakness, ataxia, dizziness). This may persist after discontinuation of therapy.

▪ **Top:** Inspect involved skin prior to and throughout course of therapy.

▪ **Lab Test Considerations:** May cause a decrease in plasma albumin.

□ Hepatic, renal, and hematologic functions should be monitored prior to and periodically throughout therapy. CBC should be monitored daily during IV therapy. Notify physician immediately if WBC <3500/mm³ or platelets <100,000/mm³. These are criteria for discontinuation of the medication. Leukopenia usually occurs in 9–14 days, nadir in 21–25 days, with recovery by day 30. May also cause thrombocytopenia (nadir 7–17 days).

POTENTIAL NURSING DIAGNOSES

- Infection, high risk for (side effects).
- Nutrition, altered: less than body requirements (side effects).
- Knowledge deficit related to medication regimen (patient/family teaching).

IMPLEMENTATION

- **General Info:** Solution should be prepared in a biologic cabinet. Wear gloves, gown, and mask while handling IV medication. Discard IV equipment in specially designated containers (see Appendix I).
- ☐ The number 5 in 5-fluorouracil is part of the drug name and does not refer to the dosage.
- **Direct IV:** Rapid IV push administration (over 1–2 min) is most effective, but there is a more rapid onset of toxicity.
- **Intermittent Infusion:** May be diluted with D5W or 0.9% NaCl.
- ☐ Use plastic IV tubing and IV bags to maintain greater stability of medication. Solution is stable for 24 hr at room temperature; do not refrigerate. Solution is colorless to faint yellow. Discard highly discolored or cloudy solution. If crystals form, dissolve by warming solution to 140°F, shaking vigorously, and cooling to body temperature.
- *Rate:* Onset of toxicity is greatly delayed by administering an infusion over 2–8 hr.
- **Syringe Compatibility:** ▪ bleomycin ▪ cisplatin ▪ cyclophosphamide ▪ doxorubicin ▪ furosemide ▪ heparin ▪ leucovorin ▪ methotrexate ▪ metoclopramide ▪ mitomycin ▪ vinblastine ▪ vincristine. Mix immediately before use.
- **Syringe Incompatibility:** ▪ droperidol.
- **Y-Site Compatibility:** ▪ bleomycin ▪ cisplatin ▪ cyclophosphamide ▪ doxorubicin ▪ fludarabine ▪ furosemide ▪ heparin ▪ hydrocortisone ▪ leucovorin ▪ methotrexate ▪ metoclopramide ▪ mitomycin ▪ potassium chlor-

ide ▪ sargramostim ▪ vinblastine ▪ vincristine.
- **Y-Site Incompatibility:** ▪ droperidol.
- **Additive Compatibility:** ▪ D5/LR ▪ bleomycin ▪ cyclophosphamide ▪ etoposide ▪ floxuridine ▪ ifosfamide ▪ leucovorin ▪ methotrexate ▪ prednisolone ▪ vincristine ▪ vitamin B complex with C.
- **Additive Incompatibility:** ▪ carboplatin ▪ cisplatin ▪ cytarabine ▪ diazepam ▪ doxorubicin.
- **Top:** Consult physician before administering topical preparations, to determine what skin preparation regimen should be followed. Tight occlusive dressings are not advised because of irritation to surrounding healthy tissue. A loose gauze dressing for cosmetic purposes is usually preferred. Wear gloves when applying medication. Do not use metallic applicator.

PATIENT/FAMILY TEACHING

- **General Info:** Instruct patient to notify physician if fever, chills, sore throat, signs of infection, yellowing of skin or eyes, abdominal pain, joint of flank pain, swelling of feet or legs, bleeding gums, bruising, petechiae, blood in urine or stool, or emesis occurs. Caution patient to avoid crowds and persons with known infections. Instruct patient to use soft toothbrush and electric razor. Patients should be cautioned not to drink alcoholic beverages or take products containing aspirin or ibuprofen.
- ☐ Advise patient to rinse mouth with clear water after eating and drinking and to avoid flossing to minimize stomatitis.
- ☐ Discuss with patient the possibility of hair loss. Explore methods of coping.
- ☐ Caution patient to use sunscreen and protective clothing to prevent phototoxicity reactions.
- ☐ Instruct patient not to receive any vaccinations without advice of physician.
- ☐ Emphasize the importance of routine

follow-up lab tests to monitor progress and to check for side effects.

☐ Review with patient the need for contraception during therapy.

■ **Top:** Instruct patient in correct application of solution or cream. Emphasize importance of avoiding the eyes; caution should also be used when applying medication near mouth and nose. If patient uses clean finger to self-administer, emphasize importance of washing hands thoroughly after application. Explain that erythema, scaling, and blistering with pruritus and burning sensation are expected. Therapy is discontinued when erosion, ulceration, and necrosis occur in 2–6 wk (10–12 wk for basal cell carcinomas). Skin heals 4–8 wk later.

EVALUATION
Effectiveness of therapy can be demonstrated by: ■ Tumor size regression ■ Removal of solar keratoses or superficial basal cell skin cancers.

FLUOXETINE
(floo-**ox**-uh-teen)
Prozac

CLASSIFICATION(S):
Antidepressant
Pregnancy Category B

INDICATIONS

■ Treatment of various forms of depression, often in conjunction with psychotherapy. **Unlabeled Use:** ■ Obsessive compulsive disorder (OCD).

ACTION

■ Inhibits the upake of serotonin in the CNS. **Therapeutic Effect:** ■ Antidepressant action.

PHARMACOKINETICS

Absorption: Well absorbed following oral administration.
Distribution: Crosses the blood–brain barrier well.

Metabolism and Excretion: Converted by the liver to norfluoxetine, another antidepressant compound; fluoxetine and norfluoxetine are mostly metabolized by the liver. 12% excreted by kidneys as unchanged fluoxetine, 7% as unchanged norfluoxetine.
Half-life: 1–3 days (norfluoxetine 5–7 days).

CONTRAINDICATIONS AND PRECAUTIONS

Contraindicated in: ■ Hypersensitivity.
Use Cautiously in: ■ Severe hepatic or renal impairment (dosage adjustment may be necessary) ■ Pregnancy, lactation, or children (safety not established) ■ History of seizures ■ Debilitated patients (increased risk of seizures) ■ Diabetes mellitus ■ Eating disorders (anorexia, bulimia).

ADVERSE REACTIONS AND SIDE EFFECTS*

CNS: SEIZURES, anxiety, nervousness, insomnia, headache, drowsiness, tremor, dizziness, fatigue, mania, hypomania, weakness, abnormal dreams.
EENT: visual disturbances, stuffy nose.
CV: palpitations, chest pain.
Endo: dysmenorrhea.
GI: anorexia, weight loss, nausea, diarrhea, dry mouth, dyspepsia, constipation, abdominal pain, abnormal taste, vomiting.
GU: urinary frequency.
Derm: rashes, excessive sweating, pruritus, flushing.
MS: back pain, arthralgia, myalgia.
Neuro: trembling.
Resp: cough.
Misc: flu-like syndrome, fever, hot flashes, sexual dysfunction, sensitivity reaction.

INTERACTIONS

Drug–Drug: ■ Additive CNS depression with **alcohol, antihistamines,** other **antidepressants, opioid analgesics,** or **sedative/hypnotics** ■ May prolong the effect of **diazepam** ■ Discontinue use of

---

*Underlines indicate most frequent; **CAPITALS** indicate life-threatening.

MAO inhibitors for 14 days prior to fluoxetine therapy; combined therapy may result in confusion, agitation, seizures, hypertension, hyperpyrexia. Fluoxetine should be discontinued for at least 5 wk before therapy is initiated
- Increased risk of side effects and adverse reactions with other **antidepressants, tryptophan,** or **phenothiazines**
- May increase effectiveness/risk of toxicity of **digitoxin, lithium,** or **oral anticoagulants**.

ROUTE AND DOSAGE

- **PO (Adults):** 20 mg/day in the morning. After several weeks, may increase by 20 mg/day at weekly intervals. Doses greater than 20 mg/day should be given in 2 divided doses, in the morning and at noon (not to exceed 80 mg/day).

AVAILABILITY

- *Capsules:* 20 mg ▪ *Liquid:* 20 mg/5 ml.

TIME/ACTION PROFILE (antidepressant effect)

	ONSET	PEAK	DURATION
PO	1–4 wk	UK	2 wk

NURSING IMPLICATIONS

ASSESSMENT

- Monitor mood changes. Inform physician if patient demonstrates significant increase in anxiety, nervousness, or insomnia.
- Assess for suicidal tendencies, especially during early therapy. Restrict amount of drug available to patient.
- Monitor appetite and nutritional intake. Weigh weekly. Notify physician of continued weight loss. Adjust diet as tolerated to support nutritional status.
- Assess patient for possible sensitivity reaction (urticaria, fever, arthralgia, edema, carpal tunnel syndrome, rash, lymphadenopathy, respiratory distress) and notify physician if present; these symptoms usually resolve by stopping fluoxetine but may require

administration of antihistamines or glucocorticoids.
- **Lab Test Considerations:** Monitor CBC and differential periodically during course of therapy. Notify physician if leukopenia, anemia, thrombocytopenia, or increased bleeding time occurs.
- Proteinuria and mild increase in AST (SGOT) may occur during sensitivity reactions.

POTENTIAL NURSING DIAGNOSES

- Coping, ineffective individual (indications).
- Injury, high risk for (side effects).
- Knowledge deficit related to medication regimen (patient/family teaching).

IMPLEMENTATION

- **PO:** Administer as a single dose in the morning. Some patients may require increased amounts, in divided doses.

PATIENT/FAMILY TEACHING

- Instruct patient to take fluoxetine exactly as directed. If a dose is missed, omit dose and return to regular dosing schedule. Do not double doses.
- May cause drowsiness, dizziness, impaired judgment, and blurred vision. Caution patient to avoid driving and other activities requiring alertness until response to the drug is known.
- Advise patient to avoid alcohol or other CNS depressant drugs during therapy and to consult with physician before taking other medications with fluoxetine.
- Inform patient that frequent mouth rinses, good oral hygiene, and sugarless gum or candy may minimize dry mouth. If dry mouth persists for more than 2 wk, consult physician or dentist regarding use of saliva substitute.
- Instruct female patient to inform physician if pregnancy is planned or suspected.
- Advise patient to notify physician if symptoms of sensitivity reaction occur. Patient should also inform physician if headache, nausea, anorexia, anxiety, or insomnia persist.

□ Emphasize the importance of follow-up examinations to monitor progress. Encourage patient participation in psychotherapy.

EVALUATION
Effectiveness of therapy can be demonstrated by: ▪ Increased sense of well-being □ Renewed interest in surroundings. May require 1–4 wk of therapy to obtain antidepressant effects.

FLUPHENAZINE
(floo-**fen**-a-zeen)
{Apo-Fluphenazine}, {Modicate}, {Moditen}, Permitil, Prolixin

CLASSIFICATION(S):
Antipsychotic (phenothiazine)
Pregnancy Category UK

INDICATIONS

▪ Treatment of acute and chronic psychoses.

ACTION

▪ Alters the effects of dopamine in the CNS ▪ Possesses anticholinergic and alpha-adrenergic blocking activity. **Therapeutic Effect:** ▪ Diminished signs and symptoms of psychoses.

PHARMACOKINETICS

Absorption: Well absorbed following oral and IM administration. Decanoate and enanthate salts in sesame oil have delayed onset and prolonged action due to delayed release from oil vehicle and subsequent delayed release from fatty tissues.
Distribution: Widely distributed. Crosses the blood–brain barrier. Crosses the placenta and enters breast milk.
Metabolism and Excretion: Highly metabolized by the liver, undergoes enterohepatic recirculation.
Half-life: Fluphenazine hydrochlo-

ride—4.7–15.3 hr; fluphenazine enanthate—3.7 days; fluphenazine decanoate—6.8–9.6 days.

CONTRAINDICATIONS AND PRECAUTIONS

Contraindicated in: ▪ Hypersensitivity ▪ Cross-sensitivity with other phenothiazines may exist ▪ Narrow-angle glaucoma ▪ Bone marrow depression ▪ Severe liver or cardiovascular disease ▪ Hypersensitivity to sesame oil (decanoate and enanthate salts).
Use Cautiously in: ▪ Elderly or debilitated patients (initial dosage reduction may be necessary) ▪ Pregnancy or lactation (safety not established) ▪ Diabetes mellitus ▪ Respiratory disease ▪ Prostatic hypertrophy ▪ CNS tumors ▪ Epilepsy ▪ Intestinal obstruction.

ADVERSE REACTIONS AND SIDE EFFECTS*

CNS: sedation, <u>extrapyramidal reactions</u>, tardive dyskinesia.
EENT: dry eyes, blurred vision, lens opacities.
CV: hypotension, tachycardia.
GI: constipation, dry mouth, ileus, anorexia, hepatitis.
GU: urinary retention.
Derm: rashes, <u>photosensitivity</u>, pigment changes.
Endo: galactorrhea.
Hemat: AGRANULOCYTOSIS, leukopenia.
Misc: allergic reactions, hyperthermia.

INTERACTIONS

Drug–Drug: ▪ Additive hypotension with **antihypertensive agents** ▪ Additive CNS depression with other **CNS depressants,** including **alcohol, antidepressants, antihistamines, MAO inhibitors, narcotic analgesics, sedative/hypnotics,** or **general anesthetics** ▪ **Phenobarbital** may increase metabolism and decrease effectiveness ▪ Concurrent use with **lithium** may produce any of the following—acute encephalopathy, decreased chlorpromazine absorption, increased excretion of lithium, increased risk of extrapyramidal reactions, or masking of the early signs of lithium toxicity ▪ **Antacids** or **adsorbent antidiarrheals (kaolin)** may decrease absorption ▪ Increased risk of agranulocytosis with **antithyroid drugs** ▪ May decrease antiparkinson activity of **levodopa** and **bromocriptine** ▪ Decreases vasopressor response to **epinephrine** and **norepinephrine** ▪ Decreases antihypertensive effect of **guanethidine** ▪ Concurrent use with **beta blockers** may result in inhibition of metabolism of one or both drugs producing an increased response ▪ Increased risk of anticholinergic effects with other **agents having anticholinergic properties,** including **antihistamines, tricyclic antidepressants, disopyramide,** or **quinidine.**

ROUTE AND DOSAGE

Fluphenazine Hydrochloride
▪ **PO (Adults):** 0.5–10 mg/day in divided doses q 6–8 hr initially, maintenance dose 1–5 mg/day. Initial dose in elderly or debilitated patients is 1–2.5 mg/day.
▪ **IM (Adults):** 1.5–2.5 mg q 6–8 hr. Initial dose in elderly or debilitated patients is 1–2.5 mg/day.

Fluphenazine Enanthate
▪ **IM, SC (Adults):** 25 mg q 2 wk. May be slowly increased as needed (not to exceed 100 mg/dose). Some patients require q 1–3 wk dosing.

Fluphenazine Decanoate
▪ **IM, SC (Adults):** 12.5–25 mg initially. May be slowly increased as needed (not to exceed 100 mg/dose). Some patients require q 4–6 wk dosing.

AVAILABILITY

▪ *Tablets:* 1 mg, 2.5 mg, 5 mg, 10 mg ▪ *Elixir:* 2.5 mg/5 ml ▪ *Concentrate:* 5 mg/ml ▪ *Injection:* hydrochloride—2.5 mg/ml, decanoate—25 mg/ml, ethanate—25 mg/ml.

TIME/ACTION PROFILE (antipsychotic activity)

	ONSET	PEAK	DURATION
PO hydrochloride	1 hr	UK	6–8 hr
IM hydrochloride	1 hr	1.5–2 hr	6–8 hr
IM enanthate	24–72 hr	UK	1–3 wk
IM decanoate	24–72 hr	UK	≥4 wk

NURSING IMPLICATIONS

ASSESSMENT
□ Assess patient's mental status (orientation, mood, behavior) prior to and periodically throughout therapy.
□ Monitor blood pressure (sitting, standing, lying), pulse, and respiratory rate prior to and frequently during the period of dosage adjustment.
□ Observe patient carefully when administering oral medication to ensure medication is actually taken and not hoarded.
□ Assess fluid intake and bowel function. Increased bulk and fluids in the diet help minimize the constipating effects of this medication.
□ Observe patient carefully for extrapyramidal symptoms (akathisia—restlessness; dystonia—muscle spasms and twisting motions; pseudoparkinsonism—mask facies, rigidity, tremors, drooling, shuffling gait, dysphagia). Notify physician if these symptoms occur, as reduction in dose or discontinuation may be necessary. Physician may also order trihexyphenidyl or diphenhydramine to control these symptoms.
□ Monitor for tardive dyskinesia (rhythmic movement of mouth, face, and extremities). Notify physician immediately if these symptoms occur, as these side effects may be irreversible.
□ Monitor for development of neuroleptic malignant syndrome (fever, respiratory distress, tachycardia, convulsions, diaphoresis, hypertension or hypotension, pallor, tiredness). No-

tify physician immediately if these symptoms occur.

- **Lab Test Considerations:** Monitor liver function tests, urine bilirubin, and bile for evidence of hepatic toxicity periodically throughout course of therapy. Urine bilirubin may be falsely elevated.
- □ May cause false-positive and false-negative pregnancy tests.
- □ May cause blood dyscrasias; monitor CBC periodically throughout course of therapy.

POTENTIAL NURSING DIAGNOSES

- Thought processes, altered (indications).
- Knowledge deficit related to medication regimen (patient/family teaching).
- Noncompliance (patient/family teaching).

IMPLEMENTATION

- **General Info:** Slight yellow to amber color does not alter potency.
- □ To prevent contact dermatitis, avoid getting liquid preparations on hands and wash hands thoroughly if spillage occurs.
- □ Injectable forms must be drawn up with a dry syringe and dry 21-gauge needle to prevent clouding of the solution.
- **PO:** Dilute concentrate just prior to administration in 120–240 ml of water, milk, carbonated beverage, soup, or tomato or fruit juice. Do not mix with beverages containing caffeine (cola, coffee); tannics (tea); or pectinates (apple juice).
- **SC:** Fluphenazine decanoate and enanthate are dissolved in sesame oil for long duration of action. They may be administered SC or IM.
- **IM:** IM dose is usually ⅓–½ of oral dose. Because fluphenazine hydrochloride has a shorter duration of action, it is used initially to determine the patient's response to the drug and to treat the acutely agitated patient.
- □ Administer deep IM using a dry syringe and 21-gauge needle into dorsal gluteal site. Instruct patient to remain recumbent for 30 min to prevent hypotension.

PATIENT/FAMILY TEACHING

- □ Advise patient to take medication exactly as directed and not to skip doses or double up on missed doses. Abrupt withdrawal may lead to gastritis, nausea, vomiting, dizziness, headache, tachycardia, and insomnia.
- □ Inform patient of possibility of extrapyramidal symptoms and tardive dyskinesia. Caution patient to report these symptoms immediately to physician.
- □ Advise patient to make position changes slowly to minimize orthostatic hypotension.
- □ Medication may cause drowsiness. Caution patient to avoid driving or other activities requiring alertness until response to medication is known.
- □ Caution patient to avoid taking alcohol or other CNS depressants concurrently with this medication.
- □ Advise patient to use sunscreen and protective clothing when exposed to the sun. Exposed surfaces may develop a blue-grey pigmentation, which may fade following discontinuation of the medication. Extremes of temperature should also be avoided, as this drug impairs body temperature regulation.
- □ Advise patient that good oral hygiene, frequent rinsing of mouth with water, and sugarless gum or candy may help relieve dry mouth. Physician or dentist should be notified if dry mouth persists beyond 2 wk.
- □ Inform patient that this medication may turn urine pink to reddish-brown.
- □ Instruct patient to notify physician promptly if sore throat, fever, unusual bleeding or bruising, skin rashes, weakness, tremors, visual disturbances, dark-colored urine, or clay-colored stools are noted.
- □ Advise patient to notify physician or dentist of medication regimen prior to treatment or surgery.

□ Emphasize the importance of routine follow-up examinations, including ocular examinations, with long-term therapy and continued participation in psychotherapy.

EVALUATION
Effectiveness of therapy can be demonstrated by: ■ Decrease in excitable, paranoic, or withdrawn behavior.

FLURAZEPAM
(flur-**az**-e-pam)
{Apo-flurazepam}, Dalmane, Durapam, {Novoflupam}, {Somnol}, {Som-Pam}

CLASSIFICATION(S):
Sedative/hypnotic (benzodiazepine)
Schedule IV
Pregnancy Category UK

INDICATIONS
■ Short-term management of insomnia (<4 wk).

ACTION
■ Depresses the CNS, probably by potentiating gamma-aminobutyric acid (GABA), an inhibitory neurotransmitter. **Therapeutic Effect:** ■ Relief of insomnia.

PHARMACOKINETICS
Absorption: Well absorbed following oral administration.
Distribution: Widely distributed, crosses blood–brain barrier. Probably crosses the placenta and enters breast milk. Accumulation of drug occurs with chronic dosing.
Metabolism and Excretion: Metabolized by the liver. Some metabolites have hypnotic activity.
Half-life: 2.3 hr (half-life of active metabolite may be 30–200 hr).

CONTRAINDICATIONS AND PRECAUTIONS
Contraindicated in: ■ Hypersensitivity ■ Cross-sensitivity with other benzodiazepines may exist ■ Pre-existing CNS depression ■ Severe uncontrolled pain ■ Narrow-angle glaucoma ■ Pregnancy or lactation.
Use Cautiously in: ■ Hepatic dysfunction (dosage reduction may be necessary) ■ Patients who may be suicidal or have been addicted to drugs previously ■ Elderly or debilitated patients (initial dosage reduction may be necessary).

ADVERSE REACTIONS AND SIDE EFFECTS*
CNS: dizziness, daytime drowsiness, lethargy, <u>hangover</u>, paradoxical excitation, confusion, mental depression, headache.
Derm: rashes.
EENT: blurred vision.
GI: nausea, vomiting, diarrhea, constipation.
Misc: tolerance, psychological dependence, physical dependence.

INTERACTIONS
Drug–Drug: ■ Concurrent use with **alcohol, antidepressants, antihistamines,** and **opioid analgesics** may result in additive CNS depression ■ **Cimetidine, oral contraceptives, disulfiram, fluoxetine, isoniazid, ketoconazole, metoprolol, propoxyphene, propranolol,** or **valproic acid** may decrease the metabolism of flurazepam, enhancing its actions ■ May decrease efficacy of **levodopa** ■ **Rifampin** or **barbiturates** may increase the metabolism and decrease effectiveness of flurazepam ■ Sedative effects may be decreased by **theophylline.**

ROUTE AND DOSAGE
■ **PO (Adults):** 15–30 mg at bedtime.
■ **PO (Elderly or Debilitated Patients):** 15 mg initially, may be increased.

AVAILABILITY
■ *Capsules:* 15 mg, 30 mg ■ {Tablets: 15 mg, 30 mg}.

F

{} = Available in Canada only.
*<u>Underlines</u> indicate most frequent; **CAPITALS** indicate life-threatening.

TIME/ACTION PROFILE (hypnotic activity)

	ONSET	PEAK	DURATION
PO	15–45 min	0.5–1 hr	7–8 hr

NURSING IMPLICATIONS

ASSESSMENT

▫ Assess sleep patterns prior to and periodically throughout course of therapy.

▫ Prolonged therapy may lead to psychological or physical dependence. Restrict amount of drug available to patient, especially if patient is depressed, suicidal, or has a history of addiction.

POTENTIAL NURSING DIAGNOSES

▪ Sleep pattern disturbance (indications).

▪ Injury, high risk for (side effects).

▪ Knowledge deficit related to medication regimen (patient/family teaching).

IMPLEMENTATION

▪ **General Info:** Supervise ambulation and transfer of patients following administration. Remove cigarettes. Side rails should be raised and call bell within reach at all times.

▪ **PO:** Capsules may be opened and mixed with food or fluids for patients having difficulty swallowing.

PATIENT/FAMILY TEACHING

▫ Advise patient to take medication exactly as directed. Discuss the importance of preparing environment for sleep (dark room, quiet, avoidance of nicotine and caffeine).

▫ Medication may cause daytime drowsiness. Caution patient to avoid driving and other activities requiring alertness until response to medication is known.

▫ Caution patient to avoid taking alcohol or other CNS depressants concurrently with this medication.

▫ Instruct patient to contact physician immediately if pregnancy is suspected.

EVALUATION

Effectiveness of therapy can be demonstrated by: ▪ Improvement in sleep patterns. Maximum hypnotic properties are apparent 2–3 nights after initiating therapy and may last 1–2 nights after therapy is discontinued.

FLURBIPROFEN
(flure-**bi**-proe-fen)
Ansaid, {Froben}, Ocufen

CLASSIFICATION(S):
Nonsteroidal anti-inflammatory agent, Ophthalmic (miotic)
Pregnancy Category C (Ophth)

INDICATIONS

▪ **PO:** Management of inflammatory disorders including: ▫ Rheumatoid arthritis ▫ Osteoarthritis ▪ **Ophth:** Used to inhibit intra-operative miosis. **Unlabeled Use:** ▪ **Ophth:** Ocular anti-inflammatory.

ACTION

▪ Inhibits prostaglandin synthesis, resulting in reduced inflammation and pain when administered orally. Inhibition of prostaglandin synthesis in the eye relaxes the iris sphincter. **Therapeutic Effects:** ▪ **PO:** Suppression of pain and inflammation ▪ **Ophth:** Suppression of miosis.

PHARMACOKINETICS

Absorption: Well absorbed following oral administration. Following ophth administration, penetration of the cornea results in systemic absorption.

Distribution: Systemic distribution following oral administration.

Metabolism and Excretion: Mostly metabolized by the liver. 20–25% excreted unchanged by the kidneys.

Half-life: 3–6 hr.

CONTRAINDICATIONS AND PRECAUTIONS

Contraindicated in: ▪ Hypersensitivity

▪ Cross-sensitivity may exist with other nonsteroidal anti-inflammatory agents, including aspirin ▪ Active GI bleeding or ulcer disease ▪ Herpes simplex keratitis (ophth form only).

Use Cautiously in: ▪ Severe cardiovascular, renal, or hepatic disease ▪ History of ulcer disease ▪ Diabetes mellitus ▪ Bleeding disorders ▪ Pregnancy, lactation, or children (safety not established).

ADVERSE REACTIONS AND SIDE EFFECTS*

CNS: *PO*—mental depression, headache, drowsiness, psychic disturbances, dizziness, insomnia.

EENT: *PO*—blurred vision, corneal opacities, tinnitus; *Ophth*—burning, stinging, itching.

CV: *PO*—edema, changes in blood pressure, palpitations.

GI: *PO*—nausea, abdominal pain, heartburn, bloated feeling, diarrhea, constipation, hepatitis, GASTRIC BLEEDING, stomatitis.

GU: *PO*—incontinence.

Derm: *PO*—rashes, increased sweating.

Hemat: *PO*—blood dyscrasias, prolonged bleeding time.

MS: *PO*—myalgia.

Misc: *PO*—allergic reactions, including ANAPHYLAXIS and STEVENS-JOHNSON SYNDROME, chills, fever.

INTERACTIONS

For oral flurbiprofen, unless indicated.

Drug–Drug: ▪ Concurrent use with **aspirin** may decrease effectiveness ▪ Additive adverse GI effects with **aspirin,** other **nonsteroidal anti-inflammatory agents, potassium supplements, glucocorticoids,** or **alcohol** ▪ Chronic use with **acetaminophen** may increase the risk of adverse renal reactions ▪ May decrease the effectiveness of **diuretics** or **antihypertensive** therapy ▪ May increase the hypoglycemic response to **insulin** or **oral hypoglycemic** agents ▪ Increases the risk of toxicity from **methotrexate** ▪ **Probenecid** increases

risk of toxicity from flurbiprofen ▪ Increased risk of bleeding with **cefamandole, cefotetan, cefoperazone, plicamycin, heparin, thrombolytic agents, valproic acid,** or **oral anticoagulants** ▪ Increased risk of adverse hematologic reactions with **antineoplastic agents** or **radiation therapy** ▪ Increased risk of nephrotoxicity with other **nephrotoxic agents** ▪ Ophthalmic **acetylcholine** or **carbachol** are not effective when administered after ophthalmic flurbiprofen ▪ Ophthalmic flurbiprofen decreases the intraocular pressure-lowering effect of ophthalmic **epinephrine.**

ROUTE AND DOSAGE

▪ **PO (Adults):** 200–300 mg daily in 2–4 divided doses (not to exceed 300 mg/day or 100 mg/dose).
▪ **Ophth (Adults):** 1 drop of 0.03% solution every 30 min beginning 2 hr prior to surgery (total of 4 drops).

AVAILABILITY

▪ *Tablets:* 50 mg, 100 mg ▪ *Ophthalmic solution:* 0.03% in 2.5-, 5-, and 10-ml bottles.

TIME/ACTION PROFILE

	ONSET	PEAK	DURATION
PO (anti-inflammatory)	few days–1 wk	1–2 wk	UK
Ophth (miosis)	UK	UK	UK

NURSING IMPLICATIONS

ASSESSMENT

▪ **General Info:** Patients who have asthma, aspirin-induced allergy, and nasal polyps are at increased risk for developing hypersensitivity reactions. Monitor for rhinitis, asthma, and urticaria.
▪ **Arthritis:** Assess pain and range of movement prior to and periodically during therapy.
▪ **Lab Test Considerations:** May cause prolonged bleeding time.

POTENTIAL NURSING DIAGNOSES

▪ Pain (indications).

---

*Underlines indicate most frequent; CAPITALS indicate life-threatening.

- Physical mobility, impaired (indications).
- Knowledge deficit related to medication regimen (patient/family teaching).

IMPLEMENTATION
- **PO:** For rapid initial effect, administer 30 min before or 2 hr after meals.
- **Ophth:** Instill 1 drop every 30 min beginning 2 hr prior to surgery, for a total of 4 drops. See Appendix H for administration of ophthalmic solution.

PATIENT/FAMILY TEACHING
- **Arthritis:** Advise patient to take this medication with a full glass of water and to remain in an upright position for 15–30 min after administration.
- Instruct patient to take medication exactly as prescribed. If a dose is missed, take as soon as remembered, but not if almost time for next dose. Do not double doses.
- This medication may cause drowsiness or dizziness. Advise patient to avoid driving or other activities requiring alertness until response to medication is known.
- Caution patient to avoid the concurrent use of alcohol, aspirin, ibuprofen, acetaminophen, or other over-the-counter medications without consulting physician or pharmacist.
- Instruct patient to notify physician if rash, itching, chills, fever, muscle aches, visual disturbances, tinnitus, weight gain, edema, black stools, or persistent headache occur.
- Advise patient to inform physician or dentist of medication regimen prior to treatment or surgery.

EVALUATION
Effectiveness of therapy can be demonstrated by: ■ Decreased pain □ Improved joint mobility. Patients who do not respond to one nonsteroidal anti-inflammatory agent may respond to another ■ Inhibition of intraoperative miosis.

FLUTAMIDE
(**floo**-ta-mide)
Eulexin

CLASSIFICATION(S):
Antineoplastic (hormone)
Pregnancy Category D

INDICATIONS
- Treatment of metastatic prostate carcinoma in conjunction with gonadotropin-releasing hormone analogs (leuprolide).

ACTION
- Antagonizes the effects of androgen (testosterone) at the cellular level. **Therapeutic Effect:** ■ Decreased growth of prostate carcinoma, an androgen-sensitive tumor.

PHARMACOKINETICS
Absorption: Well absorbed following oral administration.
Distribution: Distribution not known.
Metabolism and Excretion: Mostly metabolized by the liver. Some converted to another antiandrogenic compound.
Half-life: UK.

CONTRAINDICATIONS AND PRECAUTIONS
Contraindicated in: ■ Hypersensitivity.
Use Cautiously in: ■ Severe cardiovascular disease ■ Requires concurrent luteinizing hormone releasing hormone (LHRH) agonist therapy.

ADVERSE REACTIONS AND SIDE EFFECTS*
Side effects primarily due to LHRH antagonist.
CNS: drowsiness, confusion, anxiety, nervousness, depression.
CV: edema, hypertension.
GI: diarrhea, nausea, vomiting, other gastric disturbances, hepatitis.

---

*Underlines indicate most frequent; **CAPITALS** indicate life-threatening.

GU: loss of libido, impotence.
Derm: rash, photosensitivity.
Endo: gynecomastia.
Misc: hot flashes.

INTERACTIONS
Drug–Drug: ▪ Acts synergistically with gonadotropin-releasing hormone analogs (leuprolide).

ROUTE AND DOSAGE
▪ **PO (Adults):** 250 mg q 8 hr.

AVAILABILITY
▪ *Capsules:* 125 mg.

TIME/ACTION PROFILE

	ONSET	PEAK	DURATION
PO	UK	UK	UK

NURSING IMPLICATIONS

ASSESSMENT
▫ Monitor for diarrhea, nausea, and vomiting. Adjust diet as tolerated. Notify physician if these symptoms become severe.
▪ **Lab Test Considerations:** May cause elevated AST (SGOT), ALT (SGPT), bilirubin, and serum creatinine values.

POTENTIAL NURSING DIAGNOSES
▪ Sexual dysfunction (side effects).
▪ Knowledge deficit related to medication regimen (patient/family teaching).

IMPLEMENTATION
▪ **General Info:** Used in combination with LHRH agonist, such as leuprolide.

PATIENT/FAMILY TEACHING
▫ Explain that flutamide must be taken in conjunction with leuprolide.
▫ Warn patient that side effects such as hot flashes, loss of sex drive, impotence, and breast enlargement may be caused by the LHRH agonist. The primary side effect of flutamide alone is diarrhea, but the combination of drugs is necessary to achieve the therapeutic effect.

EVALUATION
Effectiveness of therapy can be demonstrated by: ▪ Decrease in the spread of prostate cancer.

FOLIC ACID
(foe-lik a-sid)
{Apo-Folic}, Folate, Folvite, {Novofolacid}, vitamin B₉

CLASSIFICATION(S):
Vitamin (water-soluble),
Antianemic
Pregnancy Category UK

INDICATIONS
▪ Used in the treatment of megaloblastic and macrocytic anemias ▪ Given during pregnancy to promote normal fetal development.

ACTION
▪ Required for protein synthesis and red blood cell function. Stimulates the production of red blood cells, white blood cells, and platelets. Necessary for normal fetal development. **Therapeutic Effect:** ▪ Restoration and maintenance of normal hematopoiesis.

PHARMACOKINETICS
Absorption: Well absorbed from the GI tract and IM and SC sites.
Distribution: Half of all stores are in the liver. Enters breast milk. Crosses the placenta.
Metabolism and Excretion: Converted by the liver to its active metabolite, dihydrofolate reductase. Excess amounts are excreted unchanged by the kidneys.
Half-life: UK.

CONTRAINDICATIONS AND PRECAUTIONS
Contraindicated in: ▪ Uncorrected pernicious anemia (neurologic damage will progress despite correction of hematologic abnormalities) ▪ Preparations containing benzyl alcohol should not be used in newborns.

F

Use Cautiously in: ▪ Undiagnosed anemias.

ADVERSE REACTIONS AND SIDE EFFECTS*

Derm: rashes.
Misc: fever.

INTERACTIONS

Drug–Drug: ▪ **Sulfomanides, methotrexate,** and **triamterene** prevent the activation of folic acid ▪ Absorption of folic acid is decreased by **sulfasalazine** ▪ Folic acid requirements are increased by **estrogens, phenytoin,** or **glucocorticoids**.

ROUTE AND DOSAGE

Anemia
▪ **PO, IM, IV, SC (Adults and Children):** 0.25–1.0 mg/day.

Pregnancy and Lactation
▪ **PO, IM, IV, SC (Adults):** 0.8–1.0 mg/day.

Dietary Supplement
▪ **PO, IM, IV, SC (Adults and Children):** 0.1–1 mg/day.

AVAILABILITY

▪ *Tablets:* 0.1 mg, 0.4 mg, 0.8 mg, 1 mg ▪ *Injection:* 5 mg/ml, 10 mg/ml ▪ *In combination with:* other vitamins and minerals as multiple vitamins.

TIME/ACTION PROFILE (increase in reticulocyte count)

	ONSET	PEAK	DURATION
PO, IM, SC, IV	3–5 days	5–10 days	UK

NURSING IMPLICATIONS

ASSESSMENT

□ Assess patient for signs of megaloblastic anemia (fatigue, weakness, dyspnea) prior to and periodically throughout therapy.
▪ **Lab Test Considerations:** Monitor plasma folic acid levels, hemoglobin, hematocrit, and reticulocyte count prior to and periodically during course of therapy.

□ May cause decrease in serum concentrations of vitamin B_{12} when given in high continuous doses.

POTENTIAL NURSING DIAGNOSES

▪ Nutrition, altered: less than body requirements (indications).
▪ Activity intolerance (indications).
▪ Knowledge deficit related to medication regimen (patient/family teaching).

IMPLEMENTATION

▪ **General Info:** Because of infrequency of solitary vitamin deficiencies, combinations are commonly administered (see Appendix A).
□ May be given SC, deep IM, or IV when PO route is not feasible.
▪ **IV:** Solution ranges from yellow to orange-yellow in color.
▪ **Direct IV:** Administer at a rate of 5 mg over at least 1 min.
▪ **Continuous Infusion:** May be added to hyperalimentation solution.
▪ **Y-Site Compatibility:** ▪ famotidine.
▪ **Additive Compatibility:** ▪ D20W.
▪ **Additive Incompatibility:** ▪ D50W ▪ calcium gluconate.

PATIENT/FAMILY TEACHING

□ Encourage patient to comply with physician's diet recommendations. Explain that the best source of vitamins is a well-balanced diet with foods from the 4 basic food groups. If physician is trying to diagnose folic acid deficiency without concealing pernicious anemia, a diet low in vitamin B_{12} and folate will be ordered.
□ Foods high in folic acid include vegetables, fruits, and organ meats; heat destroys folic acid in foods.
□ Patients self-medicating with vitamin supplements should be cautioned not to exceed RDA (see Appendix L). The effectiveness of megadoses for treatment of various medical conditions is unproven and may cause side effects.
□ Explain that folic acid may make urine more intensely yellow.
□ Instruct patient to notify physician if rash occurs, which may indicate hypersensitivity.

*Underlines indicate most frequent; **CAPITALS** indicate life-threatening.

□ Emphasize the importance of follow-up examinations to evaluate progress.

EVALUATION

Effectiveness of therapy may be demonstrated by: ■ Reticulocytosis 2–5 days after beginning therapy □ Resolution of symptoms of megaloblastic anemia.

FOSCARNET
(foss-**kar**-net)
Foscavir

CLASSIFICATION(S):
Antiviral
Pregnancy Category C

INDICATIONS

■ Treatment of cytomegalovirus (CMV) retinitis in patients with the acquired immunodeficiency syndrome (AIDS).

ACTION

■ Prevents viral replication by inhibiting viral DNA-polymerase and reverse transcriptase. **Therapeutic Effect:** ■ Virastatic action against susceptible viruses including CMV.

PHARMACOKINETICS

Absorption: Following IV administration absorption is essentially complete.
Distribution: Variable penetration into CSF. May concentrate in and be slowly released from bone. Remainder of distribution not known.
Metabolism and Excretion: 80–90% excreted unchanged in urine.
Half-life: 3 hr (in patients with normal renal function). A longer half-life of 90 hr may reflect release of drug from bone.

CONTRAINDICATIONS AND PRECAUTIONS

Contraindicated in: ■ Hypersensitivity.
Use Cautiously in: ■ Renal impairment (dosage reduction required if

creatinine clearance ≤50 ml/min/kg) ■ Pregnancy, lactation, or children (safety not established) ■ History of seizures.

ADVERSE REACTIONS AND SIDE EFFECTS*

CNS: SEIZURES, headache, fatigue, weakness, malaise, dizziness, depression, confusion, anxiety.
EENT: vision abnormalities, eye pain, conjunctivitis.
Resp: coughing, dyspnea.
CV: edema, chest pain, palpitations, ECG abnormalities.
GI: nausea, vomiting, diarrhea, anorexia, abdominal pain, constipation, dyspepsia, abnormal taste sensation.
GU: renal failure, albuminuria, dysuria, polyuria, urinary retention, nocturia.
Derm: rash, increased sweating, pruritus, skin ulceration.
F and E: hypocalcemia, hypomagnesemia, hypokalemia, hypophosphatemia, hyperphosphatemia.
Hemat: anemia, granulocytopenia, leukopenia.
Local: pain or inflammation at injection site.
MS: involuntary muscle contraction, back pain, arthralgia, myalgia.
Neuro: paresthesia, hypoesthesia, neuropathy, tremor, ataxia.
Misc: fever, chills, flu-like syndrome, lymphoma, sarcoma.

INTERACTIONS

Drug–Drug: ■ Concurrent use with parenteral **pentamidine** may result in severe, life-threatening hypocalcemia.

ROUTE AND DOSAGE

■ **IV (Adults):** 60 mg/kg q 8 hr for 2–3 wk initially, then 90–120 mg/kg/day as a single dose. Dosage reduction required for any degree of renal impairment.

AVAILABILITY

■ *Injection:* 24 mg/ml.

TIME/ACTION PROFILE

	ONSET	PEAK
IV	rapid	end of infusion

NURSING IMPLICATIONS

ASSESSMENT

□ Diagnosis of CMV retinitis should be determined by ophthalmoscopy prior to treatment with foscarnet.

□ Culture for CMV (urine, blood, throat) may be taken prior to administration. However, a negative CMV culture does not rule out CMV retinitis.

■ **Lab Test Considerations:** Monitor serum creatinine prior to and 2–3 times weekly during induction therapy and at least every 1–2 wk during maintenance therapy. Monitor 24-hr creatinine clearance prior to and periodically throughout therapy. If creatinine clearance drops below 0.4 ml/min/kg foscarnet may need to be discontinued.

□ Monitor serum calcium, magnesium, potassium, and phosphorous prior to and 2–3 times weekly during induction therapy and at least every 1–2 wk during maintenance therapy.

□ May cause anemia, granulocytopenia, leukopenia, and thrombocytopenia.

□ May cause elevated AST (SGOT) and ALT (SGPT) levels and abnormal A-G ratios.

POTENTIAL NURSING DIAGNOSES

■ Infection, high risk for (indications).

■ Knowledge deficit related to medication regimen (patient/family teaching).

IMPLEMENTATION

■ **General Info:** Patient should be adequately hydrated prior to and throughout infusion to prevent renal toxicity.

■ **Intermittent Infusion:** May be administered via central line in standard 24 mg/ml solution undiluted. If administered via peripheral line, *must* be diluted to 12 mg/ml concentration with D5W or 0.9% NaCl to prevent vein irritation. Do not administer solution that is discolored or contains particulate matter. Use diluted solution within 24 hr.

□ Do not administer concurrently with other solutions in IV catheter except D5W or 0.9% NaCl; precipitate will develop.

□ Dose is based on patient weight; excess solution may be discarded from bottle prior to administration to prevent overdosage.

□ Patients who experience progression of CMV retinitis during maintenance therapy may be retreated with induction therapy followed by maintenance therapy.

■ **Rate:** Induction treatment is infused over 1 hr every 8 hr for 2–3 wk depending on clinical response.

□ Maintenance treatment is infused over 2 hr.

□ Infuse solution via infusion pump to ensure accurate infusion rate.

■ **Y-Site Incompatibility:** Manufacturer recommends that foscarnet not be administered concurrently with other drugs or solutions in the same IV catheter except D5W or 0.9% NaCl; precipitate will develop.

PATIENT/FAMILY TEACHING

□ Inform patient that foscarnet is not a cure for CMV retinitis. Progression of retinitis may continue in immunocompromised patients during and following therapy. Advise patients to have regular ophthalmologic examinations.

□ Advise patient to notify nurse or physician immediately if perioral tingling or numbness in the extremities or paresthesia occur during or after infusion. If these signs of electrolyte imbalance occur during administration, stop infusion and consult physician. Lab samples for serum electrolyte concentrations should be obtained immediately.

□ Emphasize the importance of frequent follow-up examinations to monitor renal function and electrolytes.

EVALUATION

Effectiveness of therapy can be demonstrated by: ▪ Resolution of the symptoms of CMV retinitis in patients with AIDS.

FOSINOPRIL
(foss-**in**-o-pril)
Monopril

CLASSIFICATION(S):
Antihypertensive, Angiotensin converting enzyme (ACE) inhibitor
Pregnancy Category D

INDICATIONS

▪ Alone or in combination with thiazide diuretics in the management of hypertension.

ACTION

▪ Prevents the production of angiotensin II, a potent vasoconstrictor that stimulates the production of aldosterone, by blocking its conversion to the active form. Result is systemic vasodilation. **Therapeutic Effect:** ▪ Lowering of blood pressure in hypertensive patients.

PHARMACOKINETICS

Absorption: 36% absorbed following oral administration.
Distribution: Crosses the placenta and enters breast milk.
Metabolism and Excretion: Converted to fosinoprilat, the active form, of which 50% excreted in feces, 50% excreted in urine as metabolites. Minimal amounts excreted unchanged.
Half-life: 12 hr (fosinoprilat).

CONTRAINDICATIONS AND PRECAUTIONS

Contraindicated in: ▪ Hypersensitivity ▪ Cross-sensitivity with other ACE inhibitors may exist ▪ Pregnancy (may cause fetal hypotension, oliguria, renal failure, skull hypoplasia, other fetal abnormalities, and death).

Use Cautiously in: ▪ Hypovolemia, hyponatremia, concurrent diuretic therapy, elderly patients (dosage reduction required) ▪ Renal disease ▪ Aortic stenosis ▪ Cerebrovascular or cardiac insufficiency ▪ Lactation or children (safety not established) ▪ Surgery/anesthesia (hypotension may be exaggerated).
Extreme Caution in: ▪ Family history of hereditary angioedema.

ADVERSE REACTIONS AND SIDE EFFECTS*

CNS: headache, dizziness, fatigue.
EENT: ANGIOEDEMA.
Resp: cough.
CV: orthostatic hypotension.
GI: nausea, diarrhea, vomiting.
Misc: allergic reactions.

INTERACTIONS

Drug–Drug: ▪ Additive or possibly excessive hypotension with other **antihypertensives, diuretics, nitrates, phenothiazines,** and acute ingestion of **alcohol** ▪ Hyperkalemia may result with concurrent **potassium supplements, cyclosporine,** or **potassium-sparing diuretics** ▪ Antihypertensive response may be blunted by **nonsteroidal anti-inflammatory agents** ▪ May increase serum **digoxin** levels ▪ Increases blood levels and risk of toxicity from **lithium** ▪ Increased risk of hypersensitivity reactions with **allopurinol.**

ROUTE AND DOSAGE

▪ **PO (Adults):** 10 mg once daily initially, may be increased as required. Usual range 20–40 mg/day. Doses as high as 80 mg have been used.

AVAILABILITY

▪ *Tablets:* 10 mg, 20 mg.

TIME/ACTION PROFILE
(antihypertensive effect)

	ONSET	PEAK	DURATION
PO	1 hr	2–6 hr	24 hr

F

*Underlines indicate most frequent; **CAPITALS** indicate life-threatening.

NURSING IMPLICATIONS

ASSESSMENT

▫ Monitor blood pressure and pulse frequently during initial dosage adjustment and periodically throughout course of therapy. Notify physician of significant changes.

▪ **Lab Test Considerations:** Monitor BUN, creatinine, and electrolyte levels periodically. Serum potassium may be increased, and BUN and creatine transiently increased while sodium levels may be decreased.

POTENTIAL NURSING DIAGNOSES

▪ Cardiac output, decreased (indications, side effects).

▪ Knowledge deficit related to medication regimen (patient/family teaching).

▪ Noncompliance (patient/family teaching).

IMPLEMENTATION

▪ **PO:** Precipitous drop in blood pressure following first dose may occur. Discontinuing diuretic therapy 2–3 days prior to initiation of fosinopril may decrease risk of hypotension. Resume diuretics if blood pressure is not controlled with fosinopril.

PATIENT/FAMILY TEACHING

▫ Instruct patient to take fosinopril exactly as directed, even if feeling better. Missed doses should be taken as soon as remembered but not if almost time for next dose. Do not double doses. Medication controls but does not cure hypertension. Caution patients not to discontinue fosinopril therapy unless directed by the physician.

▫ Encourage patient to comply with additional interventions for hypertension (weight reduction, smoking cessation, moderation of alcohol consumption, regular exercise, and stress management).

▫ Instruct patient and family on proper technique for blood pressure monitoring. Advise them to check blood pressure at least weekly and report significant changes to physician.

▫ Caution patient to avoid salt substitutes or foods containing high levels of potassium or sodium unless directed by physician (see Appendix K).

▫ Caution patient to change positions slowly to minimize orthostatic hypotension, particularly after initial dose. Patients should also be advised that exercising or hot weather may increase hypotensive effects.

▫ Advise patient to consult physician or pharmacist before taking any over-the-counter medications, especially cold remedies. Patients should also avoid excessive amounts of tea, coffee, or cola.

▫ May cause dizziness. Caution patient to avoid driving and other activities requiring alertness until response to medication is known.

▫ Advise patient to inform physician or dentist of medication regimen prior to treatment or surgery.

▫ Instruct patient to notify physician if rash, mouth sores, sore throat, fever, swelling of hands or feet, irregular heart beat, chest pain, dry cough, swelling of face, eyes, lips, or tongue, or difficulty breathing occurs or if taste impairment persists.

▫ Emphasize the importance of follow-up examinations to monitor progress.

EVALUATION

Effectiveness of therapy can be demonstrated by: ▪ Decrease in blood pressure without appearance of side effects.

FUROSEMIDE
(fur-**oh**-se-mide)
{Apo-Furosemide}, {Furoside}, Lasix, Myrosemide, {Novosemide}, {Uritol}

CLASSIFICATION(S):
Diuretic (loop)
Pregnancy Category C

{} = Available in Canada only.

INDICATIONS

- Management of: □ Edema secondary to congestive heart failure □ Hepatic or renal disease ■ Used alone or in combination with antihypertensives in the treatment of hypertension ■ Management of hypercalcemia of malignancy.

ACTION

- Inhibits the reabsorption of sodium and chloride from the loop of Henle and distal renal tubule ■ Increases renal excretion of water, sodium, chloride, magnesium, hydrogen, and calcium ■ May have renal and peripheral vasodilatory effects ■ Effectiveness persists in impaired renal function. **Therapeutic Effects:** ■ Diuresis and subsequent mobilization of excess fluid (edema, pleural effusions) ■ Lowers blood pressure.

PHARMACOKINETICS

Absorption: Absorbed from the GI tract (60–75%) following oral administration. Also absorbed from IM sites.
Distribution: Distribution not known. Crosses the placenta and enters breast milk.
Metabolism and Excretion: Some is metabolized by the liver (30–40%). Some nonhepatic metabolism and some renal excretion as unchanged drug.
Half-life: 30–60 min (increased in renal impairment and neonates, markedly increased in hepatic impairment).

CONTRAINDICATIONS AND PRECAUTIONS

Contraindicated in: ■ Hypersensitivity ■ Cross-sensitivity with thiazides and sulfonamides may exist ■ Pregnancy or lactation.
Use Cautiously in: ■ Severe liver disease ■ Electrolyte depletion ■ Diabetes mellitus ■ Anuria or increasing azotemia.

ADVERSE REACTIONS AND SIDE EFFECTS*

CNS: dizziness, headache, encephalopathy.
EENT: hearing loss, tinnitus.

CV: hypotension.
GI: nausea, vomiting, diarrhea, constipation.
GU: frequency.
Derm: rashes, photosensitivity.
Endo: hyperglycemia.
F and E: <u>metabolic alkalosis</u>, <u>hypovolemia</u>, <u>dehydration</u>, <u>hyponatremia</u>, <u>hypokalemia</u>, <u>hypochloremia</u>, <u>hypomagnesemia</u>.
Hemat: blood dyscrasias.
Metab: hyperuricemia.
MS: muscle cramps.
Misc: increased BUN.

INTERACTIONS

Drug–Drug: ■ Additive hypotension with **antihypertensives** or **nitrates** ■ Additive hypokalemia with other **diuretics, mezlocillin, piperacillin, amphotericin B,** and **glucocorticoids** ■ Hypokalemia may increase **cardiac glycoside** toxicity ■ Decreases **lithium** excretion, may cause toxicity ■ Increased risk of ototoxicity with **aminoglycosides** ■ May increase the effectiveness of **oral anticoagulants**.

ROUTE AND DOSAGE

- **PO, IM, IV (Adults):** 20–80 mg/day initially (up to 600 mg may be necessary; doses up to 1 g/day have been used in CHF and renal failure). When maintenance dose is determined, dose may be given every other day or 2–3 times weekly.
- **PO, IM, IV (Children):** 1–2 mg/kg/day initially (up to 6 mg/kg/day); may be increased at 6–8 hr intervals.

AVAILABILITY

- **Tablets:** 20 mg, 40 mg, 80 mg ■ **Oral solution:** 40 mg/5 ml ■ **Injection:** 10 mg/ml.

TIME/ACTION PROFILE (diuretic effect)

	ONSET	PEAK	DURATION
PO	30–60 min	1–2 hr	6–8 hr
IM	10–30 min	UK	4–8 hr
IV	5 min	30 min	2 hr

F

*Underlines indicate most frequent; **CAPITALS** indicate life-threatening.

NURSING IMPLICATIONS

Assessment

◻ Assess fluid status throughout therapy. Monitor daily weight, intake and output ratios, amount and location of edema, lung sounds, skin turgor, and mucous membranes. Notify physician if thirst, dry mouth, lethargy, weakness, hypotension, or oliguria occur.

◻ Monitor blood pressure and pulse before and during administration.

◻ Assess patients receiving cardiac glycosides for anorexia, nausea, vomiting, muscle cramps, paresthesia, confusion. Patients taking cardiac glycosides are at increased risk of digitalis toxicity because of the potassium-depleting effect of the diuretic.

◻ Assess patient for tinnitus and hearing loss. Audiometry is recommended for patients receiving prolonged therapy. Hearing loss is most common following rapid or high-dose IV administration in patients with decreased renal function or those taking other ototoxic drugs.

◻ Assess for allergy to sulfonamides.

▪ **Lab Test Considerations:** Monitor electrolytes, renal and hepatic function, glucose, and uric acid prior to and periodically throughout course of therapy. May cause decreased electrolyte levels (especially potassium). May cause elevated blood glucose, BUN, and uric acid levels.

Potential Nursing Diagnoses

▪ Fluid volume excess (indications).
▪ Fluid volume deficit (side effects).
▪ Knowledge deficit related to medication regimen (patient/family teaching).

Implementation

▪ **General Info:** Administer medication in the morning to prevent disruption of sleep cycle.

◻ Do not administer discolored solution or tablets.

▪ **PO:** Administer with food or milk to minimize gastric irritation. Tablets may be crushed if patient has difficulty swallowing.

▪ **Direct IV:** Administer each 20 mg slowly over 1–2 min.

▪ **Intermittent Infusion:** Dilute large doses in D5W, D10W, D20W, D5/0.9% NaCl, D5/LR, 0.9% NaCl, 3% NaCl, ⅙ M sodium lactate, or lactated Ringer's solution. Use reconstituted solution within 24 hr.

▪ *Rate:* Administer through Y-tubing or 3-way stopcock at a rate not to exceed 4 mg/min in adults to prevent ototoxicity. Use an infusion pump to ensure accurate dosage.

▪ **Syringe Compatibility:** ▪ bleomycin ▪ cisplatin ▪ cyclophosphamide ▪ fluorouracil ▪ heparin ▪ leucovorin calcium ▪ methotrexate ▪ mitomycin ▪ vinblastine ▪ vincristine.

▪ **Syringe Incompatibility:** ▪ doxapram ▪ doxorubicin ▪ droperidol ▪ metoclopramide ▪ milrinone.

▪ **Y-Site Compatibility:** ▪ amikacin ▪ bleomycin ▪ cisplatin ▪ cyclophosphamide ▪ famotidine ▪ fludarabine ▪ fluorouracil ▪ foscarnet ▪ heparin ▪ hydrocortisone sodium succinate ▪ kanamycin ▪ leucovorin calcium ▪ methotrexate ▪ mitomycin ▪ potassium chloride ▪ tobramycin ▪ tolazoline ▪ vitamin B complex with C.

▪ **Y-Site Incompatibility:** ▪ doxorubicin ▪ droperidol ▪ esmolol ▪ gentamicin ▪ hydralazine ▪ metoclopramide ▪ milrinone ▪ morphine ▪ netilmicin ▪ ondansetron ▪ quinidine gluconate ▪ vinblastine ▪ vincristine.

Patient/Family Teaching

▪ **General Info:** Instruct patient to take furosemide exactly as directed. Missed doses should be taken as soon as remembered; do not double doses.

◻ Caution patient to make position changes slowly to minimize orthostatic hypotension. Caution patient that the use of alcohol, exercise during hot weather, or standing for long periods during therapy may enhance orthostatic hypotension.

◻ Instruct patient to consult physician regarding a diet high in potassium (see Appendix K).

- Caution patient to use sunscreen and protective clothing to prevent photosensitivity reactions.
- Advise patient to consult physician or pharmacist before taking over-the-counter medication concurrently with this therapy.
- Instruct patient to notify physician or dentist of medication regimen prior to treatment or surgery.
- Advise patient to contact physician immediately if muscle weakness, cramps, nausea, dizziness, numbness or tingling of extremities occur.
- Emphasize the importance of routine follow-up examinations.
- **Hypertension:** Advise patients on antihypertensive regimen to continue taking medication even if feeling better. Furosemide controls but does not cure hypertension.
- Reinforce the need to continue additional therapies for hypertension (weight loss, restricted sodium intake, stress reduction, regular exercise, moderation of alcohol consumption, cessation of smoking).

EVALUATION

Effectiveness of therapy can be demonstrated by: ▪ Increase in urinary output □ Decrease in edema ▪ Decrease in blood pressure ▪ Decrease in serum calcium when used to manage hypercalcemia.

GALLAMINE
(**gal**-a-meen)
Flaxedil

CLASSIFICATION(S):
Neuromuscular blocking agent
(nondepolarizing)
Pregnancy Category C

INDICATIONS

▪ Production of skeletal muscle paralysis after induction of anesthesia.

ACTION

▪ Prevents neuromuscular transmission

by blocking the effect of acetylcholine at the myoneural junction. **Therapeutic Effect:** ▪ Skeletal muscle paralysis.

PHARMACOKINETICS

Absorption: Following IV administration absorption is essentially complete.
Distribution: Distributes into extracellular space. Crosses the placenta.
Metabolism and Excretion: Excreted almost entirely unchanged by the kidneys.
Half-life: 2.5 hr.

CONTRAINDICATIONS AND PRECAUTIONS

Contraindicated in: ▪ Hypersensitivity ▪ Hypersensitivity to iodides or bisulfites.
Use Cautiously in: ▪ History of pulmonary disease ▪ Renal or liver impairment ▪ Elderly or debilitated patients ▪ Electrolyte disturbances ▪ Fractures or muscular spasm ▪ Children weighing <5 kg.
Extreme Caution in: Myasthenia gravis or myasthenic syndrome.

ADVERSE REACTIONS AND SIDE EFFECTS*

CV: tachycardia, hypertension.
Resp: wheezing, increased bronchial secretions.
Derm: skin flush, erythema, pruritus, urticaria.
Misc: allergic reactions, including ANAPHYLAXIS.

INTERACTIONS

Drug–Drug: ▪ Intensity and duration of paralysis may be prolonged by pretreatment with **succinylcholine, general anesthesia** (dosage reduction may be necessary), **aminoglycoside antibiotics, polymyxin B, colistin, clindamycin, lidocaine, quinidine, procainamide, beta-adrenergic blocking agents, potassium-losing diuretics,** and **magnesium** ▪ Additive respiratory depression with **narcotic analgesics** ▪ Neuromuscular blockade may be diminished by **azathioprine** or reversed by **calcium salts.**

*Underlines indicate most frequent; **CAPITALS** indicate life-threatening.

ROUTE AND DOSAGE

- **IV (Adults and Children):** 1 mg/kg (not to exceed 100 mg/dose), then 0.5–1 mg/kg may be given 30–40 min later if needed during prolonged procedures.

AVAILABILITY

- *Injection:* 20 mg/ml.

TIME/ACTION PROFILE (muscle relaxation)

	ONSET	PEAK	DURATION
IV	1–2 min	3–5 min	15–30 min

NURSING IMPLICATIONS

ASSESSMENT

- Assess respiratory status continuously throughout gallamine therapy. Gallamine should be used only by individuals experienced in endotracheal intubation; equipment for this procedure should be readily available.
- Neuromuscular response to gallamine should be monitored with a peripheral nerve stimulator intraoperatively. Paralysis is initially selective and usually occurs sequentially in the following muscles: levator muscles of eyelids, muscles of mastication, limb muscles, abdominal muscles, muscles of the glottis, intercostal muscles, and the diaphragm. Recovery of muscle function usually occurs in reverse order.
- Monitor heart rate and ECG throughout therapy. Tachycardia caused by gallamine occurs after doses of 500 mcg/kg. This reaches a maximum within 3 min and then declines gradually.
- Observe the patient for residual muscle weakness and respiratory distress during the recovery period.
- **Toxicity and Overdose:** If overdose occurs, use peripheral nerve stimulator to determine the degree of neuro-

muscular blockade. Maintain airway patency and ventilation until recovery of normal respirations occur.

- Administration of anticholinesterase agents (edrophonium, neostigmine, pyridostigmine) may be used to antagonize the action of gallamine. Atropine is usually administered prior to or concurrently with anticholinesterase agents to counteract the muscarinic effects.
- Administration of fluids and vasopressors may be necessary to treat severe hypotension or shock.

POTENTIAL NURSING DIAGNOSES

- Breathing pattern, ineffective (indications).
- Communication, impaired verbal (side effects).
- Fear (patient/family teaching).

IMPLEMENTATION

- **General Info:** Dose is titrated to patient response.
- Gallamine has no effect on consciousness or the pain threshold. Adequate anesthesia/analgesia should *always* be used when gallamine is used as an adjunct to surgical procedures.
- Should be refrigerated during storage.
- **Direct IV:** Administer each single dose undiluted as a bolus over 30–60 sec.
- **Syringe Incompatibility:** ■ barbiturates ■ meperidine.

PATIENT/FAMILY TEACHING

- Explain all procedures to patient receiving gallamine therapy without anesthesia, as consciousness is not affected by gallamine alone.
- Reassure patient that communication abilities will return as the medication wears off.

EVALUATION

Effectiveness of therapy can be demonstrated by: ■ Adequate suppression of the twitch response when tested with peripheral nerve stimulation and subsequent muscle paralysis.

GALLIUM NITRATE
(**gal**-ee-yum **nye**-trate)
Ganite

CLASSIFICATION(S):
Electrolyte modifier (hypocalce-mic agent)
Pregnancy Category C

INDICATIONS
▪ Management of cancer-related hyper-calcemia.

ACTION
▪ Inhibits calcium resorption from bone. **Therapeutic Effect:** ▪ Lowering of serum calcium levels.

PHARMACOKINETICS
Absorption: Administered IV only, resulting in complete bioavailability.
Distribution: Distribution not known.
Metabolism and Excretion: Mostly excreted unchanged by the kidneys.
Half-life: UK.

CONTRAINDICATIONS AND PRECAUTIONS
Contraindicated in: ▪ Severe renal impairment (serum creatinine >2.5 mg%).
Use Cautiously in: ▪ Renal impairment ▪ Pregnancy, lactation, or children (safety not established).

ADVERSE REACTIONS AND SIDE EFFECTS*
EENT: hearing loss, optic neuritis, visual impairment.
F and E: hypocalcemia, hypophosphatemia.
GU: renal toxicity.

INTERACTIONS
Drug–Drug: ▪ Increased risk of nephrotoxicity with other **nephrotoxic agents,** including **amphotericin B** and **aminoglycosides** (discontinue gallium).

ROUTE AND DOSAGE
▪ **IV (Adults):** 100–200 mg/m^2 daily for 5 days.

AVAILABILITY
▪ *Injection:* 25 mg/ml.

TIME/ACTION PROFILE (effect on serum calcium)

	ONSET	PEAK	DURATION
IV	within 24 hr	5 days	7.5 days

NURSING IMPLICATIONS
ASSESSMENT
▫ Monitor symptoms of hypercalcemia (nausea, vomiting, anorexia, lethargy, fatigue, weakness, constipation, thirst, dehydration, impaired mental status, and cardiac arrhythmias).
▫ Observe patient carefully for evidence of hypocalcemia (paresthesia, muscle twitching, laryngospasm, colic, cardiac arrhythmias, and Chvostek's or Trousseau's sign). Protect symptomatic patients by elevating and padding side rails; keep bed in low position. If hypocalcemia occurs, stop gallium nitrate therapy. Temporary calcium therapy may be needed.
▫ If patient requires other nephrotoxic drugs, discontinue gallium nitrate and continue hydration for several days following administration of potentially nephrotoxic drug. Monitor serum creatinine and urine output during and after this period.
▪ **Lab Test Considerations:** Monitor BUN and serum creatinine prior to and frequently throughout course of therapy. Gallium nitrate therapy should be discontinued if serum creatinine is >2.5 mg/dl.
▫ Monitor serum calcium daily and serum phosphate levels twice weekly to determine effectiveness of therapy. Oral phosphate therapy may be needed for hypophosphatemia. May also cause decreased serum bicarbonate concentrations.

POTENTIAL NURSING DIAGNOSES
▪ Injury, high risk for (indications).
▪ Urinary elimination, altered patterns of (adverse reactions).

Underlines indicate most frequent; CAPITALS indicate life-threatening.

IMPLEMENTATION

▪ **General Info:** Gallium nitrate should be instituted after adequate hydration with IV saline has been established. Saline promotes the renal excretion of calcium. Diuretics may also be used following correction of hypovolemia. Adequate hydration and urine output should be maintained at 2000 mg/day throughout therapy.

▪ **Continuous Infusion:** Dilute daily dose in 1000 ml of 0.9% NaCl or D5W. Solution is stable for 48 hr at room temperature and 7 days if refrigerated.

▪ *Rate:* Infuse over 24 hr.

PATIENT/FAMILY TEACHING

▢ Encourage patient to comply with physician's diet recommendations. Diet should contain adequate amounts of calcium and vitamin D (see Appendix K).

▢ Emphasize need for keeping follow-up appointments to monitor progress, even after medication is discontinued, in order to detect relapse.

EVALUATION

Effectiveness of therapy can be demonstrated by: ▪ Lowered serum calcium levels in patients with cancer-related hypercalcemia.

GANCICLOVIR
(gan-**sye**-kloe-vir)
Cytovene

CLASSIFICATION(S):
Antiviral
Pregnancy Category C

INDICATIONS

▪ Treatment of cytomegalovirus (CMV) retinitis in immunocompromised patients, including HIV-infected patients ▪ Prevention of CMV infection in transplant patients at risk.

ACTION

▪ CMV virus converts ganciclovir to its active form (ganciclovir phosphate) inside host cell, where it inhibits viral DNA polymerase. **Therapeutic Effect:** ▪ Antiviral effect directed preferentially against CMV-infected cells.

PHARMACOKINETICS

Absorption: Administered IV only, resulting in complete bioavailability.
Distribution: Enters the CSF. Remainder of distribution not known.
Metabolism and Excretion: 90% excreted unchanged by the kidneys.
Half-life: 2.9 hr (increased in renal impairment).

CONTRAINDICATIONS AND PRECAUTIONS

Contraindicated in: ▪ Hypersensitivity to ganciclovir or acyclovir.
Use Cautiously in: ▪ Renal impairment (dosage reduction required if creatinine clearance <80 ml/min) ▪ Pregnancy, lactation, or children (safety not established) ▪ Elderly patients (dosage reduction recommended) ▪ Bone marrow depression ▪ Immunosuppression.

ADVERSE REACTIONS AND SIDE EFFECTS*

CNS: malaise, abnormal dreams, confusion, dizziness, headache, coma, nervousness, headache, drowsiness.
EENT: retinal detachment.
Resp: dyspnea.
CV: arrhythmias, hypertension, hypotension, edema.
GI: nausea, vomiting, gastric bleeding, abdominal pain, increased liver enzymes.
GU: hematuria, gonadal suppression.
Derm: rash, alopecia, pruritus, urticaria.
Endo: hypoglycemia.
Hemat: <u>neutropenia</u>, <u>thrombocytopenia</u>, anemia, eosinophilia.
Local: pain, phlebitis at IV site.
Neuro: tremor, ataxia.
Misc: fever.

INTERACTIONS

Drug–Drug: ▪ Increased risk of bone marrow depression with **antineoplastic**

---

*<u>Underlines</u> indicate most frequent; **CAPITALS** indicate life-threatening.

agents, radiation therapy, or zidovudine ▪ Toxicity may be increased by probenecid ▪ Increased risk of seizures with imepenem/cilastatin.

ROUTE AND DOSAGE

CMV Treatment
▪ **IV (Adults):** 5 mg/kg q 12 hr for 14–21 days initially, then 5 mg/kg/day or 6 mg/kg for 5 days of each week. If progression occurs, increase to twice daily regimen.
▪ **Intravitreal (Adults):** 200 mcg once weekly.

CMV Prevention
▪ **IV (Adults):** 5 mg/kg q 12 hr for 7–14 days, then 5 mg/kg/day or 6 mg/kg for 5 days of each week.

AVAILABILITY
▪ *Injection:* 500 mg/vial.

TIME/ACTION PROFILE (blood levels)

	ONSET	PEAK
IV	rapid	end of infusion

NURSING IMPLICATIONS

ASSESSMENT
☐ Diagnosis of CMV retinitis should be determined by ophthalmoscopy prior to treatment with ganciclovir.
☐ Culture for CMV (urine, blood, throat) may be taken prior to administration. However, a negative CMV culture does not rule out CMV retinitis.
▪ **Lab Test Considerations:** Monitor neutrophil and platelet count at least every 2 days during bid therapy and weekly thereafter. Granulocytopenia usually occurs during the first 2 wk of treatment but may occur anytime during therapy. Do not administer if neutrophil count <500/mm³ or platelet count <25,000/mm³. Recovery begins within 3–7 days of discontinuation of therapy.
☐ Monitor serum creatinine at least once every 2 wk throughout therapy.
☐ May cause abnormal liver function test values.
☐ May cause a decrease in blood glucose.

POTENTIAL NURSING DIAGNOSES
▪ Infection, high risk for (indications, patient/family teaching).
▪ Knowledge deficit related to medication regimen (patient/family teaching).

IMPLEMENTATION
▪ **General Info:** Solution should be prepared in a biologic cabinet. Wear gloves, gown, and mask while handling medication. Discard IV equipment in specially designated containers (see Appendix I).
☐ Do not administer SC or IM, as severe tissue irritation may result.
▪ **IV:** Observe infusion site for phlebitis. Rotate infusion site to prevent phlebitis.
▪ **Intermittent Infusion:** Reconstitute 500 mg with 10 ml of Sterile Water for Injection for a concentration of 50 mg/ml. Do not reconstitute with bacteriostatic water with parabens; precipitation will occur. Shake well to dissolve completely. Discard vial if particulate matter or discoloration occurs. Reconstituted solution is stable for 12 hr at room temperature; do not refrigerate.
☐ Dilute in 100 ml of D5W, 0.9% NaCl, Ringer's or lactated Ringer's solution for a concentration not to exceed 10 mg/ml. Once diluted for infusion, solution should be used within 24 hr. Refrigerate but do not freeze.
▪ *Rate:* Administer slowly, via infusion pump, over 1 hr. Rapid administration may increase toxicity.
▪ **Y-Site Compatibility:** ▪ enalaprilat ▪ fluconazole.
▪ **Y-Site Incompatibility:** ▪ fludarabine ▪ foscarnet ▪ ondansetron ▪ sargramostim.

PATIENT/FAMILY TEACHING
☐ Inform patient that ganciclovir is not a cure for CMV retinitis. Progression of retinitis may continue in immunocompromised patients during and following therapy. Advise patients to have regular ophthalmic examinations at least every 6 wk. Duration of therapy for CMV prevention is

G

based on the duration and degree of immunosuppression.

□ Advise patient that ganciclovir may have teratogenic effects. A nonhormonal method of contraception should be used during and for at least 90 days following therapy.

□ Emphasize the importance of frequent follow-up examinations to monitor blood counts.

EVALUATION

Effectiveness of therapy can be demonstrated by: ▪ Resolution of the symptoms of CMV retinitis in immunocompromised patients ▪ Prevention of CMV retinitis in transplant patients at risk.

GEMFIBROZIL
(gem-**fye**-broe-zil)
Lopid

CLASSIFICATION(S):
Lipid-lowering agent
Pregnancy Category B

INDICATIONS
▪ Adjunct to dietary therapy in the management of hyperlipidemias associated with high triglyceride levels.

ACTION
▪ Inhibits peripheral lipolysis ▪ Decreases triglyceride (very low-density lipoprotein [VLDL]) production by the liver ▪ Decreases production of the triglyceride carrier protein ▪ Increases high-density lipoproteins (HDL). **Therapeutic Effect:** ▪ Decreased plasma triglycerides and increased HDL.

PHARMACOKINETICS
Absorption: Well absorbed following oral administration.
Distribution: Distribution not known.
Metabolism and Excretion: Some metabolism by the liver, 70% excreted by the kidneys (mostly unchanged) 6% excreted in feces.
Half-life: 1.3–1.5 hr.

CONTRAINDICATIONS AND PRECAUTIONS
Contraindicated in: ▪ Hypersensitivity ▪ Primary biliary cirrhosis.
Use Cautiously in: ▪ Gallbladder disease ▪ Liver disease ▪ Severe renal impairment ▪ Pregnancy, lactation, or children (safety not established).

ADVERSE REACTIONS AND SIDE EFFECTS*
CNS: headache, dizziness.
EENT: blurred vision.
GI: <u>abdominal pain</u>, <u>epigastric pain</u>, heartburn, gallstones, <u>diarrhea</u>, nausea, vomiting, flatulence.
Derm: rashes, urticaria, alopecia.
Hemat: leukopenia, anemia.
MS: myositis.

INTERACTIONS
Drug–Drug: ▪ May increase the effect of **oral anticoagulants** ▪ **Thiazide diuretics, methyldopa,** or **estrogens** may decrease the response to gemfibrozil ▪ Concurrent use with lovastatin may increase the risk of rhabdomyolysis.

ROUTE AND DOSAGE
▪ **PO (Adults):** 600 mg twice daily 30 min before breakfast and dinner.

AVAILABILITY
▪ *Capsules:* 300 mg, 600 mg.

TIME/ACTION PROFILE
(triglyceride—VLDL lowering effect)

	ONSET	PEAK	DURATION
PO	2–5 days	4 wk	several mos

NURSING IMPLICATIONS
ASSESSMENT
□ Obtain patient's diet history, especially regarding fat and alcohol consumption.
▪ **Lab Test Considerations:** Serum triglyceride and cholesterol levels should be monitored closely. LDL and VLDL levels should be assessed prior to and periodically throughout therapy. Medication should be dis-

continued if paradoxic increase in lipid levels occurs.

□ Liver function tests should be assessed prior to and periodically throughout therapy. May cause an increase in alkaline phosphatase, CPK, LDH, AST (SGOT), and ALT (SGPT).

□ CBC and electrolytes should be evaluated every 3–6 mo and then yearly throughout course of therapy. May cause mild decrease in hemoglobin, hematocrit, and leukocyte counts. May cause a decrease in serum potassium concentrations.

□ May cause slight increase in serum glucose.

POTENTIAL NURSING DIAGNOSES

- Knowledge deficit related to medication regimen (patient/family teaching).
- Noncompliance (patient/family teaching).

IMPLEMENTATION

- **PO:** Administer 30 min before breakfast or dinner.

PATIENT/FAMILY TEACHING

□ Instruct patient to take medication exactly as directed, not to skip doses or double up on missed doses. If a dose is missed, take as soon as remembered unless almost time for next dose.

□ Advise patient that this medication should be used in conjunction with dietary restrictions (fat, cholesterol, carbohydrates, alcohol), exercise, and cessation of smoking.

□ Instruct patient to notify physician promptly if any of the following symptoms occur: severe stomach pains with nausea and vomiting, fever, chills, sore throat. Physician should also be notified if rash, diarrhea, muscle cramping, general abdominal discomfort, or persistent flatulence occurs.

EVALUATION

Effectiveness of therapy can be demonstrated by: ■ Decrease in serum triglyceride and cholesterol levels and im-

proved high-density lipoprotein (HDL) to total cholesterol ratios. If response is not seen within 3 mo, medication is usually discontinued.

GENTAMICIN
(jen-ta-**mye**-sin)
{Alcomicin}, {Cidomycin}, Garamycin, Genoptic, Gentafair, Gentak, Gentrasul, G-Mycon, Jenamicin, Ocu-Mycin, Spectro-Genta

CLASSIFICATION(S):
Anti-infective (aminoglycoside)
Pregnancy Category C

INDICATIONS

■ **IM, IV:** Treatment of gram-negative bacillary infections and infections due to staphylococci when penicillins or other less toxic drugs are contraindicated. Especially useful in the following serious gram-negative bacillary infections: □ Bone infections □ CNS infections (intrathecal administration required) □ Respiratory tract infections □ Skin and soft tissue infections □ Abdominal infections □ Complicated urinary tract infections □ Endocarditis □ Septicemia ■ **IM, IV:** Part of a regimen for endocarditis prophylaxis in certain patient populations ■ **Top, Ophth:** Treatment of localized infections.

ACTION

■ Inhibits protein synthesis in bacteria at the level of the 30S ribosome. **Therapeutic Effect:** ■ Bactericidal action against susceptible bacteria. **Spectrum:** ■ *Pseudomonas aeruginosa* ■ *Klebsiella pneumoniae* ■ *Escherichia coli* ■ *Serratia* ■ *Acenitobacter* ■ *Staphlococcus aureus* ■ In the treatment of enterococcal infections, synergy with a penicillin is required.

PHARMACOKINETICS

Absorption: Well absorbed after IM administration. Minimal systemic ab-

G

sorption following topical, intrathecal, or intraventricular administration.

Distribution: Widely distributed in extracellular fluids following IM or IV administration. Crosses the placenta. Poor penetration into CSF.

Metabolism and Excretion: Excretion is mainly renal (>90%). Dosage adjustments are required for any decrease in renal function. Minimal amounts metabolized by the liver.

Half-life: 2–3 hr (increased in renal impairment).

CONTRAINDICATIONS AND PRECAUTIONS

Contraindicated in: ▪ Hypersensitivity ▪ Cross-sensitivity with other aminoglycosides may exist ▪ Some products contain bisulfites and should be avoided in patients with known intolerance.

Use Cautiously in: ▪ Renal impairment of any kind (dosage adjustments required) ▪ Pregnancy and lactation (safety not established) ▪ Neuromuscular diseases, such as myasthenia gravis.

ADVERSE REACTIONS AND SIDE EFFECTS*

EENT: <u>ototoxicity</u> (vestibular and cochlear).

GU: <u>nephrotoxicity</u>.

Neuro: enhanced neuromuscular blockade.

Misc: hypersensitivity reactions, superinfection.

INTERACTIONS

Drug–Drug: ▪ Inactivated by **penicillins** when coadministered to patients with renal insufficiency ▪ Possible respiratory paralysis after inhalation anesthetics (**ether, cyclopropane, halothane,** or **nitrous oxide**) or **neuromuscular blockers** (**atracurium, tubocurarine, gallamine, succinylcholine, decamethonium**) ▪ Additive possibility of neuromuscular blockade with other **aminoglycoside antibiotics** ▪ Increased incidence of ototoxicity with **loop diuretics** (**ethacrynic acid, furosemide**)

▪ Incidence of nephrotoxicity may be increased with other potentially **nephrotoxic drugs** (**cisplatin**).

ROUTE AND DOSAGE

All doses after initial loading dose should be determined by renal function/blood levels.

▪ **IM, IV (Adults):** 3–5 mg/kg/day in divided doses q 8 hr. Doses as low as 3 mg/kg/day given once daily or in divided doses q 12 hr have been used for uncomplicated urinary tract infections.

▪ **IM, IV (Children):** 6–7.5 mg/kg/day in divided doses q 8 hr.

▪ **IM, IV (Infants and Neonates):** 2.5 mg/kg q 8–16 hr.

▪ **IM, IV (Premature Infants, Neonates <1 wk):** 2.5 mg/kg q 12–24 hr.

▪ **Top (Adults and Children):** Apply cream or ointment to cleansed area 3–4 times daily.

▪ **Ophth (Adults and Children):** 1–2 drops of ophthalmic solution q 2–4 hr or ophthalmic ointment 2–3 times daily.

▪ **Intrathecal (Adults):** 4–8 mg/day as a single dose.

▪ **Intrathecal (Children and Infants >3 mo):** 1–2 mg/day as a single dose.

AVAILABILITY

▪ *Injection:* 2 mg/ml (for intrathecal use), 10 mg/ml, 40 mg/ml ▪ *Ophthalmic solution:* 0.3% ▪ *Ophthalmic ointment:* 0.3% ▪ *Topical ointment:* 0.1% ▪ *Topical cream:* 0.1%.

TIME/ACTION PROFILE (blood levels)

	ONSET	PEAK
IM	rapid	30–90 min
IV	rapid	end of infusion

NURSING IMPLICATIONS

ASSESSMENT

▫ Assess patient for infection (vital signs; appearance of wound, sputum, urine, and stool; WBC) at beginning and throughout course of therapy.

---

*<u>Underlines</u> indicate most frequent; **CAPITALS** indicate life-threatening.

□ Obtain specimens for culture and sensitivity prior to initiating therapy. First dose may be given before receiving results.

□ Evaluate eighth cranial nerve function by audiometry prior to and throughout course of therapy. Hearing loss is usually in the high-frequency range. Prompt recognition and intervention is essential in preventing permanent damage. Also monitor for vestibular dysfunction (vertigo, ataxia, nausea, vomiting). Eighth cranial nerve dysfunction is associated with persistently elevated peak gentamicin levels.

□ Monitor intake and output and daily weight to assess hydration status and renal function.

□ Assess patient for signs of superinfections (fever, upper respiratory infection, vaginal itching or discharge, increasing malaise, diarrhea). Report to physician.

■ **Lab Test Considerations:** Monitor renal function by urinalysis, specific gravity, BUN, creatinine, and creatinine clearance prior to and throughout therapy.

□ May cause increased AST (SGOT), ALT (SGPT), LDH, bilirubin, and serum alkaline phosphatase levels.

□ May cause decreased serum calcium, magnesium, sodium, and potassium levels.

■ **Toxicity and Overdose:** Blood levels should be monitored periodically during therapy. Timing of blood levels is important in interpreting results. Draw blood for peak levels 30–60 min after IM injection and immediately after IV infusion is completed. Trough levels should be drawn just prior to next dose. Acceptable peak level is 4–12 mcg/ml; trough level should not exceed 2 mcg/ml.

POTENTIAL NURSING DIAGNOSES

■ Infection, high risk for (indications).
■ Sensory-perceptual alteration: auditory (side effects).

IMPLEMENTATION

■ **General Info:** Keep patient well hydrated (1500–2000 ml/day) during therapy.

□ Solution is colorless to slightly yellow. Do not use solution that is discolored or that contains a precipitate.

■ **IM:** IM administration should be deep into a well-developed muscle.

■ **Intermittent Infusion:** Dilute each dose of gentamicin in 50–200 ml of D5W, 0.9% NaCl, or Ringer's solution to provide a concentration not to exceed 1 mg/ml (0.1%). Also available in commercially mixed piggyback injections.

■ *Rate:* Infuse slowly over 30 min–2 hr. Flush IV line with D5W or 0.9% NaCl following administration.

■ **Y-Site Compatibility:** ■ acyclovir ■ atracurium ■ cyclophosphamide ■ enalaprilat ■ esmolol ■ famotidine ■ fluconazole ■ fludarabine ■ foscarnet ■ hydromorphone ■ insulin ■ labetalol ■ hydromorphone ■ magnesium sulfate ■ meperidine ■ morphine ■ multivitamins ■ ondansetron ■ pancuronium ■ vecuronium ■ vitamin B complex with C ■ zidovudine.

■ **Y-Site Incompatibility:** ■ furosemide ■ heparin ■ hetastarch.

■ **Additive Incompatibility:** □ Manufacturer recommends administering separately; do not admix. If aminoglycosides and penicillins or cephalosporins must be administered concurrently, administer in separate sites.

■ **Ophth:** See Appendix H for administration of ophthalmic preparations.

■ **Top:** Cleanse skin prior to application. Wear gloves during application.

PATIENT/FAMILY TEACHING

■ **General Info:** Instruct patient to report signs of hypersensitivity, tinnitus, vertigo, or hearing loss.

□ Patients with a history of rheumatic heart disease or valve replacement should be taught the importance of using antimicrobial prophylaxis before invasive medical or dental procedures.

■ **Top:** Instruct patient on correct technique for application.

EVALUATION
Clinical response to therapy can be evaluated by: ▪ Resolution of the signs and symptoms of infection. Length of time for complete resolution depends on the organism and site of infection ▪ Endocarditis prophylaxis.

GLUCAGON
(gloo-ka-gon)

CLASSIFICATION(S):
Hormone (pancreatic)
Pregnancy Category B

INDICATIONS

▪ Acute management of severe hypoglycemia when administration of glucose is not feasible ▪ Used to terminate insulin shock therapy in psychiatric patients ▪ Used to facilitate radiographic examination of the GI tract.

ACTION

▪ Stimulates hepatic production of glucose from glycogen stores (glycogenolysis) ▪ Relaxes the musculature of the GI tract ▪ Has positive inotropic and chronotropic effects. **Therapeutic Effects:** ▪ Increase in blood sugar ▪ Relaxation of GI musculature, facilitating radiographic examination.

PHARMACOKINETICS

Absorption: Well absorbed following IM and SC administration.
Distribution: Distribution not known.
Metabolism and Excretion: Extensively metabolized by the liver and kidneys.
Half-life: 3–10 min.

CONTRAINDICATIONS AND PRECAUTIONS

Contraindicated in: ▪ Hypersensitivity to beef or pork protein ▪ Diluent contains glycerin and phenol—avoid use in patients with hypersensitivities to these ingredients.

Use Cautiously in: ▪ History of insulinoma or pheochromocytoma.

ADVERSE REACTIONS AND SIDE EFFECTS*

GI: nausea, vomiting.
Misc: hypersensitivity reactions.

INTERACTIONS

Drug–Drug: ▪ Large doses may enhance the effect of **oral anticoagulants** ▪ Negates the response to **insulin** or **oral hypoglycemic** agents ▪ Hyperglycemic effect is intensified and prolonged by **epinephrine**.

ROUTE AND DOSAGE
1 mg = 1 USP unit.

Hypoglycemia, Terminating Insulin Shock
▪ IV, IM, SC (Adults): 0.5–1 mg; if no response, may repeat in 20 min.
▪ IV, IM, SC (Children): 25 mcg/kg; if no response, may repeat in 20 min.

Radiographic Examination of the GI Tract
▪ IV (Adults): 0.25–1 mg.

AVAILABILITY

▪ *Injection:* 1-mg vials, 10-mg vials.

TIME/ACTION PROFILE

	ONSET	PEAK	DURATION
IV, SC (hyperglycemic action)	5–20 min	30 min	1–2 hr
IV (effect on GI musculature)	1 min	UK	9–25 min

NURSING IMPLICATIONS

ASSESSMENT
▫ Assess patient for signs of hypoglycemia (sweating, hunger, weakness, headache, dizziness, tremor, irritability, tachycardia, anxiety) prior to and periodically during course of therapy.
▫ Assess neurologic status throughout course of therapy. Institute safety precautions to protect patient from injury caused by seizures, falling, or aspira-

---

*Underlines indicate most frequent; **CAPITALS** indicate life-threatening.

tion. For insulin shock therapy, 0.5–1 mg or more is administered after 1 hr of coma; patient usually awakens in 10–25 min. If no response occurs, repeat the dose. Feed patient orally as soon as possible after awakening.

□ Assess nutritional status. Patients who lack liver glycogen stores (as in starvation, chronic hypoglycemia, and adrenal insufficiency) will require administration of glucose instead of glucagon.

□ Assess for nausea and vomiting after administration of dose. Protect patients with depressed level of consciousness from aspiration by positioning on side; ensure that a suction unit is available. Notify physician if vomiting occurs; patient will require parenteral glucose to prevent recurrent hypoglycemia.

□ Monitor serum glucose levels to determine effectiveness of therapy. Use of bedside fingerstick blood glucose determination methods is recommended for rapid results. Follow-up lab results may be ordered to validate fingerstick values, but do not delay treatment while awaiting lab results as this could result in neurologic injury or death.

POTENTIAL NURSING DIAGNOSES

- Injury, high risk for (indications).
- Knowledge deficit related to medication regimen (patient/family teaching).
- Noncompliance (patient/family teaching).

IMPLEMENTATION

- **General Info:** May be given SC, IM, or IV. Reconstitute with diluent supplied in kit by manufacturer. Inspect solution prior to use; use only clear, water-like solution. Solution is stable for 48 hr if refrigerated, 24 hr at room temperature.
- □ Administer supplemental carbohydrates IV or orally to facilitate increase of serum glucose levels.
- **IV:** With doses >2 units (2 mg), use Sterile Water for Injection instead of diluent supplied by manufacturer.

Use immediately after reconstituting. Final concentration should not exceed 1 unit (1 mg/ml).

- **Direct IV:** Administer at a rate not exceeding 1 unit (1 mg) per min. May be administered through IV line containing D5W.
- □ May be given at the same time as a bolus of dextrose.
- **Additive Incompatibility:** ■ 0.9% NaCl ■ potassium chloride ■ calcium chloride.

PATIENT/FAMILY TEACHING

- □ Teach patient and family signs and symptoms of hypoglycemia. Instruct patient to take oral glucose as soon as symptoms of hypoglycemia occur— glucagon is reserved for episodes when patient is unable to swallow due to decreased level of consciousness.
- □ Instruct family on correct technique to prepare, draw up, and administer injection. Physician must be contacted immediately after each dose for orders regarding further therapy or adjustment of insulin dose or diet.
- □ Advise family that patient should receive oral glucose when alertness returns.
- □ Instruct family to position patient on side until fully alert. Explain that glucagon may cause nausea and vomiting. Aspiration may occur if patient vomits while lying on back.
- □ Instruct patient to check expiration date monthly and to replace outdated medication immediately.
- □ Review hypoglycemic medication regimen, diet, and exercise programs.
- □ Patients with diabetes mellitus should carry a source of sugar (such as a packet of sugar or candy) and identification describing disease process and treatment regimen at all times.

EVALUATION

Effectiveness of therapy can be demonstrated by: ■ Increase of serum glucose to normal levels with improved level of consciousness ■ Smooth muscle relaxation of the stomach, duodenum, and

G

small and large intestine in patients undergoing radiologic examination of the GI tract.

GLUTETHIMIDE
(gloo-teth-i-mide)
Doriglute

CLASSIFICATION(S):
Sedative/hypnotic (miscellaneous)
Schedule II
Pregnancy Category C

INDICATIONS
- Short-term (3–7 days) management of insomnia.

ACTION
- Produces generalized CNS depression similar to barbiturates ■ Has anticholinergic properties. **Therapeutic Effect:** ■ Relief of insomnia.

PHARMACOKINETICS
Absorption: Unpredictably absorbed.
Distribution: Widely distributed, concentrates in adipose tissue. Crosses the placenta well; enters breast milk in small amounts.
Metabolism and Excretion: Highly (>95%) metabolized by the liver.
Half-life: 10–12 hr.

CONTRAINDICATIONS AND PRECAUTIONS
Contraindicated in: ■ Hypersensitivity ■ Poorly controlled pain ■ Porphyria ■ Severe renal disease ■ Patients who have been addicted to drugs previously.
Use Cautiously in: ■ Prostatic hypertrophy ■ Ulcer disease ■ GI obstruction ■ Bladder neck obstruction ■ Glaucoma ■ Cardiac arrhythmias ■ Pregnancy, lactation, or children <12 yr (safety not established) ■ Elderly patients (dosage reduction recommended).

ADVERSE REACTIONS AND SIDE EFFECTS*
CNS: hangover, paradoxical excitation, headache, vertigo.
EENT: blurred vision.
GI: gastric irritation, nausea, hiccups, dry mouth, diarrhea, hepatitis.
Hemat: blood dyscrasias, porphyria.
Derm: rashes, exfoliative dermatitis.
Neuro: peripheral neuropathy.
Misc: hypersensitivity reactions, psychological dependence, physical dependence.

INTERACTIONS
Drug–Drug: ■ Additive CNS depression with other **CNS depressants,** including **alcohol, sedative/hypnotics, opioid analgesics, tricyclic antidepressants,** and **antihistamines** ■ Additive anticholinergic effects with **tricyclic antidepressants** ■ May decrease the effectiveness of **oral anticoagulants.**

ROUTE AND DOSAGE
- **PO (Adults):** 250–500 mg at bedtime, may repeat once (not to exceed 1 g/day).
- **PO (Elderly Patients):** 250 mcg (up to 500 mg) at bedtime.

AVAILABILITY
- *Tablets:* 500 mg.

TIME/ACTION PROFILE (hypnotic effect)

	ONSET	PEAK	DURATION
PO	30 min	UK	4–8 hr

NURSING IMPLICATIONS
ASSESSMENT
□ Assess mental status, sleep patterns, and potential for abuse prior to administering this medication. Prolonged use of greater than 1 wk may lead to decreased effectiveness and physical and psychological depen-

dence. Limit amount of drug available to the patient.

▫ Assess alertness at time of peak effect. Notify physician if desired sedation does not occur or if paradoxical reaction occurs.

▫ Assess patient for pain. Medicate as needed. Untreated pain decreases sedative effects.

POTENTIAL NURSING DIAGNOSES

▪ Sleep pattern disturbance (indications).

▪ Injury, high risk for (side effects).

IMPLEMENTATION

▪ **PO:** Before administering, reduce external stimuli and provide comfort measures to increase effectiveness of medication. Administer at least 4 hr before usual time of awakening to minimize daytime drowsiness.

▫ Protect patient from injury. Place bed side rails up. Assist with ambulation. Remove cigarettes from patients with hypnotic dose.

PATIENT/FAMILY TEACHING

▫ Instruct patient to take glutethimide exactly as directed. Do not take more than the amount prescribed because of the habit-forming potential. Not recommended for use longer than 1 wk. If used for 2 wk or longer, effectiveness may decrease and abrupt withdrawal may result in convulsions, tachycardia, hallucinations, increased dreaming, muscle cramps, nausea, or vomiting.

▫ May cause daytime drowsiness or dizziness. Advise patient to avoid driving or other activities requiring alertness until response to this medication is known.

▫ Caution patient to avoid concurrent use of alcohol or other CNS depressants.

▫ Advise patient to discontinue use and notify physician if skin rash occurs.

EVALUATION

Effectiveness of therapy can be demonstrated by: ▪ Relief of insomnia.

GLYCERIN
(gli-ser-in)
Babylax, Ophthalgan, Osmoglyn, Sani-Supp

CLASSIFICATION(S):
Laxative (osmotic), Diuretic, Antiglaucoma agent
Pregnancy Category C

INDICATIONS

▪ **Rect:** Treatment of constipation ▪ **PO:** Short-term reduction of intraocular pressure ▪ **Ophth:** Management of edema of the superficial layers of the cornea. **Unlabeled Use:** ▪ **PO:** Reduction of elevated intracranial pressure.

ACTION

▪ Draws water into the lumen of the colon ▪ Osmotically draws water from extravascular spaces, including the eye, into intravascular compartment. **Therapeutic Effects:** ▪ Relief of constipation ▪ Reduction of intraocular and intracranial pressure ▪ Reduced swelling of superficial layers of the cornea.

PHARMACOKINETICS

Absorption: Not significantly absorbed from colonic mucosa. Well absorbed following oral administration.

Distribution: Remains in the intravascular space.

Metabolism and Excretion: 80% metabolized by the liver, 10–20% metabolized by the kidneys.

Half-life: 30–45 min.

CONTRAINDICATIONS AND PRECAUTIONS

Contraindicated in: ▪ Hypersensitivity ▪ Hypersensitivity to ingredients in preparations (ophthalmic solution contains chlorobutanol).

Use Cautiously in: ▪ Cardiovascular disease ▪ Mental confusion ▪ Severe dehydration ▪ Diabetes mellitus ▪ Hypervolemia ▪ Renal disease ▪ Elderly patients (increased risk of dehydration).

ADVERSE REACTIONS AND SIDE EFFECTS*

CNS: confusion, headache, SEIZURES.
GI: nausea, vomiting, diarrhea.
F and E: dehydration.
Misc: thirst.

INTERACTIONS

Drug–Drug: ▪ Diuretics increase the intraocular pressure-lowering effects of glycerin.

ROUTE AND DOSAGE

Laxative

▪ **Rect (Adults and Children >6 yr):** 2–3 g as a suppository or 5–15 ml as an enema.
▪ **Rect (Children <6 yr):** 1–1.7 g as a suppository or 2–5 ml as an enema.

Reduction of Intraocular Pressure

▪ **PO (Adults):** 1–1.5 g/kg as a single dose, may be followed by 500 mg/kg q 6 hr.
▪ **PO (Children):** 1–1.5 g/kg as a single dose, may be followed by 500 mg/kg 4–8 hr later.

Management of Superficial Edema of the Cornea

▪ **Ophth (Adults):** 1–2 drops every 3–4 hr.

AVAILABILITY

▪ *Suppositories:* Adult, pediatric
▪ *Liquid for rectal use:* 4-ml applicators ▪ *Oral solution:* 0.6 g/ml (50% v/v)
▪ *Ophthalmic solution:* 7.5-ml containers.

TIME/ACTION PROFILE

	ONSET	PEAK	DURATION
Rect (laxative effect)	UK	15–30 min	UK
PO (reduction of intraocular pressure)	10–30 min	30 min– 2 hr	4–8 hr
Ophth (reduced corneal swelling)	UK	UK	3–4 hr

NURSING IMPLICATIONS

ASSESSMENT

▪ **Laxative:** Assess patient for abdominal distension, presence of bowel sounds, and normal pattern of bowel function.
▫ Assess color, consistency, and amount of stool produced.
▪ **Lab Test Considerations:** May cause slightly elevated serum and urine glucose concentrations.

POTENTIAL NURSING DIAGNOSES

▪ Constipation (indications).
▪ Knowledge deficit related to medication regimen (patient/family teaching).

IMPLEMENTATION

▪ **PO:** Solution is clear, colorless, and syrupy, with a sweet taste.
▫ Administer 50% glycerin solution with 0.9% NaCl flavored with lemon, lime, or orange juice or commercially prepared 50% or 75% flavored solution to improve taste and to minimize nausea and vomiting. Pour over cracked ice and sip through a straw.
▫ Have patient lie down during and after administration to prevent headache from cerebral dehydration.
▫ When used to decrease intraocular pressure, do not give the patient hypotonic fluids following administration, as these will cancel the osmotic effect of glycerin.
▪ **Rect:** Glycerin suppositories or enema usually cause evacuation of the colon in 15–30 min.
▪ **Ophth:** Do not administer solution that is cloudy or discolored or that contains crystals or a precipitate.
▫ Ophthalmic solution may cause pain and eye irritation. Topical local anesthetic should be instilled shortly before administration of glycerin ophthalmic solution.
▫ See Appendix H for administration of ophthalmic solution.

PATIENT/FAMILY TEACHING

▪ **General Info:** Instruct patient to take glycerin as directed.

---

*Underlines indicate most frequent; **CAPITALS** indicate life-threatening.

- **Laxative:** Advise patient that laxatives should be used only for short-term therapy. Long-term therapy may cause electrolyte imbalance and dependence.
  □ Caution patients not to use laxatives when abdominal pain, nausea, vomiting, or fever are present.

EVALUATION
Effectiveness of therapy can be demonstrated by: ▪ Soft, formed bowel movement ▪ Reduction of intraocular pressure ▪ Reduction of corneal edema.

GLYCOPYRROLATE
(glye-koe-**pye**-roe-late)
Robinul, Robinul-Forte

CLASSIFICATION(S):
Anticholinergic
Pregnancy Category B

INDICATIONS

▪ Used as a preoperative medication to inhibit salivation and excessive respiratory secretions ▪ Used to reverse some of the secretory and vagal actions of cholinesterase inhibitors used to treat nondepolarizing neuromuscular blockade (cholinergic adjunct) ▪ Adjunct in the management of peptic ulcer disease.

ACTION

▪ Inhibits the action of acetylcholine at postganglionic sites located in smooth muscle, secretory glands, and the CNS (antimuscarinic activity) ▪ Low doses decrease sweating, salivation, and respiratory secretions ▪ Intermediate doses result in increased heart rate ▪ GI and GU tract motility are decreased at larger doses. **Therapeutic Effects:** ▪ Decreased GI and respiratory secretions.

PHARMACOKINETICS

Absorption: Incompletely absorbed following oral administration. Well absorbed following IM administration.

Distribution: Distribution not fully known. Does not significantly cross the blood–brain barrier or eye. Crosses the placenta.

Metabolism and Excretion: Eliminated primarily unchanged in the feces, via biliary excretion.

Half-life: 1.7 hr (0.6–4.6 hr).

CONTRAINDICATIONS AND PRECAUTIONS

Contraindicated in: ▪ Hypersensitivity ▪ Narrow-angle glaucoma ▪ Acute hemorrhage ▪ Tachycardia secondary to cardiac insufficiency or thyrotoxicosis ▪ Children <12 yr (for management of peptic ulcer only) ▪ Products containing benzyl alcohol should not be used in neonates.

Use Cautiously in: ▪ Elderly and the very young (increased susceptibility to adverse reactions) ▪ Patients who may have intra-abdominal infections ▪ Prostatic hypertrophy ▪ Chronic renal, hepatic, pulmonary, or cardiac disease ▪ Pregnancy and lactation (safety not established).

ADVERSE REACTIONS AND SIDE EFFECTS*

CNS: drowsiness, confusion.

EENT: dry eyes, blurred vision, mydriasis, cycloplegia.

CV: palpitations, <u>tachycardia</u>, orthostatic hypotension.

GI: <u>dry mouth</u>, constipation.

GU: <u>urinary hesitancy</u>, retention.

INTERACTIONS

Drug–Drug: ▪ Additive anticholinergic effects with other **anticholinergic compounds,** including **antihistamines, tricyclic antidepressants, quinidine,** and **disopyramide** ▪ May alter the absorption of **other orally administered drugs** by slowing motility of the GI tract ▪ **Antacids** or **adsorbent antidiarrheals** decrease the absorption of anticholinergics ▪ May increase GI mucosal lesions in patients taking **oral potassium chloride tablets.**

G

ROUTE AND DOSAGE

Control of Secretions During Surgery

- **IM (Adults and Children >2 yr):** 4.4 mcg/kg 30–60 min preop (not to exceed 0.1 mg).
- **IM (Children <2 yr):** 4.4–8.8 mcg/kg 30–60 min preop.

Cholinergic Adjunct

- **IV (Adults and Children):** 200 mcg for each 1 mg of neostigmine or 5 mg of pyridostigmine given at the same time.

Antiarrhythmic

- **IV (Adults):** 100 mcg, may be repeated q 2–3 min.
- **IV (Children):** 4.4 mcg/kg (up to 100 mcg); may be repeated q 2–3 min.

Peptic Ulcer

- **PO (Adults):** 1–2 mg 2–3 times daily.
- **IM, IV (Adults):** 100–200 mcg q 4 hr up to 4 times daily.

AVAILABILITY

- **Tablets:** 1 mg, 2 mg ▪ **Injection:** 0.2 mg/ml.

TIME/ACTION PROFILE
(anticholinergic effects)

	ONSET	PEAK	DURATION
PO	UK	UK	8–12 hr
IM	15–30 min	30–45 min	2–7 hr
IV	1 min	UK	2–7 hr

NURSING IMPLICATIONS

Assessment

- □ Assess heart rate, blood pressure, and respiratory rate prior to and periodically during parenteral therapy.
- □ Monitor intake and output ratios in elderly or surgical patients, as glycopyrrolate may cause urinary retention. Instruct patient to void prior to administration.
- □ Assess patient routinely for abdominal distention and auscultate for bowel sounds. If constipation becomes a problem, increasing fluids and adding bulk to the diet may help alleviate the constipating effects of the drug.
- □ Periodic intraocular pressure determinations should be made on patients receiving long-term therapy.
- ▪ **Lab Test Considerations:** Antagonizes effects of pentagastrin and histamine during the gastric acid secretion test. Avoid administration for 24 hr preceding the test.
- □ May cause decreased uric acid levels in patients with gout or hyperuricemia.
- ▪ **Toxicity and Overdose:** If overdosage occurs, neostigmine is the antidote.

Potential Nursing Diagnoses

- ▪ Oral mucous membranes, altered (side effects).
- ▪ Constipation (side effects).
- ▪ Knowledge deficit related to medication regimen (patient/family teaching).

Implementation

- ▪ **General Info:** Do not administer cloudy or discolored solution.
- ▪ **PO:** Administer 30–60 min before meals to maximize absorption.
- □ Do not administer within 1 hr of antacids or antidiarrheal medications.
- ▪ **IM:** May be administered undiluted or mixed and administered with D5W, D10W, or 0.9% NaCl.
- ▪ **Direct IV:** May be given undiluted through Y-site injection or 3-way stopcock.
- ▪ **Rate:** Administer at a rate of 0.2 mg over 1–2 min.
- ▪ **Syringe Compatibility:** ▪ benzquinamide ▪ chlorpromazine ▪ cimetidine ▪ codeine ▪ diphenhydramine ▪ droperidol ▪ droperidol/fentanyl ▪ hydromorphone ▪ hydroxyzine ▪ levorphanol ▪ lidocaine ▪ meperidine ▪ midazolam ▪ morphine ▪ nalbuphine ▪ neostigmine ▪ oxymorphone ▪ prochlorperazine ▪ promazine ▪ promethazine ▪ propiomazine ▪ pyridostigmine ▪ ranitidine ▪ triflupromazine ▪ trimethobenzamide.
- ▪ **Syringe Incompatibility:** ▪ chloramphenicol ▪ dexamethasone ▪ diaze-

pam ■ dimenhydrinate ■ methohexital
■ pentazocine ■ pentobarbital ■ secobarbital ■ sodium bicarbonate ■ thiopental.
- **Solution Compatibility:** ■ D5/0.45%
NaCl ■ D5W ■ 0.9% NaCl ■ Ringer's
solution. Administer immediately after admixing.
- **Additive Incompatibility:** ■ methylprednisolone sodium succinate.

PATIENT/FAMILY TEACHING

□ Instruct patient to take glycopyrrolate
exactly as directed and not to take
more than the prescribed amount.
Missed doses should be taken as
soon as remembered if not just before
next dose.
□ Medication may cause drowsiness
and blurred vision. Caution patient to
avoid driving or other activities requiring alertness until response to the
medication is known.
□ Inform patient that frequent oral
rinses, sugarless gum or candy, and
good oral hygiene may help relieve
dry mouth. Consult physician or dentist regarding use of saliva substitute
if dry mouth persists for more than
2 wk.
□ Advise patient receiving glycopyrrolate to make position changes slowly
to minimize the effects of drug-
induced orthostatic hypotension.
□ Caution patient to avoid extremes
of temperature. This medication decreases the ability to sweat and may
increase the risk of heat stroke.
□ Advise patient to notify physician
immediately if eye pain or increased
sensitivity to light occurs. Emphasize
the importance of routine eye examinations throughout therapy.
□ Advise patient to consult physician or
pharmacist prior to taking any over-
the-counter medications concurrently
with this therapy.

EVALUATION

**Effectiveness of therapy can be demon-
strated by:** ■ Mouth dryness preoperatively ■ Reversal of cholinergic medications ■ Decrease in GI motility and pain
in patients with peptic ulcer disease.

GOLD SODIUM THIOMALATE
(gold so-dee-um thye-oh-**mah**-
late)
Aurothiomalate, Myochrisine

CLASSIFICATION(S):
Anti-inflammatory agent
Pregnancy Category C

INDICATIONS

■ Treatment of progressive rheumatoid
arthritis resistant to conventional therapy.

ACTION

■ Inhibits the inflammatory process
■ Modifies the immune response (immunomodulating properties). **Therapeutic Effects:** ■ Relief of pain and inflammation and slowing of the disease
process in rheumatoid arthritis.

PHARMACOKINETICS

Absorption: Rapidly absorbed following IM administration.
Distribution: Widely distributed, appears to concentrate in arthritic joints
more than uninvolved joints. Enters
breast milk.
Metabolism and Excretion: 60–90%
slowly excreted by the kidneys (up to 15
mo). 10–40% excreted in the feces.
Half-life: Gold—26 days in blood, 40–
128 days in tissue.

CONTRAINDICATIONS AND PRECAUTIONS

Contraindicated in: ■ Hypersensitivity
■ Severe hepatic or renal dysfunction
■ Previous heavy metal toxicity ■ History
of colitis or exfoliative dermatitis ■ Uncontrolled diabetes mellitus ■ Tuberculosis ■ Congestive heart failure ■ Systemic lupus erythematosus ■ Recent
radiation therapy ■ Pregnancy or lactation ■ Debilitated patients.
Use Cautiously in: ■ History of blood
dyscrasias ■ Hypertension ■ Rashes
■ Discontinue at first sign of toxicity,
skin rash, proteinuria, or stomatitis.

G

ADVERSE REACTIONS AND SIDE EFFECTS*

CNS: <u>dizziness</u>, syncope, headache, neuropathy.
EENT: corneal gold deposition, corneal ulcerations.
Resp: pneumonitis.
CV: bradycardia.
GI: <u>metallic taste</u>, difficulty swallowing, <u>stomatitis</u>, nausea, vomiting, <u>diarrhea</u>, <u>abdominal pain</u>, <u>cramping</u>, anorexia, dyspepsia, flatulence, hepatitis.
GU: <u>proteinuria</u>, nephrotoxicity.
Derm: <u>rash</u>, <u>dermatitis</u>, pruritus, photosensitivity reactions.
Hemat: <u>thrombocytopenia</u>, APLASTIC ANEMIA, AGRANULOCYTOSIS, leukopenia, eosinophilia.
Misc: allergic reactions, including ANAPHYLAXIS, angioneurotic edema, nitritoid reactions.

INTERACTIONS

Drug–Drug: ▪ Bone marrow toxicity may be additive with other **agents capable of bone marrow depression (antineoplastics, radiation therapy)** ▪ Increased risk of renal and hematologic toxicity with **penicillamine** ▪ Increased risk of dermatitis, hepatotoxicity, or renal toxicity with **agents causing similar toxicities**.

ROUTE AND DOSAGE

- **IM (Adults):** 10 mg test dose initially, then 25 mg 1 wk later, then 25–50 mg weekly until improvement or toxicity occurs (up to 1 g total dose). Maintenance dose is 25–50 mg q 2 wk for up to 20 wk, then 25–50 mg q 3–4 wk.
- **IM (Children):** 10 mg test dose initially, then 1 wk later 1 mg/kg/wk (not to exceed 50 mg/dose) until improvement or toxicity occurs (up to 1 g total dose). Maintenance dose is 1 mg/kg q 2 wk for up to 20 wk, then 1 mg/kg q 3–4 wk.

AVAILABILITY

- **Injection:** 25 mg/ml, 50 mg/ml.

TIME/ACTION PROFILE (anti-inflammatory activity)

	ONSET	PEAK	DURATION
IM	6–8 wk	UK	mos

NURSING IMPLICATIONS

ASSESSMENT

- □ Assess patient's range of motion and degree of swelling and pain in affected joints prior to and periodically throughout therapy. Injections may be followed by joint pain for 1–2 days.
- ▪ **Lab Test Considerations:** Monitor renal, hepatic, and hematologic function and urinalysis prior to and monthly throughout therapy. Notify physician immediately if WBC $<4000/mm^3$, eosinophils $>5\%$, granulocytes $<1500/mm^3$, or platelets $<100,000/mm^3$. These values may indicate a hypersensitivity reaction and should improve upon discontinuation. Proteinuria or hematuria may necessitate discontinuation of therapy.
- □ May interfere with serum protein-bound iodine determinations during and for several weeks following discontinuation of therapy.
- ▪ **Toxicity and Overdose:** If signs of overdose occur, glucocorticoids are usually used to reverse effects. A chelating agent, dimercaprol (BAL), may be given to enhance gold excretion when glucocorticoids are ineffective.

POTENTIAL NURSING DIAGNOSES

- ▪ Physical mobility, impaired (indications).
- ▪ Diarrhea (adverse effects).
- ▪ Knowledge deficit related to medication regimen (patient/family teaching).

IMPLEMENTATION

- ▪ **General Info:** Concurrent therapy with salicylates or other nonsteroidal anti-inflammatory agents or glucocorticoids is usually necessary, especially during the first few months of gold therapy.
- □ Never administer IV.

*<u>Underlines</u> indicate most frequent; **CAPITALS** indicate life-threatening.

- **IM:** Using an 18-gauge, 1½-in. needle, inject deep into gluteal muscle. Solution is pale yellow; do not use solution that has darkened or contains a precipitate.
- ☐ Instruct patient to remain recumbent for 15 min after injection. Monitor for nitritoid (dizziness, flushing, fainting, diaphoresis, dyspnea, bradycardia, swelling of face, lips, or eyelids, thickening of tongue) or allergic reaction.

PATIENT/FAMILY TEACHING

- ☐ Patient should continue physical therapy and obtain adequate rest. Explain that joint damage will not be reversed; the goal is to slow or stop disease process.
- ☐ Emphasize the importance of good oral hygiene to reduce the incidence of stomatitis.
- ☐ Caution patient to use sunscreen and protective clothing to prevent photosensitivity reactions.
- ☐ Instruct patient to report symptoms of leukopenia (fever, sore throat, signs of infection) or thrombocytopenia (bleeding gums; bruising; petechiae; blood in stools, urine, or emesis) immediately to physician.
- ☐ Discuss the need for contraception while receiving this medication. Advise patient to notify physician promptly if pregnancy is suspected.
- ☐ Instruct patient to notify physician immediately if symptoms of gold toxicity (pruritus, skin rash, metallic taste in mouth, stomatitis, diarrhea) occur. Diarrhea may be resolved by decreasing the dose.
- ☐ Emphasize the importance of regular visits to physician to monitor progress and to evaluate blood and urine tests for side effects.

EVALUATION

Effectiveness of therapy can be demonstrated by: ▪ Decrease in swelling, pain, and stiffness of joints ☐ Increase in mobility. Continuous therapy for 3–6 mo may be required before therapeutic effects are seen.

GONADORELIN ACETATE
(goe-nad-oh-**rell**-in **ass**-e-tate)
Lutrepulse

CLASSIFICATION(S):
Hormone (gonadotropin-releasing)
Pregnancy Category B

INDICATIONS

▪ Used to produce ovulation in patients with primary hypothalamic amenorrhea.

ACTION

▪ Causes the release of luteinizing hormone and, to a smaller extent, follicle-stimulating hormone from the pituitary. When administered in a pulsatile manner, ovulation is induced ▪ If ovulation and pregnancy occur, gonadorelin helps to maintain the corpeus luteum. **Therapeutic Effects:** ▪ Induction of ovulation ▪ Maintenance of the corpeus luteum.

PHARMACOKINETICS

Absorption: IV administration results in complete bioavailability.
Distribution: UK.
Metabolism and Excretion: Rapidly metabolized to inactive compounds.
Half-life: 10–40 min.

CONTRAINDICATIONS AND PRECAUTIONS

Contraindicated in: ▪ Hypersensitivity ▪ Concurrent use with ovarian simulators ▪ Conditions that would be exacerbated by pregnancy ▪ Ovarian cysts, hormonally sensitive tumors, or other conditions worsened by reproductive hormones.
Use Cautiously in: ▪ Patients <18 yr (safety not established).

ADVERSE REACTIONS AND SIDE EFFECTS*

Endo: multiple pregnancies, ovarian hyperstimulation.
Local: inflammation, infection, mild phlebitis, hematomas at IV site.

G

*Underlines indicate most frequent; CAPITALS indicate life-threatening.

INTERACTIONS

Drug–Drug: ▪ Avoid concurrent use with other **ovarian stimulators**.

ROUTE AND DOSAGE

▪ **IV (Adults):** 5 mcg q 90 min (range 2.5–20 mcg) for 21 days. If ovulation occurs, continue for 2 wk to maintain corpeus luteum.

AVAILABILITY

▪ *Injection:* 0.8-, 3.2-mg vials for use with the Lutrepulse pump.

TIME/ACTION PROFILE (ovulation)

	ONSET	PEAK	DURATION
IV	UK	2–3 wk	UK

NURSING IMPLICATIONS

ASSESSMENT

▫ Regular physical examinations, including pelvic examination, should be performed throughout therapy.

▫ Ovarian ultrasound should be performed before therapy, on day 7 and again on day 14.

▫ Observe patient for the development of ovarian hyperstimulation syndrome (sudden ovarian enlargement, ascites, or pleural effusion). Discontinue treatment if this syndrome occurs. May proceed to fluid imbalance, ovarian rupture, or sepsis.

▪ **Lab Test Considerations:** Monitor midluteal phase serum progesterone levels.

POTENTIAL NURSING DIAGNOSES

▪ Sexual dysfunction (indications).

▪ Knowledge deficit related to medication regimen (patient/family teaching).

IMPLEMENTATION

▪ **Continuous Infusion:** Dilute each vial with 8 ml of the saline diluent immediately prior to use. Shake for a few seconds to produce a clear, colorless solution. Do not use solution if particulate matter or discoloration is present. Fill reservoir bag with reconstituted solution. The 8 ml of solution will supply 90-min pulsatile doses for approximately 7 consecutive days.

▪ *Rate:* Lutrepulse pump should be set to deliver 25 or 50 mcl of solution, based on the dose selected, over a pulse period of 1 min and a pulse frequency of 90 min.

PATIENT/FAMILY TEACHING

▫ Instruct patient regarding proper reconstitution of gonadorelin acetate and use of Lutrepulse pump.

▫ Advise patient to report any redness or inflammation at IV site.

▫ Counsel patient regarding the need for follow-up if pregnancy occurs and of the possibility of multiple pregnancies.

EVALUATION

Effectiveness of therapy can be determined by: ▪ Induction of ovulation in women with primary hypothalamic amenorrhea.

GONADORELIN HYDRO-CHLORIDE

(goe-nad-oh-**rell**-in hye-droe-**klor**-ide)
Factrel

CLASSIFICATION(S):
Hormone (gonadotropin-releasing)
Pregnancy Category B

INDICATIONS

▪ Used to assess the gonadotropin-producing capacity of the anterior pituitary.

ACTION

▪ Causes the release of gonadotropin (luteinizing hormone) from the pituitary. **Therapeutic Effect:** ▪ Increased levels of luteinizing hormone (LH).

PHARMACOKINETICS

Absorption: IV administration results in complete bioavailability.
Distribution: UK.
Metabolism and Excretion: Rapidly metabolized to inactive compounds.
Half-life: 10–40 min.

CONTRAINDICATIONS AND PRECAUTIONS

Contraindicated in: ▪ Hypersensitivity to gonadorelin or benzyl alcohol.

Use Cautiously in: ▪ Pregnancy, lactation, or children (safety not established).

ADVERSE REACTIONS AND SIDE EFFECTS*

Local: hypersensitivity reactions (multiple dose use) including ANAPHYLAXIS and antibody formation (large multiple doses).

INTERACTIONS

Drug–Drug: ▪ Concurrent use of **androgens, estrogens, progestins,** or **glucocorticoids** may alter production of gonadotropins ▪ **Digoxin** and **oral contraceptives** may decrease gonadotropin levels ▪ **Levodopa** and **spironolactone** may increase gonadotropin levels ▪ Response to gonadorelin may be decreased by **phenothiazines** and **dopamine antagonists**.

ROUTE AND DOSAGE

▪ **SC, IV (Adults):** 100 mcg.

AVAILABILITY

▪ *Injection:* 100 mcg/vial.

TIME/ACTION PROFILE (increase in LH levels)

	ONSET	PEAK	DURATION
SC (females)	within mins	30 min	more than 2 hr
SC (males)	within mins	60 min	more than 2 hr
IV (females)	within mins	30 min	more than 2 hr
IV (males)	within mins	15 min	more than 2 hr

NURSING IMPLICATIONS

ASSESSMENT

▫ Determine patient's menstrual cycle. Testing of the response to gonadorelin hydrochloride should be done during the first 7 days of the menstrual cycle.

▪ **Lab Test Considerations:** Blood for luteinizing hormone concentration levels should be drawn 15 min and immediately prior to administration of gonadorelin to determine the baseline luteinizing hormone concentration.

▫ Following administration of gonadorelin, venous blood samples should be drawn at regular intervals.

▫ Normal serum luteinizing hormone concentrations are usually 5–25 mIU/ml in postpubertal males and females and in premenopausal females.

POTENTIAL NURSING DIAGNOSES

▪ Knowledge deficit related to medication regimen (patient/family teaching).

IMPLEMENTATION

▪ **Direct IV:** Dilute the 100-mcg vial with 1 ml or the 500-mcg vial with 2 ml of the diluent provided by the manufacturer. Administer immediately after dilution. Discard unused solution or diluent.

▪ *Rate:* Administer as a bolus.

PATIENT/FAMILY TEACHING

▫ Inform patient of the purpose of this medication.

▫ Instruct patient to report the symptoms of anaphylaxis immediately (difficulty breathing, persistent flushing, hives).

EVALUATION

Effectiveness of therapy is determined by: Evaluation of the functioning of the gonadotropes of the anterior pituitary gland.

GONADOTROPIN, CHORIONIC
(goe-**nad**-oh-troe-pin, kor-ee-**on**-ik)
A.P.L., Chorex, Chorigon, Choron, Corgonject, Follutein, Glukor, Gonic, HCG, Pregnyl, Profasi

CLASSIFICATION(S):
Hormone
Pregnancy Category C

INDICATIONS

■ Treatment of: □ Cryptorchidism □ Male infertility (secondary to hypogonadism) □ Female infertility (to induce ovulation in patients who do not respond to clomiphene) □ Male infertility (induction of spermatogenesis) ■ To induce ovulation in patients undergoing *in vitro* fertilization. **Unlabeled Uses:** ■ Diagnosis of male hypogonadism ■ Treatment of corpus luteum dysfunction.

ACTION

■ Has action similar to that of luteinizing hormone—causes ovulation ■ Stimulates androgen production by the testes. **Therapeutic Effects:** ■ Promotion of androgen production by the testes and subsequent descent ■ Ovulation.

PHARMACOKINETICS

Absorption: Destroyed in the GI tract, necessitating IM administration.
Distribution: Distributed primarily to the ovaries in females and to the testes in males.
Metabolism and Excretion: 10–12% excreted in urine in first 24 hr.
Half-life: 23 hr.

CONTRAINDICATIONS AND PRECAUTIONS

Contraindicated in: ■ Previous hypersensitivity reactions ■ Precocious puberty ■ Carcinoma of the prostate or other androgen-sensitive tumor.
Use Cautiously in: ■ Asthma ■ History of seizures ■ Migraine headaches ■ Renal disease ■ Cardiac disease.

ADVERSE REACTIONS AND SIDE EFFECTS*

CNS: headache, irritability, restlessness, depression, fatigue.
CV: edema, fluid retention, ascites (with menotropins), pleural effusion (with menotropins), thromboembolism (with menotropins).
Endo: gynecomastia (males), precocius puberty (prepubertal males), ovarian enlargement (with menotropins), rupture of ovarian cyst (with menotropins), ovarian hyperstimulation syndrome.
Local: pain at IM site.
Misc: multiple pregnancy (with menotropins).

INTERACTIONS

Drug–Drug: ■ None significant.

ROUTE AND DOSAGE

Hypogonadism/Male Infertility
■ **IM (Adults):** 500–4000 units 2–3 times/wk.

Induction of Ovulation
■ **IM (Adults):** 5000–10,000 units 1 day after last dose of menotropins or urofollitropin or 5–9 days following clomiphene.

Prepubertal Cryptorchidism
■ **IM (Children):** 500–4000 units 2–3 times/wk (not to exceed 6 wk of treatment). Up to 5000 units every other day for 4 doses.

AVAILABILITY

■ *Injection:* 200 units/ml, 500 units/ml, 1000 units/ml, 2000 units/ml.

TIME/ACTION PROFILE (ovulation)

	ONSET	PEAK	DURATION
IM	UK	18 hr	UK

NURSING IMPLICATIONS

ASSESSMENT

■ **General Info:** Assess blood pressure prior to and periodically throughout therapy.
□ Monitor intake and output ratios and weekly weight. Report significant discrepancies or steady weight gain to physician.
■ **Cryptorchidism:** Monitor for development of precocious puberty (acne, sudden increase in height, secondary

sex characteristics—pubic, axillary, or facial hair, voice changes, penile growth. Notify physician; therapy should be discontinued.

- **Anovulatory Infertility:** An ultrasound examination should be conducted prior to therapy to determine number of follicles and degree of development. A pelvic examination to determine ovarian size should be completed prior to course of therapy and daily for 2 wk after chorionic gonadotropin injection. Cervical mucus should be monitored to determine whether ovulation has occurred.
- **Lab Test Considerations:** May cause false results in pregnancy testing. May cause false elevations in tests of urinary steroid excretion.
- **Female Infertility:** Estrogen excretion or serum estrogen level should be monitored prior to administration of chorionic gonadotropin. Levels should be assessed daily beginning 1 wk after course of menotropins.
- **Male Infertility:** Sperm count and motility should be evaluated prior to and after course of therapy.

POTENTIAL NURSING DIAGNOSES
- Sexual dysfunction (indications).
- Body image disturbance (indications).
- Knowledge deficit related to medication regimen (patient/family teaching).

IMPLEMENTATION
- **General Info:** Female infertility—chorionic gonadotropin is usually administered 1 day following a course of human menotropins.
- **IM:** Reconstitute powder with 10-ml vial of normal saline for injection provided by manufacturer. Withdraw sterile air from vial that contains powder, inject air into diluent vial, withdraw same volume of diluent, and inject into vial containing powder. Shake gently until powder fully dissolved. Stable for 90 days when refrigerated.

PATIENT/FAMILY TEACHING
- **General Info:** Advise patient to report

signs and symptoms of fluid retention (swelling of ankles and feet, weight gain); thromboembolic disorders (pain, swelling, tenderness in extremities, headache, chest pain, blurred vision); and abdominal or pelvic pain or bloating to physician.

- **Cryptorchidism:** Review symptoms of precocious puberty with parents; instruct them to notify physician immediately if these symptoms occur.
- **Female Infertility:** Instruct patient in the correct method for measuring basal body temperature. A record of the daily basal body temperature should be maintained prior to and throughout course of therapy.
□ Reinforce physician's instructions regarding timing of sexual intercourse (usually daily beginning 1 day after administration of chorionic gonadotropin).
□ Emphasize the importance of close monitoring by physician throughout course of therapy.
□ Inform patient prior to therapy of the potential for multiple pregnancy.
□ Instruct patient to notify physician immediately if pregnancy is suspected (menses do not occur when expected and basal body temperature is biphasic) or if signs and symptoms of ovarian hyperstimulation syndrome (severe abdominal pain; indigestion; moderate to severe bloating; decreased amount of urine; continuing or severe nausea, vomiting, or diarrhea; severe pelvic pain; rapid weight gain; dyspnea; swelling of lower legs) occur.

EVALUATION
Effectiveness of therapy can be demonstrated by: ■ Testicular descent in boys (age 4–9) with cryptorchidism ■ Ovulation 18 hr after therapy in women with anovulatory cycles, with subsequent pregnancy ■ Increase in spermatogenesis. Therapy may be discontinued in boys with cryptorchidism if testicular descent is progressing poorly after 8 wk of therapy or in infertile woman if ovulation does not occur after 3–6 menstrual cycles.

GOSERELIN
(**goe**-se-rel-lin)
Zoladex

CLASSIFICATION(S):
Antineoplastic (hormone)
Pregnancy Category X

INDICATIONS
- Treatment (palliative) of prostate cancer in patients who will not tolerate orchiectomy or estrogen therapy.

ACTION
- Acts as a synthetic form of leuteinizing hormone releasing hormone (LHRH, GnRH). Inhibits the production of gonadotropins by the pituitary gland. Initially, levels of luteinizing hormone (LH), follicle stimulating hormone (FSH), and testosterone increase. Continued administration leads to decreased production, particularly of testosterone. **Therapeutic Effect:** • Decreased spread of cancer of the prostate.

PHARMACOKINETICS
Absorption: Well absorbed from SC implant. Absorption is slower in first 8 days, then is faster and continuous for remainder of 28-day dosing cycle.
Distribution: Distribution not known.
Metabolism and Excretion: Metabolism and excretion not known.
Half-life: 4.2 hr.

CONTRAINDICATIONS AND PRECAUTIONS
Contraindicated in: • Hypersensitivity • Pregnancy.
Use Cautiously in: • Lactation or children <18 yr (safety not established).

ADVERSE REACTIONS AND SIDE EFFECTS*
CNS: weakness, anxiety, depression, dizziness, headache, insomnia, fatigue.
Resp: dyspnea.
CV: chest pain, palpitations, hyperten-

sion, MYOCARDIAL INFARCTION, CEREBROVASCULAR ACCIDENT.
GI: constipation, diarrhea, anorexia, nausea, vomiting, ulcer.
GU: renal insufficiency, urinary obstruction.
Derm: rashes.
Endo: decreased libido, impotence, breast tenderness, breast swelling, infertility.
F and E: peripheral edema.
Hemat: anemia.
Metab: hyperglycemia, gout.
MS: increased bone pain, arthralgia.
Misc: hot flashes, chills, fever, weight gain.

INTERACTIONS
Drug–Drug: • None significant.

ROUTE AND DOSAGE
- **SC (Adults):** 3.6 mg every 28 days (as an implant).

AVAILABILITY
- *Implant:* 3.6 mg.

TIME/ACTION PROFILE (decrease in serum testosterone levels)

	ONSET	PEAK	DURATION
SC	UK	2–4 wk	length of therapy

NURSING IMPLICATIONS

ASSESSMENT
- ☐ Monitor patients with vertebral metastases for increased back pain and decreased sensory/motor function.
- ☐ Monitor intake and output ratios and assess for bladder distention in patients with urinary tract obstruction during initiation of therapy.
- ☐ Initially increases then decreases luteinizing hormone (LH), follicle stimulating hormone (FSH). This leads to castration levels of testosterone in males 2–4 wk after initial increase in concentrations.

POTENTIAL NURSING DIAGNOSES
- Sexual dysfunction (side effects).
- Knowledge deficit related to medica-

*Underlines indicate most frequent; **CAPITALS** indicate life-threatening.

tion regimen (patient/family teaching).

IMPLEMENTATION

- **SC:** Implant is inserted in upper SC tissue of abdominal wall every 28 days.

PATIENT/FAMILY TEACHING

□ Advise patient that bone pain may increase at initiation of therapy. This will resolve with time. Patient should discuss use of analgesics to control pain with physician.

□ Advise patient that medication may cause hot flashes. Notify physician if these become bothersome.

□ Instruct patient to notify physician promptly if difficulty urinating occurs.

EVALUATION

Effectiveness of therapy can be demonstrated by: ▪ Decrease in the spread of prostate cancer.

GRISEOFULVIN
(gris-ee-oh-**ful**-vin)
Fulvicin P/G, Fulvicin-U/F,
Grifulvin V, Grisactin, Grisactin
Ultra, {Grisovin-FP}, Gris-PEG

CLASSIFICATION(S):
Antifungal
Pregnancy Category UK

INDICATIONS

▪ Treatment of various Tinea (ringworm) infections, including: □ *Tinea barbae* □ *Tinea capitis* □ *Tinea corporis* □ *Tinea cruris* □ *Tinea pedis* □ *Tinea unguium,* caused by one or a combination of susceptible □ *Trichophyton* □ *Microsporum* □ *Epidermatophyton* ▪ Should not be used for superficial infections that may respond to topical antifungals.

ACTION

▪ Inhibits mitosis of fungal cells. Deposits in precursor cells of hair, skin,

and nails, making them resistant to fungal invasion. **Therapeutic Effect:** ▪ Growth of new cells that are resistant to invasion by fungi.

PHARMACOKINETICS

Absorption: Microsize (Grisactin, Grisovin-FP, Grifulvin V, Fulvicin-U/F, Grifulvin V) preparations are variably (25–70%) absorbed following oral administration. Ultramicrosize products (Fulvicin P/G, Grisactin Ultra, Gris-PEG) are almost completely absorbed.

Distribution: Mostly deposited in keratin layer of skin. Also found in liver, fat, and skeletal muscle.

Metabolism and Excretion: Metabolized by the liver, some excreted in feces and perspiration.

Half-life: 9–24 hr.

CONTRAINDICATIONS AND PRECAUTIONS

Contraindicated in: ▪ Hypersensitivity ▪ Severe liver disease or porphyria.

Use Cautiously in: ▪ Pregnancy or lactation (safety not established) ▪ Possible cross-sensitivity with penicillin.

ADVERSE REACTIONS AND SIDE EFFECTS*

CNS: headache, dizziness.

EENT: hearing loss.

GI: epigastric distress, nausea, vomiting, extreme thirst, flatulence, diarrhea.

Derm: photosensitivity, rashes.

Hemat: leukopenia.

Misc: hypersensitivity reactions, including serum sickness, lupus-like syndrome.

INTERACTIONS

Drug–Drug: ▪ Tachycardia, flushing, and increased CNS depression may result if taken concurrently with **alcohol** ▪ **Phenobarbital** decreases blood levels and may decrease effectiveness ▪ May decrease the effectiveness of **oral anticoagulants** ▪ May decrease the effectiveness of **oral contraceptive agents.**

Drug–Food: ▪ Absorption is increased by **fatty foods.**

{} = Available in Canada only.
*<u>Underlines</u> indicate most frequent; **CAPITALS** indicate life-threatening.

ROUTE AND DOSAGE

Microsize
- **PO (Adults):** 250–500 mg q 12 hr or 500 mg once daily.
- **PO (Children):** 10 mg/kg/day, single or divided doses.

Ultramicrosize
- **PO (Adults):** 330–375 mg/day in 1–2 divided doses.
- **PO (Children >2 yr):** 5.5–7.3 mg/kg/day, single or divided doses.

AVAILABILITY

- *Microsize tablets:* 250 mg, 500 mg
- *Microsize capsules:* 125 mg, 250 mg
- *Oral suspension:* 125 mg/5 ml
- *Ultramicrosize tablets:* 125 mg, 165 mg, 250 mg, 330 mg.

TIME/ACTION PROFILE (antifungal activity)

	ONSET	PEAK	DURATION
PO	4 hr	24 hr	2 days

NURSING IMPLICATIONS

ASSESSMENT
- ☐ Assess skin at site of fungal infection routinely throughout course of therapy.
- ☐ Assess patient for allergy to penicillin; potential cross-sensitivity exists.
- ▪ **Lab Test Considerations:** Hematologic, hepatic, and renal functions should be monitored periodically throughout treatment.

POTENTIAL NURSING DIAGNOSES
- ▪ Skin integrity, impaired (indications).
- ▪ Infection, high risk for (indications, side effects).
- ▪ Knowledge deficit related to medication regimen (patient/family teaching).

IMPLEMENTATION
- ▪ **General Info:** Concurrent use of a topical agent is usually required.
- ☐ Ultramicrosize griseofulvin 250 mg provides serum concentration equal

to that of microsize griseofulvin 500 mg.
- ▪ PO: Administer with or after meals, preferably meals with high fat content, to minimize GI irritation and increase absorption.

PATIENT/FAMILY TEACHING
- ☐ Instruct patient to complete full course of therapy; several weeks of therapy may be necessary. If a dose is missed, take as soon as remembered, but do not take if almost time for next dose.
- ☐ Instruct patient on hygiene to control sources of infection or reinfection.
- ☐ Griseofulvin may cause dizziness. Caution patient to avoid driving or other activities requiring alertness until response to medication is known.
- ☐ Advise patient to wear sunscreen and protective clothing to prevent photosensitivity reaction.
- ☐ Caution patient not to drink alcohol while taking this medication.
- ☐ Advise patient to use a nonhormonal form of contraception and to notify physician if pregnancy is planned or suspected.
- ☐ Advise patient to notify physician if rash, sore throat, fever, diarrhea, or soreness of mouth or tongue occurs.
- ☐ Emphasize importance of follow-up examinations to monitor progress of therapy.

EVALUATION
Effectiveness of therapy can be demonstrated by: ▪ Resolution of signs and symptoms of fungal infection. To prevent relapse, treatment may take weeks to months.

GUAIFENESIN
(gwye-**fen**-e-sin)
Amonidrin, Anti-tuss, {Balminil Expectorant}, Breonesin, Fenesin, Gena-tuss, Gee-Gee, GG-Cen, Glyate, glyceryl guaiacolate, Gly-

cotuss, Glytuss, Guiatuss, Halotussin, Humibid L.A., Humibid Sprinkle, Hytuss, Hytuss-2X, Malotuss, Mytussin, Naldecon Senior Ex, Nortassin, {Neo-Spec}, {Resyl}, Robafen, Robitussin, Scot-tussin Expectorant, Sinumist-SR Caplets, Unitussin

CLASSIFICATION(S):
Expectorant
Pregnancy Category C

INDICATIONS

- Symptomatic management of coughs associated with viral upper respiratory tract infections.

ACTION

- Reduces viscosity of tenacious secretions by increasing respiratory tract fluid. **Therapeutic Effect:** ▪ Mobilization and subsequent expectoration of mucus.

PHARMACOKINETICS

Absorption: Well absorbed after oral administration.
Distribution: Distribution not known.
Metabolism and Excretion: Metabolism or excretion not known.
Half-life: UK.

CONTRAINDICATIONS AND PRECAUTIONS

Contraindicated in: ▪ Hypersensitivity.
Use Cautiously in: ▪ Cough lasting >1 wk or accompanied by fever, rash, or headache (if self-medicating, physician should be consulted) ▪ Pregnancy—although safety has not been established, guaifenesin has been used without adverse effects ▪ Patients receiving disulfiram (liquid products may contain alcohol) ▪ Diabetics (products may contain sugar).

ADVERSE REACTIONS AND SIDE EFFECTS*

CNS: drowsiness.
GI: nausea, vomiting, diarrhea, stomach pain.

INTERACTIONS

Drug–Drug: ▪ None significant.

ROUTE AND DOSAGE

- **PO (Adults):** 100–400 mg q 4 hr or 600–1200 mg q 12 hr as extended-release product (not to exceed 2400 mg/day).
- **PO (Children 6–12 yr):** 100–200 mg q 4 hr or 600 mg q 12 hr as extended-release product (not to exceed 1200 mg/day).
- **PO (Children 2–6 yr):** 50–100 mg q 4 hr (not to exceed 600 mg/day).

AVAILABILITY

- *Syrup:* 100 mg/5 ml ▪ *Liquid:* 200 mg/5 ml ▪ Capsules: 200 mg ▪ *Sustained-release capsules:* 300 mg ▪ *Tablets:* 100 mg, 200 mg ▪ *Sustained-release tablets:* 600 mg.

TIME/ACTION PROFILE (expectorant action)

	ONSET	PEAK	DURATION
PO	30 min	UK	4–6 hr
PO-ER	UK	UK	12 hr

G

NURSING IMPLICATIONS

ASSESSMENT

▫ Assess lung sounds, frequency and type of cough, and character of bronchial secretions periodically throughout therapy. Maintain fluid intake of 1500–2000 ml/day to decrease viscosity of secretions.

POTENTIAL NURSING DIAGNOSES

- Airway clearance, ineffective (indications).
- Knowledge deficit related to medication regimen (patient/family teaching).

IMPLEMENTATION

- **PO:** Do not give fluids immediately after administering liquid preparations, to prevent dilution of the vehicle.
▫ Sustained-release tablets should be swallowed whole; do not crush, break, or chew.

*Underlines indicate most frequent; **CAPITALS** indicate life-threatening.

□ Instruct patient to cough effectively. Patient should sit upright and take several deep breaths before attempting to cough.
□ Inform patient that drug may occasionally cause drowsiness. Avoid driving or other activities requiring alertness until response to drug is known.
□ Advise patient to limit talking, stop smoking, maintain moisture in environmental air, and take some sugarless gum or hard candy to help alleviate the discomfort caused by a chronic nonproductive cough.
□ Instruct patient to contact physician if cough persists longer than 1 wk or is accompanied by fever or chest pain.

EVALUATION
Effectiveness of therapy can be demonstrated by: ▪ Decreased frequency of a dry, nonproductive cough. Thick, viscous secretions are thinned, which allows easier expectoration.

GUANABENZ
(**gwahn**-a-benz)
Wytensin

CLASSIFICATION(S):
Antihypertensive (centrally acting alpha₂-adrenergic agonist)
Pregnancy Category C

INDICATIONS
▪ Used alone and with other antihypertensives in the management of hypertension.

ACTION
▪ Stimulates CNS alpha$_2$-adrenergic receptors, resulting in decreased sympathetic outflow. Result is decreased peripheral resistance, a slight decrease in heart rate, and no change in cardiac output. **Therapeutic Effect:** ▪ Lowering of blood pressure.

PHARMACOKINETICS
Absorption: 70–80% absorbed following oral administration.
Distribution: Appears to be widely distributed.
Metabolism and Excretion: >95% metabolized by the liver.
Half-life: 4–14 hr.

CONTRAINDICATIONS AND PRECAUTIONS
Contraindicated in: ▪ Hypersensitivity.
Use Cautiously in: ▪ Serious cardiac, cerebrovascular disease, renal or hepatic insufficiency ▪ Elderly patients (more prone to adverse reactions) ▪ Pregnancy, lactation, or children <12 yr (safety not established) ▪ Do not discontinue abruptly.

ADVERSE REACTIONS AND SIDE EFFECTS*
CNS: <u>drowsiness</u>, <u>dizziness</u>, <u>weakness</u>, headache, irritability, nervousness.
EENT: nasal congestion, blurred vision, dry eyes, miosis.
Resp: dyspnea.
CV: chest pain, bradycardia, edema, arrhythmias, palpitations, hypotension.
GI: <u>dry mouth</u>, nausea, abdominal pain, diarrhea, vomiting, anorexia, constipation, abnormal taste.
GU: frequency, impotence.
Derm: rashes, pruritus, sweating.
Endo: gynecomastia.
MS: painful extremities, backache.
Misc: <u>withdrawal phenomenon</u>.

INTERACTIONS
Drug–Drug: ▪ Additive sedation with **CNS depressants,** including **alcohol, antihistamines, opioid analgesics,** and **sedative/hypnotics** ▪ **Tricyclic antidepressants** and **nonsteroidal antiinflammatory agents** may decrease antihypertensive effects ▪ **MAO inhibitors** decrease effectiveness ▪ Additive hypotension with other **antihypertensives, nitrates,** and acute ingestion of **alcohol.**

*<u>Underlines</u> indicate most frequent; **CAPITALS** indicate life-threatening.

ROUTE AND DOSAGE

- **PO (Adults):** 4 mg bid; may increase q 1–2 wk in 4–8 mg increments (range 8–16 mg/day; not to exceed 32 mg/day).

AVAILABILITY

- *Tablets:* 4 mg, 8 mg.

TIME/ACTION PROFILE
(antihypertensive effect)*

	ONSET	PEAK	DURATION
PO	1 hr	2–7 hr	6–12 hr

*After single dose.

NURSING IMPLICATIONS

ASSESSMENT

- Monitor blood pressure (lying and standing) and pulse frequently during initial dosage adjustment and periodically throughout course of therapy. Notify physician of significant changes.
- Monitor intake and output ratios and daily weight; assess for edema daily.
- **Lab Test Considerations:** With chronic use, may decrease serum cholesterol and triglyceride levels.

POTENTIAL NURSING DIAGNOSES

- Injury, high risk for (side effects).
- Knowledge deficit related to medication regimen (patient/family teaching).
- Noncompliance (patient/family teaching).

IMPLEMENTATION

- **PO:** Administer last dose at bedtime to minimize daytime sedation.
- May be used in conjunction with a thiazide diuretic in patients who fail to respond to diet, exercise, and initial antihypertensive drug therapy.

PATIENT/FAMILY TEACHING

- Emphasize the importance of continuing to take this medication as directed, even if feeling well. Medication controls but does not cure hypertension. Instruct patient to take medication at the same time each day. If a dose is missed, take as soon as remembered; do not double doses. Instruct patient to inform physician if more than 1 consecutive dose is missed. Do not discontinue abruptly; may cause sympathetic overstimulation (nervousness, anxiety, rebound hypertension).
- Encourage patient to comply with additional interventions for hypertension (weight reduction, low-sodium diet, discontinuation of smoking, moderation of alcohol consumption, regular exercise, and stress management).
- Instruct patient and family on proper technique for blood pressure monitoring. Advise them to check blood pressure at least weekly and report significant changes to physician.
- Patients should also weigh themselves twice weekly and assess feet and ankles for fluid retention.
- Guanabenz may cause drowsiness or dizziness. Caution patient to avoid driving or other activities requiring alertness until response to the medication is known.
- Advise patient to consult physician or pharmacist before taking any cough, cold, or allergy remedies. Patients should also avoid excessive amounts of coffee, tea, and cola.
- Frequent mouth rinses, good oral hygiene, and sugarless gum or candy may minimize dry mouth. If dry mouth persists for more than 2 wk, consult dentist regarding use of saliva substitute.
- Advise women of childbearing age to use contraception and notify the physician if pregnancy is suspected or planned.
- Instruct patient to notify physician or dentist of medication regimen prior to treatment or surgery.
- Advise patient to notify physician if frequent dizziness or weakness, irritability or nervousness, slow heart rate, pinpoint pupils, unusual tiredness, or persistent dry mouth occur.
- Emphasize the importance of follow-up examinations to evaluate effectiveness of medication.

G

EVALUATION
Effectiveness of therapy can be demonstrated by: ▪ Decrease in blood pressure without appearance of excessive side effects.

GUANADREL
(**gwahn**-a-drel)
Hylorel

CLASSIFICATION(S):
Antihypertensive (peripherally acting antiadrenergic)
Pregnancy Category B

INDICATIONS
▪ Treatment of moderate to severe hypertension, usually in combination with at least one other agent, most commonly a diuretic.

ACTION
▪ Prevents the release of norepinephrine from adrenergic nerve endings and the adrenal medulla in response to sympathetic (adrenergic) stimulation ▪ Depletes norepinephrine from nerve endings. Result is decreased sympathetically mediated vasoconstriction. **Therapeutic Effect:** ▪ Lowering of blood pressure.

PHARMACOKINETICS
Absorption: Well absorbed following oral administration.
Distribution: Widely distributed. CNS penetration is minimal.
Metabolism and Excretion: 50% metabolized by the liver, 50% excreted unchanged by the kidneys.
Half-life: 10–12 hr.

CONTRAINDICATIONS AND PRECAUTIONS
Contraindicated in: ▪ Hypersensitivity ▪ Congestive heart failure ▪ Pheochromocytoma ▪ Lactation.

Use Cautiously in: ▪ Asthma ▪ Cardiovascular or cerebrovascular insufficiency ▪ Peptic ulcer disease ▪ Pregnancy, lactation, or children <18 yr (safety not established) ▪ Elderly patients and patients with renal failure (increased dosing interval recommended if CCr <60 ml/min) ▪ Discontinue 2–3 days prior to surgical procedures if possible.

ADVERSE REACTIONS AND SIDE EFFECTS*
CNS: drowsiness, fatigue, confusion, headaches, sleep disturbances, dizziness, fainting, depression, anxiety.
EENT: nasal stuffiness, chest pain, palpitations, visual disturbances.
Resp: cough, shortness of breath.
CV: orthostatic hypotension, edema, palpitations.
GI: diarrhea, gas pain, indigestion, constipation, dry mouth, anorexia, nausea, abdominal pain.
GU: ejaculation disturbances, impotence, nocturia, frequency.
MS: leg cramps, aching limbs.
Neuro: paresthesia.

INTERACTIONS
Drug–Drug: ▪ Additive hypotension with other **antihypertensives, levodopa, nitrates,** or acute ingestion of **alcohol** ▪ **Tricyclic antidepressants, phenothiazines, MAO inhibitors,** or **ephedrine** may block the antihypertensive effect of guanadrel (MAO inhibitors should be stopped at least 7 days prior to guanadrel) ▪ May potentiate the pressor and mydriatic effects of **norepinephrine, amphetamines,** or **phenylephrine** ▪ Rapid withdrawal of concurrent **tricyclic antidepressant** therapy will potentiate the hypotensive response.

ROUTE AND DOSAGE
▪ **PO (Adults):** 5 mg bid, increased weekly or monthly as needed. Usual daily dose is 20–75 mg given in 2 divided doses. Higher doses may be given 3–4 times daily.

*Underlines indicate most frequent; **CAPITALS** indicate life-threatening.

AVAILABILITY

- **Tablets:** 10 mg, 25 mg.

TIME/ACTION PROFILE*
(antihypertensive effect)

	ONSET	PEAK	DURATION
PO	2 hr	4–6 hr	9 hr

*Following single dose.

NURSING IMPLICATIONS

ASSESSMENT

- Monitor blood pressure (lying and standing) and pulse prior to administration, frequently during initial dosage adjustment, and periodically throughout course of therapy. Notify physician of significant changes.
- Monitor intake and output ratios and daily weight; assess for edema daily, especially at beginning of therapy.
- Monitor frequency and consistency of stools. Notify physician if excessive diarrhea occurs.

POTENTIAL NURSING DIAGNOSES

- Injury, high risk for (side effects).
- Knowledge deficit related to medication regimen (patient/family teaching).
- Noncompliance (patient/family teaching).

IMPLEMENTATION

- **General Info:** Dosage adjustments should not be made unless there is no decrease in blood pressure when taken supine and after standing for 10 min.
- May be administered concurrently with diuretics to minimize tolerance and fluid retention.

PATIENT/FAMILY TEACHING

- Emphasize the importance of continuing to take this medication as directed, even if feeling well. Medication controls but does not cure hypertension. Instruct patient to take medication at the same time each day. If a dose is missed, take as soon as remembered; do not double doses.
- Encourage patient to comply with additional interventions for hypertension (weight reduction, low-sodium diet, smoking cessation, moderation of alcohol consumption, regular exercise, and stress management).
- Instruct patient and family on proper technique for blood pressure monitoring. Advise them to check blood pressure at least weekly and report significant changes to physician.
- Patients should weigh themselves twice weekly and assess feet and ankles for fluid retention.
- Inform patient that severity of side effects is usually reduced after the initial 8 wk of therapy.
- Guanadrel may cause drowsiness or dizziness. Advise patient to avoid driving or other activities requiring alertness until response to the medication is known.
- Caution patient to avoid sudden changes in position, especially upon arising in the morning, to minimize orthostatic hypotension. Alcohol and other CNS depressants, standing for long periods, hot showers, and exercising in hot weather should be avoided because of enhanced orthostatic effects.
- Advise patient to consult physician or pharmacist before taking any cough, cold, or allergy remedies. Patient should also avoid excessive amounts of tea, coffee, and cola.
- Instruct patient to notify physician or dentist of medication regimen prior to any surgery.
- Advise patient to notify physician if severe diarrhea, frequent dizziness or fainting, fever, or swelling of feet or lower legs occurs.
- Emphasize the importance of follow-up examinations to evaluate effectiveness of medication.

EVALUATION

Effectiveness of therapy can be demonstrated by: ■ Decrease in blood pressure without appearance of excessive side effects.

GUANETHIDINE
(gwahn-**eth**-i-deen)
{Apo-Guanethidine}, Ismelin

CLASSIFICATION(S):
Antihypertensive (peripherally
acting antiadrenergic)
Pregnancy Category C

INDICATIONS

- Treatment of moderate to severe hypertension, usually in combination with at least one other agent, usually a diuretic.

ACTION

- Prevents the release of norepinephrine from adrenergic nerve endings in response to sympathetic stimulation
- Depletes norepinephrine from nerve endings. Result is decreased sympathetically mediated vasoconstriction.
Therapeutic Effect: • Gradual and prolonged fall in blood pressure.

PHARMACOKINETICS

Absorption: Incompletely absorbed (3–50%) from the GI tract following oral administration.
Distribution: Widely distributed to storage sites, including adrenergic neurons. Minimal amounts enter breast milk. Does not appreciably cross the blood–brain barrier.
Metabolism and Excretion: Partially metabolized by the liver.
Half-life: 5 days.

CONTRAINDICATIONS AND PRECAUTIONS

Contraindicated in: • Hypersensitivity • Congestive heart failure • Pheochromocytoma.
Use Cautiously in: • Asthma • Cardiovascular or cerebrovascular insufficiency • Peptic ulcer disease • Pregnancy, lactation, or children (safety not established) • Discontinue 3–4 wk prior to surgical procedures if possible

- Impaired renal function (dosage reduction required).

ADVERSE REACTIONS AND SIDE EFFECTS*

CNS: drowsiness, fatigue, confusion, headaches, sleep disturbances, dizziness, fainting, depression, anxiety.
EENT: nasal stuffiness, chest pain, palpitations, visual disturbances.
Resp: cough, shortness of breath.
CV: orthostatic hypotension, edema, palpitations.
GI: diarrhea, gas pain, indigestion, constipation, dry mouth, anorexia, nausea, abdominal pain.
GU: ejaculation disturbances, impotence, nocturia, urinary frequency.
MS: leg cramps, aching limbs.

INTERACTIONS

Drug–Drug: • Additive hypotension with other **antihypertensives**, acute ingestion of **alcohol, levodopa, nitrates,** or acute ingestion of **alcohol** • Additive bradycardia with **reserpine** or **cardiac glycosides** • **Tricyclic antidepressants, phenothiazines, nonsteroidal anti-inflammatory agents,** and **oral contraceptives** may block antihypertensive action of guanethidine • Concurrent use with MAO inhibitors may result in hypertension (MAO inhibitors should be stopped at least 7 days prior to guanethidine) • May potentiate the pressor and mydriatic effects of **norepinephrine, amphetamines, phenylephrine,** and **metaraminol.**

ROUTE AND DOSAGE

- **PO (Adults):** 10 mg/day initially; may be increased every 5–7 days by 10–12.5 mg/day. Usual maintenance dose is 25–50 mg/day. In hospitalized patients, initial dose may be 25–50 mg, increased by 25–50 mg daily or every other day as needed.
- **PO (Children):** 0.2 mg/kg/day (6 mg/m^2/day); may be increased every 7–10 days by 0.2 mg/kg (6 mg/m^2) as needed.

{} = Available in Canada only.
*Underlines indicate most frequent; **CAPITALS** indicate life-threatening.

AVAILABILITY

- **Tablets:** 10 mg, 25 mg ▪ **In combination with:** hydrochlorothiazide (Esimil). See Appendix A.

TIME/ACTION PROFILE
(antihypertensive effect; more rapid effect is achieved with loading regimen)

	ONSET	PEAK	DURATION
PO	1–3 wk	1–3 wk	1–3 wk

NURSING IMPLICATIONS

ASSESSMENT

- ◻ Monitor blood pressure (lying and standing) and pulse frequently during initial dosage adjustment and periodically throughout course of therapy. Notify physician of significant changes.
- ◻ Monitor intake and output ratios and daily weight and assess for edema daily, especially at beginning of therapy.
- ◻ Monitor frequency and consistency of stools. Notify physician if excessive diarrhea occurs.
- ▪ **Lab Test Considerations:** Renal function should be evaluated periodically during prolonged therapy.

POTENTIAL NURSING DIAGNOSES

- ▪ Injury, high risk for (side effects).
- ▪ Knowledge deficit related to medication regimen (patient/family teaching).
- ▪ Noncompliance (patient/family teaching).

IMPLEMENTATION

- ▪ **General Info:** Dosage adjustments should not be made unless there is no decrease in blood pressure when taken supine and after standing for 10 min.
- ◻ Usually administered concurrently with diuretics to minimize tolerance and fluid retention.
- ▪ **PO:** Tablet may be crushed prior to administration and taken with fluid of patient's choice for patients with difficulty swallowing.

PATIENT/FAMILY TEACHING

- ◻ Emphasize the importance of continuing to take this medication, even if feeling well. Instruct patient to take medication at the same time each day. If a dose is missed, take as soon as remembered; do not double doses. If 2 doses in a row are missed, consult physician. Guanethidine controls but does not cure hypertension. Do not discontinue medication without consulting physician.
- ◻ Encourage patient to comply with additional interventions for hypertension (weight reduction, low-sodium diet, smoking cessation, moderation of alcohol consumption, regular excr cise, and stress management).
- ◻ Instruct patient and family on proper technique for blood pressure monitoring. Advise them to check blood pressure at least weekly and report significant changes to physician.
- ◻ Patients should weigh themselves twice weekly and assess feet and ankles for fluid retention.
- ◻ Guanethidine may occasionally cause drowsiness. Advise patient to avoid driving or other activities requiring alertness until response to medication is known.
- ◻ Caution patient to avoid sudden changes in position to minimize orthostatic hypotension, especially upon arising in the morning. Alcohol or other CNS depressants, standing for long periods, hot showers, and exercising in hot weather should be avoided because of enhanced orthostatic effects.
- ◻ If dry mouth occurs, frequent mouth rinses, good oral hygiene, and sugarless gum or candy may decrease effect. If dry mouth persists for more than 2 wk, consult dentist regarding use of saliva substitute.
- ◻ Advise patient to consult physician or pharmacist before taking any cough, cold, or allergy remedies. Patient should also avoid excessive amounts of tea, coffee, and cola.
- ◻ Instruct patient to notify physician or

G

dentist of medication regimen prior to treatment or surgery.

□ Advise patient to notify physician if severe diarrhea, frequent dizziness, or fainting occur.

□ Emphasize the importance of follow-up examinations to evaluate effectiveness of medication.

EVALUATION

Effectiveness of therapy can be demonstrated by: ▪ Decrease in blood pressure without excessive side effects.

GUANFACINE
(gwahn-fa-seen)
Tenex

CLASSIFICATION(S):
Antihypertensive (centrally acting alpha-adrenergic agonist)
Pregnancy Category B

INDICATIONS

▪ Used with thiazide-type diuretics in the management of hypertension.

ACTION

▪ Stimulates CNS alpha-adrenergic receptors, resulting in decreased sympathetic outflow. Overall result is decrease in peripheral resistance, a slight decrease in heart rate, and no change in cardiac output. **Therapeutic Effect:** ▪ Lowering of blood pressure.

PHARMACOKINETICS

Absorption: Well absorbed (80%) following oral administration.
Distribution: Appears to be widely distributed.
Metabolism and Excretion: 50% metabolized by the liver, 50% excreted unchanged by the kidneys.
Half-life: 17 hr.

CONTRAINDICATIONS AND PRECAUTIONS

Contraindicated in: ▪ Hypersensitivity.

Use Cautiously in: ▪ Severe coronary artery disease or recent myocardial infarction ▪ Cerebrovascular disease ▪ Severe renal or liver disease ▪ Pregnancy, lactation, or children <12 yr (safety not established) ▪ Do not discontinue abruptly.

ADVERSE REACTIONS AND SIDE EFFECTS*

CNS: drowsiness, weakness, fatigue, dizziness, headache, insomnia, depression.
EENT: tinnitus.
Resp: dyspnea.
CV: bradycardia, palpitations, chest pain, rebound hypertension.
GI: dry mouth, constipation, abdominal pain, nausea.
GU: impotence.

INTERACTIONS

Drug–Drug: ▪ Additive hypotension with other **antihypertensive agents, nitrates,** and acute ingestion of **alcohol** ▪ Additive CNS depression may occur with other **CNS depressants,** including **alcohol, antihistamines, opioid analgesics, tricyclic antidepressants,** and **sedative/hypnotics.**

ROUTE AND DOSAGE

▪ **PO (Adults):** 1 mg daily given at bedtime, may be increased if necessary at 3–4-wk intervals up to 3 mg/day.

AVAILABILITY

▪ *Tablets:* 1 mg.

TIME/ACTION PROFILE
(antihypertensive effect)

	ONSET	PEAK	DURATION
PO (single dose)	UK	8–12 hr	24 hr
PO (multiple doses)	within 1 wk	1–3 mo	UK

NURSING IMPLICATIONS

ASSESSMENT

□ Monitor blood pressure (lying and standing) and pulse frequently dur-

---

*Underlines indicate most frequent; **CAPITALS** indicate life-threatening.

ing initial dosage adjustment and periodically throughout course of therapy. Notify physician of significant changes.

- **Lab Test Considerations:** May cause temporary, clinically insignificant increase in plasma growth hormone levels.
- May cause decrease in urinary catecholamines and vanillylmandelic acid levels.

POTENTIAL NURSING DIAGNOSES

- Injury, high risk for (side effects).
- Knowledge deficit related to medication regimen (patient/family teaching).
- Noncompliance (patient/family teaching).

IMPLEMENTATION

- **General Info:** Administer daily dose at bedtime to minimize daytime sedation.

PATIENT/FAMILY TEACHING

- Emphasize the importance of continuing to take medication as directed, even if feeling well. Medication controls but does not cure hypertension. Instruct patient to take medication at the same time each day. If a dose is missed, take as soon as remembered; do not double doses. If 2 or more doses are missed, consult physician. Do not discontinue abruptly; may cause sympathetic overstimulation (nervousness, anxiety, rebound hypertension). These effects may occur 2–7 days after discontinuation, although rebound hypertension is rare and more likely to occur with high doses.
- Encourage patient to comply with additional interventions for hypertension (weight reduction, low-sodium diet, discontinuation of smoking, moderation of alcohol consumption, regular exercise, and stress management).
- Instruct patient and family on proper technique for blood pressure monitoring. Advise them to check blood pressure at least weekly and to report significant changes to physician.

- Guanfacine may cause drowsiness or dizziness. Advise patient to avoid driving or other activities requiring alertness until response to the medication is known.
- Caution patient to avoid alcohol and over-the-counter medications without consulting physician or pharmacist.
- Advise patient to notify physician if dry mouth or constipation persists. Frequent mouth rinses, good oral hygiene, and sugarless gum or candy may minimize dry mouth. Increase in fluid and fiber intake and exercise may decrease constipation.
- Instruct patient to notify physician or dentist of medication regimen prior to treatment or surgery.
- Advise patient to notify physician if dizziness, prolonged drowsiness, fatigue, weakness, depression, headache, sexual dysfunction, or sleep pattern disturbance occur.
- Emphasize the importance of follow-up examinations to evaluate effectiveness of medication.

EVALUATION

Effectiveness of therapy can be demonstrated by: • Decrease in blood pressure without excessive side effects.

H

HALAZEPAM
(hal-**az**-e-pam)
Paxipam

CLASSIFICATION(S):
Sedative/hypnotic
(benzodiazepine)
Schedule IV
Pregnancy Category D

INDICATIONS

- Adjunct in the management of anxiety.

ACTION

- Depresses the CNS, probably by potentiating gamma-aminobutyric acid (GABA), an inhibitory neurotransmitter. **Therapeutic Effect:** • Relief of anxiety.

PHARMACOKINETICS

Absorption: Well absorbed following oral administration.

Distribution: Widely distributed. Crosses the placenta and enters breast milk.

Metabolism and Excretion: Mostly metabolized by the liver (some conversion to desmethyldiazepam, an active sedative compound). <1% excreted unchanged by the kidneys.

Half-life: 2 hr (desmethyldiazepam 30–100 hr).

CONTRAINDICATIONS AND PRECAUTIONS

Contraindicated in: ▪ Hypersensitivity ▪ Cross-sensitivity with other benzodiazepines may exist ▪ Comatose patients ▪ Pre-existing CNS depression ▪ Uncontrolled severe pain ▪ Narrow-angle glaucoma ▪ Pregnancy or lactation.

Use Cautiously in: ▪ Hepatic dysfunction ▪ Severe renal impairment ▪ Patients who may be suicidal or who may have been addicted to drugs previously ▪ Elderly or debilitated patients (initial dosage reduction required).

ADVERSE REACTIONS AND SIDE EFFECTS*

CNS: <u>dizziness</u>, <u>drowsiness</u>, <u>lethargy</u>, hangover, paradoxical excitation, mental depression, headache.

EENT: blurred vision.

Resp: respiratory depression.

GI: nausea, vomiting, diarrhea, constipation, dry mouth.

Derm: rashes.

Misc: tolerance, psychological dependence, physical dependence.

INTERACTIONS

Drug–Drug: ▪ Additive CNS depression with other **CNS depressants,** including **alcohol, antihistamines, antidepressants, opioid analgesics,** and other **sedative/hypnotics** ▪ **Cimetidine, oral contraceptives, disulfiram, fluoxetine, isoniazid, ketoconazole, metoprolol, propoxyphene, propranolol,** or **valproic acid** may decrease metabolism and increase CNS depression ▪ May decrease the efficacy of **levodopa** ▪ **Rifampin** or **barbiturates** may increase metabolism and decrease effectiveness.

ROUTE AND DOSAGE

▪ **PO (Adults):** 20–40 mg 3–4 times daily.

▪ **PO (Elderly/Debilitated Patients):** 20 mg 1–2 times daily initially.

AVAILABILITY

▪ *Tablets:* 20 mg, 40 mg.

TIME/ACTION PROFILE (antianxiety effect)

	ONSET	PEAK	DURATION
PO	UK	UK	UK

NURSING IMPLICATIONS

ASSESSMENT

▢ Assess degree and manifestations of anxiety and mental status prior to and periodically throughout therapy.

▢ Assess patient for drowsiness, light-headedness, and dizziness. These symptoms usually disappear as therapy progresses. Dosage should be reduced if these symptoms persist.

▢ Prolonged high-dose therapy may lead to psychological or physical dependence. Restrict the amount of drug available to patient.

POTENTIAL NURSING DIAGNOSES

▪ Anxiety (indications).

▪ Injury, high risk for (side effects).

▪ Knowledge deficit related to medication regimen (patient/family teaching).

IMPLEMENTATION

▪ **PO:** Tablets may be crushed and taken with food or fluids if patient has difficulty swallowing.

PATIENT/FAMILY TEACHING

▢ Instruct patient to take medication exactly as directed; do not skip or double up on missed doses. If a dose is missed, it can be taken within 1 hr, otherwise skip the dose and return to

---

*<u>Underlines</u> indicate most frequent; **CAPITALS** indicate life-threatening.

the regular schedule. If medication is less effective after a few weeks, check with physician; do not increase dose. Abrupt withdrawal of halazepam may cause sweating, vomiting, muscle cramps, tremors, and convulsions.

▫ Halazepam may cause drowsiness or dizziness. Caution patient to avoid driving and other activities requiring alertness until response to the medication is known.

▫ Advise patient to avoid the use of alcohol or other CNS depressants concurrently with this medication. Instruct patient to consult physician or pharmacist before taking over-the-counter medications concurrently with this medication.

▫ Inform patient that frequent mouth rinses, good oral hygiene, and sugarless gum or candy may minimize dry mouth.

EVALUATION
Effectiveness of therapy can be demonstrated by: ▪ Decreased sense of anxiety ▫ Increased ability to cope. Treatment with this medication should not continue without periodic re-evaluation of the patient's need for the drug.

HALOPERIDOL
(ha-loe-**per**-i-dole)
{Apo-Haloperidol}, Haldol, Haldol Decanoate, {Haldol L.A.}, {Novoperidol}, {Peridol}

CLASSIFICATION(S):
Antipsychotic (butyrophenone)
Pregnancy Category C (decanoate salt only, others UK)

INDICATIONS
▪ Treatment of acute and chronic psychoses ▪ Used to control Tourette's disorder and severe behavioral problems in children.

ACTION
▪ Alters the effects of dopamine in the CNS ▪ Also has anticholinergic and alpha-adrenergic blocking activity. **Therapeutic Effect:** ▪ Diminished signs and symptoms of psychoses.

PHARMACOKINETICS
Absorption: Well absorbed following oral and IM administration. Decanoate salt is slowly absorbed and has a long duration of action.
Distribution: Distribution not fully known. High concentrations in the liver. Crosses the placenta. Enters breast milk.
Metabolism and Excretion: Mostly metabolized by the liver.
Half-life: 21–24 hr.

CONTRAINDICATIONS AND PRECAUTIONS
Contraindicated in: ▪ Hypersensitivity ▪ Narrow-angle glaucoma ▪ Bone marrow depression ▪ CNS depression ▪ Severe liver disease ▪ Severe cardiovascular disease ▪ Some injectables contain parabens, sesame oil, or benzyl alcohol and should be avoided in patients with known intolerance or hypersensitivity.
Use Cautiously in: ▪ Elderly or debilitated patients (dosage reduction required) ▪ Pregnancy and lactation (safety not established) ▪ Cardiac disease ▪ Severely ill patients and diabetics ▪ Respiratory insufficiency ▪ Prostatic hypertrophy ▪ CNS tumors ▪ Intestinal obstruction ▪ History of seizures.

ADVERSE REACTIONS AND SIDE EFFECTS*
CNS: sedation, extrapyramidal reactions, tardive dyskinesia, restlessness, confusion, seizures.
EENT: dry eyes, blurred vision.
Resp: respiratory depression.
CV: hypotension, tachycardia.
GI: constipation, ileus, anorexia, dry mouth, hepatitis.

H

GU: urinary retention.
Derm: rashes, photosensitivity, diaphoresis.
Endo: galactorrhea.
Hemat: anemia, leukopenia.
Metab: hyperpyrexia.
Misc: hypersensitivity reactions, NEUROLEPTIC MALIGNANT SYNDROME.

INTERACTIONS

Drug–Drug: ▪ Additive hypotension with **antihypertensives, nitrates,** or acute ingestion of **alcohol** ▪ Additive anticholinergic effects with **drugs having anticholinergic properties,** including **antihistamines, antidepressants, atropine, phenothiazines, quinidine,** and **disopyramide** ▪ Additive CNS depression with other **CNS depressants,** including **alcohol, antihistamines, opioid analgesics,** and **sedative/hypnotics** ▪ Concurrent use with **epinephrine** may result in severe hypotension and tachycardia ▪ May decrease therapeutic effects of **levodopa** ▪ Acute encephalopathic syndrome may occur when used with **lithium** ▪ Dementia may occur with **methyldopa.**

ROUTE AND DOSAGE

Haloperidol
▪ **PO (Adults):** 0.5–5 mg 2–3 times daily. Patients with severe symptoms may require up to 100 mg/day.
▪ **PO (Children 3–12 yr or 15–40 kg):** *Psychotic disorders*—50–150 mcg/kg/day in 2–3 divided doses. *Nonpsychotic disorders and Tourette's syndrome*—50–75 mcg/kg/day in 1–3 divided doses.
▪ **IM (Adults):** 2–5 mg q 1–8 hr, not to exceed 100 mg/day.
▪ **IV (Adults):** 0.5–50 mg, may be repeated in 30 min.

Haloperidol Decanoate
▪ **IM (Adults):** 10–15 times the previous daily PO dose, but not to exceed 100 mg initially, given monthly (not to exceed 300 mg/mo).

AVAILABILITY
▪ *Tablets:* 0.5 mg, 1 mg, 2 mg, 5 mg, 10 mg, 20 mg ▪ *Oral concentrate:* 2 mg/ml

▪ *Injection:* 5 mg/ml ▪ *Long-acting injection:* 50 mg/ml, 100 mg/ml.

TIME/ACTION PROFILE
(antipsychotic activity)

	ONSET	PEAK	DURATION
PO	2 hr	2–6 hr	8–12 hr
IM	20–30 min	30–45 min	4–8 hr*
IM (decanoate)	3–9 days	UK	1 mo

*Effect may persist for several days.

NURSING IMPLICATIONS

ASSESSMENT
▫ Assess patient's mental status (orientation, mood, behavior) prior to and periodically throughout therapy.
▫ Monitor blood pressure (sitting, standing, lying) and pulse prior to and frequently during the period of dosage adjustment.
▫ Observe patient carefully when administering medication, to ensure that medication is actually taken and not hoarded.
▫ Monitor intake and output ratios and daily weight. Assess patient for signs and symptoms of dehydration (decreased thirst, lethargy, hemoconcentration).
▫ Assess fluid intake and bowel function. Increased bulk and fluids in the diet help minimize the constipating effects of this medication.
▫ Observe patient carefully for extrapyramidal symptoms (pill-rolling motions, drooling, tremors, rigidity, shuffling gait), tardive dyskinesia (uncontrolled movements of face, mouth, tongue, or jaw and involuntary movements of extremities), and neuroleptic malignant syndrome (pale skin, hyperthermia, skeletal muscle rigidity, autonomic dysfunction, altered consciousness, leukocytosis, elevated liver function tests, elevated CPK). Notify physician immediately at the onset of these symptoms.
▪ **Lab Test Considerations:** CBC and liver function tests should be evalu-

ated periodically throughout course of therapy.

POTENTIAL NURSING DIAGNOSES

- Thought processes, altered (indications).
- Knowledge deficit related to medication regimen (patient/family teaching).

IMPLEMENTATION

- **PO:** Administer with food or full glass of water or milk to minimize GI irritation.
- Use calibrated measuring device for accurate dosage. Do not dilute concentrate with coffee or tea; may cause precipitation. Should be given undiluted, but if necessary may dilute in at least 60 ml of liquid.
- **IM:** Inject slowly using 2-in., 21-gauge needle into well-developed muscle. Do not exceed 3 ml per injection site. Slight yellow color does not indicate altered potency. Keep patient recumbent for at least 30 min following injection to minimize hypotensive effects.
- **Syringe Incompatibility:** ▪ heparin.
- **Y-Site Compatibility:** ▪ fludarabine ▪ ondansetron.
- **Y-Site Incompatibility:** ▪ fluconazole ▪ foscarnet ▪ heparin ▪ sargramostim.

PATIENT/FAMILY TEACHING

- Advise patient to take medication exactly as directed. Missed doses should be taken as soon as remembered, with remaining doses evenly spaced throughout the day. May require several weeks to obtain desired effects. Do not increase dose or discontinue medication without consulting physician. Abrupt withdrawal may cause dizziness, nausea, vomiting, GI upset, trembling, or uncontrolled movements of mouth, tongue, or jaw.
- Inform patient of possibility of extrapyramidal symptoms and tardive dyskinesia. Caution patient to report these symptoms immediately to physician.
- Advise patient to make position changes slowly to minimize orthostatic hypotension.
- Medication may cause drowsiness. Caution patient to avoid driving or other activities requiring alertness until response to medication is known.
- Caution patient to avoid taking alcohol or other CNS depressants concurrently with this medication.
- Advise patient to use sunscreen and protective clothing when exposed to the sun to prevent photosensitivity reactions. Extremes of temperature should also be avoided, as this drug impairs body temperature regulation.
- Instruct patient to use frequent mouth rinses, good oral hygiene, and sugarless gum or candy to minimize dry mouth.
- Instruct patient to notify physician promptly if weakness, tremors, visual disturbances, dark-colored urine or clay-colored stools, sore throat, or fever is noted.
- Emphasize the importance of routine follow-up examinations.

EVALUATION

Effectiveness of therapy can be demonstrated by: ▪ Decrease in hallucinations, insomnia, agitation, hostility, and delusions ▪ Decreased tics and vocalization in Tourette's syndrome. If no therapeutic effects are seen in 2–4 wk, dosage may be increased.

H

HEPARIN
(hep-a-rin)
{Calcilean}, Calciparine, {Hepalean}, {Heparin Leo}, Liquaemin
HEPARIN LOCK FLUSH
Hep-Lock, Hep-Lock U/P

CLASSIFICATION(S):
Anticoagulant
Pregnancy Category C

INDICATIONS

▪ Prophylaxis and treatment of various thromboembolic disorders including: □ Venous thromboembolism □ Pulmonary emboli □ Atrial fibrillation with embolization □ Acute and chronic consumptive coagulopathies □ Peripheral arterial thromboembolism ▪ Used in very low doses (10–100 units) to maintain patency of IV catheters ("heparin flush").

ACTION

▪ Potentiates the effects of antithrombin III ▪ In low doses prevents the conversion of prothrombin to thrombin by its effects on factor X_a ▪ Higher doses neutralize thrombin, preventing the conversion of fibrinogen to fibrin. **Therapeutic Effects:** ▪ Prevention of thrombus formation ▪ Prevention of extension of existing thrombi.

PHARMACOKINETICS

Absorption: Destroyed by enzymes in the GI tract, necessitating parenteral administration. Well absorbed following SC administration.
Distribution: Does not cross the placenta or enter breast milk.
Metabolism and Excretion: Appears to be removed by the reticuloendothelial system (lymph nodes, spleen).
Half-life: 1–2 hr (increases with increasing dosage).

CONTRAINDICATIONS AND PRECAUTIONS

Contraindicated in: ▪ Hypersensitivity ▪ Hypersensitivity to pig or beef proteins (some products are derived from pig intestinal mucosa, others from beef lung) ▪ Uncontrolled bleeding ▪ Open wounds ▪ Severe liver or kidney disease ▪ Products containing benzyl alcohol should not be used in premature infants.
Use Cautiously in: ▪ Untreated hypertension ▪ Ulcer disease ▪ Spinal cord or brain injury ▪ Malignancy ▪ May be used during pregnancy, but use with caution during the last trimester and in the immediate postpartum period.

ADVERSE REACTIONS AND SIDE EFFECTS*

GI: hepatitis.
Hemat: BLEEDING, thrombocytopenia.
Derm: rashes, urticaria.
Misc: hypersensitivity, fever.

INTERACTIONS

Drug–Drug: ▪ Risk of bleeding may be increased by concurrent use of **drugs that affect platelet function,** including **aspirin, nonsteroidal anti-inflammatory agents, dipyridamole,** some **penicillins,** and **dextran** ▪ Risk of bleeding may be increased by concurrent use of **drugs that cause hypoprothrombinemia,** including **quinidine, cefamandole, cefmetazole, cefoperazone, cefotetan, moxalaxtam,** and **plicamycin** ▪ Concurrent use of **thrombolytic agents** increases the risk of bleeding ▪ Heparin affects the prothrombin time used in assessing the response to **warfarin** ▪ **Probenecid** increases the intensity and duration of the action of heparin.

ROUTE AND DOSAGE

Therapeutic Anticoagulation
Dosage depends on results of PTT.
▪ **Intermittent IV Bolus (Adults):** 10,000 units, followed by 5000–10,000 units q 4–6 hr.
▪ **Intermittent IV Bolus (Children):** 50 units/kg, followed by 50–100 units/kg q 4 hr.
▪ **IV Infusion (Adults):** 5000 units (35–70 units/kg), followed by 20,000–40,000 units infused over 24 hr (approx. 1000 units/hr).
▪ **IV Infusion (Children):** 50 units/kg, followed by 20,000 units/m^2/24 hr.
▪ **SC (Adults):** 5000 units IV, followed by initial SC dose of 10,000–20,000 units, then 8000–10,000 units q 8 hr, or 15,000–20,000 units q 12 hr.

Prophylaxis of Thromboembolic Events
▪ **SC (Adults):** 5000 units q 8–12 hr (may be started 2 hr prior to surgery).

*Underlines indicate most frequent; **CAPITALS** indicate life-threatening.

Heparin Flush
- **IV (Adults and Children):** 10–100 units.

AVAILABILITY
Heparin Sodium
- *Injection:* 10 units/ml, 100 units/ml, 1000 units/ml, 5000 units/ml, 10,000 units/ml, 20,000 units/ml, 40,000 units/ml.

Heparin Calcium
- *Injection:* 5000 units/0.2 ml.

TIME/ACTION PROFILE
(anticoagulant effect)

	ONSET	PEAK	DURATION
SC	20–60 min	2 hr	8–12 hr
IV	immediate	5–10 min	2–6 hr

NURSING IMPLICATIONS
Assessment
- **General Info:** Assess patient for signs of bleeding and hemorrhage (bleeding gums, nose bleed, unusual bruising, black tarry stools, hematuria, fall in hematocrit or blood pressure, guaiac-positive stools). Notify physician if these occur.
- Assess patient for evidence of additional or increased thrombosis. Symptoms will depend on area of involvement.
- Monitor patient for hypersensitivity reactions (chills, fever, urticaria). Report signs to physician.
- **SC:** Observe injection sites for hematomas or ecchymosis or inflammation.
- **Lab Test Considerations:** Activated partial thromboplastin time (aPTT) and hematocrit should be monitored prior to and periodically throughout course of therapy. When intermittent IV therapy is used, draw aPTT levels 30 min before next dose. During continuous administration, blood for aPTT levels can be drawn 1.5–2 hr after initiation of heparin therapy.
- Monitor platelet count every 2–3 days throughout course of therapy. May cause mild thrombocytopenia, which appears on fourth day and resolves

despite continued heparin therapy. Thrombocytopenia, which necessitates discontinuing medication, may develop on eighth day of therapy. Patients who have received a previous course of heparin may be at higher risk for severe thrombocytopenia for several months after the initial course.
- May cause prolonged PT levels, false elevations of serum thyroxine, T_3 resin, sulfobromopthalein (BSP), and false-negative ^{125}I fibrinogen uptake tests.
- May cause decreased serum triglyceride and cholesterol levels and increased plasma free fatty acid concentrations.
- May also cause elevated AST (SGOT) and ALT (SGPT) levels.
- **Toxicity and Overdose:** Protamine sulfate is the antidote. However, because of the short half-life of heparin, overdose can often be treated by withdrawing the drug.

Potential Nursing Diagnoses
- Tissue perfusion, altered (indications).
- Injury, high risk for (side effects).
- Knowledge deficit related to medication regimen (patient/family teaching).

Implementation
- **General Info:** Inform all personnel caring for patient of anticoagulant therapy. Venipunctures and injection sites require application of pressure to prevent bleeding or hematoma formation. IM injections of other medications should be avoided, as hematomas may develop.
- In patients requiring long-term anticoagulation, oral anticoagulant therapy should be instituted 4–5 days prior to discontinuing heparin therapy.
- Solution is colorless to slightly yellow.
- **SC:** Administer deep into SC tissue with a small-gauge (25–27), ⅜–⅝-in. needle. Check dosage for accuracy with another licensed nurse prior to

H

administration. Inject into lower abdomen (preferred site); do not aspirate or massage. Rotate sites frequently. Do not administer IM, because of the danger of hematoma formation.

- **Direct IV:** Loading dose usually precedes continuous infusion.
- **Rate:** May be given undiluted over at least 1 min.
- **Intermittent/Continuous Infusion:** Dilute in prescribed amount of 0.9% NaCl, D5W, or Ringer's solution for injection and give as a continuous or intermittent infusion. Ensure adequate mixing of heparin in solution by inverting container at least 6 times initially and periodically mixing during infusing.
- **Rate:** Infusion may be administered over 4–24 hr. Use an infusion pump to ensure accuracy. See infusion rate table in Appendix D.
- **Heparin Lock:** To prevent clot formation in intermittent infusion (heparin lock) sets, inject dilute heparin solution of 10–100 units/0.5–1 ml after each medication injection or every 8–12 hr. To prevent incompatibility of heparin with medication, flush heparin lock set with Sterile Water or 0.9% NaCl for Injection before and after medication is administered.
- **Y-Site Compatibility:** ▪ acyclovir ▪ aminophylline ▪ ampicillin ▪ atracurium ▪ atropine ▪ betamethasone ▪ bleomycin ▪ calcium gluconate ▪ cephalothin ▪ cephapirin ▪ chlordiazepoxide ▪ chlorpromazine ▪ cimetidine ▪ cisplatin ▪ cyancobalamin ▪ cyclophosphamide ▪ dexamethasone ▪ digoxin ▪ diphenhydramine ▪ dopamine ▪ edrophonium ▪ enalaprilat ▪ epinephrine ▪ esmolol ▪ conjugated estrogens ▪ ethacrynate ▪ famotidine ▪ fentanyl ▪ fluconazole ▪ fludarabine ▪ fluorouracil ▪ foscarnet ▪ furosemide ▪ hydralazine ▪ insulin ▪ isoproterenol ▪ kanamycin ▪ labetalol ▪ leucovorin ▪ lidocaine ▪ magnesium sulfate ▪ menadiol sodium ▪ meperidine ▪ methicillin ▪ methotrexate ▪ methoxamine ▪ methylergonovine ▪ met-oclopramide ▪ minocycline ▪ mitomycin ▪ morphine ▪ neostigmine ▪ norepinephrine ▪ ondansetron ▪ oxacillin ▪ oxytocin ▪ pancuronium ▪ penicillin G potassium ▪ pentazocine ▪ phytonadione ▪ prednisolone ▪ procainamide ▪ prochlorperazine ▪ propranolol ▪ pyridostigmine ▪ ranitidine ▪ sargramostim ▪ scopolamine ▪ sodium bicarbonate ▪ streptokinase ▪ succinylcholine ▪ trimethophan camsylate ▪ trimethobenzamide ▪ vecuronium ▪ vinblastine ▪ vincristine ▪ zidovudine.

- **Y-Site Incompatibility:** ▪ alteplase ▪ ciprofloxacin ▪ dacarbazine ▪ diazepam ▪ dobutamine ▪ doxorubicin ▪ ergotamine tartrate ▪ gentamicin ▪ haloperidol ▪ methotrimeprazine ▪ phenytoin ▪ promethazine ▪ tobramycin ▪ triflupromazine.

- **Additive Compatibility:** ▪ amphotericin ▪ calcium gluconate ▪ cephalothin ▪ cephapirin ▪ chloramphenicol ▪ clindamycin ▪ colistimethate ▪ dimenhydrinate ▪ erythromycin glucceptate ▪ furosemide ▪ methyldopate ▪ methylprednisolone ▪ nafcillin ▪ octreotide ▪ potassium chloride ▪ prednisolone ▪ promazine ▪ ranitidine ▪ sodium bicarbonate ▪ verapamil ▪ vitamin B complex ▪ vitamin B complex with C. Also compatible with TPN solutions or fat emulsion.

- **Additive Incompatibility:** ▪ amikacin ▪ erythromycin lactobionate ▪ gentamicin ▪ kanamycin ▪ meperidine ▪ methadone ▪ morphine ▪ polymyxin B ▪ streptomycin.

PATIENT/FAMILY TEACHING

- □ Caution patient to avoid IM injections and activities leading to injury and to use a soft toothbrush and electric razor during heparin therapy.
- □ Advise patient to report any symptoms of unusual bleeding or bruising to physician immediately.
- □ Instruct patient not to take medications containing aspirin or ibuprofen while on heparin therapy.
- □ Advise patient to inform physician and dentist of medication regimen prior to treatment or surgery.

□ Patients on anticoagulant therapy should carry an identification card with this information at all times.

EVALUATION

Clinical response to therapy is indicated by: ▪ Prolonged PTT of 1.5–2.5 times the control, without signs of hemorrhage ▪ Prevention of thromboembolism ▪ Patency of IV catheters.

HEPATITIS B IMMUNE GLOBULIN
(hep-a-**tite**-iss B i-**myoon** **glo**-byoo-lin)
H-BIG, Hep-B-Gammagee, HyperHep

CLASSIFICATION(S):
Serum (immune globulin)
Pregnancy Category UK

INDICATIONS

▪ Prevents hepatitis B infection in patients who are known to have been exposed, including neonates born to HBsAg-positive women, by providing passive immunity.

ACTION

▪ An immune gamma-globulin fraction containing high titers of antibodies to the hepatitis B surface antigen. Confers passive immunity to hepatitis B infection. **Therapeutic Effect:** ▪ Prevention of hepatitis B infection.

PHARMACOKINETICS

Absorption: Slowly absorbed following IM administration.
Distribution: Distribution not known. Probably crosses the placenta.
Metabolism and Excretion: Metabolism and excretion not known.
Half-life: 21 days.

CONTRAINDICATIONS AND PRECAUTIONS

Contraindicated in: ▪ Hypersensitivity to immune globulins, glycine, or thimerosol.

Use Cautiously in: ▪ Thrombocytopenia ▪ IgA deficiency ▪ Lactation ▪ Has been used during pregnancy.

ADVERSE REACTIONS AND SIDE EFFECTS*

CNS: faintness, dizziness, weakness, malaise.
Derm: rashes, urticaria, pruritus.
MS: joint pain.
Local: pain, swelling, tenderness, erythema at IM site.
Misc: allergic reactions, including angioedema and ANAPHYLACTIC SHOCK.

INTERACTIONS

Drug–Drug: ▪ May interfere with the immune response to **live vaccines**.

ROUTE AND DOSAGE

▪ **IM (Adults):** 0.06 ml/kg (usual dose 3–5 ml).
▪ **IM (Neonates):** 0.5 ml.

AVAILABILITY

▪ *Injection:* 0.5 ml prefilled syringes; 1-, 4-, 5-ml vials.

TIME/ACTION PROFILE (development of anti-HBs antibodies)

	ONSET	PEAK	DURATION
IM	1–6 days	3–11 days	2–6 mo

H

NURSING IMPLICATIONS

ASSESSMENT

□ For passive immunity, determine the date of exposure to infection. Hepatitis B immune globulin should be administered preferably within 24 hr but not later than 7 days of exposure to hepatitis B.
□ Assess patient for signs of anaphylaxis (hypotension, flushing, chest tightness, wheezing, fever, dizziness, nausea, vomiting, diaphoresis) following administration. Epinephrine and antihistamines should be available for treatment of anaphylactic reactions.

POTENTIAL NURSING DIAGNOSES

▪ Infection, high risk for (indications).

*Underlines indicate most frequent; CAPITALS indicate life-threatening.

- Knowledge deficit related to medication regimen (patient/family teaching).

IMPLEMENTATION
- **General Info:** Solution for injection is clear, slightly amber, and viscous. Solution should be refrigerated.
- If administered with hepatitis B virus vaccine, do not administer via same syringe or into same injection site.
- **IM:** Administer hepatitis B immune globulin (HBIG) in adults and children into the deltoid muscle or anterolateral thigh. The gluteal site should be used only in adults with injections of large volumes or when large volumes are divided into multiple doses.
- Do not administer IV.

PATIENT/FAMILY TEACHING
- Explain to patient the use and purpose of hepatitis B immune globulin therapy.
- Advise patient to report symptoms of anaphylaxis immediately.
- Inform patient that pain, tenderness, swelling, and erythema at the injection site may occur following IM injections.

EVALUATION
Effectiveness of immune globulin therapy can be demonstrated by: ■ Prevention of hepatitis B infection in exposed patients by providing passive immunity.

HETASTARCH
Hespan

CLASSIFICATION(S):
Volume expander
Pregnancy Category UK

INDICATIONS
- Adjunct for fluid replacement and volume expansion in the early management of shock or impending shock due to: □ Burns □ Hemorrhage □ Surgery □ Sepsis □ Trauma.

ACTION
- A synthetic molecule that acts as a colloidal osmotic agent similar to albumin. **Therapeutic Effect:** ■ Plasma volume expansion.

PHARMACOKINETICS
Absorption: Administered IV only, resulting in complete bioavailability.
Distribution: Not known.
Metabolism and Excretion: Molecules with a molecular weight of 50,000 or less are excreted unchanged by the kidneys. Larger molecules are slowly degraded before excretion.
Half-life: 90% has half-life of 17 days, remaining 10% has half-life of 48 days.

CONTRAINDICATIONS AND PRECAUTIONS
Contraindicated in: ■ Hypersensitivity ■ Severe bleeding disorders ■ Congestive heart failure ■ Pulmonary edema ■ Oliguric or anuric renal failure ■ Early pregnancy.
Use Cautiously in: ■ Thrombocytopenia ■ Elderly patients ■ Lactation or children (safety not established).

ADVERSE REACTIONS AND SIDE EFFECTS*
CNS: headache.
CV: pulmonary edema, congestive heart failure.
GI: vomiting.
Hemat: decreased platelet function, decreased hematocrit.
Derm: pruritus, urticaria.
F and E: fluid overload, peripheral edema of the lower extremities.
MS: mylagia.
Misc: hypersensitivity reactions, including ANAPHYLACTOID REACTIONS, chills, fever, parotid and submaxillary gland enlargement.

INTERACTIONS
Drug–Drug: ■ No known interactions.

---

*Underlines indicate most frequent; **CAPITALS** indicate life-threatening.

ROUTE AND DOSAGE
- **IV (Adults):** 30–60 g (500–1000 ml of 6% solution), may be repeated, not to exceed 90 g (1500 ml/day). In acute hemorrhagic shock, up to 20 ml/kg/hr may be used.

AVAILABILITY
- *Injection:* 6 g/100 ml in 0.9% saline 500-ml infusion bottles.

TIME/ACTION PROFILE (volume expansion)

	ONSET	PEAK	DURATION
IV	rapid	end of infusion	24 hr or longer

NURSING IMPLICATIONS

ASSESSMENT
- ☐ Monitor vital signs, CVP, cardiac output, pulmonary capillary wedge pressure, and urinary output prior to and frequently throughout therapy. Assess patient for signs of vascular overload (elevated CVP, rales/crackles, dyspnea, hypertension, jugular venous distention) during and following administration.
- ☐ If fever, wheezing, flu-like symptoms, urticaria, periorbital edema, or submaxillary and parotid gland enlargement occur, stop infusion and notify physician immediately. Antihistamines, epinephrine, glucocorticoids, and airway management may be required to suppress this response.
- ☐ Assess surgical patients for increased bleeding following administration caused by interference with platelet function and clotting factors.
- **Lab Test Considerations:** Monitor CBC with differential, hemoglobin, hematocrit, platelet count, prothrombin time, partial thromboplastin time, and clotting time throughout course of therapy. Large volumes of hetastarch may cause hemodilution; do not allow hematocrit to drop below 30% by volume. May cause increased erythrocyte sedimentation rate; prolonged bleeding time; and prolonged prothrombin, partial thromboplastin, and clotting times.

- ☐ May cause elevated indirect serum bilirubin and amylase concentrations.

POTENTIAL NURSING DIAGNOSES
- Tissue perfusion, altered (indications).
- Fluid volume deficit (indications).
- Fluid volume excess (side effects).

IMPLEMENTATION
- **General Info:** Available in a 6% solution diluted with 0.9% NaCl. Solution should be clear pale yellow to amber; do not administer solution that is cloudy or that contains a precipitate. Store at room temperature. Discard unused solution.
- ☐ There is no danger of serum hepatitis or AIDS from hetastarch. Crossmatching is not required.
- **Continuous Infusion:** Administer hetastarch undiluted by IV infusion.
- **Rate:** Rate of administration is determined by blood volume, indication, and patient response.
- ☐ In acute hemorrhagic shock hetastarch may be administered up to 1.2 g/kg (20 ml/kg) per hr. Slower rates are generally used with burns and septic shock.
- **Y-site Compatibility:** ■ cimetidine ■ enalaprilat.
- **Y-site Incompatibility:** ■ amikacin ■ cefamandole ■ cefoperazone ■ cefotaxime ■ cefoxitin ■ gentamicin ■ theophylline ■ tobramycin.

PATIENT/FAMILY TEACHING
- ☐ Explain to patient the rationale for use of this solution.
- ☐ Instruct patient to notify physician or nurse if dyspnsea, itching, or flu-like symptoms occur.

EVALUATION
Effectiveness of therapy can be demonstrated by: ■ Increase in blood pressure, blood volume, and urinary output when used to treat shock and burns.

H

HISTRELIN
(hiss-tre-linn)
Supprelin

> **CLASSIFICATION(S):**
> Hormone (gonadotropin-releasing)
> **Pregnancy Category X**

INDICATIONS

■ Management of central precocious puberty in girls <8 yr or boys <9.5 yr.

ACTION

■ Daily administration decreases production of gonadotropins. **Therapeutic Effect:** ■ Regression of secondary sexual characteristics in children with precocious puberty.

PHARMACOKINETICS

Absorption: UK.
Distribution: UK.
Metabolism and Excretion: UK.
Half-life: UK.

CONTRAINDICATIONS AND PRECAUTIONS

Contraindicated in: ■ Hypersensitivity ■ Pregnancy or lactation.
Use Cautiously in: ■ Children <2 yr (safety not established).

ADVERSE REACTIONS AND SIDE EFFECTS*

CNS: headache, mood changes, nervousness, dizziness, depression, libido changes, insomnia, anxiety, cognitive changes, syncope, lethargy, SEIZURES, conduct disorders.
EENT: epistaxis, hearing loss, visual disturbances, photophobia.
Resp: respiratory congestion, cough, asthma, rhinorrhea, hyperventilation.
CV: vasodilation, edema, palpitations, tachycardia.
GI: abdominal pain, nausea, vomiting, diarrhea, flatulence, dyspepsia, cramps, constipation, gastritis.
GU: vaginal dryness, leukorrhea, tenderness of female genitalia, vaginal bleeding, irritation of female genitalia, polyuria, dysuria, urinary frequency, incontinence, hematuria, nocturia.
Derm: purpura, pallor.

Endo: breast pain, breast discharge, decreased breast size, metrorrhagia, goiter, hyperlipidemia.
Hemat: anemia.
Local: redness, swelling, itching at injection site, acne, sweating, rash, urticaria, erythema, pruritus, keratoderma, alopecia, skin discoloration.
MS: arthralgia, joint stiffness, muscle cramps, muscle stiffness, myalgia.
Neuro: paresthesia, tremors, hyperkinesia.
Misc: fever, chills, malaise, glycosuria, decreased appetite, thirst.

INTERACTIONS

Drug–Drug: ■ None known.

ROUTE AND DOSAGE

■ **SC (Children):** 10 mcg/kg/day.

AVAILABILITY

■ *Injection:* 120 mcg/0.6 ml, 300 mcg/0.6 ml, 600 mcg/0.6 ml.

TIME/ACTION PROFILE (decrease in LH, FSH, and sex-steroid levels)

	ONSET	PEAK	DURATION
SC	within 3 mo	UK	UK

NURSING IMPLICATIONS

ASSESSMENT

□ Prior to therapy, a complete physical and endocrinologic examination, including height, weight, hand and wrist x-ray, total sex steroid level (estradiol or testosterone), adrenal steroid level, beta human chorionic gonadotropin level, GnRH stimulation test, pelvic/adrenal/testicular ultrasound, and computerized tomography of the head must be performed. These parameters are monitored after 3 mo and every 6–12 mo during therapy.

□ Assess patient for signs of precocious puberty (menses, breast development, testicular growth) periodically throughout therapy.

□ Monitor patient for signs of hypersensitivity (angioedema, urticaria, hypo-

---

*Underlines indicate most frequent; **CAPITALS** indicate life-threatening.

tension, tachycardia, loss of consciousness, bronchospasm, dyspnea, flushing, pruritus). Therapy should be discontinued if any of these symptoms occur.

□ Histrelin is discontinued when the onset of normal puberty is desired. Monitor the onset of normal puberty and assess menstrual cycle, reproductive function, and final adult height.

POTENTIAL NURSING DIAGNOSES
▪ Sexual dysfunction (indications).
▪ Knowledge deficit related to medication regimen (patient/family teaching).

IMPLEMENTATION
▪ **SC:** Histrelin is given as a single daily injection.

PATIENT/FAMILY TEACHING
□ Instruct patient and family on the proper technique for SC injection. Emphasize the importance of administering the medication at the same time each day. Unused vials should be refrigerated. Medication should be allowed to reach room temperature before administration. Explain that vials should be used once and discarded. Rotate injection sites daily.
□ Inform patient and parents that if injections are not given daily pubertal process may be reactivated.
□ Advise patient and parents that during initial agonistic phase (1–3 wk) the patient may have transient increases in breast tissue, moodiness, vaginal secretions, or testicular volume. Girls may also experience a light menstrual flow during the first month of therapy.
□ Inform patient and parents that redness or swelling may occur at the injection site. Notify physician if this reaction is severe or does not go away.
□ Instruct patient and parents to discontinue medication and contact physician at the first sign of skin rash, urticaria, rapid heartbeat, difficulty swallowing or breathing, or any

swelling that may suggest angioedema.

EVALUATION
Clinical response to therapy can be determined by: ▪ Resolution of the signs of precocious puberty.

HYDRALAZINE
(hyr-**dral**-a-zeen)
Alazine, Apresoline, Dralzine, {Novo-Hylazin}, Rolzine

CLASSIFICATION(S):
Antihypertensive (vasodilator)
Pregnancy Category C

INDICATIONS
▪ In combination with a diuretic in the management of moderate to severe hypertension ▪ Treatment of congestive heart failure unresponsive to conventional therapy with cardiac glycosides and diuretics.

ACTION
▪ Direct-acting peripheral arteriolar vasodilator. **Therapeutic Effects:** ▪ Lowering of blood pressure in hypertensive patients and decreased afterload in patients with congestive heart failure.

PHARMACOKINETICS
Absorption: Rapidly absorbed following oral administration. Well absorbed from IM sites.
Distribution: Widely distributed. Crosses the placenta. Enters breast milk in minimal concentrations.
Metabolism and Excretion: Mostly metabolized by the GI mucosa and liver.
Half-life: 2–8 hr.

CONTRAINDICATIONS AND PRECAUTIONS
Contraindicated in: ▪ Hypersensitivity ▪ Some products contain tartrazine (FDC yellow dye #5)—avoid use in pa-

H

tients with tartrazine hypersensitivity.

Use Cautiously in: ▪ Cardiovascular or cerebrovascular disease ▪ Severe renal and hepatic disease ▪ Pregnancy, lactation, or children (safety not established).

ADVERSE REACTIONS AND SIDE EFFECTS*

CNS: headache, peripheral neuropathy, dizziness, drowsiness.

CV: <u>tachycardia</u>, angina, arrhythmias, orthostatic hypotension, edema.

GI: nausea, vomiting, diarrhea.

Derm: rashes.

F and E: <u>sodium retention</u>.

MS: arthritis, arthralgias.

Neuro: peripheral neuropathy.

Misc: <u>drug-induced lupus syndrome</u>.

INTERACTIONS

Drug–Drug: ▪ Additive hypotension with other **antihypertensive agents,** acute ingestion of **alcohol,** or **nitrates** ▪ **MAO inhibitors** may exaggerate hypotension ▪ May reduce the pressor response to **epinephrine** ▪ **Nonsteroidal anti-inflammatory agents** may decrease antihypertensive response ▪ **Beta-adrenergic blockers** decrease tachycardia from hydralazine (therapy may be combined for this reason).

ROUTE AND DOSAGE

▪ **PO (Adults):** 40–400 mg/day in 4 divided doses.
▪ **PO (Children):** 0.75 mg/kg/day (25 mg/m^2) in 2–4 divided doses; may increase gradually to 7.5 mg/kg/day (300 mg/day) in 4 divided doses (unlabeled).
▪ **IM, IV (Adults):** 10–40 mg repeated as needed.
▪ **IM, IV (Children):** 1.7–3.5 mg/kg/day or 50–100 mg/m^2/day in 4–6 divided doses (unlabeled).

AVAILABILITY

▪ **Tablets:** 10 mg, 25 mg, 50 mg, 100 mg
▪ **Injection:** 20 mg/ml ▪ **In combination with:** hydrochlorothiazide and reserpine. See Appendix A.

TIME/ACTION PROFILE
(antihypertensive effect)

	ONSET	PEAK	DURATION
PO	20–30 min	2 hr	6–12 hr
IM	10–30 min	1 hr	4–6 hr
IV	5–20 min	10–80 min	4–6 hr

NURSING IMPLICATIONS

ASSESSMENT

▫ Monitor blood pressure and pulse frequently during initial dosage adjustment and periodically throughout course of therapy. Notify physician of significant changes.
▪ **Lab Test Considerations:** CBC, electrolytes, LE cell prep, and antinuclear antibody (ANA) titer should be monitored prior to and periodically during prolonged therapy.
▫ May cause a positive direct Coombs' test.

POTENTIAL NURSING DIAGNOSES

▪ Tissue perfusion, altered (indications).
▪ Knowledge deficit related to medication regimen (patient/family teaching).
▪ Noncompliance (patient/family teaching).

IMPLEMENTATION

▪ **General Info:** IM or IV route should be used only when drug cannot be given orally.
▫ May be administered concurrently with diuretics or beta-adrenergic blocking agents to permit lower doses and minimize side effects.
▪ **PO:** Administer with meals consistently to enhance absorption.
▫ Pharmacist may prepare oral solution from hydralazine injection for patients with difficulty swallowing.
▪ **Direct IV:** Inject undiluted through Y-tubing or 3-way stopcock.
▫ Use solution as quickly as possible after drawing through needle into syringe. Hydralazine changes color after contact with a metal filter.
▪ **Rate:** Administer at a rate of 10 mg

---

*<u>Underlines</u> indicate most frequent; **CAPITALS** indicate life-threatening.

over at least 1 min. Monitor blood pressure and pulse frequently after injection.

- **Y-Site Compatibility:** ▪ heparin ▪ hydrocortisone sodium succinate ▪ potassium chloride ▪ verapamil ▪ vitamin B complex with C.
- **Y-Site Incompatibility:** ▪ aminophylline ▪ ampicillin ▪ diazoxide ▪ furosemide.
- **Solution Compatibility:** dextrose/saline combinations ▪ dextrose/Ringer's solution combinations ▪ D5/LR ▪ D5W ▪ D10W ▪ D10/LR ▪ 0.45% NaCl ▪ 0.9% NaCl ▪ Ringer's or lactated Ringer's solution.

PATIENT/FAMILY TEACHING

□ Emphasize the importance of continuing to take this medication, even if feeling well. Instruct patient to take medication at the same time each day; last dose of the day should be taken at bedtime. If a dose is missed, take as soon as remembered; do not double doses. If more than 2 doses in a row are missed, consult physician. Must be discontinued gradually to avoid sudden increase in blood pressure. Hydralazine controls but does not cure hypertension.

□ Encourage patient to comply with additional interventions for hypertension (weight reduction, low-sodium diet, discontinuation of smoking, moderation of alcohol intake, regular exercise, and stress management). Instruct patient and family on proper technique for blood pressure monitoring. Advise them to check blood pressure at least weekly and report significant changes to physician.

□ Patients should weigh themselves twice weekly and assess feet and ankles for fluid retention.

□ Hydralazine may occasionally cause drowsiness. Advise patient to avoid driving or other activities requiring alertness until response to medication is known.

□ Caution patient to avoid sudden

changes in position to minimize orthostatic hypotension.

□ Advise patient to consult physician or pharmacist before taking any cough, cold, or allergy remedies. Patient should also avoid excessive amounts of tea, coffee, and cola.

□ Instruct patient to notify physician or dentist of medication prior to treatment or surgery.

□ Advise patient to notify physician immediately if general tiredness, fever, muscle or joint aching, chest pain, skin rash, sore throat or numbness, tingling, pain, or weakness of hands and feet occur. Vitamin B_6 (pyridoxine) may be used to treat peripheral neuritis.

□ Emphasize the importance of follow-up examinations to evaluate effectiveness of medication.

EVALUATION

Effectiveness of therapy can be demonstrated by: ▪ Decrease in blood pressure without appearance of side effects ▪ Decreased afterload in patients with congestive heart failure.

HYDROCHLOROTHIAZIDE   H
(hye-droe-klor-oh-**thye**-a-zide)
{Apo-Hydro}, {Diuclor H}, Esidrex, Ezide, HCTZ, HydroDIURIL, Hydro-Par, {Natrimax}, {Neo-Codema}, Novo-Hydrazide, Oretic, {Urozide}

CLASSIFICATION(S):
Diuretic (thiazide), Antihypertensive
Pregnancy Category B

INDICATIONS

▪ Used alone or in combination with other agents in the management of mild to moderate hypertension ▪ Used alone or in combination in the treatment of edema associated with: □ Congestive heart failure □ Renal dysfunction □ Cirrhosis □ Glucocorticoid therapy □ Estrogen therapy.

ACTION

■ Increases excretion of sodium and water by inhibiting sodium reabsorption in the distal tubule ■ Promotes excretion of chloride, potassium, magnesium, and bicarbonate ■ May produce arteriolar dilation. **Therapeutic Effects:** ■ Lowering of blood pressure in hypertensive patients and diuresis with subsequent mobilization of edema.

PHARMACOKINETICS

Absorption: Variably absorbed from the GI tract following oral administration.
Distribution: Distributed into extracellular space. Crosses the placenta and enters breast milk.
Metabolism and Excretion: Excreted mainly unchanged by the kidneys.
Half-life: 6–15 hr.

CONTRAINDICATIONS AND PRECAUTIONS

Contraindicated in: ■ Hypersensitivity ■ Cross-sensitivity with other thiazides or sulfonamides may exist ■ Anuria ■ Lactation.
Use Cautiously in: ■ Renal or severe hepatic impairment ■ Pregnancy (jaundice or thrombocytopenia may be seen in the newborn).

ADVERSE REACTIONS AND SIDE EFFECTS*

CNS: drowsiness, lethargy, dizziness, weakness.
CV: hypotension.
Derm: rashes, photosensitivity.
Endo: hyperglycemia.
F and E: hypokalemia, hypochloremic alkalosis, hyponatremia, hypercalcemia, hypophosphatemia, hypomagnesemia, dehydration, hypovolemia.
GI: anorexia, nausea, vomiting, cramping, hepatitis.
Hemat: blood dyscrasias.
Metab: hyperuricemia, elevated lipids.

MS: muscle cramps.
Misc: pancreatitis.

INTERACTIONS

Drug–Drug: ■ Additive hypotension with other **antihypertensive agents,** acute ingestion of **alcohol,** or **nitrates** ■ Additive hypokalemia with **glucocorticoids, amphotericin B, mezlocillin, piperacillin,** or **ticarcillin** ■ Hypokalemia increases the risk of **cardiac glycoside** toxicity ■ Decreases the excretion of **lithium** and may cause toxicity ■ **Cholestyramine** or **colestipol** decreases absorption □ May potentiate the effects of **general anesthetics** or **neuromuscular blocking agents.**
Drug–Food: ■ **Food** may increase extent of absorption.

ROUTE AND DOSAGE

In the treatment of hypertension, daily dose should not exceed 50 mg.
■ **PO (Adults):** 25–100 mg/day in 1–2 doses (up to 200 mg/day). As a diuretic, may be given every other day or 3–5 days/wk.
■ **PO (Children >6 mo):** 1–2 mg/kg (30–60 mg/m²/day) in 1–2 divided doses.
■ **PO (Children <6 mo):** up to 3.3 mg/kg/day in 2 divided doses.

AVAILABILITY

■ *Tablets:* 25 mg, 50 mg, 100 mg ■ *In combination with:* potassium-sparing diuretics and various antihypertensives. See Appendix A.

TIME/ACTION PROFILE

	ONSET	PEAK	DURATION
PO (diuretic)	2 hr	3–6 hr	6–12 hr
PO (antihypertensive)	3–4 days	7–14 days	7 days

NURSING IMPLICATIONS

ASSESSMENT

□ Monitor blood pressure, intake and output, and daily weight; assess feet, legs, and sacral area for edema daily.

---

*Underlines indicate most frequent; **CAPITALS** indicate life-threatening.

□ Assess patient for anorexia, nausea, vomiting, muscle cramps, paresthesia, and confusion, especially if patient is taking cardiac glycosides. Patients on cardiac glycosides are at increased risk of digitalis toxicity because of the potassium-depleting effect of the diuretic.

□ Assess patient for allergy to sulfonamides.

■ **Lab Test Considerations:** Monitor electrolytes (especially potassium), blood glucose, BUN, and serum uric acid levels prior to and periodically throughout course of therapy.

□ May cause increase in serum and urine glucose in diabetic patients.

□ May cause an increase in serum bilirubin, calcium, and uric acid and a decrease in serum magnesium, potassium, and sodium levels.

□ May cause increased serum cholesterol, low-density lipoprotein, and triglyceride concentrations.

POTENTIAL NURSING DIAGNOSES

■ Fluid volume excess (indications).
■ Fluid volume deficit (side effects).
■ Knowledge deficit related to medication regimen (patient/family teaching).

IMPLEMENTATION

■ **General Info:** Administer in the morning to prevent disruption of sleep cycle.

■ **PO:** May give with food or milk to minimize GI irritation. Tablets may be crushed and mixed with fluid for patients with difficulty swallowing.

□ Intermittent dose schedule may be used for continued control of edema.

PATIENT/FAMILY TEACHING

□ Instruct patient to take this medication at the same time each day. If a dose is missed, take as soon as remembered but not just before next dose is due. Do not double doses. Advise patients using hydrochlorothiazide for hypertension to continue taking the medication even if feeling well. Medication controls but does not cure hypertension.

□ Encourage patient to comply with ad-

ditional interventions for hypertension (weight reduction, low-sodium diet, regular exercise, smoking cessation, moderation of alcohol consumption, and stress management).

□ Instruct patient to monitor weight biweekly and to notify physician of significant changes. Instruct patients with hypertension in correct technique for monitoring weekly blood pressure.

□ Caution patient to make position changes slowly to minimize orthostatic hypotension. This may be potentiated by alcohol.

□ Advise patient to use sunscreen (avoid those containing PABA) and protective clothing when in the sun to prevent photosensitivity reactions.

□ Instruct patient to follow a diet high in potassium (see Appendix K).

□ Advise patient to consult physician or pharmacist before taking alcohol or over-the-counter medication concurrently with this therapy.

□ Advise patient to report muscle weakness, cramps, nausea, or dizziness to the physician.

□ Instruct patient to notify physician or dentist of medication regimen prior to treatment or surgery.

□ Emphasize the importance of routine follow-up examinations.

EVALUATION

Effectiveness of therapy can be demonstrated by: ■ Decrease in blood pressure ■ Increase in urine output □ Decrease in edema.

H

HYDROCODONE

(hye-droe-**koe**-done)
Hycodan, (U.S. antitussive formulations contains homatropine)

CLASSIFICATION(S):
Opioid analgesic (agonist),
Antitussive
Schedule III (in combination)
Pregnancy Category C

INDICATIONS

■ Alone and in combination with non-opioid analgesics in the management of moderate to severe pain ■ Antitussive (usually in combination products with decongestants).

ACTION

■ Binds to opiate receptors in the CNS. Alters the perception of and response to painful stimuli while producing generalized CNS depression. **Therapeutic Effects:** ■ Decrease in severity of moderate pain ■ Suppression of the cough reflex.

PHARMACOKINETICS

Absorption: Well absorbed following oral administration.
Distribution: Distribution not known.
Metabolism and Excretion: Mostly metabolized by the liver.
Half-life: 3.8 hr.

CONTRAINDICATIONS AND PRECAUTIONS

Contraindicated in: ■ Hypersensitivity ■ Pregnancy or lactation (avoid chronic use) ■ Products may contain tartrazine, sulfites, or alcohol; avoid use in hypersensitive patients.
Use Cautiously in: ■ Head trauma ■ Increased intracranial pressure ■ Severe renal, hepatic, or pulmonary disease ■ Hypothyroidism ■ Adrenal insufficiency ■ Alcoholism ■ Elderly or debilitated patients (dosage reduction required) ■ Patients with undiagnosed abdominal pain ■ Prostatic hypertrophy ■ Pregnancy and lactation (safety not established).

ADVERSE REACTIONS AND SIDE EFFECTS*

CNS: <u>sedation</u>, <u>confusion</u>, headache, euphoria, floating feeling, unusual dreams, hallucinations, dysphoria.
CV: <u>hypotension</u>, bradycardia.
EENT: miosis, diplopia, blurred vision.
Resp: respiratory depression.
GI: nausea, vomiting, <u>constipation</u>.
GU: urinary retention.
Derm: sweating, flushing.

Misc: tolerance, physical dependence, psychological dependence.

INTERACTIONS

Drug–Drug: ■ Use with extreme caution in patients receiving **MAO inhibitors** (may produce severe, unpredictable reactions—reduce initial dose of hydrocodone to 25% of usual dose) ■ Additive CNS depression with **alcohol, antihistamines,** and **sedative/hypnotics** ■ Administration of **partial-antagonist opioid analgesics** may precipitate opioid withdrawal in physically dependent patients ■ **Nalbuphine** or **pentazocine** may decrease analgesia.

ROUTE AND DOSAGE

Analgesic
■ **PO (Adults):** 5–10 mg q 4–6 hr as needed.

Antitussive
■ **PO (Adults):** 5–10 mg q 4–6 hr as needed (not to exceed 15 mg/dose) or 10 mg q 12 hr as long-acting preparation.
■ **PO (Children):** 0.6 mg/kg/day (20 mg/m²/day) in 3–4 divided doses (not to exceed 10 mg/single dose in children >12 yr; 5 mg/single dose in children 2–12 yr or 1.25 mg/single dose in children <2 yr) or 5 mg q 12 hr as extended-release preparation in children 6–12 yr (not to exceed 10 mg/day).

AVAILABILITY

■ *Tablets:* 2.5 mg, 5 mg, 7.5 mg, 10 mg ■ *In combination with:* aspirin or acetaminophen. See Appendix A ■ *Liquids, syrups, suspensions:* containing 1.67–10 mg hydrocodone/5 ml in combination with antihistamine and decongestants.

TIME/ACTION PROFILE

	ONSET	PEAK	DURATION
PO (analgesic)	10–30 min	30–60 min	4–6 hr
PO (antitussive)	UK	UK	4–6 hr

*<u>Underlines</u> indicate most frequent; **CAPITALS** indicate life-threatening.

NURSING IMPLICATIONS

ASSESSMENT

□ Assess blood pressure, pulse, and respiratory rate before and periodically during administration.

□ Assess bowel function routinely. Increased intake of fluids and bulk, stool softeners, and laxatives may minimize constipating effects.

■ **Pain:** Assess type, location, and intensity of pain prior to and 60 min following administration.

□ Prolonged use may lead to physical and psychological dependence and tolerance. This should not prevent patient from receiving adequate analgesia. Most patients who receive hydrocodone for medical reasons do not develop psychological dependence. Potential for dependence is less than that of morphine. Progressively higher doses may be required to relieve pain with long-term therapy.

■ **Cough:** Assess cough, sputum, and lung sounds during antitussive use.

■ **Lab Test Considerations:** May increase plasma amylase and lipase levels.

■ **Toxicity and Overdose:** If overdosage occurs, naloxone (Narcan) is the antidote.

POTENTIAL NURSING DIAGNOSES

■ Pain (indications).

■ Sensory-perceptual alteration: visual, auditory (side effects).

■ Injury, high risk for (side effects).

IMPLEMENTATION

■ **General Info:** Explain therapeutic value of medication prior to administration to enhance the analgesic effect.

□ Regularly administered doses may be more effective than prn administration. Analgesic is more effective if given before pain becomes severe.

□ Medication should be discontinued gradually after long-term use to prevent withdrawal symptoms.

■ **PO:** May be administered with food or milk to minimize GI irritation.

PATIENT/FAMILY TEACHING

□ Instruct patient on how and when to ask for pain medication.

□ Medication may cause drowsiness or dizziness. Advise patient to call for assistance when ambulating or smoking. Caution patient to avoid driving or other activities requiring alertness until response to the medication is known.

□ Advise patient to make position changes slowly to minimize orthostatic hypotension.

□ Caution patient to avoid concurrent use of alcohol or other CNS depressants with this medication.

□ Encourage patient to turn, cough, and breathe deeply every 2 hr to prevent atelectasis.

EVALUATION

Effectiveness of therapy can be demonstrated by: ■ Decrease in severity of pain without a significant alteration in level of consciousness or respiratory status ■ Suppression of nonproductive cough.

HYDROCORTISONE
(hye-droe-**kor**-ti-sone)

H

systemic (oral/parenteral)
A-Hydro-Cort, Cortef, Hydrocortone, Solu-Cortef

rectal
Anusol-HC, Cort-Dome, Cortenema, Corticaine, Cortifoam, {Cortiment}, Proctocort, Proctofoam-HC, {Rectocort}

CLASSIFICATION(S):
Glucocorticoid (short-acting)
Pregnancy Category UK

INDICATIONS

■ Management of adrenocortical insufficiency ■ Short-term management of a variety of inflammatory and allergic conditions, including asthma and ulcerative colitis ■ Chronic use is limited

---

due to mineralocorticoid activity ▪ Not suitable for alternate-day therapy.

ACTION

▪ Replaces cortisol in deficiency states ▪ Suppresses the normal immune response and inflammation ▪ Has additional profound and varied metabolic effects ▪ Potent mineralocorticoid (sodium retention) ▪ Suppresses adrenal function with chronic use at doses >20 mg/day. **Therapeutic Effects:** ▪ Replacement of cortisol in deficiency states ▪ Suppression of inflammation.

PHARMACOKINETICS

Absorption: Well absorbed following oral administration. Phosphate and succinate salts are rapidly absorbed following IM administration. The acetate salt provides slower absorption and a longer duration of action. Some systemic absorption may occur with chronic use of topical preparations.
Distribution: Widely distributed. Crosses the placenta and probably enters breast milk.
Metabolism and Excretion: Metabolized by the liver.
Half-life: 80–120 min.

CONTRAINDICATIONS AND PRECAUTIONS

Contraindicated in: ▪ Serious infections—except for some forms of meningitis ▪ Do not administer live vaccines to patients receiving more than 20 mg/day ▪ Some products contain bisulfites and should be avoided in patients with known intolerance.
Use Cautiously in: ▪ Children— chronic use may lead to growth suppression ▪ Chronic treatment with doses greater than 20 mg/day (results in adrenal suppression) ▪ Do not discontinue abruptly ▪ Periods of stress (infections, surgery), additional doses may be needed ▪ May mask signs of infection ▪ Use lowest possible dose for shortest period of time ▪ Pregnancy or lactation (safety not established).

ADVERSE REACTIONS AND SIDE EFFECTS*

CNS: psychoses, depression, euphoria.
EENT: cataracts, increased intraocular pressure.
CV: edema, hypertension, congestive heart failure, thromboembolism.
GI: nausea, vomiting, increased appetite, weight gain, GI bleeding, peptic ulceration.
Derm: petechiae, ecchymoses, fragility, decreased wound healing, hirsutism, acne.
Endo: menstrual irregularities, hyperglycemia, decreased growth in children, adrenal suppression.
F and E: hypokalemia, sodium retention, metabolic alkalosis, hypocalcemia.
Local: atrophy at IM sites (sustained-release dosage forms).
MS: weakness, myopathy, aseptic necrosis of joints, osteoporosis.
Misc: increases susceptibility to infections, pancreatitis, Cushingoid appearance (moon face, buffalo hump).

INTERACTIONS

Drug–Drug: ▪ Additive hypokalemia with **amphotericin B, mezlocillin, piperacillin, ticarcillin,** or **diuretics** ▪ Hypokalemia may increase the risk of **cardiac glycoside** toxicity ▪ May increase requirements for **insulin** or **oral hypoglycemic agents** ▪ **Phenytoin, phenobarbital,** and **rifampin** stimulate metabolism; may decrease effectiveness ▪ **Oral contraceptives** may block metabolism ▪ May decrease antibody response to **live virus vaccines** and increase the risk of adverse reactions.

ROUTE AND DOSAGE

▪ **PO (Adults):** 10–320 mg/day in 1–4 divided doses.
▪ **PO (Children):** 0.56 mg/kg/day (15– 20 mg/m^2/day) for adrenal insufficiency. For other uses doses range from 2–8 mg/kg/day (60–240 mg/m^2/ day).
▪ **IM, IV (Adults):** 100–500 mg q 2–6

---

*Underlines indicate most frequent; **CAPITALS** indicate life-threatening.

hr (succinate) (range 100–8000 mg/
day). 15–240 mg (phosphate) q 12 hr.
- **IM, IV (Children):** 0.186–0.28 mg/
kg/day (10–12 mg/m²/day in 3 divided
doses for adrenal insufficiency. For
other uses doses range from 0.666–4
mg/kg (20–120 mg/m²) q 12–24 hr
(phosphate or succinate).
- **Intra-Articular (Adults):** 5–75 mg
(acetate).
- **Rectal (Adults):** 100 mg/day as enema or 90 mg 1–2 times daily as foam
or 10–25 mg daily as suppositories.

AVAILABILITY

- *Tablets:* 5 mg, 10 mg, 20 mg ▪ *Oral
suspension:* 10 mg/5 ml ▪ *Injection
(suspension):* 25 mg/ml ▪ *Injection
(sodium phosphate):* 50 mg/ml ▪ *Injection (sodium succinate):* 100 mg,
250 mg, 500 mg, 1 g ▪ *Enema:* 100
mg/60 ml ▪ *Rectal foam:* 90 mg/
applicatorful ▪ *Rectal ointment:* 0.75%
▪ *Suppositories:* 10 mg, 25 mg, {40 mg}.

TIME/ACTION PROFILE (anti-inflammatory activity)

	ONSET	PEAK	DURATION
PO	6 hr	UK	1.25–1.5 days
IM	rapid	UK	1.25–1.5 days
IV	rapid	UK	1.25–1.5 days

NURSING IMPLICATIONS

ASSESSMENT

- **General Info:** This drug is indicated
for many conditions. Assess involved
systems prior to and periodically
throughout course of therapy.
- ▫ Assess patient for signs of adrenal insufficiency (hypotension, weight
loss, weakness, nausea, vomiting,
anorexia, lethargy, confusion, restlessness) prior to and periodically
throughout course of therapy.
- ▫ Monitor intake and output ratios and
daily weights. Observe patient for
the appearance of peripheral edema,
steady weight gain, rales/crackles, or
dyspnea. Notify physician if these occur.
- ▫ Children should have periodic evaluations of growth.

- **Intra-articular:** Monitor pain, edema,
and range of motion of affected joints.
- **Lab Test Considerations:** Patients on
prolonged courses of therapy should
routinely have hematologic values,
serum electrolytes, and serum and
urine glucose evaluated. May cause
decreased WBC counts. May cause
hyperglycemia, especially in persons
with diabetes. May decrease serum
potassium and calcium and increase
serum sodium concentrations.
- ▫ Promptly report presence of guaiac-
positive stools.
- ▫ May increase serum cholesterol and
lipid values. May decrease serum
protein–bound iodine and thyroxine
concentrations.
- ▫ Suppresses reactions to allergy skin
tests.
- ▫ Periodic adrenal function tests may
be ordered to assess degree of hypothalamic-pituitary-adrenal (HPA) axis
suppression.

POTENTIAL NURSING DIAGNOSES

- Infection, high risk for (side effects).
- Knowledge deficit related to medication regimen (patient/family teaching).

IMPLEMENTATION

- ▫ If dose is ordered daily, administer in
the morning to coincide with the
body's normal secretion of cortisol.
- **PO:** Administer with meals to minimize gastric irritation.
- **Direct IV:** Reconstitute with provided
solution (i.e., Act-O-Vials) or 2 ml of
Bacteriostatic Water or Saline for Injection.
- **Rate:** Administer each 100 mg over at
least 30 sec. Doses 500 mg and larger
should be infused over at least 10
min.
- **Intermittent IV:** May be added to 50–
1000 ml of D5W, 0.9% NaCl, or
D5/0.9% NaCl. Administer infusions
at prescribed rate. Diluted solutions
should be used within 24 hr.

Hydrocortisone Sodium Phosphate

- **Syringe Compatibility:** ▪ fluconazole
▪ fludarabine ▪ metoclopramide.

H

- **Additive Compatibility:** ■ amphotericin B ■ bleomycin ■ dacarbazine.

Hydrocortisone Sodium Succinate

- **Syringe Compatibility:** ■ metoclopramide ■ thiopental.
- **Y-Site Compatibility:** ■ acyclovir ■ aminophylline ■ ampicillin ■ amrinone ■ atracurium ■ atropine ■ betamethasone ■ calcium gluconate ■ cephalothin ■ cephapirin ■ chlordiazepoxide ■ chlorpromazine ■ cyanocobalamin ■ dexamethasone ■ digoxin ■ diphenhydramine ■ dopamine ■ droperidol ■ edrophonium ■ enalaprilat ■ epinephrine ■ esmolol ■ conjugated estrogens ■ ethacrynate ■ famotidine ■ fentanyl ■ fentanyl/droperidol ■ fludarabine ■ fluorouracil ■ foscarnet ■ furosemide ■ hydralazine ■ insulin ■ isoproterenol ■ kanamycin ■ lidocaine ■ magnesium sulfate ■ menadiol ■ methicillin ■ methoxamine ■ methylergonovine ■ minocycline ■ morphine ■ neostigmine ■ norepinephrine ■ ondansetron ■ oxacillin ■ oxytocin ■ pancuronium ■ penicillin G potassium ■ pentazocine ■ phytonadione ■ prednisolone ■ procainamide, prochlorperazine ■ propranolol ■ pyridostigmine ■ scopolamine ■ sodium bicarbonate ■ succinylcholine ■ trimethobenzamide ■ trimethaphan camsylate ■ vecuronium.
- **Y-Site Incompatibility:** ■ diazepam ■ ergotamine tartrate ■ phenytoin ■ sargramostim.
- **Additive Compatibility:** ■ aminophylline ■ amphotericin ■ daunorubicin ■ mitoxantrone ■ potassium chloride.
- **Additive Incompatibility:** ■ bleomycin ■ doxorubicin.
- **Rect:** Applicator is provided by manufacturer. Do not insert aerosol container into rectum. Instructions are provided for correct usage of applicator. Clean applicator after each use.

PATIENT/FAMILY TEACHING

□ Instruct patient on correct technique of administration for prescribed form. Patient should take medication exactly as directed and not skip doses or double up on missed doses. Stopping the medication suddenly may result in adrenal insufficiency (anorexia, nausea, fatigue, weakness, hypotension, dyspnea, and hypoglycemia). If these signs appear, notify physician immediately. This can be life-threatening.

□ Encourage patients on long-term therapy to eat a diet high in protein, calcium, and potassium and low in sodium and carbohydrates (see Appendix K for foods included).

□ This drug causes immunosuppression and may mask symptoms of infection. Instruct patient to avoid people with known contagious illnesses and to report possible infections.

□ Review side effects with patient. Instruct patient to inform physician promptly if severe abdominal pain or tarry stools occur. Patient should also report unusual swelling, weight gain, tiredness, bone pain, bruising, nonhealing sores, visual disturbances, or behavior changes.

□ Instruct patient to inform physician if symptoms of underlying disease return or worsen.

□ Advise patient to carry identification in the event of an emergency in which patient cannot relate medical history.

□ Advise parents not to administer topical preparations to a child <2 yr unless directed by physician.

□ Caution patient to avoid vaccinations without consulting physician.

□ Emphasize the importance of follow-up examinations to monitor progress and side effects.

EVALUATION

Effectiveness of therapy can be demonstrated by: ■ Suppression of the inflammatory and immune responses in autoimmune disorders and allergic reactions.

HYDROMORPHONE
(hye-droe-**mor**-fone)
dihydromorphinone, Dilaudid, Dilaudid-HP

INDICATIONS

▪ Used alone and in combination with nonopioid analgesics (acetaminophen or aspirin) in the management of moderate to severe pain ▪ Used as an antitussive in lower doses.

ACTION

▪ Binds to opiate receptors in the CNS ▪ Alters the perception of and response to painful stimuli while producing generalized CNS depression. **Therapeutic Effects:** ▪ Decrease in moderate to severe pain ▪ Suppression of cough.

PHARMACOKINETICS

Absorption: Well absorbed following oral, Rect, SC, and IM administration.
Distribution: Widely distributed. Crosses the placenta and enters breast milk.
Metabolism and Excretion: Mostly metabolized by the liver.
Half-life: 2–4 hr.

CONTRAINDICATIONS AND PRECAUTIONS

Contraindicated in: ▪ Hypersensitivity ▪ Avoid chronic use during pregnancy or lactation.
Use Cautiously in: ▪ Head trauma ▪ Increased intracranial pressure ▪ Severe renal, hepatic, or pulmonary disease ▪ Hypothyroidism ▪ Adrenal insufficiency ▪ Alcoholism ▪ Elderly or debilitated patients (dosage reduction recommended) ▪ Undiagnosed abdominal pain ▪ Prostatic hypertrophy.

ADVERSE REACTIONS AND SIDE EFFECTS*

CNS: sedation, confusion, headache, euphoria, floating feeling, unusual dreams, hallucinations, dysphoria, dizziness.
EENT: miosis, diplopia, blurred vision.
Resp: respiratory depression.
CV: hypotension, bradycardia.
GI: nausea, vomiting, constipation.
GU: urinary retention.
Derm: sweating, flushing.
Misc: tolerance, physical dependence, psychological dependence.

INTERACTIONS

Drug–Drug: ▪ Use with extreme caution in patients receiving **MAO inhibitors** (may produce severe, unpredictable reactions—reduce initial dose of hydromorphone to 25% of usual dose) ▪ Additive CNS depression with **alcohol, antidepressants, antihistamines,** and **sedative/hypnotics** ▪ Administration of **partial-antagonist opioid analgesics** may precipitate opioid withdrawal in physically dependent patients ▪ **Nalbuphine** or **pentazocine** may decrease analgesia.

ROUTE AND DOSAGE

As tolerance develops, larger doses may be required.

Analgesic
▪ **PO (Adults):** 2 mg q 3–6 hr as needed; may be increased to 4 mg q 4–6 hr.
▪ **IM, SC (Adult):** 1–2 mg q 3–6 hr as needed; may be increased to 3–4 mg q 4–6 hr.
▪ **IV (Adults):** 0.5–1 mg q 3 hr as needed.
▪ **Rect (Adults):** 3 mg q 4–8 hr as needed.

Antitussive
▪ **PO (Adults):** 1 mg q 3–4 hr.
▪ **PO (Children 6–12 yr):** 0.5 mg q 3–4 hr.

AVAILABILITY

▪ *Tablets:* 1 mg, 2 mg, 3 mg, 4 mg ▪ *Injection:* 2 mg/ml, 3 mg/ml, 4 mg/ml, 10 mg/ml ▪ *Suppositories:* 3 mg ▪ *In combination with:* guaifenesin and alcohol (Dilaudid Cough Syrup). See Appendix A.

H

*Underlines indicate most frequent; CAPITALS indicate life-threatening.

TIME/ACTION PROFILE (analgesic effect)

	ONSET	PEAK	DURATION
PO	15–30 min	30–90 min	4–5 hr
SC	15–30 min	30–90 min	4–5 hr
IM	15–30 min	30–90 min	4–5 hr
IV	10–15 min	15–30 min	2–3 hr
Rect	15–30 min	30–90 min	4–5 hr

NURSING IMPLICATIONS

ASSESSMENT

- **General Info:** Assess blood pressure, pulse, and respiratory rate before and periodically during administration.
- Assess bowel function routinely. Increased intake of fluids and bulk, stool softeners, and laxatives may minimize constipating effects.
- **Pain:** Assess type, location, and intensity of pain prior to and 30 min following administration.
- Prolonged use may lead to physical and psychological dependence and tolerance. This should not prevent patient from receiving adequate analgesia. Most patients who receive hydromorphone for medical reasons do not develop psychological dependence. Progressively higher doses may be required to relieve pain with long-term therapy.
- **Cough:** Assess cough and lung sounds during antitussive use.
- **Lab Test Considerations:** May increase plasma amylase and lipase concentrations.
- **Toxicity and Overdose:** If overdosage occurs, naloxone (Narcan) is the antidote. Monitor patient closely; dose may need to be repeated or naloxone infusion administered.

POTENTIAL NURSING DIAGNOSES

- Pain (indications).
- Sensory-perceptual alteration: visual, auditory (side effects).
- Injury, high risk for (side effects).

IMPLEMENTATION

- **General Info:** Explain therapeutic value of medication prior to administration to enhance the analgesic effect.

- Regularly administered doses may be more effective than prn administration. Analgesic is more effective if given before pain becomes severe.
- Coadministration with nonopioid analgesics may have additive analgesic effects and permit lower opioid doses.
- Medication should be discontinued gradually after long-term use to prevent withdrawal symptoms.
- **PO:** May be administered with food or milk to minimize GI irritation.
- **Direct IV:** Dilute with at least 5 ml of Sterile Water or 0.9% NaCl for Injection.
- **Rate:** Administer slowly, at a rate not to exceed 2 mg over 3–5 min. Rapid administration may lead to increased respiratory depression, hypotension, and circulatory collapse. Do not use IV without antidote available.
- **Syringe Compatibility:** • atropine • chlorpromazine • cimetidine • diphenhydramine • fentanyl • glycopyrrolate • hydroxyzine • midazolam • pentazocine • pentobarbital • promethazine • ranitidine • scopolamine • thiethylperazine • trimethobenzamide.
- **Y-Site Compatibility:** • acyclovir • amikacin • ampicillin • cefamandole • cefazolin • cefoperazone • ceforanide • cefotaxime • cefoxitin • ceftizoxime • cefuroxime • cephalothin • cephapirin • chloramphenicol • clindamycin • doxycycline • erythromycin lactobionate • fludarabine • foscarnet • gentamicin • kanamycin • metronidazole • mezlocillin • moxalactam • nafcillin • ondansetron • oxacillin • penicillin G potassium • piperacillin • ticarcillin • tobramycin • trimethoprim/sulfamethoxazole • vancomycin.
- **Y-Site Incompatibility:** • minocycline • sargramostim.
- **Additive/Solution Compatibility:** • D5W • D5/0.45% NaCl • D5/0.9% NaCl • D5/LR • D5/Ringer's solution • 0.45% NaCl • 0.9% NaCl • Ringer's and lactated Ringer's solution.
- **Additive Incompatibility:** • sodium bicarbonate • thiopental.

PATIENT/FAMILY TEACHING

▫ Instruct patient on how and when to ask for pain medication.

▫ Medication may cause drowsiness or dizziness. Advise patient to call for assistance when ambulating or smoking. Caution patient to avoid driving or other activities requiring alertness until response to medication is known.

▫ Advise patient to make position changes slowly to minimize orthostatic hypotension.

▫ Instruct patient to avoid concurrent use of alcohol or other CNS depressants.

▫ Encourage patient to turn, cough, and breathe deeply every 2 hr to prevent atelectasis.

EVALUATION

Effectiveness of therapy can be demonstrated by: ▪ Decrease in severity of pain without a significant alteration in level of consciousness or respiratory status ▪ Suppression of cough.

HYDROXYCHLOROQUINE
(hye-drox-ee-**klor**-oh-kwin)
Plaquenil

CLASSIFICATION(S):
Antimalarial, Antiarthritic
Pregnancy Category UK

INDICATIONS

▪ Suppression and chemoprophylaxis of malaria ▪ Treatment of severe rheumatoid arthritis and systemic lupus erythematosus.

ACTION

▪ Inhibits protein synthesis in susceptible organisms by inhibiting DNA and RNA polymerase. **Therapeutic Effects:** ▪ Death of plasmodia responsible for causing malaria ▪ Also has anti-inflammatory properties.

PHARMACOKINETICS

Absorption: Appears to be well absorbed following oral administration.

Distribution: Appears to be widely distributed; high tissue concentrations achieved (especially liver). Probably enters breast milk.

Metabolism and Excretion: Partially metabolized by the liver, partially excreted unchanged by the kidneys.

Half-life: 72–120 hr.

CONTRAINDICATIONS AND PRECAUTIONS

Contraindicated in: ▪ Hypersensitivity to hydroxychloroquine or chloroquine ▪ Patients with visual damage caused by hydroxychloroquine or chloroquine.

Use Cautiously in: ▪ Patients receiving other hepatotoxic drugs ▪ Patients with liver disease ▪ Alcoholism ▪ G6-PD deficiency ▪ Psoriasis ▪ Bone marrow depression ▪ Obese patients (dose should be determined by ideal body weight).

ADVERSE REACTIONS AND SIDE EFFECTS*

CNS: headache, fatigue, nervousness, anxiety, apathy, irritability, agitation, aggressiveness, confusion, personality changes, psychoses, SEIZURES.

EENT: visual disturbances, keratopathy, retinopathy, ototoxicity, tinnitus.

CV: hypotension, ECG changes.

GI: epigastric discomfort, anorexia, nausea, vomiting, abdominal cramps, diarrhea.

Derm: dermatoses.

Hemat: leukopenia, thrombocytopenia, AGRANULOCYTOSIS, APLASTIC ANEMIA.

Neuro: peripheral neuritis, neuromyopathy.

INTERACTIONS

Drug–Drug: ▪ May increase the risk of hepatotoxicity when administered with **hepatotoxic drugs** ▪ May increase the risk of hematologic toxicity when administered with **penicillamine** ▪ May increase risk of dermatitis when admin-

H

*Underlines indicate most frequent; CAPITALS indicate life-threatening.

istered with other **agents having dermatologic toxicity** ■ May decrease serum titers of rabies antibody when given concurrently with **human diploid-cell rabies vaccine** ■ **Urinary acidifiers** may increase renal excretion ■ May increase serum levels of **digoxin**.

ROUTE AND DOSAGE
Doses expressed as mg of hydroxychloroquine base: 155 mg of hydroxychloroquine base = 200 mg hydroxychloroquine sulfate.

Malaria (Suppression or Chemoprophylaxis)
■ **PO (Adults):** 310 mg once weekly; start 1–2 wk prior to entering malarious area; continue for 4 wk after leaving area.
■ **PO (Children):** 5 mg/kg once weekly; start 1–2 wk prior to entering malarious area; continue for 4 wk after leaving area.

Malaria (Treatment)
■ **PO (Adults):** 620 mg initially, then 310 mg at 6 hr, 24 hr, and 48 hr after initial dose.
■ **PO (Children):** 10 mg/kg initially, then 5 mg/kg at 6 hr, 24 hr, and 48 hr after initial dose.

Rheumatoid Arthritis, Systemic Lupus Erythematosus
■ **PO (Adults):** 5 mg/kg/day.

AVAILABILITY
■ *Tablets:* 200 mg (155-mg base).

TIME/ACTION PROFILE (blood levels)

	ONSET	PEAK	DURATION
PO	rapid	1–2 hr	days–wk

NURSING IMPLICATIONS
ASSESSMENT
■ **General Info:** Assess deep tendon reflexes periodically to determine muscle weakness. Therapy may be discontinued should this occur.
▢ Patients on prolonged high-dose therapy should have eye examinations prior to and every 3 mo during therapy to detect retinal damage.
■ **Malaria or Lupus Erythematosus:** As-

sess patient for improvement in signs and symptoms of condition daily throughout course of therapy.
■ **Rheumatoid Arthritis:** Assess patient monthly for pain, swelling, and range of motion.
■ **Lab Test Considerations:** Monitor CBC and platelet count periodically throughout therapy. May cause decreased RBC, WBC, and platelet counts.

IMPLEMENTATION
■ **PO:** Administer with milk or meals to minimize GI distress. Tablets may be crushed and placed inside empty capsules for patients with difficulty swallowing. Contents of capsules may also be mixed with a teaspoonful of jam, jelly, or jello prior to administration.
■ **Malaria Prophylaxis:** Hydroxychloroquine therapy should be started 2 wk prior to potential exposure and continued for 6 wk after leaving the area.

PATIENT/FAMILY TEACHING
▢ Instruct patient to take medication exactly as directed and continue full course of therapy even if feeling better. Missed doses should be taken as soon as remembered except with regimens requiring doses more than once a day, for which missed doses should be taken within 1 hr or omitted. Do not double doses.
▢ Review methods of minimizing exposure to mosquitos with patients receiving hydroxychloroquine prophylactically (use repellant, wear long-sleeved shirt and long trousers, use screen or netting).
▢ Hydroxychloroquine may cause dizziness or lightheadedness. Caution patient to avoid driving or other activities requiring alertness until response to medication is known.
▢ Advise patients to avoid use of alcohol while taking hydroxychloroquine.
▢ Caution patient to keep hydroxychloroquine out of reach of children; fatalities have occurred with ingestion of 3 or 4 tablets.
▢ Advise patient that the risk of ocular

damage may be decreased by the use of dark glasses in bright light. Protective clothing and sunscreen should also be used to reduce risk of dermatoses.

▫ Advise patient to notify physician promptly if sore throat, fever, unusual bleeding or bruising, blurred vision, visual changes, ringing in the ears, difficulty hearing, or muscle weakness occurs.

▫ Instruct patient to contact physician if no improvement is noticed within a few days. Treatment for rheumatoid arthritis may require up to 6 mo for full benefit.

EVALUATION

Effectiveness of therapy may be demonstrated by: ▪ Prevention or resolution of malaria ▪ Improvement in signs and symptoms of rheumatoid arthritis ▪ Improvement in symptoms of lupus erythematosus.

HYDROXYPROGESTERONE

(hye-drox-ee-pro-**jess**-te-rone)
Delalutin, Duralutin, Gesterol LA, Hylutin, Hyprogest, Hyproval PA, Pro-Depo, Prodrox

CLASSIFICATION(S):
Hormone (progestin)
Pregnancy Category D

INDICATIONS

▪ Treatment of amenorrhea and functional uterine bleeding associated with hormonal imbalance ▪ Production of secretory endometrium and desquamation ▪ Diagnostic agent for endogenous estrogen production ▪ Treatment of uterine carcinoma.

ACTION

▪ A synthetic analog of progesterone ▪ Produces secretory changes in the endometrium ▪ Increases basal temperature ▪ Produces changes in the vaginal epithelium ▪ Relaxes uterine smooth muscle ▪ Stimulates mammary alveolar growth ▪ Inhibits pituitary function ▪ Produces withdrawal bleeding (requires estrogen). **Therapeutic Effects:** ▪ Restoration of normal hormonal balance ▪ Decreased tumor growth.

PHARMACOKINETICS

Absorption: Systemic absorption follows IM administration.
Distribution: Distribution not known.
Metabolism and Excretion: Metabolism and excretion not known.
Half-life: UK.

CONTRAINDICATIONS AND PRECAUTIONS

Contraindicated in: ▪ Hypersensitivity ▪ Hypersensitivity to castor oil, sesame oil, or benzyl alcohol ▪ Pregnancy, lactation, or children ▪ Thromboembolic disorders ▪ Undiagnosed vaginal bleeding ▪ Missed abortion ▪ Severe liver disease ▪ Breast carcinoma.
Use Cautiously in: ▪ Cardiac disease ▪ Renal dysfunction ▪ Asthma ▪ Seizures ▪ Migraine headaches ▪ Diabetes mellitus.

ADVERSE REACTIONS AND SIDE EFFECTS*

CNS: depression, cerebral thrombosis.
Resp: coughing, dyspnea.
CV: thrombophlebitis, PULMONARY EMBOLISM, edema.
GI: cholestatic jaundice.
GU: breakthrough bleeding, amenorrhea, cervical changes.
Derm: rashes, increased pigmentation.
Misc: weight changes, allergic reactions.

INTERACTIONS

Drug–Drug: ▪ Interferes with the effects of **bromocriptine** (causes amenorrhea or galactorrhea).

ROUTE AND DOSAGE

Amenorrhea and Uterine Bleeding, Production of Secretory Endometrium
▪ **IM (Adults):** 375 mg q 4 wk. May be followed by cyclic therapy consisting

H

of 20 mg estradiol valerate on day 1, then 250 mg of hydroxyprogesterone with 5 mg estradiol valerate are given on day 15, repeated at 4-wk intervals.

Uterine Carcinoma
- **IM (Adults):** 1 g/1–7 times/wk.

AVAILABILITY

- *Injection:* 125 mg/ml, 250 mg/ml.

TIME/ACTION PROFILE (hormonal effects)

	ONSET	PEAK	DURATION
IM	UK	UK	7–14 days

NURSING IMPLICATIONS

ASSESSMENT

- ☐ Blood pressure should be monitored periodically throughout therapy.
- ☐ Monitor intake and output ratios and weekly weight. Report significant discrepancies or steady weight gain to physician.
- ☐ Monitor pattern and amount of vaginal bleeding (pad count).
- **Lab Test Considerations:** Monitor hepatic function prior to and periodically throughout therapy.
- ☐ May cause increased serum glucose and alkaline phosphatase levels. May decrease pregnandiol excretion concentrations.
- ☐ May alter thyroid hormone assays.

POTENTIAL NURSING DIAGNOSES

- Sexual dysfunction (indications).
- Knowledge deficit related to medication regimen (patient/family teaching).

IMPLEMENTATION

- **IM:** Administer deep IM. Use dry needle and syringe to prevent clouding of solution.

PATIENT/FAMILY TEACHING

- **General Info:** Advise patient to report signs and symptoms of fluid retention (swelling of ankles and feet, weight gain), thromboembolic disorders (pain, swelling, tenderness in extremities, headache, chest pain, blurred vision), depression, or hepatic dysfunction (yellowed skin or eyes, pruritus, dark urine, light-colored stools) to physician.
- ☐ Instruct patient to notify physician if change in vaginal bleeding pattern or spotting occurs.
- ☐ Instruct patient to stop taking medication and notify physician if pregnancy is suspected.
- ☐ Caution patient to use sunscreen and protective clothing to prevent increased pigmentation.
- ☐ Advise patient to notify physician or dentist of medication regimen prior to treatment or surgery.
- ☐ Emphasize the importance of routine follow-up physical examinations, including blood pressure; breast, abdomen, and pelvic examinations; and PAP smears.
- **Amenorrhea or Functional Uterine Bleeding:** Explain 28-day cyclic dosage schedule. Cyclic therapy begins after 4 days of desquamation from initial dose or 21 days after injection if bleeding did not occur. Explain that several months of estrogen therapy may be required before menstruation occurs.

EVALUATION

Effectiveness of therapy can be demonstrated by: ▪ Development of normal cyclic menses ▪ Control of the spread of advanced metastatic uterine cancer.

HYDROXYUREA
(hye-drox-ee-yoo-**ree**-ah)
Hydrea

CLASSIFICATION(S):
Antineoplastic (antimetabolite)
Pregnancy Category UK

INDICATIONS

▪ Treatment of head and neck carcinoma ▪ Treatment of ovarian carcinoma ▪ Treatment of resistant chronic myelogenous leukemia ▪ Treatment of melanoma.

ACTION

- Interferes with DNA synthesis (cell cycle-S phase specific). **Therapeutic Effect:** ▪ Death of rapidly replicating cells, particularly malignant ones.

PHARMACOKINETICS

Absorption: Well absorbed following oral administration.
Distribution: Crosses the blood–brain barrier.
Metabolism and Excretion: 50% excreted unchanged by the kidneys, 50% metabolized by the liver and eliminated as respiratory CO_2.
Half-life: 3–4 hr.

CONTRAINDICATIONS AND PRECAUTIONS

Contraindicated in: ▪ Hypersensitivity ▪ Pregnancy or lactation ▪ Some products contain tartrazine (FDC yellow dye #5) and should be avoided in patients with known hypersensitivity.
Use Cautiously in: ▪ Patients with childbearing potential ▪ Active infections ▪ Decreased bone marrow reserve ▪ Other chronic debilitating illness ▪ Obese patients or patients with edema (dose should be determined using ideal body weight).

ADVERSE REACTIONS AND SIDE EFFECTS*

CNS: drowsiness (large doses).
GI: stomatitis, anorexia, nausea, vomiting, diarrhea, constipation, hepatitis.
GU: dysuria, renal tubular dysfunction, gonadal suppression.
Derm: rashes, erythema, pruritus, alopecia.
Hemat: leukopenia, thrombocytopenia, anemia.
Metab: hyperuricemia.
Misc: fever, chills, malaise.

INTERACTIONS

Drug–Drug: ▪ Additive bone marrow depression with **agents that depress bone marrow,** including **radiation therapy.**

ROUTE AND DOSAGE

Head and Neck Cancer, Ovarian Cancer, Malignant Melanoma
- **PO (Adults):** 60–80 mg/kg (2–3 g/m^2) as a single daily dose q 3 days or 20–30 mg/kg/day.

Resistant Chronic Myelogenous Leukemia
- **PO (Adults):** 20–30 mg/kg/day in 1–2 divided doses.

AVAILABILITY

- *Capsules:* 50 mg.

TIME/ACTION PROFILE (effects on blood counts)

	ONSET	PEAK	DURATION
PO	7 days	10 days	21 days

NURSING IMPLICATIONS

ASSESSMENT

□ Assess for fever, sore throat, and signs of infection. If these symptoms occur, notify physician immediately.
□ Anemia may occur. Monitor for increased fatigue, dyspnea, and orthostatic hypotension.
□ Assess for bleeding (bleeding gums; bruising; petechiae; guaiac stools, urine, and emesis). Avoid IM injections and rectal temperatures. Hold pressure on all venipuncture sites for at least 10 min.
□ Monitor intake and output, appetite, and nutritional intake. Adjust diet as tolerated to maintain nutritional status.
- **Lab Test Considerations:** Monitor CBC and differential prior to and weekly during course of therapy. The onset of leukopenia occurs within 10 days of beginning therapy. Recovery usually occurs within 30 days. Notify physician if WBC <2500 mm^3 or if a precipitous drop occurs. Institute thrombocytopenia precautions if platelet count <100,000/mm^3. May cause temporary increase in mean corpuscular volume (MCV).

H

*Underlines indicate most frequent; **CAPITALS** indicate life-threatening.

□ Monitor renal (BUN, creatinine, and uric acid) and liver function tests (AST [SGOT], ALT [SGPT], bilirubin and LDH) prior to and periodically during course of therapy. May cause increased BUN, creatinine, and uric acid concentrations.

POTENTIAL NURSING DIAGNOSES
▪ Injury, high risk for (side effects).
▪ Infection, high risk for (side effects).
▪ Knowledge deficit related to medication regimen (patient/family teaching).

IMPLEMENTATION
▪ PO: Capsules may be opened and contents mixed into a glass of water and taken immediately if patient has difficulty swallowing. Some inert powder may float on the surface.

PATIENT/FAMILY TEACHING
▪ General Info: Instruct patient to take medication exactly as directed, even if nausea, vomiting, or diarrhea is a problem. Consult physician if vomiting occurs shortly after dose is taken. If a dose is missed, do not take at all; do not double doses.
□ Instruct patient to notify physician if fever, chills, sore throat, signs of infection, loss of appetite, nausea, vomiting, diarrhea, bleeding gums, bruising, petechiae, or blood in urine, stool, or emesis occurs. Caution patient to avoid crowds and persons with known infections. Instruct patient to use soft toothbrush and electric razor. Patients should be cautioned not to drink alcoholic beverages or take products containing aspirin or ibuprofen.
□ Instruct patient to inspect oral mucosa for erythema and ulceration. If ulceration occurs, advise patient to use sponge brush and rinse mouth with water after eating and drinking. Consult physician if mouth pain interferes with eating.
□ Discuss possibility of drowsiness with patients receiving large doses. Advise patient to avoid driving or other activities until response to drug is known.
□ Review with patient the need for contraception during therapy. Women need to use contraception even if amenorrhea occurs.
□ Instruct patient not to receive any vaccinations without advice of physician.
□ Discuss need for lab tests and follow-up visits to monitor progress and detect side effects.
▪ Leukemia: Encourage fluid intake of 2000–3000 ml/day. Physician may also order allopurinol and alkalinization of the urine to help prevent urate stone formation.

EVALUATION
Effectiveness of therapy can be demonstrated by: ▪ Decrease in size and spread of tumors ▪ Improved hematologic values in leukemia. Therapy is held if leukocytes are less than 2500/mm^3 or platelets less than 100,000/mm^3 and resumed when these values begin to return to normal limits, usually within 3 days.

HYDROXYZINE
(hye-**drox**-i-zeen)
Anxanil, {Apo-Hydroxyzine}, Atarax, E-Vista, Hydroxacen, Hyzine, {Multipax}, {Novohydroxyzine}, Quiess, Vistaject, Vistaquel, Vistaril, Vistazine

CLASSIFICATION(S):
Sedative/hypnotic, Antihistamine
Pregnancy Category UK

INDICATIONS
▪ Treatment of anxiety ▪ Preoperative sedation ▪ Antiemetic ▪ Antipruritic ▪ Often combined with opioid analgesics.

ACTION
▪ Acts as a CNS depressant at the subcortical level of the CNS ▪ Has anticho-

linergic, antihistaminic, and antiemetic properties. **Therapeutic Effects:** ▪ Sedation ▪ Relief of anxiety ▪ Relief of nausea and vomiting ▪ Relieves allergic symptoms associated with release of histamine, including pruritus.

PHARMACOKINETICS

Absorption: Well absorbed following oral or IM administration.
Distribution: Distribution not known.
Metabolism and Excretion: Completely metabolized by the liver. Eliminated in the feces via biliary excretion.
Half-life: 3 hr.

CONTRAINDICATIONS AND PRECAUTIONS

Contraindicated in: ▪ Hypersensitivity ▪ Pregnancy.
Use Cautiously in: ▪ Severe hepatic dysfunction ▪ Elderly patients (dosage reduction recommended) ▪ Has been used during labor ▪ Lactation (safety not established).

ADVERSE REACTIONS AND SIDE EFFECTS*

CNS: excess sedation, <u>drowsiness</u>, dizziness, ataxia, weakness, headache, paradoxical agitation.
Resp: wheezing.
GI: <u>dry mouth</u>, bitter taste, nausea, constipation.
GU: urinary retention.
Derm: flushing.
Local: <u>pain</u> at IM site, abscesses at IM sites.
Misc: chest tightness.

INTERACTIONS

Drug–Drug: ▪ Additive CNS depression with other **CNS depressants,** including **alcohol, antidepressants, antihistamines, opioid analgesics,** and **sedative/hypnotics** ▪ Additive anticholinergic effects with other **drugs possessing anticholinergic properties,** including **antihistamines, antidepressants, atropine, haloperidol, phenothiazines, quinidine,** and **disopyramide.**

ROUTE AND DOSAGE

Antianxiety
▪ **PO (Adults):** 50–100 mg single dose.
▪ **PO (Children):** 0.6 mg/kg single dose.
▪ **IM (Adults):** 50–100 mg q 4–6 hr.

Sedative/Hypnotic
▪ **PO (Adults):** 50–100 mg single dose.
▪ **PO (Children):** 0.6 mg/kg single dose.
▪ **IM (Adults):** 50 mg single dose.

Antiemetic
▪ **PO (Adults):** 25–100 mg 3–4 times daily.
▪ **PO (Children):** 0.5 mg/kg (15 mg/m^2) q 6 hr.
▪ **IM (Adults):** 25–100 mg.
▪ **IM (Children):** 1 mg/kg (30 mg/m^2).

Antipruritic
▪ **PO (Adults):** 25–100 mg 3–4 times daily.
▪ **PO (Children):** 0.5 mg/kg (15 mg/m^2) q 6 hr.

Adjunct to Opioid Analgesics
▪ **IM (Adults):** 25–100 mg.
▪ **IM (Children):** 1 mg/kg (30 mg/m^2).

AVAILABILITY

▪ *Tablets:* 10 mg, 25 mg, 50 mg, 100 mg ▪ *Capsules:* 25 mg, 50 mg, 100 mg ▪ *Syrup:* 100 mg/5 ml ▪ *Oral suspension:* 25 mg/5 ml ▪ *Injection:* 25 mg/ml, 50 mg/ml.

TIME/ACTION PROFILE
(antihistaminic, sedative, antiemetic effects)

	ONSET	PEAK	DURATION
PO	15–30 min	2–4 hr	4–6 hr
IM	15–30 min	2–4 hr	4–6 hr

NURSING IMPLICATIONS

ASSESSMENT
▪ **General Info:** Assess patient for profound sedation and provide safety precautions as indicated (side rails up, bed in low position, call bell within reach, supervision of ambulation and transfer).

*<u>Underlines</u> indicate most frequent; **CAPITALS** indicate life-threatening.

- **Anxiety:** Assess mental status, mood, and behavior.
- **Nausea and Vomiting:** Assess degree of nausea and frequency and amount of emesis.
- **Pruritus:** Assess degree of itching and character of involved skin.
- **Lab Test Considerations:** May cause false-negative skin tests using allergen extracts. Discontinue hydroxyzine at least 72 hr prior to test.

POTENTIAL NURSING DIAGNOSES
- Anxiety (indications).
- Skin integrity, impaired (indications).
- Injury, high risk for (side effects).

IMPLEMENTATION
- **PO:** Tablets may be crushed and capsules opened and administered with food or fluids for patients having difficulty swallowing.
- Shake suspension well before administration.
- **IM:** Administer IM deep into well-developed muscle, preferably with Z-track technique. Do not use deltoid site. Significant tissue damage, necrosis, and sloughing may result from SC or intra-arterial injections. Hemolysis may result from IV injections. Rotate injection sites frequently.
- **Syringe Compatibility:** ■ atropine ■ benzquinamide ■ buprenorphine ■ butorphanol ■ chlorpromazine ■ cimetidine ■ codeine ■ diphenhydramine ■ doxapram ■ droperidol ■ fentanyl ■ glycopyrrolate ■ hydromorphone ■ lidocaine ■ meperidine ■ methotrimeprazine ■ metoclopramide ■ midazolam ■ morphine ■ nalbuphine ■ oxymorphone ■ pentazocine ■ procaine ■ prochlorperazine ■ promazine ■ promethazine ■ scopolamine.
- **Syringe Incompatibility:** ■ aminophylline ■ chloramphenicol ■ dimenhydrinate ■ heparin ■ penicillin G potassium ■ pentobarbital ■ phenobarbital ■ phenytoin.

PATIENT/FAMILY TEACHING
- Instruct patient to take medication exactly as directed. Missed doses should be taken as soon as remembered unless almost time for next dose; do not double doses.
- Medication may cause drowsiness or dizziness. Caution patient to avoid driving or other activities requiring alertness until response to medication is known.
- Advise patient to avoid concurrent use of alcohol or other CNS depressants with this medication.
- Inform patient that frequent mouth rinses, good oral hygiene, and sugarless gum or candy may help decrease dry mouth. If dry mouth persists for more than 2 wk, consult dentist regarding saliva substitute.

EVALUATION
Effectiveness of therapy can be demonstrated by: ■ Decrease in anxiety ■ Relief of nausea and vomiting ■ Relief of pruritus ■ Sedation when used as a sedative/hypnotic.

IBUPROFEN
(eye-byoo-**proe**-fen)
Aches-N-Pain, {Actiprofen}, Advil, {Amersol}, {Apo-Ibuprofen}, Children's Motrin, Excedrin IB, Genpril, Haltran, Ibuprin, Ibuprohm, Ibu-Tab, Medipren, Midol 200, Motrin, Motrin IB, {Novoprofen}, Nuprin, Pamprin-IB, Rufen, Saleto, Trendar

CLASSIFICATION(S):
Nonsteroidal anti-inflammatory agent, Nonopioid analgesic, Antipyretic
Pregnancy Category UK

INDICATIONS

- Used as an analgesic in the treatment of mild to moderate pain or dysmenor-

---

{} = Available in Canada only.

rhea ▪ Management of inflammatory disorders including: □ Rheumatoid arthritis □ Osteoarthritis ▪ Lowering of fever.

ACTION

▪ Inhibits prostaglandin synthesis. **Therapeutic Effects:** ▪ Suppression of pain and inflammation ▪ Reduction of fever.

PHARMACOKINETICS

Absorption: Well absorbed from the GI tract.
Distribution: Distribution not known. Probably crosses the placenta. Does not appear to enter breast milk.
Metabolism and Excretion: Mostly metabolized by the liver. Small amounts (10%) excreted unchanged by the kidneys.
Half-life: 2–4 hr.

CONTRAINDICATIONS AND PRECAUTIONS

Contraindicated in: ▪ Hypersensitivity ▪ Cross-sensitivity may exist with other nonsteroidal anti-inflammatory agents, including aspirin ▪ Active GI bleeding or ulcer disease.
Use Cautiously in: ▪ Severe cardiovascular, renal, or hepatic disease ▪ History of ulcer disease ▪ Pregnancy, lactation, or children (safety not established).

ADVERSE REACTIONS AND SIDE EFFECTS*

CNS: headache, drowsiness, psychic disturbances, dizziness.
EENT: blurred vision, tinnitus, amblyopia.
CV: edema, arrhythmias.
GI: nausea, dyspepsia, vomiting, constipation, GI BLEEDING, discomfort, HEPATITIS.
GU: renal failure, hematuria, cystitis.
Derm: rashes.
Hemat: blood dyscrasias, prolonged bleeding time.
Misc: allergic reactions, including ANAPHYLAXIS.

INTERACTIONS

Drug–Drug: ▪ Concurrent use with **aspirin** may decrease effectiveness ▪ Additive adverse GI side effects with **aspirin,** other **nonsteroidal anti-inflammatory agents, potassium supplements, glucocorticoids,** or **alcohol** ▪ Chronic use with **acetaminophen** may increase the risk of adverse renal reactions ▪ May decrease the effectiveness of **diuretics** or **antihypertensive** therapy ▪ May increase the hypoglycemic effects of **insulin** or **oral hypoglycemic agents** ▪ May slightly increase serum **digoxin** levels ▪ May increase serum **lithium** levels and increase the risk of toxicity ▪ Increases the risk of toxicity from **methotrexate** ▪ **Probenecid** increases risk of toxicity from ibuprofen ▪ Increased risk of bleeding with **cefamandole, cefotetan, cefoperazone, valproic acid** or **plicamycin, thrombolytic agents,** or **anticoagulants** ▪ Increased risk of adverse hematologic reactions with **antineoplastic agents** or **radiation therapy** ▪ Increased risk of nephrotoxicity with **cyclosporine.**

ROUTE AND DOSAGE

Analgesia
▪ **PO (Adults):** 200–400 mg q 4–6 hr (not to exceed 3200 mg/day).

Anti-inflammatory
▪ **PO (Adults):** 300–800 mg 3–4 times daily (not to exceed 3200 mg/day).
▪ **PO (Children):** 30–40 mg/kg/day in 3–4 divided doses; not to exceed 50 mg/kg/day.

Antipyretic
▪ **PO (Children 6 mo–12 yr):** 5 mg/kg for temperature <102.5°F or 10 mg/kg for temperature >102.5°F (not to exceed 40 mg/kg/day); may be repeated q 4–6 hr.

AVAILABILITY

▪ *Tablets:* 200 mg, 300 mg, 400 mg, 600 mg, 800 mg ▪ *Oral suspension:* 100 mg/5 ml ▪ *In combination with:* decongestants. See Appendix A.

TIME/ACTION PROFILE

	ONSET	PEAK	DURATION
PO (analgesic)	30 min	1–2 hr	4–6 hr
PO (anti-inflammatory)	7 days	1–2 wk	UK

NURSING IMPLICATIONS

ASSESSMENT

- **General Info:** Patients who have asthma, aspirin-induced allergy, and nasal polyps are at increased risk for developing hypersensitivity reactions. Assess for rhinitis, asthma, and urticaria.
- **Pain:** Assess pain (note type, location, and intensity) prior to and 1–2 hr following administration.
- **Arthritis:** Assess pain and range of motion prior to and 1–2 hr following administration.
- **Fever:** Monitor temperature; note signs associated with fever (diaphoresis, tachycardia, malaise).
- **Lab Test Considerations:** BUN, serum creatinine, CBC, and liver function tests should be evaluated periodically in patients receiving prolonged courses of therapy.
  - Serum potassium, BUN, serum creatinine, AST (SGOT), and ALT (SGPT) tests may show increased levels. Blood glucose, hemoglobin, and hematocrit concentrations and creatinine clearance may be decreased.
  - May cause prolonged bleeding time, which may persist for 2 days following discontinuation of therapy.

POTENTIAL NURSING DIAGNOSES

- Pain (indications).
- Physical mobility, impaired (indications).
- Knowledge deficit related to medication regimen (patient/family teaching).

IMPLEMENTATION

- **General Info:** Coadministration with opioid analgesics may have additive analgesic effects and may permit lower opioid doses.
- **PO:** For rapid initial effect, adminis-

ter 30 min before or 2 hr after meals. May be administered with food, milk, or antacids to decrease GI irritation. Food slows but does not reduce the extent of absorption. Tablets may be crushed and mixed with fluids or food. 800-mg tablet can be dissolved in water.
- **Dysmenorrhea:** Administer as soon as possible after the onset of menses. Prophylactic treatment has not been shown to be effective.

PATIENT/FAMILY TEACHING

- Advise patients to take this medication with a full glass of water and to remain in an upright position for 15–30 min after administration.
- Instruct patient to take medication exactly as prescribed. If dose is missed, it should be taken as soon as remembered but not if almost time for next dose. Do not double doses.
- This medication may cause drowsiness or dizziness. Advise patient to avoid driving or other activities requiring alertness until response to medication is known.
- Caution patient to avoid the concurrent use of alcohol, aspirin, acetaminophen, or other over-the-counter medications without consultation with physician or pharmacist.
- Advise patient to inform physician or dentist of medication regimen prior to treatment or surgery.
- Instruct patients not to take the over-the-counter ibuprofen preparations for more than 10 days for pain or 3 days for fever and to consult physician if symptoms persist or worsen.
- Instruct patient to notify physician if rash, itching, chills, fever, muscle aches, visual disturbances, weight gain, edema, black stools, or persistent headache occurs.

EVALUATION

Effectiveness of therapy can be demonstrated by: ▪ Decrease in severity of pain ▪ Improved joint mobility. Partial arthritic relief is usually seen within 7 days, but maximum effectiveness may require 1–2 wk of continuous therapy

- Reduction in fever. Patients who do not respond to one nonsteroidal anti-inflammatory agent may respond to another.

IDARUBICIN
(eye-da-**roo**-bi-sin)
Idamycin

CLASSIFICATION(S):
Antineoplastic agent (anthra-cycline)
Pregnancy Category D

INDICATIONS

- As part of combination chemotherapy in the treatment of acute myelogenous leukemia in adults.

ACTION

- Inhibits nucleic acid synthesis. **Therapeutic Effect:** - Death of rapidly replicating cells, particularly malignant ones.

PHARMACOKINETICS

Absorption: IV administration results in complete bioavailability.
Distribution: Rapidly distributed with extensive tissue binding. High degree of cellular uptake.
Metabolism and Excretion: Extensive hepatic and extrahepatic metabolism. One metabolite is active (idarubicinol). Primarily eliminated via biliary excretion.
Half-life: 22 hr (range 4–46 hr).

CONTRAINDICATIONS AND PRECAUTIONS

Contraindicated in: - Pregnancy or lactation.
Use Cautiously in: - Children (safety not established) - Patients with child-bearing potential - Active infection - Decreased bone marrow reserve - Other chronic debilitating illnesses - Hepatic impairment (dosage reduction may be required; avoid if bilirubin ≥5 mg/dl) - Renal impairment - Pre-existing cardiac disease - Previous daunorubicin or doxorubicin therapy.

ADVERSE REACTIONS AND SIDE EFFECTS*

CNS: headache, mental status changes.
Resp: pulmonary toxicity, pulmonary allergic reactions.
CV: CARDIOTOXICITY, CONGESTIVE HEART FAILURE, ARRHYTHMIAS.
GI: nausea, vomiting, abdominal cramps, diarrhea, mucositis.
Derm: alopecia, rashes.
Endo: gonadal suppression.
Hemat: anemia, leukopenia, thrombo-cytopenia, BLEEDING.
Local: phlebitis at IV site.
Metab: hyperuricemia.
Neuro: peripheral neuropathy.
Misc: fever.

INTERACTIONS

Drug–Drug: - Additive myelosuppression with other **antineoplastic agents** or **radiation therapy** - May decrease antibody response to and increase risk of adverse reactions from **live virus vaccines.**

ROUTE AND DOSAGE

- **IV (Adults):** 12 mg/m² daily for 3 days in combination with cytarabine.

AVAILABILITY

- *Injection:* 5-mg, 10-mg vials.

TIME/ACTION PROFILE (effects on blood counts)

	ONSET	PEAK	DURATION
IV	UK	UK	UK

NURSING IMPLICATIONS

ASSESSMENT

- Monitor blood pressure, pulse, respiratory rate, and temperature frequently during administration. Notify physician of significant changes.
- Assess for fever, chills, sore throat, and signs of infection. Notify physician if these symptoms occur.

I

▢ Monitor platelet count throughout therapy. Assess for bleeding (bleeding gums, bruising, petechiae; guaiac stools, urine, and emesis). Avoid IM injections and rectal temperatures. Apply pressure to venipuncture sites for 10 min.

▢ Anemia may occur. Monitor for increased fatigue, dyspnea, and orthostatic hypotension.

▢ Monitor intake and output ratios and inform physician if significant discrepancies occur. Encourage fluid intake of 2000–3000 ml/day. Physician may also order allopurinol and alkalinization of the urine to decrease serum uric acid levels and to help prevent urate stone formation.

▢ Severe and protracted nausea and vomiting may occur as early as 1 hr after therapy and may last 24 hr. Parenteral antiemetic agents should be administered 30–45 min prior to therapy and routinely around the clock for the next 24 hr as indicated. Monitor amount of emesis and notify physician if emesis exceeds guidelines to prevent dehydration.

▢ Monitor for development of signs of myocardial toxicity manifested by life-threatening arrhythmias, cardiomyopathy, and congestive heart failure (peripheral edema, dyspnea, rales/crackles, weight gain).

▢ Assess injection site frequently for redness, irritation, or inflammation. Medication may infiltrate painlessly. If extravasation occurs, infusion must be stopped and restarted elsewhere to avoid damage to SC tissue. Treatment of extravasation includes intermittent ice packs (apply for 30 min immediately and 30 min qid for 3 days). If pain, erythema, or vesication occurs, plastic surgery may be warranted.

▪ **Lab Test Considerations:** Monitor CBC, differential, and renal and hepatic function prior to and frequently throughout therapy. May cause hyperuricemia.

POTENTIAL NURSING DIAGNOSES

▪ Infection, high risk for (adverse reactions).

▪ Nutrition; altered: less than body requirements (adverse reactions).

▪ Knowledge deficit related to medication regimen (patient/family teaching).

IMPLEMENTATION

▪ **General Info:** Solution should be prepared in a biologic cabinet. Wear gloves, gown, and mask while handling medication. Discard IV equipment in specially designated containers (see Appendix I).

▢ See cytarabine monograph for specific information on administration of cytarabine with idarubicin.

▪ **Direct IV:** Reconstitute 5-mg and 10-mg vials with 5 ml and 10 ml, respectively, of 0.9% NaCl (nonbacteriostatic) for injection for a concentration of 1 mg/ml. Vial contents are under pressure, use care when inserting needle.

▢ Reconstituted medication is stable for 72 hr at room temperature and 7 days if refrigerated.

▪ *Rate:* Administer each dose slowly over 10–15 min through Y-site or 3-way stopcock of a free-flowing infusion of 0.9% NaCl or D5W. Tubing may be attached to a butterfly needle and injected into a large vein.

▪ **Syringe Incompatibility:** ▪ heparin.

▪ **Y-Site Incompatibility:** ▪ sargramostim.

PATIENT/FAMILY TEACHING

▢ Instruct patient to notify physician promptly if fever, sore throat, signs of infection, bleeding gums, bruising, petechiae; or blood in stools, urine, or emesis; increased fatigue, dyspnea, or orthostatic hypotension occur. Caution patient to avoid crowds and persons with known infections. Instruct patient to use soft toothbrush and electric razor and to avoid falls. Patients should be cautioned not to drink alcoholic beverages or take medication containing aspirin or ibuprofen as these may precipitate gastric bleeding.

▢ Instruct patient to report pain at injection site immediately.

□ Instruct patient to inspect oral mucosa for erythema and ulceration. If ulceration occurs, advise patient to use sponge brush, rinse mouth with water after eating and drinking, and confer with physician if mouth pain interferes with eating. Further courses of idarubicin should be withheld until recovery from mucositis, and subsequent doses should be decreased by 25%.

□ Advise patient that this medication may have teratogenic effects. Contraception should be practiced during and for at least 4 mo after therapy is concluded.

□ Instruct patient to notify physician immediately if irregular heart beat, shortness of breath, or swelling of lower extremities occurs.

□ Discuss with patient the possibility of hair loss. Explore methods of coping.

□ Instruct patient not to receive any vaccinations without advice of physician.

□ Emphasize the need for periodic lab tests to monitor for side effects.

EVALUATION

Effectiveness of therapy can be demonstrated by: ▪ Improvement of hematologic status in leukemias.

IFOSFAMIDE
(**eye**-foss-fam-ide)
Ifex

CLASSIFICATION(S):
Antineoplastic agent (alkylating agent)
Pregnancy Category D

INDICATIONS

▪ In combination with other agents in the treatment of germ cell testicular carcinoma ▪ Used in combination with mesna, which prevents ifosfamide-induced hemorrhagic cystitis.

ACTION

▪ Following conversion to active compounds, interferes with DNA replication and RNA transcription, ultimately disrupting protein synthesis (cell cycle-phase nonspecific). **Therapeutic Effect:** ▪ Death of rapidly replicating cells, particularly malignant ones.

PHARMACOKINETICS

Absorption: Administered IV only, inactive prior to conversion to metabolites.
Distribution: Excreted in breast milk.
Metabolism and Excretion: Metabolized by the liver to active antineoplastic compounds.
Half-life: 15 hr.

CONTRAINDICATIONS AND PRECAUTIONS

Contraindicated in: ▪ Hypersensitivity ▪ Pregnancy, lactation, or children.
Use Cautiously in: ▪ Patients with childbearing potential ▪ Active infections ▪ Decreased bone marrow reserve ▪ Other chronic debilitating illness ▪ Impaired renal function.

ADVERSE REACTIONS AND SIDE EFFECTS*

CNS: <u>CNS toxicity</u> (somnolence, confusion, hallucinations, coma), dizziness, disorientation, cranial nerve dysfunction.
CV: cardiotoxicity.
GI: <u>nausea</u>, <u>vomiting</u>, anorexia, diarrhea, constipation, liver dysfunction.
GU: <u>hemorrhagic cystitis</u>, renal toxicity, dysuria, gonadal suppression.
Derm: <u>alopecia</u>.
Hemat: leukopenia, thrombocytopenia, anemia.
Local: phlebitis.
Misc: allergic reactions.

INTERACTIONS

Drug–Drug: ▪ Additive myelosuppression with other **antineoplastic agents** or **radiation therapy** ▪ May decrease antibody response to and increase risk

I

of adverse reactions from live virus vaccines.

ROUTE AND DOSAGE

- **IV (Adults):** 1.2 g/m²/day for 5 days, coadminister with mesna. May repeat cycle q 3 wk.

AVAILABILITY

- *Injection:* 1-g, 3-g vials.

TIME/ACTION PROFILE (effects on blood counts)

	ONSET	PEAK	DURATION
IV	UK	UK	UK

NURSING IMPLICATIONS

ASSESSMENT

- **General Info:** Monitor blood pressure, pulse, respiratory rate, and temperature frequently during administration. Notify physician of significant changes.
- Monitor urinary output frequently throughout therapy. Notify physician if hematuria occurs. To reduce the risk of hemorrhagic cystitis, fluid intake should be at least 3000 ml/day for adults and 1000–2000 ml/day for children. Mesna is given concurrently to prevent hemorrhagic cystitis.
- Monitor neurologic status. Inform physician if lethargy, confusion, or hallucinations occurs.
- Assess nausea, vomiting, and appetite. Weigh weekly. Confer with physician about premedication with an antiemetic to minimize GI effects. Adjust diet as tolerated.
- Assess for fever, chills, sore throat, and signs of infection. Notify physician if these symptoms occur.
- Monitor platelet count throughout therapy. Assess for bleeding (bleeding gums; bruising; petechiae; guaiac stools, urine, and emesis). Avoid IM injections and rectal temperatures. Apply pressure to venipuncture sites for 10 min.
- **Lab Test Considerations:** Monitor CBC and differential prior to and periodically throughout course of therapy. Withhold dose and notify physician if WBC <2,000/mm³ or platelets <50,000/mm³.
- Urinalysis should be evaluated before each dose. Withhold dose and notify physician if urinalysis shows >10 RBCs per high power field.
- May cause elevation in liver enzymes and serum bilirubin.

POTENTIAL NURSING DIAGNOSES

- Infection, high risk for (side effects).
- Body image disturbance (side effects).
- Knowledge deficit related to medication regimen (patient/family teaching).

IMPLEMENTATION

- **General Info:** Solution should be prepared in a biologic cabinet. Wear gloves, gown, and mask while handling IV medication. Discard IV equipment in specially designated containers (see Appendix I).
- **IV:** Prepare solution by diluting each 1-g vial with 20 ml of Sterile Water or Bacteriostatic Water for Injection containing parabens. Use solution prepared without bacteriostatic water within 6 hr. Solution prepared with bacteriostatic water is stable for 1 wk at 30°C or 6 wk at 5°C.
- **Intermittent Infusion:** May be further diluted to a concentration of 0.6 to 20 mg/ml in D5W, 0.9% NaCl, lactated Ringer's solution, or Sterile Water for Injection.
- *Rate:* Administer over 30 min.
- **Syringe Compatibility:** ▪ mesna.
- **Y-Site Compatibility:** ▪ fludarabine ▪ ondansetron ▪ sargramostim.
- **Additive Compatibility:** ▪ carboplatin ▪ cisplatin ▪ etoposide ▪ fluorouracil ▪ mesna.

PATIENT/FAMILY TEACHING

- Emphasize need for adequate fluid intake throughout course of therapy. Patient should void frequently to decrease bladder irritation from metabolites excreted by the kidneys. Physician should be notified immediately if hematuria is noted.
- Instruct patient to notify physician

promptly if fever, sore throat, signs of infection, bleeding gums, bruising, petechiae, or blood in urine, stool, or emesis, or confusion occurs.

□ Caution patient to avoid crowds and persons with known infections. Instruct patient to use soft toothbrush, electric razor, and to avoid falls. Patients should also be cautioned not to drink alcoholic beverages or to take products containing aspirin or ibuprofen, as these may precipitate GI hemorrhage.

□ Review with patient the need for contraception during therapy.

□ Discuss with patient the possibility of hair loss. Explore methods of coping.

□ Instruct patient not to receive any vaccinations without advice of physician.

EVALUATION
Effectiveness of therapy can be demonstrated by: ■ Decrease in size or spread of malignant germ cell testicular carcinoma.

IMIPENEM/CILASTATIN
(i-me-**pen**-em/sye-la-**stat**-in)
Primaxin

CLASSIFICATION(S):
Anti-infective (*miscellaneous penicillin*)
Pregnancy Category C

INDICATIONS

■ Treatment of the following serious infections: □ Lower respiratory tract infections □ Urinary tract infections □ Abdominal infections □ Gynecologic infections □ Skin and skin structure infections □ Bone and joint infections □ Bacteremia □ Endocarditis □ Polymicrobic infections.

ACTION

■ Imipenem binds to bacterial cell wall, resulting in cell death ■ Combination with cilastatin prevents renal inactiva-tion of imipenem, resulting in high urinary concentrations ■ Imipenem resists the actions of many enzymes that degrade most other penicillins and penicillin-like anti-infectives. **Therapeutic Effect:** ■ Bactericidal action against susceptible bacteria. **Spectrum:** ■ Spectrum is broad ■ Active against most gram-positive aerobic cocci: □ *Streptococcus pneumoniae* □ Group A beta-hemolytic streptococci □ *Enterococcus* □ *Staphylococcus aureus* ■ Active against many gram-negative bacillary organisms: □ *Escherichia coli* □ *Klebsiella* □ *Acinetobacter* □ *Proteus* □ *Serratia* □ *Pseudomonas aeruginosa* ■ Also displays activity against: □ *Salmonella* □ *Shigella* □ *Neisseria gonorrhoeac* □ Numerous anaerobes.

PHARMACOKINETICS

Absorption: Administered IV only, resulting in complete bioavailability.
Distribution: Widely distributed. Crosses the placenta. Enters breast milk.
Metabolism and Excretion: 70% excreted unchanged by the kidneys.
Half-life: 1 hr (prolonged in renal impairment).

CONTRAINDICATIONS AND PRECAUTIONS

Contraindicated in: ■ Hypersensitivity ■ Cross-sensitivity may exist with penicillins and cephalosporins.
Use Cautiously in: ■ Previous history of multiple hypersensitivity reactions ■ Seizure disorders ■ Renal impairment (dosage reduction required if creatinine clearance ≤ 70 ml/min/1.73 m^2) ■ Pregnancy, lactation, or children (safety not established).

ADVERSE REACTIONS AND SIDE EFFECTS*

CNS: SEIZURES, dizziness, somnolence.
CV: hypotension.
GI: nausea, diarrhea, vomiting.
Derm: rash, pruritus, urticaria, sweating.
Hemat: eosinophilia.

I

*Underlines indicate most frequent; **CAPITALS** indicate life-threatening.

Local: phlebitis at IV site.
Misc: allergic reaction, including ANA-PHYLAXIS, fever, superinfection.

INTERACTIONS

Drug–Drug: ▪ May antagonize the action of **penicillins** and **cephalosporins** ▪ Do not admix with **aminoglycosides** (inactivation may occur) ▪ **Probenecid** decreases renal excretion and increases blood levels ▪ Increased risk of seizures with **ganciclovir** (avoid concurrent use).

ROUTE AND DOSAGE

▪ **IV (Adults):** 250 mg–1 g q 6 hr or 500 mg–1 g q 8 hr.
▪ **IM (Adults):** 500–750 mg q 12 hr.

AVAILABILITY

▪ *Injection (IV):* 250 mg imipenem/250 mg cilastatin, 500 mg imipenem/500 mg cilastatin ▪ *Injection (IM):* 500 mg imipenem/500 mg cilastatin, 750 mg imipenem/750 mg cilastatin.

TIME/ACTION PROFILE (blood levels)

	ONSET	PEAK
IV	rapid	end of infusion

NURSING IMPLICATIONS

ASSESSMENT

▫ Assess patient for infection (vital signs; appearance of wound, sputum, urine, and stool; WBC) at beginning and throughout course of therapy.
▫ Obtain a history before initiating therapy to determine previous use of and reactions to penicillins. Persons with a negative history of penicillin sensitivity may still have an allergic response.
▫ Obtain specimens for culture and sensitivity prior to initiating therapy. First dose may be given before receiving results.
▫ Observe patient for signs and symptoms of anaphylaxis (rash, pruritus, laryngeal edema, wheezing). Discontinue the drug and notify the physician immediately if these occur. Have epinephrine, an antihistamine, and

resuscitative equipment close by in the event of an anaphylactic reaction.
▪ **Lab Test Considerations:** BUN, AST (SGOT), ALT (SGPT), LDH, serum alkaline phosphatase, bilirubin, and creatinine may be transiently increased.
▫ Hemoglobin and hematocrit concentrations may be decreased.
▫ May cause positive direct Coombs' test.

POTENTIAL NURSING DIAGNOSES

▪ Infection, high risk for (indications, side effects).
▪ Knowledge deficit related to medication regimen (patient/family teaching).

IMPLEMENTATION

▪ **IM:** Reconstitute 500-mg vial with 2 ml and 750-mg vial with 3 ml of lidocaine without epinephrine. Shake well to form a suspension. Withdraw and inject entire contents of vial IM.
▪ **Intermittent Infusion:** Reconstitute each 250- or 500-mg vial with 10 ml of compatible diluent and shake well. Transfer the resulting suspension to not less than 100 ml of compatible diluent. Add an additional 10 ml to each previously reconstituted vial and shake well to ensure all medication is used. Transfer the remaining contents of the vial to the infusion container. Do not administer suspension by direct injection.
▫ Reconstitute 120 ml infusion bottles with 100 ml of a compatible diluent. Shake well until clear.
▫ *Compatible diluents* include 0.9% NaCl, D5W, D10W, D5/0.2% sodium bicarbonate, D5/0.9% NaCl, D5/0.45% NaCl, D5/0.225% NaCl, or mannitol 2.5%, 5%, or 10%. Solution may range from clear to yellow in color. Do not administer cloudy solutions. Solution is stable for 4 hr at room temperature and 24 hr if refrigerated.
▪ *Rate:* Administer each 250- or 500-mg dose over 20–30 min and each 1-g dose over 40–60 min. Administer over 15–20 min for pediatric patients. Do not administer direct IV.

□ Rapid infusion may cause nausea, vomiting, hypotension, dizziness, or sweating. If these symptoms develop, slow infusion. Discontinuation of medication may be necessary.

- **Y-Site Compatibility:** ▪ acyclovir ▪ famotidine ▪ fludarabine ▪ foscarnet ▪ insulin ▪ ondansetron ▪ zidovudine.
- **Y-Site Incompatibility:** ▪ fluconazole ▪ meperidine ▪ sargramostim.
- **Additive Incompatibility:** Do not admix with other antibiotics.

PATIENT/FAMILY TEACHING

□ Advise patient to report the signs of superinfection (black, furry overgrowth on the tongue, vaginal itching or discharge, loose or foul-smelling stools) and allergy.

EVALUATION

Clinical response can be evaluated by: ▪ Resolution of the signs and symptoms of infection. Length of time for complete resolution depends on the organism and site of infection.

IMIPRAMINE
(im-ip-ra-meen)
{Apo-Imipramine}, {Impril}, Janimine, {Nono-Pramine}, SK-Pramine, Tipramine, Tofranil, Tofranil PM

CLASSIFICATION(S):
Antidepressant (tricyclic)
Pregnancy Category C

INDICATIONS

▪ Treatment of various forms of depression, often in conjunction with psychotherapy ▪ Management of enuresis in children. **Unlabeled Uses:** ▪ Adjunct in the management of chronic pain, migraine prophylaxis, and cluster headache.

ACTION

▪ Potentiates the effect of serotonin and norepinephrine ▪ Has significant anticholinergic properties. **Therapeutic Ef-** fect: ▪ Antidepressant action that develops slowly over several weeks.

PHARMACOKINETICS

Absorption: Well absorbed from the GI tract.
Distribution: Widely distributed. Appears to cross the placenta and enter breast milk.
Metabolism and Excretion: Extensively metabolized by the liver, much of it on its first pass through the liver. Some is converted to active compounds. Undergoes enterohepatic recirculation and secretion into gastric juices.
Half-life: 8–16 hr.

CONTRAINDICATIONS AND PRECAUTIONS

Contraindicated in: ▪ Hypersensitivity ▪ Cross-sensitivity with other antidepressants may exist ▪ Narrow-angle glaucoma ▪ Pregnancy and lactation ▪ Hypersensitivity to tartrazine or sulfites (in some preparations).
Use Cautiously in: ▪ Elderly patients (more susceptible to adverse reaction) ▪ Pre-existing cardiovascular disease ▪ Elderly men with prostatic hypertrophy (more susceptible to urinary retention) ▪ Seizures or history of seizure disorder.

ADVERSE REACTIONS AND SIDE EFFECTS*

CNS: <u>drowsiness</u>, <u>sedation</u>, <u>fatigue</u>, confusion, agitation, hallucinations, insomnia.
CV: <u>hypotension</u>, ECG changes, ARRHYTHMIAS.
Derm: photosensitivity.
EENT: <u>dry mouth</u>, <u>dry eyes</u>, <u>blurred vision</u>.
Endo: gynecomastia.
GI: <u>constipation</u>, paralytic ileus, nausea.
GU: urinary retention.
Hemat: blood dyscrasias.

INTERACTIONS

Drug–Drug: ▪ May cause hypotension and tachycardia when used with MAO

I

inhibitors (avoid concurrent use—discontinue 2 wk prior to imipramine) ▪ May prevent therapeutic response to most **antihypertensives** ▪ May cause severe hypertension when used with **clonidine** (avoid concurrent use) ▪ Additive CNS depression with other **CNS depressants,** including **alcohol, antihistamines, opioid analgesics,** and **sedative/hypnotics** ▪ **Adrenergic** and **anticholinergic** side effects may be additive with other agents having these properties ▪ **Cimetidine, fluoxetine, phenothiazines,** or **oral contraceptives** may increase levels and may cause toxicity ▪ May produce organic brain syndrome with **disulfiram** ▪ **Smoking** may increase metabolism and decrease effectiveness.

ROUTE AND DOSAGE
Antidepressant
▪ **PO (Adults):** 25–50 mg 3–4 times daily (not to exceed 300 mg/day or 100 mg/day in elderly patients); total daily dose may be given at bedtime.
▪ **PO (Elderly):** 25 mg at bedtime initially, up to 100 mg/day in divided doses.
▪ **PO (Adolescents):** 25–50 mg/day in divided doses (not to exceed 100 mg/day).
▪ **PO (Children 6–12 yr):** 10–30 mg/day in 2 divided doses.
▪ **IM (Adults):** 100 mg/day in divided doses (not to exceed 300 mg/day).

Enuresis
▪ **PO (Children >6 yr):** 25 mg once daily 1 hr before bedtime; increase if necessary by 25 mg at weekly intervals to 50 mg in children <12 yr, up to 75 mg in children >12 yr.

AVAILABILITY
▪ *Tablets:* 10 mg, 25 mg, 50 mg ▪ *Capsules:* 75 mg, 100 mg, 125 mg, 150 mg ▪ *Injection:* 25 mg/2 ml.

TIME/ACTION PROFILE
(antidepressant effect)

	ONSET	PEAK	DURATION
PO	hr	2–6 wk	wk
IM	hr	2–6 wk	wk

NURSING IMPLICATIONS
ASSESSMENT
▪ **General Info:** Monitor blood pressure and pulse rate prior to and during initial therapy.
▫ Monitor baseline and periodic ECGs in elderly or patients with heart disease and before increasing dosage with children treated for enuresis. May cause prolonged PR and QT intervals and may flatten T waves.
▪ **Depression:** Assess mental status frequently. Confusion, agitation, and hallucinations may occur during initiation of therapy and may require dosage reduction. Monitor mood changes. Assess for suicidal tendencies, especially during early therapy. Restrict amount of drug available to patient.
▪ **Pain:** Assess location, duration, and severity of pain periodically throughout therapy.
▪ **Lab Test Considerations:** Assess leukocyte and differential blood counts and renal and hepatic functions prior to and periodically during prolonged or high-dose therapy.
▫ Serum levels may be monitored in patients who fail to respond to usual therapeutic dose. Therapeutic plasma concentration range is 200–350 ng/ml.
▫ May cause alterations in blood glucose levels.
▪ **Toxicity and Overdose:** Symptoms of acute overdose include disturbed concentration, confusion, restlessness, agitation, convulsions, drowsiness, mydriasis, arrhythmias, fever, hallucinations, vomiting, and dyspnea.
▫ Treatment of overdose includes gastric lavage, activated charcoal, and a stimulant cathartic. Maintain respiratory and cardiac function (monitor ECG for at least 5 days) and temperature. Medications may include digoxin for congestive heart failure, antiarrhythmics, anticonvulsants, and physostigmine to help reverse anticholinergic effects.

POTENTIAL NURSING DIAGNOSES
▪ Coping, ineffective individual (indications).

- Urinary elimination, altered (indications).
- Knowledge deficit related to medication regimen (patient/family teaching).

IMPLEMENTATION
- **General Info:** May be given as a single dose at bedtime to minimize sedation during the day.
- **PO:** Administer medication with or immediately following a meal to minimize gastric irritation.
- **IM:** May be slightly yellow or red in color. Crystals may develop if solution is cool; place ampule under warm running water for 1 min to dissolve.

PATIENT/FAMILY TEACHING
- **General Info:** Instruct patient to take medication exactly as directed. Do not skip or double up on missed doses. Inform patient that at least 2 wk are needed before drug effects may be noticed. Abrupt discontinuation may cause nausea, headache, and malaise.
- May cause drowsiness and blurred vision. Caution patient to avoid driving and other activities requiring alertness until response to drug is known.
- Instruct patient to notify physician if visual changes occur. Inform patient that periodic glaucoma testing may be needed during long-term therapy.
- Caution patient to make position changes slowly to minimize orthostatic hypotension.
- Advise patient to avoid alcohol or other CNS depressant drugs during therapy and for at least 3–7 days after therapy has been discontinued.
- Instruct patient to notify physician if urinary retention or uncontrolled movements occur or if dry mouth or constipation persists. Sugarless candy or gum may diminish dry mouth, and an increase in fluid intake or bulk may prevent constipation.
- Caution patient to use sunscreen and protective clothing to prevent photosensitivity reactions.

- Inform patient of need to monitor dietary intake, as possible increase in appetite may lead to undesired weight gain.
- Advise patient to notify physician or dentist of medication regimen prior to treatment or surgery.
- Therapy for depression is usually prolonged. Emphasize the importance of follow-up examinations to evaluate progress.
- **Children:** Inform parents that the side effects most likely to occur include nervousness, insomnia, unusual tiredness, and mild nausea and vomiting. Notify physician if these symptoms become pronounced.
- Advise parents to keep medication out of reach of children to prevent inadvertent overdose.

EVALUATION
Effectiveness of therapy can be demonstrated by: ■ Increased sense of well-being □ Renewed interest in surroundings □ Increased appetite □ Improved energy level □ Improved sleep ■ Control of bedwetting in children >6 yr ■ Prevention and management of chronic neurogenic pain. Patients may require 2–6 wk of therapy before full therapeutic effects of medication are noticeable.

IMMUNE GLOBULIN
(im-**myoon glo**-byoo-lin)
gamma globulin, IG, ISG, immune serum globulin
IMMUNE GLOBULIN IM
Gamastan, Gammar, IGIM
IMMUNE GLOBULIN IV
Gamimune N, Gammagard, Gammar-IV, IG IV, Iveegam, Sandoglobulin, Venoglobulin-I

CLASSIFICATION(S):
Serum (immune globulin)
Pregnancy Category UK

I

INDICATIONS

- **IM:** Provides passive immunity to a variety of infections including: □ Hepatitis A □ Measles (rubeola) when immune sera are unavailable or there is insufficient time for active immunization to take place ▪ **IV:** Useful in patients with immunodeficiency syndromes who are unable to produce IgG-type antibodies ▪ **IV:** Prevention of bacterial infections in patients with B-cell chronic lymphocytic leukemia (Gammagard only) ▪ Treatment of idiopathic thrombocytopenic purpura.

ACTION

▪ A human serum fraction containing gamma globulin antibodies (IgG). **Therapeutic Effect:** ▪ Provision of passive immunity against many infections.

PHARMACOKINETICS

Absorption: Well absorbed following IM administration.
Distribution: Rapidly and evenly distributed.
Metabolism and Excretion: Removed by redistribution, tissue binding, and catabolism.
Half-life: 21–24 days.

CONTRAINDICATIONS AND PRECAUTIONS

Contraindicated in: ▪ Hypersensitivity to immune globulins or additives (maltose, thimerisol, glycine, polyethylene glycol, albumin) ▪ Selective IgA deficiency.
Use Cautiously in: ▪ IM form should be used cautiously in patients with thrombocytopenia ▪ Gamimune N product should be used cautiously in patients with acid-base disorders ▪ Agammaglobulinemia or hypogammaglobulinemia (increased risk of hypotension and anaphylaxis following rapid IV administration) ▪ Has been used during pregnancy, though safety is not established.

ADVERSE REACTIONS AND SIDE EFFECTS*

CNS: faintness, lightheadedness, headache, malaise.

Resp: dyspnea, wheezing.
CV: chest pain.
GI: nausea.
GU: diuresis (if maltose in preparation), nephrotic syndrome.
Derm: urticaria, cyanosis.
Local: <u>pain</u>, <u>tenderness</u>, <u>muscle stiffness at IM site</u>, local inflammation, urticaria at site, phlebitis.
MS: hip pain, back pain, arthralgia.
Misc: allergic reactions, including ANAPHYLAXIS, angioedema, fever, chills, sweating.

INTERACTIONS

Drug–Drug: ▪ May interfere with the normal immune response to some **live vaccines,** including **measles, mumps,** and **rubella virus vaccine** (do not administer within 3 mo of immune globulin).

ROUTE AND DOSAGE

Pre- and Postexposure Hepatitis A Prophylaxis
▪ **IM (Adults and Children):** 0.02 ml/kg (for pre-exposure prophylaxis, higher doses—0.06 ml/kg q 4–6 mo are used if exposure will last >3 mo).

Postexposure Measles Prophylaxis
▪ **IM (Adults and Children):** 0.25 ml/kg (0.5 ml/kg if immunosuppressed). Not to exceed 15 ml.

Immunodeficiency Syndrome
▪ **IV (Adults and Children):** 200–400 mg/kg/mo (other regimens have been used).

Idiopathic Thrombocytopenic Purpura
▪ **IV (Adults and Children):** 400 mg/kg/day for 2–5 days or 1 g/kg/day for 1–2 days (other regimens have been used).

AVAILABILITY

▪ *Injection (IM):* 2-ml, 10-ml vials ▪ *Injection (IV):* 5% solution, 0.5-g, 1-g, 2.5-g, 3-g, 6-g, 10-g vials.

*<u>Underlines</u> indicate most frequent; **CAPITALS** indicate life-threatening.

TIME/ACTION PROFILE (antibody levels)

	ONSET	PEAK	DURATION
IM	UK	2 days	UK
IV	immediate	UK	UK

NURSING IMPLICATIONS

ASSESSMENT

□ For passive immunity, determine the date of exposure to infection. Immune globulin should be administered within 2 wk of exposure to hepatitis A, within 6 days after exposure to measles, and within 7 days after exposure to hepatitis B.

□ Monitor vital signs continuously during infusion of immune globulin IV and assess patient for signs of anaphylaxis (hypotension, flushing, chest tightness, wheezing, fever, dizziness, nausea, vomiting, diaphoresis) for 1 hr following initiation of infusion. Epinephrine and antihistamines should be available for treatment of anaphylactic reactions.

□ Patients receiving repeated injections of immune globulin IM should be monitored for sensitization (fever, chills, sweating).

□ Monitor platelet counts in patients being treated for idiopathic thrombocytopenic purpura.

■ **Leukemia:** Monitor patient for signs of infection (vital signs, WBC) throughout therapy.

POTENTIAL NURSING DIAGNOSES

■ Infection, high risk for (indications).

■ Knowledge deficit related to medication regimen (patient/family teaching).

IMPLEMENTATION

■ **IM:** Administer immune globulin IM (IGIM) in adults and children into the deltoid muscle or anterolateral thigh. Volumes greater than 10 ml should be divided into several injections to minimize local pain. Avoid IM administration of doses exceeding 20 ml. Use of the gluteal site should be reserved only for volumes >3 ml or when large volumes are divided into multiple injections to prevent damage to the sciatic nerve. Do not administer SC, intradermally, or IV. Solution of IGIM should be transparent or opalescent and may be colorless or brownish in color.

■ **Intermittent Infusion:** Immune globulin IV (IGIV) should be administered by IV infusion using separate tubing. Powder and diluent should be brought to room temperature prior to reconstitution. Use transfer device provided by the manufacturer for preparation. Do not shake. Do not mix with other drugs or solutions If adverse reactions occur during infusion, decrease the rate of infusion or stop the infusion until the adverse reactions subside. The infusion may then be resumed at a rate of tolerance for the individual. Do not use turbid solution. Do not administer IGIV SC or IM.

□ *Gamimune N* should be diluted with D5W and infused at a rate of 0.01–0.02 ml/kg/min for 30 min. If no adverse reactions occur, the infusion rate may be gradually increased to a maximum of 0.08 ml/kg/hr. Solutions of *Gamimune N* should be refrigerated but not frozen. Discard solution that has been frozen.

□ *Gammagard* should be reconstituted with Sterile Water for Injection for a solution containing 50 mg protein per ml. Administer solution as soon as possible within 2 hr of reconstitution. Infuse via the administration set containing an integral airway and 15 micron filter provided by the manufacturer. Infuse at a rate of 0.5 ml/kg/hr initially. If no adverse reactions occur, the rate of infusion may be increased gradually to a maximum of 4 ml/kg/hr.

□ *Gammar-IV* should be administered initially at a rate of 0.01 ml/kg/min of the 50 mg/ml solution for 15–30 min. The rate may then be increased to 0.02 ml/kg/min. If patient does not ex-

I

perience discomfort, rate may gradually be increased to 0.03–0.06 ml/kg/min. Store at room temperature. Avoid freezing. Discard unused solution.

□ Administer the 5% solution of *Iveegam* at a rate of 1–2 ml/min. Lower doses diluted in 0.9% NaCl or D5W have been used in patients with severe immunodeficiency who have not been treated previously. Refrigerate but do not freeze.

□ *Sandoglobulin* should be reconstituted with the 0.9% NaCl provided by the manufacturer for a solution containing 30 or 60 mg of protein per ml. For patients with agammaglobulinemia or hypogammaglobulinemia, use a solution containing 30 mg/ml for the initial dose. Infuse at an initial rate of 0.5–1 ml/min. After 15–30 min, the rate may be increased to 1.5–2.5 ml/min, and subsequent infusions may be given at a rate of 2–2.5 ml/min. When infusing the solution containing 60 mg/ml, the initial rate should be 1–1.5 ml/min and increased to a maximum of 2.5 ml/min after 15–30 minutes. Solutions of *Sandoglobulin* should be stored at room temperature.

□ The 50 mg/ml solution of *Venoglobulin-I* should be administered at a rate of 0.01–0.02 ml/kg/min for 30 min. If patient does not experience discomfort, the rate may be gradually increased to 0.04 ml/kg/min. If patient tolerates higher rate, subsequent doses may be administered at the higher rate. Store at room temperature.

PATIENT/FAMILY TEACHING

□ Explain the use and purpose of immune globulin therapy to the patient.

□ Advise patient to report symptoms of anaphylaxis immediately.

□ Inform patients that pain, tenderness, and muscle stiffness at the injection site may occur following IM injections of immune globulin. These may persist for several hours following administration.

EVALUATION

Effectiveness of therapy can be demonstrated by: ▪ Prevention of certain infectious diseases by provision of passive immunity in patients exposed to the infections or patients with immunodeficiency diseases ▪ Increased platelet counts in patients with idiopathic thrombocytopenic purpura ▪ Prevention of bacterial infections in patients with hypogammaglobulinemia associated with B-cell chronic lymphocytic leukemia.

INDAPAMIDE
(in-**dap**-a-mide)
{Lozide}, Lozol

CLASSIFICATION(S):
Diuretic (thiazide-like), Antihypertensive
Pregnancy Category B

INDICATIONS

▪ Used alone or with other agents in the management of mild to moderate hypertension ▪ Used alone or with other agents in the treatment of edema associated with congestive heart failure and other causes.

ACTION

▪ Increases excretion of sodium and water by inhibiting sodium reabsorption in the distal tubule ▪ Promotes excretion of chloride, potassium, magnesium, and bicarbonate ▪ May produce arteriolar dilation. **Therapeutic Effects:** ▪ Lowering of blood pressure in hypertensive patients and diuresis with subsequent mobilization of edema.

PHARMACOKINETICS

Absorption: Well absorbed from the GI tract following oral administration.
Distribution: Widely distributed.
Metabolism and Excretion: Mostly metabolized by the liver. Small

amounts (7%) excreted unchanged by the kidneys.

Half-life: 14–18 hr.

CONTRAINDICATIONS AND PRECAUTIONS

Contraindicated in: ▪ Hypersensitivity ▪ Cross-sensitivity with sulfonamides may exist ▪ Anuria ▪ Lactation.

Use Cautiously in: ▪ Renal or severe hepatic impairment ▪ Pregnancy or children (safety not established) ▪ Elderly patients (increased sensitivity).

ADVERSE REACTIONS AND SIDE EFFECTS*

CNS: drowsiness, lethargy, dizziness.
CV: hypotension, arrhythmias.
GI: anorexia, nausea, vomiting, cramping.
Derm: rashes, photosensitivity.
Endo: hyperglycemia.
F and E: <u>hypokalemia</u>, hypochloremic alkalosis, hyponatremia, dehydration, hypovolemia.
Metab: <u>hyperuricemia</u>.
MS: muscle cramps.

INTERACTIONS

Drug–Drug: ▪ Additive hypotension with other **antihypertensives, nitrates,** or acute ingestion of **alcohol** ▪ Additive hypokalemia with **glucocorticoids, amphotericin B, mezlocillin, piperacillin,** or **ticarcillin** ▪ Decreases the excretion of **lithium;** may cause toxicity ▪ Hypokalemia may increase risk of **cardiac glycoside toxicity.**

ROUTE AND DOSAGE

Hypertension
▪ **PO (Adults):** 1.25–5 mg daily in the morning; may be increased at 4-wk intervals up to 5 mg/day.

Edema Secondary to Congestive Heart Failure
▪ **PO (Adults):** 2.5 mg daily in the morning; may be increased after 1 wk to 5 mg/day.

AVAILABILITY
▪ **Tablets:** 1.25 mg, 2.5 mg.

TIME/ACTION PROFILE
(antihypertensive effect)

	ONSET	PEAK	DURATION
PO (single dose)	UK	24 hr	UK
PO (multiple dose)	1–2 wk	8–12 wk	up to 8 wk

NURSING IMPLICATIONS

ASSESSMENT
☐ Monitor blood pressure, intake and output, and daily weight and assess feet, legs, and sacral area for edema daily.
☐ Assess patient, especially if taking cardiac glycosides, for anorexia, nausea, vomiting, muscle cramps, paresthesia, and confusion. Notify physician if these signs of electrolyte imbalance occur. Patients taking cardiac glycosides have an increased risk of digitalis toxicity due to the potassium-depleting effect of the diuretic.
☐ Assess patient for allergy to sulfonamides.
▪ **Lab Test Considerations:** Monitor electrolytes (especially potassium), blood glucose, BUN, and serum creatinine and uric acid levels prior to and periodically throughout course of therapy. May cause decreased potassium, sodium, and chloride concentrations. May increase serum glucose; diabetic patients may require increased oral hypoglycemic or insulin dosage. Increases uric acid level an average of 1.0 mg/100 ml; may precipitate an episode of gout.

POTENTIAL NURSING DIAGNOSES
▪ Fluid volume excess (indications).
▪ Fluid volume deficit (side effects).
▪ Knowledge deficit related to medication regimen (patient/family teaching).

IMPLEMENTATION
▪ **General Info:** Administer in the morning to prevent disruption of sleep cycle.

I

*<u>Underlines</u> indicate most frequent; **CAPITALS** indicate life-threatening.

□ Intermittent dose given on alternate days for 3–4 days with rest periods of 1–2 days may be used for continued control of edema.
▪ **PO:** May be given with food or milk to minimize GI irritation.

PATIENT/FAMILY TEACHING

▪ **General Info:** Instruct patient to take this medication at the same time each day. If a dose is missed, take as soon as remembered, but not just before next dose is due. Do not double doses. Advise patients using indapamide for hypertension to continue taking the medication even if feeling well. Indapamide controls but does not cure hypertension.
□ Caution patient to make position changes slowly to minimize orthostatic hypotension. This may be potentiated by alcohol.
□ Advise patient to use sunscreen (avoid those containing PABA) and protective clothing when in the sun to prevent photosensitivity reactions.
□ Instruct patient to follow a diet high in potassium (see Appendix K).
□ Advise patient to report muscle weakness, cramps, nausea, or dizziness to physician.
□ Advise patient to consult physician or pharmacist before taking over-the-counter medication concurrently with this therapy.
□ Emphasize the importance of routine follow-up examinations.
▪ **Hypertension:** Instruct patient and family on proper technique of blood pressure monitoring. Advise them to check blood pressure at least weekly and to report significant changes to physician.
□ Encourage patient to comply with additional interventions for hypertension (weight reduction, low-sodium diet, regular exercise, smoking cessation, moderation of alcohol consumption, and stress management).

EVALUATION

Effectiveness of therapy can be demonstrated by: ▪ Control of hypertension ▪ Decrease in edema secondary to congestive heart failure.

INDOMETHACIN
(in-doe-**meth**-a-sin')
{Apo-Indomethacin}, Indameth, {Indocid}, Indocin, Indocin I.V., {Indocin PDA}, Indocin SR, {Novomethacin}

CLASSIFICATION(S):
Nonsteroidal anti-inflammatory agent
Pregnancy Category UK

INDICATIONS
▪ **PO, Rect:** Management of inflammatory disorders including: □ Rheumatoid arthritis □ Gouty arthritis □ Osteoarthritis ▪ **IV:** Alternative to surgery in the management of patent ductus arteriosus in premature neonates.

ACTION
▪ Inhibits prostaglandin synthesis. **Therapeutic Effects:** ▪ **PO:** Suppression of pain and inflammation ▪ **IV:** Closure of patent ductus arteriosus.

PHARMACOKINETICS
Absorption: Well absorbed from the GI tract.
Distribution: Crosses the blood–brain barrier and the placenta. Enters breast milk.
Metabolism and Excretion: Mostly metabolized by the liver.
Half-life: 2.6–11 hr (prolonged in neonates—up to 60 hr, average range 12–21 hr).

CONTRAINDICATIONS AND PRECAUTIONS
Contraindicated in: ▪ Hypersensitivity ▪ Known alcohol intolerance (suspension) ▪ Cross-sensitivity may exist with other nonsteroidal anti-inflammatory agents, including aspirin ▪ Active GI bleeding ▪ Ulcer disease ▪ Proctitis or a recent history of rectal bleeding.

{} = Available in Canada only.

Use Cautiously in: ▪ Severe cardiovascular, renal, or hepatic disease ▪ History of ulcer disease ▪ Pregnancy or lactation.

ADVERSE REACTIONS AND SIDE EFFECTS*

CNS: <u>headache</u>, <u>drowsiness</u>, <u>psychic disturbances</u>, <u>dizziness</u>.
CV: edema, arrhythmias.
Derm: rashes.
EENT: blurred vision, tinnitus.
F and E: hyperkalemia.
GI: PO—<u>nausea</u>, <u>dyspepsia</u>, <u>vomiting</u>, <u>constipation</u>, GI BLEEDING, discomfort, HEPATITIS; Rect—rectal irritation, tenesmus.
GU: renal failure, hematuria, cystitis.
Hemat: blood dyscrasias, prolonged bleeding time.
Local: phlebitis at IV site (IV only).
Misc: allergic reactions, including ANAPHYLAXIS.

INTERACTIONS

Drug–Drug: ▪ Concurrent use with **aspirin** may decrease effectiveness ▪ Additive adverse GI effects with **aspirin**, other **nonsteroidal anti-inflammatory agents, potassium supplements, glucocorticoids,** or **alcohol** ▪ Chronic use with **acetaminophen** may increase the risk of adverse renal reactions ▪ May decrease the effectiveness of **diuretics** or **antihypertensive** therapy ▪ May increase hypoglycemia from **insulin** or **oral hypoglycemia agents** ▪ May increase serum levels and risk of toxicity from **lithium** or **zidovudine** (concurrent use with zidovudine should be avoided) ▪ Increases the risk of toxicity from **methotrexate** ▪ **Probenecid** increases risk of toxicity from indomethacin ▪ Increased risk of bleeding with **cefamandole, cefotetan, cefoperazone, valproic acid** or **plicamycin, thrombolytic agents,** or **anticoagulants** ▪ Increased risk of adverse hematologic reactions with **antineoplastic agents** or **radiation therapy** ▪ Increased risk of nephrotoxicity with **cyclosporine.**

ROUTE AND DOSAGE

Anti-Inflammatory
▪ **PO, Rect (Adults):** 25–50 mg 2–4 times daily or 75 mg extended-release capsule once or twice daily (not to exceed 200 mg or 150 mg of SR/day). For gout, initial PO dose of 100 mg may be used. For arthritis, up to 100 mg PO given at bedtime.
▪ **PO, Rect (Children):** 1.5–2.5 mg/kg/day in 3–4 divided doses (not to exceed 4 mg/kg/day or 150–200 mg/day).

Closure of Patent Ductus Arteriosus
▪ **IV, PO (Neonates):** 0.2 mg/kg initially, then 2 subsequent doses at 12–24 hr intervals of 0.1 mg/kg if age <48 hr at time of inital dose, 0.2 mg/kg if 2–7 days at initial dose, 0.25 mg/kg if >7 days at initial dose.

AVAILABILITY

▪ *Capsules:* 25 mg, 50 mg ▪ *Sustained-release capsules:* 75 mg ▪ *Suppositories:* ▪ 50 mg ▪ *Oral suspension:* 25 mg/5 ml ▪ *Injection:* 1-mg vials.

TIME/ACTION PROFILE

	ONSET	PEAK	DURATION
PO (analgesic)	30 min	0.5–2 hr	4–6 hr
PO-ER (analgesic)	30 min	UK	4–6 hr
PO (anti-inflammatory)	up to 7 days	1–2 wk	UK
PO-ER (anti-inflammatory)	up to 7 days	1–2 wk	UK
IV (closure of PDA)	up to 48 hr	UK	UK

NURSING IMPLICATIONS

ASSESSMENT
▪ **General Info:** Patients who have asthma, aspirin-induced allergy, and nasal polyps are at increased risk for developing hypersensitivity reactions. Monitor for rhinitis, asthma, and urticaria.
▪ **Arthritis:** Assess limitation of move-

I

---

*<u>Underlines</u> indicate most frequent; **CAPITALS** indicate life-threatening.

ment and pain—note type, location, and intensity prior to and 1–2 hr following administration.

- **Patent Ductus Arteriosus:** Monitor respiratory status and heart sounds routinely throughout therapy.
- ▢ Monitor intake and output. Fluid restriction is usually instituted throughout therapy.
- **Lab Test Considerations:** BUN, serum creatinine, CBC, serum potassium levels, and liver function tests should be evaluated periodically in patients receiving prolonged courses of therapy.
- ▢ Serum potassium, BUN, serum creatinine, AST (SGOT), and ALT (SGPT) tests may show increased levels. Blood glucose concentrations may be altered.
- ▢ Urine glucose and urine protein concentrations may be increased. May cause decreased creatinine clearance; serum sodium concentrations; urine chloride, potassium, and sodium concentrations; urine osmolality; and urine volume.
- ▢ Leukocyte and platelet count may be decreased. Bleeding time may be prolonged for 1 day after discontinuation.

POTENTIAL NURSING DIAGNOSES

- Pain (indications).
- Physical mobility, impaired (indications).
- Knowledge deficit related to medication regimen (patient/family teaching).

IMPLEMENTATION

- **PO:** Administer after meals or with food or administer antacids to decrease GI irritation. Do not crush, break, or chew sustained-release capsules.
- ▢ Shake suspension prior to administration. Do not mix with antacid or any other liquid.
- **Direct IV:** Reconstitute with 1 or 2 ml of preservative-free 0.9% NaCl or preservative-free sterile water for a concentration of 0.1 mg/ml or 0.05

mg/ml, respectively. Reconstitute immediately prior to use and discard any unused solution. Do not dilute further or admix.

- **_Rate:_** Administer over 5–10 sec. Avoid extravasation, as solution is irritating to tissues.
- **Rect:** Encourage patient to retain suppository for 1 hr following administration.

PATIENT/FAMILY TEACHING

- **General Info:** Advise patient to take this medication with a full glass of water and to remain in an upright position for 15–30 min after administration.
- ▢ Instruct patient to take medication exactly as directed. Missed doses should be taken as soon as remembered if not almost time for next dose. Do not double doses.
- ▢ May cause drowsiness or dizziness. Advise patient to avoid driving or other activities requiring alertness until response to medication is known.
- ▢ Caution patient to avoid the concurrent use of alcohol, aspirin, ibuprofen, acetaminophen, or other over-the-counter medications without consulting physician or pharmacist.
- ▢ Instruct patient to notify physician if rash, itching, chills, fever, muscle aches, visual disturbances, weight gain, edema, abdominal pain, black stools, or persistent headache occur.
- ▢ Advise patient to inform physician or dentist of medication regimen prior to treatment or surgery.
- **Patent Ductus Arteriosus:** Explain to parents the purpose of medication and the need for frequent monitoring.

EVALUATION

Effectiveness of therapy can be demonstrated by: ▪ Decrease in severity of moderate pain ▢ Improved joint mobility. Partial arthritic relief is usually seen within 2 wk, but maximum effectiveness may require up to 1 mo of continuous therapy ▪ Successful closure of patent ductus arteriosus.

INSULIN
(in-su-lin)

Rapid-acting Insulins
regular (Actrapid, Humulin R, Iletin I, Iletin II, Iletin II U-500 [concentrated], Novolin R, Velosulin)
prompt zinc suspension (Semilente, Semilente Iletin, Semitard)

Intermediate-acting Insulins
isophane suspension (Humulin N, Iletin II, Insultard NPH, Lentard, Novolin N, NPH, NPH Purified)
zinc suspension (Humulin L, Lente, Lente Iletin, Monotard, Novolin L)

Long-acting Insulins
extended zinc suspension (Humulin U, Ultralente, Ultralente Iletin, Ultratard)

Insulin Mixture
regular plus NPH (Humulin 70/30, Mixtard 70/30, Novolin 70/30)

CLASSIFICATION(S):
Hormone (pancreatic)
Pregnancy Category UK

INDICATIONS

■ Treatment of insulin-dependent diabetes mellitus (IDDM, type I) ■ Management of noninsulin-dependent diabetes mellitus (NIDDM, type II) unresponsive to treatment with diet and/or oral hypoglycemic agents ■ Concentrated insulin U-500 is only for use in patients with insulin requirements >200 units/day.

ACTION

■ Lowers blood glucose by increasing transport into cells and promoting the conversion of glucose to glycogen ■ Promotes the conversion of amino acids to proteins in muscle and stimulates triglyceride formation ■ Inhibits the release of free fatty acids ■ Sources include beef, pork, beef/pork combinations, semisynthetic, and human insulin prepared by recombinant DNA technology. **Therapeutic Effect:** ■ Control of blood sugar in diabetic patients.

PHARMACOKINETICS

Absorption: Rapidly absorbed from SC administration sites. Absorption rate is determined by type of insulin, injection site, volume of injectate, and other factors.

Distribution: Widely distributed.

Metabolism and Excretion: Metabolized by liver, kidney, and muscle.

Half-life: 9 min (prolonged in diabetics).

CONTRAINDICATIONS AND PRECAUTIONS

Contraindicated in: ■ Allergy or hypersensitivity to a particular type of insulin, preservatives, or other additives.

Use Cautiously in: ■ Stress, pregnancy, and infection (temporarily increase insulin requirements).

ADVERSE REACTIONS AND SIDE EFFECTS*

Derm: urticaria.

Endo: HYPOGLYCEMIA, rebound hyperglycemia (Somogyi effect).

Local: lipodystrophy, lipohypertrophy, itching, swelling, redness.

Misc: allergic reactions, including ANAPHYLAXIS.

INTERACTIONS

Drug–Drug: ■ **Beta-adrenergic blocking agents** may block some of the signs and symptoms of hypoglycemia and delay recovery from hypoglycemia ■ **Thiazide diuretics, glucocorticoids, diltiazem, dobutamine, thyroid preparations, estrogens, smoking,** and **rifampin** may increase insulin requirements ■ **Anabolic steroids (testosterone), alcohol, clofibrate, guanethidine, MAO inhibitors,** most **NSAIAs, fenfluramine, sulfinpyrazone, tetracyclines, phenylbutazone,** and **oral anticoagulants** may decrease insulin requirements.

I

*Underlines indicate most frequent; CAPITALS indicate life-threatening.

ROUTE AND DOSAGE
Dose depends on blood sugar, response, and many other factors.

Ketoacidosis—Regular Insulin Only
- **IV (Adults):** 0.1 unit/kg/hr as a continuous infusion.
- **IV (Children):** Individualized on the basis of patient's size.

Maintenance Therapy
- **SC (Adults and Children):** 0.5–1 unit/kg/day.
- **SC (Adolescents During Rapid Growth):** 0.8–1.2 units/kg/day.

AVAILABILITY
- *Insulin injection:* 100 units/ml, 400 units/ml, 500 units/ml.

TIME/ACTION PROFILE
(hypoglycemic effect)

	ONSET	PEAK	DURATION
regular IV	10–30 min	15–30 min	30–60 min
regular SC	0.5–1 hr	2–4 hr	5–7 hr
Semilente SC	1–3 hr	2–8 hr	12–16 hr
NPH SC	1–4 hr	6–12 hr	18–28 hr
Lente SC	1–3 hr	8–12 hr	18–28 hr
Ultralente SC	4–6 hr	18–24 hr	36 hr

NURSING IMPLICATIONS

ASSESSMENT
- Assess patient for signs and symptoms of hypoglycemia (anxiety, chills, cold sweats, confusion, cool pale skin, difficulty in concentration, drowsiness, excessive hunger, headache, irritability, nausea, nervousness, rapid pulse, shakiness, unusual tiredness or weakness) and hyperglycemia (drowsiness, flushed dry skin, fruit-like breath odor, frequent urination, loss of appetite, tiredness, unusual thirst) periodically throughout therapy.
- Monitor body weight periodically. Changes in weight may necessitate changes in insulin dosage.
- **Lab Test Considerations:** May cause decreased serum inorganic phosphate, magnesium, and potassium levels.

- Monitor blood glucose or urine glucose and ketones every 6 hr throughout course of therapy, more frequently in ketoacidosis and times of stress. Glycosylated hemoglobin may also be monitored to determine effectiveness of therapy.
- **Toxicity and Overdose:** Overdose is manifested by symptoms of hypoglycemia. Mild hypoglycemia may be treated by ingestion of oral glucose. Severe hypoglycemia is a life-threatening emergency; treatment consists of IV glucose, glucagon, or epinephrine.

POTENTIAL NURSING DIAGNOSES
- Knowledge deficit related to medication regimen (patient/family teaching).
- Noncompliance (patient/family teaching).

IMPLEMENTATION
- **General Info:** Available in different types and strengths and from different species. Check type, species source, dose, and expiration date with another licensed nurse. Do not interchange insulins without physician's order.
- Use *only* insulin syringes to draw up dose. The unit markings on the insulin syringe must match the insulin's units/ml. Special syringes for doses <50 units are available. Prior to withdrawing dose, rotate vial between palms to ensure uniform solution; do not shake.
- When mixing insulins, draw regular insulin into syringe first to avoid contamination of regular insulin vial.
- Insulin should be stored in a cool place but does not need to be refrigerated.
- **IV:** Regular insulin is the ONLY insulin that can be administered IV. Do not use if cloudy, discolored, or unusually viscous.
- Regular insulin U-500 is not intended for IV route.
- **Direct IV:** May be administered IV undiluted directly into vein or through Y-site injection or 3-way stopcock.

- **Rate:** Administer up to 50 units over 1 min.
- **Continuous Infusion:** May be diluted in commonly used IV solutions as an infusion; however, insulin potency may be reduced by at least 20–80% by the plastic or glass container or tubing before reaching the venous system.
- **Rate:** When administered as an infusion, rate should be ordered by physician, and infusion should be placed on an IV pump for accurate administration.
- Rate of administration should be decreased when serum glucose level reaches 250 mg/100 ml.
- **Y-Site Compatibility:** ▪ ampicillin ▪ ampicillin/sulbactam ▪ aztreonam ▪ cefazolin ▪ cefotetan ▪ dobutamine ▪ famotidine ▪ gentamicin ▪ heparin ▪ imipenem/cilastatin ▪ magnesium sulfate ▪ meperidine ▪ morphine ▪ oxytocin ▪ pentobarbital ▪ potassium chloride ▪ ritodrine ▪ sodium bicarbonate ▪ terbutalin ▪ ticarcillin ▪ ticarcillin/clavulonate ▪ tobramycin ▪ vancomycin ▪ vitamin B complex with C.
- **Additive Compatibility:** May be added to TPN solutions.

PATIENT/FAMILY TEACHING

- Instruct patient on proper technique for administration. Include type of insulin, equipment (syringe, cartridge pens, alcohol swabs), storage, and where to discard syringes. Discuss the importance of not changing brands of insulin or syringes, selection and rotation of injection sites, and compliance with therapeutic regimen.
- Demonstrate technique for mixing insulins by drawing up regular insulin first and rolling intermediate-acting insulin vial between palms to mix, rather than shaking (may cause inaccurate dose).
- Explain to patient that this medication controls hyperglycemia but does not cure diabetes. Therapy is long-term.
- Instruct patient in proper testing of serum glucose or urine glucose and

ketones. Stress the importance of double-voided specimens for accuracy. These tests should be closely monitored during periods of stress or illness and physician notified if significant changes occur.

- Emphasize the importance of compliance with diabetic diet and exchange system for meals and regular exercise as directed by physician.
- Advise patient to consult physician or pharmacist prior to using alcohol or other medications concurrently with insulin.
- Advise patient to notify physician or dentist of medication regimen prior to treatment or surgery.
- Advise patient to notify physician if nausea, vomiting, or fever develops, if unable to eat regular diet, or if blood sugar levels are not controlled.
- Instruct patient on signs and symptoms of hypoglycemia and hyperglycemia and what to do if they occur.
- Advise patient to notify physician if pregnancy is planned or suspected.
- Patients with diabetes mellitus should carry a source of sugar (candy, sugar packets) and identification describing their disease and treatment regimen at all times.

EVALUATION
Effectiveness of therapy can be demonstrated by: ▪ Control of blood glucose levels without the appearance of hypoglycemic or hyperglycemic episodes.

I

INTERFERON ALFA-2a
(in-ter-**feer**-on)
Roferon-A

CLASSIFICATION(S):
Antineoplastic (miscellaneous)
Pregnancy Category C

INDICATIONS

- Treatment of hairy cell leukemia
- Treatment of AIDS-associated Kaposi's sarcoma.

ACTION

- A protein produced by recombinant DNA techniques that modulates the immune response and has an antiproliferative action against tumor cells
- Antiviral activity. **Therapeutic Effects:**
- Antineoplastic and antiproliferative activity.

PHARMACOKINETICS

Absorption: Not absorbed orally. Well absorbed (>80%) following IM and SC administration.
Distribution: Distribution not known.
Metabolism and Excretion: Filtered by the kidneys and subsequently degraded in the renal tubule.
Half-life: 3.7–8.5 hr.

CONTRAINDICATIONS AND PRECAUTIONS

Contraindicated in: ▪ Hypersensitivity to interferon alfa-2a, human serum albumin, or phenol ▪ Pregnancy.
Use Cautiously in: ▪ Severe cardiovascular, renal, or hepatic disease ▪ Active infections ▪ Decreased bone marrow reserve ▪ Previous or concurrent radiation therapy ▪ Other debilitating illnesses ▪ Patients with childbearing potential ▪ Lactation and children <18 yr (safety not established).

ADVERSE REACTIONS AND SIDE EFFECTS*

Most reactions are dose-dependent.
CNS: fatigue, depression, decreased mental status, sleep disturbances, SEIZURES, nervousness, confusion, gait disturbances, coordination difficulties, speech difficulties.
EENT: conjunctivitis.
Resp: bronchospasm.
CV: hypotension, edema, hypertension, chest pain, arrhythmias, palpitations.
GI: nausea, anorexia, diarrhea, vomiting, abdominal fullness, hypermotility, hepatitis, dry mouth, altered taste.
GU: impotence, gonadal suppression.
Derm: rash, pruritus, alopecia, sweating, dry skin.

Hemat: anemia, leukopenia, thrombocytopenia.
MS: myalgia.
Neuro: paresthesia, numbness, peripheral neuropathy.
Misc: flu-like syndrome, fever, chills, weight loss.

INTERACTIONS

Drug–Drug: ▪ Additive myelosuppression with other **antineoplastic agents** or **radiation therapy** ▪ May decrease metabolism and increase blood levels and toxicity of **aminophylline**.

ROUTE AND DOSAGE

Hairy Cell Leukemia

- **IM, SC (Adults):** 3 million IU/day for 16–24 wk. If severe adverse reactions occur, reduce dosage by 50%. Maintenance dose 3 million IU 3 times weekly.

Kaposi's Sarcoma

- **IM, SC (Adults):** 36 million IU/day for 10–12 wk or 3 million IU/day for 3 days, then 9 million IU/day for next 3 days, then 18 million IU/day for next 3 days, then 36 million IU/day for rest of 10–12 wk course. If severe adverse reactions occur, reduce dosage by 50%. Maintenance dose 36 million IU 3 times weekly.

AVAILABILITY

- *Injection:* 3 million IU/ml, 6 million IU/ml, 36 million IU/ml.

TIME/ACTION PROFILE

	ONSET	PEAK	DURATION
IM, SC (effects on blood counts)	UK	17–19 days	several wk
IM, SC (clinical response)	1–3 mo	UK	UK

NURSING IMPLICATIONS

ASSESSMENT

- **General Info:** Monitor vital signs prior to and periodically throughout course of therapy. Hypotension may occur up to 2 days after therapy.

□ Assess patient for development of flu-like syndrome (fever, chills, myalgia, headache). Symptoms often appear suddenly 3–6 hr after therapy. Symptoms tend to decrease, even with continued therapy. Confer with physician regarding acetaminophen for control of these symptoms.

□ Monitor cardiac status, especially in patients with underlying cardiac disease or advanced malignancy. Assess heart sounds and chest pain, auscultate lung sounds for rales/crackles, and assess for edema. Physician may order periodic ECGs.

□ Assess for fever, sore throat, and signs of infection. Notify physician if these symptoms occur.

□ Assess for bleeding (bleeding gums; bruising; petechiae; guaiac stools, urine, and emesis). Avoid other IM injections and rectal temperatures. Hold pressure on venipuncture sites for at least 10 min.

□ May cause nausea and vomiting. Confer with physician regarding prophylactic use of an antiemetic. Monitor intake and output, daily weight, and appetite. Adjust diet as tolerated for anorexia. Encourage fluid intake of at least 2 liters/day.

□ Monitor neurologic status throughout course of therapy. Notify physician if confusion, decreased coordination, dizziness, gait disturbances, paresthesia, difficulty with speech, or psychological disturbances occur.

■ **Kaposi's Sarcoma:** Monitor number, size, and character of lesions prior to and throughout therapy.

■ **Lab Test Considerations:** Monitor CBC and differential prior to and periodically throughout course of therapy. May cause leukopenia, neutropenia, thrombocytopenia, and decreased hemoglobin and hematocrit. The nadir of leukopenia occurs in 22–38 days and the nadir of thrombocytopenia in 17–19 days. Recovery of leukopenia and thrombocytopenia occur

a few weeks after withdrawal of interferon alfa-2a.

□ Monitor liver function tests (AST [SGOT], ALT [SGPT], LDH, bilirubin) and renal function tests (BUN, creatinine, urinalysis) prior to and periodically throughout therapy.

□ May cause increased uric acid; monitor levels periodically during therapy.

■ **Hairy Cell Leukemia:** Monitor number of peripheral blood hairy cells and bone marrow hairy cells prior to and during therapy.

POTENTIAL NURSING DIAGNOSES
■ Injury, high risk for (side effects).
■ Infection, high risk for (side effects).
■ Knowledge deficit related to medication regimen (patient/family teaching).

IMPLEMENTATION
■ **General Info:** Solution should be prepared in a biologic cabinet. Wear gloves, gown, and mask while handling medication. Discard equipment in specially designated containers (see Appendix I).

□ The 36 million IU/ml vial is for use in patients with AIDS-related Kaposi's sarcoma and should not be used for hairy cell leukemia.

■ **SC/IM:** SC route is preferred for patients with a platelet count <50,000/mm^3.

□ Interferon alfa-2a is available in solution or as a powder requiring reconstitution. Reconstitute the 18-million-IU vial with 3 ml of diluent provided. Refrigerate after reconstitution and use within 30 days.

PATIENT/FAMILY TEACHING
□ Advise patient to take medication exactly as directed. If a dose is missed, omit dose and return to the regular schedule. The patient should notify the physician if more than 1 dose is missed.

■ **Home Care Issues:** Instruct patient and family on preparation and correct technique for administration of injection and care and disposal of equipment. Explain to patient that brands should not be switched without physician's approval, as this may result in a change of dosage.

□ Discuss possibility of flu-like reaction 3–6 hr after dose. Physician may recommend that patient take acetaminophen prior to injection and every 3–4 hr afterward as needed to control symptoms.

□ Review side effects with patient. Physician may temporarily discontinue interferon or decrease dose by 50% if serious side effects occur.

□ Advise patient to notify physician if fever, chills, sore throat, signs of infection, bleeding gums, bruising, petechiae, or blood in urine, stool, or emesis occurs. Caution patient to avoid crowds and persons with known infections. Instruct patient to use soft toothbrush, avoid flossing, and use electric razor. Caution patient not to drink alcoholic beverages or take products containing aspirin or ibuprofen. Caution patient against use of CNS depressants concurrently with this medication.

□ Discuss with patient the possibility of hair loss. Explore coping strategies.

□ Explain to patient that fertility may be impaired and that contraception is needed throughout course of treatment to prevent potential harm to the fetus.

□ Instruct patient not to receive any vaccinations without advice of physician.

□ Emphasize need for periodic lab tests to monitor for side effects.

EVALUATION

Effectiveness of therapy can be demonstrated by: ■ Normalized blood parameters (hemoglobin, neutrophils, platelets, monocytes, and bone marrow and peripheral hairy cells) in hairy cell leukemia. Response may not be seen for 1–3 mo ■ Decrease in the size and number of lesions in Kaposi's sarcoma. Six months of therapy may be required before full response is seen. Therapy is discontinued when there is no further clinical improvement and parameters have stabilized for 3 mo.

INTERFERON ALFA-2b
(in-ter-**feer**-on)
a-2-interferon, Intron A

CLASSIFICATION(S):
Antineoplastic (miscellaneous)
Pregnancy Category C

INDICATIONS

■ Treatment of hairy cell leukemia ■ Treatment of AIDS-associated Kaposi's sarcoma ■ Treatment of condylomata acuminata (intralesional) ■ Treatment of chronic hepatitis non-A, non-B/C ■ Treatment of chronic hepatitis B.

ACTION

■ A protein produced by recombinant DNA techniques that modulates the immune response and has an antiproliferative action against tumor cells ■ Antiviral activity. **Therapeutic Effects:** ■ Antineoplastic and antiproliferative activity ■ Improvement in liver function in patients with chronic hepatitis non-A, non-B/C.

PHARMACOKINETICS

Absorption: Not absorbed orally. Well absorbed (>80%) following IM and SC administration.
Distribution: Distribution not known.
Metabolism and Excretion: Filtered by the kidneys and subsequently degraded in the renal tubule.
Half-life: 2–3 hr.

CONTRAINDICATIONS AND PRECAUTIONS

Contraindicated in: ■ Hypersensitivity to interferon alfa-2b, human serum albumin ■ Pregnancy.
Use Cautiously in: ■ Severe cardiovascular, renal, or hepatic disease ■ Active infections ■ Decreased bone marrow reserve (dosage reduction required) ■ Previous or concurrent radiation therapy ■ Other debilitating illnesses ■ Patients with childbearing potential ■ Lactation and children <18 yr (safety not established) ■ Any adverse reaction (decrease dose by 50%).

ADVERSE REACTIONS AND SIDE EFFECTS*

CNS: fatigue, depression, decreased mental status, sleep, seizures, disturbances, nervousness, gait disturbances, coordination difficulties, speech difficulties.
EENT: conjunctivitis.
Resp: bronchospasm.
CV: hypotension, edema, hypertension, chest pain, arrhythmias, palpitations.
GI: nausea, anorexia, diarrhea, vomiting, abdominal fullness, hypermotility, hepatitis, dry mouth, altered taste.
GU: impotence, gonadal suppression.
Derm: rash, pruritus, alopecia, sweating.
Hemat: anemia, leukopenia, thrombocytopenia.
MS: myalgia.
Neuro: paresthesia, numbness.
Misc: flu-like syndrome, fever, chills, weight loss.

INTERACTIONS

Drug–Drug: ▪ Additive myelosuppression with other **antineoplastic agents** or **radiation therapy** ▪ May decrease metabolism and increase blood levels and toxicity of **aminophylline** ▪ Increases the risk of neutropenia associated with **zidovudine** therapy.

ROUTE AND DOSAGE

Hairy Cell Leukemia
▪ **IM, SC (Adults):** 2 million IU/m² 3 times weekly.

Kaposi's Sarcoma
▪ **IM, SC (Adults):** 30 million IU/m² 3 times weekly.

Condylomata Acuminata
▪ **Intralesional (Adults):** 1 million IU/lesion 3 times weekly for 3 wk, treat only 5 lesions per course.

Chronic Hepatitis Non-A/Non-B/C
▪ **IM, SC (Adults):** 3 million IU 3 times weekly.

Chronic Hepatitis B
▪ **IM, SC (Adults):** 5 million IU/day or 10 million IU 3 times weekly.

AVAILABILITY

▪ *Injection:* 3 million units, 5 million units, 10 million units, 18 million units, 25 million units, 50 million units per vial.

TIME/ACTION PROFILE
(IM, SC-CR = clinical response,
IM, SC-BC = effects on platelet counts,
IM, SC-LFT = effects on liver function in patients with hepatitis.
Intralesional = regression of lesions)

	ONSET	PEAK	DURATION
IM, SC-CR	1–3 mo	UK	UK
IM, SC-BC	UK	3–5 days	3–5 days
IM, SC-LFT	2 wk	UK	UK
Intralesional	UK	4–8 wk	UK

NURSING IMPLICATIONS

ASSESSMENT
▪ **General Info:** Monitor vital signs prior to and periodically throughout course of therapy. Hypotension may occur up to 2 days after therapy.
▫ Assess patient for development of flu-like syndrome (fever, chills, myalgia, headache). Symptoms often appear suddenly 3–6 hr after therapy. Symptoms tend to decrease, even with continued therapy. Confer with physician regarding acetaminophen for control of these symptoms.
▫ Monitor cardiac status, especially in patients with underlying cardiac disease or advanced malignancy. Assess heart sounds and chest pain, auscultate lung sounds for rales/crackles, and assess for edema. Physician may order periodic ECGs.
▫ Assess for fever, sore throat, and signs of infection. Notify physician if these symptoms occur.
▫ Assess for bleeding (bleeding gums; bruising; petechiae; guaiac stools, urine, and emesis). Avoid other IM injections and rectal temperatures. Hold pressure on venipuncture sites for at least 10 min.
▫ May cause nausea and vomiting. Confer with physician regarding prophy-

I

*Underlines indicate most frequent; CAPITALS indicate life-threatening.

lactic use of an antiemetic. Monitor intake and output, daily weight, and appetite. Adjust diet as tolerated for anorexia. Encourage fluid intake of at least 2 liters/day.

☐ Monitor neurologic status throughout course of therapy. Notify physician if confusion, decreased coordination, dizziness, gait disturbances, paresthesia, difficulty with speech, or psychologic disturbances occur.

■ **Kaposi's Sarcoma:** Monitor number, size, and character of lesions prior to and throughout therapy.

■ **Lab Test Considerations:** Monitor CBC and differential prior to and periodically throughout course of therapy. May cause leukopenia, neutropenia, thrombocytopenia, and decreased hemoglobin and hematocrit. The nadirs of leukopenia and thrombocytopenia occur in 3–5 days, with recovery 3–5 days after withdrawal of interferon alfa-2b. If granulocyte count <750 mm³ or platelet count <50,000/mm³, reduce interferon alfa-2b dose by 50%. If granulocyte count <500/mm³ or platelet count <30,000/mm³, discontinue interferon alfa-2b until platelet or granulocyte counts return to normal or baseline levels, then reinstitute at up to 100% of dose.

☐ Monitor liver function tests (AST [SGOT], ALT [SGPT], LDH, bilirubin) and renal function tests (BUN, creatinine, urinalysis) prior to and periodically throughout therapy.

☐ May cause increased uric acid; monitor levels periodically during therapy.

■ **Intralesional Route:** Monitor CBC and liver function tests. May cause mild to moderate leukopenia and elevated AST (SGOT).

POTENTIAL NURSING DIAGNOSES

■ Injury, high risk for (side effects).
■ Infection, high risk for (side effects).
■ Knowledge deficit related to medication regimen (patient/family teaching).

IMPLEMENTATION

■ **General Info:** Solution should be prepared in a biologic cabinet. Wear gloves, gown, and mask while handling medication. Discard equipment in specially designated containers (see Appendix I).

■ **SC/IM:** SC route is preferred for patients with a platelet count <50,000/mm³.

☐ Reconstitute 3-, 5-, and 50-million-IU vials with 1 ml, 10-million-IU dose with 2 ml, 18-million-IU vial with 3.8 ml, and 25-million-IU vial with 5 ml of diluent provided by manufacturer (Bacteriostatic Water for Injection). Agitate gently. Solution may be colorless to light yellow. Refrigerate after reconstitution. Stable for 1 mo.

■ **Intralesional:** Reconstitute 10-million-IU vial with 1 ml of Bacteriostatic Water for Injection. Use a TB syringe with 25–30-gauge needle to administer. Each 0.1-ml dose is injected into the center of the base of the wart using the intradermal injection approach. As many as 5 lesions can be treated at one time.

PATIENT/FAMILY TEACHING

☐ Advise patient to take medication exactly as directed. If a dose is missed, skip the next dose and return to the regular schedule. The patient should notify the physician if more than 1 dose is missed.

■ **Home Care Issues:** Instruct patient and family on preparation and correct technique for administration of injection and care and disposal of equipment. Explain to patient that brands should not be switched without physician's approval, as this may result in a change of dosage.

☐ Discuss possibility of flu-like reaction 3–6 hr after dose. Physician may recommend that patient take acetaminophen prior to injection and every 3–4 hr afterward as needed to control symptoms.

☐ Review side effects with patient. Physician may temporarily discontinue interferon or decrease dose by 50% if serious side effects occur.

☐ Advise patient to notify physician if fever, chills, sore throat, signs of infection, bleeding gums, bruising, petechiae, or blood in urine, stool, or emesis occurs. Caution patient to avoid crowds and persons with known infections. Instruct patient to use soft toothbrush, avoid flossing, and use electric razor. Caution patient not to drink alcoholic beverages or take products containing aspirin or ibuprofen. Caution patient against use of CNS depressants concurrently with this medication.

□ Caution patients to use sunscreen and protective clothing to prevent photosensitivity reactions.

□ Discuss with patient the possibility of hair loss. Explore coping strategies.

□ Explain to patient that fertility may be impaired and that contraception is needed throughout course of treatment to prevent potential harm to the fetus.

□ Instruct patient not to receive any vaccinations without advice of physician.

□ Emphasize need for periodic lab tests to monitor for side effects.

EVALUATION
Effectiveness of therapy can be demonstrated by: ■ Normalized blood parameters (hemoglobin, neutrophils, platelets, monocytes, and bone marrow and peripheral hairy cells) in hairy cell leukemia. Six months or more of therapy may be required before full response is seen ■ Decrease in the size and number of lesions in Kaposi's sarcoma ■ Disappearance of or decrease in size and number of genital warts. Condylomata acuminata usually respond in 4–8 wk. The course of therapy may need to be extended to 16 wk; a second course may be required if genital warts persist and laboratory values remain in acceptable limits.

INTERFERON BETA-1b
(in-ter-**feer**-on)
Betaseron

CLASSIFICATION(S):
Immune modifier
Pregnancy Category C

INDICATIONS
■ Management of relapsing-remitting multiple sclerosis in ambulatory patients.

ACTION
■ Has antiviral and immunoregulatory properties produced by interacting with specific receptor sites on cell surfaces ■ Produced by recombinant DNA technology. **Therapeutic Effect:** ■ Reduced incidence of relapse (neurologic dysfunction) in patients with multiple sclerosis.

PHARMACOKINETICS
Absorption: 50% absorbed following SC administration.
Distribution: Distribution not known.
Metabolism and Excretion: Metabolism and excretion are not known.
Half-life: 8 min–4.3 hr.

CONTRAINDICATIONS AND PRECAUTIONS
Contraindicated in: ■ Hypersensitivity to natural or recombinant interferon beta or human albumin.
Use Cautiously in: ■ Patients with a history of suicide or depression ■ Patients with childbearing potential ■ Pregnancy, lactation, or children <18 yr (safety not established).

ADVERSE REACTIONS AND SIDE EFFECTS*
CNS: depression, suicidal ideation, confusion, anxiety, emotional lability, depersonalization, somnolence.
EENT: laryngitis.
Resp: dyspnea.
CV: palpitations, hypertension, peripheral vascular disorders.
GI: GI disorders, elevated liver function studies.
GU: cystitis, pelvic pain.

*Underlines indicate most frequent; CAPITALS indicate life-threatening.

Endo: <u>menstrual disorders</u>, spontaneous abortion, breast pain, menorrhagia.
Hemat: <u>neutropenia</u>.
Local: <u>injection-site reactions</u>, injection-site necrosis.
Misc: <u>flu-like symptoms</u>.

INTERACTIONS
Drug–Drug: ▪ None known.

ROUTE AND DOSAGE
▪ **SC (Adults):** 0.25 mg (8 million IU) every other day.

AVAILABILITY
▪ *Injection:* 0.3 mg (9.6 million IU)/vial.

TIME/ACTION PROFILE (serum interferon levels)

	ONSET	PEAK	DURATION
SC	Rapid	1–8 hr	UK

NURSING IMPLICATIONS
ASSESSMENT
□ Assess frequency of exacerbations of symptoms of multiple sclerosis periodically throughout therapy.
□ Monitor patient for signs of depression throughout therapy. If depression occurs, notify physician immediately.
▪ **Lab Test Considerations:** Monitor hemoglobin, WBC, platelets, and blood chemistries including liver function tests prior to and periodically throughout therapy. Therapy may be temporarily discontinued if the absolute neutrophil count is <750/mm^3, AST (SGOT) or ALT (SGPT) exceeds 10 times the upper limit of normal, or if serum bilirubin exceeds 5 times the upper limit of normal. Once the absolute neutrophil count is >750/mm^3 or the hepatic enzymes have returned to normal, therapy can be restarted at 50% the original dose.

POTENTIAL NURSING DIAGNOSES
▪ Knowledge deficit related to medication regimen (patient/family teaching).

IMPLEMENTATION
▪ **SC:** To reconstitute, inject 1.2 ml of diluent supplied into interferon beta-1b vial for a concentration of 0.25 mg (8 million IU)/ml. Swirl gently to dissolve completely, do not shake. Do not use solutions that are discolored or contain particulate matter. Keep reconstituted solution refrigerated; inject within 3 hr of reconstitution.
□ Following reconstitution, withdraw 1 ml into a syringe with a 27-gauge needle and inject SC into arms, abdomen, hips, or thighs. Discard unused portion; vials are for single dose only.

PATIENT/FAMILY TEACHING
▪ **Home Care Issues:** Instruct patient in correct technique for injection and care and disposal of equipment. Caution patient not to reuse needles or syringes and provide patient with a puncture-resistant container for disposal.
□ Instruct patient to take medication as directed; do not change dosage or schedule without consulting physician.
□ Inform patient that flu-like symptoms may occur during therapy. Acetaminophen may be used for relief of symptoms.
□ Advise patient to notify physician if pregnancy is planned or suspected. Interferon beta-1b may cause spontaneous abortion.

EVALUATION
Effectiveness of therapy can be demonstrated by: ▪ Decrease in the frequency of relapse (neurologic dysfunction) in patients with relapsing-remitting multiple sclerosis.

INTERFERON GAMMA-1B
(in-ter-**feer**-on)
Actimmune

CLASSIFICATION(S):
Immune modifier
Pregnancy Category C

INDICATIONS
▪ Diminished severity and frequency

of infectious complications of chronic granulomatous disease.

ACTION

- A protein produced by recombinant DNA technology that is capable of activating phagocytes, enhancing their ability to kill pathogens, including: □ *Staphylococcus aureus* □ *Toxoplasma gondii* □ *Leishmania donovani* □ *Listeria monocytogenes* □ *Myobacterium avium intracellulare*.
Therapeutic Effects: ■ Decreased incidence and severity of infection in patients with chronic granulomatous disease.

PHARMACOKINETICS

Absorption: Slowly absorbed following SC administration.
Distribution: Distribution not known.
Metabolism and Excretion: Metabolism and excretion not known.
Half-life: 5.9 hr.

CONTRAINDICATIONS AND PRECAUTIONS

Contraindicated in: ■ Hypersensitivity to interferon gamma, *E. coli*-derived products, mannitol, or polysorbate.
Use Cautiously in: ■ Pregnancy, lactation, or children <1 yr (safety not established) ■ Cardiovascular disease ■ Bone marrow depression.

ADVERSE REACTIONS AND SIDE EFFECTS*

CNS: <u>headache</u>, decreased mental status, dizziness.
GI: <u>nausea</u>, <u>vomiting</u>, abdominal pain.
Derm: <u>rash</u>.
Hemat: neutropenia, thrombocytopenia.
Local: <u>edema or tenderness at injection site</u>.
MS: <u>myalgia</u>, <u>arthralgia</u>, back pain.
Neuro: gait disturbances.
Misc: <u>fever</u>, <u>chills</u>.

INTERACTIONS

Drug–Drug: ■ May have additive bone marrow depressing effects with **antineoplastic agents** or **radiation therapy**.

ROUTE AND DOSAGE

Body Surface Area >0.5 m²
- **SC (Adults):** 50 mcg/m² (1.5 million units/m²) 3 times weekly.

Body Surface Area ≤0.5 m²
- **SC (Adults and Children >1 yr):** 1.5 mcg/kg 3 times weekly.

AVAILABILITY

- *Injection:* 100 mcg (3 million units)/ vial.

TIME/ACTION PROFILE (blood levels)

	ONSET	PEAK	DURATION
SC	UK	4 hr	UK

NURSING IMPLICATIONS

ASSESSMENT

□ Assess patient for signs and symptoms of infection prior to and throughout therapy. Flu-like syndrome (fever, headache, chills, myalgia, fatigue) is a frequent side effect that may decrease in severity as treatment continues. Side effects may be minimized by administering at bedtime. Headache and fever may be treated with acetaminophen. If adverse reactions are severe, dose may be reduced by 50% or discontinued.
- **Lab Test Considerations:** Monitor CBC with differential, platelet count, blood chemistries including liver and kidney function, and urinalysis prior to and every 3 mo throughout therapy.

POTENTIAL NURSING DIAGNOSES

- Infection, high risk for (indications).
- Knowledge deficit related to medication regimen (patient/family teaching).

IMPLEMENTATION

- **General Info:** Vial must be refrigerated; do not freeze. If left at room temperature for more than 12 hr, discard vial. Vials do not contain a preservative and are for single use only. Do not shake.
- **SC:** Administer in the right or left arm or anterior thigh.

I

PATIENT/FAMILY TEACHING
- **Home Care Issues:** Instruct patient or family on proper technique for administering injection and care and disposal of equipment. Provide a puncture-proof container for disposal of needles.
- Advise patient of the need for contraception throughout therapy.

EVALUATION
Effectiveness of therapy can be demonstrated by: ■ Decrease in frequency and severity of infections in patients with chronic granulomatous disease.

IPECAC SYRUP
(ip-e-kak)

CLASSIFICATION(S):
Emetic
Pregnancy Category C

INDICATIONS
■ Used to induce vomiting in the early management of overdose or poisoning of noncaustic substances in conscious patients.

ACTION
■ Stimulates the chemoreceptor trigger zone in the CNS and irritates the gastric mucosa. **Therapeutic Effect:** ■ Induction of emesis in overdose situations.

PHARMACOKINETICS
Absorption: Absorption is minimal.
Distribution: Distribution not known.
Metabolism and Excretion: Metabolism and excretion not known.
Half-life: UK.

CONTRAINDICATIONS AND PRECAUTIONS
Contraindicated in: ■ Semicomatose, inebriated, unconscious, or seizing patients ■ Shock ■ Patients who may not have a gag reflex ■ Ingestion of caustic substances ■ Alcohol intolerance.
Use Cautiously in: ■ Pregnancy, lactation, or children <6 mo (safety not es-

tablished) ■ Do not confuse syrup with fluidextract, which is 14 times more concentrated.

ADVERSE REACTIONS AND SIDE EFFECTS*
CNS: sedation.
CV: <u>arrhythmias</u>, MYOCARDITIS (if drug is absorbed or overdosage ingested).
GI: diarrhea.

INTERACTIONS
Drug–Drug: ■ Should not be given concurrently with **antiemetics** or **activated charcoal** (may reduce emetic efficacy).
Drug–Food: ■ Concurrent administration with **milk** decreases effectiveness ■ Avoid concurrent use of **carbonated beverages** (causes abdominal distention).

ROUTE AND DOSAGE
- **PO (Adults):** 15–30 ml. May be repeated in 30 min.
- **PO (Children ≥1 yr):** 15 ml. May be repeated in 30 min.
- **PO (Children <1 yr):** 5–10 ml.

AVAILABILITY
- *Syrup:* 7% in 15 ml, 30 ml, pts, and gallons.

TIME/ACTION PROFILE (onset of emesis)

	ONSET	PEAK	DURATION
PO	20–30 min	UK	20–25 min

NURSING IMPLICATIONS
ASSESSMENT
- A history is essential in determining treatment and antidotes for accidental poisoning. Do not induce vomiting if patient has ingested petroleum distillates, volatile oils, or caustic substances.
- Assess level of consciousness prior to administration. Do not administer ipecac if patient is unconscious, semiconscious, or convulsing.

POTENTIAL NURSING DIAGNOSES
- Injury, high risk for (indications).
- Knowledge deficit related to medica-

tion regimen (patient/family teaching).

IMPLEMENTATION

- **General Info:** If vomiting does not occur within 30 min, dose may be repeated. If vomiting does not occur within 20 min after second dose, gastric lavage must be performed to recover the medication.
- □ Administer activated charcoal only after vomiting has been induced and completed.
- **PO:** Have patient sit up with head forward prior to administration. Ipecac syrup may not work on an empty stomach. Administer syrup followed immediately by adequate amounts of water (3–4 glasses for adults, 1–2 glasses for children over 1 yr and ½–1 glass for children younger than 1 yr).
- □ Do not administer concurrently with milk, as it decreases the effectiveness of ipecac, or carbonated beverages, as they cause stomach distention.

PATIENT/FAMILY TEACHING

- **Home Care Issues:** Advise parents with children >1 yr to keep a small amount of ipecac syrup on hand for emergency use. If child ingests a dangerous substance, the parents should contact a poison control center, physician, or emergency department for advice before administering this medication.
- □ Caution parents to avoid inducing emesis if child swallowed caustic substances, volatile oils, or petroleum distillates or if child is unconscious, semiconscious, or convulsing. Instruct parent to position child to avoid aspiration.
- □ Advise parents that the drug has a 1-yr shelf life and therefore needs to be replaced yearly. Advise parents to check expiration date of product before purchasing.

EVALUATION

Effectiveness of therapy can be demonstrated by: ▪ Emesis within 30 min of administration.

IPRATROPIUM
(i-pra-**troe**-pee-um)
Atrovent

CLASSIFICATION(S):
Bronchodilator (anticholinergic)
Pregnancy Category B

INDICATIONS
▪ Bronchodilator in maintenance therapy of reversible airway obstruction due to asthma or COPD.

ACTION
▪ Inhibits cholinergic receptors in bronchial smooth muscle, resulting in decreased concentrations of cyclic guanosine monophosphate (cGMP). Decreased levels of cGMP produce local bronchodilation. **Therapeutic Effect:**
▪ Bronchodilation without systemic anticholinergic properties.

PHARMACOKINETICS
Absorption: Minimal systemic absorption.
Distribution: Does not appear to cross the blood–brain barrier.
Metabolism and Excretion: Small amounts absorbed are metabolized by the liver.
Half-life: 2 hr.

CONTRAINDICATIONS AND PRECAUTIONS
Contraindicated in: ▪ Hypersensitivity to ipratropium, atropine, belladonna alkaloids, bromide, or fluorocarbons ▪ Avoid use during acute bronchospasm.
Use Cautiously in: ▪ Patients with bladder neck obstruction, prostatic hypertrophy, glaucoma, or urinary retention ▪ Elderly patients (may be more sensitive to effects).

ADVERSE REACTIONS AND SIDE EFFECTS*
CNS: nervousness, dizziness, headache.
EENT: blurred vision, sore throat.

I

*Underlines indicate most frequent; CAPITALS indicate life-threatening.

Resp: cough, bronchospasm.
CV: palpitations, hypotension.
GI: nausea, GI irritation.
Derm: rash.

INTERACTIONS

Drug–Drug: ▪ Potential additive fluorocarbon toxicity when used with other **inhalation bronchodilators having a fluorocarbon propellant.**

ROUTE AND DOSAGE

▪ **Inhalation (Adults):** 1–2 inhalation 3–4 times daily (not to exceed 12 inhalations/24 hr). During initial therapy, up to 4 inhalations may be repeated.

AVAILABILITY

▪ *Aerosol inhaler:* 18 mcg/actuation— 200 inhalations/14-g cannister ▪ {*Inhalation solution:* 0.025%}.

TIME/ACTION PROFILE
(bronchodilation)

	ONSET	PEAK	DURATION
Inhaln	5–15 min	1–2 hr	3–4 hr (up to 6 hr)

NURSING IMPLICATIONS

ASSESSMENT

□ Assess respiratory status (rate, breath sounds, degree of dyspnea, pulse) before administration and at peak of medication. Confer with physician about alternative medication if severe bronchospasm is present, because onset of action is too slow for patients in acute distress. If paradoxical bronchospasm (wheezing) occurs, withhold medication and notify physician immediately.

□ Assess for allergy to atropine and belladonna alkaloids; patients with these allergies may also be sensitive to ipratropium.

POTENTIAL NURSING DIAGNOSES

▪ Airway clearance, ineffective (indications).
▪ Activity intolerance (indications).

▪ Knowledge deficit related to medication regimen (patient/family teaching).

IMPLEMENTATION

▪ **Inhalation:** See Appendix H for administration of inhalation medications.
□ When ipratropium is administered concurrently with other inhalation medications, administer ipratropium first.

PATIENT/FAMILY TEACHING

□ Instruct patient on proper use of inhaler. Instruct patient to take medication as directed. If a dose is missed, take as soon as remembered unless almost time for the next dose. Do not double doses.

□ Caution patient not to exceed 12 doses within 24 hr. Patient should notify physician if symptoms do not improve within 30 min after administration of medication or if condition worsens.

□ Explain need for pulmonary function tests prior to and periodically throughout therapy to determine effectiveness of medication.

□ Caution patient to avoid spraying medication in eyes; may cause blurring of vision or irritation.

□ Advise patient that rinsing mouth after using inhaler, good oral hygiene, and sugarless gum or candy may minimize dry mouth. Physician should be notified if stomatitis occurs or if dry mouth persists for more than 2 wk.

□ Advise patient to inform physician if cough, nervousness, headache, dizziness, nausea, or GI distress occurs.

EVALUATION

Effectiveness of therapy can be demonstrated by: ▪ Decreased dyspnea □ Improved breath sounds.

IRON DEXTRAN
(**eye**-ern **dex**-tran)
{Imferon}, InFed

INDICATIONS

▪ Treatment and prevention of iron-deficiency anemia in patients who are unable to tolerate oral iron preparations.

ACTION

▪ Enters the bloodstream and organs of the reticuloendothelial system (liver, spleen, bone marrow), where iron is separated from the dextran complex and becomes part of the body's iron stores. **Therapeutic Effect:** ▪ Prevention and treatment of iron deficiency.

PHARMACOKINETICS

Absorption: Well absorbed following IM administration.
Distribution: Remains in the body for many months. Crosses the placenta and enters breast milk.
Metabolism and Excretion: Lost slowly from the body through desquamation or blood loss.
Half-life: 6 hr.

CONTRAINDICATIONS AND PRECAUTIONS

Contraindicated in: ▪ Hypersensitivity ▪ All other types of anemias.
Use Cautiously in: ▪ Autoimmune disorders and arthritis (more susceptible to allergic reactions).

ADVERSE REACTIONS AND SIDE EFFECTS*

CNS: headache, dizziness, SEIZURES, syncope.
EENT: bad taste.
CV: hypotension, tachycardia.
GI: nausea, vomiting.
Derm: urticaria, flushing.
Local: pain at IM site, staining at IM site, phlebitis at IV site.
MS: arthralgia.
Misc: allergic reactions, including ANAPHYLAXIS, fever, lymphadenopathy.

INTERACTIONS

Drug–Drug: ▪ **Chloramphenicol** and **vitamin E** may impair the normal hematologic response to parenteral iron.

ROUTE AND DOSAGE

Test dose of 0.5 ml (25 mg) is given prior to therapy.
Iron Deficiency Anemia
▪ **IM, IV (Adults and Children >15 kg):** Total dose (ml) $= 0.0476 \times$ weight (kg) $\times$ (14.8-hemoglobin) $+ 1$ ml/5 kg weight up to 14 ml for iron stores. Divided up and given in small daily doses until total is reached; not to exceed 250 mg (5 ml)/day IM or 100 mg (2 ml) IV/day. *Unlabeled*—Total dose may be diluted and infused over 4–5 hr following a test dose of 10 drops.
▪ **IM, IV (Children 5–15 kg):** $0.0476 \times$ weight (kg) $\times$ (12-hemoglobin) $+$ iron stores. Not to exceed 50–100 mg (1–2 ml)/day IM.
Blood Loss
▪ **IM, IV (Adults and Children):** Dose $(ml) = \dfrac{\text{Blood loss (ml)} \times \text{hematocrit}}{50}$

AVAILABILITY

▪ *Injection:* 50 mg/ml.

TIME/ACTION PROFILE (effects on reticulocyte counts)

	ONSET	PEAK	DURATION
IV	4 days	1–2 wk	wk–mos
IM	4 days	1–2 wk	wk–mos

I

NURSING IMPLICATIONS

ASSESSMENT

▫ Assess patient's nutritional status and dietary history to determine possible cause of anemia and need for patient teaching.
▫ Monitor blood pressure and heart rate frequently following IV administration until stable. Rapid infusion rate may cause hypotension and flushing.
▫ Assess patient for signs and symptoms of anaphylaxis (rash, pruritus,

*Underlines indicate most frequent; **CAPITALS** indicate life-threatening.*

laryngeal edema, wheezing). Notify physician immediately if these occur. Keep epinephrine and resuscitation equipment close by in the event of an anaphylactic reaction.

- **Lab Test Considerations:** Monitor hemoglobin, hematocrit, reticulocyte values, transferrin, ferritin, total iron-binding capacity, and plasma iron concentrations periodically throughout therapy. Serum ferritin levels peak in 7–9 days and return to normal in 3 wk. Serum iron determinations may be inaccurate for 1–2 wk after therapy with large doses, therefore hemoglobin and hematocrit are used to gauge initial response.
□ May impart a brownish hue to blood drawn within 4 hr of administration. May cause false increase in serum bilirubin and false decrease in serum calcium values. Prolonged PTT may be calculated when blood sample is anticoagulated with citrate dextrose solution; use sodium citrate instead.

POTENTIAL NURSING DIAGNOSES
- Activity intolerance (indications).
- Knowledge deficit related to medication and dietary regimen (patient/family teaching).

IMPLEMENTATION
- **General Info:** Oral iron preparations should be discontinued prior to parenteral administration.
□ The 2-ml ampule may be used for IM or IV administration; the 10-ml multidose vials may be used only for IM administration.
□ Prior to initial IM or IV dose, a test dose of 25 mg should be given by the same route as the dose is to be given, to determine reaction. The IV test dose should be administered over 5 min. The IM dose should be administered in same injection site and by same technique as the therapeutic dose. The remaining portion may be administered after 1 hr, if no adverse symptoms have occurred.
- **IM:** Inject deeply via Z-track technique into upper outer quadrant of buttock, never into arm or other exposed areas. Use a 2–3 in, 19-gauge or 20-gauge needle. Change needles between withdrawal from container and injection to minimize staining of subcutaneous tissues. Stains are usually permanent.
- **Direct IV:** Give undiluted at a rate of 50 mg over at least 1 min.
□ Following IV administration, patient should remain recumbent for at least 30 min to prevent orthostatic hypotension.
- **Continuous Infusion:** May be diluted in 500 ml of D5W.
- *Rate:* Administer over 4–5 hr following a test dose of 10 drops/min for 10 min.

PATIENT/FAMILY TEACHING
□ Delayed reaction may occur 1–2 days after administration and last 3–4 days if IV route used, 3–7 days with IM route. Instruct patient to contact physician if fever, chills, malaise, muscle and joint aches, nausea, vomiting, dizziness, and backache occur.
□ Instruct patient to follow a diet high in iron (organ meat, leafy green vegetables, dried beans and peas, dried fruit, cereals).

EVALUATION
Clinical response can be determined by: - Increase in hemoglobin, hematocrit, and plasma iron levels. The diagnosis of iron-deficiency anemia should be reconfirmed if hemoglobin has not increased by 1 g/100 ml in 2 wk.

ISONIAZID
(eye-soe-**nye**-a-zid)
INH, {Isotamine}, Laniazid, Nydrazid, {PMS Isoniazid}, Tubizid

CLASSIFICATION(S):
Antitubercular
Pregnancy Category UK

INDICATIONS

- Used as a first-line antitubercular in combination with other agents in the treatment of active disease ▪ Prevention of tuberculosis in patients exposed to active disease.

ACTION

- Inhibits mycobacterial cell wall synthesis and interferes with metabolism. **Therapeutic Effect:** ▪ Bacteriostatic or bactericidal action against susceptible mycobacteria.

PHARMACOKINETICS

Absorption: Well absorbed following oral and IM administration.

Distribution: Widely distributed to many body tissues and fluids. Readily crosses the blood–brain barrier. Crosses the placenta and enters breast milk in concentrations equal to plasma.

Metabolism and Excretion: 50% metabolized by the liver at rates that vary widely among individuals. Remainder is excreted unchanged by the kidneys.

Half-life: 1–4 hr.

CONTRAINDICATIONS AND PRECAUTIONS

Contraindicated in: ▪ Hypersensitivity ▪ Acute liver disease ▪ Previous hepatitis from isoniazid.

Use Cautiously in: ▪ History of liver damage or chronic alcohol ingestion ▪ Pregnancy and lactation (although safety is not established, isoniazid has been used with ethambutol to treat tuberculosis in pregnant women without harm to the fetus) ▪ Severe renal impairment (dosage reduction may be necessary) ▪ Malnourished patients, diabetics, or chronic alcoholics (increased risk of neuropathy).

ADVERSE REACTIONS AND SIDE EFFECTS*

CNS: <u>peripheral neuropathy</u>, seizures, psychosis.

EENT: visual disturbances.

GI: nausea, vomiting, HEPATITIS.

Derm: rashes.

Endo: gynecomastia.

Hemat: blood dyscrasias.

Misc: fever.

INTERACTIONS

Drug–Drug: ▪ Additive CNS toxicity with other antituberculars ▪ **BCG vaccine** may not be effective during isoniazid therapy ▪ Isoniazid inhibits the metabolism of **phenytoin** ▪ **Aluminum-containing antacids** may decrease absorption ▪ Psychotic reactions and coordination difficulties may result with **disulfiram** ▪ Concurrent administration of **pyridoxine** may prevent neuropathy ▪ Increased risk of hepatotoxicity with other **hepatotoxic agents** ▪ Concurrent use with **carbamazepine** increases carbamazepine blood levels and risk of hepatotoxicity.

Drug–Food: ▪ Severe reactions may occur with ingestion of foods containing high concentrations of **tyramine** (see Appendix K).

ROUTE AND DOSAGE

- **PO, IM (Adults):** 5–10 mg/kg/day (usually 300 mg) or 15 mg/kg 2–3 times weekly after 2 mo at 300 mg/day.
- **PO, IM (Children):** 10–20 mg/kg/day (up to 300 mg/day).

AVAILABILITY

- ***Tablets:*** 100 mg, 300 mg ▪ ***Syrup:*** 50 mg/5 ml ▪ ***Injection:*** 100 mg/ml ▪ ***In combination with:*** rifampin (Rifamate).

TIME/ACTION PROFILE (blood levels)

	ONSET	PEAK
PO	rapid	1–2 hr
IM	rapid	1–2 hr

NURSING IMPLICATIONS

ASSESSMENT

- ▢ Mycobacterial studies and susceptibility tests should be performed prior to and periodically throughout therapy to detect possible resistance.
- ▪ **Lab Test Considerations:** May cause

*<u>Underlines</u> indicate most frequent; **CAPITALS** indicate life-threatening.

false-positive test results for copper sulfate urine glucose tests (Clinitest). Diabetic patients should test urine glucose with enzymatic tests (Ketodiastix, Clinistix, Tes-Tape).

□ Hepatic function should be evaluated prior to and monthly throughout therapy. Increased AST (SGOT), ALT (SGPT), and serum bilirubin may indicate drug-induced hepatitis. Patients over 50 yr are at highest risk. The risk is lower in children; therefore liver function tests are usually ordered less frequently for children.

▪ **Toxicity and Overdose:** If isoniazid overdosage occurs, treatment with pyridoxine (vitamin B_6) is instituted.

POTENTIAL NURSING DIAGNOSES
▪ Infection, high risk for (indications).
▪ Knowledge deficit related to medication regimen (patient/family teaching).
▪ Noncompliance (patient/family teaching).

IMPLEMENTATION
▪ **PO:** Administer medication on an empty stomach, at least 1 hr before or 2 hr after meals. If GI irritation becomes a problem, may be administered with food, although food decreases absorption of isoniazid. Antacids may also be taken 1 hr prior to administration.
▪ **IM:** Medication may cause discomfort at injection site. Massage site after administration and rotate injection sites.

PATIENT/FAMILY TEACHING
□ Advise patient to take medication exactly as directed, not to skip doses or double up on missed doses. Emphasize the importance of continuing therapy even after symptoms have subsided.
□ Advise patient to notify physician promptly if signs and symptoms of hepatitis (yellow eyes and skin, nausea, vomiting, anorexia, dark urine, unusual tiredness, or weakness) or peripheral neuritis (numbness, tingling, paresthesia) occur. Pyridoxine may be used concurrently to prevent neuropathy. Any changes in visual acuity, eye pain, or blurred vision should also be reported to the physician immediately.

□ Caution patient to avoid the use of alcohol during this therapy, as this may increase the risk of hepatotoxicity. Ingestion of Swiss or Cheshire cheeses, fish (tuna, skipjack, and Sardinella), and possibly tyramine-containing foods (see Appendix K) should also be avoided, as they may result in redness or itching of the skin, hot feeling, rapid or pounding heart beat, sweating, chills, cold clammy feeling, headache, or lightheadedness.

□ Emphasize the importance of regular follow-up physical and ophthalmologic examinations to monitor progress and to check for side effects.

EVALUATION
Effectiveness of therapy can be demonstrated by: ▪ Resolution of signs and symptoms of tuberculosis □ Negative sputum cultures ▪ Prevention of activation of tuberculosis in persons known to be exposed.

ISOPROTERENOL
(eye-soe-proe-ter-e-nole)
Aerolone, Isuprel, Medihaler-Iso, Vapo-Iso

CLASSIFICATION(S):
Bronchodilator (beta-adrenergic agonist), Antiarrhythmic, Inotropic agent
Pregnancy Category UK

INDICATIONS
▪ **Inhalation:** Used as a bronchodilator in reversible airway obstruction due to asthma or COPD ▪ **IV, SL, Rect:** Management of ventricular arrhythmias due to AV nodal block ▪ **IV:** Treatment of shock associated with decreased cardiac output and vasoconstriction.

ACTION
▪ A beta-adrenergic agonist that results in the accumulation of cyclic adenosine

monophosphate (cAMP) ▪ Results of increased levels of cAMP at beta-adrenergic receptors include bronchodilation, CNS and cardiac stimulation, diuresis, and gastric acid secretion ▪ Stimulates both beta$_1$ (myocardial) and beta$_2$ (pulmonary) receptors. **Therapeutic Effects:** ▪ Bronchodilation ▪ Increased heart rate ▪ Increased cardiac output.

PHARMACOKINETICS

Absorption: Rapidly absorbed following oral inhalation and from parenteral sites. Orally administered isoproterenol is rapidly metabolized. Sublingual and rectal absorption is erratic and unreliable.
Distribution: Distribution not known.
Metabolism and Excretion: If swallowed, metabolized in the GI tract. Following other routes of administration, drug is metabolized by the lung, liver, and other tissues. 50% excreted unchanged by the kidneys following IV administration.
Half-life: UK.

CONTRAINDICATIONS AND PRECAUTIONS

Contraindicated in: ▪ Hypersensitivity to adrenergic amines or any ingredients in preparations (fluorocarbons in inhalers, bisulfites in injection and SL tablets).
Use Cautiously in: ▪ Elderly patients (more susceptible to adverse reactions; may require dosage reduction) ▪ Lactation (safety not established) ▪ Cardiac disease ▪ Hypertension ▪ Hyperthyroidism ▪ Diabetes ▪ Glaucoma ▪ Pregnancy (near term).

ADVERSE REACTIONS AND SIDE EFFECTS*

CNS: <u>nervousness</u>, <u>restlessness</u>, insomnia, <u>tremor</u>, headache.
Resp: paradoxical bronchospasm (with excessive use).
CV: hypertension, arrhythmias, angina.
GI: nausea, vomiting.
Endo: hyperglycemia.

INTERACTIONS

Drug–Drug: ▪ Additive adrenergic effects with other **adrenergic (sympathomimetic) agents** ▪ Use with **MAO inhibitors** may lead to hypertensive crisis ▪ **Beta-adrenergic blockers** may block therapeutic effect ▪ Arrhythmias may be increased with **cyclopropane** or **halothane-type anesthesia**.

ROUTE AND DOSAGE

Bronchodilation
▪ **Inhalation (Adults and Children):** *Metered-dose inhaler*—1–2 inhalations 4–6 times daily. *Nebulization*—6–12 inhalations q 15 min for 3 treatments up to 8 times/day. *IPPB* (Adults): up to 5 times/day. *IPPB* (Children): up to 5 times/day.
▪ **SL (Adults):** 10–20 mg (not to exceed 60 mg/day, not to be administered more than 3 times daily or more often than q 3–4 hr).
▪ **SL (Children):** 5–10 mg (not to exceed 30 mg/day, not to be administered more than 3 times daily or more often than q 3–4 hr).
▪ **IV (Adults):** For bronchodilation during anesthesia—10–20 mcg.

Cardiac Standstill and Arrhythmias
See infusion rate table in Appendix D.
▪ **IV Bolus (Adults):** 20–60 mcg (may follow with 10–200 mcg).
▪ **IV Infusion (Adults):** 5 mcg/min (range 2–20 mcg/min).
▪ **SC (Adults):** 200 mcg (may follow with 150–200 mcg).
▪ **SL (Adults):** 10 mg initially, followed by 5–50 mg as needed.
▪ **Rect (Adults):** 5 mg followed by 5–15 mg as needed.

Shock
▪ **IV Infusion (Adults):** 0.5–5 mcg/min.

AVAILABILITY

▪ *Sublingual tablets:* 10 mg, 15 mg ▪ *Solution for inhalation:* 0.25%, 0.5%, 1% ▪ *Aerosol:* 131 mcg/mist spray in 80 mcg/metered dose ▪ *Injection:* 0.2 mg/ml (1:5000) ▪ *In combination with:* phenylephrine (Duo-Medihaler).

I

---

*<u>Underlines</u> indicate most frequent; **CAPITALS** indicate life-threatening.

TIME/ACTION PROFILE
(Inhaln = bronchodilation,
IV = cardiovascular effects)

	ONSET	PEAK	DURATION
Inhaln	rapid	UK	1 hr
IV	rapid	UK	min
SL	UK	UK	2 hr
Rect	UK	UK	2–4 hr

NURSING IMPLICATIONS

ASSESSMENT

- **General Info:** Assess blood pressure, pulse, respiratory pattern, lung sounds, arterial blood gases, and character of secretions frequently during course of therapy. ECG, hemodynamic parameters, and urine output should be monitored continuously during IV administration.
- ▢ Monitor for chest pain, arrhythmias, heart rate >110 bpm, and hypertension. Consult physician for parameters of pulse, blood pressure, and ECG changes for adjusting dosage or discontinuing medication.
- **Bronchospasm:** Observe patient for appearance of drug tolerance and rebound bronchospasm. Patients requiring more than 3 aerosol treatments within 24 hr should be under close supervision. If minimal or no relief is seen after 3–5 aerosol treatments within 6–12 hr, further treatment with aerosol alone is not recommended.
- **Shock:** Assess volume status. Hypovolemia should be corrected prior to administering isoproterenol IV.
- **Lab Test Considerations:** May cause decreased serum potassium concentrations.

POTENTIAL NURSING DIAGNOSES

- Airway clearance, ineffective (indications).
- Cardiac output, decreased (indications).
- Knowledge deficit related to medication regimen (patient/family teaching).

IMPLEMENTATION

- **General Info:** In treatment of heart block, SL tablet may be administered rectally.
- **Direct IV:** May be administered by diluting 0.2 mg (1 ml) of a 1:5000 solution with 10 ml of 0.9% NaCl for injection, or D5W to make a 1:50,000 solution. Do not use if solution is pinkish to brownish or contains a precipitate.
- *Rate:* Administer each 1 ml of 1:50,000 solution (0.02 mg) over 1 min.
- **Continuous Infusion:** Prepare by adding 2 mg (10 ml) of a 1:5000 solution to 500 ml of D5W, D10W, 0.9% NaCl, 0.45% NaCl, dextrose/saline combinations, dextrose/Ringer's or lactated Ringer's combinations, Ringer's or lactated Ringer's solution for a 1:250,000 solution (4 mcg = 1 ml).
- *Rate:* Administer at a rate of 1 ml/min, adjusting according to patient response and parameters for blood pressure, hemodynamic values, and urine output specified by physician. Administer via infusion pump to ensure delivery of precise amounts of medication. See Infusion Rate Table in Appendix D.
- **Y-Site Compatibility:** ▪ amrinone ▪ atracurium ▪ bretyllium ▪ famotidine ▪ heparin ▪ hydrocortisone sodium succinate ▪ pancuronium ▪ potassium chloride ▪ vecuronium ▪ vitamin B complex with C.
- **Inhalation:** For aerosol administration, dilute ordered dose in sterile water or 0.45% or 0.9% NaCl. Administer aerosol medications over 10–20 min.

PATIENT/FAMILY TEACHING

- **General Info:** Instruct patient to take medication exactly as directed. Taking more often than prescribed may lead to tolerance or paradoxical bronchospasm.
- **SL:** Instruct patient to hold SL tablet under tongue until completely dissolved. Do not chew or swallow. Encourage patient to rinse mouth frequently between doses and to practice good oral hygiene.

- **Inhalation:** Review correct administration technique (aerosolization, IPPB, metered-dose inhaler) with patient. See Appendix H for administration with metered-dose inhaler. Wait 1–5 min before administering next dose. Mouthpiece should be washed after each use. Medication should be discarded if pinkish to brownish or if it contains a precipitate.
- □ Patients taking inhalation glucocorticoids concurrently with isoproterenol should be advised to take isoproterenol first and to allow 15 min to elapse between using the 2 aerosols, unless directed by physician.
- □ Inform patient that medication may tinge sputum pink or red.
- □ Advise patient to maintain an adequate fluid intake (2000–3000 ml/day) to help liquify tenacious secretions.
- □ Advise patient to consult physician if respiratory symptoms are not relieved or worsen after treatment. Patient should also inform physician if chest pain, headache, severe dizziness, palpitations, nervousness, or weakness occurs.

EVALUATION
Effectiveness of therapy can be demonstrated by: ■ Decrease in bronchoconstriction and bronchospasm □ Increase in ease of breathing ■ Increase in heart rate ■ Increase in cardiac output.

ISOSORBIDE DINITRATE
(eye-soe-**sor**-bide dye-**nye**-trate)
{Apo-ISDN}, {Cedocard-SR}, {Coronex}, Dilatrate-SR, ISDN, Iso-Bid, Isonate, Isorbid, Isordil, Isotrate, {Novosorbide}, Sorbitrate

ISOSORBIDE MONONITRATE
(eye-soe-**sor**-bide mo-noe-**nye**-trate)
Imdur, ISMO, Monoket

CLASSIFICATION(S):
Vasodilator (nitrate), Antianginal
Pregnancy Category C

INDICATIONS

■ Acute treatment of anginal attacks (SL, chewable dinitrate only) ■ Long-term prophylactic management of angina pectoris (dinitrate and mononitrate) ■ Treatment of chronic congestive heart failure (dinitrate).

ACTION

■ Produces vasodilation (venous greater than arterial) ■ Decreases left ventricular end-diastolic pressure and left ventricular end-diastolic volume (preload). Net effect is reduced myocardial oxygen consumption ■ Increases coronary blood flow by dilating coronary arteries and improving collateral flow to ischemic regions. **Therapeutic Effect:** Relief of anginal attacks and increased cardiac output.

PHARMACOKINETICS

Absorption: Well absorbed following oral and sublingual administration.
Distribution: Distribution not known.
Metabolism and Excretion: Mostly metabolized by the liver.
Half-life: dinitrate—50 min, mononitrate—5 hr.

CONTRAINDICATIONS AND PRECAUTIONS

Contraindicated in: ■ Hypersensitivity ■ Severe anemia.
Use Cautiously in: ■ Head trauma or cerebral hemorrhage ■ Pregnancy (may compromise maternal/fetal circulation) ■ Children or lactation (safety not established).

ADVERSE REACTIONS AND SIDE EFFECTS*

CNS: <u>headache</u>, apprehension, weakness, <u>dizziness</u>.

I

{} = Available in Canada only.
*<u>Underlines</u> indicate most frequent; **CAPITALS** indicate life-threatening.

CV: hypotension, tachycardia, syncope, paradoxical bradycardia.
GI: nausea, vomiting, abdominal pain.
Misc: flushing, tolerance, cross-tolerance.

INTERACTIONS

Drug–Drug: ▪ Additive hypotension with **antihypertensives,** acute ingestion of **alcohol, beta-adrenergic blocking agents, calcium channel blockers,** and **phenothiazines**.

ROUTE AND DOSAGE

Isosorbide Dinitrate
Acute Attack of Angina Pectoris
▪ **SL, Chew, or Intrabuccal (Adults):** 2.5–10 mg may be repeated q 5–10 min for 3 doses in 15–30 min (initial dose of chewable tablet should not exceed 5 mg).

Prophylaxis of Angina Pectoris
▪ **SL, Chew, or Intrabuccal (Adults):** 2.5–10 mg may be repeated q 2–3 hr (initial dose of chewable tablet should not exceed 5 mg).
▪ **PO (Adults):** 5–20 mg initially. Usual maintenance dose is 10–40 mg q 6 hr or 40–80 mg q 8–12 hr as sustained-release form.

Isosorbide Mononitrate
▪ **PO (Adults):** 20 mg twice daily, 7 hr apart (ISMO, Monoket) or 30–60 mg once daily, may increase to 120 mg once daily (Imdur).

AVAILABILITY

Isosorbide Dinitrate
▪ *Sublingual tablets:* 2.5 mg, 5 mg, 10 mg ▪ *Chewable tablets:* 5 mg, 10 mg ▪ *Tablets:* 5 mg, 10 mg, 20 mg, 30 mg, 40 mg ▪ *Sustained-release tablets:* 40 mg.

Isosorbide Mononitrate
▪ *Tablets:* 20 mg.

TIME/ACTION PROFILE
(cardiovascular effects)

	ONSET	PEAK	DURATION
ISDN-SL, Chew	2–5 min	UK	1–2 hr
ISDN-PO	15–40 min	UK	4 hr
ISDN-PO-ER	30 min	UK	up to 12 hr
ISMN-PO	30–60 min	UK	UK
ISMN-ER	UK	UK	12 hr

NURSING IMPLICATIONS

ASSESSMENT
▫ Assess location, duration, intensity, and precipitating factors of anginal pain.
▫ Monitor blood pressure and pulse routinely during period of dosage adjustment.

POTENTIAL NURSING DIAGNOSES
▪ Tissue perfusion, altered (indications).
▪ Activity intolerance (indications).
▪ Knowledge deficit related to medication regimen (patient/family teaching).

IMPLEMENTATION
Isosorbide Dinitrate
▪ **PO:** Administer 1 hr before or 2 hr after meals with a full glass of water for faster absorption.
▫ Chewable tablets should be chewed well before swallowing and held in mouth for 2 min. Do not swallow whole.
▫ Extended-release tablets and capsules should be swallowed whole. Do not crush, break, or chew.
▪ **SL:** SL tablets should be held under tongue until dissolved.
▫ Avoid eating, drinking, or smoking until tablet is dissolved. Replace tablet if inadvertently swallowed.

Isosorbide Mononitrate

- **PO:** Administer twice daily, once upon awakening and the second dose 7 hr later. Medication should be taken on an empty stomach with a full glass of water.

PATIENT/FAMILY TEACHING

□ Instruct patient to take medication exactly as directed, even if feeling better. If a dose is missed, take as soon as remembered; doses of isosorbide dinitrate should be taken at least 2 hr apart (6 hr with extended-release preparations); daily doses of isosorbide mononitrate should be taken 7 hr apart. Do not double doses. Do not discontinue abruptly.

□ Caution patient to make position changes slowly to minimize orthostatic hypotension.

□ May cause dizziness. Caution patient to avoid driving or other activities requiring alertness until response to medication is known.

□ Advise patient to avoid concurrent use of alcohol with this medication. Patients should also consult physician or pharmacist before taking over-the-counter medications while taking isosorbide mononitrate.

□ Inform patient that headache is a common side effect that should decrease with continuing therapy. Aspirin or acetaminophen may be ordered to treat headache. Notify physician if headache is persistent or severe. Do not alter dose to avoid headache.

□ Advise patient to notify physician if dry mouth or blurred vision occurs.

EVALUATION

Effectiveness of therapy can be demonstrated by: ■ Decrease in frequency and severity of anginal attacks □ Increase in activity tolerance.

ISOTRETINOIN

(eye-soe-**tret**-i-noyn)
Accutane, {Accutane Roche}

CLASSIFICATION(S):
Antiacne agent
Pregnancy Category X

INDICATIONS

■ Management of cystic acne resistant to more conventional therapy, including topical therapy and systemic antibiotics.

ACTION

■ A metabolite of vitamin A (retinol); reduces sebaceous gland size and differentiation. **Therapeutic Effects:** ■ Diminution and resolution of severe acne. May also prevent abnormal keratinization.

PHARMACOKINETICS

Absorption: 23–25% absorbed following oral administration.
Distribution: Appears to be widely distributed. Probably crosses the placenta.
Metabolism and Excretion: Mostly metabolized by the liver.
Half-life: 10–20 hr.

CONTRAINDICATIONS AND PRECAUTIONS

Contraindicated in: ■ Hypersensitivity to retinoids, glycerin, soybean oil, or parabens ■ Pregnant patients ■ Women of childbearing age who may become or intend to become pregnant ■ Lactation ■ Patients planning to donate blood.
Use Cautiously in: ■ Pre-existing hypertriglyceridemia ■ Diabetes mellitus ■ Alcoholics ■ Obese patients ■ Inflammatory bowel disease.

ADVERSE REACTIONS AND SIDE EFFECTS*

CNS: pseudotumor cerebrii.
EENT: epistaxis, conjunctivitis, dry eyes, cornea opacities, blurred vision, decreased night vision.
CV: edema.
GI: cheilitis, dry mouth, anorexia, nausea, vomiting, abdominal pain, increased appetite, hepatitis.

{} = Available in Canada only.
*Underlines indicate most frequent; **CAPITALS** indicate life-threatening.

Derm: <u>pruritus</u>, thinning of hair, palmar desquamation, skin infections, photosensitivity.
Hemat: <u>decreased hemoglobin</u>, <u>decreased hematocrit</u>.
Metab: <u>hypertriglyceridemia</u>, <u>hypercholesterolemia</u>, <u>decreased high-density lipoproteins</u>, hyperglycemia, hyperuricemia.
MS: <u>bone pain</u>, <u>arthralgia</u>, hyperostosis.
Misc: thirst.

INTERACTIONS

Drug–Drug: ▪ Additive toxicity with **vitamin A** and **related compounds** ▪ Increased risk of pseudotumor cerebreii with **tetracycline** or **minocycline** ▪ Concurrent use with **alcohol** increases hypertriglyceridemia ▪ Drying effects increased by concurrent use of **benzoyl peroxide, sulfur, tretinoin,** and **other topical agents**.
Drug–Food: ▪ Excessive ingestion of **foods high in vitamin A content** may result in additive toxicity.

ROUTE AND DOSAGE

▪ **PO (Adults):** 0.5–1 mg/kg/day (up to 2 mg/kg/day) in 2 divided doses for 15–20 wk. Once discontinued, if relapse occurs, therapy may be reinstituted after an 8-wk rest period.

AVAILABILITY

▪ *Capsules:* 10 mg, 20 mg, 40 mg.

TIME/ACTION PROFILE (diminution of acne)

	ONSET	PEAK	DURATION
PO	UK	up to 8 wk	UK

NURSING IMPLICATIONS

Assessment

□ Assess skin prior to and periodically during therapy. Transient worsening of acne may occur at initiation of therapy. Note number and severity of cysts, degree of skin dryness, erythema, and itching.
□ Assess for allergy to parabens, as

capsules contain parabens as a preservative.
▪ **Lab Test Consideration:** Monitor liver function (AST [SGOT], ALT [SGPT], and LDH) prior to therapy, after 1 mo of therapy, and periodically thereafter. Inform physician if these values become elevated; therapy may need to be discontinued.
□ Monitor blood lipids (cholesterol, high-density lipoproteins, triglycerides) prior to beginning therapy, after 1 mo, and periodically thereafter. Inform physician of increase in cholesterol and triglyceride levels or decrease in high-density lipoproteins.
□ Obtain baseline and periodic CBC, urinalysis, and SMA-12. May cause increased blood glucose, CPK, platelet counts, and sedimentation rate. May decrease RBC and WBC parameters. May cause proteinuria, red and white blood cells in urine, and elevated uric acid.

Potential Nursing Diagnoses

▪ Skin integrity, impaired (indications, side effects).
▪ Body image disturbance (indications).
▪ Knowledge deficit related to medication regimen (patient/family teaching).

Implementation

▪ **PO:** Administer with meals. Do not crush or open capsules.

Patient/Family Teaching

□ Instruct patient to take isotretinoin exactly as directed. Do not take more than the amount prescribed. If a dose is missed, take as soon as remembered if not almost time for next dose. Do not double doses.
□ Explain to patient that a temporary worsening of acne may occur at beginning of therapy.
□ Instruct female patients to use contraception 1 mo before therapy, throughout therapy, and for at least 1 mo after discontinuation of drug. This drug is contraindicated during pregnancy and may cause birth defects. Physician may order pregnancy

test 2 wk prior to initiation of therapy. Patient should discontinue medication and inform physician immediately if pregnancy is suspected. Recommended consent form prepared by manufacturer stresses fetal risk. Parents of minors should also read and sign form.

□ May cause sudden decrease in night vision. Caution patient to avoid driving at night until response to the medication is known.

□ Advise patient to consult with physician before using other acne preparations while taking isotretinoin. Soaps, cosmetics, and shaving lotion may also worsen dry skin.

□ Inform patient that dry skin and chapped lips will occur. Lubricant to lips may help cheilitis.

□ Instruct patient that oral rinses, good oral hygiene, and sugarless gum or candy may help minimize dry mouth. Notify physician if dry mouth persists for more than 2 wk.

□ Discuss possibility of excessively dry eyes with patients who wear contact lenses. Patient should contact physician about eye lubricant. Patient may need to switch to glasses during course of therapy and for up to 2 wk following discontinuation.

□ Advise patient to avoid alcoholic beverages while taking isotretinoin, as this may further increase triglyceride levels.

□ Caution patient to use sunscreen and protective clothing to prevent photosensitivity reactions. Physician should be consulted about sunscreen, as some sunscreens may worsen acne.

□ Instruct patient not to take vitamin A supplements and to avoid excessive ingestion of foods high in vitamin A (liver, fish liver oils, egg yolks, yellow-orange fruits and vegetables, dark green leafy vegetables, whole milk, vitamin A-fortified skim milk, butter, margarine) while taking isotretinoin; this may result in hypervitaminosis.

□ Advise patient not to donate blood while receiving this medication. After discontinuing isotretinoin, wait at least 1 mo before donating blood to prevent the possibility of a pregnant patient receiving the blood.

□ Instruct patient to report burning of eyes, visual changes, rash, abdominal pain, diarrhea, headache, nausea, and vomiting to physician.

□ Inform patient of need for medical follow-up. Physician may order periodic lab tests.

EVALUATION

Effectiveness of therapy can be demonstrated by: ■ Decrease in the number and severity of cysts in severe acne. Therapy may take 4–5 mo before full effects are seen. Therapy is discontinued when the number of cysts is reduced by 70% or after 5 mo. Improvement may occur after discontinuation of therapy; therefore, a delay of at least 8 wk is recommended before a second course of therapy is considered.

ISRADIPINE
(is-**ra**-di-peen)
DynaCirc

CLASSIFICATION(S):
Calcium channel blocker, Antihypertensive
Pregnancy Category C

I

INDICATIONS

■ Management of hypertension, alone or in combination with thiazide-type diuretics.

ACTION

■ Inhibits the transport of calcium into vascular smooth muscle cells, resulting in the inhibition of excitation-contraction coupling and subsequent contraction. Net result is vasodilation. **Therapeutic Effect:** ■ Lowering of blood pressure.

PHARMACOKINETICS

Absorption: Well absorbed following oral administration, but large amounts

are rapidly metabolized, resulting in decreased bioavailability.
Distribution: Distribution not known. 95% bound to plasma proteins.
Metabolism and Excretion: Mostly metabolized by the liver.
Half-life: 8 hr.

CONTRAINDICATIONS AND PRECAUTIONS

Contraindicated in: ▪ Hypersensitivity ▪ Sick sinus syndrome, 2nd- or 3rd-degree heart block (without a pacemaker) ▪ Severe hypotension.
Use Cautiously in: ▪ Severe hepatic disease (dosage reduction may be required) ▪ Congestive heart failure ▪ Pregnancy, lactation, or children (safety not established) ▪ Elderly patients (increased sensitivity).

ADVERSE REACTIONS AND SIDE EFFECTS*

CNS: <u>headache</u>, fatigue, dizziness.
Resp: shortness of breath.
CV: <u>peripheral edema</u>, palpitations, angina, tachycardia.
GI: nausea, diarrhea, abdominal discomfort, vomiting.
Derm: rashes, flushing.

INTERACTIONS

Drug–Drug: ▪ **Beta-adrenergic blockers** may increase the risk of myocardial depression and other adverse cardiovascular reactions ▪ **Fentanyl** increases the risk of hypotension.

ROUTE AND DOSAGE

▪ **PO (Adults):** 2.5 mg twice daily, may be increased at 2–4 wk intervals by 5 mg/day (not to exceed 20 mg/day).

AVAILABILITY

▪ *Capsules:* 2.5 mg, 5 mg.

TIME/ACTION PROFILE
(antihypertensive effect)*

	ONSET	PEAK	DURATION
PO	<2 hr	2–3 hr	12 hr

*Maximum antihypertensive effects may require 2–4 wk of therapy.

NURSING IMPLICATIONS

ASSESSMENT

□ Monitor blood pressure and pulse prior to and periodically throughout therapy. Monitor ECG periodically in patients receiving prolonged therapy.
□ Monitor intake and output ratios and daily weight. Assess patient for signs of congestive heart failure (peripheral edema, rales/crackles, dyspnea, weight gain, jugular venous distention).
▪ **Lab Test Considerations:** Monitor hepatic function periodically in patients receiving long-term therapy. May cause elevated liver function tests.

POTENTIAL NURSING DIAGNOSES

▪ Cardiac output, decreased (indications).
▪ Knowledge deficit related to medication regimen (patient/family teaching).

IMPLEMENTATION

▪ **PO:** Administration with food significantly increases the time to peak effects by about 1 hr, but has no effect on the total bioavailability of isradipine.

PATIENT/FAMILY TEACHING

□ Advise patient to take medication exactly as directed, not to skip or double up on missed doses. Isradipine may need to be discontinued gradually.
□ Caution patients to make position changes slowly to minimize orthostatic hypotension.
□ Isradipine may cause dizziness. Advise patient to avoid driving or other activities requiring alertness until response to the medication is known.
□ Instruct patient to avoid concurrent use of alcohol or over-the-counter medications without consulting physician or pharmacist.
□ Advise patient to notify the physician if irregular heart beats, dyspnea, swelling of hands and feet, pronounced dizziness, nausea, constipation, or hypotension occur.

*<u>Underlines</u> indicate most frequent; **CAPITALS** indicate life-threatening.

EVALUATION
Effectiveness of therapy can be demonstrated by: ▪ Decrease in blood pressure. Antihypertensive response may be seen in 2–3 hr, but maximal response may require 2–4 wk.

ITRACONAZOLE
(it-tra-**kon**-a-zole)
Sporanox

CLASSIFICATION(S):
Antifungal
Pregnancy Category C

INDICATIONS
▪ Treatment of histoplasmosis and blastomycosis.

ACTION
▪ Inhibits enzymes necessary for integrity of the fungal cell wall. **Spectrum:** ▪ Active against *Histoplasma capsulatum, Blastomyces dermatidis, Cryptococcus neoformans, Aspergillus fumigatus,* and *Candida* sp. **Therapeutic Effects:** ▪ Fungistatic effects against susceptible organisms.

PHARMACOKINETICS
Absorption: Absorption following oral administration is enhanced by food.
Distribution: Tissue concentrations are higher than plasma concentrations. Does not enter CSF. Enters breast milk.
Metabolism and Excretion: Mostly metabolized by the liver and excreted in feces. Hydroxyitraconazole, the major metabolite, has antifungal activity.
Half-life: 21 hr.

CONTRAINDICATIONS AND PRECAUTIONS
Contraindicated in: ▪ Hypersensitivity. Cross-sensitivity with other azole antifungals (miconazole, ketoconazole) may occur ▪ Lactation.
Use Cautiously in: ▪ Patients with hepatic impairment (dosage reduction may be required).

ADVERSE REACTIONS AND SIDE EFFECTS*
CNS: fatigue, malaise, headache, somnolence, dizziness.
EENT: tinnitus.
CV: hypertension, edema.
GI: nausea, vomiting, elevated liver enzymes, hepatitis, anorexia, flatulence, diarrhea, abdominal pain.
GU: decreased libido, albuminuria, impotence.
Derm: toxic epidermal necrolysis, rash, pruritus.
Endo: adrenal insufficiency.
F and E: hypokalemia.
MS: rhabdomyolysis.
Misc: fever.

INTERACTIONS
Drug–Drug: ▪ **Phenytoin, phenobarbital, isoniazid, rifampin,** and **carbamazepine** increase metabolism of itraconzole. Increased dosage may be necessary ▪ Itraconazole decreases metabolism and may increase effects of **phenytoin, cyclosporine, oral hypoglycemic agents, warfarin,** and **digoxin** ▪ May increase the risk of arrhythmias with **astemizole** or **terfenadine** ▪ If hypokalemia occurs, the risk of **cardiac glycoside** toxicity is increased.
Drug–Food: ▪ Food increases absorption.

ROUTE AND DOSAGE
▪ **PO (Adults):** 200 mg tid for the first 3 days, then 200–400 mg/day as a single daily dose. Daily doses >200 mg should be given in 2 divided doses.

AVAILABILITY
▪ *Capsules:* 100 mg.

TIME/ACTION PROFILE (blood levels)

	ONSET	PEAK
PO	rapid	4 hr

NURSING IMPLICATIONS
ASSESSMENT
▫ Assess patient for signs and symptoms of infection (vital signs, lung

sounds, sputum, WBC) prior to and periodically throughout therapy.

□ Specimens for culture should be taken prior to instituting therapy. Therapy may be started before results are obtained.

■ **Lab Test Considerations:** Hepatic function tests should be monitored prior to and periodically throughout course of therapy, especially in patients with pre-existing hepatic function abnormalities.

POTENTIAL NURSING DIAGNOSES

■ Infection, high risk for (indications).
■ Knowledge deficit related to medication regimen (patient/family teaching).

IMPLEMENTATION

■ **PO:** Administer with a meal or snack to minimize nausea and vomiting.

PATIENT/FAMILY TEACHING

□ Instruct patient to take medication exactly as directed, even if feeling better. Doses should be taken at the same time each day.

□ May occasionally cause drowsiness. Caution patient to avoid driving or other activities requiring alertness until response to medication is known.

□ Instruct patient to notify physician if signs and symptoms of liver dysfunction (unusual fatigue, anorexia, nausea, vomiting, jaundice, dark urine, or pale stools) occur.

EVALUATION

Effectiveness of therapy can be demonstrated by: ■ Resolution of clinical and laboratory indications of fungal infections. Minimal treatment for systemic fungal infections is 3 mo. Inadequate period of treatment may lead to recurrence of active infection.

KANAMYCIN
(kan-a-**mye**-sin)
Kantrex

CLASSIFICATION(S):
Anti-infective (aminoglycoside)
Pregnancy Category D

INDICATIONS

■ Treatment of gram-negative bacillary infections and infections due to staphylococci when penicillins or other less toxic drugs are contraindicated ■ Treatment of the following infections due to susceptible organisms: □ Bone infections □ Respiratory tract infections □ Skin and soft tissue infections □ Abdominal infections □ Complicated urinary tract infections □ Endocarditis □ Septicemia ■ Treatment of enterococcal infections requires synergy with a penicillin ■ Adjunct therapy in the management of hepatic encephalopathy.

ACTION

■ Inhibits protein synthesis in bacteria at the level of the 30S ribosome. **Therapeutic Effect:** ■ Bactericidal action against susceptible bacteria. **Spectrum:** ■ *Pseudomonas aeruginosa* ■ *Klebsiella pneumoniae* ■ *Escherichia coli* ■ *Proteus* ■ *Serratia* ■ *Acenitobacter.*

PHARMACOKINETICS

Absorption: Poorly absorbed following oral administration. Well absorbed after IM administration. Some absorption follows intraperitoneal instillation.

Distribution: Widely distributed into extracellular fluids following IM or IV administration. Crosses the placenta. Poor penetration into CSF.

Metabolism and Excretion: Excretion is mainly (>90%) renal. Minimal amounts metabolized by the liver.

Half-life: 2–4 hr (increased in renal impairment).

CONTRAINDICATIONS AND PRECAUTIONS

Contraindicated in: ■ Hypersensitivity ■ Cross-sensitivity with other aminoglycosides may exist ■ Hypersensitivity to bisulfites (parenteral only).

Use Cautiously in: ■ Renal impairment of any kind (dosage adjustments necessary) ▪ Pregnancy and lactation (safety not established) ▪ Neuromuscular diseases, such as myasthenia gravis.

ADVERSE REACTIONS AND SIDE EFFECTS*

EENT: <u>ototoxicity</u> (vestibular and cochlear).
GU: <u>nephrotoxicity</u>.
Neuro: enhanced neuromuscular blockade.
Misc: hypersensitivity reactions.

INTERACTIONS

Drug–Drug: ▪ Inactivated by penicillins when coadministered to patients with renal insufficiency ▪ Possible respiratory paralysis after **inhalation anesthetics (ether, cyclopropane, halothane,** or **nitrous oxide)** or **neuromuscular blockers (tubocurarine, succinylcholine, decamethonium)** ▪ Increased incidence of ototoxicity with **loop diuretics (ethacrynic acid, furosemide)** ▪ Increased incidence of nephrotoxicity with other **nephrotoxic drugs**.

ROUTE AND DOSAGE

Not to exceed 1.5 g/day by any route.
▪ **IM, IV (Adults, Children, Infants):** 15 mg/kg/day in divided doses q 6–12 hr.
▪ **PO (Adults):** 4–6 g/day in divided doses for preoperative intestinal antisepsis; 8–12 g/day in divided doses for hepatic encephalopathy.

AVAILABILITY

▪ *Capsules:* 500 mg ▪ *Injection:* 75 mg/2 ml, 500 mg/2 ml, 1 g/3 ml.

TIME/ACTION PROFILE (blood levels)

	ONSET	PEAK
IM	rapid	0.5–2 hr
IV	rapid	end of infusion

NURSING IMPLICATIONS

ASSESSMENT

▫ Assess patient for infection (vital signs; appearance of wound, sputum, urine, and stool; WBC) at beginning and throughout course of therapy.

▫ Obtain specimens for culture and sensitivity prior to initiating therapy. First dose may be given before receiving results.

▫ Evaluate eighth cranial nerve function by audiometry prior to and throughout course of therapy. Hearing loss is usually of the high-frequency type. Prompt recognition and intervention is essential in preventing permanent damage. Also monitor for vestibular dysfunction (vertigo, ataxia, nausea, vomiting). Eighth cranial nerve dysfunction is associated with persistently elevated peak kanamycin levels.

▫ Monitor intake and output and daily weight to assess hydration status and renal function.

▫ Assess patient for signs of superinfection (fever, upper respiratory infection, vaginal itching or discharge, increasing malaise, diarrhea). Report to physician.

▪ **Lab Test Considerations:** Monitor renal function by urinalysis, specific gravity, BUN, creatinine, and creatinine clearance prior to and throughout therapy.

▫ May cause increased AST (SGOT), ALT (SGPT), LDH, bilirubin, and serum alkaline phosphatase levels.

▫ May cause decreased serum calcium, magnesium, sodium, and potassium levels.

▪ **Toxicity and Overdose:** Blood levels should be monitored periodically during therapy. Timing of blood levels is important in interpreting results. Draw blood for peak levels 30–60 min after IM injection and immediately after IV infusion is completed. Trough levels should be drawn just prior to next dose. Acceptable peak level is 15–30 mcg/ml; trough level should not exceed 5–10 mcg/ml.

POTENTIAL NURSING DIAGNOSES

▪ Infection, high risk for (indications).

K

- Sensory-perceptual alteration: auditory (side effects).
- Knowledge deficit related to medication regimen (patient/family teaching).

IMPLEMENTATION

- **General Info:** Keep patient well-hydrated (1500–2000 ml/day) during therapy.
- **PO:** May be taken without regard to meals.
- **IM:** Administration should be deep into a well-developed muscle.
- **Intermittent Infusion:** Dilute each 500 mg of kanamycin in 100–200 ml or each 1 g in 200–400 ml of D5W, D10W, D5/0.9% NaCl, 0.9% NaCl, or lactated Ringer's solution. Darkening of solution does not alter potency.
- **Rate:** Infuse slowly over 30–60 min. Flush IV line with D5W or 0.9% NaCl following administration.
- **Y-Site Compatibility:** ■ cyclophosphamide ■ furosemide ■ hydromorphone ■ magnesium sulfate ■ meperidine ■ morphine ■ perphenazine ■ potassium chloride.
- **Additive Incompatibility:** Manufacturer does not recommend admixing with other antibacterial agents.

PATIENT/FAMILY TEACHING

- **General Info:** Instruct patient to report signs of hypersensitivity, tinnitus, vertigo, or hearing loss.
- **PO:** Instruct patient to take kanamycin as directed. Missed doses should be taken as soon as remembered if not almost time for next dose; do not double doses.

EVALUATION

Clinical response can be evaluated by:
■ Resolution of the signs and symptoms of infection. If no response is seen within 3–5 days, new cultures should be taken. Length of time for resolution depends on the organism and site of infection.

KAOLIN/PECTIN
(**kay**-oh-lin **pek**-tin)
{Donnagel-MB}, K-C, K-P, K-Pek, {Kao-Con}, Kao-Spen, Kaotin, Kapectolin

CLASSIFICATION(S):
Antidiarrheal
Pregnancy Category UK

INDICATIONS

■ Adjunctive therapy in the treatment of mild to moderate diarrhea.

ACTION

■ Acts as an adsorbent and protectant
■ Decreases stool fluid content, although total water loss does not change. **Therapeutic Effect:** ■ Relief of diarrhea.

PHARMACOKINETICS

Absorption: Action is local, not systemically absorbed.
Distribution: Distribution not known.
Metabolism and Excretion: Pectin decomposes in the GI tract.
Half-life: UK.

CONTRAINDICATIONS AND PRECAUTIONS

Contraindicated in: ■ Severe abdominal pain of unknown cause, especially when associated with fever ■ Children <3 yr.
Use Cautiously in: ■ Elderly patients (>60 yr) ■ Diarrhea continuing >48 hr (physician should be consulted).

ADVERSE REACTIONS AND SIDE EFFECTS*

GI: constipation.

INTERACTIONS

Drug–Drug: ■ Decreases the absorption of **digoxin** and **chloroquine**.

{} = Available in Canada only.
*<u>Underlines</u> indicate most frequent; **CAPITALS** indicate life-threatening.

ROUTE AND DOSAGE

Kaolin/pectin suspension contains 0.65–0.98 g kaolin/5 ml and 21.7–43.5 mg pectin/5 ml. Concentrated suspension contains 1.46 g kaolin/5 ml and 32.4 mg pectin/5 ml.

- **PO (Adults):** 60–120 ml (45–90 ml concentrate) after each loose stool.
- **PO (Children 6–11 yr):** 30–60 ml (15 ml concentrate) after each loose stool.
- **PO (Children 3–6 yr):** 15–30 ml (7.5 ml concentrate) after each loose stool.

AVAILABILITY

- **Suspension:** 5.2 g kaolin plus 260 mg pectin/30 ml, 5.85 g kaolin plus 130 mg pectin/30 ml ■ {**Concentrated suspension:** 8.8 g kaolin plus 195 mg pectin/30 ml} ■ **In combination with:** paregoric (Parepectolin), bismuth, carboxymethycellulose, and others. See Appendix A.

TIME/ACTION PROFILE (relief of diarrhea)

	ONSET	PEAK	DURATION
PO	30 min	UK	4–6 hr

NURSING IMPLCATIONS

ASSESSMENT
- Assess the frequency and consistency of stools and bowel sounds prior to and throughout course of therapy.
- Assess fluid and electrolyte balance and skin turgor for dehydration.

POTENTIAL NURSING DIAGNOSES
- Diarrhea (indications).
- Constipation (side effects).
- Knowledge deficit related to medication regimen (patient/family teaching).

IMPLEMENTATION
- **General Info:** Administer after each loose bowel movement until diarrhea is controlled.
- **PO:** Shake suspension well prior to administration.

PATIENT/FAMILY TEACHING
- Instruct patient to notify physician if diarrhea persists longer than 48 hr or if fever or abdominal pain develops.

EVALUATION
Effectiveness of therapy can be demonstrated by: ■ Decrease in frequency of loose stools □ Return to soft, formed stools.

KETAMINE
(**ket**-a-meen)
Ketalar

CLASSIFICATION(S):
Anesthetic (general)
Pregnancy Category UK

INDICATIONS

- Provides anesthesia for short-term procedures ■ As induction prior to the use of other anesthetics ■ As a supplement to other anesthetics.

ACTION

- Blocks afferent impulses of pain perception ■ Suppresses spinal cord activity ■ Effects CNS transmitter systems. **Therapeutic Effect:** ■ Anesthesia with profound analgesia, minimal respiratory depression, and minimal skeletal muscle relaxation.

PHARMACOKINETICS

Absorption: Rapidly absorbed following IM administration.
Distribution: Rapidly distributed, enters the CNS. Crosses the placenta.
Metabolism and Excretion: Mostly metabolized by the liver. Some conversion to another active compound.
Half-life: 2.5 hr.

CONTRAINDICATIONS AND PRECAUTIONS

Contraindicated in: ■ Hypersensitivity ■ Psychiatric disturbances ■ Hypertension ■ Pregnancy or lactation.
Use Cautiously in: ■ Cardiovascular disease ■ Procedures involving larynx, pharynx, or bronchial tree (muscle relaxants required) ■ History of alcohol

K

abuse ▪ Cerebral trauma ▪ Intracerebral mass or hemorrhage ▪ Hyperthyroidism ▪ History of psychiatric problems ▪ Increased CSF pressure ▪ Increased intraocular pressure ▪ Severe eye trauma.

ADVERSE REACTIONS AND SIDE EFFECTS*

CNS: emergence reactions.
EENT: diplopia, nystagmus, increased intraocular pressure.
Resp: respiratory depression and apnea (rapid IV administration of large doses), laryngospasm.
CV: hypertension, tachycardia, hypotension, bradycardia, arrhythmias.
GI: nausea, vomiting, excessive salivation.
Derm: erythema, rash.
Local: pain at injection site.
MS: increased skeletal muscle tone.

INTERACTIONS

Drug–Drug: ▪ Use with barbiturates or opioid analgesics may result in prolonged recovery time ▪ Use with halothane may result in decreased blood pressure, cardiac output, and heart rate ▪ Use with tubocurarine or nondepolarizing neuromuscular blocking agents may result in prolonged respiratory depression ▪ Concurrent use with thyroid hormone increases the risk of tachycardia and hypertension ▪ Concurrent administration with diazepam may decrease the incidence of emergence reaction ▪ Concurrent administration with atropine may increase the incidence of unpleasant dreams.

ROUTE AND DOSAGE

▪ IV (Adults and Children): Induction—1–4.5 mg/kg—2 mg produces 5–10 min of surgical anesthesia or 1–2 mg/kg (at rate of 0.5 mg/kg/min). May be used with concurrent diazepam. Maintenance—½ to the full induction dose may be repeated as needed to maintain anesthesia. If given with concurrent diazepam, an infusion of 0.1–0.5 mg/min may be

used, augmented by 2–5 mg doses of diazepam.
▪ IM (Adults and Children): 5–10 mg/kg (10 mg/kg produces 12–25 min of surgical anesthesia).

AVAILABILITY

▪ Injection: 10 mg/ml, 50 mg/ml, 100 mg/ml.

TIME/ACTION PROFILE (anesthesia)

	ONSET	PEAK	DURATION
IV	30 sec	UK	5–10 min
IM	3–4 min	UK	12–25 min

NURSING IMPLICATIONS

ASSESSMENT

▫ Assess level of consciousness frequently throughout therapy. Ketamine produces a dissociative state. The patient does not appear to be asleep and experiences a feeling of dissociation from the environment.

▫ Monitor blood pressure, ECG, and respiratory status frequently throughout therapy. May cause hypertension and tachycardia. May cause increased cerebrospinal fluid pressure and increased intraocular pressure.

▪ Toxicity and Overdose: Respiratory depression or apnea may be treated with mechanical ventilation or analeptics.

POTENTIAL NURSING DIAGNOSES

▪ Injury, high risk for (side effects).
▪ Sensory-perceptual alteration (adverse reactions).
▪ Knowledge deficit related to medication regimen (patient/family teaching).

IMPLEMENTATION

▪ General Info: Administer on an empty stomach to prevent vomiting and aspiration.

▫ May be administered concurrently with a drying agent (atropine, scopolamine), as ketamine increases salivary and tracheobronchial mucous gland secretions. Atropine may also increase the incidence of unpleasant dreams.

▫ Patients may experience a state of confusion (emergence delirium) during recovery from ketamine. Administration of a benzodiazepine and minimizing verbal, tactile, and visual stimulation may prevent emergence delirium. Severe emergence delirium may be treated with short- or ultra-short-acting barbiturates.

■ **Direct IV:** Dilute 100 mg/ml concentration with equal parts of Sterile Water for Injection, 0.9% NaCl, or D5W.

■ *Rate:* Administer over 60 sec unless a rapid-sequence induction technique is indicated. More rapid administration may cause respiratory depression, apnea, and hypertension.

■ **Continuous Infusion:** Dilute 10 ml of 50 mg/ml concentration or 5 ml of 100 mg/ml concentration with 500 ml of 0.9% NaCl or D5W and mix well, for a concentration of 1 mg/ml. Dilution with 250 ml may be used if fluid restriction is needed.

■ *Rate:* Administer at a rate of 1–2 mg/min. Dosage must be titrated according to individual patient requirements. Tonic-clonic movements during anesthesia do not indicate the need for more ketamine.

■ **Syringe Compatibility:** ■ benzquinamide.

■ **Syringe Incompatibility:** ■ barbiturates ■ diazepam ■ doxipram.

PATIENT/FAMILY TEACHING

▫ Psychomotor impairment may last for 24 hr following anesthesia. Caution patient to avoid driving or other activities requiring alertness until response to medication is known.

▫ Advise patient to avoid alcohol or other CNS depressants for 24 hr following anesthesia.

EVALUATION

Effectiveness of therapy can be demonstrated by: ■ Sense of dissociation and general anesthesia without muscle relaxation.

KETOCONAZOLE
(kee-toe-**koe**-na-zole)
Nizoral

CLASSIFICATION(S):
Antifungal
Pregnancy Category C

INDICATIONS

■ **PO:** Treatment of the following fungal infections: ▫ Candidiasis (disseminated and mucocutaneous) ▫ Chromomycosis ▫ Coccidiomycosis ▫ Histoplasmosis ▫ Paracoccidiomycosis ■ **Top:** Treatment of fungal dermatologic infections caused by: ▫ *Tinea corporis* ▫ *Tinea cruris* ▫ *Tinea versicolor* ■ **Shampoo:** Treatment of seborrheic dermatitis and dandruff due to *Pityrosporum ovale.* **Unlabeled Uses:** ■ **PO:** Treatment of advanced prostate cancer ■ Treatment of Cushing's syndrome.

ACTION

■ Disrupts fungal cell wall ■ Interferes with fungal metabolism ■ Also inhibits the production of adrenal steroids. **Therapeutic Effect:** ■ Fungistatic or fungicidal action against susceptible organisms, depending on organism and site of infection. **Spectrum:** ■ Active against many pathogenic fungi, including: ▫ Blastomycoses ▫ *Candida* ▫ *Coccidioides* ▫ *Cryptococcus* ▫ *Histoplasma* ▫ Many dermatophytes.

PHARMACOKINETICS

Absorption: Absorption from the GI tract is pH dependent; increasing pH decreases absorption. Negligible absorption following topical administration.

Distribution: Widely distributed. CNS penetration is unpredictable and minimal. Crosses the placenta and enters breast milk.

Metabolism and Excretion: Partially metabolized by the liver. Excreted in feces via biliary excretion.

Half-life: 8 hr.

K

CONTRAINDICATIONS AND PRECAUTIONS

Contraindicated in: ▪ Hypersensitivity ▪ Pregnancy or lactation ▪ Cream contains sulfite and should be avoided in patients with known intolerance.
Use Cautiously in: ▪ History of liver disease ▪ Achlorhydria ▪ Alcoholism.

ADVERSE REACTIONS AND SIDE EFFECTS*

Unless noted, adverse reactions listed are for oral ketoconazole.
CNS: dizziness, drowsiness.
EENT: photophobia.
GI: HEPATITIS, nausea, vomiting, abdominal pain, flatulence, constipation, diarrhea.
Derm: PO—rashes; Top—stinging, burning, irritation; Shampoo—increased hair loss, altered hair or scalp texture.
Endo: gynecomastia.

INTERACTIONS

For oral ketoconazole, unless indicated.
Drug–Drug: ▪ Drugs that increase gastric pH, including **antacids, nizatadine, famotidine, ranitidine, cimetidine,** or **omeprazole** may decrease absorption ▪ Additive hepatoxicity with other **hepatotoxic agents,** including **alcohol** ▪ **Rifampin** or **isoniazid** may decrease serum levels and effectiveness ▪ May enhance the activity of **oral anticoagulants** ▪ May increase blood levels and toxicity of **cyclosporine** or **glucocorticoids** ▪ May alter the metabolism of **phenytoin** ▪ May decrease serum levels and effectiveness of **theophylline** ▪ Increased risk of arrhythmias with **terfenadine** or **astemizole.**

ROUTE AND DOSAGE

▪ **PO (Adults):** 200–400 mg/day, single dose.
▪ **PO (Children >2 yr):** 3.3–6.6 mg/kg/day, single dose.
▪ **Top (Adults and Children):** 2% cream applied 1–2 times daily.
▪ **Shampoo (Adults):** Massage 2% shampoo into scalp for 1 min, rinse, then reapply for 3 min, then rinse and dry. Shampoo twice weekly for 4 wk waiting at least 3 days between treatments.

AVAILABILITY

▪ *Tablets:* 200 mg ▪ *Cream:* 2% ▪ *Shampoo:* 2%.

TIME/ACTION PROFILE (blood levels)

	ONSET	PEAK
PO	rapid	1–4 hr

NURSING IMPLICATIONS

ASSESSMENT

▫ Assess infected area prior to and periodically throughout therapy.
▫ Specimens for culture should be taken prior to instituting therapy. Therapy may be started before results are obtained.
▪ **Lab Test Considerations:** Hepatic function tests should be monitored prior to and periodically throughout course of therapy. May cause increased AST (SGOT), ALT (SGPT), serum alkaline phosphatase, and bilirubin concentrations.
▫ May cause decreased serum testosterone concentrations.

POTENTIAL NURSING DIAGNOSES

▪ Infection, high risk for (indications).
▪ Knowledge deficit related to medication regimen (patient/family teaching).

IMPLEMENTATION

▪ **PO:** Administer with meals or snacks to minimize nausea and vomiting.
▫ Shake suspension well prior to administration.
▫ Do not administer histamine H_2 antagonists or antacids within 2 hr of ketoconazole.
▫ For patients with achlorhydria, dissolve each tablet in 4 ml of aqueous solution of 0.2 N hydrochloric acid. Use a glass or plastic straw to avoid contact with teeth and follow with a glass of water, swished in mouth and

swallowed. Patients with AIDS may be at increased risk for achlorhydria.

- **Top:** Apply enough medication to cover affected and surrounding areas and rub in gently.

PATIENT/FAMILY TEACHING

- **General Info:** Instruct patient to take medication exactly as directed, even if feeling better. Doses should be taken at the same time each day. If a dose is missed, take as soon as remembered; if almost time for next dose, space missed dose and next dose 10–12 hr apart.
- May cause dizziness or drowsiness. Caution patient to avoid driving or other activities requiring alertness until response to medication is known.
- Advise patient to avoid taking over-the-counter antacids within 2 hr of ketoconazole.
- Caution patient to wear sunglasses and to avoid prolonged exposure to bright light to prevent photophobic reactions.
- Advise patient to avoid concurrent use of alcohol while taking ketoconazole.
- Instruct patient to notify physician if abdominal pain, fever, or diarrhea become pronounced or if signs and symptoms of liver dysfunction (unusual fatigue, anorexia, nausea, vomiting, jaundice, dark urine, or pale stools) occur.
- **Top:** Caution patient to avoid contact of medication with eyes.
- Advise patient to use a bland, absorbent or antifungal powder on the skin between administration times for cream.
- Instruct patient with tinea cruris to wear loose-fitting cotton underwear and to avoid tight-fitting or synthetic clothing.
- Instruct patient with tinea pedis to dry feet, especially between toes, after bathing. Sandals or well-ventilated shoes with cotton socks should be worn and socks changed daily or

more often if feet perspire excessively. Avoid wool or synthetic socks.

- Advise patient to notify physician if skin irritation develops or if no improvement is seen in 2–4 wk.
- **Shampoo:** Moisten hair and scalp with water and apply enough shampoo to lather scalp and hair. Gently massage over entire scalp for 1 min. Rinse thoroughly with warm water. Repeat, leaving shampoo on scalp for an additional 3 min and rinse.
- Shampoo twice weekly for 4 wk with at least 3 days between shampooing, then intermittently prn.
- Advise patient that shampoo may remove curl from permanently waved hair.

EVALUATION

Effectiveness of therapy can be demonstrated by: ■ Resolution of clinical and laboratory indications of fungal infections □ Minimal treatment for candidiasis is 1–2 wk and for other systemic mycoses is 6 mo □ Chronic mucocutaneous candidiasis usually requires maintenance therapy □ Tinea infections should be treated for at least 2–4 wk ■ Reduction of scaling due to dandruff.

KETOPROFEN
(kee-toe-**proe**-fen)
Orudis, {Orudis-E}, Oruvail

CLASSIFICATION(S):
Nonsteroidal anti-inflammatory
agent, Nonopioid analgesic
Pregnancy Category B

INDICATIONS

■ Management of inflammatory disorders, including: □ Rheumatoid arthritis □ Osteoarthritis ■ Management of mild to moderate pain, including dysmenorrhea.

ACTION

■ Inhibits prostaglandin synthesis. **Therapeutic Effects:** ■ Suppression of pain and inflammation.

K

PHARMACOKINETICS

Absorption: Well absorbed from the GI tract.
Distribution: Distribution not known.
Metabolism and Excretion: Mostly (60%) metabolized by the liver. Some renal excretion.
Half-life: 2–4 hr.

CONTRAINDICATIONS AND PRECAUTIONS

Contraindicated in: ▪ Hypersensitivity ▪ Cross-sensitivity may exist with other nonsteroidal anti-inflammatory agents, including aspirin ▪ Active GI bleeding ▪ Ulcer disease.
Use Cautiously in: ▪ Severe cardiovascular, renal, or hepatic disease ▪ History of ulcer disease ▪ Pregnancy, lactation, or children (safety not established) ▪ Renal impairment (dosage reduction suggested) ▪ Extended-release product should not be used in elderly patients, patients of small stature, or patients with renal impairment.

ADVERSE REACTIONS AND SIDE EFFECTS*

CNS: headache, drowsiness, dizziness.
EENT: blurred vision, tinnitus.
CV: edema.
GI: nausea, dyspepsia, vomiting, diarrhea, constipation, GI BLEEDING, discomfort, HEPATITIS, flatulence, anorexia.
GU: renal failure, hematuria, cystitis.
Derm: rashes, photosensitivity.
Endo: gynecomastia.
Hemat: blood dyscrasias, prolonged bleeding time.
MS: myalgia.
Misc: allergic reactions, including ANAPHYLAXIS, fever.

INTERACTIONS

Drug–Drug: ▪ Aspirin alters distribution, metabolism, and excretion of ketoprofen (concurrent use not recommended) ▪ Additive adverse GI effects with other **nonsteroidal anti-inflammatory agents, potassium supplements,** **glucocorticoids,** or **alcohol** ▪ Chronic use with **acetaminophen** may increase the risk of adverse renal reactions ▪ May decrease the effectiveness of **diuretics** or **antihypertensive** therapy ▪ May increase the hypoglycemic effects of **insulin** or **oral hypoglycemic agents** ▪ May increase serum **lithium** levels and increase the risk of toxicity ▪ Increases the risk of toxicity from **methotrexate** ▪ **Probenecid** increases risk of toxicity from ketoprofen (concurrent use not recommended) ▪ Increased risk of bleeding with **cefamandole, cefotetan, cefoperazone, valproic acid** or **plicamycin, heparin, thrombolytic agents,** or **oral anticoagulants** ▪ Increased risk of adverse hematologic reactions with **antineoplastic agents** or **radiation therapy.**

ROUTE AND DOSAGE

Anti-inflammatory
▪ **PO (Adults):** 150–300 mg/day in 3–4 divided doses or 200 mg once daily as extended-release product.

Analgesic
▪ **PO (Adults):** 25–50 mg q 6–8 hr.

AVAILABILITY

▪ *Capsules:* 25 mg, 50 mg, 75 mg.

TIME/ACTION PROFILE

	ONSET	PEAK	DURATION
PO (analgesic)	1–2 days	UK	UK
PO (anti-inflammatory)	few days– 1 wk	UK	UK

NURSING IMPLICATIONS

ASSESSMENT
▪ **General Info:** Patients who have asthma, aspirin-induced allergy, and nasal polyps are at increased risk for developing hypersensitivity reactions. Assess for rhinitis, wheezing, and urticaria.
▪ **Arthritis:** Assess pain and range of motion prior to and 1 hr following administration.

*Underlines indicate most frequent; **CAPITALS** indicate life-threatening.

- **Pain:** Assess pain (note type, location, and intensity) prior to and 1 hr following administration.
- **Lab Test Considerations:** BUN, serum creatinine, CBC, and liver function tests should be evaluated periodically in patients receiving prolonged courses of therapy.
- May prolong bleeding time by 3–4 min.
- May cause decreased hemoglobin and hematocrit.
- May cause increased AST (SGOT), ALT (SGPT), LDH, and serum alkaline phosphatase.

POTENTIAL NURSING DIAGNOSES
- Pain (indications).
- Physical mobility, impaired (indications).
- Knowledge deficit related to medication regimen (patient/family teaching).

IMPLEMENTATION
- **General Info:** Coadministration with opioid analgesics may have additive analgesic effects and may permit lower opioid doses.
- Analgesic is more effective if given before pain becomes severe.
- **PO:** For rapid initial effect, administer 30 min before or 2 hr after meals. Capsules may be administered with food, milk, or antacids containing aluminum hydroxide and magnesium hydroxide to decrease GI irritation. Food slows but does not reduce the extent of absorption.
- **Dysmenorrhea:** Administer as soon as possible after the onset of menses. Prophylactic treatment has not been proved effective.

PATIENT/FAMILY TEACHING
- Advise patient to take this medication with a full glass of water and to remain in an upright position for 15–30 min after administration.
- Instruct patient to take medication exactly as directed. If a dose is missed, it should be taken as soon as remembered but not if almost time for the next dose. Do not double doses.

- Medication may occasionally cause drowsiness or dizziness. Advise patient to avoid driving or other activities requiring alertness until response to medication is known.
- Caution patient to avoid the concurrent use of alcohol, aspirin, ibuprofen, acetaminophen, or other over-the-counter medications without consulting a physician.
- Advise patient to wear sunscreen and protective clothing to prevent photosensitivity reactions.
- Instruct patient to notify physician if rash, itching, chills, fever, muscle aches, visual disturbances, weight gain, edema, black stools, or persistent headache occurs.
- Advise patient to notify physician or dentist of medication regimen prior to treatment or surgery.

EVALUATION
Effectiveness of therapy can be demonstrated by: ▪ Improved joint mobility ▪ Decrease in severity of moderate pain. Improvement in arthritis may be seen in a few days to 1 wk; 2–3 wk may be required for maximum effectiveness. Patients who do not respond to one nonsteroidal anti-inflammatory agent may respond to another.

KETOROLAC
(kee-**toe**-role-ak)
Toradol

CLASSIFICATION(S):
Nonopioid analgesic, Nonsteroidal anti-inflammatory agent
Pregnancy Category B

K

INDICATIONS
- **PO, IM:** Short-term (not to exceed 5 days for IM) management of pain
- **Ophth:** Management of ocular itching due to seasonal allergic conjunctivitis.

ACTION
- Inhibits prostaglandin synthesis producing peripherally mediated analge-

sia ▪ Also has antipyretic and anti-inflammatory properties. **Therapeutic Effects:** ▪ **PO, IM:** Decreased pain ▪ **Ophth:** Decreased ocular itching.

PHARMACOKINETICS

Absorption: Rapidly and completely absorbed following IM administration.
Distribution: Enters breast milk in low concentrations. >99% bound to plasma proteins.
Metabolism and Excretion: <50% metabolized by the liver. Ketorolac and its metabolites are excreted primarily by the kidneys (92%). 6% excreted in feces.
Half-life: 4.5 hr (range 3.8–6.3; increased in elderly patients and patients with impaired renal function).

CONTRAINDICATIONS AND PRECAUTIONS

Contraindicated in: ▪ Hypersensitivity ▪ Cross-sensitivity with other nonsteroidal anti-inflammatory agents may exist ▪ Known alcohol intolerance (injection only) ▪ Patients wearing soft contact lenses (ophth only).
Use Cautiously in: ▪ Pregnancy and children (use not recommended) ▪ Lactation (use with caution) ▪ History of GI bleeding ▪ Renal impairment (dosage reduction may be required) ▪ Cardiovascular disease.

ADVERSE REACTIONS AND SIDE EFFECTS*

Unless noted, adverse reactions are listed for PO/IM ketorolac.

CNS: <u>drowsiness</u>, dizziness, headache, abnormal thinking, euphoria.
EENT: abnormal vision.
Resp: dyspnea, asthma.
CV: edema, vasodilation, pallor.
GI: abnormal taste, dry mouth, nausea, dyspepsia, GI pain, diarrhea, BLEEDING.
GU: urinary frequency, oliguria, renal toxicity.
Hemat: prolonged bleeding time.
Derm: sweating, pruritus, urticaria, purpura.

Local: injection site pain.
Neuro: paresthesia.

INTERACTIONS

Drug–Drug: ▪ Concurrent use with **aspirin** may decrease effectiveness ▪ Additive adverse GI effects with **aspirin**, other **nonsteroidal anti-inflammatory agents, potassium supplements, glucocorticoids** or **alcohol** ▪ Chronic use with **acetaminophen** may increase the risk of adverse renal reactions ▪ May decrease the effectiveness of **diuretics** or **antihypertensive** therapy ▪ May increase serum **lithium** levels and increase the risk of toxicity ▪ Increases the risk of toxicity from **methotrexate** ▪ Increased risk of bleeding with **cefamandole, cefotetan, cefoperazone, valproic acid** or **plicamycin, thrombolytic agents,** or **anticoagulants** ▪ Increased risk of adverse hematologic reactions with **antineoplastic agents** or **radiation therapy** ▪ May increase the risk of nephrotoxicity from **cyclosporine**.

ROUTE AND DOSAGE

▪ **PO (Adults):** 10 mg q 4–6 hr as needed (not to exceed 40 mg/day).
▪ **IM (Adults):** 30–60 mg initially, followed by 15–30 mg q 6 hr (not to exceed 150 mg/day on first day or 120 mg/day thereafter; not to exceed 5 days).
▪ **IM (Elderly Patients):** 30 mg initially, then 15 mg q 6 hr (not to exceed 5 days).
▪ **Ophth (Adults):** 1 drop qid for up to 1 wk.

AVAILABILITY

▪ *Tablets:* 10 mg ▪ *Injection:* 15 mg/ml, 30 mg/ml ▪ *Ophthalmic solution:* 0.5%.

TIME/ACTION PROFILE (analgesic effects)

	ONSET	PEAK	DURATION
IM	about 10 min	75–150 min	3–6 hr
Ophth	UK	UK	UK

*Underlines indicate most frequent; **CAPITALS** indicate life-threatening.

NURSING IMPLICATIONS

ASSESSMENT

- **General Info:** Patients who have asthma, aspirin-induced allergy, and nasal polyps are at increased risk for developing hypersensitivity reactions. Assess for rhinitis, asthma, and urticaria.
- **Pain:** Assess pain (note type, location, and intensity) prior to and 1–2 hr following administration.
- **Ophth:** Assess patient for ocular itching prior to and during therapy.
- **Lab Test Considerations:** Liver function tests, especially AST (SGOT) and ALT (SGPT) should be evaluated periodically in patients receiving prolonged courses of therapy. May cause increased levels.
- □ May cause prolonged bleeding time that may persist for 24–48 hr following discontinuation of therapy.

POTENTIAL NURSING DIAGNOSES

- Pain (indications).
- Knowledge deficit related to medication regimen (patient/family teaching).

IMPLEMENTATION

- □ Coadministration with opioid analgesics may have additive analgesic effects and may permit lower opioid doses.
- □ Ketorolac may be administered on a routine or prn schedule depending on the type and severity of the pain.
- **Ophth:** See Appendix H for instillation of ophthalmic medications.

PATIENT/FAMILY TEACHING

- **General Info:** Instruct patient on how and when to ask for pain medication.
- **Home Care Issues:** Instruct patients taking medication at home on correct technique for IM injection. Instruct patient to take medication exactly as directed. If dose is missed it should be taken as soon as remembered but not if almost time for next dose. Do not double dose.
- □ This medication may cause drowsiness or dizziness. Advise patient to avoid driving or other activities requiring alertness until response to the medication is known.
- □ Caution patient to avoid the concurrent use of alcohol, aspirin, ibuprofen, acetaminophen, or other over-the-counter medications without consultating with physician or pharmacist.
- □ Advise patient to inform physician or dentist of medication regimen prior to treatment or surgery.
- □ Instruct patient to notify physician if rash, itching, visual disturbances, weight gain, edema, black stools, or persistent headache occur.
- **Ophth:** Advise patients with hydrogel soft contact lenses that ketorolac may cause redness and burning.

EVALUATION

Effectiveness of therapy can be demonstrated by: ■ Decrease in severity of pain. Patients who do not respond to one nonsteroidal anti-inflammatory agent may respond to another ■ Relief of ocular itching due to seasonal allergic conjunctivitis.

LABETALOL
(la-**bet**-a-lole)
Normodyne, Trandate

CLASSIFICATION(S):
Beta-adrenergic blocker (nonselective), Antihypertensive
Pregnancy Category C

INDICATIONS

- **PO:** Used alone or in combination with other agents in the treatment of hypertension ■ **IV:** Treatment of severe hypertension. **Unlabeled Uses:** ■ **PO:** Angina pectoris ■ **IV:** Production of controlled hypotension during surgery.

ACTION

- Blocks stimulation of beta$_1$ (myocardial) and beta$_2$ (pulmonary, vascular, or uterine) receptor sites ■ Has alpha-adrenergic blocking activity, which results in peripheral vasodilation and orthostatic hypotension. **Therapeutic**

Effects: ▪ Decreased heart rate and blood pressure.

PHARMACOKINETICS

Absorption: Although absorbed following oral administration, rapid metabolism results in low systemic bioavailability (25%).
Distribution: Moderate penetration of the CNS. Crosses the placenta and enters breast milk.
Metabolism and Excretion: Undergoes extensive hepatic metabolism.
Half-life: 3–8 hr.

CONTRAINDICATIONS AND PRECAUTIONS

Contraindicated in: ▪ Hypersensitivity to labetolol ▪ Hypersensitivity to parabens (IV only) ▪ Uncompensated congestive heart failure ▪ Pulmonary edema ▪ Cardiogenic shock ▪ Bradycardia ▪ Heart block ▪ Pregnancy or lactation (may cause apnea, low Apgar scores, bradycardia, and hypoglycemia in the newborn) ▪ Patients wearing soft contact lenses (ophth only).
Use Cautiously in: ▪ Thyrotoxicosis or hypoglycemia (may mask symptoms) ▪ Do not withdraw abruptly ▪ Renal impairment (dosage reduction recommended) ▪ Children (safety not established).

ADVERSE REACTIONS AND SIDE EFFECTS*

CNS: fatigue, weakness, dizziness, depression, memory loss, mental changes, nightmares.
CV: BRADYCARDIA, CONGESTIVE HEART FAILURE, PULMONARY EDEMA, orthostatic hypotension, peripheral vasoconstriction.
EENT: dry eyes, blurred vision; Ophth only: transient burning, stinging, irritation.
GI: constipation, diarrhea, nausea, change in taste.
GU: impotence, diminished libido, urinary retention.
Derm: rash, itching.
Endo: hyperglycemia, hypoglycemia.

MS: joint pain, arthralgia.
Resp: bronchospasm, wheezing.

INTERACTIONS

Drug–Drug: ▪ **Halothane** anesthesia may produce severe myocardial depression ▪ Additive bradycardia may occur with concurrent use of **cardiac glycosides** ▪ Additive hypotension may occur with other **antihypertensive agents, nitrates,** and acute ingestion of **alcohol** ▪ Concurrent **thyroid** administration may decrease effectiveness ▪ May antagonize **beta-adrenergic bronchodilators** ▪ **Cimetidine** decreases metabolism and may increase toxicity ▪ **Glutethimide** may decrease the effects of labetolol ▪ May blunt tachycardia produced by **nitroglycerin** ▪ Avoid concurrent **MAO inhibitor** therapy (may produce hypertension for up to 14 days following discontinuation of MAO inhibitor).
Drug–Food: ▪ Food increases oral absorption.

ROUTE AND DOSAGE

▪ **PO (Adults):** 100 mg bid, increase by 100 mg bid q 2–3 days until desired response is obtained. Usual maintenance dose is 200–400 mg bid.
▪ **IV (Adults):** 20 mg, may give an additional 40–80 mg at 10-min intervals until desired response is obtained or 2-mg/min infusion (total dose should not exceed 300 mg).

AVAILABILITY

▪ *Tablets:* 100 mg, 200 mg, 300 mg
▪ *Injection:* 5 mg/vial.

TIME/ACTION PROFILE
(antihypertensive effect)

	ONSET	PEAK	DURATION
PO	20 min–2 hr	1–4 hr	8–12 hr
IV	2–5 min	5–15 min	2–4 hr (up to 24 hr)

NURSING IMPLICATIONS

ASSESSMENT

▫ Monitor blood pressure and pulse frequently during period of adjustment

---

*Underlines indicate most frequent; **CAPITALS** indicate life-threatening.

and periodically throughout therapy. Confer with physician prior to giving drug if pulse is <50 bpm.

□ Patients receiving labetolol IV must be supine during and for 3 hr after administration. Vital signs should be monitored every 5–15 min during and for several hours after administration. Assess for orthostatic hypotension when assisting patient up from supine position.

□ Monitor intake and output ratios and daily weight. Assess patient routinely for evidence of congestive heart failure (peripheral edema, dyspnea, rales/ crackles, fatigue, weight gain, jugular venous distension).

■ **Lab Test Considerations:** Hepatic and renal function and CBC should be monitored routinely in patients receiving prolonged therapy.

□ May cause elevations in serum potassium, uric acid, LDH, AST (SGOT), ALT (SGPT), alkaline phosphatase, ANA titers, BUN, serum lipoprotein, and triglyceride concentrations.

POTENTIAL NURSING DIAGNOSES

■ Cardiac output, decreased (indications, adverse reactions).

■ Knowledge deficit related to medication regimen (patient/family teaching).

■ Noncompliance (patient/family teaching).

IMPLEMENTATION

■ **PO:** Administer with meals or directly after eating to enhance absorption.

■ **IV:** Solution ranges from clear, colorless to slight yellow in color.

■ **Direct IV:** Administer by injecting 20 mg over 2 min; increase dose to 40–80 mg every 10 min until desired response is achieved.

■ **Continuous Infusion:** Add 200 mg to 160 ml of diluent (1 mg/1 ml solution) or 200 mg to 250 ml of diluent (2 mg/ 3 ml solution). Compatible diluents include D5W, 0.9% NaCl, D5/0.25% NaCl, D5/0.9% NaCl, D5/Ringer's solution, D5/LR, Ringer's and lactated Ringer's solution.

■ *Rate:* Administer at a rate of 2 mg/ min and titrate for desired response. Infuse via infusion pump to ensure accurate dosage of medication.

■ **Y-Site Compatibility:** ■ amikacin ■ aminophylline ■ ampicillin ■ butorphanol ■ calcium gluconate ■ cefazolin ■ ceftazidine ■ ceftizoxime ■ chloramphenicol ■ cimetidine ■ clindamycin ■ dopamine ■ enalaprilat ■ erythromycin lactobionate ■ famotidine ■ fentanyl ■ gentamicin ■ heparin ■ lidocaine ■ magnesium sulfate ■ meperidine ■ metronidazole ■ morphine ■ oxycillin ■ penicillin G potassium ■ piperacillin ■ potassium chloride ■ potassium phosphate ■ ranitidine ■ sodium acetate ■ tobramycin ■ trimethoprim/sulfamethoxazole ■ vancomycin.

■ **Y-Site Incompatibility:** ■ cefoperazone ■ nafcillin.

■ **Additive Incompatibility:** ■ sodium bicarbonate.

PATIENT/FAMILY TEACHING

□ Instruct patient to take medication exactly as directed, even if feeling better. If a dose is missed, take as soon as remembered up to 8 hr before next dose. Abrupt withdrawal may precipitate a severe reaction and result in arrhythmias, hypertension, or myocardial ischemia. Labetalol controls but does not cure hypertension.

□ Teach patient and family how to check pulse and blood pressure. Instruct them to take pulse daily and blood pressure biweekly. Advise patient to hold dose and contact physician if pulse is <50 bpm or blood pressure changes significantly.

□ Caution patient to make position changes slowly and to avoid standing in a stationary position for long periods to minimize orthostatic hypotension. Patient should also be instructed to call for assistance when ambulating during period of dose adjustment.

□ Reinforce need to continue additional therapies for hypertension (weight loss, restricted sodium intake, stress reduction, regular exercise, modera-

L

tion of alcohol consumption, and cessation of smoking).

□ Caution patient that this medication may cause increased sensitivity to cold.

□ Advise patient to consult physician or pharmacist before taking any over-the-counter drugs concurrently with this medication.

□ Diabetics should monitor serum glucose closely, especially if weakness, fatigue, or irritability occurs.

□ Advise patient to notify physician if weight gain, peripheral edema, dyspnea, or fatigue occur.

□ Instruct patient to notify physician or dentist of medication regimen prior to treatment or surgery.

□ Advise patient to carry identification describing disease process and medication regimen at all times.

EVALUATION
Effectiveness of therapy can be demonstrated by: ▪ Decrease in blood pressure.

LACTULOSE
(**lak**-tyoo-lose)
Cephulac, Cholac, Chronulac, Constilac, Constulose, Duphalac, Emulose, Enulose, {Lactulax}

CLASSIFICATION(S):
Laxative (hyperosmotic)
Pregnancy Category B

INDICATIONS
▪ Treatment of chronic constipation in adults and in the elderly ▪ Adjunct in the management of hepatic encephalopathy.

ACTION
▪ Increases water content and softens the stool ▪ Lowers the pH of the colon, which inhibits the diffusion of ammonia from the colon into the blood, thereby reducing blood ammonia levels. **Therapeutic Effects:** ▪ Relief of constipation and decreased blood ammonia levels.

PHARMACOKINETICS
Absorption: Less than 3% absorbed following oral administration.
Distribution: Distribution not known.
Metabolism and Excretion: Absorbed lactulose is excreted unchanged in the urine. Unabsorbed lactulose is metabolized by colonic bacteria to lactic, acetic, and formic acids.
Half-life: UK.

CONTRAINDICATIONS AND PRECAUTIONS
Contraindicated in: ▪ Patients on low-galactose diets.
Use Cautiously in: ▪ Diabetes mellitus ▪ Pregnancy, lactation, or children (safety not established) ▪ Excessive or prolonged use (may lead to dependence).

ADVERSE REACTIONS AND SIDE EFFECTS*
GI: <u>cramps</u>, <u>distention</u>, <u>flatulence</u>, <u>belching</u>, diarrhea.
Endo: hyperglycemia (diabetic patients).

INTERACTIONS
Drug–Drug: ▪ Should not be used with **other laxatives** in the treatment of hepatic encephalopathy (leads to inability to determine optimal dose of lactulose) ▪ **Anti-infectives** may diminish effectiveness in hepatic encephalopathy ▪ **Antacids** may decrease the effect of lactulose on colonic pH.

ROUTE AND DOSAGE
Constipation
▪ **PO (Adults):** 15–30 ml/day up to 60 ml/day.
Hepatic Encephalopathy
▪ **PO (Adults):** 30–45 ml 3–4 times/day.
▪ **Rect (Adults):** 300 ml diluted and administered as a retention enema q 4–6 hr.

{} = Available in Canada only.
*<u>Underlines</u> indicate most frequent; **CAPITALS** indicate life-threatening.

AVAILABILITY

- **Syrup:** 10 g lactulose/15 ml.

TIME/ACTION PROFILE (relief of constipation)

	ONSET	PEAK	DURATION
PO	24–48 hr	UK	UK

NURSING IMPLICATIONS

ASSESSMENT

- **General Info:** Assess patient for abdominal distention, presence of bowel sounds, and normal pattern of bowel function.
- Assess color, consistency, and amount of stool produced.
- **Hepatic Encephalopathy:** Assess mental status (orientation, level of consciousness) prior to and periodically throughout course of therapy.
- **Lab Test Considerations:** Decreases blood ammonia concentrations by 25–50%.
- May cause increased blood glucose levels in diabetic patients.
- Monitor serum electrolytes periodically when used chronically. May cause diarrhea with resulting hypokalemia and hypernatremia.

POTENTIAL NURSING DIAGNOSES

- Constipation (indications).
- Knowledge deficit related to medication regimen (patient/family teaching).

IMPLEMENTATION

- **General Info:** Darkening of solution does not alter potency.
- **PO:** Mix with fruit juice, water, milk, or carbonated citrus beverage to improve flavor. Administer with a full glass of water or juice. May be administered on an empty stomach for more rapid results.
- **Rect:** To administer enema, use rectal balloon catheter. Mix 300 ml of lactulose with 700 ml of water or 0.9% NaCl. Enema should be retained for 30–60 min. If inadvertently evacuated, may repeat administration.

PATIENT/FAMILY TEACHING

- Encourage patients to utilize other forms of bowel regulation, such as increasing bulk in the diet, increasing fluid intake, increasing mobility. Normal bowel habits are individualized and may vary from 3 times/day to 3 times/wk.
- Caution patients that this medication may cause belching, flatulence, or abdominal cramping. Physician should be notified if this becomes bothersome or if diarrhea occurs.

EVALUATION

Effectiveness of therapy can be demonstrated by: ■ Passage of a soft, formed bowel movement, usually within 24–48 hr ■ Clearing of confusion, apathy, and irritation and improved mental status in hepatic encephalopathy. When used in hepatic encephalopathy, dosage will be adjusted until patient averages 2–3 soft bowel movements per day. Improvement may occur within 2 hr following enema and 24–48 hr following oral administration.

LEUCOVORIN CALCIUM
(loo-koe-**vor**-in)
Citrovorum factor, 5-formyl tetrahydrofolate, folinic acid, Wellcovorin

CLASSIFICATION(S):
Antidote (for methotrexate and folic acid antagonists), Vitamin (folic acid analog)
Pregnancy Category C

INDICATIONS

- Used to minimize the hematologic effects of high-dose methotrexate therapy ("leucovorin rescue") ■ In combination with 5-fluorouracil in the management of advanced colorectal carcinoma ■ Management of overdoses of folic acid antagonists (pyrimethamine or trimethoprim) ■ Treatment of folic acid deficiency unresponsive to oral replacement.

L

ACTION

- The reduced form of folic acid that serves as a cofactor in the synthesis of DNA and RNA. **Therapeutic Effects:**
- Reversal of toxic effects of folic acid antagonists, such as methotrexate and trimethoprim ■ Reversal of folic acid deficiency.

PHARMACOKINETICS

Absorption: Rapidly absorbed following oral administration. Bioavailability decreases with increasing dose. Oral absorption is saturated at doses >25 mg.

Distribution: Widely distributed. Concentrates in the CNS and liver.

Metabolism and Excretion: Extensively converted to tetrahydrofolic derivatives, including 5-methyltetrahydrofolate, a major storage form.

Half-life: 3.5 hr.

CONTRAINDICATIONS AND PRECAUTIONS

Contraindicated in: ■ Hypersensitivity ■ Preparations containing benzyl alcohol should not be used in neonates.

Use Cautiously in: ■ Undiagnosed anemia (may mask the progression of pernicious anemia) ■ Pregnancy and lactation (safety not established but has been used safely to treat megaloblastic anemia in pregnancy) ■ Coadministration with high-dose methotrexate requires crucial timing of dosing and knowledge of methotrexate levels ■ Ascites ■ Renal failure ■ Dehydration ■ Pleural effusions ■ Urine pH <7.

ADVERSE REACTIONS AND SIDE EFFECTS*

Hemat: thrombocytosis (intra-arterial methotrexate only).

Misc: allergic reactions (rash, urticaria, wheezing).

INTERACTIONS

Drug–Drug: ■ May decrease the anticonvulsant effect of **barbiturates, phenytoin,** or **primidone.**

ROUTE AND DOSAGE

High-Dose Methotrexate-Leucovorin Rescue (Must start within 24 hr of methotrexate)

- **PO, IM, IV (Adults and Children):** 10 mg/m^2, followed by 10 mg/m^2 q 6 hr for 72 hr. If serum creatinine at 24 hr is 100% greater than premethotrexate level, dosage should be increased to 100 mg/m^2 q 3 hr until serum methotrexate level is <5 × 10^{-8} M. Many other rescue protocols are used.

Advanced Colorectal Cancer

- **IV (Adults):** 200 mg/m^2 followed by 5-fluorouracil 370 mg/m^2 or leucovorin 20 mg/m^2 is followed by 5-fluorouracil 425 mg/m^2. Regimen is given daily for 5 days q 4–5 wk.

Treatment of Hematologic Toxicity of other Folic Acid Antagonists

- **PO, IM (Adults and Children):** 5–15 mg.

Prevention of Hematologic Toxicity of other Folic Acid Antagonists

- **PO, IM (Adults and Children):** 0.4–5 mg with each dose of folic acid antagonist.

Megaloblastic Anemia

- **PO, IM, IV (Adults and Children):** up to 1 mg/day.

AVAILABILITY

- **Tablets:** 5 mg, 10 mg, 15 mg, 25 mg.

TIME/ACTION PROFILE (serum folate levels)

	ONSET	PEAK	DURATION
PO	<5 min	UK	3–6 hr
IM	<5 min	UK	3–6 hr
IV	<5 min	UK	3–6 hr

NURSING IMPLICATIONS

ASSESSMENT

- **General Info:** Assess patient for nausea and vomiting secondary to methotrexate therapy or folic acid antagonists (pyrimethamine and trimethoprim) overdose; if present, no-

---

*Underlines indicate most frequent; **CAPITALS** indicate life-threatening.

tify physician. Parenteral route may be necessary to ensure that patient receives dose.

□ Monitor for development of allergic reactions (rash, urticaria, wheezing). Notify physician if these occur.

■ **Megaloblastic Anemia:** Assess degree of weakness and fatigue.

LAB TEST CONSIDERATIONS

■ **Leucovorin Rescue:** Monitor serum methotrexate levels to determine dosage and effectiveness of therapy. Leucovorin calcium levels should be equal to or greater than methotrexate level. Rescue continues until serum methotrexate level is $<5 \times 10^{-8}$ M.

□ Monitor creatinine clearance and serum creatinine prior to and every 24 hr during therapy to detect methotrexate toxicity. An increase $>50\%$ over the pretreatment concentration at 24 hr is associated with severe renal toxicity.

□ Monitor urine pH every 6 hr throughout therapy. pH should be maintained >7 to decrease nephrotoxic effects of high-dose methotrexate. Sodium bicarbonate or acetazolamide may be ordered to alkalinize urine.

■ **Megaloblastic Anemia:** Monitor plasma folic acid levels, hemoglobin, hematocrit, and reticulocyte count prior to and periodically during course of therapy.

POTENTIAL NURSING DIAGNOSES

■ Injury, high risk for (indications).
■ Nutrition, altered: less than body requirements (indications).
■ Knowledge deficit related to medication regimen (patient/family teaching).

IMPLEMENTATION

■ **General Info:** Make sure leucovorin calcium is available before administering high-dose methotrexate. Administration must be initiated within 24 hr of methotrexate therapy.

□ Administer as soon as possible after toxic dose of folic acid antagonists (pyrimethamine and trimethoprim). Effectiveness of therapy begins to decrease 1 hr after overdose.

■ **IM:** IM route is preferred for treatment of megaloblastic anemia. Ampules of leucovorin calcium injection for IM use do not require reconstitution.

■ **IV:** To reconstitute 50-mg vial of leucovorin calcium for injection, add 5 ml of Bacteriostatic Water or Sterile Water for Injection, to yield a concentration of 10 mg/ml. Use 10-ml diluent for 100-mg vial. If dose is >10 mg/m^2, do not use product containing benzyl alcohol. Use immediately if reconstituted with Sterile Water for Injection. Stable for 7 days when reconstituted with bacteriostatic water.

■ **Direct IV:** Rate of direct IV infusion should not exceed 160 mg/min (16 ml of 10 mg/ml solution per min).

■ **Intermittent Infusion:** May be diluted in 100–500 ml of D5W, D10W, 0.9% NaCl, Ringer's or lactated Ringer's solution. Stable for 24 hr.

■ **Syringe Compatibility:** ■ bleomycin ■ cisplatin ■ cyclophosphamide ■ doxorubicin ■ fluorouracil ■ furosemide ■ heparin ■ methotrexate ■ metoclopramide ■ mitomycin ■ vinblastine ■ vincristine.

■ **Syringe Incompatibility:** ■ droperidol.

■ **Y-Site Compatibility:** ■ bleomycin ■ cisplatin ■ cyclophosphamide ■ doxorubicin ■ fluconazole ■ fluorouracil ■ furosemide ■ heparin ■ methotrexate ■ metoclopramide ■ mitomycin ■ vinblastine ■ vincristine.

■ **Y-Site Incompatibility:** ■ droperidol ■ foscarnet.

■ **Additive Compatibility:** ■ floxuridine ■ fluorouracil.

PATIENT/FAMILY TEACHING

■ **General Info:** Explain purpose of medication to patient. Emphasize need to take exactly as ordered. Advise patient to contact physician if a dose is missed.

■ **Leucovorin Rescue:** Instruct patient to drink at least 3 liters of fluid each day during leucovorin rescue.

■ **Folic Acid Deficiency:** Encourage patient to eat a diet high in folic acid (meat proteins, bran, dried beans, and green leafy vegetables).

L

EVALUATION

Effectiveness of therapy can be demonstrated by: ▪ Reversal of bone marrow and GI toxicity in patients receiving methotrexate or in overdose of folic acid antagonists ▪ Increased sense of wellbeing and increased production of normoblasts in patients with megaloblastic anemia.

LEUPROLIDE
(loo-**proe**-lide)
Leupron DepoPed, Lupron,
Lupron Depot

CLASSIFICATION(S):
Antineoplastic (hormone)
Pregnancy Category X (depot only)

INDICATIONS

▪ **SC:** Palliative treatment of advanced prostate cancer in patients who are unable to tolerate orchiectomy or estrogen therapy (may be used in combination with flutamide) ▪ **IM:** Treatment of endometriosis (depot form only) ▪ **SC, IM:** Management of central precocious puberty (CPP).

ACTION

▪ A synthetic analogue of luteinizing hormone releasing hormone (LHRH) ▪ Initially causes a transient increase in testosterone; however, with continuous administration, testosterone levels are decreased ▪ Reduces gonadotropins, testosterone, and estradiol to prepubertal levels in children with CPP. **Therapeutic Effects:** ▪ Decreased testosterone levels and resultant decrease in spread of prostate cancer ▪ Reduction of pain and lesions in endometriosis ▪ Delayed puberty.

PHARMACOKINETICS

Absorption: Rapidly and almost completely absorbed following SC administration. More slowly absorbed following IM administration of depot form.

Distribution: Distribution not known.
Metabolism and Excretion: Metabolism and elimination not known.
Half-life: 3 hr.

CONTRAINDICATIONS AND PRECAUTIONS

Contraindicated in: ▪ Intolerance to synthetic analogs of LHRH (GnRH) ▪ Pregnancy or lactation (depot form).
Use Cautiously in: ▪ Hypersensitivity to benzyl alcohol (results in induration and erythema at SC site).

ADVERSE REACTIONS AND SIDE EFFECTS*

CNS: dizziness, headache, syncope; *depot only*—personality disorder, somnolence; *SC only*—anxiety, blurred vision, memory disorder, lethargy, mood swings.
EENT: blurred vision; *SC only*—hearing disorder.
Resp: hemoptysis; *depot only*—throat nodules, epistaxis; *SC injection only*—cough, pleural rub, pulmonary fibrosis, pulmonary infiltrate.
CV: angina, cardiac arrhythmias, MYOCARDIAL INFARCTION, PULMONARY EMBOLI; *depot only*—vasodilation; *SC only*—transient ischemic attack/stroke.
GI: diarrhea, dysphagia, anorexia, nausea, vomiting; *depot only*—gingivitis; *SC only*—GI bleeding, rectal polyps, peptic ulcer, hepatic dysfunction, taste disorders.
GU: dysuria, testicular pain, incontinence; *depot only*—cervix disorder; *SC only*—bladder spasm, urinary obstruction, penile swelling, prostate pain.
Derm: *depot only*—hair growth, rash; *SC injection only*—dry skin, skin cancer, hair loss, pigmentation, skin lesions.
Endo: breast swelling, breast tenderness, diabetes.
F and E: lower extremity edema, increased serum calcium.
Local: burning, itching, swelling at injection site.

Underlines indicate most frequent; **CAPITALS indicate life-threatening.*

Metab: *depot only*—increased uric acid, increased bone density.

MS: transient increase in bone pain (prostate cancer only); *SC only*—joint pain, ankylosing spondylitis, pelvic fibrosis, temporal bone pain.

Neuro: *SC only*—peripheral neuropathy.

Misc: <u>hot flashes</u>, decreased libido, fever, chills; *depot only*—body odor, epistaxis, accelerated sexual maturity.

INTERACTIONS

Drug–Drug: ▪ Additive antineoplastic effects with **antiandrogens (megestrol, flutamide).**

ROUTE AND DOSAGE

Prostate Carcinoma
▪ **SC (Adults):** 1 mg/day.

Endometriosis/Prostate Carcinoma
▪ **IM (Adults):** 7.5 mg once monthly.

Central Precocious Puberty
▪ **SC (Children):** 50 mcg/kg/day, may be increased by 10 mcg/kg/day as required.
▪ **IM (Children):** 0.3 mg/kg/4 wk. Dose should not be less than 7.5 mg and may be increased by 3.75 mg q 4 wk.

AVAILABILITY

▪ *Injection:* 5 mg/ml ▪ *Depot injection:* 3.75 mg, 7.5 mg ▪ *Pediatric depot injection:* 7.5 mg, 11.25 mg, 15 mg kits.

TIME/ACTION PROFILE (decline in serum testosterone concentrations)

	ONSET	PEAK	DURATION
SC	1–2 wk*	2–4 wk	UK

*Follows a transient increase in the first week of therapy.

NURSING IMPLICATIONS

Assessment
▪ **Prostate Cancer:** Assess patient for an increase in bone pain, especially during the first few weeks of therapy. Monitor patients with vertebral metastases for increased back pain and decreased sensory/motor function.
□ Monitor intake and output ratios, assess for bladder distention in patients with urinary tract obstruction during initiation of therapy.
▪ **Endometriosis:** Assess patient for endometrial pain prior to and periodically throughout therapy.
▪ **Central Precocious Puberty (CPP):** Prior to therapy, diagnosis of CPP should be confirmed by onset of secondary sex characteristics in females <8 yr or males <9 yr, and a complete physical and endocrinologic examination, including height, weight, hand and wrist x-ray, total sex steroid level (estradiol or testosterone), adrenal steroid level, beta human chorionic gonadotropin level, GnRH stimulation test, and computerized tomography of the head must be performed. These parameters are monitored after 1–2 mo and every 6–12 mo during therapy.
□ Assess patient for signs of precocious puberty (menses, breast development, testicular growth) periodically throughout therapy. Dose is increased until no progression of the disease is noted either clinically or by lab test parameters, then usually maintained throughout therapy. Discontinuation of therapy should be considered before age 11 in females and age 12 in males.
▪ **Lab Test Considerations:** Initially increases, then decreases luteinizing hormone (LH) and follicle stimulating hormone (FSH). This leads to castration levels of testosterone in males 2–4 wk after initial increase in concentrations.
□ Monitor acid phosphate to evaluate response to therapy. Transient increase in levels may occur during the first month of therapy for prostate cancer.

Potential Nursing Diagnoses
▪ Sexual dysfunction (side effects).
▪ Knowledge deficit related to medication regimen (patient/family teaching).

Implementation
▪ **SC/IM:** Use syringe supplied by manufacturer. Rotate sites.

L

□ Leuprolide depot is *only* for IM injection.

□ To reconstitute a single vial, use 22-g needle and withdraw 1 ml of diluent and inject into vial to mix. To mix 2 or more vials, withdraw 0.5 ml and inject into each vial for a total volume of 1 ml. Shake each vial well, suspension will appear milky. Withdraw entire contents of all vials into syringe and inject immediately. Patients may store medication at room temperature.

PATIENT/FAMILY TEACHING

■ **General Info:** Advise patient that medication may cause hot flashes. Notify physician if these become bothersome.

■ **Prostate Cancer:** Instruct patient and family on SC injection technique. Review patient insert provided with leuprolide patient-administration kit.

□ Instruct patient to take medication exactly as directed. If a dose is missed, take as soon as remembered unless not remembered until next day.

□ Advise patient that bone pain may increase at initiation of therapy. This will resolve with time. Patient should discuss with physician use of analgesics to control pain.

□ Instruct patient to notify physician promptly if difficulty urinating, weakness, or numbness occurs.

■ **Endometriosis:** Advise patient to use a form of contraception other than oral contraceptives during therapy. Inform patient that amenorrhea is expected but does not guarantee contraception.

■ **Central Precocious Puberty:** Instruct patient and family on the proper technique for SC injection. Emphasize the importance of administering the medication at the same time each day. Rotate injection sites periodically.

□ Inform patient and parents that if injections are not given daily pubertal process may be reactivated.

□ Advise patient and parents that during the first 2 mo of therapy patient may experience a light menstrual flow or spotting. Physician should be noti-

fied if this continues beyond second month.

□ Instruct patient and parents to notify physician immediately if irritation at the injection site or unusual signs or symptoms occur.

EVALUATION

Effectiveness of therapy can be demonstrated by: ■ Decrease in the spread of prostate cancer ■ Decrease in lesions and pain in endometriosis ■ Resolution of the signs of central precocious puberty.

LEVAMISOLE
(lee-**vam**-i-sole)
Ergamisole

CLASSIFICATION(S):
Antineoplastic (immunomodulator)
Pregnancy Category C

INDICATIONS

■ Adjunctive treatment following surgery of Dukes C colorectal carcinoma (with fluorouracil). **Unlabeled Use:** ■ Advanced malignant melanoma.

ACTION

■ Restores depressed immune function including formation of antibodies, T-cell response, phagocytosis, and chemotaxis ■ Also has cholinergic activity. **Therapeutic Effect:** ■ Enhanced immunologic response to presence of tumor when used in conjunction with fluorouracil.

PHARMACOKINETICS

Absorption: Rapidly absorbed following oral administratin.
Distribution: Distribution not known.
Metabolism and Excretion: Extensively metabolized by the liver.
Half-life: 3–4 hr.

CONTRAINDICATIONS AND PRECAUTIONS

Contraindicated in: ■ Hypersensitivity ■ Pregnancy.

Use Cautiously in: ■ Bone marrow depression ■ Other chronic debilitating illnesses ■ Patients with childbearing potential ■ Lactation or children (safety not established).

ADVERSE REACTIONS AND SIDE EFFECTS*

As occurring in combination with fluorouracil.

CNS: fatigue, dizziness, headache, somnolence, depression, nervousness, insomnia, anxiety, forgetfulness.
EENT: altered sense of smell, abnormal tearing, conjunctivitis, blurred vision.
GI: nausea, vomiting, stomatitis, diarrhea, anorexia, abdominal pain, flatulence, dyspepsia, abnormal taste.
Derm: dermatitis, alopecia, pruritis, skin discoloration.
Hemat: anemia, leukopenia, thrombocytopenia, AGRANULOCYTOSIS.
MS: arthralgia, myalgia.
Neuro: paresthesia, ataxia.
Misc: fever, chills.

INTERACTIONS

Drug–Drug: ■ Increased bone marrow depression with other **antineoplastic agents** or **radiation therapy** ■ Ingestion of **alcohol** may produce disulfiram-like reaction ■ May increase blood levels and risk of toxicity with **phenytoin**.

ROUTE AND DOSAGE

■ **PO (Adults):** 50 mg q 8 hr for 3 days every 2 wk with fluorouracil 450 mg/m²/day for 5 days initially then followed 28 days later by fluorouracil 450 mg/m² once weekly.

AVAILABILITY

■ *Tablets:* 50 mg.

TIME/ACTION PROFILE (blood levels)

	ONSET	PEAK	DURATION
PO	UK	1.5–2 hr	UK

NURSING IMPLICATIONS

ASSESSMENT

□ Assess mucous membranes, number and consistency of stools, and frequency of vomiting. Assess for fever, chills, sore throat, and signs of infection. Assess for bleeding (bleeding gums, bruising, petechiae; guaiac stools, urine, and emesis). Avoid IM injections and rectal temperatures. Apply pressure to venipuncture sites for 10 min. Notify physician if symptoms of toxicity (stomatitis, uncontrollable vomiting, diarrhea, gastrointestinal bleeding, leukocyte count of less than 3500/mm³, platelet count <100,000/mm³, or hemorrhage from any site) occur as drug will need to be discontinued.

■ **Lab Test Considerations:** Hematologic functions should be monitored prior to and throughout therapy. CBC with differential and platelets, electrolytes, and liver function tests should be performed on the first day of therapy with levamisole and fluorouracil. Then, a CBC with differential should be performed weekly prior to each treatment with fluorouracil. Electrolytes and liver function should be monitored every 3 mo for 1 yr. If WBC is 2500–3500/mm³, withhold fluorouracil until WBC >3500/mm³; if WBC <2500/mm³ withhold fluorouracil until WBC >3500/mm³ and decrease dose by 20%; if WBC remains <2500/mm³ for >10 days despite withholding fluorouracil, discontinue levamisole. Withhold both levamisole and fluorouracil if platelet count <100,000/mm³. Neutropenia is usually reversible upon discontinuation of therapy.

POTENTIAL NURSING DIAGNOSES

■ Infection, high risk for (side effects).
■ Nutrition, altered: less than body requirements (side effects).
■ Knowledge deficit related to medication regimen (patient/family teaching).

IMPLEMENTATION

■ **General Info:** Levamisole therapy should be initiated no earlier than 7 days and no later than 30 days fol-

L

lowing surgery. Fluorouracil therapy should be initiated no earlier than 21 days and no later than 35 days following surgery in patients who are out of the hospital, ambulatory, maintaining oral nutrition, have well-healed wounds, and are fully recovered from postoperative complications. If levamisole has been initiated 7–20 days postoperatively, begin fluorouracil therapy with the second course of levamisole therapy; if levamisole is initiated 21–30 days postoperatively, initiate fluorouracil with first course of levamisole therapy.

□ Refer to fluorouracil monograph for specific information on administration of fluorouracil.

▪ **PO:** Administer levamisole every 8 hr for 3 days. Repeat course every 14 days for 1 yr.

PATIENT/FAMILY TEACHING

□ Instruct patient to notify physician immediately if flu-like symptoms or malaise occurs. Physician should also be notified if fever, chills, sore throat, signs of infection, bleeding gums, bruising, petechiae, or blood in urine, stool, or emesis occurs. Caution patient to avoid crowds and persons with known infections. Instruct patient to use soft toothbrush and electric razor. Patients should be cautioned not to take products containing aspirin or ibuprofen.

□ Caution patient that concurrent use of alcohol may cause a disulfiram-like reaction (abdominal cramps, nausea, headache, flushing, hypoglycemia).

□ Advise patient to rinse mouth with clear water after eating and drinking and to avoid flossing to minimize stomatitis. Consult physician if mouth pain interferes with eating.

□ Discuss with patient the possibility of hair loss. Explore methods of coping.

□ Instruct patient not to receive any vaccinations without advice of physician.

□ Review with patient the need for contraception during therapy.

□ Emphasize the importance of routine follow-up lab tests to monitor progress and check for side effects.

EVALUATION
Effectiveness of therapy can be demonstrated by: ▪ Enhanced immunologic response to presence of tumor when used in conjunction with fluorouracil.

LEVODOPA
(**lee**-voe-doe-pa)
Dopar, Larodopa, L-Dopa

CLASSIFICATION(S):
Antiparkinsonian (dopamine agonist)
Pregnancy Category UK

INDICATIONS

▪ Treatment of Parkinson's syndrome. Not useful for drug-induced extrapyramidal reactions.

ACTION

▪ Levodopa is converted to dopamine in the CNS, where it serves as a neurotransmitter. **Therapeutic Effect:** ▪ Relief of tremor and rigidity in Parkinson's syndrome.

PHARMACOKINETICS

Absorption: Well absorbed following oral administration.
Distribution: Widely distributed. When administered alone, enters the CNS in small concentrations. Enters breast milk.
Metabolism and Excretion: Mostly metabolized by the GI tract and liver.
Half-life: 1 hr.

CONTRAINDICATIONS AND PRECAUTIONS

Contraindicated in: ▪ Hypersensitivity ▪ Narrow-angle glaucoma ▪ Patients receiving MAO inhibitors ▪ Malignant melanoma ▪ Undiagnosed skin lesions ▪ Lactation.
Use Cautiously in: ▪ History of cardiac, psychiatric, or ulcer disease

- Pregnancy or children <18 yr (safety not established).

ADVERSE REACTIONS AND SIDE EFFECTS*

CNS: involuntary movements, memory loss, anxiety, psychiatric problems, hallucinations, dizziness.
EENT: mydriasis, blurred vision.
CV: hypertension, hypotension.
GI: nausea, vomiting, anorexia, dry mouth, hepatotoxicity.
Derm: melanoma.
Hemat: hemolytic anemia, leukopenia.
Misc: darkening of sweat or urine.

INTERACTIONS

Drug–Drug: ■ Use with **MAO inhibitors** may result in hypertensive reactions ■ **Phenothiazines, haloperidol, papaverine, phenytoin,** and **reserpine** may antagonize the beneficial effect of levodopa ■ Large doses of **pyridoxine** may reverse the effect of levodopa ■ Concurrent use with **methyldopa** may alter the effectiveness of levodopa and increase the risk of CNS side effects ■ Additive hypotension may result with concurrent **antihypertensives** ■ **Anticholinergics** may decrease absorption of levodopa ■ Increased risk of adverse reactions (dyskinesias, nausea, hypotension, confusion, hallucinations) with **selegiline** (decrease dose of levodopa) ■ Increased risk of arrhythmias with **cocaine.**
Drug–Food: ■ Ingestion of foods containing large amounts of **pyridoxine** may reverse the effect of levodopa.

ROUTE AND DOSAGE

- **PO (Adults):** 500–1000 mg/day given in divided doses q 6–12 hr initially. Increase by 100–750 mg/day q 3–7 days until response occurs or 8000 mg/day is reached. Usual maintenance dose is 2000–8000 mg/day.

AVAILABILITY

- *Tablets:* 100 mg, 250 mg, 500 mg
- *Capsules:* 100 mg, 250 mg, 500 mg.

TIME/ACTION PROFILE
(antiparkinson effects)

	ONSET	PEAK	DURATION
PO	10–15 min	UK	5–24 hr or more

NURSING IMPLICATIONS

ASSESSMENT

□ Assess parkinsonian symptoms (akinesia, rigidity, tremors, gait, facial expression, and drooling) prior to and throughout course of therapy. "On-off phenomena" may cause symptoms to appear or to improve suddenly.
□ Assess blood pressure and pulse frequently during period of dose adjustment.
■ **Lab Test Considerations:** May cause false-positive Coombs' test, serum and urine uric acid, serum gonadotropin, urine norepinephrine, and urine protein concentrations.
□ May interfere with results of urine glucose and urine ketone tests. Copper reduction method (Clinitest) of testing urine glucose and dipstick (Ketostix) for urine ketones may reveal false-positive results. Glucose enzymatic tests (Tes-Tape) of testing urine glucose may yield false-negative results.
□ Patients on long-term therapy should have hepatic and renal functions and CBC monitored periodically. May cause elevated BUN, AST (SGOT), ALT (SGPT), bilirubin, alkaline phosphatase, LDH, and serum protein-bound iodine.
■ **Toxicity and Overdose:** Assess for signs of toxicity (involuntary muscle twitching, facial grimacing, spasmodic eye winking, exaggerated protrusion of tongue, or behavioral changes). Consult physician promptly if these symptoms occur.

POTENTIAL NURSING DIAGNOSES

- Physical mobility, impaired (indications).

L

---

*Underlines indicate most frequent; **CAPITALS** indicate life-threatening.

- Injury, high risk for (indications).
- Knowledge deficit related to medication regimen (patient/family teaching).

IMPLEMENTATION

- **General Info:** In preoperative patients or patients who are NPO, confer with physician regarding continuing medication administration.
- □ Wait 8 hr after last levodopa dose before switching patient to carbidopa/levodopa. Carbidopa reduces the need for levodopa by 75%. Administering carbidopa shortly after a full dose of levodopa may result in toxicity.
- **PO:** Administer food shortly after medication to minimize GI irritation; taking food before or concurrently may retard levodopa's effects but may be necessary to minimize GI irritation. If patient has difficulty swallowing, confer with pharmacist.

PATIENT/FAMILY TEACHING

- □ Instruct patient to take this drug exactly as directed. If a dose is missed, take as soon as remembered unless next scheduled dose is within 2 hr; do not double doses.
- □ Explain that gastric irritation may be decreased by taking food shortly after medication but that high-protein meals may impair levodopa's effects. Dividing the daily protein intake between all meals may help ensure adequate protein intake and drug effectiveness. Do not drastically alter diet during levodopa therapy without consulting physician.
- □ May cause drowsiness or dizziness. Advise patient to avoid driving or other activities that require alertness until response to drug is known.
- □ Caution patient to make position changes slowly to minimize orthostatic hypotension. Physician should be notified if orthostatic hypotension occurs.
- □ Instruct patient that frequent rinsing of mouth, good oral hygiene, and sugarless gum or candy may decrease dry mouth.
- □ Advise patient to confer with physician or pharmacist prior to taking over-the-counter medications, especially cold remedies. Patients receiving only levodopa should avoid multivitamins. Large amounts of vitamin B_6 (pyridoxine) may interfere with levodopa's action.
- □ Inform patient that harmless darkening of urine or sweat may occur.
- □ Advise patient to notify physician if palpitations, urinary retention, involuntary movements, behavioral changes, severe nausea and vomiting, or new skin lesions occur.

EVALUATION

Effectiveness of therapy can be demonstrated by: • Resolution of parkinsonian signs and symptoms. Therapeutic effects usually become evident after 2–3 wk of therapy but may require up to 6 mo. Patients who take this medication for several years may experience a decrease in the effectiveness of this drug. Effectiveness of therapy may sometimes be restored after a "drug holiday."

LEVORPHANOL
(lee-**vor**-fan-ole)
Levo-Dromoran, levorphan

CLASSIFICATION(S):
Opioid analgesic (agonist)
Schedule II
Pregnancy Category UK

INDICATIONS

- Management of moderate to severe pain.

ACTION

- Binds to opiate receptors in the CNS, altering perception of and response to pain • Produces generalized CNS depression. **Therapeutic Effect:** • Decreased pain.

PHARMACOKINETICS

Absorption: Well absorbed following oral and SC administration.
Distribution: Distribution not known.

Metabolism and Excretion: Mostly metabolized by the liver.
Half-life: 12–16 hr.

CONTRAINDICATIONS AND PRECAUTIONS

Contraindicated in: ▪ Hypersensitivity ▪ Avoid chronic use during pregnancy or lactation ▪ Hypersensitivty to phenol or parabens (injection only).
Use Cautiously in: ▪ Head trauma ▪ Increased intracranial pressure ▪ Severe renal, hepatic, or pulmonary disease ▪ Hypothyroidism ▪ Adrenal insufficiency ▪ Alcoholism ▪ Undiagnosed abdominal pain ▪ Prostatic hypertrophy ▪ Elderly or debilitated patients (dosage reduction suggested).

ADVERSE REACTIONS AND SIDE EFFECTS*

CNS: sedation, confusion, headache, euphoria, floating feeling, unusual dreams, hallucinations, dysphoria.
EENT: miosis, diplopia, blurred vision.
Resp: respiratory depression.
CV: hypotension, bradycardia.
GI: nausea, vomiting, constipation, dry mouth.
GU: urinary retention.
Derm: sweating, flushing.
Misc: tolerance, physical dependence, psychological dependence.

INTERACTIONS

Drug–Drug: ▪ Use with extreme caution in patients receiving **MAO inhibitors** (may result in unpredictable, severe reactions—decrease initial dose of levorphanol to 25% of usual dose) ▪ Additive CNS depression with **alcohol, antihistamines, antidepressants,** and **sedative/hypnotics** ▪ Administration of **partial-antagonist opioid analgesics** may precipitate withdrawal in physically dependent patients ▪ **Nalbuphine** or **pentazocine** may decrease analgesia.

ROUTE AND DOSAGE

Larger doses may be required during chronic use.
▪ **PO (Adults):** 2 mg initially q 4–5 hr, may be increased to 3–4 mg if necessary.
▪ **SC, IV (Adults):** 2 mg q 4–5 hr, may be increased to 3 mg if pain is severe.

AVAILABILITY

▪ *Tablets:* 2 mg ▪ *Injection:* 2 mg/ml.

TIME/ACTION PROFILE (analgesic effect)

	ONSET	PEAK	DURATION
PO	10–60 min	90–120 min	4–5 hr
SC	UK	60–90 min	4–5 hr
IV	UK	within 20 min	4–5 hr

NURSING IMPLICATIONS

ASSESSMENT
□ Assess type, location, and intensity of pain prior to and 60 min following administration.
□ Assess blood pressure, pulse, and respiratory rate before and periodically during administration.
□ Prolonged use may lead to physical and psychological dependence and tolerance. This should not prevent patient from receiving adequate analgesia. Most patients who receive levorphanol for medical reasons do not develop psychological dependence. Progressively higher doses may be required to relieve pain with long-term therapy.
□ Assess bowel function routinely. Increased intake of fluids and bulk, stool softeners, and laxatives may minimize constipating effects.
□ Monitor intake and output ratios. If significant discrepancies occur, assess for urinary retention and inform physician.
▪ **Lab Test Considerations:** May increase plasma amylase and lipase levels.
▪ **Toxicity and Overdose:** If overdosage occurs, naloxone (Narcan) is the antidote.

POTENTIAL NURSING DIAGNOSES
▪ Pain (indications).

L

*Underlines indicate most frequent; **CAPITALS** indicate life-threatening.

- Sensory-perceptual alteration: visual, auditory (side effects).
- Injury, high risk for (side effects).

IMPLEMENTATION
- **General Info:** Explain therapeutic value of medication prior to administration to enhance the analgesic effect.
  □ Regularly administered doses may be more effective than prn administration. Analgesic is more effective if given before pain becomes severe.
  □ Coadministration with nonopioid analgesics may have additive analgesic effects and permit lower opioid doses.
  □ Encourage patient to turn, cough, and breathe deeply every 2 hr to prevent atelectasis.
  □ Medication should be discontinued gradually after long-term use to prevent withdrawal symptoms.
- **PO:** May be administered with food or milk to minimize GI irritation.
- **SC, IV:** Patients receiving parenteral therapy should be lying down and remain recumbent to minimize side effects for at least 30–60 min.
- **Direct IV:** Administer slowly, over 3–5 min. Rapid administration may lead to increased respiratory depression, hypotension, and circulatory collapse. Do not use IV administration without antidote available.
- **Syringe Compatibility:** ■ glycopyrrolate.

PATIENT/FAMILY TEACHING
- □ Instruct patient on how and when to ask for pain medication.
- □ Instruct patient to take levorphanol exactly as directed. If dose is less effective after a few weeks, do not increase dose without consulting physician.
- □ Medication may cause drowsiness or dizziness. Advise patient to call for assistance when ambulating or smoking. Caution patient to avoid driving or other activities that require alertness until response to the medication is known.
- □ Advise patient to make position

changes slowly to minimize orthostatic hypotension.
- □ Caution patient to avoid concurrent use of alcohol or other CNS depressants.
- □ Advise ambulatory patients that nausea and vomiting may be decreased by lying down.

EVALUATION
Effectiveness of therapy can be demonstrated by: ■ Decrease in severity of pain without a significant alteration in level of consciousness, respiratory status, or blood pressure.

LEVOTHYROXINE
(lee-voe-thye-**rox**-een)
{Eltroxin}, Levothroid, Levoxine, Synthroid, T_4

CLASSIFICATION(S):
Hormone (thyroid)
Pregnancy Category A

INDICATIONS
- Replacement or substitution therapy in diminished or absent thyroid function of many causes. Provides a standardized and predictable effect.

ACTION
- Principal effect is increasing metabolic rate of body tissues ■ Promotes gluconeogenesis, increases utilization and mobilization of glycogen stores, and stimulates protein synthesis ■ Promotes cell growth and differentiation and aids in the development of the brain and CNS. **Therapeutic Effects:** ■ Replacement in deficiency states ■ Restoration of normal hormonal balance.

PHARMACOKINETICS
Absorption: Variably (50–80%) absorbed from the GI tract.
Distribution: Distributed into most body tissues. Thyroid hormones do not readily cross the placenta; minimal amounts enter breast milk.

{} = Available in Canada only.

Metabolism and Excretion: Metabolized by the liver. Undergoes enterohepatic recirculation. Excreted in the feces via the bile.

Half-life: 6–7 days.

CONTRAINDICATIONS AND PRECAUTIONS

Contraindicated in: ▪ Hypersensitivity ▪ Recent myocardial infarction ▪ Thyrotoxicosis.

Use Cautiously in: ▪ Cardiovascular disease ▪ Severe renal insufficiency ▪ Uncorrected adrenocortical disorders ▪ Elderly and myxedematous patients (extremely sensitive to thyroid hormones; initial dosage should be markedly reduced) ▪ Has been used safely in pregnancy.

ADVERSE REACTIONS AND SIDE EFFECTS*

CNS: irritability, insomnia, nervousness, headache.

CV: tachycardia, arrhythmias, increased cardiac output, angina pectoris, increased blood pressure, CARDIOVASCULAR COLLAPSE, hypotension.

GI: diarrhea, cramps, vomiting.

Derm: increased sweating, hair loss (children only).

Endo: menstrual irregularities.

Metab: weight loss, heat intolerance.

MS: accelerated bone maturation in children.

INTERACTIONS

Drug–Drug: ▪ **Cholestyramine** and **colestipol** decrease oral absorption ▪ **IV phenytoin** causes the release of thyroid hormone ▪ Thyroid hormones increase the effect of **oral anticoagulants** ▪ May cause an increase in the requirement for **insulin** or **oral hypoglycemic agents** in diabetics ▪ Additive CNS and cardiac stimulation with **sympathomimetic agents (amphetamines, vasopressors, decongestants)** ▪ May decrease some effects of **beta-adrenergic blockers**.

ROUTE AND DOSAGE

Hypothyroidism

▪ **PO (Adults):** 12.5–50 mcg as a single

daily dose initially, may be increased q 2–4 wk. Usual maintenance dose 75–125 mcg/day.
▪ **PO (Children >12 yr):** 2–3 mcg/kg/day as a single daily dose.
▪ **PO (Children 6–12 yr):** 4–5 mcg/kg/day as a single daily dose.
▪ **PO (Children 1–5 yr):** 5–6 mcg/kg/day as a single dose.
▪ **PO (Children 6–12 mo):** 6–8 mcg/kg/day as a single daily dose.
▪ **PO (Children 0–6 mo):** 8–10 mcg/kg/day as a single dose.
▪ **IM, IV (Adults):** 50–100 mcg/day as a single dose.
▪ **IM, IV (Children):** 75% of the calculated oral dose.

Myxedema Coma

▪ **IV (Adults):** 200–500 mcg, if no response in 24 hr, may give additional 100–300 mcg. Maintenance dose, 50–100 mcg/day.

AVAILABILITY

▪ ***Tablets:*** 0.025 mg, 0.05 mg, 0.075 mg, 0.088 mg, 0.1 mg, 0.112 mg, 0.125 mg, 0.15 mg, 0.175 mg, 0.2 mg, 0.3 mg ▪ ***Injection:*** 50 mcg, 200 mcg, 500 mcg.

TIME/ACTION PROFILE (effects on thyroid function testing)

	ONSET	PEAK	DURATION
PO	UK	1–3 wk	1–3 wk
IV	6–8 hr	24 hr	UK

NURSING IMPLICATIONS

ASSESSMENT

▪ **General Info:** Assess apical pulse and blood pressure prior to and periodically during therapy. Assess for tachyarrhythmias and chest pain.
▪ **Children:** Monitor height, weight, and psychomotor development.
▪ **Lab Test Considerations:** Thyroid function studies should be monitored prior to and throughout course of therapy.
▫ Monitor blood and urine glucose in diabetic patients. Insulin or oral hypoglycemic dose may need to be increased.

L

*Underlines indicate most frequent; **CAPITALS** indicate life-threatening.

- **Toxicity and Overdose:** Overdose is manifested as hyperthyroidism (tachycardia, chest pain, nervousness, insomnia, diaphoresis, tremors, weight loss). Usual treatment is to withhold dose for 2–6 days. Acute overdose is treated by induction of emesis or gastric lavage, followed by activated charcoal. Sympathetic overstimulation may be controlled by antiadrenergic drugs, such as propranolol. Oxygen and supportive measures to control symptoms such as fever are also used.

POTENTIAL NURSING DIAGNOSES

- Knowledge deficit related to medication regimen (patient/family teaching).

IMPLEMENTATION

- **General Info:** Administer as a single dose, preferably before breakfast to prevent insomnia.
- **IV:** For IV levothyroxine, dilute each 500 mcg in 5 ml of 0.9% NaCl without preservatives (diluent usually provided), for a concentration of 100 mcg/ml. Shake well to dissolve completely. Administer solution immediately after preparation; discard unused portion.
- *Rate:* Administer at a rate of 100 mcg over 1 min. Do not add to IV infusions; may be administered through Y-tubing or a 3-way stopcock.

PATIENT/FAMILY TEACHING

- **General Info:** Instruct patient to take medication exactly as directed at the same time each day. If a dose is missed, take as soon as remembered unless almost time for next dose. If more than 2–3 doses are missed, notify physician. Do not discontinue without consulting physician.
- Instruct patient and family on correct technique for checking pulse. Dose should be withheld and physician notified if resting pulse >100 bpm.
- Explain to patient that levothyroxine does not cure hypothyroidism, it provides a thyroid hormone; therapy is lifelong.
- Caution patient not to change brands of this medication, as this may effect drug bioavailability.
- Advise patient to notify physician if headache, nervousness, diarrhea, excessive sweating, heat intolerance, chest pain, increased pulse rate, palpitations, weight loss >2 lb/wk, or any unusual symptoms occur.
- Caution patient to avoid taking other medications concurrently with levothyroxine unless instructed by physician.
- Instruct patient to inform physician or dentist of thyroid therapy.
- Emphasize importance of follow-up examinations to monitor effectiveness of therapy. Thyroid function tests are performed at least yearly.
- **Children:** Discuss with parents need for routine follow-up studies to ensure correct development. Inform patient that partial hair loss may be experienced by children on thyroid therapy. This is usually temporary.

EVALUATION

Clinical response can be evaluated by:
- Resolution of symptoms of hypothyroidism. Response includes: □ Diuresis □ Weight loss □ Increased sense of wellbeing □ Increased energy, pulse rate, appetite, psychomotor activity □ Normalization of skin texture and hair □ Correction of constipation □ Increased T_3 and T_4 levels ■ In children, effectiveness of therapy is determined by: □ Appropriate physical and psychomotor development.

LIDOCAINE
(lye-doe-kane)
Anestacon, Baylocaine, L-Caine, LidoPen, Xylocaine, {Xylogard}

CLASSIFICATION(S):
Antiarrhythmic (group IB), Anesthetic (local)
Pregnancy Category B

{} = Available in Canada only.

INDICATIONS

• **IV:** Acute treatment of ventricular arrhythmias • **IM:** Given as a self-injection or when IV unavailable (during transport to hospital facilities) • **Local:** Used as a local or infiltration anesthetic.

ACTION

• **IV, IM:** Suppresses automaticity of conduction tissue and spontaneous depolarization of the ventricles during diastole by altering the flux of sodium ions across cell membranes. Has little or no effect on heart rate • **Topical/Local:** Produces local anesthesia by inhibiting transport of ions across neuronal membranes, thereby preventing initiation and conduction of normal nerve impulses. **Therapeutic Effects:** • Control of ventricular arrhythmias • Local anesthetic activity.

PHARMACOKINETICS

Absorption: Well absorbed following IM administration into the deltoid muscle. Some absorption may follow topical application.
Distribution: Widely distributed. Concentrates in adipose tissue. Crosses the blood–brain barrier and placenta.
Metabolism and Excretion: Mostly metabolized by the liver.
Half-life: Biphasic—initial phase 7–30 min; terminal phase—90–120 min.

CONTRAINDICATIONS AND PRECAUTIONS

Contraindicated in: • Hypersensitivity • Advanced AV block.
Use Cautiously in: • Liver disease, congestive heart failure, patients weighing <50 kg, and elderly patients (reduce bolus and/or maintenance dose) • Respiratory depression, shock, or heart block • Pregnancy or lactation (safety not established).

ADVERSE REACTIONS AND SIDE EFFECTS*

CNS: <u>drowsiness</u>, dizziness, lethargy, <u>confusion</u>, nervousness, SEIZURES, tremor.

CV: hypotension, arrhythmias, bradycardia, CARDIAC ARREST.
GI: nausea, vomiting.
Local: burning, stinging, erythema (Top or infiltration use).

INTERACTIONS

Drug–Drug: • Additive cardiac depression and toxicity with **phenytoin, quinidine, procainamide,** or **propranolol** • **Cimetidine** and **beta-adrenergic blockers** may decrease metabolism and increase risk of toxicity.

ROUTE AND DOSAGE

See infusion rate table in Appendix D.

• **IV (Adults):** 50–100 mg (1 mg/kg) bolus (may be repeated in 5 min), then 1–4 mg/min (20–50 mcg/kg/min) infusion (up to 200–300 mg in 1 hr).
• **IV (Children):** 1 mg/kg bolus, followed by 30 mcg/kg/min infusion.
• **IM (Adults):** 300 mg (4.3 mg/kg), may be repeated in 60–90 min.
• **Top (Adults and Children):** Apply to affected area as needed (increased amount and frequency of use increases likelihood of systemic absorption and adverse reactions).

AVAILABILITY

• *IM injection:* 300 mg/3 ml automatic injection device • *Direct IV injection:* 10 mg/ml (1%), 20 mg/ml (2%) • *For IV admixture:* 40 mg/ml (4%), 100 mg/ml (10%), 200 mg/ml (20%) • *For IV infusion:* 2 mg/ml (0.2%), 4 mg/ml (0.4%), 8 mg/ml (0.8%) • *Topical ointment:* 2.5%, 5% • *Topical cream:* 0.5% • *Spray:* 10% • *Solution:* 2%, 4% • *Viscous solution:* 2% • *Jelly:* 2% • *Injection for local infiltration:* 0.5%, 1% • *In combination with:* epinephrine for local infiltration.

TIME/ACTION PROFILE (IV, IM = antiarrhythmic effects, Top = local anesthetic effects)

	ONSET	PEAK	DURATION
IV	immediate	immediate	10–20 min
IM	5–15 min	20–30 min	60–90 min
Top	UK	2–5 min	30–60 min

*Underlines indicate most frequent; **CAPITALS** indicate life-threatening.

NURSING IMPLICATIONS

ASSESSMENT

- **Antiarrhythmic:** Monitor ECG continuously and blood pressure and respiratory status frequently throughout administration.
- **Anesthetic:** Assess degree of numbness of affected part. If spray or viscous lidocaine was used on the throat, assess gag reflex before giving food or fluids.
- **Lab Test Considerations:** Serum electrolyte levels should be monitored periodically throughout prolonged therapy.
  - ▫ IM administration may cause increased CPK levels.
- **Toxicity and Overdose:** Serum lidocaine levels should be monitored periodically throughout prolonged or high-dose therapy. Therapeutic serum lidocaine levels range from 1.5 to 5 mcg/ml.
  - ▫ Signs and symptoms of toxicity include confusion, excitation, blurred or double vision, nausea, vomiting, ringing in ears, tremors, twitching, convulsions, difficulty breathing, severe dizziness or fainting, and unusually slow heart rate.
  - ▫ If symptoms of overdose occur, stop infusion and monitor patient closely.

POTENTIAL NURSING DIAGNOSES

- Cardiac output, decreased (indications).
- Pain (indications).
- Knowledge deficit related to medication regimen (patient/family teaching).

IMPLEMENTATION

- **IM:** IM injections are recommended only when ECG monitoring is not available and physician feels benefits outweigh risks. Administer IM injections only into deltoid muscle while frequently aspirating to prevent IV injection.
- **IV:** Only 1% and 2% solutions are used for direct IV injection.
- **Direct IV:** Administer undiluted IV loading dose of 1 mg/kg at a rate of 25–50 mg over 1 min. May repeat dose after 5 min. Follow by IV infusion. Do not use lidocaine with preservatives or other medications, such as epinephrine, for IV injection.
- **Continuous Infusion:** To prepare for IV infusion add 1 g lidocaine to 250, 500, or 1000 ml of D5W. Solution is stable for 24 hr. Other compatible solutions include D5/LR, D5/0.45% NaCl, D5/0.9% NaCl, 0.45% NaCl, 0.9% NaCl, and lactated Ringer's solution.
- *Rate:* Administer via infusion pump for accurate dose at a rate of 1–4 mg/min (see Appendix D for infusion rate table).
- **Y-Site Compatibility:** ▪ altaplase ▪ amrinone ▪ cefazolin ▪ dobutamine ▪ enalaprilat ▪ famotidine ▪ labetalol ▪ nitroglycerin ▪ nitroprusside ▪ potassium chloride ▪ streptokinase ▪ vitamin B complex with C.
- **Infiltration:** Lidocaine with epinephrine may be used to minimize systemic absorption and prolong local anesthesia.

PATIENT/FAMILY TEACHING

- **General Info:** May cause drowsiness and dizziness. Advise patient to call for assistance during ambulation and transfer.
- **IM:** Available in LidoPen Auto-Injector for use outside the hospital setting. Advise patient to telephone physician immediately if symptoms of a heart attack occur. Do not administer unless instructed by physician. To administer, remove safety cap and place back end on thickest part of thigh or deltoid muscle. Press hard until needle prick is felt. Hold in place for 10 sec, then massage area for 10 sec. Do not drive after administration unless absolutely necessary.

EVALUATION

Effectiveness of therapy can be demonstrated by: ▪ Decrease in ventricular arrhythmias ▪ Local anesthesia.

LIDOCAINE/PRILOCAINE
(lye-doe-kane/pri-loe-kane)
EMLA

CLASSIFICATION(S):
Local anesthetic combination
Pregnancy Category B

INDICATIONS
- Produces local anesthesia when applied to normal intact skin.

ACTION
- Produces local anesthesia by inhibiting transport of ions across neuronal membranes, thereby preventing initiation and conduction of normal nerve impulses. The two anesthetics are applied as a system consisting of a cream under an occlusive dressing. Active drug is released into the dermal and epidermal skin layers, resulting in accumulation of local anesthetic in the regions of dermal pain receptors and nerve endings. **Therapeutic Effect:** • Anesthetic action localized to the area of the application.

PHARMACOKINETICS
Absorption: Small amounts are systemically absorbed during 4-hr placement of EMLA system.
Distribution: Small amounts absorbed are widely distributed and cross the placenta and blood–brain barrier.
Metabolism and Excretion: Lidocaine is mostly metabolized by the liver. Prilocaine is metabolized by the liver and kidneys.
Half-life: Lidocaine—7–30 min first phase, 90–120 min terminal phase; prilocaine—10–50 min.

CONTRAINDICATIONS AND PRECAUTIONS
Contraindicated in: • Hypersensitivity to lidocaine, prilocaine, or any other amide-type local anesthetic • Hypersensitivity to any other product in the formulation • Should not be applied to middle ear • Congenital or idiopathic methemoglobinemia • Infants <6 mo who are receiving methemoglobin-inducing agents • Infants <1 mo.
Use Cautiously in: • Repeated use or use on large areas of skin (more likely to result in systemic absorption) • Severe liver disease • Any conditions associated with methemoglobinemia (including glucose-6-phosphate dehydrogenase deficiency) • Lactation.

ADVERSE REACTIONS AND SIDE EFFECTS*
Local: blanching, redness, alteration in temperature sensation, edema, itching, rash.
Misc: allergic reactions, including ANAPHYLAXIS.

INTERACTIONS
Drug–Drug: • Concurrent use with **group 1 antiarrhythmic drugs (tocainide, mexiletine)** may result in adverse cardiovascular effects • Concurrent use with **other local anesthetics** may result in additive toxicity.

ROUTE AND DOSAGE
Minor Dermal Procedures (Venipuncture, IV Cannulation)
- Topical (Adults and Children): 2.5 g applied to 20–25 cm^2 (2 in. by 2 in.) area of skin, covered with an occlusive dressing for at least 1 hr. Area covered should not be >100 cm^2 in children weighing <10 kg, or 600 cm^2 in children weighing 10–20 kg.

Major Dermal Procedures (Split-Thickness Skin Graft Harvesting)
- Topical (Adults and Children): 2 g/10 cm^2 area of skin, covered with an occlusive dressing for at least 2 hr.

AVAILABILITY
- *Cream:* 2.5% lidocaine with 2.5% prilocaine in 5-g and 30-g tubes.

TIME/ACTION PROFILE (local anesthesia)

	ONSET	PEAK	DURATION*
Top	1–3 hr	3 hr	1–2 hr

*Following removal of occlusive dressing.

L

NURSING IMPLICATIONS

ASSESSMENT

□ Assess application site for open wounds. Apply only to intact skin.

□ Assess application site for anesthesia following removal of system and prior to procedure.

POTENTIAL NURSING DIAGNOSES

■ Pain [acute] (indications).

■ Knowledge deficit related to medication regimen (patient/family teaching).

IMPLEMENTATION

■ **Topical:** When used for minor dermal procedures (venipuncture, IV cannulation), apply the 2.5-g tube of cream (½ of the 5-g tube) to each 2 in. by 2 in. area of skin in a thick layer at the site of the impending procedure. Remove the center cut-out piece from an occlusive dressing (supplied with the 5-g tube) and peel the paper liner from the paper framed dressing. Cover the lidocaine/prilocaine cream so that there is a thick layer of cream underneath the occlusive dressing. Do not spread out the cream. Smooth the dressing edges carefully and ensure it is secure to avoid leakage. Remove the paper frame and mark the time of application on the occlusive dressing. Lidocaine/prilocaine cream must be applied at least 1 hr before the start of a minor dermal procedure (venipuncture, IV cannulation). Remove the occlusive dressing and wipe off the lidocaine/prilocaine cream. Clean the entire area with antiseptic solution and prepare the patient for the procedure.

□ For major dermal procedures (skin graft harvesting), follow the above procedure using larger amounts of lidocaine/prilocaine cream and the appropriate size occlusive dressing. Lidocaine/prilocaine cream must be applied 2 hr before major dermal procedures.

PATIENT/FAMILY TEACHING

□ Explain the purpose of cream and oc-

clusive dressing to patient and parents. Inform the patient that lidocaine/prilocaine cream may block all sensations in the treated skin. Caution patient to avoid trauma to the area from scratching, rubbing, or exposure to extreme heat or cold temperatures until all sensation has returned.

EVALUATION

Clinical response to therapy can be determined by: ■ Anesthesia in the area of application.

LINDANE
(lin-dane)
Bio-well, Gamma benzene hexachloride, GBH, G-well, Kwell, {Kwellada}, Kwildane, Scabene, Thionex

CLASSIFICATION(S):
Antiparasitic
Pregnancy Category B

INDICATIONS

■ Treatment of: □ Scabies □ Head lice □ Body lice □ Crab lice.

ACTION

■ Causes seizures and death in parasitic arthropods. **Therapeutic Effect:** ■ Cure of infestation by parasitic arthropods (scabies and lice).

PHARMACOKINETICS

Absorption: Significant systemic absorption (9–13%) occurs slowly following topical application.

Distribution: Stored in fat.

Metabolism and Excretion: Metabolized by the liver.

Half-life: 18 hr (infants and children).

CONTRAINDICATIONS AND PRECAUTIONS

Contraindicated in: ■ Hypersensitivity ■ Neonates ■ History of seizures.

Use Cautiously in: ■ Children (increased risk of systemic absorption and CNS side effects) ▪ Pregnancy or lactation (do not exceed recommended dose; do not use >2 courses of therapy).

ADVERSE REACTIONS AND SIDE EFFECTS*

CNS: SEIZURES.
Derm: local irritation, contact dermatitis.

INTERACTIONS
Drug–Drug: ▪ Simultaneous topical use of **skin, scalp,** or **hair preparations** may increase systemic absorption.

ROUTE AND DOSAGE
Scabies
▪ **Top (Adults and Children):** 1% cream or lotion applied to all skin surfaces from neck to toes. Treatment may be repeated in 1 wk.

Lice
▪ **Top (Adults and Children):** 1% cream or lotion applied to hairy affected and adjacent areas. Treatment may be repeated in 1 wk.

Head Lice
▪ **Top (Adults and Children):** 15–30 ml of 1% shampoo, apply and lather for 4–5 min (may need 60 ml for long hair), rinse thoroughly. Treatment may be repeated in 1 wk.

AVAILABILITY
▪ **Cream:** 1% ▪ **Lotion:** 1% ▪ **Shampoo:** 1%.

TIME/ACTION PROFILE (antiparasitic action)

	ONSET	PEAK	DURATION
Top	rapid	rapid	190 min

NURSING IMPLICATIONS
ASSESSMENT
▫ Assess skin and hair for signs of infestation before and after treatment.
▫ Examine family members and close contacts for infestation. When used in treatment of pediculosis pubis or scabies, sexual partners should receive concurrent therapy.

POTENTIAL NURSING DIAGNOSES
▪ Skin integrity, impaired (indications).
▪ Knowledge deficit related to medication regimen (patient/family teaching).

IMPLEMENTATION
▪ **Top:** When applying medication to another person, wear gloves to prevent systemic absorption.
▫ Do not apply to open wounds (scratches, cuts, sores on skin or scalp) to minimize systemic absorption. Avoid contact with the eyes. If eye contact occurs, flush thoroughly with water and notify physician.
▫ Institute appropriate isolation techniques.
▪ **Cream/Lotion:** Instruct patient to bathe with soap and water. Dry skin well and allow to cool prior to application. Apply cream or lotion in amount sufficient to cover entire body surface with a thin film from neck down (60 ml for an adult). Leave medication on for 8–12 hr, then remove by washing. If rash, burning, or itching develops, wash off medication and notify physician.
▪ **Shampoo:** Use a sufficient amount of shampoo to wet hair and scalp (30 ml for short hair, 45 ml for medium hair, 60 ml for long hair). Rub thoroughly into hair and scalp and leave in place for 4 min. Then use enough water to work up a good lather; follow with thorough rinsing and drying. When hair is dry, use fine-toothed comb to remove remaining nits or nit shells. Shampoo may also be used on combs and brushes to prevent spread of infestation.

PATIENT/FAMILY TEACHING
▪ **General Info:** Instruct patient on application technique. Patient should repeat therapy only at the recommendation of the physician. Discuss hygienic measures to prevent and to control infestation. Discuss potential

L

*Underlines indicate most frequent; **CAPITALS** indicate life-threatening.

for infectious contacts with patient. Explain why household members should be examined and sexual partners treated simultaneously.

☐ Instruct patient to wash all recently worn clothing and used bed linens and towels in very hot water or to dry clean to prevent reinfestation or spreading.

☐ Instruct patient not to apply other oils or creams during therapy, as these increase the absorption of lindane and may lead to toxicity.

☐ Explain to patient that itching may persist after treatment; repeat treatment is necessary only if live mites are found.

▪ **Shampoo:** Advise patient that shampoo should not be used as a regular shampoo in the absence of infestation. Emphasize need to avoid eye contact.

▪ **Children:** Advise parents to monitor young children closely for evidence of CNS toxicity during and immediately after treatment.

EVALUATION

Effectiveness of therapy can be demonstrated by: ▪ Resolution of signs of infestation with scabies or lice.

LIOTHYRONINE
(lye-oh-**thye**-roe-neen)
Cytomel, L-triiodothyronine, T$_{3r}$
Triostat

CLASSIFICATION(S):
Hormone (thyroid)
Pregnancy Category A

INDICATIONS

▪ Replacement or substitution therapy in diminished or absent thyroid function of many causes.

ACTION

▪ Principal effect is increasing metabolic rate of body tissues ▪ Promotes gluconeogenesis, increases utilization and mobilization of glycogen stores, and stimulates protein synthesis ▪ Promotes cell growth and aids in the development of the brain and CNS. **Therapeutic Effects:** ▪ Replacement in deficiency states ▪ Restoration of normal hormonal balance.

PHARMACOKINETICS

Absorption: 95% absorbed following oral administration.

Distribution: Distributed into many body tissues. Thyroid hormones do not readily cross the placenta; minimal amounts enter breast milk.

Metabolism and Excretion: Metabolized by the liver and other tissues.

Half-life: 1–2 days (increased in hypothyroidism).

CONTRAINDICATIONS AND PRECAUTIONS

Contraindicated in: ▪ Hypersensitivity ▪ Recent myocardial infarction ▪ Thyrotoxicosis.

Use Cautiously in: ▪ Cardiovascular disease ▪ Severe renal insufficiency ▪ Uncorrected adrenocortical disorders ▪ Elderly and myxedematous patients (extremely sensitive to thyroid hormones, initial dosage should be markedly reduced) ▪ Cretinism (may not enter brain in sufficient amounts).

ADVERSE REACTIONS AND SIDE EFFECTS*

CNS: <u>irritability</u>, <u>nervousness</u>, <u>insomnia</u>, headache.

CV: <u>tachycardia</u>, <u>arrhythmias</u>, increased cardiac output, angina pectoris, increased blood pressure, CARDIOVASCULAR COLLAPSE, hypotension.

GI: diarrhea, cramps, vomiting.

Derm: increased sweating, hair loss (in children).

Endo: menstrual irregularities.

Metab: <u>weight loss</u>, heat intolerance.

MS: accelerated bone maturation in children.

*<u>Underlines</u> indicate most frequent; **CAPITALS** indicate life-threatening.

INTERACTIONS

Drug–Drug: ▪ **Colestipol** and **cholestyramine** decrease absorption ▪ **IV phenytoin** causes release of thyroid hormone ▪ May increase the effectiveness of **oral anticoagulants** ▪ May alter the requirements for **insulin** or **oral hypoglycemic agents** in diabetics ▪ Additive CNS and cardiac stimulation with **sympathomimetic agents (amphetamines, vasopressors, decongestants)** ▪ May decrease some cardiac effects of **beta-adrenergic blockers**.

ROUTE AND DOSAGE

Mild Hypothyroidism

▪ **PO (Adults):** 25 mcg once daily, may increase by 12.5–25 mcg/day at 1–2 wk intervals; usual maintenance dose is 25–50 mcg/day.

Severe Hypothyroidism, Myxedema

▪ **PO (Adults):** 5 mcg once daily initially, increase by 5 mcg/day at 1–2 wk intervals.

Simple Goiter

▪ **PO (Adults):** 5 mcg once daily initially, increase by 5–10 mcg/day at 1–2-wk intervals until daily dose is 25 mcg, then increase by 12.5–25 mcg/day at 1-wk intervals until effect is obtained.

T_3 Suppression Test

▪ **PO (Adults):** 75–100 mcg daily for 7 days. Radioactive I^{131} is administered before and after 7-day course.

Myxedema Coma/Precoma

▪ **IV (Adults):** 25–50 mcg initially. If cardiovascular disease is present, start with 10–20 mcg. At least 65 mcg/day should be given initially. Space doses 4–12 hr apart. Use 5 mcg initial dose in elderly patients.

AVAILABILITY

▪ *Tablets:* 5 mcg, 25 mcg, 50 mcg ▪ *Injection:* 10 mcg/ml.

TIME/ACTION PROFILE (effects on thyroid function tests)

	ONSET	PEAK	DURATION
PO, IV	UK	24–72 hr	72 hr

NURSING IMPLICATIONS

ASSESSMENT

▪ **General Info:** Assess apical pulse and blood pressure prior to and periodically during therapy. Assess for tachyarrhythmias and chest pain.

▫ Thyroid function studies should be monitored prior to and throughout course of therapy.

▫ Monitor blood and urine glucose in diabetic patients; insulin or oral hypoglycemic dose may need to be increased.

▪ **Toxicity and Overdose:** Overdose is manifested as hyperthyroidism (tachycardia, chest pain, nervousness, insomnia, diaphoresis, tremors, weight loss). Usual treatment is to withhold dose for 2–6 days.

POTENTIAL NURSING DIAGNOSES

▪ Knowledge deficit related to medication regimen (patient/family teaching).

IMPLEMENTATION

▪ **PO:** Administer as a single dose, preferably before breakfast to prevent insomnia.

▫ Initial dose is low, especially in elderly and cardiac patients. Dosage is increased gradually based on thyroid function tests. Side effects occur more rapidly with liothyronine because of its rapid onset of effect.

▪ **IV:** Liothyronine injection is for IV use only. Do not give IM or SC. Administer doses at least 4 hr and not more than 12 hr apart. Base doses on continuous monitoring of patient and response to therapy.

▫ Resume PO therapy as soon as patient is stable and able to take PO medication. When switching to PO therapy, discontinue IV liothyronine and initiate PO at low dose, increasing gradually according to patient's response.

PATIENT/FAMILY TEACHING

▪ **General Info:** Instruct patient to take medication exactly as directed at the same time each day. If a dose is missed, take as soon as remembered, unless almost time for next dose. If more than 2–3 doses are missed,

L

notify physician. Do not discontinue without consulting physician.

□ Instruct patient and family on correct technique for checking pulse. Dose should be withheld and physician notified if resting pulse >100 bpm.

□ Explain to patient that liothyronine does not cure hypothyroidism, it provides a thyroid hormone; therapy is lifelong.

□ Advise patient to notify physician if headache, nervousness, diarrhea, excessive sweating, heat intolerance, chest pain, increased pulse rate, palpitations, weight loss >2 lb/wk, or any unusual symptoms occur.

□ Caution patient to avoid taking other medications concurrently with levothyroxine unless instructed by physician.

□ Instruct patient to inform physician or dentist of thyroid therapy.

□ Emphasize importance of follow-up examinations to monitor effectiveness of therapy. Thyroid function tests are performed at least yearly.

EVALUATION

Clinical response can be determined by: ▪ Resolution of symptoms of hypothyroidism. Response includes: □ Diuresis □ Weight loss □ Increased sense of well-being □ Increased energy, pulse rate, appetite, psychomotor activity □ Normalization of skin texture and hair □ Correction of constipation □ Increased T_3 and T_4 levels.

LIOTRIX
(lye-oh-trix)
Euthroid, T_3/T_4, Thyrolar

CLASSIFICATION(S):
Hormone (thyroid)
Pregnancy Category A

INDICATIONS

▪ Replacement or substitution therapy in diminished or absent thyroid function of many causes.

ACTION

▪ A synthetic mixture of T_3 (liothyronine) and T_4 (levothyroxine) in a fixed ratio ▪ Principal effect is increasing metabolic rate of body tissues ▪ Promotes gluconeogenesis, increases utilization and mobilization of glycogen stores, and stimulates protein synthesis ▪ Promotes cell growth and aids in the development of the brain and CNS.
Therapeutic Effects: ▪ Replacement in deficiency states ▪ Restoration of normal hormonal balance.

PHARMACOKINETICS

Absorption: Liothyronine (T_3) is 95% absorbed following oral administration; levothyroxine (T_4) is variably (50–80%) absorbed following oral administration.
Distribution: Distributed into many body tissues. Thyroid hormones do not readily cross the placenta; minimal amounts enter breast milk.
Metabolism and Excretion: Metabolized by the liver and other tissues.
Half-life: Liothyronine 1–2 days; levothyroxine 6–7 days (increased in hypothyroidism).

CONTRAINDICATIONS AND PRECAUTIONS

Contraindicated in: ▪ Hypersensitivity ▪ Recent myocardial infarction ▪ Thyrotoxicosis.
Use Cautiously in: ▪ Cardiovascular disease ▪ Severe renal insufficiency ▪ Uncorrected adrenocortical disorders ▪ Elderly and myxedematous patients (extremely sensitive to thyroid hormones; initial dosage should be markedly reduced) ▪ Has been used safely in pregnancy.

ADVERSE REACTIONS AND SIDE EFFECTS*

CNS: <u>irritability</u>, <u>nervousness</u>, <u>insomnia</u>, headache.

---

*<u>Underlines</u> indicate most frequent; **CAPITALS** indicate life-threatening.

CV: tachycardia, arrhythmias, increased cardiac output, angina pectoris, increased blood pressure, CARDIO-VASCULAR COLLAPSE, hypotension.
Derm: increased sweating, hair loss in children.
Endo: menstrual irregularities.
GI: diarrhea, cramps, vomiting.
Metab: weight loss, heat intolerance.

INTERACTIONS

Drug–Drug: ▪ Colestipol and cholestyramine decrease absorption ▪ IV phenytoin causes release of thyroid hormone ▪ May increase the effectiveness of **oral anticoagulants** ▪ May alter the requirements for **insulin** or **oral hypoglycemic agents** in diabetic patients ▪ Additive CNS and cardiac stimulation with **sympathomimetic agents (amphetamines, vasopressors, decongestants)** ▪ May decrease some cardiac effects of **beta-adrenergic blockers**.

ROUTE AND DOSAGE

Thyrolar contains T_3 and T_4 in fixed ratios, representing thyroid hormone equivalents (ex: Thyrolar ½ contains the equivalent of ½ gr or 30 mg of thyroid hormone)

Product	Thyroid equivalent (mg)	T_3 (mcg)	T_4 (mcg)
Euthroid ½	30	7.5	30
Euthroid 1	60	15	60
Euthroid 2	120	30	120
Euthroid 3	180	45	180
Thyrolar ¼	15	3.1	12.5
Thyrolar ½	30	6.25	25
Thyrolar 1	60	12.5	50
Thyrolar 2	120	25	100
Thyrolar 3	180	37.5	150

Hypothyroidism

▪ **PO (Adults and Children):** Thyrolar–¼, Thyrolar–½, or Euthroid–½ initially; dosage may be increased at 2–3 wk intervals. Use smaller doses in patients with myxedema or cardiovascular disease.

AVAILABILITY

▪ **Euthroid tablets:** ½ gr, 1 gr, 2 gr, 3 gr
▪ **Thyrolar tablets:** ¼ gr, ½ gr, 1 gr, 2 gr, 3 gr.

TIME/ACTION PROFILE (effects on thyroid function testing)

	ONSET	PEAK	DURATION
PO (liothyronine)	UK	24–72 hr	72 hr
PO (levothyroxine)	UK	1–3 wk	1–3 wk

NURSING IMPLICATIONS

ASSESSMENT

▪ **General Info:** Assess apical pulse and blood pressure prior to and periodically during therapy. Assess for tachyarrhythmias and chest pain.
▫ Thyroid function studies should be monitored prior to and throughout course of therapy.
▫ Monitor blood and urine glucose in diabetic patients; insulin or oral hypoglycemic dose may need to be increased.
▪ **Children:** Monitor height, weight, and psychomotor development.
▪ **Toxicity and Overdose:** Overdose is manifested as hyperthyroidism (tachycardia, chest pain, nervousness, insomnia, diaphoresis, tremors, weight loss). Usual treatment is to withhold dose for 2–6 days.

POTENTIAL NURSING DIAGNOSES

▪ Knowledge deficit related to medication regimen (patient/family teaching).

IMPLEMENTATION

▪ **General Info:** Administer as a single dose, preferably before breakfast, to prevent insomnia.
▫ Initial dose is low, especially in elderly patients and patients with cardiovascular disease. Dosage is increased in small increments based on thyroid function test results.

PATIENT/FAMILY TEACHING

▪ **General Info:** Instruct patient to take medication exactly as directed at the

L

same time each day. If a dose is missed, take as soon as remembered, unless almost time for next dose. If more than 2–3 doses are missed, notify physician. Do not discontinue without consulting physician.

□ Instruct patient and family on correct technique for checking pulse. Dose should be withheld and physician notified if resting pulse >100 bpm.

□ Explain to patient that liotrix does not cure hypothyroidism but provides a thyroid hormone; therapy is lifelong.

□ Caution patient not to change brands of this medication, as this may affect drug bioavailability.

□ Advise patient to notify physician if headache, nervousness, diarrhea, excessive sweating, heat intolerance, chest pain, increased pulse rate, palpitations, weight loss >2 lb/wk, or any unusual symptoms occur.

□ Caution patient to avoid taking other medications concurrently with liotrix unless instructed by physician.

□ Instruct patient to inform physician or dentist of thyroid therapy.

□ Emphasize importance of follow-up examinations to monitor effectiveness of therapy. Thyroid function tests are performed at least yearly.

■ **Children:** Discuss with parents need for routine follow-up studies to ensure correct development. Inform parents that partial hair loss may be experienced by children on thyroid therapy. This is usually temporary.

EVALUATION

Clinical response is indicated by:
■ Resolution of symptoms of hypothyroidism. Response includes: □ Diuresis □ Weight loss □ Increased sense of well-being □ Increased energy, pulse rate, appetite, psychomotor activity □ Normalization of skin texture and hair □ Correction of constipation □ Increased T_3 and T_4 levels □ Normal thyroid stimulating hormone (TSH) levels. In children effectiveness of therapy is determined by ■ Appropriate physical and psychomotor development.

LISINOPRIL
(lyse-**in**-oh-pril)
Prinivil, Zestril

CLASSIFICATION(S):
Antihypertensive (angiotensin converting enzyme [ACE] inhibitor)
Pregnancy Category C (first trimester), D (second and third trimesters)

INDICATIONS

■ Used alone or in combination with other antihypertensives in the management of hypertension ■ In combination with other agents in the management of congestive heart failure.

ACTION

■ Prevents the production of angiotensin II, a potent vasoconstrictor that stimulates the production of aldosterone by blocking its conversion to the active form. Result is systemic vasodilation. **Therapeutic Effects:** ■ Lowering of blood pressure in hypertensive patients ■ Decreased preload and afterload in patients with congestive heart failure.

PHARMACOKINETICS

Absorption: 25% absorbed following oral administration; much variability.
Distribution: Distribution not known.
Metabolism and Excretion: Excreted entirely unchanged by the kidneys.
Half-life: 12 hr.

CONTRAINDICATIONS AND PRECAUTIONS

Contraindicated in: ■ Hypersensitivity ■ Pregnancy (may cause fetal malformation or death; hypotension, oliguria, or hypokalemia may occur in newborn).
Use Cautiously in: ■ Renal impairment (dosage reduction required if creatinine clearance ≤30 ml/min) ■ Lactation or children (safety not established) ■ Surgery/anesthesia (hypotension may be exaggerated) ■ Aortic stenosis, cerebrovascular or cardiac insufficiency

- Patients with childbearing potential
- Hyponatremia or concurrent diuretic therapy (initial dosage reduction recommended).

ADVERSE REACTIONS AND SIDE EFFECTS*

CNS: <u>headache</u>, <u>dizziness</u>, <u>fatigue</u>, insomnia.
Resp: cough, dyspnea.
CV: hypotension, tachycardia, angina pectoris.
GI: anorexia, diarrhea, nausea, altered taste, stomatitis.
GU: impotence, increased BUN.
Derm: rashes.
F and E: hyperkalemia.
Hemat: neutropenia.
Neuro: paresthesias.
Misc: fever, ANGIODEMA with laryngospasm.

INTERACTIONS

Drug–Drug: ▪ Additive hypotension with other **antihypertensives, nitrates,** or acute ingestion of **alcohol** ▪ Hyperkalemia may result with concurrent **potassium supplements, cyclosporine,** or **potassium-sparing diuretics** ▪ Antihypertensive response may be blunted by **nonsteroidal anti-inflammatory agents** ▪ Incidence of hypersensitivity reactions may be increased with **allopurinol** ▪ May increase serum **lithium** or **digoxin** levels and risk of toxicity ▪ Concurrent use with **capsaicin** may increase the incidence of cough.
Drug–Food: ▪ Hyperkalemia may result from a **high-potassium** diet.

ROUTE AND DOSAGE

Hypertension
- **PO (Adults):** 10 mg once daily (5 mg if on diuretics), can be increased up to 20–40 mg day.

Congestive Heart Failure
- **PO (Adults):** 2.5–5 mg/once daily initially; range 5–20 mg once daily.

AVAILABILITY
- **Tablets:** 5 mg, 10 mg, 20 mg, 40 mg.

TIME/ACTION PROFILE (antihypertensive effect)

	ONSET	PEAK	DURATION
PO	1 hr	7 hr	24 hr

NURSING IMPLICATIONS

ASSESSMENT
- Monitor blood pressure and pulse frequently during initial dosage adjustment and periodically throughout course of therapy. Notify physician of significant changes.
- Monitor weight and assess patient routinely for resolution of fluid overload (peripheral edema, rales/crackles, dyspnea, weight gain).
- **Lab Test Considerations:** Monitor BUN, creatinine, and electrolyte levels periodically. Serum potassium may be increased and BUN and creatinine transiently increased, while sodium levels may be decreased.
- Monitor CBC periodically during therapy. May cause a decrease in hemoglobin and hematocrit.
- May cause elevated liver enzymes, serum bilirubin, uric acid, and glucose.
- Periodic assessments of urine protein may be ordered, because proteinuria and nephrotic syndrome may occur.

POTENTIAL NURSING DIAGNOSES
- Cardiac output, decreased (indications, side effects).
- Knowledge deficit related to medication regimen (patient/family teaching).
- Noncompliance (patient/family teaching).

IMPLEMENTATION
- **General Info:** Precipitous drop in blood pressure during first 1–3 hr following first dose may require volume expansion with normal saline but is not normally considered an indication for stopping therapy. Patients treated with diuretics should discontinue diuretic therapy for 2–3 days, if possible, prior to initial dose of lisin-

opril to prevent hypotension. If this is not possible, decreased dose of lisinopril may be necessary.

□ If blood pressure is not controlled with lisinopril, diuretic therapy may be added.

PATIENT/FAMILY TEACHING

■ **General Info:** Instruct patient to take lisinopril exactly as directed, even if feeling well. Advise patients not to discontinue lisinopril therapy unless directed by physician.

□ Instruct patient and family on proper technique for blood pressure monitoring. Advise them to check blood pressure at least weekly and to report significant changes to physician.

□ Caution patient to avoid salt substitutes or foods containing high levels of potassium or sodium, unless directed by physician (see Appendix K).

□ Advise patient that lisinopril may cause an impairment of taste, which generally reverses itself within 8–12 wk.

□ Caution patient to change position slowly to minimize orthostatic hypotension, particularly after initial dose. Patient should also be advised that exercising or hot weather may increase hypotensive effects.

□ Advise patient to consult physician or pharmacist before taking any over-the-counter medications, especially cold remedies. Patient should also avoid excessive amounts of tea, coffee, or cola.

□ Instruct patient to notify physician if pregnancy is planned or suspected.

□ Advise patient to inform physician or dentist of medication regimen prior to treatment or surgery.

□ Instruct patient to notify physician if cough, rash, mouth sores, sore throat, fever, swelling of hands or feet, irregular heart beat, chest pain, swelling of face, eyes, lips, or tongue, persistent fatigue, headache, or difficulty breathing occurs.

□ Emphasize the importance of follow-up examinations to monitor progress.

■ **Hypertension:** Encourage patient to comply with additional interventions for hypertension (low-sodium diet, weight reduction, discontinuation of smoking, moderation of alcohol consumption, regular exercise, and stress management).

EVALUATION
Effectiveness of therapy can be demonstrated by: ■ Decrease in blood pressure without appearance of side effects. ■ Decrease in signs and symptoms of congestive heart failure. Several weeks may be necessary before full effects of the drug are recognized.

LITHIUM
(lith-ee-um)
{Carbolith}, Cibalith-S, Duralith, Eskalith, Eskalith-CR, Lithane, {Lithizine}, Lithonate, Lithotabs

CLASSIFICATION(S):
Antimanic
Pregnancy Category D

INDICATIONS

■ Treatment of a variety of psychiatric disorders, particularly bipolar affective disorders, both to treat acute manic episodes and as prophylaxis against their recurrence.

ACTION

■ Alters cation transport in nerve and muscle ■ May also influence re-uptake of neurotransmitters. **Therapeutic Effects:** ■ Antimanic and antidepressant properties.

PHARMACOKINETICS

Absorption: Completely absorbed following oral administration.
Distribution: Widely distributed into

many tissues and fluids; CSF levels are 50% of plasma levels. Crosses the placenta and enters breast milk.

Metabolism and Excretion: Excreted almost entirely unchanged by the kidneys.

Half-life: 20–27 hr.

CONTRAINDICATIONS AND PRECAUTIONS

Contraindicated in: ▪ Hypersensitivity ▪ Severe cardiovascular or renal disease ▪ Dehydrated or debilitated patients ▪ Pregnancy or lactation ▪ Should be used only where therapy, including blood levels, may be closely monitored ▪ Known alcohol intolerance (some liquid products).

Use Cautiously in: ▪ Elderly or debilitated patients (initial dosage reduction recommended) ▪ Any degree of cardiac, renal, or thyroid disease ▪ Diabetes mellitus ▪ Children (safety not established).

ADVERSE REACTIONS AND SIDE EFFECTS*

CNS: <u>tremors</u>, <u>headache</u>, <u>impaired memory</u>, <u>lethargy</u>, <u>fatigue</u>, drowsiness, confusion, seizures, ataxia, dizziness, psychomotor retardation, restlessness, stupor.

EENT: tinnitus, blurred vision, dysarthria, aphasia.

CV: <u>ECG changes</u>, hypotension, arrhythmias, edema.

GI: <u>nausea</u>, <u>anorexia</u>, <u>epigastric bloating</u>, <u>diarrhea</u>, <u>abdominal pain</u>, dry mouth, metallic taste.

GU: <u>polyuria</u>, nephrogenic diabetes insipidus, glycosuria, renal toxicity.

Derm: <u>acneiform erruption</u>, <u>folliculitis</u>, pruritis, diminished sensation, alopecia.

Endo: <u>hypothyroidism</u>, goiter, hyperglycemia, hyperthyroidism.

F and E: hyponatremia.

Hemat: <u>leukocytosis</u>.

Metab: weight gain.

MS: <u>muscle weakness</u>, rigidity, hyperirritability.

INTERACTIONS

Drug–Drug: ▪ May prolong the action of **neuromuscular blocking agents** ▪ Neurologic toxicity may occur with **haloperidol** or **molindine** ▪ **Diuretics, methyldopa, probenecid, fluoxetine,** and **nonsteroidal anti-inflammatory agents** may increase the risk of toxicity ▪ **Aminophylline, phenothiazines, sodium bicarbonate,** and **sodium chloride** may hasten excretion and lead to decreased effect ▪ Lithium may decrease the effects of **chlorpromazine** ▪ **Chlorpromazine** may mask early signs of lithium toxicity ▪ Hypothyroid effects may be additive with **potassium iodide** or **antithyroid drugs** ▪ Drugs containing large amounts of **sodium (ticarcillin)** may increase the renal elimination and decrease the effectiveness of lithium.

Drug–Food: ▪ Large changes in **sodium** intake may alter the renal elimination of lithium. Increasing sodium intake will increase renal excretion.

ROUTE AND DOSAGE

300 mg lithium carbonate contains 8–12 mEq lithium.

▪ **PO (Adults):** 900–1200 mg/day in 3–4 divided doses (usual dose 300 mg 3–4 times daily). Blood level monitoring necessary to determine proper dose. Extended-release dosage forms (Eskalith-CR, Duralith, Lithizine) may be given 2–3 times daily.

▪ **PO (Children):** 15–20 mg (0.4–0.5 mEq)/kg/day in 2–3 divided doses.

AVAILABILITY

▪ *Capsules:* 300 mg, 600 mg ▪ *Tablets:* 300 mg ▪ *Controlled-release tablets:* 450 mg ▪ {*Slow-release capsules:* 150 mg, 300 mg} ▪ *Syrup:* 8 mEq lithium/5 ml.

L

---

*<u>Underlines</u> indicate most frequent; **CAPITALS** indicate life-threatening.

TIME/ACTION PROFILE (antimanic effects)

	ONSET	PEAK	DURATION
PO	5–7 days	10–21 days	days
PO liquid	5–7 days	10–21 days	days
PO-ER caps	5–7 days	10–21 days	days

NURSING IMPLICATIONS

ASSESSMENT

□ Assess mood, ideation, and behaviors frequently. Initiate suicide precautions if indicated.

□ Monitor intake and output ratios. Notify physician of significant changes in totals. Unless contraindicated, fluid intake of at least 2000–3000 ml/day should be maintained. Weight should also be monitored at least every 3 mo.

■ **Lab Test Considerations:** Renal and thyroid function, WBC with differential, serum electrolytes, and glucose should be evaluated periodically throughout therapy.

■ **Toxicity and Overdose:** Serum lithium levels should be monitored twice weekly during initiation of therapy and every 2–3 mo during chronic therapy. Blood samples should be drawn in the morning immediately prior to next dose. Therapeutic levels range from 0.5 to 1.5 mEq/liter.

□ Assess patient for signs and symptoms of lithium toxicity (vomiting, diarrhea, slurred speech, decreased coordination, drowsiness, muscle weakness, or twitching). If these occur, inform physician prior to administering next dose.

POTENTIAL NURSING DIAGNOSES

■ Thought processes, altered (indications).

■ Violence, high risk for: directed at self/others (indications).

■ Knowledge deficit related to medication regimen (patient/family teaching).

■ Noncompliance (patient/family teaching).

IMPLEMENTATION

■ **PO:** Administer with food or milk to minimize GI irritation. Extended-release preparations should be swallowed whole; do not break, crush, or chew.

PATIENT/FAMILY TEACHING

□ Instruct patient to take medication exactly as directed, even if feeling well. If a dose is missed, take as soon as remembered unless within 2 hr of next dose (6 hr if extended-release).

□ Medication may cause dizziness or drowsiness. Caution patient to avoid driving or other activities requiring alertness until response to medication is known.

□ Low sodium levels may predispose patient to toxicity. Advise patient to drink 2000–3000 ml fluid each day and eat a diet with liberal sodium intake. Excessive amounts of coffee, tea, and cola should be avoided because of diuretic effect. Avoid activities that cause excess sodium loss (heavy exertion, exercise in hot weather, saunas). Notify physician of fever, vomiting, and diarrhea, which also cause sodium loss.

□ Advise patient that weight gain may occur. Review principles of a low-calorie diet.

□ Instruct patient to consult physician or pharmacist prior to taking over-the-counter medications concurrently with this therapy.

□ Advise patient to use contraception and to consult physician if pregnancy is suspected.

□ Review side effects and symptoms of toxicity with patient. Instruct patient to stop medication and report signs of toxicity to physician promptly.

□ Explain to patients with cardiovascular disease or over 40 yr the need for ECG evaluation prior to and periodically during therapy. Patient should inform physician if fainting, irregular pulse, or difficulty breathing occurs.

□ Emphasize the importance of periodic lab tests to monitor for lithium toxicity.

EVALUATION

Effectiveness of therapy can be demonstrated by: ▪ Resolution of the symptoms of mania (hyperactivity, pressured speech, poor judgment, need for little sleep) ▪ Decreased incidence of mood swings in bipolar disorders ▪ Improved affect in unipolar disorders. Improvement in condition may require 1–3 wk.

LOMEFLOXACIN
(loe-me-**flox**-a-sin)
Maxaquin

CLASSIFICATION(S):
Anti-infective (fluoroquinolone)
Pregnancy Category C

INDICATIONS

▪ Treatment of the following infections due to susceptible organisms □ Lower respiratory tract infections, including acute exacerbations of chronic bronchitis (unless *Streptococcus pneumoniae* is suspected) □ Uncomplicated urinary tract infections □ As a preoperative prophylactic anti-infective before transurethral procedures.

ACTION

▪ Inhibits bacterial DNA synthesis by inhibiting DNA gyrase. **Therapeutic Effects:** ▪ Death of susceptible bacteria. **Spectrum:** ▪ Includes activity against the following gram-negative organisms: *Aeromonas* sp., *Citrobacter* sp., *Enterobacter* sp., *Escherichia coli*, *Hemophilus influenzae*, *Klebsiella* sp., *Legionella* sp., *Moraxella catarrhalis*, *Morganella morganii*, *Proteus vulgaris*, *Proteus mirabilis*, *Providencia alcalifaciens*, *Providencia rettgeri*, *Pseudomonas aeruginosa*, and *Serratia* sp. Susceptible gram-positive organisms include *Staphylococcus aureus*, *epidermidis*, and *saprophyticus* (including methicillin-resistant strains).

PHARMACOKINETICS

Absorption: Well absorbed following oral administration (95–98% bioavailability).
Distribution: Widely distributed to body tissue and fluids.
Metabolism and Excretion: 65% excreted unchanged by the kidneys. 10% excreted unchanged in feces.
Half-life: 8 hr (increased in renal impairment).

CONTRAINDICATIONS AND PRECAUTIONS

Contraindicated in: ▪ Hypersensitivity to lomefloxacin or other fluoroquinolones ▪ Children ▪ Pregnancy.
Use Cautiously in: ▪ Underlying CNS pathology ▪ Lactation (high milk concentrations achieved, safety not established) ▪ Renal impairment (dosage reduction required if creatinine clearance <40 ml/min).

ADVERSE REACTIONS AND SIDE EFFECTS*

CNS: <u>headache</u>, <u>dizziness</u>, SEIZURES.
GI: <u>nausea</u>, <u>diarrhea</u>, PSEUDOMEMBRANOUS COLITIS, increased liver enzymes.
Derm: <u>photosensitivity</u>, rash.
Hemat: anemia.

INTERACTIONS

Drug–Drug: ▪ Increases serum **theophylline** levels and may lead to toxicity ▪ Administration with **antacids, iron salts, sucralfate,** or **zinc salts** decreases absorption of fluoroquinolones ▪ May increase the effects of **oral anticoagulants** ▪ **Cimetidine** decreases metabolism of quinolones ▪ Concurrent use with **antineoplastic agents** may result in decreased fluoroquinolone levels ▪ **Probenecid** decreases urinary excretion of lomefloxacin.

ROUTE AND DOSAGE

▪ **PO (Adults):** 400 mg once daily.

AVAILABILITY

▪ *Tablets:* 400 mg.

L

TIME/ACTION PROFILE (blood levels)

	ONSET	PEAK
PO	rapid	UK

NURSING IMPLICATIONS

ASSESSMENT

□ Assess patient for infection (vital signs, urinalysis, frequency and urgency of urination, WBC, fever, cloudy or foul-smelling urine) at beginning and throughout course of therapy.

□ Obtain specimens for culture and sensitivity prior to initiating therapy. First dose may be given before receiving results.

■ **Lab Test Considerations:** Monitor hematologic, hepatic, and renal functions periodically during prolonged therapy. May cause increased BUN, AST (SGOT), ALT (SGPT), and serum bilirubin and alkaline phosphatase. May cause decreased hemoglobin and hematocrit concentrations.

POTENTIAL NURSING DIAGNOSES

■ Infection, high risk for (indications, side effects).

■ Knowledge deficit related to medication regimen (patient/family teaching).

■ Noncompliance related to medication regimen (patient/family teaching).

IMPLEMENTATION

■ **PO:** Administer once daily without regard to meals, with a full glass of water.

PATIENT/FAMILY TEACHING

□ Instruct patient to take medication as directed and to finish the drug completely, even if feeling better. If a dose is missed, take as soon as remembered unless almost time for next dose; do not double doses. Advise patient that sharing of this medication may be dangerous.

□ Encourage patient to maintain a fluid intake of at least 1200–1500 ml/day to prevent crystalluria.

□ Advise patient that antacids or medications containing iron or zinc will decrease absorption and should not be taken within 4 hr before or 2 hr after taking this medication.

□ May cause dizziness. Caution patient to avoid driving or other activities requiring alertness until response to medication is known.

□ Caution patient to use sunscreen and protective clothing to prevent photosensitivity reactions.

□ Instruct patient to notify physician immediately if rash occurs or if symptoms do not improve within a few days of therapy.

EVALUATION

Clinical response can be evaluated by:

■ Resolution of the signs and symptoms of infection. Length of time for complete resolution depends on organism and site of infection.

LOMUSTINE
(loe-**mus**-teen)
CCNU, CeeNu

CLASSIFICATION(S):
Antineoplastic agent (nitrosourea)
Pregnancy Category UK

INDICATIONS

■ Used alone or with other treatment modalities in the management of primary and metastatic brain tumors and Hodgkin's disease. **Unlabeled Uses:** ■ Bronchogenic carcinoma ■ Non-Hodgkin's lymphoma ■ Malignant melanoma ■ Breast carcinoma ■ Renal cell carcinoma ■ GI tract carcinoma.

ACTION

■ Inhibits DNA and RNA synthesis by alkylation (cell cycle phase-nonspecific. **Therapeutic Effect:** ■ Death of rapidly replicating cells, particularly malignant ones.

PHARMACOKINETICS

Absorption: Rapidly absorbed following oral administration.
Distribution: Widely distributed. Active metabolites enter the CSF well. Enters breast milk.
Metabolism and Excretion: Mostly metabolized by the liver. Some metabolites are active antineoplastic agents.
Half-life: 1–2 days.

CONTRAINDICATIONS AND PRECAUTIONS

Contraindicated in: ▪ Hypersensitivity ▪ Pregnancy or lactation.
Use Cautiously in: ▪ Patients with childbearing potential ▪ Active infections ▪ Decreased bone marrow reserve (dosage reduction required) ▪ Other chronic debilitating illnesses ▪ Impaired liver function.

ADVERSE REACTIONS AND SIDE EFFECTS*

CNS: disorientation, lethargy, ataxia, dysarthria.
GI: <u>nausea</u>, <u>vomiting</u>, stomatitis, hepatotoxicity, anorexia.
GU: azotemia, renal failure.
Endo: gonadal suppression.
Hemat: anemia, <u>leukopenia</u>, <u>thrombocytopenia</u>.
Metab: hyperuricemia.
Resp: pulmonary infiltrates, fibrosis, secondary malignancy (long-term use).

INTERACTIONS

Drug–Drug: ▪ Additive bone marrow depression with other **antineoplastic agents** or **radiation therapy** ▪ May decrease antibody response to **live virus vaccines** and increase risk of adverse reactions.

ROUTE AND DOSAGE

▪ **PO (Adults and Children):** 100–130 mg/m^2 as a single dose every 6 wk. Dosage adjustments are required for concurrent therapy or decreased blood counts.

AVAILABILITY

▪ *Capsules:* 10 mg, 40 mg, 100 mg.

TIME/ACTION PROFILE (effects on blood counts)

	ONSET	PEAK	DURATION
PO	UK	4–7 wk	1–2 wk

NURSING IMPLICATIONS

Assessment

□ Assess for fever, sore throat, and signs of infection. Notify physician if these symptoms occur.
□ Assess for bleeding (bleeding gums; bruising; petechiae; guaiac stools, urine, and emesis). Avoid IM injections and rectal temperatures. Apply pressure to venipuncture sites for 10 min.
□ Assess for nausea and vomiting, which usually begins within 3 hr of administration and persists for 24 hr. Confer with physician regarding prophylactic use of an antiemetic. Monitor intake and output, daily weight, and appetite. Adjust diet as tolerated for anorexia.
▪ **Lab Test Considerations:** Monitor CBC and differential prior to and periodically throughout therapy. The nadir of leukopenia occurs in 6 wk. Notify physician if leukocyte count is <4000/mm^3. The nadir of thrombocytopenia occurs in 4 wk. Notify physician if platelet count is <100,000/mm^3. Recovery of leukopenia and thrombocytopenia occurs in 1–2 wk. Myelosuppression is cumulative; subsequent courses of therapy should be delayed until recovery occurs.
□ Monitor liver function studies (AST [SGOT], ALT [SGPT], LDH, bilirubin) and renal function studies (BUN, creatinine) prior to and periodically throughout therapy to detect hepatotoxicity and nephrotoxicity.
□ May cause increased uric acid. Monitor periodically during therapy.

L

---

*<u>Underlines</u> indicate most frequent; **CAPITALS** indicate life-threatening.

POTENTIAL NURSING DIAGNOSES
- Infection, high risk for (side effects).
- Nutrition, altered: less than body requirements (side effects).
- Knowledge deficit related to medication regimen (patient/family teaching).

IMPLEMENTATION
- **PO:** Administer on empty stomach at bedtime. Preadministration of an antiemetic and a hypnotic may help control nausea.

PATIENT/FAMILY TEACHING
- Instruct patient to take lomustine exactly as directed, even if nausea and vomiting occurs. If vomiting occurs shortly after dose is taken, consult physician.
- Inform patient that several different types of capsules may be found in medication container. Patient should take all the capsules at one time in order to receive the correct dose.
- Advise patient to notify physician promptly if fever, chills, sore throat, signs of infection, bleeding gums, bruising, petechiae, or blood in urine, stool, or emesis occur. Caution patient to avoid crowds and persons with known infections. Instruct patient to use soft toothbrush and electric razor. Patient should be cautioned not to drink alcoholic beverages or take products containing aspirin or ibuprofen.
- Instruct patient to notify physician if abdominal pain, yellow skin, weakness, cough, slurred speech, or decreased urine output occurs.
- Instruct patient to inspect oral mucosa for redness and ulceration. If ulceration occurs, advise patient to use sponge brush and rinse mouth with water after eating and drinking. Viscous lidocaine swishes may be used if pain interferes with eating.
- Discuss with patient the possibility of hair loss. Explore coping strategies.
- Advise patient that although lomustine may cause infertility, contraception is necessary because of potential teratogenic effects in the fetus.

- Instruct patient not to receive any vaccinations without advice of physician.
- Emphasize need for periodic lab tests to monitor for side effects.

EVALUATION
Effectiveness of therapy can be demonstrated by: ▪ Decrease in size and spread of malignant tissue.

LOPERAMIDE
(loe-**per**-a-mide)
Imodium, Imodium A-D, Kaopectate II Caplets, Maalox Antidiarrheal Caplets, Pepto Diarrhea Control

CLASSIFICATION(S):
Antidiarrheal
Pregnancy Category B

INDICATIONS

▪ Adjunctive therapy in the treatment of acute diarrhea ▪ Treatment of chronic diarrhea associated with inflammatory bowel disease ▪ Used to decrease the volume of ileostomy drainage.

ACTION

▪ Inhibits peristalsis and prolongs transit time by a direct effect on nerves in the intestinal muscle wall ▪ Reduces fecal volume, increases fecal viscosity and bulk while diminishing loss of fluid and electrolytes. **Therapeutic Effect:** ▪ Relief of diarrhea.

PHARMACOKINETICS

Absorption: Not well absorbed following oral administration.
Distribution: Distribution not known. Does not cross the blood–brain barrier.
Metabolism and Excretion: Metabolized partially by the liver, undergoes enterohepatic recirculation. 30% eliminated in the feces. Minimal excretion in the urine.
Half-life: 10.8 hr.

CONTRAINDICATIONS AND PRECAUTIONS

Contraindicated in: ▪ Hypersensitivity ▪ Patients in whom constipation must be avoided ▪ Abdominal pain of unknown cause, especially if associated with fever. Alcohol intolerance (liquid only).

Use Cautiously in: ▪ Hepatic dysfunction ▪ Pregnancy, lactation, or children <2 yr (safety not established).

ADVERSE REACTIONS AND SIDE EFFECTS*

CNS: <u>drowsiness</u>, dizziness.
GI: <u>constipation</u>, <u>nausea</u>, dry mouth.

INTERACTIONS

Drug–Drug: ▪ Additive CNS depression with other **CNS depressants,** including **alcohol, antihistamines, narcotics,** and **sedative/hypnotics** ▪ Additive anticholinergic properties with other **drugs having anticholinergic properties,** including **antidepressants** and **antihistamines**.

ROUTE AND DOSAGE

▪ **PO (Adults):** 4 mg initially, then 2 mg after each loose stool. Maintenance dose usually 4–8 mg/day in divided doses (not to exceed 16 mg/day).

▪ **PO (Children 8–12 yr or >30 kg):** 2 mg, may be repeated 3 times in first 24 hr, then 0.1 mg/kg after each loose stool or 2 mg initially, then 1 mg with each loose stool (not to exceed 6 mg/24 hr).

▪ **PO (Children 5–8 yr or 20–30 kg):** 2 mg, may be repeated twice in first 24 hr, then 0.1 mg/kg after each loose stool or 2 mg initially then 1 mg with each loose stool (not to exceed 4 mg/24 hr).

▪ **PO (Children 2–5 yr or 13–20 kg):** 1 mg, may be repeated 3 times in first 24 hr, then 0.1 mg/kg after each loose stool (not to exceed 3 mg/24 hr).

AVAILABILITY

▪ *Tablets:* 2 mg ▪ *Capsules:* 2 mg ▪ *Liquid:* 1 mg/5 ml.

TIME/ACTION PROFILE (relief of diarrhea)

	ONSET	PEAK	DURATION
PO	1 hr	2.5–5 hr	10 hr

NURSING IMPLICATIONS

ASSESSMENT

▫ Assess frequency and consistency of stools and bowel sounds prior to and throughout course of therapy.

▫ Assess fluid and electrolyte balance and skin turgor for dehydration.

POTENTIAL NURSING DIAGNOSES

▪ Diarrhea (indications).
▪ Injury, high risk for (side effects).
▪ Knowledge deficit related to medication regimen (patient/family teaching).

IMPLEMENTATION

▪ **PO:** Administer with clear fluids to help prevent dehydration, which may accompany diarrhea.

PATIENT/FAMILY TEACHING

▫ Instruct patient to take medication exactly as directed. Do not take missed doses, and do not double doses. In acute diarrhea, medication may be ordered after each unformed stool. Advise patient not to exceed the maximum number of doses.

▫ Medication may cause drowsiness. Advise patient to avoid driving or other activities requiring alertness until response to drug is known.

▫ Advise patient that frequent mouth rinses, good oral hygiene, and sugarless gum or candy may relieve dry mouth.

▫ Caution patient to avoid using alcohol and other CNS depressants concurrently with this medication.

▫ Instruct patient to notify physician if diarrhea persists or if fever, abdominal pain, or distention occurs.

L

*<u>Underlines</u> indicate most frequent; **CAPITALS** indicate life-threatening.

EVALUATION
Effectiveness of therapy can be determined by: ▪ Decrease in diarrhea □ In acute diarrhea, treatment should be discontinued if no improvement is seen in 48 hr □ In chronic diarrhea, if no improvement has occurred after at least 10 days of treatment with maximum dose, loperamide is unlikely to be effective.

LORACARBEF
(lor-a-**kar**-beff)
Lorabid

CLASSIFICATION(S):
Anti-infective (second-generation cephalosporin)
Pregnancy Category B

INDICATIONS

▪ Useful in the treatment of the following infections due to susceptible organisms: □ Respiratory tract infections, including acute bronchitis and acute exacerbations of chronic bronchitis and pneumonia □ Acute maxillary sinusitis □ Acute otitis media (suspension only) □ Pharyngitis/tonsillitis □ Skin and skin structure infections □ Urinary tract infections.

ACTION

▪ Binds to bacterial cell wall membrane, causing cell death. **Therapeutic Effect:** ▪ Bactericidal action against susceptible bacteria. **Spectrum:** ▪ Many gram-positive cocci including *Streptococcus pneumoniae,* group A beta-hemolytic streptococci and penicillinase producing staphylococci. In addition has increased activity against several other important gram-negative pathogens including *Haemophilus influenzae* (including beta-lactamase-producing strains), *Escherichia coli, Klebsiella* sp. and *Moraxella catarrhalis.* Has

no activity against methicillin-resistant staphylococci or enterococcus.

PHARMACOKINETICS

Absorption: Well absorbed following oral administration (90%).
Distribution: Enters blister fluid and middle ear fluid in levels that are 50% of plasma. Crosses the placenta and enters breast milk in low concentrations.
Metabolism and Excretion: >90% excreted unchanged by the kidneys.
Half-life: 1 hr (increased up to 32 hr in renal impairment).

CONTRAINDICATIONS AND PRECAUTIONS

Contraindicated in: ▪ Hypersensitivity to cephalosporins ▪ Serious hypersensitivity to penicillins.
Use Cautiously in: ▪ Renal impairment (dosage modification required if creatinine clearance is <50 ml/min) ▪ Pregnancy, lactation, and children <6 mo (safety not established).

ADVERSE REACTIONS AND SIDE EFFECTS*

CNS: headache, somnolence.
GI: <u>nausea, vomiting,</u> anorexia, <u>diarrhea,</u> PSEUDOMEMBRANOUS COLITIS.
Derm: <u>rashes,</u> urticaria.
Misc: superinfection, allergic reactions including ANAPHYLAXIS and serum sickness.

INTERACTIONS

Drug–Drug: ▪ None significant.

ROUTE AND DOSAGE

▪ **PO (Adults and Children ≥13 yr):** 200–400 mg q 12 hr. 200 mg q 24 hr for uncomplicated cystitis.
▪ **PO (Infants and Children 6 mo–12 yr):** 15–30 mg/kg/day in divided doses q 12 hr.

AVAILABILITY

▪ *Capsules:* 200 mg ▪ *Oral suspension:* 100 mg/5 ml, 200 mg/5 ml.

TIME/ACTION PROFILE (blood levels)

	ONSET	PEAK
PO	rapid	0.8–1.2 hr

NURSING IMPLICATIONS

ASSESSMENT

- □ Assess patient for infection (vital signs; appearance of wound, sputum, urine and stool; WBC; earache) at beginning and throughout therapy.
- □ Obtain a history before initiating therapy to determine previous use of and reactions to penicillins or cephalosporins. Persons with a negative history of penicillin sensitivity may still have an allergic response.
- □ Obtain specimens for culture and sensitivity prior to initiating therapy. First dose may be given before receiving results.
- □ Observe patient for signs and symptoms of anaphylaxis (rash, pruritis, laryngeal edema, wheezing). Discontinue the drug and notify the physician immediately if these occur. Keep epinephrine, an antihistamine, and resuscitation equipment close by in the event of an anaphylactic reaction.
- ■ **Lab Test Considerations:** May cause false-positive results for Coombs' test and urine glucose when tested with copper sulfate method (Clinitest). Use glucose enzymatic tests (Clinistix or Tes-Tape) to test urine glucose.

POTENTIAL NURSING DIAGNOSES

- ■ Infection, high risk for (indications, side effects).
- ■ Diarrhea (adverse reactions).
- ■ Knowledge deficit related to medication regimen (patient/family teaching).

IMPLEMENTATION

- ■ **PO:** Administer 1 hr before or 2 hr after meals.
- □ Shake suspension well before administering. Suspension is stable for 14 days at room temperature.

PATIENT/FAMILY TEACHING

- □ Instruct patient to take loracarbef on an empty stomach and to finish the drug completely, even if feeling better. Advise patient that sharing of this medication may be dangerous.
- □ Instruct patients receiving suspension on the correct method for measuring liquid.
- □ Advise patient to report the signs of superinfection (furry overgrowth on the tongue, vaginal itching or discharge, loose or foul-smelling stools) and allergy.
- □ Instruct patient to notify physician if fever and diarrhea develop, especially if stool contains blood, pus, or mucus. Advise patient not to treat diarrhea without consulting physician or pharmacist.

EVALUATION

Clinical response to therapy can be evaluated by: ■ Resolution of the signs and symptoms of infection. Length of time for complete resolution depends on the organism and site of infection.

LORATIDINE
(lor-**a**-ti-deen)
Claritin

CLASSIFICATION(S):
Antihistamine
Pregnancy Category B

INDICATIONS

- ■ Relief of nasal and nonnasal symptoms of seasonal allergies.

ACTION

- ■ Blocks peripheral effects of histamine released during allergic reactions. **Therapeutic Effect:** ■ Decreased symptoms of allergic reactions (nasal stuffiness, red swollen eyes).

PHARMACOKINETICS

Absorption: Rapidly absorbed following oral administration (80%).
Distribution: UK.
Metabolism and Excretion: Rapidly and extensively metabolized during first pass through the liver. Much is

converted to descarboethoxyloratidine, an active metabolite.

Half-life: loratidine—7.8–11 hr; descarboethoxyloratidine—20 hr.

CONTRAINDICATIONS AND PRECAUTIONS

Contraindicated in: ▪ Hypersensitivity.

Use Cautiously in: ▪ Patients with hepatic impairment (dosage reduction to 10 mg every other day is recommended) ▪ Patients receiving drugs known to affect hepatic metabolism of drugs ▪ Pregnancy or lactation. Safe use in children <12 yr has not been established.

ADVERSE REACTIONS AND SIDE EFFECTS*

(Incidence 2% or less)

CNS: dizziness, migraine headache, tremors, vertigo, anxiety, depression, agitation, amnesia, impaired concentration, confusion, nervousness, abnormal dreams.

EENT: altered lacrimation, conjunctivitis, blurred vision, earache, eye pain, tinnitus, blepharospasm, dysphonia, nasal dryness, epistaxis, pharyngitis, nasal congestion, rhinitis, sinusitis, sneezing.

Resp: cough, hemoptysis, dyspnea, bronchospasm, bronchitis, laryngitis.

CV: chest pain, hypotension, hypertension, palpitation, syncope, tachycardia.

GI: altered salivation, abdominal distress, gastritis, diarrhea, constipation, nausea, vomiting, flatulence, altered taste, increased appetite, anorexia, dyspepsia, stomatitis, toothache.

GU: impotence, decreased libido, menorrhagia, dysmenorrhea, vaginitis, discolored urine, altered micturation.

Derm: increased sweating, flushing, dermatitis, dry hair, dry skin, urticaria, rash, pruritus, photosensitivity, purpura.

Endo: breast pain.

Neuro: hypoesthesia, paresthesia.

MS: leg cramps, back pain, hyperkinesia, arthralgia, myalgia.

Misc: thirst, rigors, fever, increased allergy symptoms, ANGIONEUROTIC EDEMA.

INTERACTIONS

Drug–Drug: ▪ None significant.

Drug–Food: ▪ Food increases absorption.

ROUTE AND DOSAGE

▪ **PO (Adults):** 10 mg once daily.

AVAILABILITY

▪ *Tablets:* 10 mg.

TIME/ACTION PROFILE
(antihistaminic effects)

	ONSET	PEAK	DURATION
PO	1–3 hr	8–12 hr	>24 hr

NURSING IMPLICATIONS

ASSESSMENT

▫ Assess allergy symptoms (rhinitis, conjunctivitis, hives) prior to and periodically throughout course of therapy.

▫ Assess lung sounds and character of bronchial secretions. Maintain fluid intake of 1500–2000 ml/day to decrease viscosity of secretions.

POTENTIAL NURSING DIAGNOSES

▪ Airway clearance, ineffective (indications).

▪ Injury, high risk for (adverse reactions).

▪ Knowledge deficit related to medication regimen (patient/family teaching).

IMPLEMENTATION

▪ **PO:** Administer once daily on an empty stomach.

PATIENT/FAMILY TEACHING

▫ Instruct patient to take medication 1 hr before or 2 hr after eating.

▫ May cause dizziness. Caution patient to avoid driving or other activities requiring alertness until response to medication is known.

▫ Discuss possibility of increased appetite. Patients on chronic therapy

---

*Underlines indicate most frequent; **CAPITALS** indicate life-threatening.

may need to limit caloric intake and increase activity to avoid undesired weight gain.
□ Caution patient to use sunscreen and protective clothing to prevent photosensitivity reactions.
□ Instruct patient to contact physician if symptoms persist.

EVALUATION
Effectiveness of therapy may be determined by: ▪ Decrease in allergic symptoms.

LORAZEPAM
(lor-**az**-e-pam)
Alzapam, {Apo-Lorazepam}, Ativan, Loraz, {Novolorazrem}

CLASSIFICATION(S):
Sedative/hypnotic (benzodiazepine), Antianxiety agent
Schedule IV
Pregnancy Category D—parenteral only, UK for oral

INDICATIONS
▪ Adjunct in the management of anxiety or insomnia ▪ Provides preoperative sedation ▪ Relieves preoperative anxiety and provides amnesia.

ACTION
▪ Depresses the CNS, probably by potentiating gamma-aminobutyric acid (GABA), an inhibitory neurotransmitter. **Therapeutic Effects:** ▪ Sedation ▪ Relief of anxiety.

PHARMACOKINETICS
Absorption: Well absorbed following oral administration. Rapidly and completely absorbed following IM administration. Sublingual absorption is more rapid than oral and is similar to IM.
Distribution: Widely distributed. Crosses the blood–brain barrier. Crosses the placenta and enters breast milk.

Metabolism and Excretion: Highly metabolized by the liver.
Half-life: 10–20 hr.

CONTRAINDICATIONS AND PRECAUTIONS
Contraindicated in: ▪ Hypersensitivity ▪ Cross-sensitivity with other benzodiazepines may exist ▪ Comatose patients or those with pre-existing CNS depression ▪ Uncontrolled severe pain ▪ Narrow-angle glaucoma ▪ Pregnancy and lactation.
Use Cautiously in: ▪ Severe hepatic or renal impairment ▪ Patients who may be suicidal or who may have been addicted to drugs previously ▪ Elderly or debilitated patients (dosage reduction recommended) ▪ Hypnotic use—should be short-term ▪ Children <18 yr (safety not established).

ADVERSE REACTIONS AND SIDE EFFECTS*
CNS: dizziness, drowsiness, lethargy, hangover, paradoxical excitation, headache, mental depression.
EENT: blurred vision.
Resp: respiratory depression.
GI: nausea, vomiting, diarrhea, constipation.
Derm: rashes.
Misc: tolerance, psychological dependence, physical dependence.

INTERACTIONS
Drug–Drug: ▪ Additive CNS depression with other **CNS depressants,** including **alcohol, antihistamines, antidepressants, opioid analgesics,** and other **sedative/hypnotics** ▪ May decrease the efficacy of **levodopa** ▪ **Smoking** may increase metabolism and decrease effectiveness ▪ **Probenecid** may decrease metabolism of lorazepam, enhancing its actions.

ROUTE AND DOSAGE
Anxiety
▪ **PO (Adults):** 1–3 mg 2–3 times daily (up to 10 mg/day).

- **PO (Elderly):** 0.5–2 mg/day in divided doses initially.

Insomnia
- **PO (Adults):** 2–4 mg at bedtime.
- **PO (Elderly):** 1–2 mg initially, increased as needed.

Preoperative Sedation
- **IM (Adults):** 50 mcg/kg 2 hr before surgery (not to exceed 4 mg).
- **IV (Adults):** 44 mcg/kg (not to exceed 2 mg) 15–20 min before surgery.

Operative Amnesia
- **IV (Adults):** up to 50 mcg/kg (not to exceed 4 mg).

AVAILABILITY

- **Tablets:** 0.5 mg, 1 mg, 2 mg ▪ **Concentrated solution:** 0.2 mg/ml ▪ **Injection:** 2 mg/ml, 4 mg/ml.

TIME/ACTION PROFILE (sedation)

	ONSET	PEAK*	DURATION
PO	15–45 min	1–6 hr	up to 48 hr
IM	15–30 min	1–1.5 hr	up to 48 hr
IV	5–15 min	UK	up to 48 hr

*Peak plasma levels.

NURSING IMPLICATIONS

ASSESSMENT
- Assess degree and manifestations of anxiety prior to and periodically throughout therapy.
- Prolonged high-dose therapy may lead to psychological or physical dependence. Restrict amount of drug available to patient.
- **Lab Test Considerations:** Patients on high-dose therapy should receive routine evaluation of renal, hepatic, and hematologic function.

POTENTIAL NURSING DIAGNOSES
- Anxiety (indications).
- Injury, high risk for (indications, side effects).
- Knowledge deficit related to medication regimen (patient/family teaching).

IMPLEMENTATION
- **General Info:** Following parenteral administration, keep patient supine for at least 8 hr and observe closely.
- **PO:** Tablet may also be given sublingually (unlabeled) for more rapid onset.
- **IM:** Administer IM doses deep into muscle mass at least 2 hr before surgery for optimum effect.
- **Direct IV:** Dilute immediately before use with an equal amount of Sterile Water, D5W, or 0.9% NaCl for Injection. Do not use if solution is colored or contains a precipitate.
- **Rate:** Administer direct IV, through Y-site or via 3-way stopcock at a rate of 2 mg over 1 min. Rapid IV administration may result in apnea, hypotension, bradycardia, or cardiac arrest.
- **Syringe Compatibility:** ▪ cimetidine.
- **Y-Site Compatibility:** ▪ acyclovir ▪ atracurium ▪ fludarabine ▪ pancuronium ▪ vecuronium ▪ zidovudine.
- **Y-Site Incompatibility:** ▪ ondansetron ▪ sargramostim.

PATIENT/FAMILY TEACHING
- Instruct patient to take medication exactly as directed, not to skip or double up on missed doses. Abrupt withdrawal may cause tremors, nausea, vomiting, and abdominal and muscle cramps.
- Medication may cause drowsiness or dizziness. Advise patient to avoid driving or other activities requiring alertness until response to medication is known.
- Caution patient to avoid taking alcohol or other CNS depressants concurrently with this medication.
- Instruct patient to contact physician immediately if pregnancy is suspected or planned.
- Emphasize the importance of follow-up examinations to determine effectiveness of the medication.

EVALUATION
Effectiveness of therapy can be demonstrated by: ▪ Increase in sense of well-being □ Decrease in subjective feelings of anxiety without excessive sedation ▪ Reduction of preoperative anxiety ▪ Postoperative amnesia.

LOVASTATIN
(loe-va-sta-tin)
Mevacor

CLASSIFICATION(S):
Lipid-lowering agent
Pregnancy Category X

INDICATIONS

- Adjunct to dietary therapy in the management of primary hypercholesterolemia.

ACTION

- Inhibits the enzyme (HMG CoA reductase) responsible for catalyzing an early step in the synthesis of cholesterol. **Therapeutic Effect:** Lowering of total and LDL cholesterol. Slightly increases HDL and decreases VLDL cholesterol and triglycerides.

PHARMACOKINETICS

Absorption: Poorly and variably absorbed following oral administration.
Distribution: Crosses the blood–brain barrier and placenta.
Metabolism and Excretion: Highly metabolized by the liver. Excreted in bile and feces. Small amounts (10%) excreted unchanged by the kidneys.
Half-life: UK.

CONTRAINDICATIONS AND PRECAUTIONS

Contraindicated in: ▪ Hypersensitivity ▪ Pregnancy or lactation ▪ Active liver disease.

Use Cautiously in: ▪ History of liver disease ▪ Alcoholism ▪ Severe acute infection ▪ Hypotension ▪ Major surgery ▪ Trauma ▪ Severe metabolic, endocrine, or electrolyte problems ▪ Uncontrolled seizures ▪ Visual disturbances ▪ Children (safety not established).

ADVERSE REACTIONS AND SIDE EFFECTS*

CNS: dizziness, headache.
EENT: blurred vision.
GI: constipation, diarrhea, dyspepsia, flatus, abdominal cramps, heartburn, nausea, hepatitis, altered taste.
Derm: rashes, pruritus.
MS: muscle cramps, myalgia, myopathy.

INTERACTIONS

Drug–Drug: ▪ Cholesterol-lowering effect may be additive with **bile acid sequestrants (cholestyramine, colestipol)** ▪ Increased risk of myopathy with concurrent **niacin, erythromycin, gemfibrozil,** or **cyclosporine**.
Drug–Food: Food enhances blood levels of lovastatin.

ROUTE AND DOSAGE

- **PO (Adults):** 20 mg once daily with evening meal. Dosage may be increased at 4-wk intervals to a maximum of 80 mg/day in single or divided doses.

AVAILABILITY

- *Tablets:* 20 mg, 40 mg.

TIME/ACTION PROFILE (cholesterol-lowering effect)

	ONSET	PEAK	DURATION
PO	2 wk	4–6 wk	UK

NURSING IMPLICATIONS

ASSESSMENT

- Obtain a diet history, especially in regard to fat consumption.
- Ophthalmic examinations are recommended prior to and yearly throughout therapy.
- **Lab Test Considerations:** Serum cholesterol and triglyceride levels should be evaluated before initiating and periodically throughout course of therapy.
- Liver function tests, including AST (SGOT), should be monitored prior to and every 4–6 wk during the first 3 mo of therapy, every 6–8 wk for the remainder of the first year, and then every 6 mo. If AST (SGOT) levels increase to 3 times normal, lovastatin therapy should be discontinued.

L

*Underlines indicate most frequent; **CAPITALS** indicate life-threatening.

□ If patient develops muscle tenderness during therapy, CPK levels should be monitored. If CPK levels are markedly increased or myopathy occurs, lovastatin therapy should be discontinued.

POTENTIAL NURSING DIAGNOSES
- Knowledge deficit related to diet and medication regimen (patient/family teaching).
- Noncompliance (patient/family teaching).

IMPLEMENTATION
- **PO:** Administer lovastatin with food. Administration on an empty stomach decreases absorption by approximately 30%. Initial once-daily dose is administered with the evening meal.

PATIENT/FAMILY TEACHING
□ Instruct patient to take medication exactly as directed, not to skip doses or double up on missed doses. Lovastatin helps control but does not cure elevated serum cholesterol levels. Consult physician prior to discontinuing lovastatin therapy; serum lipid levels may increase significantly. Therapy may be long-term.
□ Advise patient that this medication should be used in conjunction with diet restrictions (fat, cholesterol, carbohydrates, alcohol), exercise, and cessation of smoking.
□ Instruct patient to notify physician if unexplained muscle pain, tenderness, or weakness occur, especially if accompanied by fever or malaise.
□ Instruct female patients to notify physician promptly if pregnancy is planned or suspected.
□ Advise patient to notify physician or dentist of medication regimen prior to treatment or surgery.
□ Emphasize the importance of follow-up examinations to determine effectiveness and to monitor for side effects.

EVALUATION
Effectiveness of therapy can be demonstrated by: ■ Decrease in serum LDL, VLDL, and total cholesterol levels ■ Increase in HDL cholesterol levels ■ Decrease in triglyceride levels.

LOXAPINE
(**lox**-a-peen)
{Loxapac}, Loxitane, Loxitane-C, Loxitane IM

CLASSIFICATION(S):
Antipsychotic
Pregnancy Category C

INDICATIONS
- Management of psychoses. **Unlabeled Use:** ■ Management of depression and anxiety associated with depression.

ACTION
- Appears to block dopamine at postsynaptic receptors sites in the CNS. **Therapeutic Effect:** ■ Diminution of psychotic behavior.

PHARMACOKINETICS
Absorption: Well absorbed following oral or IM administration.
Distribution: Distribution in humans not known.
Metabolism and Excretion: Extensively metabolized by the liver. Some conversion to active antipsychotic compounds.
Half-life: 19 hr.

CONTRAINDICATIONS AND PRECAUTIONS
Contraindicated in: ■ Hypersensitivity or intolerance to loxapine or amoxapine ■ Coma ■ CNS depression ■ Pregnancy or lactation.
Use Cautiously in: ■ Glaucoma ■ Elderly men or patients with prostatic hypertrophy (more prone to urinary retention) ■ Elderly patients (more susceptible to adverse reactions) ■ Intestinal obstruction ■ History of seizures ■ Alcoholism ■ Cardiovascular disease ■ Impaired liver function ■ Children <16 yr (safety not established).

ADVERSE REACTIONS AND SIDE EFFECTS*

CNS: <u>drowsiness</u>, extrapyramidal syndromes, including NEUROLEPTIC MALIGNANT SYNDROME, tardive dyskinesia, insomnia, <u>dizziness</u>, lethargy, <u>lightheadedness</u>, syncope, headache, ataxia, weakness, <u>confusion</u>.
EENT: nasal congestion, <u>blurred vision</u>, lens opacities.
CV: tachycardia, <u>hypotension</u>.
GI: constipation, dry mouth, hepatitis, nausea, vomiting, ileus.
GU: urinary retention.
Derm: rashes, dermatitis, facial photosensitivity, edema, seborrhea, pigment changes.
Endo: galactorrhea.
Hemat: AGRANULOCYTOSIS.
Misc: allergic reactions, NEUROLEPTIC MALIGNANT SYNDROME.

INTERACTIONS

Drug–Drug: ▪ Decreases the antihypertensive effects of **guanethidine** or **guanadrel** ▪ Blocks the alpha-adrenergic effects of **epinephrine** (may result in hypotension and tachycardia) ▪ Additive CNS depression with other **CNS depressants,** including **alcohol, antihistamines, opioid analgesics,** and **sedative/hypnotics** ▪ **Antacids** or **adsorbent antidiarrheals** may decrease absorption ▪ Use with **antidepressants** or **MAO inhibitors** may result in prolonged CNS depression and increased anticholinergic effects.

ROUTE AND DOSAGE

▪ **PO (Adults):** 10 mg bid, may be increased gradually over the first 7–10 days as needed and tolerated. Usual maintenance dose is 15–25 mg 2–4 times daily. Severely ill patients may require up to 50 mg/day initially and maintenance doses up to 250 mg/day.
▪ **IM (Adults):** 12.5–50 mg q 4–6 hr as needed and tolerated (up to 250 mg/day).

AVAILABILITY

▪ **Capsules:** 5 mg, 10 mg, 25 mg, 50 mg

▪ **Oral concentrate:** 25 mg/ml ▪ **Injection:** 50 mg/ml.

TIME/ACTION PROFILE
(antipsychotic effect)

	ONSET	PEAK	DURATION
PO	30 min	1.5–3 hr	12 hr
IM	UK	UK	UK

NURSING IMPLICATIONS

ASSESSMENT

▢ Monitor patient's mental status (delusions, hallucinations, and behavior) prior to and periodically throughout therapy.
▢ Monitor blood pressure (sitting, standing, lying) and pulse rate prior to and frequently during the period of dosage adjustment.
▢ Observe patient carefully when administering medication to ensure medication is actually taken and not hoarded.
▢ Monitor patient for onset of extrapyramidal side effects (akathisia—restlessness; dystonia—muscle spasms and twisting motions; or pseudoparkinsonism—mask facies, rigidity, tremors, drooling, shuffling gait, dysphagia). Notify physician if these symptoms occur, as reduction in dosage or discontinuation of medication may be necessary. Physician may also order trihexyphenidyl or diphenhydramine to control these symptoms.
▢ Monitor for tardive dyskinesia (rhythmic movement of mouth, face, and extremities). Notify physician immediately if these symptoms occur, as these side effects may be irreversible.
▢ Monitor frequency and consistency of bowel movements. Increasing bulk and fluids in the diet may help minimize constipation.
▢ Loxapine lowers the seizure threshold. Institute seizure precautions for patients with history of seizures.
▢ Monitor for development of neuroleptic malignant syndrome (fever, respiratory distress, tachycardia, convulsions, diaphoresis, hypertension or

L

hypotension, pallor, tiredness). Notify physician immediately if these symptoms occur.

- **Lab Test Considerations:** Monitor CBC and differential prior to and periodically throughout therapy.
□ Monitor liver function studies prior to and periodically during therapy.
- **Toxicity and Overdose:** Antiemetic effects of loxapine may block the action of ipecac. Overdose is treated by gastric lavage, barbiturates to control seizures, and supportive care for fluctuations in body temperature. Hypotension may be corrected by use of IV fluids, norepinephrine, or phenylephrine. Avoid use of epinephrine, as it may worsen hypotension.

POTENTIAL NURSING DIAGNOSES
- Thought processes, altered (indications).
- Injury, high risk for (side effects).
- Knowledge deficit related to medication regimen (patient/family teaching).

IMPLEMENTATION
- **PO:** Administer capsules with food or milk to decrease gastric irritation.
□ Dilute oral solution with orange or grapefruit juice immediately prior to administration. Measure dose with provided dropper.
- **IM:** Do not inject SC. Inject slowly into deep, well-developed muscle. Light amber color does not alter potency of solution. Do not administer solution that is markedly discolored or that contains a precipitate.
□ Keep patient recumbent for at least 30 min following parenteral administration to minimize hypotensive effects.

PATIENT/FAMILY TEACHING
□ Instruct patient on need to take medication exactly as directed. If a dose is missed, it should be taken as soon as remembered, up to 1 hr before next scheduled dose. Patients on long-term high-dose therapy may need to discontinue gradually to avoid withdrawal symptoms (dyskinesia, tremors, dizziness, nausea, and vomiting).
□ Instruct patient receiving oral solu-

tion on correct method of measuring dose with provided dropper.
□ Inform patient of possibility of extrapyramidal symptoms and tardive dyskinesia. Instruct patient to report these symptoms immediately to physician.
□ Advise patient to make position changes slowly to minimize orthostatic hypotension.
□ May cause drowsiness. Caution patient to avoid driving or other activities requiring alertness until response to the medication is known.
□ Caution patient to use sunscreen and protective clothing to prevent photosensitivity reactions.
□ Caution patient to avoid concurrent use of alcohol, other CNS depressants, and over-the-counter medications without consulting physician or pharmacist.
□ Instruct patient to use frequent mouth rinses, good oral hygiene, and sugarless gum or candy to minimize dry mouth. Consult physician or dentist if dry mouth continues >2 wk.
□ Advise patient to notify physician or dentist of medication regimen prior to treatment or surgery.
□ Instruct patient to notify physician promptly if sore throat, fever, unusual bleeding or bruising, rash, weakness, tremors, visual disturbances, dark-colored urine, or clay-colored stools occur.
□ Advise patient of need for continued medical follow-up for psychotherapy, eye examinations, and laboratory tests.

EVALUATION
Effectiveness of therapy can be demonstrated by: ■ Decreased psychotic ideation.

LYMPHOCYTE IMMUNE GLOBULIN
(**lim**-foe-site im-**myoon glo**-byoo-lin)
ATG, Atgam

INDICATIONS

▪ Management of allograft rejection in renal transplant patients ▪ Treatment of aplastic anemia in patients who are not candidates for bone marrow transplantation.

ACTION

▪ Decreases the circulating number of T-lymphocytes, which are involved in both cell-mediated and humoral immunity. **Therapeutic Effects:** ▪ Resolution of rejection of renal allografts ▪ Remission of aplastic anemia.

PHARMACOKINETICS

Absorption: IV administration results in complete bioavailability.
Distribution: UK.
Metabolism and Excretion: UK.
Half-life: 5.7 days.

CONTRAINDICATIONS AND PRECAUTIONS

Contraindicated in: ▪ History of hypersensitivity during previous courses of therapy ▪ Hypersensitivity to thimerisol ▪ Hypersensitivity to equine gamma globuline preparations.
Use Cautiously in: ▪ Pregnancy or lactation (safety not established).

ADVERSE REACTIONS AND SIDE EFFECTS*

CNS: headache.
Resp: dyspnea.
CV: chest pain, hypotension.
GI: diarrhea, nausea, vomiting, stomatitis.
Derm: dermatologic reactions, itching, erythema.
Hemat: leukopenia, thrombocytopenia, hemolysis, anemia.
Local: phlebitis at IV site, pain at IV site.
MS: arthralgia.
Misc: allergic reactions including ANA-

PHYLAXIS, chills, fever, clotted AV fistula, night sweats, serum sickness-like reactions.

INTERACTIONS

Drug–Drug: ▪ Concurrent use of **glucocorticoids** and **immunosuppressants** may mask some adverse reactions to antilymphocyte globulin.

ROUTE AND DOSAGE

Skin Test
▪ **Intradermal (Adults):** 0.1 ml of 1 : 1000 dilution (5 mcg of horse serum).

Renal Allograft Recipients
▪ **IV (Adults):** 10–30 mg/kg/day for 14 days, then every other day for 14 days.
▪ **IV (Children):** 5–25 mg/kg/day for 14 days, then every other day for 14 days.

Aplastic Anemia
▪ **IV (Adults):** 10–20 mg/kg/day for 8–14 days, then every other day for 21 doses total.

AVAILABILITY
▪ *Injection:* 50 mg/ml.

TIME/ACTION PROFILE (decreased circulating T-lymphocytes)

	ONSET	PEAK	DURATION
IV	rapid	UK	UK

NURSING IMPLICATIONS

ASSESSMENT
▢ Assess patient for hypersensitivity reaction (respiratory distress, hypotension, pain in chest, flank, or back) continuously throughout administration. Keep epinephrine, antihistamines, glucocorticoids, syringes, and an airway at bedside at all times. If a reaction occurs, stop infusion immediately, administer 0.3 ml aqueous epinephrine 1 : 1000 IM. Administer glucocorticoids and resuscitative measures as needed. Do not resume therapy.
▢ Monitor vital signs frequently throughout administration. Medication frequently causes chills, fever, itching,

L

and erythema. Prophylactic administration of antihistamines and glucocorticoids usually controls these
symptoms.
- **Lab Test Considerations:** Monitor
CBC and platelets throughout therapy.
May cause leukopenia and thrombocytopenia. Thrombocytopenia is usually transient and does not normally
require discontinuation of therapy or
transfusion.
▫ May also cause hemolysis. Treatment
includes transfusion of erythrocytes
and administration of mannitol, furosemide, sodium bicarbonate, and
fluids if necessary.

POTENTIAL NURSING DIAGNOSES
- Infection, high risk for (indications,
side effects).
- Knowledge deficit related to medication regimen (patient/family teaching).

IMPLEMENTATION
- **General Info:** Medication should be
used only by physicians experienced
in immunosuppressive therapy and
management of renal transplant patients and administered only in facilities equipped and staffed with
adequate laboratory and medical resources.
▫ Patients with aplastic anemia may
need a transfusion of platelets prior
to administration to maintain platelets at a clinically acceptable level
due to potential thrombocytopenia.
- **Test Dose:** Administer an intradermal
injection of 0.1 ml of a 1:1000 dilution in 0.9% NaCl and a 0.9% NaCl
control. If a wheal or erythema >10
mm or both with or without a pseudo-
pod forms, and itching or a marked
local swelling occurs, administer infusion with caution. If a systemic reaction (generalized rash, tachycardia,
dyspnea, hypotension, anaphylaxis)
occurs, do not administer infusion.
Allergic reactions may occur in patients with a negative reaction to test
dose.

- **Intermittent Infusion:** Dilute total
daily dose in 0.45% NaCl or 0.9%
NaCl prior to infusion for a concentration not to exceed 1 mg/ml. Invert
IV saline bottle so that undiluted
drug does not come in contact with
the air inside. May be infused through
an in-line filter with a pore size of
0.2–1 micron. Refrigerate diluted solution if prepared prior to administration. Do not freeze; discard if frozen.
Stable for 24 hr, including infusion
time, if refrigerated.
▫ Administer through high-flow veins
to minimize phlebitis and thrombosis.
- *Rate:* Administer over at least 4 hr.

PATIENT/FAMILY TEACHING
▫ Explain the purpose of the medication
to the patient.
▫ Instruct patient to notify nurse or physician immediately if signs of hypersensitivity reaction occur.

EVALUATION
**Effectiveness of therapy can be deter-
mined by:** ▪ Prevention or management
of allograft rejection in renal transplant
patients ▪ Treatment of moderate to severe aplastic anemia.

MAGALDRATE
(**mag**-al-drate)
{Antiflux}, Lowsium, Riopan,
Riopan Extra Strength

CLASSIFICATION(S):
Antacid
Pregnancy Category UK

INDICATIONS
- Adjunctive therapy in the treatment of
peptic ulcer pain and to promote healing of duodenal and gastric ulcers
- Also useful in a variety of GI complaints including: ▫ Hyperacidity ▫ Indigestion ▫ Reflux esophagitis.

ACTION

- A chemically combined form of magnesium and aluminum ■ Neutralizes gastric acid following dissolution in gastric contents. Inactivates pepsin if pH >4. **Therapeutic Effect:** ■ Neutralization of gastric acid with subsequent healing of ulcers and diminution of associated pain.

PHARMACOKINETICS

Absorption: In general, during routine use, antacids are nonabsorbable. With chronic use, 15–30% of magnesium and smaller amounts of aluminum may be absorbed.
Distribution: Small amounts of magnesium and aluminum are widely distributed, cross the placenta and enter breast milk. Aluminum concentrates in the CNS.
Metabolism and Excretion: Excreted by the kidneys.
Half-life: UK.

CONTRAINDICATIONS AND PRECAUTIONS

Contraindicated in: ■ Severe abdominal pain of unknown cause, especially if accompanied by fever.
Use Cautiously in: ■ Magnesium-containing antacids should be used cautiously in patients with renal insufficiency.

ADVERSE REACTIONS AND SIDE EFFECTS*

GI: constipation (aluminum salts), diarrhea (magnesium salts).
F and E: hypermagnesemia (magnesium), hypophosphatemia (aluminum).

INTERACTIONS

Drug–Drug: ■ Magnesium and aluminum salts change the absorptive characteristics of many orally administered drugs ■ Absorption of tetracyclines, phenothiazines, iron salts, ketoconazole, fluoroquinolones, and isoniazid may be decreased by concurrent magaldrate ■ If urine pH is increased by large doses, **salicylate** blood levels may be decreased, **quinidine, flecainide,** and **amphetamine** blood levels may be increased.

ROUTE AND DOSAGE

Dosages vary depending on concentration of ingredients in product chosen. Generally 5–30 ml or 1–2 tab is given 1 and 3 hr after meals and at bedtime. In the early healing phase of peptic ulcer more frequent administration may be necessary.
- **PO (Adults):** 480–1080 mg between meals and at bedtime (40–160 mEq neutralizing capacity dose).

AVAILABILITY

■ *Tablets:* 480 mg ■ *Chewable tablets:* 480 mg ■ *Suspension:* 540 mg/5 ml ■ *Liquid:* 1080 mg/5 ml ■ *In combination with:* simethizone.

TIME/ACTION PROFILE (acid neutralization)

ONSET	PEAK	DURATION	
		Empty Stomach	After Meals
Aluminum	30 min	30–60 min	3 hr
Magnesium	30 min	30–60 min	3 hr

NURSING IMPLICATIONS

ASSESSMENT
□ Assess for heartburn; indigestion; and location, duration, character, and precipitating factors of gastric pain.

POTENTIAL NURSING DIAGNOSES
- Pain (indications).
- Knowledge deficit related to medication regimen (patient/family teaching).

IMPLEMENTATION
- **General Info:** Some tablets must be chewed thoroughly before swallowing (Lowsium, Riopan); others are designed to be swallowed whole (Riopan). Follow with half full glass of water. Shake suspension well.
- **PO:** Administer between meals and at bedtime.

M

*Underlines indicate most frequent; CAPITALS indicate life-threatening.

PATIENT/FAMILY TEACHING
- Caution patient to consult physician before taking antacids for more than 2 wk or if problem is recurring. Advise patient to consult physician if relief is not obtained or if symptoms of gastric bleeding (black tarry stools, coffeeground emesis) occur.

EVALUATION
Effectiveness of therapy can be demonstrated by: ▪ Relief of gastric pain and irritation.

MAGNESIUM CITRATE
(mag-**nee**-zhum **si**-trate)
Citrate of Magnesia, Citroma, {Citromag}, Citro-Nesia, Evac-Q-Mag

CLASSIFICATION(S):
Laxative (saline)
Pregnancy Category UK

INDICATIONS
▪ Used as a laxative and to evacuate the bowel in preparation for surgical or radiographic procedures.

ACTION
▪ Is osmotically active in GI tract, drawing water into the lumen and causing peristalsis. **Therapeutic Effect:** ▪ Evacuation of the colon.

PHARMACOKINETICS
Absorption: 15–30% of magnesium may be absorbed orally.
Distribution: Magnesium is widely distributed. Crosses the placenta and is present in breast milk.
Metabolism and Excretion: Magnesium is excreted primarily by the kidneys.
Half-life: UK.

CONTRAINDICATIONS AND PRECAUTIONS
Contraindicated in: ▪ Hypermagnese-

mia ▪ Hypocalcemia ▪ Anuria ▪ Heart block ▪ Active labor.
Use Cautiously in: ▪ Any degree of renal insufficiency.

ADVERSE REACTIONS AND SIDE EFFECTS*
Non-GI adverse reactions are seen only in patients who receive large doses over prolonged periods and/or have underlying renal disease.

CNS: drowsiness.
Resp: decreased respiratory rate.
CV: bradycardia, arrhythmias, hypotension.
GI: diarrhea.
Derm: flushing, sweating.
Metab: hypothermia.
Neuro: decreased deep-tendon reflexes, PARALYSIS.

INTERACTIONS
Drug–Drug: ▪ If systemic absorption occurs, may potentiate **neuromuscular blocking agents**.

ROUTE AND DOSAGE
Contains 77 mEq magnesium/100 ml.
▪ **PO (Adults):** 100–300 ml.
▪ **PO (Children 6–12 yr):** 30–100 ml.

AVAILABILITY
▪ *Oral solution:* 1.55–1.9 g magnesium citrate/100 ml.

TIME/ACTION PROFILE (laxative effect)

	ONSET	PEAK	DURATION
PO	3–6 hr	UK	UK

NURSING IMPLICATIONS
ASSESSMENT
- Assess patient for abdominal distention, presence of bowel sounds, and usual pattern of bowel function.
- Assess color, consistency, and amount of stool produced.

POTENTIAL NURSING DIAGNOSES
▪ Constipation (indications).

- Knowledge deficit related to medication regimen (patient/family teaching).

IMPLEMENTATION

- **General Info:** Refrigerate magnesium citrate solution to increase palatability. May be served over ice. An open container of magnesium citrate may become flat upon standing; this will not affect potency but may decrease palatability.
- For laxative effect, administer on empty stomach for more rapid results. Follow all oral laxative doses with a full glass of liquid to prevent dehydration and for faster effect. Do not administer at bedtime or late in the day.

PATIENT/FAMILY TEACHING

- Advise patients that laxatives should be used only for short-term therapy. Long-term therapy may cause electrolyte imbalance and dependence.
- If administered as part of a bowel preparation kit, explain the schedule in regard to other laxatives, suppository, and diet modification.
- Encourage patient to utilize other forms of bowel regulation, such as increasing bulk in the diet, increasing fluid intake, increasing mobility. Normal bowel habits are individualized and may vary from 3 times/day to 3 times/wk.
- Advise patient to notify physician if unrelieved constipation, rectal bleeding, or symptoms of electrolyte imbalance (muscle cramps or pain, weakness, dizziness, etc.) occur.

EVALUATION
Effectiveness of therapy can be demonstrated by: ■ Evacuation of colon ■ Passage of a soft, formed bowel movement.

MAGNESIUM HYDROXIDE
(mag-**nee**-zhum hye-**drox**-ide)
Magnesia tablets, Milk of Magnesia, MOM

CLASSIFICATION(S):
Laxative (saline), Antacid
Pregnancy Category UK

INDICATIONS

- Used as a laxative and to evacuate the bowel in preparation for surgical or radiographic procedures ■ Has also been used as an antacid.

ACTION

- Is osmotically active in GI tract, drawing water into the lumen and causing peristalsis ■ Also has acid-neutralizing activity. **Therapeutic Effects:** ■ Evacuation of the colon ■ Neutralization of gastric acid.

PHARMACOKINETICS
Absorption: 15–30% of magnesium may be absorbed orally.
Distribution: Magnesium is widely distributed. Crosses the placenta and is present in breast milk.
Metabolism and Excretion: Magnesium is excreted primarily by the kidneys.
Half-life: UK.

CONTRAINDICATIONS AND PRECAUTIONS
Contraindicated in: ■ Hypermagnesemia ■ Hypocalcemia ■ Anuria ■ Heart block ■ Active labor.
Use Cautiously in: ■ Any degree of renal insufficiency.

ADVERSE REACTIONS AND SIDE EFFECTS*
Non-GI adverse reactions are seen only in patients who receive large doses over prolonged periods and/or have underlying renal disease.
CNS: drowsiness.
Resp: decreased respiratory rate.
CV: bradycardia, arrhythmias, hypotension.
GI: diarrhea.
Derm: flushing, sweating.
Metab: hypothermia.
Neuro: decreased deep-tendon reflexes, PARALYSIS.

M

*Underlines indicate most frequent; **CAPITALS** indicate life-threatening.

INTERACTIONS

Drug–Drug: ▪ If systemically absorbed, may potentiate **neuromuscular blocking agents** ▪ May decrease absorption of **fluoroquinolones**.

ROUTE AND DOSAGE

Laxative

(82 mEq magnesium/30 ml Milk of Magnesia)

▪ **PO (Adults):** 30–60 ml/day as Milk of Magnesia as a single dose or in divided doses or 10–20 ml of Milk of Magnesia concentrate.

▪ **PO (Children 6–11 yr):** 15–30 ml as Milk of Magnesia as a single dose or in divided doses.

▪ **PO (Children 2–5 yr):** 5–15 ml as Milk of Magnesia as a single dose or in divided doses.

Antacid

▪ **PO (Adults and Children >12 yr):** 5–15 ml liquid or 650–1300 mg as tablets 4 times daily.

AVAILABILITY

▪ *Liquid:* 395 mg/5 ml (7–8.5% suspension) ▪ *Concentrated liquid:* 1.2 g/5 ml (25% suspension) ▪ *Chewable Tablets:* 300 mg, 600 mg.

TIME/ACTION PROFILE (laxative effect)

	ONSET	PEAK	DURATION
PO	3–6 hr	UK	UK

NURSING IMPLICATIONS

ASSESSMENT

▪ **Laxative:** Assess patient for abdominal distention, presence of bowel sounds, and usual pattern of bowel function.

▫ Assess color, consistency, and amount of stool produced.

▪ **Antacid:** Assess for heartburn; indigestion; and location, duration, character, and precipitating factors of gastric pain.

POTENTIAL NURSING DIAGNOSES

▪ Constipation (indications).

▪ Pain (indications).

▪ Knowledge deficit related to medication regimen (patient/family teaching).

IMPLEMENTATION

▪ **Antacid:** Tablet must be chewed thoroughly before swallowing to prevent entering small intestine in undissolved form. Follow with half full glass of water.

▫ Shake suspension well before administration.

▪ **Laxative:** For more rapid results, administer on empty stomach and follow dose with a full glass of liquid to prevent dehydration. Do not administer at bedtime or late in the day when used for laxative effect.

PATIENT/FAMILY TEACHING

▪ **General Info:** Advise patient not to take this medication within 2 hr of other medications.

▪ **Laxative:** Advise patient that laxatives should be used only for short-term therapy. Long-term therapy may cause electrolyte imbalance and dependence.

▫ Encourage patient to utilize other forms of bowel regulation, such as increasing bulk in the diet, increasing fluid intake, increasing mobility. Normal bowel habits are individualized and may vary from 3 times/day to 3 times/wk.

▫ Advise patient to notify physician if unrelieved constipation, rectal bleeding, or symptoms of electrolyte imbalance (muscle cramps or pain, weakness, dizziness) occur.

▪ **Antacid:** Caution patient to consult physician before taking antacids for more than 2 wk or if problem is recurring. Advise patient to consult physician if relief is not obtained or if symptoms of gastric bleeding (black tarry stools, coffee-ground emesis) occur.

EVALUATION

Effectiveness of therapy can be demonstrated by: ▪ Relief of gastric pain and irritation ▪ Passage of a soft, formed bowel movement, usually within 3–6 hr.

MAGNESIUM HYDROXIDE/ ALUMINUM HYDROXIDE

(mag-**nee**-zhum hye-**drox**-ide/ a-**loo**-mi-num hye-**drox**-ide) Alamag, Alumid, {Amphogel 500}, {Diovol}, {Diovol Ex}, Gelamal, {Gelusil Extra Strength}, Kudrox Double Strength, Maalox, Maalox No. 1, Maalox No. 2, Maalox TC, Magmalin, Mylanta-II Plain, {Neutralca-S}, Rulox, Rulox No. 1, Rulox No. 2, {Univol}, WinGel

CLASSIFICATION(S):
Antacid, Antiulcer
Pregnancy Category UK

INDICATIONS

▪ Adjunctive therapy in the treatment of peptic ulcer pain and to promote healing of duodenal and gastric ulcers ▪ Useful in a variety of GI complaints, including: □ Hyperacidity □ Indigestion □ Reflux esophagitis.

ACTION

▪ Neutralize gastric acid following dissolution in gastric contents. Pepsin is inactivated if pH ≥4. **Therapeutic Effect:** ▪ Neutralization of gastric acid with subsequent healing of ulcers and diminution of associated pain.

PHARMACOKINETICS

Absorption: In general, during routine use, antacids are nonabsorbable. With chronic use, 15–30% of magnesium and smaller amounts of aluminum may be absorbed.
Distribution: Small amounts of magnesium and aluminum absorbed are widely distributed, cross the placenta and enter breast milk. Aluminum concentrates in the CNS.
Metabolism and Excretion: Excreted by the kidneys.
Half-life: UK.

CONTRAINDICATIONS AND PRECAUTIONS

Contraindicated in: ▪ Severe abdominal pain of unknown cause, especially if accompanied by fever ▪ Magnesium is contraindicated in anuria ▪ Products containing tartrazine or sugar should be avoided in patients with known intolerance.
Use Cautiously in: ▪ Magnesium-containing antacids should be used cautiously in patients with any degree of renal insufficiency.

ADVERSE REACTIONS AND SIDE EFFECTS*

GI: constipation (aluminum salts), diarrhea (magnesium salts).
F and E: hypermagnesemia (magnesium), hypophosphatemia (aluminum).

INTERACTIONS

Drug–Drug: ▪ Magnesium and aluminum salts change the absorptive characteristics of **many orally administered drugs** ▪ The absorption of **tetracyclines, phenothiazines, iron salts, isoniazid,** and **fluoroquinolones** may be decreased ▪ If urine pH is increased by large doses, **salicylate** blood levels may be decreased and **quinidine, flecainide,** and **amphetamine** levels may be increased.

ROUTE AND DOSAGE

Dosages vary depending on concentration of ingredients in product chosen. Generally 5–30 ml or 1–2 tab is given 1 and 3 hr after meals and at bedtime. In the early healing phase of peptic ulcer more frequent administration may be necessary.

Duodenal Ulcer
▪ **PO (Adults):** 80–160 mEq neutralizing capacity/dose.

Gastric Ulcer
▪ **PO (Adults):** 40–80 mEq neutralizing capacity/dose.

M

AVAILABILITY

■ *Chewable tablets:* 200 mg aluminum hydroxide with 200 mg magnesium hydroxide, 400 mg aluminum hydroxide ■ *Liquid:* 200 mg aluminum hydroxide with 200 mg magnesium hydroxide/5 ml, 400 mg magnesium hydroxide with 400 mg/5 ml ■ *In combination with:* magnesium trisilicate, calcium carbonate, simethicone. See Appendix A.

TIME/ACTION PROFILE (acid neutralization)

ONSET	PEAK	DURATION	
		Empty Stomach	After Meals
aluminum PO (slightly delayed)	30 min	30 min– 1 hr	3 hr
magnesium PO (immediate)	30 min	30 min– 1 hr	3 hr

NURSING IMPLICATIONS

ASSESSMENT

□ Assess for heartburn; indigestion; and location, duration, character, and precipitating factors of gastric pain.

POTENTIAL NURSING DIAGNOSES

■ Pain (indications).

■ Knowledge deficit related to medication regimen (patient/family teaching).

IMPLEMENTATION

■ **General Info:** Magnesium and aluminum are combined as antacids to balance the constipating effects of aluminum with the diarrheal effects of magnesium.

□ Liquid forms are considered more effective.

■ **PO:** Tablet must be chewed thoroughly before swallowing to prevent entering small intestine in undissolved form. Follow with half full glass of water.

□ Shake suspensions well before administration.

□ For an antacid effect, administer 1–3 hr after meals and at bedtime.

PATIENT/FAMILY TEACHING

□ Caution patient to consult physician before taking antacids for more than 2 wk or if problem is recurring. Advise patient to consult physician if relief is not obtained or if symptoms of gastric bleeding (black tarry stools, coffee-ground emesis) occur.

□ Advise patient not to take this medication within 2 hr of other medication.

□ Some antacids contain large amounts of sodium. Caution patients on a sodium-restricted diet to check sodium content when on long-term, high-dose therapy.

EVALUATION

Effectiveness of therapy can be demonstrated by: ■ Relief of gastric pain and irritation.

MAGNESIUM SULFATE

(mag-**nee**-zhum sul-fate)
Epsom salt

CLASSIFICATION(S):

Electrolyte modifier (magnesium supplement), Laxative (saline), Anticonvulsant
Pregnancy Category A (anticonvulsant)

INDICATIONS

■ Treatment and prevention of hypomagnesemia ■ As an anticonvulsant in severe eclampsia or pre-eclampsia ■ Used as a laxative and to evacuate the bowel in preparation for surgical or radiographic procedures.

ACTION

■ Essential for the activity of many enzymes ■ Plays an important role in neurotransmission and muscular excitability ■ Is osmotically active in GI tract, drawing water into the lumen and causing peristalsis. **Therapeutic Effects:** ■ Replacement in deficiency states, resolution of eclampsia, and evacuation of the colon.

PHARMACOKINETICS

Absorption: 15–30% may be absorbed orally. Well absorbed from IM sites.
Distribution: Widely distributed. Crosses the placenta and is present in breast milk.
Metabolism and Excretion: Excreted primarily by the kidneys.
Half-life: UK.

CONTRAINDICATIONS AND PRECAUTIONS

Contraindicated in: ▪ Hypermagnesemia ▪ Hypocalcemia ▪ Anuria ▪ Heart block ▪ Active labor.
Use Cautiously in: ▪ Any degree of renal insufficiency (dosage reduction required).

ADVERSE REACTIONS AND SIDE EFFECTS*

Serious reactions are associated with parenteral use only.

CNS: drowsiness.
Resp: decreased respiratory rate.
CV: bradycardia, arrhythmias, hypotension.
GI: diarrhea.
Derm: flushing, sweating.
Metab: hypothermia.
Neuro: decreased deep-tendon reflexes, PARALYSIS.

INTERACTIONS

Drug–Drug: ▪ Potentiates **neuromuscular blocking agents** ▪ Orally administered magnesium decreases absorption of **fluoroquinolones**.

ROUTE AND DOSAGE

Each gram of magnesium sulfate contains 8 mEq magnesium.

Hypomagnesemia
▪ **PO (Adults):** 3 g q 6 hr for 4 doses.
▪ **IM (Adults):** 1 g q 6 hr for 4 doses, up to 250 mg/kg over a 4-hr period.
▪ **IV (Adults):** up to 5 g diluted and infused slowly over 3 hr.

Eclampsia, Pre-Eclampsia
▪ **IV (Adults):** 4 g or 4–5 g as an infusion.
▪ **IM (Adults):** 4–5 g q 4 hr.

Laxative
▪ **PO (Adults):** 10–30 g.
▪ **PO (Children 6–11 yr):** 5–10 g.
▪ **PO (Children 2–5 yr):** 2.5–5 g.

AVAILABILITY

▪ *Powder for oral use* ▪ *Epsom salts*
▪ *Injection:* 10%, 12.5%, 25%, 50%.

TIME/ACTION PROFILE
(PO = laxative effect;
IM, IV = anticonvulsant effect)

	ONSET	PEAK	DURATION
PO	3–6 hr	UK	UK
IM	60 min	UK	3–4 hr
IV	immediate	UK	30 min

NURSING IMPLICATIONS

ASSESSMENT
▪ **General Info:** Serum magnesium levels and renal function should be monitored periodically throughout administration of parenteral magnesium sulfate.
▪ **Hypomagnesemia/Anticonvulsant:** Monitor pulse, blood pressure, respirations, and ECG frequently throughout administration of parenteral magnesium sulfate. Respirations should be at least 16/min prior to each dose.
▫ Monitor neurologic status prior to and throughout therapy. Institute seizure precautions. Patellar reflex (knee jerk) should be tested before each parenteral dose of magnesium sulfate. If response is absent, no additional doses should be administered until positive response is obtained.
▫ Monitor newborn for hypotension, hyporeflexia, and respiratory depression if mother has received magnesium sulfate.
▫ Monitor intake and output ratios. Urine output should be maintained at a level of at least 100 ml every 4 hr.

M

- **Laxative:** Assess patient for abdominal distention, presence of bowel sounds, and usual pattern of bowel function.
□ Assess color, consistency, and amount of stool produced.
- **Toxicity and Overdose:** Toxicity is manifested by a prolonged P-Q and widened QRS interval, loss of deep tendon reflexes, heart block, respiratory paralysis, and cardiac arrest. Treatment includes IV calcium gluconate to antagonize the effects of magnesium.

POTENTIAL NURSING DIAGNOSES
- Injury, high risk for (indications, side effects).
- Constipation (indications).
- Knowledge deficit related to medication regimen (patient/family teaching).

IMPLEMENTATION
- **PO:** For laxative effect, administer on empty stomach for more rapid results. Dissolve magnesium sulfate in a full glass of water; may use lemon-flavored carbonated beverage to mask bitter taste. Follow with a full glass of liquid to prevent dehydration and for faster effect. May be given as a single dose or several divided doses. Do not administer at bedtime or late in the day.
- **IM:** Administer deep IM using gluteal sites. Administer subsequent injections in alternate sides.
□ Use 25–50% concentrations for adults, 20% concentrations for children <14 yr.
- **Direct IV:** Administer undiluted at a rate of 1.5 ml of a 10% solution (or its equivalent) over 1 min.
- **Continuous Infusion:** *Eclampsia*—Dilute 4 g in 250 ml of D5W or 0.9% NaCl.
- *Rate:* Administer at a rate not to exceed 4 ml/min.
□ *Hypomagnesemia*—Dilute 5 g in 1 liter of D5W, 0.9% NaCl, Ringer's or lactated Ringer's solution and administer slowly over 3 hr.

□ Use infusion pump to regulate rate accurately.
- **Y-Site Compatibility:** ■ acyclovir ■ amikacin ■ ampicillin ■ cefamandole ■ cefazolin ■ cefoperazone ■ ceforanide ■ cefotaxime ■ cefoxitin ■ cephalothin ■ cephapirin ■ chloramphenicol ■ clindamycin ■ dobutamine ■ doxycycline ■ enalaprilat ■ erythromycin lactobionate ■ esmolol ■ famotidine ■ fludarabine ■ gentamicin ■ heparin ■ hydrocortisone ■ insulin ■ kanamycin ■ labetalol ■ metronidazole ■ minocycline ■ nafcillin ■ ondansetron ■ oxacillin ■ penicillin G potassium ■ piperacillin ■ potassium chloride ■ sargramostim ■ ticarcillin ■ tobramycin ■ trimethoprim/sulfamethoxazole ■ vancomycin ■ vitamin B complex with C.
- **Additive Compatibility:** ■ calcium gluconate ■ cephalothin ■ chloramphenicol ■ cisplatin ■ hydrocortisone sodium succinate ■ methyldopate ■ penicillin G potassium ■ potassium phosphate ■ verapamil.
- **Additive Incompatibility:** ■ calcium gluceptate ■ polymyxin ■ sodium bicarbonate ■ tobramycin.

PATIENT/FAMILY TEACHING
- **Laxative:** Advise patient that laxatives should be used only for short-term therapy. Long-term therapy may cause electrolyte imbalance and dependence.
□ Encourage patient to utilize other forms of bowel regulation, such as increasing bulk in the diet, increasing fluid intake, increasing mobility. Normal bowel habits are individualized and may vary from 3 times/day to 3 times/wk.
□ Advise patient to notify physician if unrelieved constipation, rectal bleeding, or symptoms of electrolyte imbalance (muscle cramps or pain, weakness, dizziness) occur.

EVALUATION
Effectiveness of therapy can be demonstrated by: ■ Normal serum magnesium concentrations ■ Control of seizures as-

sociated with toxemias of pregnancy
■ Passage of a soft, formed bowel movement, usually within 3–6 hr.

MANNITOL
(man-i-tol)
Osmitrol

CLASSIFICATION(S):
Diuretic (osmotic)
Pregnancy Category C

INDICATIONS

■ **IV:** Adjunct in the treatment of acute oliguric renal failure □ Adjunct in the treatment of edema □ Reduction of intracranial or intraocular pressure □ To promote the excretion of certain toxic substances ■ **GU irrigant:** Used as an irrigant during transurethral procedures.

ACTION

■ Increases the osmotic pressure of the glomerular filtrate, thereby inhibiting reabsorption of water and electrolytes ■ Causes excretion of: □ Water □ Sodium □ Potassium □ Chloride □ Calcium □ Phosphorus □ Magnesium □ Urea □ Uric acid.

PHARMACOKINETICS

Absorption: Administered IV only, resulting in cómplete bioavailability. Some absorption may occur during use as a GU irrigant.
Distribution: Confined to the extracellular space. Does not usually cross the blood–brain barrier or eye.
Metabolism and Excretion: Excreted by the kidneys. Minimal metabolism by the liver.
Half-life: 100 min.

CONTRAINDICATIONS AND PRECAUTIONS

Contraindicated in: ■ Hypersensitivity ■ Anuria ■ Dehydration ■ Active intracranial bleeding.

Use Cautiously in: ■ Pregnancy and lactation (safety not established).

ADVERSE REACTIONS AND SIDE EFFECTS*

CNS: headache, confusion.
EENT: blurred vision, rhinitis.
CV: transient volume expansion, tachycardia, chest pain, congestive heart failure, pulmonary edema.
GI: thirst, nausea, vomiting.
GU: renal failure, urinary retention.
F and E: hyponatremia, hypernatremia, hypokalemia, hyperkalemia, dehydration.
Local: phlebitis at IV site.

INTERACTIONS

Drug–Drug: ■ Enhances **lithium** excretion; may decrease effectiveness.

ROUTE AND DOSAGE

Edema, Oliguric Renal Failure
■ **IV (Adults):** 50–100 g as a 5–25% solution. May precede with a test dose of 0.2 g/kg over 3–5 min.
■ **IV (Children):** 0.25–2 g/kg as a 15–20% solution over 2–6 hr. May precede with a test dose of 0.2 g/kg over 3–5 min.

Reduction of Intracranial or Intraocular Pressure
■ **IV (Adults):** 0.25–2 g/kg as 15–25% solution over 30–60 min.
■ **IV (Children):** 1–2 g/kg (30–60 g/m²) as a 15–20% solution over 30–60 min (500 mg/kg may be sufficient in small or debilitated patients).

Diuresis in Drug Intoxications
■ **IV (Adults):** 50–200 g as a 5–25% solution titrated to maintain urine flow of 100–500 ml/hr.
■ **IV (Children):** up to 2 g/kg (60 g/m²) as a 5–10% solution.

AVAILABILITY

■ *IV injection:* 5%, 10%, 15%, 20%
■ *GU irrigant:* 5% and in combination with sorbital.

M

*Underlines indicate most frequent; **CAPITALS** indicate life-threatening.*

TIME/ACTION PROFILE (diuretic effect)

	ONSET	PEAK	DURATION
IV	30–60 min	1 hr	6–8 hr

NURSING IMPLICATIONS

ASSESSMENT

- **General Info:** Monitor vital signs, urine output, CVP, and pulmonary artery pressures (PAP) prior to and hourly throughout administration. Assess patient for signs and symptoms of dehydration (decreased skin turgor, fever, dry skin and mucous membranes, thirst) or signs of fluid overload (increased CVP, dyspnea, rales/crackles, edema).
- ◻ Assess patient for anorexia, muscle weakness, numbness, tingling, paresthesia, confusion, and excessive thirst. Notify physician promptly if these signs of electrolyte imbalance occur.
- **Increased Intracranial Pressure:** Monitor neurologic status and intracranial pressure readings in patients receiving this medication to decrease cerebral edema.
- **Increased Intraocular Pressure:** Monitor for persistent or increased eye pain or decreased visual acuity.
- **Lab Test Considerations:** Renal function and serum electrolytes should be monitored routinely throughout course of therapy.

POTENTIAL NURSING DIAGNOSES

- Fluid volume excess (indications).
- Fluid volume deficit, high risk for (side effects).

IMPLEMENTATION

- **General Info:** Observe infusion site frequently for infiltration. Extravasation may cause tissue irritation and necrosis.
- ◻ Do not administer electrolyte-free mannitol solution with blood. If blood must be administered simultaneously with mannitol, add at least 20 mEq NaCl to each liter of mannitol.
- ◻ Confer with physician regarding placement of an indwelling foley catheter (except when used to decrease intraocular pressure).
- **IV:** Administer by IV infusion undiluted. If solution contains crystals, warm bottle in hot water and shake vigorously. Do not administer solution in which crystals remain undissolved. Cool to body temperature. Use an in-line filter for 15%, 20%, and 25% infusions.
- **Test Dose:** Administer over 3–5 min to produce a urine output of 30–50 ml/hr. If urine flow does not increase, administer second test dose. If urine output is not at least 30–50 ml/hr for 2–3 hr after second test dose, patient should be re-evaluated.
- **Oliguria:** Administration rate should be titrated to produce a urine output of 30–50 ml/hr.
- **Increased Intracranial Pressure:** Infuse dose over 30–60 min.
- **Intraocular Pressure:** Administer dose over 30 min. When used preoperatively, administer 60–90 min prior to surgery.
- **Y-Site Compatability:** ▪ fludarabine ▪ ondansetron ▪ sargramostim.
- **Irrigation:** Add contents of two 50-ml vials of 25% mannitol to 900 ml of Sterile Water for Injection for a 2.5% solution for irrigation. Use only clear solutions.

PATIENT/FAMILY TEACHING

- ◻ Explain purpose of therapy to patient.

EVALUATION

Effectiveness of therapy can be demonstrated by: ▪ Urine output of at least 30–50 ml/hr or an increase in urine output in accordance with parameters set by physician ▪ Reduction in intracranial pressure ▪ Reduction of intraocular pressure ▪ Excretion of certain toxic substances ▪ Irrigation during transurethral prostate resection.

MAPROTILINE
(ma-**proe**-ti-leen)
Ludiomil

INDICATIONS

- Treatment of various forms of depression and anxiety associated with depression, often in conjunction with psychotherapy.

ACTION

- Potentiates the effects of serotonin and norepinephrine ■ Has significant anticholinergic properties. **Therapeutic Effect:** ■ Antidepressant action, which may develop only over several weeks.

PHARMACOKINETICS

Absorption: Slowly but completely absorbed from the GI tract.
Distribution: Widely distributed. Probably crosses the placenta. Enters breast milk in concentrations similar to those in plasma.
Metabolism and Excretion: Slowly and extensively metabolized by the liver. Some conversion to active compounds. 30% excreted in the feces.
Half-life: 51 hr.

CONTRAINDICATIONS AND PRECAUTIONS

Contraindicated in: ■ Narrow-angle glaucoma ■ Pregnancy and lactation ■ Acute myocardial infarction ■ Seizure disorders (may lower seizure threshold) ■ Some products contain tartrazine and should be avoided in patients with known intolerance.
Use Cautiously in: ■ Elderly patients (increased risk of adverse reactions, dosage reduction suggested) ■ Patients with pre-existing cardiovascular disease ■ Elderly men with prostatic hypertrophy (more susceptible to urinary retention).

ADVERSE REACTIONS AND SIDE EFFECTS*

CNS: drowsiness, sedation, lethargy, fatigue, confusion, agitation, hallucinations, SEIZURES.
EENT: dry mouth, dry eyes, blurred vision.
CV: hypotension, ECG changes, ARRHYTHMIAS.
GI: constipation, paralytic ileus.
GU: urinary retention.
Derm: photosensitivity.
Endo: gynecomastia.
Hemat: blood dyscrasias.

INTERACTIONS

Drug–Drug: ■ May cause hyperpyrexia, seizures, hypertension and death when used with **MAO inhibitors** (avoid concurrent use—discontinue 2 wk prior to maprotiline) ■ May prevent the therapeutic response to **antihypertensives** ■ Additive CNS depression with other **CNS depressants,** including **alcohol, antihistamines, opioid analgesics, clonidine,** and **sedative/hypnotics** ■ Adrenergic effects may be additive with other **adrenergic agents,** including **vasoconstrictors** and **decongestants** ■ Additive anticholinergic effects with other **drugs possessing anticholinergic properties,** including **antihistamines, atropine, haloperidol, phenothiazines, quinidine,** and **disopyramide** ■ **Cimetidine, fluoxetine,** or **oral contraceptives** increase levels and may cause toxicity ■ **Sympathomimetics** increase risk of adverse cardiovascular reactions ■ Increased risk of seizures with **phenothiazines.**

ROUTE AND DOSAGE

- **PO (Adults):** 75 mg/day initially, may increase by 25 mg q 2 wk to a maximum of 150 mg/day. Some patients may require up to 225 mg/day. May be given in 3 divided doses or single daily dose.
- **PO (Elderly patients):** 25 mg/day initially. Maintenance dose 50–75 mg/day.

AVAILABILITY

- **Tablets:** 25 mg, 50 mg, 75 mg.

M

686MAST CELL STABILIZERS

TIME/ACTION PROFILE
(antidepressant effect)

	ONSET	PEAK	DURATION
PO	3–7 days	2–3 wk	UK

NURSING IMPLICATIONS

ASSESSMENT
□ Assess mental status frequently. Confusion, agitation, and hallucinations may occur during initiation of therapy and may require dosage reduction. Monitor mood changes. Assess for suicidal tendencies, especially during early therapy. Restrict amount of drug available to patient.
□ Monitor blood pressure and pulse rate periodically during initial therapy. Notify physician of significant changes.
□ Monitor for seizure activity in patients with a history of convulsions or alcohol abuse. Institute seizure precautions.
■ Lab Test Considerations: Assess CBC and hepatic function prior to and periodically during therapy.

POTENTIAL NURSING DIAGNOSES
■ Coping, ineffective individual (indications).
■ Anxiety (indications).
■ Knowledge deficit related to medication regimen (patient/family teaching).

IMPLEMENTATION
■ General Info: May be given as a single dose at bedtime to minimize excessive drowsiness or dizziness.

PATIENT/FAMILY TEACHING
□ Instruct patient to take medication exactly as directed. If a dose is missed, take as soon as remembered; if almost time for next dose, skip missed dose and return to regular schedule. If single bedtime dose regimen is used, do not take missed dose in morning, but consult physician.
□ May cause drowsiness and blurred vision. Caution patient to avoid driving and other activities requiring alert-

ness until response to drug is known.
□ Caution patient to make position changes slowly to minimize orthostatic hypotension.
□ Advise patient to avoid alcohol or other CNS depressant drugs during and for at least 3–7 days after therapy has been discontinued.
□ Advise patient to notify physician if dry mouth, urinary retention, or constipation occurs. Frequent rinses, good oral hygiene, and sugarless candy or gum may diminish dry mouth. An increase in fluid intake, fiber, and exercise may prevent constipation.
□ Caution patient to use sunscreen and protective clothing to prevent photosensitivity reactions.
□ Advise patient to consult physician or pharmacist before taking any over-the-counter cold remedies with this medication.
□ Advise patient to notify physician or dentist of medication regimen prior to treatment or surgery.
□ Therapy for depression may be prolonged. Emphasize the importance of follow-up examination to monitor effectiveness and side effects.

EVALUATION
Effectiveness of therapy can be demonstrated by: ■ Resolution of the symptoms of depression: □ Increased sense of well-being □ Renewed interest in surroundings □ Increased appetite □ Improved energy level □ Improved sleep ■ Decrease in anxiety associated with depression. Therapeutic effects are sometimes seen in 3–7 days, although 2–3 wk is usually necessary before improvement is observed.

MAST CELL STABILIZERS
cromolyn
(kroe-moe-lin)
cromoglycate, {Fivent}, Intal,

Gastrochrom, {Nalcrom}, Nasalcrom, Opticrom, {Rynocrom}, {Vistacrom}

nedocromil
(ne-doe-**kroe**-mil)

CLASSIFICATION(S):
Antihistamine (mast cell stabilizer)
Pregnancy Category B

INDICATIONS

■ **PO:** Treatment of mastocytosis ■ **Inhalation, ophth, nasal:** Adjunct in the prophylaxis of allergic disorders including rhinitis, conjunctivitis, and asthma ■ Inhalation product also has been used in the prevention of exercise-induced bronchospasm.

ACTION

■ Prevents the release of histamine and slow reacting substance of anaphylaxis (SRS-A) from sensitized mast cells. **Therapeutic Effects:** ■ Decreased symptoms of mastocytosis (diarrhea, flushing, headache, vomiting, urticaria, abdominal pain, nausea, itching) ■ Decreased frequency and intensity of allergic reactions, including rhinitis, conjunctivitis, and asthma.

PHARMACOKINETICS

Absorption: *Cromolyn*—Poorly absorbed following all routes of administration; action is local. Small amounts may reach systemic circulation after inhalation, even less from other routes. *Nedocromil*—90% of the inhaled dose is swallowed. 2.5–3% of swallowed drug is absorbed. Inhaled drug that reaches the lung is completely absorbed (total bioavailability is 6–9%).
Distribution: Because only small amounts are absorbed, distribution is not known. Does not cross biologic membranes well.
Metabolism and Excretion: Small amounts absorbed are excreted unchanged in bile and urine.

Half-life: *Cromolyn*—80 min; *Nedocromil*—1.5–2.3 hr.

CONTRAINDICATIONS AND PRECAUTIONS

Contraindicated in: ■ Hypersensitivity ■ Acute attacks of asthma.
Use Cautiously in: ■ Pregnancy and lactation (safety not established) ■ *Cromolyn*—Children <2 yr (oral use reserved for severe mastocytosis) ■ *Nedocromil*—Children <12 yr (safety not established) ■ Will not relieve and may worsen acute attacks of bronchospasm (inhalation).

ADVERSE REACTIONS AND SIDE EFFECTS*

CNS: all routes: headache; **PO:** irritability, trouble sleeping.
EENT: nasal: <u>nasal irritation</u>, sneezing; **ophth:** <u>ocular burning</u>, stinging, unpleasant taste.
GI: PO: diarrhea, abdominal pain; **nedocromil:** <u>unpleasant taste</u>.
Resp: inhalation: <u>irritation of the throat and trachea</u>, cough, bronchospasm.
Derm: all routes: rash, erythema, urticaria.
MS: PO: myalgia.
Misc: allergic reactions, including ANAPHYLAXIS or worsening of conditions being treated.

INTERACTIONS

Drug–Drug: ■ None significant.

ROUTE AND DOSAGE

Cromolyn
■ **PO (Adults):** 200 mg 4 times daily.
■ **PO (Children 2–12 yr):** 100 mg 4 times daily.
■ **PO (Children up to 2 yr):** 20 mg/kg/day in 4 divided doses, dose may be increased up to 30 mg/kg/day.
■ **Inhalation (Adult and Children >5 yr):** 20-mg inhaler capsules or nebulizer solution or 2 sprays as aerosol 4 times daily. For prevention of bronchospasm, use 2 aerosol sprays 10–

M

15 min before exposure to known precipitating situation.

- **Nasal (Adults and Children >6 yr):** 1 spray each nostril 3–4 times daily (up to 6 times daily).
- **Ophth (Adults and Children >4 yr):** 1 drop each eye 4–6 times daily.

Nedocromil
- **Inhalation (Adults and Children ≥12 yr):** 2 inhalations 4 times daily.

AVAILABILITY

Cromolyn
- **Oral capsules:** 100 mg **■ Capsules for inhalation:** 20 mg **■ Solution for nebulization:** 20 mg/2 ml **■ Aerosol spray for inhalation:** 800 mcg/spray in 8.1-g (112 sprays) or 14.2-g (≥200 sprays) container **■ Nasal solution:** 40 mg/ml (5.2 mg/spray) in 13-ml (≥100 sprays) or 26-ml (≥200 sprays) container **■ Ophthalmic solution:** 4% in 10-ml dropper bottle.

Nedocromil
- **Aerosol for inhalation:** 1.75 mg/spray in 16.2-g cannister (at least 112 inhalations).

TIME/ACTION PROFILE (effects on diminishing symptoms)

	ONSET	PEAK	DURATION
cromolyn—PO	UK	2–3 wk	UK
cromolyn—inhalation	<1 wk	2–4 wk	UK
cromolyn—nasal	<1 wk	2–4 wk	UK
cromolyn—Ophth	<1 wk	2–4 wk	UK
nedocromil—inhalation	within 2 wk	UK	UK

NURSING IMPLICATIONS

ASSESSMENT
- **General Info:** Assess patint for signs of mastocytosis (diarrhea, flushing, headaches, vomiting, urticaria, abdominal pain, nausea, and itching) prior to and periodically throughout therapy.
- **Inhalation:** Pulmonary function testing should be evaluated prior to initiating therapy in asthmatics.
- Assess lung sounds and respiratory function prior to and periodically throughout therapy.
- **Ophth:** Assess eye for redness, tearing, and irritation.
- **Nasal Spray:** Assess for symptoms of rhinitis (stuffiness, rhinorrhea).

POTENTIAL NURSING DIAGNOSES
- Airway clearance, ineffective (indications).
- Knowledge deficit related to medication regimen (patient/family teaching).

IMPLEMENTATION
- **General Info:** Reduction in dosage of other asthma medications may be possible after 2–4 wk of therapy.
- **PO:** Administer at regular intervals 30 min before meals and at bedtime. Dose may be reduced once therapeutic response is achieved.
- To prepare, open capsule(s) and pour into a glass half full of hot water. Stir until completely dissolved and solution is clear. Add an equal quantity of cold water while stirring. Do not mix with fruit juice, milk, or foods. Patient should drink all of the liquid.
- **Inhalation:** Medication should be used prophylactically, not for use during acute asthma attacks or status asthmaticus.
- Pretreatment with bronchodilator may be required to increase delivery of inhalation product.
- **Ophth:** See Appendix H for instillation of ophthalmic medications.

PATIENT/FAMILY TEACHING
- **General Info:** Medication must be used routinely. If a dose is missed, take as soon as remembered and space other doses at regular intervals. Do not double doses. Do not discontinue therapy without consulting physician, or exacerbation of symptoms may occur.
- If cromolyn is prescribed before contact with known allergen or exercise, explain that it should be administered 10–15 min, and no earlier than 60 min, in advance.
- **PO:** Emphasize the importance of tak-

ing at least 30 min before meals; not mixing with fruit juice, milk, or food; and drinking all of the liquid to prevent relapse.

- **Inhalation:** Inform patient that *Intal* capsules for inhalation are to be used for Spinhaler device only.
- Instruct patient in the proper use of the metered-dose inhaler. See Appendix H for instructions.
- Advise patient that gargling and rinsing the mouth after each dose helps to decrease dryness of mouth, throat irritation, and hoarseness.
- Caution patient to notify physician if asthmatic symptoms recur.
- **Ophth:** Instruct patient on correct technique for instillation of eye drops. Advise patient to notify physician if eye irritation increases; a mild, transient burning immediately following administration is not unusual.
- **Nasal Spray:** Instruct patient to clear nasal passages prior to administration and to inhale through nose during administration.

EVALUATION

Therapeutic effects, observable within 2–4 wk after beginning therapy, are demonstrated by: ▪ Decrease in symptoms of mastocytosis ▪ Reduction in symptoms of asthma ▪ Decrease in the symptoms of conjunctivitis ▪ Decrease in the symptoms of rhinitis.

MEBENDAZOLE
(me-**ben**-da-zole)
{Nemasole}, Vermox

CLASSIFICATION(S):
Antihelmintic
Pregnancy Category C

INDICATIONS

▪ Treatment of: □ Whipworm (trichuriasis) □ Pinworm (enterobiasis) □ Roundworm (ascariasis) □ Hookworm (uncinariasis) infections.

ACTION

▪ Inhibits the uptake of glucose and other nutrients by susceptible helminths. **Therapeutic Effect:** ▪ Death of parasites, eggs, and hydatid cysts (vermicidal and ovacidal).

PHARMACOKINETICS

Absorption: Minimally (2–10%) absorbed following oral administration.
Distribution: Distribution not known.
Metabolism and Excretion: >95% eliminated in feces. Absorbed drug is mostly metabolized by the liver; small amounts excreted unchanged by the kidneys.
Half-life: 2.5–9 hr (increased in liver impairment).

CONTRAINDICATIONS AND PRECAUTIONS

Contraindicated in: ▪ Hypersensitivity.
Use Cautiously in: ▪ Pregnancy, lactation, or children <2 yr (safety not established) ▪ Impaired liver function ▪ Crohn's ileitis ▪ Ulcerative colitis.

ADVERSE REACTIONS AND SIDE EFFECTS*

Most side effects and adverse reactions are seen with high-dose therapy only.

CNS: headache, dizziness.
EENT: tinnitus.
GI: diarrhea, abdominal pain, nausea, vomiting.
Hemat: reversible myelosuppression (leukopenia, thrombocytopenia).
Neuro: numbness.
Misc: fever.

INTERACTIONS

Drug–Drug: ▪ **Carbamazepine** and **phenytoin** may increase the metabolism and decrease effectiveness of therapy in patients receiving high-dose therapy.
Drug–Food: ▪ Absorption may be increased by **fatty foods**.

M

ROUTE AND DOSAGE

Enterobiasis

- **PO (Adults and Children >2 yr):** 100 mg as a single dose. May repeat in 2–3 wk.

Trichuriasis, Ascariasis, Hookworm, or Mixed Infections

- **PO (Adults and Children >2 yr):** 200 mg/day in 2 divided doses for 3 days. If not cured in 3–4 wk, a second course is given.

AVAILABILITY

- **Chewable tablets:** 100 mg.

TIME/ACTION PROFILE

	ONSET	PEAK	DURATION
PO	UK	UK	UK

NURSING IMPLICATIONS

ASSESSMENT

- **Pinworm:** Perianal examinations should be performed to detect the presence of adult worms in the perianal area, and cellophane tape swabs of the perianal area should be taken prior to and starting 1 wk following treatment to detect the presence of ova. Swabs should be taken each morning prior to defecation or bathing for at least 3 days. Patients are not considered cured unless perianal swabs have been negative for 7 days.
- **Roundworm:** Stool examinations should be monitored prior to and 1–3 wk following treatment.
- **Lab Test Considerations:** May cause transient increase in serum BUN, AST (SGOT), ALT (SGPT), and alkaline phosphatase levels.
- □ CBC should be monitored prior to therapy and 2–3 times a week from day 10–25 and weekly thereafter in patients receiving high-dose therapy. Mebendazole may cause reversible leukopenia and thrombocytopenia.
- □ May cause decreased serum hemoglobin concentrations.

POTENTIAL NURSING DIAGNOSES

- Infection, high risk for (indications).

- Home maintenance management, impaired (indications).
- Knowledge deficit related to disease process and medication regimen (patient/family teaching).

IMPLEMENTATION

- **General Info:** No special diets, fasting, laxatives, or enemas are required prior to administration of mebendazole.
- **PO:** Mebendazole tablet may be chewed, swallowed whole, or crushed and mixed with food. Patients on high-dose therapy should take tablets with high-fat meals to increase absorption.
- **Pinworm:** All members of the household should be treated concurrently, with treatment repeated in 2–3 wk.
- **Hookworm and Whipworm:** Patient may be required to take an iron supplement daily during treatment and for 6 mo following treatment if anemia occurs.

PATIENT/FAMILY TEACHING

- **General Info:** Instruct patient to take medication exactly as directed and to continue medication for full course of therapy, even if feeling better. If a dose is missed, take as soon as remembered; if on 2 doses/day schedule, space missed dose and next dose 4–5 hr apart or double next dose. A second course of therapy may be required.
- □ Advise patient of hygienic precautions to minimize reinfection (wash hands with soap prior to eating and after using the toilet, disinfect toilet daily, keep hands away from mouth, wash all fruits and vegetables, wear shoes).
- □ Medication may cause dizziness. Caution patient to avoid driving or activities requiring alertness until response to medication is known.
- □ Advise patient to consult physician if no improvement is seen within a few days.
- □ Emphasize the importance of follow-up examinations to determine effec-

tiveness, especially with high-dose therapy.

- **Pinworm:** Instruct patient to wash (do not shake) all bedding, undergarments, towels, and nightclothes after treatment to prevent reinfection.

EVALUATION

Effectiveness of therapy can be demonstrated by: ▪ Resolution of the signs and symptoms of infection or when stool specimens and perianal swabs are negative. Length of time for complete resolution depends on the parasite.

MECHLORETHAMINE
(me-klor-**eth**-a-meen)
Mustargen, Nitrogen mustard

CLASSIFICATION(S):
Antineoplastic (alkylating agent)
Pregnancy Category UK

INDICATIONS

▪ As part of combination therapy of Hodgkin's disease and malignant lymphomas ▪ Used palliatively in: □ Bronchogenic carcinoma □ Breast carcinoma □ Ovarian carcinoma □ Leukemias ▪ Administered into cavities (pleural, peritoneal) to prevent reaccumulation of malignant effusions.

ACTION

▪ Interferes with DNA and RNA synthesis by cross-linking strands (cell cyclephase nonspecific). **Therapeutic Effect:** ▪ Death of rapidly replicating cells, particularly malignant ones.

PHARMACOKINETICS

Absorption: Administered IV and intracavitary only. Some absorption occurs following intracavitary instillation.
Distribution: Distribution not known.
Metabolism and Excretion: Rapidly degraded in body tissues and fluids.
Half-life: UK.

CONTRAINDICATIONS AND PRECAUTIONS

Contraindicated in: ▪ Hypersensitivity ▪ Pregnancy or lactation.
Use Cautiously in: ▪ Patients with childbearing potential ▪ Infections ▪ Decreased bone marrow reserve ▪ Other chronic debilitating illnesses ▪ Prior radiotherapy (dosage reduction required).

ADVERSE REACTIONS AND SIDE EFFECTS*

CNS: weakness, headache, drowsiness, vertigo, seizures.
GI: nausea, vomiting, diarrhea, anorexia.
GU: gonadal suppression.
Hemat: anemia, leukopenia, thrombocytopenia.
Derm: rashes, alopecia.
Local: phlebitis at IV site, tissue necrosis.
Metab: hyperuricemia.
Misc: reactivation of herpes zoster.

INTERACTIONS

Drug–Drug: ▪ Additive myelosuppression with other **antineoplastic agents** or **radiation therapy** ▪ May decrease antibody response to **live virus vaccines** and increase the risk of adverse reactions.

ROUTE AND DOSAGE

- **IV (Adults and Children):** 0.4 mg/kg as single dose or divided over 2–4 days. May be repeated q 3–6 wk.
- **Intracavitary (Adults):** 10–20 mg (range 200–400 mcg/kg).

AVAILABILITY

- *Injection:* 10-mg vials.

TIME/ACTION PROFILE (effects on blood counts)

	ONSET	PEAK	DURATION
WBCs	24 hr	7–14 days	10–21 days
Platelets	UK	9–16 days	20 days

M

---

*Underlines indicate most frequent; **CAPITALS** indicate life-threatening.

NURSING IMPLICATIONS

ASSESSMENT

▢ Monitor blood pressure, pulse, and respiratory rate frequently during administration. Notify physician if significant changes occur.

▢ Assess injection site frequently for redness, irritation, or inflammation. If extravasation occurs, infusion must be stopped and restarted elsewhere to avoid damage to SC tissue. Infiltrate affected area promptly with isotonic sodium thiosulfate 1% or lidocaine and apply ice compresses for 6–12 hr as directed by physician.

▢ Monitor intake and output, appetite, and nutritional intake. Nausea and vomiting may occur 1–3 hr after therapy. Vomiting may persist for 8 hr; nausea may last 24 hr. Parenteral antiemetic agents should be administered 30–45 min prior to therapy and routinely around the clock for the next 24 hr as indicated. Adjust diet as tolerated to help maintain fluid and electrolyte balance and nutritional status.

▢ Assess for fever, chills, sore throat, and signs of infection. Notify physician if these symptoms occur.

▢ Assess for bleeding (bleeding gums; bruising; petechiae; guaiac stools, urine, and emesis). Avoid IM injections and rectal temperatures. Apply pressure to venipuncture sites for 10 min.

▢ Anemia may occur. Monitor for increased fatigue and dyspnea.

▢ Monitor for symptoms of gout (increased uric acid, joint pain, edema). Encourage patient to drink at least 2 liters of fluid each day. Allopurinol may be given to decrease uric acid levels. Alkalinization of urine may be ordered to increase excretion of uric acid.

▪ **Lab Test Considerations:** Monitor CBC and differential prior to and periodically throughout therapy. The nadir of leukopenia occurs in 7–14 days. Notify physician if leukocyte count is <1000/mm^3. The nadir of

thrombocytopenia occurs in 9–16 days. Notify physician if platelet count is <75,000/mm^3. Recovery of leukopenia and thrombocytopenia occurs in 20 days.

▢ Monitor liver function studies (AST [SGOT], ALT [SGPT], LDH, bilirubin) and renal function studies (BUN, creatinine) prior to and periodically throughout therapy to detect hepatotoxicity and nephrotoxicity.

▢ May cause increased uric acid levels.

POTENTIAL NURSING DIAGNOSES

▪ Infection, high risk for (adverse reactions).

▪ Nutrition, altered: less than body requirements (adverse reactions).

▪ Knowledge deficit related to medication regimen (patient/family teaching).

IMPLEMENTATION

▪ **General Info:** Solution should be prepared in a biologic cabinet. Wear gloves, gown, and mask while handling medication. All equipment in contact with this medication must be decontaminated prior to disposal. Soak gloves, IV tubing, syringes, etc. in solution of 5% sodium thiosulfate and 5% sodium bicarbonate for 45 min. Unused portions of the drug must be mixed with equal amounts of this solution.

▢ Discard all contaminated equipment in specially designated containers. If medication comes in contact with skin, flush with large volume of water for 15 min, followed by a 2% sodium thiosulfate solution. If eye contact occurs, flush eye with 0.9% NaCl and notify physician immediately (see Appendix I.)

▪ **Direct IV:** Discard vial if droplets of water appear to be present prior to reconstitution. Dilute each 10 mg with 10 ml of 0.9% NaCl or Sterile Water for Injection. Do not remove the needle from the vial stopper prior to agitating solution. Allow solution to dissolve completely. Reconstituted solution decomposes in 15 min. Administer immediately. Do not use a discolored solution or one that contains precipitates.

- **Rate:** Withdraw desired amount of drug and administer over 3–5 min via Y-tubing or 3-way stopcock into a free-flowing solution of 0.9% NaCl.
- **Y-Site Compatibility:** ▪ fludarabine ▪ ondansetron ▪ sargramostim.
- **Intracavitary:** May be further diluted in 100 ml of 0.9% NaCl. Assist physician in paracentesis prior to instillation of mechlorethamine. Confer with physician regarding analgesia and schedule for repositioning patient to ensure mechlorethamine comes in contact with entire cavity surface. Remaining fluid may be removed after 24–36 hr.

PATIENT/FAMILY TEACHING

- ▢ Advise patient to notify physician if fever, chills, sore throat, signs of infection, bleeding gums, bruising, petechiae, or blood in urine, stool, or emesis occurs. Caution patient to avoid crowds and persons with known infections. Instruct patient to use soft toothbrush and electric razor. Caution patient not to drink alcoholic beverages or take products containing aspirin or ibuprofen.
- ▢ This drug may cause irreversible gonadal suppression; however, patient should still use birth control during and for at least 4 mo after therapy, as it may have teratogenic effects.
- ▢ Discuss with patient the possibility of hair loss. Explore methods of coping.
- ▢ Instruct patient not to receive any vaccinations without advice of physician.
- ▢ Instruct patient to notify physician if skin rash occurs. Rash may indicate idiosyncratic reaction or reactivation of herpes zoster.
- ▢ Emphasize the need for periodic lab tests to monitor for side effects.

EVALUATION

Effectiveness of therapy can be demonstrated by: ▪ Decrease in size or spread of malignancies in solid tumors ▪ Improvement of hematologic status in leukemias.

MECLIZINE
(**mek**-li-zeen)
Antivert, Antrizine, {Bonamine}, Bonine, Dizmiss, D-Vert, Meni-D, Ru-vert M

CLASSIFICATION(S):
Antiemetic, Antihistamine
Pregnancy Category B

INDICATIONS

▪ Management and prevention of motion sickness ▪ Used to treat labyrinthitis or Meniere's disease.

ACTION

▪ Has central anticholinergic, CNS depressant, and antihistaminic properties ▪ Decreases excitability of the middle ear labyrinth and depresses conduction in middle ear vestibular-cerebellar pathways. **Therapeutic Effects:** ▪ Decreased motion sickness ▪ Decreased vertigo due to vestibular pathology.

PHARMACOKINETICS

Absorption: Appears to be absorbed following oral administration.
Distribution: Distribution not known.
Metabolism and Excretion: Metabolism and excretion not known.
Half-life: 6 hr.

CONTRAINDICATIONS AND PRECAUTIONS

Contraindicated in: ▪ Hypersensitivity ▪ Pregnancy.
Use Cautiously in: ▪ Prostatic hypertrophy ▪ Narrow-angle glaucoma ▪ Children or lactation (safety not established).

ADVERSE REACTIONS AND SIDE EFFECTS*

CNS: drowsiness, fatigue.
EENT: blurred vision.
GI: dry mouth.

M

INTERACTIONS

Drug–Drug: ▪ Additive CNS depression with other **CNS depressants,** including **alcohol,** other **antihistamines, opioid analgesics,** and **sedative/ hypnotics** ▪ Additive anticholinergic effects with other **drugs possessing anticholinergic properties,** including **antihistamines, antidepressants, atropine, haloperidol, phenothiazines, quinidine,** and **disopyramide.**

ROUTE AND DOSAGE

Motion Sickness
▪ **PO (Adults):** 25–50 mg 1 hr before exposure, may repeat in 24 hr.

Labyrinthitis or Meniere's Disease
▪ **PO (Adults):** 25–100 mg/day in divided doses.

AVAILABILITY

▪ *Tablets:* 12.5 mg, 25 mg, 50 mg
▪ *Chewable tablets:* 25 mg ▪ *Capsules:* 25 mg.

TIME/ACTION PROFILE
(antihistaminic effects)

	ONSET	PEAK	DURATION
PO	1 hr	UK	8–24 hr

NURSING IMPLICATIONS

ASSESSMENT
▪ **General Info:** Assess patient for level of sedation following administration.
▪ **Motion Sickness:** Assess patient for nausea and vomiting prior to and 60 min following administration.
▪ **Vertigo:** Assess degree of vertigo periodically in patients receiving meclizine for labyrinthitis.
▪ **Lab Test Considerations:** May cause false-negative results in skin tests using allergen extracts. Discontinue meclizine 72 hr prior to testing.

POTENTIAL NURSING DIAGNOSES
▪ Injury, high risk for (side effects).
▪ Knowledge deficit related to medication regimen (patient/family teaching).

IMPLEMENTATION
▪ **PO:** Administer oral doses with food, water, or milk to minimize GI irritation. Chewable tablet may be chewed or swallowed whole.

PATIENT/FAMILY TEACHING
▪ **General Info:** Meclizine may cause drowsiness. Caution patient to avoid driving or other activities requiring alertness until response to the medication is known.
▫ Advise patient that frequent mouth rinses, good oral hygiene, and sugarless gum or candy may decrease dryness of mouth.
▫ Caution patient to avoid concurrent use of alcohol and other CNS depressants with this medication.
▪ **Motion Sickness:** When used as prophylaxis for motion sickness, advise patient to take medication at least 1 hr prior to exposure to conditions that may cause motion sickness.

EVALUATION
Effectiveness of therapy can be demonstrated by: ▪ Prevention and relief of symptoms in motion sickness ▪ Prevention and treatment of vertigo due to vestibular pathology.

MECLOFENAMATE
(me-kloe-**fen**-am-ate)
Meclofen, Meclomen

CLASSIFICATION(S):
Nonsteroidal anti-inflammatory agent, Nonopioid analgesic
Pregnancy Category UK

INDICATIONS

▪ Management of inflammatory disorders, including: ▫ Rheumatoid arthritis ▫ Osteoarthritis ▪ Management of mild to moderate pain, including dysmenorrhea ▪ Management of excessive menstrual blood loss.

ACTION

▪ Inhibits prostaglandin synthesis. **Therapeutic Effect:** ▪ Suppression of pain and inflammation.

PHARMACOKINETICS

Absorption: Well absorbed from the GI tract.
Distribution: Distribution not known.
Metabolism and Excretion: Mostly metabolized by the liver.
Half-life: 40 min–2 hr.

CONTRAINDICATIONS AND PRECAUTIONS

Contraindicated in: ▪ Hypersensitivity ▪ Cross-sensitivity may exist with other nonsteroidal anti-inflammatory agents, including aspirin ▪ Active GI bleeding or ulcer disease.
Use Cautiously in: ▪ Severe cardiovascular, renal, or hepatic disease ▪ History of ulcer disease ▪ Pregnancy, lactation, or children (safety not established).

ADVERSE REACTIONS AND SIDE EFFECTS*

CNS: <u>headache</u>, drowsiness, <u>dizziness</u>.
EENT: visual disturbances, tinnitus.
CV: edema.
GI: <u>nausea</u>, <u>dyspepsia</u>, <u>vomiting</u>, <u>diarrhea</u>, constipation, GI BLEEDING, discomfort, HEPATITIS, flatulence, anorexia, stomatitis.
GU: renal failure.
Derm: hives, itching.
Hemat: blood dyscrasias, prolonged bleeding time.
Misc: allergic reactions, including ANAPHYLAXIS and STEVENS-JOHNSON SYNDROME, drug-induced systemic lupus erythematosus-like syndrome.

INTERACTIONS

Drug–Drug: ▪ Concurrent use with **aspirin** may decrease meclofenamate blood levels and may decrease effectiveness ▪ May increase risk of bleeding with **anticoagulants, thrombolytics, cefamandole, cefoperazone, cefotetan, valproic acid,** or **plicamycin** ▪ Additive adverse GI side effects with **aspirin, alcohol, glucocorticoids, potassium supplements,** and other **nonsteroidal anti-inflammatory agents** ▪ **Probenecid** increases blood levels and may increase toxicity ▪ Chronic use with **acetamino-**

phen or **gold compounds** may increase the risk of adverse renal reactions ▪ May decrease the effectiveness of **antihypertensive agents** or **diuretics** ▪ May increase hypoglycemia from **oral hypoglycemic agents** or **insulin** ▪ Increased risk of hematologic adverse reactions with **antineoplastic agents** or **radiation therapy** ▪ May increase blood levels and toxicity of **lithium** or **methotrexate** ▪ Increased risk of nephrotoxicity with **cyclosporine.**

ROUTE AND DOSAGE

Anti-inflammatory
▪ **PO (Adults):** 200–300 mg/day in 3–4 divided doses (not to exceed 400 mg/day).

Analgesic
▪ **PO (Adults):** 50–100 mg q 4–6 hr.

Dysmenorrhea/Excessive Menstrual Blood Loss
▪ **PO (Adults):** 100 mg tid.

AVAILABILITY

▪ *Capsules:* 50 mg, 100 mg.

TIME/ACTION PROFILE (anti-inflammatory activity)

	ONSET	PEAK	DURATION
PO	days	2–3 wk	days

NURSING IMPLICATIONS

ASSESSMENT
▪ **General Info:** Patients who have asthma, aspirin-induced allergy, and nasal polyps are at increased risk for developing hypersensitivity reactions. Monitor for rhinitis, asthma, and urticaria.
▪ **Arthritis:** Assess pain and range of movement prior to and periodically during therapy.
▪ **Pain:** Assess location, duration, and intensity of pain prior to and 1 hr following administration.
▪ **Lab Test Considerations:** Serum BUN, creatinine, potassium, AST (SGOT), ALT (SGPT), LDH, and alkaline phosphatase concentrations may be increased.

M

*<u>Underlines</u> indicate most frequent; CAPITALS indicate life-threatening.

□ May cause decreased hemoglobin and hematocrit levels.

POTENTIAL NURSING DIAGNOSES
- Pain (indications).
- Physical mobility, impaired (indications).
- Knowledge deficit related to medication regimen (patient/family teaching).

IMPLEMENTATION
- PO: For rapid initial effect, administer 30 min before or 2 hr after meals. May be administered with food, milk, or antacids to decrease GI irritation. Food slows but does not reduce the extent of absorption.
- **Dysmenorrhea:** Administer as soon as possible after the onset of menses. Prophylactic treatment has not been shown to be effective.

PATIENT/FAMILY TEACHING
□ Advise patients to take this medication with a full glass of water and to remain in an upright position for 15–30 min after administration.
□ Instruct patient to take medication exactly as directed. If a dose is missed, take as soon as remembered but not if almost time for next dose. Do not double doses.
□ This medication may occasionally cause drowsiness or dizziness. Advise patient to avoid driving or other activities requiring alertness until response to the medication is known.
□ Caution patient to avoid the concurrent use of alcohol, aspirin, ibuprofen, acetaminophen, or other over-the-counter medications without consulting physician or pharmacist.
□ Instruct patient to notify physician if rash, itching, chills, fever, visual disturbances, tinnitus, weight gain, edema, black stools, persistent or severe diarrhea, or persistent headache occur.
□ Advise patient to inform physician or dentist of medication regimen prior to treatment or surgery.

EVALUATION
Effectiveness of therapy can be demonstrated by: ▪ Decrease in severity of

pain ▪ Improved joint mobility. Partial arthritic relief is usually seen within a few days, but maximum effectiveness may require 2–3 wk of continuous therapy. Patients who do not respond to one nonsteroidal anti-inflammatory agent may respond to another ▪ Decrease in menstrual blood loss.

MEDROXYPROGESTERONE
(me-**drox**-ee-proe-jess-te-rone)
Amen, Curretab, Cycrin, Depo-Provera, Provera

CLASSIFICATION(S):
Hormone (progestin), Antineoplastic agent (hormone), Contraceptive
Pregnancy Category UK

INDICATIONS
▪ Treatment of secondary amenorrhea and abnormal uterine bleeding caused by hormonal imbalance ▪ Treatment of advanced unresponsive endometrial or renal carcinoma ▪ Long-acting contraceptive. **Unlabeled Uses:** ▪ Obesity-hypoventilation (Pickwickian) syndrome ▪ Sleep apnea ▪ Hypersomnolence.

ACTION
▪ A synthetic form of progesterone—actions include secretory changes in the endometrium, increases in basal body temperature, histologic changes in vaginal epithelium, relaxation of uterine smooth muscle, mammary alveolar tissue growth, pituitary inhibition, and withdrawal bleeding in the presence of estrogen. **Therapeutic Effect:** ▪ Restoration of hormonal balance with control of uterine bleeding.

PHARMACOKINETICS
Absorption: UK.
Distribution: Enters breast milk.
Metabolism and Excretion: UK.
Half-life: UK.

CONTRAINDICATIONS AND PRECAUTIONS

Contraindicated in: ▪ Hypersensitivity ▪ Hypersensitivity to parabens (IM suspension only) ▪ Pregnancy ▪ Missed abortion ▪ Thromboembolic disease ▪ Cerebrovascular disease ▪ Severe liver disease ▪ Breast or genital cancer ▪ Porphyria.

Use Cautiously in: ▪ History of liver disease ▪ Renal disease ▪ Cardiovascular disease ▪ Seizure disorders ▪ Mental depression.

ADVERSE REACTIONS AND SIDE EFFECTS*

CNS: depression.
EENT: retinal thrombosis.
CV: THROMBOEMBOLISM, PULMONARY EMBOLISM, thrombophlebitis.
GI: gingival bleeding, hepatitis.
GU: cervical erosions.
Endo: breakthrough bleeding, spotting, amenorrhea, breast tenderness, galactorrhea, changes in menstrual flow.
Derm: rashes, melasma, chloasma.
F and E: edema.
Misc: weight gain, weight loss, allergic reactions, including ANAPHYLAXIS and ANGIOEDEMA.

INTERACTIONS

Drug-Drug: ▪ May decrease the effectiveness of **bromocriptine** when used concurrently for galactorrhea/amenorrhea ▪ Concurrent use with aminogluthimide may decrease contraceptive effectiveness.

ROUTE AND DOSAGE

Secondary Amenorrhea
▪ **PO (Adults):** 5–10 mg/day for 5–10 days, start at any time in cycle.

Functional Uterine Bleeding
▪ **PO (Adults):** 5–10 mg/day for 5–10 days, start on calculated day 16 or day 21 of menstrual cycle.

Renal or Endometrial Carcinoma
▪ **IM (Adults):** 400–1000 mg, may be repeated weekly; if improvement oc-

curs, attempt to decrease dosage to 400 mg monthly.

Contraceptive
▪ **IM (Adults):** 150 mg every 3 mo, to be started within 5 days of onset of normal menstrual period or within 5 days of delivery if not breast feeding. If breast feeding, initiate at 6 wk.

AVAILABILITY

▪ *Tablets:* 2.5 mg, 5 mg, 10 mg ▪ *Depot injection:* 100 mg/ml, 150 mg/ml, 400 mg/ml.

TIME/ACTION PROFILE (IM = antineoplastic effects)

	ONSET	PEAK	DURATION
PO	UK	UK	UK
IM	wks–mos	mo	UK

NURSING IMPLICATIONS

ASSESSMENT
▪ **General Info:** Monitor blood pressure periodically throughout therapy.
▢ Assess patient's usual menstrual history. Administration of drug may begin on any day of cycle in patients with amenorrhea and on day 16 or 21 of cycle in patients with dysfunctional bleeding.
▢ Monitor intake and output ratios and weekly weight. Report significant discrepancies or steady weight gain to physician.
▪ **Lab Test Considerations:** Monitor hepatic function prior to and periodically throughout therapy.
▢ May cause increased alkaline phosphatase, prothrombin, and factors VII, IX, and X levels. May decrease pregnanediol excretion concentrations.
▢ May cause increased serum concentrations of low-density lipoproteins and decreased concentrations of high-density lipoproteins.
▢ May alter thyroid hormone assays.

POTENTIAL NURSING DIAGNOSES
▪ Sexual dysfunction (indications).

M

- Tissue perfusion, altered (side effects).
- Knowledge deficit related to medication regimen (patient/family teaching).

IMPLEMENTATION

- **IM:** Shake vial before preparing IM dose. Administer deep IM.
- □ In patients with cancer, IM dose may initially be required weekly. Once stabilized, IM dose may be required only monthly.
- □ As a contraceptive, IM dose may need to be administered only every 3 mo.

PATIENT/FAMILY TEACHING

- **General Info:** Explain the dosage schedule. Instruct patient to take medication at the same time each day. If a dose is missed, patient should make up dose as soon as remembered, but do not double doses.
- □ Advise patients receiving medroxyprogesterone for menstrual dysfunction to anticipate withdrawal bleeding 3–7 days after discontinuing medication.
- □ Review patient package insert (PPI) with patient. Emphasize the importance of notifying physician if the following side effects occur: visual changes, sudden weakness, incoordination, difficulty with speech, headache, leg or calf pain, shortness of breath, chest pain, changes in vaginal bleeding pattern, yellow skin, swelling of extremities, depression, or rash. Patients receiving medroxyprogesterone for cancer may not receive PPI.
- □ Advise patient to keep a 1-mo supply of medroxyprogesterone available at all times.
- □ Instruct patient in correct method of monthly breast self-examination. Increased breast tenderness may occur.
- □ Advise patient that gingival bleeding may occur. Instruct patient to use good oral hygiene and to receive regular dental care and examinations.
- □ Instruct patient to notify physician if menstrual period is missed or if pregnancy is suspected. Patient should not attempt conception for 3 mo after discontinuing medication, in order to decrease risk to fetus.
- □ Medroxyprogesterone may cause melasma (brown patches of discoloration) on face when patient is exposed to sunlight. Advise patient to avoid sun exposure and to wear sunscreen or protective clothing when outdoors.
- □ Emphasize the importance of routine follow-up physical examinations, including blood pressure; breast, abdomen, and pelvic examinations; and PAP smears every 6–12 mo.

EVALUATION

Effectiveness of therapy can be demonstrated by: ▪ Regular menstrual periods ▪ Prevention of pregnancy ▪ Control of the spread of endometrial or renal cancer.

MEGESTROL
(me-**jess**-trole)
Megace

CLASSIFICATION(S):
Antineoplastic agent (hormone)
Pregnancy Category UK

INDICATIONS

▪ Palliative treatment of endometrial and breast carcinoma, either alone or with surgery or radiation ▪ Treatment of anorexia, weight loss, and cachexia associated with AIDS.

ACTION

▪ Antineoplastic effect may result from inhibition of pituitary function. **Therapeutic Effects:** ▪ Regression of tumor ▪ Increased appetite and weight gain in patients with AIDS.

PHARMACOKINETICS

Absorption: Well absorbed from the GI tract.
Distribution: Distribution not known.
Metabolism and Excretion: Completely metabolized by the liver.
Half-life: UK.

CONTRAINDICATIONS AND PRECAUTIONS

Contraindicated in: ▪ Hypersensitivity ▪ Pregnancy, missed abortion, or lactation ▪ Undiagnosed vaginal bleeding ▪ Severe liver disease.

Use Cautiously in: ▪ Diabetes ▪ Mental depression ▪ Renal disease ▪ History of thrombophlebitis ▪ Cardiovascular disease ▪ Seizure disorders.

ADVERSE REACTIONS AND SIDE EFFECTS*

GI: GI irritation.
Derm: alopecia.
Hemat: thrombophlebitis.
MS: carpal tunnel syndrome.

INTERACTIONS

Drug–Drug: ▪ None significant.

ROUTE AND DOSAGE

Breast Carcinoma
▪ **PO (Adults):** 40 mg 4 times daily.

Endometrial and Ovarian Carcinoma
▪ **PO (Adults):** 40–320 mg/day in divided doses.

Anorexia associated with AIDS
▪ **PO (Adults):** 40 mg qid.

AVAILABILITY

▪ *Tablets:* 20 mg, 40 mg ▪ *Oral suspension:* 40 mg/ml.

TIME/ACTION PROFILE
(antineoplastic activity)

	ONSET	PEAK	DURATION
PO	wk–mos	2 mo	UK

NURSING IMPLICATIONS

ASSESSMENT

▪ **General Info:** Assess patient for swelling, pain, or tenderness in legs. Notify physician if these signs of deep vein thrombophlebitis occur.
▪ **Anorexia:** Monitor weight, appetite, and nutritional intake in patients with AIDS.

POTENTIAL NURSING DIAGNOSES

▪ Knowledge deficit related to medication regimen (patient/family teaching).

IMPLEMENTATION

▪ **General Info:** Because of high dose, suspension is most convenient form for patients with AIDS.
▪ **PO:** May be administered with meals if GI irritation becomes a problem.

PATIENT/FAMILY TEACHING

☐ Instruct patient to take medication exactly as directed; do not skip or double up on missed doses. Missed doses may be taken as long as it is not right before next dose.
☐ Advise patient to report to physician any unusual vaginal bleeding.
☐ Advise patient that this medication may have teratogenic effects. Contraception should be used during therapy and for at least 4 mo after therapy is completed.
☐ Discuss with patient the possibility of hair loss. Explore methods of coping.

EVALUATION

Effectiveness of therapy can be demonstrated by: ▪ Slowing or arresting the spread of endometrial or breast malignancy. Therapeutic effects usually occur within 2 mo of initiating therapy ▪ Increased appetite and weight gain in patients with AIDS.

MELPHALAN
(mel-fa-lan)
Alkeran, L-PAM, L-Sarcolysin, Phenylalanine mustard

CLASSIFICATION(S):
Antineoplastic agent (alkylating agent)
Pregnancy Category UK

INDICATIONS

▪ Used alone or with other treatment modalities in the management of:
☐ Multiple myeloma ☐ Ovarian cancer.

M

Unlabeled Uses: ▪ Breast cancer ▪ Prostate cancer ▪ Testicular carcinoma ▪ Chronic myelogenous leukemia ▪ Osteogenic sarcoma.

ACTION

▪ Inhibits DNA and RNA synthesis by alkylation (cell cycle-phase nonspecific). **Therapeutic Effects:** ▪ Death of rapidly replicating cells, particularly malignant ones ▪ Also has immunosuppressive properties.

PHARMACOKINETICS

Absorption: Incompletely and variably absorbed following oral administration. **Distribution:** Rapidly distributed throughout total body water. **Metabolism and Excretion:** Rapidly metabolized in the bloodstream. Small amounts (10%) excreted unchanged by the kidneys. **Half-life:** 1.5 hr.

CONTRAINDICATIONS AND PRECAUTIONS

Contraindicated in: ▪ Hypersensitivity to melphelan or chlorambucil ▪ Pregnancy or lactation.
Use Cautiously in: ▪ Patients with childbearing potential ▪ Active infections ▪ Decreased bone marrow reserve ▪ Other chronic debilitating illnesses ▪ Impaired renal function (dose reduction recommended if BUN ≥30 mg/dl) ▪ Children (safety not established).

ADVERSE REACTIONS AND SIDE EFFECTS*

Resp: pulmonary fibrosis, bronchopulmonary dysplasia.
GI: nausea, vomiting, stomatitis, diarrhea.
GU: gonadal suppression.
Derm: rashes, pruritus, alopecia.
Endo: menstrual irregularities.
Hemat: leukopenia, thrombocytopenia, anemia.
Metab: hyperuricemia.
Misc: allergic reactions, including ANAPHYLAXIS.

INTERACTIONS

Drug–Drug: ▪ Additive bone marrow depression with other **antineoplastic agents** or **radiation therapy** ▪ May decrease antibody response to **live virus vaccines** and increase the risk of adverse reactions ▪ May increase the risk of pulmonary toxicity with **carmustine** ▪ Concurrent IV use with **cyclosporine** may increse the risk of renal failure ▪ Risk of enterocolitis may be increased with concurrent **nalidixic acid**.

ROUTE AND DOSAGE

Multiple Myeloma
▪ **PO (Adults):** 150 mcg/kg/day for 7 days, followed by 3-wk rest, then 50 mcg/kg/day maintenance dose or 100–150 mcg/kg/day for 2–3 wk followed by 2–4-wk rest, then 2–4 mg/day maintenance dose. Other regimens are used.

Ovarian Carcinoma
▪ **IV (Adults):** 16 mg/m^2 q 2 wk for 4 doses, then q 4 wk.
▪ **PO (Adults):** 0.2 mg/kg/day for 5 days given every 4–5 wk.

AVAILABILITY

▪ *Tablets:* 2 mg ▪ *Injection:* 50 mg.

TIME/ACTION PROFILE (effects on blood counts)

	ONSET	PEAK	DURATION
PO	5 days	2–3 wk	5–6 wk

NURSING IMPLICATIONS

ASSESSMENT
▫ Assess for fever, sore throat, and signs of infection. Notify physician if these symptoms occur.
▫ Assess for bleeding (bleeding gums; bruising; petechiae; guaiac stools, urine, and emesis). Avoid IM injections and rectal temperatures. Apply pressure to venipuncture sites for 10 min.
▫ May cause nausea and vomiting. Monitor intake and output, appetite,

---

*Underlines indicate most frequent; **CAPITALS** indicate life-threatening.

and nutritional intake. Confer with physician regarding prophylactic use of an antiemetic. Adjust diet as tolerated.

□ Monitor for symptoms of gout (increased uric acid, joint pain, edema). Encourage patient to drink at least 2 liters of fluid per day. Allopurinol may be given to decrease uric acid levels.

□ Anemia may occur. Monitor for increased fatigue and dyspnea.

□ Assess patient for allergy to chlorambucil. Patients may have cross-sensitivity.

■ **Lab Test Considerations:** Monitor CBC and differential weekly throughout therapy. The nadir of leukopenia occurs in 2–3 wk. Notify physician if leukocyte count is <3000/mm^3. The nadir of thrombocytopenia occurs in 2–3 wk. Notify physician if platelet count is <100,000/mm^3. Recovery of leukopenia and thrombocytopenia occurs in 5–6 wk.

□ Monitor liver function studies (AST [SGOT], ALT [SGPT], LDH, bilirubin) and renal function studies (BUN, creatinine) prior to and periodically throughout therapy to detect hepatotoxicity and nephrotoxicity.

□ May cause increased uric acid. Monitor periodically during therapy.

□ May cause elevated 5-hydroxyindole-acetic acid (5-HIAA) concentrations as a result of tumor breakdown.

POTENTIAL NURSING DIAGNOSES

■ Injury, high risk for (side effects).
■ Infection, high risk for (side effects).
■ Knowledge deficit related to medication regimen (patient/family teaching).

IMPLEMENTATION

■ **General Info:** Solution should be prepared in a biologic cabinet. Wear gloves, gown, and mask while handling medication. Discard IV equipment in specially designated container (see Appendix I).

□ If solution contacts skin or mucosa, immediately wash skin or mucosa with soap and water.

■ **PO:** May be ordered in divided doses or as a single daily dose.

■ **Intermittent Infusion:** Reconstitute with 10 ml of diluent supplied for a concentration of 5 mg/ml and shake vigorously until solution is clear. Dilute dose immediately with 0.9% NaCl for a concentration of ≤0.45 mg/ml. Administer within 60 min of reconstitution.

■ **Rate:** Administer over 15–20 min.

PATIENT/FAMILY TEACHING

□ Instruct patient to take melphalan exactly as directed, even if nausea and vomiting occur. If vomiting occurs shortly after dose is taken, consult physician. If a dose is missed, do not take at all.

□ Advise patient to notify physician if fever, chills, dyspnea, persistent cough, sore throat, signs of infection, bleeding gums, bruising, petechiae, or blood in urine, stool, or emesis occurs. Caution patient to avoid crowds and persons with known infections. Instruct patient to use soft toothbrush and electric razor. Caution patient not to drink alcoholic beverages or take products containing aspirin or ibuprofen.

□ Instruct patient to notify physician if rash, itching, joint pain, or swelling occurs.

□ Instruct patient to inspect oral mucosa for redness and ulceration. If ulceration occurs, advise patient to use sponge brush and to rinse mouth with water after eating and drinking. Consult physician if pain interferes with eating.

□ Advise patient that although fertility may be decreased, contraception should be used during melphalan therapy because of potential teratogenic effects on the fetus.

□ Instruct patient not to receive any vaccinations without advice of physician.

□ Emphasize need for periodic lab tests to monitor for side effects.

EVALUATION

Effectiveness of therapy can be demon-

M

strated by: ▪ Decrease in size and spread of malignant tissue.

MENOTROPINS
(men-oh-**troe**-pins)
HMG, Pergonal

CLASSIFICATION(S):
Hormone (gonadotropin)
Pregnancy Category UK

INDICATIONS
▪ Used in conjunction with chorionic gonadotropin to stimulate ovulation in patients with ovarian dysfunction and resultant infertility ▪ Used in conjunction with chorionic gonadotropin to stimulate spermatogenesis in male patients with hypogonadotropic hypogonadism and resultant infertility.

ACTION
▪ A purified form of human pituitary gonadotropins consisting of follicle-stimulating hormone (FSH) and luteinizing hormone (LH). In females, FSH causes growth and maturation of the ovarian follicle. LH causes ovulation and development of the corpeus luteum. In male patients, LH causes spermatogenesis. **Therapeutic Effect:** ▪ Ovulation or spermatogenesis, with resultant fertility.

PHARMACOKINETICS
Absorption: Appears to be well absorbed following IM administration.
Distribution: Distribution not known.
Metabolism and Excretion: 8% excreted unchanged in the urine.
Half-life: FSH—70 hr; LH—4 hr.

CONTRAINDICATIONS AND PRECAUTIONS
Contraindicated in: ▪ Vaginal bleeding of unknown cause ▪ Uterine fibroid tumors ▪ Ovarian cysts.
Use Cautiously in: ▪ Asthma ▪ Cardiovascular disease ▪ Seizure disorders ▪ Migraine headaches ▪ Polycystic ova-

ries ▪ Pituitary hypertrophy or tumor ▪ Severe renal impairment.

ADVERSE REACTIONS AND SIDE EFFECTS*
CV: thrombophlebitis, THROMBOEMBOLISM, PULMONARY EMBOLISM.
GI: bloating, abdominal pain, nausea, vomiting, diarrhea.
GU: pelvic pain, ovarian enlargement, multiple pregnancies.
Endo: gynecomastia (males).
F and E: edema.
Misc: fever.

INTERACTIONS
Drug–Drug: ▪ None significant.

ROUTE AND DOSAGE
Induction of Ovulation
▪ **IM (Adults):** 75 IU FSH and 75 IU LH daily for 7 or more days, followed by chorionic gonadotropin. Course may be repeated 2 more times. If pregnancy does not occur, dosage can be increased to 150 IU FSH and 150 IU LH.

Stimulation of Spermatogenesis
▪ **IM (Adults):** Following pretreatment with chorionic gonadotropins, 75 IU FSH and 75 IU LH 3 times weekly with chorionic gonadotropins; therapy is continued for at least 4 mo. If there is no evidence of increased spermatogenesis after 4 mo, dosage may be increased to 150 IU FSH and 150 IU LH with chorionic gonadotropins.

AVAILABILITY
▪ *Injection:* 75 IU FSH activity and 75 IU LH activity/2 ml, 150 IU FSH activity and 150 IU LH activity/2 ml.

TIME/ACTION PROFILE (females— peak = ovulation after chorionic gonadotropins; males—peak = increased spermatogenesis)

	ONSET	PEAK	DURATION
IM (females)	UK	18 hr	UK
IM (males)	UK	4 mo	UK

---

*Underlines indicate most frequent; **CAPITALS** indicate life-threatening.

NURSING IMPLICATIONS

ASSESSMENT

- **Female Infertility:** A gynecologic and endocrine examination to determine the cause of infertility should be completed prior to course of therapy. The patient's partner should also be evaluated for possible decreased fertility. An endometrial biopsy should be done in older patients to rule out the presence of endometrial carcinoma.
- **Male Infertility:** A urologic and endocrine examination to determine the cause of infertility should be completed prior to the course of therapy.
- **Lab Test Considerations:** In female infertility, cervical mucus volume and character, urinary excretion of estrogen or serum estrogen levels, and ultrasound may be used to determine whether follicular maturation has occurred.
- In male infertility, serum testosterone and sperm count and motility should be evaluated prior to and after course of therapy.

POTENTIAL NURSING DIAGNOSES

- Sexual dysfunction (indications).
- Body image disturbance (indications).
- Knowledge deficit related to medication regimen (patient/family teaching).

IMPLEMENTATION

- **General Info:** *Female infertility*—chorionic gonadotropin is usually administered 1 day following course of human menotropins. *Male infertility*—chorionic gonadotropin is administered alone until secondary sex characteristics develop, then administered concurrently with menotropins.
- **IM:** Reconstitute powder with 2-ml vial of 0.9% NaCl for injection provided by manufacturer. Use immediately; discard any unused portion of dose.

PATIENT/FAMILY TEACHING

- **General Info:** Instruct patient in correct technique for medication reconstitution and administration of IM injection. Ensure that patient understands medication administration schedule.
- **Female Infertility:** Instruct patient in the correct method for measuring basal body temperature. A record of the daily basal body temperature should be maintained prior to and throughout course of therapy.
- Reinforce physician's instructions regarding timing of sexual intercourse (usually daily beginning 1 day after administration of chorionic gonadotropin).
- Emphasize the importance of close monitoring by the physician throughout course of therapy (daily pelvic examinations are indicated after estrogen levels rise and for 2 wk after chorionic gonadotropin therapy).
- Inform patient prior to therapy of the potential for multiple births.
- Instruct patient to notify physician immediately if pregnancy is suspected (menses do not occur when expected and basal body temperature is biphasic).
- Advise patient to report to physician signs and symptoms of fluid retention (swelling of ankles and feet, weight gain), thromboembolic disorders (pain, swelling, tenderness in extremities, headache, chest pain, blurred vision), or abdominal or pelvic pain or bloating.
- **Male Infertility:** Inform patient that breast enlargement may occur. Physician should be consulted if this is problematic.

EVALUATION

Effectiveness of therapy can be demonstrated by: ■ Follicular maturation in females. Menotropin therapy is followed by human chorionic gonadotropin, which should lead to ovulation with subsequent pregnancy ■ Increased spermatogenesis after 4 mo of therapy in males.

M

MEPERIDINE
(me-**per**-i-deen)
Demerol, Pethadol, pethidine

CLASSIFICATION(S):
Opioid analgesic (agonist)
Schedule II
Pregnancy Category UK

INDICATIONS

▪ Used alone and in combination with nonopioid analgesics in the management of moderate to severe pain ▪ Has been used as: □ An adjunct to anesthesia □ An analgesic during labor □ Preoperative sedation.

ACTION

▪ Binds to opiate receptors in the CNS. Alters the perception of and response to painful stimuli, while producing generalized CNS depression. **Therapeutic Effect:** ▪ Decrease in severity of pain.

PHARMACOKINETICS

Absorption: Moderately absorbed (50%) from the GI tract. Well absorbed from IM sites. Oral and parenteral doses are not equal.
Distribution: Widely distributed. Crosses the placenta and enters breast milk.
Metabolism and Excretion: Mostly metabolized by the liver. Some converted to normeperidine, which has a long half-life (15–20 hr), and CNS stimulatory effects. 5% excreted unchanged by the kidneys.
Half-life: 3–8 hr (prolonged in impaired renal or hepatic function).

CONTRAINDICATIONS AND PRECAUTIONS

Contraindicated in: ▪ Hypersensitivity ▪ Hypersensitivity to bisulfites (some injectable products) ▪ Pregnancy or lactation (chronic use) ▪ Recent (14–21 days) MAO inhibitor therapy.
Use Cautiously in: ▪ Head trauma ▪ Increased intracranial pressure ▪ Severe renal, hepatic, or pulmonary disease ▪ Hypothyroidism ▪ Adrenal insufficiency ▪ Alcoholism ▪ Elderly or debilitated patients (dosage reduction suggested) ▪ Undiagnosed abdominal pain or prostatic hypertrophy ▪ Labor (respiratory depression may occur in the newborn) ▪ Patients with renal impairments, extensive burns ▪ Children (increased risk of seizures due to accumulation of normeperidine).

ADVERSE REACTIONS AND SIDE EFFECTS*

CNS: <u>sedation</u>, <u>confusion</u>, headache, euphoria, floating feeling, unusual dreams, hallucinations, dysphoria, SEIZURES.
EENT: miosis, diplopia, blurred vision.
CV: <u>hypotension</u>, bradycardia.
GI: <u>nausea</u>, <u>vomiting</u>, <u>constipation</u>.
GU: urinary retention.
Derm: sweating, flushing.
Resp: respiratory depression.
Misc: tolerance, physical dependence, psychological dependence.

INTERACTIONS

Drug–Drug: ▪ Use with extreme caution in patients receiving **MAO inhibitors** or **procarbazine** (may result in unpredictable fatal reaction—contraindicated within 14–21 days of MAO inhibitor therapy) ▪ Additive CNS depression with **alcohol, antihistamines,** and **sedative/hypnotics** ▪ Administration of **partial-antagonist opioid analgesics** may precipitate opioid withdrawal in physically dependent patients ▪ **Nalbuphine** or **pentazocine** may decrease analgesia.

ROUTE AND DOSAGE

Analgesia
▪ **PO, IM, SC (Adults):** 50–150 mg q 3–4 hr.
▪ **PO, IM, SC (Children):** 1–1.8 mg/kg q 3–4 hr (not to exceed 100 mg dose).
▪ **IV (Adults):** 15–35 mg/hr as a continuous infusion.

Analgesia During Labor
▪ **IM, SC (Adults):** 50–100 mg when

contractions become regular, may repeat q 1–3 hr.

Preoperative Sedation

- **IM, SC (Adults):** 50–100 mg 30–90 min before anesthesia.
- **IM, SC (Children):** 1–2.2 mg/kg 30–90 min before anesthesia (not to exceed adult dose).

AVAILABILITY

- **Tablets:** 50 mg, 100 mg ▪ **Syrup:** 50 mg/ml ▪ **Injection:** 10 mg/ml, 50 mg/ml, 75 mg/ml, 100 mg/ml ▪ **In combination with:** promethazine (Mepergan) and octropine. See Appendix A.

TIME/ACTION PROFILE (analgesia)

	ONSET	PEAK	DURATION
PO	15 min	60 min	2–4 hr
IM	10–15 min	30–50 min	2–4 hr
SC	10–15 min	40–60 min	2–4 hr
IV	immediate	5–7 min	2–4 hr

NURSING IMPLICATIONS

ASSESSMENT

- ▢ Assess blood pressure, pulse, and respiratory rate before and periodically during administration.
- ▢ Assess type, location, and intensity of pain prior to and 30–60 min following administration.
- ▢ Prolonged use may lead to physical and psychological dependence and tolerance. This should not prevent patient from receiving adequate analgesia. Most patients who receive meperidine for medical reasons do not develop psychological dependence. Progressively higher doses may be required to relieve pain with long-term therapy.
- ▢ Assess bowel function routinely. Increased intake of fluids and bulk, stool softeners, and laxatives may minimize constipating effects.
- ▢ Monitor patients on chronic or high-dose therapy for CNS stimulation (restlessness, irritability, seizures) due to accumulation of normeperidine metabolite.
- ▪ **Lab Test Considerations:** May increase plasma amylase and lipase concentrations.
- ▪ **Toxicity and Overdose:** If overdosage occurs, naloxone (Narcan) is the antidote. Monitor patient closely; dose may need to be repeated or naloxone infusion administered.

POTENTIAL NURSING DIAGNOSES

- ▪ Pain (indications).
- ▪ Sensory-perceptual alteration: visual, auditory (side effects).
- ▪ Injury, high risk for (side effects).

IMPLEMENTATION

- ▪ **General Info:** Explain therapeutic value of medication prior to administration to enhance the analgesic effect.
- ▢ Regularly administered doses may be more effective than prn administration. Analgesic is more effective if given before pain becomes severe.
- ▢ Coadministration with nonopioid analgesics may have additive analgesic effects and permit lower doses.
- ▢ Oral dose is <50% as effective as parenteral. When changing to oral administration, dose may need to be increased (see Appendix B).
- ▢ Medication should be discontinued gradually after long-term use to prevent withdrawal symptoms.
- ▢ May be administered via patient-controlled analgesia (PCA) pump.
- ▪ **PO:** Doses may be administered with food or milk to minimize GI irritation. Syrup should be diluted in half full glass of water.
- ▪ **IM:** IM is the preferred parenteral route for repeated doses. SC administration may cause local irritation.
- ▪ **Direct IV:** Dilute for IV administration to a concentration of 10 mg/ml with Sterile Water or 0.9% NaCl for Injection.
- ▪ **Rate:** Administer slowly, at a rate not to exceed 25 mg over 1 min. Rapid administration may lead to increased respiratory depression, hypotension, and circulatory collapse. Do not use IV without antidote available.
- ▪ **Continuous Infusion:** Dilute to a concentration of 1 mg/ml with D5W,

M

D10W, dextrose/saline combinations, dextrose/Ringer's or lactated Ringer's injection combinations, 0.45% NaCl, 0.9% NaCl, Ringer's or lactated Ringer's solution. Administer via infusion pump. Titrate according to patient needs.

- **Syringe Compatibility:** ▪ atropine ▪ benzquinamide ▪ butorphanol ▪ chlorpromazine ▪ cimetidine ▪ dimenhydrinate ▪ diphenhydramine ▪ droperidol ▪ fentanyl ▪ glycopyrrolate ▪ hydroxyzine ▪ metoclopramide ▪ midazolam ▪ pentazocine ▪ perphenazine ▪ prochlorperazine ▪ promazine ▪ promethazine ▪ ranitidine ▪ scopolamine.
- **Syringe Incompatibility:** ▪ heparin ▪ morphine ▪ pentobarbital.
- **Y-Site Compatibility:** ▪ amikacin ▪ ampicillin ▪ ampicillin/sulbactam ▪ bumetanide ▪ cefamandole ▪ cefazolin ▪ ceforanide ▪ cefotaxime ▪ cefotetan ▪ cefoxitin ▪ ceftizoxime ▪ ceftriaxone ▪ cefuroxime ▪ cephalothin ▪ cephapirin ▪ chloramphenicol ▪ clindamycin ▪ dexamethasone ▪ diphenhydramine ▪ dobutamine ▪ dopamine ▪ doxycycline ▪ droperidol ▪ erythromycin lactobionate ▪ famotidine ▪ fluconazole ▪ fludarabine ▪ gentamicin ▪ heparin ▪ hydrocortisone sodium succinate ▪ insulin ▪ kanamycin ▪ labetalol ▪ lidocaine ▪ methyldopate ▪ methylprednisolone ▪ metoclopramide ▪ metoprolol ▪ metronidazole ▪ mezlocillin ▪ minocycline ▪ ondansetron ▪ oxacillin ▪ oxytocin ▪ penicillin G potassium ▪ piperacillin ▪ potassium chloride ▪ propranolol ▪ ranitidine ▪ sargramostim ▪ ticarcillin ▪ ticarcillin/clavulanate ▪ tobramycin ▪ trimethoprim/sulfamethoxazole ▪ vancomycin ▪ verapamil.
- **Y-Site Incompatibility:** ▪ cefoperazone ▪ imipenem/cilastatin ▪ mezlocillin ▪ minocycline.
- **Additive Compatibility:** ▪ scopolamine ▪ triflupromazine.

PATIENT/FAMILY TEACHING
- ▢ Instruct patient on how and when to ask for pain medication.

- ▢ Medication may cause drowsiness or dizziness. Advise patient to call for assistance when ambulating or smoking. Caution patient to avoid driving or other activities requiring alertness until response to medication is known.
- ▢ Advise patient to make position changes slowly to minimize orthostatic hypotension.
- ▢ Instruct patient to avoid concurrent use of alcohol or other CNS depressants.
- ▢ Encourage patient to turn, cough, and breathe deeply every 2 hr to prevent atelectasis.

EVALUATION
Effectiveness of therapy can be demonstrated by: ▪ Decrease in severity of pain without a significant alteration in level of consciousness or respiratory status.

MEPROBAMATE
(me-proe-**ba**-mate)
{Apo-Meprobamate}, Equanil, {Meditran}, Meprospan, Miltown, Neuramate, {Novomepro}, Sedabamate, Trancot

CLASSIFICATION(S):
Sedative/hypnotic, Antianxiety agent
Schedule IV
Pregnancy Category UK

INDICATIONS
▪ Used as a sedative in the management of anxiety disorders.

ACTION
▪ Produces CNS depression by acting at multiple sites in the CNS. **Therapeutic Effect:** ▪ Sedation.

PHARMACOKINETICS
Absorption: Well absorbed following oral administration.
Distribution: Widely distributed. Crosses the placenta and enters breast milk in high concentrations.

{} = Available in Canada only.

Metabolism and Excretion: Metabolized by the liver.
Half-life: 6–16 hr.

CONTRAINDICATIONS AND PRECAUTIONS

Contraindicated in: ▪ Hypersensitivity ▪ Comatose patients or those with pre-existing CNS depression ▪ Uncontrolled severe pain ▪ Pregnancy and lactation.
Use Cautiously in: ▪ Hepatic dysfunction or severe renal impairment ▪ Patients who may be suicidal or who may have been addicted to drugs previously ▪ Elderly patients (dosage reduction suggested).

ADVERSE REACTIONS AND SIDE EFFECTS*

CNS: drowsiness, ataxia.
EENT: blurred vision.
CV: hypotension.
GI: anorexia, nausea, vomiting, diarrhea.
Derm: pruritus, urticaria, rashes.
Misc: hypersensitivity reactions, tolerance, psychological dependence, physical dependence.

INTERACTIONS

Drug–Drug: ▪ Additive CNS depression with other **CNS depressants,** including **alcohol, antihistamines, opioid analgesics,** and other **sedative/hypnotics.**

ROUTE AND DOSAGE

▪ **PO (Adults):** 1200–1600 mg/day in 2–4 divided doses or 800–1600 mg/day in 2 divided doses as extended-release capsules (maximum 2400 mg/day).
▪ **PO (Children 6–12 yr):** 100–200 mg 2–3 times daily or 200 mg as extended-release capsules bid. 600-mg tablet should not be used in children.

AVAILABILITY

▪ **Tablets:** 200 mg, 400 mg, 600 mg
▪ **Sustained-release capsules:** 200 mg, 400 mg ▪ **In combination with:** aspirin

(Equagesic, Equazine M, Meprogesic Q) and benactyzine (Deprol). See Appendix A.

TIME/ACTION PROFILE (sedation)

	ONSET	PEAK	DURATION
PO	<1 hr	1–3 hr	6–12 hr
PO-ER	UK	UK	12 hr

NURSING IMPLICATIONS

ASSESSMENT

▫ Assess degree and manifestations of anxiety prior to and periodically throughout therapy.
▫ Monitor blood pressure and pulse rate prior to and during initial therapy.
▫ Prolonged high-dose therapy may lead to psychological or physical dependence. Restrict amount of drug available to patient.
▪ **Lab Test Considerations:** Assess CBC periodically during course of therapy.
▫ May cause false elevations in urinary steroid concentrations.

POTENTIAL NURSING DIAGNOSES

▪ Anxiety (indications).
▪ Injury, high risk for (side effects).
▪ Knowledge deficit related to medication regimen (patient/family teaching).

IMPLEMENTATION

▪ **PO:** May be administered with food to minimize GI irritation.
▫ Do not crush, break, or chew sustained-release capsules.

PATIENT/FAMILY TEACHING

▫ Instruct patient to take medication exactly as directed. If a dose is missed, take if remembered within 1 hr; if remembered later, do not take. Do not double doses. Abrupt discontinuation may precipitate pre-existing symptoms or withdrawal reactions within 12–48 hr (vomiting, ataxia, muscle twitching, confusion, hallucinations, convulsions). Symptoms usually subside within 12–48 hr.
▫ Meprobamate may cause drowsiness

M

*Underlines indicate most frequent; **CAPITALS** indicate life-threatening.

and blurred vision. Caution patient to avoid driving and other activities requiring alertness until effects of drug are known.
□ Caution patient to make position changes slowly to minimize orthostatic hypotension.
□ Advise patient to avoid concurrent use of alcohol or other CNS depressants.
□ Instruct patient to notify physician if pregnancy is planned or suspected.
□ Advise patient to notify physician if skin rash, sore throat, or fever occurs.
□ Emphasize the importance of participation in psychotherapy if ordered by physician and follow-up examinations to evaluate progress.

EVALUATION
Effectiveness of therapy can be demonstrated by: ■ Decrease in the signs and symptoms of anxiety ■ Sedation. Medication's efficacy should be reassessed periodically. Therapy is generally of less than 4 mo duration.

MERCAPTOPURINE
(mer-kap-toe-**pyoor**-een)
6-MP, Purinethol

CLASSIFICATION(S):
Antineoplastic (antimetabolite)
Pregnancy Category D

INDICATIONS
■ Used in combination regimens in the treatment of leukemias. **Unlabeled Uses:** ■ Treatment of: □ Some lymphomas □ Polycythemia vera □ Inflammatory bowel disease □ Psoriatic arthritis.

ACTION
■ Disrupts DNA and RNA synthesis (cell cycle-S phase specific). **Therapeutic Effects:** ■ Death of rapidly proliferating cells, especially malignant ones ■ Also has immunosuppressant properties.

PHARMACOKINETICS
Absorption: Variably and incompletely (5–50%) absorbed after oral administration.
Distribution: Widely distributed throughout total body water.
Metabolism and Excretion: Mostly metabolized by liver. Some metabolism by the GI mucosa. Small amounts excreted unchanged by the kidneys.
Half-life: UK.

CONTRAINDICATIONS AND PRECAUTIONS
Contraindicated in: ■ Hypersensitivity ■ Pregnancy or lactation ■ Severe liver disease.
Use Cautiously in: ■ Patients with childbearing potential ■ Infections ■ Decreased bone marrow reserve ■ Other chronic debilitating illnesses.

ADVERSE REACTIONS AND SIDE EFFECTS*
CNS: weakness.
Derm: hyperpigmentation, rashes.
Endo: gonadal suppression.
GI: nausea, vomiting, anorexia, diarrhea, HEPATOTOXICITY.
GU: gonadal suppression.
Hemat: anemia, leukopenia, thrombocytopenia.
Metab: hyperuricemia.
Misc: fever.

INTERACTIONS
Drug–Drug: ■ **Allopurinol** decreases the metabolism and increases the potential of toxicity from mercaptopurine (reduce dosage of mercaptopurine to 25–33% of the usual dose) ■ Additive hepatotoxicity with other **hepatotoxic agents** ■ Additive bone marrow depression with **trimethoprim/sulfamethoxazole, other antineoplastic agents,** or **radiation therapy** ■ May alter the effect of **warfarin** (increase or decrease effectiveness) ■ Decreases the antibody response to **live virus vaccines** and increases the risk of adverse reactions.

---

*Underlines indicate most frequent; **CAPITALS** indicate life-threatening.

ROUTE AND DOSAGE

- **PO (Adults):** 1.5–2.5 mg/kg/day (up to 5 mg/kg/day) single dose or divided doses.
- **PO (Children):** 2.5 mg/kg/day (75 mg/m²) single dose or divided doses.

AVAILABILITY

- *Tablets:* 50 mg.

TIME/ACTION PROFILE (effects on blood counts)

	ONSET	PEAK	DURATION
PO	7–10 days	14 days	21 days

NURSING IMPLICATIONS

ASSESSMENT

- Monitor blood pressure, pulse, respiratory rate, and temperature frequently during course of therapy. Notify physician of significant changes.
- Assess for fever, chills, sore throat, and signs of infection. Notify physician if these symptoms occur.
- Assess for bleeding (bleeding gums; bruising; petechiae; guaiac stools, urine, and emesis). Avoid IM injections and rectal temperatures. Apply pressure to venipuncture sites for 10 min.
- Monitor intake and output ratios and inform physician if significant discrepancies occur. Encourage fluid intake of 2000–3000 ml/day. Physician may also order allopurinol and alkalinization of the urine to decrease serum uric acid levels and to help prevent urate stone formation.
- Assess patient's nutritional status. Anorexia and weight loss can be decreased by feeding light, frequent meals. Nausea and vomiting can be minimized by administering an antiemetic at least 1 hr prior to receiving medication.
- Anemia may occur. Monitor for increased fatigue and dyspnea.
- **Lab Test Considerations:** CBC and differential should be monitored prior to and weekly throughout course

of therapy. May cause leukopenia, thrombocytopenia, and anemia. Notify physician if a sudden drop in values occurs.

- Monitor hepatic function (serum transaminase, alkaline phosphatase, and bilirubin) weekly throughout therapy.
- May cause increased uric acid. Monitor levels periodically during therapy.
- Serum glucose and uric acid levels may show false increases when sequential multiple analyzer is used to determine values.

POTENTIAL NURSING DIAGNOSES

- Infection, high risk for (adverse reactions).
- Nutrition, altered: less than body requirements (adverse reactions).
- Knowledge deficit related to medication regimen (patient/family teaching).

IMPLEMENTATION

- **General Info:** The dose of mercaptopurine should be reduced to ⅓–¼ the usual dose in patients receiving concurrent allopurinol to decrease the risk of toxic effects of mercaptopurine.
- **PO:** Administer medication with meals. Tablets may be crushed if patient has difficulty swallowing.

PATIENT/FAMILY TEACHING

- Instruct patient to take medication exactly as directed. If a dose is missed, it should be omitted.
- Advise patient to notify physician if fever, chills, sore throat, signs of infection, bleeding gums, bruising, petechiae, or blood in urine, stool, or emesis occurs. Caution patient to avoid crowds and persons with known infections. Instruct patient to use soft toothbrush and electric razor. Patient should be cautioned not to drink alcoholic beverages or take products containing aspirin or ibuprofen, as these may precipitate gastric bleeding.
- Instruct patient to report yellowing of skin or eyes, dark-colored urine, clay-colored stools, abdominal pain, flank

M

or joint pain, or swelling of feet or legs to physician promptly.

▫ Advise patient that this medication may have teratogenic effects. Contraception should be used by both men and women during therapy and for at least 4 mo after therapy is concluded.

▫ Instruct patient not to receive any vaccinations without advice of physician.

▫ Emphasize the need for periodic lab tests to monitor for side effects.

EVALUATION

Effectiveness of therapy can be demonstrated by: ■ Remission of acute leukemia. Patients may receive subsequent doses if hematologic profiles are within normal ranges and patients do not demonstrate serious side effects.

MESALAMINE
(me-**sal**-a-meen)
Asacol, Pentasa, Rowasa,
{Salofalk}

CLASSIFICATION(S):
Gastrointestinal anti-inflammatory
Pregnancy Category B

INDICATIONS

■ Management of: ▫ Active ulcerative colitis ▫ Proctitis ▫ Proctosigmoiditis.

ACTION

■ Locally acting anti-inflammatory in the colon, where activity is probably due to inhibition of prostaglandin synthesis. **Therapeutic Effect:** ■ Reduction of symptoms of ulcerative colitis, proctitis, or proctosigmoiditis.

PHARMACOKINETICS

Absorption: 28% absorbed following oral administration. 10–30% absorbed from the colon, depending on retention time, following rectal administration.
Distribution: Distribution not known.

Metabolism and Excretion: Some metabolism occurs, site unknown. Mostly eliminated unchanged in the feces.
Half-life: PO—12 hr (range 2–15 hr); Rectal—0.5–1.5 hr.

CONTRAINDICATIONS AND PRECAUTIONS

Contraindicated in: ■ Hypersensitivity to mesalamine ■ Hypersensitivity to bisulfites (enema only) ■ Cross-sensitivity with sulfonamides or salicylates may exist.
Use Cautiously in: ■ Renal impairment ■ Previous hypersensitivity to sulfasalazine ■ Pregnancy, lactation, or children (safety not established).

ADVERSE REACTIONS AND SIDE EFFECTS*

CV: pericarditis.
CNS: malaise, <u>headache</u>, weakness, dizziness.
EENT: pharyngitis.
GI: eructation (PO), flatulence, nausea, diarrhea, vomiting.
GU: renal failure, interstitial nephritis.
Derm: hair loss, rash.
Local: anal irritation (enema, suppository).
MS: back pain.
Misc: acute intolerance syndrome, ANAPHYLAXIS, fever.

INTERACTIONS

Drug–Drug: ■ None significant.

ROUTE AND DOSAGE

■ **PO (Adults):** 800 mg 3 times daily for 6 wk as delayed-release tablets or 1 g 4 times daily as controlled-release capsules.
■ **Rect (Adults):** 4-g enema (60 ml) at bedtime, retained for 8 hr for 3–6 wk or 500-mg suppository 2–3 times daily.

AVAILABILITY

■ *Delayed-release tablets:* 400 mg ■ *Suppositories:* 500 mg ■ *Rectal suspension:* 4 g/60 ml.

{} = Available in Canada only.
*<u>Underlines</u> indicate most frequent; **CAPITALS** indicate life-threatening.

TIME/ACTION PROFILE (signs of improvement)

	ONSET	PEAK	DURATION
Rect	3–21 days	UK	UK
PO	UK	UK	UK

NURSING IMPLICATIONS

ASSESSMENT

□ Assess abdominal pain and frequency, quantity, and consistency of stools at the beginning of and throughout therapy.

□ Assess patient for allergy to sulfonamides and salicylates. Patients allergic to sulfasalazine may take mesalamine without difficulty, but therapy should be discontinued if rash or fever occurs.

- **Lab Test Considerations:** Monitor urinalysis, BUN, and serum creatinine closely for signs of renal toxicity.

POTENTIAL NURSING DIAGNOSES

- Pain (indications).
- Diarrhea (indications).
- Knowledge deficit related to medication regimen (patient/family teaching).

IMPLEMENTATION

- **PO:** Tablets should be swallowed whole; do not break the outer coating, which is designed to remain intact to protect the active ingredient. Intact or partially intact tablets may occasionally be found in the stool. If this occurs repeatedly, advise patient to notify physician.
- **Rect:** Avoid excessive handling of suppository. Remove foil wrapper and insert pointed end first into rectum with gentle pressure. Suppository should be retained for 1–3 hr or more for maximum benefit. Administer 60-ml retention enema once daily at bedtime. Solution should be retained for approximately 8 hr.
- □ Prior to administration, shake bottle well and remove the protective cap. Have patient lie on left side with the lower leg extended and the upper leg

flexed for support or place the patient in knee-chest position. Gently insert the applicator tip into the rectum, pointing toward the umbilicus. Squeeze the bottle steadily to discharge most of the preparation.

PATIENT/FAMILY TEACHING

□ Instruct patient on the correct method of administration for mesalamine. Advise patient to take medication as directed, even if feeling better.

□ Advise patient to notify physician if hives, itching, wheezing, rash, or fever occurs.

□ Instruct patient to notify physician if symptoms worsen or do not improve. If symptoms of acute intolerance (cramping, acute abdominal pain, bloody diarrhea, fever, headache, rash) occur, discontinue therapy and notify physician immediately.

□ Inform patient that proctoscopy and sigmoidoscopy may be required periodically during treatment to determine response.

EVALUATION

Clinical response can be evaluated by:
- Decrease in diarrhea and abdominal pain □ Return to normal bowel pattern. Effects may be seen within 3–21 days. The usual course of therapy is 3–6 wk.

MESNA
(**mes**-na)
Mesnex, {Urometexan}

CLASSIFICATION(S):
Antidote (ifosfamide detoxifying agent)
Pregnancy Category B

INDICATIONS

- Prevention of ifosfamide-induced hemorrhagic cystitis. **Unlabeled Use:**
- May also prevent hemorrhagic cystitis from cyclophosphamide.

ACTION

- Binds to the toxic metabolites of ifos-

M

famide in the kidneys, thereby preventing hemorrhagic cystitis.

PHARMACOKINETICS

Absorption: Administered IV only, resulting in complete bioavailability.
Distribution: Distribution not known.
Metabolism and Excretion: Rapidly converted to mesna disulfide, then converted back to mesna in the kidneys, where it is able to bind to the toxic metabolites of ifosfamide.
Half-life: Mesna—0.36 hr; mesna disulfide—1.17 hr.

CONTRAINDICATIONS AND PRECAUTIONS

Contraindicated in: ▪ Hypersensitivity to mesna or other thiol (rubber) compounds.
Use Cautiously in: ▪ Pregnancy or lactation (safety not established).

ADVERSE REACTIONS AND SIDE EFFECTS*

GI: nausea, vomiting, diarrhea, unpleasant taste.

INTERACTIONS

Drug–Drug: ▪ None significant.

ROUTE AND DOSAGE

▪ **IV (Adults):** Give a dose of mesna equal to 20% of the ifosfamide dose at the same time as ifosfamide and 4 and 8 hr later.

AVAILABILITY

▪ *Injection:* 100 mg/ml.

TIME/ACTION PROFILE (detoxifying action)

	ONSET	PEAK	DURATION
IV	rapid	UK	4 hr

NURSING IMPLICATIONS

ASSESSMENT

▫ Monitor for development of hemorrhagic cystitis in patients receiving ifosfamide.
▪ **Lab Test Considerations:** Causes a false-positive result when testing urinary ketones.

POTENTIAL NURSING DIAGNOSES

▪ Knowledge deficit related to medication regimen (patient/family teaching).

IMPLEMENTATION

▪ **General Info:** Initial bolus is to be given at time of ifosfamide administration, second dose is given 4 hr later, third dose is given 8 hr after initial dose. This schedule must be repeated with each subsequent dose of ifosfamide.
▪ **Direct IV:** Available in 2-, 4-, and 10-ml ampules, each containing a concentration of 100 mg/ml. Dilute in 8 ml, 16 ml, or 50 ml, respectively, of D5W, 0.9% NaCl, D5/0.9% NaCl, or lactated Ringer's solution, to yield a final concentration of 20 mg/ml. Refrigerate to store. Use within 6 hr.
▪ **Syringe Compatibility:** ▪ ifosfamide.
▪ **Y-Site Compatibility:** ▪ fludarabine ▪ ondansetron ▪ sargramostim.
▪ **Additive Compatibility:** ▪ hydroxyzine ▪ ifosfamide.
▪ **Additive Incompatibility:** ▪ carboplatin ▪ cisplatin.

PATIENT/FAMILY TEACHING

▫ Inform patient that unpleasant taste may occur during administration.
▫ Advise patient to notify physician if nausea, vomiting, or diarrhea persists or is severe.

EVALUATION

Effectiveness of therapy can be demonstrated by: ▪ Prevention of hemorrhagic cystitis associated with ifosfamide therapy.

MESORIDAZINE
(mez-oh-**rid**-a-zeen)
Serentil

CLASSIFICATION(S):
Antipsychotic (phenothiazine)
Pregnancy Category UK

*Underlines indicate most frequent; **CAPITALS** indicate life-threatening.

INDICATIONS
- Treatment of acute and chronic psychoses.

ACTION
- Alters the effects of dopamine in the CNS ▪ Possesses anticholinergic and alpha-adrenergic blocking activity. **Therapeutic Effect:** ▪ Diminished signs and symptoms of psychoses.

PHARMACOKINETICS
Absorption: Appears to be well absorbed following oral administration. **Distribution:** Widely distributed. Crosses the placenta. Crosses the blood–brain barrier and probably enters breast milk. **Metabolism and Excretion:** Mostly metabolized by the liver. **Half-life:** UK.

CONTRAINDICATIONS AND PRECAUTIONS
Contraindicated in: ▪ Hypersensitivity ▪ Cross-sensitivity with other phenothiazines may exist ▪ Narrow-angle glaucoma ▪ Bone marrow depression ▪ Severe liver or cardiovascular disease ▪ Known alcohol intolerance (oral concentrate only).
Use Cautiously in: ▪ Elderly, emaciated, or debilitated patients (initial dosage reduction may be necessary) ▪ Pregnancy or lactation (safety not established) ▪ Diabetes mellitus ▪ Respiratory disease ▪ Prostatic hypertrophy ▪ CNS tumors ▪ Epilepsy ▪ Intestinal obstruction.

ADVERSE REACTIONS AND SIDE EFFECTS*
CNS: sedation, extrapyramidal reactions, tardive dyskinesia, NEUROLEPTIC MALIGNANT SYNDROME.
EENT: dry eyes, blurred vision, lens opacities.
CV: hypotension, tachycardia.
GI: constipation, dry mouth, ileus, anorexia, hepatitis.
GU: urinary retention.

Derm: rashes, photosensitivity, pigment changes.
Endo: galactorrhea.
Hemat: AGRANULOCYTOSIS, leukopenia.
Misc: allergic reactions, hyperthermia.

INTERACTIONS
Drug–Drug: ▪ Additive hypotension with acute ingestion of **alcohol, antihypertensive agents,** or **nitrates** ▪ Additive CNS depression with other **CNS depressants,** including **alcohol, antidepressants, antihistamines, MAO inhibitors, opioid analgesics, sedative/hypnotics,** or **general anesthetics** ▪ Concurrent use with **lithium** may produce any of the following—acute encephalopathy, decreased mesoridazine absorption, increased excretion of lithium, increased risk of extrapyramidal reactions, or masking of the early signs of lithium toxicity ▪ **Antacids** or **adsorbent antidiarrheals (kaolin/attapulgite)** may decrease absorption ▪ Increased risk of agranulocytoses with **antithyroid drugs** ▪ May decrease antiparkinson activity of **levodopa** and **bromocriptine** ▪ Decreases vasopressor response to **epinephrine** and **norepinephrine** ▪ Decreases antihypertensive effect of **guanethidine** ▪ Concurrent use with **beta blockers** may result in inhibition of metabolism of one or both drugs producing an increased response ▪ Increased risk of anticholinergic effects with other **agents having anticholinergic properties,** including **antihistamines, tricyclic antidepressants, quinidine,** or **disopyramide.**

ROUTE AND DOSAGE
- **PO (Adults and Children >12 yr):** 30–150 mg/day in 2–3 divided doses.
- **IM (Adults):** 25 mg, may be repeated in 30 min–1 hr if needed and tolerated (range 25–200 mg/day).

AVAILABILITY
- **Tablets:** 10 mg, 25 mg, 50 mg, 100 mg
- **Oral concentrate:** 25 mg/ml ▪ **Injection:** 25 mg/ml.

M

---

*Underlines indicate most frequent; **CAPITALS** indicate life-threatening.

TIME/ACTION PROFILE

	ONSET	PEAK	DURATION
PO	UK	UK	UK

NURSING IMPLICATIONS

ASSESSMENT

□ Monitor patient's mental status (orientation to reality, anxiety, and behavior) prior to and periodically throughout therapy.

□ Monitor blood pressure (sitting, standing, lying), pulse, and respiratory rate prior to and frequently during the period of dosage adjustment.

□ Observe patient carefully when administering oral medication to ensure medication is actually taken and not hoarded.

□ Assess patient for level of sedation following administration.

□ Monitor patient for onset of extrapyramidal side effects (akathisia—restlessness, dystonia—muscle spasms and twisting motions, or pseudoparkinsonism—mask facies, rigidity, tremors, drooling, shuffling gait, dysphagia). Risk of extrapyramidal effects is lower with mesoridazine than with most phenothiazines. Notify physician if these symptoms occur, as reduction in dosage or discontinuation of medication may be necessary. Physician may also order trihexyphenidyl or diphenhydramine to control these symptoms.

□ Monitor for tardive dyskinesia (rhythmic movement of mouth, face, and extremities). Notify physician immediately if these symptoms occur, as these side effects may be irreversible.

□ Monitor for development of neuroleptic malignant syndrome (fever, respiratory distress, tachycardia, convulsions, diaphoresis, hypertension or hypotension, pallor, tiredness). Notify physician immediately if these symptoms occur.

■ **Lab Test Considerations:** Monitor CBC and differential prior to and periodically throughout therapy. May cause blood dyscrasias.

□ Monitor liver function studies prior to and periodically during therapy.

□ May cause increased serum prolactin levels.

POTENTIAL NURSING DIAGNOSES

■ Thought processes, altered (indications).

■ Injury, high risk for (side effects).

■ Knowledge deficit related to medication regimen (patient/family teaching).

IMPLEMENTATION

■ **General Info:** To prevent contact dermatitis, avoid getting liquid preparations on hands, and wash hands thoroughly if spillage occurs.

□ Phenothiazines should be discontinued 48 hr before and not resumed for 24 hr following metrizamide myelography, because they lower the seizure threshold.

■ **PO:** Administer capsules with food or milk to decrease gastric irritation.

□ Dilute oral solution with 120 ml of acidified water, distilled water, or orange or grapefruit juice. Measure dose with provided dropper. Use just after diluting.

■ **IM:** Should be administered deep into well-developed muscle. Do not use if precipitate is present; solution may be slightly yellow.

PATIENT/FAMILY TEACHING

□ Instruct patient receiving parenteral mesoridazine to remain supine for 30 min after administration. Position changes should be made slowly to prevent orthostatic hypotension.

□ Instruct patient on need to take medication exactly as directed. If a dose is missed, medication should be taken as soon as remembered unless almost time for next dose. Patients on long-term high-dose therapy may need to discontinue medication gradually to avoid withdrawal symptoms (dyskinesia, tremors, dizziness, nausea, and vomiting).

□ Instruct patient receiving oral solution on correct method of measuring dose with provided dropper.

□ Drowsiness may occur. Caution patient to avoid driving or other activities requiring alertness until response to medication is known.

□ Advise patient that good oral hygiene, frequent rinsing of mouth with water, and sugarless gum or candy may help relieve dryness of mouth. Physician or dentist should be notified if dryness persists beyond 2 wk.

□ Caution patient to use sunscreen and protective clothing to prevent photosensitivity reactions.

□ Caution patient to avoid concurrent use of alcohol, other CNS depressants, and over-the-counter medications without consulting physician or pharmacist.

□ Instruct patient to notify physician promptly if sore throat, fever, unusual bleeding or bruising, skin rashes, weakness, tremors, visual disturbances, dark-colored urine, or clay-colored stools are noted.

□ Advise patient to notify physician or dentist of medication regimen prior to treatment or surgery.

□ Inform patient of possibility of extrapyramidal symptoms and tardive dyskinesia. Caution patient to report these symptoms to physician immediately.

□ Caution patient to avoid exercising in hot weather and taking very hot baths or showers.

□ Inform patient that increasing bulk and fluids in the diet and exercising regularly may minimize the constipating effects of this medication.

□ Advise patient of need for continued medical follow-up for psychotherapy, eye examinations, and laboratory tests.

EVALUATION

Effectiveness of therapy can be demonstrated by: ▪ Decreased psychotic ideation.

METAPROTERENOL
(met-a-pro-**ter**-e-nole)
Alupent, Arm-a-Med Metaproterenol, Metaprel

CLASSIFICATION(S):
Bronchodilator (beta-adrenergic agonist)
Pregnancy Category C

INDICATIONS

▪ Used as a bronchodilator in reversible airway obstruction due to asthma or COPD.

ACTION

▪ A beta-adrenergic agonist that results in the accumulation of cyclic adenosine monophosphate (cAMP) ▪ Results of increased levels of cAMP at beta-adrenergic receptors include bronchodilation, CNS and cardiac stimulation, diuresis, and gastric acid secretion. Relatively selective for beta$_2$ (pulmonary) receptors. **Therapeutic Effect:** ▪ Bronchodilation.

PHARMACOKINETICS

Absorption: Well absorbed following oral administration, but rapidly undergoes extensive metabolism.
Distribution: Distribution not known.
Metabolism and Excretion: Extensively metabolized by the liver and other tissues.
Half-life: UK.

CONTRAINDICATIONS AND PRECAUTIONS

Contraindicated in: ▪ Hypersensitivity to adrenergic amines or any ingredients that may be bisulfites in preparations (fluorocarbons, parabens, edetate sodium and benzalkonium chloride).
Use Cautiously in: ▪ Elderly patients (more susceptible to adverse reactions; dosage reduction suggested) ▪ Pregnancy or lactation (safety not established) ▪ Cardiac disease ▪ Hypertension ▪ Hyperthyroidism ▪ Diabetes

M

mellitus ▪ Glaucoma ▪ Excessive use of inhalers (may lead to tolerance and paradoxical bronchospasm).

ADVERSE REACTIONS AND SIDE EFFECTS*

CNS: <u>nervousness</u>, <u>restlessness</u>, insomnia, <u>tremor</u>, headache.
CV: hypertension, arrhythmias, angina.
Endo: hyperglycemia.
GI: nausea, vomiting.

INTERACTIONS

Drug–Drug: ▪ Additive adrenergic effects with other **adrenergic amines (sympathomimetics)** ▪ Use with **MAO inhibitors** may lead to hypertensive crisis ▪ Beta-adrenergic blockers may block therapeutic effect.

ROUTE AND DOSAGE

▪ **PO (Adults and Children >9 yr and >27 kg):** 20 mg 3–4 times daily.
▪ **PO (Children 6–9 yr and <27 kg):** 10 mg 3–4 times daily.
▪ **Inhalation (Adults and Children >12 yr):** *Metered-dose inhaler—* 2–3 inhalations q 3–4 hr (not to exceed 12 inhalations/day. *Hand-bulb nebulizer—*5–15 inhalations of undiluted 5% solution 3–4 times daily (not to exceed q 4 hr use). *IPPB—*0.2– 0.3 ml of 5% solution or 2.5 ml of 0.4% or 0.6% solution for nebulization 3–4 times daily (not to exceed q 4 hr use).

AVAILABILITY

▪ *Tablets:* 10 mg, 20 mg ▪ *Syrup:* 10 mg/5 ml ▪ *Aerosol for inhalation:* 0.65 mg/inhalation in 5-ml inhaler (100 inhalations) or 10-ml inhaler (200 inhalations) ▪ *Solution for inhalation:* 0.4%, 0.6%, 5%.

TIME/ACTION PROFILE
(bronchodilation)

	ONSET	PEAK	DURATION
PO	15 min	1 hr	4 hr
Inhaln	1–5 min	1 hr	3–4 hr

NURSING IMPLICATIONS

ASSESSMENT

□ Assess blood pressure, pulse, respiratory pattern, lung sounds, and character of secretions prior to and after treatment.
□ Observe patient for appearance of drug tolerance and rebound bronchospasm.
▪ **Lab Test Considerations:** May cause decreased serum potassium concentrations.

POTENTIAL NURSING DIAGNOSES

▪ Airway clearance, ineffective (indications).
▪ Knowledge deficit related to medication regimen (patient/family teaching).
▪ Noncompliance (patient/family teaching).

IMPLEMENTATION

▪ **PO:** Administer oral preparations with food if GI irritation becomes a problem.
▪ **Inhalation:** For IPPB administration, dilute each dose in 2.5 ml of 0.9% NaCl. Do not use if solution is brown or darker than slightly yellow, pinkish, or if it contains a precipitate.

PATIENT/FAMILY TEACHING

▪ **General Info:** Instruct patient to take medication exactly as directed. Taking more often than prescribed may lead to paradoxical bronchospasm. If a dose is missed, take right away if remembered within 1 hr; do not take if remembered later. Do not double doses.
□ Advise patient to maintain adequate fluid intake to help liquify tenacious secretions.
□ Advise patient to consult physician if respiratory symptoms are not relieved or worsen after treatment. Patient should also inform physician if chest pain, headache, severe dizziness, palpitations, nervousness, or weakness occurs.
▪ **Inhalation:** Instruct patient on proper use of inhaler. See Appendix H.

*<u>Underlines</u> indicate most frequent; **CAPITALS** indicate life-threatening.

□ Patient taking inhalant glucocorticoids concurrently with metaproterenol should be advised to use metaproterenol first and to allow 5 min to elapse between using the 2 aerosols, unless directed by physician.

EVALUATION

Effectiveness of therapy can be demonstrated by: ▪ Decrease in bronchospasm □ Increased ease of breathing.

METHADONE
(meth-a-done)
Dolophine, Methadose

CLASSIFICATION(S):
Opioid analgesic (agonist)
Schedule II
Pregnancy Category UK

INDICATIONS

▪ Used alone and in combination with nonopioid analgesics (acetaminophen or aspirin) in the management of severe pain ▪ Replaces heroin or other opioid analgesics in detoxification/maintenance programs.

ACTION

▪ Binds to opiate receptors in the CNS ▪ Alters the perception of and response to painful stimuli, while producing generalized CNS depression. Therapeutic Effects: ▪ Decrease in severity of pain ▪ Heroin detoxification/maintenance.

PHARMACOKINETICS

Absorption: Well absorbed from the GI tract and IM and SC sites.
Distribution: Widely distributed. Crosses the placenta and enters breast milk.
Metabolism and Excretion: Mostly metabolized by the liver.
Half-life: 25 hr.

CONTRAINDICATIONS AND PRECAUTIONS

Contraindicated in: ▪ Hypersensitivity

▪ Hypersensitivity to chlorobutanol (injection only) ▪ Known alcohol intolerance (some oral solutions) ▪ Pregnancy or lactation (chronic use).
Use Cautiously in: ▪ Head trauma ▪ Increased intracranial pressure ▪ Severe renal, hepatic, or pulmonary disease ▪ Hypothyroidism ▪ Adrenal insufficiency ▪ Alcoholism ▪ Elderly or debilitated patients (dosage reduction suggested) ▪ Undiagnosed abdominal pain ▪ Prostatic hypertrophy.

ADVERSE REACTIONS AND SIDE EFFECTS*

CNS: sedation, confusion, headache, euphoria, floating feeling, unusual dreams, hallucinations, dysphoria, dizziness.
EENT: miosis, diplopia, blurred vision.
Resp: respiratory depression.
CV: hypotension, bradycardia.
GI: nausea, vomiting, constipation.
GU: urinary retention.
Derm: sweating, flushing.
Misc: tolerance, physical dependence, psychological dependence.

INTERACTIONS

Drug–Drug: ▪ Use with extreme caution in patients receiving MAO inhibitors (may result in severe, unpredictable reactions—reduce initial dose of methadone to 25% of usual dose) ▪ Additive CNS depression with alcohol, antihistamines, and sedative/hypnotics ▪ Administration of partial-antagonist opioid analgesics may precipitate opioid withdrawal in physically dependent patients ▪ Nalbuphine or pentazocine may decrease analgesia.

ROUTE AND DOSAGE

Larger doses may be required for analgesics during chronic therapy.

Analgesia
▪ PO, IM, SC (Adults): 2.5–10 mg q 3–4 hr, up to 5–20 mg q 6–12 hr.

Detoxification
▪ PO (Adults): 15–40 mg/day initially for 2–3 days, then decreased every 2 days.

M

*Underlines indicate most frequent; CAPITALS indicate life-threatening.

Maintenance

▪ **PO (Adults):** 20–120 mg/day.

AVAILABILITY

▪ *Tablets:* 5 mg, 10 mg ▪ *Dispensible tablets:* 40 mg ▪ *Oral solution:* 5 mg/5 ml, 10 mg/5 ml ▪ *Oral concentrate:* 10 mg/ml.

TIME/ACTION PROFILE (analgesic effect)

	ONSET	PEAK	DURATION
PO	30–60 min	90–120 min	4–12 hr
IM	10–20 min	60–120 min	4–6 hr
SC	10–20 min	60–120 min	4–6 hr

NURSING IMPLICATIONS

ASSESSMENT

□ Assess type, location, and intensity of pain prior to and 60 min after administration. Cumulative effects of this medication may require periodic dosage adjustments.

□ Assess blood pressure, pulse, and respiratory rate before and periodically during administration.

□ Prolonged use may lead to physical and psychological dependence and tolerance. This should not prevent patient from receiving adequate analgesia. Most patients who receive methadone for medical reasons do not develop psychological dependence.

□ Assess bowel function routinely. Increased intake of fluids and bulk, stool softeners, and laxatives may minimize constipating effects.

▪ **Lab Test Considerations:** May increase plasma amylase and lipase levels.

▪ **Toxicity and Overdose:** If overdosage occurs, naloxone (Narcan) is the antidote.

POTENTIAL NURSING DIAGNOSES

▪ Pain (indications).

▪ Sensory-perceptual alteration: visual, auditory (side effects).

▪ Injury, high risk for (side effects).

IMPLEMENTATION

▪ **General Info:** Explain therapeutic value of medication prior to administration to enhance the analgesic effect.

□ Regularly administered doses may be more effective than prn administration. Analgesic is more effective if administered before pain becomes severe.

□ Coadministration with nonopioid analgesics may have additive analgesic effects and may permit lower doses.

□ Medication should be discontinued gradually after long-term use to prevent withdrawal symptoms.

□ Diskette (dispersible tablets) are to be dissolved and used for detoxification and maintenance treatment only.

▪ **PO:** Doses may be administered with food or milk to minimize GI irritation.

□ For patients in chronic severe pain the oral solution containing 5 or 10 mg/5 ml is recommended on a fixed dosage schedule.

□ Dilute each dose of 10 mg/ml oral concentrate with at least 30 ml of water or other liquid prior to administration.

▪ **IM, SC:** IM is the preferred parenteral route for repeated doses. SC administration may cause tissue irritation.

PATIENT/FAMILY TEACHING

□ Instruct patient on how and when to ask for pain medication.

□ Methadone may cause drowsiness or dizziness. Advise patient to call for assistance when ambulating or smoking and to avoid driving or other activities requiring alertness until response to medication is known.

□ Advise patient to make position changes slowly to minimize orthostatic hypotension.

□ Caution patient to avoid concurrent use of alcohol or other CNS depressants with this medication.

□ Encourage patient to turn, cough, and breathe deeply every 2 hr to prevent atelectasis.

EVALUATION

Effectiveness of therapy can be demonstrated by: ▪ Decrease in severity of pain without a significant alteration in level of consciousness or respiratory status ▪ Prevention of withdrawal symptoms in detoxification from heroin and other opioid analgesics.

METHICILLIN
(meth-i-sill-in)
Staphcillin

CLASSIFICATION(S):
Anti-infective (penicillinase-resistant penicillin)
Pregnancy Category B

INDICATIONS

▪ Treatment of the following infections due to susceptible strains of penicillinase-producing staphylococci: □ Respiratory tract infections □ Skin and skin structure infections □ Bone and joint infections □ Urinary tract infections □ Endocarditis □ Septicemia □ Meningitis.

ACTION

▪ Binds to bacterial cell wall, leading to cell death ▪ Resists the action of penicillinase, an enzyme capable of inactivating penicillin. **Therapeutic Effect:** ▪ Bactericidal action against susceptible bacteria. **Spectrum:** ▪ Active against most gram-positive aerobic cocci, but less so than penicillin ▪ Spectrum is notable for activity against penicillinase-producing strains of: □ *Staphylococcus aureus* □ *Staphyloccoccus epidermidis*.

PHARMACOKINETICS

Absorption: Poorly absorbed from the GI tract. Well absorbed from IM sites.
Distribution: Widely distributed. Penetration into CSF is minimal but sufficient in the presence of inflamed meninges. Crosses the placenta and enters breast milk.
Metabolism and Excretion: Excreted unchanged by the kidneys.
Half-life: 20–30 min (increased in renal impairment).

CONTRAINDICATIONS AND PRECAUTIONS

Contraindicated in: ▪ Hypersensitivity to penicillins.
Use Cautiously in: ▪ Severe renal impairment (dosage reduction recommended if creatinine clearance ≤10 ml/min) ▪ Pregnancy or lactation (safety not established) ▪ Previous hypersensitivity reactions.

ADVERSE REACTIONS AND SIDE EFFECTS*

CNS: SEIZURES (high doses).
Derm: rashes, urticaria.
GI: nausea, vomiting, diarrhea, hepatitis.
GU: interstitial nephritis.
Hemat: blood dyscrasias.
Local: phlebitis at IV site, pain at IM site.
Misc: superinfection, allergic reactions, including ANAPHYLAXIS and serum sickness.

INTERACTIONS

Drug–Drug: ▪ **Probenecid** decreases renal excretion and increases blood levels ▪ May alter the effect of **oral anticoagulants**.

ROUTE AND DOSAGE

1 g contains 2.6–3.1 mEq of sodium.
▪ **IM (Adults):** 1 g q 4–6 hr (up to 24 g/day).
▪ **IM (Children):** 25 mg/kg q 6 hr (up to 300 mg/kg/day).
▪ **IV (Adults):** 1–2 g q 4 hr (up to 24 g/day).
▪ **IV (Children):** 100–300 mg/kg/day in divided doses q 4–6 hr.
▪ **IM, IV (Children >7 days and >2000 g):** 100 mg/kg/day in divided doses q 6 hr. Up to 200 mg/kg/day for meningitis.
▪ **IM, IV (Children <7 days and >2000 g):** 75 mg/kg/day in divided doses q 8 hr. Up to 150 mg/kg/day for meningitis.
▪ **IM, IV (Children <7 days and <2000 g):** 50 mg/kg/day in divided

M

*Underlines indicate most frequent; **CAPITALS** indicate life-threatening.

doses q 12 hr. Up to 100 mg/kg/day for meningitis.

AVAILABILITY

- *Injection:* 1-g, 4-g, 6-g, 10-g vials.

TIME/ACTION PROFILE (blood levels)

	ONSET	PEAK	DURATION
IM	rapid	30–60 min	4–6 hr
IV	rapid	end of infusion	4–6 hr

NURSING IMPLICATIONS

ASSESSMENT

- Assess patient for infection (vital signs; appearance of wound, sputum, urine, and stool; WBC) at beginning and throughout course of therapy.
- Obtain a history before initiating therapy to determine previous use of and reactions to penicillins or cephalosporins. Persons with a negative history of penicillin sensitivity may still have an allergic response.
- Obtain specimens for culture and sensitivity prior to initiating therapy. First dose may be given before receiving results.
- Observe patient for signs and symptoms of anaphylaxis (rash, pruritus, laryngeal edema, wheezing). Discontinue the drug and notify physician immediately if these occur. Keep epinephrine, an antihistamine, and resuscitation equipment close by in the event of an anaphylactic reaction.
- Assess vein for signs of irritation and phlebitis. Change IV site every 48 hr to prevent phlebitis.
- **Lab Test Considerations:** Renal function tests should be monitored periodically during prolonged therapy.
- May cause positive direct Coombs' test result.

POTENTIAL NURSING DIAGNOSES

- Infection, high risk for (indications, side effects).
- Knowledge deficit related to medication regimen (patient/family teaching).

IMPLEMENTATION

- **General Info:** To reconstitute for IM or IV use add 1.5 ml of Sterile Water or 0.9% NaCl for Injection to each 1-g vial, 5.7 ml to each 4-g vial, and 8.6 ml to each 6-g vial for a concentration of 500 mg/ml. Solution is straw-colored.
- **IM:** Administer slowly by deep intragluteal injection.
- **Direct IV:** Each ml (500 mg) of reconstituted solution should be further diluted in 20–25 ml of Sterile Water or 0.9% NaCl for Injection.
- *Rate:* Administer at a rate of 10 ml over 1 min.
- **Intermittent Infusion:** Dilute in 0.9% NaCl, D5W, D10W, D5/0.9% NaCl, D5/LR, Ringer's or lactated Ringer's solution. Diluted concentrations of 2–60 mg/ml are stable for 8 hr at room temperature.
- *Rate:* Infuse over 30 min–8 hr.
- **Y-Site Compatibility:** ▪ heparin ▪ hydrocortisone sodium succinate ▪ potassium chloride ▪ verapamil ▪ vitamin B complex with C.
- **Additive Incompatibility:** Manufacturer recommends that methicillin not be admixed with other drugs.

PATIENT/FAMILY TEACHING

- Advise patient to report signs of superinfection (black, furry overgrowth on the tongue, vaginal itching or discharge, loose or foul-smelling stools) and allergy to physician promptly.
- Instruct patient to notify physician if fever and diarrhea develop, especially if stool contains blood, pus, or mucus. Advise patient not to treat diarrhea without consulting physician or pharmacist.

EVALUATION

Clinical response can be evaluated by:
- Resolution of the signs and symptoms of infection. Length of time for complete resolution depends on the organism and site of infection.

METHIMAZOLE
(meth-**im**-a-zole)
Tapazole

CLASSIFICATION(S):
Antithyroid agent
Pregnancy Category D

INDICATIONS
- Palliative treatment of hyperthyroidism ▪ Used as an adjunct to control hyperthyroidism in preparation for thyroidectomy or radioactive iodine therapy.

ACTION
▪ Inhibits the synthesis of thyroid hormones. **Therapeutic Effect:** ▪ Decreased signs and symptoms of hyperthyroidism.

PHARMACOKINETICS
Absorption: Rapidly absorbed following oral administration.
Distribution: Crosses the placenta and enters breast milk in high concentrations.
Metabolism and Excretion: Mostly metabolized by the liver, <10% eliminated unchanged by the kidneys.
Half-life: 3–5 hr.

CONTRAINDICATIONS AND PRECAUTIONS
Contraindicated in: ▪ Hypersensitivity ▪ Lactation.
Use Cautiously in: ▪ Patients with decreased bone marrow reserve ▪ Pregnancy (may be used cautiously; however, thyroid problems may result in the fetus) ▪ Patients >40 yr (increased risk of agranulocytosis).

ADVERSE REACTIONS AND SIDE EFFECTS*
CNS: headache, drowsiness, vertigo.
GI: diarrhea, nausea, vomiting, hepatitis, parotitis, loss of taste.
Hemat: AGRANULOCYTOSIS, anemia, leukopenia, thrombocytopenia.

Derm: rash, urticaria, skin discoloration.
MS: arthralgia.
Misc: fever, lymphadenopathy.

INTERACTIONS
Drug–Drug: ▪ Additive bone marrow depression with **antineoplastic agents** or **radiation therapy** ▪ Antithyroid effect may be intensified by **potassium iodide** or **lithium** ▪ Increased risk of agranulocytosis with **phenothiazines**.

ROUTE AND DOSAGE
- **PO (Adults):** 15–60 mg/day single dose or 2 divided doses for 6–8 wk (15–20 mg q 4 hr for first 24 hr in thyrotoxicosis). Maintenance dose 15–30 mg/day single dose or 2 divided doses.
- **PO (Children):** 400 mcg/kg/day single dose or 2 divided doses initially, then 200 mcg/kg/day in 1–2 divided doses.

AVAILABILITY
- *Tablets:* 5 mg, 10 mg.

TIME/ACTION PROFILE (effect on thyroid status)

	ONSET	PEAK	DURATION
PO	1 wk	4–10 wk	wks

NURSING IMPLICATIONS
ASSESSMENT
▫ Monitor response for symptoms of hyperthyroidism or thyrotoxicosis (tachycardia, palpitations, nervousness, insomnia, fever, diaphoresis, heat intolerance, tremors, weight loss, diarrhea).
▫ Assess patient for development of hypothyroidism (intolerance to cold, constipation, dry skin, headache, listlessness, tiredness, or weakness). Dosage adjustment may be required.
▫ Assess patient for skin rash or swelling of cervical lymph nodes. Treatment may be discontinued if this occurs.

M

*Underlines indicate most frequent; **CAPITALS** indicate life-threatening.

- **Lab Test Considerations:** Thyroid function studies should be monitored prior to therapy, monthly during initial therapy, and every 2–3 mo throughout therapy.
- WBC and differential counts should be monitored periodically throughout course of therapy. Agranulocytosis may develop rapidly; it usually occurs during the first 2 mo and is more common in patients over 40 yr and those receiving >40 mg/day. This necessitates discontinuation of therapy.
- May cause increased AST (SGOT), ALT (SGPT), LDH, alkaline phosphatase, serum bilirubin, and prothrombin time.

POTENTIAL NURSING DIAGNOSES
- Knowledge deficit related to medication regimen (patient/family teaching).
- Noncompliance (patient/family teaching).

IMPLEMENTATION
- **PO:** Administer at same time in relation to meals every day. Food may either increase or decrease absorption.

PATIENT/FAMILY TEACHING
- Instruct patient to take medication exactly as directed, around the clock. If a dose is missed, take as soon as remembered; take both doses together if almost time for next dose; check with physician if more than 1 dose is missed. Consult physician prior to discontinuing medication.
- Instruct patient to monitor weight 2–3 times weekly. Notify physician of significant changes.
- May cause drowsiness. Caution patient to avoid driving or other activities requiring alertness until response to medication is known.
- Advise patient to consult physician regarding dietary sources of iodine (iodized salt, shellfish).
- Advise patient to report sore throat, fever, chills, headache, malaise, weakness, yellowing of eyes or skin, unusual bleeding or bruising, rash, or symptoms of hyperthyroidism or hypothyroidism to physician promptly.

- Instruct patient to consult physician or pharmacist before taking any over-the-counter medications.
- Advise patient to carry identification describing medication regimen at all times.
- Advise patient to notify physician or dentist of medication regimen prior to treatment or surgery.
- Emphasize the importance of routine examinations to monitor progress and to check for side effects.

EVALUATION
Effectiveness of therapy can be demonstrated by: ▪ Decrease in severity of symptoms of hyperthyroidism (lowered pulse rate and weight gain) ▪ Return of thyroid function studies to normal ▪ May be used as short-term adjunctive therapy to prepare patient for thyroidectomy or radiation therapy or may be used in treatment of hyperthyroidism. Treatment of 6 mo to several years may be necessary, usually averaging 1 yr.

METHOCARBAMOL
(meth-oh-**kar**-ba-mole)
Delaxin, Marbaxin, Robaxin, Robomol

CLASSIFICATION(S):
Skeletal muscle relaxant (centrally acting)
Pregnancy Category UK

INDICATIONS
▪ Adjunct to rest and physical therapy in the treatment of muscle spasm associated with acute painful musculoskeletal conditions ▪ Adjunct in the management of tetanus.

ACTION
▪ Skeletal muscle relaxation, probably due to CNS depression. **Therapeutic Effect:** ▪ Skeletal muscle relaxation.

PHARMACOKINETICS
Absorption: Rapidly absorbed from the GI tract.

Distribution: Widely distributed. Crosses the placenta.
Metabolism and Excretion: Metabolized by the liver.
Half-life: 1–2 hr.

CONTRAINDICATIONS AND PRECAUTIONS

Contraindicated in: ▪ Hypersensitivity ▪ Hypersensitivity to polyethylene glycol (parenteral only) ▪ Renal impairment (parenteral form).
Use Cautiously in: ▪ Pregnancy, lactation, and children (safety not established) ▪ Seizure disorders (parenteral form).

ADVERSE REACTIONS AND SIDE EFFECTS*

CNS: SEIZURES (IV, IM only), drowsiness, dizziness, lightheadedness.
EENT: blurred vision, nasal congestion.
CV: IV—hypotension, bradycardia.
GI: nausea, anorexia, GI upset.
GU: brown, black, or green urine.
Derm: urticaria, pruritis, rashes, flushing (IV only).
Local: pain at IM site, phlebitis at IV site.
Misc: fever, allergic reactions including ANAPHYLAXIS (IM, IV use only).

INTERACTIONS

Drug–Drug: ▪ Additive CNS depression with other **CNS depressants**, including **alcohol, antihistamines, opioid analgesics,** and **sedative/hypnotics.**

ROUTE AND DOSAGE

Muscle Spasm
▪ **PO (Adults):** 1.5 g qid initially (up to 8 g/day), for 2–3 days then 4–4.5 g/day in 3–6 divided doses.
▪ **IM, IV (Adults):** 1 g, if PO not feasible can give up to 1 g q 8 hr for up to 3 days.

Tetanus
▪ **PO (Adults):** up to 24 g/day in divided doses.
▪ **IV (Adults):** 1–2 g, additional 1–2 g may be given (total initial dose not

to exceed 3 g), repeat 1–2 g q 6 hr until nasogastric tube is inserted, then change to PO.
▪ **IV (Children):** 15 mg/kg, may be repeated q 6 hr.

AVAILABILITY

▪ *Tablets:* 500 mg, 750 mg ▪ *Injection:* 100 mg/ml ▪ *In combination with:* aspirin (Robaxisol).

TIME/ACTION PROFILE (skeletal muscle relaxation)

	ONSET	PEAK	DURATION
PO	30 min	2 hr	UK
IM	rapid	UK	UK
IV	immediate	end of infusion	UK

NURSING IMPLICATIONS

ASSESSMENT
▫ Assess patient for pain, muscle stiffness, and range of motion prior to and periodically throughout therapy.
▫ Monitor pulse and blood pressure every 15 min during parenteral administration.
▫ Assess patient for allergic reactions (skin rash, asthma, hives, wheezing, hypotension) following parenteral administration. Keep epinephrine and oxygen on hand in the event of a reaction.
▫ Monitor IV site. Injection is hypertonic and may cause thrombophlebitis. Avoid extravasation.
▪ **Lab Test Considerations:** Monitor renal function periodically during prolonged parenteral therapy (>3 days), as polyethylene glycol 300 vehicle is nephrotoxic.

POTENTIAL NURSING DIAGNOSES
▪ Pain (indications).
▪ Physical mobility, impaired (indications).
▪ Injury, high risk for (side effects).

IMPLEMENTATION
▪ **General Info:** Provide safety measures as indicated. Supervise ambulation and transfer of patients.
▪ **PO:** May be administered with food to

M

minimize GI irritation. Tablets may be crushed and mixed with food or liquids to facilitate swallowing. For administration via nasogastric tube, crush tablet and suspend in water or saline.

- **IM:** Do not administer SC. IM injections should contain no more than 5 ml (500 mg) in the gluteal region at a time.
- **Direct IV:** May be given undiluted at a rate of 3 ml (300 mg) over 1 min.
- **Intermittent Infusion:** Dilute each dose in no more than 250 ml of 0.9% NaCl or D5W for injection. Do not refrigerate after dilution.
- □ Have patient remain recumbent during and for at least 10–15 min following infusion to avoid orthostatic hypotension.

PATIENT/FAMILY TEACHING
- □ Advise patient to take medication exactly as directed. Missed doses should be taken within 1 hr, if not, return to regular dosing schedule. Do not double doses.
- □ Encourage patient to comply with additional therapies prescribed for muscle spasm (rest, physical therapy, heat).
- □ Medication may cause dizziness, drowsiness, and blurred vision. Advise patient to avoid driving and other activities requiring alertness until response to drug is known.
- □ Instruct patient to make position changes slowly to minimize orthostatic hypotension.
- □ Advise patient to avoid concurrent use of alcohol and other CNS depressants while taking this medication.
- □ Inform patient that urine may turn black, brown, or green, especially if left standing.
- □ Instruct patient to notify physician if skin rash, itching, fever, or nasal congestion occurs.
- □ Emphasize the importance of routine follow-up examinations to monitor progress.

EVALUATION
Effectiveness of therapy can be demonstrated by: ▪ Decreased musculoskeletal pain and muscle spasticity □ Increased range of motion.

METHOHEXITAL
(meth-o-**hex**-i-tal)
Brevital, {Brietal}

CLASSIFICATION(S):
Anesthetic (general), Barbiturate (ultra-short-acting)
Schedule IV
Pregnancy Category C

INDICATIONS
▪ Induction of general anesthesia ▪ Sole anesthesia in short (<15 min), minimally painful procedures ▪ Supplement with other anesthetic agents ▪ To produce unconsciousness during balanced anesthesia.

ACTION
▪ Produces anesthesia by depressing the CNS, probably by potentiating gamma-aminobutyric acid (GABA), an inhibitory neurotransmitter. **Therapeutic Effects:** ▪ Unconsciousness and general anesthesia.

PHARMACOKINETICS
Absorption: Well absorbed following IM administration.
Distribution: Accumulates and may be slowly re-released from lipoid tissues. Excreted in breast milk following large doses.
Metabolism and Excretion: Mostly metabolized by the liver. Some metabolism in kidneys and brain.
Half-life: 4 hr (increased in elderly patients).

CONTRAINDICATIONS AND PRECAUTIONS
Contraindicated in: ▪ Hypersensitivity ▪ Porphyria ▪ Lactation.

{} = Available in Canada only.

Use Cautiously in: ▪ Addison's disease ▪ Severe anemia ▪ Severe cardiovascular or hepatic disease ▪ Myxedema ▪ Shock or hypotension ▪ Pulmonary disease ▪ Elderly or debilitated patients ▪ Obesity ▪ Pregnancy (safety not established).

ADVERSE REACTIONS AND SIDE EFFECTS*

CNS: SEIZURES, restlessness, anxiety, headache, emergence delerium.
EENT: rhinitis.
Resp: coughing, LARYNGOSPASM, APNEA, respiratory depression, dyspnea, bronchospasm.
CV: CARDIORESPIRATORY ARREST, hypotension.
GI: hiccoughs, salivation, nausea, vomiting, abdominal pain.
Derm: erythema, pruritus, urticaria.
MS: muscle twitching.
Local: phlebitis at IV site, pain at IM site.
Misc: shivering, allergic reactions.

INTERACTIONS

Drug–Drug: ▪ Additive CNS depression with **alcohol, antihistamines, opioid analgesics,** and **sedative/hypnotics.**

ROUTE AND DOSAGE

All doses must be individualized.

Induction
▪ **IV (Adults and Children):** 1–2 mg/kg.
▪ **IM (Children):** 5–10 mg/kg as needed.

Maintenance
▪ **IV (Adults):** 0.25–1 mg/kg as needed or continuous infusion of 0.2% solution, usually at rate of 3 ml/min (6 mg/min), with additional doses of 20–40 mg q 4–7 min as needed.

Basal Anesthesia in Children
▪ **Rect (Children):** 15–30 mg/kg as a 5–10% solution (decrease dosage in inactive or debilitated patients). Rectal product not commercially available, must be compounded.

AVAILABILITY

▪ *Injection:* 500 mg, 2.5 g, 5 g.

TIME/ACTION PROFILE (anesthesia)

	ONSET	PEAK	DURATION
IM	UK	UK	UK
IV	within 60 sec	UK	5–7 min

NURSING IMPLICATIONS

ASSESSMENT
▫ Assess blood pressure, ECG, heart rate, and respiratory status continuously throughout methohexital therapy. Methohexital should be used only by individuals qualified to administer anesthesia and experienced in endotracheal intubation. Equipment for this procedure should be immediately available. Apnea may occur immediately after IV injection, especially in the presence of opioid premedication.
▫ Monitor IV site carefully. Extravasation may cause pain, swelling, ulceration, and necrosis. Intra-arterial injection may cause arteritis, vasospasm, edema, thrombosis, and gangrene of the extremity.
▪ **Toxicity and Overdose:** Overdose may occur from rapid injection (drop in blood pressure, possibly to shock levels) or excessive or repeated injections (respiratory distress, laryngospasm, apnea).

POTENTIAL NURSING DIAGNOSES
▪ Breathing pattern, ineffective (side effects).
▪ Injury, high risk for (side effects).

IMPLEMENTATION
▪ **General Info:** Dose is individualized according to depth of anesthesia desired; concurrent use of other medications and/or nitrous oxide; patient's condition, age, weight, and sex.
▫ Middle-aged or elderly patients may require smaller doses than young patients. Tolerance may develop with repeated use, such as for burns. Indi-

M

*Underlines indicate most frequent; **CAPITALS** indicate life-threatening.

viduals tolerant to alcohol or barbiturates may require higher doses.

- **Rect:** May be administered via rectal suspension. To prepare a 10% rectal solution, dissolve the appropriate amount of methohexital in warm tap water. Discard solution that is cloudy or that contains a precipitate.
- **IV:** Repeated doses or continuous infusion of methohexital may cause prolonged somnolence and respiratory and circulatory depression. If the patient requires a second anesthetic in the same day, reduction in the dose of methohexital may be required.
- □ Methohexital may be given in doses sufficient to produce deep surgical anesthesia, but such doses may cause dangerous respiratory and circulatory depression.
- □ Premedication with anticholinergics (atropine, glycopyrrolate) may be used to decrease mucus secretions. Opioid analgesics may be administered pre-operatively to enhance the poor analgesic effects of methohexital. Preoperative medications should be given so that peak effect is attained shortly before induction of anesthesia. Muscle relaxants, if required, should be administered separately.
- □ Dilute methohexital with Sterile Water for Injection, D5W, or 0.9% NaCl. Solution should be freshly prepared and used within 24 hr of reconstitution. Refrigerate and keep sealed. Do not administer solution containing a precipitate.
- **Direct IV:** Induction dose is administered at a rate not to exceed 1 ml (10 mg) over 5 sec. Anesthesia is maintained by intermittent injections every 4–7 min or by continuous infusion.
- **Continuous Infusion:** To prepare a 1% (10 mg/ml) solution, reconstitute each 2.5-g vial with 15 ml or each 5-g vial with 30 ml of sterile water, D5W, or 0.9% NaCl. Initial solution will be yellow. Further dilute the 2.5-g vial in 250 ml and the 5-g vial in 500 ml. Solution should be used only if clear and colorless.
- □ To prepare a 0.2% solution, dilute 500

mg in 250 ml of D5W or 0.9% NaCl. Do not dilute with sterile water to avoid hypotonicity.
- □ Solution is stable for 24 hr.
- **Syringe Incompatibility:** ▪ glycopyrrolate.
- **Additive Incompatibility:** ▪ atropine ▪ chlorpromazine ▪ cimetidine ▪ clindamycin ▪ droperidol ▪ fentanyl ▪ hydralazine ▪ kanamycin ▪ lidocaine ▪ mechlorethamine ▪ metaraminol ▪ methicillin ▪ methyldopate ▪ metocurine ▪ oxytetracycline ▪ pancuronium ▪ penicillin G potassium ▪ pentazocine ▪ prochlorperazine ▪ promazine ▪ promethazine ▪ propiomazine ▪ scopolamine ▪ succinylcholine ▪ streptomycin ▪ tetracycline ▪ tubocurarine.

PATIENT/FAMILY TEACHING

- □ Methohexital may cause psychomotor impairment for 24 hr following administration. Caution patient to avoid driving or other activities requiring alertness for 24 hr.
- □ Advise patient to avoid use of alcohol or other CNS depressants for 24 hr following anesthesia, unless directed by physician or dentist.

EVALUATION

Effectiveness of therapy can be demonstrated by: ▪ Loss of consciousness ▪ Maintenance of desired level of anesthesia without complications.

METHOTREXATE
(meth-o-**trex**-ate)
Amethopterin, Folex, Folex PFS, Rheumatrex

CLASSIFICATION(S):
Antineoplastic (antimetabolite),
Immunosuppressant
Pregnancy Category X

INDICATIONS

- ▪ Alone or in combination with other treatment modalities (other antineoplastic agents, surgery, or radiation therapy) in the treatment of: □ Trophoblastic neoplasms (choriocarcinoma, chorioadenoma destruens, hydatidiform mole) □ Leukemias □ Breast carcinoma □ Head carcinoma □ Neck carcinoma □ Lung carcinoma ▪ Treatment of severe psoriasis and rheumatoid arthritis unresponsive to conventional therapy ▪ Treatment of mycosis fungoides.

ACTION

▪ Interferes with folic acid metabolism. Result is inhibition of DNA synthesis and cell reproduction (cell cycle-S phase specific) ▪ Also has immunosuppressive activity. **Therapeutic Effects:** ▪ Death of rapidly replicating cells, particularly malignant ones, and immunosuppression.

PHARMACOKINETICS

Absorption: Small doses are well absorbed from the GI tract. Larger doses incompletely absorbed.
Distribution: Actively transported across cell membranes, widely distributed. Does not reach therapeutic concentrations in the CSF. Crosses the placenta. Enters breast milk in low concentrations.
Metabolism and Excretion: Excreted mostly unchanged by the kidneys.
Half-life: 2–4 hr (increased in renal impairment).

CONTRAINDICATIONS AND PRECAUTIONS

Contraindicated in: ▪ Hypersensitivity ▪ Pregnancy or lactation.
Use Cautiously in: ▪ Renal impairment (creatinine clearance must be ≥60 ml/min prior to therapy) ▪ Patients with childbearing potential ▪ Active infections ▪ Decreased bone marrow reserve ▪ Other chronic debilitating illnesses.

ADVERSE REACTIONS AND SIDE EFFECTS*

CNS: arachnoiditis (IT use only), headaches, blurred vision, drowsiness, malaise, dizziness.
GI: stomatitis, anorexia, nausea, vomiting, hepatotoxicity.

GU: gonadal suppression.
Derm: rashes, urticaria, photosensitivity, pruritus, alopecia.
Hemat: anemia, leukopenia, thrombocytopenia.
Metab: hyperuricemia.
Misc: nephropathy, chills, fever.

INTERACTIONS

Drug–Drug: ▪ The following drugs may increase the toxicity of methotrexate: high-dose **salicylates, nonsteroidal anti-inflammatory agents, sulfonylureas (oral hypoglycemic agents), phenytoin, phenylbutazone, tetracyclines, probenecid,** and **chloramphenicol** ▪ Additive hepatotoxicity with other **hepatotoxic drugs** ▪ Additive nephrotoxicity with other **nephrotoxic drugs** ▪ Additive bone marrow depression with other **antineoplastic agents** or **radiation therapy** ▪ May decrease antibody response to **live virus vaccines** and increase the risk of adverse reactions ▪ Increased risk of neurologic reactions with **acyclovir** (IT methotrexate only) ▪ **Asparaginase** may decrease effects of methotrexate.

ROUTE AND DOSAGE

Trophoblastic Neoplasms

▪ **PO, IM (Adults):** 15–30 mg/day for 5 days, repeat after 1 or more weeks for 3–5 courses.

Leukemia—Induction

▪ **PO (Adults and Children):** 3.3 mg/m^2/day, usually with prednisone.
▪ **IT (Adults and Children):** 12 mg/m^2 or 15 mg.

Leukemia—Maintenance

▪ **PO, IM (Adults and Children):** 10–15 mg/m^2 twice weekly every 2 wk or 30 mg/m^2/wk.
▪ **IV (Adults and Children):** 2.5 mg/kg q 2 wk.

Osteosarcoma

▪ **IV (Adults and Children):** 12 g/m^2 as a 4-hr infusion followed by leucovorin rescue, usually as part of a combination chemotherapeutic regimen.

M

*Underlines indicate most frequent; **CAPITALS** indicate life-threatening.

Psoriasis

(Precede therapy with 5–10 mg test dose.)

- **PO (Adults):** 2.5–5 mg q 12 hr for 3 doses once weekly, or q 8 hr for 4 doses; may increase by 2.5 mg/wk up to 20 mg/wk.
- **PO, IM, IV (Adults):** 10 mg once weekly; may be increased up to 25 mg/weekly.

Arthritis

(Precede therapy with 5–10 mg test dose.)

- **PO (Adults):** 7.5 mg weekly (2.5 mg q 12 hr for 3 doses; not to exceed 20 mg/wk).

Mycosis Fungoides

- **PO (Adults):** 2.5–10 mg/day for several weeks to months.
- **IM (Adults):** 50 mg once weekly or 25 mg twice weekly.

AVAILABILITY

- **Tablets:** 2.5 mg ▪ **Injection:** 2.5 mg/ml, 25 mg/ml, 20 mg, 50 mg, 100 mg, 250 mg, 1 g ▪ **Preservative-free injection:** 25 mg/ml.

TIME/ACTION PROFILE (effects on blood counts)

	ONSET	PEAK	DURATION
PO, IM, IV	4–7 days	7–14 days	21 days

NURSING IMPLICATIONS

Assessment

- **General Info:** Monitor blood pressure, pulse, and respiratory rate periodically during administration. Notify physician of significant changes.
- Monitor for abdominal pain, diarrhea, or stomatitis. Inform physician if these occur, as therapy may need to be discontinued.
- Assess for fever, sore throat, and signs of infection. If these symptoms occur, notify physician immediately.
- Assess for bleeding (bleeding gums; bruising; petechiae; guaiac stools, urine, emesis). Avoid IM injections and rectal temperatures. Hold pres-sure on all venipuncture sites for at least 10 min.
- Monitor intake and output ratios and daily weights. Notify physician if significant changes in totals occur.
- Monitor for symptoms of gout (increased uric acid, joint pain, edema). Encourage patient to drink at least 2 liters of fluid each day. Allopurinol and alkalinization of urine may be used to decrease uric acid levels.
- Assess patient's nutritional status. Administering an antiemetic prior to and periodically throughout therapy and adjusting diet as tolerated may help maintain fluid and electrolyte balance and nutritional status.
- Anemia may occur. Monitor for increased fatigue, dyspnea, and orthostatic hypotension.
- **IT:** Assess for development of nuchal rigidity, headache, fever, confusion, drowsiness, dizziness, weakness, or seizures.
- **Lab Test Considerations:** Monitor CBC and differential prior to and frequently throughout therapy. The nadir of leukopenia and thrombocytopenia occurs in 7–14 days. Leukocyte and thrombocyte counts usually recover 7 days after the nadirs. Notify physician of any sudden drop in values.
- Renal (BUN and creatinine) and hepatic function (AST [SGOT], ALT [SGPT], bilirubin, and LDH) should be monitored prior to and routinely throughout course of therapy. Urine pH should be monitored prior to high-dose methotrexate therapy and every 6 hr during leucovorin rescue. Urine pH should be kept above 7.0 to prevent renal damage.
- May cause elevated serum uric acid concentrations, especially during initial treatment of leukemia and lymphoma.
- **Toxicity and Overdose:** Serum methotrexate levels should be monitored every 12–24 hr during high-dose therapy until levels are $<5 \times 10^{-8}$ M. This monitoring is essential to plan correct leucovorin dose and deter-

mine duration of rescue therapy
- □ With high-dose therapy, patient must receive folinic acid or citrovorum factor (leucovorin rescue) exactly when ordered to prevent fatal toxicity.

POTENTIAL NURSING DIAGNOSES

- Infection, high risk for (adverse reactions).
- Nutrition, altered: less than body requirements (adverse reactions).
- Knowledge deficit related to medication regimen (patient/family teaching).

IMPLEMENTATION

- **General Info:** Solution for injection should be prepared in a biologic cabinet. Wear gloves, gown, and mask while handling medication. Discard equipment in specially designated containers (see Appendix I).
- **PO:** Administer doses 1 hr before or 2 hr after meals.
- **Direct IV:** Reconstitute each vial with 2–10 ml of Sterile Preservative-free 0.9% NaCl for Injection. Do not use preparations that are discolored or that contain a precipitate. Reconstitute immediately before use. Discard unused portion.
- **Rate:** Administer at a rate of 10 mg/min into Y-site or 3-way stopcock of a free-flowing IV.
- **Intermittent/Continuous Infusion:** May be diluted in D5W, D5/0.9% NaCl, or 0.9% NaCl and infused as intermittent or continuous infusion.
- **Syringe Compatibility:** bleomycin cisplatin cyclophosphamide doxapram doxorubicin fluorouracil furosemide leucovorin mitomycin vinblastine vincristine.
- **Syringe Incompatibility:** droperidol ranitidine.
- **Y-Site Compatibility:** bleomycin cisplatin cyclophosphamide doxorubicin fludarabine fluorouracil furosemide heparin leucovorin metoclopramide mitomycin ondansetron sargramostim vancomycin vinblastine vincristine.
- **Y-Site Incompatibility:** droperidol.

- **Additive Compatibility:** cyclophosphamide cytarabine fluorouracil mercaptopurine sodium bicarbonate vincristine.
- **Additive Incompatibility:** bleomycin prednisolone.
- **IT:** Reconstitute preservative-free methotrexate with preservative-free 0.9% NaCl, Elliot's B solution, or patient's CSF to a concentration of 1 mg/ml. May be administered via lumbar puncture or Ommaya reservoir. To prevent bacterial contamination use immediately.

PATIENT/FAMILY TEACHING

- □ Instruct patient to take medication exactly as directed. If a dose is missed, it should be omitted. Physician should be consulted if vomiting occurs shortly after a dose is taken.
- □ Caution patient to avoid crowds and persons with known infections. Physician should be informed immediately if symptoms of infection occur.
- □ Instruct patient to report unusual bleeding. Advise patient of thrombocytopenia precautions (use soft toothbrush and electric razor; avoid falls; do not drink alcoholic beverages or take medication containing aspirin or ibuprofen, as these may precipitate gastric bleeding).
- □ Instruct patient to inspect oral mucosa for erythema and ulceration. If ulceration occurs, advise patient to use sponge brush and to rinse mouth with water after eating and drinking. Viscous lidocaine swishes may be used if mouth pain interferes with eating.
- □ Instruct patient to avoid the use of over-the-counter drugs without first consulting physician or pharmacist.
- □ Advise patient that this medication may have teratogenic effects. Contraception should be used during therapy and for at least 3 mo for males and 1 ovulatory cycle for females after completion of therapy.
- □ Discuss the possibility of hair loss with patient. Explore methods of coping.

M

□ Instruct patient not to receive any vaccinations without advice of physician.
□ Caution patient to use sunscreen and protective clothing to prevent photosensitivity reactions.
□ Emphasize the need for periodic lab tests to monitor for side effects.

EVALUATION
Effectiveness of therapy can be demonstrated by: ■ Improvement of hematopoietic values in leukemia □ Decrease in symptoms of meningeal involvement in leukemia ■ Decrease in size and spread of non-Hodgkin's lymphomas and other solid cancers ■ Resolution of skin lesions in severe psoriasis ■ Decreased joint pain and swelling □ Improved mobility in patients with rheumatoid arthritis ■ Regression of lesions in mycosis fungoides.

METHOTRIMEPRAZINE
(meth-oh-try-**mep**-ra-zeen)
{Nozinan}, Levoprome

CLASSIFICATION(S):
Nonopioid analgesic (phenothiazine)
Pregnancy Category UK

INDICATIONS
■ Management of moderate to severe pain in patients who are not ambulatory ■ Used as an obstetric analgesic in situations where respiratory depression should not occur ■ Used as a preoperative sedative. **Unlabeled Uses:** ■ Treatment of psychotic disorders.

ACTION
■ Alters the effects of dopamine in the CNS ■ Suppresses sensory impulses resulting in increased pain threshold ■ Produces amnesia ■ Has alpha-adrenergic blocking activity that results in orthostatic hypotension. **Therapeutic Effects:** ■ Reduction in severity of pain ■ Sedation.

PHARMACOKINETICS
Absorption: Well absorbed following IM administration.
Distribution: Enters CSF and crosses the placenta. Minimal amounts enter breast milk.
Metabolism and Excretion: Mostly metabolized by the liver. Some metabolites are active. 1% excreted unchanged by the kidneys.
Half-life: 15–30 hr.

CONTRAINDICATIONS AND PRECAUTIONS
Contraindicated in: ■ Hypersensitivity to methotrimeprazine, benzyl alcohol, or sulfites ■ Comatose patients ■ Severe renal, cardiac, or hepatic disease ■ Patients who have overdosed on CNS depressants ■ Premature labor.
Use Cautiously in: ■ History of seizures ■ Children or lactation (safety not established) ■ Prolonged use (>30 days) ■ Elderly or debilitated patients (initial dosage reduction recommended).

ADVERSE REACTIONS AND SIDE EFFECTS*
CNS: drowsiness, excess sedation, amnesia, disorientation, euphoria, headache, weakness, slurred speech, extrapyramidal reactions, SEIZURES.
EENT: nasal congestion.
CV: orthostatic hypotension, tachycardia, bradycardia, palpitations.
GI: abdominal discomfort, dry mouth, nausea, vomiting.
GU: difficulty in urination.
Local: pain at injection site.
Misc: chills.

INTERACTIONS
Drug–Drug: ■ Additive CNS depression with other **CNS depressants** including **alcohol, antihistamines, antidepressants, opioid analgesics,** or **sedative/hypnotics** ■ Additive anticholinergic effects with **antihistamines, antidepressants, phenothiazines, quinidine, disopyramide, atropine,** or **scopolamine** (reduce doses of concur-

rent atropine or scopolamine) ▪ Reverses vasopressor effects of **epinephrine** (avoid concurrent use—if vasopressor required use phenylephrine, methoxamine, or norepinephrine) ▪ Additive hypotension with acute ingestion of **alcohol, nitrates, MAO inhibitors,** or **antihypertensives**.

ROUTE AND DOSAGE

Analgesia
- **IM (Adults):** 10–20 mg q 4–6 hr. For postoperative pain, 2.5–7.5 mg.
- **IM (Elderly Patients):** 5–10 mg initial dose q 4–6 hr. May be increased as tolerated.

Preoperative Sedation
- **IM (Adults):** 2–20 mg 45 min–3 hr before surgery, if also used postoperatively, initial dose should be 2.5–7.5 mg.

Obstetric Analgesia
- **IM (Adults):** 15–20 mg.

AVAILABILITY
- *Injection:* 20 mg/ml.

TIME/ACTION PROFILE (analgesia)

	ONSET	PEAK	DURATION
IM	UK	20–40 min	4 hr

NURSING IMPLICATIONS

ASSESSMENT
- Assess type, location, and intensity of pain prior to and 30 min following administration.
- Monitor blood pressure frequently following injection. Orthostatic hypotension, fainting, syncope, and weakness frequently occur from 10 min to 12 hr after administration. Patient should remain supine for 6–12 hr following injection.
- Observe patient carefully for extrapyramidal symptoms (pill-rolling motions, drooling, tremors, rigidity, shuffling gait).
- **Lab Test Considerations:** CBC and liver function tests should be evaluated periodically throughout long-term (>30 days) therapy.

POTENTIAL NURSING DIAGNOSES
- Pain (indications).
- Injury, high risk for (side effects).
- Knowledge deficit related to medication regimen (patient/family teaching).

IMPLEMENTATION
- **General Info:** To prevent contact dermatitis avoid getting solution on hands.
- Phenothiazines should be discontinued 48 hr before and not resumed for 24 hr following metrizamide myelography as they lower the seizure threshold.
- **IM:** Do not inject SC or IV. Inject slowly into deep, well-developed muscle. Rotate injection sites.
- **Syringe Compatibility:** ▪ atropine ▪ hydroxyzine ▪ metoclopramide ▪ scopolamine.
- **Syringe Incompatibility:** ▪ ranitidine. Manufacturer does not recommend mixing other drugs in syringe with methotrimeprazine.

PATIENT/FAMILY TEACHING
- Instruct patient on how and when to ask for pain medication.
- Advise patients to make position changes slowly and to remain recumbent for 6–12 hr after administration to minimize orthostatic hypotension.
- Medication may cause drowsiness. Caution patient to request assistance with ambulation and transfer and to avoid driving or other activities requiring alertness until response to the medication is known.
- Caution patient to avoid taking alcohol or other CNS depressants concurrently with this medication.
- Instruct patient to use frequent mouth rinses, good oral hygiene, and sugarless gum or candy to minimize dry mouth.
- Instruct patient to notify physician promptly if sore throat, fever, unusual bleeding or bruising, rash, weakness, tremors, dark-colored urine, or clay-colored stools occur.

EVALUATION
Effectiveness of therapy can be demon-

strated by: ▪ Decrease in severity of pain ▪ Sedation.

METHYLDOPA (oral)
(meth-ill-**doe**-pa)
Aldomet, Amodopar, {Apo-Methyldopa}, {Dopamet}, {Novamedopa}

METHYLDOPATE
(intravenous)
(meth-ill-**doe**-pate)
Aldomet

CLASSIFICATION(S):
Antihypertensive (centrally acting alpha-adrenergic agonist)
Pregnancy Category UK

INDICATIONS

▪ Used in combination with other antihypertensives in the management of moderate to severe hypertension ▪ Due to delayed onset, parenteral form should not be used in emergencies.

ACTION

▪ Stimulates central alpha-adrenergic receptors, resulting in decreased sympathetic outflow. Result is inhibition of cardioacceleration and vasoconstrictor center ▪ Overall effect is decrease in total peripheral resistance, with little change in heart rate or cardiac output. **Therapeutic Effect:** ▪ Lowering of blood pressure.

PHARMACOKINETICS

Absorption: 50% absorbed from the GI tract. Parenteral form, methyldopate hydrochloride, is slowly converted to methyldopa.
Distribution: Crosses the blood–brain barrier. Crosses the placenta and small amounts enter breast milk.
Metabolism and Excretion: Partially metabolized by the liver, partially excreted unchanged by the kidneys.
Half-life: 1.7 hr.

CONTRAINDICATIONS AND PRECAUTIONS

Contraindicated in: ▪ Hypersensitivity ▪ Active liver disease ▪ Known alcohol or bisulfite intolerance (oral suspension only).
Use Cautiously in: ▪ Previous history of liver disease ▪ Pregnancy (has been used safely) ▪ Lactation.

ADVERSE REACTIONS AND SIDE EFFECTS*

CNS: <u>sedation</u>, depression, decreased mental acuity.
EENT: nasal stuffiness.
CV: orthostatic hypotension, bradycardia, MYOCARDITIS, edema.
GI: diarrhea, dry mouth, HEPATITIS.
GU: <u>impotence</u>.
Hemat: hemolytic anemia.
Misc: fever.

INTERACTIONS

Drug–Drug: ▪ Additive hypotension with other **antihypertensive agents,** acute **ingestion of alcohol,** and **nitrates** ▪ **Amphetamines, tricyclic antidepressants, nonsteroidal anti-inflammatory agents,** and **phenothiazines** may decrease antihypertensive effect of methyldopa ▪ May increase **lithium** toxicity ▪ Additive hypotension and CNS toxicity with **levodopa.**

ROUTE AND DOSAGE

▪ **PO (Adults):** 500–2000 mg/day in 2–3 divided doses (not to exceed 750 mg/day for first 2 days, not to exceed 3000 mg/24 hr maintenance).
▪ **PO (Children):** 10–65 mg/kg/day in 2–4 divided doses (not to exceed 3000 mg/24 hr).
▪ **IV (Adults):** 250–1000 mg q 6 hr.
▪ **IV (Children):** 20–40 mg/kg/24 hr given in divided doses q 6 hr (not to exceed 3000 mg/24 hr).

AVAILABILITY

▪ **Tablets:** 125 mg, 250 mg, 500 mg ▪ **Oral suspension:** 250 mg/5 ml ▪ **In-**

jection: 250 mg/5 ml ▪ *In combination with:* hydrochlorothiazide (Aldoril) or chlorothiazide (Aldochlor). See Appendix A.

TIME/ACTION PROFILE
(antihypertensive effect)

	ONSET	PEAK	DURATION
PO	12–24 hr	4–6 hr	24–48 hr
IV	4–6 hr	UK	10–16 hr

NURSING IMPLICATIONS

ASSESSMENT

▢ Monitor blood pressure and pulse frequently during initial dosage adjustment and periodically throughout course of therapy. Notify physician of significant changes.

▢ Monitor intake and output ratios and weight and assess for edema daily, especially at beginning of therapy. Notify physician if weight gain or edema occurs, as sodium and water retention may be treated with diuretics.

▢ Assess patient for depression or other alterations in mental status. Notify physician promptly if these symptoms develop.

▪ **Lab Test Considerations:** Renal and hepatic function and CBC should be monitored prior to and periodically throughout therapy.

▢ May cause a positive direct Coombs' test, rarely associated with hemolytic anemia.

▢ May cause increased BUN, serum potassium, sodium, prolactin, uric acid, AST (SGOT), ALT (SGPT), alkaline phosphatase, and bilirubin concentrations.

▢ May interfere with serum creatinine and AST (SGOT) measurements.

▪ **Toxicity and Overdose:** If overdose occurs, monitor blood pressure frequently. Treatment includes elevation of legs, replacement of volume with IV fluids, and administration of vasopressors if hypotension is severe.

POTENTIAL NURSING DIAGNOSES

▪ Injury, high risk for (side effects).

▪ Knowledge deficit related to medication regimen (patient/family teaching).

▪ Noncompliance (patient/family teaching).

IMPLEMENTATION

▪ **General Info:** Fluid retention and expanded volume may cause tolerance to develop within 2–3 mo after initiation of therapy. Diuretics may be added to regimen at this time to maintain control.

▢ Dosage increases should be made with the evening dose to minimize drowsiness.

▢ When changing from IV to oral forms, dosage should remain consistent.

▪ **PO:** Shake suspension prior to administration.

▪ **Intermittent Infusion:** Dilute in 100 ml of D5W, 0.9% NaCl, D5/0.9% NaCl, 5% sodium bicarbonate, or Ringer's solution.

▪ *Rate:* Infuse slowly over 30–60 min.

▪ **Y-Site Compatibility:** ▪ esmolol ▪ meperidine ▪ morphine.

PATIENT/FAMILY TEACHING

▢ Emphasize the importance of continuing to take this medication, even if feeling well. Instruct patient to take medication at the same time each day; last dose of the day should be taken at bedtime. If a dose is missed, take as soon as remembered, but not if almost time for next dose. Do not double doses. Methyldopa controls but does not cure hypertension.

▢ Encourage patient to comply with additional interventions for hypertension (weight reduction, low-sodium diet, smoking cessation, moderation of alcohol consumption, regular exercise, and stress management).

▢ Instruct patient and family on proper technique for monitoring blood pressure. Advise them to check blood pressure at least weekly and to report significant changes to physician.

▢ Inform patient that urine may darken or turn red-black when left standing.

▢ Methyldopa may cause drowsiness. Advise patient to avoid driving or

M

other activities requiring alertness until response to medication is known. Drowsiness usually subsides after 7–10 days of continuous use.

- ▢ Caution patient to avoid sudden changes in position to decrease orthostatic hypotension.
- ▢ Advise patient that frequent mouth rinses, good oral hygiene, and sugarless gum or candy may minimize dry mouth. Notify physician or dentist if dry mouth continues for >2 wk.
- ▢ Caution patient to avoid concurrent use of alcohol or other CNS depressants.
- ▢ Advise patient to consult physician or pharmacist before taking any cough, cold, or allergy remedies. Patient should also avoid excessive amounts of coffee, tea, and cola.
- ▢ Advise patient to notify physician or dentist of medication regimen prior to treatment or surgery.
- ▢ Instruct patient to notify physician if fever, muscle aches, or flu-like syndrome occurs.

EVALUATION

Effectiveness of therapy can be demonstrated by: ▪ Decrease in blood pressure without appearance of side effects.

METHYLERGONOVINE
(meth-ill-er-goe-**noe**-veen)
Methergine, methylergometrine

CLASSIFICATION(S):
Oxytocic
Pregnancy Category C

INDICATIONS

▪ Prevention and treatment of postpartum or postabortion hemorrhage caused by uterine atony or subinvolution.

ACTION

▪ Directly stimulates uterine and vascular smooth muscle. **Therapeutic Effect:** ▪ Uterine contraction.

PHARMACOKINETICS

Absorption: Well absorbed following oral or IM administration.
Distribution: Distribution not known. Enters breast milk in small quantities.
Metabolism and Excretion: Metabolic fate unknown. Probably metabolized by the liver.
Half-life: 30–120 min.

CONTRAINDICATIONS AND PRECAUTIONS

Contraindicated in: ▪ Hypersensitivity ▪ Hypersensitivity to tartaric acid (injection only) ▪ Should not to be used to induce labor.
Use Cautiously in: ▪ Hypertensive or eclamptic patients (more susceptible to hypertensive and arrhythmogenic side effects) ▪ Severe hepatic or renal disease ▪ Sepsis.
Extreme Caution in: ▪ Third stage of labor.

ADVERSE REACTIONS AND SIDE EFFECTS*

CNS: dizziness, headache.
EENT: tinnitus.
Resp: dyspnea.
CV: palpitations, HYPOTENSION, chest pain, hypertension, arrhythmias.
GI: nausea, vomiting.
GU: cramps.
Derm: diaphoresis.
Misc: allergic reactions.

INTERACTIONS

Drug–Drug: ▪ Excessive vasoconstriction may result when used with heavy cigarette smoking (**nicotine**) or other **vasopressors,** such as **dopamine.**

ROUTE AND DOSAGE

- ▪ **PO (Adults):** 200–400 mcg q 6–12 hr for 2–7 days.
- ▪ **IM, IV (Adults):** 200 mcg q 2–4 hr for up to 5 doses.

AVAILABILITY

▪ *Tablets:* 0.2 mg ▪ *Injection:* 0.2 mg/ml.

---

*Underlines indicate most frequent; **CAPITALS** indicate life-threatening.

TIME/ACTION PROFILE (effects on uterine contractions)

	ONSET	PEAK	DURATION
PO	5–15 min	UK	3 hr
IM	2–5 min	UK	3 hr
IV	immediate	UK	45 min–3 hr

NURSING IMPLICATIONS

ASSESSMENT

□ Monitor blood pressure, heart rate, and uterine response frequently during medication administration. Notify physician promptly if uterine relaxation becomes prolonged or character of vaginal bleeding changes.

□ Assess for signs of ergotism (cold, numb fingers and toes; chest pain; nausea; vomiting; headache; muscle pain; weakness).

■ Lab Test Considerations: If no response to methylergonovine, calcium levels may need to be assessed. Effectiveness of medication is decreased with hypocalcemia.

□ May cause decreased serum prolactin levels.

POTENTIAL NURSING DIAGNOSES

■ Pain (side effects).

■ Knowledge deficit related to medication regimen (patient/family teaching).

IMPLEMENTATION

■ IV: IV administration is used for emergencies only. Oral and IM routes are preferred.

■ Direct IV: May be given undiluted or diluted in 5 ml of 0.9% NaCl and administered through Y-site or 3-way stopcock. Do not add to IV solutions. Do not mix in syringe with any other drug. Refrigerate; stable for storage at room temperature for 60 days; deteriorates with age. Only use solution that is clear and colorless and that contains no precipitate.

■ Rate: Administer at a rate of 0.2 mg over 1 min.

■ Y-Site Compatibility: ■ heparin ■ hydrocortisone sodium succinate ■ potassium chloride ■ vitamin B complex with C.

PATIENT/FAMILY TEACHING

□ Instruct patient to take medication as directed; do not skip or double up on missed doses. If a dose is missed, omit it and return to regular dosage schedule.

□ Advise patient that medication may cause menstrual-like cramps.

□ Caution patient to avoid smoking, as nicotine constricts blood vessels.

□ Instruct patient to notify physician if infection develops, as this may cause increased sensitivity to the medication.

EVALUATION

Effectiveness of therapy can be demonstrated by: ■ Contractions that maintain uterine tone and prevent postpartum hemorrhage.

METHYLPHENIDATE
(meth-ill-**fen**-i-date)
Ritalin, Ritalin-SR

CLASSIFICATION(S):
CNS stimulant
Schedule II
Pregnancy Category UK

INDICATIONS

■ Adjunct in the treatment of: □ Attention deficit disorder (ADD) □ Hyperkinetic syndrome of childhood □ Minimal brain dysfunction ■ Symptomatic treatment of narcolepsy.

ACTION

■ Produces CNS and respiratory stimulation with weak sympathomimetic activity. **Therapeutic Effects:** ■ Increased attention span in ADD ■ Increased motor activity, mental alertness, and diminished fatigue in narcoleptic patients.

PHARMACOKINETICS

Absorption: Well absorbed following oral administration, although absorption of extended-release tablet (SR) is delayed.

Distribution: Distribution not known.

M

Metabolism and Excretion: Mostly metabolized (80%) by the liver.
Half-life: 1–3 hr.

CONTRAINDICATIONS AND PRECAUTIONS

Contraindicated in: ▪ Hypersensitivity ▪ Pregnancy or lactation ▪ Hyperexcitable states ▪ Hyperthyroidism ▪ Patients with psychotic personalities, suicidal or homicidal tendencies ▪ Glaucoma ▪ Motor tics.
Use Cautiously in: ▪ History of cardiovascular disease ▪ Hypertension ▪ Diabetes mellitus ▪ Elderly or debilitated patients ▪ Continual use (may result in psychological or physical dependence) ▪ Seizure disorders (may lower seizure threshold).

ADVERSE REACTIONS AND SIDE EFFECTS*

CNS: restlessness, tremor, hyperactivity, insomnia, irritability, dizziness, headache.
EENT: blurred vision.
CV: tachycardia, palpitations, hypertension, hypotension.
GI: nausea, vomiting, anorexia, dry mouth, cramps, diarrhea, constipation, metallic taste.
Derm: rashes.
Neuro: akathisia, dyskinesia.
Misc: hypersensitivity reactions, fever.

INTERACTIONS

Drug–Drug: ▪ Additive sympathomimetic effects with other **sympathomimetics,** including **vasoconstrictors** and **decongestants** ▪ Use with **MAO inhibitors** or **vasopressors** may result in hypertensive crisis ▪ May antagonize the hypotensive effect of **guanethidine** ▪ Metabolism of **oral anticoagulants, anticonvulsants,** and **tricyclic antidepressants** may be inhibited and effects increased ▪ Avoid concurrent use with **pimozide** (cause of tics may be masked).
Drug–Food: ▪ Excessive use of **caffeine**-containing foods or beverages

(coffee, cola, tea) may cause additive CNS stimulation.

ROUTE AND DOSAGE

▪ **PO (Adults):** 5–20 mg 2–3 times daily. When maintenance dose is determined, may change to sustained-release formulation 20 mg 1–3 times daily at 8-hr intervals.
▪ **PO (Children >6 yr):** 5 mg before breakfast and lunch, increase by 5–10 mg at weekly intervals (not to exceed 60 mg/day). When maintenance dose is determined, may change to sustained-release formulation 20 mg 1–3 times daily at 8-hr intervals.

AVAILABILITY

▪ *Tablets:* 5 mg, 10 mg, 20 mg ▪ *Sustained-release tablets:* 20 mg.

TIME/ACTION PROFILE (CNS stimulation)

	ONSET	PEAK	DURATION
PO	UK	1–3 hr	4–6 hr
PO-ER	UK	UK	up to 8 hr

NURSING IMPLICATIONS

Assessment

▪ **General Info:** Monitor blood pressure, pulse, and respiration before administering and periodically throughout course of therapy.
□ Monitor growth, both height and weight, in children on long-term therapy.
□ May produce a false sense of euphoria and well-being. Provide frequent rest periods and observe patient for rebound depression after the effects of the medication have worn off.
□ Methylphenidate has high dependence and abuse potential. Tolerance to medication occurs rapidly; do not increase dose.
▪ **Attention Deficit Disorders:** Assess attention span, impulse control, and interactions with others in children. Therapy may be interrupted at intervals to determine if symptoms are sufficient to continue therapy.

---

*Underlines indicate most frequent; **CAPITALS** indicate life-threatening.

- **Narcolepsy:** Observe and document frequency of episodes.
- **Lab Test Considerations:** Monitor CBC, differential, and platelet count periodically in patients receiving prolonged therapy.

POTENTIAL NURSING DIAGNOSES

- Thought processes, altered (side effects).
- Knowledge deficit related to medication regimen (patient/family teaching).

IMPLEMENTATION

- **PO:** Administer 30–45 min before meals. Extended-release tablets should be swallowed whole; do not crush, break, or chew.

PATIENT/FAMILY TEACHING

- **General Info:** Instruct patient to take medication exactly as directed. If a dose is missed, take the remaining doses for that day at regularly spaced intervals; do not double doses. Take the last dose before 6 PM to minimize the risk of insomnia. Instruct patient not to alter dosage without consulting physician. Abrupt cessation with high doses may cause extreme fatigue and mental depression.
- Advise patient to check weight 2–3 times weekly and report weight loss to physician.
- May cause dizziness or blurred vision. Caution patient to avoid driving or activities requiring alertness until response to medication is known.
- Advise patient to avoid using caffeine-containing beverages concurrently with this therapy.
- Advise patient to notify physician if nervousness, insomnia, palpitations, vomiting, skin rash, or fever occur.
- Inform patient that physician may order periodic holidays from the drug to assess progress and to decrease dependence.
- Emphasize the importance of routine follow-up examinations to monitor progress.
- **Attention Deficit Disorder:** Advise parents to notify school nurse of medication regimen.

EVALUATION

Effectiveness of therapy can be demonstrated by: ▪ Decreased frequency of narcoleptic symptoms ▪ Improved attention span and social interactions.

METHYLPREDNISOLONE
(meth-ill-pred-**niss**-oh-lone)
Medrol

METHYLPREDNISOLONE ACETATE
dep Medalone, Depoject, Depo-Medrol, Depopred, D-Med, Duralone, Medralone, M-Prednisol, Rep-Pred

METHYLPREDNISOLONE SODIUM SUCCINATE
A-Methapred, Solu-Medrol

CLASSIFICATION(S):
Glucocorticoid (intermediate-acting)
Pregnancy Category UK

INDICATIONS

- Used systemically and locally in a wide variety of: □ Chronic inflammatory diseases □ Allergic diseases □ Hematologic diseases □ Neoplastic diseases □ Autoimmune diseases ▪ Suitable for alternate-day dosing.

ACTION

▪ Suppresses inflammation and the normal immune response ▪ Has numerous intense metabolic effects ▪ Suppresses adrenal function at chronic doses of 4 mg/day ▪ Practically devoid of mineralocorticoid (sodium-retaining) activity.
Therapeutic Effects: ▪ Suppression of inflammation and modification of the normal immune response.

PHARMACOKINETICS

Absorption: Well absorbed following oral and IM administration. Chronic high-dose topical application may also lead to systemic absorption. IM acetate salt is long-acting.
Distribution: Widely   distributed.

M

Crosses the placenta, and small amounts enter breast milk.

Metabolism and Excretion: Mostly metabolized by the liver; small amounts excreted unchanged by the kidneys.

Half-life: 80–190 min. Adrenal suppression lasts 1.25–1.5 days.

CONTRAINDICATIONS AND PRECAUTIONS

Contraindicated in: ▪ Active untreated infections, except for some forms of meningitis ▪ Lactation (avoid chronic use) ▪ Products containing benzyl alcohol should not be used in neonates.

Use Cautiously in: ▪ Chronic treatment (will lead to adrenal suppression) ▪ Should never be abruptly discontinued ▪ Stress (surgery, infection)— supplemental doses needed during chronic therapy ▪ Pregnancy or lactation (safety not established) ▪ Children (chronic use will result in decreased growth) ▪ Infections (may mask fever, inflammation).

ADVERSE REACTIONS AND SIDE EFFECTS*

CNS: headache, restlessness, psychoses, depression, euphoria, personality changes, increased intracranial pressure (children only).

EENT: cataracts, increased intraocular pressure.

CV: hypertension.

GI: nausea, vomiting, anorexia, peptic ulceration.

Hemat: thromboembolism, thrombophlebitis.

Derm: decreased wound healing, petechiae, ecchymoses, fragility, hirsutism, acne.

Endo: adrenal suppression, hyperglycemia.

F and E: hypokalemia, hypokalemic alkalosis, fluid retention (long-term high doses).

Metab: weight loss, weight gain.

MS: muscle wasting, muscle pain, aseptic necrosis of joints, osteoporosis.

Misc: increased susceptibility to infec-tion, cushingoid appearance (moon face, buffalo hump).

INTERACTIONS

Drug–Drug: ▪ Additive hypokalemia with **diuretics, amphotericin B, mezlocillin, piperacillin,** or **ticarcillin** ▪ Hypokalemia may increase the risk of **cardiac glycoside** toxicity ▪ May increase requirement for **insulin** or **hypoglycemic agents** ▪ May decrease antibody response to **live virus vaccines** and increase the risk of adverse reactions.

ROUTE AND DOSAGE

▪ **PO (Adults):** 4–48 mg/day single dose or divided doses. If used chronically, when dose is stabilized, daily dose may be doubled and given every other day.

▪ **PO (Children):** *Adrenal insufficiency*—117 mcg/kg/day in 3 divided doses. *Other uses*—4.7 mcg/kg–1.67 mg/kg/day in 3–4 divided doses.

▪ **IM, IV (Adults):** *Methylprednisolone sodium succinate*—10–40 mg. High-dose therapy of 30 mg/kg may be given IV q 4–6 hr for up to 72 hr. For multiple sclerosis 160 mg/day for 7 days, then 64 mg every other day for 1 mo.

▪ **IM, IV (Infants and Children):** *Methylprednisolone sodium succinate—Adrenal insufficiency*—117 mcg/kg/day in 3 divided doses. *Other uses*—139–835 mcg/kg q 12–24 hr.

▪ **IM (Adults):** *Methylprednisolone acetate*—40–120 mg daily, weekly or every 2 wk.

▪ **Intra-articular, Intralesional (Adults):** *Methylprednisolone acetate*—4–80 mg q 1–5 wk.

AVAILABILITY

Methylprednisolone
▪ *Tablets:* 2 mg, 4 mg, 8 mg, 16 mg, 24 mg, 32 mg.

Methylprednisolone Sodium Succinate
▪ *Injection:* 40 mg, 125 mg, 500 mg, 1 g, 2 g.

*Underlines indicate most frequent; CAPITALS indicate life-threatening.

Methylprednisolone Acetate
- *Suspension for injection:* 20 mg/ml, 40 mg/ml, 80 mg/ml.

TIME/ACTION PROFILE (anti-inflammatory activity)

	ONSET	PEAK	DURATION
PO	hr	1–2 hr	1.25–1.5 days
IM acetate	6–48 hr	4–8 days	1–4 wk
IM succinate	rapid	UK	UK
IV succinate	rapid	UK	UK
IA, IL acetate	very slow	7 days	1–5 wk

NURSING IMPLICATIONS

ASSESSMENT
- **General Info:** This drug is indicated for many conditions. Assess involved systems prior to and periodically throughout course of therapy.
- Assess patient for signs of adrenal insufficiency (hypotension, weight loss, weakness, nausea, vomiting, anorexia, lethargy, confusion, restlessness) prior to and periodically throughout course of therapy.
- Monitor intake and output ratios and daily weights. Observe patient for the appearance of peripheral edema, steady weight gain, rales/crackles, or dyspnea. Notify physician should these occur.
- Children should also have periodic evaluations of growth.
- **Intra-articular:** Monitor pain, edema, and range of motion of affected joints.
- **Intralesional:** Assess affected skin prior to and daily during therapy. Note degree of inflammation, pruritus, lesion characteristics, and size.
- **Lab Test Considerations:** Patients on prolonged courses of therapy should routinely have hematologic values, serum electrolytes, serum, and urine glucose evaluated. May cause decreased WBC counts. May cause hyperglycemia, especially in persons with diabetes. May decrease serum potassium and calcium and increase serum sodium concentrations.
- Promptly report presence of guaiac-positive stools.
- Periodic adrenal function tests may be ordered to assess degree of hypothalamic-pituitary-adrenal (HPA) axis suppression in systemic and chronic topical therapy.
- May increase serum cholesterol and lipid values.
- May decrease serum protein-bound iodine and thyroxine concentrations.
- Suppresses reactions to allergy skin tests.

POTENTIAL NURSING DIAGNOSES
- Infection, high risk for (side effects).
- Knowledge deficit related to medication regimen (patient/family teaching).

IMPLEMENTATION
- **General Info:** If dose is ordered daily or every other day, administer in the morning to coincide with the body's normal secretion of cortisol.
- **PO:** Administer with meals to minimize gastric irritation.
- **IM:** Shake suspension well before drawing up. IM doses should not be administered when rapid effect is desirable.
- **Direct IV:** Reconstitute with provided solution (Act-O-Vials, Univials, ADD-Vantage vials) or 2 ml of Bacteriostatic Water (with benzyl alcohol) for Injection.
- *Rate:* May be administered direct IV push over 1 to several minutes.
- **Intermittent/Continuous Infusion:** May be diluted further in D5W, 0.9% NaCl, or D5/0.9% NaCl and administered as intermittent or continuous infusion at the prescribed rate. Solution may form a haze upon dilution.

Methylprednisolone Sodium Succinate
- **Syringe Compatibility:** ▪ metoclopramide.
- **Y-Site Compatibility:** ▪ acyclovir ▪ amrinone ▪ enalaprilat ▪ famotidine ▪ fludarabine ▪ meperidine ▪ morphine ▪ vitamin B complex with C.
- **Y-Site Incompatibility:** ▪ ondansetron ▪ sargramostim.

M

- **Additive Compatibility:** ■ heparin ■ theophylline.

PATIENT/FAMILY TEACHING

▢ Instruct patient on correct technique of administration for prescribed form. Patient should take medication exactly as directed and not skip doses or double up on missed doses. Stopping the medication suddenly may result in adrenal insufficiency (anorexia, nausea, fatigue, weakness, hypotension, dyspnea, and hypoglycemia). If these signs appear, notify physician immediately. This can be life-threatening.

▢ Encourage patient on long-term therapy to eat a diet high in protein, calcium, and potassium, and low in sodium and carbohydrates (see Appendix K for foods included).

▢ This drug causes immunosuppression and may mask symptoms of infection. Instruct patient to avoid people with known contagious illnesses and to report possible infections.

▢ Review side effects with patient. Instruct patient to inform physician promptly if severe abdominal pain or tarry stools occur. Patient should also report unusual swelling, weight gain, tiredness, bone pain, bruising, nonhealing sores, visual disturbances, or behavior changes.

▢ Instruct patient to inform physician if symptoms of underlying disease return or worsen.

▢ Advise patient to carry identification in the event of an emergency in which patient cannot relate medical history.

▢ Caution patient to avoid vaccinations without consulting physician.

▢ Emphasize the importance of follow-up examinations to monitor progress and side effects.

EVALUATION

Effectiveness of therapy can be demonstrated by: ■ Suppression of the inflammatory and immune responses in autoimmune disorders and allergic reactions ■ Resolution of the symptoms of adrenal insufficiency.

METHYSERGIDE
(meth-i-**ser**-jide)
Sansert

CLASSIFICATION(S):
Vascular headache suppressant
Pregnancy Category UK

INDICATIONS

■ Prevention of vascular headaches, including migraine headaches and cluster headaches.

ACTION

■ Antiserotonin activity on smooth muscle produces direct vasoconstriction. **Therapeutic Effect:** ■ Prevention of vascular headaches.

PHARMACOKINETICS

Absorption: Rapidly absorbed following oral administration.
Distribution: Widely distributed. Probably enters breast milk.
Metabolism and Excretion: Metabolized by the liver. Some conversion to methylergonovine (an active compound).
Half-life: 10 hr.

CONTRAINDICATIONS AND PRECAUTIONS

Contraindicated in: ■ Hypersensitivity ■ Hypersensitivity to tartrazine (FDC yellow dye #5) ■ Pulmonary disease ■ Severe cardiovascular disease ■ Valvular heart disease ■ Sepsis ■ Peripheral vascular disease ■ Pregnancy, lactation, or children.
Use Cautiously in: ■ Impaired renal or hepatic function ■ Peptic ulcer disease ■ Pruritus ■ Rheumatoid arthritis and related conditions.

ADVERSE REACTIONS AND SIDE EFFECTS*

CNS: insomnia, drowsiness, mild euphoria, lethargy, depression, vertigo, dizziness, ataxia, lightheadedness, restlessness, nervousness, rapid speech, confusion, hallucinations, psychoses.

*<u>Underlines</u> indicate most frequent; **CAPITALS** indicate life-threatening.

EENT: visual disturbances.
Resp: pulmonary fibrosis.
CV: myocardial fibrosis, peripheral vasoconstriction, hypotension, tachycardia, edema.
GI: GI irritation.
Derm: flushing, rashes, dermatitis, thickened skin, itching.
Neuro: peripheral neuropathy.
Misc: retroperitoneal fibrosis.

INTERACTIONS

Drug–Drug: ▪ Additive vasoconstriction with **cocaine,** other **vasopressors,** and heavy **cigarette smoking.**

ROUTE AND DOSAGE

▪ **PO (Adults):** 4–8 mg/day in divided doses (not to be given for more than 6 mo without a 3–4 wk rest period).

AVAILABILITY

▪ *Tablets:* 2 mg.

TIME/ACTION PROFILE (headache prophylaxis)

	ONSET	PEAK	DURATION
PO	1–2 days	UK	1–2 days

NURSING IMPLICATIONS

ASSESSMENT

▫ Assess frequency, location, duration, and characteristics (pain, nausea, vomiting, visual disturbances) of chronic headaches.

▫ Monitor blood pressure and peripheral pulses periodically during therapy. Inform physician if signs of vascular insufficiency or peripheral neuropathy occur.

▫ Assess for signs of ergotism (cold, numb fingers and toes; nausea; vomiting; headache; muscle pain; weakness).

POTENTIAL NURSING DIAGNOSES

▪ Pain [acute] (indications).
▪ Injury, high risk for (side effects).
▪ Knowledge deficit related to medication regimen (patient/family teaching).

IMPLEMENTATION

▪ **PO:** Administer with milk or meals to minimize GI irritation.

PATIENT/FAMILY TEACHING

▫ Instruct patient to take methysergide exactly as directed. If a dose is missed, omit; do not double doses.

▫ Do not discontinue without consulting with physician, as gradual withdrawal over 2–3 wk may be required to prevent rebound headaches. Methysergide should not be used continuously for more than 6 mo. A drug-free interval of 3–4 wk is required with each 6 mo course of therapy.

▫ Methysergide may cause dizziness, lightheadedness, or drowsiness. Caution patient to avoid driving or other activities requiring alertness until response to medication is known.

▫ Instruct patient to report signs of infection to physician promptly.

▫ Advise patient to make position changes slowly to minimize dizziness or lightheadedness.

▫ Caution patient not to smoke and to avoid exposure to cold, as these vasoconstrictors may further impair peripheral circulation.

▫ Advise patient to avoid alcohol, as it may precipitate vascular headaches.

▫ Caution patient to monitor calorie intake; methylsergide may cause weight gain.

EVALUATION

Effectiveness of therapy can be demonstrated by: ▪ Prevention of vascular headaches.

METOCLOPRAMIDE
(met-oh-kloe-**pra**-mide)
{Emex}, Clopra, {Maxeran}, Maxolon, Octamide, Reclomide, Reglan

CLASSIFICATION(S):
Antiemetic, GI stimulant
Pregnancy Category B

M

{} = Available in Canada only.

INDICATIONS

▪ Prevention of chemotherapy-induced emesis ▪ Treatment of postsurgical and diabetic gastric stasis ▪ Facilitation of small bowel intubation in radiographic procedures ▪ Management of esophageal reflux ▪ Treatment and prevention of postoperative nausea and vomiting when nasogastric suctioning is undesirable.

ACTION

▪ Blocks dopamine receptors in chemoreceptor trigger zone of the CNS ▪ Stimulates motility of the upper GI tract and accelerates gastric emptying. **Therapeutic Effects:** ▪ Decreased nausea and vomiting ▪ Decreased symptoms of gastric stasis.

PHARMACOKINETICS

Absorption: Well absorbed from the GI tract, from rectal mucosa and from IM sites.

Distribution: Widely distributed into body tissues and fluids. Crosses blood–brain barrier and placenta. Enters breast milk in concentrations greater than plasma.

Metabolism and Excretion: Partially metabolized by the liver. 25% eliminated unchanged in the urine.

Half-life: 2.5–5 hr.

CONTRAINDICATIONS AND PRECAUTIONS

Contraindicated in: ▪ Hypersensitivity ▪ Possible GI obstruction or hemorrhage ▪ History of seizure disorders ▪ Pheochromocytoma ▪ Parkinson's disease.

Use Cautiously in: ▪ Children and the elderly (increased incidence of extrapyramidal reactions) ▪ Pregnancy and lactation (safety not established) ▪ Patients with a history of depression.

ADVERSE REACTIONS AND SIDE EFFECTS*

CNS: <u>restlessness</u>, <u>drowsiness</u>, <u>fatigue</u>, <u>extrapyramidal reactions</u>, depression, tardive dyskinesia, irritability, anxiety.

CV: arrhythmias.
GI: constipation, diarrhea, nausea, dry mouth.
Endo: gynecomastia.

INTERACTIONS

Drug–Drug: ▪ Additive CNS depression with other **CNS depressants,** including **alcohol, antidepressants, antihistamines, opioid analgesics,** and **sedative/hypnotics** ▪ Diabetics may require adjustments in **insulin** dosing ▪ May affect the GI absorption of other **orally administered drugs** as a result of effect on GI motility ▪ May exaggerate hypotension during **general anesthesia** ▪ Increased risk of extrapyramidal reactions with agents such as **haloperidol** or **phenothiazines** ▪ **Opioid analgesics** and **anticholinergics** may antagonize the GI effects of metoclopramide ▪ May increase absorption and risk of toxicity from **cyclosporine** ▪ Use cautiously with **MAO inhibitors** (causes release of catechol amines) ▪ May increase neuromuscular blockade from **succinylcholine.**

ROUTE AND DOSAGE

Prevention of Chemotherapy-Induced Vomiting
▪ **IV (Adults):** 1–2 mg/kg 30 min prior to chemotherapy. Additional doses of 1–2 mg/kg may be given q 2 hr for 2 doses, then q 3 hr for 3 additional doses.

Facilitation of Small Bowel Intubation (Stimulation of Peristalsis, Improvement of Gastric Emptying)
▪ **IV (Adults):** 10 mg.
▪ **IV (Children 6–14 yr):** 2.5–5 mg (dose should not exceed 0.5 mg/kg).
▪ **IV (Children <6 yr):** 0.1 mg/kg.

Diabetic Gastroparesis
▪ **PO, IM, IV (Adults):** 10 mg 30 min before meals and at bedtime.
▪ **Rectal (Adults):** 25 mg 30–60 min before meals and at bedtime.

Gastroesophageal Reflux
▪ **PO (Adults):** 10–15 mg 30 min before meals and at bedtime (up to 4 times daily, not to exceed 0.5 mg/kg/day).

*<u>Underlines</u> indicate most frequent; **CAPITALS** indicate life-threatening.

Postoperative Nausea/Vomiting
- **IM (Adults):** 10–20 mg.

AVAILABILITY
- **Tablets:** 5 mg, 10 mg ▪ **Syrup:** 5 mg/5 ml ▪ **Injection:** 5 mg/ml.

TIME/ACTION PROFILE (effects on peristalsis)

	ONSET	PEAK	DURATION
PO	30–60 min	UK	1–2 hr
IM	10–15 min	UK	1–2 hr
IV	1–3 min	immediate	1–2 hr

NURSING IMPLICATIONS

ASSESSMENT
- Assess patient for nausea, vomiting, abdominal distention, and bowel sounds prior to and following administration.
- Assess patient for extrapyramidal effects (involuntary movements, facial grimacing, rigidity, shuffling walk, trembling of hands) periodically throughout course of therapy. Extrapyramidal effects are more common in children and the elderly. May be treated with 50 mg of IM diphenhydramine.
- Monitor for tardive dyskinesia (involuntary rhythmic movements of the tongue, face, mouth or jaw, and sometimes extremities). Notify physician immediately if these symptoms occur, as these side effects may be irreversible.
- Assess patient for signs of depression periodically throughout therapy.

POTENTIAL NURSING DIAGNOSES
- Nutrition, altered: less than body requirements (indications).
- Injury, high risk for (side effects).
- Knowledge deficit related to medication regimen (patient/family teaching).

IMPLEMENTATION
- **PO:** Administer doses 30 min before meals and at bedtime.
- **IM:** For prevention of postoperative nausea and vomiting, inject IM near the end of surgery.
- **Rect:** Suppositories may be made by pharmacist. Administer 1 suppository 30–60 min before each meal and at bedtime.
- **Direct IV:** Administer IV dose 30 min prior to administration of chemotherapeutic agent.
- **Rate:** Doses may be given slowly over 1–2 min. Rapid administration causes a transient but intense feeling of anxiety and restlessness followed by drowsiness.
- **Intermittent Infusion:** May be diluted for IV infusion in 50 ml of D5W, 0.9% NaCl, D5/0.45% NaCl, Ringer's solution, or lactated Ringer's solution. Diluted solution is stable for 48 hr if protected from light, or 24 hr under normal light.
- **Rate:** Infuse slowly over at least 15 min.
- **Syringe Compatibility:** ▪ bleomycin ▪ cisplatin ▪ cyclophosphamide ▪ cytarabine ▪ dexamethasone ▪ dimenhydrinate ▪ diphenhydramine ▪ doxorubicin ▪ droperidol ▪ fluorouracil ▪ heparin ▪ hydrocortisone ▪ leucovorin ▪ magnesium sulfate ▪ meperidine ▪ methotrimeprazine ▪ methylprednisolone sodium succinate ▪ midazolam ▪ mitomycin ▪ morphine ▪ vinblastine ▪ vincristine.
- **Syringe Incompatibility:** ▪ calcium gluconate ▪ furosemide ▪ sodium bicarbonate.
- **Y-Site Compatibility:** ▪ acyclovir ▪ bleomycin ▪ cisplatin ▪ cyclophosphamide ▪ doxorubicin ▪ droperidol ▪ famotidine ▪ fluconazole ▪ fludarabine ▪ fluorouracil ▪ foscarnet ▪ heparin ▪ leucovorin ▪ meperidine ▪ methotrexate ▪ mitomycin ▪ morphine ▪ ondansetron ▪ sargramostim ▪ vinblastine ▪ vincristine ▪ zidovudine.
- **Y-Site Incompatibility:** ▪ furosemide.
- **Additive Incompatibility:** ▪ cisplatin.

PATIENT/FAMILY TEACHING
- Instruct patient to take metoclopramide exactly as directed. If a dose is missed, take as soon as remembered if not almost time for next dose.
- Metoclopramide may cause drowsiness. Caution patient to avoid driv-

M

ing or other activities requiring alertness until response to medication is known.
□ Advise patient to avoid concurrent use of alcohol and other CNS depressants while taking this medication.
□ Advise patient to notify physician immediately if involuntary movement of eyes, face, or limbs occurs.

EVALUATION
Effectiveness of therapy can be demonstrated by: ▪ Prevention or relief of nausea and vomiting ▪ Decreased symptoms of gastric stasis ▪ Facilitation of small bowel intubation ▪ Decreased symptoms of esophageal reflux.

METOCURINE
(me-toe-**cure**-een)
Metubine

CLASSIFICATION(S):
Neuromuscular blocking agent
(nondepolarizing)
Pregnancy Category C

INDICATIONS
▪ Production of skeletal muscle paralysis after induction of anesthesia in surgical procedures ▪ Adjunct to electroconvulsive therapy.

ACTION
▪ Prevents neuromuscular transmission by blocking the effect of acetylcholine at the myoneural junction. **Therapeutic Effect:** ▪ Skeletal muscle paralysis. Has no anxiolytic or analgesic effects.

PHARMACOKINETICS
Absorption: Administered IV only, resulting in complete bioavailability.
Distribution: Extensively distributed. Crosses the placenta.
Metabolism and Excretion: 50% excreted unchanged in urine.
Half-life: 3.6 hr.

CONTRAINDICATIONS AND PRECAUTIONS
Contraindicated in: ▪ Hypersensitivity to metocurine, iodides, or phenol.
Use Cautiously in: ▪ History of pulmonary disease, renal or hepatic impairment ▪ Elderly patients (recovery time may be increased, dosage requirements may vary) ▪ Myasthenia gravis or myasthenic syndromes (prolonged respiratory paralysis).

ADVERSE REACTIONS AND SIDE EFFECTS*
EENT: excess salivation.
Resp: bronchospasm, APNEA.
CV: hypotension, arrhythmias.
GI: decreased GI tone, decreased GI motility.
MS: muscle weakness.
Misc: allergic reactions.

INTERACTIONS
Drug–Drug: ▪ Intensity and duration of paralysis may be prolonged by pretreatment with **succinylcholine, general anesthesia, aminoglycoside antibiotics, polymixin B, colistin, clindamycin, lidocaine, quinidine, procainamide, beta-adrenergic blocking agents, potassium-losing diuretics,** and **magnesium** ▪ **Ether, methoxyflurane, halothane, enflurane,** or **isoflurane** increase intensity and duration of action (dosage reduction of 33–50% recommended) ▪ **Doxapram** masks residual effects.

ROUTE AND DOSAGE
Surgery
▪ **IV (Adults):** 150–400 mcg/kg initially, may give additional doses of 0.5–1 mg.

Adjunct to Electroconvulsive Therapy
▪ **IV (Adults):** 2–3 mg (range 1.75–5.5 mg).

AVAILABILITY
▪ *Injection:* 2 mg/ml.

---

*Underlines indicate most frequent; **CAPITALS** indicate life-threatening.

TIME/ACTION PROFILE (skeletal muscle paralysis)

	ONSET	PEAK	DURATION
IV	within min	6 min	25–90 min*

*Total recovery of function may take several hr.

NURSING IMPLICATIONS

ASSESSMENT

□ Assess respiratory status continuously throughout metocurine therapy. Metocurine should be used only by individuals experienced in endotracheal intubation, and equipment for this procedure should be immediately available.

□ Neuromuscular response to metocurine should be monitored with a peripheral nerve stimulator. Paralysis is initially selective and usually occurs consecutively in the following muscles: levator muscles of eyelids, muscles of mastication, limb muscles, abdominal muscles, muscles of the glottis, intercostal muscles, and the diaphragm. Recovery of muscle function usually occurs in reverse order.

□ Observe the patient for residual muscle weakness and respiratory distress during the recovery period.

▪ **Toxicity and Overdose:** If overdose occurs use peripheral nerve stimulator to determine the degree of neuromuscular blockade. Maintain airway patency and ventilation until recovery of normal respirations occurs.

□ Administration of anticholinesterase agents (edrophonium, neostigmine, pyridostigmine) may be used to antagonize the action of metocurine. Atropine is usually administered prior to or concurrently with anticholinesterase agents to counteract the muscarinic effects.

□ Administration of fluids and vasopressors may be necessary to treat severe hypotension or shock.

POTENTIAL NURSING DIAGNOSES

▪ Breathing pattern, ineffective (indications).

▪ Communication, impaired verbal (side effects).

▪ Fear (side effects).

IMPLEMENTATION

▪ **General Info:** Dose is titrated to patient response.

□ Metocurine has no effect on consciousness or the pain threshold. Adequate anesthesia should *always* be used when metocurine is used as an adjunct to surgical procedures.

▪ **Direct IV:** Administer over 30–60 sec. Relaxation from initial dose lasts 25–90 min (average 60 min), administer supplemental doses of 0.5–1 mg as needed.

▪ **Syringe Incompatibility:** ▪ barbiturates ▪ meperidine ▪ morphine ▪ sodium bicarbonate.

PATIENT/FAMILY TEACHING

□ Explain all procedures to patient receiving metocurine therapy without anesthesia, as consciousness is not affected by metocurine alone.

□ Reassure patient that communication abilities will return as the medication wears off.

EVALUATION

Effectiveness of therapy can be demonstrated by: ▪ Adequate suppression of the twitch response when tested with peripheral nerve stimulation and subsequent muscle paralysis.

METOLAZONE
(me-**tole**-a-zone)
Mykrox, Zaroxolyn

CLASSIFICATION(S):
Diuretic (thiazide-like), Antihypertensive
Pregnancy Category B

INDICATIONS

▪ Used alone or in combination with other agents in the management of mild to moderate hypertension ▪ Used alone or in combination in the treatment of

M

edema associated with congestive heart failure or the nephrotic syndrome (Zaroxolyn only).

ACTION

- Increases excretion of sodium and water by inhibiting sodium reabsorption in the distal tubule - Promotes excretion of chloride, potassium, magnesium, and bicarbonate - May produce arteriolar dilation. **Therapeutic Effects:** - Lowering of blood pressure in hypertensive patients - Diuresis with subsequent mobilization of edema. Effect may continue in renal impairment.

PHARMACOKINETICS

Absorption: Absorption is more rapid and more complete with prompt tablet (Mykrox). Absorption is more variable with extended tablet (Zaroxolyn).
Distribution: Distribution not known.
Metabolism and Excretion: Excreted mainly unchanged by the kidneys.
Half-life: Extended tablet—8 hr, prompt tablet—14 hr.

CONTRAINDICATIONS AND PRECAUTIONS

Contraindicated in: - Hypersensitivity - Cross-sensitivity with other sulfonamides may exist - Anuria - Lactation.
Use Cautiously in: - Severe hepatic impairment - Pregnancy or children (safety not established) - Elderly patients (increased sensitivity).

ADVERSE REACTIONS AND SIDE EFFECTS*

CNS: drowsiness, lethargy.
CV: hypotension, palpitations, chest pain.
Derm: rashes, photosensitivity.
Endo: hyperglycemia.
F and E: hypokalemia, hypochloremic alkalosis, hyponatremia, hypercalcemia, hypophosphatemia, hypomagnesemia, dehydration, hypovolemia.
GI: anorexia, nausea, vomiting, cramping, hepatitis, bloating.
Hemat: blood dyscrasias.
Metab: hyperuricemia.

MS: muscle cramps.
Misc: pancreatitis, chills.

INTERACTIONS

Drug–Drug: - Additive hypotension with **nitrates, acute ingestion of alcohol** or other **antihypertensives** - Additive hypokalemia with **glucocorticoids, amphotericin B, azlocillin, mezlocillin, piperacillin,** or **ticarcillin** - By causing hypokalemia, may increase the risk of **cardiac glycoside** toxicity - Decreases the excretion of **lithium,** may cause toxicity - May decrease the effectiveness of **methenamine**.
Drug–Food: - **Food** may increase extent of absorption.

ROUTE AND DOSAGE

Mykrox
- PO (Adults): 0.5–1 mg/day.

Zaroxolyn
- PO (Adults): *hypertension*—2.5–5 mg/day, *edema*—5–20 mg/day.

AVAILABILITY

- *Mykrox tablets:* 0.5 mg - *Zaroxolyn tablets:* 2.5 mg, 5 mg, 10 mg.

TIME/ACTION PROFILE (noted for diuretic effect, full antihypertensive effect may take days–wk)

	ONSET	PEAK	DURATION
PO (extended tab)	1 hr	2 hr	12–24 hr
PO (prompt tab)	UK	2 hr	12–24 hr

NURSING IMPLICATIONS

ASSESSMENT

- Monitor blood pressure, intake and output, and daily weight and assess feet, legs, and sacral area for edema daily.
- Assess patient, especially if taking cardiac glycosides, for anorexia, nausea, vomiting, muscle cramps, paresthesia, and confusion. Patients receiving cardiac glycosides are at increased risk of digitalis toxicity due to the potassium-depleting effect of the diuretic.

*Underlines indicate most frequent; CAPITALS indicate life-threatening.

□ Assess patient for allergy to sulfon-amides.

■ **Lab Test Considerations:** Monitor electrolytes (especially potassium), blood glucose, BUN, and serum uric acid levels prior to and periodically throughout course of therapy.

□ May cause increase in serum and urine glucose in diabetic patients.

□ May cause an increase in serum bili-rubin, calcium, and uric acid and a decrease in serum magnesium, potas-sium, and sodium levels.

POTENTIAL NURSING DIAGNOSES

■ Fluid volume excess (indications).
■ Fluid volume deficit (side effects).
■ Knowledge deficit related to medica-tion regimen (patient/family teach-ing).

IMPLEMENTATION

■ **General Info:** Administer in the morn-ing to prevent disruption of sleep cycle.

□ Intermittent dose schedule may be used for continued control of edema.

□ Extended (Zaroxolyn) and prompt (Mykrox) metolazone tablets are not equal. Do not substitute.

■ **PO:** May give with food or milk to minimize GI irritation.

PATIENT/FAMILY TEACHING

□ Instruct patient to take this medica-tion at the same time each day. If a dose is missed, take as soon as re-membered, but not just before next dose is due. Do not double doses. Ad-vise patients using metolazone for hypertension to continue taking the medication even if feeling better. Medication controls but does not cure hypertension.

□ Encourage patient to comply with ad-ditional interventions for hyperten-sion (weight reduction, low sodium diet, regular exercise, smoking cessa-tion, moderation of alcohol consump-tion, and stress management).

□ Instruct patient to monitor weight biweekly and to notify physician of significant changes. Instruct patients with hypertension in correct tech-nique for monitoring weekly blood pressure.

□ Caution patient to make position changes slowly to minimize ortho-static hypotension. This may be po-tentiated by alcohol.

□ Advise patient to use sunscreen (avoid those containing PABA) and protective clothing when in the sun to prevent photosensitivity reactions.

□ Instruct patient to follow a diet high in potassium (see Appendix K).

□ Advise patient to consult physician or pharmacist before taking over-the-counter medication concurrently with this therapy.

□ Advise patient to report muscle weak-ness, cramps, nausea, or dizziness to the physician.

□ Instruct patient to notify physician or dentist of medication regimen prior to treatment or surgery.

□ Emphasize the importance of routine follow-up examinations.

EVALUATION

Effectiveness of therapy can be demon-strated by: ■ Decrease in blood pressure ■ Increase in urine output □ Decrease in edema.

METOPROLOL
(me-**toe**-proe-lole)
{Apo-Metoprolol}, {Betaloc}, {Betaloc Durules}, Lopressor, {Lopressor SR}, {Novometoprol}, Toprol XL

CLASSIFICATION(S):
Antihypertensive, Antianginal, Beta-adrenergic blocker (selective)
Pregnancy Category C

INDICATIONS

■ **PO:** Used alone or in combination with other agents in the treatment of hypertension and angina pectoris ■ **PO, IV:** Treatment of myocardial infarction.

M

Unlabeled Uses: ▪ Prophylaxis and treatment of arrhythmias ▪ Treatment of hypertrophic cardiomyopathy ▪ Tremors ▪ Symptomatic treatment of pheochromocytoma ▪ Prevention of vascular headaches.

ACTION

▪ Blocks stimulation of beta$_1$ (myocardial) adrenergic receptors with less effect on beta$_2$ (pulmonary, vascular, or uterine) receptor sites. **Therapeutic Effects:** ▪ Decreased heart rate ▪ Decreased blood pressure.

PHARMACOKINETICS

Absorption: Well absorbed following oral administration.
Distribution: Crosses the blood–brain barrier. Crosses the placenta, and small amounts enter breast milk.
Metabolism and Excretion: Mostly metabolized by the liver, mostly on first pass through.
Half-life: 3–7 hr.

CONTRAINDICATIONS AND PRECAUTIONS

Contraindicated in: ▪ Uncompensated congestive heart failure ▪ Pulmonary edema ▪ Cardiogenic shock ▪ Bradycardia or heart block.
Use Cautiously in: ▪ Pregnancy (may cause apnea, low Apgar scores, bradycardia, and hypoglycemia in the newborn) ▪ Hyperthyroidism (may mask symptoms) ▪ Diabetes mellitus (may mask signs of hypoglycemia) ▪ Lactation or children (safety not established) ▪ Patients with a history of severe allergic reactions (intensity of reactions may be increased).

ADVERSE REACTIONS AND SIDE EFFECTS*

CNS: <u>fatigue</u>, <u>weakness</u>, dizziness, <u>depression</u>, memory loss, mental changes, nightmares.
EENT: blurred vision.

Resp: bronchospasm, wheezing.
CV: BRADYCARDIA, CONGESTIVE HEART FAILURE, PULMONARY EDEMA, peripheral vasoconstriction.
GI: constipation, diarrhea, nausea.
GU: impotence, diminished libido.
Endo: hyperglycemia, hypoglycemia.

INTERACTIONS

Drug–Drug: ▪ **General anesthesia, IV phenytoin,** and **verapamil** may cause additive myocardial depression ▪ Additive bradycardia may occur with concurrent use of **cardiac glycosides** ▪ Additive hypotension may occur with other **antihypertensive agents,** acute ingestion of **alcohol,** or **nitrates** ▪ Concurrent use with **amphetamines, cocaine, ephedrine, epinephrine, norepinephrine, phenylephrine,** or **pseudoephedrine** may result in excess alpha-adrenergic stimulation, hypertension, and bradycardia ▪ May produce hypertension within 14 days of **MAO inhibitor** therapy ▪ May negate the beneficial beta$_1$ cardiac effects of **dopamine** or **dobutamine** ▪ Concurrent **thyroid** administration may decrease effectiveness ▪ Use with **insulin** may result in prolonged hypoglycemia.

ROUTE AND DOSAGE

Chronic Treatment of Hypertension, Angina

▪ **PO (Adults):** 100–450 mg/day— single dose or bid. Extended-release tablets (Toprol XL) are given once daily.

Myocardial Infarction Prophylaxis—Acute Treatment

▪ **IV, PO (Adults):** 5 mg q 2 min IV for 3 doses. 15 min after last IV dose, start 50 mg PO q 6 hr for 48 hr, then 100 mg bid.

AVAILABILITY

▪ *Tablets:* 50 mg, 100 mg ▪ *Extended-release tablets (Toprol XL):* 50 mg, 100 mg, 200 mg ▪ *Injection:* 1 mg/ml.

---

*<u>Underlines</u> indicate most frequent; **CAPITALS** indicate life-threatening.

TIME/ACTION PROFILE (PO = hypotensive effects, IV = beta-adrenergic blockade)

	ONSET	PEAK	DURATION
PO*	15 min	UK hr	6–12 hr
PO-ER	UK	UK	24 hr
IV	immediate	20 min	5–8 hr

*Maximal effects on blood pressure during chronic therapy may not occur for 1 wk. Hypotensive effects may persist for up to 4 wk after discontinuation.

NURSING IMPLICATIONS

ASSESSMENT

- **General Info:** Monitor intake and output ratios and daily weight. Assess patient routinely for evidence of congestive heart failure (peripheral edema, dyspnea, rales/crackles, fatigue, weight gain, jugular venous distention).
- **Hypertension:** Monitor blood pressure and pulse frequently during period of adjustment and periodically throughout therapy. Confer with physician prior to giving drug if pulse is <50 bpm. Vital signs and ECG should be monitored every 5–15 min during and for several hours after parenteral administration. If heart rate <40 bpm, especially if cardiac output is also decreased, administer atropine 0.25–0.5 mg IV.
- **Angina:** Assess frequency and duration of episodes of chest pain throughout therapy.
- **Lab Test Considerations:** May occasionally cause elevations in serum potassium, uric acid, lipoprotein levels, and BUN.
- Hepatic and renal function and CBC should be monitored periodically in patients receiving prolonged therapy. May cause elevated serum transaminase, alkaline phosphatase, and LDH.

POTENTIAL NURSING DIAGNOSES

- Cardiac output, decreased (indications, adverse reactions).
- Knowledge deficit related to medication regimen (patient/family teaching).

- Noncompliance (patient/family teaching).

IMPLEMENTATION

- **PO:** Administer medication with meals or directly after eating.
- Extended release tablets should be swallowed whole; do not crush, break, or chew.
- **Direct IV:** May be administered by injecting 5 mg slowly over 2 min.
- **Y-Site Compatibility:** ■ meperidine ■ morphine.

PATIENT/FAMILY TEACHING

- Instruct patient to take medication exactly as directed, even if feeling well. If a dose is missed, it may be taken as soon as remembered up to 4 hr before next dose. Abrupt withdrawal may result in life-threatening arrhythmias, hypertension, or myocardial ischemia.
- Teach patient and family how to check pulse and blood pressure. Instruct them to take pulse daily and blood pressure biweekly. Advise patient to withhold dose and contact physician if pulse is <50 bpm or blood pressure changes significantly.
- Reinforce need to continue additional therapies for hypertension (weight loss, restricted sodium intake, stress reduction, regular exercise, moderation of alcohol consumption, and cessation of smoking). Metoprolol controls but does not cure hypertension.
- Caution patient that this medication may cause increased sensitivity to cold.
- Advise patient to consult physician before taking any over-the-counter drugs, especially cold remedies, concurrently with this medication. Patients on antihypertensive therapy should also avoid excessive amounts of coffee, tea, and cola.
- Diabetics should monitor serum glucose closely, especially if weakness, fatigue, or irritability occurs. Medication does not block sweating as a sign of hypoglycemia.
- Metoprolol may cause dizziness, drowsiness, or blurred vision. Cau-

M

tion patient to avoid driving or other activities requiring alertness until response to medication is known.

▫ Instruct patient to inform physician or dentist of this therapy prior to treatment or surgery.

▫ Advise patient to carry identification describing medication regimen at all times.

▫ Instruct patient to notify physician if slow pulse rate, dizziness, lightheadedness, depression, rash, fever, sore throat, unusual bleeding or brusing, or signs of congestive heart failure occur.

EVALUATION
Effectiveness of therapy can be demonstrated by: ▪ Decrease in blood pressure ▪ Reduction in frequency of anginal attacks and improved exercise tolerance ▪ Prevention of myocardial infarction.

METRONIDAZOLE
(me-troe-**ni**-da-zole)
{Apo-Metronidazole}, Flagyl, Metizol, Metric 21, MetroGel, Metro IV, Metryl, Metryl IV, {Neo-Metric}, {Novonidazol}, {PMS Metronidazole}, Protostat, Satric, {Trikacide}

CLASSIFICATION(S):
Anti-infective
Pregnancy Category B

INDICATIONS

▪ **PO, IV:** Treatment of the following anaerobic infections: ▫ Intra-abdominal infections ▫ Gynecologic infections ▫ Skin and skin structure infections ▫ Lower respiratory tract infections ▫ Bone and joint infections ▫ CNS infections ▫ Septicemia ▫ Endocarditis ▪ **IV:** Perioperative prophylactic agent in colorectal surgery ▪ **PO:** Amebicode in the management of amebic dysentery, amebic liver abscess, and trichomoniasis ▪ **Topical:** Treatment of

acne rosacea ▪ **Vaginal:** Management of bacterial vaginosis. **Unlabeled Use:** ▪ Giardiasis.

ACTION

▪ Disrupts DNA and protein synthesis in susceptible organisms. **Therapeutic Effects:** ▪ Bactericidal, trichomonacidal, or amebicidal action. **Spectrum:** ▪ Most notable for activity against anaerobic bacteria, including: ▫ *Bacteroides* ▫ *Clostridium* ▪ In addition, is active against: ▫ *Trichomonas vaginalis* ▫ *Entamoeba histolytica* ▫ *Giardia lambdia.*

PHARMACOKINETICS

Absorption: 80% absorbed following oral administration. Minimal absorption following topical vaginal application.
Distribution: Widely distributed into most tissues and fluids, including CSF. Crosses the placenta and enters breast milk in concentrations equal to plasma levels.
Metabolism and Excretion: Partially metabolized by the liver (30–60%), partially excreted unchanged in the urine, 6–15% eliminated in the feces.
Half-life: 6–8 hr.

CONTRAINDICATIONS AND PRECAUTIONS

Contraindicated in: ▪ Hypersensitivity ▪ Hypersensitivity to parabens (topical only) ▪ First trimester of pregnancy.
Use Cautiously in: ▪ History of blood dyscrasias ▪ Children (safe use of IV form not established; safety of oral form for infections other than amebiasis in children not established) ▪ Pregnancy (although safety not established, has been used to treat trichomoniasis in second- and third-trimester pregnancy—but not as single-dose regimen) ▪ Lactation (if needed, use single dose and interrupt nursing for 24 hr thereafter) ▪ History of seizures or neurologic problems ▪ Severe hepatic impairment (dosage reduction suggested).

{} = Available in Canada only.

ADVERSE REACTIONS AND SIDE EFFECTS*

CNS: <u>headache</u>, vertigo, SEIZURES, <u>dizziness</u>.

EENT: tearing (top only).

GI: <u>nausea</u>, <u>vomiting</u>, <u>abdominal pain</u>, anorexia, dry mouth, <u>diarrhea</u>, unpleasant taste, furry tongue, glossitis.

Derm: transient redness, mild dryness, burning, skin irritation (top only), urticaria, rashes.

Hemat: leukopenia.

Local: phlebitis at IV site.

Neuro: peripheral neuropathy.

Misc: superinfection.

INTERACTIONS

Drug–Drug: ▪ **Cimetidine** may decrease the metabolism of metronidazole ▪ **Phenobarbital** increases metabolism and may decrease effectiveness ▪ Metronidazole increases the effects of **oral anticoagulants** ▪ Disulfiram-like reaction may occur with **alcohol** ingestion ▪ May cause acute psychosis and confusion with **disulfiram** ▪ Increased risk of leukopenia with **fluorouracil** or **azathioprine**.

ROUTE AND DOSAGE

Flagyl IV RTU contains 14 mEq of sodium/500 mg metronidazole.

Anaerobic Infections

▪ **PO (Adults):** 7.5 mg/kg q 6 hr (not to exceed 4 g/day).

▪ **IV (Adults):** Initial dose 15 mg/kg, then 7.5 mg/kg q 6 hr (not to exceed 4 g/day).

Trichomoniasis

▪ **PO (Adults):** 250 mg q 8 hr for 7 days (single 2-g dose or 1 g bid for 1 day may be used).

▪ **PO (Children):** 15 mg/kg/day in 3 divided doses q 8 hr for 7–10 days.

Perioperative Prophylaxis

▪ **IV (Adults):** Initial dose 15 mg/kg 1 hr prior to surgery, then 7.5 mg/kg 6 and 12 hr later.

Amebiasis

▪ **PO (Adults):** 500–750 mg q 8 hr for 5–10 days.

▪ **PO (Children):** 35–50 mg/kg/day in 3 divided doses q 8 hr for 5–10 days.

▪ **IV (Adults):** 500–750 mg q 8 hr for 5–10 days.

Acne Rosacea

▪ **Top (Adults):** Apply thin film to affected area bid.

Bacterial Vaginosis

▪ **Vaginal:** 5 g bid for 5 days.

AVAILABILITY

▪ *Tablets:* 250 mg, 500 mg ▪ *Injection:* 500 mg ▪ *Topical gel:* 0.75% ▪ *Vaginal gel:* 0.75%.

TIME/ACTION PROFILE

(PO, IV = blood levels,
Top = improvement in rosacea)

	ONSET	PEAK
PO	rapid	1–3 hr
IV	rapid	end of infusion
Top	3 wk	9 wk

NURSING IMPLICATIONS

ASSESSMENT

▪ **General Info:** Assess patient for infection (vital signs; appearance of wound, sputum, urine, and stool; WBC) at beginning and throughout course of therapy.

▫ Obtain specimens for culture and sensitivity prior to initiating therapy. First dose may be given before receiving results.

▫ Monitor neurologic status during and after IV infusions. Inform physician if numbness, paresthesia, weakness, ataxia, or convulsions occur.

▫ Monitor intake and output and daily weight, especially for patients on sodium restriction. Each 500 mg of Flagyl IV for dilution contains 5 mEq of sodium; each 500 mg of Flagyl RTU contains 14 mEq of sodium.

▪ **Giardiasis:** Monitor 3 stool samples taken several days apart beginning 1–2 wk following treatment.

▪ **Lab Test Considerations:** May cause low serum AST (SGOT) levels.

M

*Underlines indicate most frequent; **CAPITALS** indicate life-threatening.

POTENTIAL NURSING DIAGNOSES
- Infection, high risk for (indications).
- Diarrhea (indications).
- Knowledge deficit related to medication regimen (patient/family teaching).

IMPLEMENTATION
- **PO:** Administer with food or milk to minimize GI irritation. Tablets may be crushed for patients with difficulty swallowing.
- **Intermittent Infusion:** Flagyl IV RTU is prediluted and ready to use (5 mg/ml). Prefilled plastic minibags should not be used in series connections, as air embolism may result. Crystals may form during refrigeration but will dissolve when warmed to room temperature.
- □ Preparation of Flagyl IV requires a specific process. Do not use aluminum needles or hubs; color will turn orange/rust. Add 4.4 ml of Sterile or Bacteriostatic Sterile Water, or 0.9% or bacteriostatic 0.9% NaCl for Injection (100 mg/ml). Solution should be clear, pale yellow-green. Do not use cloudy or precipitated solution. Dilute further to at least 8 mg/ml with 0.9% NaCl, D5W, or lactated Ringer's solution. Neutralize solution with 5 mEq sodium bicarbonate for each 500 mg. Mix thoroughly. Carbon dioxide gas will be generated and may require venting. Do not refrigerate. Stable for 24 hr at room temperature.
- **Rate:** Administer IV doses as a slow infusion, each single dose over 1 hr.
- **Y-Site Incompatibility:** Manufacturer recommends discontinuing primary IV during metronidazole infusion.
- **Additive Incompatibility:** Do not admix with other medications.
- **Top:** Cleanse affected area prior to application. Apply and rub in a thin film twice daily, morning, and evening. Avoid contact with eyes.

PATIENT/FAMILY TEACHING
- □ Instruct patient to take medication exactly as directed with evenly spaced times between doses, even if feeling better. Do not skip doses or double up on missed doses. If a dose is missed, take as soon as remembered if not almost time for next dose.
- □ Advise patients treated for trichomoniasis that sexual partners may be asymptomatic sources of reinfection and should be treated concurrently. Patient should also refrain from intercourse or use a condom to prevent reinfection.
- □ Caution patients to avoid intake of alcoholic beverages or alcohol-containing preparations during and for at least 1 day following treatment with metronidazole, including vaginal gel. May cause a disulfiram-like reaction (flushing, nausea, vomiting, headache, abdominal cramps).
- □ May cause dizziness or lightheadedness. Caution patient to avoid driving or other activities requiring alertness until response to medication is known.
- □ Inform patient that medication may cause an unpleasant metallic taste.
- □ Advise patient not to take over-the-counter medications concurrently without advice of the physician or pharmacist.
- □ Advise patient that frequent mouth rinses, good oral hygiene, and sugarless gum or candy may minimize dry mouth. Notify physician or dentist if dry mouth persists for more than 2 wk.
- □ Advise patient to inform physician if pregnancy is suspected prior to taking this medication.
- □ Inform patient that medication may cause urine to turn dark.
- □ Advise patient to consult physician if no improvement in a few days or if signs and symptoms of superinfection (black, furry overgrowth on tongue; vaginal itching or discharge; loose or foul-smelling stools) develop.
- **Vag:** Instruct patient in correct technique for intravaginal instillation. Advise patient to avoid intercourse during treatment with vaginal gel.
- **Top:** Instruct patient on correct technique for application of topical gel.

Cosmetics may be used following application of gel.

EVALUATION

Effectiveness of therapy can be demonstrated by: ▪ Resolution of the signs and symptoms of infection. Length of time for complete resolution depends on organism and site of infection ◻ Significant results should be seen in 3 wk of application of topical gel. Application may be continued for 9 wk.

MEXILETINE
(mex-il-e-teen)
Mexitil

CLASSIFICATION(S):
Antiarrhythmic (group IB)
Pregnancy Category C

INDICATIONS

▪ Prophylaxis and treatment of serious ventricular arrhythmias, including VT and PVCs.

ACTION

▪ Decreases the duration of the action potential and effective refractory period in cardiac conduction tissue by altering transport of sodium across myocardial cell membranes ▪ Has little or no effect on heart rate. **Therapeutic Effect:** ▪ Control of ventricular arrhythmias.

PHARMACOKINETICS

Absorption: Well absorbed from the GI tract.

Distribution: Enters breast milk in concentrations similar to plasma.

Metabolism and Excretion: Mostly metabolized by the liver. 10% excreted unchanged by the kidneys.

Half-life: 10–12 hr.

CONTRAINDICATIONS AND PRECAUTIONS

Contraindicated in: ▪ Hypersensitivity ▪ Cardiogenic shock ▪ 2nd- or 3rd-degree heart block (if a pacemaker has not been inserted) ▪ Lactation.

Use Cautiously in: ▪ Sinus node or intraventricular conduction abnormalities ▪ Hypotension ▪ Congestive heart failure ▪ Severe hepatic impairment (dosage reduction suggested) ▪ Pregnancy or children (safety not established).

ADVERSE REACTIONS AND SIDE EFFECTS*

CNS: dizziness, lightheadedness, nervousness.

EENT: blurred vision, tinnitus.

CV: arrhythmias, palpitations, chest pain, headache, change in sleep habits, fatigue, confusion, edema.

GI: HEPATIC NECROSIS, nausea, vomiting, heartburn.

Derm: rashes.

Hemat: blood dyscrasias.

Neuro: tremor, coordination difficulties, paresthesia.

Resp: dyspnea.

INTERACTIONS

Drug–Drug: ▪ **Opioid analgesics, atropine,** and **antacids** may slow absorption ▪ **Metoclopramide** may speed absorption ▪ **Phenytoin, rifampin, cigarette smoking,** or **phenobarbital** may increase metabolism and decrease effectiveness ▪ **Cimetidine** may slow metabolism and increase toxicity ▪ Additive cardiac effects may occur with other **antiarrythmics** ▪ **Drugs that drastically alter urine pH** may alter blood levels (alkalinization increases reabsorption and blood levels; acidification increases excretion and decreases blood levels).

Drug–Food: ▪ **Foods that drastically alter urine pH** (see Appendix K) may alter blood levels. Alkalinization increases reabsorption and increases blood levels. Acidification increases excretion and may decrease effectiveness (see Appendix K).

ROUTE AND DOSAGE

▪ **PO (Adults):** 400 mg loading dose initially, then 200 mg 8 hr later, then 200–400 mg q 8 hr. If controlled on

M

*Underlines indicate most frequent; **CAPITALS** indicate life-threatening.

≤300 mg q 8 hr, can give same daily dose at 12-hr intervals (not to exceed 1200 mg/day). Some patients may require q 6 hr dosing.

AVAILABILITY

- *Capsules:* 150 mg, 200 mg, 250 mg.

TIME/ACTION PROFILE (antiarrhythmic effects, provided a loading dose has been given)

	ONSET	PEAK	DURATION
PO	30 min–2 hr	2–3 hr	8–12 hr

NURSING IMPLICATIONS

ASSESSMENT

- ▢ Monitor pulse, blood pressure, and ECG periodically throughout course of therapy. Continuous Holter monitoring and chest x-ray examinations may be necessary to determine efficacy and aid in dosage adjustment.
- Lab Test Considerations: May occasionally cause a positive ANA test result.
- ▢ May cause a transient increase in AST (SGOT) concentrations.
- ▢ May cause thrombocytopenia within a few days after initiation of therapy. Blood counts usually return to normal within 1 mo after discontinuation of therapy.
- Toxicity and Overdose: Serum mexiletine concentrations may be determined during dosage adjustment. Incidence of side effects is greater with concentrations >2 mcg/ml.

POTENTIAL NURSING DIAGNOSES

- Cardiac output, decreased (indications).
- Knowledge deficit related to medication regimen (patient/family teaching).

IMPLEMENTATION

- General Info: When changing from other antiarrhythmic therapy, give the first dose of mexiletine 6–12 hr after the last dose of quinidine, 3–6 hr after last dose of procainamide, or 8–12 hr after last dose of tocainide. When changing from parenteral lidocaine,

decrease lidocaine dose or discontinue lidocaine 1–2 hr after administration of mexiletine or administer lower initial doses of mexiletine.
- ▢ Transfer of patients with life-threatening arrhythmias from other antiarrhythmic agents to mexiletine should be managed in the hospital.
- PO: Administer with food or antacids to minimize GI irritation.

PATIENT/FAMILY TEACHING

- ▢ Advise patient to take medication exactly as directed, at evenly spaced intervals, even if feeling well. Missed doses should be taken within 4 hr or omitted. Do not skip or double up on missed doses.
- ▢ Teach patients to monitor pulse. Advise patient to contact physician if pulse rate is <50 bpm or becomes irregular.
- ▢ Mexiletine may cause dizziness and lightheadedness. Caution patient to avoid driving and other activities requiring alertness until response to medication is known.
- ▢ Instruct patient to avoid changes in diet that may drastically acidify or alkalinize the urine (see Appendix K for foods included).
- ▢ Advise patient to notify physician or dentist of disease process and medication regimen prior to treatment or surgery.
- ▢ Advise patient to notify physician if general tiredness, yellowing of the skin or eyes, fever, sore throat, or persistent side effects occur.
- ▢ Patient should carry identification describing disease process and medication regimen at all times.

EVALUATION

Effectiveness of therapy can be demonstrated by: ■ Decrease in frequency or resolution of serious ventricular arrhythmias.

MEZLOCILLIN
(mez-loe-**sill**-in)
Mezlin

INDICATIONS

- Treatment of serious infections due to susceptible organisms, including: □ Skin and skin structure infections □ Bone and joint infections □ Septicemia □ Respiratory tract infections □ Intra-abdominal, gynecologic, and urinary tract infections ▪ Combination with an aminoglycoside may be synergistic against *Pseudomonas* ▪ Has been combined with other antibiotics in the treatment of infections in immunosuppressed patients.

ACTION

- Binds to bacterial cell wall membrane, causing cell death. **Therapeutic Effect:** ▪ Bactericidal against susceptible bacteria. **Spectrum:** ▪ Spectrum similar to penicillin but greatly extended to include several important gram-negative aerobic pathogens, notably: □ *Pseudomonas aeruginosa* □ *Escherichia coli* □ *Proteus mirabilis* □ *Providencia rettgeri* ▪ Also active against some anaerobic bacteria, including *Bacteroides* ▪ Not active against penicillinase-producing staphylococci or beta-lactamase–producing Enterobacteriaceae.

PHARMACOKINETICS

Absorption: Well absorbed from IM sites.
Distribution: Widely distributed. Enters CSF well only when meninges are inflamed. Crosses the placenta and enters breast milk in low concentrations.
Metabolism and Excretion: 55–60% excreted unchanged by the kidneys. Small amounts metabolized by the liver. 15–30% excreted in the bile.
Half-life: 0.7–1.3 hr (increased in renal impairment).

CONTRAINDICATIONS AND PRECAUTIONS

Contraindicated in: ▪ Hypersensitivity to penicillins or cephalosporins.
Use Cautiously in: ▪ Severe renal impairment (increase dosing interval if creatinine clearance <30 ml/min) ▪ Pregnancy and lactation (safety not established) ▪ Severe liver disease.

ADVERSE REACTIONS AND SIDE EFFECTS*

CNS: confusion, lethargy, SEIZURES (high doses).
CV: congestive heart failure, arrhythmias.
GI: nausea, diarrhea.
GU: hematuria (children only).
Derm: rashes, urticaria.
F and E: hypokalemia, hypernatremia.
Hemat: bleeding, blood dyscrasias, increased bleeding time.
Local: phlebitis at IV site, pain at IM site.
Metab: metabolic alkalosis.
Misc: superinfection, hypersensitivity reactions, including ANAPHYLAXIS and serum sickness.

INTERACTIONS

Drug–Drug: ▪ **Probenecid** decreases renal excretion and increases blood levels ▪ May alter excretion of **lithium** ▪ **Diuretics** may increase the risk of hypokalemia ▪ Hypokalemia increases the risk of **cardiac glycoside** toxicity.

ROUTE AND DOSAGE

Contains 1.85 mEq sodium/g.

- **IV (Adults):** 3–4 g q 4–6 hr.
- **IM (Adults):** 1.5–2 g q 6 hr.
- **IV (Children 1 mo–12 yr):** 60 mg/kg q 4 hr.
- **IM, IV (Children 1 mo–12 yr):** 50 mg/kg q 4 hr.
- **IM, IV (Neonates ≥7 days and ≥2 kg):** 75 mg/kg q 6 hr.
- **IM, IV (Neonates ≥7 days and <2 kg):** 75 mg/kg q 8 hr.
- **IM, IV (Neonates 0–7 days):** 75 mg/kg q 12 hr.

M

*Underlines indicate most frequent; CAPITALS indicate life-threatening.

AVAILABILITY

▪ *Injection:* 1 g, 2 g, 3 g, 4 g, 20 g.

TIME/ACTION PROFILE (blood levels)

	ONSET	PEAK
IM	rapid	45–90 min
IV	rapid	end of infusion

NURSING IMPLICATIONS

ASSESSMENT

□ Assess patient for infection (vital signs; appearance of wound, sputum, urine, and stool; WBC) at beginning and throughout course of therapy.

□ Obtain a history before initiating therapy to determine previous use of and reactions to penicillins or cephalosporins. Persons with a negative history of penicillin sensitivity may still have an allergic response.

□ Obtain specimens for culture and sensitivity prior to initiating therapy. First dose may be given before receiving results.

□ Observe patient for signs and symptoms of anaphylaxis (rash, pruritus, laryngeal edema, wheezing). Discontinue the drug and notify the physician immediately if these occur. Keep epinephrine, an antihistamine, and resuscitation equipment close by in the event of an anaphylactic reaction.

▪ **Lab Test Considerations:** Renal and hepatic function, CBC, and serum potassium should be evaluated prior to and routinely throughout course of therapy.

□ May cause false-positive urine protein test results.

□ May cause elevated serum creatinine, AST (SGOT), ALT (SGPT), bilirubin, and alkaline phosphatase. May also cause elevated serum sodium and decreased serum potassium levels.

□ May cause positive direct Coombs' test result.

POTENTIAL NURSING DIAGNOSES

▪ Infection, high risk for (indications, side effects).

▪ Knowledge deficit related to medication regimen (patient/family teaching).

IMPLEMENTATION

▪ **General Info:** Reconstituted solution is stable for 48 hr at room temperature and 72 hr if refrigerated. Solution is colorless to pale yellow; darkened solution does not affect potency.

▪ **IM:** To constitute for IM use, add 3–4 ml of Sterile Water for Injection or 0.5 or 1% lidocaine hydrochloride injection (without epinephrine) to each 1-g vial and shake vigorously. Inject deep into a well-developed muscle mass over 12–15 sec to minimize discomfort and massage well. IM injections should not exceed 2 g at each site.

▪ **IV:** The initial reconstitution is made with at least 10 ml of Sterile Water for Injection, 0.9% NaCl or D5W.

□ Change IV sites every 48 hr to prevent phlebitis.

▪ **Direct IV:** Inject slowly, 1 g over 3–5 min to minimize vein irritation.

▪ **Intermittent Infusion:** Dilute in 50–100 ml of 0.9% NaCl, D5W, D10W, D5/0.25% NaCl, D5/0.45% NaCl, Ringer's or lactated Ringer's solution.

▪ *Rate:* Administer over 30 min.

▪ **Y-Site Incompatibility:** Manufacturer recommends temporarily discontinuing primary infusion during mezlocillin infusion.

▪ **Additive Incompatibility:** Incompatible with aminoglycosides; do not admix, if penicillins and aminoglycosides must be administered concurrently, administer in separate sites.

PATIENT/FAMILY TEACHING

□ Advise patient to report the signs of superinfection (black, furry overgrowth on the tongue; vaginal itching or discharge; loose or foul-smelling stools) and allergy.

□ Advise patient to notify physician if fever and diarrhea develop, especially if stool contains blood, pus, or mucus. Instruct patient not to treat diarrhea without consulting physician or pharmacist.

EVALUATION
Clinical response can be evaluated by:
■ Resolution of the signs and symptoms of infection. Length of time for complete resolution depends on the organism and site of infection.

MICONAZOLE
(mi-**kon**-a-zole)
Micatin, Monistat

CLASSIFICATION(S):
Antifungal
Pregnancy Category UK

INDICATIONS

■ **IV:** Treatment of severe fungal infections, such as: □ Pulmonary infections □ Disseminated infections ■ **IV, Intrathecal:** Meningitis ■ **IV, Bladder Irrigation:** Candida bladder infections caused by susceptible organisms.

ACTION

■ Alters permeability of fungal cell membrane and function of fungal enzymes. **Therapeutic Effect:** ■ Fungistatic or fungicidal action. **Spectrum:** ■ Active against all pathogenic fungi and gram-positive bacteria ■ Spectrum notable for activity against: □ *Aspergillus* □ *Coccidioides* □ *Cryptococcus* □ *Candida albicans* □ *Histoplasma* □ *Dermatophytes*.

PHARMACOKINETICS

Absorption: Poorly (50%) absorbed following oral administration.
Distribution: Following IV administration is widely distributed. CSF penetration is poor, necessitating intrathecal administration in the treatment of meningitis.
Metabolism and Excretion: Mostly metabolized by the liver.
Half-life: 24 hr.

CONTRAINDICATIONS AND PRECAUTIONS

Contraindicated in: ■ Hypersensitivity

■ Hypersensitivity to castor oil or parabens (IV only).
Use Cautiously in: ■ Pregnancy, lactation, or children <1 yr (safety not established).

ADVERSE REACTIONS AND SIDE EFFECTS*

All adverse reactions listed except local irritation are for IV dosage form.
CNS: drowsiness, dizziness, anxiety, headache.
EENT: blurred vision, dry eyes.
CV: arrhythmias.
GI: nausea, vomiting, diarrhea, bitter taste.
F and E: hyponatremia.
Hemat: anemia.
Local: IV—phlebitis, pruritus.
Misc: hyperlipidemia, fever, increased libido, allergic reaction, including ANA-PHYLAXIS.

INTERACTIONS

Drug-Drug: ■ Parenteral miconazole enhances the anticoagulant effect of **warfarin** ■ Concurrent use with **rifampin** or **isoniazid** decreases blood levels and effectiveness of miconazole.

ROUTE AND DOSAGE

■ **IV (Adults):** 200–3600 mg/day in divided doses q 8 hr.
■ **IV (Children 1–12 yr):** 20–40 mg/kg/day in divided doses q 8 hr (not to exceed 15 mg/kg/dose).
■ **IV (Children <1 yr):** 15–30 mg/kg/day in divided doses q 8 hr.
■ **Intrathecal (Adults):** 20 mg q 3–7 days.
■ **Bladder Instillation (Adults):** 200 mg q 6–12 hr by continuous irrigation.

AVAILABILITY

■ *Injection:* 10 mg/ml.

TIME/ACTION PROFILE (blood levels)

	ONSET	PEAK
IV	rapid	end of infusion

M

*Underlines indicate most frequent; **CAPITALS** indicate life-threatening.

NURSING IMPLICATIONS

ASSESSMENT

□ Assess patient for infection prior to and throughout course of therapy.

□ Obtain specimens for culture prior to treatment. First dose may be given before receiving results.

□ Monitor IV site closely for phlebitis.

▪ **Lab Test Considerations:** Hemoglobin, hematocrit, serum electrolytes, and lipids should be monitored periodically throughout IV therapy.

□ May cause abnormalities in tests of serum lipid concentrations.

POTENTIAL NURSING DIAGNOSES

▪ Infection, high risk for (indications).

▪ Skin integrity, impaired (indications).

▪ Knowledge deficit related to medication regimen (patient/family teaching).

IMPLEMENTATION

▪ **Intermittent Infusion:** Dilute each dose in at least 200 ml of 0.9% NaCl or D5W. Solution is stable at room temperature for 48 hr. Darkened color of solution shows deterioration; discard. Manufacturer does not recommend admixing miconazole with other medications.

□ Initial dose of 200 mg should be administered under physician's supervision to determine hypersensitivity.

▪ *Rate:* Administer over 30–60 min. Rapid administration may cause transient tachycardia or arrhythmias.

□ Nausea and vomiting may be minimized by reducing dose, slowing infusion rate, avoiding administration at mealtime, or administering antiemetics or antihistamines prior to IV miconazole infusion.

▪ **Y-Site Compatibility:** ▪ foscarnet ▪ ondansetron ▪ sargramostim.

▪ **Y-Site Incompatibility:** ▪ fludarabine.

▪ **Bladder Irrigation:** Bladder irrigation may be used concurrently with IV administration for bladder mycoses.

PATIENT/FAMILY TEACHING

□ Explain purpose of medication to patient.

EVALUATION

Effectiveness of therapy can be demonstrated by: ▪ Resolution of the signs and symptoms of infection.

MIDAZOLAM
(mid-**ay**-zoe-lam)
Versed

CLASSIFICATION(S):
Sedative/hypnotic (benzo-diazepine)
Schedule IV
Pregnancy Category D

INDICATIONS

▪ Used to produce sedation preoperatively and amnesia postoperatively
▪ To aid in the induction of anesthesia
▪ Provides conscious sedation before diagnostic or radiographic procedures.

ACTION

▪ Acts at many levels of the CNS to produce generalized CNS depression
▪ Effects may be mediated by gamma-aminobutyric acid (GABA), an inhibitory neurotransmitter. **Therapeutic Effects:** ▪ Short-term sedation ▪ Postoperative amnesia.

PHARMACOKINETICS

Absorption: Well absorbed following IM administration.

Distribution: Crosses the blood–brain barrier and placenta.

Metabolism and Excretion: Almost exclusively metabolized by the liver.

Half-life: 1–12 hr (increased in renal impairment or congestive heart failure).

CONTRAINDICATIONS AND PRECAUTIONS

Contraindicated in: ▪ Hypersensitivity ▪ Cross-sensitivity with other benzodiazepines may exist ▪ Shock ▪ Comatose patients or those with pre-existing CNS depression ▪ Uncontrolled severe pain ▪ Pregnancy or lactation.

Use Cautiously in: ▪ Pulmonary disease ▪ Congestive heart failure ▪ Renal impairment ▪ Severe hepatic impairment ▪ Elderly or debilitated patients (more susceptible to depressant effects; dosage reduction required) ▪ Children (safety not established).

ADVERSE REACTIONS AND SIDE EFFECTS*

CNS: headache, excess sedation, drowsiness, agitation.
EENT: blurred vision.
Resp: coughing, LARYNGOSPASM, bronchospasm, RESPIRATORY DEPRESSION, APNEA.
CV: arrhythmias, CARDIAC ARREST.
GI: hiccoughs, nausea, vomiting.
Derm: rashes.
Local: pain at IM site, phlebitis at IV site.

INTERACTIONS

Drug–Drug: ▪ Additive CNS depression with **alcohol, antihistamines, opioid analgesics,** and **sedative/hypnotics** (decrease midazolam dose by 30–50% if used concurrently) ▪ Increased risk of hypotension with **antihypertensives,** acute ingestion of **alcohol,** or **nitrates**.

ROUTE AND DOSAGE

Dosage must be individualized, taking caution to reduce dosage in elderly patients and those who are already sedated.

Preoperative Sedation/Memory Impairment

▪ **IM (Adults):** 70–80 mcg/kg 1 hr before surgery (usual dose 5 mg).

Conscious Sedation for Short Procedure

▪ **IV (Adults):** 1–2.5 mg initially, dosage may be increased further as needed, doses >5 mg are rarely needed. In elderly (>60 yr) or debilitated patients, initial dose should not exceed 1.5 mg with doses >3.5 mg rarely needed.

Induction of Anesthesia

▪ **IV (Adults):** 200–350 mcg/kg initially. May give additional dose of 25% of initial dose if needed up to 600 mcg/kg total. If >55 yr, initial dose should be 150–300 mcg/kg. For seriously ill or debilitated patients, initial dose may be 150–250 mcg/kg. If patient is premedicated, initial dose should be further reduced.

AVAILABILITY

▪ *Injection:* 1 mg/ml, 5 mg/ml.

TIME/ACTION PROFILE (sedation)

	ONSET	PEAK	DURATION
IM	15 min	30–60 min	2–6 hr
IV	1.5–5 min	rapid	2–6 hr

NURSING IMPLICATIONS

ASSESSMENT

▫ Assess level of sedation and level of consciousness throughout and for 2–6 hr following administration.
▫ Monitor blood pressure, pulse, and respiration continuously throughout IV administration. Oxygen and resuscitative equipment should be immediately available.
▪ **Toxicity and Overdose:** If overdose occurs, monitor pulse, respiration, and blood pressure continuously. Maintain patent airway and assist ventilation as needed. If hypotension occurs, treatment includes IV fluids, repositioning, and vasopressors.
▫ The effects of midazolam can be reversed with flumazenil (Romazicon).

POTENTIAL NURSING DIAGNOSES

▪ Breathing pattern, ineffective (adverse reactions).
▪ Injury, high risk for (side effects).
▪ Knowledge deficit related to medication regimen (patient/family teaching).

IMPLEMENTATION

▪ **IM:** Administer IM doses deep into muscle mass.
▪ **Direct IV:** Administer undiluted or diluted with D5W, 0.9% NaCl, or lactated Ringer's injection through Y-site or 3-way stopcock.
▫ When administered concurrently with

M

*Underlines indicate most frequent; **CAPITALS** indicate life-threatening.

opioid analgesics, dose should be reduced by 30–50%.

- **Rate:** Administer each dose slowly over at least 2 min. Monitor IV site closely to avoid extravasation. Titrate dose to patient response.
- **Syringe Compatibility:** ▪ atropine ▪ benzquinamide ▪ buprenorphine ▪ butorphanol ▪ chlorpromazine ▪ cimetadine ▪ diphenhydramine ▪ droperidol ▪ fentanyl ▪ glycopyrrolate ▪ hydromorphone ▪ hydroxyzine ▪ meperidine ▪ metoclopramide ▪ morphine ▪ nalbuphine ▪ promazine ▪ promethazine ▪ scopolamine ▪ thiethylperazine ▪ trimethobenzamide.
- **Syringe Incompatibility:** ▪ dimenhydrinate ▪ pentobarbital ▪ perphenazine ▪ prochlorperazine ▪ ranitidine.
- **Y-Site Compatibility:** ▪ atracurium ▪ famotidine ▪ fluconazole ▪ pancuronium ▪ vecuronium.
- **Y-Site Incompatibility:** ▪ foscarnet.

PATIENT/FAMILY TEACHING
- ☐ Inform patient that this medication will decrease mental recall of the procedure.
- ☐ Medication may cause drowsiness or dizziness. Advise patient to request assistance prior to ambulation and transfer and to avoid driving or other activities requiring alertness for 24 hr following administration.
- ☐ Instruct patient to inform physician prior to administration if pregnancy is suspected.
- ☐ Advise patient to avoid alcohol or other CNS depressants for 24 hr following administration of midazolam.

EVALUATION
Effectiveness of therapy can be demonstrated by: ▪ Sedation during and amnesia following surgical, diagnostic, and radiologic procedures.

MILRINONE
(**mill**-ri-none)
Primacor

CLASSIFICATION(S):
Inotropic agent
Pregnancy Category C

INDICATIONS
- Short-term treatment of congestive heart failure unresponsive to conventional therapy with cardiac glycosides, diuretics, and vasodilators.

ACTION
- Increases myocardial contractility
- Decreases preload and afterload by a direct dilating effect on vascular smooth muscle. **Therapeutic Effect:** Increased cardiac output (inotropic effect).

PHARMACOKINETICS
Absorption: IV administration results in complete bioavailability.
Distribution: Distribution of milrinone is not known.
Metabolism and Excretion: 80–90% of milrinone is excreted unchanged by the kidneys.
Half-life: 2.3 hr (increased in renal impairment).

CONTRAINDICATIONS AND PRECAUTIONS
Contraindicated in: ▪ Hypersensitivity ▪ Patients with severe aortic or pulmonic valvular heart disease ▪ Patients with hypertrophic subaortic stenosis (may increase outflow tract obstruction).
Use Cautiously in: ▪ Patients with a history of arrhythmias, electrolyte abnormalities, abnormal digoxin levels, or insertion of vascular catheters (increased risk of ventricular arrhythmias) ▪ Patients with renal impairment (reduction of infusion rate is recommended if creatinine clearance is <50 ml/min) ▪ Pregnancy, lactation, or children (safety not established).

ADVERSE REACTIONS AND SIDE EFFECTS*
CNS: headache, tremor.
CV: VENTRICULAR ARRHYTHMIAS, su-

---

*<u>Underlines</u> indicate most frequent; **CAPITALS** indicate life-threatening.

praventricular arrhythmias, hypotension, angina pectoris, chest pain.
F and E: hypokalemia.
Hemat: thrombocytopenia.

INTERACTIONS
Drug–Drug: ▪ None significant.

ROUTE AND DOSAGE
▪ **IV (Adults):** *Loading dose*—50 mcg/kg followed by *infusion* at 0.50 mcg/kg/min (range 0.375–0.75 mcg/kg/min).

AVAILABILITY
▪ *Injection:* 1 mg/ml.

TIME/ACTION PROFILE
(hemodynamic effects)

	ONSET	PEAK	DURATION
IV	5–15 min	UK	UK

NURSING IMPLICATIONS
Assessment
▫ Monitor heart rate and blood pressure continuously during administration. Milrinone should be slowed or discontinued if blood pressure drops excessively.
▫ Monitor intake and output and daily weight. Assess patient for resolution of signs and symptoms of congestive heart failure (peripheral edema, dyspnea, rales/crackles, weight gain) and improvement in hemodynamic parameters (increase in cardiac output, decrease in pulmonary capillary wedge pressure). The effects of previous aggressive diuretic therapy should be corrected to allow for optimal filling pressure.
▫ Monitor ECG continuously during infusion. Arrhythmias are common and may be life-threatening. The risk of ventricular arrhythmias is increased in patients with a history of arrhythmias, electrolyte abnormalities, abnormal digoxin levels, or insertion of vascular catheters.
▪ **Lab Test Considerations:** Monitor electrolytes and renal fuction frequently during administration. Hypo-

kalemia should be corrected prior to administration to decrease the risk of arrhythmias.
▫ Monitor platelet count during therapy.
▪ **Toxicity and Overdose:** Overdose manifests as hypotension. Dosage should be decreased or discontinued. Supportive measures may be necessary.

Implementation
▪ **Direct IV:** Loading dose may be administered undiluted.
▪ *Rate:* Administer the loading dose over 10 min.
▪ **Continuous Infusion:** The 20-mg vial may be diluted with 180 ml of diluent for a concentration of 100 mcg/ml, with 113 ml of diluent for a concentration of 150 mcg/ml, or with 80 ml of diluent for a concentration of 200 mcg/ml. Compatible diluents include 0.45% NaCl, 0.9% NaCl, and D5W. Do not use solutions that are discolored or contain particulate matter.
▪ *Rate:* Infusion rate is titrated according to hemodynamic and clinical response. See infusion rate table in Appendix D.
▪ **Y-Site Incompatibility:** ▪ furosemide.

Patient/Family Teaching
▫ Inform patient and family of reasons for administration. Milrinone is not a cure but is a temporary measure to control the symptoms of congestive heart failure.

Evaluation
Clinical response to therapy can be determined by: ▪ Decrease in the signs and symptoms of congestive heart failure ▫ Improvement in hemodynamic parameters.

MINERAL OIL
Agoral Plain, Fleet Mineral Oil, {Kondremul}, Kondremul Plain, Liqui-doss, Milkinol, {Lansoyl}, Neo-Cultol, Nujol, Petrogalar, Zymenol

M

{} = Available in Canada only.

CLASSIFICATION(S):
Laxative (lubricant)
Pregnancy Category UK

INDICATIONS

- Used to soften impacted feces in the management of constipation.

ACTION

- Coats surface of stool and intestine with lubricant film to allow passage of stool through intestine ▪ Improves water retention of stool. **Therapeutic Effect:**
- Softening of fecal mass and subsequent passage.

PHARMACOKINETICS

Absorption: Minimally absorbed following oral administration.

Distribution: Distributes into mesenteric lymph nodes, intestinal mucosa, liver, and spleen.

Metabolism and Excretion: Metabolism and excretion not known. Action is primarily local; unabsorbed mineral oil is passed with fecal mass.

Half-life: UK.

CONTRAINDICATIONS AND PRECAUTIONS

Contraindicated in: ▪ Hypersensitivity ▪ Children <6 yr (oral) ▪ Children <2 yr (rect).

Use Cautiously in: ▪ Children, elderly or debilitated patients (increased risk of lipid pneumonia) ▪ Pregnancy (chronic use decreases absorption of fat-soluble vitamins, may cause hypoprothrombinemia in newborn).

ADVERSE REACTIONS AND SIDE EFFECTS*

Resp: lipid pneumonia.

GI: rectal seepage of mineral oil, anal irritation.

INTERACTIONS

Drug–Drug: ▪ Decreases absorption of fat-soluble vitamins (A, D, E, K).

Drug–Food: ▪ Decreases absorption of fat-soluble vitamins (A, D, E, K).

ROUTE AND DOSAGE

- **PO (Adults and Children >12 yr):** 5–45 ml as a single dose or divided doses.
- **PO (Children 6–12 yr):** 5–20 ml as a single dose or divided doses.
- **Rect (Adults and Children >12 yr):** 60–150 ml as a single dose.
- **Rect (Children 2–11 yr):** 30–60 ml as a single dose.

AVAILABILITY

▪ *Liquid* ▪ *Jelly* ▪ *Emulsion* ▪ *In combination with:* magnesium hydroxide (Haley's M-O), cascara, glyceron, and phenolphthalein. See Appendix A.

TIME/ACTION PROFILE (laxation)

	ONSET	PEAK	DURATION
PO	6–8 hr	UK	UK
Rect	2–15 min	UK	UK

NURSING IMPLICATIONS

ASSESSMENT

▢ Assess patient for abdominal distention, presence of bowel sounds, and usual pattern of bowel function.

▢ Assess color, consistency, and amount of stool produced.

POTENTIAL NURSING DIAGNOSES

- Constipation (indications).
- Knowledge deficit related to medication regimen (patient/family teaching).

IMPLEMENTATION

- **General Info:** This medication does not stimulate intestinal peristalsis.

▢ Administer carefully to bedridden patients or children to prevent lipid pneumonia from aspiration of mineral oil. Do not administer to patients in a reclining position.

- **PO:** Usually administered at bedtime. Do not administer within 2 hr of meals; may interfere with absorption of nutrients and vitamins.

▢ Do not administer within 2 hr of stool softeners; may cause increased absorption of mineral oil.

---

*Underlines indicate most frequent; **CAPITALS** indicate life-threatening.

- **Rect:** Do not lubricate suppositories containing mineral oil, as this may interfere with the action of the suppository. Moisten with water by placing under tap for 30 sec or in a cup of water for at least 10 sec prior to insertion.

PATIENT/FAMILY TEACHING
- Advise patients that laxatives should be used only for short-term therapy. Long-term therapy may interfere with absorption of nutrients and vitamins A, D, E, and K.
- Advise patient not to take this medication within 2 hr of food or other medications.
- Encourage patients to use other forms of bowel regulation, such as increasing bulk in the diet, increasing fluid intake, increasing mobility. Normal bowel habits are variable and may vary from 3 times/day to 3 times/wk.
- Instruct patients with cardiac disease to avoid straining during bowel movements (Valsalva maneuver).
- Advise patients that large doses of mineral oil may cause leakage of mineral oil from the rectum; protection of clothing may be necessary. This may be prevented by reducing or dividing the dose or by administering in emulsified form.
- Advise patient not to use laxatives when abdominal pain, nausea, vomiting, or fever is present.

EVALUATION
Effectiveness of therapy can be demonstrated by: ▪ Soft, formed bowel movement, usually within 6–8 hr □ Results are usually obtained from rectal doses in 2–15 min.

MINOCYCLINE
(min-oh-**sye**-kleen)
Minocin

CLASSIFICATION(S):
Anti-infective (tetracycline)
Pregnancy Category UK

INDICATIONS
▪ Used most commonly in the treatment of infections due to unusual (atypical) organisms, including: □ *Mycoplasma* □ *Chlamydia* □ *Rickettsia* ▪ Treatment of gonorrhea in patients who cannot tolerate conventional therapy.

ACTION
▪ Inhibits bacterial protein synthesis at the level of the 30S ribosome. **Therapeutic Effect:** ▪ Bacteriostatic action against susceptible bacteria. **Spectrum:** ▪ Active against a wide variety of gram-positive, gram-negative, and atypical organisms, including: □ *Neisseria meningitidis* □ *Neisseria gonorrhea* □ *Treponema pallidum* □ *Chlamydia trachomatis* □ *Ureaplasma urealyticum* □ *Mycoplasma pneumoniae* □ Norcardia.

PHARMACOKINETICS
Absorption: Well absorbed from the GI tract.
Distribution: Widely distributed, some penetration into CSF. Crosses the placenta and enters breast milk.
Metabolism and Excretion: 5–20% excreted unchanged by the urine. Some metabolism by the liver with enterohepatic circulation and excretion in bile and feces.
Half-life: 11–26 hr.

CONTRAINDICATIONS AND PRECAUTIONS
Contraindicated in: ▪ Hypersensitivity ▪ Children <8 (permanent staining of teeth) ▪ Pregnancy or lactation.
Use Cautiously in: ▪ Cachectic or debilitated patients ▪ Hepatic or renal disease.

ADVERSE REACTIONS AND SIDE EFFECTS*
CNS: lightheadedness, dizziness, vertigo.
EENT: vestibular reactions.
GI: nausea, vomiting, diarrhea, pancreatitis, hepatotoxicity.
Derm: rashes, photosensitivity.

M

*Underlines indicate most frequent; **CAPITALS** indicate life-threatening.

Hemat: blood dyscrasias.
Local: phlebitis at IV site.
Misc: superinfection, hypersensitivity reactions.

INTERACTIONS

Drug–Drug: ▪ May enhance the effect of **oral anticoagulants** ▪ May decrease the effectiveness of **oral contraceptives** ▪ **Calcium, iron,** and **magnesium** form chelates and may decrease absorption ▪ **Adsorbent antidiarrheals** may decrease absorption.

ROUTE AND DOSAGE

Treatment of Infections

▪ **PO, IV (Adults):** 100–200 mg initially, then 100 mg q 12 hr or 50 mg q 6 hr.
▪ **PO, IV (Children >8 yr):** 4 mg/kg initially, then 2 mg/kg q 12 hr.

AVAILABILITY

▪ *Capsules:* 50 mg, 100 mg ▪ *Tablets:* 50 mg, 100 mg ▪ *Oral suspension:* 50 mg/5 ml ▪ *Injection:* 100 mg.

TIME/ACTION PROFILE (blood levels)

	ONSET	PEAK
PO	rapid	2–3 hr
IV	rapid	end of infusion

NURSING IMPLICATIONS

ASSESSMENT

□ Assess patient for infection (vital signs; appearance of wound, sputum, urine, and stool; WBC) at beginning and throughout course of therapy.
□ Obtain specimens for culture and sensitivity prior to initiating therapy. First dose may be given before receiving results.
▪ **Lab Test Considerations:** May cause increased AST (SGOT), ALT (SGPT), serum alkaline phosphatase, bilirubin, and amylase concentrations.

POTENTIAL NURSING DIAGNOSES

▪ Infection, high risk for (indications, side effects).
▪ Knowledge deficit related to medication regimen (patient/family teaching).

▪ Noncompliance related to medication regimen (patient/family teaching).

IMPLEMENTATION

▪ **General Info:** May cause yellow-brown discoloration and softening of teeth and bones if administered prenatally or prior to 8 yr of age.
▪ **PO:** Administer around the clock. May be taken with food or milk. Take with a full glass of liquid and take at least 1 hr before going to bed. Use calibrated measuring for liquid preparations. Shake liquid preparations well.
□ Do not administer within 1–3 hr of other medications.
□ Avoid administration of calcium salts, antacids, magnesium-containing medications, or iron supplements within 1–3 hr of oral minocycline.
▪ **SC, IM:** Do not administer SC or IM.
▪ **Intermittent Infusion:** Dilute each 100 mg with 5–10 ml of Sterile Water for Injection. Dilute further in 500–1000 ml of 0.9% NaCl, D5W, D5/0.9% NaCl, Ringer's or lactated Ringer's solution. Solution is stable for 24 hr at room temperature.
▪ *Rate:* Administer over 6 hr immediately following dilution. Avoid rapid infusions. May cause thrombophlebitis; avoid extravasation.
▪ **Y-Site Compatibility:** ▪ cyclophosphamide ▪ fludarabine ▪ heparin ▪ hydrocortisone sodium succinate ▪ magnesium sulfate ▪ perphenazine ▪ potassium chloride ▪ sargramostim ▪ vitamin B complex with C.
▪ **Y-Site Incompatibility:** ▪ hydromorphone ▪ meperidine ▪ morphine.

PATIENT/FAMILY TEACHING

□ Instruct patients to take medication around the clock and to finish the drug completely as directed, even if feeling better. Missed doses should be taken as soon as remembered unless almost time for next dose. Advise patients that sharing of this medication may be dangerous.
□ Commonly causes dizziness, lightheadedness, or unsteadiness. Caution patient to avoid driving or other activities requiring alertness until re-

sponse to medication is known. Notify physician if these symptoms occur.

- Caution patient to use sunscreen and protective clothing to prevent photosensitivity reactions.

- Advise patient to use a nonhormonal method of contraception while taking minocycline.

- Instruct patient to notify physician or dentist of medication regimen prior to treatment or surgery.

- Advise patient to report the signs of superinfection (black, furry overgrowth on the tongue; vaginal itching or discharge; loose or foul-smelling stools). Skin rash, pruritus, and urticaria also should be reported.

- Instruct the patient to notify the physician if symptoms do not improve.

- Caution patient to discard outdated or decomposed products, as they may be toxic.

EVALUATION

Clinical response can be evaluated by:
■ Resolution of the signs and symptoms of infection. Length of time for complete resolution depends on the organism and site of infection.

MINOXIDIL
(mi-**nox**-i-dill)
Loniten, Minodyl, Rogaine

CLASSIFICATION(S):
Antihypertensive (vasodilator),
Hair growth stimulant
Pregnancy Category C (PO)

INDICATIONS

■ **PO:** Management of severe symptomatic hypertension or hypertension associated with end-organ damage that has failed to respond to combinations of more conventional therapy ■ **Top:** Management of androgenic alopecia.

ACTION

■ Directly relaxes vascular smooth muscle, probably by inhibiting the enzyme phosphodiesterase. Results in vasodilation, which is more pronounced on arterioles than veins ■ Hair regrowth may be due to increased cutaneous blood flow or stimulation of hair follicles from resting phase to growing phase. **Therapeutic Effects:** ■ Lowering of blood pressure ■ Hair regrowth.

PHARMACOKINETICS

Absorption: Well absorbed from the GI tract following oral administration. Minimal absorption follows topical use (<2%), but is enhanced by increasing dose or applying to larger surface area.
Distribution: Widely distributed. Enters breast milk.
Metabolism and Excretion: 90% metabolized by the liver.
Half-life: 4.2 hr.

CONTRAINDICATIONS AND PRECAUTIONS

Contraindicated in: ■ Hypersensitivity ■ Pheochromocytoma ■ Patients currently receiving guanethidine.
Use Cautiously in: ■ PO: Recent myocardial infarction ■ Pregnancy or lactation (safety not established) ■ Severe renal impairment (can be used in moderate renal impairment) ■ **Top:** Cardiovascular disease ■ Abraded or irritated skin (increased risk of systemic absorption).

ADVERSE REACTIONS AND SIDE EFFECTS*

CNS: PO—headache.
Resp: PO—pulmonary edema.
CV: PO—edema, CONGESTIVE HEART FAILURE, tachycardia, ECG changes (alteration in T waves), pericardial effusion, angina.
GI: PO—nausea.
Derm: PO—hypertrichosis, pigment changes, rashes; Top—burning or itching of scalp, skin rash, swelling of face.
Endo: PO—breast tenderness, gynecomastia, menstrual irregularities.
F and E: PO—sodium and water retention.
Misc: PO—intermittent claudication.

M

*Underlines indicate most frequent; CAPITALS indicate life-threatening.

INTERACTIONS

For oral minoxidil, unless indicated.

Drug–Drug: ▪ Additive hypotensive effects with other **antihypertensive agents,** acute ingestion of **alcohol,** or **nitrates** ▪ Severe hypotension may occur with **guanethidine** ▪ **Nonsteroidal antiinflammatory agents** may decrease the antihypertensive effectiveness of minoxidil ▪ Top: Topical **glucocorticoids, petrolatum,** or **retinoids** may enhance absorption and lead to systemic side effects.

ROUTE AND DOSAGE

Hypertension

▪ **PO (Adults and Children >12 yr):** 5 mg once daily initially, increase at 3-day intervals (for rapid control with careful monitoring, doses may be adjusted q 6 hr) to 10 mg/day, then 20 mg/day, then 40 mg/day given in 2 divided doses. Usual dose required is 10–40 mg/day. Doses up to 100 mg have been used.

▪ **PO (Children <12 yr):** 0.2 mg/kg/day (5 mg maximum) initially, may be gradually increased at 3-day intervals in increments of 50–100% until response is obtained. Usual dose required is 0.25–1 mg/kg/day in 1–2 divided doses. For rapid control, doses may be adjusted q 6 hr (daily dose not to exceed 50 mg).

Alopecia

▪ **Top (Adults):** Apply 1 ml of 2% solution to affected area bid (up to 2 ml/day).

AVAILABILITY

▪ *Tablets:* 2.5 mg, 10 mg ▪ *Topical solution:* 20 mg/ml.

TIME/ACTION PROFILE
(PO = antihypertensive effect,
Top = hair regrowth)

	ONSET	PEAK	DURATION
PO	30 min	2–8 hr	2–5 days
Top	4 mo	UK	3–4 mo

NURSING IMPLICATIONS

ASSESSMENT

▪ **Hypertension:** Monitor blood pressure and pulse frequently during initial dosage adjustment and periodically throughout therapy. Notify physician of significant changes.

▫ Monitor intake and output ratios and daily weight and assess for edema daily, especially at beginning of therapy. Notify physician of weight gain or edema, as sodium and water retention may be treated with diuretics.

▪ **Top:** Assess patient for systemic effects of minoxidil at least 1 mo after starting and at least every 6 mo thereafter. Topical minoxidil should be discontinued if systemic effects occur.

▪ **Lab Test Considerations:** Renal and hepatic function, CBC, and electrolytes should be monitored prior to and periodically throughout therapy.

▫ May cause increased BUN, serum creatinine, alkaline phosphatase, and sodium levels. May also cause decreased RBC, hemoglobin, and hematocrit counts.

POTENTIAL NURSING DIAGNOSES

▪ Tissue perfusion, altered (indications).

▪ Body image disturbance (indications, side effects).

▪ Knowledge deficit related to medication regimen (patient/family teaching).

IMPLEMENTATION

▪ **Hypertension:** Medication may need to be discontinued gradually to prevent rebound hypertension.

▫ Minoxidil is given concurrently with a diuretic unless patient is on hemodialysis.

▫ Dosage adjustments should not be made more frequently than every 3 days to allow for maximum effectiveness, unless rapid control is necessary.

▪ **PO:** May be administered without regard to meals or food.

- **Top:** The same 1-ml dose is used regardless of the size of the balding area. More than 2 ml/day does not speed up process of hair growth and may increase side effects.
- Available with pump spray, extended tip, or rub-on applicators.

PATIENT/FAMILY TEACHING

- **Hypertension:** Emphasize the importance of continuing to take this medication, even if feeling well. Instruct patient to take medication at the same time each day. If a dose is missed, take as soon as remembered if within a few hours; otherwise omit dose and return to regular dosage schedule. Do not double doses. Advise patient not to discontinue minoxidil or other antihypertensive medications without consulting physician. Minoxidil helps control but does not cure hypertension.
- Encourage patient to comply with additional interventions for hypertension (weight reduction, low-sodium diet, smoking cessation, moderation of alcohol consumption, regular exercise, and stress management).
- Instruct patient and family on proper technique for pulse and blood pressure monitoring. Advise them to check blood pressure at least weekly and to report significant changes to physician. Physician should also be notified if resting pulse increases more than 20 bpm above baseline.
- Advise patient to check weight daily and to notify physician of rapid weight gain of >5 lb or if signs of fluid retention occur.
- Caution patient to make position changes slowly to minimize orthostatic hypotension.
- Advise patient to consult physician or pharmacist before taking any cough, cold, or allergy remedies. Patient should also avoid excessive amounts of coffee, tea, or cola.
- Inform patient that depilatory creams may minimize increased hair growth. This is temporary and is reversible within 1–6 mo following discontinuation of minoxidil.
- Advise patient to notify physician if unusual swelling of face, extremities or abdomen; difficulty breathing especially when lying down, new or aggravated angina, severe indigestion, dizziness, lightheadedness, or fainting occurs.

- **Top:** Instruct patient to use minoxidil exactly as directed. Do not use more medication or more frequently to avoid systemic side effects. Missed doses should be applied as soon as remembered if not almost time for next dose.
- Instruct patient to apply only to scalp, not to other parts of the body, to minimize side effects. Do not use with other topical scalp medications or if scalp is sunburned. Hair should be dry prior to application.
- Inform patient that first hair growth may be soft, colorless, and barely visible. With further treatment hair should be same color and thickness as other hair on scalp.
- Caution patient that if treatment is stopped, new hair may be shed within months.
- Shampoo hair each morning before first daily application. Apply to affected area beginning at center of balding area. Wash hands immediately after application. Do not use hairdryer to speed drying. Do not lie down within 30 min of application to prevent transfer of medication to pillow.
- Advise patient to avoid contact of minoxidil with eyes, nose, or mouth. Flush area with water if accidental contact occurs.
- Advise patient to notify physician if itching, burning, or redness occurs.

EVALUATION

Effectiveness of therapy can be demonstrated by: ▪ Decrease in blood pressure without appearance of serious side effects ▪ Hair regrowth in androgenic alo-

M

pecia. Evidence of hair growth usually requires 4 mo or longer.

MISOPROSTOL
(mye-soe-**prost**-ole)
Cytotec

CLASSIFICATION(S):
Gastrointestinal (antiulcer)
Pregnancy Category X

INDICATIONS

■ Prevention of gastric mucosal injury from nonsteroidal anti-inflammatory agents, including aspirin, in high-risk patients (elderly or debilitated patients, or those with a history of ulcers). **Unlabeled Use:** ■ Treatment of duodenal ulcers.

ACTION

■ Acts as a prostaglandin analog, decreasing gastric acid secretion (antisecretory effect) and increasing the production of protective mucus (cytoprotective effect). **Therapeutic Effect:** ■ Prevention of gastic ulceration from nonsteroidal anti-inflammatory agents.

PHARMACOKINETICS

Absorption: Well absorbed following oral administration and rapidly converted to its active form (misoprostol acid).
Distribution: Distribution not known.
Metabolism and Excretion: Undergoes some metabolism and is then excreted by the kidneys.
Half-life: 20–40 min.

CONTRAINDICATIONS AND PRECAUTIONS

Contraindicated in: ■ Hypersensitivity to prostaglandins ■ Pregnancy or lactation.
Use Cautiously in: ■ Patients with child-bearing potential ■ Children <18 yr (safety not established).

ADVERSE REACTIONS AND SIDE EFFECTS*

CNS: headache.
GI: <u>diarrhea</u>, <u>abdominal pain</u>, nausea, flatulence, dyspepsia, vomiting, constipation.
GU: menstrual disorders, <u>miscarriage</u>.

INTERACTIONS

Drug–Drug: ■ Increased risk of diarrhea with **magnesium-containing antacids**.

ROUTE AND DOSAGE

■ **PO (Adults):** 200 mcg 4 times daily with or after meals and at bedtime, or 400 mcg twice daily, last dose at bedtime. If intolerance occurs, dosage may be decreased to 100 mcg.

AVAILABILITY

■ *Tablets:* 100 mcg, 200 mcg.

TIME/ACTION PROFILE (effect on gastic-acid secretion)

	ONSET	PEAK	DURATION
PO	30 min	UK	3 hr

NURSING IMPLICATIONS

ASSESSMENT
□ Assess patient routinely for epigastric or abdominal pain and frank or occult blood in the stool, emesis, or gastric aspirate.
□ Assess women of childbearing age for pregnancy. Medication is usually begun on second or third day of menstrual period following a negative pregnancy test.

POTENTIAL NURSING DIAGNOSES
■ Pain (indications).
■ Knowledge deficit related to medication regimen (patient/family teaching).

IMPLEMENTATION
■ **PO:** Administer medication with meals and at bedtime to reduce severity of diarrhea.

---

*<u>Underlines</u> indicate most frequent; **CAPITALS** indicate life-threatening.

PATIENT/FAMILY TEACHING

- □ Instruct patient to take medication as directed for the full course of therapy, even if feeling better. Emphasize that sharing of this medication may be dangerous.
- □ Inform patient that misoprostol will cause spontaneous abortion. Women of childbearing age must be informed of this effect through verbal and written information and must use contraception throughout therapy. If pregnancy is suspected, the woman should stop taking misoprostol and immediately notify her physician.
- □ Inform patient that diarrhea may occur. The physician should be notified if diarrhea persists for more than 1 wk. Also advise patient to report onset of black, tarry stools or severe abdominal pain.
- □ Advise patient to avoid alcohol and foods that may cause an increase in GI irritation.

EVALUATION

Effectiveness of therapy can be demonstrated by: ▪ The prevention of gastric ulcers in patients receiving chronic nonsteroidal anti-inflammatory drug therapy.

MITOMYCIN
(mye-toe-**mye**-sin)
Mutamycin

CLASSIFICATION(S):
Antineoplastic agent (antitumor antibiotic)
Pregnancy Category UK

INDICATIONS

▪ Used with other agents in the management of disseminated adenocarcinoma of the stomach or pancreas. **Unlabeled Uses:** ▪ Palliative treatment of: □ Carcinoma of the colon or breast □ Head and neck tumors □ Advanced biliary, lung, and cervical squamous cell carcinomas.

ACTION

▪ Primarily inhibits DNA synthesis by causing cross-linking, also inhibits RNA and protein synthesis (cell cycle-phase nonspecific, but is most active in S and G phases). **Therapeutic Effect:** ▪ Death of rapidly replicating cells, particularly malignant ones.

PHARMACOKINETICS

Absorption: Administered IV only, resulting in complete bioavailability.
Distribution: Widely distributed, concentrates in tumor tissue. Does not enter CSF.
Metabolism and Excretion: Mostly metabolized by the liver. Small amounts (<10%) excreted unchanged by the kidneys and in bile.
Half-life: 50 min.

CONTRAINDICATIONS AND PRECAUTIONS

Contraindicated in: ▪ Hypersensitivity ▪ Pregnancy or lactation.
Use Cautiously in: ▪ Patients with childbearing potential ▪ Active infections ▪ Decreased bone marrow reserve ▪ Other chronic debilitating illnesses ▪ Impaired liver function ▪ History of pulmonary problems.

ADVERSE REACTIONS AND SIDE EFFECTS*

Resp: pulmonary toxicity (hemoptysis, dyspnea, coughing, pneumonia).
CV: edema.
GI: nausea, vomiting, anorexia, stomatitis.
GU: renal failure, gonadal suppression.
Derm: alopecia, desquamation.
Hemat: anemia, leukopenia, thrombocytopenia.
Local: phlebitis at IV site.
Misc: prolonged malaise, fever, HEMOLYTIC UREMIC SYNDROME.

INTERACTIONS

Drug–Drug: ▪ Additive bone marrow depression with other **antineoplastic**

M

---

*Underlines indicate most frequent; CAPITALS indicate life-threatening.

agents or **radiation therapy** ■ May decrease antibody response to **live virus vaccines** and increase the risk of adverse reactions ■ Concurrent or sequential use with **vinca alkaloids** may result in respiratory toxicity.

ROUTE AND DOSAGE

■ **IV (Adults):** 10–20 mg/m^2 every 6–8 wk.

AVAILABILITY

■ *Injection:* 5-mg, 20-mg, 40-mg vials.

TIME/ACTION PROFILE (effects on blood counts)

	ONSET	PEAK	DURATION
IV	3–8 wk	4–8 wk	up to 3 mo

NURSING IMPLICATIONS

ASSESSMENT

□ Monitor vital signs periodically during administration.

□ Assess for fever, sore throat, and signs of infection due to leukopenia. Notify physician if these symptoms occur.

□ Assess for bleeding (bleeding gums; bruising; petechiae; guaiac stools, urine, and emesis) due to thrombocytopenia. Avoid IM injections and rectal temperatures. Apply pressure to venipuncture sites for 10 min.

□ Monitor intake and output, appetite, and nutritional intake. Nausea and vomiting usually occur within 1–2 hr. Vomiting may stop within 3–4 hr; nausea may persist for 2–3 days. Physician may order prophylactic use of an antiemetic. Adjust diet as tolerated to help maintain fluid and electrolyte balance and nutritional status.

□ Assess respiratory status and chest x-ray examination prior to and periodically throughout course of therapy. Notify physician if cough, bronchospasm, or dyspnea develops.

□ Monitor for potentially fatal hemolytic uremia syndrome in patients receiving long-term therapy. Symptoms include microangiopathic hemolytic anemia, thrombocytopenia, renal failure, and hypertension.

■ **Lab Test Considerations:** Monitor CBC and differential prior to and periodically throughout course of therapy and for several months following therapy.

□ The nadir of leukopenia occurs in 4 wk. Notify physician if leukocyte count is <4000/mm^3. The nadir of thrombocytopenia occurs in 4 wk. Notify physician if the platelet count is <150,000/mm^3 or is progressively declining. Recovery of leukopenia and thrombocytopenia occurs within 10 wk after cessation of therapy. Myelosuppression is cumulative and may be irreversible. Repeat courses of therapy are held until leukocyte count is >3000/mm^3 and platelet count is >75,000/mm^3.

□ Monitor liver function studies AST [SGOT], ALT [SGPT], LDH, bilirubin) and renal function studies (BUN, creatinine) prior to and periodically throughout therapy to detect hepatotoxicity and nephrotoxicity. Notify physician if creatinine is greater than 1.7 mg/dl.

POTENTIAL NURSING DIAGNOSES

■ Injury, high risk for (side effects).
■ Infection, high risk for (side effects).
■ Body image disturbance (side effects).

IMPLEMENTATION

■ **General Info:** Solution should be prepared in a biologic cabinet. Wear gloves, gown, and mask while handling medication. Discard equipment in designated containers (see Appendix I).

□ Ensure patency of IV. Extravasation may cause severe tissue necrosis. If patient complains of discomfort at IV site, discontinue immediately and restart infusion at another site. Promptly notify physician of extravasation.

■ **Direct IV:** Reconstitute 5-mg vial with 10 ml and 10-mg vial with 40 ml of Sterile Water for Injection. Shake the vial; may need to stand at room temperature for additional time to dissolve. Final solution is blue-gray. Reconstituted solution is stable for 7 days at room temperature, 14 days if refrigerated.

- *Rate:* May be administered IV push over 5–10 min through free-flowing IV of 0.9% NaCl or D5W.
- **Syringe Compatibility:** ▪ bleomycin ▪ cisplatin ▪ cyclophosphamide ▪ doxorubicin ▪ droperidol ▪ fluorouracil ▪ furosemide ▪ heparin ▪ leucovorin ▪ methotrexate ▪ metoclopramide ▪ vinblastine ▪ vincristine.
- **Y-Site Compatibility:** ▪ bleomycin ▪ cisplatin ▪ cyclophosphamide ▪ doxorubicin ▪ droperidol ▪ fluorouracil ▪ furosemide ▪ heparin ▪ leucovorin ▪ methotrexate ▪ metoclopramide ▪ ondansetron ▪ vinblastine ▪ vincristine.
- **Y-Site Incompatibility:** ▪ sargramostim.
- **Additive Compatibility:** ▪ sodium lactate.
- **Additive Incompatibility:** ▪ bleomycin.

PATIENT/FAMILY TEACHING

- ▢ Advise patient to notify physician promptly if fever, chills, sore throat, signs of infection, bleeding gums, bruising, petechiae, or blood in urine, stool, or emesis occurs. Caution patient to avoid crowds and persons with known infections. Instruct patient to use soft toothbrush and electric razor. Patients should be cautioned not to drink alcoholic beverages or take products containing aspirin or ibuprofen.
- ▢ Instruct patient to notify physician if decreased urine output, edema in lower extremities, shortness of breath, skin ulceration, or persistent nausea occurs.
- ▢ Instruct patient to inspect oral mucosa for redness and ulceration. If ulceration occurs, advise patient to use sponge brush and rinse mouth with water after eating and drinking. Viscous lidocaine swishes may be used if pain interferes with eating.
- ▢ Discuss with patient the possibility of hair loss. Explore coping strategies.
- ▢ Advise patient that although mitomycin may cause infertility, contraception during therapy is necessary because of teratogenic effects.
- ▢ Instruct patient not to receive any vaccinations without advice of physician.
- ▢ Emphasize need for periodic lab tests to monitor for side effects.

EVALUATION
Effectiveness of therapy can be demonstrated by: ▪ Decrease in size and spread of malignant tissue.

MITOTANE
(**mye**-toe-tane)
o, p'-DDD, Lysodren

CLASSIFICATION(S):
Antineoplastic agent (miscellaneous)
Pregnancy Category C

INDICATIONS

▪ Treatment of carcinoma of the adrenal cortex. **Unlabeled Use:** ▪ Cushing's syndrome due to pituitary disorders.

ACTION

▪ Suppresses the adrenal function ▪ Has a direct cytotoxic effect on adrenal tumors ▪ Structurally related to DDT (an insecticide). **Therapeutic Effect:** ▪ Regression of adrenal cortical tumors.

PHARMACOKINETICS

Absorption: 30–40% absorbed following oral administration.
Distribution: Widely distributed to all body tissues. Accumulates in fatty tissue.
Metabolism and Excretion: Slowly released from fatty tissue. Mostly metabolized by the liver. 10% excreted by the kidneys. 15% excreted in bile.
Half-life: 18–159 days.

M

CONTRAINDICATIONS AND PRECAUTIONS

Contraindicated in: ▪ Hypersensitivity. **Use Cautiously in:** ▪ Pregnancy or lactation (especially first trimester; safety not established) ▪ Obesity (increased risk of adverse reactions).

ADVERSE REACTIONS AND SIDE EFFECTS*

CNS: brain damage, functional impairment (high-dose, long-term therapy), lethargy, somnolence, dizziness, vertigo, mental depression, headache, irritability, tremors, weakness, fatigue.
EENT: blurred vision, diplopia, lens opacities, optic neuritis, toxic retinopathy, decreased hearing.
Resp: wheezing, shortness of breath.
CV: hypotension, hypertension.
GI: anorexia, nausea, vomiting, diarrhea, increased salivation.
GU: hemorrhagic cystitis, hematuria, albuminuria.
Derm: maculopapular rash, flushing.
Endo: adrenal suppression, gynecomastia.
Metab: hypouricemia, hypercholesterolemia.
MS: arthralgia, myalgia, aching.
Misc: fever.

INTERACTIONS

Drug–Drug: ▪ Stimulates hepatic drug–metabolizing enzymes, which may decrease the effectiveness of **drugs that are highly metabolized (warfarin, phenytoin)** ▪ Additive CNS depression with other **CNS depressants,** including **alcohol, antihistamines, antidepressants, opioid analgesics,** or **sedative/ hypnotics** ▪ Spironolactone may block the effects of mitotane in Cushing's disease.

ROUTE AND DOSAGE

Adrenocortical Carcinoma

▪ **PO (Adults):** 8–10 g/day in 3–4 divided doses, may be increased as tolerated (range 2–16 g/day).
▪ **PO (Children):** 100–500 mcg/kg/day or 1–2 g/day in divided doses. May be

increased gradually to 5–7 g/day in divided doses.

Cushing's Syndrome

▪ **PO (Adults):** 3–6 g/day in 3–4 divided doses initially, decreased to maintenance dose of 500 mg twice weekly–2 g/day.

AVAILABILITY

▪ *Tablets:* 500 mg.

TIME/ACTION PROFILE
(onset = inhibition of adrenocortical function, peak = tumor response)

	ONSET	PEAK	DURATION
PO	2–4 wk	6 wk	UK

NURSING IMPLICATIONS

ASSESSMENT

▫ Monitor for symptoms of adrenal insufficiency (anorexia, nausea and vomiting, diarrhea, fatigue, weakness, hypotension, darkening of skin). Obese patients are at increased risk for this side effect.
▫ Monitor for development of dose-limiting side effects (severe nausea, vomiting, anorexia, or diarrhea). Physician may order an antiemetic. Adjust diet as tolerated to maintain nutritional intake and fluid and electrolyte balance.
▫ Monitor neurologic status; report depression, lethargy, and complaints of dizziness.
▪ **Lab Test Considerations:** 8-hr plasma cortisol concentrations and 24-hr urine tests for 17-hydroxycorticosteroid (OHCS) concentrations should be obtained prior to and periodically throughout therapy to determine degree of adrenal suppression.
▫ May decrease serum uric acid and protein bound iodine (PBI) concentrations.

POTENTIAL NURSING DIAGNOSES

▪ Knowledge deficit related to medication regimen (patient/family teaching).

*Underlines indicate most frequent; **CAPITALS** indicate life-threatening.

IMPLEMENTATION

- **PO:** Premedication with an antiemetic may be necessary.

PATIENT/FAMILY TEACHING

☐ Instruct patient to take medication exactly as directed. If a dose is missed, it should be taken as soon as remembered unless almost time for next dose. Notify physician of missed doses.

☐ Explain to patient that this drug suppresses the adrenal glands and therefore impairs the body's ability to cope with stress. Concurrent glucocorticoid and mineralocorticoid therapy may be ordered to ensure that adequate amounts of adrenal hormones are present. The physician should be notified if an infection, illness, or injury occurs because supplemental steroids may be necessary or mitotane may need to be discontinued in the event of severe trauma or shock.

☐ Advise patient to carry identification describing medication regimen in the event of an emergency in which patient cannot relate medical history.

☐ Mitotane may cause drowsiness. Caution patient to avoid driving or other activities requiring alertness until response to medication is known.

☐ Instruct patient to notify physician if depression; lethargy; dizziness; or persistent nausea, vomiting, or diarrhea occurs; or if skin rashes develop.

☐ Caution patient to avoid taking alcohol or other CNS depressants with this medication.

☐ Advise patient to use a nonhormonal form of contraception throughout therapy.

☐ Explain need for continued medical follow-up, including neurologic examination to assess effectiveness and possible side effects of medication.

EVALUATION

Effectiveness of therapy can be demonstrated by: ▪ Decrease in the size and spread of adrenal malignancy, decrease in pain and symptoms of excess adrenal function.

MITOXANTRONE
(mye-toe-**zan**-trone)
Novantrone

CLASSIFICATION(S):
Antineoplastic (antitumor antibiotic)
Pregnancy Category D

INDICATIONS

▪ Used in combination with other antineoplastic agents in the treatment of acute nonlymphocytic leukemia (ANLL) in adults. **Unlabeled Uses:** ▪ Breast cancer, liver cancer, and non-Hodgkin's lymphoma.

ACTION

▪ Inhibits DNA synthesis (cell cycle-phase nonspecific). **Therapeutic Effect:** ▪ Death of rapidly replicating cells, particularly malignant ones.

PHARMACOKINETICS

Absorption: Administered IV only, resulting in complete bioavailability.
Distribution: Widely distributed. Limited penetration of CSF.
Metabolism and Excretion: Small amounts (<10%) excreted unchanged by the kidneys. Mostly eliminated by hepatobiliary clearance.
Half-life: 5.8 days.

CONTRAINDICATIONS AND PRECAUTIONS

Contraindicated in: ▪ Hypersensitivity ▪ Pregnancy or lactation.
Use Cautiously in: ▪ Previous cardiac disease ▪ Patients with childbearing potential ▪ Active infections ▪ Depressed bone marrow reserve ▪ Previous mediastinal radiation ▪ Other chronic debilitating illness ▪ Children (safety not established) ▪ Impaired hepatobiliary function or decreased blood counts (dosage reduction required).

ADVERSE REACTIONS AND SIDE EFFECTS*

CNS: headache, SEIZURES.

EENT: conjunctivitis, blue-green sclera.
Resp: <u>cough</u>, <u>dyspnea</u>.
CV: cardiotoxicity, ECG changes, arrhythmias.
GI: <u>nausea</u>, <u>vomiting</u>, <u>diarrhea</u>, <u>abdominal pain</u>, <u>stomatitis</u>, <u>hepatic toxicity</u>.
GU: renal failure, gonadal suppression, blue-green urine.
Derm: <u>alopecia</u>, rashes.
Hemat: <u>anemia</u>, <u>leukopenia</u>, <u>thrombocytopenia</u>.
Metab: hyperuricemia.
Misc: <u>fever</u>, hypersensitivity reactions.

INTERACTIONS

Drug–Drug: ▪ Additive bone marrow depression with other **antineoplastics** or **radiation therapy** ▪ Risk of cardiomyopathy increased by previous **anthracycline antineoplastic** therapy or **mediastinal radiation** ▪ May decrease antibody response to **live virus vaccines** and increase the risk of adverse reactions.

ROUTE AND DOSAGE

▪ **IV (Adults):** *Induction*—12 mg/m^2/day for 3 days as IV infusion (usually given with cytosine arabinoside 100 mg/m^2/day for 7 days as continuous IV infusion); if incomplete remission occurs, a second induction may be given. *Consolidation*—12 mg/m^2/day for 2 days as IV infusion (usually given with cytosine arabinoside 100 mg/m^2/day for 5 days as continuous IV infusion), given 6 wk after induction, with another course 4 wk later.

AVAILABILITY

▪ *Injection:* 2 mg/ml.

TIME/ACTION PROFILE (effects on blood counts)

	ONSET	PEAK	DURATION
IV	UK	10–14 days	28 days

NURSING IMPLICATIONS

ASSESSMENT

□ Monitor for hypersensitivity reaction (rash, urticaria, bronchospasm, tachycardia, hypotension). If these occur, stop infusion and notify physician. Keep epinephrine, an antihistamine, and resuscitation equipment close by in the event of an anaphylactic reaction.

□ Assess for fever, sore throat, and signs of infection caused by leukopenia. Notify physician if these symptoms occur.

□ Assess for bleeding (bleeding gums; bruising; petechiae; guaiac stools, urine, and emesis) caused by thrombocytopenia. Avoid IM injections and rectal temperatures. Apply pressure to venipuncture sites for 10 min.

□ Monitor intake and output, appetite, and nutritional intake. Assess patient for nausea and vomiting. Confer with physician regarding prophylactic use of an antiemetic. Adjust diet as tolerated to help maintain fluid and electrolyte balance and nutritional status.

□ May cause cardiotoxicity, especially in patients who have received daunorubicin or doxorubicin. Assess for rales/crackles, dyspnea, edema, jugular vein distention, ECG changes, arrhythmias, and chest pain.

□ Monitor for symptoms of gout (increased uric acid levels and joint pain and swelling). Encourage patient to drink at least 2 liters of fluid per day. Allopurinol may be given to decrease serum uric acid levels.

▪ **Lab Test Considerations:** Monitor CBC and differential prior to and periodically throughout therapy.

□ Monitor liver function studies AST [SGOT], ALT [SGPT], LDH, bilirubin) and renal function studies (BUN, creatinine) prior to and periodically throughout therapy to detect hepatotoxicity and nephrotoxicity.

□ May cause increased uric acid. Monitor periodically during therapy.

POTENTIAL NURSING DIAGNOSES

▪ Injury, high risk for (side effects).
▪ Infection, high risk for (side effects).
▪ Body image disturbance (side effects).

IMPLEMENTATION

▪ **General Info:** Solution should be prepared in a biologic cabinet. Wear gloves, gown, and mask while handling medication. Discard equipment in designated containers (see Appendix I).

□ Avoid contact with skin. Use Luer Loc tubing to prevent accidental leakage. If contact with skin occurs, immediately wash skin with soap and water.

□ Clean all spills with an aqueous solution of calcium hypochlorite. Mix solution by adding 5.5 parts (per weight) of calcium hypochlorite to 13 parts water.

- **IV:** Monitor IV site. If extravasation occurs, discontinue IV and restart at another site. Mitoxantrone is not a vesicant.

- **Direct IV:** Dilute solution in at least 50 ml of 0.9% NaCl or D5W. Discard unused solution appropriately.

- **Rate:** Administer slowly over at least 3 min into the tubing of a free-flowing IV of 0.9% NaCl or D5W.

- **Intermittent IV:** May be further diluted in D5W, 0.9% NaCl, or D5/0.9% NaCl and used immediately.

- **Y-Site Compatibility:** ■ fludarabine ■ ondansetron ■ sargramostim.

- **Additive Compatibility:** ■ hydrocortisone sodium succinate.

- **Additive Incompatibility:** ■ heparin.

PATIENT/FAMILY TEACHING

□ Advise patient to notify physician promptly if fever, chills, sore throat, signs of infection, bleeding gums, bruising, petechiae, or blood in urine, stool, or emesis occurs.

□ Caution patient to avoid crowds and persons with known infections. Instruct patient to use soft toothbrush and electric razor. Patients should be cautioned not to drink alcoholic beverages or take products containing aspirin or ibuprofen.

□ Instruct patient to notify physician if abdominal pain, yellow skin, cough, diarrhea, or decreased urine output occurs.

□ Inform patient that medication may cause the urine and sclera to turn blue-green.

□ Instruct patient to inspect oral mucosa for redness and ulceration. If mouth sores occur, advise patient to use sponge brush and rinse mouth with water after eating and drinking. Viscous lidocaine swishes may be used if pain interferes with eating.

□ Discuss with patient the possibility of hair loss. Explore coping strategies.

□ Advise patient that although mitoxantrone may cause infertility, contraception during therapy is necessary because of possible teratogenic effects.

□ Instruct patient not to receive any vaccinations without advice of physician.

□ Emphasize need for periodic lab test to monitor for side effects.

EVALUATION
Effectiveness of therapy can be demonstrated by: ■ Decrease in the production and spread of leukemic cells.

MIVACURIUM
(mi-va-**kure**-ee-um)
Mivacron

CLASSIFICATION(S):
Neuromuscular blocking agent (nondepolarizing)
Pregnancy Category C

INDICATIONS

■ Used to produce skeletal muscle paralysis during surgical procedures in conjunction with general anesthesia. Also used to facilitate endotracheal intubation (succinylcholine is preferred because its onset is quicker) and to facilitate compliance during mechanical ventilation.

ACTION

■ Mivacurium prevents neuromuscular transmission by blocking the effect of acetylcholine at the myoneural junction. It has no anxiolytic or analgesic properties. **Therapeutic Effect:** ■ Skeletal muscle paralysis.

PHARMACOKINETICS

Absorption: IV administration results in complete bioavailability.

Distribution: Tissue distribution is limited.

Metabolism and Excretion: Mivacurium is rapidly metabolized by cholinesterases in plasma.

Half-life: 2 hr.

CONTRAINDICATIONS AND PRECAUTIONS

Contraindicated in: ▪ Hypersensitivity to mivacurium. Cross-sensitivity with other similar agents may occur.

Use Cautiously in: ▪ Patients with a history of pulmonary disease, renal or liver impairment, or elderly or debilitated patients (increased sensitivity to drug effects; smaller maintenance doses may be used) ▪ Patients with electrolyte disturbances or who are receiving cardiac glycosides (increased risk of arrhythmias) ▪ Obese patients (more prone to hypotension; dosage should be based on ideal body weight) ▪ Pregnancy, lactation, or children <2 yr (safety not established) ▪ Children (may require larger doses at more frequent intervals than adults).

Use with Extreme Caution in: ▪ Patients with myasthenia gravis or myasthenic syndromes (prolonged respiratory paralysis may occur) ▪ Patients homozygous for atypical plasma cholinesterase (extreme sensitivity to these agents).

ADVERSE REACTIONS AND SIDE EFFECTS*

CNS: dizziness.

Resp: bronchospasm, wheezing, hypoxemia.

CV: tachycardia, bradycardia, arrhythmias, hypotension.

Derm: flushing, rash, urticaria, erythema.

Local: phlebitis.

MS: muscle spasms.

INTERACTIONS

Drug–Drug: ▪ Intensity and duration of paralysis may be prolonged by pretreatment with **succinylcholine, general anesthesia, aminoglycoside antibiotics, polymyxin, colistin, clindamycin, lidocaine, quinidine, procainamide, beta-adrenergic blocking agents, potassium-losing diuretics, magnesium, demecarium, echothiophate,** and **isoflurophate**. If used concurrently with **enflurane** or **isoflurane** decrease dose by 25%.

ROUTE AND DOSAGE

Initial Intubation Dose

▪ **IV (Adults):** 150–200 mcg/kg.
▪ **IV (Children 2–12 yr):** 200–250 mcg/kg.

Maintenance Dose

▪ **IV (Adults):** 0.1 mg/kg as bolus doses every 15 min or as a continuous infusion at 9–10 mcg/kg/min. If infusion is begun at the same time as initial dose, start with rate of 4 mcg/kg/min. Infusion rates may range from 1–15 mcg/kg/min.
▪ **IV (Children 2–12 yr):** 14 mcg/kg/min (range 5–31 mcg/kg/min).

AVAILABILITY

▪ *Injection:* 0.5 mg/ml premixed infusion in D5W, 2 mg/ml, 5-, and 10-ml vials.

TIME/ACTION PROFILE (skeletal paralysis)*

	ONSET	PEAK	DURATION
IV—adults	rapid	3.3 min	26 min
IV—children	rapid	1.9 min	19 min

*When used in conjunction with general anesthesia.

NURSING IMPLICATIONS

ASSESSMENT

▫ Assess respiratory status continuously throughout mivacurium therapy. Notify physician of significant changes immediately.
▫ Neuromuscular response to mivacurium should be monitored with a peripheral nerve stimulator. Paralysis is initially selective and usually occurs

*Underlines indicate most frequent; **CAPITALS** indicate life-threatening.

sequentially in the following muscles: levator muscles of eyelids, muscles of mastication, limb muscles, abdominal muscles, muscles of the glottis, intercostal muscles, and the diaphragm. Recovery of muscle function usually occurs in reverse order.

□ Monitor ECG, heart rate, and blood pressure throughout the use of mivacurium.

□ Observe the patient for residual muscle weakness and respiratory distress during the recovery period. Monitor effects with peripheral nerve stimulator.

■ **Toxicity and Overdose:** If overdose occurs, use peripheral nerve stimulator to determine the degree of neuromuscular blockade. Maintain airway patency and ventilation until recovery of normal respirations occur.

□ Administration of anticholinesterase agents (edrophonium, neostigmine, pyridostigmine) may be used to antagonize the action of mivacurium. Atropine is usually administered prior to or concurrently with anticholinesterase agents to counteract the muscarinic effects. Administration of fluids and vasopressors may be necessary to treat severe hypotension or shock.

POTENTIAL NURSING DIAGNOSES

■ Breathing pattern, ineffective (indications).
■ Communication, impaired verbal (side effects).
■ Fear (patient/family teaching).

IMPLEMENTATION

□ Mivacurium should be used only by individuals experienced in endotracheal intubation, and equipment for this procedure should be readily available.

□ Mivacurium has no effect on consciousness or the pain threshold. Adequate anesthesia and analgesia should *always* be used when mivacurium is used as an adjunct to surgical procedures or when painful procedures are performed. Benzodiazepines and/or analgesics should be adminstered concurrently when prolonged mivacurium therapy is used for ventilator patients, because patient is awake and able to feel all sensations.

□ If eyes remain open throughout prolonged administration, protect corneas with artificial tears.

■ **Direct IV:** May be administered undiluted.

■ *Rate:* Administer over 5–15 min.

■ **Continuous Infusion:** May be diluted to 0.5 mg/ml in D5W, D5/0.9% NaCl, 0.9% NaCl, lactated Ringer's solution, or D5/LR. Solution is stable for 24 hr at room temperature. Discard unused portion after each use. Also available in premixed infusion of D5W.

■ *Rate:* Titrate rate according to patient response and peripheral nerve stimulator.

■ **Y-Site Compatibility:** ■ alfentanil ■ droperidol ■ fentanyl ■ midazolam ■ sufentanil.

■ **Y-Site Incompatibility:** ■ barbiturates.

PATIENT/FAMILY TEACHING

□ Explain all procedures to patient receiving mivacurium therapy without anesthesia, as consciousness is not affected by mivacurium alone. Provide emotional support.

□ Reassure patient that communication abilities will return as the medication wears off.

EVALUATION

Effectiveness of therapy can be determined by: ■ Adequate suppression of the twitch response when tested with the peripheral nerve stimulator and subsequent muscle paralysis.

MOLINDONE
(moe-lin-done)
Moban

CLASSIFICATION(S):
Antipsychotic
Pregnancy Category UK

M

INDICATIONS

- Treatment of schizophrenia.

ACTION

- Blocks the effects of dopamine in the reticular activating and limbic systems in the brain. **Therapeutic Effect:** ▪ Diminished psychoses associated with schizophrenic behavior.

PHARMACOKINETICS

Absorption: Rapidly absorbed following oral administration.

Distribution: Appears to be widely distributed; probably enters the CNS and enters breast milk.

Metabolism and Excretion: Mainly (>90%) metabolized by the liver. Small (<3%) amounts excreted unchanged by the kidneys.

Half-life: 1.5 hr.

CONTRAINDICATIONS AND PRECAUTIONS

Contraindicated in: ▪ Hypersensitivity to molindone ▪ Cross-sensitivity with other antipsychotics may exist ▪ Hypersensitivity to bisulfites, parabens, or alcohol (in liquid).

Use Cautiously in: ▪ Elderly or debilitated patients (lower doses recommended) ▪ Diabetes mellitus ▪ Respiratory disease ▪ Prostatic hypertrophy ▪ CNS tumors ▪ Epilepsy ▪ Intestinal obstruction ▪ Pregnancy, lactation, or children (safety not established).

ADVERSE REACTIONS AND SIDE EFFECTS*

CNS: <u>sedation</u>, extrapyramidal reactions, tardive dyskinesia, headache, dizziness, insomnia, depression, euphoria, NEUROLEPTIC MALIGNANT SYNDROME.

EENT: dry eyes, blurred vision, nasal congestion.

CV: hypotension, tachycardia.

GI: <u>constipation</u>, <u>dry mouth</u>, nausea, anorexia, hepatitis.

Derm: rashes, photosensitivity.

Endo: galactorrhea, irregular menses, increased libido.

Misc: allergic reactions.

INTERACTIONS

Drug–Drug: ▪ Calcium in the formulation may decrease absorption of **phenytoin** or **tetracycline** ▪ Additive CNS depression with other **CNS depressants,** including **alcohol, antihistamines, antidepressants, MAO inhibitors, opioid analgesics,** and **sedative/ hypnotics** ▪ Additive anticholinergic properties with **agents having anticholinergic effects,** including **phenothiazines, haloperidol, antihistamines, MAO inhibitors,** or **disopyramide** ▪ Encephalopathy may occur with **lithium** ▪ Molindone may mask early signs of **lithium** toxicity ▪ May negate the beneficial effects of **levodopa.**

ROUTE AND DOSAGE

- **PO (Adults):** 50–75 mg/day in 3–4 divided doses initially in acute schizophrenia. Dosage may be increased to 100 mg/day after 3–4 days. Usual maintenance dose is 5–25 mg 3–4 times daily. (Doses up to 225 mg/ day in divided doses have been used in severe psychoses.)

AVAILABILITY

- **Tablets:** 5 mg, 10 mg, 25 mg, 50 mg, 100 mg ▪ **Concentrate:** 20 mg/ml.

TIME/ACTION PROFILE
(peak = blood levels, duration = antipsychotic effects)

	ONSET	PEAK	DURATION
PO	UK	1.5 hr	24–36 hr

NURSING IMPLICATIONS

ASSESSMENT

- ☐ Assess patient's mental status (orientation, mood, behavior, degree of sedation) prior to and periodically throughout therapy.
- ☐ Observe patient carefully when administering medication to ensure medication is actually taken and not hoarded.

*<u>Underlines</u> indicate most frequent; **CAPITALS** indicate life-threatening.

□ Assess fluid intake and bowel function. Increased bulk and fluids in the
diet help minimize the constipating
effects of this medication.

□ Observe patient carefully for extrapyramidal symptoms (pill-rolling motions, drooling, tremors, rigidity,
shuffling gait) and tardive dyskinesia
(uncontrolled movements of face,
mouth, tongue, or jaw and involuntary movements of extremities). Notify
physician immediately at the onset of
these symptoms.

□ Monitor patient for akathisia (restlessness or need to keep moving).
This may appear during first few days
of treatment and may increase with
increase in dosage. Elderly patients
are more susceptible to akathisia.
Treatment may include antiparkinsonian agents, propranolol, diazepam,
or decrease in molindone dosage.

□ Molindone may lower seizure threshold. Institute seizure precautions for
patients with a history of a seizure
disorder.

□ Monitor patient for development of
neuroleptic malignant syndrome (fever, respiratory distress, tachycardia,
convulsions, diaphoresis, hypertension or hypotension, pallor, tiredness). Notify physician immediately
if these symptoms occur.

□ Ocular examinations may be required
periodically during high-dose or prolonged therapy to monitor for deposition of particulate matter on the lens
or cornea.

▪ **Lab Test Considerations:** Monitor
WBC periodically throughout therapy. WBC may be increased or decreased, but molindone therapy may
be continued unless clinical symptoms of leukocytosis or leukopenia
occur. However, if the WBC is <4000
without clinical symptoms, it is recommended that therapy be discontinued until WBC increases. Therapy
should then be re-evaluated.

□ Liver function tests should be monitored periodically during therapy.

□ May cause alterations in BUN, RBC
counts, and serum glucose. These
alterations are not clinically significant.

□ May cause elevated serum prolactin
concentrations during chronic use.

POTENTIAL NURSING DIAGNOSES

▪ Thought processes, altered (indications).

▪ Constipation (side effects).

▪ Knowledge deficit related to medication regimen (patient/family teaching).

IMPLEMENTATION

▪ **PO:** Administer molindone with food
or a full glass of milk or water to minimize gastric irritation. Liquid form
may be administered undiluted or
mixed with water, milk, fruit juice, or
carbonated beverage.

PATIENT/FAMILY TEACHING

□ Instruct patient to take medication exactly as directed and not to take more
or less than prescribed. If a dose is
missed, take as soon as remembered
but not within 2 hr of next dose; do
not double up on missed doses. Consult physician prior to discontinuing
molindone; gradual withdrawal may
be necessary.

□ Inform patient of possibility of extrapyramidal symptoms and tardive dyskinesia. Caution patient to report
these symptoms immediately to physician.

□ Instruct patient not to take molindone
within 2 hr of antacids or medications
for treating diarrhea.

□ Advise patient to make position
changes slowly to minimize orthostatic hypotension. Exercise, hot
weather, or hot baths may increase
hypotensive effects.

□ Medication may cause drowsiness.
Caution patient to avoid driving or
other activities requiring alertness
until response to medication is
known.

□ Caution patient to avoid taking alcohol or other CNS depressants concurrently with this medication.

□ Advise patient to use frequent mouth

M

rinses, good oral hygiene, and sugarless gum or candy to minimize dry mouth.
□ Advise patient to use sunscreen and protective clothing to prevent photosensitivity reactions.
□ Instruct patient to notify physician promptly if tremors, involuntary muscle twitching, or visual disturbances occur.
□ Emphasize the importance of routine follow-up examinations.

Evaluation
Effectiveness of therapy can be demonstrated by: ▪ Decrease in hallucinations, insomnia, agitation, hostility, and delusions. May require several weeks of therapy to obtain optimal effects.

MONOAMINE OXIDASE (MAO) INHIBITORS

isocarboxazid
(eye-soe-kar-**box**-a-zid)
Marplan

phenelzine
(**fen**-el-zeen)
Nardil

tranylcypromine
(tran-ill-**sip**-roe-meen)
Parnate

CLASSIFICATIONS:
Antidepressants
Pregnancy Category UK

INDICATIONS
▪ Treatment of neurotic or atypical depression, usually in conjunction with psychotherapy, in patients who may not tolerate other more conventional modes of therapy (tricyclic antidepressants or electroconvulsive therpy).

ACTION
▪ Inhibits the enzyme monoamine oxidase, resulting in an accumulation of various neurotransmitters (dopamine, epinephrine, norepinephrine, and serotonin) in the body. **Therapeutic Effect:**
▪ Improved mood in depressed patients.

PHARMACOKINETICS
Absorption: All are well absorbed from the GI tract.
Distribution: All cross the placenta and probably enter breast milk.
Metabolism and Excretion: All are mostly metabolized by the liver.
Half-life: UK

CONTRAINDICATIONS AND PRECAUTIONS
Contraindicated in: ▪ Hypersensitivity ▪ Liver disease ▪ Severe renal disease ▪ Cerebrovascular disease ▪ Pheochromocytoma ▪ Congestive heart failure ▪ History of headache ▪ Patients >60 yr ▪ Concurrent meperidine, fluoxetine, paroxetine, or sertraline administration.
Use Cautiously in: ▪ Patients who may be suicidal or have a history of drug dependency ▪ Symptomatic cardiovascular disease ▪ Hyperthyroidism ▪ Seizure disorders ▪ Pregnancy, lactation, or children (safety not established) ▪ Surgery (should be discontinued several weeks prior to surgery if possible due to increased risk of unpredictable reactions).

ADVERSE REACTIONS AND SIDE EFFECTS*
CNS: restlessness, insomnia, dizziness, headache, confusion, SEIZURES, weakness, drowsiness.
EENT: glaucoma, nystagmus, blurred vision.
CV: HYPERTENSIVE CRISIS, orthostatic hypotension, arrhythmias, edema.
GI: constipation, anorexia, nausea, vomiting, diarrhea, abdominal pain, dry mouth.
GU: dysuria, urinary incontinence, urinary retention.
Derm: rashes.
Endo: hypoglycemia.
MS: arthralgia.

*Underlines indicate most frequent; **CAPITALS** indicate life-threatening.

INTERACTIONS

Drug–Drug: ▪ Hypertensive crisis may occur with **amphetamines, methyldopa, levodopa, dopamine, epinephrine, norepinephrine, desipramine, imipramine, guanethidine, reserpine,** or **vasoconstrictors** ▪ Hypertension or hypotension, coma, convulsions, and death may occur with **opioid analgesics** (avoid use of meperidine within 14–21 days of MAO inhibitor therapy—decrease initial dose of other agents to 25% of usual dose) ▪ Additive hypotension with **antihypertensives** or **spinal anesthesia** ▪ Additive hypoglycemia with **insulin** or **oral hypoglycemic agents** ▪ Serious adverse reactions may occur with **fluoxetine, paroxetine,** or **sertraline.** Avoid using within 2 wk of each other (wait 5 wk from end of fluoxetine therapy).

Drug–Food: ▪ Hypertensive crisis may occur with ingestion of foods containing high concentrations of **tyramine** (see Appendix K).

ROUTE AND DOSAGE

Isocarboxazid
▪ **PO (Adults):** 30 mg/day initially in single or divided doses (up to 60 mg/day). Maintenance dose 10–20 mg/day.

Phenelzine
▪ **PO (Adults):** 15 mg 3 times daily, increase to 60–90 mg/day in divided doses, then gradually reduce to smallest effective dose (15 mg/day or every other day). Elderly patients should be started on 15 mg/day with slow-dose titration. For panic attacks, use 15 mg/day, increase over 2 wk to 15 mg 3–4 times daily.

Tranylcypromine
▪ **PO (Adults):** 30 mg/day in 2 divided doses (morning and afternoon); after 2 wk can increase by 10 mg/day, at 1–3 wk intervals, up to 60 mg/day. In elderly patients, start with 2.5–5 mg/day, increase every 3–4 days up to 45 mg/day. For panic attacks, 10 mg/day initially, increased over 2 wk to 20–30 mg/day.

AVAILABILITY

Isocarboxazid
▪ **Tablets:** 10 mg.

Phenelzine
▪ **Tablets:** 15 mg.

Tranylcypromine
▪ **Tablets:** 10 mg.

TIME/ACTION PROFILE
(antidepressant effect)

	ONSET	PEAK	DURATION
Isocarboxazid	1–4 wk	3–4 wk	2 wk
Phenelzine	1–4 wk	2–6 wk	2 wk
Tranylcypromine	several days	2–3 wk	3–5 days

NURSING IMPLICATIONS

ASSESSMENT

▫ Assess mental status and mood changes and anxiety level frequently. Assess for suicidal tendencies, especially during early therapy. Restrict amount of drug available to patient.

▫ Monitor blood pressure and pulse rate prior to and frequently throughout therapy. Notify physician promptly of significant changes.

▫ Monitor intake and output ratios and daily weight. Assess patient for peripheral edema and urinary retention.

▪ **Lab Test Considerations:** Assess hepatic function periodically during prolonged or high-dose therapy.

▫ Monitor serum or urine glucose closely in diabetic patients; hypoglycemia may occur.

▪ **Toxicity and Overdose:** Concurrent ingestion of tyramine-rich foods and many medications may result in a life-threatening hypertensive crisis. Signs and symptoms of hypertensive crisis include chest pain, severe headache, nausea and vomiting, photosensitivity, and enlarged pupils. Treatment includes IV phentolamine.

▫ Symptoms of overdose include anxiety, irritability, tachycardia, hypertension or hypotension, respiratory distress, dizziness, drowsines, hallu-

M

cinations, confusion, seizures, fever, and diaphoresis. Treatment includes induction of vomiting or gastric lavage and supportive therapy as symptoms arise.

POTENTIAL NURSING DIAGNOSES

- Coping, ineffective individual (indications).
- Knowledge deficit related to medication regimen (patient/family teaching).
- Noncompliance (patient/family teaching).

IMPLEMENTATION

- **General Info:** Do not administer these medications in the evening because the psychomotor stimulating effects may cause insomnia or other sleep disturbances.
- **PO:** Tablets may be crushed and mixed with food or fluids for patients with difficulty swallowing.

PATIENT/FAMILY TEACHING

- □ Instruct patient to take medication exactly as directed. If a dose is missed, take if remembered within 2 hours; otherwise omit and return to regular dosage schedule. Medication should not be abruptly discontinued as withdrawal symptoms (confusion, hallucinations, nightmares, headache, nausea, diaphoresis, shivering, tachycardia, slurred speech, unsteady gait) may occur.
- □ Caution patient to avoid alcohol, CNS depressants, over-the-counter drugs, and foods or beverages containing tyramine (see Appendix K) during and for at least 2 wk after therapy has been discontinued; they may precipitate a hypertensive crisis. Contact physician immediately if symptoms of hypertensive crisis develop.
- □ Medication may cause dizziness or drowsiness. Caution patient to avoid driving and other activities requiring alertness until response to medication is known.
- □ Caution patient to make position changes slowly to minimize orthostatic hypotension. Elderly patients

are at increased risk for this side effect.

- □ Advise patient to notify physisican if dry mouth, urinary retention, or constipation occurs. Frequent rinses, good oral hygiene, and sugarless candy or gum may diminish dry mouth. An increase in fluid intake, fiber, and exercise may prevent constipation.
- □ Instruct patient to notify physician of severe headache, skin rash, diarrhea, pale stools, darkening of the urine, jaundice, swelling of feet, palpitations, or increased nervousness.
- □ Advise patient to notify physician or dentist of medication regimen prior to treatment or surgery. If possible, therapy should be discontinued at least 2 wk prior to surgery.
- □ Instruct patient to carry identification describing medication regimen at all times.
- □ Emphasize the importance of participation in psychotherapy if ordered by physician and follow-up examinations to evaluate progress. Ophthalmic testing should also be done periodically during long-term therapy.

EVALUATION

Effectiveness of therapy can be demonstrated by: ■ Improved mood in depressed patients □ Decreased anxiety □ Increased appetite □ Improved energy level □ Improved sleep. Patients may require 1–4 wk of therapy before therapeutic effects of medication are seen.

MORICIZINE
(more-i-siz-een)
Ethmozine

CLASSIFICATION(S):
Antiarrhythmic (group I)
Pregnancy Category B

INDICATIONS

■ Treatment of life-threatening ventricular arrhythmias, including sustained ventricular tachycardia.

ACTION

- Suppresses abnormal automaticity and prolongs PR and QRS interval by blocking fast sodium channel in myocardial tissue ▪ Also has membrane stabilizing and local anesthetic properties. **Therapeutic Effect:** ▪ Suppression of life-threatening arrhythmias.

PHARMACOKINETICS

Absorption: Well absorbed, but rapidly metabolized following oral administration.
Distribution: 95% bound to plasma proteins. Enters breast milk.
Metabolism and Excretion: Extensively metabolized, <1% excreted unchanged in the urine. Metabolites may be active.
Half-life: 1.5–3.5 hr.

CONTRAINDICATIONS AND PRECAUTIONS

Contraindicated in: ▪ Hypersensitivity ▪ Cardiogenic shock ▪ 2nd- or 3rd-degree AV block or bundle branch block (unless a pacemaker has been placed).
Use Cautiously in: ▪ Electrolyte disturbances ▪ Severe renal or hepatic impairment (dosage reduction may be necessary) ▪ Pregnancy, lactation, or children (safety not established) ▪ Congestive heart failure.
Extreme Caution in: ▪ Sick-sinus syndrome.

ADVERSE REACTIONS AND SIDE EFFECTS*

CNS: <u>dizziness</u>, <u>headache</u>, <u>fatigue</u>, weakness, nervousness, sleep disorders.
EENT: blurred vision.
Resp: dyspnea.
CV: ARRHYTHMIAS, chest pain, congestive heart failure, palpitations.
GI: <u>nausea</u>, vomiting, dyspepsia, diarrhea, dry mouth.
Derm: sweating.
MS: musculoskeletal pain.
Neuro: paresthesia.
Misc: drug fever.

INTERACTIONS

Drug–Drug: ▪ Decreases blood levels of **theophylline** ▪ **Cimetidine** increases blood levels of moricizine.

ROUTE AND DOSAGE

- **PO (Adults):** 600–900 mg/day given q 8–12 hr. Within this range dosage may be adjusted by 150 mg/day every 3 days as required and tolerated.

AVAILABILITY

- *Tablets:* 200 mg, 250 mg, 300 mg.

TIME/ACTION PROFILE (arrhythmia suppression)

	ONSET	PEAK	DURATION
PO	UK	0.5–2 hr	8–12 hr

NURSING IMPLICATIONS

ASSESSMENT

- Monitor ECG or Holtor monitor prior to and periodically throughout therapy. May cause PR prolongation and QT prolongation.
- Monitor blood pressure and pulse periodically during course of therapy.
- Monitor intake and output ratios and daily weight. Assess patient for signs of congestive heart failure (peripheral edema, rales/crackles, dyspnea, weight gain, jugular venous distension).
- **Lab Test Considerations:** Renal, pulmonary, and hepatic function, and CBC should be evaluated periodically on patients receiving long-term therapy.

POTENTIAL NURSING DIAGNOSES

- Cardiac output, decreased (indications).
- Knowledge deficit related to medication regimen (patient/family teaching).

IMPLEMENTATION

- **General Info:** Moricizine therapy should be initiated in a hospital with facilities for cardiac rhythm monitoring.
- Previous antiarrhythmic therapy

M

*<u>Underlines</u> indicate most frequent; **CAPITALS** indicate life-threatening.

should be withdrawn 1–2 half-lives before starting moricizine.

□ Dosage adjustments should be at least 3 days apart due to the long half-life of moricizine.

□ Pre-existing hypokalemia, hyperkalemia, or hypomagnesemia should be corrected prior to instituting therapy.

▪ **PO:** Tablets are usually administered every 8 hr. Total daily dose may be divided and administered every 12 hr for greater compliance, but risk of adverse reactions is greater with higher single dose.

PATIENT/FAMILY TEACHING

□ Instruct patient to take medication around the clock exactly as directed, even if feeling better. Missed doses should be taken as soon as remembered if within 6 hr; omit if remembered later. Gradual dosage reduction may be necessary.

□ Medication may cause dizziness or visual disturbances. Caution patient to avoid driving and other activities requiring alertness until response to medication is known.

□ Advise patient to notify physician or dentist of medication regimen prior to treatment or surgery.

□ Instruct patient to notify physician if chest pain, shortness of breath, fever, or diaphoresis occurs.

□ Advise patient to carry identification describing disease process and medication regimen at all times.

□ Emphasize the importance of follow-up examinations to monitor progress.

EVALUATION

Effectiveness of therapy can be demonstrated by: ▪ Decrease in frequency of ventricular arrhythmias.

MORPHINE
(mor-feen)
Astramorph PF, Duramorph, {Epimorph}, {Morphine H.P.}, {Morphitec}, {M.O.S.}, {M.O.S.-

S.R.}, MS, MSO₄, MS Contin, MSIR, MSIR Capsules, OMS Concentrate, Oramorph SR, RMS, Roxanol, Roxanol SR, {Statex}

CLASSIFICATION(S):
Opioid analgesic (agonist)
Schedule II
Pregnancy Category C

INDICATIONS

▪ Management of severe pain ▪ Management of pulmonary edema ▪ Management of pain associated with myocardial infarction.

ACTION

▪ Binds to opiate receptors in the CNS. Alters the perception of and response to painful stimuli, while producing generalized CNS depression. **Therapeutic Effect:** ▪ Decrease in severity of pain.

PHARMACOKINETICS

Absorption: Variably absorbed following oral administration. More reliably absorbed from rectal, SC, and IM sites.
Distribution: Widely distributed. Crosses the placenta and enters breast milk in small amounts.
Metabolism and Excretion: Mostly metabolized by the liver.
Half-life: 2–3 hr.

CONTRAINDICATIONS AND PRECAUTIONS

Contraindicated in: ▪ Hypersensitivity ▪ Pregnancy or lactation (avoid chronic use) ▪ Some products contain bisulfites and should be avoided in patients with known hypersensitivity.

Use Cautiously in: ▪ Head trauma ▪ Increased intracranial pressure ▪ Severe renal, hepatic, or pulmonary disease ▪ Hypothyroidism ▪ Adrenal insufficiency ▪ Alcoholism ▪ Elderly or debilitated patients (dosage reduction suggested) ▪ Undiagnosed abdominal pain ▪ Prostatic hypertrophy ▪ During labor (has been used to relieve pain; may cause respiratory depression in the newborn).

{} = Available in Canada only.

ADVERSE REACTIONS AND SIDE EFFECTS*

CNS: <u>sedation</u>, <u>confusion</u>, headache, euphoria, floating feeling, unusual dreams, hallucinations, dysphoria, dizziness.
EENT: miosis, diplopia, blurred vision.
Resp: respiratory depression.
CV: <u>hypotension</u>, bradycardia.
GI: nausea, vomiting, <u>constipation</u>.
GU: urinary retention.
Derm: sweating, flushing.
Misc: tolerance, physical dependence, psychological dependence.

INTERACTIONS

Drug–Drug: ▪ Use with **extreme caution** in patients receiving **MAO inhibitors** (may result in unpredictable, severe reactions—decrease initial dose of morphine to 25% of usual dose) ▪ Additive CNS depression with **alcohol, sedative/hypnotics,** and **antihistamines** ▪ Administration of **partial-antagonist opioid analgesics** may precipitate opioid withdrawal in physically dependent patients ▪ **Nalbuphine** or **pentazocine** may decrease analgesia.

ROUTE AND DOSAGE

Larger doses may be required during chronic therapy.

- ▪ **PO (Adults):** 10–30 mg q 4 hr or 30 mg q 8–12 hr initially as extended-release or sustained-release preparations.
- ▪ **IM, SC (Adults):** 5–20 mg q 4 hr as needed.
- ▪ **SC (Children):** 100–200 mcg/kg q 4 hr (not to exceed 15 mg/dose).
- ▪ **IV (Adults):** 2.5–15 mg q 4 hr or IV infusion initiated with a loading dose of 15 mg followed by infusion at 0.8–10 mg/hr, rate increased as needed. Doses of 20–150 mg/hr have been used.
- ▪ **IM, IV (Children):** 50–100 mcg/kg (not to exceed 10 mg/dose initially).
- ▪ **Rect (Adults):** 10–30 mg q 4 hr.
- ▪ **Epidural (Adults):** 2–10 mg/day (initially) or 2–4 mg/day as a continuous infusion.
- ▪ **Intrathecal (Adults):** 0.2–1 mg as a single dose.

AVAILABILITY

▪ *Soluble tablets:* 10 mg, 15 mg, 30 mg ▪ *Tablets:* 15 mg, 30 mg ▪ *Controlled-release tablets:* 30 mg, 60 mg, 100 mg, 200 mg ▪ *Sustained-release tablets:* 15 mg, 30 mg, 60 mg, 100 mg ▪ *Immediate-release capsules:* 15 mg, 30 mg ▪ *Oral solution:* 10 mg/5 ml, 20 mg/5 ml, 20 mg/ml, 100 mg/5 ml ▪ *Rectal suppositories:* 5 mg, 10 mg, 20 mg, 30 mg ▪ *Injection:* 0.5 mg/ml, 1 mg/ml, 2 mg/ml, 3 mg/ml, 4 mg/ml, 5 mg/ml, 8 mg/ml, 15 mg/ml, 25 mg/ml, 50 mg/ml ▪ *In combination with:* atropine.

TIME/ACTION PROFILE (analgesia)

	ONSET	PEAK	DURATION
PO	UK	60 min	4–5 hr
PO-ER	UK	UK	8–12 hr
IM	10–30 min	30–60 min	4–5 hr
SC	20 min	50–90 min	4–5 hr
Rect	UK	20–60 min	4–5 hr
IV	rapid	20 min	4–5 hr
Epidural	6–30 min	UK	up to 24 hr
IT	rapid (min)	UK	up to 24 hr

NURSING IMPLICATIONS

ASSESSMENT

- ▢ Assess type, location, and intensity of pain prior to and 30–60 min following administration.
- ▢ Assess blood pressure, pulse, and respiratory rate before and periodically during administration.
- ▢ Prolonged use may lead to physical and psychological dependence and tolerance. This should not prevent patient from receiving adequate analgesia. Most patients who receive morphine for medical reasons do not develop psychological dependence. Progressively higher doses may be required to relieve pain with long-term therapy.

M

*<u>Underlines</u> indicate most frequent; **CAPITALS** indicate life-threatening.

- Assess bowel function routinely. Increased intake of fluids and bulk, stool softeners, and laxatives may minimize constipating effects.
- Monitor intake and output ratios. If significant discrepancies occur, assess for urinary retention and inform physician.
- **Lab Test Considerations:** May increase plasma amylase and lipase levels.
- **Toxicity and Overdose:** If overdosage occurs, naloxone (Narcan) is the antidote. Monitor patient closely; dose may need to be repeated or may need to be administered as an infusion.

POTENTIAL NURSING DIAGNOSES
- Pain (indications).
- Sensory-perceptual alteration: visual, auditory (side effects).
- Injury, high risk for (side effects).
- Knowledge deficit related to medication regimen (patient/family teaching).

IMPLEMENTATION
- **General Info:** Explain therapeutic value of medication prior to administration to enhance the analgesic effect.
- Regularly administered doses may be more effective than prn administration. Analgesic is more effective if given before pain becomes severe.
- Coadministration with nonopioid analgesics may have additive analgesic effects and may permit lower doses.
- When transferring from other opioids or other forms of morphine to extended-release tablets, administer a total daily dose of oral morphine equivalent to previous daily dose (see Appendix B) and divided every 8 hr (Roxanol SR) or every 12 hr (MS Contin, Oramorph SR).
- Medication should be discontinued gradually after long-term use, to prevent withdrawal symptoms.
- **Rect:** *MS Contin* has been administered rectally.
- **PO:** Doses may be administered with food or milk to minimize GI irritation.
- Extended-release and controlled-release tablets should be swallowed whole; do not crush, break, or chew.
- Solution may be diluted in a glass of fruit juice just prior to administration to improve taste.
- MSIR capsules may be swallowed whole or opened, and the contents sprinkled on cool food (pudding, applesauce). As the coated beads inside capsule will not affect taste of food, the capsule may be opened and the contents added to liquid (i.e., juice) and administered immediately, or the capsule contents may be delivered via gastric or nasogastric tube by adding to or following with liquid. Coated beads inside capsule will not stick to tubes.
- **SC, IM:** Use IM route for repeated doses, as morphine is irritating to SC tissues.
- **IV:** Solution is colorless; do not administer discolored solution.
- **Direct IV:** Dilute with at least 5 ml of Sterile Water or 0.9% NaCl for Injection.
- **Rate:** Administer 2.5–15 mg over 4–5 min. Rapid administration may lead to increased respiratory depression, hypotension, and circulatory collapse.
- Do not use IV administration without antidote available.
- **Continuous Infusion:** May be added to D5W, D10W, 0.9% NaCl, 0.45% NaCl, Ringer's or lactated Ringer's solution, dextrose/saline solution, or dextrose/Ringer's or lactated Ringer's solution in a concentration of 0.1–1 mg/ml or greater for continuous infusion.
- **Rate:** Administer via infusion pump to control the rate. Dose should be titrated to ensure adequate pain relief without excessive sedation, respiratory depression, or hypotension.
- May be administered via patient-controlled analgesia (PCA) pump.
- **Syringe Compatibility:** ▪ atropine ▪benzquinamide▪butorphanol▪chlorpromazine ▪ cimetidine ▪ dimenhydrinate ▪ diphenhydramine ▪ droperidol ▪ fentanyl ▪ glycopyrrolate ▪ hydroxy-

zine ▪ metoclopramide ▪ midazolam ▪ milrinone ▪ perphenazine ▪ promazine ▪ ranitidine ▪ scopolamine.
▪ **Syringe Incompatibility:** ▪ meperidine ▪ thiopental.
▪ **Y-Site Compatibility:** ▪ amikacin ▪ aminophylline ▪ ampicillin ▪ ampicillin/sulbactam ▪ atenolol ▪ atracurium ▪ aztreonam ▪ bumetanide ▪ calcium chloride ▪ cefamandole ▪ cefazolin ▪ cefoperazone ▪ ceforanide ▪ cefotaxime ▪ cefotetan ▪ cefoxitin ▪ ceftazidime ▪ ceftizoxime ▪ ceftriaxone ▪ cefuroxime ▪ cephalothin ▪ cephapirin ▪ chloramphenicol ▪ clindamycin ▪ dexamethasone sodium phosphate ▪ digoxin ▪ dopamine ▪ doxycycline ▪ enalaprilat ▪ erythromycin lactobionate ▪ esmololol ▪ famotidine ▪ fluconazole ▪ fludarabine ▪ foscarnet ▪ gentamicin ▪ heparin ▪ hydrocortisone sodium succinate ▪ insulin ▪ kanamycin ▪ labetalol ▪ lidocaine ▪ methyldopate ▪ methylprednisolone ▪ metoclopramide ▪ metoprolol ▪ metronidazole ▪ mezlocillin ▪ nafcillin ▪ ondansetron ▪ oxacillin ▪ oxytocin ▪ pancuronium ▪ penicillin G potassium ▪ piperacillin ▪ potassium chloride ▪ propranolol ▪ ranitidine ▪ sodium bicarbonate ▪ ticarcillin ▪ ticarcillin/clavulanate ▪ tobramycin ▪ trimethoprim/sulfamethoxazole ▪ vancomycin ▪ vecuronium ▪ vitamin B complex with C ▪ zidovudine.
▪ **Y-Site Incompatibility:** ▪ furosemide ▪ minocycline ▪ sargramostim.

PATIENT/FAMILY TEACHING
▫ Instruct patient on how and when to ask for pain medication.
▫ Medication may cause drowsiness or dizziness. Caution patient to call for assistance when ambulating or smoking, and to avoid driving or other activities requiring alertness until response to medication is known.
▫ Advise patient to make position changes slowly to minimize orthostatic hypotension.
▫ Caution patient to avoid concurrent use of alcohol or other CNS depressants with this medication.

▫ Encourage patient to turn, cough, and breathe deeply every 2 hr to prevent atelectasis.

EVALUATION
Effectiveness of therapy can be demonstrated by: ▪ Decrease in severity of pain without a significant alteration in level of consciousness, respiratory status, or blood pressure.

MULTIPLE VITAMINS—ORAL
Adavite, Dayalets, LKV Drops, Multi-75, Multi-Day, One-A-Day, Optilets, Poly-Vi-Sol, Quintabs, Ru-lets, Sesame Street Vitamins, Siytab, Tab-A-Vite, Therabid, Theragenerix, Theragram, Theravess, Theravim, Therems, Unicaps, Vita-Bob, Vita-Kid, Zymacaps

MULTIVITAMIN INFUSION
Berocca Parenteral Nutrition, M.V.C. 9 + 3, M.V.C. Plus, M.V.I.-12, M.V.I. Pediatric

CLASSIFICATION(S):
Vitamins (multiple, parenteral),
Vitamins (multiple, oral)
Pregnancy Category UK

INDICATIONS
▪ **PO:** Treatment and prevention of vitamin deficiencies. Special formulations are available for patients with particular needs, including: ▫ Prenatal multiple vitamins (with larger doses of folic acid) ▫ Multiple vitamins with iron ▫ Multiple vitamins with fluoride ▫ Multiple vitamins with minerals or trace elements ▪ **IV:** Treatment and prevention of vitamin deficiencies in patients who are unable to ingest oral feedings or vitamins.

ACTION
▪ Contain fat-soluble vitamins (A, D, and E) and most water-soluble vitamins (B-complex vitamins B_1, B_2, B_3, B_5, B_6, B_{12}, vitamin C, biotin, and folic acid).

M

These vitamins are a diverse group of compounds necessary for normal growth and development. Many act as coenzymes or catalysts in numerous metabolic processes. **Therapeutic Effects:** ▪ **PO:** Prevention of deficiency or replacement in patients whose nutritional status is questionable ▪ **IV:** Replacement in patients who are unable to ingest oral feedings or vitamins.

PHARMACOKINETICS

Absorption: Well absorbed from the GI tract following oral administration; some processes are active, some are passive. Absorption of water-soluble vitamins generally increases in deficiency states. Absorption of some lipid-soluble vitamins may require bile acids. **Distribution:** Widely distributed, cross the placenta and enter breast milk. Fat-soluble vitamins (A, D, and E) are stored in fatty tissues and the liver. **Metabolism and Excretion:** Utilized in various biologic processes. Excess amounts of water-soluble vitamins (B vitamins, vitamin C, and folic acid) are excreted unchanged by the kidneys. **Half-life:** UK.

CONTRAINDICATIONS AND PRECAUTIONS

Contraindicated in: ▪ Hypersensitivity to preservatives, colorants, or additives, including tartrazine, saccharin, and aspartame (oral forms) ▪ Hypersensitivity to preservatives, including polysorbates, propylene glycol, EDTA, or benzyl alcohol (parenteral forms).

ADVERSE REACTIONS AND SIDE EFFECTS*

In recommended doses, adverse reactions are extremely rare.

Misc: allergic reactions to preservatives, additives, or colorants.

INTERACTIONS

Drug–Drug: ▪ Large amounts of vitamin B_6 may interfere with the beneficial effect of **levodopa**.

ROUTE AND DOSAGE

▪ **PO (Adults and Children):** 1 dosage unit (tablet/capsule/dropperful)/day or amount recommended by individual manufacturer.

▪ **IV (Adults and Children):** Amount sufficient to meet RDA (Recommended Daily Allowances—see Appendix L) for age group. Usually added to large volume parenteral or total parenteral nutrition (hyperalimentation) solution.

AVAILABILITY

▪ *Tablets:* ▪ *Capsules* ▪ *Liquids* ▪ *Drops* ▪ *Injection* ▪ *In combination with:* fluoride, minerals, and trace elements.

TIME/ACTION PROFILE

	ONSET	PEAK	DURATION
PO	UK	UK	UK
IV	UK	UK	UK

NURSING IMPLICATIONS

ASSESSMENT

▫ Assess patient for signs of nutritional deficiency prior to and throughout therapy. Patients at risk include those who are elderly, debilitated, burned, unable to take oral nutrition, and those with malabsorption syndromes or chronic alcoholism.

▪ **Toxicity and Overdose:** Toxicity rarely occurs with multivitamin preparations due to the small amounts per unit of fat-soluble vitamins. For symptoms, see individual vitamin entries.

▫ If overdose occurs, treatment includes induction of emesis or gastric lavage, calcium gluconate IV if hypocalcemic, and maintenance of high urine output.

POTENTIAL NURSING DIAGNOSES

▪ Nutrition, altered: less than body requirements (indications).
▪ Knowledge deficit related to dietary

---

*Underlines indicate most frequent; **CAPITALS** indicate life-threatening.

needs and medication regimen (patient/family teaching).

IMPLEMENTATION

- **General Info:** Vitamins are usually given orally but may be given parenterally to patients in whom oral administration is not feasible.
- ▫ Combinations with >1 mg folic acid require a prescription.
- **PO:** Forms are not standardized.
- ▫ Chewable tablets should be crushed or chewed prior to swallowing.
- ▫ Liquid preparations may be dropped directly into mouth or mixed with juice or cereal.
- **IV:** Administer multivitamin infusion by infusion only; do not use direct IV injection.
- ▫ Solution is bright yellow and will color IV solutions.
- **Continuous Infusion:** Dilute each 5- or 10-ml ampule in 500–1000 ml of D5/LR, D5/0.9% NaCl, D5W, D10W, D20W, lactated Ringer's injection, 0.9% NaCl, 3% NaCl, or ⅙ M sodium lactate. Do not administer solution that has crystallized.
- **Y-Site Compatibility:** ▪ acyclvoir ▪ ampicillin ▪ cefazolin ▪ cephalothin ▪ cephapirin ▪ erythromycin lactobionate ▪ fludarabine ▪ gentamicin.
- **Additive Compatibility:** ▪ cefoxitin ▪ isoproterenol ▪ methyldopate ▪ metoclopramide ▪ netilmicin ▪ norepinephrine ▪ sodium bicarbonate ▪ verapamil.
- **Additive Incompatibility:** Incompatible in solution with many antibiotics.

PATIENT/FAMILY TEACHING

- ▫ Encourage patient to comply with physician's recommendations. Explain that the best source of vitamins is a well-balanced diet with foods from the 4 basic food groups.
- ▫ Advise parents not to refer to chewable multivitamins for children as candy.

EVALUATION

Effectiveness of therapy can be demonstrated by: ▪ Prevention or decrease in the symptoms of vitamin deficiency.

MUPIROCIN

(myoo-**peer**-oh-sin)
Bactroban, Pseudomonic acid A

CLASSIFICATION(S):
Anti-infective (topical)
Pregnancy Category B

INDICATIONS

- ▪ Treatment of impetigo.

ACTION

- ▪ Inhibits bacterial protein synthesis.

Therapeutic Effect: ▪ Inhibition of bacterial growth and reproduction.
Spectrum: ▪ Greatest activity against gram-positive organisms, including:
▫ *Staphylococcus aureus* ▫ Beta hemolytic streptococci.

PHARMACOKINETICS

Absorption: Minimal systemic absorption.

Distribution: Remains in the stratum corneum for prolonged periods of time (72 hr).

Metabolism and Excretion: Metabolized in the skin, removed by desquamation.

Half-life: UK.

CONTRAINDICATIONS AND PRECAUTIONS

Contraindicated in: ▪ Hypersensitivity to mupirocin or polyethylene glycol.

Use Cautiously in: ▪ Pregnancy or lactation (safety not established).

ADVERSE REACTIONS AND SIDE EFFECTS*

Derm: burning, stinging, pain, erythema, dry skin, tenderness, contact dermatitis, increased exudate.

GI: nausea.

INTERACTIONS

Drug–Drug: ▪ None known.

M

*Underlines indicate most frequent; **CAPITALS** indicate life-threatening.

ROUTE AND DOSAGE
- **Top (Adults and Children):** Apply ointment tid.

AVAILABILITY
- *Ointment:* 2%.

TIME/ACTION PROFILE (resolution of lesions)

	ONSET	PEAK	DURATION
Top	UK	3–5 days	72 hr

NURSING IMPLICATIONS

ASSESSMENT
☐ Assess lesions prior to and daily during therapy.

POTENTIAL NURSING DIAGNOSES
- Skin integrity, impaired (indications).
- Infection, high risk for (indications, patient/family teaching).
- Knowledge deficit related to medication regimen (patient/family teaching).

IMPLEMENTATION
- **Top:** Apply a small amount of mupirocin ointment to the affected area tid. Treated area may be covered with gauze if desired.

PATIENT/FAMILY TEACHING
☐ Instruct patient on the correct application of mupirocin. Advise patient to apply medication exactly as directed for the full course of therapy.
☐ Teach patient and family appropriate hygienic measures to prevent spread of impetigo.
☐ Instruct parents to notify school nurse for screening and prevention of transmission.
☐ Patient should consult physician if symptoms have not improved in 3–5 days.

EVALUATION
Effectiveness of therapy can be demonstrated by: ▪ Healing of skin lesions. If no clinical response is seen in 3–5 days, condition should be re-evaluated.

MUROMONAB-CD3
(myoor-oh-**mon**-ab CD3)
Orthoclone OKT3

CLASSIFICATION(S):
Immunosuppressant (monoclonal antibody)
Pregnancy Category C

INDICATIONS
▪ Treatment of acute renal allograft rejection reactions in transplant patients that have occurred despite conventional antirejection therapy ▪ Treatment of acute steroid-resistant hepatic or cardiac allograft rejection reactions.

ACTION
▪ A purified immunoglobulin antibody that acts as an immunosuppressant by interfering with normal T-cell function. **Therapeutic Effect:** ▪ Reversal of graft rejection in transplant patients.

PHARMACOKINETICS
Absorption: Administered IV only, resulting in complete bioavailability.
Distribution: UK.
Metabolism and Excretion: UK.
Half-life: UK.

CONTRAINDICATIONS AND PRECAUTIONS
Contraindicated in: ▪ Hypersensitivity to muromonab-CD3, murine (mouse) proteins, or polysorbate ▪ Previous muromonab therapy ▪ Fluid overload ▪ Fever >37.8°C or 110°F ▪ Chickenpox or recent exposure to chickenpox ▪ Herpes zoster.
Use Cautiously in: ▪ Active infections ▪ Depressed bone marrow reserve ▪ Chronic debilitating illnesses ▪ Congestive heart failure ▪ Pregnancy, lactation, or children <2 yr (safety not established).

ADVERSE REACTIONS AND SIDE EFFECTS*
CNS: <u>tremor</u>, aseptic meningitis, dizziness.

---

*<u>Underlines</u> indicate most frequent; **CAPITALS** indicate life-threatening.

Resp: dyspnea, shortness of breath, wheezing, PULMONARY EDEMA.
CV: chest pain.
GI: vomiting, nausea, diarrhea.
Misc: fever, chills, INFECTIONS, increased risk of lymphoma, hypersensitivity reactions, CYTOKINE RELEASE SYNDROME.

INTERACTIONS

Drug–Drug: ▪ Additive immunosuppression with other **immunosuppressive agents** ▪ Concurrent **prednisone** and **azathioprine** dosages should be reduced during muromonab therapy (increased risk of infection and lymphoproliferative disorders) ▪ **Cyclosporine** should be reduced or discontinued during muromonab-CD3 therapy (increased risk of infection and lymphoproliferative disorders) ▪ Increased risk of adverse CNS reactions with **indomethacin.**

ROUTE AND DOSAGE

▪ **IV (Adults):** 5 mg/day for 10–14 days (pretreatment with glucocorticoids, acetaminophen, and/or antihistamines recommended).
▪ **IV (Children):** 100 mcg/kg/day for 10–14 days.

AVAILABILITY

▪ *Injection:* 5 mg/5 ml.

TIME/ACTION PROFILE (noted as levels of circulating CD3-positive T cells)

	ONSET	PEAK	DURATION
IV	min	2–7 days	1 wk

NURSING IMPLICATIONS

ASSESSMENT

□ Assess for fluid overload (monitor weight and intake and output, assess for edema and rales/crackles). Notify physician if patient has experienced 3% or more weight gain in the previous week. Chest x-ray examination should be obtained within 24 hr prior to beginning therapy. Fluid-overloaded patients are at high risk of developing pulmonary edema. Monitor vital signs and breath sounds closely.

□ Assess for fever and chills, headache, nausea and vomiting, chest pain, muscle and joint pain, generalized weakness, shortness of breath, dizziness, abdominal pain, malaise, diarrhea, and trembling of hands. The severity of this cytokine release syndrome (CRS) reaction is greatest with initial dose. Reaction occurs within 30–60 min and may persist for up to 6 hr. Prophylactic glucocorticoids (methylprednisolone sodium succinate 8 mg/kg IV), antihistamines, and acetaminophen may be ordered 1–4 hr prior to administration of muromonab-CD3, especially with the initial doses.

□ Assess patient for hypersensitivity reaction. May appear similar to CRS or anaphylaxis (cardiovascular collapse, loss of consciousness, shock, tachycardia, hypotension, angioedema, dyspnea, bronchospasm, urticaria, pruritus). Usually occurs within 10 min of administration. Discontinue drug immediately and do not resume therapy. Keep epinephrine, antihistamines, and resuscitative equipment on hand in case of a reaction.

□ Monitor for infection (fever, chills, rash, sore throat, purulent discharge, dysuria). Notify physician immediately if these symptoms occur, as they may necessitate discontinuation of therapy.

□ Monitor for development of aseptic meningitis. Onset is usually within 3 days of beginning therapy. Assess for fever, headache, nuchal rigidity, and photophobia.

▪ **Lab Test Considerations:** Monitor CBC and differential, platelet count, BUN, creatinine, serum transaminases, alkaline phosphatase, and bilirubin prior to and periodically throughout therapy.

□ Monitor assays of T cell with CD3 antigen daily; target is CD3 positive T cells <25 cells/mm^3 or plasma lev-

M

els as determined by ELISA; target levels should be ≥800 ng/ml.

□ Test for human-mouse antibody titers; a titer of ≥1 : 1000 is a contraindication for use.

POTENTIAL NURSING DIAGNOSES

- Infection, high risk for (side effects).
- Fluid volume excess (side effects).
- Knowledge deficit related to medication regimen (patient/family teaching).

IMPLEMENTATION

- **General Info:** Physician will reduce dosage of glucocorticoids and azathioprine and discontinue cyclosporine during 10–14 day course of muromonab-CD3. Cyclosporine may be resumed 3 days before end of therapy.
- □ Initial dose is administered during hospitalization; patient should be monitored closely for 48 hr. Subsequent doses may be administered on outpatient basis.
- □ Keep medication refrigerated at 2–8°C. Do not shake vial.
- **Direct IV:** Draw solution into syringe via low-protein-binding 0.2- or 22-micrometer filter to ensure removal of translucent protein particles that may be present. Discard filter and attach 20-gauge needle for IV administration.
- □ Do not administer as an infusion; do not admix; do not administer in IV line containing other medications.
- **Rate:** Administer IV push over <1 min.

PATIENT/FAMILY TEACHING

- □ Explain purpose of medication to patient. Inform patient of possible initial-dose side effects, which are markedly reduced in subsequent doses. Explain that patient will need to resume lifelong therapy with other immunosuppressive drugs after completion of muromonab course.
- □ Instruct patient not to receive any vaccinations and to avoid contact with persons receiving oral polio vaccine without advice of physician.
- □ Instruct patient to continue to avoid crowds and persons with known infections, as this drug also suppresses the immune system.

EVALUATION

Effectiveness of therapy can be demonstrated by: ■ Reversal of the symptoms of acute organ rejection.

NABUMETONE
(na-**byoo**-me-tone)
Relafen

CLASSIFICATION(S):
Nonsteroidal anti-inflammatory agent
Pregnancy Category C

INDICATIONS

- Treatment of the signs and symptoms of rheumatoid arthritis and osteoarthritis.

ACTION

- Inhibits prostaglandin synthesis. **Therapeutic Effect:** ■ Suppression of pain and inflammation.

PHARMACOKINETICS

Absorption: Well absorbed following oral administration (80%). 35% is rapidly converted to 6-methoxy-2-naphylacetic acid (6MNA), which is the active metabolite.

Distribution: Distribution is not known.

Metabolism and Excretion: 6-MNA is metabolized by the liver to inactive compounds.

Half-life: 24 hr (increased in severe renal impairment).

CONTRAINDICATIONS AND PRECAUTIONS

Contraindicated in: ■ Hypersensitivity ■ Cross-sensitivity may occur with other nonsteroidal anti-inflammatory agents, including aspirin ■ Active GI bleeding or ulcer disease.

Use Cautiously in: ■ Severe cardiovascular, renal, or hepatic disease ■ History of ulcer disease ■ Pregnancy, lactation, or children (safety not established).

ADVERSE REACTIONS AND SIDE EFFECTS*

CNS: dizziness, headache, fatigue, insomnia, nervousness, somnolence, weakness, agitation, anxiety, confusion, depression, malaise, tremor, vertigo.
EENT: tinnitus, abnormal vision.
Resp: dyspnea, hypersensitivity pneumonitis.
CV: fluid retention, edema, vasculitis.
GI: abnormal liver function tests, diarrhea, dyspepsia, abdominal pain, constipation, flatulence, nausea, dry mouth, gastritis, stomatitis, vomiting, cholestatic jaundice, anorexia, duodenal ulcer, GI BLEEDING, gastroenteritis, increased appetite, melena.
GU: albuminuria, azotemia, interstitial nephritis.
Derm: photosensitivity, increased sweating, pruritus, rash.
Hemat: prolonged bleeding time.
Neuro: paresthesia.
Misc: allergic reactions including ANAPHYLAXIS, weight gain, ANGIONEUROTIC EDEMA.

INTERACTIONS

Drug–Drug: ▪ Additive adverse GI effects with **aspirin**, other **nonsteroidal anti-inflammatory agents, potassium supplements, glucocorticoids,** or **alcohol** ▪ Chronic use with **acetaminophen** may increase the risk of adverse renal reactions ▪ May decrease the effectiveness of **diuretics** or **antihypertensive** therapy ▪ May increase the hypoglycemic effects of **insulin** or **oral hypoglycemic agents** ▪ Increases the risk of toxicity from **methotrexate** ▪ Increased risk of bleeding with **cefamandole, cefotetan, cefoperazone, valproic acid** or **plicamycin, heparin, thrombolytic agents** or **oral anticoagulants** ▪ Increased risk of adverse hematologic reactions with **antineoplastic agents** or **radiation therapy** ▪ Concurrent use with **cyclosporine** may increase the risk of renal toxicity.

ROUTE AND DOSAGE

▪ **PO (Adults):** 1000–2000 mg/day as a single dose or divided dose twice daily. Use lowest effective dose during chronic therapy.

AVAILABILITY

▪ *Tablets:* 500 mg, 750 mg.

TIME/ACTION PROFILE
(analgesia/anti-inflammatory effects)

	ONSET	PEAK	DURATION
PO	1–2 days	few days–2 wk	UK

NURSING IMPLICATIONS

ASSESSMENT

▢ Patients who have asthma, aspirin-induced allergy, and nasal polyps are at increased risk for developing hypersensitivity reactions. Monitor for rhinitis, asthma, and urticaria.
▢ Assess pain and range of motion prior to and periodically throughout therapy.
▪ **Lab Test Considerations:** Liver function tests should be evaluated periodically in patients receiving prolonged courses of therapy. Serum alkaline phosphatase, LDH, AST (SGOT), and ALT (SGPT) levels may be increased.

POTENTIAL NURSING DIAGNOSES

▪ Pain (indications).
▪ Physical mobility, impaired (indications).
▪ Knowledge deficit related to medication regimen (patient/family teaching).

IMPLEMENTATION

▪ **PO:** Administer with meals or antacids to decrease GI irritation and increase absorption.

PATIENT/FAMILY TEACHING

▢ Advise patient to take this medication with a full glass of water and to remain in an upright position for 15–30 min after administration.
▢ Instruct patient to take medication exactly as directed. If a dose is missed, it should be taken as soon as remembered but not if almost time for the next dose. Do not double doses.
▢ Nabumetone may cause drowsiness, dizziness, lightheadedness, or visual

N

disturbances. Advise patient to avoid driving or other activities requiring alertness until response to the medication is known.

□ Advise patient to use sunscreen and protective clothing to prevent photosensitivity reactions.

□ Caution patient to avoid the concurrent use of alcohol, aspirin, ibuprofen, acetaminophen, or other over-the-counter medications without consultation with physician or pharmacist.

□ Advise patient to notify physician or dentist of medication regimen prior to treatment or surgery.

□ Instruct patient to notify physician if rash, itching, muscle aches, visual disturbances, edema, black stools, difficulty breathing, jaundice, blisters or hives, mental depression, weight gain, difficulty swallowing, or bloody or cloudy urine occur.

EVALUATION
Effectiveness of therapy can be demonstrated by: ■ Decreased pain and improved joint mobility. Partial arthritic relief is usually seen within 1 wk, but maximum effectiveness may require 2 wk or more of continuous therapy. Patients who do not respond to one nonsteroidal anti-inflammatory agent may respond to another.

NADOLOL
(nay-doe-lole)
Corgard

CLASSIFICATION(S):
Beta-adrenergic blocker (nonselective), Antihypertensive, Antianginal
Pregnancy Category C

INDICATIONS

■ Used alone or in combination with other agents in the treatment of hypertension ■ Used alone or with other agents in the management of angina pectoris. Unlabeled Uses: ■ Treatment of: □ Tachyarrhythmias □ Anxiety □ Aggressive behavior □ Tremors □ Rebleeding of esophageal vances □ Migraine prophylaxis.

ACTION

■ Blocks stimulation of beta$_1$ (myocardial) and beta$_2$ (pulmonary, vascular, or uterine) receptor sites. Therapeutic Effects: ■ Decreased heart rate and blood pressure.

PHARMACOKINETICS

Absorption: Variably (30%) absorbed following oral administration.
Distribution: Minimal penetration of the CNS. Crosses the placenta and enters breast milk.
Metabolism and Excretion: 70% excreted unchanged by the kidneys.
Half-life: 10–24 hr (increased in renal failure).

CONTRAINDICATIONS AND PRECAUTIONS

Contraindicated in: ■ Uncompensated congestive heart failure ■ Pulmonary edema ■ Cardiogenic shock ■ Bradycardia ■ Heart block ■ COPD or asthma.
Use Cautiously in: ■ Thyrotoxicosis or hypoglycemia (may mask symptoms) ■ Renal impairment (increased dosage interval recommended if CCr <50 ml/min) ■ Pregnancy or lactation (may cause apnea, low Apgar scores, bradycardia, and hypoglycemia in the newborn) ■ Children (safety not established) ■ History of severe allergic reactions (intensity of reactions may be increased).

ADVERSE REACTIONS AND SIDE EFFECTS*

CNS: fatigue, weakness, depression, memory loss, mental change, drowsiness.
EENT: dry eyes, blurred vision, nasal stuffiness.
Resp: bronchospasm, wheezing.
CV: BRADYCARDIA, CONGESTIVE HEART FAILURE, PULMONARY EDEMA, hypotension, peripheral vasoconstriction.

---

*Underlines indicate most frequent; CAPITALS indicate life-threatening.

GI: constipation, diarrhea, nausea, vomiting.
GU: impotence, diminished libido.
Derm: rash, itching.
Endo: hyperglycemia, hypoglycemia.
Misc: Raynaud's phenomenon.

INTERACTIONS

Drug–Drug: ▪ **General anesthesia, IV phenytoin,** or **verapamil** may cause additive myocardial depression ▪ Additive bradycardia may occur with concurrent use of **cardiac glycosides** ▪ Additive hypotension may occur with other **antihypertensive agents,** acute ingestion of **alcohol,** or **nitrates** ▪ May negate the beneficial effects of **beta-adrenergic bronchodilators, dopamine,** or **dobutamine** ▪ **Nonsteroidal anti-inflammatory agents** or **thyroid** may decrease effectiveness ▪ Concurrent use of **amphetamines, cocaine, ephedrine, epinephrine, norepinephrine, phenylephrine,** or **pseudoephedrine** may cause excess alpha-adrenergic stimulation, hypertension, and bradycardia ▪ Use with **insulin** may produce prolonged hypoglycemia ▪ May produce hypertension when used within 14 days of **MAO inhibitor** therapy.

ROUTE AND DOSAGE

▪ **PO (Adults):** 40–80 mg once daily (doses up to 240 mg/day for angina have been used; 320 mg/day have been used for hypertension).

AVAILABILITY

▪ *Tablets:* 20 mg, 40 mg, 80 mg, 120 mg, 160 mg.

TIME/ACTION PROFILE
(antihypertensive effect)

	ONSET	PEAK	DURATION
PO	up to 5 days	6–9 days	24 hr

NURSING IMPLICATIONS

ASSESSMENT

▪ **General Info:** Monitor blood pressure and pulse frequently during period of adjustment and periodically through-

out therapy. Confer with physician prior to giving drug if pulse is <50 bpm. Assess for orthostatic hypotension when assisting patient up from supine position.
▫ Monitor intake and output ratios and daily weight. Assess patient routinely for evidence of congestive heart failure (peripheral edema, dyspnea, rales/crackles, fatigue, weight gain, jugular venous distention).
▪ **Angina:** Assess frequency and duration of episodes of chest pain periodically throughout therapy.
▪ **Lab Test Considerations:** Hepatic and renal function and CBC should be monitored routinely in patients receiving prolonged therapy.
▫ May cause elevations in serum potassium, uric acid, triglyceride, LDH, alkaline phosphatase levels, and BUN.

POTENTIAL NURSING DIAGNOSES

▪ Cardiac output, decreased (indications, adverse reactions).
▪ Knowledge deficit related to medication regimen (patient/family teaching).
▪ Noncompliance (patient/family teaching).

IMPLEMENTATION

▪ **PO:** May be administered with food or on an empty stomach. May be crushed and mixed with food or fluid if patient has difficulty swallowing.

PATIENT/FAMILY TEACHING

▫ Instruct patient to take medication exactly as directed, even if feeling well. If a dose is missed, it may be taken as soon as remembered up to 8 hr before next dose. Abrupt withdrawal may result in life-threatening arrhythmias, hypertension, or myocardial ischemia.
▫ Teach patient and family how to check pulse and blood pressure. Instruct them to take pulse daily and blood pressure biweekly. Advise patient to withhold dose and contact physician if pulse is <50 bpm or blood pressure changes significantly.
▫ Reinforce need to continue additional therapies for hypertension (weight

N

loss, restricted sodium intake, stress reduction, regular exercise, moderation of alcohol consumption, smoking cessation). Nadolol helps control but does not cure hypertension.

□ May occasionally cause drowsiness. Caution patient to avoid driving or other activities that require alertness until response to drug is known.

□ Caution patient that nadolol may cause increased sensitivity to cold.

□ Advise patient to consult physician or pharmacist before taking any over-the-counter drugs, especially cold remedies, concurrently with this medication. Patient should also avoid excessive amounts of coffee, tea, and cola.

□ Diabetic patients should monitor serum glucose closely, especially if weakness, fatigue, or irritability occurs. Nadolol may mask tachycardia and increased blood pressure as signs of hypoglycemia, but dizziness and sweating may still occur.

□ Instruct patient to inform physician or dentist of this therapy prior to treatment or surgery.

□ Advise patient to carry identification describing medication regimen at all times.

□ Instruct patient to notify physician if slow pulse rate, depression, or skin rash occurs.

EVALUATION

Effectiveness of therapy can be demonstrated by: ■ Decrease in blood pressure ■ Reduction in frequency of anginal attacks □ Improved exercise tolerance. May require up to 5 days before therapeutic effects are seen.

NAFARELIN
(na-**fare**-e-lin)
Synarel

CLASSIFICATION(S):
Hormone (gonadotropin-releasing hormone)
Pregnancy Category X

INDICATIONS

■ Management of endometriosis ■ Management of central precocious puberty (gonadotropin-dependent) in children.

ACTION

■ Acts as a synthetic analogue of gonadotropin-releasing hormone (GnRH). Initially increases pituitary production of luteinizing hormone (LH) and follicle-stimulating hormone (FSH), which cause ovarian steroid production. Chronic administration leads to decreased production of gonadotropins. Endometriotic lesions are sensitive to ovarian hormones. **Therapeutic Effects:** ■ Reduction in lesions and associated pain in endometriosis ■ Arrest and regression of puberty in children with central precocious puberty.

PHARMACOKINETICS

Absorption: Well absorbed following intranasal administration.
Distribution: Distribution not known.
Metabolism and Excretion: 20–40% excreted in feces. 3% excreted unchanged by the kidneys.
Half-life: 3 hr.

CONTRAINDICATIONS AND PRECAUTIONS

Contraindicated in: ■ Hypersensitivity to gonadotropin-releasing hormone, its analogues, benzalkonium chloride, galcial acetic acid, or sorbitol ■ Pregnancy or lactaion.
Use Cautiously in: ■ Rhinitis.

ADVERSE REACTIONS AND SIDE EFFECTS*

CNS: <u>headaches</u>, <u>emotional instability</u>, insomnia, depression.
EENT: <u>nasal irritation</u>.
CV: edema.
GU: <u>vaginal dryness</u>.
Derm: <u>acne</u>, seborrhea, hirsutism.
Endo: <u>reduced breast size</u>, <u>impaired fertility</u>, <u>cessation of menses</u>.
MS: myalgia, decreased bone density.
Misc: <u>hot flashes</u>, <u>decreased libido</u>, weight gain, hypersensitivity reactions.

---

*<u>Underlines</u> indicate most frequent; **CAPITALS** indicate life-threatening.

INTERACTIONS

Drug–Drug: ■ Concurrent **topical nasal decongestants** may reduce absorption of nafarelin (administer decongestant at least 2 hr after nafarelin).

ROUTE AND DOSAGE

Endometriosis

■ **Intranasal (Adults):** 1 spray (200 mcg) in one nostril in the morning and 1 spray in the other nostril in the evening (400 mcg/day). May be increased to 1 spray in each nostril in the morning and evening (800 mcg/day).

Central Precocious Puberty

■ **Intranasal (Children):** 2 sprays in each nostril in the morning and in the evening (1600 mcg/day; may be increased up to 1800 mcg/day).

AVAILABILITY

■ **Nasal spray:** 2 mg/ml 10-ml bottle (200 mcg/spray).

TIME/ACTION PROFILE (decreased ovarian steroid production)

	ONSET	PEAK	DURATION
Intranasal	UK	4 wk	UK

NURSING IMPLICATIONS

ASSESSMENT

■ **Endometriosis:** Assess patient for endometriotic pain periodically throughout therapy.
■ **Central Precocious Puberty:** Prior to therapy a complete physical and endocrinologic examination, including height, weight, hand and wrist x-ray, total sex steroid level (estradiol or testosterone), adrenal steroid level, beta human chorionic gonadotropin level, GnRH stimulation test, pelvic/adrenal/testicular ultrasound, and computerized tomography of the head must be performed. These parameters are monitored after 6–8 wk and every 3–6 mo during therapy.
□ Assess patient for signs of precocious puberty (menses, breast development, testicular growth) periodically throughout therapy.
□ Nafarelin is discontinued when the onset of normal puberty is desired. Monitor the onset of normal puberty and assess menstrual cycle, reproductive function, and final adult height.

POTENTIAL NURSING DIAGNOSES

■ Pain (indications).
■ Sexual dysfunction (indications, side effects).
■ Knowledge deficit related to medication regimen (patient/family teaching).

IMPLEMENTATION

■ **Endometriosis:** Treatment should be started between days 2 and 4 of the menstrual cycle and continued for up to 6 mo.

PATIENT/FAMILY TEACHING

■ **General Info:** Instruct patient on the correct technique for nasal spray, the head should be tilted back slightly; wait 30 sec between sprays.
□ Advise patient to consult physician if rhinitis occurs during therapy. If a topical decongestant is needed, do not use decongestant until 2 hr after nafarelin dosing. If possible, avoid sneezing during and immediately after nafarelin dose.
■ **Endometriosis:** Inform patient that 1 spray should be administered into one nostril in the morning and 1 spray into the other nostril in the evening for the 400 mcg/dose. If dose is increased to 800 mcg/day, administer 1 spray to each nostril (2 sprays) morning and evening. 1 bottle should provide a 30-day supply at the 400 mcg/day dose.
□ Advise patient to use a form of contraception other than oral contraceptives during therapy. Inform patient that amenorrhea is expected. Instruct patient to notify physician if regular menstruation persists or if successive doses are missed.
□ Advise patient that medication may cause hot flashes. Notify physician if these become bothersome.

N

- **Central Precocious Puberty:** Instruct patient on correct timing and number of sprays. The 1600 mcg/day dose is achieved by 2 sprays to each nostril in the morning (4 sprays) and 2 sprays to each nostril in the evening (4 sprays) for a total of 8 sprays. The 1800 mcg/day dose is achieved by 3 sprays into alternating nostrils 3 times per day for a total of 9 sprays. Inform patient and parents that if doses are not taken as directed pubertal process may be reactivated. 1 bottle should provide a 7-day supply at the 1600 mcg/day dose.
- Advise patient and parents that during first month of therapy some signs of puberty (vaginal bleeding, breast enlargement) may occur. These should resolve after the first month of therapy. If these signs persist after the second month of therapy, notify physician.

EVALUATION
Clinical response to therapy can be determined by: ▪ Reduction in lesions and associated pain in endometriosis ▪ Resolution of the signs of precocious puberty.

NAFCILLIN
(naf-**sill**-in)
Nafcil, Nallpen, Unipen

CLASSIFICATION(S):
Anti-infective (penicillinase-resistant penicillin)
Pregnancy Category B

INDICATIONS
▪ Treatment of the following infections due to susceptible strains of penicillinase-producing staphylococci: ▫ Respiratory tract infections ▫ Skin and skin structure infections ▫ Bone and joint infections ▫ Urinary tract infections ▫ Endocarditis ▫ Septicemia ▫ Meningitis.

ACTION
▪ Binds to bacterial cell wall, leading to cell death ▪ Resists the action of penicillinase, an enzyme capable of inactivating penicillin. **Therapeutic Effect:** ▪ Bactericidal action against susceptible bacteria. **Spectrum:** ▪ Active against most gram-positive aerobic cocci, but less so than penicillin ▪ Notable for activity against penicillinase-producing strains of: ▫ *Staphylococcus aureus* ▫ *Staphylococcus epidermidis* ▪ Not active against methicillin-resistant staphylococci.

PHARMACOKINETICS
Absorption: Poorly and erratically absorbed from the GI tract. Well absorbed from IM sites.
Distribution: Widely distributed. Penetration into CSF is minimal but sufficient in the presence of inflamed meninges. Crosses the placenta and enters breast milk.
Metabolism and Excretion: Excreted unchanged by the kidneys.
Half-life: 30–90 min (increased in renal impairment).

CONTRAINDICATIONS AND PRECAUTIONS
Contraindicated in: ▪ Hypersensitivity to penicillins.
Use Cautiously in: ▪ Severe renal impairment (dosage reduction required) ▪ Pregnancy or lactation (safety not established) ▪ History of previous hypersensitivity reactions.

ADVERSE REACTIONS AND SIDE EFFECTS*
CNS: SEIZURES (high doses).
GI: <u>nausea</u>, <u>vomiting</u>, <u>diarrhea</u>, hepatitis.
GU: interstitial nephritis.
Derm: <u>rashes</u>, urticaria.
Hemat: blood dyscrasias.
Local: phlebitis at IV site, pain at IM site.
Misc: superinfection, <u>allergic reactions</u>, including ANAPHYLAXIS and serum sickness.

*<u>Underlines</u> indicate most frequent; **CAPITALS** indicate life-threatening.

INTERACTIONS

Drug–Drug: ▪ **Probenecid** decreases renal excretion and increases blood levels ▪ May alter the effect of **oral anticoagulants**.

Drug–Food: ▪ **Food, acidic juices,** or **carbonated beverages** decrease absorption of nafcillin.

ROUTE AND DOSAGE

Parenteral nafcillin contains 2.9 mEq sodium/g.

- ▪ **PO (Adults):** 250–1000 mg q 4–6 hr.
- ▪ **PO (Children and Infants):** 25–50 mg/kg/day in divided doses q 6 hr.
- ▪ **PO (Neonates):** 30–40 mg/kg/day in divided doses q 6–8 hr.
- ▪ **IM (Adults):** 500 mg q 4–6 hr.
- ▪ **IM (Children and Infants):** 25 mg/kg q 12 hr.
- ▪ **IM (Neonates):** 10–20 mg/kg q 12 hr.
- ▪ **IV (Adults):** 500–1500 mg q 4 hr.
- ▪ **IV (Children and Neonates):** 10–20 mg/kg q 4 hr or 20–40 mg/kg q 8 hr (up to 200 mg/kg/day).

AVAILABILITY

- ▪ *Tablets:* 500 mg ▪ *Capsules:* 250 mg
- ▪ *Oral solution:* 250 mg/5 ml ▪ *Injection:* 1 g, 2 g, 10 g.

TIME/ACTION PROFILE (blood levels)

	ONSET	PEAK
PO	30 min	1–2 hr
IM	30 min	1–2 hr
IV	rapid	end of infusion

NURSING IMPLICATIONS

ASSESSMENT

- ▢ Assess patient for infection (vital signs; appearance of wound, sputum, urine, and stool; WBC) at beginning and throughout course of therapy.
- ▢ Obtain a history before initiating therapy to determine previous use of and reactions to penicillins or cephalosporins. Persons with a negative history of penicillin sensitivity may still have an allergic response.
- ▢ Obtain specimens for culture and sensitivity prior to initiating therapy.

First dose may be given before receiving results.

- ▢ Observe patient for signs and symptoms of anaphylaxis (rash, pruritus, laryngeal edema, wheezing). Discontinue the drug and notify physician immediately if these occur. Keep epinephrine, an antihistamine, and resuscitation equipment close by in the event of an anaphylactic reaction.
- ▪ **Lab Test Considerations:** May cause positive direct Coombs' test results.

POTENTIAL NURSING DIAGNOSES

- ▪ Infection, high risk for (indications, side effects).
- ▪ Knowledge deficit related to medication regimen (patient/family teaching).
- ▪ Noncompliance related to medication regimen (patient/family teaching).

IMPLEMENTATION

- ▪ **PO:** Administer around the clock on an empty stomach, at least 1 hr before or 2 hr after meals. Take with a full glass of water; acidic juices or carbonated beverages may decrease absorption of penicillins. Use calibrated measuring device for liquid preparations. Shake well. Solution is stable for 14 days if refrigerated.
- ▪ **IM, IV:** To reconstitute, add 1.7–1.8 ml of Sterile Water or Bacteriostatic Water for Injection to each 500-mg vial, 3.4 ml to each 1-g vial, or 6.6–6.8 ml to each 2-g vial, for a concentration of 250 mg/ml. Stable for 2–7 days if refrigerated.
- ▪ **Direct IV:** Dilute reconstituted solution with 15–30 ml of Sterile Water or 0.9% NaCl for Injection.
- ▪ *Rate:* Administer over 5–10 min.
- ▪ **Intermittent Infusion:** Dilute to a concentration of 2–40 mg/ml with Sterile Water for Injection, 0.9% NaCl, D5W, D10W, D5/0.25% NaCl, D5/0.45% NaCl, D5/0.9% NaCl, D5/LR, Ringer's or lactated Ringer's solution. Stable for 24 hr at room temperature, 96 hr if refrigerated.
- ▪ *Rate:* Infuse over at least 30–60 min to avoid vein irritation.

N

- **Syringe Compatibility:** ▪ cimetidine ▪ heparin.
- **Y-Site Compatibility:** ▪ acyclovir ▪ atropine ▪ cyclophosphamide ▪ diazepam ▪ enalaprilat ▪ esmolol ▪ famotidine ▪ fentanyl ▪ fluconazole ▪ foscarnet ▪ hydromorphone ▪ magnesium sulfate ▪ morphine ▪ perphenazine ▪ zidovudine.
- **Y-Site Incompatibility:** ▪ droperidol ▪ droperidol/fentanyl ▪ insulin ▪ labetalol ▪ nalbuphine ▪ pentazocine ▪ verapamil. Incompatible with aminoglycosides. If penicillins and aminoglycosides must be administered concurrently, administer at separate sites.
- **Additive Compatibility:** ▪ dexamethasone ▪ heparin ▪ sodium bicarbonate ▪ sodium lactate.
- **Additive Incompatibility:** ▪ ascorbic acid ▪ bleomycin ▪ cytarabine ▪ gentamicin ▪ hydrocortisone sodium succinate ▪ methylprednisolone sodium succinate.

PATIENT/FAMILY TEACHING

▢ Instruct patient to take medication around the clock and to finish the drug completely as directed, even if feeling better. If a dose is missed, it should be taken as soon as remembered. Advise patient that sharing of this medication may be dangerous.

▢ Advise patient to report the signs of superinfection (black, furry overgrowth on the tongue; vaginal itching or discharge; loose or foul-smelling stools) and allergy to physician promptly.

▢ Instruct patient to notify physician if symptoms do not improve.

EVALUATION

Clinical response can be evaluated by:
▪ Resolution of the signs and symptoms of infection. Length of time for complete resolution depends on the organism and site of infection.

NALBUPHINE
(**nal**-byoo-feen)
Nubain

> ### CLASSIFICATION(S):
> Opioid analgesic (agonist/antagonist)
> **Pregnancy Category C**

INDICATIONS

▪ Management of moderate to severe pain ▪ Also used as an analgesic during labor, as a sedative prior to surgery, and as a supplement in balanced anesthesia.

ACTION

▪ Binds to opiate receptors in the CNS ▪ Alters the perception of and response to painful stimuli, while producing generalized CNS depression ▪ In addition, has partial antagonist properties, which may result in opioid withdrawal in physically dependent patients. **Therapeutic Effect:** ▪ Decrease in moderate to severe pain.

PHARMACOKINETICS

Absorption: Well absorbed following IM and SC administration.
Distribution: Probably crosses the placenta and enters breast milk.
Metabolism and Excretion: Mostly metabolized by the liver and eliminated in the feces via biliary excretion. Minimal amounts excreted unchanged by the kidneys.
Half-life: 5 hr.

CONTRAINDICATIONS AND PRECAUTIONS

Contraindicated in: ▪ Hypersensitivity to nalbuphine or bisulfites ▪ Opioid-dependent patients.
Use Cautiously in: ▪ Head trauma ▪ Increased intracranial pressure ▪ Severe renal, hepatic, or pulmonary disease ▪ Hypothyroidism ▪ Adrenal insufficiency ▪ Alcoholism ▪ Elderly or debilitated patients (dosage reduction suggested) ▪ Undiagnosed abdominal pain ▪ Prostatic hypertrophy ▪ Pregnancy (has been used during labor but may cause respiratory depression in the newborn) ▪ Lactation or children (safety not established).

ADVERSE REACTIONS AND SIDE EFFECTS*

CNS: <u>sedation</u>, confusion, <u>headache</u>, euphoria, floating feeling, unusual dreams, hallucinations, dysphoria, <u>dizziness</u>, <u>vertigo</u>.

EENT: miosis (high doses), blurred vision, diplopia.

Resp: respiratory depression.

CV: orthostatic hypotension, hypertension, palpitations.

GI: <u>nausea</u>, <u>vomiting</u>, constipation, ileus, <u>dry mouth</u>.

GU: urinary urgency.

Derm: <u>sweating</u>, <u>clammy feeling</u>.

Misc: tolerance, physical dependence, psychological dependence.

INTERACTIONS

Drug–Drug: ▪ Use with extreme caution in patients receiving **MAO inhibitors** (may result in unpredictable, severe reactions—reduce initial dose of nalbuphine to 25% of usual dose) ▪ Additive CNS depression with **alcohol, antihistamines,** and **sedative/hypnotics** ▪ May precipitate opioid withdrawal in patients who are physically dependent on **opioid analgesic-agonists** ▪ Avoid concurrent use with other **opioid analgesic-agonists** (may diminish analgesic effect).

ROUTE AND DOSAGE

Analgesia

▪ **IM, SC, IV (Adults):** Usual dose is 10 mg q 3–6 hr (single dose not to exceed 20 mg, total daily dose not to exceed 160 mg).

Supplement To Balanced Anesthesia

▪ **IV (Adults):** 0.3–3 mg/kg over 10–15 min initially. Maintenance dose 0.25–0.5 mg/kg as needed.

AVAILABILITY

▪ *Injection:* 10 mg/ml, 20 mg/ml.

TIME/ACTION PROFILE (analgesia)

	ONSET	PEAK	DURATION
IM	<15 min	60 min	3–6 hr
SC	<15 min	UK	3–6 hr
IV	2–3 min	30 min	3–6 hr

NURSING IMPLICATIONS

ASSESSMENT

▫ Assess type, location, and intensity of pain prior to and 60 min following IM and 30 min following IV administration.

▫ Assess blood pressure, pulse, and respirations before and periodically during administration. Nalbuphine produces respiratory depression, but this does not markedly increase with increased doses.

▫ Although this drug has a low potential for dependence, prolonged use may lead to physical and psychological dependence and tolerance. This should not prevent patient from receiving adequate analgesia. Most patients who receive nalbuphine for medical reasons do not develop psychological dependence. If tolerance develops, changing to an opioid agonist may be required to relieve pain.

▫ Assess prior analgesic history. Antagonistic properties may induce withdrawal symptoms (vomiting, restlessness, abdominal cramps, increased blood pressure, and temperature) in opioid-dependent patients.

▪ **Lab Test Considerations:** May cause elevated serum amylase and lipase levels.

▪ **Toxicity and Overdose:** If overdose occurs, respiratory depression may be reversed by naloxone (Narcan), the antidote.

POTENTIAL NURSING DIAGNOSES

▪ Pain (indications).

▪ Injury, high risk for (side effects).

▪ Sensory-perceptual alteration: visual, auditory (side effects).

IMPLEMENTATION

▪ **General Info:** Explain therapeutic value of medication prior to administration to enhance the analgesic effect.

▫ Regularly administered doses may be more effective than prn administration. Analgesic is more effective if administered before pain becomes severe.

*<u>Underlines</u> indicate most frequent; **CAPITALS** indicate life-threatening.

N

- Coadministration with nonopioid analgesics may have additive effects and permit lower opioid doses.
- **IM:** Administer deep into well-developed muscle. Rotate sites of injections.
- **Direct IV:** May give IV undiluted.
- *Rate:* Administer slowly, each 10 mg over 3–5 min.
- **Syringe Compatibility:** ▪ atropine ▪ cimetidine ▪ diphenhydramine ▪ droperidol ▪ glycopyrrolate ▪ hydroxyzine ▪ lidocaine ▪ midazolam ▪ prochlorperazine ▪ ranitidine ▪ scopolamine ▪ trimethobenzamide.
- **Syringe Incompatibility:** ▪ diazepam ▪ pentobarbital.
- **Y-Site Compatibility:** ▪ fludarabine.
- **Y-Site Incompatibility:** ▪ nafcillin ▪ sargramostim.

PATIENT/FAMILY TEACHING

- Instruct patient on how and when to ask for pain medication.
- Nalbuphine may cause drowsiness or dizziness. Advise patient to call for assistance when ambulating and to avoid driving or other activities requiring alertness until response to the medication is known.
- Caution patient to make position changes slowly to minimize orthostatic hypotension.
- Advise patient that frequent mouth rinses, good oral hygiene, and sugarless gum or candy may decrease dry mouth.
- Encourage patient to turn, cough, and breathe deeply every 2 hr to prevent atelectasis.
- Advise patient to avoid concurrent use of alcohol or other CNS depressants with this medication.

EVALUATION

Effectiveness of therapy can be demonstrated by: ▪ Decrease in severity of pain without a significant alteration in level of consciousness or respiratory status.

NALOXONE
(nal-**ox**-one)
Narcan

CLASSIFICATION(S):
Antidote (for opioids)
Pregnancy Category B

INDICATIONS

▪ Reversal of CNS depression and respiratory depression due to suspected opioid overdosage ▪ Management of refractory circulatory shock.

ACTION

▪ Competitively blocks the effects of opioids, including CNS and respiratory depression, without producing any agonist (opioid-like) effects. **Therapeutic Effect:** ▪ Reversal of signs of opioid excess.

PHARMACOKINETICS

Absorption: Well absorbed following IM or SC administration.
Distribution: Rapidly distributed to tissues. Crosses the placenta.
Metabolism and Excretion: Metabolized by the liver.
Half-life: 60–90 min (up to 3 hr in neonates).

CONTRAINDICATIONS AND PRECAUTIONS

Contraindicated in: ▪ Hypersensitivity.
Use Cautiously in: ▪ Cardiovascular disease ▪ Patients physically dependent on opioids (may precipitate severe withdrawal) ▪ Pregnancy (may cause withdrawal in mother and fetus if mother is opioid-dependent) ▪ Lactation (safety not established) ▪ Neonates of opioid-dependent mothers.

ADVERSE REACTIONS AND SIDE EFFECTS*

CV: ventricular tachycardia, ventricular fibrillation, hypotension, hypertension.
GI: nausea, vomiting.

---

*Underlines indicate most frequent; **CAPITALS** indicate life-threatening.

INTERACTIONS

Drug–Drug: ▪ Can precipitate withdrawal in patients who are physically dependent on **opioid analgesics** ▪ Antagonizes postoperative **analgesia**.

ROUTE AND DOSAGE

Opioid-Induced Respiratory or CNS Depression

▪ **IV, IM, SC (Adults):** 0.4 mg may repeat q 2–3 min (IV route is preferred); some patients may require up to 2 mg. If patient is suspected of being opioid-dependent, initial dose should be decreased to 0.1–0.2 mg. May also be given by IV infusion at rate adjusted to patient's response.

▪ **IV, IM, SC (Children):** 0.01 mg/kg q 2–3 min.

Postoperative Respiratory Depression

▪ **IV (Adults):** 0.1–0.2 mg q 2–3 min until response obtained, may repeat q 1–2 hr later if needed (0.5 mcg/kg dose will not interfere with analgesia).

▪ **IV (Children):** 5–10 mcg, may repeat q 2–3 min until response obtained.

AVAILABILITY

▪ *Injection:* 0.4 mg/ml, 1 mg/ml ▪ *Neonatal injection:* 0.02 mg/ml ▪ *In combination with:* pentazocine (Talcoin NX). See Appendix A.

TIME/ACTION PROFILE (reversal of opioid effects)

	ONSET	PEAK	DURATION
IV	1–2 min	UK	45 min
IM, SC	2–5 min	UK	>45 min

NURSING IMPLICATIONS

ASSESSMENT

▫ Monitor respiratory rate, rhythm, and depth, pulse, ECG, blood pressure, and level of consciousness frequently until opioid effects wear off. The effects of some opioids may last longer than the effects of naloxone, and repeat doses may be necessary.

▫ Assess patient for level of pain following administration when used to treat postoperative respiratory depression. Naloxone decreases respiratory depression but also reverses analgesia.

▫ Assess patient for signs and symptoms of opioid withdrawal (vomiting, restlessness, abdominal cramps, increased blood pressure, and temperature). Symptoms may occur within a few minutes to 2 hr. Severity depends on dose of naloxone, opioid involved, and degree of physical dependence.

▫ Lack of significant improvement indicates that symptoms are due to a disease process or to other nonopioid CNS depressants not affected by naloxone.

POTENTIAL NURSING DIAGNOSES

▪ Breathing pattern, ineffective (indications).

▪ Coping, ineffective individual (indications).

▪ Pain (interactions).

IMPLEMENTATION

▪ **General Info:** Larger doses of naloxone may be necessary when used to antagonize the effects of buprenorphine, butorphanol, nalbuphine, pentazocine, and propoxyphene.

▫ Resuscitation equipment, oxygen, vasopressors, and mechanical ventilation should be available to supplement naloxone therapy as needed.

▪ **Direct IV:** Administer undiluted at a rate of 0.1–0.4 mg over 15 sec. Titrate to patient response. Supplemental doses administered SC or a continuous infusion may provide longer-lasting effects.

▫ Doses should be titrated carefully in postoperative patients to avoid interference with control of postoperative pain.

▪ **Continuous Infusion:** Dilute in D5W or 0.9% NaCl for injection. Naloxone 2 mg in 500 ml equals a concentration of 4 mcg/ml. Mixture is stable for 24 hr; discard unused solution.

▪ *Rate:* Titrate dose according to patient response.

▪ **Additive Incompatibility:** Incompatible with preparations containing bi-

N

sulfite, sulfite, and solutions with an alkaline pH.

PATIENT/FAMILY TEACHING

▢ As medication becomes effective, explain purpose and effects of naloxone to patient.

EVALUATION

Clinical response can be demonstrated by: ▪ Adequate ventilation ▢ Alertness without significant pain ▪ Management of refractory shock.

NAPROXEN
(na-**prox**-en)
{Apo-Naproxen}, Naprosyn, {Naxen}, {Novonaprox}

NAPROXEN SODIUM
(na-**prox**-en **soe**-dee-um)
Anaprox, Anaprox DS, {Apo-Napro-Na}, {Novonaprox Sodium}, {Synflex}

CLASSIFICATION(S):
Nonopioid analgesic, Nonsteroidal anti-inflammatory agent
Pregnancy Category C

INDICATIONS

▪ Management of mild to moderate pain ▪ Treatment of dysmenorrhea ▪ Management of inflammatory disorders, including: ▢ Rheumatoid arthritis ▢ Osteoarthritis.

ACTION

▪ Inhibits prostaglandin synthesis. **Therapeutic Effects:** ▪ Suppression of inflammation ▪ Decreased pain.

PHARMACOKINETICS

Absorption: Completely absorbed from the GI tract. Sodium salt (Anaprox) is more rapidly absorbed.
Distribution: Crosses the placenta and enters breast milk in low concentrations.
Metabolism and Excretion: Mostly metabolized by the liver.
Half-life: 10–20 hr.

CONTRAINDICATIONS AND PRECAUTIONS

Contraindicated in: ▪ Hypersensitivity ▪ Cross-sensitivity may exist with other nonsteroidal anti-inflammatory agents, including aspirin ▪ Active GI bleeding ▪ Ulcer disease.
Use Cautiously in: ▪ Severe cardiovascular, renal, or hepatic disease ▪ History of ulcer disease ▪ Pregnancy or lactation (safety not established).

ADVERSE REACTIONS AND SIDE EFFECTS*

CNS: headache, drowsiness, dizziness.
CV: edema, palpitations, tachycardia.
EENT: tinnitus.
Resp: dyspnea.
GI: nausea, dyspepsia, vomiting, diarrhea, constipation, GI BLEEDING, discomfort, HEPATITIS, flatulence, anorexia.
GU: renal failure, hematuria, cystitis.
Derm: rashes, sweating, photosensitivity.
Hemat: blood dyscrasias, prolonged bleeding time.
Misc: allergic reactions, including ANAPHYLAXIS.

INTERACTIONS

Drug–Drug: ▪ Concurrent use with **aspirin** decreases naproxen blood levels and may decrease effectiveness ▪ Increased risk of bleeding with **anticoagulants, thrombolytic agents, cefamandole, cefotetan, cefoperazone, valproic acid,** or **plicamycin** ▪ Additive adverse GI side effects with **aspirin, glucocorticoids,** and other **nonsteroidal anti-inflammatory agents** ▪ **Probenecid** increases blood levels and may increase toxicity ▪ Increased risk of photosensitivity with other **photosensitizing agents** ▪ May increase the risk of toxicity from **methotrexate, antineoplastic agents,** or **radiation therapy** ▪ May increase serum levels and risk of toxicity from **lithium** ▪ Increased risk of adverse renal effects with **cyclosporine** or chronic use of **acetaminophen** ▪ May

---

{} = Available in Canada only.
*Underlines indicate most frequent; **CAPITALS** indicate life-threatening.

decrease response to **antihypertensives** or **diuretics** ▪ May increase risk of hypoglycemia with **insulin** or **oral hypoglycemic agents**.

ROUTE AND DOSAGE
275 mg naproxen sodium is equivalent to 250 mg naproxen.

Anti-inflammatory
▪ **PO (Adults):** 250–500 mg naproxen bid or 275 mg naproxen sodium in the morning and 550 mg in the evening.
▪ **PO (Children):** 10 mg/kg/day of naproxen in 2 divided doses.

Analgesic
▪ **PO (Adults):** 500 mg naproxen initially followed by 250 mg q 6–8 hr, or 550 mg naproxen sodium initially followed by 275 mg q 6–8 hr (not to exceed 1.25 g naproxen or 1.375 g naproxen sodium/day).

AVAILABILITY
Naproxen
▪ *Tablets:* 250 mg, 375 mg, 500 mg
▪ *Oral suspension:* 125 mg/5 ml.

Napoxen sodium
▪ *Tablets:* 275 mg, 550 mg.

TIME/ACTION PROFILE

	ONSET	PEAK	DURATION
PO (analgesic)	1 hr	UK	up to 7 hr
PO (anti-inflammatory)	14 days	4 wk	UK

NURSING IMPLICATIONS
ASSESSMENT
▪ **General Info:** Patients who have asthma, aspirin-induced allergy, and nasal polyps are at increased risk for developing hypersensitivity reactions. Assess for rhinitis, asthma, and urticaria.
▪ **Pain:** Assess pain (note type, location, and intensity) prior to and 1–2 hr following administration.
▪ **Arthritis:** Assess pain and range of motion prior to and 1–2 hr following administration.
▪ **Lab Test Considerations:** BUN, serum creatinine, CBC, and liver function tests should be evaluated periodically in patients receiving prolonged courses of therapy.
▫ Serum potassium, BUN, serum creatinine, AST (SGOT), and ALT (SGPT) may show increased levels.
▫ Bleeding time may be prolonged up to 4 days following discontinuation of therapy.

POTENTIAL NURSING DIAGNOSES
▪ Pain (indications).
▪ Physical mobility, impaired (indications).
▪ Knowledge deficit related to medication regimen (patient/family teaching).

IMPLEMENTATION
▪ **General Info:** Coadministration with opioid analgesics may have additive analgesic effects and may permit lower opioid doses. Analgesic is more effective if administered before pain becomes severe.
▪ **PO:** For rapid initial effect, administer 30 min before or 2 hr after meals. May be administered with food, milk, or antacids to decrease GI irritation. Food slows but does not reduce the extent of absorption. Do not mix suspension with antacid or other liquid prior to administration.
▪ **Dysmenorrhea:** Administer as soon as possible after the onset of menses. Prophylactic treatment has not been shown to be effective.

PATIENT/FAMILY TEACHING
▫ Advise patient to take this medication with a full glass of water and to remain in an upright position for 15–30 min after administration.
▫ Instruct patient to take medication exactly as directed. If a dose is missed, it should be taken as soon as remembered but not if almost time for the next dose. Do not double doses.
▫ Naproxen may cause drowsiness or dizziness. Advise patient to avoid driving or other activities requiring alertness until response to the medication is known.

N

□ Caution patient to avoid the concurrent use of alcohol, aspirin, ibuprofen, acetaminophen, or other over-the-counter medications without consulting physician or pharmacist.

□ Advise patient to use sunscreen and protective clothing to prevent photosensitivity reactions.

□ Advise patient to inform physician or dentist of medication regimen prior to treatment or surgery.

□ Instruct patient to notify physician if rash, itching, muscle aches, tinnitus, weight gain, edema, black stools, or persistent headache occurs.

EVALUATION
Effectiveness of therapy may be determined by: ▪ Relief of pain ▪ Improved joint mobility. Partial arthritic relief is usually seen within 2 wk, but maximum effectiveness may require 2–4 wk of continuous therapy. Patients who do not respond to one nonsteroidal anti-inflammatory agent may respond to another.

NEOMYCIN
(nee-oh-**mye**-sin)
Mycifradin, Myciguent

CLASSIFICATION(S):
Anti-infective (aminoglycoside)
Pregnancy Category D

INDICATIONS

▪ **PO:** Used to prepare the GI tract for surgery or to decrease the population of ammonia-producing bacteria in the management of hepatic encephalopathy ▪ **Top:** Treatment of minor skin infections.

ACTION

▪ Inhibits protein synthesis in bacteria at the level of the 30S ribosome. **Therapeutic Effect:** ▪ Bactericidal action against susceptible bacteria.

PHARMACOKINETICS

Absorption: Minimally absorbed (<3%) following topical administration.

Distribution: Distribution not known.

Metabolism and Excretion: If systemically absorbed, eliminated unchanged by the kidneys. Orally administered neomycin is eliminated unchanged in the feces.

Half-life: 2–3 hr.

CONTRAINDICATIONS AND PRECAUTIONS

Contraindicated in: ▪ Hypersensitivity ▪ Cross-sensitivity with other aminoglycosides may exist ▪ Renal impairment (chronic use of high-dose oral therapy). **Use Cautiously in:** ▪ Renal impairment of any degree (dosage reduction required) ▪ Pregnancy and lactation (safety not established) ▪ Neuromuscular diseases, such as myasthenia gravis.

ADVERSE REACTIONS AND SIDE EFFECTS*

EENT: ototoxicity (vestibular and cochlear).

GU: nephrotoxicity.

Derm: Top—rashes.

Neuro: enhanced neuromuscular blockade (parenteral).

Misc: hypersensitivity reactions.

INTERACTIONS

Drug–Drug: ▪ Possible respiratory paralysis after **inhalation anesthetics (ether, cyclopropane, halothane, or nitrous oxide)** or **neuromuscular blockers (tubocurarine, succinylcholine, decamethonium)** ▪ Increased risk of ototoxicity with **loop diuretics (ethacrynic acid, furosemide)** ▪ Increased risk of nephrotoxicity with other **nephrotoxic drugs (cisplatin)**.

ROUTE AND DOSAGE

Preparation for GI Surgery

▪ **PO (Adults):** 1 g q hr for 4 hr, then 1 g q 4 hr for 24 hr prior to surgery or 1 g

---

*Underlines indicate most frequent; **CAPITALS** indicate life-threatening.

given 19 hr, 18 hr, and 9 hr prior to surgery.

- **PO (Children):** 88 mg/kg/day in divided doses q 4 hr for 24 hr prior to surgery.

Hepatic Encephalopathy

- **PO (Adults):** 4–12 g/day in divided doses q 6 hr.
- **PO (Children):** 40–100 mg/kg/day in divided doses q 4–6 hr.

Minor Skin Infections

- **Top (Adults and Children):** 0.5% cream or ointment 1–3 times daily.

AVAILABILITY

- **Tablets:** 500 mg ▪ **Oral solution:** 125 mg/5 ml ▪ **In combination with:** other anti-infectives and glucocorticoids in various topical preparations. See Appendix A.

TIME/ACTION PROFILE (blood levels)

	ONSET	PEAK	DURATION
IM	rapid	1–4 hr	6–8 hr

NURSING IMPLICATIONS

ASSESSMENT

- **General Info:** Assess patient for infection (vital signs; appearance of infected skin) at beginning and throughout course of therapy.
- ◻ Obtain specimens for culture and sensitivity prior to initiating therapy. First dose may be given before receiving results.
- **Hepatic Encephalopathy:** Monitor neurologic status. Prior to administering oral medication assess patient's ability to swallow.
- **Lab Test Considerations:** Monitor urinalysis, specific gravity, BUN, creatinine, and creatinine clearance prior to and throughout prolonged therapy.

POTENTIAL NURSING DIAGNOSES

- Infection, high risk for (indications).
- Knowledge deficit related to medication regimen (patient/family teaching).

IMPLEMENTATION

- **Preoperative Bowel Prep:** Usually used in conjunction with erythromycin, a low-residue diet, and a cathartic or enema.

PATIENT/FAMILY TEACHING

- **General Info:** Advise patient to take medication for full course of therapy, even if feeling better.
- ◻ Instruct patient to inform physician if rash, diarrhea, tinnitus, vertigo, or hearing loss occurs.
- **Top Therapy:** Instruct patient to wash affected skin gently and pat dry. Apply a thin film of ointment. Apply occlusive dressing only if ordered by physician. Patient should assess skin and inform physician if skin irritation develops or infection worsens.

EVALUATION

Effectiveness of therapy can be demonstrated by: ▪ Prevention of infection in intestinal surgery ▪ Improved neurologic status in hepatic encephalopathy ▪ Resolution of the signs and symptoms of infection.

NEOSTIGMINE
(nee-oh-**stig**-meen)
Prostigmin

CLASSIFICATION(S):
Cholinergic (anticholinesterase agent)
Pregnancy Category C

INDICATIONS

- Used to increase muscle strength in symptomatic treatment of myasthenia gravis ▪ Prevention and treatment of postoperative bladder distention and urinary retention or ileus ▪ Reversal of nondepolarizing neuromuscular blockers.

ACTION

- Inhibits the breakdown of acetylcholine so that it accumulates and has a prolonged effect ▪ Effects include miosis, increased intestinal and skeletal muscle tone, bronchial and ureteral constriction, bradycardia, increased sal-

N

ivation, lacrimation, and sweating. **Therapeutic Effects:** ▪ Improved muscular function in patients with myasthenia gravis, bladder emptying in patients with urinary retention, or reversal of nondepolarizing neuromuscular blockers.

PHARMACOKINETICS

Absorption: Poorly absorbed following oral administration, necessitating large oral doses as compared to parenteral doses.
Distribution: Does not appear to cross the placenta or enter breast milk.
Metabolism and Excretion: Metabolized by plasma cholinesterases and the liver.
Half-life: PO, IV—40–60 min; IM—50–90 min.

CONTRAINDICATIONS AND PRECAUTIONS

Contraindicated in: ▪ Hypersensitivity ▪ Mechanical obstruction of the GI or GU tract.
Use Cautiously in: ▪ History of asthma ▪ Ulcer disease ▪ Cardiovascular disease ▪ Epilepsy ▪ Hyperthyroidism ▪ Pregnancy (may cause uterine irritability after IV administration near term; newborns may display muscle weakness) ▪ Lactation.

ADVERSE REACTIONS AND SIDE EFFECTS*

CNS: dizziness, weakness, SEIZURES.
EENT: miosis, lacrimation.
Resp: excess secretions, bronchospasm.
CV: bradycardia, hypotension.
GI: abdominal cramps, nausea, vomiting, diarrhea, excess salivation.
Derm: rashes, sweating.

INTERACTIONS

Drug–Drug: ▪ Action may be antagonized by **drugs possessing anticholinergic properties,** including **antihistamines, antidepressants, atropine, haloperidol, phenothiazines, quinidine,** and **disopyramide** ▪ Prolongs action of **depolarizing muscle-relaxing agents (succinylcholine, decamethonium).**

ROUTE AND DOSAGE
Myasthenia Gravis
▪ **PO (Adults):** 15 mg q 3–4 hr initially, increase at daily intervals until optimal response is achieved. Usual maintenance dose is 150 mg/day (up to 375 mg/day may be needed).
▪ **PO (Children):** 2 mg/kg/day in 3–4 divided doses.
▪ **SC, IM (Adults):** 0.5 mg.
▪ **SC, IM (Children):** 10–40 mcg/kg, may give with 10 mcg/kg atropine.

Bladder Atony, Abdominal Distention: Prevention
▪ **IM, SC (Adults):** 250 mcg q 4–6 hr for 2–3 days.

Bladder Atony, Abdominal Distention: Treatment
▪ **IM, SC (Adults):** 500 mcg, may repeat q 3 hr for 5 doses after bladder has been emptied.

Antidote for Nondepolarizing Neuromuscular Blockers
▪ **IV (Adults):** 0.5–2 mg slowly; pretreat with 0.6–1.2 mg atropine IV (may be repeated to a total dose of 5 mg).
▪ **IV (Children):** 40 mcg/kg with 20 mcg/kg atropine.

AVAILABILITY
▪ *Tablets:* 15 mg ▪ *Injection:* 1 : 1000, 1 : 2000, 1 : 4000 ▪ *In combination with:* atropine (Neostigmine Methylsulfate Min-I-Mix).

TIME/ACTION PROFILE (cholinergic effects, increased muscle tone)

	ONSET	PEAK	DURATION
PO	45–75 min	UK	2–4 hr
IM	10–30 min	20–30 min	2–4 hr
IV	10–30 min	20–30 min	2–4 hr

NURSING IMPLICATIONS
ASSESSMENT
▪ **General Info:** Assess pulse, respiratory rate, and blood pressure prior to

---

*Underlines indicate most frequent; **CAPITALS** indicate life-threatening.

administration. Notify physician of significant changes in heart rate.

- **Myasthenia Gravis:** Assess neuromuscular status, including vital capacity, ptosis, diplopia, chewing, swallowing, hand grasp, and gait, prior to administering and at peak effect. Patients with myasthenia gravis may be advised to keep a daily record of their condition and the effects of this medication.

□ Assess patient for overdosage and underdosage or resistance. Both have similar symptoms (muscle weakness, dyspnea, dysphagia), but symptoms of overdosage usually occur within 1 hr of administration, whereas underdosage symptoms occur 3 or more hr after administration. Overdosage (cholinergic crisis) symptoms may also include increased respiratory secretions and saliva, bradycardia, nausea, vomiting, cramping, diarrhea, and diaphoresis. A Tensilon test (edrophonium chloride) may be used to distinguish between overdosage and underdosage.

- **Postoperative Ileus:** Monitor abdominal status (assess for distention, auscultate bowel sounds). A rectal tube may be inserted to facilitate expulsion of flatus.

- **Postoperative Urinary Retention:** Assess for bladder distention. Monitor intake and output. If patient is unable to void within 1 hr of neostigmine administration, confer with physician about catheterization.

- **Antidote to Nondepolarizing Neuromuscular Blocking Agents:** Monitor reversal of effects of neuromuscular blocking agents with a peripheral nerve stimulator. Recovery usually occurs consecutively in the following muscles: diaphragm, intercostal muscles, muscles of the glottis, abdominal muscles, limb muscles, muscles of mastication, and levator muscles of the eyelids. Closely observe the patient for residual muscle weakness and respiratory distress throughout the recovery period. Maintain airway

patency and ventilation until recovery of normal respirations occurs.

- **Toxicity and Overdose:** If overdose occurs, atropine is the antidote.

POTENTIAL NURSING DIAGNOSES

- Physical mobility, impaired (indications).
- Breathing pattern, ineffective (indications).
- Knowledge deficit related to medication regimen (patient/family teaching).

IMPLEMENTATION

- **General Info:** Oral and parenteral doses are not interchangeable.

□ When used as an antidote to nondepolarizing neuromuscular blocking agents, atropine may be ordered prior to or currently with neostigmine to prevent or treat bradycardia.

- **PO:** Administer with food or milk to minimize side effects. For patients who have difficulty chewing, neostigmine may be taken 30 min before meals.

- **Direct IV:** Administer doses undiluted. May be given through Y-site or 3-way stopcock of an IV of D5W, 0.9% NaCl, Ringer's solution, or lactated Ringer's solution.

- *Rate:* Administer each 0.5 mg over 1 min.

- **Syringe Compatibility:** ■ glycopyrrolate ■ heparin ■ pentobarbital ■ thiopental.

- **Y-Site Compatibility:** ■ heparin ■ hydrocortisone sodium succinate ■ potassium chloride ■ vitamin B complex with C.

PATIENT/FAMILY TEACHING

□ Instruct patient to take medication exactly as directed. Do not skip or double up on missed doses. Patients with a history of dysphagia should have a nonelectric or battery-operated backup alarm clock to remind them of exact dose time. Patients with dysphagia may not be able to swallow the medication if the dose is not taken exactly on time. Taking the dose late may result in myasthenic crisis. Tak-

N

ing the dose early may result in a cholinergic crisis. Patients with myasthenia gravis must continue this regimen as a lifelong therapy.
□ Instruct patient with myasthenia gravis to space activities to avoid fatigue.
□ Advise patient to carry identification describing disease and medication regimen at all times.

EVALUATION
Effectiveness of therapy can be demonstrated by: ■ Relief of ptosis and diplopia □ Improved chewing, swallowing, extremity strength, and breathing without the appearance of cholinergic symptoms in myasthenia gravis ■ Relief or prevention of postoperative gastrointestinal ileus ■ Relief of nonobstructive postoperative urinary retention ■ Reversal of nondepolarizing neuromuscular blocking agents in general anesthesia.

NETILMICIN
(ne-till-**mye**-sin)
Netromycin

CLASSIFICATION(S):
Anti-infective (aminoglycoside)
Pregnancy Category D

INDICATIONS
■ Useful in the treatment of gram-negative bacillary infections and infections due to staphylococci when penicillins or other less toxic drugs are contraindicated or resistance to other aminoglycosides has occurred ■ Used in the treatment of the following infections due to susceptible organisms: □ Bone infection □ Respiratory tract infections □ Skin and soft tissue infections □ Abdominal infections □ Complicated urinary tract infections □ Septicemia.

ACTION
■ Inhibits protein synthesis in bacteria at the level of the 30S ribosome. **Therapeutic Effect:** ■ Bactericidal action against susceptible bacteria. **Spectrum:**

■ Especially useful in serious gram-negative bacillary infections due to *Pseudomonas aeruginosa* and many Enterobacteriaceae, including: □ *Citrobacter diversus* □ *C. freundii* □ *Enterobacter aerogenes* □ *E. cloacae* □ *Escherichia coli* □ *Klebsiella* □ *Morganella morganii* □ *Proteus* □ *Providencia* □ *Salmonella* □ *Shigella*.

PHARMACOKINETICS
Absorption: Well absorbed after IM administration.
Distribution: Widely distributed in extracellular fluids following IM or IV administration. Crosses the placenta. Enters breast milk. Poor penetration into CSF.
Metabolism and Excretion: Excretion is mainly (>90%) renal. Dosage adjustments are required for any decrease in renal function. Minimal amounts metabolized by the liver.
Half-life: 2–3.4 hr (increased in renal impairment).

CONTRAINDICATIONS AND PRECAUTIONS
Contraindicated in: ■ Hypersensitivity to netilmicin, bisulfites, or benzyl alcohol ■ Cross-sensitivity with other aminoglycosides may exist.
Use Cautiously in: ■ Renal impairment of any degree (dosage reduction required) ■ Pregnancy and lactation (safety not established) ■ Neuromuscular diseases, such as myasthenia gravis ■ Obese patients (base dose on ideal body weight) ■ Patients with poor nutritional status (increased risk of hypomagnesemia).

ADVERSE REACTIONS AND SIDE EFFECTS*
EENT: ototoxicity (vestibular and cochlear).
F and E: hypomagnesemia.
GU: nephrotoxicity.
Neuro: enhanced neuromuscular blockade.
Misc: hypersensitivity reactions, superinfection.

*Underlines indicate most frequent; **CAPITALS** indicate life-threatening.

INTERACTIONS

Drug–Drug: ■ Inactivated by **penicillins** when coadministered to patients with renal insufficiency ■ Possible respiratory paralysis after **general anesthetics** or **neuromuscular blockers (tubocurarine, succinylcholine, decamethonium)** ■ Increased risk of ototoxicity with **loop diuretics** ■ Risk of nephrotoxicity may be increased with other potentially **nephrotoxic drugs (cisplatin)**.

ROUTE AND DOSAGE

All doses after initial loading dose should be determined by renal function/blood level monitoring.

■ **IM, IV (Adults):** 4–6.5 mg/kg/day individual doses q 8–12 hr (3–4 mg/kg/day in divided doses q 12 hr for urinary tract infection).

■ **IM, IV (Children 6 wk–12 yr):** 1.8–2.7 mg/kg q 8 hr or 2.7–4 mg/kg q 12 hr (up to 12 mg/kg/day in cystic fibrosis patients).

■ **IM, IV (Premature or Full-Term Neonates <6 wk):** 2–3.25 mg/kg q 12 hr.

AVAILABILITY

■ *Injection:* 100 mg/dl.

TIME/ACTION PROFILE (blood levels)

	ONSET	PEAK
IM	rapid	30–90 min
IV	rapid	end of infusion

NURSING IMPLICATIONS

ASSESSMENT

□ Assess patient for infection (vital signs; wound appearance, sputum, urine, and stool; WBC) at beginning and throughout course of therapy.

□ Obtain specimens for culture and sensitivity prior to initiating therapy. First dose may be given before receiving results.

□ Evaluate eighth cranial nerve function by audiometry prior to and throughout course of therapy. Hearing loss is usually in the high-frequency range. Prompt recognition and intervention is essential in preventing permanent damage. Also monitor for vestibular dysfunction (vertigo, ataxia, nausea, vomiting). Eighth cranial nerve dysfunction is associated with persistently elevated peak netilmicin levels.

□ Monitor intake and output and daily weight to assess hydration status and renal function.

□ Assess patient for signs of superinfection (fever, upper respiratory infection, vaginal itching or discharge, increasing malaise, diarrhea). Report to physician.

■ **Lab Test Considerations:** Monitor renal function by urinalysis, specific gravity, BUN, creatinine, and creatinine clearance prior to and throughout therapy.

□ May cause increased serum BUN, AST (SGOT), ALT (SGPT), LDH, alkaline phosphatase, bilirubin, and creatinine concentrations.

□ May cause decreased serum calcium, magnesium, potassium, and sodium concentrations.

■ **Toxicity and Overdose:** Blood levels should be monitored periodically during therapy. Timing of blood levels is important in interpreting results. Draw blood for peak levels 1 hr after IM injection and 15–30 min after IV infusion is completed. Trough levels should be drawn just prior to next dose. Acceptable peak level is 6–10 mcg/ml; trough level should not exceed 4 mcg/ml.

POTENTIAL NURSING DIAGNOSES

■ Infection, high risk for (indications).

■ Sensory-perceptual alteration: auditory (side effects).

IMPLEMENTATION

■ **General Info:** Keep patient well hydrated (1500–2000 ml/day) during therapy.

□ Solution is clear and colorless to pale yellow.

■ **Intermittent Infusion:** Dilute each dose in 50–200 ml of D5/LR, D5/0.9% NaCl, D5W, D10W, Ringer's or lactated Ringer's solution, 0.9% NaCl,

N

3% NaCl, or 5% NaCl. Dilute in a proportionately smaller volume for pediatric patients. Stable for 72 hr at room temperature.
- **Rate:** Infuse slowly over 30 min–2 hr.
- **Y-Site Compatibility:** ■ aminophylline ■ calcium gluconate ■ fludarabine ■ sargramostim.
- **Y-Site Incompatibility:** ■ furosemide ■ heparin. If aminoglycosides and penicillins or cephalosporins must be administered concurrently, administer in separate sites.
- **Additive Compatibility:** ■ aminocaproic acid ■ clindamycin ■ dexamethasone sodium phosphate ■ fibrinolysin and deoxyribonuclease ■ hydrocortisone sodium succinate ■ metronidazole ■ multivitamins ■ potassium chloride ■ vitamin B complex with C.

PATIENT/FAMILY TEACHING
□ Instruct patient to report signs of hypersensitivity, tinnitus, vertigo, or hearing loss.

EVALUATION
Clinical response can be evaluated by:
- Resolution of the signs and symptoms of infection. Length of time for complete resolution depends on the organism and site of infection. If no response is seen within 3–5 days, new cultures should be obtained.

NIACIN
(**nye**-a-sin)
Nia-Bid, Niac, Niacels, Niacor, Nico-400, Nicobid, Nicolar, Nicotinex, Nicotinic acid, Slo-Niacin, {Tri-B3}, vitamin B₃

NIACINAMIDE
(nye-a-**sin**-a-mide)
nicotinamide

CLASSIFICATION(S):
Lipid-lowering agent, Vitamin (water-soluble)
Pregnancy Category C

INDICATIONS
- Treatment and prevention of niacin deficiency (pellagra) ■ Adjunctive therapy in certain hyperlipidemias (niacin only).

ACTION
- Required as coenzymes (for lipid metabolism, glycogenolysis, and tissue respiration) ■ Large doses decrease lipoprotein and triglyceride synthesis by inhibiting the release of free fatty acids from adipose tissue and decreasing hepatic lipoprotein synthesis (niacin only) ■ Causes peripheral vasodilation in large doses (niacin only). **Therapeutic Effects:** ■ Decreased blood lipids (niacin only) ■ Supplementation in deficiency states.

PHARMACOKINETICS
Absorption: Well absorbed following oral administration.
Distribution: Widely distributed following conversion to niacinamide. Enters breast milk.
Metabolism and Excretion: Amounts required for metabolic processes are converted to niacinamide. Large doses of niacin are excreted unchanged in the urine.
Half-life: 45 min.

CONTRAINDICATIONS AND PRECAUTIONS
Contraindicated in: ■ Hypersensitivity to niacin ■ Some products may contain tartrazine (FDC yellow dye #5) and should be avoided in patients with aspirin allergy ■ Hypersensitivity to chlorobutanol (parenteral niacinamide) ■ Alcohol intolerance (Nicotinex only).
Use Cautiously in: ■ Liver disease ■ Arterial bleeding ■ History of peptic ulcer disease ■ Gout ■ Glaucoma ■ Diabetes mellitus.

ADVERSE REACTIONS AND SIDE EFFECTS*
Adverse reactions and side effects refer to IV administration or doses used to treat hyperlipidemias.

{} = Available in Canada only.
*Underlines indicate most frequent; **CAPITALS** indicate life-threatening.

CNS: nervousness, panic.
CV: orthostatic hypotension.
EENT: toxic amblyopia, blurred vision, proptosis, loss of central vision.
GI: metallic taste (IV only), <u>GI upset</u>, nausea, bloating, flatulence, hunger pains, heartburn, diarrhea, dry mouth, peptic ulceration, hepatotoxicity (SR oral form only).
Derm: <u>flushing of the face and neck</u>, <u>pruritus</u>, burning, stinging or tingling of skin, increased sebaceous gland activity, rashes, hyperpigmentation, dry skin.
Hemat: activation of fibrinolysis (IV only).
Metab: hyperuricemia, hyperglycemia, glycosuria.
Misc: ANAPHYLACTIC SHOCK (IV only).

INTERACTIONS

Drug–Drug: ▪ Increased risk of myopathy with concurrent use of **lovastatin** ▪ Additive hypotension with **ganglionic blocking agents (guanethidine, guanedrel)** ▪ Large doses may decrease the uricosuric effects of **probenecid** or **sulfinpyrazone.**

ROUTE AND DOSAGE

Niacin—Dietary Supplementation
▪ **PO (Adults and Children):** 10–20 mg/day.

Niacin—Hyperlipidemias
▪ **PO (Adults):** 500 mg/day initially, increase up to 2 g tid.

Niacin—Deficiency
▪ **PO (Adults):** up to 500 mg/day in divided doses.
▪ **PO (Children):** up to 300 mg/day in divided doses.
▪ **IM, SC (Adults):** 50–100 mg 5 or more times daily.
▪ **IV (Adults):** 25–100 mg 2 or more times daily.

Niacinamide
▪ **PO (Adults):** 50 mg 3–10 times daily.

AVAILIBILITY

Niacin
▪ *Tablets:* 25 mg, 50 mg, 100 mg, 250 mg, 500 mg ▪ *Timed-release tablets:* 250 mg, 500 mg, 750 mg ▪ *Timed-release capsules:* 125 mg, 250 mg, 300 mg, 400 mg, 500 mg ▪ *Elixir:* 50 mg/5 ml ▪ *Injection:* 100 mg/ml.

Niacinamide
▪ *Tablets:* 50 mg, 100 mg, 125 mg, 250 mg, 500 mg.

TIME/ACTION PROFILE (effects on blood lipids)

	ONSET	PEAK	DURATION
PO (cholesterol)	several days	UK	UK
PO (triglycerides)	several hr	UK	UK
IV	UK	UK	UK

NURSING IMPLICATIONS

ASSESSMENT

▪ **Vitamin Deficiency:** Assess patient for signs of niacin deficiency (pellagra—dermatitis, stomatitis, glossitis, anemia, nausea, and vomiting, confusion, memory loss, and delirium) prior to and periodically throughout therapy.

▪ **Hyperlipidemia:** Obtain a diet history, especially in regard to fat consumption.

▪ **Lab Test Considerations:** Serum glucose and uric acid levels and hepatic function tests should be monitored periodically during prolonged high-dose therapy. Notify physician if AST (SGOT), ALT (SGPT), or LDH becomes elevated. May increase prothrombin times and decrease serum albumin.

□ High-dose therapy may cause elevated serum glucose and uric acid levels. May also cause falsely elevated urine glucose when measured with copper sulfate method (Clinitest) and catecholamine levels during high-dose therapy. Use glucose enzymatic tests (Tes-Tape) to measure urine glucose.

□ When niacin is used as a lipid-lowering agent, serum cholesterol and triglyceride levels should be monitored prior to and periodically throughout course of therapy.

N

POTENTIAL NURSING DIAGNOSES
- Nutrition, altered: less than body requirements (indications).
- Knowledge deficit related to medication regimen (patient/family teaching).
- Noncompliance (patient/family teaching).

IMPLEMENTATION
- **General Info:** Because of infrequency of single B-vitamin deficiencies, combinations are commonly administered.
- **PO:** Administer with meals or milk to minimize GI irritation.
- □ Timed-release tablet and capsules should be swallowed whole, without crushing, breaking, or chewing. Use calibrated measuring device to ensure accurate dosage of solution.
- **Direct IV:** Dilute to a strength of 2 mg/ml.
- **Rate:** Administer at a rate not exceeding 2 mg/min.
- **Intermittent/Continuous Infusion:** Add to 500 ml of 0.9% NaCl.
- **Rate:** Administer at a rate not exceeding 2 mg/min.
- **Additive Compatibility:** ▪ TPN solutions.
- **Additive Incompatibility:** ▪ erythromycin ▪ kanamycin ▪ streptomycin ▪ alkalis ▪ strong acids.

PATIENT/FAMILY TEACHING
- **General Info:** Inform patient that cutaneous flushing and a sensation of warmth, especially in the face, neck, and ears, itching or tingling, and headache may occur within the first 2 hr after taking the drug (immediately after IV doses). These effects are usually transient and subside with continued therapy. If flushing is distressing or persistent, aspirin 325 mg given 30 mg before each dose or slow upward titration of dose may decrease flushing.
- □ Emphasize the importance of follow-up examinations to evaluate progress.
- □ Advise patient to make position changes slowly to minimize orthostatic hypotension.
- ▪ **Vitamin Deficiency:** Encourage patient to comply with diet recommendations of physician. Explain that the best source of vitamins is a well-balanced diet with foods from the 4 basic food groups.
- □ Foods high in niacin include meats, eggs, milk, and dairy products; little is lost during ordinary cooking.
- □ Patients self-medicating with vitamin supplements should be cautioned not to exceed RDA (see Appendix L). The effectiveness of megadoses for treatment of various medical conditions is unproven and may cause side effects.
- **Hyperlipidemia:** Advise patient that this medication should be used in conjunction with diet restrictions (fat, cholesterol, carbohydrates, alcohol), exercise, and cessation of smoking.

EVALUATION
Effectiveness of therapy can be demonstrated by: ▪ Prevention and treatment of niacin deficiency ▪ Decrease in serum cholesterol and triglyceride levels.

NICARDIPINE
(nye-**kar**-de-peen)
Cardene, Cardene SR

CLASSIFICATION(S):
Calcium channel blocker,
Antianginal, Coronary vasodilator, Antihypertensive
Pregnancy Category C

INDICATIONS
▪ Management of angina pectoris (immediate release only) ▪ Alone or with other agents in the management of hypertension.

ACTION
▪ Inhibits the transport of calcium into myocardial and vascular smooth muscle cells, resulting in inhibition of excitation-contraction coupling and subsequent contraction. **Therapeutic Effects:** ▪ Coronary vasodilation and subsequent decrease in frequency and sever-

ity of attacks of angina pectoris ▪ Lowering of blood pressure.

PHARMACOKINETICS

Absorption: Well absorbed following oral administration. Large amounts are rapidly metabolized, resulting in decreased bioavailability (35%).
Distribution: Distribution not known.
Metabolism and Excretion: Mostly metabolized by the liver. Negligible amounts excreted by the kidneys.
Half-life: 2–4 hr.

CONTRAINDICATIONS AND PRECAUTIONS

Contraindicated in: ▪ Hypersensitivity ▪ Aortic stenosis ▪ Lactation.
Use Cautiously in: ▪ Hepatic or renal impairment (initial dosage reduction recommended) ▪ Congestive heart failure ▪ Pregnancy or children (safety not established).

ADVERSE REACTIONS AND SIDE EFFECTS*

CNS: <u>dizziness</u>, <u>lightheadedness</u>, <u>headache</u>, nervousness, somnolence, weakness.
Resp: dyspnea.
CV: <u>peripheral edema</u>, palpitations, angina, tachycardia, orthostatic hypotension.
GI: nausea, abdominal pain, dry mouth, constipation.
Derm: <u>flushing</u>, rash.
Neuro: paresthesia.

INTERACTIONS

Drug–Drug: ▪ Increased risk of bradycardia, conduction defects, or congestive heart failure when used with **beta-adrenergic blockers, disopyramide,** or **digoxin** ▪ **Phenytoin** and **phenobarbital** may hasten metabolism and decrease effectiveness ▪ **Cimetidine** and **propranolol** may slow metabolism and lead to toxicity ▪ May increase blood levels and toxicity of **cyclosporine** ▪ Antihypertensive effect may be decreased by **nonsteroidal anti-inflammatory agents** ▪ Additive hypertension with acute ingestion of **alcohol, nitrates,** and other **antihypertensives**.
Drug–Food: ▪ Absorption may be decreased by concurrent administration with a **high-fat** meal.

ROUTE AND DOSAGE

▪ **PO (Adults):** 20 mg tid, may be increased at 3-day intervals (range 20–40 mg tid) or 30 mg twice daily as sustained-release form (up to 60 mg twice daily).

AVAILABILITY

▪ **Capsules:** 20 mg, 30 mg ▪ **Sustained-release capsules:** 30 mg, 45 mg, 60 mg.

TIME/ACTION PROFILE (on blood pressure)

	ONSET	PEAK	DURATION
PO	20 min	1–2 hr	8 hr
PO-ER	UK	2–6	up to 12 hr

NURSING IMPLICATIONS

ASSESSMENT

▪ **Angina:** Assess location, duration, intensity, and precipitating factors of patient's anginal pain.
▪ **Hypertension:** Monitor blood pressure and pulse before administering medication. Measurements taken 1–2 hr following administration demonstrate peak effectiveness; measurements 8 hr after administration demonstrate adequacy of dose.
▫ Monitor intake and output ratios and daily weight. Assess patient for peripheral edema periodically throughout therapy

POTENTIAL NURSING DIAGNOSES

▪ Cardiac output, decreased (indications).
▪ Pain (indications).
▪ Knowledge deficit related to medication regimen (patient/family teaching).

IMPLEMENTATION

▪ **General Info:** Dosage adjustments should be made no more frequently than every 3 days.

*<u>Underlines</u> indicate most frequent; **CAPITALS** indicate life-threatening.

N

- **PO:** Administer on an empty stomach, 1 hr before or 3 hr after meals. Food with especially high-fat content decreases absorption. Do not crush, break, or chew sustained-release capsule.

PATIENT/FAMILY TEACHING

- **General Info:** Advise patient to take medication exactly as directed, not to skip or double up on missed doses.
- ▫ May cause dizziness and drowsiness. Advise patient to avoid driving or other activities requiring alertness until response to the medication is known.
- ▫ Instruct patient to avoid concurrent use of alcohol or over-the-counter medications without consulting physician or pharmacist.
- ▫ Advise patient to notify physician if irregular heartbeat, dyspnea, swelling of hands and feet, pronounced dizziness, nausea, constipation, or hypotension occurs.
- **Angina:** Inform patient that anginal attacks may occur 30 min after administration due to reflex tachycardia. This is usually temporary and is not an indication for discontinuation.
- ▫ Instruct patient on concurrent nitrate or beta-blocker therapy to continue taking both medications as ordered and using SL nitroglycerin as needed for anginal attacks.
- ▫ Advise patient to contact physician if chest pain does not improve or worsens after therapy or is accompanied by diaphoresis or shortness of breath or if severe, persistent headache occurs.
- **Hypertension:** Encourage patient to comply with additional interventions for hypertension (weight reduction, low-sodium diet, smoking cessation, moderation of alcohol consumption, regular exercise, stress management).

EVALUATION

Effectiveness of therapy can be demonstrated by: ▪ Decrease in frequency and severity of anginal attacks ▫ Decrease in need for nitrate therapy ▫ Increase in activity tolerance and sense of well-being ▪ Decrease in blood pressure.

NICOTINE POLACRILEX CHEWING GUM
(nik-o-teen)
Nicorette, Nicorette DS

NICOTINE TRANSDERMAL
Habitrol, Nicoderm, Nicotrol, Prostep

CLASSIFICATION(S):
Smoking deterrent
**Pregnancy Category X (gum),
D (transdermal)**

INDICATIONS

- Adjunct therapy (with behavior modification) in the management of nicotine withdrawal in patients desiring to give up cigarette smoking.

ACTION

- Provides a source of nicotine during controlled withdrawal from cigarette smoking. **Therapeutic Effect:** ▪ Lessened sequelae of nicotine withdrawal (irritability, insomnia, somnolence, headache, and increased appetite).

PHARMACOKINETICS

Absorption: *Chewing gum*—Slowly absorbed from buccal mucosa during chewing. *Transdermal*—68% of nicotine released from the system is absorbed through the skin (Nicoderm).

Distribution: Enters breast milk.

Metabolism and Excretion: Mostly metabolized by the liver. Small amounts are metabolized by kidneys and lungs. 10–20% excreted unchanged by kidneys.

Half-life: 1–2 hr.

CONTRAINDICATIONS AND PRECAUTIONS

Contraindicated in: ▪ Severe cardiovascular disease ▪ Temporomandibular joint disease (gum only) ▪ Children.

Use Cautiously in: ▪ Cardiovascular

disease including hypertension ▪ Diabetes mellitus ▪ Pheochromocytoma ▪ Peripheral vascular diseases ▪ Pregnancy (cessation of all nicotine is preferred; safety not established) ▪ Skin disorders (transdermal only) ▪ Dental disorders (gum only) ▪ Esophagitis, pharyngitis, or stomatitis (gum only) ▪ Hyperthyroidism ▪ Lactation (potential for adverse effects in the newborn) ▪ Hepatic disease ▪ Patients <50 kg or who smoke <10 cigarettes/day (use lower initial dose).

ADVERSE REACTIONS AND SIDE EFFECTS*

CNS: <u>headache</u>, <u>insomnia</u>, abnormal dreams, nervousness, dizziness, drowsiness, impaired concentration, weakness.
EENT: sinusitus; *gum*—<u>pharyngitis</u>.
Resp: increased cough.
CV: chest pain, hypertension, atrial fibrillation, <u>tachycardia</u>.
GI: diarrhea, dyspepsia, constipation, nausea, abdominal pain, vomiting, dry mouth, abnormal taste; *gum*—<u>oral injury</u>, <u>belching</u>, <u>sore mouth</u>, <u>increased salivation</u>, <u>increased appetite</u>, hiccups.
Derm: *transdermal*—<u>erythema</u>, <u>pruritus</u>, <u>burning at patch site</u>, cutaneous hypersensitivity, rash, sweating.
Endo: dysmenorrhea.
MS: back pain, myalgia, arthralgia; *gum*—<u>jaw muscle ache</u>.
Neuro: paresthesia.
Misc: pain, allergy.

INTERACTIONS

Drug–Drug: ▪ **Insulin** requirements may decrease during nicotine withdrawal ▪ Effects of **acetaminophen, furosemide, caffeine, imipramine, oxazepam, pentazocine, propranolol,** or **theophylline** may be increased during nicotine withdrawal (decreased metabolism).

ROUTE AND DOSAGE

Transdermal Habitrol, Nicoderm
▪ **Transdermal (Adults):** 21 mg/day for 6 wk, 14 mg/day for 2 wk, 7 mg/day for 2 wk (8–12 wk total).

Transdermal Nicotrol
▪ **Transdermal (Adults):** 15 mg/day for first 12 wk, 10 mg/day for next 2–4 wk, 5 mg/day for last 2–4 wk (14–20 wk total). System is removed at bedtime.

Prostep
▪ **Transdermal (Adults):** 22 mg/day for 4–8 wk, 11 mg/day for 2–4 wk (6–12 wk total). Patients <50 kg start with 11 mg/day dose.

Chewing Gum
▪ **Chew (Adults):** 2 or 4 mg (1 piece of gum) as needed, amount needed determined by smoking urge or rate of chewing, or on a fixed schedule every 1–2 hr. Usual initial requirement 20 mg (not to exceed 60 mg/day as 2-mg strength or 80 mg/day as 4-mg strength).

AVAILABILITY

Nicorette
▪ *Chewing gum:* 2 mg, 4 mg.

Habitrol, Nicoderm
▪ *Transdermal patch:* 7 mg/day, 14 mg/day, 21 mg/day.

Nicotrol
▪ *Transdermal patch:* 5 mg/day, 10 mg/day, 15 mg/day.

Prostep
▪ *Transdermal patch:* 11 mg/day, 22 mg/day.

TIME/ACTION PROFILE (nicotine blood levels)

	ONSET	PEAK	DURATION
Nicorette— chew	rapid	15–30 min	UK
Nicoderm— TD	rapid	2–4 hr	UK
Habitrol— TD	rapid	6–12 hr	UK
Prostep— TD	rapid	9 hr	UK

NURSING IMPLICATIONS

ASSESSMENT
▪ **General Info:** Prior to therapy, assess

---

*Underlines indicate most frequent; **CAPITALS** indicate life-threatening.

N

smoking history (number of cigarettes smoked daily, smoking patterns, nicotine content of preferred brand, degree to which patient inhales smoke).

▫ Assess patient for symptoms of smoking withdrawal (irritability drowsiness, fatigue, headache, nicotine craving) periodically throughout therapy.

▫ Evaluate progress in smoking cessation periodically during therapy.

▪ **Gum:** Assess patient for history of temporomandibular joint pain or dysfunction.

▪ **Toxicity and Overdose:** Monitor for nausea, vomiting, diarrhea, increased salivation, abdominal pain, headache, dizziness, auditory and visual disturbances, weakness, dyspnea, hypotension, and irregular pulse.

POTENTIAL NURSING DIAGNOSES

▪ Coping, ineffective individual (indications).

▪ Knowledge deficit related to medication regimen (patient/family teaching).

IMPLEMENTATION

▪ **Gum:** Protect gum from light; exposure to light causes gum to turn brown.

▪ **Transdermal:** Determine whether patch is to be worn for 16 or 24 hr. *Nicotrol* system should be applied upon awakening and removed at bedtime.

PATIENT/FAMILY TEACHING

▪ **General Info:** Explain to patient the necessity of immediate cessation of smoking upon initiation and throughout therapy.

▫ Encourage patient to participate in a smoking cessation program while using this product.

▫ Emphasize the importance of regular visit to physician to monitor progress of smoking cessation.

▪ **Gum:** Explain purpose of nicotine gum to patient. The patient should chew 1 piece of gum whenever a craving for nicotine occurs or according to a fixed schedule (every 1–2 hr while awake) as directed. The gum should

be chewed slowly until a tingling sensation is felt (after about 15 chews). Then, patient should stop chewing and store the gum between the cheek and gums until the tingling sensation disappears (after about 1 min). The process of stopping then resuming chewing should be repeated for approximately 30 min. Rapid, vigorous chewing may result in side effects similar to those of smoking too many cigarettes (headache, dizziness, nausea, increased salivation, heartburn, and hiccoughs).

▫ Inform patient that the gum has a slight tobacco/pepperlike taste. Many patients initially find it unpleasant and slightly irritating to the mouth. This usually resolves after several days of therapy.

▫ Advise patient to avoid eating or drinking acidic beverages (coffee, juices, wine, soft drinks) for 15 min before and during chewing of nicotine gum; these interfere with buccal absorption of nicotine.

▫ The gum usually can be chewed by denture wearers. Contact dentist if the gum adheres to bridgework.

▫ Use of the gum may be discontinued when 1–2 pieces/day is sufficient to control the craving for nicotine. Gradual reduction of dose can be accomplished by decreasing daily dose by 1 or more every 4–7 days, decreasing chewing time with each piece from 30 min to 10–15 min for 4–7 days and then decreasing number of pieces per day; substituting 1 or more pieces of sugarless gum for pieces of nicotine gum; increasing number of doses substituted every 4–7 days; replacing 4-mg dose with 2-mg dose; or applying any of the above suggestions. The duration of treatment is limited to 6 mo because physical and psychological dependence can occur. Discontinuing the gum too soon may result in withdrawal symptoms (anxiety, irritability, GI distress, headache, drowsiness, or tobacco craving).

▫ Instruct patient not to swallow gum.

▫ Emphasize need to keep nicotine gum

out of the reach of children. Dispose of the gum by wrapping in wrapper to prevent ingestion by children and animals. Call the poison control center, emergency department, or physician immediately if a child ingests the gum.

□ Emphasize the need to discontinue the gum, and inform the physician if pregnancy occurs.

□ Review the patient instruction sheet enclosed in the package of gum.

▪ **Transdermal:** Instruct patient in application and use of patch. Apply patch at the same time each day. Keep patch in sealed pouch until ready to apply. Apply to clean dry skin of upper arm or torso free of oil, hair, scars, cuts, burns, or irritation. Press patch firmly in place with palm for 10 sec; making sure there is good contact, especially around the edges. Keep patch in place during showering, bathing, or swimming; replace patches that have fallen off. Wash hands with plain water after handling patches; soap will increase absorption of nicotine. Do not trim or cut patch. Alternate application sites. Dispose of used patches by folding adhesive sides together and replacing in protective pouch or aluminum foil.

□ Advise patient that redness, itching, and burning at application site usually subside within 1 hr. Instruct patient to notify physician and not apply new patch if signs of allergic reaction (urticaria, generalized rash, hives) or if persistent local skin reactions (severe erythema, pruritus, edema) occur.

□ May cause drowsiness or dizziness. Caution patient to avoid driving or other activities requiring alertness until response to medication is known.

EVALUATION
Effectiveness of therapy can be determined by: ▪ Smoking cessation ▪ Decrease in nicotine withdrawal symptoms in patients participating in a supervised smoking cessation program. Therapy with nicotine gum is limited to 6 mo; most patients begin a gradual withdrawal after 3 mo of therapy. Nicotine transdermal should be discontinued if patient is unable to stop smoking by fourth week of therapy, as patient is unlikely to quit on that attempt. Therapy with nicotine transdermal should not be used for longer than 20 wk.

NIFEDIPINE
(nye-**fed**-i-pccn)
Adalat, Adalat CC, {Adalat P. A.}, {Apo-Nifed}, {Novo-Nifedin}, {Nu-Nifed}, Procardia, Procardia XL

CLASSIFICATION(S):
Calcium channel blocker, Antianginal, Coronary vasodilator, Antihypertensive
Pregnancy Category C

INDICATIONS
▪ **PO:** Management of angina pectoris due to coronary insufficiency or vasospasm (Prinzmetal's angina) ▪ Treatment of hypertension. **Unlabeled Uses:** ▪ **SL:** Acute treatment of hypertension ▪ **PO:** Management of migraine headache, Raynaud's syndrome, and congestive heart failure.

ACTION
▪ Acts on slow calcium channels in vascular smooth muscle and myocardium, producing coronary vasodilation. **Therapeutic Effects:** ▪ Coronary vasodilation and subsequent decrease in frequency and severity of attacks of angina pectoris ▪ Lowering of blood pressure.

PHARMACOKINETICS
Absorption: Well absorbed after oral administration, but large amounts are rapidly metabolized, resulting in decreased bioavailability (45–70%). Bioavailability increased with long-acting (CC, PA, XL) forms (80%).
Distribution: Distribution not known.

N

Metabolism and Excretion: Mostly metabolized by the liver.
Half-life: 2–5 hr.

CONTRAINDICATIONS AND PRECAUTIONS

Contraindicated in: ▪ Hypersensitivity ▪ Severe hypotension.
Use Cautiously in: ▪ Severe hepatic disease (dosage reduction required) ▪ Congestive heart failure ▪ Edema ▪ Aortic stenosis ▪ Pregnancy, lactation, or children (safety not established).

ADVERSE REACTIONS AND SIDE EFFECTS*

CNS: dizziness, lightheadedness, giddiness, headache, nervousness.
EENT: nasal congestion, sore throat.
Resp: dyspnea, cough, wheezing.
CV: hypotension, syncope, CONGESTIVE HEART FAILURE, MYOCARDIAL INFARCTION, ventricular arrhythmias, tachycardia.
GI: nausea, heartburn, abdominal discomfort, hepatitis, diarrhea, constipation, flatulence.
MS: muscle cramps.
Derm: flushing, warmth, rashes, sweating.
Misc: fever.

INTERACTIONS

Drug–Drug: ▪ Increased risk of bradycardia, conduction defects, or congestive heart failure when used with **beta-adrenergic blockers, disopyramide,** or **digoxin** ▪ **Cimetidine** may slow metabolism and lead to toxicity ▪ Severe hypotension may occur when used with **fentanyl** ▪ Additive hypotension with **antihypertensives,** acute ingestion of **alcohol,** or **nitrates** ▪ May increase blood levels and risk of toxicity with **digoxin** ▪ **NSAIDs** may decrease antihypertensive effects.

ROUTE AND DOSAGE

▪ **PO (Adults):** 10–30 mg 3 times daily (not to exceed 180 mg/day) or 30–90 mg once daily as sustained release (CC, PA, XL) form (not to exceed 90–120 mg/day).
▪ **SL (Adults):** 10 mg, repeated in 15 min (unlabeled).

AVAILABILITY

▪ *Capsules:* {5 mg}, 10 mg, 20 mg
▪ *Sustained-release tablets:* 30 mg, 60 mg, 90 mg.

TIME/ACTION PROFILE (effects on blood pressure)

	ONSET	PEAK	DURATION
PO	20 min	UK	6–8 hr
PO-XL, CC, PA	UK	UK	24 hr

NURSING IMPLICATIONS

ASSESSMENT

▪ **General Info:** Monitor blood pressure and pulse before administering medication. Monitor ECG periodically in patients receiving prolonged therapy. Blood pressure should be monitored closely when nifedipine is administered for hypertension.
▫ Monitor intake and output ratios and daily weight. Assess patient for signs of congestive heart failure (peripheral edema, rales/crackles, dyspnea, weight gain, jugular venous distention).
▫ Patients receiving cardiac glycosides concurrently with nifedipine should have routine serum digitalis levels and be monitored for signs and symptoms of cardiac glycoside toxicity.
▪ **Angina:** Assess location, duration, intensity, and precipitating factors of patient's anginal pain.
▪ **Lab Test Considerations:** Monitor renal and hepatic function periodically in patients receiving long-term therapy. May cause elevated alkaline phosphatase, CPK, LDH, AST (SGOT), and ALT (SGPT) levels.
▫ May cause positive direct Coombs' test results.

POTENTIAL NURSING DIAGNOSES

▪ Cardiac output, decreased (indications).

*Underlines indicate most frequent; **CAPITALS** indicate life-threatening.

- Pain (indications).
- Knowledge deficit related to medication regimen (patient/family teaching).

IMPLEMENTATION

- **PO:** May be administered with meals if gastric irritation becomes a problem. Capsules and sustained release tablets (XL, CC, PA) should be swallowed whole; do not crush, break, or chew. Empty tablets that appear in stool are not significant.
- **SL:** May be administered by puncturing the capsule with a sterile needle and squeezing to administer the liquid into the buccal pouch. The dose used is the same as the oral dose. Chewing or puncturing and swallowing capsule has shown similar effectiveness as SL route for hypertensive emergencies.

PATIENT/FAMILY TEACHING

- **General Info:** Advise patient to take medication exactly as directed, not to skip or double up on missed doses. May need to be discontinued gradually.
- Caution patient to make position changes slowly to minimize orthostatic hypotension.
- May cause dizziness. Advise patient to avoid driving or other activities requiring alertness until response to the medication is known.
- Instruct patient to avoid concurrent use of alcohol or over-the-counter medications without consulting physician or pharmacist.
- Advise patient to notify physician if irregular heartbeat, dyspnea, swelling of hands and feet, pronounced dizziness, nausea, constipation, or hypotension occur.
- **Angina:** Inform patient that anginal attacks may occur 30 min after administration due to reflex tachycardia. This is usually temporary and is not an indication for discontinuation.
- Instruct patient on concurrent nitrate or beta-blocker therapy to continue taking both medications as ordered

and using SL nitroglycerin as needed for anginal attacks.

- Advise patient to contact physician if chest pain does not improve or worsens after therapy or is accompanied by diaphoresis or shortness of breath or if severe, persistent headache occurs.
- **Hypertension:** Encourage patient to comply with additional interventions for hypertension (weight reduction, low-sodium diet, smoking cessation, moderation of alcohol consumption, regular exercise, stress management).

EVALUATION

Effectiveness of therapy can be demonstrated by: ■ Decrease in frequency and severity of anginal attacks □ Decrease in need for nitrate therapy □ Increase in activity tolerance and sense of well-being ■ Decrease in blood pressure.

NIMODIPINE
(ni-**moe**-dip-een)
Nimotop

CLASSIFICATION(S):
Calcium channel blocker
Pregnancy Category C

INDICATIONS

■ Prevention of cerebral vasospasm in the management of subarachnoid hemorrhage following ruptured congenital intracranial aneurysm.

ACTION

■ Acts on slow calcium channels in vascular smooth muscle, producing vasodilation ■ High CNS concentrations may have specific spasmolytic effect on cerebral arteries. **Therapeutic Effect:** ■ Prevention of vascular spasm after subarachnoid hemorrhage, resulting in decreased neurologic impairment.

PHARMACOKINETICS

Absorption: Although well absorbed following oral administration, rapid hepatic metabolism leads to decreased bioavailability.

N

Distribution: Crosses the blood–brain barrier. Remainder of distribution not known.
Metabolism and Excretion: Mostly metabolized by the liver.
Half-life: 1–2 hr.

CONTRAINDICATIONS AND PRECAUTIONS

Contraindicated in: ▪ Hypersensitivity.
Use Cautiously in: ▪ Severe hypertension ▪ Hepatic impairment (decrease initial doses by 50%) ▪ Geriatric patients (may be more sensitive).

ADVERSE REACTIONS AND SIDE EFFECTS*

CNS: psychiatric disturbances, headache, dizziness.
Resp: shortness of breath, dyspnea, wheezing.
CV: hypotension, tachycardia, bradycardia, peripheral edema.
GI: nausea, constipation, hepatitis, abdominal discomfort.
Derm: dermatitis, rash, flushing.
Hemat: thrombocytopenia.
MS: muscle cramps.

INTERACTIONS

Drug–Drug: ▪ Additive hypotension with **antihypertensive agents,** acute ingestion of **alcohol,** or **nitrates** ▪ May produce additive myocardial depression with **beta-adrenergic blockers** ▪ May result in severe hypotension with **fentanyl.**

ROUTE AND DOSAGE

▪ **PO (Adults):** 60 mg q 4 hr for 21 days; therapy should be started within 96 hr of subarachnoid hemorrhage.

AVAILABILITY

▪ *Capsules:* 30 mg.

TIME/ACTION PROFILE (blood levels)

	ONSET	PEAK	DURATION
PO	UK	within 1 hr	UK

NURSING IMPLICATIONS

ASSESSMENT

▫ Assess patient's neurologic status (level of consciousness, movement) prior to and periodically following administration.
▫ Monitor blood pressure before and during administration of medication.
▫ Monitor intake and output ratios and daily weight. Assess patient for peripheral edema periodically throughout therapy.
▪ **Lab Test Considerations:** May occasionally cause decreased platelet count.
▫ May cause elevated alkaline phosphatase, LDH, ALT (SGPT), and serum glucose levels.

POTENTIAL NURSING DIAGNOSES

▪ Injury, high risk for (indications).
▪ Knowledge deficit related to medication regimen (patient/family teaching).

IMPLEMENTATION

▪ **General Info:** Begin administration within 96 hr of subarachnoid hemorrhage and continue every 4 hr for 21 consecutive days.
▪ **PO:** If patient is unable to swallow capsule, make a hole in both ends of the capsule with a sterile 18-gauge needle and extract the contents into a syringe. Empty contents into water or nasogastric tube and flush with 30 ml normal saline.

PATIENT/FAMILY TEACHING

▫ Advise patient to take medication exactly as directed, not to skip or double up on missed doses.
▫ Caution patients to make position changes slowly to minimize orthostatic hypotension.
▫ Advise patient to notify physician if irregular heartbeat, dyspnea, swelling of hands and feet, pronounced dizziness, nausea, constipation, hypotension, or persistent headache occurs.

*Underlines indicate most frequent; **CAPITALS** indicate life-threatening.

EVALUATION
Effectiveness of therapy can be demonstrated by: ▪ Improvement in neurologic deficits due to vasospasm following subarachnoid hemorrhage.

NITROFURANTOIN
(nye-troe-fyoor-**an**-toyn)
{Apo-Nitrofurantoin}, Furadantin, Furalan, Macpac, Macrobid, Macrodantin, {Nephronex}, Nitrofuracot, {Novofuran}

CLASSIFICATION(S):
Anti-infective (miscellaneous)
Pregnancy Category UK

INDICATIONS
▪ Treatment of urinary tract infections due to susceptible organisms. Not effective in systemic bacterial infections ▪ Chronic suppressive therapy of urinary tract infections.

ACTION
▪ Interferes with bacterial enzymes. **Therapeutic Effect:** ▪ Bactericidal or bacteriostatic action against susceptible organisms. **Spectrum:** ▪ Many gram-negative and some gram-positive organisms, specifically: □ *Citrobacter* □ *Corynebacterium* □ *Enterobacter* □ *Escherichia coli* □ *Klebsiella* □ *Neisseria* □ *Salmonella* □ *Shigella* □ *Staphylococcus aureus* □ *Staphylococcus epidermidis* □ *Enterococcus*.

PHARMACOKINETICS
Absorption: Readily absorbed following oral administration. Absorption is slower, but more complete with macrocrystals (Macrodantin).
Distribution: Crosses the placenta and enters breast milk.
Metabolism and Excretion: Partially metabolized by the liver. 30–50% excreted unchanged by the kidneys.
Half-life: 20 min (increased in renal impairment).

CONTRAINDICATIONS AND PRECAUTIONS
Contraindicated in: ▪ Hypersensitivity ▪ Hypersensitivity to parabens (suspension) ▪ Oliguria or anuria ▪ Infants <1 mo and pregnancy near term (increased risk of hemolytic anemia in newborn) ▪ Glucose-6-phosphate dehydrogenase (G6-PD) deficiency.
Use Cautiously in: ▪ Diabetics or debilitated patients (neuropathy may be more common) ▪ Pregnancy and lactation (although safety not established, has been used in pregnant women).

ADVERSE REACTIONS AND SIDE EFFECTS*
CNS: dizziness, headache, drowsiness.
EENT: nystagmus.
Resp: pneumonitis.
CV: chest pain.
GI: nausea, vomiting, anorexia, diarrhea, abdominal pain, hepatitis.
GU: rust/brown discoloration of urine.
Derm: photosensitivity.
Hemat: blood dyscrasias, hemolytic anemia.
Neuro: peripheral neuropathy.

INTERACTIONS
Drug–Drug: ▪ **Probenecid** and **sulfinpyrazone** prevent high urinary concentrations, may decrease effectiveness ▪ **Antacids** may decrease absorption ▪ Increased risk of neurotoxicity with **neurotoxic drugs** ▪ Increased risk of hepatotoxicity with **hepatotoxic drugs** ▪ Increased risk of pneumonitis with **drugs having pulmonary toxicity** ▪ Nitrofurantoin decreases the anti-infective action of **fluoroquinolones.**

ROUTE AND DOSAGE
Active Infection
▪ **PO (Adults):** 50–100 mg q 6–8 hr or 100 mg q 12 hr as extended-release product.
▪ **PO (Children >1 mo):** 7 mg/kg/day in divided doses q 6 hr.

{} = Available in Canada only.
*Underlines indicate most frequent; **CAPITALS** indicate life-threatening.

N

Chronic Suppression
- **PO (Adults):** 50–100 mg, single evening dose.
- **PO (Children):** 1 mg/kg/day as a single dose.

AVAILABILITY
- **Tablets:** 50 mg, 100 mg □ **Capsules:** 50 mg, 100 mg ■ **Oral suspension:** 25 mg/5 ml ■ **Macrocrystal capsules:** 25 mg, 50 mg, 100 mg ■ **Extended-release capsule:** 100 mg.

TIME/ACTION PROFILE (urine levels)

	ONSET	PEAK
PO	UK	30 min

NURSING IMPLICATIONS

ASSESSMENT
□ Assess patient for signs and symptoms of urinary tract infection (frequency, urgency, pain, and burning on urination; fever; cloudy or foul-smelling urine) prior to and periodically throughout course of therapy.
□ Obtain specimens for culture and sensitivity prior to and during drug administration.
□ Monitor intake and output ratios. Notify physician of significant discrepancies in totals.
■ **Lab Test Considerations:** CBC should be routinely monitored with patients on prolonged therapy.
□ May cause elevated serum glucose, bilirubin, alkaline phosphatase, BUN, and creatinine.
□ May cause a false-positive result with copper sulfate urine glucose tests (Clinitest). Use glucose enzymatic test method (Ketodiastix or Tes-Tape) to test for urine glucose.

POTENTIAL NURSING DIAGNOSES
■ Infection, high risk for (indications).
■ Pain (indications).
■ Knowledge deficit related to medication regimen (patient/family teaching).

IMPLEMENTATION
■ **PO:** Administer with food or milk to minimize GI irritation, to delay and increase absorption, to increase peak concentration, and to prolong duration of therapeutic concentration in the urine.
□ Do not crush tablets or open capsules.
□ Administer liquid preparations with calibrated measuring device. Shake well prior to administration. Oral suspension may be mixed with water, milk, fruit juices, or infant's formula. Rinse mouth with water following administration of oral suspension to avoid staining teeth.

PATIENT/FAMILY TEACHING
□ Instruct patient to take medication around the clock, exactly as directed. If a dose is missed, take as soon as remembered and space next dose 2–4 hr apart. Do not skip or double up on missed doses.
□ May cause dizziness or drowsiness. Caution patient to avoid driving or other activities requiring alertness until response to medication is known.
□ Inform patient that medication may cause a rust-yellow to brown discoloration of urine, which is not significant.
□ Advise patient to notify physician if fever, chills, cough, chest pain, dyspnea, skin rash, numbness or tingling of the fingers or toes, or intolerable GI upset occurs. Signs of superinfection (milky, foul-smelling urine; perineal irritation; dysuria) should also be reported.
□ Instruct patient to consult physician if no improvement is seen within a few days after initiation of therapy.

EVALUATION
Effectiveness of therapy can be demonstrated by: ■ Resolution of the signs and symptoms of infection. Therapy should be continued for a minimum of 7 days and for at least 3 days after the urine has become sterile ■ Decrease in the frequency of infections in chronic suppressive therapy.

NITROGLYCERIN
(nye-tro-**gli**-ser-in)

nitroglycerin extended-release capsules
Nitrobid, Nitrocap T.D., Nitrocine, Nitroglyn, Nitrolin

nitroglycerin extended-release tablets
Klavikordal, Niong, Nitronet, Nitrong

nitroglycerin extended-release buccal tablets
Nitrogard, {Nitrogard SR}

nitroglycerin intravenous
Nitro-bid, Tridil

nitroglycerin lingual spray
Nitrolingual

nitroglycerin ointment
Nitro-bid, Nitrol, Nitrong

nitroglycerin sublingual
Nitrostat

nitroglycerin transdermal system
Deponit, Minitran, Nitrodisc, Nitro-Dur, Nitro-Dur II, NTS, Transderm-Nitro

CLASSIFICATION(S):
Vasodilator (nitrate), Antianginal, Coronary vasodilator
Pregnancy Category C

INDICATIONS

■ **Lingual, SL:** Acute treatment of angina pectoris ■ **Lingual, SL, extended-release tablet, buccal tablet, capsules, ointment, transdermal:** Long-term prophylactic management of angina pectoris ■ **PO, transdermal, ointment:** Adjunct treatment of congestive heart failure ■ **IV:** Adjunct treatment of acute myocardial infarction ■ **IV:** Production of controlled hypotension during surgical procedures.

ACTION

■ Increases coronary blood flow by dilating coronary arteries and improv-

ing collateral flow to ischemic regions ■ Produces vasodilation (venous greater than arterial) ■ Decreases left ventricular end-diastolic pressure and left ventricular end-diastolic volume (preload) ■ Reduces myocardial oxygen consumption. **Therapeutic Effects:** ■ Relief or prevention of anginal attacks ■ Increased cardiac output.

PHARMACOKINETICS

Absorption: Well absorbed following oral, buccal, and sublingual administration. Also absorbed through skin. Orally administered nitroglycerin is rapidly metabolized, leading to decreased bioavailability.
Distribution: Distribution not known.
Metabolism and Excretion: Undergoes rapid and almost complete metabolism by the liver. Also metabolized by enzymes in bloodstream.
Half-life: 1–4 min.

CONTRAINDICATIONS AND PRECAUTIONS

Contraindicated in: ■ Hypersensitivity ■ Severe anemia ■ Pericardial tamponade ■ Constrictive pericarditis ■ Alcohol intolerance (large IV doses only).
Use Cautiously in: ■ Head trauma or cerebral hemorrhage ■ Pregnancy (may compromise maternal/fetal circulation) ■ Children or lactation (safety not established) ■ Glaucoma ■ Hypertrophic cardiomyopathy ■ Severe liver impairment ■ Malabsorption or hypermotility (PO) ■ Hypovolemia (IV) ■ Normal or decreased pulmonary capillary wedge pressure (IV) ■ Cardioversion (remove transdermal patch prior to).

ADVERSE REACTIONS AND SIDE EFFECTS*

CNS: headache, apprehension, weakness, dizziness, lightheadedness, restlessness.
EENT: blurred vision.
CV: hypotension, tachycardia, syncope.
GI: nausea, vomiting, abdominal pain.

{} = Available in Canada only.
*Underlines indicate most frequent; **CAPITALS** indicate life-threatening.

N

Derm: contact dermatitis (transdermal or oint).

Misc: flushing, tolerance, cross-tolerance, alcohol intoxication (large IV doses only).

INTERACTIONS

Drug–Drug: ▪ Additive hypotension with **antihypertensives,** acute ingestion of **alcohol, beta-adrenergic blocking agents, calcium channel blockers, haloperidol,** or **phenothiazines** ▪ Agents having anticholinergic properties (**tricyclic antidepressants, antihistamines, phenothiazines**) may decrease absorption of sublingual or buccal nitroglycerin.

ROUTE AND DOSAGE

- **SL (Adults):** 0.15–0.6 mg, may repeat q 5 min for 15 min for acute attack.
- **Lingual Spray (Adults):** (0.4 mg/spray) 1–2 sprays, may be repeated q 5 min for 15 min.
- **Buccal (Adults):** 1 mg q 3–5 hr; dosage and frequency may be increased as needed.
- **PO (Adults):** 2.5–9 mg q 8–12 hr as extended-release capsules or 1.3–6.5 mg q 8–12 hr as extended-release tablet. Up to 26 mg 4 times daily has been used.
- **IV (Adults):** 5 mcg/min, increase by 5 mcg/min q 3–5 min to 20 mcg/min, then increase by 10–20 mcg/min q 3–5 min (dosing determined by hemodynamic parameters).
- **Oint (Adults):** (1 in. = 15 mg) 1–2 in. q 8 hr (up to 5 in. q 4 hr).
- **Transdermal Patch:** 0.1–0.6 mg/hr, up to 0.8 mg/hr. Patch should be worn 12–14 hr/day.

AVAILABILITY

▪ **Sustained-release tablets:** 2.6 mg, 6.5 mg, 9 mg ▪ **Sustained-release capsules:** 2.5 mg, 6.5 mg, 9 mg, 13 mg ▪ **Sublingual tablets:** 0.15 mg (¹⁄₄₀₀ gr), 0.3 mg (¹⁄₂₀₀ gr), 0.4 mg (¹⁄₁₅₀ gr), 0.6 mg (¹⁄₁₀₀ gr) ▪ **Translingual spray:** 0.4 mg/spray in 14.5-g cannister (200 doses) ▪ **Transmucosal (con-**trolled-release buccal tablets):** 1 mg, 2 mg, 3 mg ▪ **Transdermal systems:** 0.1 mg/hr, 0.2 mg/hr, 0.3 mg/hr, 0.4 mg/hr, 0.6 mg/hr ▪ **Transdermal ointment:** 2% ▪ **Injection:** 0.5 mg/ml, 5 mg/ml ▪ **Injection solution:** 25 mg/250 ml, 50 mg/250 ml, 50 mg/500 ml, 100 mg/250 ml, 200 mg/500 ml.

TIME/ACTION PROFILE
(cardiovascular effects)

	ONSET	PEAK	DURATION
SL	1–3 min	UK	30–60 min
Buccal-ER	UK	UK	5 hr
PO	40–60 min	UK	8–12 hr
Oint	20–60 min	UK	4–8 hr
TD-Patch	40–60 min	UK	8–24 hr
IV	immediate	UK	several min

NURSING IMPLICATIONS

ASSESSMENT

▫ Assess location, duration, intensity, and precipitating factors of patient's anginal pain.

▫ Monitor blood pressure and pulse prior to and following administration. Patients receiving IV nitroglycerin require continuous ECG and blood pressure monitoring. Additional hemodynamic parameters may be ordered.

▪ **Lab Test Considerations:** May cause increased urine catecholamine and urine vanillylmandelic concentrations.

▫ Excessive doses may cause increased methemoglobin concentrations.

▫ May cause falsely elevated serum cholesterol levels.

POTENTIAL NURSING DIAGNOSES

▪ Pain (indications).

▪ Tissue perfusion, altered (indications).

▪ Knowledge deficit related to medication regimen (patient/family teaching).

IMPLEMENTATION

▪ **PO:** Administer dose 1 hr before or 2 hr after meals with a full glass of water for faster absorption. Sustained-release preparations should be swallowed whole; do not crush, break, or chew.

- **SL:** Tablet should be held under tongue until dissolved. Avoid eating, drinking, or smoking until tablet is dissolved.
- **Buccal:** Place tablet under upper lip or between cheek and gum. Onset of action may be increased by touching the tablet with the tongue or by drinking hot liquids.
- **IV:** Doses must be diluted and administered as an infusion. Standard infusion sets made of polyvinyl-chloride (PVC) plastic may absorb up to 80% of the nitroglycerin in solution. Use glass bottles only and special tubing provided by manufacturer.
- **Continuous Infusion:** Dilute in D5W or 0.9% NaCl in a concentration of 25–40 mcg/ml, dependent upon patient fluid tolerance (see Appendix D for infusion rate chart). Solution is stable for 48 hr at room temperature. Solution is not explosive either before or after dilution.
- *Rate:* Administer via infusion pump to ensure accurate rate. Titrate rate according to patient response.
- **Syringe Compatibility:** ▪ heparin.
- **Y-Site Compatibility:** ▪ amrinone ▪ atracurium ▪ dobutamine ▪ dopamine ▪ famotidine ▪ lidocaine ▪ nitroprusside ▪ pancuronium ▪ ranitidine ▪ streptokinase ▪ vecuronium.
- **Y-Site Incompatibility:** ▪ alteplase.
- **Additive Incompatibility:** Manufacturer recommends that nitroglycerin not be admixed with other medications.
- **Top:** Sites of topical application should be rotated to prevent skin irritation. Remove patch or ointment from previous site before application.
- ▫ Doses may be increased to the highest dose that does not cause symptomatic hypotension.
- ▫ Apply ointment by using dose-measuring application papers supplied with ointment. Squeeze ointment onto measuring scale printed on paper. Use paper to spread ointment onto nonhairy area of skin (chest, abdo-

men, thighs; avoid distal extremities) in a thin, even layer, covering a 2–3-in. area. Do not allow ointment to come in contact with hands. Do not massage or rub in ointment, as this will increase absorption and interfere with sustained action. Apply occlusive dressing if ordered.
- ▫ Transdermal patches may be applied to any hairless site (avoid distal extremities or areas with cuts or callouses). Apply firm pressure over patch to ensure contact with skin, especially around edges. Apply a new dosage unit if the first one becomes loose or falls off. Units are waterproof and not affected by showering or bathing. Do not cut or trim system to adjust dosage. Do not alternate between brands of transdermal products; dosage may not be equivalent. Remove patches before cardioversion or defibrillation to prevent patient burns. Physician may recommend wearing patch for 12–14 hr and removing patch for 10–12 hr at night to prevent development of tolerance.

PATIENT/FAMILY TEACHING

- **General Info:** Instruct patient to take medication exactly as directed, even if feeling better. If a dose is missed, take as soon as remembered unless next dose is scheduled within 2 hr (6 hr with extended-release preparations). Do not double doses. Do not discontinue abruptly; gradual dosage reduction may be necessary to prevent rebound angina.
- ▫ Caution patient to make position changes slowly to minimize orthostatic hypotension.
- ▫ Advise patient to avoid concurrent use of alcohol with this medication. Patient should also consult physician or pharmacist before taking over-the-counter medications while taking nitroglycerin.
- ▫ Inform patient that headache is a common side effect that should decrease with continuing therapy. Aspirin or acetaminophen may be ordered to treat headache. Notify physician if headache is persistent or severe.

N

□ Advise patient to notify physician if dry mouth or blurred vision occurs.

- **Acute Anginal Attacks:** Advise patient to sit down and use medication at first sign of attack. Relief usually occurs within 5 min. Dose may be repeated if pain is not relieved in 5–10 min. Call physician or go to nearest emergency room if anginal pain is not relieved by 3 tablets in 15 min.

- **SL:** Inform patient that tablets should be kept in original glass container or in specially made metal containers, with cotton removed to prevent absorption. Tablets lose potency in containers made of plastic or cardboard or when mixed with other capsules or tablets. Exposure to air, heat, and moisture also causes loss of potency. Instruct patient not to open bottle frequently, handle tablets, or keep bottle of tablets next to body (i.e., shirt pocket) or in automobile glove compartment. Advise patient that tablets should be replaced 6 mo after opening to maintain potency.

- **Lingual Spray:** Instruct patient to lift tongue and spray dose under tongue.

EVALUATION
Effectiveness of therapy can be demonstrated by: ■ Decrease in frequency and severity of anginal attacks □ Increase in activity tolerance. During chronic therapy, tolerance may be minimized by intermittent administration of 12 hr on/12 hr off intervals ■ Controlled hypotension during surgical procedures.

NITROPRUSSIDE
(nye-troe-**pruss**-ide)
Nitropress

CLASSIFICATION(S):
Antihypertensive (vasodilator)
Pregnancy Category C

INDICATIONS

- Management of hypertensive crises
- Production of controlled hypotension

during anesthesia ■ Treatment of cardiac pump failure or cardiogenic shock (alone or with dopamine).

ACTION

- Produces peripheral vasodilation by direct action on venous and arteriolar smooth muscle. **Therapeutic Effects:** ■ Rapid lowering of blood pressure ■ Decreased cardiac preload and afterload.

PHARMACOKINETICS

Absorption: Administered IV only, resulting in complete bioavailability.
Distribution: Distribution not known.
Metabolism and Excretion: Rapidly metabolized in RBCs and tissues to cyanide and subsequently by the liver to thiocyanate.
Half-life: UK.

CONTRAINDICATIONS AND PRECAUTIONS

Contraindicated in: ■ Hypersensitivity ■ Decreased cerebral perfusion.
Use Cautiously in: ■ Renal disease (increased risk of thiocyanate accumulation) ■ Hepatic disease (increased risk of cyanide accumulation) ■ Elderly patients (increased sensitivity) ■ Hypothyroidism ■ Hyponatremia ■ Pregnancy or lactation (safety not established) ■ Vitamin B_{12} deficiency.

ADVERSE REACTIONS AND SIDE EFFECTS*

CNS: <u>headache</u>, <u>dizziness</u>, restlessness.
EENT: tinnitus, blurred vision.
CV: palpitations, dyspnea, excessive hypotension.
GI: <u>nausea</u>, vomiting, <u>abdominal pain</u>.
F and E: acidosis.
Local: phlebitis at IV site.
Misc: thiocyanate toxicity, cyanide toxicity.

INTERACTIONS

Drug–Drug: ■ Increased hypotensive effect with **ganglionic blocking agents, general anesthetics,** and other **antihypertensives.**

---

*<u>Underlines</u> indicate most frequent; **CAPITALS** indicate life-threatening.

ROUTE AND DOSAGE

- **IV (Adults and Children):** 0.3–10 mcg/kg/min. Not to exceed 10 min of therapy at 10 mcg/kg/min infusion rate.

AVAILABILITY

- *Injection:* 50 mg/vial.

TIME/ACTION PROFILE (hypotensive effect)

	ONSET	PEAK	DURATION
IV	immediate	rapid	1–10 min

NURSING IMPLICATIONS

ASSESSMENT

- ☐ Monitor blood pressure, heart rate, and ECG frequently throughout course of therapy; continuous monitoring is preferred. Consult physician for parameters. Monitor for rebound hypertension following discontinuation of nitroprusside.
- ☐ Pulmonary capillary wedge pressure (PCWP) may be monitored in patients with myocardial infarction or congestive heart failure.
- **Lab Test Considerations:** May cause decrease in bicarbonate concentrations, pCO_2, and pH.
- ☐ May cause increased lactate concentrations.
- ☐ May cause increased serum cyanide and thiocyanate concentrations.
- ☐ Monitor serum methemoglobin concentrations in patients receiving >10 mg/kg and who exhibit signs of impaired oxygen delivery despite adequate cardiac output and arterial pO_2 (blood is chocolate brown without change on exposure to air). Treatment of methemoglobinemia is 1–2 mg/kg of methylene blue IV administered over several minutes.
- **Toxicity and Overdose:** If severe hypotension occurs, drug effects are quickly reversed by decreasing rate or temporarily discontinuing infusion.
- ☐ Plasma thiocyanate levels should be monitored every 24 hr in patients receiving prolonged infusions at a rate

>3 mcg/kg/min. Levels should not exceed 1 millimole/liter.

- ☐ Signs and symptoms of thiocyanate toxicity include tinnitus, blurred vision, dyspnea, dizziness, headache, syncope, and metabolic acidosis.
- ☐ Treatment may include amyl nitrite inhalation and infusions of sodium nitrite and sodium thiosulfate.

POTENTIAL NURSING DIAGNOSES

- Tissue perfusion, altered (indications).

IMPLEMENTATION

- **General Info:** If infusion of 10 mcg/kg/min for 10 min does not produce adequate reduction in blood pressure, manufacturer recommends nitroprusside be discontinued.
- ☐ May be administered in left ventricular congestive heart failure concurrently with an inotropic agent (dopamine, dobutamine) when effective doses of nitroprusside restore pump function and cause excessive hypotension.
- **Continuous Infusion:** Reconstitute each 50 mg with 2–3 ml of D5W for injection. Dilute further in 250–1000 ml of D5W. Do not use other diluents for reconstitution or infusion. Wrap infusion bottle in aluminum foil to protect from light; administration set tubing need not be covered. Freshly prepared solution has a slight brownish tint; discard if solution is dark brown, orange, blue, green, or dark red. Solution must be used within 24 hr of preparation.
- ☐ Avoid extravasation.
- *Rate:* Administer via infusion pump to ensure accurate dosage rate (see Appendix D for dosage rate chart).
- **Syringe Compatibility:** ▪ heparin.
- **Y-Site Compatibility:** ▪ amrinone ▪ atracurium ▪ dobutamine ▪ dopamine ▪ enalaprilat ▪ famotidine ▪ lidocaine ▪ nitroglycerin ▪ pancuronium ▪ vecuronium.
- **Additive Incompatibility:** Do not admix with other medications.

PATIENT/FAMILY TEACHING

- ☐ Advise patient to report the onset of

N

tinnitus, dyspnea, dizziness, headache, or blurred vision immediately.

EVALUATION

Effectiveness of therapy is indicated by: ▪ Decrease in blood pressure without the appearance of side effects ▪ Treatment of cardiac pump failure or cardiogenic shock.

NIZATIDINE
(ni-**za**-ti-deen)
Axid

CLASSIFICATION(S):
Histamine H₂ antagonist,
Antiulcer
Pregnancy Category C

INDICATIONS

▪ Short-term treatment and maintenance preventive treatment of active duodenal ulcers ▪ Management of gastroesophageal reflux disease (GERD). **Unlabeled Use:** ▪ Short-term treatment of benign gastric ulcers.

ACTION

▪ Inhibits the action of histamine at the H_2 receptor site located primarily in gastric parietal cells ▪ Inhibits gastric acid secretion. **Therapeutic Effects:** ▪ Healing and prevention of ulcers ▪ Decreased symptoms of gastroesophageal reflux.

PHARMACOKINETICS

Absorption: Well absorbed following oral administration.
Distribution: Distribution not known. Probably enters breast milk.
Metabolism and Excretion: 60% excreted unchanged by the kidneys. Some hepatic metabolism; one metabolite is active.
Half-life: 1.6 hr (increased in renal failure).

CONTRAINDICATIONS AND PRECAUTIONS

Contraindicated in: ▪ Hypersensitivity.

Use Cautiously in: ▪ Pregnancy, lactation, or children (safety not established) ▪ Impaired liver function ▪ Elderly patients (increased risk of adverse reactions) ▪ Renal impairment (increased dosing interval recommended if CCr <50 ml/min).

ADVERSE REACTIONS AND SIDE EFFECTS*

CNS: somnolence, dizziness.
CV: arrhythmias.
Derm: sweating, urticaria.
GI: hepatitis.
Metab: hyperuricemia.

INTERACTIONS

Drug–Drug: ▪ May increase salicylate serum levels in patients on high-dose (>3900 mg/day) **aspirin** therapy ▪ Concurrently administered **antacids** may decrease absorption of nizatidine.

ROUTE AND DOSAGE

Active Duodenal Ulcers
▪ **PO (Adults):** 150 mg bid or 300 mg at bedtime.

Prophylaxis of Duodenal Ulcers
▪ **PO (Adults):** 150 mg at bedtime.

GERD
▪ **PO (Adults):** 150 mg twice daily.

AVAILABILITY

▪ *Capsules:* 150 mg, 300 mg.

TIME/ACTION PROFILE (inhibition of gastric acid secretion)

	ONSET	PEAK	DURATION
PO	UK	UK	8–12 hr

NURSING IMPLICATIONS

ASSESSMENT

▫ Assess patient routinely for epigastric or abdominal pain and frank or occult blood in the stool, emesis, or gastric aspirate.
▪ **Lab Test Considerations:** Monitor liver function test periodically throughout therapy.
▫ May cause elevated AST (SGOT), ALT

---

*Underlines indicate most frequent; **CAPITALS** indicate life-threatening.

(SGPT), and alkaline phosphatase concentrations.

□ May cause false-positive tests for urobilinogen.

POTENTIAL NURSING DIAGNOSES

- Pain (indications).
- Knowledge deficit related to medication regimen (patient/family teaching).

IMPLEMENTATION

- **General Info:** Diagnosis of malignant GI neoplasm should be ruled out prior to initiation of nizatidine therapy.
- □ If antacids are used concurrently with nizatidine for relief of pain, avoid administration within 1 hr of nizatidine, as they decrease the absorption of nizatidine.
- **PO:** Usually administered once daily at bedtime to prolong effect. May also be divided into 2 daily doses.

PATIENT/FAMILY TEACHING

- □ Instruct patient to take medication as directed for the full course of therapy, even if feeling better. If a dose is missed, it should be taken as soon as remembered, but not if almost time for next dose. Do not double doses. Nizatidine therapy is not recommended for >8 wk.
- □ Inform patient that smoking interferes with the action of nizatidine. Encourage patient to quit smoking or at least not to smoke after last dose of the day.
- □ Nizatidine may cause drowsiness. Caution patient to avoid driving or other activities requiring alertness until response to drug is known.
- □ Advise patient to avoid alcohol, products containing aspirin or ibuprofen, and foods that may cause an increase in GI irritation.
- □ Advise patient to report onset of black, tarry stools or dizziness to physician promptly.

EVALUATION

Effectiveness of therapy can be demonstrated by: ■ Decrease in abdominal pain ■ Prevention of gastric irritation and bleeding □ Healing of duodenal ul-

cers is demonstrated by x-rays or endoscopy ■ Decrease in the symptoms of gastroesophageal reflux disease (GERD).

NOREPINEPHRINE
(nor-ep-i-nef-rin)
Levarterenol, Levophed

CLASSIFICATION(S):
Vasopressor
Pregnancy Category C

INDICATIONS

- Produces vasoconstriction and myocardial stimulation, which may be required after adequate fluid replacement in the treatment of shock.

ACTION

- Stimulates alpha-adrenergic receptors located mainly in blood vessels causing constriction of both capacitance and resistance vessels ■ Also has minor $beta_1$-adrenergic activity (myocardial stimulation). **Therapeutic Effects:** ■ Increased blood pressure ■ Increased cardiac output.

PHARMACOKINETICS

Absorption: Administered IV only, resulting in complete bioavailability.

Distribution: Concentrates in sympathetic nervous tissue. Does not cross the blood–brain barrier, but readily crosses the placenta.

Metabolism and Excretion: Taken up and metabolized rapidly by sympathetic nerve endings.

Half-life: UK.

CONTRAINDICATIONS AND PRECAUTIONS

Contraindicated in: ■ Vascular, mesenteric, or peripheral thrombosis ■ Pregnancy (reduces uterine blood flow) ■ Hypoxia ■ Hypercarbia ■ Hypotension secondary to hypovolemia ■ Hypersensitivity to bisulfites.

Use Cautiously in: ■ Hypertension ■ Hyperthyroidism ■ Cardiovascular disease ■ Lactation (safety not established).

N

ADVERSE REACTIONS AND SIDE EFFECTS*

CNS: headache, anxiety, dizziness, weakness, tremor, restlessness, insomnia.
Resp: dyspnea.
CV: bradycardia, hypertension, arrhythmias, chest pain.
GU: decreased urine output, renal failure.
Endo: hyperglycemia.
F and E: metabolic acidosis.
Local: phlebitis at IV site.
Misc: fever.

INTERACTIONS

Drug–Drug: ▪ Use with **cyclopropane** or **halothane anesthesia, bretylium, cardiac glycosides, doxapram,** or **local use of cocaine** may result in increased myocardial irritability ▪ Use with **MAO inhibitors, guanethidine, methyldopa, doxapram,** or **tricyclic antidepressants** may result in severe hypertension ▪ **Alpha-adrenergic blockers** can prevent pressor responses ▪ **Beta-adrenergic blockers** may exaggerate hypertension or block cardiac stimulation ▪ Concurrent use with **ergot alkaloids (ergotamine, ergonovine, methylergonovine, methysergide)** or **oxytocin** may result in enhanced vasoconstriction.

ROUTE AND DOSAGE

▪ **IV (Adults):** 8–12 mcg/min initially, then 2–4 mcg/min maintenance infusion rate, titrated by blood pressure response.
▪ **IV (Children):** 2 mcg/min initially or 2 mcg/m^2/min maintenance infusion rate, titrated by blood pressure response. In severe hypotension during cardiac arrest, use initial dose of 0.1 mcg/kg/min; maintenance infusion rate titrated by blood pressure response.

AVAILABILITY

▪ *Injection:* 1 mg/ml.

TIME/ACTION PROFILE (effects on blood pressure)

	ONSET	PEAK	DURATION
IV	immediate	rapid	1–2 min

NURSING IMPLICATIONS

ASSESSMENT

□ Monitor blood pressure every 2–3 min until stabilized and every 5 min thereafter. Systolic blood pressure is usually maintained at 80–100 mmHg or 30–40 mmHg below the previously existing systolic pressure in previously hypertensive patients. Consult physician for parameters. Continue to monitor blood pressure frequently for hypotension following discontinuation of norepinephrine.
□ ECG should be monitored continuously. CVP, intra-arterial pressure, pulmonary artery diastolic pressure, pulmonary capillary wedge pressure (PCWP), and cardiac output may also be monitored.
□ Monitor urine output and notify physician if it decreases to <30 ml/hr.
□ Assess IV site frequently throughout infusion. The antecubital or other large vein should be used to minimize risk of extravasation, which may cause tissue necrosis. Phentolamine 5–10 mg may be added to each liter of solution to prevent sloughing of tissue in extravasation. If extravasation occurs, the site should be infiltrated promptly with 10–15 ml of 0.9% NaCl solution containing 5–10 mg of phentolamine to prevent necrosis and sloughing. If prolonged therapy is required or blanching along the course of the vein occurs, change injection sites to provide relief from vasoconstriction.

POTENTIAL NURSING DIAGNOSES

▪ Cardiac output, decreased (indications).
▪ Tissue perfusion, altered (indications).

*Underlines indicate most frequent; **CAPITALS** indicate life-threatening.

IMPLEMENTATION

- **General Info:** Volume depletion should be corrected, if possible, prior to initiation of norepinephrine.
- Heparin may be added to each 500 ml of solution to prevent thrombosis in the infused vein, perivenous reactions, and necrosis in patients with severe hypotension following myocardial infarction.
- Norepinephrine may deplete plasma volume and cause ischemia of vital organs, resulting in hypotension when discontinued, if used for prolonged periods. Prolonged or large doses may also decrease cardiac output.
- Infusion should be discontinued gradually, upon adequate tissue perfusion and maintenance of blood pressure, to prevent hypotension. Do not resume therapy unless blood pressure falls to 70–80 mmHg.
- **Continuous Infusion:** Dilute 4 mg in 1000 ml of D5W or D5/0.9% NaCl, for a concentration of 4 mcg/ml. Do not dilute in 0.9% NaCl without dextrose. Do not use discolored solutions (pink, yellow, brown) or those containing a precipitate.
- *Rate:* Titrate infusion rate according to patient response, using slowest possible rate to correct hypotension (see Appendix D for infusion rate chart). Administer via infusion pump to ensure accurate dosage.
- **Y-Site Compatibility:** ▪ amrinone ▪ famotidine ▪ heparin ▪ hydrocortisone sodium succinate ▪ potassium chloride ▪ vitamin B complex with C.

PATIENT/FAMILY TEACHING

- Instruct patient to report headache, dizziness, dyspnea, chest pain, or pain at infusion site promptly.

EVALUATION

Effectiveness of therapy can be demonstrated by: ▪ Increase in blood pressure to normal range ▫ Increased tissue perfusion.

NORFLOXACIN

(nor-**flox**-a-sin)

Chibroxin, Noroxin

CLASSIFICATION(S):

Anti-infective (fluoroquinolone)

Pregnancy Category C

INDICATIONS

- **PO:** Treatment of urinary tract infections due to susceptible organisms
- **PO:** Treatment of uncomplicated gonorrhea ▪ **Ophth:** Treatment of superficial occular infections due to susceptible organisms.

ACTION

- Inhibits bacterial DNA synthesis by inhibiting DNA gyrase. **Therapeutic Effect:** ▪ Bactericidal action against susceptible organisms. **Spectrum:** ▪ Broad spectrum of activity includes many gram-positive pathogens: ▫ Staphylococci (including *Staphylococcus epidermidis* and methicillin-resistant strains of *Staphylococcus aureus*) ▫ Group D streptococci ▪ Gram-negative spectrum notable for activity against: ▫ *E. coli* ▫ *Klebsiella pneumoniae* ▫ *Enterobacter cloacae* ▫ *Neisseria gonorrhoeae* ▫ *Proteus mirabilis* ▫ Indole positive *Proteus* (including *P. vulgaris*, *Providencia retgerii*, and *Morganella morganii*) ▫ *Pseudomonas aeruginosa* ▫ *Citrobacter freundii*.

PHARMACOKINETICS

Absorption: 30–40% absorbed following oral administration.

Distribution: High urinary concentrations are achieved.

Metabolism and Excretion: Small amount (10%) metabolized by the liver. 30% excreted unchanged by the kidneys, 30% excreted in feces.

Half-life: 6.5 hr (increased in renal disease).

N

CONTRAINDICATIONS AND PRECAUTIONS

Contraindicated in: ▪ Hypersensitivity ▪ Cross-sensitivity with other fluoroquinolones may exist ▪ Pregnancy, lactation, or children <18 yr.

Use Cautiously in: ▪ Underlying CNS pathology ▪ History of seizure disorders ▪ Severe renal impairment (dosage reduction recommended if CCr ≤30 ml/min).

ADVERSE REACTIONS AND SIDE EFFECTS*

Listed for oral norfloxacin, unless indicated.

CNS: <u>dizziness</u>, <u>headache</u>, somnolence, fatigue, depression, SEIZURES.

EENT: tinnitus, photophobia; *Ophth*— conjunctival hyperemia, conjunctival edema, photophobia.

GI: <u>nausea</u>, abdominal pain, dyspepsia, constipation, flatulence, heartburn, dry mouth, diarrhea, vomiting; *Ophth*— bitter taste in mouth.

GU: crystalluria.

Derm: rash, erythema.

MS: joint swelling, tendinitis.

Misc: fever.

INTERACTIONS

Listed for oral norfloxacin.

Drug–Drug: ▪ Concurrent use with **probenecid** decreases urinary levels of norfloxacin ▪ **Nitrofurantoin** may negate the anti-infective activity of norfloxacin ▪ **Agents that akalinize the urine** may increase the risk of crystalluria ▪ **Antacids, sucralfate, iron salts,** or **zinc salts** decrease absorption; do not use concurrently ▪ May increase serum **theophylline** levels ▪ May increase the effects of **oral anticoagulants**.

ROUTE AND DOSAGE

▪ **PO (Adults):** 400 mg q 12 hr for 3–10 days in uncomplicated infections; continue for 10–21 days in complicated infections. For uncomplicated gonorrhea, a single 800-mg dose is used.

▪ **Ophth (Adults and Children >1**

yr): 1 drop 4 times daily. For severe infections, 1 drop q 2 hr while awake.

AVAILABILITY

▪ *Tablets:* 400 mg ▪ *Ophthalmic solution:* 3 mg/ml in 5-ml dropper bottle.

TIME/ACTION PROFILE (urine levels)

	ONSET	PEAK
PO	UK	2–3 hr

NURSING IMPLICATIONS

ASSESSMENT

▪ **Urinary Tract Infections:** Assess patient for infection (vital signs, urinalysis, frequency and urgency of urination, WBC, fever, cloudy or foul-smelling urine) at beginning and throughout course of therapy.

▫ Obtain specimens for culture and sensitivity prior to initiating therapy. First dose may be given before receiving results

▪ **Ophth:** Assess patient for conjunctival swelling, redness, and pain prior to and throughout therapy.

▪ **Lab Test Considerations:** May cause increased serum BUN, AST (SGOT), ALT (SGPT), LDH, alkaline phosphatase, and creatinine concentrations.

▫ May cause decreased WBC, neutrophils, and hematocrit concentrations.

POTENTIAL NURSING DIAGNOSES

▪ Infection, high risk for (indications, side effects).

▪ Knowledge deficit related to medication regimen (patient/family teaching).

▪ Noncompliance related to medication regimen (patient/family teaching).

IMPLEMENTATION

▪ **PO:** Administer around the clock on an empty stomach, at least 1 hr before or 2 hr after meals, with a full glass of water.

▪ **Ophth:** See Appendix H for instillation of ophthalmic medications.

PATIENT/FAMILY TEACHING

▪ **PO:** Instruct patient to take medication around the clock and to finish the

*<u>Underlines</u> indicate most frequent; **CAPITALS** indicate life-threatening.*

drug completely as directed, even if feeling better. If a dose is missed, take as soon as remembered unless almost time for next dose; do not double doses. Advise patient that sharing of this medication may be dangerous.

▫ Encourage patient to maintain a fluid intake of at least 1200–1500 ml/day to prevent crystalluria.

▫ Advise patient that antacids will decrease absorption and should not be taken within 2 hr of this medication.

▫ May cause dizziness and drowsiness. Caution patient to avoid driving or other activities requiring alertness until response to medication is known.

▫ Caution patient to use sunglasses and avoid prolonged exposure to bright light to prevent photophobia.

▫ Advise patient that frequent mouth rinses, good oral hygiene, and sugarless gum or candy may minimize dry mouth.

▫ Instruct patient to notify physician if symptoms do not improve within a few days of therapy.

▪ **Ophth:** Instruct patient on correct technique for instillation of eye drops (see Appendix H).

EVALUATION

Clinical response can be evaluated by:
▪ Resolution of the signs and symptoms of urinary tract infection ▫ Negative urine culture ▪ Resolution of the signs and symptoms of ophthalmic infections.

NORTRIPTYLINE
(nor-**trip**-ti-leen)
Aventyl, Pamelor

CLASSIFICATION(S):
Antidepressant (tricyclic)
Pregnancy Category UK

INDICATIONS

▪ Treatment of various forms of depression, often in conjunction with psychotherapy. **Unlabeled Use:** ▪ Adjunct in

the management of chronic neurogenic pain.

ACTION

▪ Potentiates the effect of serotonin and norepinephrine ▪ Has significant anticholinergic properties. **Therapeutic Effect:** ▪ Antidepressant action that develops slowly over several weeks.

PHARMACOKINETICS

Absorption: Well absorbed following oral administration.

Distribution: Widely distributed. Enters breast milk in small amounts. Probably crosses the placenta.

Metabolism and Excretion: Extensively metabolized by the liver, much of it on its first pass through the liver. Some is converted to active compounds. Undergoes enterohepatic recirculation and secretion into gastric juices.

Half-life: 18–28 hr.

CONTRAINDICATIONS AND PRECAUTIONS

Contraindicated in: ▪ Hypersensitivity ▪ Narrow-angle glaucoma ▪ Pregnancy and lactation ▪ Alcohol intolerance (solution only).

Use Cautiously in: ▪ Elderly patients (more susceptible to adverse reactions; dosage reduction recommended) ▪ Pre-existing cardiovascular disease ▪ Elderly men with prostatic hypertrophy (more susceptible to urinary retention) ▪ Seizures or history of seizure disorder ▪ Asthma.

ADVERSE REACTIONS AND SIDE EFFECTS*

CNS: drowsiness, sedation, lethargy, fatigue, confusion, agitation, hallucinations, insomnia, headache, extrapyramidal reactions.

CV: hypotension, ECG changes, AR-RHYTHMIAS.

Derm: photosensitivity.

EENT: dry mouth, dry eyes, blurred vision.

Endo: gynecomastia.

GI: constipation, paralytic ileus, nausea, unpleasant taste.

*Underlines indicate most frequent; **CAPITALS** indicate life-threatening.

N

GU: urinary retention.
Hemat: blood dyscrasias, weight gain.

INTERACTIONS

Drug–Drug: ▪ May cause hypertension, hyperpyrexia, seizures, and death when used with **MAO inhibitors** (avoid concurrent use—discontinue 2 wk prior to nortriptyline) ▪ May prevent the therapeutic response to most **antihypertensives** ▪ Hypertensive crisis may occur with **clonidine** ▪ Additive CNS depression with other **CNS depressants,** including **alcohol, antihistamines, opioid analgesics,** and **sedative/hypnotics** ▪ Sympathomimetic effects may be additive with other **adrenergic agents,** including **vasoconstrictors** and **decongestants** ▪ Additive anticholinergic effects with other **drugs possessing anticholinergic properties,** including **antihistamines, antidepressants, atropine, haloperidol, phenothiazines, quinidine,** and **disopyramide** ▪ **Cimetidine** or **oral contraceptives** increase blood levels and risk of toxicity ▪ Increased risk of agranulocytosis with **antithyroid agents** ▪ **Fluoxetine** increases risk of toxicity.

ROUTE AND DOSAGE

▪ **PO (Adults):** 25 mg 3–4 times daily, up to 150 mg/day.
▪ **PO (Elderly or Adolescent Patients):** 30–50 mg/day as a single dose or in divided doses.

AVAILABILITY

▪ *Capsules:* 10 mg, 25 mg, 50 mg, 75 mg ▪ *Oral solution:* 10 mg/5 ml.

TIME/ACTION PROFILE
(antidepressant effect)

	ONSET	PEAK	DURATION
PO	2–3 wk	6 wk	UK

NURSING IMPLICATIONS

ASSESSMENT
▪ **General Info:** Monitor mental status and affect. Assess for suicidal tendencies, especially during early therapy. Restrict amount of drug available to patient.
▫ Monitor blood pressure and pulse rate prior to and during initial therapy. Notify physician of significant decreases in blood pressure or a sudden increase in pulse rate.
▫ Monitor baseline and periodic ECGs in elderly patients or patients with heart disease. May cause prolonged PR and QT intervals and may flatten T waves.
▪ **Pain:** Assess type, location, and severity of pain prior to and periodically throughout therapy
▪ **Lab Test Considerations:** Assess leukocyte and differential blood counts and renal and hepatic functions prior to and periodically during prolonged or high-dose therapy.
▫ Serum levels may be monitored in patients who fail to respond to usual therapeutic dose. Therapeutic plasma concentration range is 50–150 ng/ml.
▫ May cause alterations in blood glucose levels.

POTENTIAL NURSING DIAGNOSES
▪ Coping, ineffective individual (indications).
▪ Injury, high risk for (side effects).
▪ Knowledge deficit related to medication regimen (patient/family teaching).

IMPLEMENTATION
▪ **PO:** Administer medication with meals to minimize gastric irritation.
▫ May be given as a single dose at bedtime to minimize sedation during the day. Dose increases should be made at bedtime because of sedation.

PATIENT/FAMILY TEACHING
▫ Instruct patient to take medication exactly as prescribed. Do not skip or double up on missed doses. If a dose is missed, it should be taken as soon as remembered unless almost time for next dose. Inform patient that at least 2 wk are needed before drug effects may be noticed. Abrupt discontinuation after long-term therapy

may cause nausea, headache, vivid dreams, and malaise.

□ May cause drowsiness and blurred vision. Caution patient to avoid driving and other activities requiring alertness until response to drug is known.

□ Instruct patient to notify physician if visual changes occur. Inform patient that physician may order periodic glaucoma testing during long-term therapy.

□ Caution patient to make position changes slowly to minimize orthostatic hypotension. (This side effect is less pronounced with this medication than with other tricyclic antidepressants.)

□ Advise patient to avoid alcohol or other CNS depressant drugs during therapy and for at least 3–7 days after therapy has been discontinued.

□ Instruct patient to notify physician if urinary retention, uncontrolled movements, or fever occurs or if dry mouth or constipation persists. Sugarless candy or gum may diminish dry mouth, and an increase in fluid intake or bulk may prevent constipation.

□ Caution patient to use sunscreen and protective clothing to prevent photosensitivity reactions.

□ Advise patient to notify physician or dentist of medication regimen prior to treatment or surgery.

□ Therapy for depression is usually prolonged. Emphasize the importance of follow-up examinations and participation in prescribed psychotherapy.

EVALUATION

Effectiveness of therapy can be demonstrated by: ▪ Increased sense of well-being □ Renewed interest in surroundings □ Increased appetite □ Improved energy level □ Improved sleep ▪ Decrease in severity of chronic neurogenic pain. Patients may require 2–6 wk of therapy before full therapeutic effects of medication are seen.

NYSTATIN
(nye-**stat**-in)
Mycostatin, {Nadostine}, {Nyaderm}, Nystex

CLASSIFICATION(S):
Antifungal
Pregnancy Category A (Vaginal), UK (Others)

INDICATIONS

▪ Local treatment of *Candida* infections
▪ Treatment of intestinal candidiasis
▪ Preparation of bowel for GI surgery.

ACTION

▪ Binds to fungal cell membrane, allowing leakage of cellular contents. **Therapeutic Effect:** ▪ Fungistatic or fungicidal action. **Spectrum:** ▪ Active against most pathogenic *Candida* species, including *Candida albicans*.

PHARMACOKINETICS

Absorption: Poorly absorbed. Action is local. Not absorbed through intact skin or mucous membranes.
Distribution: Distribution not known.
Metabolism and Excretion: Excreted unchanged in the feces following oral administration.
Half-life: UK.

CONTRAINDICATIONS AND PRECAUTIONS

Contraindicated in: ▪ Hypersensitivity ▪ Some products may contain povidone, propylene glycol, alcohol, parabens, or benzyl alcohol—avoid use in patients who may be hypersensitive or intolerant to these additives.
Use Cautiously in: ▪ Children <5 yr (lozenges, pastilles, troches) ▪ Denture wearers (dentures require soaking in nystatin suspension).

ADVERSE REACTIONS AND SIDE EFFECTS*

GI: PO—nausea, vomiting, diarrhea, stomach pain (large doses).

{} = Available in Canada only.
*Underlines indicate most frequent; **CAPITALS** indicate life-threatening.

N

INTERACTIONS

Drug–Drug: ▪ None significant.

ROUTE AND DOSAGE

Oral Monilia

- **PO (Adults and Children):** 400,000–600,000 units 4 times daily as oral suspension or 200,000–400,000 units 4–5 times daily as pastilles (lozenges).
- **PO (Infants):** 200,000 units 4 times daily.
- **PO (Premature and Low-Birth-Weight Infants):** 100,000 units 4 times daily.

Intestinal Infections

- **PO (Adults):** 500,000–1,000,000 units 3 times daily.
- **PO (Children):** 500,000 units 4 times daily.

AVAILABILITY

- **Oral suspension:** 100,000 units/ml
- **Oral pastilles (lozenges, troches):** 200,000 units troche ▪ **Powder for oral suspension:** ⅛ tsp = 500,000 units
- **Oral tablets:** 500,000 units.

TIME/ACTION PROFILE (antifungal effects)

	ONSET	PEAK	DURATION
PO	rapid	UK	6–12 hr

NURSING IMPLICATIONS

ASSESSMENT

- Inspect mucous membranes prior to and frequently throughout course of therapy. Increased irritation of mucous membranes may indicate need to discontinue medication.

POTENTIAL NURSING DIAGNOSES

- Skin integrity, impaired: actual (indications).
- Infection, high risk for (indications).
- Knowledge deficit related to medication regimen (patient/family teaching).

IMPLEMENTATION

- **PO:** Suspension should be administered by placing ½ of dose in each side of mouth. Patient should hold suspension in mouth or swish throughout mouth for several minutes prior to swallowing. Use calibrated measuring device for liquid doses. Shake well prior to administration.
- Nystatin Vaginal tablets can be administered orally for treatment of oral candidiasis.

PATIENT/FAMILY TEACHING

- Instruct patient to take medication as directed. If a dose is missed, take as soon as remembered, but not if almost time for next dose. Do not double doses.
- Advise patient to report increased irritation of mucous membranes or lack of therapeutic response to physician.

EVALUATION

Effectiveness of therapy can be demonstrated by: ▪ Decrease in stomatitis ▪ To prevent relapse following oral therapy, therapy should be continued for 48 hr after symptoms have disappeared and cultures are negative ▫ Therapy for a period of 2 wk is usually sufficient, but more prolonged therapy may be necessary.

OCTREOTIDE
(ok-**tree**-oh-tide)
Sandostatin

CLASSIFICATION(S):
Hormone (gastrointestinal),
Antidiarrheal
Pregnancy Category B

INDICATIONS

▪ Treatment of severe diarrhea and flushing episodes in patients with GI endocrine tumors including metastatic carcinoid tumors and Vasoactive Intestinal Peptide Tumors (VIPomas). **Unlabeled Use:** ▪ Relief of symptoms and suppressed tumor growth in patients with pituitary tumors associated with acromegaly.

ACTION

▪ Suppresses secretion of serotonin and gastroenterohepatic peptides ▪ Increases absorption of fluid and electrolytes from the GI tract and increases transit time ▪ Decreased levels of serotonin metabolites ▪ Also suppresses growth hormone, insulin, and glucagon. **Therapeutic Effect:** ▪ Control of severe flushing and diarrhea associated with GI endocrine tumors.

PHARMACOKINETICS

Absorption: Well absorbed following SC administration.
Distribution: Distribution not known.
Metabolism and Excretion: 32% excreted unchanged in urine.
Half-life: 1.5 hr.

CONTRAINDICATIONS AND PRECAUTIONS

Contraindicated in: ▪ Hypersensitivity.
Use Cautiously in: ▪ Gallbladder disease (increased risk of stone formation) ▪ Renal impairment (dosage reduction may be necessary) ▪ Pregnancy or lactation (safety not established) ▪ Hyperglycemia or hypoglycemia (changes in blood sugar may occur) ▪ Fat malabsorption (may be aggravated).

ADVERSE REACTIONS AND SIDE EFFECTS*

CNS: headache, dizziness, fatigue, weakness, drowsiness.
EENT: visual disturbances.
CV: edema, palpitations, orthostatic hypotension.
GI: nausea, diarrhea, abdominal pain, vomiting, fat malabsorption, cholelithiasis.
Derm: flushing.
Endo: hyperglycemia, hypoglycemia.
Local: injection site pain.

INTERACTIONS

Drug–Drug: ▪ May alter requirements for **insulin** or **oral hypoglycemic agents** ▪ May reduce blood levels of **cyclosporine.**

ROUTE AND DOSAGE

Carcinoid Tumors
▪ **SC (Adults):** 50 mcg initially, then

100–600 mcg/day in 2–4 divided doses during first 2 wk of therapy (range 50–1500 mcg/day).

VIPomas
▪ **SC (Adults):** 50 mcg initially, then 100–200 mcg/day in 2–4 divided doses during first 2 wk of therapy (range 150–750 mcg/day).

Antidiarrheal (GI Tumors)
▪ **SC (Adults):** 50 mcg 1–2 times daily.

AVAILABILITY

▪ *Injection:* 0.05 mg/ml, 0.1 mg/ml, 0.5 mg/ml.

TIME/ACTION PROFILE (control of symptoms)

	ONSET	PEAK	DURATION
SC	UK	UK	up to 12 hr

NURSING IMPLICATIONS

ASSESSMENT
▫ Assess frequency and consistency of stools and bowel sounds throughout therapy.
▫ Monitor pulse and blood pressure prior to and periodically throughout therapy.
▫ Assess patient's fluid and electrolyte balance and skin turgor for dehydration.
▫ Monitor diabetic patients for signs of hypoglycemia. May require reduction in requirements for insulin and sulfonylureas and treatment with diazoxide.
▫ Assess patient for gallbladder disease; assess for pain and monitor ultrasound examinations of gallbladder and bile ducts prior to and periodically throughout prolonged therapy.
▪ **Lab Test Considerations:** Monitor 5-HIAA (urinary 5-hydroxyindole acetic acid), plasma serotonin, plasma substance P in patients with carcinoid; VIP (plasma vasoactive intestinal peptide) in patients with VIPoma; and free T_4, and serum glucose concentrations prior to and periodically throughout therapy in all patients taking octreotide.

*Underlines indicate most frequent; **CAPITALS** indicate life-threatening.

□ Monitor quantitative 72-hr fecal fat and serum carotene determinations periodically for possible drug-induced aggravations of fat malabsorption.

□ May cause a slight increase in liver enzymes.

POTENTIAL NURSING DIAGNOSES

▪ Diarrhea (indications).

▪ Knowledge deficit related to medication regimen (patient/family teaching).

IMPLEMENTATION

▪ **General Info:** Do not use solution that is discolored or contains particulate matter. Ampules should be refrigerated but may be stored at room temperature for the days they will be used.

▪ **SC:** Rotate injection sites; avoid multiple injections in same site within short periods of time.

▪ **IV:** Bolus injections have been used under emergency conditions.

PATIENT/FAMILY TEACHING

□ May cause dizziness, drowsiness, or visual disturbances. Caution patient to avoid driving or other activities requiring alertness until response to medication is known.

□ Advise patient to make position changes slowly to minimize orthostatic hypotension.

▪ **Home Care Issues:** Instruct patients administering octreotide at home on correct technique for injection, storage, and disposal of equipment.

EVALUATION

Effectiveness of therapy can be demonstrated by: ▪ Decrease in severity of diarrhea and improvement of electrolyte imbalances in patients with carcinoid or VIP-secreting tumors.

OFLOXACIN
(o-**flox**-a-sin)
Floxin, Ocuflox

INDICATIONS

▪ **PO, IV:** Treatment of the following infections due to susceptible organisms: □ Lower respiratory infections □ Skin and skin structure infections □ Urinary tract infections □ Prostatitis □ Sexually transmitted diseases including gonorrhea, nongonococcal cervicitis, and urethritis ▪ **Ophth:** Conjunctivitis caused by susceptible organisms.

ACTION

▪ Inhibits bacterial DNA synthesis by inhibiting DNA gyrase. **Therapeutic Effect:** ▪ Death of susceptible bacteria. **Spectrum:** ▪ Broad activity includes many gram-positive pathogens: staphylococci (including *Staphylococcus epidermidis* and methicillin-resistant strains of *Staphylococcus aureus*), *Streptococcus pyogenes*, and *Streptococcus pneumoniae* ▪ Gram-negative spectrum notable for activity against *E. coli,* Klebsiella sp., Enterobacter, Salmonella, Shigella, *Proteus vulgaris, Proteus mirabilis, Providencia stuartii, Providencia retgerii, Morganella morganii, Pseudomonas aeruginosa,* Serratia, Haemophilus sp., Acenitobacter, *Neisseria gonorrhea* and *meningitidis, Branhamella catarrhalis,* Yersinia, Vibrio, Brucella, Campylobacter, and Aeromonas sp. Active against the following anaerobic pathogens: *Bacteroides fragilis* and *intermedius, Clostridium perfrigens* and *welchii, Gardnerella vaginalis, Peptococcus niger, Peptostreptococcus* sp. Additional spectrum includes *Chlamydia pneumoniae* and *trachomatis, Legionella pneumoniae, Mycobacterium tuberculosis, Mycoplasma pneumoniae* and *Urea urealyticum* ▪ Not active against *T. pallidum.*

PHARMACOKINETICS

Absorption: Well absorbed following oral administration (89% bioavail-

ability). IV administration results in complete bioavailability. Minimal absorption follows ophthalmic administration.
Distribution: Widely distributed to body tissue and fluids. Levels in breast milk are similar to those in plasma.
Metabolism and Excretion: 70–80% excreted unchanged by the kidneys.
Half-life: 5–7 hr (increased in renal disease).

CONTRAINDICATIONS AND PRECAUTIONS

Contraindicated in: ▪ Hypersensitivity to ofloxacin or other quinolones ▪ Children <18 yr (PO and IV) ▪ Pregnancy.
Use Cautiously in: ▪ Underlying CNS pathology ▪ Lactation (high milk concentrations achieved, safety not established) ▪ Children <1 yr (Ophth form only; safety not established) ▪ Renal impairment (dosage reduction of PO and IV forms required if creatinine clearance ≤50 ml/min).

ADVERSE REACTIONS AND SIDE EFFECTS*

For PO and IV ofloxacin unless noted.

CNS: tremors, restlessness, confusion, sleep disorders, nervousness, drowsiness, hallucinations, SEIZURES, dizziness.
EENT: photophobia; *Ophth only* —local burning, stinging, itching, tearing, dryness.
CV: chest pain, vasodilation.
GI: nausea, diarrhea, vomiting, abdominal pain, unpleasant taste, decreased appetite, dry mouth.
GU: cylinduria, hematuria, vaginal discharge, genital pruritus.
Derm: rash, phototoxicity.

INTERACTIONS

For oral and IV ofloxacin.

Drug–Drug: ▪ Increases serum **theophylline** levels and may lead to toxicity ▪ Administration with **antacids, iron salts, bismuth subsalicylate, sucralfate,** or **zinc salts** decreases absorption of ofloxacin ▪ May increase the effects of

oral anticoagulants ▪ Serum levels of ofloxacin may be decreased by **antineoplastic agents** ▪ **Cimetidine** may interfere with elimination of ofloxacin.

ROUTE AND DOSAGE

▪ **PO, IV (Adults):** 200–400 mg q 12 hr for 3–10 days. For uncomplicated gonorrhea, 400 mg single dose.
▪ **Ophth (Adults and Children >1 yr):** 1–2 drops q 2–4 hr for first 2 days, then 4 times daily for up to 5 days.

AVAILABILITY

▪ *Tablets:* 200 mg, 300 mg, 400 mg
▪ *Injection:* 200 mg, 400 mg ▪ *Ophthalmic solution:* 0.3%.

TIME/ACTION PROFILE (blood levels)

	ONSET	PEAK
PO	rapid	1–2 hr
IV	rapid	end of infusion

NURSING IMPLICATIONS

ASSESSMENT
▫ Assess patient for infection (vital signs; appearance of wound, sputum, urine, and stool; WBC) at beginning and throughout course of therapy.
▫ Obtain specimens for culture and sensitivity prior to initiating therapy. First dose may be given before receiving results.
▪ **Lab Test Considerations:** Ofloxacin may cause increased serum AST (SGOT) and ALT (SGPT).
▫ May also cause decreased WBC; increased or decreased serum glucose; and glucosuria, hematuria, proteinuria, and albuminuria.

POTENTIAL NURSING DIAGNOSES
▪ Infection, high risk for (indications).
▪ Knowledge deficit related to medication regimen (patient/family teaching).

IMPLEMENTATION
▪ **PO:** Administer on an empty stomach 1 hr before or 2 hr after meals with a full glass of water. Magnesium- or

*<u>Underlines</u> indicate most frequent; **CAPITALS** indicate life-threatening.

aluminum-containing antacids, iron, or zinc preparations should not be taken within 2 hr before or 2 hr after administration of ofloxacin.

- **Intermittent Infusion:** Dilute to a concentration of 4 mg/ml with 0.9% NaCl, D5W, D5/0.9% NaCl, D5/LR, 5% sodium bicarbonate, D5/Plasmalyte 56, or sodium lactate. Also available in premixed bottles and flexible containers with D5W that need no further dilution. Discard unused solution.
- *Rate:* Administer by infusion only over at least 60 min.
- **Ophth:** See Appendix H for instillation of ophthalmic medications.

PATIENT/FAMILY TEACHING

□ Instruct patient to take medication as directed and to finish drug completely, even if feeling better. Missed doses should be taken as soon as possible, unless almost time for next dose. Do not double doses.

□ Encourage patient to maintain a fluid intake of at least 1200–1500 ml/day to prevent crystalluria.

□ Ofloxacin may cause dizziness and drowsiness. Caution patient to avoid driving or other activities requiring alertness until response to medication is known.

□ Caution patient to use sunglasses and avoid prolonged exposure to bright light to prevent photophobia and to use sunscreen and protective clothing to prevent phototoxicity reactions.

□ Advise patient that frequent mouth rinses, good oral hygiene, and sugarless gum or candy may minimize dry mouth.

EVALUATION

Clinical response to therapy can be determined by: ■ Resolution of the signs and symptoms of infection. Time for complete resolution depends on organism and site of infection.

OLSALAZINE
(ole-**sal**-a-zeen)
Dipentum

CLASSIFICATION(S):
Gastrointestinal (anti-inflammatory)
Pregnancy Category C

INDICATIONS

- Management of ulcerative colitis in patients who cannot tolerate sulfasalazine.

ACTION

- Locally acting anti-inflammatory in the colon, where activity is probably due to inhibition of prostaglandin synthesis. **Therapeutic Effect:** ■ Reduction of symptoms of ulcerative colitis, proctitis, or proctosigmoiditis.

PHARMACOKINETICS

Absorption: Acts locally in colon where 98–99% is converted to mesalamine (5-aminosalicylic acid).

Distribution: Action is primarily local and remains in the colon.

Metabolism and Excretion: 2% absorbed into systemic circulation is rapidly metabolized. Mostly eliminated as mesalamine in the feces.

Half-life: 0.9 hr.

CONTRAINDICATIONS AND PRECAUTIONS

Contraindicated in: ■ Hypersensitivity to mesalamine, olsalazine, or salicylates.

Use Cautiously in: ■ Renal impairment (increased risk of renal tubular damage) ■ Pregnancy, lactation, or children (safety not established).

ADVERSE REACTIONS AND SIDE EFFECTS*

CNS: vertigo, depression.
GI: diarrhea, exacerbation of colitis,

---

*Underlines indicate most frequent; **CAPITALS** indicate life-threatening.

hepatitis, abdominal pain, loss of appetite, nausea, vomiting.
Hemat: blood dyscrasias.
Derm: rash, itching.

INTERACTIONS

Drug–Drug: ▪ None significant.

ROUTE AND DOSAGE

▪ **PO (Adults):** 500 mg twice daily.

AVAILABILITY

▪ *Capsules:* 250 mg.

TIME/ACTION PROFILE
(concentration)

	ONSET	PEAK	DURATION
PO	UK	1hr* (4–8 hr†)	UK

*For olsalazine.
†For mesalamine.

NURSING IMPLICATIONS

ASSESSMENT

▫ Assess abdominal pain and frequency, quantity, and consistency of stools at the beginning and throughout therapy.
▫ Assess patient for allergy to salicylates. Patients allergic to sulfasalazine may take olsalazine without difficulty, but therapy should be discontinued if rash or fever occur.
▪ **Lab Test Considerations:** Monitor urinalysis, BUN, and serum creatinine closely for signs of renal toxicity.
▫ May cause elevated AST (SGOT) and ALT (SGPT) levels.

POTENTIAL NURSING DIAGNOSES

▪ Pain (indications).
▪ Diarrhea (indications).
▪ Knowledge deficit related to medication regimen (patient/family teaching).

IMPLEMENTATION

▪ **PO:** Administer with food in evenly divided doses every 12 hr.

PATIENT/FAMILY TEACHING

▫ Instruct patient to take medication as directed, even if feeling better.
▫ Advise patient to notify physician if

hives, itching, wheezing, rash, or fever occur.
▫ Instruct patient to notify physician if symptoms worsen or do not improve or if diarrhea occurs.
▫ Inform patient that proctoscopy and sigmoidoscopy may be required periodically during treatment to determine response.

EVALUATION

Clinical response can be evaluated by:
▪ Decrease in diarrhea and abdominal pain ▫ Return to normal bowel pattern.

OMEPRAZOLE
(o-**mep**-ra-zole)
{Losec}, Prilosec

CLASSIFICATION(S):
Gastrointestinal (antiulcer),
Gastric acid pump inhibitor
Pregnancy Category C

INDICATIONS

▪ Treatment of gastroesophageal reflux disease (GERD) which has not responded to conventional therapy with histamine H_2-receptor blocking agents
▪ Short-term management of active duodenal ulcers ▪ Treatment of gastric hypersecretory conditions associated with Zollinger-Ellison Syndrome, systemic mastocytosis, or multiple endocrine adenomas.

ACTION

▪ Binds to an enzyme on gastric parietal cells in the presence of acidic gastric pH, preventing the final transport of hydrogen ions into the gastric lumen.
Therapeutic Effects: ▪ Diminished accumulation of acid in the gastric lumen with lessened gastroesophageal reflux
▪ Healing of duodenal ulcers.

PHARMACOKINETICS

Absorption: Rapidly absorbed following oral administration.
Distribution: Good distribution into gastric parietal cells.

Metabolism and Excretion: Extensively metabolized by the liver.
Half-life: 0.5–1 hr (increased in liver disease).

CONTRAINDICATIONS AND PRECAUTIONS

Contraindicated in: ▪ Hypersensitivity.
Use Cautiously in: ▪ Pregnancy, lactation, or children (safety not established).

ADVERSE REACTIONS AND SIDE EFFECTS*

CNS: weakness, dizziness, headache, somnolence, fatigue.
CV: chest pain.
GI: <u>abdominal pain</u>, acid regurgitation, constipation, diarrhea, flatulence, nausea, vomiting.
Derm: rash, itching.

INTERACTIONS

Drug–Drug: ▪ Decreases metabolism and may increase effects of **phenytoin, diazepam,** and **warfarin** ▪ May interfere with absorption of drugs requiring acidic gastric pH including **ketoconazole,** esters of **ampicillin,** and **iron salts** ▪ Has been used safely with **antacids.**

ROUTE AND DOSAGE

Gastroesophageal Reflux Disease/ Duodenal Ulcer

▪ **PO (Adults):** 20 mg once daily for 4–8 wk (up to 40 mg/day).

Gastric Hypersecretory Conditions

▪ **PO (Adults):** 60 mg once daily initially, may be increased up to 120 mg 3 times daily. Doses >80 mg/day should be given in divided doses.

AVAILABILITY

▪ *Sustained-release capsules:* 20 mg.

TIME/ACTION PROFILE (antisecretory effects)

	ONSET	PEAK	DURATION
PO	within 1 hr	within 2 hr	72–96 hr

NURSING IMPLICATIONS

ASSESSMENT

▢ Assess patient routinely for epigastric or abdominal pain and frank or occult blood in the stool, emesis, or gastric aspirate.
▪ **Lab Test Considerations:** CBC with differential should be monitored periodically throughout therapy.
▢ May cause elevated AST (SGOT), ALT (SGPT), alkaline phosphatase, and bilirubin.

POTENTIAL NURSING DIAGNOSES

▪ Pain (indications).
▪ Knowledge deficit related to medication regimen (patient/family teaching).

IMPLEMENTATION

▪ **PO:** Administer doses before meals, preferably in the morning. Capsules should be swallowed whole; do not crush, open, or chew.
▢ May be administered concurrently with antacids.

PATIENT/FAMILY TEACHING

▢ Instruct patient to take medication as directed for the full course of therapy, even if feeling better. If a dose is missed it should be taken as soon as remembered, but not if almost time for next dose. Do not double doses.
▢ May cause drowsiness or dizziness. Caution patient to avoid driving or other activities requiring alertness until response to medication is known.
▢ Advise patient to avoid alcohol, products containing aspirin or ibuprofen, and foods that may cause an increase in GI irritation.
▢ Advise patient to report onset of black tarry stools, diarrhea, abdominal pain, or persistent headache to the physician promptly.

EVALUATION

Effectiveness of therapy can be demonstrated by: ▪ Decrease in abdominal pain or prevention of gastric irritation and bleeding. Healing of duodenal ulcers can be seen on x-ray examination

*Underlines indicate most frequent; **CAPITALS** indicate life-threatening.

or endoscopy ▪ Decrease in symptoms of gastroesophageal reflux disease (GERD). Therapy is continued for 4–8 wk after initial episode.

ONDANSETRON
(on-**dan**-se-tron)
Zofran

CLASSIFICATION(S):
Antiemetic (*miscellaneous*)
Pregnancy Category B

INDICATIONS

▪ **PO, IV:** Prevention of nausea and vomiting associated with chemotherapy. Oral form to be used only for moderately emetogenic chemotherapy and not for high-dose regimens ▪ **IV:** Prevention of postoperative nausea and vomiting.

ACTION

▪ Blocks the effects of serotonin at 5-HT$_3$ receptor sites (selective antagonist) located in vagal nerve terminals and the chemoreceptor trigger zone in the CNS. **Therapeutic Effect:** ▪ Decreased incidence and severity of nausea and vomiting following chemotherapy or surgery.

PHARMACOKINETICS

Absorption: IV administration results in complete bioavailability. Bioavailability of oral form is diminished.
Distribution: Distribution not known.
Metabolism and Excretion: Extensively metabolized by the liver. 5% excreted unchanged by the kidneys.
Half-life: 3.5–5.5 hr.

CONTRAINDICATIONS AND PRECAUTIONS

Contraindicated in: ▪ Hypersensitivity.
Use Cautiously in: ▪ Pregnancy, lactation, or children ≤3 yr (safety not established).

ADVERSE REACTIONS AND SIDE EFFECTS*

CNS: headache, dizziness, weakness.

GI: diarrhea, constipation, dry mouth, abdominal pain.
Neuro: extrapyramidal reactions.

INTERACTIONS

Drug–Drug: ▪ None significant.

ROUTE AND DOSAGE

Prevention of Chemotherapy-induced Nausea/Vomiting

▪ **PO (Adults):** 8 mg 30 min prior to chemotherapy, repeated 4 and 8 hr later. 8 mg 3 times daily may be given for 1–2 days following chemotherapy.
▪ **PO (Children 4–12 yr):** 4 mg 3 times daily.
▪ **IV (Adults):** 0.15 mg/kg 15–30 min prior to chemotherapy, repeated 4 and 8 hr later or 32 mg single dose 30 min prior to chemotherapy.

Prevention of Postoperative Nausea/Vomiting
▪ **IV (Adults):** 4 mg.

AVAILABILITY

▪ *Tablets:* 4 mg, 8 mg ▪ *Injection:* 2 mg/ml.

TIME/ACTION PROFILE (antiemetic effect)

	ONSET	PEAK	DURATION
PO, IV	rapid	15–30 min	4 hr

NURSING IMPLICATIONS

ASSESSMENT
▫ Assess patient for nausea, vomiting, abdominal distention, and bowel sounds prior to and following administration.
▫ Assess patient for extrapyramidal effects (involuntary movements, facial grimacing, rigidity, shuffling walk, trembling of hands) periodically throughout course of therapy.
▪ **Lab Test Considerations:** May cause transient elevations in AST (SGOT) and ALT (SGPT) levels.

POTENTIAL NURSING DIAGNOSES
▪ Nutrition, altered: less than body requirements (indications).

*Underlines indicate most frequent; **CAPITALS** indicate life-threatening.

- Diarrhea or Constipation (side effects).
- Knowledge deficit related to medication regimen (patient/family teaching).

IMPLEMENTATION

- **PO:** Administer the first dose 30 min prior to start of emetogenic chemotherapy and subsequent doses 4 and 8 hr after the first dose. May also be administered every 8 hr for 1–2 days after completion of chemotherapy.
- **Direct IV:** Administer 4 mg undiluted immediately before induction of anesthesia or postoperatively if nausea and vomiting occurs shortly after surgery.
- **Rate:** Administer over at least 30 sec and preferably over 2–5 min.
- **Intermittent Infusion:** Dilute in 50 ml of D5W or 0.9% NaCl. Stable for 48 hr following dilution.
- **Rate:** Administer each of 3 doses as IV infusion over 15 min. Infuse first dose 30 min prior to start of emetogenic chemotherapy. Administer subsequent doses 4 and 8 hr after first dose. May also be given as a single dose 30 min prior to chemotherapy.
- **Y-Site Compatibility:** amikacin ▪ aztreonam ▪ bleomycin ▪ carboplatin ▪ carmustine ▪ cefazolin ▪ ceforanide ▪ cefotaxime ▪ cefoxitin ▪ ceftazidime ▪ ceftizoxime ▪ cefuroxime ▪ chlorpromazine ▪ cimetidine ▪ cisplatin ▪ clindamycin ▪ cyclophosphamide ▪ cytarabine ▪ dacarbazine ▪ dactinomycin ▪ daunorubicin ▪ dexamethasone sodium phosphate ▪ diphenhydramine ▪ doxorubicin ▪ doxycycline ▪ droperidol ▪ etoposide ▪ famotidine ▪ floxuridine ▪ fluconazole ▪ fludarabine ▪ gentamicin ▪ haloperidol ▪ heparin ▪ hydrocortisone sodium succinate ▪ hydromorphone ▪ hydroxyzine ▪ ifosfamide ▪ imipenem/cilastatin ▪ magnesium sulfate ▪ mannitol ▪ mechlorethamine ▪ meperidine ▪ mesna ▪ methotrexate ▪ metoclopramide ▪ miconazole ▪ mitomycin ▪ mitoxantrone ▪ morphine ▪ pentostatin ▪ potassium chloride ▪ pro-
chlorperazine edisylate ▪ ranitidine ▪ streptozocin ▪ teniposide ▪ ticarcillin ▪ ticarcillin/clavulanate ▪ vancomycin ▪ vinblastine ▪ vincristine ▪ zidovudine.
- **Y-Site Incompatibility:** acyclovir ▪ aminophylline ▪ amphotericin B ▪ ampicillin ▪ ampicillin/sulbactam ▪ cefoperazone ▪ furosemide ▪ ganciclovir ▪ lorazepam ▪ methylprednisolone sodium succinate ▪ mezlocillin ▪ piperacillin ▪ sargramostim ▪ sodium bicarbonate.
- **Solution Compatibility:** May also be diluted with D5/0.9% NaCl, D5/0.45% NaCl, and 3% NaCl.

PATIENT/FAMILY TEACHING

▫ Advise patient to notify physician immediately if involuntary movement of eyes, face, or limbs occurs.

EVALUATION

Effectiveness of therapy can be demonstrated by: ▪ Prevention of nausea and vomiting associated with initial and repeat courses of emetogenic cancer chemotherapy ▪ Prevention of postoperative nasuea and vomiting.

OPHTHALMIC AGENTS

ANESTHETICS

proparacaine (proe-**par**-a-kane)
AK-Taine, Alcaine, I-Paracine, Kainair, Ophthaine, Ophthetic

tetracaine (tet-ra-kane)
Pontocaine

ARTIFICIAL TEARS

Adsorbotear, Akwa Tears, Hypotears, I-Liqui Tears, Ultra Tears, Isopto Plain, Just Tears, Lacril, Lacrisert, Liquifilm Forte, Liquifilm Tears, Moisture Drops, Murine, Murocel, Muro Tears, Neo-Tears, Refresh, TearGard, Tears Naturale, Tears Naturale II, Tears Plus, Tears Renewed

OCULAR LUBRICANTS

Akwa Tears Ointment, Artificial Tears Ointment, Dey-Lube, Duolube, Duratears Naturale, Hypotears Ointment, Lacrilube NP, Lacri-Lube S.O.P., Lipo-Tears, Refresh PM

OPHTHALMIC ALPHA-ADRENERGIC BLOCKER

dapiprazole (da-**pip**-ra-zole)
Rev-Eyes

OPHTHALMIC ANTI-INFECTIVES

idoxuridine
(eye-dox-**yoor**-i-deen)
Herplex, Stoxil

natamycin (nat-a-**mye**-sin)
Natacyn

sulfacetamide
(sul-fa-**seet**-a-mide)
AK-Sulf, Bleph, Ophthacet, Sodium Sulamyd, SOSS, Sulten, Isopto Cetamide, Sulfair

trifluridine (trye-**floor**-i-deen)
Viroptic

OPHTHALMIC BETA BLOCKERS

levobunolol
(lee-voe-**byoo**-no-lole)
Betagan

metipranolol
(me-tee-**pra**-no-lole)
OptiPranolol

OPHTHALMIC CHOLINERGIC AGENTS

DIRECT-ACTING CHOLINERGICS

carbachol (**kar**-ba-kole)
Iosopto Carbachol, Miostat

pilocarpine (pye-loe-**kar**-peen)
Adsorbocarpine, Akarpine, Isopto Carpine, Ocu-Carpine, Pilagan, Pilocar, Piloptic, Pilostat, Pilopto-Carpine, Ocusert-Pilo

CHOLINESTERASE INHIBITORS

demecarium
(dem-e-**kare**-ee-um)
Humorsol

ecothiophate
(ek-oh-**thye**-oh-fate)
Ecostigmine Iodide, Phospholine Iodide

isoflurophate
(eye-soe-**floor**-oh-fate)
Floropryl

OPHTHALMIC CYCLOPLEGIC MYDRIATICS

cyclopentolate
(sye-kloe-**pen**-toe-late)
AK-Pentolate, Cyclogly, I-Pentolate

homatropine
(home-**a**-troe-peen)
AK Homatropine, I-Homatrine, Isopto Homatropine, {Minims Homatropine}, Spectro-Homatropine

tropicamide (troe-**pik**-a-mide)
Mydriacyl, Tropicacyl, I-Picamide

OPHTHALMIC GLUCOCOCORTICOIDS

fluoromethalone
(floor-oh-**meth**-alone)
FML, Fluor-Op

medrysone (**me**-dri-sone)
HMS

OPHTHALMIC NONSTEROIDAL ANTI-INFLAMMATORY AGENTS

suprofen (soo-**proe**-fen)
Profenal

OPHTHALMIC SYMPATHO-MIMETICS

apraclonidine
(a-pra-**klon**-i-deen)
Iopidine

dipivefrin (dye-**pi**-vef-rin)
Propine

Pregnancy Category B (dapiprazole, dipivefrin); C (apraclonidine, cyclopentolate, ecothipate, glucocorticoids, levobunalol, metipranolol, pilocarpine, proparacaine, suprofen, tetracaine); X (demecarium, isoflurophate)

INDICATIONS

▪ Used for local effect for a variety of ophthalmic conditions.

{} = Available in Canada only.

ACTION/INDICATIONS

• *Alpha-adrenergic blocker*—Reverses mydriasis from phenylephrine or tropicamide • *Anesthetics*—Provide local anesthesia of short duration, which allows for short procedures, examinations, or removal of foreign bodies • *Antiglaucoma agents*—Work by decreasing the formation of aqueous humor (beta blockers) or facilitating the outflow of aqueous humor (cholinergics, anticholinesterases) • *Artificial tears*—Keep the eye moist with isotonic solutions and wetting agents for the management of eyes that are dry or irritated due to lack of tears. Also provide lubrication for artificial eyes. Ocular insert (Lacrisert) thickens existing tears and prevents their breakdown • *Cycloplegic mydriatics*—Anticholinergics that dilate the pupil (mydriasis) and paralyze accommodation (cycloplegia). Used to allow cycloplegic refraction and to treat inflammatory disorders of the iris • *Glucocorticoids*—Local relief of inflammatory conditions • *Anti-infectives/ Antivirals*—Local treatment of ocular infections • *Nonsteroidal anti-inflammatory agents*—Inhibit intraoperative miosis and are also used to treat ocular inflammatory conditions • *Ocular lubricants*—Provide ocular lubrication and protection in a variety of conditions including □ Exposure keratitis □ Decreased corneal sensitivity □ Corneal erosions □ Keratitis sicca □ During and following surgery □ Following removal of a foreign body • *Sympathomimetics*—Reduce intraocular pressure. Apraclonidine is used to prevent increases in intraocular pressure that accompany some types of laser eye surgery. Dipivefrin is used to control intraocular pressure in chronic open-angle glaucoma. **Therapeutic Effects:** • Local action for a variety of ophthalmic conditions, while minimizing systemic effects.

PHARMACOKINETICS

Absorption: Although absorption is usually minimal, systemic side effects may occur and are most significant for anticholinesterase/cholinergic agents, sympathomimetics (adrenergics), and beta blockers.

Distribution: If systemic absorption occurs, then distribution to various body tissue may follow, including crossing the placenta and entering breast milk.

Metabolism and Excretion: Local removal through tears is usual method of elimination, but if systemic absorption occurs, the liver and kidneys may be involved in metabolism and excretion.

Half-life: Brief unless agent is inherently long acting. See **TIME/ACTION PROFILE**.

CONTRAINDICATIONS AND PRECAUTIONS

Contraindicated in: • Hypersensitivity to active ingredients, additives, preservatives or other components in individual formulations. Cross-sensitivity with similar ophthalmic or systemic agents may occur. Anesthetics are only recommended for short-term use. Cycloplegic mydriatics are contraindicated in patients with tendency for glaucoma or hypersensitivity to belladonna alkaloids. Dapiprazole should not be used in patients with acute iritis. Dipivefrin should not be used in patients with narrow-angle glaucoma.

Use Cautiously in: • Safe use of tetracaine in children has not been established • Patients with asthma or congestive heart failure (beta blockers) • Cycloplegic mydriatics should be used cautiously in children (increased risk of adverse reactions) • Glucocorticoids should be used cautiously in infectious processes • Ophthalmic anti-infectives may sensitize patients to later course of similar systemic anti-infectives • Apraclonidine should be used cautiously in patients with a history of cardiovascular disease.

ADVERSE REACTIONS AND SIDE EFFECTS*

Anesthetics
EENT: local irritation, stinging, burning, photophobia, chemosis, conjunctival redness.
Misc: systemic toxicity (CNS and cardiovascular depression—tetracaine only).

Anti-infectives/Antifungals/Antivirals
EENT: local irritation.

Artificial Tears
EENT: photophobia, edema of eyelids, stinging (insert only), temporarily blurred vision.

Beta Blockers
EENT: ocular stinging, conjunctivitis, erythema, decreased visual acuity, blepharitis.
Resp: bronchospasm.
CV: bradycardia, pulmonary edema.
Derm: rashes.

Cholinergics
EENT: brow ache, transient lens opacities, blurred vision, impaired night vision.
Resp: dyspnea.
CV: bradycardia, hypotension.
GI: abdominal cramping.
Derm: flushing, sweating.

Cycloplegia Mydriatics
CNS: psychotic reactions, behavioral disturbances (children), restlessness, hallucinations.
CV: CARDIORESPIRATORY ARREST (tropicamide—children only).
EENT: increased intraocular pressure, burning, stinging, edema, conjunctivitis, exudate, blurred vision, photosensitivity.

Dapiprazole
CNS: headache.
EENT: corneal edema, punctate keratitis (irritation of the clear part of the

eye), burning, conjunctivitis, blurred vision, brow ache, ptosis, lid erythema, photophobia, itching, dry eyes, tearing.

Glucocorticoids
EENT: local irritation, stinging, burning.

Nonsteroidal Anti-inflammatory Agents
EENT: local irritation, dendritic keratitis.

Ocular Lubricants
EENT: blurred vision, eye discomfort.

Sympathomimetics
EENT: apraclonidine—upper lid elevation, conjunctival blanching, mydriasis; dipivefrin—local irritation.

DRUG–DRUG INTERACTIONS

Ocular Lubricants
▪ May alter the affects of concurrently administered **ophthalmic medications**.

Ophthalmic Anti-infectives/Antifungals/Antivirals
▪ Concurrent use of **idoxuridine** or **natamycin** with **glucocorticoids** may increase the spread of infection ▪ **Sulfacetamide** is incompatible with **silver nitrate** ▪ **Gentamicin** may antagonize the effectiveness of **sulfacetamide**.

Ophthalmic Anticholinesterases
▪ Long-acting **cholinesterase inhibitors** (demecarium, ecothiophate, isofluorphate) may prolong and intensify neuromuscular blockade from **succinylcholine** (respiratory and cardiovascular collapse may occur) ▪ Additive effects will occur with systemic anticholinesterases.

Ophthalmic Beta Blockers
▪ Additive cardiovascular and systemic side effects with **systemic beta blockers** and other **cardiovascular agents** (antiarrhythmics, antihypertensives) ▪ Concurrent use with **ophthalmic epinephrine** may result in decreased effectiveness of hypertension.

Ophthalmic Cholinergics
▪ **Carbachol** may not be effective when used with **ophthalmic flurbiprofen**.

*Underlines indicate most frequent; **CAPITALS** indicate life-threatening.

Ophthalmic Cycloplegic Mydriatics

- **Cyclopentolate** or **homatropine** may antagonize the antiglaucoma effects of **pilocarpine**, or **carbachol**. However, these combinations may be used therapeutically ▪ **Cyclopentolate** or **homatropine** may also decrease the antiglaucoma effect of **demecarium, ecothiophate,** or **isofluorphate**.

Ophthalmic Nonsteroidal Antiinflammatory Agents

- Concurrent use may decrease effectiveness of **carbachol** or **acetylcholine**.

Ophthalmic Sympathomimetics

- If significant systemic absorption occurs, adverse reactions may occur with **drugs having cardiovascular effects**.

ROUTE AND DOSAGE

Apraclonidine
- **Ophth (Adults):** 1 drop 1 hr before surgery, another drop when surgery is completed.

Artificial Tears
- **Ophth Solution (Adults and Children):** 1–2 drops 3–4 times daily as needed.
- **Ophth Insert (Adults):** 1 insert 1–2 times daily.

Carbachol
- **Ophth (Adults):** 1–2 drops q 4–8 hr.

Cyclopentolate
- **Ophth (Adults):** 1 drop, repeated in 5–10 min.
- **Ophth (Children):** 1 drop, repeated in 5 min (do not use solutions >1%).

Dapiprazole
- **Ophth (Adults):** 2 drops, followed 5 min later by 2 more drops in each eye (not to be used more than once a week).

Demecarium
- **Ophth (Adults):** 1–2 drops twice a week, up to 1–2 drops twice a day.

Dipivefrin
- **Ophth (Adults):** 1 drop q 12 hr.

Ecothiophate
- **Ophth (Adults and Children):** 1–2 drops twice daily.

Fluoromethalone
- **Ophth (Adults):** 1–2 drops every hour during the day, and every 2 hr at night or thin coating of ointment every 3–4 hr. Frequency may be decreased as condition improves.

Homatropine
- **Ophth (Adults):** For refraction, 1–2 drops; may be repeated in 5–10 min. For uveitis, 1–2 drops q 3–4 hr.

Idoxuridine
- **Ophth (Adults):** *Solution*—1 drop every hour during the day and every 2 hr at night, decreased to 1 drop every 2 hr during the day and every 4 hr at night as healing occurs, continued for 3–5 days after healing is complete. *Ointment*—Instill 5 times daily, every 4 hours; continue for 3–5 days after healing is complete.

Isofluorphate
- **Ophth (Adults):** ¼ in. strip of ointment into eye q 8–72 hr.

Levobunolol
- **Ophth (Adults):** 1 drop 1–2 times daily.

Medrysone
- **Ophth (Adults):** 1–2 drops every hour during the day and every 2 hr at night. Frequency may be decreased as condition improves.

Metipranolol
- **Ophth (Adults):** 1 drop twice daily.

Ocular Lubricants
- **Ophth (Adults):** Small amount instilled into conjunctiva several times daily.

Pilocarpine
- **Ophth (Adults):** 1–2 drops up to 6 times daily or 0.5-in. ribbon of gel at bedtime, or 20–40 mcg/hr system inserted into eye once weekly.

Proparacaine
- **Ophth (Adults):** 1–2 drops 2–3 min before procedure or removal of foreign body. For deeper anesthesia, use 1 drop q 5–10 min for 5–7 doses.

Sulfacetamide
- **Ophth (Adults):** 1–3 drops every 2–3

hr or small amount of ointment 1–4 times daily.

Suprofen
- **Ophth (Adults):** 2 drops 3, 2, and 1 hr prior to surgery and/or 2 drops every 4 hr on the day before surgery.

Tetracine
- **Ophth (Adults):** 1–2 drops or ½–1 in. of ointment.

Trifluridine
- **Ophth (Adults):** 1 drop every 2 hr. When healing starts, decrease to 1 drop every 4 hr (minimum of 5 drops) for 7 more days.

Tropicamide
- **Ophth (Adults):** 1–2 drops, may be repeated in 5 min.

AVAILABILITY

Apraclonidine
- *Ophthalmic solution:* 1%.

Artificial Tears
- *Ophthalmic solutions:* A variety of products isotonic saline, buffers, preservatives, and agents to increase viscosity and ocular contact time • *Ocular insert:* 5 mg hydropropyl cellulose.

Carbachol
- *Ophthalmic solution:* 0.75%, 1.5%, 2.25%, 3%.

Cyclopentolate
- *Ophthalmic solution:* 0.5%, 1%, 2% • *In combination with:* phenylephrine (Cyclomydril). See Appendix A.

Dapiprazole
- *Ophthalmic solution:* 0.5%.

Demecarium
- *Ophthalmic solution:* 0.125%, 0.25%.

Dipivefrin
- *Ophthalmic solution:* 0.1%.

Ecothiophate
- *Ophthalmic solution:* 0.03%, 0.06%, 0.125%, 0.25%.

Fluoromethalone
- *Ophthalmic suspension:* 0.25% • *Ophthalmic ointment:* 0.1%.

Homatropine
- *Ophthalmic solution:* 2.5%, 5%.

Idoxuridine
- *Ophthalmic solution:* 0.1% • *Ophthalmic ointment:* 0.5%.

Isoflurophate
- *Ophthalmic ointment:* 0.025%.

Levobunolol
- *Ophthalmic solution:* 0.25%, 0.5%.

Medrysone
- *Ophthalmic suspension:* 1%.

Ocular Lubricants
- *Ophthalmic ointments:* A variety of products containing sterile petrolatum and mineral oil and/or other emollients.

Pilocarpine
- *Ophthalmic solution:* 0.25%, 0.5%, 1%, 2%, 3%, 4%, 6%, 8%, 10% • *Ophthalmic gel:* 4% • *Ocular therapeutic system:* 20 mcg/hr system, 40 mcg/hr system.

Proparacaine
- *Ophthalmic solution:* 0.5% • *In combination with:* fluorescein (Fluorocaine, I-Parascein). See Appendix A.

Sulfacetamide
- *Ophthalmic solution:* 10%, 15%, 30% • *Ophthalmic ointment:* 10%.

Suprofen
- *Ophthalmic solution:* 1%.

Tetracaine
- *Ophthalmic solution:* 0.5% • *Ophthalmic ointment:* 0.5%.

Trifluridine
- *Ophthalmic solution:* 1%.

Tropicamide
- *Ophthalmic solution:* 0.5%, 1%.

TIME/ACTION PROFILE (ophthalmic effects)

	ONSET	PEAK	DURATION
Apraclonidine	within 1 hr	3–5 hr	UK
Artificial tears	immediate	UK	6–8 hr
Artificial tear insert	rapid	UK	12 hr
Carbachol	10–20 min	<4 hr	4–8 hr
Cyclopentolate	rapid	30–60 min	24 hr
Cyclopentolate	rapid	25–75 min	6–24 hr

	ONSET	PEAK	DURATION
Dapiprazole	within min	UK	UK
Demecarium	15–60 min	UK	3–10 days
Demecarium	UK	24 hr	7–28 days
Dipivefrin	30 min	1 hr	12 hr
Ecothiophate	10–30 min	UK	1–4 wk
Ecothiophate	4–8 hr	UK	7–28 days
Fluoromethalone	rapid	UK	UK
Homatropine	rapid	40–60 min	24–72 hr
Homatropine	rapid	30–60 min	24–72 hr
Idoxuridine	rapid	UK	UK
Isoflurophate	5–10 min	UK	1–4 wk
Isoflurophate	UK	24 hr	1 wk
Levobunolol	<60 min	2–6 hr	12–24 hr
Medrysone	rapid	UK	UK
Metipranolol	30 min	2 hr	24 hr
Natamycin	rapid	UK	UK
Ocular lubricants	rapid	UK	UK
Pilocarpine solution	45–60 min	1.25 hr	4–14 hr
Pilocarpine gel	1 hr	3–12 hr	18–24 hr
Pilocarpine system	1 hr	1.5–2 hr	7 days
Proparacaine	15–20 sec	UK	15–20 min
Sulfacetamide	rapid	UK	UK
Suprofen	1–2 hr	UK	4–6 hr
Tetracaine	15–20 sec	UK	15–20 min
Trifluridine	rapid	UK	UK
Tropicamide	rapid	20–40 min	6 hr
Tropicamide	rapid	20–35 min	6 hr

NURSING IMPLICATIONS

ASSESSMENT

- **Alpha-Adrenergic Blockers:** Assess pupil size prior to and following administration.
- **Anti-infectives / Antifungals / Antivirals:** Assess eye lesions daily prior to and throughout therapy.
- Assess eyes for signs of infection (redness, purulent discharge, pain) prior to and periodically throughout therapy. Report purulent eye discharge to physician; sulfacetamide is inactivated by purulent exudate.
- Assess patient for allergy to sulfonamides (sulfacetamide).
- **Artificial Tears and Ocular Lubricants:** Monitor patient for changes in vision and eye irritation and inflammation.
- **Beta Blockers:** Intraocular pressure should be monitored periodically during therapy.
- Monitor heart rate and blood pressure periodically throughout therapy. May reduce cardiac output if systemically absorbed.
- **Cholinergic Agents:** Monitor pulse, blood pressure, and lung sounds. Inform physician if hypotension, bradycardia, or bronchospasm occurs.
- Assess for symptoms of systemic absorption (nausea, vomiting, diarrhea, abdominal cramping, increased urge to urinate, shortness of breath, increased sweating, salivation). Notify physician if these symptoms occur.
- **Cycloplegic Mydriatics:** Assess for symptoms of systemic absorption (tachycardia, flushed face, dry mouth, drowsiness, or confusion). Notify physician if these symptoms occur.
- **Children:** Assess for psychotic response (ataxia, incoherent speech, disorientation, hallucinations, restlessness, tachycardia) in children taking cyclopentolate. Notify physician immediately if these symptoms occur.
- **Glucocorticoids:** Monitor patient for changes in vision, eye irritation, or persistent headache. Notify physician if signs of infection develop.
- **Nonsteroidal Anti-inflammatory Agents:** Monitor patient for changes in vision, pupil size, and conjunctival irritation periodically during therapy.
- Patients sensitive to aspirin and other nonsteroidal anti-inflammatory agents are at increased risk for developing hypersensitivity reactions. Monitor for rhinitis, asthma, and urticaria.
- **Sympathomimetics:** Monitor pulse

and blood pressure. Systemic absorption may cause slight decrease in pulse or blood pressure.

- **Lab Test Considerations:** Physician may obtain culture prior to therapy with *anti-infectives* or *antifungals*.
- □ *Nonsteroidal anti-inflammatory agents* may prolong bleeding time if systemically absorbed.
- □ *Beta blockers* may cause increased or decreased blood glucose levels.
- **Toxicity and Overdose:** Systemic effects of *cholinergic agents* are manifested by systemic symptoms and may be reversed with atropine.
- □ If symptoms of atropine toxicity occur with use of *cycloplegic mydriatics,* physostigmine IV is the antidote.

POTENTIAL NURSING DIAGNOSES

- Sensory-perceptual alteration: visual (indications, side effects).
- Infection, high risk for (indications).
- Knowledge deficit related to medication regimen (patient/family teaching).

IMPLEMENTATION

- **Solution:** Wash hands. Instruct patient to lie down or tilt head back and look at ceiling. Pull down on lower lid, creating a small pocket. Place drop in pocket. Instruct patient to close lids gently and roll eyes around in all directions to ensure even distribution. After instillation, maintain gentle pressure on the inner canthus for 1 min to avoid systemic absorption of the drug. Wait 5 min between each drop and before applying other prescribed eyedrops. Do not touch cap or tip of container to eye, fingers, or any surface. Discard solution if it becomes cloudy.
- **Ointment:** Prior to instilling ointment, hold in hand for several minutes to warm before use. Have patient lie down or tilt head back and look at ceiling. Squeeze small amount of ointment (¼–½ in.) inside lower lid. Have patient close eye gently and roll eye in all directions while eye is closed. May cause temporary blurring of vision. Allow 10 min before administration of any other eye ointments. Ointment may be refrigerated or kept for 8 wk at room temperature.

- **Anesthetics:** Cover eye with patch for protection because blink reflex is temporarily eliminated following administration.
- □ Protect solution from light; do not use discolored solutions.
- **Dapiprazole:** To prepare solution, tear off seals and remove rubber plugs from drug and diluent. Pour diluent into drug vial and shake for several minutes to ensure mixing. Stable at room temperature for 21 days. Discard solution that is not clear and colorless.
- □ Do not use more frequently than once per week.
- **Dipivefrin:** If miotic agent is ordered concurrently, administer miotic first.
- □ If dipivefrin is the sole antiglaucoma agent, to switch from epinephrine, just administer dipivefrin when next epinephrine dose is due. To switch from other antiglaucoma agents, continue other drug for the first day of dipivefrin therapy.
- **Levobunolol:** When using levobunolol to replace other antiglaucoma agents, discontinue administration of single-agent antiglaucoma therapy. If beta blockers are used with multiple agents, discontinue beta blocker before starting levobunolol therapy. To control intraocular pressure, levobunolol may be used concurrently with cholinergic agents (pilocarpine, echothiophate, carbachol), beta agonists (ophthalmic epinephrine, dipivefrin), and/or systemic carbonic anhydrase inhibitors (acetazolamide).

PATIENT/FAMILY TEACHING

- **General Info:** Instruct patient in correct method of application of ophthalmic preparation. If a dose is missed, it should be instilled as soon as remembered. Patient should confer with physician before wearing contact lenses. Do not discontinue without consulting physician; therapy for glaucoma may be lifelong.

□ Instruct patient to notify physician if eye irritation or discomfort increases or if blurred vision persists.

□ Advise patient of the need for regular eye examinations to monitor response to treatment.

□ Advise patient that anesthetics, anti-infectives, antivirals, antifungals, beta blockers, cycloplegic mydriatics, dapiprazole, glucocorticoids, and suprofen may cause burning or stinging upon instillation.

□ Emphasize the importance of follow-up examinations to determine progress.

■ **Anesthetics:** Instruct patient to use sparingly and only as directed; anesthetics may slow wound healing.

□ Caution patient not to touch or rub eye until anesthesia has completely worn off to prevent inadvertent damage to the cornea and conjunctiva.

■ **Anti-infective/Antifungal/Antiviral:** Instruct patient to instill medication exactly as directed, even if feeling better or if procedure is inconvenient. Herpetic keratitis may recur if trifluridine or idoxuridine are discontinued before microscopic staining with fluorescein has cleared. Do not use more frequently or for longer than directed.

□ Emphasize the importance of hand-washing to prevent the spread of infection.

□ Idoxuridine ointment may temporarily cause blurred vision. Caution patient not to drive until vision has cleared.

□ Advise patient to wear sunglasses and to avoid prolonged exposure to bright light to prevent photophobic reactions.

□ Burning on instillation or failure to respond to treatment may suggest deterioration of idoxuridine solution. Notify physician if this occurs.

□ Advise patient to consult physician if no improvement after 1 wk of therapy, if condition worsens, or if irritation persists.

■ **Artificial Tears and Ocular Lubricants:** Medication may cause blurred vision. Caution patient to avoid driving until response to medication is known. Increased sensitivity to light may occur; sunglasses may provide relief.

□ Discuss the possibility of matting of eyelashes. Instruct patient in correct technique for washing lids from inner to outer canthus.

□ Advise patients using over-the-counter preparations to seek medical help if condition does not resolve within 3 days.

■ **Insert (Lacrisert):** 2 applicators are provided in the box. Instruct patient to insert deep within the lower conjunctival sac. If the original falls out, instruct patient to replace it with a new one in order to prevent contamination of eye. Removing the insert a few hours after instillation may prevent blurred vision in patients prone to this side effect. Another insert may be placed later.

■ **Beta Blockers:** Inform diabetic patient that levobunolol may mask some signs of hypoglycemia and may cause decreased or increased blood glucose levels if systemically absorbed.

■ **Cholinergic Agents:** Explain to patient that pupil size will decrease. This may cause blurred vision and eye or brow ache. Night vision will be impaired, so patient should not drive at night until response to medication is known. To prevent injury at night, patient should use a night light and keep environment uncluttered.

□ Instruct patient to notify physician if visual changes, eye or brow ache, or headache persist or if symptoms of systemic absorption occur.

□ Instruct patient to avoid use of pesticides with carbamate and organophosphate bases during therapy.

□ Advise patient to inform physician or dentist of medication regimen prior to surgery as interaction with anesthetic agents may occur.

■ **Insert (Ocusert):** Instruct patient on correct method of using pilocarpine ocular system (Ocusert). Store Ocusert in refrigerator prior to use. New system is inserted once a week at bedtime. Bedtime application minimizes initial visual effects (myopia). Ocusert may be placed in upper- or lower-conjunctival sac. The system is less likely to fall out at night if placed in upper-conjunctival sac. The system may be removed from eye by gently pressing Ocusert through closed lids or by directly pushing it with clean hands. If Ocusert falls out, it may be washed with cool tap water and reinserted. Do not insert if contaminated or damaged. If an Ocusert is lost, patient wearing bilateral Ocuserts may replace both systems to maintain similar changing schedule. Review systemic side effects and instruct patient to remove system and notify physician if these occur.

- **Cycloplegic Mydriatics:** Advise patient that ophthalmic preparations temporarily may impair ability to judge distances. Dark glasses may be needed to protect eyes from bright light.

EVALUATION

Effectiveness of therapy can be demonstrated by: ■ Corneal anesthesia (anesthetics) ■ Increased tear film in dry eye conditions (artificial tears and ocular lubricants) ■ Restoration of pupillary function following ophthalmic examination (dapiprazole) ■ Resolution of cyc lesions in herpetic keratitis. Treatment is usually not continued for more than 21 days or 3–5 days after healing has occurred, except in chronic cases or infections that are difficult to cure (trifluridine, idoxuridine) ■ Resolution of the signs and symptoms of infection (anti-infectives, antifungals) ■ Decreased intraocular pressure (beta blockers, cholinergic agents, dipivefrin) ■ Reversal of mydriatic agents (pilocarpine) ■ Mydriasis and cycloplegia (cycloplegic mydriatics) ■ Suppression of ocular inflammation (glucocorticoids) ■ Inhibition of intraoperative miosis (suprofen) ■ Prevention of increased intraocular pressure dur-

ing and after ocular laser surgery (apraclonidine).

O

ORAL HYPOGLYCEMIC AGENTS

acetohexamide
(a-set-oh-**hex**-a-mide)
{Dimelor}, Dymelor

chlorpropamide
(klor-**proe**-pa-mide)
{Apo-Chlorpropamide}, Diabinese, Glucamide, {Novopropamide}

glipizide
(**glip**-i-zide)
Glucotrol

glyburide
(**glye**-byoo-ride)
DiaBeta, {Euglucon}, Glynase PresTab, Micronase

tolazamide
(tole-**az**-a-mide)
Tolamide, Tolinase

tolbutamide
(tole-**byoo**-ta-mide)
{Apo-Tolbutamide}, {Mobenol}, {Novobutamide}, Oramide, Orinase

CLASSIFICATION(S):
*Oral hygoglycemic agents
(sulfonylureas)*
**Pregnancy Category C
(glyburide-B)**

INDICATIONS

■ **PO:** Control blood sugar in adult onset, noninsulin-dependent (NIDDM) diabetes mellitus when diet therapy fails. Require some pancreatic function ■ **IV:** Tolbutamide is used in the diagnosis of pancreatic islet cell adenomas. **Unlabeled Use:** ■ Chloropramide is used to treat central partial diabetes insipidus.

ACTION

■ Lower blood sugar by stimulating the release of insulin from the pancreas and increasing the sensitivity to insulin at receptor sites ▪ May also decrease hepatic glucose production. Chlorpropamide potentiates the effects of antidiuretic hormone. **Therapeutic Effect:** ▪ Lowering of blood sugar in diabetic patients.

PHARMACOKINETICS

Absorption: Well absorbed following oral administration. IV administration of tolbutamide results in complete bioavailability.

Distribution: Glyburide reaches high concentrations in bile and crosses the placenta. Chlorpropamide enters breast milk.

Metabolism and Excretion: Mostly metabolized by the liver. Acetohexamide and tolazamide are converted to metabolites with hypoglycemic activity.

Half-life: *Acetohexamide*—1.3 hr (active metabolite—6 hr); *chlorpropamide*—36 hr (range 25–60 hr); *glipizide*—2.1–2.6 hr; *glyburide*—10 hr; *tolazamide*—7 hr; *tolbutamide*—7 hr (range 4–25 hr).

CONTRAINDICATIONS AND PRECAUTIONS

Contraindicated in: ▪ Hypersensitivity ▪ Cross-sensitivity with sulfonamides may occur ▪ Insulin-dependent (type 1, juvenile onset, ketosis prone, brittle) diabetics ▪ Diabetic coma or ketoacidosis ▪ Severe renal, hepatic, thyroid, or other endocrine disease ▪ Uncontrolled infection, serious burns or trauma.

Use Cautiously in: ▪ Severe cardiovascular or hepatic disease ▪ Elderly patients (increased sensitivity, dosage reduction may be required) ▪ Severe renal disease (increased risk of hypoglycemia) ▪ Infection, stress, or changes in diet may alter requirements for control of blood sugar ▪ Impaired thyroid, pituitary or adrenal function ▪ Malnutrition, high fever, prolonged nausea or vomiting ▪ Congestive heart failure or fluid retention (chlorpropamide only) ▪ Pregnancy or lactation (safety not established).

ADVERSE REACTIONS AND SIDE EFFECTS*

CNS: headache, weakness, dizziness, mild drowsiness.

Derm: photosensitivity, rashes.

Endo: hypoglycemia; *chlorpropamide*—Syndrome of inappropriate secretion of antidiuretic hormone (SIADH).

F and E: hyponatremia.

GI: nausea, vomiting, diarrhea, cramps, hepatitis, constipation, heartburn, increased appetite.

Hemat: APLASTIC ANEMIA, agranulocytosis, leukopenia, pancytopenia, thrombocytopenia.

INTERACTIONS

Drug–Drug: ▪ Ingestion of **alcohol** may result in disulfiram-like reaction ▪ **Glucocorticoids, rifampin, diclofenac,** and **thiazides** may decrease effectiveness ▪ **Alcohol, androgens (testosterone), chloramphenicol, clofibrate, guanethidine, MAO inhibitors, nonsteroidal anti-inflammatory agents** (except diclofenac), **salicylates, sulfonamides,** and **warfarin** may increase the risk of hypoglycemia ▪ **Beta-adrenergic blockers** may alter the response to oral hypoglycemic agents (increase or decrease requirements; nonselective agents may cause prolonged hypoglycemia).

ROUTE AND DOSAGE

Acetohexamide
▪ **PO (Adults):** 250 mg once daily (not to exceed 1.5 g/day; doses >1 g/day should be given as divided doses). Elderly patients should be started on 125–250 mg/day initially.

Chlorpropamide
▪ **PO (Adults):** 250–500 mg/day in 1–2 divided doses (range 100–750 mg/day). Antidiuretic dose is 100–250 mg/day.

Glipizide
▪ **PO (Adults):** 5 mg/day initially (range 2.5–40 mg/day). Doses >15 mg/day should be given as 2 divided doses.

*Underlines indicate most frequent; **CAPITALS** indicate life-threatening.

Elderly patients should be started on 2.5 mg/day.

Glyburide

- **PO (Adults):** *DiaBeta/Micronase*—2.5–5 mg once daily initially (range 1.25–20 mg/day). Elderly patients should be started on 1.25 mg/day initially. *Glynase PresTab*—1.5–3 mg/day initially (range 0.75–12 mg/day; doses >6 mg/day should be given as divided doses).

Tolazamide

- **PO (Adults):** 100–250 mg/day (range 100–1000 mg/day; doses >500 mg/day should be given as divided doses). Elderly patients should receive 100 mg/day initially.

Tolbutamide

- **PO (Adults):** 500–2000 mg/day in divided doses (range 250–3000 mg/day).
- **IV (Adults):** 1 g as part of the Fajans Test.

AVAILABILITY

Acetohexamide
- *Tablets:* 250 mg, 500 mg.

Chlorpropamide
- *Tablets:* 100 mg, 250 mg.

Glipizide
- *Tablets:* 5 mg, 10 mg.

Glyburide
- *Tablets:* 1.25 mg, 5 mg ▪ *Micronized tablets:* 1.5 mg, 3 mg, 6 mg.

Tolazamide
- *Tablets:* 100 mg, 250 mg, 500 mg.

Tolbutamide
- *Tablets:* 250 mg, 500 mg ▪ *Injection:* 1 g.

TIME/ACTION PROFILE
(hypoglycemic activity)

	ONSET	PEAK	DURATION
Acetohexamide	60 min	UK	12–24 hr
Chlorpropamide	60 min	3–6 hr	24 hr
Glipizide	15–30 min	1–2 hr	up to 24 hr
Glyburide	45–60 min	1.5–3 hr	24 hr

	ONSET	PEAK	DURATION
Tolazamide	60 min	1–6 hr	12–24 hr
Tolbutamide PO	60 min	4–6 hr	6–12 hr
Tolbutamide IV*	rapid	30–45 min	120–210 min

*Normal subjects.

NURSING IMPLICATIONS

ASSESSMENT

- ▫ Observe patient for signs and symptoms of hypoglycemic reactions (sweating, hunger, weakness, dizziness, tremor, tachycardia, anxiety). Long half-life of chlorpropamide increases the risk of recurrent hypoglycemia. Monitor patients who experience a hypoglycemic episode closely for 3–5 days if taking chlorpropamide.
- ▫ Assess patient for allergy to sulfonamides.
- ▫ Monitor intake and output ratios and daily weight in patients taking chlorpropamide. Notify physician promptly if peripheral edema, rales/crackles, or a significant discrepancy in totals develops.
- ▪ **Lab Test Considerations:** Serum glucose and glycosylated hemoglobin should be monitored periodically throughout therapy to evaluate effectiveness of treatment.
- ▫ Monitor CBC periodically throughout therapy. Notify physician promptly if decrease in blood counts occur.
- ▫ May cause an increase in AST (SGOT), LDH, BUN, and serum creatinine.
- ▫ Serum sodium levels and plasma osmolarity should be monitored periodically throughout therapy in patients taking chlorpropamide.
- ▪ **Toxicity and Overdose:** Overdose is manifested by symptoms of hypoglycemia. Mild hypoglycemia may be treated with administration of oral glucose. Severe hypoglycemia should be treated with IV D5W followed by continuous IV infusion of more dilute dextrose solution at a rate sufficient

to keep serum glucose at approximately 100 mg/dl.

POTENTIAL NURSING DIAGNOSES

- Nutrition, altered: more than body requirements (indications).
- Knowledge deficit related to medication regimen (patient/family teaching).
- Noncompliance (patient/family teaching).

IMPLEMENTATION

- **General Info:** Patients stabilized on a diabetic regimen who are exposed to stress, fever, trauma, infection, or surgery may require administration of insulin.
- To convert from other oral hypoglycemic agents or insulin dosage of less than 20 units/day, change can be made without gradual dosage adjustment. Patients taking 20–40 units/day should convert gradually by receiving tolbutamide and a 25–50% reduction in insulin dose the first day with gradual insulin dosage reduction as tolerated. Patients taking glyburide may discontinue insulin immediately. Patients taking greater than 40 units/day should use a 20–50% reduction in insulin dose the first day with a gradual insulin dosage adjustment as tolerated. Monitor serum or urine glucose and ketones at least 3 times/day during conversion.
- **PO:** May be administered once in the morning or divided into 2 doses. Administer with meals to ensure best diabetic control and minimize gastric irritation. Do not administer after last meal of the day.
- Tablets may be crushed and taken with fluids if patient has difficulty swallowing.

PATIENT/FAMILY TEACHING

- Instruct patient to take medication at same time each day. If a dose is missed, take as soon as remembered unless almost time for next dose. Do not take if unable to eat.
- Explain to patient that this medication controls hyperglycemia but does not cure diabetes. Therapy is long-term.
- Review signs of hypoglycemia and hyperglycemia with patient. If hypoglycemia occurs, advise patient to take a glass of orange juice or 2–3 tsp of sugar, honey, or corn syrup dissolved in water and notify physician.
- Encourage patient to follow prescribed diet, medication, and exercise regimen to prevent hypoglycemic or hyperglycemia episodes.
- Instruct patient in proper testing of serum glucose or urine glucose and ketones. Stress the importance of double-voided urine specimens for accuracy. These tests should be closely monitored during periods of stress or illness and physician notified if significant changes occur.
- May occasionally cause dizziness or drowsiness. Caution patient to avoid driving or other activities requiring alertness until response to medication is known.
- Caution patient to avoid other medications, especially aspirin and alcohol, while on this therapy without consulting physician or pharmacist.
- Concurrent use of alcohol may cause a disulfiram-like reaction (abdominal cramps, nausea, flushing, headaches, and hypoglycemia).
- Insulin is the preferred method of controlling blood sugar during pregnancy. Counsel female patients to use a form of contraception other than oral contraceptives and to notify physician promptly if pregnancy is planned or suspected.
- Caution patient to use sunscreen and protective clothing to prevent photosensitivity reactions.
- Advise patient to inform physician or dentist of medication regimen prior to treatment or surgery.
- Advise patient to carry a form of sugar (sugar packets, candy) and identification describing disease process and medication regimen at all times.
- Advise patient to notify physician promptly if unusual weight gain,

swelling of ankles, drowsiness, shortness of breath, muscle cramps, weakness, sore throat, rash, or unusual
bleeding or bruising occurs.
□ Emphasize the importance of routine
follow-up examinations.

EVALUATION
**Effectiveness of therapy can be demon-
strated by:** ▪ Control of blood glucose
levels without the appearance of hypoglycemic or hyperglycemic episodes.

OXACILLIN
(ox-a-**sill**-in)
Bactocill, Prostaphlin

CLASSIFICATION(S):
*Anti-infective (penicillinase-
resistant penicillin)*
Pregnancy Category B

INDICATIONS
▪ Treatment of the following infections due to susceptible strains of
penicillinase-producing staphylococci:
□ Respiratory tract infections □ Skin and
skin structure infections □ Bone and
joint infections □ Urinary tract infections □ Endocarditis □ Septicemia
□ Meningitis.

ACTION
▪ Binds to bacterial cell wall, leading to
cell death ▪ Resists the action of penicillinase, an enzyme capable of inactivating penicillin. **Therapeutic Effect:**
▪ Bactericidal action against susceptible bacteria. **Spectrum:** ▪ Active
against most gram-positive aerobic
cocci, but less so than penicillin ▪ Notable for activity against penicillinase-
producing strains of: □ *Staphylococcus
aureus* □ *Staphylococcus epidermidis*
▪ Not active against methicillin-resistant staphylococci.

PHARMACOKINETICS
Absorption: Rapidly but incompletely
absorbed from the GI tract. Well absorbed from IM sites.

Distribution: Widely distributed. Penetration into CSF is minimal but sufficient in the presence of inflamed meninges. Crosses the placenta and enters
breast milk.
Metabolism and Excretion: Partially
metabolized by the liver (49%), partially
excreted unchanged by the kidneys.
Half-life: 20–50 min (increased in severe hepatic impairment).

CONTRAINDICATIONS AND PRECAUTIONS
Contraindicated in: ▪ Hypersensitivity
to penicillins.
Use Cautiously in: ▪ Severe hepatic
impairment (dosage reduction recommended) ▪ Seriously ill patients or patients who are experiencing nausea or
vomiting (use parenteral dosage form)
▪ Pregnancy or lactation (safety not established) ▪ History of previous hypersensitivity reactions.

ADVERSE REACTIONS AND SIDE EFFECTS*
CNS: SEIZURES (high doses).
GI: nausea, vomiting, diarrhea, hep-
atitis.
GU: interstitial nephritis.
Derm: rashes, urticaria.
Hemat: blood dyscrasias.
Local: phlebitis at IV site, pain at IM
site.
Misc: superinfection, allergic reac-
tions, including ANAPHYLAXIS and se-
rum sickness.

INTERACTIONS
Drug–Drug: ▪ Probenecid decreases
renal excretion and increases blood levels ▪ May alter the effects of **oral anticoagulants**.
Drug–Food: ▪ **Food, acidic juices,** or
carbonated beverages decrease absorption.

ROUTE AND DOSAGE
Injection contains 2.5–3.1 mEq so-
dium/g.
▪ **PO (Adults and Children >20 kg):**
500 mg q 4–6 hr, up to 1 g q 4–6 hr.

*Underlines indicate most frequent; **CAPITALS** indicate life-threatening.

- **PO (Children <20 kg):** 50 mg/kg/day in divided doses q 6 hr, up to 100 mg/kg/day or more in divided doses q 4–6 hr.
- **IM, IV (Adults and Children ≥40 kg):** 250–2000 mg or more q 4–6 hr (up to 12–20 g/day).
- **IM, IV (Children <40 kg):** 100 mg/kg/day or more in divided doses q 4–6 hr (up to 300 mg/kg/day).

AVAILABILITY

- *Capsules:* 250 mg, 500 mg ▪ *Oral solution:* 250 mg/5 ml ▪ *Injection:* 250 mg, 500 mg, 1 g, 2 g, 4 g, 10 g.

TIME/ACTION PROFILE (blood levels)

	ONSET	PEAK
PO	rapid	30–60 min
IM	rapid	30 min
IV	rapid	end of infusion

NURSING IMPLICATIONS

ASSESSMENT

□ Assess patient for infection (vital signs; appearance of wound, sputum, urine, and stool; WBC) at beginning and throughout course of therapy.

□ Obtain a history before initiating therapy to determine previous use of and reactions to penicillins or cephalosporins. Persons with a negative history of penicillin sensitivity may still have an allergic response.

□ Obtain specimens for culture and sensitivity prior to initiating therapy. First dose may be given before receiving results.

□ Observe patient for signs and symptoms of anaphylaxis (rash, pruritus, laryngeal edema, wheezing). Discontinue the drug and notify physician immediately if these occur. Keep epinephrine, an antihistamine, and resuscitation equipment close by in the event of an anaphylactic reaction.

- **Lab Test Considerations:** CBC, BUN, creatinine, urinalysis, and liver function tests should be monitored periodically during therapy.

□ May cause elevations in AST (SGOT) and ALT (SGPT).

□ May cause positive direct Coombs' test results.

POTENTIAL NURSING DIAGNOSES

- Infection, high risk for (indications, side effects).
- Knowledge deficit related to medication regimen (patient/family teaching).
- Noncompliance related to medication regimen (patient/family teaching).

IMPLEMENTATION

- **PO:** Administer around the clock on an empty stomach, at least 1 hr before or 2 hr after meals. Take with a full glass of water; acidic juices or carbonated beverages may decrease absorption of penicillins.

□ Use calibrated measuring device for liquid preparations. Shake well. Solution is stable for 14 days if refrigerated.

- **IM, IV:** To reconstitute for IM or IV use, add 1.4 ml of Sterile Water for Injection to each 250-mg vial, 2.7–2.8 ml to each 500-mg vial, 5.7 ml to each 1-g vial, 11.4–11.5 ml to each 2-g vial, and 21.8–23 ml to each 4-g vial, for a concentration of 250 mg/1.5 ml. Stable for 3 days at room temperature or 7 days if refrigerated.
- **Direct IV:** Further dilute each reconstituted 250-mg or 500-mg vial with 5 ml of Sterile Water or 0.9% NaCl for Injection, 10 ml for each 1-g vial, 20 ml for each 2-g vial, and 40 ml for each 4-g vial.
- *Rate:* Administer slowly over 10 min.
- **Intermittent Infusion:** Dilute to a concentration of 0.5–40 mg/ml with 0.9% NaCl, D5W, D5/0.9% NaCl, or lactated Ringer's solution.
- *Rate:* May be infused for up to 6 hr.
- **Y-Site Compatibility:** ▪ acyclovir ▪ cyclophosphamide ▪ famotidine ▪ fluconazole ▪ foscarnet ▪ heparin ▪ hydrocortisone sodium succinate ▪ hydromorphone ▪ labetalol ▪ magnesium sulfate ▪ meperidine ▪ morphine ▪ perphenazine ▪ potassium chloride ▪ vitamin B complex with C ▪ zidovudine.
- **Y-Site Incompatibility:** ▪ verapamil.

- **Additive Compatibility:** ▪ cephapirin ▪ chloramphenicol ▪ potassium chloride.
- **Additive Incompatibility:** ▪ cytarabine.

PATIENT/FAMILY TEACHING

▢ Instruct patient to take medication around the clock and to finish the drug completely as directed, even if feeling better. If a dose is missed, it should be taken as soon as remembered. Advise patient that sharing of this medication may be dangerous.

▢ Advise patient to report signs of superinfection (black, furry overgrowth on the tongue; vaginal itching or discharge; loose or foul-smelling stools) and allergy promptly to physician.

▢ Instruct patient to notify physician if symptoms do not improve.

EVALUATION

Clinical response can be evaluated by:
▪ Resolution of the signs and symptoms of infection. Length of time for complete resolution depends on the organism and site of infection.

OXAPROZIN
(ox-a-**proe**-zin)
Daypro

CLASSIFICATION(S):
Nonsteroidal anti-inflammatory agent
Pregnancy Category C

INDICATIONS

▪ Treatment of the signs and symptoms of rheumatoid arthritis and osteoarthritis.

ACTION

▪ Inhibits prostaglandin synthesis. **Therapeutic Effect:** ▪ Suppression of pain and inflammation.

PHARMACOKINETICS

Absorption: Well absorbed following oral administration (80%). 35% is rapidly converted to an active metabolite.
Distribution: Distribution is not known.
Metabolism and Excretion: The active metabolite is metabolized by the liver to inactive compounds.
Half-life: 42–50 hr.

CONTRAINDICATIONS AND PRECAUTIONS

Contraindicated in: ▪ Hypersensitivity ▪ Cross-sensitivity may exist with other nonsteroidal anti-inflammatory agents, including aspirin ▪ Active GI bleeding or ulcer disease.
Use Cautiously in: ▪ Severe cardiovascular, renal, or hepatic disease ▪ History of ulcer disease ▪ Pregnancy, lactation, or children (safety not established).

ADVERSE REACTIONS AND SIDE EFFECTS*

CNS: dizziness, headache, fatigue, insomnia, nervousness, somnolence, weakness, agitation, anxiety, confusion, depression, malaise, tremor, vertigo, lightheadedness.
EENT: tinnitus, abnormal vision.
Resp: dyspnea, hypersensitivity pneumonitis.
CV: fluid retention, edema, vasculitis.
GI: abnormal liver function tests, diarrhea, dyspepsia, abdominal pain, constipation, flatulence, nausea, dry mouth, gastritis, stomatitis, vomiting, cholestatic jaundice, anorexia, duodenal ulcer, GI BLEEDING, gastroenteritis, increased appetite, melana.
GU: albuminuria, azotemia, interstitial nephritis.
Derm: photosensitivity, increased sweating, pruritus, rash.
Hemat: prolonged bleeding time.
Neuro: paresthesia.
Misc: allergic reactions including ANAPHYLAXIS, weight gain, ANGIONEUROTIC EDEMA.

*Underlines indicate most frequent; CAPITALS indicate life-threatening.

INTERACTIONS

Drug–Drug: ▪ Additive adverse GI effects and toxicity with **aspirin**, other **nonsteroidal anti-inflammatory agents, potassium supplements, glucocorticoids,** or **alcohol** ▪ Chronic use with **acetaminophen** may increase the risk of adverse renal reactions ▪ May decrease the effectiveness of **diuretics** or **antihypertensive** therapy ▪ May increase the hypoglycemic effects of **insulin** or **oral hypoglycemic agents** ▪ Increases the risk of toxicity from **methotrexate** ▪ Increased risk of bleeding with **cefamandole, cefotetan, cefoperazone, plicamycin, heparin, thrombolytic agents,** or **oral anticoagulants** ▪ Increased risk of adverse hematologic reactions with **antineoplastic agents** or **radiation therapy.**

ROUTE AND DOSAGE

▪ **PO (Adults):** 1200 mg once daily. Osteoarthritis patients with low body weight or mild disease may be started at 600 mg/day. Not to exceed 1800 mg/day (or 26 mg/kg/day, whichever is lower) in divided doses.

AVAILABILITY

▪ *Tablets:* 600 mg.

TIME/ACTION PROFILE
(antirheumatic action)

	ONSET	PEAK	DURATION
PO	within 7 days	UK	UK

NURSING IMPLICATIONS

ASSESSMENT

□ Patients who have asthma, aspirin-induced allergy, and nasal polyps are at increased risk for developing hypersensitivity reactions. Monitor for rhinitis, asthma, and urticaria.
□ Assess pain and range of motion prior to and periodically throughout therapy.
▪ **Lab Test Considerations:** May cause prolonged bleeding time, which may persist for up to 2 wk following discontinuation of therapy.
□ Liver function tests should be evalu-

ated periodically in patients receiving prolonged courses of therapy. Serum alkaline phosphatase, LDH, AST (SGOT), and ALT (SGPT) levels may be increased.

POTENTIAL NURSING DIAGNOSES
▪ Pain (indications).
▪ Knowledge deficit related to medication regimen (patient/family teaching).

IMPLEMENTATION
▪ **PO:** Administer with food or antacids to decrease GI irritation.

PATIENT/FAMILY TEACHING
□ Advise patient to take this medication with a full glass of water and to remain in an upright position for 15–30 min after administration.
□ Instruct patient to take medication exactly as directed. If a dose is missed, it should be taken as soon as remembered but not if almost time for the next dose. Do not double doses.
□ This medication may cause drowsiness, dizziness, and lightheadedness. Advise patient to avoid driving or other activities requiring alertness until response to the medication is known.
□ Caution patient to avoid the concurrent use of alcohol, aspirin, ibuprofen, acetaminophen, or other over-the-counter medications without consultation with physician or pharmacist.
□ Advise patient to notify physician or dentist of medication regimen prior to treatment or surgery. Oxaprozin should be discontinued 2 wk prior to surgery.
□ Caution patient to use sunscreen and protective clothing to prevent photosensitivity reactions.
□ Instruct patient to notify physician if rash, itching, muscle aches, edema, black stools, difficulty breathing, jaundice, mental depression, or weight gain occurs.

EVALUATION
Effectiveness of therapy can be demonstrated by: ▪ Decreased pain and improved joint mobility. Maximum effectiveness may require 2 wk or more of

continuous therapy. Patients who do not respond to one nonsteroidal anti-inflammatory agent may respond to another.

OXAZEPAM
(ox-**az**-e-pam)
{Apo-Oxazepam}, {Novoxapam},
{Ox-Pam}, Serax, {Zapex}

CLASSIFICATION(S):
Sedative/hypnotic (benzodiazepine), Antianxiety agent
Schedule IV
Pregnancy Category D

INDICATIONS

■ Management of anxiety ■ Symptomatic treatment of alcohol withdrawal.

ACTION

■ Depresses the CNS, probably by potentiating gamma-aminobutyric acid (GABA), an inhibitory neurotransmitter. **Therapeutic Effects:** ■ Relief of anxiety ■ Diminished symptoms of alcohol withdrawal.

PHARMACOKINETICS

Absorption: Well absorbed following oral administration. Absorption is slower than with other benzodiazepines.
Distribution: Widely distributed. Crosses the blood–brain barrier. May cross the placenta and enter breast milk.
Metabolism and Excretion: Metabolized by the liver to inactive compounds.
Half-life: 5–15 hr.

CONTRAINDICATIONS AND PRECAUTIONS

Contraindicated in: ■ Hypersensitivity ■ Cross-sensitivity with other benzodiazepines may exist ■ Comatose pa-

tients or those with pre-existing CNS depression ■ Uncontrolled severe pain ■ Narrow-angle glaucoma ■ Pregnancy and lactation.
Use Cautiously in: ■ Hepatic dysfunction ■ Patients who may be suicidal or who may have been addicted to drugs previously ■ Elderly or debilitated patients (dosage reduction recommended) ■ Severe chronic obstructive pulmonary disease ■ Myasthenia gravis.

ADVERSE REACTIONS AND SIDE EFFECTS*

CNS: dizziness, drowsiness, lethargy, confusion, impaired memory, hangover, paradoxical excitation, mental depression, headache, slurred speech.
EENT: blurred vision.
Resp: respiratory depression.
CV: tachycardia.
GI: nausea, vomiting, diarrhea, constipation, hepatitis.
GU: urinary problems.
Hemat: leukopenia.
Derm: rashes.
Misc: tolerance, psychological dependence, physical dependence.

INTERACTIONS

Drug–Drug: ■ Additive CNS depression with other **CNS depressants**, including **alcohol, antihistamines, antidepressants, opioid analgesics,** and other **sedative/hypnotics** ■ May decrease the therapeutic effectiveness of **levodopa** ■ **Oral contraceptives** or **phenytoin** may decrease effectiveness ■ **Theophylline** may decrease sedative effects of oxazepam.

ROUTE AND DOSAGE

■ **PO (Adults):** 10–30 mg 3–4 times daily. In older patients, initial dose should be 5 mg 1–2 times daily or 10 mg 3 times daily.

AVAILABILITY

■ *Capsules:* 10 mg, 15 mg, 30 mg
■ *Tablets:* 15 mg.

{} = Available in Canada only.
*Underlines indicate most frequent; **CAPITALS** indicate life-threatening.

TIME/ACTION PROFILE (sedation)

	ONSET	PEAK	DURATION
PO	45–90 min	UK	6–12 hr

NURSING IMPLICATIONS

ASSESSMENT

□ Assess patient for anxiety and level of sedation (ataxia, dizziness, slurred speech) periodically throughout course of therapy.

□ Prolonged high-dose therapy may lead to psychological or physical dependence. Restrict the amount of drug available to patient.

■ **Lab Test Considerations:** Monitor CBC and liver function tests periodically during prolonged therapy.

□ May cause an increase in serum bilirubin, AST (SGOT), and ALT (SGPT).

POTENTIAL NURSING DIAGNOSES

■ Anxiety (indications).

■ Injury, high risk for (side effects).

■ Knowledge deficit related to medication regimen (patient/family teaching).

IMPLEMENTATION

■ **General Info:** Medication should be tapered at the completion of therapy. Sudden cessation of medication may lead to withdrawal (insomnia, irritability, nervousness, tremors).

■ **PO:** Administer with food if GI irritation becomes a problem.

PATIENT/FAMILY TEACHING

□ Instruct patient to take oxazepam exactly as directed. Missed doses should be taken within 1 hr; if remembered later, omit and return to regular dosing schedule. Do not double or increase doses. If dose is less effective after a few weeks, notify physician.

□ Oxazepam may cause drowsiness or dizziness. Caution patient to avoid driving or other activities requiring alertness until response to medication is known.

□ Advise patient to avoid the use of alcohol and to consult physician or pharmacist prior to the use of over-the-counter preparations that contain antihistamines or alcohol.

□ Advise patient to inform physician if pregnancy is planned or suspected.

EVALUATION

Effectiveness of therapy can be demonstrated by: ■ Decreased sense of anxiety □ Increased ability to cope ■ Prevention or relief of acute agitation, tremor, and hallucinations during alcohol withdrawal.

OXTRIPHYLLINE
(ox-**trye**-fi-lin)
{Apo-Oxtriphylline}, Choledyl, Choledyl SA, {Novotriphyl}

CLASSIFICATION(S):
Bronchodilator (phosphodiesterase inhibitor)
Pregnancy Category C

INDICATIONS

■ Bronchodilator in reversible airway obstruction due to asthma or COPD.

ACTION

■ Inhibits phosphodiesterase, producing increased tissue concentrations of cyclic adenosine monophosphate (cAMP). Increased levels of cAMP result in bronchodilation, CNS stimulation, positive inotropic and chronotropic effects, diuresis, and gastric acid secretion ■ Oxtriphylline is the choline salt of theophylline and releases theophylline following administration. **Therapeutic Effect:** ■ Bronchodilation.

PHARMACOKINETICS

Absorption: Well absorbed following oral administration. Absorption of enteric-coated and sustained-release forms may be delayed, unpredictable, or unreliable.

Distribution: Widely distributed as theophylline. Crosses the placenta.

Breast milk concentrations are 70% of plasma levels.

Metabolism and Excretion: Mostly metabolized by the liver (90%), some conversion to caffeine. Metabolites are renally excreted. 10% excreted unchanged by the kidneys (up to 50% in neonates).

Half-life: 3–13 hr (theophylline). Increased in the elderly (>60 yr), neonates, and patients with congestive heart failure or liver disease. Shortened in cigarette smokers and children.

CONTRAINDICATIONS AND PRECAUTIONS

Contraindicated in: ▪ Uncontrolled arrhythmias ▪ Hyperthyroidism ▪ Alcohol intolerance (small oral liquids).

Use Cautiously in: ▪ Elderly patients (>60 yr) ▪ CHF or liver disease—decrease dosage ▪ Pregnancy (although safety not established, has been used safely during pregnancy) ▪ Lactation (may cause irritability in the newborn) ▪ Alcohol intolerance (Choledyl elixir only).

ADVERSE REACTIONS AND SIDE EFFECTS*

CNS: <u>nervousness</u>, <u>anxiety</u>, headache, insomnia, SEIZURES.

CV: <u>tachycardia</u>, palpitations, arrhythmias, angina pectoris.

GI: <u>nausea</u>, <u>vomiting</u>, anorexia, cramps.

Neuro: tremor.

INTERACTIONS

Drug–Drug: ▪ Additive CV and CNS side effects with **adrenergic agents** ▪ May decrease the therapeutic effect of **lithium** ▪ Smoking, adrenergic agents, **phenobarbital, rifampin, ketoconazole, phenytoin,** and **carbamazepine** increase metabolism and may decrease effectiveness ▪ **Erythromycin, beta blockers, cimetidine, influenza vaccination, oral contraceptives, glucocorticoids, disulfiram, interferon, mexiletine, thiabendazole, fluoroquinolones,** and large doses of **allopurinol** decrease

metabolism and may lead to toxicity ▪ Increased risk of arrhythmias with **halothane**.

Drug–Food: ▪ Large amounts of **caffeine (cola, chocolate, coffee, tea)** may increase serum theophylline levels and risk of toxicity ▪ Chronic ingestion of **charcoal-broiled beef** may increase metabolism and decrease effectiveness.

ROUTE AND DOSAGE
Dosage should be determined by theophylline serum level monitoring. Dosage expressed in mg of oxtriphylline. Oxtriphylline contains 64% theophylline.

▪ **PO (Adults):** 4.7 mg/kg q 8 hr. If daily dose is 800 or 1200 mg, may be given as sustained-action tablets q 12 hr.

▪ **PO (Adult Smokers and Children 9–16 yr):** 4.7 mg/kg q 6 hr. If daily dose is 800 or 1200 mg, may be given as sustained-action tablets q 12 hr.

▪ **PO (Children 1–9 yr):** 6.2 mg/kg q 6 hr.

AVAILABILITY

▪ *Tablets:* 100 mg, 200 mg ▪ *Sustained-action tablets:* 400 mg, 600 mg ▪ *Syrup:* 50 mg/5 ml ▪ *Elixir:* 100 mg/5 ml ▪ *In combination with:* guaifenesin (Brondelate elixir). See Appendix A.

TIME/ACTION PROFILE
(onset = onset of bronchodilation, peak = peak plasma levels, duration = duration of bronchodilation)

	ONSET	PEAK	DURATION
PO (liquid)	UK	1 hr	UK
PO (tab)	15–60 min	5 hr	6–8 hr
PO-SA tab	UK	4–7 hr	12 hr

NURSING IMPLICATIONS

ASSESSMENT

□ Assess blood pressure, pulse, respiration, and lung sounds before administering medication and throughout therapy.

□ Monitor intake and output ratios for an increase in diuresis.

*<u>Underlines</u> indicate most frequent; **CAPITALS** indicate life-threatening.

□ Patients with cardiovascular problems should be monitored for ECG changes.

■ **Lab Test Considerations:** Caffeine ingestion may falsely elevate drug concentration levels.

■ **Toxicity and Overdose:** Observe patient closely for drug toxicity (anorexia, nausea, vomiting, restlessness, insomnia, tachycardia, arrhythmias, seizures). Notify physician immediately if these occur.

□ Monitor drug levels routinely. Peak levels should be evaluated 1–2 hr after rapid-acting forms and 4–12 hr after extended-release forms.

□ Therapeutic plasma levels range from 10–20 mcg/ml. Drug levels >20 mcg/ml are associated with toxicity.

POTENTIAL NURSING DIAGNOSES

■ Airway clearance, ineffective (indications).

■ Activity intolerance (indications).

■ Knowledge deficit related to medication regimen (patient/family teaching).

IMPLEMENTATION

■ **General Info:** Administer around the clock to maintain therapeutic plasma levels.

□ Determine if patient has had another form of theophylline prior to administering loading dose.

■ **PO:** Administer with food or a full glass of water to minimize GI irritation. Food slows but does not reduce the extent of absorption. Do not crush, break, or chew enteric-coated or extended-release tablets.

PATIENT/FAMILY TEACHING

□ Emphasize the importance of taking only the prescribed dose at the prescribed time intervals. Missed doses should be taken as soon as remembered unless almost time for the next dose.

□ Encourage patient to drink adequate liquids (2000 ml/day minimum) to decrease the viscosity of the airway secretions.

□ Advise patient to avoid over-the-counter cough, cold, or breathing preparations without consulting physician or pharmacist. These medications may increase side effects and cause arrhythmias.

□ Encourage patients not to smoke. A change in smoking habits may necessitate a change in dosage.

□ Advise patient to minimize intake of xanthine-containing foods or beverages (cola, coffee, chocolate) and not to eat charcoal-broiled foods daily.

□ Instruct patient not to change brands or dosage forms without consulting physician.

□ Advise patient to contact physician promptly if the usual dose of medication fails to produce the desired results, symptoms worsen after treatment, or toxic effects occur.

□ Emphasize the importance of having serum levels routinely tested every 6–12 mo.

EVALUATION

Effectiveness of therapy can be demonstrated by: ■ Increased ease in breathing □ Clearing of lung fields on auscultation.

OXYBUTYNIN
(ox-i-**byoo**-ti-nin)
Ditropan

CLASSIFICATION(S):
Antispasmodic (urinary)
Pregnancy Category UK

INDICATIONS

■ Treatment of the following urinary symptoms that may be associated with neurogenic bladder: □ Frequent urination □ Urgency ■ Nocturia □ Incontinence.

ACTION

■ Inhibits the action of acetylcholine at postganglionic receptors ■ Has direct spasmolytic action on smooth muscle, including smooth muscle lining the GU tract, without affecting vascular smooth muscle. **Therapeutic Effects:**

O

• Increased bladder capacity • Delayed desire to void.

PHARMACOKINETICS
Absorption: Rapidly absorbed following oral administration.
Distribution: Distribution not known.
Metabolism and Excretion: Metabolism and excretion not known.
Half-life: UK.

CONTRAINDICATIONS AND PRECAUTIONS
Contraindicated in: • Hypersensitivity • Glaucoma • Intestinal obstruction or atony • Toxic megacolon • Paralytic ileus • Severe colitis • Myasthenia gravis • Acute hemorrhage with shock • Obstructive uropathy.
Use Cautiously in: • Pregnancy or children <5 yr (safety not established) • Lactation (may inhibit lactation) • Cardiovascular disease • Reflux esophagitis.

ADVERSE REACTIONS AND SIDE EFFECTS*
CNS: drowsiness, dizziness, insomnia, weakness, hallucinations.
EENT: blurred vision, mydriasis, increased intraocular pressure, cycloplegia, photophobia.
CV: tachycardia, palpitations.
GI: dry mouth, nausea, vomiting, bloated feeling, constipation.
GU: urinary hesitancy, urinary retention, impotence.
Derm: decreased sweating, urticaria.
Endo: suppressed lactation.
Metab: hyperthermia.
Misc: allergic reactions, hot flashes, fever.

INTERACTIONS
Drug–Drug: • Additive anticholinergic effects with other **agents having anticholinergic properties,** including **antidepressants, phenothiazine, disopyramide,** and **haloperidol** • Additive CNS depression with other **CNS depressants,** including **alcohol, antihistamines, antidepressants, opioid anal-**

gesics, and **sedative/hypnotics** • Concurrent use with **haloperidol** may result in tardive dyskinesia, worsening of schizophrenia, and decreased haloperidol levels • May increase serum **digoxin** levels.

ROUTE AND DOSAGE
• **PO (Adults):** 5 mg 2–3 times daily (not to exceed 20 mg/day).
• **PO (Children >5 yr):** 5 mg 2–3 times daily (not to exceed 15 mg/day).

AVAILABILITY
• *Tablets:* 5 mg • *Syrup:* 5 mg/5 ml.

TIME/ACTION PROFILE (urinary spasmolytic effect)

	ONSET	PEAK	DURATION
PO	30–60 min	3–6 hr	6–10 hr

NURSING IMPLICATIONS
ASSESSMENT
▫ Monitor voiding pattern and intake and output ratios and assess abdomen for bladder distention prior to and periodically throughout therapy. Physician may order catheterization to assess postvoid residual. Cystometry, to diagnose type of bladder dysfunction, is usually performed prior to prescription of oxybutynin.

POTENTIAL NURSING DIAGNOSES
• Urinary elimination, altered patterns of (indications).
• Pain (indications).
• Knowledge deficit related to medication regimen (patient/family teaching).

IMPLEMENTATION
• **PO:** May be administered on an empty stomach or with meals or milk to prevent gastric irritation.

PATIENT/FAMILY TEACHING
▫ Instruct patient to take medication exactly as directed. If a dose is missed, it should be taken as soon as remembered unless almost time for next dose.
▫ Medication may cause drowsiness or

---

*Underlines indicate most frequent; **CAPITALS** indicate life-threatening.

blurred vision. Advise patient to avoid driving and other activities requiring alertness until response to medication is known.
▢ Advise patient to avoid concurrent use of alcohol and other CNS depressants while taking this medication.
▢ Instruct patient that frequent rinsing of mouth, good oral hygiene, and sugarless gum or candy may decrease dry mouth. Physician or dentist should be notified if mouth dryness persists >2 wk.
▢ Inform patient that oxybutynin decreases the body's ability to perspire. The patient should avoid strenuous activity in a warm environment because overheating may occur.
▢ Advise patient to wear sunglasses when out in bright sunlight, as increased sensitivity to light may occur.
▢ Advise patient to notify physician if urinary retention occurs or if constipation persists. Discuss with patient methods of preventing constipation, such as increasing bulk in the diet, increasing fluid intake, and increasing mobility.
▢ Discuss need for continued medical follow-up. Physician may order periodic cystometry to evaluate effectiveness of medication and periodic ophthalmic examinations to detect glaucoma, especially in patients over 40 yr of age.

EVALUATION
Effectiveness of therapy can be demonstrated by: ▪ Relief of bladder spasm and associated symptoms (frequency, urgency, nocturia, and incontinence) in patients with a neurogenic bladder.

OXYCODONE
(ox-i-**koe**-done)
Roxicodone, {Supeudol}

OXYCODONE/ACETAMINO-PHEN
{Endocet}, {Oxycocet}, Percocet, Roxicet, Roxilox, Tylox

OXYCODONE/ASPIRIN
{Endodan}, {Oxycodan}, Percodan, Percodan-Demi, Roxiprin

CLASSIFICATION(S):
Opioid analgesic (agonist)
Schedule II
Pregnancy Category UK

For information on acetaminophen or aspirin, see individual monographs.

INDICATIONS
▪ Used alone and in combination with nonopioid analgesics in the management of moderate to severe pain.

ACTION
▪ Binds to opiate receptors in the CNS
▪ Alters the perception of and response to painful stimuli, while producing generalized CNS depression. **Therapeutic Effect:** ▪ Decreased pain.

PHARMACOKINETICS
Absorption: Well absorbed from the GI tract.
Distribution: Widely distributed. Crosses the placenta and enters breast milk.
Metabolism and Excretion: Mostly metabolized by the liver.
Half-life: 2–3 hr.

CONTRAINDICATIONS AND PRECAUTIONS
Contraindicated in: ▪ Hypersensitivity ▪ Pregnancy or lactation (avoid chronic use) ▪ Some products contain alcohol or bisulfites and should be avoided in patients with known intolerance or hypersensitivity.
Use Cautiously in: ▪ Head trauma ▪ Increased intracranial pressure ▪ Severe renal, hepatic, or pulmonary disease ▪ Hypothyroidism ▪ Adrenal insufficiency ▪ Alcoholism ▪ Elderly or debilitated patients (dosage reduction recommended) ▪ Undiagnosed abdominal pain ▪ Prostatic hypertrophy.

{} = Available in Canada only.

ADVERSE REACTIONS AND SIDE EFFECTS*

CNS: <u>sedation</u>, <u>confusion</u>, headache, euphoria, floating feeling, unusual dreams, hallucinations, dysphoria, dizziness.
EENT: miosis, diplopia, blurred vision.
Resp: respiratory depression.
CV: orthostatic hypotension.
GI: nausea, vomiting, <u>constipation</u>, dry mouth.
GU: urinary retention.
Derm: sweating, flushing.
Misc: tolerance, physical dependence, psychological dependence.

INTERACTIONS

Drug–Drug: ▪ Use with caution in patients receiving **MAO inhibitors** (may result in unpredictable reactions—decrease initial dose of oxycodone to 25% of usual dose) ▪ Additive CNS depression with **alcohol, antihistamines,** and **sedative/hypnotics** ▪ Administration of **partial-antagonist opioid analgesics** may precipitate withdrawal in physically dependent patients ▪ **Nalbuphine** or **pentazocine** may decrease analgesia.

ROUTE AND DOSAGE

Larger doses may be required during chronic therapy.
▪ **PO (Adults):** 5 mg q 3–6 hr as needed or 10 mg 3–4 times daily as needed.

AVAILABILITY

Oxycodone
▪ *Tablets:* 5 mg ▪ *Concentrated oral solution:* 20 mg/ml ▪ {*Suppositories:* 10 mg, 20 mg}.

Oxycodone/Acetaminophen
▪ *Tablets:* 5 mg oxycodone with 325 mg acetaminophen ▪ *Capsules:* 5 mg oxycodone with 500 mg acetaminophen ▪ *Oral solution:* 5 mg oxycodone with 325 mg acetaminophen/5 ml.

Oxycodone/Aspirin
▪ *Tablets:* 2.44 mg oxycodone with 325 mg aspirin, 4.88 mg oxycodone with 325 mg aspirin.

TIME/ACTION PROFILE (analgesic effects)

	ONSET	PEAK	DURATION
PO	10–15 min	60–90 min	3–6 hr

NURSING IMPLICATIONS

ASSESSMENT
◻ Assess type, location, and intensity of pain prior to and 60 min following administration.
◻ Assess blood pressure, pulse, and respiratory rate before and periodically during administration.
◻ Prolonged use may lead to physical and psychological dependence and tolerance. This should not prevent patient from receiving adequate analgesia. Most patients who receive oxycodone for medical reasons do not develop psychological dependence. Progressively higher doses may be required to relieve pain with long-term therapy.
◻ Assess bowel function routinely. Increased intake of fluids and bulk, stool softeners, and laxatives may minimize constipating effects.
▪ **Lab Test Considerations:** May increase plasma amylase and lipase levels.
▪ **Toxicity and Overdose:** If overdose occurs, naloxone (Narcan) is the antidote.

POTENTIAL NURSING DIAGNOSES
▪ Pain (indications).
▪ Sensory-perceptual alteration: visual, auditory (side effects).
▪ Injury, high risk for (side effects).

IMPLEMENTATION
▪ **General Info:** Explain therapeutic value of medication prior to administration to enhance the analgesic effect.
◻ Regularly administered doses may be more effective than prn administration. Analgesic is more effective if given before pain becomes severe.
◻ Coadministration with nonopioid analgesics may have additive anal-

---

*<u>Underlines</u> indicate most frequent; **CAPITALS** indicate life-threatening.

gesic effects and may permit lower doses.

□ Medication should be discontinued gradually after long-term use to prevent withdrawal symptoms.

▪ **PO:** May be administered with food or milk to minimize GI irritation.

PATIENT/FAMILY TEACHING

□ Instruct patient on how and when to ask for pain medication.

□ Medication may cause drowsiness or dizziness. Advise patient to call for assistance when ambulating or smoking. Caution patient to avoid driving and other activities requiring alertness until response to medication is known.

□ Advise patient to make position changes slowly to minimize orthostatic hypotension.

□ Advise patient to avoid concurrent use of alcohol or other CNS depressants with this medication.

□ Encourage patient to turn, cough, and breathe deeply every 2 hr to prevent atelectasis.

EVALUATION

Effectiveness of therapy can be demonstrated by: ▪ Decrease in severity of pain without a significant alteration in level of consciousness or respiratory status.

OXYMORPHONE
(ox-i-**mor**-fone)
Numorphan

CLASSIFICATION(S):
Opioid analgesic (agonist)
Schedule II
Pregnancy Category UK

INDICATIONS

▪ Used in the management of moderate to severe pain ▪ As a supplement in balanced anesthesia.

ACTION

▪ Binds to opiate receptors in the CNS

▪ Alters the perception of and response to painful stimuli, while producing generalized CNS depression. **Therapeutic Effect:** ▪ Decrease in pain.

PHARMACOKINETICS

Absorption: Well absorbed following IM, SC, or rectal administration.

Distribution: Widely distributed. Crosses the placenta and enters breast milk.

Metabolism and Excretion: Mostly metabolized by the liver.

Half-life: 2.6–4 hr.

CONTRAINDICATIONS AND PRECAUTIONS

Contraindicated in: ▪ Hypersensitivity ▪ Pregnancy or lactation (avoid chronic use) ▪ Children <12 yr.

Use Cautiously in: ▪ Head trauma ▪ Increased intracranial pressure ▪ Severe renal, hepatic, or pulmonary disease ▪ Hypothyroidism ▪ Adrenal insufficiency ▪ Alcoholism ▪ Elderly or debilitated patients (dosage reduction recommended) ▪ Undiagnosed abdominal pain ▪ Prostatic hypertrophy.

ADVERSE REACTIONS AND SIDE EFFECTS*

CNS: <u>sedation</u>, <u>confusion</u>, headache, euphoria, floating feeling, unusual dreams, hallucinations, dysphoria, dizziness.

EENT: miosis, diplopia, blurred vision.

Resp: respiratory depression.

CV: orthostatic hypotension.

GI: nausea, vomiting, <u>constipation</u>, dry mouth.

GU: urinary retention.

Derm: sweating, flushing.

Misc: tolerance, physical dependence, psychological dependence.

INTERACTIONS

Drug–Drug: ▪ Use with caution in patients receiving **MAO inhibitors** (may result in unpredictable reactions—decrease initial dose of oxymorphone to 25% of usual dose) ▪ Additive CNS depression with **alcohol, antihista-**

---

*<u>Underlines</u> indicate most frequent; **CAPITALS** indicate life-threatening.

mines, and sedative/hypnotics ▪ Administration of partial-antagonist opioid analgesics may precipitate withdrawal in physically dependent patients ▪ Nalbuphine or pentazocine may decrease analgesia.

ROUTE AND DOSAGE

Larger doses may be required during chronic therapy.

Analgesia—Moderate to Severe Pain

- **SC, IM (Adults):** 1–1.5 mg q 3–6 hr as needed.
- **IV (Adults):** 0.5 mg q 3–6 hr as needed, increase as needed.
- **Rect (Adults):** 5 mg q 4–6 hr as needed.

Analgesia During Labor

- **IM (Adults):** 0.5–1 mg.

AVAILABILITY

▪ *Injection:* 1 mg/ml, 1.5 mg/ml ▪ *Suppositories:* 5 mg.

TIME/ACTION PROFILE (analgesic effects)

	ONSET	PEAK	DURATION
IM	10–15 min	30–90 min	3–6 hr
IV	5–10 min	15–30 min	3–4 hr
SC	10–20 min	UK	3–6 hr
Rect	15–30 min	120 min	3–6 hr

NURSING IMPLICATIONS

ASSESSMENT

- ☐ Assess type, location, and intensity of pain prior to and 60 min following administration.
- ☐ Assess blood pressure, pulse, and respiratory rate before and periodically during administration.
- ☐ Prolonged use may lead to physical and psychological dependence and tolerance. This should not prevent patient from receiving adequate analgesia. Most patients who receive oxymorphone for medical reasons do not develop psychological dependence. Progressively higher doses may be required to relieve pain with long-term therapy.
- ☐ Assess bowel function routinely. Increased intake of fluids and bulk, stool softeners, and laxatives may minimize constipating effects.
- ▪ **Lab Test Considerations:** May increase plasma amylase and lipase levels.
- ▪ **Toxicity and Overdose:** If overdose occurs, naloxone (Narcan) is the antidote.

POTENTIAL NURSING DIAGNOSES

- ▪ Pain (indications).
- ▪ Sensory-perceptual alteration: visual, auditory (side effects).
- ▪ Injury, high risk for (side effects).

IMPLEMENTATION

- ▪ **General Info:** Explain therapeutic value of medication prior to administration to enhance the analgesic effect.
- ☐ Regularly administered doses may be more effective than prn administration. Analgesic is more effective if given before pain becomes severe.
- ☐ Coadministration with nonopioid analgesics may have additive analgesic effects and may permit lower doses.
- ☐ Medication should be discontinued gradually after long-term use to prevent withdrawal symptoms.
- ▪ **Rect:** Suppositories should be stored in the refrigerator.
- ▪ **Direct IV:** Administer undiluted over 2–3 min.
- ▪ **Y-Site Compatibility:** ▪ glycopyrrolate hydroxyzine ▪ ranitidine.

PATIENT/FAMILY TEACHING

- ☐ Instruct patient on how and when to ask for pain medication.
- ☐ Medication may cause drowsiness or dizziness. Advise patient to call for assistance when ambulating or smoking. Caution patient to avoid driving and other activities requiring alertness until response to medication is known.
- ☐ Advise patient to make position changes slowly to minimize orthostatic hypotension.
- ☐ Advise patient to avoid concurrent use of alcohol or other CNS depressants with this medication.

□ Encourage patient to turn, cough, and breathe deeply every 2 hr to prevent atelectasis.

EVALUATION
Effectiveness of therapy can be demonstrated by: ▪ Decrease in severity of pain without a significant alteration in level of consciousness or respiratory status.

OXYTOCIN
(ox-i-**toe**-sin)
Pitocin, Syntocinon

CLASSIFICATION(S):
Hormone (oxytocic)
Pregnancy Category UK

INDICATIONS

▪ Induction of labor at term ▪ Facilitation of uterine contractions at term ▪ Facilitation of threatened abortion ▪ Postpartum control of bleeding after expulsion of the placenta ▪ Nasal preparation used to promote milk letdown in lactating women. **Unlabeled Use:** ▪ Evaluation of fetal competence (fetal stress test).

ACTION

▪ Stimulates uterine smooth muscle, producing uterine contractions similar to those in spontaneous labor ▪ Stimulates mammary gland smooth muscle, facilitating lactation ▪ Has vasopressor and antidiuretic effects. **Therapeutic Effects:** ▪ Induction of labor (IV) ▪ Milk letdown (intranasal).

PHARMACOKINETICS

Absorption: Well absorbed from the nasal mucosa.
Distribution: Widely distributed in extracellular fluid. Small amounts reach fetal circulation.
Metabolism and Excretion: Rapidly metabolized by liver and kidneys.
Half-life: 3–9 min.

CONTRAINDICATIONS AND PRECAUTIONS

Contraindicated in: ▪ Hypersensitivity ▪ Hypersensitivity to chlorobutanol (IV only) ▪ Anticipated nonvaginal delivery ▪ Pregnancy (intranasal).
Use Cautiously in: ▪ First and second stages of labor.

ADVERSE REACTIONS AND SIDE EFFECTS*

Maternal adverse reactions are noted for IV use only.
CNS: *Maternal*—SEIZURES, COMA; *fetal*—INTRACRANIAL HEMORRHAGE.
Resp: *Fetal*—hypoxia, ASPHYXIA.
CV: *Maternal*—hypotension, *fetal*—arrhythmias.
F and E: *Maternal*—water intoxication, hyponatremia, hypochloremia.
Misc: *Maternal*—abruptio placenta, hypersensitivity, painful contractions, decreased uterine blood flow, increased uterine motility.

INTERACTIONS

Drug–Drug: ▪ Severe hypertension may occur if oxytocin follows administration of **vasopressors** ▪ Concurrent use with **cyclopropane anesthesia** may result in excessive hypotension.

ROUTE AND DOSAGE

Induction/Stimulation of Labor
▪ **IV (Adults):** 0.5–2 milliunits/min, increase by 1–2 milliunits q 15–60 min until pattern established (maximum 20 milliunits/min), then decrease dose.

Postpartum Hemorrhage
▪ **IV (Adults):** 10 units infused at 20–40 milliunits/min.
▪ **IM (Adults):** 10 units after delivery of placenta.

Incomplete/Inevitable Abortion
▪ **IV (Adults):** 10 units at a rate of 20–40 milliunits/min.

Promotion of Milk Letdown
▪ **Intranasal (Adults):** 1 spray in one or both nostrils 2–3 min before breast feeding or pumping breasts.

---

*Underlines indicate most frequent; **CAPITALS** indicate life-threatening.

Fetal Stress Test
- **IV (Adults):** 0.5 milliunits/min, may be increased q 20 min until 3 moderate contractions occur in one 10-min period, to a maximum of 20 milliunits with maternal/fetal monitoring.

AVAILABILITY
- *Injection:* 10 units/ml ▪ *Nasal spray:* 40 units/ml.

TIME/ACTION PROFILE (IV = uterine contractions, intranasal = milk letdown)

	ONSET	PEAK	DURATION
IV	immediate	UK	1 hr
IM	3–5 min	UK	30–60 min
Intranasal	few min	UK	20 min

NURSING IMPLICATIONS

ASSESSMENT
- Fetal maturity, presentation, and pelvic adequacy should be assessed prior to administration of oxytocin for induction of labor.
- Assess character, frequency, and duration of uterine contractions; resting uterine tone; and fetal heart rate frequently throughout administration. If contractions occur <2 min apart and are >50–65 mmHg on monitor, if they last 60–90 sec or longer, or if a significant change in fetal heart rate develops, stop infusion and turn patient on her left side to prevent fetal anoxia. Notify physician immediately.
- Monitor maternal blood pressure and pulse frequently and fetal heart rate continuously throughout administration.
- This drug occasionally causes water intoxication. Monitor patient for signs and symptoms (drowsiness, listlessness, confusion, headache, anuria) and notify physician if they occur.
- Monitor maternal electrolytes. Water retention may result in hypochloremia or hyponatremia.

POTENTIAL NURSING DIAGNOSES
- Knowledge deficit related to medication regimen (patient/family teaching).

IMPLEMENTATION
- **Continuous Infusion:** Rotate infusion container to ensure thorough mixing. Store solution in refrigerator, but do not freeze.
- Infuse via infusion pump for accurate dosage. Oxytocin should be connected via Y-site injection or 3-way stopcock to an IV of 0.9% NaCl for use during adverse reactions.
- Magnesium sulfate should be available if needed for relaxation of the myometrium.
- **Induction of Labor:** Dilute 1 ml (10 units) in 1 liter of compatible infusion fluid for a concentration of 10 milliunits/ml.
- *Rate:* Begin infusion at 1–2 milliunits/min (0.1–0.2 ml), increase in increments of 1–2 milliunits/min at 15–30 min intervals until contractions simulate normal labor.
- **Postpartum Bleeding:** For control of postpartum bleeding, dilute 1–4 ml (10–40 units) in 1 liter of compatible infusion fluid (10–40 milliunits/ml).
- *Rate:* Begin infusion at a rate of 10–40 milliunits/min to control uterine atony. Adjust rate as indicated.
- **Incomplete or Inevitable Abortion:** For incomplete or inevitable abortion, dilute 1 ml (10 units) in 500 ml of compatible infusion fluid, for a concentration of 20 milliunits/ml.
- *Rate:* Infuse at a rate of 10–40 milliunits/min.
- **Y-Site Compatibility:** ▪ heparin ▪ hydrocortisone sodium succinate ▪ insulin ▪ meperidine ▪ morphine ▪ potassium chloride ▪ vitamin B complex with C.
- **Solution Compatibility:** ▪ dextrose/Ringer's or lactated Ringer's combinations ▪ dextrose/saline combinations ▪ Ringer's or lactated Ringer's injection ▪ D5W ▪ D10W ▪ 0.45% NaCl ▪ 0.9% NaCl.
- **Intranasal:** Hold squeeze bottle upright while patient is in sitting position. Patient should clear nasal passages prior to administration.

PATIENT/FAMILY TEACHING
- **General Info:** Advise patient to expect contractions similar to menstrual cramps after administration has started.
- **Nasal Spray:** Advise patient to administer nasal spray 2–3 min prior to planned breast feeding. Patient should notify physician if milk drips from non-nursed breast or if uterine cramps occur.

EVALUATION
Effectiveness of therapy can be demonstrated by: ▪ Onset of effective contractions ▪ Increase in uterine tone ▪ Effective letdown reflex.

PACLITAXEL
(pa-kli-**tax**-el)
Taxol

CLASSIFICATION(S):
Antineoplastic (antimicrotubule agent)
Pregnancy Category D

INDICATIONS
- Used in the management of ovarian cancer that has been unresponsive to first-line or other therapy.

ACTION
- Paclitaxel interferes with the normal cellular microtubule function that is required for interphase and mitosis. **Therapeutic Effect:** ▪ Death of rapidly replicating cells, particularly malignant ones.

PHARMACOKINETICS
Absorption: IV administration results in complete bioavailability.
Distribution: Distribution of paclitaxel is not known.
Metabolism and Excretion: Although not extensively studied, paclitaxel appears to be highly metabolized by the liver.
Half-life: 5.3–17.4 hr.

CONTRAINDICATIONS AND PRECAUTIONS
Contraindicated in: ▪ Patients with hypersensitivity to paclitaxel or to castor oil (vehicle contains polyoxethylated castor oil) ▪ Known alcohol intolerance ▪ Pregnancy or lactation ▪ Patients with WBCs ≤1500/mm^3.
Use Cautiously in: ▪ Patients with severe hepatic impairment, childbearing potential, active infections, decreased bone marrow reserve, or chronic debilitating illnesses ▪ Children (safety not established).

ADVERSE REACTIONS AND SIDE EFFECTS*
CNS: <u>bradycardia</u>, <u>hypotension</u>, <u>abnormal ECG</u>.
GI: <u>nausea</u>, <u>vomiting</u>, <u>diarrhea</u>, <u>stomatitis</u>, <u>abnormal liver function tests</u>.
Derm: <u>alopecia</u>.
Hemat: <u>anemia</u>, <u>leukopenia</u>, <u>thrombocytopenia</u>.
MS: <u>myalgia</u>, <u>arthralgia</u>.
Neuro: <u>peripheral neuropathy</u>.
Misc: <u>hypersensitivity reactions</u> including ANAPHYLAXIS.

INTERACTIONS
Drug–Drug: ▪ Ketoconazole may inhibit the metabolism of paclitaxel and increase the risk of serious toxicity; concurrent use should be undertaken with caution ▪ Increased risk of myelosuppression with **cisplatin**.

ROUTE AND DOSAGE
Other regimens have been used.
- **IV (Adults):** 135 mg/m^2 over 24 hr every 3 wk. (Canadian labeling recommends a dose of 170 mg/m^2.)

AVAILABILITY
- *Injection:* 30 mg/5-ml vials.

TIME/ACTION PROFILE (effect on WBC counts)

ONSET	PEAK	DURATION
UK	11 days	3 wk

---

*<u>Underlines</u> indicate most frequent; CAPITALS indicate life-threatening.

NURSING IMPLICATIONS

ASSESSMENT

▫ Monitor vital signs frequently especially during first hour of 24-hr infusion.

▫ Monitor for hypersensitivity reactions. These occur frequently (19%) during administration of paclitaxel. Most common manifestations are dyspnea, hypotension, and chest pain. If these occur, stop infusion and notify physician. Treatment may include bronchodilators, epinephrine, antihistamines, and glucocorticoids. Keep these agents and resuscitative equipment close by in the event of an anaphylactic reaction. Other manifestations of hypersensitivity reactions include flushing and rash. Pretreatment is recommended for *all* patients and should include a glucocorticoid (dexamethasone), diphenhydramine, and an H_2 antagonist (cimetidine or ranitidine).

▫ Monitor cardiovascular status. Hypotension and bradycardia are common but usually do not require treatment. Continuous ECG monitoring is recommended only for patients with serious underlying conduction abnormalities.

▫ Assess for fever, chills, sore throat, and signs of infection throughout therapy. Notify physician if these occur.

▫ Monitor platelet count during therapy. Assess for bleeding (bleeding gums; bruising; petechiae; guaiac stools, urine, and emesis). Avoid IM injections and rectal temperatures. Apply pressure to venipuncture sites for 10 min.

▫ Anemia may occur. Monitor for increased fatigue, dyspnea, and orthostatic hypotension.

▫ Assess for development of peripheral neuropathy. If severe symptoms occur, subsequent dosage should be reduced by 20%.

▫ Monitor intake and output, appetite, and nutritional intake. Paclitaxel causes nausea and vomiting in 60% of patients. Confer with physician regarding prophylactic use of an antiemetic. Adjust diet as tolerated to help maintain fluid and electrolyte balance and nutritional status.

▪ **Lab Test Considerations:** Monitor CBC and differential prior to and periodically throughout therapy. The nadir of leukopenia occurs in 11 days. Notify physician if the leukocyte count is less than 1500/mm³. Notify physician if the platelet count is less than 75,000/mm³.

▫ Monitor liver function studies (AST [SGOT], ALT [SGPT], LDH, bilirubin) prior to and periodically throughout therapy to detect hepatotoxicity.

POTENTIAL NURSING DIAGNOSES

▪ Infection, high risk for (adverse reactions).

▪ Injury, high risk for (adverse reactions).

▪ Knowledge deficit related to medication regimen (patient/family teaching).

IMPLEMENTATION

▪ **Continuous Infusion:** Paclitaxel must be diluted prior to injection. Dilute contents of 5-ml (30-mg) vials to a concentration of 0.3–1.2 mg/ml with the following diluents: 0.9% NaCl, D5W, D5/0.9% NaCl, or dextrose in Ringer's solution. Although haziness in the solution is normal, inspect for particulate matter or discoloration before use. Use an in-line filter of not greater than 0.22 micron pore size. Solutions are stable for 27 hr at room temperature and lighting. Do not use PVC containers or administration sets.

▪ **Rate:** Dose is administered as a 24-hour infusion.

PATIENT/FAMILY TEACHING

▫ Advise patient to notify physician if fever, chills, sore throat, signs of infection, bleeding gums, bruising, petechiae, or blood in urine, stool, or emesis occurs. Caution patient to avoid crowds and persons with known infections. Instruct patient to use soft toothbrush and electric razor.

▫ Patient should be cautioned not to

drink alcoholic beverages or take products containing aspirin or ibuprofen.

▫ Instruct patient to notify physician if abdominal pain, yellow skin, weakness, paresthesia, gait disturbances, or joint or muscle aches occur.

▫ Instruct patient to inspect oral mucosa for redness and ulceration. If mouth sores occur, advise patient to use sponge brush and rinse mouth with water after eating and drinking.

▫ Discuss with patient the possibility of hair loss. Explore coping strategies.

▫ Advise patient to use a nonhormonal method of contraception.

▫ Instruct patient not to receive any vaccinations without advise of physician.

▫ Emphasize the need for periodic lab tests to monitor for side effects.

EVALUATION

Effectiveness of therapy is determined by: ▪ Decrease in size or spread of malignancy.

PAMIDRONATE
(pa-**mid**-roe-nate)
Aredia

CLASSIFICATION(S):
Electrolyte modifier (hypocalcemic), Bone-resorption inhibitor, Hypocalcemic (biphosphonate)
Pregnancy Category C

INDICATIONS

▪ Used in the management of moderate to severe hypercalcemia associated with malignancy.

ACTION

▪ Inhibits resorption of bone. **Therapeutic Effect:** ▪ Decreased serum calcium.

PHARMACOKINETICS

Absorption: IV administration results in complete bioavailability.

Distribution: Rapidly absorbed by bone. Reaches high concentrations in bone, liver, spleen, teeth, and tracheal cartilage. Approximately 50% of a dose is retained by bone and then slowly released.

Metabolism and Excretion: 50% is excreted unchanged in the urine.

Half-life: Elimination half-life from plasma is biphasic—first phase 1.6 hr, second phase 27.2 hr. Elimination half-life from bone is 300 days.

CONTRAINDICATIONS AND PRECAUTIONS

Contraindicated in: ▪ Patients who have hypersensitivity to pamidronate, to other biphosphonates, or to mannitol.

Use Cautiously in: ▪ Patients with underlying cardiovascular disease, especially congestive heart failure (initiate saline hydration cautiously) ▪ Pregnancy, lactation, or children (safety not established) ▪ Renal impairment (dosage reduction recommended).

ADVERSE REACTIONS AND SIDE EFFECTS*

CNS: fatigue.

EENT: rhinitis.

CV: fluid overload, hypertension, arrhythmias, tachycardia, syncope.

Resp: rales.

GI: anorexia, abdominal pain, constipation, nausea, vomiting.

F and E: hypocalcemia, hypomagnesemia, hypokalemia, hypophosphatemia.

Hemat: anemia.

Metab: hypothyroidism.

MS: bone pain.

Local: phlebitis at injection site.

Misc: fever, generalized pain.

INTERACTIONS

Drug–Drug: ▪ Hypokalemia and hypomagnesemia may increase the risk of **cardiac glycoside** toxicity.

ROUTE AND DOSAGE

▪ **IV (Adults):** 60 mg (range 30–90 mg).

AVAILABILITY

▪ *Injection:* 30 mg/vial.

---

*Underlines indicate most frequent; **CAPITALS** indicate life-threatening.

TIME/ACTION PROFILE (effect on serum calcium)

ONSET	PEAK	DURATION
24 hr	7 days	UK

NURSING IMPLICATIONS

ASSESSMENT

□ Monitor intake/output ratios and blood pressure frequently during therapy. Assess for signs of fluid overload (edema, rales/crackles).

□ Monitor symptoms of hypercalcemia (nausea, vomiting, anorexia, weakness, constipation, thirst, and cardiac arrhythmias).

□ Observe for evidence of hypocalcemia (paresthesia, muscle twitching, laryngospasm, and Chvostek's or Trousseau's sign). Protect symptomatic patients by elevating and padding side rails; keep bed in low position.

□ Monitor IV site for phlebitis (pain, redness, swelling). Symptomatic treatment should be used if this occurs.

□ Assess patient for bone pain. Treatment with nonopioid or opioid analgesics may be necessary.

■ **Lab Test Considerations:** Electrolytes (including calcium, phosphorous, and magnesium), hemoglobin, and creatinine should be monitored closely. CBC and platelet count should be monitored during the first 2 wk of therapy.

IMPLEMENTATION

■ **General Info:** Vigorous saline hydration, maintaining a urine output of 2000 ml/24 hr, should be undertaken concurrently with pamidronate therapy. Initiate saline hydration cautiously in patients with underlying cardiovascular disease, especially congestive heart failure.

□ Patients with severe hypercalcemia should be started at the 90-mg dose.

■ **Continuous Infusion:** Reconstitute by adding 10 ml of Sterile Water for Injection to each vial for a concentration of 30 mg/10 ml. Allow drug to dissolve before withdrawing. Dilute further in 1000 ml of 0.45% NaCl, 0.9% NaCl or D5W. Solution is stable for 24 hours at room temperature.

■ *Rate:* Administer over 24 hr.

■ **Additive Incompatibility:** ■ calcium-containing solutions, such as Ringer's solution.

PATIENT/FAMILY TEACHING

□ Advise patient to report signs of hypercalcemic relapse (bone pain, anorexia, nausea, vomiting, thirst, lethargy) to the physician promptly.

□ Advise patient to notify nurse of pain at the infusion site.

□ Encourage patient to comply with dietary recommendations. Diet should contain adequate amounts of calcium and vitamin D (see Appendix K).

□ Advise patient to notify physician if bone pain is severe or persistent.

□ Emphasize the need for keeping follow-up appointments to monitor progress, even after medication is discontinued, in order to detect relapse.

EVALUATION

Effectiveness of therapy can be determined by: ■ Lowered serum calcium levels.

PANCRELIPASE
(pan-kree-li-pase)
Catozym, Cotazym-S, Cotazym-65 B, Cotazym E.C.S. 8, Cotazym E.C.S. 20, Enzymase-16, Ilozyme, Ku-Zyme HP, Pancrease, Pancrease MT 4, Pancrease MT 10, Pancoate, Pancrease MT 16, Protilase, Ultrase MT 12, Ultrase MT 12, Ultrase MT 20, Ultrase MT 24, Viokase, Zymase

CLASSIFICATION(S):
Pancreatic
Pregnancy Category C

INDICATIONS

■ Treatment of pancreatic insufficiency associated with: □ Chronic pancreatitis □ Pancreatectomy □ Cystic fibrosis □ GI bypass surgery □ Ductal obstruction secondary to tumor.

ACTION

- Contains lipolytic, amylolytic, and proteolytic activity. **Therapeutic Effect:**
- Increased digestion of fats, carbohydrates, and proteins in the GI tract.

PHARMACOKINETICS

Absorption: Absorption not known.
Distribution: Distribution not known.
Metabolism and Excretion: Metabolism and excretion not known.
Half-life: UK.

CONTRAINDICATIONS AND PRECAUTIONS

Contraindicated in: ▪ Hypersensitivity to hog proteins.
Use Cautiously in: ▪ Pregnancy or lactation (safety not established).

ADVERSE REACTIONS AND SIDE EFFECTS*

EENT: nasal stuffiness.
Resp: shortness of breath, wheezing, dyspnea.
GI: <u>diarrhea</u>, <u>nausea</u>, <u>stomach cramps</u>, <u>abdominal pain</u> (high doses only), oral irritation.
GU: hematuria.
Derm: rash, hives.
Metab: hyperuricemia.
Misc: allergic reactions.

INTERACTIONS

Drug–Drug: ▪ **Antacids (calcium carbonate** or **magnesium hydroxide)** may decrease effectiveness of pancrelipase ▪ May decrease the absorption of concurrently administered **iron preparations.**
Drug–Food: ▪ **Alkaline foods** destroy coating on enteric-coated products.

ROUTE AND DOSAGE

- **PO (Adults):** 1–3 capsule(s) before or with meals, dosage may be increased as needed (up to 8 capsules may be needed), or 1–2 delayed-release capsule(s) or 0.7 g powder.
- **PO (Children):** 1–3 capsule(s) before or with meals, dosage may be increased as needed, or 1–2 delayed-release capsule(s) or 0.7 g powder.

AVAILABILITY

▪ **Capsules:** 8000 units lipase/30,000 units protease and amylase ▪ **Delayed-release capsules:** 4000 units lipase/12,000 units protease and amylase; 4000 units lipase/25,000 units protease/20,000 units amylase; 5000 units lipase/20,000 units protease and amylase; {8000 units lipase/30,000 units protease and amylase}; 10,000 units lipase/30,000 units protease and amylase; 12,000 units lipase/24,000 units protease and amylase; 12,000 units lipase/39,000 units protease and amylase; 16,000 units lipase/48,000 units protease and amylase; {20,000 units lipase/55,000 units protease and amylase}; 20,000 units lipase/65,000 units protease and amylase; 24,000 units lipase/78,000 units protease and amylase ▪ **Powder:** 16,800 units lipase/70,000 units protease and amylase.

TIME/ACTION PROFILE (digestant effects)

	ONSET	PEAK	DURATION
PO	rapid	UK	UK

NURSING IMPLICATIONS

ASSESSMENT

- ▢ Assess patient's nutritional status (height, weight, skin-fold thickness, arm muscle circumference, and lab values) prior to and periodically throughout therapy.
- ▢ Monitor stools for high fat content (steatorrhea). Stools will be foul-smelling and frothy.
- ▢ Assess patient for allergy to pork; sensitivity to pancrelipase may exist.
- ▪ **Lab Test Considerations:** May cause elevated serum and urine uric acid concentrations.

POTENTIAL NURSING DIAGNOSES

- ▪ Nutrition, altered: less than body requirements (indications).
- ▪ Knowledge deficit related to medication regimen (patient/family teaching).

*<u>Underlines</u> indicate most frequent; **CAPITALS** indicate life-threatening.

IMPLEMENTATION

- **PO:** Administer immediately before or with meals and snacks.
  - □ Capsules may be opened and sprinkled on foods. Capsules filled with enteric-coated beads should not be chewed (sprinkle on soft foods that can be swallowed without chewing, such as apple sauce or jello).
  - □ Pancrelipase is destroyed by acid. Physician may order concurrent sodium bicarbonate or aluminum-containing antacids with nonenteric-coated preparations to neutralize gastric pH. Enteric-coated beads are designed to withstand the acid pH of the stomach. These medications should not be chewed or mixed with alkaline foods prior to ingestion or coating will be destroyed.

PATIENT/FAMILY TEACHING

- □ Encourage patients to comply with diet recommendations of physician (generally high-calorie, high-protein, low-fat). Dosage should be adjusted for fat content of diet. Usually 300 mg of pancrelipase is necessary to digest every 17 g of dietary fat. If a dose is missed, it should be omitted.
- □ Instruct patient not to chew tablets and to swallow them quickly with plenty of liquid to prevent mouth and throat irritation. Patient should be sitting upright to enhance swallowing. Eating immediately after taking medication helps further assure that the medication is swallowed and does not remain in contact with mouth and esophagus for a prolonged period. Patient should avoid sniffing powdered contents of capsules, as sensitization of nose and throat may occur (nasal stuffiness or respiratory distress).
- □ Instruct patient to notify physician if joint pain, swelling of legs, gastric distress, or rash occurs.

EVALUATION

Effectiveness of therapy can be demonstrated by: ■ Improved nutritional status in patients with pancreatic insufficiency □ Normalization of stools in patients with steatorrhea.

PANCURONIUM
(pan-cure-**oh**-nee-yum)
Pavulon

CLASSIFICATION(S):
Neuromuscular blocking agent (nondepolarizing)
Pregnancy Category C

INDICATIONS

■ Production of skeletal muscle paralysis and facilitation of intubation after induction of anesthesia in surgical procedures ■ Used during mechanical ventilation to increase pulmonary compliance

ACTION

■ Prevents neuromuscular transmission by blocking the effect of acetylcholine at the myoneural junction ■ Has no analgesic or anxiolytic effects. **Therapeutic Effect:** ■ Skeletal muscle paralysis.

PHARMACOKINETICS

Absorption: Administered IV only, resulting in complete bioavailability.
Distribution: Rapidly distributes into extracellular fluid. Small amounts cross the placenta.
Metabolism and Excretion: Excreted mostly unchanged by the kidneys; small amounts are eliminated in bile.
Half-life: 2 hr.

CONTRAINDICATIONS AND PRECAUTIONS

Contraindicated in: ■ Hypersensitivity to pancuronium or benzyl alcohol ■ Avoid use of benzyl alcohol-containing preparations in neonates.
Use Cautiously in: ■ Patients with any history of pulmonary disease or renal or liver impairment ■ Elderly or debilitated patients ■ Electrolyte disturbances ■ Patients receiving cardiac glycosides ■ Pregnancy (has been used during cesarean section).
Extreme Caution in: Myasthenia gravis or myasthenic syndromes.

ADVERSE REACTIONS AND SIDE EFFECTS*

Almost all adverse reactions to pancuronium are extensions of pharmacologic effects.

CV: mild tachycardia.
EENT: excessive salivation (children).
Resp: apnea, wheezing.
Local: burning sensation along vein.
MS: muscle weakness.
Derm: excessive sweating (children), rashes.
Misc: allergic reactions.

INTERACTIONS

Drug–Drug: ▪ Intensity and duration of paralysis may be prolonged by pretreatment with **succinylcholine, general anesthesia, aminoglycoside antibiotics, polymyxin B, colistin, clindamycin, lidocaine, quinidine, procainamide, beta-adrenergic blocking agents, potassium-losing diuretics,** and **magnesium.**

ROUTE AND DOSAGE

▪ **IV (Adults and Children >1 mo):** 40–100 mcg/kg initially, supplemental doses of 10 mcg/kg may be given q 20–60 min to maintain paralysis or 15 mcg/kg to allow mechanical ventilation.

AVAILABILITY

▪ *Injection:* 1 mg/ml, 2 mg/ml.

TIME/ACTION PROFILE (skeletal muscle paralysis)

	ONSET	PEAK	DURATION
IV	30–45 sec	3–4.5 min	35–45 min

NURSING IMPLICATIONS

ASSESSMENT

□ Assess respiratory status continuously throughout pancuronium therapy. Pancuronium should be used only for intubated patients. Assess patient for increased respiratory secretions; suction as necessary.

□ Neuromuscular response to pancuronium should be monitored with a peripheral nerve stimulator intraoperatively. Monitor deep tendon reflexes during prolonged administration. Paralysis is initially selective and usually occurs consecutively in the following muscles: levator muscles of eyelids, muscles of mastication, limb muscles, abdominal muscles, muscles of the glottis, intercostal muscles, and diaphragm. Recovery of muscle function usually occurs in reverse order.

□ Monitor heart rate, ECG, and blood pressure periodically throughout pancuronium therapy. May cause a slight increase in heart rate and blood pressure.

□ Observe patient for residual muscle weakness and respiratory distress during the recovery period.

▪ **Toxicity and Overdose:** If overdose occurs, use peripheral nerve stimulator to determine the degree of neuromuscular blockade. Maintain airway patency and ventilation until recovery of normal respirations occurs.

□ Administration of anticholinesterase agents (edrophonium, neostigmine, pyridostigmine) may be used to antagonize the action of pancuronium. Atropine is usually administered prior to or concurrently with anticholinesterase agents.

POTENTIAL NURSING DIAGNOSES

▪ Breathing pattern, ineffective (indications).
▪ Communication, impaired verbal (side effects).
▪ Fear (patient/family teaching).

IMPLEMENTATION

▪ **General Info:** Pancuronium has no effect on consciousness or the pain threshold. Adequate anesthesia should *always* be used when pancuronium is used as an adjunct to surgical procedures or when painful

*Underlines indicate most frequent; **CAPITALS** indicate life-threatening.

procedures are performed. Benzodiazepines and/or analgesics should be administered concurrently when prolonged pancuronium therapy is used for ventilator patients, as patient is awake and able to feel all sensations.

□ If eyes remain open throughout prolonged administration, protect corneas with artificial tears.

□ To prevent absorption by plastic, pancuronium should not be stored in plastic syringes. May be administered in plastic syringes.

■ **Direct IV:** Incremental doses may be administered every 20–60 min as needed. Dose is titrated to patient response.

■ **Intermittent Infusion:** May be diluted in 0.9% NaCl, D5W, D5/0.9% NaCl, and lactated Ringer's injection. Solution is stable for 48 hr.

■ *Rate:* Titrate rate according to patient response.

■ **Syringe Compatibility:** ■ heparin.

■ **Y-Site Compatibility:** ■ aminophylline ■ cefazolin ■ cefuroxime ■ cimetidine ■ dobutamine ■ dopamine ■ epinephrine ■ esmolol ■ fentanyl ■ gentamicin ■ heparin ■ hydrocortisone sodium succinate ■ isoproterenol ■ lorazepam ■ midazolam ■ morphine ■ nitroglycerin ■ nitroprusside ■ ranitidine ■ trimethoprim/sulfamethoxazole ■ vancomycin.

■ **Y-Site Incompatibility:** ■ diazepam.

PATIENT/FAMILY TEACHING

□ Explain all procedures to patient receiving pancuronium therapy without anesthesia, as consciousness is not affected by pancuronium alone. Provide emotional support.

□ Reassure patient that communication abilities will return as the medication wears off.

EVALUATION

Effectiveness of therapy can be demonstrated by: ■ Adequate suppression of the twitch response when tested with peripheral nerve stimulation and subsequent muscle paralysis.

PAPAVERINE
(pa-**pav**-er-een)
Cerespan, Genabid, Pavabid, Pavabid HP, Pavacels, Pavacot, Pavagen, Pava Par, Pavarine, Pavased, Pavasule, Pavatine, Pavatym, Paverolan

CLASSIFICATION(S):
Vasodilator
Pregnancy Category C

INDICATIONS

■ Although FDA-designated as ineffective for these indications, has been used in the following: □ Management of cerebral and peripheral ischemia, usually associated with arterial spasm □ Treatment of myocardial ischemia complicated by arrhythmias □ Improvement of collateral circulation in acute vascular occlusion □ Management of ureteral, biliary, or GI colic. **Unlabeled Use:** ■ Adjunct treatment (with alpha-adrenergic blockers) in the management of male impotence due to organic causes (intracavernosal injection).

ACTION

■ Claimed to dilate coronary, cerebral, pulmonary, and peripheral arteries by a direct spasmolytic action on vascular smooth muscle. **Therapeutic Effect:** ■ Claimed arterial vasodilation.

PHARMACOKINETICS

Absorption: Variably (50%) absorbed following oral administration, absorption from timed-release formulations may be less. Slowly absorbed following intracavernosal administration.

Distribution: Distribution not known.

Metabolism and Excretion: Mainly metabolized by the liver.

Half-life: 0.5–2 hr (highly variable—may be as long as 24 hr).

CONTRAINDICATIONS AND PRECAUTIONS

Contraindicated in: ■ Hypersensitivity or complete AV block.

Use Cautiously in: ▪ Glaucoma ▪ Depressed cardiac conduction ▪ Priapism ▪ Sickle cell disease ▪ Impaired liver function ▪ Severe coagulation defects ▪ Pregnancy, lactation, or children (safety not established).

ADVERSE REACTIONS AND SIDE EFFECTS*

CNS: depression, dizziness, vertigo, headache, drowsiness, sedation.
CV: arrhythmias (IV only), hypotension, slight hypertension.
Derm: flushing, sweating.
EENT: dry throat, visual changes.
GI: dry mouth, constipation, nausea, diarrhea, abdominal distress, anorexia, hepatitis.
GU: priapism (intracavernosal only).
Local: thrombosis at IV site.
Resp: APNEA (IV only).

INTERACTIONS

Drug–Drug: ▪ May prevent response to **levodopa** in patients with Parkinson's disease ▪ **Alpha-adrenergic agonists (metaraminol, epinephrine,** or **phenylephrine)** or **cigarette smoking** may reverse the vasodilating effects of papaverine.

ROUTE AND DOSAGE

▪ **PO (Adults):** 100–300 mg 3–5 times daily or 150 mg of timed-release formulation q 8–12 hr or 300 mg of timed-release formulation q 12 hr.
▪ **IM, IV (Adults):** 30 mg initially, 30–120 mg may be repeated q 3 hr if necessary.
▪ **Intracavernosal (Adults):** 30 mg with 0.5–1 mg of phentolamine or 60 mg alone (not to exceed 60 mg/dose, not to be repeated more than 3 times/wk).

AVAILABILITY

▪ *Tablets:* 30 mg, 60 mg, 100 mg, 150 mg, 200 mg, 300 mg ▪ *Timed-release tablets:* 200 mg ▪ *Timed-release capsules:* 150 mg ▪ *Injection:* 30 mg/ml, {32.5 mg/ml}.

TIME/ACTION PROFILE (PO, IM, IV = vasodilating effects, intracavernosal = penile erection)

	ONSET	PEAK	DURATION
PO	UK	UK	4–8 hr
PO-ER	UK	UK	8–12 hr
IM	UK	UK	3 hr
IV	UK	UK	3 hr
Intracavernosal	10 min	UK	4 hr

NURSING IMPLICATIONS

ASSESSMENT

▫ Monitor blood pressure and pulse prior to and periodically throughout course of therapy.
▫ Monitor ECG in patients receiving IV papaverine. Withhold dose and notify physician if AV block is present.
▫ Monitor IV site for thrombosis (erythema, pain, edema).
▪ **Lab Test Considerations:** Monitor liver function studies. May cause elevated AST (SGOT), ALT (SGPT), alkaline phosphatase, and bilirubin levels. Notify physician of these symptoms of hepatic sensitivity. Eosinophils may also be elevated.

POTENTIAL NURSING DIAGNOSES

▪ Tissue perfusion, altered (indications).
▪ Knowledge deficit related to medication regimen (patient/family teaching).

IMPLEMENTATION

▪ **PO:** Tablets may be administered with milk, meals, or antacids if nausea occurs.
▫ The timed-release form should not be crushed or chewed.
▪ **Direct IV:** Solution should be clear to light yellow. Do not refrigerate.
▪ *Rate:* Administer dose undiluted over at least 2 min. Rapid administration may cause hypotension, tachycardia, dizziness, and facial flushing.
▪ **Syringe Compatibility:** ▪ phentolamine.
▪ **Solution/Additive   Compatibility:** ▪ 0.9% NaCl ▪ 0.45% NaCl ▪ D5W ▪ D10W ▪ D5/0.9% NaCl ▪ D5/0.45%

---

*Underlines indicate most frequent; **CAPITALS** indicate life-threatening.

NaCl ■ D5/0.25% NaCl ■ Ringer's injection ■ phentolamine.
- **Solution/Additive   Incompatibility:** ■ lactated Ringer's injection ■ aminophylline ■ alkaline solutions ■ bromides ■ iodides.
- **Impotence:** Has been used with phentolamine to treat men with impotence associated with spinal cord injury. This method requires special training. Produces an erection following injection into corpus cavernosum. Risk of priapism exists.

PATIENT/FAMILY TEACHING
☐ Instruct patient to take medication as ordered. If a dose is missed, patient should take dose as soon as remembered, but not if almost time for next dose. Do not double doses. Instruct patient not to discontinue medication without conferring with physician.
☐ Encourage patient not to smoke, as nicotine will cause vasoconstriction.
☐ May cause dizziness or drowsiness. Advise patient to avoid driving or other activities requiring alertness until response to medication is known.
☐ Caution patient to make position changes slowly to minimize orthostatic hypotension.
☐ Instruct patient to notify physician if dizziness, drowsiness, jaundice, or vision changes occur.
☐ Advise patients with a history of glaucoma to have regular eye examinations.

EVALUATION
Effectiveness of therapy can be demonstrated by: ■ Absence of symptoms of cerebral, peripheral, or myocardial ischemia ■ Relief of ureteral, biliary, or GI colic ■ Erection in men with impotence, beginning 10 min after injection into corpus cavernosum and sustained for up to 4 hr.

PAREGORIC
(par-e-**gor**-ik)
Camphorated tincture of opium

CLASSIFICATION(S):
Antidiarrheal
Schedule III
Pregnancy Category UK

INDICATIONS
- Symptomatic treatment of diarrhea.

ACTION
- Morphine contained in paregoric inhibits normal GI peristalsis. **Therapeutic Effect:** ■ Decreased frequency of bowel movements in patients with diarrhea.

PHARMACOKINETICS
Absorption: Variably absorbed from the GI tract.
Distribution: Distribution not known. Small amounts of morphine probably cross the placenta and enter breast milk.
Metabolism and Excretion: Morphine is metabolized by the liver.
Half-life: Morphine—2–3 hr.

CONTRAINDICATIONS AND PRECAUTIONS
Contraindicated in: ■ Hypersensitivity ■ Severe undiagnosed abdominal pain, especially when accompanied by fever ■ Alcohol intolerance.
Use Cautiously in: ■ Asthma ■ Severe prostatic hypertrophy ■ Severe liver disease ■ History of drug dependence (prolonged use may result in physical dependence).

ADVERSE REACTIONS AND SIDE EFFECTS*
CNS: drowsiness, dizziness, lightheadedness (high dose).
CV: hypotension (high dose).
GI: constipation.
GU: urinary retention.

INTERACTIONS
Drug–Drug: ■ Additive CNS depression with other **CNS depressants,** including **alcohol, antihistamines, opioid analgesics,** and **sedative/hypnotics.**

---

*Underlines indicate most frequent; **CAPITALS** indicate life-threatening.

ROUTE AND DOSAGE

Contains 2 mg anhydrous morphine/5 ml.

- **PO (Adults):** 5–10 ml 1–4 times daily.
- **PO (Children):** 0.25–0.5 ml/kg 1–4 times daily.

AVAILABILITY

- *Liquid:* 2 mg morphine/5 ml.

TIME/ACTION PROFILE (antidiarrheal effects)

	ONSET	PEAK	DURATION
PO	1–2 hr	2–4 hr	4–6 hr

NURSING IMPLICATIONS

ASSESSMENT

- □ Assess frequency and consistency of stools and bowel sounds prior to and throughout course of therapy.
- □ Assess fluid and electrolyte balance and skin turgor for dehydration.
- □ Monitor respiratory rate, especially in infants and elderly and severely ill patients, as respiratory depression may occur.
- ■ **Lab Test Considerations:** May cause elevations in serum amylase and lipase levels.

POTENTIAL NURSING DIAGNOSES

- ■ Diarrhea (indications).
- ■ Injury, high risk for (side effects).
- ■ Knowledge deficit related to medication regimen (patient/family teaching).

IMPLEMENTATION

- ■ **General Info:** The effect of 4 ml of paregoric is similar to that of 2.5 mg of diphenoxylate.
- □ Do not confuse with deodorized opium tincture, which is 25 times more potent.
- ■ **PO:** Administer with food or meals if GI irritation occurs. Shake well. Mix with enough water to facilitate passage to stomach. Mixture will be milky in appearance. Do not refrigerate.

PATIENT/FAMILY TEACHING

- □ Instruct patient to take medication exactly as directed. If a dose is missed, it should be taken as soon as remembered unless almost time for next dose. Dosage may need to be gradually reduced after prolonged therapy to prevent withdrawal symptoms (tachycardia, irritability, tremors, difficulty sleeping, diaphoresis, shivering, stomach cramps, nausea, or vomiting). Physical or psychological dependence may occur.
- □ Caution patient to make position changes slowly to minimize orthostatic hypotension.
- □ Paregoric may cause drowsiness in large doses. Advise patient to avoid driving or other activities requiring alertness until response to drug is known.
- □ Caution patient to avoid using alcohol and other CNS depressants concurrently with this medication.
- □ Instruct patient to notify physician if diarrhea persists or if fever occurs.

EVALUATION

Effectiveness of therapy can be demonstrated by: ■ Decrease in diarrhea □ Return to normal bowel habits.

PAROXETINE
(par-**ox**-e-teen)
Paxil

CLASSIFICATION(S):
Antidepressant
Pregnancy Category B

INDICATIONS

- ■ Used in the treatment of depression, often in conjunction with psychotherapy.

ACTION

- ■ Inhibits neuronal reuptake of serotonin in the CNS, thus potentiating the activity of serotinin. Has little effect on norepinephrine or dopamine. **Therapeutic Effect:** ■ Antidepressant action.

PHARMACOKINETICS

Absorption: Well absorbed following oral administration.

Distribution: Widely distributed throughout body fluids and tissues, including the CNS. Enters breast milk.
Metabolism and Excretion: Highly metabolized by the liver. Minimal (2%) renal excretion of unchanged drug.
Half-life: 21 hr.

CONTRAINDICATIONS AND PRECAUTIONS

Contraindicated in: ▪ Hypersensitivity ▪ Concurrent MAO inhibitor therapy (may result in serious, potentially fatal reactions).
Use Cautiously in: ▪ Patients with severe renal or hepatic impairment, elderly or debilitated patients (start with smaller doses; daily dose should not be >40 mg) ▪ Patients with history of mania ▪ Pregnancy, lactation, or children (safety not established) ▪ Patients at risk for suicide.

ADVERSE REACTIONS AND SIDE EFFECTS*

CNS: <u>somnolence</u>, <u>dizziness</u>, <u>insomnia</u>, <u>tremor</u>, <u>nervousness</u>, <u>anxiety</u>, <u>headache</u>, <u>weakness</u>, malaise, agitation, "drugged" feeling, CNS stimulation, confusion, amnesia, impaired concentration, depression, emotional lability, vertigo.
EENT: oropharyngeal disorder, rhinitis, blurred vision.
Resp: respiratory disorders, yawning, pharyngitis, increased cough.
CV: chest pain, palpitations, vasodilation, postural hypotension, hypertension, syncope, tachycardia, edema.
GI: <u>nausea</u>, <u>dry mouth</u>, <u>constipation</u>, diarrhea, <u>ejaculatory disturbance</u>, <u>male genital disorders</u>, urinary frequency, urinary disorders, female genital disorders, decreased appetite, flatulence, vomiting, abdominal pain, dyspepsia, increased appetite, taste disturbances.
GU: decreased libido.
Derm: <u>sweating</u>, rash, pruritus.
Metab: weight gain, weight loss.
MS: back pain, myopathy, myalgia, myasthenia.
Neuro: paresthsia, myoclonus.

Misc: fever, chills.

INTERACTIONS

Drug–Drug: ▪ Serious, potentially fatal reactions (hyperthermia, rigidity, myoclonus, autonomic instability, with fluctuating vital signs and extreme agitation, which may proceed to delirium and coma) may occur with concurrent **MAO inhibitor** therapy. MAO inhibitors should be stopped at least 14 days prior to paroxetine therapy. Paroxetine should be stopped at least 14 days prior to MAO inhibitor therapy ▪ Paroxetine may decrease the metabolism and increase the effects of certain drugs that are metabolized by the liver including other **antidepressants, phenothiazines, group IC antiarrhythmics, procyclidine,** and **quinidine.** Concurrent use should be undertaken with caution ▪ **Cimetidine** increases paroxetine blood levels ▪ **Phenobarbital** and **phenytoin** may decrease the effectiveness of paroxetine ▪ Concurrent use with **alcohol** is not recommended ▪ Paroxetine may decrease the effectiveness of **digoxin** ▪ Concurrent use with **tryptophan** may result in headache, nausea, sweating, and dizziness ▪ May increase the risk of bleeding with **warfarin** without altering prothrombin time.

ROUTE AND DOSAGE

▪ **PO (Adults):** 20 mg as a single dose in the morning, may be increased by 10 mg/day at weekly intervals (range 20–50 mg). Initial dose in elderly or debilitated patients or patients with severe hepatic or renal impairment should be 10 mg/day and should not exceed 40 mg/day.

AVAILABILITY

▪ *Tablets:* 20 mg, 30 mg.

TIME/ACTION PROFILE
(antidepressant action)

	ONSET	PEAK	DURATION
PO	1–4 wk	UK	UK

*<u>Underlines</u> indicate most frequent; **CAPITALS** indicate life-threatening.

NURSING IMPLICATIONS

ASSESSMENT

□ Monitor mood changes. Inform physician if patient demonstrates significant increase in anxiety, nervousness, or insomnia.

□ Assess for suicidal tendencies, especially during early therapy. Restrict amount of drug available to patient.

□ Monitor appetite and nutritional intake. Weigh weekly. Notify physician of continued weight loss. Adjust diet as tolerated to support nutritional status.

■ **Lab Test Considerations:** Monitor CBC and differential periodically during course of therapy. Notify physician if leukopenia or anemia occurs.

POTENTIAL NURSING DIAGNOSES

■ Coping, ineffective individual (indications).

■ Injury, high risk for (side effects).

■ Knowledge deficit related to medication regimen (patient/family teaching).

IMPLEMENTATION

■ **PO:** Administer as a single dose in the morning.

PATIENT/FAMILY TEACHING

□ Instruct patient to take paroxetine exactly as directed. If a dose is missed, omit dose and return to regular dosing schedule. Do not double doses.

□ May cause drowsiness or dizziness. Caution patient to avoid driving and other activities requiring alertness until response to the drug is known.

□ Advise patient to avoid alcohol or other CNS-depressant drugs during therapy and to consult with physician before taking other medications with paroxetine.

□ Inform patient that frequent mouth rinses, good oral hygiene, and sugarless gum or candy may minimize dry mouth. If dry mouth persists for more than 2 wk, consult physician or dentist regarding use of saliva substitute.

□ Instruct female patient to inform physician if pregnancy is planned or suspected or if she is breastfeeding.

□ Advise patient to notify physician if headache, weakness, nausea, anorexia, anxiety, or insomnia persists.

□ Emphasize the importance of follow-up examinations to monitor progress. Encourage patient participation in psychotherapy.

EVALUATION

Effectiveness of therapy can be demonstrated by: ■ Increased sense of well-being □ Renewed interest in surroundings. May require 1–4 wk of therapy to obtain antidepressant effects.

PEMOLINE
(**pem**-oh-leen)
Cylert

CLASSIFICATION(S):
CNS stimulant
Schedule IV
Pregnancy Category B

INDICATIONS

■ Adjunct in the management of attention deficit disorder (ADD) in children >6 yr. **Unlabeled Uses:** ■ Treatment of fatigue or mental depression ■ Schizophrenia ■ As a stimulant in geriatric patients.

ACTION

■ Produces CNS stimulation, which may be mediated by dopamine ■ Causes increased motor activity and mental alertness, decreased fatigue, mild euphoria, and decreased appetite. **Therapeutic Effect:** ■ Increased attention span in children with attention deficit disorder.

PHARMACOKINETICS

Absorption: Absorbed from the GI tract.

Distribution: Distribution not known.

Metabolism and Excretion: Partially (50%) metabolized by the liver. 40% excreted unchanged by the kidneys.

Half-life: 9–14 hr.

CONTRAINDICATIONS AND PRECAUTIONS

Contraindicated in: ■ Hypersensitivity ■ Liver disease.

Use Cautiously in: ▪ Renal impairment ▪ Pregnancy or lactation (safety not established) ▪ Unstable emotional status or psychoses ▪ History of seizure disorders ▪ Tics.

ADVERSE REACTIONS AND SIDE EFFECTS*

CNS: <u>insomnia</u>, SEIZURES, dyskinetic movements, dizziness, headache, depression, irritability, nervousness (large doses).
CV: tachycardia (large doses).
GI: <u>anorexia</u>, hepatitis.
Derm: rash, sweating.
Metab: weight loss.
Misc: fever.

INTERACTIONS

Drug–Drug: ▪ May have additive CNS stimulation with other **CNS stimulants** or **adrenergics,** including **decongestants.**

ROUTE AND DOSAGE

▪ **PO (Children >6 yr):** 37.5 mg initially as single morning dose, may be increased by 18.75 mg at weekly intervals until optimum response is achieved. Range 56.25–75 mg/day; not to exceed 112.5 mg/day.

AVAILABILITY

▪ *Tablets:* 18.75 mg, 37.5 mg, 75 mg
▪ *Chewable tablets:* 37.5 mg.

TIME/ACTION PROFILE
(ADD = effects in attention deficit disorder)

	ONSET	PEAK	DURATION
PO (ADD)	days–wks	2–3 wk	days
PO (CNS stimulation)	UK	4 hr	8 hr

NURSING IMPLICATIONS

ASSESSMENT

▫ Assess attention span, impulse control, and interactions with others in children with attention deficit disorders. Therapy may be interrupted at intervals to determine if symptoms are sufficient to continue therapy.
▫ Monitor growth, both height and weight, in children on long-term therapy. Inform physician if growth inhibition occurs.
▪ **Lab Test Considerations:** Hepatic function should be monitored prior to and periodically throughout course of therapy. May cause elevated LDH, alkaline phosphatase, AST (SGOT), ALT (SGPT) levels.

POTENTIAL NURSING DIAGNOSES

▪ Sleep pattern disturbance (side effects).
▪ Knowledge deficit related to medication regimen (patient/family teaching).

IMPLEMENTATION

▪ **General Info:** Administer daily dose in the morning. Chewable tablets must be chewed well before swallowing.

PATIENT/FAMILY TEACHING

▪ **General Info:** Instruct patient to take medication in morning to avoid sleep disturbances. If a dose is missed, take as soon as remembered; if remembered the next day, omit and continue on dosage schedule. Do not double doses. Pemoline has a high dependence and abuse potential. Tolerance occurs rapidly; do not increase dose. Consult physician before discontinuing. In long-term therapy, dosage should be reduced gradually to prevent withdrawal symptoms. Abrupt cessation of high doses may cause extreme fatigue and mental depression.
▫ Pemoline may cause dizziness. Caution patient to avoid driving or other activities requiring alertness until response to medication is known.
▫ Advise patient to avoid intake of large amounts of caffeine.
▫ Advise patient to notify physician if yellow skin or sclera, pale stools or dark urine, palpitations, sweating, fever, or uncontrolled tremors develop or if nervousness, restlessness, in-

P

*<u>Underlines</u> indicate most frequent; **CAPITALS** indicate life-threatening.

somnia, dizziness, or anorexia becomes severe.

□ Inform patient that physician may order periodic holidays from the drug to assess progress and to decrease dependence.

□ Emphasize the importance of routine follow-up examinations to monitor progress.

■ **Attention Deficit Disorder:** Advise parents to notify school nurse of medication regimen.

EVALUATION

Effectiveness of therapy can be demonstrated by: ■ Calming effect with decreased hyperactivity and prolonged attention span in children with an attention deficit disorder. Significant beneficial effects may not be evident until the third or fourth week of therapy, because clinical improvement is gradual.

PENBUTOLOL
(pen-**byoo**-toe-lole)
Levatol

CLASSIFICATION(S):
Antihypertensive, Beta-adrenergic blocker (nonselective)
Pregnancy Category C

INDICATIONS

■ Alone or with other agents in the treatment of hypertension.

ACTION

■ Blocks stimulation of beta$_1$ (myocardial) and beta$_2$ (pulmonary, vascular, or uterine) receptor sites. Has minor intrinsic sympathomimetic activity (ISA), which may result in less bradycardia. **Therapeutic Effects:** ■ Decreased heart rate ■ Decreased blood pressure.

PHARMACOKINETICS

Absorption: Well absorbed following oral administration.
Distribution: Distribution not known.

Metabolism and Excretion: Mostly metabolized by the liver.
Half-life: 5 hr.

CONTRAINDICATIONS AND PRECAUTIONS

Contraindicated in: ■ Uncompensated congestive heart failure ■ Pulmonary edema ■ Cardiogenic shock ■ Bradycardia ■ Heart block ■ COPD or asthma.
Use Cautiously in: ■ Thyroxicosis or hypoglycemia (may mask symptoms) ■ Liver disease ■ Pregnancy or lactation (may cause apnea, low Apgar scores, bradycardia, and hypoglycemia in the newborn) ■ Children (safety not established) ■ Patients with a history of severe allergic reactions (intensity of reactions may be increased).

ADVERSE REACTIONS AND SIDE EFFECTS*

CNS: fatigue, weakness, depression, memory loss, mental change.
EENT: dry eyes, blurred vision, nasal stuffiness.
Resp: bronchospasm, wheezing.
CV: BRADYCARDIA, CONGESTIVE HEART FAILURE, PULMONARY EDEMA, hypotension, peripheral vasoconstriction.
GI: constipation, diarrhea, nausea, vomiting.
GU: impotence, diminished libido.
Derm: rash, itching.
Endo: hyperglycemia, hypoglycemia.
Misc: Raynaud's phenomenon.

INTERACTIONS

Drug–Drug: ■ **General anesthesia, IV phenytoin,** or **verapamil** may cause additive myocardial depression ■ Concurrent use with **amphetamines, cocaine, ephedrine, norepinephrine, phenylephrine,** or **pseudoephedrine** may result in excess alpha-adrenergic stimulation, hypertension, and bradycardia ■ Additive bradycardia may occur with concurrent use of **cardiac glycosides** ■ Additive hypotension may occur with other **antihypertensive agents,** acute ingestion of **alcohol,** and **nitrates** ■ Concurrent **thyroid** administration may

*Underlines indicate most frequent; CAPITALS indicate life-threatening.

decrease effectiveness ▪ May antagonize **beta-adrenergic bronchodilators** ▪ **Non-steroidal anti-inflammatory agents** may decrease antihypertensive effectiveness ▪ May prolong **insulin**-induced hypoglycemia ▪ May negate the beneficial beta₁ cardiac effects of **dopamine** or **dobutamine** ▪ May produce hypertension within 14 days of **MAO inhibitor** therapy.

ROUTE AND DOSAGE

▪ **PO (Adults):** 20 mg/day (range 10–40 mg).

AVAILABILITY

▪ *Tablets:* 20 mg.

TIME/ACTION PROFILE (full antihypertensive effect)

	ONSET	PEAK	DURATION
PO	UK	2–6 wk	UK

NURSING IMPLICATIONS

ASSESSMENT

□ Monitor blood pressure and pulse frequently during period of adjustment and periodically throughout therapy. Confer with physician prior to giving drug if pulse is <50 bpm.
□ Monitor intake and output ratios and daily weight. Assess patient routinely for evidence of fluid overload (peripheral edema, dyspnea, rales/crackles, fatigue, weight gain, jugular venous distension).

POTENTIAL NURSING DIAGNOSES

▪ Cardiac output, decreased (indications, adverse reactions).
▪ Knowledge deficit related to medication regimen (patient/family teaching).
▪ Noncompliance (patient/family teaching).

IMPLEMENTATION

▪ **PO:** Administered as a single daily dose. Doses >20 mg do not usually increase effectiveness.

PATIENT/FAMILY TEACHING

□ Instruct patient to take medication exactly as directed, even if feeling well.

If a dose is missed, it may be taken as soon as remembered up to 4 hr before next dose. Abrupt withdrawal may result in life-threatening arrhythmias, hypertension, or myocardial ischemia.
□ Teach patient and family how to check pulse and blood pressure. Instruct them to take pulse daily and blood pressure biweekly. Advise patient to withhold dose and contact physician if pulse is <50 bpm or blood pressure changes significantly.
□ Reinforce need to continue additional therapies for hypertension (weight loss, restricted sodium intake, stress reduction, regular exercise, moderation of alcohol consumption, and cessation of smoking). Penbutolol controls but does not cure hypertension.
□ Caution patient that this medication may cause increased sensitivity to cold.
□ Advise patient to consult physician before taking any over-the-counter drugs, especially cold remedies, concurrently with this medication. Patients on antihypertensive therapy should also avoid excessive amounts of coffee, tea, and cola.
□ Diabetics should monitor serum glucose closely, especially if weakness, fatigue, or irritability occur. Penbutolol may mask tachycardia and increased blood pressure as signs of hypoglycemia, but dizziness and sweating may still occur.
□ Instruct patient to inform physician or dentist of this therapy prior to treatment or surgery.
□ Advise patient to carry identification describing medication regimen at all times.
□ Instruct patient to notify physician if slow pulse rate, depression, or skin rash occurs.

EVALUATION

Effectiveness of therapy can be demonstrated by: ▪ Decrease in blood pressure. Maximum antihypertensive effects are usually seen by the end of second week. Full effects of lower doses may not be seen for 4–6 wk.

PENICILLAMINE
(pen-i-sill-a-meen)
Cuprimine, Depen

CLASSIFICATION(S):
Anti-inflammatory agent, Chelating agent, Antiurolithic
Pregnancy Category UK

INDICATIONS

▪ Treatment of progressive rheumatoid arthritis resistant to conventional therapy ▪ Prophylaxis and treatment of copper deposition in Wilson's disease ▪ Management of recurrent cystine calculi. **Unlabeled Use:** ▪ Adjunct in the treatment of heavy metal poisoning.

ACTION

▪ Antirheumatic effect, probably due to enhanced lymphocyte function ▪ Chelates heavy metals, including copper, mercury, lead, and iron, into complexes that are excreted by the kidneys ▪ Forms a soluble complex with cystine that is readily excreted by the kidneys. **Therapeutic Effects:** ▪ Decreased disease progression in rheumatoid arthritis ▪ Decreased copper deposition in Wilson's disease ▪ Decreased cystine renal calculi formation.

PHARMACOKINETICS

Absorption: Well absorbed following oral administration.
Distribution: Crosses the placenta.
Metabolism and Excretion: Some excreted in urine as heavy metal-penicillamine complex, some excreted in urine as cystine-penicillamine complex, some metabolized by the liver.
Half-life: UK.

CONTRAINDICATIONS AND PRECAUTIONS

Contraindicated in: ▪ Hypersensitivity ▪ Cross-sensitivity with penicillin may exist ▪ Patients currently receiving gold salts, antimalarials, antineoplastic agents, oxyphenbutazone, or phenyl-butazone ▪ Concurrent use of iron supplements.
Use Cautiously in: ▪ Elderly patients (increased risk of hematologic toxicity; dosage reduction recommended) ▪ Renal impairment (increased risk of adverse renal reactions in patients with rheumatoid arthritis) ▪ Pregnancy (limit daily dose to <1 g. If cesarean section is planned, decrease daily dose to 250 mg for last 6 wk of pregnancy and until incision is healed) ▪ History of aplastic anemia due to penicillamine ▪ Lactation (safety not established) ▪ Patients requiring surgery (may impair wound healing).

ADVERSE REACTIONS AND SIDE EFFECTS*

EENT: eye pain, blurred vision.
Resp: coughing, wheezing, shortness of breath.
GI: oral ulceration, anorexia, nausea, vomiting, epigastric pain, dyspepsia, diarrhea, decreased taste sensation, hepatic dysfunction, cholestatic jaundice, pancreatitis.
GU: proteinuria.
Derm: pemphigus, rashes, hives, itching, ecchymoses, wrinkling.
Hemat: APLASTIC ANEMIA, leukopenia, thrombocytopenia, eosinophilia, thrombocytosis, anemia.
MS: arthralgia, migratory polyarthritis.
Neuro: myasthenia gravis syndrome.
Misc: allergic reactions, fever, lymphadenopathy, systemic lupus erythematosus-like syndrome, GOODPASTURE'S SYNDROME (glomerulonephritis and intra-alveolar hemorrhage).

INTERACTIONS

Drug–Drug: ▪ Increased risk of adverse hematologic effects with **antineoplastic agents, immunosuppresive agents,** or **gold salts** (avoid concurrent use) ▪ Concurrent administration of **iron supplements** decreases absorption of penicillamine ▪ May decrease serum **digoxin** levels.
Drug–Food: ▪ May increase requirements for **pyridoxine** (vitamin B_6).

---

*Underlines indicate most frequent; **CAPITALS** indicate life-threatening.

ROUTE AND DOSAGE

Antirheumatic
- **PO (Adults):** 125–250 mg/day as a single dose. May be slowly increased up to 1.5 g/day.

Chelating Agent (Wilson's Disease)
- **PO (Adults and Older Children):** 250 mg qid.
- **PO (Children >6 mo):** 250 mg/day as a single dose.

Antiurolithic
- **PO (Adults):** 500 mg qid.
- **PO (Children):** 7.5 mg/kg qid.

AVAILABILITY
- *Capsules:* 125 mg, 250 mg ▪ *Tablets:* 250 mg.

TIME/ACTION PROFILE

	ONSET	PEAK	DURATION
PO (antirheumatic)	1–3 mo	UK	1–3 mo
PO (Wilson's disease)	1–3 mo	UK	UK

NURSING IMPLICATIONS

ASSESSMENT
- **General Info:** Monitor intake and output and daily weight and assess patient for edema throughout therapy. Notify physician if edema or weight gain occurs.
- **Arthritis:** Assess pain and range of motion periodically throughout course of therapy.
- **Cystinuria:** X-ray examinations for renal calculi should be monitored annually for stone formation.
- **Lab Test Considerations:** Monitor CBC with differential, platelet counts, and urinalysis (especially for protein and cells) at least every 2 wk during the first 6 mo of therapy or following dose increases, and monthly thereafter. May cause leukopenia, anemia, and thrombocytopenia.
- Monitor liver function tests every 6 mo during the first 18 mo of therapy.
- *Arthritis:* Monitor 24-hr urinary protein levels every 1–2 wk in patients with moderate proteinuria.
- *Wilson's Disease:* Monitor urinary copper levels prior to and soon after initiation of therapy and every 3 mo during continued therapy.
- *Cystinuria:* Monitor urinary cystine levels. Urinary cystine excretion should be maintained at <100 mg in patients with a history of pain or calculi, or 100–200 mg in patients without a history of calculi.

POTENTIAL NURSING DIAGNOSES
- Pain (indications).
- Knowledge deficit related to medication regimen (patient/family teaching).

IMPLEMENTATION
- **PO:** Administer on an empty stomach, at least 1 hr before or 2 hr after meals. Other medications should be administered at least 1 hr apart from penicillamine to maximize absorption.
- Do not administer concurrently with iron-containing products.
- Penicillamine increases the daily requirements for pyridoxine. Supplemental doses of pyridoxine 25 mg/day (vitamin B6) may be ordered in patients with impaired nutrition.
- **Arthritis:** Dosage adjustments may be required every 2–3 mo during therapy.
- If no improvement is seen after 3–4 mo of therapy with doses of 1–1.5 g daily, medication should be discontinued.
- **Wilson's Disease:** Sulfurated potash (10–40 mg) may be administered with meals to minimize copper absorption.

PATIENT/FAMILY TEACHING
- **General Info:** Instruct patient to take penicillamine exactly as directed. If on once-daily schedule, missed doses should be taken as soon as remembered unless remembered the next day; if on twice-daily schedule, take missed doses as soon as remembered unless almost time for next dose; if on more than twice-daily dosing schedule, take missed doses within 1 hr or omit. Do not double doses.
- Consult physician prior to discontinuation of therapy, as interruption of

therapy may cause sensitivity reactions when therapy is resumed. Therapy should be resumed starting with smaller dose and increasing gradually.

□ Inform patient that penicillamine may alter taste acuity, which may be restored by administration of copper 5–10 mg daily. Cupric sulfate 4% solution 5–10 drops may be mixed in fruit juice and taken bid. This is contraindicated in patients with Wilson's disease.

□ Advise patient to notify physician or dentist of medication regimen prior to surgery or treatment. Dose of penicillamine should be reduced until wound healing is complete.

□ Instruct patient to notify physician of skin rash, unusual bleeding or bruising, sore throat, exertional dyspnea, unexplained coughing or wheezing, fever, chills, or any unusual effects.

□ Emphasize the importance of follow-up examinations to check progress.

■ **Wilson's Disease:** Advise patient to discuss dietary restrictions with physician. A low-copper diet may be required. Chocolate, nuts, shellfish, mushrooms, liver, molasses, broccoli, and cereals enriched with copper should be avoided. If drinking water contains >100 mcg/liter of copper, distilled or demineralized water should be used.

■ **Crystinuria:** Advise patient to maintain a fluid intake of at least 2000–3000 ml/day, with increased fluids at night.

□ Advise patient to discuss dietary restrictions with physician. Low-methionine diet may be required to minimize cystine production but is contraindicated in growing children or pregnancy due to low protein content.

EVALUATION

Effectiveness of therapy can be demonstrated by: ■ Decreased pain and increased range of motion in patients with rheumatoid arthritis ■ Prevention and treatment of symptoms of Wilson's disease ■ Prevention and treatment of renal calculi in patients with excessive urinary cystine levels.

PENICILLIN G BENZATHINE
(pen-i-**sill**-in jee **ben**-za-theen)
Bicillin, Bicillin L-A, {Megacillin}, Permapen

CLASSIFICATION(S):
Anti-infective (penicillin)
Pregnancy Category B

INDICATIONS

■ Treatment of a wide variety of infections, including: □ Pneumococcal pneumonia □ Streptococcal pharyngitis □ Syphilis ■ Prevention of rheumatic fever.

ACTION

■ Binds to bacterial cell wall, resulting in cell death. **Therapeutic Effect:** ■ Bactericidal action against susceptible bacteria. **Spectrum:** ■ Active against most gram-positive organisms, including: □ Streptococci (*Streptococcus pneumoniae,* group A beta-hemolytic streptococci) □ Staphylococci (non-penicillinase-producing strains) □ Some gram-negative organisms, such as *Neisseria meningitis* and *Neisseria gonorrheae* □ Some anaerobic bacteria and spirochetes.

PHARMACOKINETICS

Absorption: IM absorption is delayed and prolonged, resulting in sustained therapeutic blood levels.

Distribution: Widely distributed, although CNS penetration is poor in the presence of uninflamed meninges. Crosses the placenta and enters breast milk.

Metabolism and Excretion: Minimally metabolized by the liver, excreted mainly unchanged by the kidneys.

Half-life: 30–60 min.

CONTRAINDICATIONS AND PRECAUTIONS

Contraindicated in: ▪ Previous hypersensitivity to penicillins ▪ Cross-sensitivity may exist with cephalosporins ▪ Hypersensitivity to benzathine.

Use Cautiously in: ▪ Severe renal insufficiency (dosage reduction recommended) ▪ Pregnancy (although safety not established, has been used safely) ▪ Lactation.

ADVERSE REACTIONS AND SIDE EFFECTS*

CNS: SEIZURES.

GI: <u>nausea</u>, <u>vomiting</u>, <u>diarrhea</u>, <u>epigastric distress</u>.

GU: interstitial nephritis.

Derm: <u>rashes</u>, urticaria.

Hemat: eosinophilia, hemolytic anemia, leukopenia.

Local: <u>pain</u> at IM site.

Misc: superinfection, allergic reactions, including ANAPHYLAXIS and serum sickness.

INTERACTIONS

Drug–Drug: ▪ **Probenecid** decreases renal excretion and increases blood levels of penicillin. Therapy may be combined for this purpose ▪ Effectiveness of penicillin may be decreased by concurrent use of **chloramphenicol** ▪ Half-life of **chloramphenicol** may be increased by concurrent use of penicillin.

ROUTE AND DOSAGE

1 mg = 1600 units.

Streptococcal Infections/Erysipeloid

▪ **IM (Adults):** 1.2 million units single dose.

▪ **IM (Children >27 kg):** 900,000–1.2 million units single dose.

▪ **IM (Children <27 kg):** 300,000–600,000 units single dose.

▪ **Neonates:** 50,000 units/dose.

Syphilis

▪ **IM (Adults):** 2.4 million units single dose (primary, secondary, or latent syphilis of <1 yr duration); repeated q wk for 3 wk (latent, cardiovascular, or late benign). Patients with neurosyphilis should be initially treated with aqueous penicillin G plus probenecid, then 2.4 million units benzathine penicillin G weekly for 3 wk.

▪ **IM (Children <2 yr):** 50,000 units/kg single dose (congenital syphilis).

Prevention of Rheumatic Fever

▪ **IM (Adults and Children):** 1.2 million units q 4 wk.

AVAILABILITY

▪ *Injection:* 300,000 units/ml, 600,000 units/dose, 1.2 million units/dose, 2.4 million units/dose ▪ *In combination with:* procaine penicillin (Bicillin CR). See Appendix A.

TIME/ACTION PROFILE (blood levels)

	ONSET	PEAK	DURATION
IM	delayed	12–24 hr	1–4 wk

NURSING IMPLICATIONS

ASSESSMENT

□ Assess patient for infection (vital signs; appearance of wound, sputum, urine, and stool; WBC) at beginning and throughout course of therapy.

□ Obtain a history before initiating therapy to determine previous use of and reactions to penicillins or cephalosporins. Persons with a negative history of penicillin sensitivity may still have an allergic response.

□ Obtain specimens for culture and sensitivity prior to initiating therapy. First dose may be given before receiving results.

□ Observe patient for signs and symptoms of anaphylaxis (rash, pruritus, laryngeal edema, wheezing). Discontinue drug and notify physician immediately if these occur. Keep epinephrine, an antihistamine, and resuscitation equipment close by in the event of an anaphylactic reaction.

▪ **Lab Test Considerations:** Patients receiving penicillin G may have false-

---

*<u>Underlines</u> indicate most frequent; **CAPITALS** indicate life-threatening.

positive results for urine glucose using the copper sulfate method (Clinitest). Use glucose enzymatic tests (Keto-Diastix, Tes-Tape) to test urine glucose.

□ May cause positive direct Coombs' test results.

POTENTIAL NURSING DIAGNOSES

■ Infection, high risk for (indications, side effects).

■ Knowledge deficit related to medication regimen (patient/family teaching).

■ Noncompliance related to medication regimen (patient/family teaching).

IMPLEMENTATION

■ **IM:** Reconstitute with Sterile Water for Injection, D5W, or 0.9% NaCl.

□ Shake medication well prior to injection. Inject deep into a well-developed muscle mass at a slow, consistent rate to prevent blockage of the needle. Massage well. Accidental injection near or into a nerve can result in severe pain and dysfunction. Do not inject SC, as this may cause pain and induration.

□ Never give penicillin G benzathine suspension IV. May cause embolism or toxic reactions.

PATIENT/FAMILY TEACHING

□ Advise patient to report the signs of superinfection (black, furry overgrowth on the tongue; vaginal itching or discharge; loose or foul-smelling stools) and allergy.

□ Instruct patient to notify the physician if symptoms do not improve.

□ Patients with an allergy to penicillin should be instructed to carry an identification card with this information at all times.

EVALUATION

Clinical response to therapy can be evaluated by: ■ Resolution of the signs and symptoms of infection. Length of time for complete resolution depends on the organism and site of infection ■ Prevention of rheumatic fever.

PENICILLIN G POTASSIUM

(pen-i-**sill**-in jee poe-**tass**-ee-um)
{Crystapen}, {Megacillin}, {Nova-pen-G}, {P-50}, Pfizerpen

CLASSIFICATION(S):
Anti-infective (penicillin)
Pregnancy Category B

INDICATIONS

■ Treatment of a wide variety of infections, including: □ Pneumococcal pneumonia □ Streptococcal pharyngitis □ Syphilis □ Gonorrhea □ Lyme disease ■ Treatment of enterococcal infections (requires the addition of an aminoglycoside) ■ Prevention of rheumatic fever.

■ **Unlabeled Use:** Treatment of Lyme disease.

ACTION

■ Binds to bacterial cell wall, resulting in cell death. **Therapeutic Effect:** ■ Bactericidal action against susceptible bacteria. **Spectrum:** ■ Active against most gram-positive organisms, including: □ Streptococci (*Streptococcus pneumoniae,* group A beta-hemolytic streptococci) □ Staphylococci (non-penicillinase-producing strains) □ Some gram-negative organisms, such as *Neisseria meningitis* and *Neisseria gonorrheae* □ Some anaerobic bacteria and spirochetes (including *Treponema pallidum* and *Borrelia burgdorferi*).

PHARMACOKINETICS

Absorption: Well absorbed following IM administration.

Distribution: Widely distributed, although CNS penetration is poor in the presence of uninflamed meninges. Crosses the placenta and enters breast milk.

Metabolism and Excretion: Minimally metabolized by the liver, excreted mainly unchanged by the kidneys.

Half-life: 30–60 min.

{} = Available in Canada only.

CONTRAINDICATIONS AND PRECAUTIONS

Contraindicated in: ▪ Previous hypersensitivity to penicillins ▪ Cross-sensitivity with cephalosporins may exist ▪ Some products may contain tartrazine (Pentids)—avoid use in patients with tartrazine (FDC yellow dye #5) hypersensitivity.

Use Cautiously in: ▪ Severe renal insufficiency (dosage reduction recommended) ▪ Pregnancy (although safety not established, has been used safely) ▪ Lactation.

ADVERSE REACTIONS AND SIDE EFFECTS*

CNS: SEIZURES.
GI: nausea, vomiting, diarrhea, epigastric distress.
GU: interstitial nephritis.
Derm: rashes, urticaria.
Hemat: eosinophilia, hemolytic anemia, leukopenia.
Local: phlebitis at IV site, pain at IM site.
Misc: superinfection, allergic reactions, including ANAPHYLAXIS and serum sickness.

INTERACTIONS

Drug–Drug: ▪ **Probenecid** decreases renal excretion and increases blood levels of penicillin. Therapy may be combined for this purpose ▪ **Cholestyramine** and **colestipol** may decrease the absorption of penicillin G ▪ Effectiveness of penicillin may be decreased by concurrent use of **chloramphenicol** ▪ Half-life of **chloramphenicol** may be increased by concurrent use of penicillin.

ROUTE AND DOSAGE

1 mg = 1600 units. Contains 1.7 mEq potassium and 0.3 mEq sodium/million units.
▪ **IM, IV (Adults):** 1 million–5 million units q 4–6 hr (up to 30 million units/day).
▪ **IM, IV (Children):** 25,000–250,000 units/kg/day in divided doses q 4 hr.

▪ **IM, IV (Infants >7 days and >2000 g):** 30,000–100,000 units/kg/day in divided doses q 6–12 hr (up to 200,000 units/kg/day for meningitis).
▪ **IM, IV (Infants >7 days and <2000 g):** 75,000 units/kg/day in divided doses q 8 hr (up to 150,000 units/kg/day for meningitis).
▪ **IM, IV (Infants <7 days and >2000 g):** 50,000 units/kg/day in divided doses q 8 hr (up to 150,000 units/kg/day for meningitis).
▪ **IM, IV, (Infants <7 days and <2000 g):** 50,000 units/kg/day in divided doses q 12 hr (up to 100,000 units/kg/day for meningitis).

AVAILABILITY

▪ *Injection:* 1 million units, 2 million units, 3 million units, 5 million units, 10 million units, 20 million units.

TIME/ACTION PROFILE (blood levels)

	ONSET	PEAK
IM	rapid	0.25–0.5 hr
IV	rapid	rapid

NURSING IMPLICATIONS

ASSESSMENT

▫ Assess patient for infection (vital signs; appearance of wound, sputum, urine, and stool; WBC) at beginning and throughout course of therapy.
▫ Obtain a history before initiating therapy to determine previous use of and reactions to penicillins or cephalosporins. Persons with a negative history of penicillin sensitivity may still have an allergic response.
▫ Obtain specimens for culture and sensitivity prior to initiating therapy. First dose may be given before receiving results.
▫ Observe patient for signs and symptoms of anaphylaxis (rash, pruritus, laryngeal edema, wheezing). Discontinue drug and notify physician immediately if these occur. Keep epinephrine, an antihistamine, and resuscitation equipment close by in the event of an anaphylactic reaction.

*Underlines indicate most frequent; **CAPITALS** indicate life-threatening.

896 PENICILLIN G POTASSIUM

- **Lab Test Considerations:** Patients receiving penicillin G may have false-positive results for urine glucose using the copper sulfate method (Clinitest). Use glucose enzymatic tests (Keto-Diastix, Tes-Tape) to test urine glucose.
- □ May cause positive direct Coombs' test results.
- □ Hyperkalemia may develop following large doses of penicillin G potassium.

POTENTIAL NURSING DIAGNOSES

- Infection, high risk for (indications, side effects).
- Knowledge deficit related to medication regimen (patient/family teaching).
- Noncompliance related to medication regimen (patient/family teaching).

IMPLEMENTATION

- **IM, IV:** Reconstitute with Sterile Water for Injection, D5W, or 0.9% NaCl.
- **IM:** Shake medication well prior to injection. Inject deep into a well-developed muscle mass at a slow, consistent rate to prevent blockage of the needle. Massage well. Accidental injection near or into a nerve can result in severe pain and dysfunction. Do not inject SC, as this may cause pain and induration.
- □ Penicillin G potassium may be diluted with lidocaine 1% or 2% (without epinephrine) to minimize pain from IM injection.
- **IV:** Change sites every 48 hr to prevent phlebitis.
- □ Administer IV form of penicillin slowly and observe patient closely for signs of hypersensitivity.
- **Intermittent Infusion:** Doses of 3 million units or less should be diluted in at least 50 ml; doses of more than 3 million units should be diluted with 100 ml of D5W, D10W, 0.45% NaCl, 0.9% NaCl, Ringer's or lactated Ringer's solution, dextrose/saline combinations, or dextrose/Ringer's or lactated Ringer's combinations.
- **Rate:** Infuse over 1–2 hr in adults, 15–30 min in children.

- **Continuous Infusion:** May be diluted and infused over 24 hr.
- **Syringe Compatibility:** ■ heparin.
- **Syringe Incompatibility:** ■ metoclopramide.
- **Y-Site Compatibility:** ■ acyclovir ■ cyclophosphamide ■ enalaprilat ■ esmolol ■ fluconazole ■ foscarnet ■ hydromorphone ■ labetalol ■ magnesium sulfate ■ meperidine ■ morphine ■ perphenazine ■ potassium chloride ■ verapamil ■ vitamin B complex with C.
- **Y-Site Incompatibility:** If aminoglycosides and penicillins must be administered concurrently, administer in separate sites.
- **Additive Compatibility:** ■ ascorbic acid ■ calcium chloride ■ calcium gluconate ■ cephapirin ■ chloramphenicol ■ cimetidine ■ clindamycin ■ colistimethate ■ corticotropin ■ erythromycin ■ hydrocortisone sodium succinate ■ kanamycin ■ magnesium sulfate ■ methicillin ■ methylprednisolone sodium succinate ■ polymyxin B ■ prednisolone sodium phosphate ■ potassium chloride ■ verapamil.
- **Additive Incompatibility:** ■ amphotericin B ■ Incompatible with aminoglycosides; do not admix.

PATIENT/FAMILY TEACHING

- □ Instruct patient to take medication around the clock and to finish the drug completely as directed, even if feeling better. Advise patient that sharing of this medication may be dangerous.
- □ Advise patient to report the signs of superinfection (black, furry overgrowth on the tongue; vaginal itching or discharge; loose or foul-smelling stools) and allergy.
- □ Instruct the patient to notify physician if symptoms do not improve.
- □ Patients with an allergy to penicillin should be instructed to carry an identification card with this information at all times.

EVALUATION

Clinical response to therapy can be evaluated by: ■ Resolution of the signs and symptoms of infection. Length of time for complete resolution depends on the organism and site of infection.

PENICILLIN G PROCAINE
(pen-i-sill-in jee **proe**-cane)
{Ayercillin}, Crysticillin A.S.,
Pfizerpen-AS, Wycillin

CLASSIFICATION(S):
Anti-infective (penicillin)
Pregnancy Category B

INDICATIONS

- Treatment of a wide variety of infections, including: □ Pneumococcal pneumonia □ Streptococcal pharyngitis □ Syphilis □ Gonorrhea ■ Treatment of enterococcal infections (requires the addition of an aminoglycoside).

ACTION

- Binds to bacterial cell wall, resulting in cell death. **Therapeutic Effect:**
- Bactericidal action against susceptible bacteria. **Spectrum:** ■ Active against most gram-positive organisms, including: □ Streptococci (*Streptococcus pneumoniae,* group A beta-hemolytic streptococci) □ Staphylococci (non-penicillinase-producing strains) □ Some gram-negative organisms, such as *Neisseria meningitis* and *Neisseria gonorrheae* □ Some anaerobic bacteria and spirochetes.

PHARMACOKINETICS

Absorption: IM absorption is delayed and prolonged, resulting in sustained therapeutic blood levels.
Distribution: Widely distributed, although CNS penetration is poor in the presence of uninflamed meninges. Crosses the placenta and enters breast milk.
Metabolism and Excretion: Minimally metabolized by the liver, excreted mainly unchanged by the kidneys.
Half-life: 30–60 min.

CONTRAINDICATIONS AND PRECAUTIONS

Contraindicated in: ■ Previous hypersensitivity to penicillins ■ Cross-sensitivity with cephalosporins may exist ■ Hypersensitivity to procaine.
Use Cautiously in: ■ Severe renal insufficiency (dosage reduction recommended) ■ Pregnancy (although safety not established, has been used safely) ■ Lactation.

ADVERSE REACTIONS AND SIDE EFFECTS*

CNS: SEIZURES.
GI: nausea, vomiting, diarrhea, epigastric distress.
GU: interstitial nephritis.
Derm: rashes, urticaria.
Hemat: eosinophilia, hemolytic anemia, leukopenia.
Local: pain at IM site.
Misc: superinfection, allergic reactions, including ANAPHYLAXIS and serum sickness.

INTERACTIONS

Drug–Drug: ■ Probenecid decreases renal excretion and increases blood levels of penicillin. Therapy may be combined for this purpose ■ Effectiveness of penicillin may be decreased by concurrent use of **chloramphenicol** ■ Half-life of **chloramphenicol** may be increased by concurrent use of penicillin.

ROUTE AND DOSAGE
1 mg = 1600 units.

Moderate to Severe Infections
- **IM (Adults and Children):** 600,000–1.2 million units/day, single dose or 2 divided doses.
- **IM (Neonates):** 50,000 units/kg/day, single dose.

Uncomplicated Gonorrhea
- **IM (Adults):** 4.8 million units divided into 2 injection sites, preceded by 1 g probenecid PO.

AVAILABILITY
- *Injection:* 300,000 units/ml, 500,000

units/ml, 600,000 units/ml, 1,200,000 units/2 ml, 2,400,000 units/4 ml ■ *In combination with:* benzathine penicillin (Bicillin CR). See Appendix A.

TIME/ACTION PROFILE (blood levels)

	ONSET	PEAK	DURATION
IM	delayed	1–4 hr	1–2 days

NURSING IMPLICATIONS

ASSESSMENT
□ Assess patient for infection (vital signs; appearance of wound, sputum, urine, and stool; WBC) at beginning and throughout course of therapy.
□ Obtain a history before initiating therapy to determine previous use of and reactions to penicillins or cephalosporins. Persons with a negative history of penicillin sensitivity may still have an allergic response.
□ Obtain specimens for culture and sensitivity prior to initiating therapy. First dose may be given before receiving results.
□ Observe patient for signs and symptoms of anaphylaxis (rash, pruritus, laryngeal edema, wheezing). Discontinue drug and notify physician immediately if these occur. Keep epinephrine, an antihistamine, and resuscitation equipment close by in the event of an anaphylactic reaction.
■ **Lab Test Considerations:** Patients receiving penicillin G may have false-positive results for urine glucose using the copper sulfate method (Clinitest). Use glucose enzymatic tests (Keto-Diastix, Tes-Tape) to test urine glucose.
□ May cause positive direct Coombs' test results.

POTENTIAL NURSING DIAGNOSES
■ Infection, high risk for (indications, side effects).
■ Knowledge deficit related to medication regimen (patient/family teaching).

IMPLEMENTATION
■ **IM:** Reconstitute with Sterile Water for Injection, D5W, or 0.9% NaCl.

□ Shake medication well prior to injection. Inject deep into a well-developed muscle mass at a slow, consistent rate to prevent blockage of the needle. Massage well. Accidental injection near or into a nerve can result in severe pain and dysfunction.
□ Patient may experience a transient toxic reaction to procaine (anxiety, confusion, agitation, combativeness, depression, seizures, hallucinations, expressed fear of impending death).
□ Never give penicillin G procaine suspension IV. May cause embolism or toxic reactions.

PATIENT/FAMILY TEACHING
□ Advise patient to report the signs of superinfection (black, furry overgrowth on the tongue; vaginal itching or discharge; loose or foul-smelling stools) and allergy.
□ Instruct patient to notify physician if symptoms do not improve.
□ Patients with an allergy to penicillin should be instructed to carry an identification card with this information at all times.

EVALUATION
Clinical response to therapy can be evaluated by: ■ Resolution of the signs and symptoms of infection. Length of time for complete resolution depends on the organism and site of infection.

PENICILLIN G SODIUM
(pen-i-**sill**-in jee **soe**-dee-um)
{Crystapen}

CLASSIFICATION(S):
Anti-infective (penicillin)
Pregnancy Category B

INDICATIONS
■ Treatment of a wide variety of infections, including: □ Pneumococcal pneumonia □ Streptococcal pharyngitis □ Syphilis □ Gonorrhea ■ Treatment of enterococcal infections (requires the addition of an aminoglycoside) ■ Prevention of rheumatic fever.

{} = Available in Canada only.

ACTION

- Binds to bacterial cell wall, resulting in cell death. **Therapeutic Effect:**
- Bactericidal action against susceptible bacteria. **Spectrum:** ■ Active against most gram-positive organisms, including: □ Streptococci (*Streptococcus pneumoniae*, group A beta-hemolytic streptococci) □ Staphylococci (non-penicillinase-producing strains) □ Some gram-negative organisms, such as *Neisseria meningitis* and *Neisseria gonorrheae* □ Some anaerobic bacteria and spirochetes.

PHARMACOKINETICS

Absorption: Well absorbed following IM administration.

Distribution: Widely distributed, although CNS penetration is poor in the presence of uninflamed meninges. Crosses the placenta and enters breast milk.

Metabolism and Excretion: Minimally metabolized by the liver, excreted mainly unchanged by the kidneys.

Half-life: 30–60 min.

CONTRAINDICATIONS AND PRECAUTIONS

Contraindicated in: ■ Previous hypersensitivity to penicillins ■ Cross-sensitivity with cephalosporins may exist.

Use Cautiously in: ■ Severe renal insufficiency (dosage reduction recommended) ■ Pregnancy (although safety not established, has been used safely) ■ Lactation.

ADVERSE REACTIONS AND SIDE EFFECTS*

CNS: SEIZURES.

GI: nausea, vomiting, diarrhea, epigastric distress.

GU: interstitial nephritis.

Derm: rashes, urticaria.

Hemat: eosinophilia, hemolytic anemia, leukopenia.

Local: phlebitis at IV site, pain at IM site.

Misc: superinfection, allergic reactions, including ANAPHYLAXIS and serum sickness.

INTERACTIONS

Drug–Drug: ■ May decrease the effectiveness of **oral contraceptive agents** ■ **Probenecid** decreases renal excretion and increases blood levels of penicillin. Therapy may be combined for this purpose ■ **Cholestyramine** and **colestipol** may decrease the absorption of penicillin G ■ Effectiveness of penicillin may be decreased by concurrent **chloramphenicol** ■ Half-life of **chloramphenicol** may be increased by concurrent penicillin.

ROUTE AND DOSAGE

1 mg = 1600 units. Contains 2 mEq sodium/million units.

- **IM, IV (Adults):** 1 million–5 million units q 4–6 hr (up to 30 million units/day).
- **IM, IV (Children):** 100,000–250,000 units/kg/day in divided doses q 4 hr.
- **IM, IV (Infants >7 days and >2000 g):** 100,000 units/kg/day in divided doses q 6 hr (up to 200,000 units/kg/day for meningitis).
- **IM, IV (Infants >7 days and <2000 g):** 75,000 units/kg/day in divided doses q 8 hr (up to 150,000 units/kg/day for meningitis).
- **IM, IV (Infants <7 days and >2000 g):** 50,000 units/kg/day in divided doses q 8 hr (up to 150,000 units/kg/day for meningitis).
- **IM, IV (Infants <7 days and <2000 g):** 50,000 units/kg/day in divided doses q 12 hr (up to 100,000 units/kg/day for meningitis).

AVAILABILITY

- *Injection:* 5 million units/vial.

TIME/ACTION PROFILE (blood levels)

	ONSET	PEAK
IM	rapid	0.25–0.5 hr
IV	rapid	rapid

*Underlines indicate most frequent; **CAPITALS** indicate life-threatening.

NURSING IMPLICATIONS

ASSESSMENT

- Assess patient for infection (vital signs; appearance of wound, sputum, urine, and stool; WBC) at beginning and throughout course of therapy.
- Obtain a history before initiating therapy to determine previous use of and reactions to penicillins or cephalosporins. Persons with a negative history of penicillin sensitivity may still have an allergic response.
- Obtain specimens for culture and sensitivity prior to initiating therapy. First dose may be given before receiving results.
- Observe patient for signs and symptoms of anaphylaxis (rash, pruritus, laryngeal edema, wheezing). Discontinue drug and notify physician immediately if these occur. Keep epinephrine, an antihistamine, and resuscitation equipment close by in the event of an anaphylactic reaction.
- **Lab Test Considerations:** Patients receiving penicillin G may have false-positive results for urine glucose using the copper sulfate method (Clinitest). Use glucose enzymatic tests (Keto-Diastix, Tes-Tape) to test urine glucose.
- May cause positive direct Coombs' test results.
- Monitor sodium concentrations in patients with hypertension or congestive heart failure. Hypernatremia may develop following large doses of penicillin G sodium.

POTENTIAL NURSING DIAGNOSES

- Infection, high risk for (indications, side effects).
- Knowledge deficit related to medication regimen (patient/family teaching).

Implementation

- **IM, IV:** Reconstitute with Sterile Water for Injection, D5W, or 0.9% NaCl.
- **IM:** Shake medication well prior to injection. Inject penicillin deep into a well-developed muscle mass at a slow, consistent rate to prevent blockage of the needle. Massage well. Accidental injection near or into a nerve can result in severe pain and dysfunction. Do not inject SC, as this may cause pain and induration.
- Penicillin G sodium may be diluted with lidocaine 1% or 2% (without epinephrine) to minimize pain from IM injection.
- **IV:** Change sites every 48 hr to prevent phlebitis.
- Administer slowly and observe patient closely for signs of hypersensitivity.
- **Intermittent Infusion:** Doses of 3 million units or less should be diluted with at least 50 ml; doses of >3 million units should be diluted with 100 ml of D5W or 0.9% NaCl.
- **Rate:** Infuse over 1–2 hr in adults, 15–30 min in children.
- **Continuous Infusion:** May be diluted and infused over 24 hr.
- **Syringe Compatibility:** ▪ chloramphenicol ▪ cimetidine ▪ colistimethate ▪ heparin ▪ lincomycin ▪ polymyxin B.
- **Additive Compatibility:** ▪ calcium chloride ▪ calcium gluconate ▪ chloramphenicol ▪ clindamycin ▪ colistimethate ▪ erythromycin lactobionate ▪ hydrocortisone sodium succinate ▪ methicillin ▪ polymyxin B ▪ prednisolone sodium phosphate.
- **Additive Incompatibility:** ▪ amphotericin B ▪ bleomycin ▪ cephalothin ▪ cytarabine ▪ methylprednisolone sodium succinate ▪ vitamin B complex with C. Incompatible with aminoglycosides; do not admix.

PATIENT/FAMILY TEACHING

- Advise patient to report the signs of superinfection (black, furry overgrowth on the tongue; vaginal itching or discharge; loose or foul-smelling stools) and allergy.
- Instruct patient to notify physician if symptoms do not improve.
- Patients with an allergy to penicillin should be instructed to carry an identification card with this information at all times.

EVALUATION
Clinical response to therapy can be evaluated by: ▪ Resolution of the signs and symptoms of infection. Length of time for complete resolution depends on the organism and site of infection.

PENICILLIN V
(pen-i-**sill**-in vee)
{Apo-Pen-VK}, Beepen-VK, Beta-pen-VK, Ledercillin VK, {Nado-pen-V}, {Novopen-VK}, Pen-Veek, {PVF K}, Robicillin-VK, {VC-K}, V-Cillin K, Veetids

CLASSIFICATION(S):
Anti-infective (penicillin)
Pregnancy Category B

INDICATIONS

▪ Treatment of a wide variety of infections, including: □ Pneumococcal pneumonia □ Erisipelas □ Skin and soft tissue infections □ Streptococcal pharyngitis ▪ Prevention of rheumatic fever.

ACTION

▪ Binds to bacterial cell wall, resulting in cell death. **Therapeutic Effect:** ▪ Bactericidal action against susceptible bacteria. **Spectrum:** ▪ Active against most gram-positive organisms, including: □ Streptococci (*Streptococcus pneumoniae*, group A beta-hemolytic streptococci) □ Staphylococci (non-penicillinase-producing strains) □ Some gram-negative organisms, such as *Neisseria meningitis* and *Neisseria gonorrheae* □ Some anaerobic bacteria and spirochetes.

PHARMACOKINETICS

Absorption: Penicillin V resists acid degradation in the GI tract and is absorbed better than penicillin G.
Distribution: Widely distributed, although CNS penetration is poor in the presence of uninflamed meninges. Crosses the placenta and enters breast milk.

Metabolism and Excretion: Minimally metabolized by the liver, excreted mainly unchanged by the kidneys.
Half-life: 30–60 min.

CONTRAINDICATIONS AND PRECAUTIONS

Contraindicated in: ▪ Previous hypersensitivity to penicillins ▪ Cross-sensitivity with cephalosporins may exist ▪ Hypersensitivity to procaine or benzathine (procaine and benzathine preparations only) ▪ Some products may contain tartrazine (Veetids 125 liquid)— avoid use in patients with tartrazine (FDC yellow dye #5) hypersensitivity.
Use Cautiously in: ▪ Severe renal insufficiency (dosage reduction recommended) ▪ Pregnancy (although safety not established, has been used safely) ▪ Lactation.

ADVERSE REACTIONS AND SIDE EFFECTS*

CNS: SEIZURES.
GI: <u>nausea</u>, <u>vomiting</u>, <u>diarrhea</u>, <u>epigastric distress</u>.
GU: interstitial nephritis.
Derm: <u>rashes</u>, urticaria.
Hemat: eosinophilia, hemolytic anemia, leukopenia.
Misc: superinfection, allergic reactions, including ANAPHYLAXIS and serum sickness.

INTERACTIONS

Drug–Drug: ▪ May decrease the effectiveness of **oral contraceptive agents** ▪ **Probenecid** decreases renal excretion and increases blood levels of penicillin. Therapy may be combined for this purpose ▪ **Neomycin** may decrease the absorption of penicillin V ▪ Effectiveness of penicillin may be decreased by concurrent use of **chloramphenicol** ▪ Half-life of **chloramphenicol** may be increased by concurrent use of penicillin.

ROUTE AND DOSAGE
1 mg = 1600 units.

{} = Available in Canada only.
*<u>Underlines</u> indicate most frequent; **CAPITALS** indicate life-threatening.

Infections Due to Susceptible Organisms
- **PO (Adults):** 125–500 mg q 6 hr.
- **PO (Children):** 25–50 mg/kg/day in divided doses q 6–8 hr.

Rheumatic Fever Prophylaxis
- **PO (Adults):** 125–250 mg q 12 hr.

AVAILABILITY
- *Tablets:* 125 mg, 250 mg, 500 mg
- *Oral solution:* 125 mg/5 ml, 250 mg/5 ml.

TIME/ACTION PROFILE (blood levels)

	ONSET	PEAK
PO	rapid	0.5–1 hr

NURSING IMPLICATIONS

ASSESSMENT
- □ Assess patient for infection (vital signs; appearance of wound, sputum, urine, and stool; WBC) at beginning and throughout course of therapy.
- □ Obtain a history before initiating therapy to determine previous use of and reactions to penicillins or cephalosporins. Persons with a negative history of penicillin sensitivity may still have an allergic response.
- □ Obtain specimens for culture and sensitivity prior to initiating therapy. First dose may be given before receiving results.
- □ Observe patient for signs and symptoms of anaphylaxis (rash, pruritus, laryngeal edema, wheezing). Discontinue drug and notify physician immediately if these occur. Keep epinephrine, an antihistamine, and resuscitation equipment close by in the event of an anaphylactic reaction.
- ▪ **Lab Test Considerations:** May cause positive direct Coombs' test results.

POTENTIAL NURSING DIAGNOSES
- ▪ Infection, high risk for (indications, side effects).
- ▪ Knowledge deficit related to medication regimen (patient/family teaching).

- ▪ Noncompliance related to medication regimen (patient/family teaching).

IMPLEMENTATION
- ▪ **PO:** Administer around the clock. Penicillin V may be administered without regard for meals.
- □ Use calibrated measuring device for liquid preparations. Solution is stable for 14 days if refrigerated.

PATIENT/FAMILY TEACHING
- □ Instruct patient to take medication around the clock and to finish the drug completely as directed, even if feeling better. Advise patient that sharing of this medication may be dangerous.
- □ Advise patient to report the signs of superinfection (black, furry overgrowth on the tongue; vaginal itching or discharge; loose or foul-smelling stools) and allergy.
- □ Instruct patient to notify physician if symptoms do not improve.
- □ Advise patients taking oral contraceptives to use additional nonhormonal methods of contraception during therapy with penicillin V and until next menstrual period.
- □ Patients with an allergy to penicillin should be instructed to carry an identification card with this information at all times.

EVALUATION
Clinical response to therapy can be evaluated by: ▪ Resolution of the signs and symptoms of infection. Length of time for complete resolution depends on the organism and site of infection. ▪ Prevention of rheumatic fever.

PENTAMIDINE
(pen-**tam**-i-deen)
Nebupent, Pentam, {Pentacarinat}, {Pneumopent}

CLASSIFICATION(S):
Anti-infective (antiprotozoal)
Pregnancy Category C

INDICATIONS

▪ **IV:** Treatment of *Pneumocystis carinii* pneumonia (PCP) ▪ **Inhalation:** Prevention of *Pneumocystis carinii* pneumonia (PCP) in AIDS or HIV-positive patients who have had PCP or who have a peripheral CD4 lymphocyte (T_4 helper/inducer) count of $\leq 200/mm^3$. **Unlabeled Use:** ▪ **Inhalation:** Treatment of *Pneumocystis carinii* pneumonia.

ACTION

▪ Appears to disrupt DNA or RNA synthesis in protozoa ▪ Also has a direct toxic effect on pancreatic islet cells. **Therapeutic Effect:** ▪ Death of susceptible protozoa.

PHARMACOKINETICS

Absorption: Minimal systemic absorption occurs following inhalation.

Distribution: Widely and extensively distributed. Does not appear to enter the CSF. Concentrates in liver, kidneys, lungs, and spleen, with prolonged storage in some tissues.

Metabolism and Excretion: 1–30% excreted unchanged by the kidneys. Remainder of metabolic fate unknown.

Half-life: 6.4–9.4 hr (increased in renal impairment).

CONTRAINDICATIONS AND PRECAUTIONS

Contraindicated in: ▪ History of previous anaphylactic reaction to pentamidine.

Use Cautiously in: ▪ Hypotension ▪ Hypertension ▪ Hypoglycemia ▪ Hyperglycemia ▪ Hypocalcemia ▪ Leukopenia ▪ Thrombocytopenia ▪ Anemia ▪ Renal impairment (dosage reduction required) ▪ Diabetes mellitus ▪ Liver impairment ▪ Pregnancy or lactation (safety not established) ▪ Cardiovascular disease ▪ Bone marrow depression, previous antineoplastic therapy, or radiation therapy.

ADVERSE REACTIONS AND SIDE EFFECTS*

For parenteral form, unless indicated.

CNS: dizziness, confusion, hallucinations, anxiety, headache.

EENT: burning in throat (inhalation only).

Resp: bronchospasm, cough (inhalation only).

CV: HYPOTENSION, ARRHYTHMIAS.

GI: nausea, vomiting, abdominal pain, unpleasant metallic taste, anorexia, PANCREATITIS, hepatitis.

GU: nephrotoxicity.

Derm: rash, pallor.

Endo: HYPOGLYCEMIA, hyperglycemia.

F and E: hypocalcemia, hyperkalemia.

Hemat: leukopenia, thrombocytopenia, anemia.

Local: phlebitis, pruritus, urticaria at IV site.

Misc: fever, chills, STEVENS-JOHNSON SYNDROME, allergic reactions, including ANAPHYLAXIS.

INTERACTIONS

Listed for parenteral administration.

Drug–Drug: ▪ Additive nephrotoxicity with other **nephrotoxic agents,** including **aminoglycosides, amphotericin B,** and **vancomycin** ▪ Additive bone marrow depression with **antineoplastic agents** or previous **radiation therapy.**

ROUTE AND DOSAGE

Pneumocystis Carinii Pneumonia—Treatment

▪ **IV (Adults and Children):** 4 mg/kg once daily for 14–21 days (longer treatment may be required in AIDS patients).

Pneumocystis Carinii Pneumonia—Prevention

▪ **Inhalation (Adults):** 300 mg q 4 wk, administered using a Respirgard II Nebulizer.

AVAILABILITY

▪ *Injection:* 300 mg/vial ▪ *Solution for aerosol use:* 300 mg/vial.

TIME/ACTION PROFILE (blood levels)

	ONSET	PEAK
IV	UK	end of infusion
Inhaln	UK	UK

*Underlines indicate most frequent; **CAPITALS** indicate life-threatening.

NURSING IMPLICATIONS

ASSESSMENT

☐ Assess patient for infection (vital signs, sputum, WBC) and monitor respiratory status (rate, character, lung sounds, dyspnea, sputum) at beginning and throughout therapy.

☐ Obtain specimens for culture and sensitivity prior to initiating therapy. First dose may be given before receiving results.

☐ Monitor blood pressure frequently during and following IM or IV administration of pentamidine. Patient should be lying down during administration. Sudden, severe hypotension may occur following a single dose. Resuscitation equipment should be immediately available.

☐ Assess patient for signs of hypoglycemia (anxiety, chills, diaphoresis, cold pale skin, headache, increased hunger, nausea, nervousness, shakiness) and hyperglycemia (drowsiness, flushed dry skin, fruit-like breath odor, increased thirst, increased urination, loss of appetite), which may occur up to several months after therapy is discontinued.

☐ Pulse and ECG should be monitored prior to and periodically during course of therapy. Fatalities due to cardiac arrhythmias, tachycardia, and cardiotoxicity have been reported.

■ **Lab Test Considerations:** Blood glucose concentrations should be monitored prior to, daily during, and for several months following course of therapy.

☐ Monitor BUN and serum creatinine prior to and daily during therapy to monitor for nephrotoxicity.

☐ Monitor CBC and platelet count prior to and periodically during therapy. Pentamidine may cause leukopenia, anemia, and thrombocytopenia.

☐ May cause elevated serum bilirubin, alkaline phosphatase, AST (SGOT) and ALT (SGPT) concentrations. These liver function tests should be monitored prior to and every 3 days during course of therapy.

☐ Serum calcium concentrations should be monitored prior to and every 3 days during therapy, as pentamidine may cause hypocalcemia.

☐ May cause elevated serum potassium concentrations.

POTENTIAL NURSING DIAGNOSES

■ Infection, high risk for (indications, side effects).

■ Knowledge deficit related to medication regimen (patient/family teaching).

IMPLEMENTATION

■ **General Info:** Pentamidine must be given on a regular schedule for the full course of therapy. If a dose is missed, administer as soon as remembered. If almost time for the next dose, skip the missed dose and return to the regular schedule. Do not double doses.

■ **Intermittent Infusion:** To reconstitute, add 3, 4, or 5 ml of Sterile Water for Injection or D5W to each 300-mg vial for a concentration of 100, 75, or 60 mg/ml, respectively. Withdraw dose and dilute further in 50–250 ml of D5W. Solution is stable for 48 hr at room temperature. Discard unused portions.

■ *Rate:* Administer slowly over at least 60 min.

■ **Y-Site Compatibility:** ■ zidovudine.

■ **Y-Site Incompatibility:** ■ fluconazole ■ foscarnet.

■ **Inhalation:** Dilute 300 mg in 6 ml of Sterile Water for Injection. Place reconstituted solution into Respirgard II nebulizer. Do not dilute with 0.9% NaCl or admix with other medications, as solution will form a precipitate. Solution is stable for 48 hr at room temperature if protected from light. Do not use Respirgard II nebulizer for other medications.

☐ Administer inhalation dose through nebulizer until chamber is empty, approximately 30–45 min.

PATIENT/FAMILY TEACHING

☐ Inform patient of the importance of completing the full course of pentamidine therapy, even if feeling better.

□ Instruct patient to notify physician promptly if fever, sore throat, signs of infection, bleeding of gums, unusual bruising, petechiae, or blood in stool, urine, or emesis occurs. Caution patient to avoid crowds and persons with known infections. Instruct patient to use soft toothbrush and electric razor and to avoid falls. Patient should not be given IM injections or rectal thermometers. Patient should be cautioned not to drink alcoholic beverages or take medication containing aspirin or ibuprofen, as these may precipitate gastric bleeding.

□ Caution patient to make position changes slowly to minimize orthostatic hypotension.

□ Advise patient that an unpleasant metallic taste may occur with pentamidine administration but is not significant.

EVALUATION

Clinical response to therapy can be evaluated by: ▪ Prevention or resolution of the signs and symptoms of *Pneumocystis carinii* pneumonia in HIV-positive patients.

PENTAZOCINE
(pen-**taz**-oh-seen)
Talwin, Talwin NX

CLASSIFICATION(S):
Opioid analgesic (agonist/antagonist)
Schedule IV
Pregnancy Category C

INDICATIONS

▪ Management of moderate to severe pain ▪ Also used as: □ Analgesic during labor □ Sedative prior to surgery □ Supplement in balanced anesthesia.

ACTION

▪ Binds to opiate receptors in the CNS ▪ Alters perception of and response to painful stimuli, while producing generalized CNS depression ▪ Has partial antagonist properties, which may result in opioid withdrawal in physically dependent patients. **Therapeutic Effect:** ▪ Decrease in moderate to severe pain.

PHARMACOKINETICS

Absorption: Well absorbed following oral, IM, and SC administration. Small amount (0.5 mg) of naloxone in tablets included to prevent parenteral abuse.

Distribution: Widely distributed. Crosses the placenta.

Metabolism and Excretion: Mostly metabolized by the liver. Small amounts excreted unchanged by the kidneys.

Half-life: 2–3 hr.

CONTRAINDICATIONS AND PRECAUTIONS

Contraindicated in: ▪ Hypersensitivity ▪ Patients who are physically dependent on opioids (may precipitate withdrawal).

Use Cautiously in: ▪ Head trauma ▪ Increased intracranial pressure ▪ Severe renal, hepatic, or pulmonary disease ▪ Hypothyroidism ▪ Adrenal insufficiency ▪ Alcoholism ▪ Elderly, debilitated patients or patients with severe liver impairment (dosage reduction recommended) ▪ Undiagnosed abdominal pain ▪ Prostatic hypertrophy ▪ Pregnancy (has been used during labor, but may cause respiratory depression in the newborn) ▪ Lactation or children (safety not established).

ADVERSE REACTIONS AND SIDE EFFECTS*

CNS: <u>sedation</u>, confusion, <u>headache</u>, <u>euphoria</u>, floating feeling, unusual dreams, <u>hallucinations</u>, dysphoria, <u>dizziness</u>, vertigo.

EENT: miosis (high doses), blurred vision, diplopia.

Resp: respiratory depression.

CV: hypotension, hypertension, palpitations.

GI: <u>nausea</u>, vomiting, constipation, ileus, dry mouth.

GU: urinary retention.

*<u>Underlines</u> indicate most frequent; **CAPITALS** indicate life-threatening.

Derm: sweating, clammy feeling.
Local: severe tissue damage at SC sites.
Misc: tolerance, physical dependence, psychological dependence.

INTERACTIONS

Drug–Drug: ▪ Use with caution in patients receiving **MAO inhibitors** (may result in unpredictable reactions—decrease initial dose of pentazocine to 25% of usual dose) ▪ Additive CNS depression with **alcohol, antihistamines,** and **sedative/hypnotics** ▪ May precipitate withdrawal in patients who are physically dependent on **opioid analgesic agonists** ▪ May diminish analgesic effects of other **opioid analgesics**.

ROUTE AND DOSAGE

Moderate to Severe Pain
▪ **PO (Adults):** 50–100 mg q 3–4 hr (not to exceed 600 mg/day).
▪ **SC, IV, IM (Adults):** 30 mg q 3–4 hr as needed (not to exceed 30 mg/dose IV or 60 mg/dose IM or SC; not to exceed 360 mg/day SC, IV, or IM).

Obstetric Use
▪ **IM, IV (Adults):** 20 mg IV or 30 mg IM. When contractions become regular, may be repeated 2–3 times at 2–3 hr intervals.

AVAILABILITY

▪ *Tablets:* 50 mg (with 0.5 mg naloxone), {50 mg} ▪ *Injection:* 30 mg/ml ▪ *In combination with:* acetaminophen (Talacen) or aspirin (Talwin compound). See Appendix A.

TIME/ACTION PROFILE (analgesia)

	ONSET	PEAK	DURATION
PO	15–30 min	1–3 hr	3 hr
IM, SC	15–20 min	1 hr	2 hr
IV	2–3 min	15 min	1 hr

NURSING IMPLICATIONS

ASSESSMENT
□ Assess type, location, and intensity of pain prior to and 60 min following IM and oral doses and 15 min following IV administration.

□ Assess blood pressure, pulse, and respirations before and periodically during administration.
□ While this drug has a low potential for dependence, prolonged use may lead to physical and psychological dependence and tolerance. This should not prevent patient from receiving adequate analgesia. Most patients receiving pentazocine for medical reasons do not develop psychological dependence. If tolerance develops, changing to an opioid agonist may be required to relieve pain.
□ Assess prior analgesic history. Antagonistic properties may induce withdrawal symptoms (vomiting, restlessness, abdominal cramps, increased blood pressure and temperature) in opioid-dependent patients.
▪ **Lab Test Considerations:** May cause elevated serum amylase and lipase levels.
▪ **Toxicity and Overdose:** If overdose occurs, naloxone (Narcan) is the antidote.

POTENTIAL NURSING DIAGNOSES
▪ Pain (indications).
▪ Injury, high risk for (side effects).
▪ Sensory-perceptual alteration: visual, auditory (side effects).

IMPLEMENTATION
▪ **General Info:** Explain therapeutic value of medication prior to administration to enhance the analgesic effect.
□ Regularly administered doses may be more effective than prn administration. Analgesic is more effective if administered before pain becomes severe.
□ Coadministration with nonopioid analgesics may have additive effects and may permit lower opioid doses.
▪ **PO:** Talwin NX contains 0.5 mg of naloxone, which has no pharmacologic activity when administered orally. If the product is abused by injection, naloxone antagonizes pentazocine. Parenteral use of oral pentazocine may lead to severe, potentially fatal reactions (pulmonary emboli,

vascular occlusion, ulceration and abscess, and withdrawal symptoms in opioid-dependent individuals).
- **IM, SC:** Administer IM injections deep into well-developed muscle. Rotate sites of injections. SC route may cause tissue damage with repeated injections.
- **Direct IV:** Manufacturer recommends diluting each 5 mg with at least 1 ml of Sterile Water for Injection.
- *Rate:* Administer slowly, each 5 mg over at least 1 minute.
- **Syringe Compatibility:** ▪ atropine ▪ benzquinamide ▪ butorphanol ▪ chlorpromazine ▪ cimetidine ▪ dimenhydrinate ▪ diphenhydramine ▪ droperidol ▪ hydroxyzine ▪ metoclopramide ▪ perphenazine ▪ prochlorperazine edisylate ▪ promazine ▪ promethazine ▪ propiomazine ▪ ranitidine ▪ scopolamine.
- **Syringe Incompatibility:** ▪ glycopyrrolate ▪ heparin ▪ pentobarbital.
- **Y-Site Compatibility:** ▪ heparin ▪ hydrocortisone sodium succinate ▪ potassium chloride ▪ vitamin B complex with C.
- **Y-Site Incompatibility:** ▪ nafcillin.
- **Additive Incompatibility:** ▪ aminophylline ▪ amobarbital ▪ pentobarbital ▪ phenobarbital ▪ secobarbital ▪ sodium bicarbonate.

PATIENT/FAMILY TEACHING
- Instruct patient on how and when to ask for pain medication.
- Medication may cause drowsiness, dizziness, or hallucinations. Advise patient to call for assistance when ambulating and to avoid driving or other activities requiring alertness until response to medication is known.
- Encourage patient to turn, cough, and breathe deeply every 2 hr to prevent atelectasis.
- Caution patient to make position changes slowly to minimize orthostatic hypotension.
- Advise patient to avoid concurrent use of alcohol and other CNS depressants.
- Advise patient that frequent mouth rinses, good oral hygiene, and sugarless gum or candy may decrease dry mouth.

EVALUATION
Effectiveness of therapy can be demonstrated by: ▪ Decrease in severity of pain without a significant alteration in level of consciousness or respiratory status.

PENTOBARBITAL
(pen-toe-**bar**-bi-tal)
Nembutal, {Novopentobarb}

CLASSIFICATION(S):
Sedative/hypnotic (barbiturate),
Anticonvulsant
Schedule II
Pregnancy Category D

INDICATIONS
▪ Hypnotic agent (short-term) ▪ Preoperative sedation and other situations where sedation is required ▪ Treatment of seizures. **Unlabeled Uses:** ▪ IV: Induction of coma in selected patients with cerebral ischemia and management of increased intracranial pressure.

ACTION
▪ Depresses the CNS, probably by potentiating gamma-aminobutyric acid (GABA), an inhibitory neurotransmitter ▪ Produces all levels of CNS depression, including the sensory cortex, motor activity, and altered cerebellar function ▪ Anticonvulsant effect due to decreased synaptic transmission and increased seizure threshold ▪ May decrease cerebral blood flow, cerebral edema, and intracranial pressure (IV only). **Therapeutic Effect:** ▪ Sedation and/or induction of sleep.

PHARMACOKINETICS
Absorption: Well absorbed following oral, rectal, or IM administration.
Distribution: Widely distributed, highest concentrations in brain and liver.

Crosses the placenta, small amounts enter breast milk.

Metabolism and Excretion: Metabolized by the liver. Minimal amounts excreted unchanged by the kidneys.

Half-life: 35–50 hr.

CONTRAINDICATIONS AND PRECAUTIONS

Contraindicated in: ▪ Hypersensitivity ▪ Hypersensitivity or known intolerance to propylene glycol ▪ Comatose patients or those with pre-existing CNS depression (unless used to induce coma) ▪ Uncontrolled severe pain ▪ Pregnancy or lactation.

Use Cautiously in: ▪ Hepatic dysfunction ▪ Severe renal impairment ▪ Patients who may be suicidal or who may have been addicted to drugs previously ▪ Elderly or debilitated patients (dosage reduction recommended) ▪ Hypnotic use should be short-term (chronic use may lead to dependence).

ADVERSE REACTIONS AND SIDE EFFECTS*

CNS: drowsiness, lethargy, vertigo, depression, <u>hangover</u>, excitation, delirium.

Resp: respiratory depression, LARYNGOSPASM (IV only), bronchospasm (IV only).

CV: hypotension (IV only).

GI: nausea, vomiting, diarrhea, constipation.

Derm: rashes, urticaria.

Local: phlebitis at IV site.

MS: myalgia, arthralgia, neuralgia.

Misc: hypersensitivity reactions, including ANGIODEDEMA and serum sickness; psychological dependence, physical dependence.

INTERACTIONS

Drug–Drug: ▪ Additive CNS depression with other **CNS depressants,** including **alcohol, antihistamines,** opioid analgesics, and other **sedative/hypnotics** ▪ May induce hepatic enzymes, which metabolize other drugs, decreasing their effectiveness, including **oral contraceptives, oral anticoagulants, chloramphenicol, cyclosporine, dacarbazine, glucocorticoids, tricyclic antidepressants,** and **quinidine** ▪ May increase the risk of hepatic toxicity of **acetaminophen** ▪ **MAO inhibitors, valproic acid,** or **divalproex** may decrease the metabolism of pentobarbital, increasing sedation.

ROUTE AND DOSAGE

Sedation

▪ **PO (Adults):** 20 mg 3–4 times daily.
▪ **PO (Children):** 2–6 mg/kg/day in divided doses.
▪ **Rect (Adults):** 30 mg 2–4 times daily.
▪ **Rect (Children):** 2 mg/kg (60 mg/m^2) 3 times daily.

Hypnotic

▪ **PO (Adults):** 100 mg at bedtime.
▪ **IM (Adults):** 150–200 mg at bedtime.
▪ **IM (Children):** 2–6 mg/kg (up to 100 mg).
▪ **IV (Adults):** 100 mg initially (up to 500 mg).
▪ **IV (Children):** 50 mg, additional, smaller doses may be given.
▪ **Rect (Adults):** 120–200 mg at bedtime.
▪ **Rect (Children 12–14 yr):** 60–120 mg at bedtime.
▪ **Rect (Children 5–12 yr):** 60 mg at bedtime.
▪ **Rect (Children 1–4 yr):** 30–60 mg at bedtime.
▪ **Rectal (Children 2 mo–1 yr):** 30 mg.

Preoperative Sedation

▪ **IM (Adults):** 150–200 mg.
▪ **IM (Children):** 2–6 mg/kg (up to 100 mg/dose).

Anticonvulsant

▪ **IV (Adults):** 100 mg initially, smaller additional doses q minute up to 500 mg total.
▪ **IV (Children):** 50 mg initially, smaller, additional doses q minute.

AVAILABILITY

▪ *Capsules:* 50 mg, 100 mg ▪ *Elixir:* 20 mg/5 ml ▪ *Suppositories:* 30 mg, 60 mg, 120 mg, 200 mg ▪ *Injection:* 50 mg/ml.

TIME/ACTION PROFILE (sedation)

	ONSET	PEAK	DURATION*
PO	15–60 min	3–4 hr	1–4 hr
Rectal	15–60 min	UK	1–4 hr
IM	10–25 min	UK	1–4 hr
IV	immediate	1 min	15 min

*Noted as hypnotic effect; sedative effects are longer-lasting.

NURSING IMPLICATIONS

ASSESSMENT

▪ **General Info:** Assess sleep patterns prior to and periodically throughout course of therapy. Hypnotic doses of pentobarbital suppress REM sleep. Patient may experience an increase in dreaming upon discontinuation of medication.

▢ Monitor respiratory status, pulse, and blood pressure frequently in patients receiving pentobarbital IV. Equipment for resuscitation and artificial ventilation should be readily available. Respiratory depression is dose-dependent.

▢ Prolonged therapy may lead to psychological or physical dependence. Restrict amount of drug available to patient, especially if depressed, suicidal, or previously addicted.

▢ Assess postoperative patients for pain. Pentobarbital may increase responsiveness to painful stimuli.

▪ **Cerebral Edema:** Monitor intracranial pressure and level of consciousness in patients in barbiturate coma.

▪ **Seizures:** Assess location, duration, and characteristics of seizure activity. Implement seizure precautions.

POTENTIAL NURSING DIAGNOSES

▪ Sleep pattern disturbance (indications).
▪ Injury, high risk for (side effects).
▪ Knowledge deficit related to medication regimen (patient/family teaching).

IMPLEMENTATION

▪ **General Info:** Supervise ambulation and transfer of patients following administration. Remove cigarettes. Side rails should be raised and call bell within reach at all times. Keep bed in low position.

▪ **PO:** Elixir may be administered undiluted or diluted in water, milk, or fruit juice. Use calibrated measuring device for accurate dosage. Do not use cloudy solutions.

▪ **IM:** Do not administer SC. IM injections should be given deep into the gluteal muscle to minimize tissue irritation. Do not inject more than 5 ml into any one site, because of tissue irritation.

▪ **Direct IV:** Doses may be given undiluted or diluted with sterile water, 0.45% NaCl, 0.9% NaCl, D5W, D10W, Ringer's or lactated Ringer's solution, dextrose/saline combinations or dextrose/Ringer's or lactated Ringer's combinations. Do not use solution that is discolored or that contains particulate matter.

▢ Solution is highly alkaline; avoid extravasation, which may cause tissue damage and necrosis. If extravasation occurs, infiltration of 5% procaine solution into affected area and application of moist heat may be ordered.

▪ *Rate:* Administer each 50 mg over at least 1 min. Titrate slowly for desired response. Rapid administration may result in respiratory depression, apnea, laryngospasm, bronchospasm, or hypertension.

▪ **Syringe Compatibility:** ▪ ephedrine ▪ hydromorphone ▪ neostigmine ▪ scopolamine.

▪ **Syringe Incompatibility:** ▪ benzquinamide ▪ butorphanol ▪ chlorpromazine ▪ cimetidine ▪ dimenhydrinate ▪ diphenhydramine ▪ droperidol ▪ fentanyl ▪ glycopyrrolate ▪ hydroxyzine ▪ meperidine ▪ midazolam ▪ nalbuphine ▪ pentazocine ▪ perphenazine ▪ prochlorperazine edisylate ▪ promazine ▪ promethazine ▪ ranitidine.

▪ **Y-Site Compatibility:** ▪ acyclovir ▪ regular insulin.

▪ **Rect:** To ensure accurate dose, do not divide rectal suppository. Suppositories should be refrigerated.

PATIENT/FAMILY TEACHING

- Advise patient to take medication exactly as prescribed. Do not increase dose of the drug without consulting physician.
- Discuss the importance of preparing environment for sleep (dark room, quiet, avoidance of nicotine and caffeine).
- Advise patients on prolonged therapy not to discontinue medication without consulting physician. Abrupt withdrawal may precipitate withdrawal symptoms.
- May cause daytime drowsiness. Caution patient to avoid driving and other activities requiring alertness until response to medication is known.
- Caution patient to avoid taking alcohol or other CNS depressants concurrently with this medication.
- Instruct patient to contact physician immediately if pregnancy is suspected.

EVALUATION

Effectiveness of therapy can be demonstrated by: ▪ Improvement in sleep pattern without excessive daytime sedation. Therapy is usually limited to a 2-wk period ▪ Prevention of cerebral anoxia ▪ Decrease or cessation of seizures without excessive sedation.

PENTOSTATIN
(**pen**-toe-sta-tin)
Nipent

CLASSIFICATION(S):
Antineoplastic agent (enzyme inhibitor)
Pregnancy Category D

INDICATIONS

▪ Treatment of hairy cell leukemia.

ACTION

▪ Inhibits adenine deaminase (ADA), an enzyme that blocks the synthesis of DNA, especially in T cells of the lymphoid system. **Therapeutic Effect:** ▪ Decreased signs/symptoms of disease (recovery of hematologic parameters, organomegaly, and lymphadenoapthy).

PHARMACOKINETICS

Absorption: IV administration results in complete bioavailability.
Distribution: Distribution is not known.
Metabolism and Excretion: Pentostatin and its metabolites are renally excreted.
Half-life: 6 hr (increased in renal impairment).

CONTRAINDICATIONS AND PRECAUTIONS

Contraindicated in: ▪ Hypersensitivity to pentostatin or mannitol.
Use Cautiously in: ▪ Patients with underlying cardiovascular disease, seizures, or pre-existing renal, hepatic, or pulmonary disease or other chronic debilitating illness ▪ Patients with childbearing potential ▪ Pregnancy, lactation, or children (safety not established).

ADVERSE REACTIONS AND SIDE EFFECTS*

CNS: SEIZURES, fatigue, headache, anxiety, confusion, depression, dizziness, insomnia, nervousness, somnolence, weakness, malaise.
EENT: abnormal vision, conjunctivitis, ear pain, eye pain.
Resp: cough, bronchitis, dypsnea, pneumonia, pharyngitis, rhinitis, sinusitis
CV: chest pain, peripheral edema, arrhythmias, abnormal ECG.
GI: anorexia, nausea, vomiting, diarrhea, constipation, flatulence, abdominal pain, stomatitis.
GU: nephrotoxicity, hematuria, dysuria.
Derm: rashes, herpes simplex, herpes zoster, pruritus, skin discoloration, seborrhea, sweating, dry skin, eczema, ecchymoses, petechia, photosensitivity.

*Underlines indicate most frequent; **CAPITALS** indicate life-threatening.

P

Hemat: anemia, leukopenia, thrombo-cytopenia, hemorrhage, thrombophle-bitis.
Metab: weight loss.
MS: back pain, myalgia, arthralgia.
Neuro: paresthesia.
Misc: lymphadenopathy, infection, pain, allergic reactions, chills, second neoplasms.

INTERACTIONS

Drug–Drug: ▪ Risk of fatal pulmonary toxicity is increased by concurrent use of **fludarabine** ▪ Effects of **vidarabine** are increased by pentostatin, which may result in increased toxicity.

ROUTE AND DOSAGE

▪ **IV (Adults):** 4 mg/m^2 every other week.

AVAILABILITY

▪ *Injection:* 10 mg/vial.

TIME/ACTION PROFILE (clinical response)

	ONSET	PEAK	DURATION
IV	4.7 mo	UK	>7.7 mo (range 1.4–35.1 mo)

NURSING IMPLICATIONS

ASSESSMENT

□ Monitor patient for CNS toxicity, which initially manifests as lethargy and may progress to seizures and coma. Dose should be withheld in patients manifesting CNS toxicity.

□ Monitor intake and output and renal function; provide adequate hydration. Administer 500–1000 ml of D5/0.45% NaCl prior to administration and 500 ml of D5W or a similar solution after administration of pentostatin.

□ Monitor patient for allergic reactions including anaphylactic reactions and rash. Therapy may be discontinued if severe rash or anaphylaxis develops. Epinephrine, an antihistamine, and resuscitation equipment should be available during therapy.

□ Assess patient for signs of infection (vital signs, WBC) throughout ther-

apy. Dose may be withheld if infection develops during therapy.

▪ **Lab Test Considerations:** Prior to initiating therapy, assess renal function by measuring serum creatinine or creatinine clearance. Serum creatinine should be measured prior to each dose. Dose may be withheld if serum creatinine is elevated.

□ Monitor CBC prior to each dose and periodically throughout therapy. Pentostatin should be temporarily withheld if the absolute neutrophil count (ANC) is less than 200 cells/mm^3 during treatment in a patient whose initial neutrophil count was greater than 500 cells/mm^3. Resume treatment when ANC returns to pretreatment levels.

□ May cause elevated liver function tests.

□ Monitor peripheral blood for hairy cells periodically throughout therapy to determine response to treatment.

□ Bone marrow aspiration and biopsies may be required every 2–3 mo to assess response to therapy.

POTENTIAL NURSING DIAGNOSES

▪ Infection, high risk for (side effects).

▪ Knowledge deficit related to medication regimen (patient/family teaching).

IMPLEMENTATION

▪ **General Info:** Pentostatin should be administered under the supervision of a physician experienced in the use of antineoplastic agents.

□ Solution should be prepared in a biologic cabinet. Wear gloves, gown, and mask while handling medication. Discard equipment in specially designated containers (see Appendix I).

□ Reconstitute by adding 5 ml of Sterile Water for Injection to each 10-mg vial for a concentration of 2 mg/ml. Shake thoroughly to ensure complete dissolution of the drug.

▪ **Direct IV:** May be administered undiluted.

▪ *Rate:* Administer as a bolus injection over 5 min.

▪ **Intermittent Infusion:** Dilute in 25–

50 ml of D5W or 0.9% NaCl. Solutions are stable for 8 hr at room temperature. Discard unused solution.

- **Rate:** Administer over 20–30 min.
- **Y-Site Compatibility:** ▪ fludarabine ▪ ondansetron ▪ sargramostim.

PATIENT/FAMILY TEACHING

☐ Instruct patient to notify physician or nurse immediately if rash or signs of anaphylaxis develop.

☐ Advise patient to notify physician promptly if fever, chills, sore throat, or signs of infection occur. Caution patient to avoid crowds and persons with known infections.

☐ Advise patient to use sunscreen and protective clothing to prevent photosensitivity reactions.

EVALUATION

Effectiveness of therapy can be determined by: ▪ Decrease in number of hairy cells in the peripheral blood and bone marrow ▪ Decreased organomegaly ▪ Decreased lymphadenopathy.

PENTOXIFYLLINE
(pen-tox-**if**-i-lin)
Trental

CLASSIFICATION(S):
Hemorrheologic agent
Pregnancy Category C

INDICATIONS

▪ Management of symptomatic peripheral vascular disease (intermittent claudication).

ACTION

▪ Increases the flexibility of red blood cells by increasing levels of cyclic adenosine monophosphate (cAMP) ▪ Decreases blood viscosity by inhibiting platelet aggregation and decreasing fibrinogen. **Therapeutic Effect:** ▪ Increased blood flow.

PHARMACOKINETICS

Absorption: Well absorbed following oral administration.
Distribution: Distribution not known.
Metabolism and Excretion: Metabolized by red blood cells and the liver.
Half-life: 25–50 min.

CONTRAINDICATIONS AND PRECAUTIONS

Contraindicated in: ▪ Hypersensitivity ▪ Intolerance to other xanthine derivatives (caffeine and theophylline).
Use Cautiously in: ▪ Coronary artery or cerebrovascular disease ▪ Pregnancy, lactation, or children (safety not established) ▪ Renal disease (lower doses may be used).

ADVERSE REACTIONS AND SIDE EFFECTS*

CNS: <u>headache</u>, <u>tremor</u>, <u>dizziness</u>, agitation, nervousness, drowsiness, insomnia.
EENT: blurred vision.
Resp: dyspnea.
CV: angina, hypotension, arrhythmias, flushing, edema.
GI: <u>dyspepsia</u>, <u>nausea</u>, <u>vomiting</u>, belching, flatus, bloating, abdominal discomfort, diarrhea.

INTERACTIONS

Drug–Drug: ▪ Additive hypotension may occur with **antihypertensives** and **nitrates** ▪ May increase the risk of bleeding with **warfarin, heparin, aspirin, nonsteroidal anti-inflammatory agents, cefamandole, cefoperazone, cefotetan, plicamycin, valproic acid,** or **thrombolytic agents** ▪ May increase the risk of theophylline toxicity ▪ **Smoking** may decrease the beneficial effects of pentoxifylline.

ROUTE AND DOSAGE

▪ **PO (Adults):** 400 mg 3 times daily.

AVAILABILITY

▪ *Controlled-release tablets:* 400 mg.

---

*<u>Underlines</u> indicate most frequent; **CAPITALS** indicate life-threatening.

TIME/ACTION PROFILE (improvement in blood flow)

	ONSET	PEAK	DURATION
PO	2–4 wk	8 wk	UK

NURSING IMPLICATIONS

ASSESSMENT
□ Assess patient for intermittent claudication prior to and periodically throughout course of therapy.
□ Monitor blood pressure periodically in patients on concurrent antihypertensive therapy.

POTENTIAL NURSING DIAGNOSES
▪ Pain (indications).
▪ Activity intolerance (indications).
▪ Knowledge deficit related to medication regimen (patient/family teaching).

IMPLEMENTATION
▪ **PO:** Administer with meals to minimize GI irritation. Tablets should be swallowed whole; do not crush, break, or chew.

PATIENT/FAMILY TEACHING
□ Instruct patient to take medication exactly as directed. If a dose is missed, it should be taken as soon as remembered unless almost time for next dose. Consult physician before discontinuing medication, because several weeks of therapy may be required before effects are seen.
□ Medication may cause dizziness and blurred vision. Caution patient to avoid driving and other activities requiring alertness until response to medication is known.
□ Advise patient to avoid smoking, as nicotine constricts blood vessels.
□ Instruct patient to notify physician if nausea, vomiting, GI upset, drowsiness, dizziness, or headache persists, as the dose may need to be reduced.

EVALUATION
Effectiveness of therapy can be demonstrated by: ▪ Relief from cramping in calf muscles, buttocks, thighs, and feet during exercise □ Improvement in walking endurance.

PERGOLIDE
(**per**-goe-lide)
Permax

CLASSIFICATION(S):
Antiparkinson agent (dopamine agonist)
Pregnancy Category B

INDICATIONS
▪ Management of Parkinson's disease in conjunction with levodopa/carbidopa.

ACTION
▪ Acts as a dopamine agonist, directly stimulating postsynaptic dopaminergic receptors in the CNS. **Therapeutic Effect:** ▪ Continued relief of symptoms of Parkinson's disease at a lower dosage of levodopa/carbidopa.

PHARMACOKINETICS
Absorption: Well absorbed following oral administration.
Distribution: Distribution not known.
Metabolism and Excretion: Highly metabolized by the liver. Metabolites are excreted by the kidneys.
Half-life: UK.

CONTRAINDICATIONS AND PRECAUTIONS
Contraindicated in: ▪ Hypersensitivity to pergolide or ergot derivatives.
Use Cautiously in: ▪ Arrhythmias ▪ Pregnancy or children (safety not established) ▪ Lactation (may inhibit lactation, safety not established).

ADVERSE REACTIONS AND SIDE EFFECTS*
CNS: hallucinations, dyskinesia, somnolence, insomnia, confusion.
EENT: rhinitis.
Resp: dyspnea.
CV: orthostatic hypotension, palpita-

---

*Underlines indicate most frequent; **CAPITALS** indicate life-threatening.

tions, arrhythmias (atrial premature contractions, sinus tachycardia).
GI: <u>nausea</u>, <u>constipation</u>, diarrhea, abdominal pain, dyspepsia, dry mouth.

INTERACTIONS

Drug–Drug: ▪ **Phenothiazines, metoclopramide,** or **haloperidol** may decrease effectiveness by antagonizing the effects of dopamine ▪ Additive hypotension may occur with **antihypertensives**.

ROUTE AND DOSAGE

▪ **PO (Adults):** 50 mcg/day in 3 divided doses for 2 days, increase by 100–150 mcg/day every third day for 12 days, then may increase by 250 mcg/day every third day until optimal response is obtained. Usual dose is 3 mg/day in divided doses tid, not to exceed 5 mg/day.

AVAILABILITY

▪ *Tablets:* 0.05 mg, 0.25 mg, 1 mg.

TIME/ACTION PROFILE
(antiparkinson effects)

	ONSET	PEAK	DURATION
PO	UK	UK	UK

NURSING IMPLICATIONS

ASSESSMENT

▫ Assess patient for signs and symptoms of Parkinson's disease (tremor, muscle weakness and rigidity, ataxic gait) prior to and throughout therapy.
▫ Assess patient for confusion or hallucinations. Notify physician if these occur.
▫ Monitor ECG frequently during dosage adjustment and periodically throughout therapy.

POTENTIAL NURSING DIAGNOSES

▪ Physical mobility, impaired (indications).
▪ Injury, high risk for (indications, side effects).
▪ Knowledge deficit related to medication regimen (patient/family teaching).

IMPLEMENTATION

▪ **PO:** An attempt to reduce the dose of levodopa/carbidopa may be made cautiously during pergolide therapy.
▫ Administer with meals to minimize nausea; usually resolves with continued therapy.

PATIENT/FAMILY TEACHING

▫ Instruct patient to take medication exactly as directed. Missed doses should be taken as soon as remembered if not almost time for next dose. Do not double doses. Consult physician before reducing dose or discontinuing medication.
▫ May cause drowsiness. Caution patient to avoid driving or other activities requiring alertness until response to medication is known.
▫ Advise patient to make position changes slowly to minimize orthostatic hypotension. Initial dose may be administered at bedtime to minimize this effect.
▫ Inform patient that frequent mouth rinses, good oral hygiene, and sugarless gum or candy may minimize dry mouth. Advise patient to consult physician or dentist if dry mouth persists for longer than 2 wk.

EVALUATION

Effectiveness of therapy can be demonstrated by: ▪ Improved response to levodopa/carbidopa in patients with Parkinson's disease.

PERMETHRIN
(per-**meth**-rin)
Elimite, Nix, Nix Dermal Cream

CLASSIFICATION(S):
Anti-infective (pediculocide)
Pregnancy Category B

INDICATIONS

▪ **1% lotion:** Eradication of *Pediculus humanus capitis* (head lice and their eggs) ▪ **5% cream:** Eradication of *Sarcoptes scabiei* (scabies).

ACTION

- Causes repolarization and paralysis in lice by disrupting normal nerve cell-sodium transport. **Therapeutic Effect:**
- Death of parasites.

PHARMACOKINETICS

Absorption: Small amounts (<2%) systemically absorbed. Remains on hair for 10 days.
Distribution: Distribution not known.
Metabolism and Excretion: Rapidly inactivated by enzymes.
Half-life: UK.

CONTRAINDICATIONS AND PRECAUTIONS

Contraindicated in: ▪ Hypersensitivity to permethrins, pyrethrins (insecticides or veterinary pesticides), chrysanthemums, or isopropyl alcohol.
Use Cautiously in: ▪ Pregnancy or lactation ▪ Children <2 yr (1% lotion) ▪ Children <2 mo (5% cream).

ADVERSE REACTIONS AND SIDE EFFECTS*

Derm: itching, redness, swelling, rash, stinging, burning.
Neuro: numbness, tingling.

INTERACTIONS

Drug–Drug: ▪ No significant interactions.

ROUTE AND DOSAGE

Head Lice

- **Top (Adults and Children >2 yr):** 1% lotion applied to the hair, left on for 10 min, then rinsed, for 1 application.

Scabies

- **Top (Adults and Children):** Massage 5% cream into all skin surfaces. Leave on for 8–14 hr, then wash off.
- **Top (Infants >2 mo):** Massage 5% cream into hairline, scalp, neck, temple, and forehead. Leave on for 8–14 hr, then wash off.

AVAILABILITY

- *Liquid cream rinse (lotion):* 1%
- *Cream:* 5%.

TIME/ACTION PROFILE
(pediculocidal action)

	ONSET	PEAK	DURATION
Top	10 min	UK	14 days

P

NURSING IMPLICATIONS

ASSESSMENT

- **Head Lice:** Assess scalp for presence of lice and their ova (nits) prior to and 1 wk after application of permethrin.
- **Scabies:** Assess skin for scabies prior to and following therapy.

POTENTIAL NURSING DIAGNOSES

- Home maintenance management, impaired (indications).
- Self-care deficit (indications).
- Knowledge deficit related to medication regimen (patient/family teaching).

IMPLEMENTATION

- **Top:** For topical application only.

PATIENT/FAMILY TEACHING

- **General Info:** Instruct patient to notify physician if scalp itching, numbness, redness, or rash occurs.
- □ Instruct patient to avoid getting Elimite cream in eyes. If this occurs, eyes should be flushed thoroughly with water. Physician should be contacted if eye irritation persists.
- □ Advise patient that others residing in the home should also be checked for lice.
- □ Instruct patient on methods of preventing reinfestation. All clothes, including outdoor apparel and household linens, should be machine-washed using very hot water and dried for at least 20 min in a hot dryer. Dry clean nonwashable clothes. Brushes and combs should be soaked in hot (130°F), soapy water for 5–10 min. Remind patient that brushes and combs should not be shared. Wigs and hairpieces should be shampooed. Rugs and upholstered furniture should be vacuumed. Toys should be washed in hot, soapy water. Items that cannot be washed

should be sealed in a plastic bag for 2 wk.

▫ If patient is a child, instruct parents to notify school nurse or day care center so that classmates and playmates can be checked.

▪ **Head Lice:** Instruct patient to wash hair with regular shampoo, rinse, and towel dry. Each container holds enough medication for one treatment. The patient should use as much of the solution as needed to coat entire head of hair, then discard remainder of solution. Shake the container well. Thoroughly wet scalp and hair with the lotion. Allow lotion to remain on hair for 10 min, then thoroughly rinse hair and towel dry with a clean towel. Comb hair with a fine-toothed comb to remove dead lice and eggs.

▫ Explain to patient that permethrin will protect from reinfestation for 2 wk. These effects continue even when the patient resumes regular shampooing.

▪ **Scabies:** Instruct patient to massage thoroughly into the skin from head to soles of feet. Treat infants on the hairline, neck, scalp, temple, and forehead. Remove the cream by washing after 8–14 hr. Usually 30 g (½ tube) is sufficient for adults. One application is curative.

EVALUATION

Effectiveness of therapy can be demonstrated by: ▪ Absence of lice and nits 1 wk after therapy ▪ Eradication of scabies following one application.

PERPHENAZINE
(per-**fen**-a-zeen)
{Apo-Perphenazine}, {Phenazine}, {PMS Perphenazine}, Trilafon

CLASSIFICATION(S):
Antipsychotic (phenothiazine), Antiemetic
Pregnancy Category UK

INDICATIONS
▪ Treatment of acute and chronic psychoses ▪ Management of nausea and vomiting or intractable hiccoughs.

ACTION
▪ Alters the effects of dopamine in the CNS ▪ Possesses significant anticholinergic and alpha-adrenergic blocking activity ▪ Blocks dopamine in the chemoreceptor trigger zone (CTZ). **Therapeutic Effects:** ▪ Diminished signs and symptoms of psychoses ▪ Decreased nausea and vomiting.

PHARMACOKINETICS
Absorption: Absorption from tablet is variable; may be better with oral liquid formulations. Well absorbed following IM administration.
Distribution: Widely distributed, high concentrations in the CNS. Crosses the placenta and enters breast milk.
Metabolism and Excretion: Highly metabolized by the liver and GI mucosa. Some conversion to active compounds.
Half-life: UK.

CONTRAINDICATIONS AND PRECAUTIONS
Contraindicated in: ▪ Hypersensitivity ▪ Hypersensitivity to bisulfites (injection only) ▪ Known alcohol intolerance (concentrate only) ▪ Cross-sensitivity with other phenothiazines may occur ▪ Narrow-angle glaucoma ▪ Bone marrow depression ▪ Severe liver or cardiovascular disease ▪ Intestinal obstruction.
Use Cautiously in: ▪ Elderly, emaciated, or debilitated patients (lower initial dose recommended) ▪ Pregnancy or lactation or children <12 yr (safety not established) ▪ Diabetes mellitus ▪ Respiratory disease ▪ Prostatic hypertrophy ▪ CNS tumors ▪ History of seizure disorder.

ADVERSE REACTIONS AND SIDE EFFECTS*
CNS: sedation, extrapyramidal reac-

tions, tardive dyskinesia, NEUROLEPTIC MALIGNANT SYNDROME.

CV: hypotension, tachycardia.

EENT: dry eyes, blurred vision, lens opacities.

GI: constipation, dry mouth, ileus, anorexia, hepatitis.

GU: urinary retention.

Derm: rashes, photosensitivity, pigment changes.

Endo: galactorrhea.

Hemat: AGRANULOCYTOSIS, leukopenia.

Metab: hyperthermia.

Misc: allergic reactions.

INTERACTIONS

Drug–Drug: ▪ Additive hypotension with **antihypertensive agents**, acute ingestion of **alcohol**, or **nitrates** ▪ Additive CNS depression with **MAO inhibitors** or other **CNS depressants**, including **alcohol, antihistamines, opioid analgesics, sedative/hypnotics**, and **general anesthetics** ▪ Additive anticholinergic effects with other **drugs possessing anticholinergic properties**, including **antihistamines, antidepressants, atropine, disopyramide, haloperidol**, and **other phenothiazines** ▪ Hypotension and tachycardia may occur with **epinephrine** ▪ Increased risk of agranulocytosis with **antithyroid agents** ▪ Increased risk of extrapyramidal reactions with **lithium** ▪ May mask **lithium** toxicity ▪ **Antacids** or **lithium** may decrease absorption of perphenazine ▪ May decrease antiparkinson effect of **levodopa**.

ROUTE AND DOSAGE

Psychoses
▪ **PO (Adults):** 4–16 mg 2–4 times daily (not to exceed 64 mg/day).
▪ **IM (Adults):** 5–10 mg initially, may repeat q 6 hr (not to exceed 15 mg/day).

Nausea and Vomiting
▪ **PO (Adults):** 8–16 mg/day in divided doses (up to 24 mg/day).
▪ **IM (Adults):** 5–10 mg initially, then 5 mg q 6 hr (not to exceed 15–30 mg/day).

Severe Nausea, Vomiting, or Hiccoughs
▪ **IV (Adults):** 1 mg at 1–2-min intervals to a total of 5 mg or as an infusion at a rate not to exceed 1 mg/min.

AVAILABILITY

▪ *Tablets:* 2 mg, 4 mg, 8 mg, 16 mg
▪ *Oral concentrate:* 16 mg/5 ml ▪ *Injection:* 5 mg/ml ▪ *In combination with:* amitriptyline (Etrafon, Triavil). See Appendix A.

TIME/ACTION PROFILE (PO, IM = antipsychotic effect,* IV = antiemetic effect)

	ONSET	PEAK	DURATION
PO	2–6 hr	UK	6–12 hr
IM	2–6 hr	UK	6–12 hr
IV	rapid	UK	UK

*Optimal antipsychotic response may not occur for several wk.

NURSING IMPLICATIONS

ASSESSMENT
▪ **General Info:** Assess patient's mental status (orientation, mood, behavior) prior to and periodically throughout therapy.
□ Monitor blood pressure (sitting, standing, lying), pulse, and respiratory rate prior to and frequently during the period of dosage adjustment.
□ Observe patient carefully when administering medication to ensure that medication is actually taken and not hoarded.
□ Observe patient carefully for extrapyramidal symptoms (akathesia—restlessness; dystonia—muscle spasm and twisting motions; or pseudoparkinsonism—mask facies, pill-rolling motions, drooling, tremors, rigidity, shuffling gait, dysphagia). Notify physician immediately at the onset of these symptoms, as a reduction of dosage or discontinuation of medication may be necessary. Trihexylphenidyl or diphenhydramine may be used to control these symptoms.
□ Monitor for tardive dyskinesia (uncontrolled movements of face, mouth,

tongue, or jaw and involuntary movements of extremities). Notify physician immediately if these symptoms occur, as these side effects may be irreversible.

☐ Monitor for development of neuroleptic malignant syndrome (fever, respiratory distress, tachycardia, convulsions, diaphoresis, hypertension or hypotension, pallor, tiredness). Notify physician immediately if these symptoms occur.

■ **Antiemetic:** Assess nausea and vomiting prior to and following perphenazine administration.

☐ Monitor intake and output. Patients with severe nausea and vomiting may require IV fluids with electrolytes in addition to antiemetics.

■ **Lab Test Considerations:** May cause false-positive and false-negative pregnancy tests.

☐ May cause blood dyscrasias; monitor CBC periodically throughout course of therapy.

☐ Monitor liver function tests, urine bilirubin, and bile for evidence of hepatic toxicity periodically throughout course of therapy. Urine bilirubin may be falsely elevated.

POTENTIAL NURSING DIAGNOSES

■ Thought processes, altered (indications).

■ Knowledge deficit related to medication regimen (patient/family teaching).

■ Noncompliance (patient/family teaching).

IMPLEMENTATION

■ **General Info:** To prevent contact dermatitis, avoid getting liquid preparations on hands, and wash hands thoroughly if spillage occurs.

■ **PO:** Dilute concentrate just prior to administration in 120 ml of water, milk, carbonated beverage, soup, or tomato or fruit juice. Do not mix with beverages containing caffeine (cola, coffee), tannics (tea), or pectinates (apple juice).

■ **IM:** Inject deep into well-developed muscle. Keep patient in recumbent position and monitor for at least 30 min following injection. Slight yellow color will not alter potency; do not use if solution is dark or contains a precipitate.

■ **Direct IV:** Dilute to a concentration of 0.5 mg/ml with 0.9% NaCl.

■ *Rate:* Administer each 1 mg over at least 1 min.

■ **Syringe Compatibility:** ■ atropine ■ butorphanol ■ chlorpromazine ■ cimetidine ■ dimenhydrinate ■ diphenhydramine ■ droperidol ■ fentanyl ■ meperidine ■ metoclopramide ■ morphine ■ pentazocine ■ prochlorperazine ■ promethazine ■ ranitidine ■ scopolamine.

■ **Syringe Incompatibility:** ■ midazolam ■ pentobarbital ■ thiethylperazine.

■ **Y-Site Compatibility:** ■ acyclovir ■ amikacin ■ ampicillin ■ azlocillin ■ cefamandole ■ cefazolin ■ ceforanide ■ cefotaxime ■ cefoxitin ■ cefuroxime ■ cephalothin ■ cephapirin ■ chloramphenicol ■ clindamycin ■ doxycycline ■ erythromycin lactobionate ■ famotidine ■ gentamicin ■ kanamycin ■ metronidazole ■ mezlocillin ■ minocycline ■ nafcillin ■ oxacillin ■ penicillin G potassium ■ piperacillin ■ ticarcillin ■ ticarcillin/clavulanate ■ tobramycin ■ trimethoprim/sulfamethoxazole ■ vancomycin.

■ **Y-Site Incompatibility:** ■ cefoperazone.

PATIENT/FAMILY TEACHING

☐ Advise patient to take medication exactly as directed and not to skip doses or double up on missed doses. If a dose is missed, it should be taken as soon as remembered unless almost time for the next dose. If more than 2 doses a day are ordered, the missed dose should be taken within 1 hr of the scheduled time or omitted. Abrupt withdrawal may lead to gastritis, nausea, vomiting, dizziness, headache, tachycardia, and insomnia.

□ Inform patient of possibility of extrapyramidal symptoms and tardive dyskinesia. Caution patient to report these symptoms immediately to physician.

□ Advise patient to make position changes slowly to minimize orthostatic hypotension.

□ Medication may cause drowsiness. Caution patient to avoid driving or other activities requiring alertness until response to medication is known.

□ Caution patient to avoid taking alcohol or other CNS depressants concurrently with this medication.

□ Advise patient to use sunscreen and protective clothing when exposed to the sun. Exposed surfaces may develop a blue-gray pigmentation, which may fade following discontinuation of the medication. Extremes in temperature should also be avoided, as this drug impairs body temperature regulation.

□ Instruct patient to notify physician if urinary retention, uncontrolled movements, rash, fever, or yellow coloration of skin occurs or if dry mouth or constipation persists. Sugarless candy or gum may diminish dry mouth, and an increase in fluid intake, bulk, or exercise may prevent constipation.

□ Advise patient to notify physician or dentist of medication regimen prior to treatment or surgery.

□ Inform patient that this medication may turn urine pink to reddish-brown.

□ Emphasize the importance of routine follow-up examinations, including ocular examinations, with long-term therapy and continued participation in psychotherapy.

EVALUATION

Effectiveness of therapy can be demonstrated by: ▪ Decrease in excitable, paranoic, or withdrawn behavior ▪ Relief of nausea and vomiting ▪ Relief of intractable hiccoughs.

P

PHENAZOPYRIDINE
(fen-az-oh-**peer**-i-deen)
Azo-Standard, Baridium, Eridium, Geridium, {Phenazo}, Phenazodine, Pyridiate, Pyridium, Urodine, Urogesic, Viridium

CLASSIFICATION(S):
Nonopioid analgesic (urinary tract analgesic)
Pregnancy Category B

INDICATIONS

▪ Provides relief from the following urinary tract symptoms, which may occur in association with infection or following urologic procedures: □ Pain □ Itching □ Burning □ Urgency □ Frequency.

ACTION

▪ Acts locally on the urinary tract mucosa to produce analgesic or local anesthetic effects ▪ Has no antimicrobial activity. **Therapeutic Effect:** Diminished urinary tract discomfort.

PHARMACOKINETICS

Absorption: Appears to be well absorbed following oral administration.
Distribution: Distribution not known. Small amounts cross the placenta.
Metabolism and Excretion: Rapidly excreted unchanged in the urine.
Half-life: UK.

CONTRAINDICATIONS AND PRECAUTIONS

Contraindicated in: ▪ Hypersensitivity ▪ Glomerulonephritis ▪ Pregnancy or lactation ▪ Severe hepatitis, uremia, or renal failure ▪ Renal insufficiency ▪ G6PD deficiency.
Use Cautiously in: ▪ Hepatitis.

{} = Available in Canada only.

ADVERSE REACTIONS AND SIDE EFFECTS*

CNS: headache, vertigo.
GI: nausea, hepatotoxicity.
GU: renal failure, <u>bright-orange urine</u>.
Derm: rash.
Hemat: methemoglobinemia, hemolytic anemia.

INTERACTIONS

Drug–Drug: ▪ None significant.

ROUTE AND DOSAGE

▪ **PO (Adults):** 200 mg tid for 2 days.
▪ **PO (Children):** 12 mg/kg/day in 3 divided doses for 2 days.

AVAILABILITY

▪ **Tablets:** 95 mg, 100 mg, 200 mg ▪ **In combination with:** hyoscyamine and butalbital (Pyridium Plus), sulfamethoxazole (Azo-Gantanol, Azo-Sulfamethoxazole, {Uro-Gantanol}; and sulfisoxazole {Azo-Cheragan, Azo-Gantrisin, Azo-Sulfisoxazole, Azo-Truxazole). See Appendix A.

TIME/ACTION PROFILE (urinary analgesia)

	ONSET	PEAK	DURATION
PO	UK	5–6 hr	6–8 hr

NURSING IMPLICATIONS

ASSESSMENT

□ Assess patient for urgency, frequency, and pain on urination prior to and throughout therapy.
▪ **Lab Test Considerations:** Renal function should be monitored periodically during course of therapy.
□ Interferes with urine tests based on color reactions (glucose, ketones, bilirubin, steroids, protein). Use Clinitest to test urine glucose concentration.

POTENTIAL NURSING DIAGNOSES

▪ Pain (indications).
▪ Urinary elimination, altered patterns of (indications).
▪ Knowledge deficit related to medication regimen (patient/family teaching).

IMPLEMENTATION

▪ **General Info:** Medication should be discontinued after pain or discomfort is relieved (usually 2 days for treatment of urinary tract infection). Concurrent antibiotic therapy should continue for full prescribed duration.
▪ **PO:** Administer medication with or following meals to decrease GI irritation. Do not crush or chew tablet.

PATIENT/FAMILY TEACHING

□ Instruct patient to take medication exactly as directed. If a dose is missed, take as soon as remembered unless almost time for next dose.
□ Advise patient that while phenazopyridine administration is stopped once pain or discomfort is relieved, concurrent antibiotic therapy must be continued for full duration of therapy.
□ Inform patient that drug causes reddish-orange discoloration of urine that may stain clothing or bedding. Sanitary napkin may be worn to avoid clothing stains. May also cause staining of contact lenses.
□ Instruct patient to notify physician if rash, skin discoloration, or unusual tiredness occurs.

EVALUATION

Effectiveness of therapy can be demonstrated by: ▪ Decrease in pain and burning on urination.

PHENOBARBITAL

(fee-noe-**bar**-bi-tal)
Barbita, Luminal, Solfoton

CLASSIFICATION(S):
Anticonvulsant (barbiturate),
Sedative/hypnotic
Schedule IV
Pregnancy Category D

INDICATIONS

▪ Anticonvulsant in tonic-clonic (grand mal), partial, and febrile seizures in

---

children • Preoperative sedative and in other situations in which sedation may be required • Hypnotic. **Unlabeled Uses:** • Prevention and treatment of hyperbilirubinemia.

ACTION

• Produces all levels of CNS depression • Depresses the sensory cortex, decreases motor activity, and alters cerebellar function • Inhibits transmission in the nervous system and raises the seizure threshold • Capable of inducing (speeding up) enzymes in the liver that metabolize drugs, bilirubin, and other compounds. **Therapeutic Effects:** • Anticonvulsant activity • Sedation.

PHARMACOKINETICS

Absorption: Absorption is slow but relatively complete (70–90%).
Distribution: Distribution not known.
Metabolism and Excretion: 75% metabolized by the liver, 25% excreted unchanged by the kidneys.
Half-life: 2–6 days.

CONTRAINDICATIONS AND PRECAUTIONS

Contraindicated in: • Hypersensitivity • Comatose patients or those with pre-existing CNS depression • Uncontrolled severe pain • Lactation • Known alcohol intolerance (elixir only).

Use Cautiously in: • Pregnancy (chronic use results in drug dependency in the infant; may result in coagulation defects and fetal malformation; acute use at term may result in respiratory depression in the newborn) • Hepatic dysfunction • Severe renal impairment • Patients who may be suicidal or who may have been addicted to drugs previously • Elderly patients (dosage reduction recommended) • Hypnotic use should be short-term. Chronic use may lead to dependence.

ADVERSE REACTIONS AND SIDE EFFECTS*

CNS: drowsiness, lethargy, vertigo, depression, hangover, excitation, delirium.

Resp: respiratory depression, LARYNGOSPASM (IV only), bronchospasm (IV only).
CV: hypotension (IV only).
GI: nausea, vomiting, diarrhea, constipation.
Derm: rashes, urticaria, photosensitivity.
Local: phlebitis at IV site.
MS: mylagia, arthralgia, neuralgia.
Misc: hypersensitivity reactions, including ANGIOEDEMA and serum sickness; physical dependence, psychological dependence.

INTERACTIONS

Drug–Drug: • Additive CNS depression with other CNS **depressants,** including **alcohol, antihistamines, opioid analgesics,** and other **sedative/hypnotics** • May induce hepatic enzymes that metabolize other drugs, decreasing their effectiveness, including **oral contraceptives, oral anticoagulants, chloramphenicol, cyclosporine, dacarbazine, glucocorticoids, tricyclic antidepressants,** and **quinidine** • May increase the risk of hepatic toxicity of **acetaminophen** • MAO inhibitors, val**proic acid,** or **divalproex** may decrease the metabolism of phenobarbital, increasing sedation • May increase the risk of hemotologic toxicity with **cyclophosphamide**.

ROUTE AND DOSAGE

Anticonvulsant

• **PO (Adults):** 60–250 mg/day, single dose or 2–3 divided doses.
• **PO (Children):** 1–6 mg/kg/day, single dose or divided doses.
• **IV (Adults):** 100–320 mg as needed initially (total of 600 mg/24-hr period). 10–20 mg/kg has been used for status epilepticus.
• **IV (Children):** 10 20 mg initially, followed by 1–6 mg/kg/day. 15–20 mg/kg has been used for status epilepticus.

Sedation

• **PO (Adults):** 30–120 mg/day in 2–3 divided doses.

*Underlines indicate most frequent; **CAPITALS** indicate life-threatening.

- **PO (Children):** 2 mg/kg 3 times daily.
- **IM (Adults):** 30–120 mg/day in 2–3 divided doses.

Preoperative Sedation
- **IM (Adults):** 130–200 mg 60–90 min preop.
- **PO, IM, IV (Children):** 1–3 mg/kg.

Hypnotic
- **PO (Adults):** 100–320 mg at bedtime.
- **IV, IM (Adults):** 100–325 mg at bedtime.

Hyperbilirubinemia
- **PO (Adults):** 30–60 mg 3 times daily.
- **PO (Children up to 12 yr):** 1–4 mg/kg 3 times daily.
- **PO, IM (Neonates):** 5–10 mg/kg/day.

AVAILABILITY

- **Tablets:** 8 mg, 16 mg, 32 mg, 65 mg, 100 mg ▪ **Capsules:** 15 mg ▪ **Elixir:** 15 mg/ml ▪ **Injection:** 30 mg/ml, 60 mg/ml, 65 mg/ml, 120 mg/amp, 130 mg/ml ▪ **In combination with:** phenytoin.

TIME/ACTION PROFILE (noted as sedation; full anticonvulsant effects occur after 2–3 wk of chronic dosing)

	ONSET	PEAK	DURATION
PO	30–60 min	UK	>6 hr
IM, SC	10–30 min	UK	4–6 hr
IV	5 min	30 min	4–6 hr

NURSING IMPLICATIONS

ASSESSMENT
- **General Info:** Monitor respiratory status, pulse, and blood pressure frequently in patients receiving phenobarbital IV. Equipment for resuscitation and artificial ventilation should be readily available. Respiratory depression is dose-dependent.
- □ Prolonged therapy may lead to psychological or physical dependence. Restrict amount of drug available to patient, especially if depressed, suicidal, or has a history of addiction.
- **Seizures:** Assess location, duration, and characteristics of seizure activity.
- **Sedation:** Assess level of consciousness and anxiety when used as a preoperative sedative.

- □ Assess postoperative patients for pain. Phenobarbital may increase responsiveness to painful stimuli.
- **Lab Test Considerations:** Patients on prolonged therapy should have hepatic and renal function and CBC evaluated periodically.
- **Toxicity and Overdose:** Serum phenobarbital levels may be monitored when used as an anticonvulsant. Therapeutic blood levels are 10–40 mcg/ml. Symptoms of toxicity include confusion, drowsiness, dyspnea, slurred speech, and staggering.

POTENTIAL NURSING DIAGNOSES
- Injury, high risk for (indications, side effects).
- Knowledge deficit related to medication regimen (patient/family teaching).

IMPLEMENTATION
- **General Info:** Supervise ambulation and transfer of patients following administration. Remove cigarettes. Side rails should be raised and call bell within reach at all times. Keep bed in low position. Institute seizure precautions.
- □ When changing from phenobarbital to another anticonvulsant, gradually decrease phenobarbital dose while concurrently increasing dose of replacement medication to maintain anticonvulsant effects.
- **PO:** Tablets may be crushed and mixed with food or fluids (do not administer dry) for patients with difficulty swallowing. Oral solution may be taken undiluted or mixed with water, milk, or fruit juice. Use calibrated measuring device for accurate measurement of liquid doses.
- **SC:** *Sterile* phenobarbital sodium may be administered SC after reconstitution, but phenobarbital sodium *injection* is not recommended for SC use.
- **IM:** Injections should be given deep into the gluteal muscle to minimize tissue irritation. Do not inject >5 ml into any one site, because of tissue irritation.

- **IV:** Doses may require 15–30 min to reach peak concentrations in the brain. Administer minimal dose and wait for effectiveness before administering second dose to prevent cumulative barbiturate-induced depression.
- **Direct IV:** Reconstitute sterile powder for IV dose with a minimum of 10 ml of Sterile Water for Injection. Dilute further with 10 ml of sterile water. Do not use solution that is not absolutely clear within 5 min after reconstitution or that contains a precipitate. Discard powder or solution that has been exposed to air for longer than 30 min.
- □ Solution is highly alkaline; avoid extravasation, which may cause tissue damage and necrosis. If extravasation occurs, injection of 5% procaine solution into affected area and application of moist heat may be ordered.
- *Rate:* Administer each 60 mg over at least 1 min. Titrate slowly for desired response. Rapid administration may result in respiratory depression.
- **Syringe Compatibility:** ▪ heparin.
- **Syringe Incompatibility:** ▪ benzquinamide ▪ dimenhydrinate ▪ diphenhydramine ▪ erythromycin glucceptate ▪ hydroxyzine ▪ kanamycin ▪ phenytoin ▪ prochlorperazine ▪ promazine ▪ promethazine ▪ ranitidine.

PATIENT/FAMILY TEACHING

- □ Advise patient to take medication exactly as directed. If a dose is missed, take as soon as remembered if not almost time for next dose; do not double doses.
- □ Advise patients on prolonged therapy not to discontinue medication without consulting physician. Abrupt withdrawal may precipitate seizures or status epilepticus.
- □ Medication may cause daytime drowsiness. Caution patient to avoid driving and other activities requiring alertness until response to medication is known. Do not resume driving until physician gives clearance based on control of seizure disorder.
- □ Caution patient to avoid taking alcohol or other CNS depressants concurrently with this medication.

- □ Instruct patient to contact physician immediately if pregnancy is suspected.
- □ Advise patient to notify physician if fever, sore throat, mouth sores, unusual bleeding or bruising, nosebleeds, or petechiae occur.

EVALUATION

Effectiveness of therapy can be demonstrated by: ▪ Decrease or cessation of seizure activity without excessive sedation. Several weeks may be required to achieve maximum anticonvulsant effects ▪ Preoperative sedation ▪ Improvement in sleep patterns ▪ Decrease in serum bilirubin levels.

PHENOLPHTHALEIN

(fee-nole-**thay**-leen)
Alophen Pills, No. 973, Correctol, Espotabs, Evac-U-Gen, Evac-U-Lax, Ex-Lax, Ex-Lax Pills, Feen-a-Mint, Feen-a-Mint Gum, Lax-Pills, Modane, Medilax, Phenolax, Prulet

CLASSIFICATION(S):
Laxative (stimulant)
Pregnancy Category UK

INDICATIONS

- ▪ Treatment of constipation (short-term).

ACTION

- ▪ Initiates peristalsis by acting directly on mucosa, stimulating myenteric plexus ▪ Alters fluid and electrolyte transport, producing fluid accumulation in the small intestine ▪ Action requires the presence of bile. **Therapeutic Effect:** ▪ Evacuation of the colon.

PHARMACOKINETICS

Absorption: 15% absorbed following oral administration. Action is primarily local in intestine.
Distribution: Small amounts excreted in breast milk.

Metabolism and Excretion: Eliminated by kidneys and in feces.
Half-life: UK.

CONTRAINDICATIONS AND PRECAUTIONS

Contraindicated in: ▪ Hypersensitivity ▪ Abdominal pain of unknown cause, especially if associated with fever ▪ Rectal fissures ▪ Ulcerated hemorrhoids. **Use Cautiously in:** ▪ Chronic use (may lead to laxative dependence) ▪ Pregnancy or lactation (safety not established) ▪ Possibility of intestinal obstruction.

ADVERSE REACTIONS AND SIDE EFFECTS*

GI: nausea, abdominal cramps, diarrhea, rectal burning.
MS: muscle weakness (chronic use).
F and E: hypokalemia (chronic use).
Misc: protein-losing enteropathy, tetany (chronic use).

INTERACTIONS

Drug–Drug: ▪ May decrease the absorption of other **orally administered drugs** because of increased motility and decreased transit time.

ROUTE AND DOSAGE

▪ **PO (Adults and Children >12 yr):** 30–270 mg/day as a single dose or in divided doses.
▪ **PO (Children 6–11 yr):** 30–60 mg/day as a single dose or in divided doses.
▪ **PO (Children 2–5 yr):** 15–30 mg/day as a single dose or in divided doses.

AVAILABILITY

▪ **Tablets:** 60 mg, 90 mg, 97.2 mg, 130 mg ▪ **Chewable tablets:** 65 mg, 90 mg, 97.2 mg, 120 mg ▪ **Wafers:** 64.8 mg ▪ **Chewable wafers:** 80 mg ▪ **Gum:** 97.2 mg ▪ **In combination with:** docusate, cascara, and mineral oil. See Appendix A.

TIME/ACTION PROFILE (laxative effect)

	ONSET	PEAK	DURATION
PO	6–10 hr	UK	several days

NURSING IMPLICATIONS

ASSESSMENT
▫ Assess patient for abdominal distention, presence of bowel sounds, and usual pattern of bowel function.
▫ Assess color, consistency, and amount of stool produced.

POTENTIAL NURSING DIAGNOSES
▪ Constipation (indications).
▪ Diarrhea (side effects).
▪ Knowledge deficit related to medication regimen (patient/family teaching).

IMPLEMENTATION
▪ **PO:** Take with a full glass of water. Administer at bedtime for bowel movement 6–12 hr later. Administer on an empty stomach for more rapid results.
▫ Chewable tablets should not be swallowed whole. Chew well before swallowing.

PATIENT/FAMILY TEACHING
▫ Advise patient that laxatives should be used only for short-term therapy. Long-term therapy may cause electrolyte imbalance and dependence.
▫ Encourage patient to utilize other forms of bowel regulation, such as increasing bulk in the diet, fluid intake, and mobility. Normal bowel habits are individualized and may vary from 3 times/day to 3 times/wk.
▫ Inform patient that this medication may cause a color change in feces and urine to pink, red, yellow, or brown.
▫ Instruct patient with cardiac disease to avoid straining during bowel movements (Valsalva maneuver).
▫ Advise patient not to use laxatives when abdominal pain, nausea, vomiting, or fever is present.

*Underlines indicate most frequent; **CAPITALS** indicate life-threatening.

EVALUATION
Effectiveness of therapy can be demonstrated by: ▪ Soft, formed bowel movement. Laxative effects may last for up to 3 days.

PHENOXYBENZAMINE
(fen-ox-ee-**ben**-za-meen)
Dibenzyline

CLASSIFICATION(S):
Antihypertensive (alpha-adrenergic blocking agent)
Pregnancy Category C

INDICATIONS

▪ Management of symptoms of pheochromocytoma (particularly hypertension and sweating) due to adrenergic (sympathomimetic) excess ▪ Treatment of hypertension associated with adrenergic excess, including that produced by tyramine-containing foods in patients receiving MAO inhibitor therapy. **Unlabeled Use:** ▪ Treatment of peripheral vascular disease.

ACTION

▪ Produces long-lasting blockade of alpha-adrenergic receptors in smooth muscle and exocrine glands ▪ Blocks epinephrine- and norepinephrine-induced vasoconstriction, resulting in hypotension and tachycardia. **Therapeutic Effect:** ▪ Reduction of symptoms of pheochromocytoma.

PHARMACOKINETICS

Absorption: Variably absorbed from the GI tract.
Distribution: Distribution not known.
Metabolism and Excretion: Mostly metabolized by the liver.
Half-life: 24 hr.

CONTRAINDICATIONS AND PRECAUTIONS

Contraindicated in: ▪ Shock (if fluid deficits have not been corrected).
Use Cautiously in: ▪ Coronary or cerebral arteriosclerosis ▪ Renal impairment ▪ Pregnancy (although safety not established, has been used safely in the third trimester of pregnancy) ▪ Lactation or children ▪ Elderly patients (more susceptible to hypotensive effects; dosage reduction recommended) ▪ Peptic ulcer disease ▪ Respiratory infection.

ADVERSE REACTIONS AND SIDE EFFECTS*

CNS: drowsiness, sedation, tiredness, weakness, malaise, confusion, headache, dizziness.
EENT: miosis, nasal congestion.
CV: hypotension, tachycardia, congestive heart failure, angina.
GI: nausea, vomiting, diarrhea, dry mouth.
GU: inhibition of ejaculation.

INTERACTIONS

Drug–Drug: ▪ Antagonizes the effects of **alpha-adrenergic stimulants** ▪ May decrease the pressor response to **ephedrine, phenylephrine,** or **methoxamine** ▪ Hypotension, vasodilation, and tachycardia may be exaggerated by **drugs that stimulate both alpha and beta receptors,** such as **epinephrine** ▪ Use with **guanethidine** or **guanadrel** may result in exaggerated hypotension and bradycardia ▪ Decreases peripheral vasoconstriction from high doses of **dopamine** ▪ Additive CNS depression may occur with concurrent use of **antihistamines, antidepressants, alcohol, opioid analgesics,** or **sedative/hypnotics.**

ROUTE AND DOSAGE
Dosage requires individual titration.

▪ **PO (Adults):** 10 mg once daily, increase by 10 mg/day at 2-day intervals. Usual maintenance dose is 20–40 mg, 2–3 times daily.
▪ **PO (Children):** 0.2 mg/kg or 6 mg/m^2 daily (not to exceed 10 mg); dosage increments may be made at 4-day intervals. Usual maintenance dose is 0.4–1.2 mg/kg/day (12–36 mg/m^2/day) in 3–4 divided doses.

---

*Underlines indicate most frequent; **CAPITALS** indicate life-threatening.

AVAILABILITY

- **Capsules:** 10 mg.

TIME/ACTION PROFILE (alpha-adrenergic blockade)

	ONSET	PEAK	DURATION
PO	1–4 hr	1 wk	3–4 days

NURSING IMPLICATIONS

ASSESSMENT

- Monitor blood pressure (sitting and lying), pulse, respiratory status, and diaphoretic episodes frequently, especially during initiation of therapy.
- **Lab Test Considerations:** Urinary catecholamine measurements should be made periodically to determine maximal dose.

POTENTIAL NURSING DIAGNOSES

- Tissue perfusion, altered (indications).
- Injury, high risk for (side effects).
- Knowledge deficit related to medication regimen (patient/family teaching).

IMPLEMENTATION

- **General Info:** Concurrent use of a beta-adrenergic blocker may be necessary to control reflex tachycardia.
- **PO:** May be administered with meals or milk if GI irritation becomes a problem. Dosage reduction may be required.

PATIENT/FAMILY TEACHING

- Instruct patient to take medication exactly as directed at the same time each day. Do not skip or double up on missed doses. Consult physician prior to discontinuation.
- Medication may cause drowsiness or dizziness. Caution patient to avoid driving or other activities requiring alertness until response to medication is known.
- Caution patient to make position changes slowly to minimize orthostatic hypotension. Standing for long periods or exercising during hot weather may also induce orthostatic hypotension.
- Inform patient that good oral hygiene, frequent mouth rinses, and sugarless gum or candy may reduce dryness of mouth. The physician or dentist should be notified if dryness persists >2 wk. Regular dental care is recommended, as a dry mouth may increase risk of caries and periodontal disease.
- Advise patient to avoid use of alcohol or over-the-counter cold preparations without consulting physician or pharmacist.
- Inform patient that medication may cause nasal congestion, inhibition of ejaculation, and constriction of pupils, which may interfere with night vision. These effects usually decrease with continued therapy. Notify physician if these side effects persist.
- Advise patient to inform physician or dentist of medication regimen prior to treatment or surgery.

EVALUATION

Effectiveness of therapy can be demonstrated by: ■ Decrease in blood pressure, pulse, and sweating in patients with pheochromocytoma ■ Decrease in blood pressure due to adrenergic excess. May require 1 wk of therapy for full therapeutic effects to be apparent.

PHENTOLAMINE
(fen-**tole**-a-meen)
Regitine, {Rogitine}

CLASSIFICATION(S):
Alpha-adrenergic blocking agent
Pregnancy Category C

INDICATIONS

- Treatment of hypertension associated with pheochromocytoma or adrenergic (sympathetic) excess, such as administration of phenylephrine, tyramine-containing foods in patients on MAO inhibitor therapy, or clonidine withdrawal ■ Control of blood pressure during surgical removal of a pheochromocytoma ■ Prevention and treatment of dermal necrosis and sloughing following extravasation of norepinephrine, phenylephrine, or dopamine. **Unlabeled Use:** ■ Adjunct therapy of impotence (intracavernosal).

ACTION

■ Produces incomplete and short-lived blockade of alpha-adrenergic receptors located primarily in smooth muscle and exocrine glands ■ Induces hypotension by direct relaxation of vascular smooth muscle and by alpha blockade. **Therapeutic Effects:** ■ Reduction of blood pressure in situations in which hypertension is due to adrenergic (sympathetic) excess ■ When infiltrated locally, reverses vasoconstriction caused by norepinephrine or dopamine.

PHARMACOKINETICS

Absorption: Well absorbed following IM administration.
Distribution: Distribution not known.
Metabolism and Excretion: 10% excreted unchanged by kidneys.
Half-life: UK.

CONTRAINDICATIONS AND PRECAUTIONS

Contraindicated in: ■ Hypersensitivity ■ Coronary or cerebral arteriosclerosis ■ Renal impairment.
Use Cautiously in: ■ Pregnancy or lactation (safety not established) ■ Peptic ulcer disease ■ Elderly patients (more susceptible to hypotensive effects; dosage reduction recommended).

ADVERSE REACTIONS AND SIDE EFFECTS*

CNS: CEREBROVASCULAR SPASM, weakness, dizziness.
CV: HYPOTENSION, tachycardia, arrhythmias, angina, MYOCARDIAL INFARCTION.
Derm: flushing.
EENT: nasal stuffiness.

GI: abdominal pain, nausea, vomiting, diarrhea, aggravation of peptic ulcer.

INTERACTIONS

Drug–Drug: ■ Antagonizes the effects of **alpha-adrenergic stimulants** ■ May decrease the pressor response to **ephedrine, phenylephrine,** or **mefaraminol** ■ Severe hypotension may occur with concurrent use of **epinephrine** or **methoxamine.** Use with **guanethidine** or **guanadrel** may result in exaggerated hypotension and bradycardia ■ Decreases peripheral vasoconstriction from high doses of **dopamine.**

ROUTE AND DOSAGE

Diagnosis of Pheochromocytoma
■ **IV (Adults):** 5 mg.
■ **IV, IM (Children):** 1 mg or 0.1 mg/kg (3 mg/m²).

Hypertension Associated with Pheochromocytoma— Before/During Surgery
■ **IV, IM (Adults):** 5 mg given 1–2 hr preop, repeated as necessary. May be infused at a rate of 0.5–1 mg/min during surgery.
■ **IV, IM (Children):** 1 mg or 0.1 mg/kg (3 mg/m²) given 1–2 hr preop, repeated IV as necessary during surgery.

Prevention of Dermal Necrosis Following Extravasation of Norepinephrine, Phenylephrine, or Dopamine
■ **Infiltrate:** 5–10 mg.

Prevention of Dermal Necrosis During Infusion of Norepinephrine
■ Add 10 mg phentolamine to every 1000 ml of fluid containing norepinephrine.

Adjunct Therapy of Impotence
■ **Intracavernosal (Adults):** 0.5–1 mg with 30 mg papaverine (not to exceed 3 treatments/wk).

AVAILABILITY
■ *Injection:* 5 mg/ml.

*Underlines indicate most frequent; CAPITALS indicate life-threatening.

TIME/ACTION PROFILE (IM, IV = alpha-adrenergic blockade, Intracavernosal = erection)

	ONSET	PEAK	DURATION
IM	UK	20 min	30–45 min
IV	immediate	2 min	15–30 min
Intra-cavernosal	UK	within 10 min	4 hr

NURSING IMPLICATIONS

ASSESSMENT

□ Monitor blood pressure, pulse, and ECG every 2 min until stable during IV administration. If hypotensive crisis occurs, epinephrine is contra-indicated and may cause paradoxical further decrease in blood pressure; norepinephrine may be used.

POTENTIAL NURSING DIAGNOSES

■ Tissue perfusion, altered (indications).
■ Injury, high risk for (indications).
■ Knowledge deficit related to medication regimen (patient/family teaching).

IMPLEMENTATION

■ **General Info:** Patient should remain supine throughout parenteral administration.
■ **IV:** Reconstitute each 5 mg with 1 ml of Sterile Water for Injection or 0.9% NaCl. Discard unused solution.
■ **Direct IV:** Inject each 5 mg over 1 min.
■ **Continuous Infusion:** Dilute 5–10 mg in 500 ml of D5W.
■ *Rate:* Titrate infusion rate according to patient response.
□ May also add 10 mg to every 1000 ml of fluid containing norepinephrine for prevention of dermal necrosis and sloughing. Does not affect pressor effect of norepinephrine.
■ **Syringe Compatibility:** ■ papaverine.
■ **Additive Compatibility:** ■ dobutamine ■ verapamil.
■ **Infiltration:** Dilute 5–10 mg of phentolamine in 5–10 ml of 0.9% NaCl. Infiltrate site of extravasation promptly. Must be given within 12 hr of extravasation to be effective.

■ **Impotence:** Has been used with papaverine to treat men with impotence, usually associated with spinal cord injury. This method requires special training. Administration is by injection into the corpus cavernosum, producing an erection. Risk of priapism exists.

PATIENT/FAMILY TEACHING

□ Advise patient to make position changes slowly to minimize orthostatic hypotension.
□ Instruct patient to notify physician if chest pain occurs during IV infusion.

EVALUATION

Clinical response to therapy is indicated by: ■ Decrease in blood pressure ■ Prevention of dermal necrosis and sloughing in extravasation of norepinephrine, dopamine, and phenylephrine ■ Erection in men with impotence, beginning 10 min after injection into corpus cavernosum and sustained for up to 4 hr.

PHENYLEPHRINE
(fen-il-**eff**-rin)

PHENYLEPHRINE NASAL
Alconefrin, Coricidin Nasal Mist, Doktors, Duration, Neo-Synephrine, Nostril, Rhinall, Sinex

PHENYLEPHRINE OPHTHALMIC
Ak-Dilate, Ak-Nefrin, Dilatair, I-Phrine, Isopto Frin, {Minims Phenylephrine}, Mydfrin, Neo-Synephrine, Ocugestrin, Ocu-Phrin, Prefrin Liquifilm, Relief, {Spersafrin}

PHENYLEPHRINE PARENTERAL
Neo-Synephrine

CLASSIFICATION(S):
Vasopressor (alpha-adrenergic agonist), Decongestant, Ophthalmic (mydriatic)
Pregnancy Category C (Ophth, Parenteral)

{} = Available in Canada only.

INDICATIONS

• **SC, IM, IV:** Adjunct in the treatment of shock—to correct hypotension that may persist after adequate fluid replacement • **Ophth:** Mydriatic • **Nasal, Ophth:** Decongestant • As an adjunct in spinal anesthesia (to prolong duration of anesthesia) • As an adjunct in regional anesthesia (to localize effect).

ACTION

• Constricts blood vessels by stimulating alpha-adrenergic receptors. **Therapeutic Effects:** • **SC, IM, IV:** Increased blood pressure • **Ophth:** Mydriasis • **Nasal, Ophth:** Decreased congestion.

PHARMACOKINETICS

Absorption: Well absorbed from IM sites. Minimal absorption following nasal and ophthalmic application.
Distribution: Distribution not known.
Metabolism and Excretion: Metabolized by the liver and other tissues.
Half-life: UK.

CONTRAINDICATIONS AND PRECAUTIONS

Contraindicated in: • Uncorrected fluid volume deficits • Tachyarrhythmias • Pheochromocytoma • Angle-closure glaucoma • Hypersensitivity to bisulfites (parenteral) • Hypersensitivity to bisulfites, camphor, eucalyptol, thimerisol (nasal and ophthalmic).
Use Cautiously in: • Occlusive vascular disease • Cardiovascular disease • Elderly patients • Hyperthyroidism • Pregnancy and lactation (safety not established) • Diabetes mellitus.

ADVERSE REACTIONS AND SIDE EFFECTS*

Seen mainly with parenteral administration.

CNS: dizziness, trembling, restlessness, anxiety, nervousness, weakness, dizziness, tremor, insomnia, headache.
EENT: Ophth—burning, stinging, browache, photophobia, lacrimation, irritation; Nasal—burning, stinging, dry nasal mucosa, rebound congestion.

Resp: respiratory distress, dyspnea.
CV: tachycardia, ARRHYTHMIAS, hypertension, chest pain, bradycardia, vasoconstriction.
Derm: blanching, piloerection, pallor, sweating.
Local: phlebitis, sloughing at IV sites.

INTERACTIONS

Drug–Drug: • Use with **MAO inhibitors, ergot alkaloids (ergonovine, methylergonovine),** or **oxytocics** results in severe hypertension • Use with **general anesthetics** may result in myocardial irritability • **Alpha-adrenergic blockers (phenoxybenzamine, phentolamine)** may antagonize vasopressor effects • **Atropine** blocks bradycardia from phenylephrine and enhances pressor effects.

ROUTE AND DOSAGE

Hypotension
• **SC, IM (Adults):** 2–5 mg, may repeat q 10–15 min (initial dose not to exceed 5 mg).
• **SC (Children):** 100 mcg/kg, may repeat in 1–2 hr.
• **IV (Adults):** 200 mcg, may repeat q 10–15 min (initial dose not to exceed 500 mcg) or as an infusion at 100–180 mcg/min initially, 40–60 mcg/min maintenance.

Mydriasis
• **Ophth (Adult):** 1 drop of 2.5% or 10% solution. May be repeated in 1 hr (not to exceed 3 drops/day).

Decongestant
• **Ophth (Adults and Children >2 yr):** 1 drop of 0.08%–0.12% solution q 3–4 hr.
• **Nasal (Adults):** 2–3 drops or 1–2 sprays in each nostril q 3–4 hr (1% solution no more frequently than q 4 hr).
• **Nasal (Children 6–12 yr):** 2–3 drops or 1–2 sprays of 0.25% solution q 3–4 hr as needed.
• **Nasal (Children 2–6 yr):** 2–3 drops of 0.125% solution q 3–4 hr as needed or 2–3 drops of 0.16% solution q 4 hr as needed.

*Underlines indicate most frequent; CAPITALS indicate life-threatening.

- **Nasal (Children >6 mo and <2 yr):** 1–2 drops of 0.16% solution q 3 hr as needed or 2–3 drops of 0.125% solution q 3–4 hr.

AVAILABILITY

- *Injection:* 1% (10 mg/ml) ▪ *Nasal solution:* 0.125%, 0.16%, 0.25%, 0.5%, 1% ▪ *In combination with:* pyrilamine (Myci-Spray, Dristan Nasal), pyrilamine and naphazoline (4-way Fast Acting Original) ▪ *Ophthalmic solution:* 0.12%, 2.5%, 10%.

TIME/ACTION PROFILE (IV, IM, SC = vasopressor effects, Ophth = mydriasis, Nasal = decongestant action)

	ONSET	PEAK	DURATION
IV	immediate	UK	15–20 min
IM	10–15 min	UK	1–2 hr
SC	10–15 min	UK	50–60 min
Nasal	UK	UK	30 min–4 hr
Ophth	several mins	10–90 min	3–7 hr

NURSING IMPLICATIONS

ASSESSMENT

- **Hypotension:** Monitor blood pressure every 2–3 min until stabilized and every 5 min thereafter during IV administration.
- ▫ Monitor ECG continuously for arrhythmias during IV administration.
- ▫ Assess IV site frequently throughout infusion. Antecubital or other large vein should be used to minimize risk of extravasation, which may cause tissue necrosis. If extravasation occurs, the site should be infiltrated promptly with 10–15 ml of 0.9% NaCl solution containing 5–10 mg of phentolamine to prevent necrosis and sloughing.
- **Decongestant:** Assess patient for allergic symptoms prior to and periodically throughout therapy. Chronic, excessive use can lead to rebound congestion.

POTENTIAL NURSING DIAGNOSES

- Cardiac output, decreased (indications).
- Tissue perfusion, altered (indications).
- Knowledge deficit related to medication regimen (patient/family teaching).

IMPLEMENTATION

- **General Info:** Available in several concentrations. Carefully check label for percentage of solution prior to administration.
- **IV:** Blood volume depletion should be corrected, if possible, prior to initiation of IV phenylephrine.
- **Direct IV:** Dilute each 1 mg with 9 ml of Sterile Water for Injection.
- *Rate:* Administer each single dose over 1 min.
- **Continuous Infusion:** Dilute 10 mg in 500 ml of dextrose/Ringer's or lactated Ringer's combination, dextrose/saline combinations, D5W, D10W, Ringer's or lactated Ringer's solution, 0.45% NaCl, or 0.9% NaCl to provide a 1:50,000 solution.
- *Rate:* Titrate rate according to patient response. Infuse via infusion pump to ensure accurate dosage rate. See Infusion Rate Table (Appendix D).
- **Y-Site Compatibility:** ▪ amrinone ▪ famotidine ▪ zidovudine.
- **Additive Compatibility:** ▪ chloramphenicol ▪ dobutamine ▪ lidocaine ▪ potassium chloride ▪ sodium bicarbonate.
- **Anesthesia:** Phenylephrine 2–5 mg may be added to spinal anesthetic solution to prolong anesthesia.
- ▫ Phenylephrine 1 mg may be added to each 20 ml of local anesthetic to produce vasoconstriction.

PATIENT/FAMILY TEACHING

- **IV:** Instruct patient to report headache, dizziness, dyspnea, or pain at IV infusion site promptly.
- **Ophth:** Instruct patient on correct procedure to instill ophthalmic preparations (see Appendix H). Solution may cause stinging or burning.
- ▫ Inform patient that ophthalmic preparations will dilate pupils and may make eyes more sensitive to light.

Dark glasses will minimize this sensitivity.

- **Nasal:** Instruct patient to blow nose gently prior to instilling nasal preparations. For instillation of nasal drops, instruct patient to tilt head back or lie on bed and hang head over the side. After instillation, remain in this position to allow medication to be distributed throughout nose. After using, wash dropper in hot water and dry with clean tissues.
  - For nasal spray, hold head upright and squeeze bottle quickly and firmly. Wait 3–5 min, blow nose, and repeat.
  - Solution that is brown or has formed a precipitate has lost potency and should be discarded.
  - Advise patient that prolonged or excessive use may cause rebound congestion. Use the weakest strength that is effective. Use only as directed.

EVALUATION
Effectiveness of therapy can be demonstrated by: ▪ Increase in blood pressure to normal range ▪ Mydriasis ▪ Decongestant effects in nose and eyes ▪ Prolonged duration of spinal anesthesia ▪ Localization of regional anesthesia.

PHENYLPROPANOLAMINE
(fen-il-proe-pa-**nole**-a-meen)
Acutrim, Control, Dex-A-Diet, Dexatrim, Diet-Aid, Eped-II Yellow, Phenxyldrine, PPA, Prolamine, Propagest, Rhinedecon, Stay-Trim, Unitrol

CLASSIFICATION(S):
Appetite suppressant, Decongestant
Pregnancy Category UK

INDICATIONS
- Short-term adjunct therapy in the management of exogenous obesity in conjunction with behavior modification, diet, and exercise ▪ Short-term management of nasal congestion.

ACTION
- Acts as an agonist of dopamine and norepinephrine ▪ Suppresses appetite by depressing CNS appetite control center ▪ Stimulates alpha-adrenergic receptors in nasal mucosa, producing vasoconstriction. **Therapeutic Effects:** ▪ Decreased appetite ▪ Nasal decongestion.

PHARMACOKINETICS
Absorption: Well absorbed following oral administration.
Distribution: Distribution not known.
Metabolism and Excretion: 80–90% excreted unchanged by the kidneys. Small amounts metabolized by the liver.
Half-life: 3–4 hr.

CONTRAINDICATIONS AND PRECAUTIONS
Contraindicated in: ▪ Hypersensitivity ▪ Children <12 yr (appetite suppressant use only) ▪ Pregnancy or lactation.
Use Cautiously in: ▪ Glaucoma ▪ Prostatic hypertrophy ▪ Hyperthyroidism ▪ Cardiovascular disease, including hypertension ▪ Diabetes mellitus.

ADVERSE REACTIONS AND SIDE EFFECTS*
CNS: nervousness, restlessness, insomnia, dizziness, headache, drowsiness.
EENT: rebound congestion (decongestant use).
CV: chest pain, arrhythmias, hypertension.
GI: nausea.
Misc: tachyphylaxis (decongestant use).

INTERACTIONS
Drug–Drug: ▪ Additive sympathomimetic effects with other **adrenergic (sympathomimetic) agents** ▪ Vasopressor effects are increased by concurrent

---

*Underlines indicate most frequent; **CAPITALS** indicate life-threatening.

administration of **MAO inhibitors** ▪ Increased risk of arrhythmias with **some general anesthetics** ▪ Increased risk of hypertension with **rauwolfia alkaloids (reserpine), tricyclic antidepressants,** or **ganglionic blocking agents**.

ROUTE AND DOSAGE

Appetite Suppressant
▪ **PO (Adults):** 25 mg tid or 75 mg of extended or precision-release preparation once daily.

Decongestant
▪ **PO (Adults):** 25 mg q 4 hr (not to exceed 150 mg/day) or 75 mg of extended-release preparation q 12 hr.
▪ **PO (Children 6–12 yr):** 12.5 mg q 4 hr (not to exceed 75 mg/day).
▪ **PO (Children 2–6 yr):** 6.25 mg q 4 hr (not to exceed 37.5 mg/day).

AVAILABILITY

Appetite Suppressants
▪ *Tablets:* 25 mg ▪ *Timed-release tablets:* 75 mg ▪ *Precision-release tablets:* 75 mg ▪ *Capsules:* 37.5 mg ▪ *Timed-release capsules:* 25 mg, 75 mg ▪ *Gum:* 8.3 mg ▪ *In combination with:* vitamins and/or grapefruit extract.

Decongestants
▪ *Tablets:* 25 mg, 50 mg ▪ *Timed-release capsules:* 75 mg ▪ *In combination with:* antihistamines, other decongestants, antipyretics, expectorants, and cough suppressants in a wide variety of cough and cold preparations.

TIME/ACTION PROFILE (nasal decongestion)

	ONSET	PEAK	DURATION
PO	15–30 min	UK	3 hr
PO-ER	UK	UK	12–16 hr

NURSING IMPLICATIONS

ASSESSMENT
▪ **Obesity:** Monitor patient's weight and nutritional intake periodically throughout therapy.

▪ **Nasal Congestion:** Assess patient for nasal congestion periodically throughout therapy.

POTENTIAL NURSING DIAGNOSES
▪ Nutrition, altered: more than body requirements (indications).
▪ Knowledge deficit related to medication regimen (patient/family teaching).

IMPLEMENTATION
▪ **General Info:** Administer last dose a few hours prior to sleep (12 hr with timed-release forms) to minimize insomnia.
▪ **PO:** Administer timed-release tablets once daily, in the morning after breakfast. Timed-release tablets should be swallowed whole; do not crush or chew.
▪ **Obesity:** Do not administer to children under 12 yr. Administer to children 12–18 yr according to physician's recommendations.

PATIENT/FAMILY TEACHING
▪ **General Info:** Instruct patient to take only as directed. Do not take more medication or for a longer time than directed; tolerance may develop.
▫ Advise patient not to drink large amounts of coffee, tea, or colas containing caffeine.
▪ **Obesity:** Instruct patient on modification of caloric intake and exercise program.
▪ **Nasal Decongestant:** Missed doses should be taken as soon as remembered if within 2 hr (12 hr with timed-release tablets) of next scheduled dose. Do not double doses.
▫ Advise patient to consult physician if symptoms do not improve within 7 days or if a fever is present.

EVALUATION
Effectiveness of therapy can be demonstrated by: ▪ Decrease in appetite and subsequent decrease in weight when used for obesity. Should be used no longer than a few weeks for obesity ▪ Decrease in nasal congestion.

PHENYTOIN
(**fen**-i-toyn)
diphenylhydantoin, DPH, Dilantin, Diphenylan

CLASSIFICATION(S):
Anticonvulsant (hydantoin),
Antiarrhythmic (group IB)
Pregnancy Category UK

INDICATIONS

■ Treatment and prevention of tonic–clonic (grand mal) seizures and complex partial seizures. **Unlabeled Uses:** ■ As an antiarrhythmic, particularly for arrhythmias associated with cardiac glycoside toxicity ■ Management of painful syndromes, including trigeminal neuralgia.

ACTION

■ Limits seizure propagation by altering ion transport ■ Antiarrhythmic properties as a result of improvement in AV conduction ■ May also decrease synaptic transmission. **Therapeutic Effects:** ■ Diminished seizure activity ■ Control of arrhythmias ■ Decreased pain.

PHARMACOKINETICS

Absorption: Absorbed slowly from the GI tract. Erratically and unreliably absorbed from IM sites. Bioavailability differs among products. Only Dilantin preparation is considered to be extended release. Other products are considered to be prompt release.

Distribution: Distribution not known. Crosses the placenta and enters breast milk. Preferentially distributes into fatty tissue.

Metabolism and Excretion: Mostly metabolized by the liver; minimal amounts excreted in the urine.

Half-life: 22 hr.

CONTRAINDICATIONS AND PRECAUTIONS

Contraindicated in: ■ Hypersensitivity ■ Hypersensitivity to propylene glycol (injection only) ■ Alcohol intolerance (injection only) ■ Sinus bradycardia and heart block (antiarrhythmic use).

Use Cautiously in: ■ Severe liver disease (dosage reduction recommended) ■ Pregnancy (safety not established; may result in fetal hydantoin syndrome if used chronically or hemorrhage in the newborn if used at term) ■ Lactation (safety not established) ■ Elderly patients or those with severe cardiac or respiratory disease (parenteral use—increased risk of serious adverse reactions) ■ Obese patients (initial dose should be based on ideal body weight + 1.33 times excess weight).

ADVERSE REACTIONS AND SIDE EFFECTS*

CNS: nystagmus, ataxia, diplopia, drowsiness, lethargy, coma, dizziness, headache, nervousness, dyskinesia.
EENT: gingival hyperplasia.
CV: hypotension (IV only).
GI: nausea, vomiting, anorexia, weight loss, constipation, hepatitis.
GU: pink, red, reddish-brown discoloration of urine.
Derm: hypertrichosis, rashes, exfoliative dermatitis.
F and E: hypocalcemia.
Hemat: APLASTIC ANEMIA, AGRANULOCYTOSIS, leukopenia, thrombocytopenia, megaloblastic anemia.
MS: osteomalacia.
Misc: lymphadenopathy, fever, allergic reactions, including STEVENS–JOHNSON SYNDROME.

INTERACTIONS

Drug–Drug: ■ **Phenylbutazone, disulfiram, isoniazid, chloramphenicol, influenza vaccine, sulfonamides, benzodiazepines, omeprazole, metronidazole, ketoconazole, fluconazole, miconazole, succinamides, felbamate,** and **cimetidine** may decrease phenytoin metabolism and increase blood levels ■ **Barbiturates, chronic ingestion of alcohol,** and **warfarin** may stimulate phenytoin metabolism and decrease blood levels ■ Phenytoin may stimulate the metabolism and decrease the effectiveness of **digitoxin methadone, theophylline, cyclosporine,** and **oral contraceptives** ▪ IV phenytoin and **dopamine** may cause additive hypotension ▪ Additive CNS depression with other **CNS depressants,** including **alcohol, antihistamines, antidepressants, opioid analgesics,** and **sedative/hypnotics** ▪ Phenytoin may alter the effect of **oral anticoagulants** ▪ **Antacids** may decrease absorption of orally administered phenytoin ▪ May decrease therapeutic effect of **streptozocin** ▪ Phenytoin may decrease absorption and effectiveness of **theophylline** ▪ Additive cardiac depression may occur with **propranol** or **lidocaine** ▪ **Valproic acid** or **carbamazepine** may increase or decrease phenytoin plasma levels ▪ **Calcium** decreases phenytoin absorption ▪ Phenytoin decreases **felbamate** levels.

Drug–Food: ▪ Phenytoin may decrease absorption of **folic acid.**

ROUTE AND DOSAGE

IM administration should be a last resort. Dosage should be increased by 50% over previously established daily oral dosage.

Anticonvulsant

▪ **PO (Adults):** Loading dose 1 g or 20 mg/kg as extended-release capsules in 3 divided doses at 2-hr intervals. Maintenance dose 300–400 mg/day. May be given once daily as extended-release capsules (Dilantin Kapseals) or in 3 divided doses. Usual maximum dose 600 mg/day.

▪ **PO (Elderly Patients):** 3 mg/kg/day in divided doses.

▪ **PO (Children):** Initially 5 mg/kg, maintenance dose 4–8 mg/kg/day in 2–3 divided doses (not to exceed 300 mg/day).

Status Epilepticus

▪ **IV (Adults):** 15–20 mg/kg. Rate not to exceed 25–50 mg/min, followed by 100 mg q 6–8 hr.

▪ **IV (Children):** 15–20 mg/kg (250 mg/m^2) at 1–3 mg/kg/min.

Antiarrhythmic

▪ **IV (Adults):** 100 mg q 5 min or 50–100 mg q 10–15 min until arrhyth-

mia is abolished, 15 mg/kg has been given, or toxicity occurs.

Antineuralgia

▪ **PO (Adults):** 200–600 mg/day in divided doses.

AVAILABILITY

▪ *Chewable tablets:* 50 mg ▪ *Oral suspension:* 30 mg/5 ml, 125 mg/5 ml ▪ *Prompt-release capsules:* 30 mg, 100 mg ▪ *Extended-release capsules:* 100 mg ▪ *Injection:* 50 mg/ml ▪ *In combination with:* phenobarbital.

TIME/ACTION PROFILE
(anticonvulsant effect)

	ONSET*	PEAK	DURATION
PO	2–24 hr (1 wk)	1.5–3 hr	6–12 hr
PO-ER	2–24 hr (1 wk)	4–12 hr	12–36 hr
IV	1–2 hr (1 wk)	rapid	12–24 hr
IM	UK (erratic)	erratic	12–24 hr

*( ) = time required for onset of action without a loading dose.

NURSING IMPLICATIONS

ASSESSMENT

▪ **General Info:** Assess oral hygiene. Vigorous cleaning beginning within 10 days of initiation of phenytoin therapy may help control gingival hyperplasia.

▪ **Seizures:** Assess location, duration, and characteristics of seizure activity.

▪ **Arrhythmias:** Monitor ECG continuously during treatment of arrhythmias.

▪ **Neuralgia:** Assess pain (location, duration, intensity, precipitating factors) prior to and periodically throughout therapy.

▪ **Lab Test Considerations:** CBC and platelet count, serum calcium, urinalysis, and hepatic and thyroid function tests should be monitored prior to and monthly for the first several months, then periodically throughout course of therapy.

▫ May cause increased serum alkaline phosphatase and glucose levels.

▪ **Toxicity and Overdose:** Serum phenytoin levels should be routinely monitored. Therapeutic blood levels are 10–20 mcg/ml.

□ Progressive signs and symptoms of phenytoin toxicity include nystagmus, ataxia, confusion, nausea, slurred speech, and dizziness.

POTENTIAL NURSING DIAGNOSES

■ Injury, high risk for (indications).

■ Oral mucous membranes, altered (side effects).

■ Knowledge deficit related to medication regimen (patient/family teaching).

IMPLEMENTATION

■ General Info: Implement seizure precautions.

□ When transferring from phenytoin to another anticonvulsant, dosage adjustments are made gradually over several weeks.

■ PO: Administer with or immediately after meals to minimize GI irritation. Shake liquid preparations well before pouring. Use a calibrated measuring device for accurate dosage. Chewable tablets must be crushed or chewed well before swallowing. Capsules may be opened and mixed with food or fluids for patients with difficulty swallowing. To prevent direct contact of alkaline drug with mucosa, have patient swallow a liquid first, follow with mixture of medication, then follow with a full glass of water, milk, or with food.

□ Do not interchange 100-mg tablets with capsules, as capsules contain 92 mg of phenytoin and are not equal to two 50-mg tablets or capsules.

□ Capsules labeled "extended" may be used for once-a-day dosage (Dilantin Kapseals only); those labeled "prompt" may result in toxic serum levels if used for once-a-day dosage.

■ IV: Slight yellow color will not alter solution potency. If refrigerated, may form precipitate, which dissolves after warming to room temperature. Discard solution that is not clear.

■ Direct IV: Administer at a rate not to exceed 50 mg over 1 min (25 mg/min in elderly patients; 1–3 mg/kg/min in neonates). Rapid administration may result in severe hypotension or CNS depression.

■ Intermittent Infusion: Administer by mixing with 0.9% NaCl in a concentration of 1–10 mg/ml. Administer immediately following admixture. Use tubing with a 0.22-micron in-line filter.

□ To prevent precipitation and minimize local venous irritation, follow infusion with 0.9% NaCl. Avoid extravasation; phenytoin is caustic to tissues.

■ *Rate:* Complete infusion within 4 hr at a rate not to exceed 50 mg/min. Monitor cardiac function and blood pressure throughout infusion.

■ Y-Site Compatibility: ■ esmolol ■ famotidine ■ fluconazole ■ foscarnet.

■ Y-Site Incompatibility: ■ enalaprilat ■ potassium chloride ■ vitamin B complex with C.

■ Additive Incompatibility: Do not admix with other solutions or medications, especially dextrose, as precipitation will occur.

PATIENT/FAMILY TEACHING

□ Instruct patient to take medication every day exactly as directed. Consult physician if doses are missed for 2 consecutive days. Abrupt withdrawal may lead to status epilepticus.

□ Phenytoin may cause drowsiness or dizziness. Caution patient to avoid driving or other activities requiring alertness until response to medication is known. Do not resume driving until physician gives clearance based on control of seizure disorder.

□ Caution patient to avoid taking alcohol or over-the-counter medications concurrently with phenytoin without consulting physician or pharmacist.

□ Instruct patient on importance of maintaining good dental hygiene and seeing dentist frequently for teeth cleaning to prevent tenderness, bleeding, and gingival hyperplasia. Institution of oral hygiene program within 10 days of initiation of phenytoin therapy may minimize growth rate and severity of gingival enlargement. Patients under 23 yrs of age and those taking doses >500 mg/day are at increased risk for gingival hyperplasia.

▫ Advise patient that brands of phenytoin may not be equivalent. Check with physician or pharmacist if brand or dosage form is changed.

▫ Inform patient that phenytoin may color urine pink, red, or reddish brown, but color change is not significant.

▫ Advise diabetic patients to monitor urine glucose carefully and to notify physician of significant changes.

▫ Instruct patient to notify physician or dentist of medication regimen prior to treatment or surgery.

▫ Advise patient not to take phenytoin within 2–3 hr of antacids.

▫ Advise patient to carry identification describing disease process and medication regimen at all times.

▫ Advise patient to notify physician if skin rash, severe nausea or vomiting, drowsiness, slurred speech, unsteady gait, swollen glands, bleeding or tender gums, yellow skin or eyes, joint pain, fever, sore throat, unusual bleeding or bruising, persistent headache, or pregnancy occurs.

▫ Emphasize the importance of routine examinations to monitor progress. Patient should have routine physical examinations, especially monitoring skin and lymph nodes, and EEG testing.

EVALUATION
Effectiveness of therapy can be demonstrated by: ▪ Decrease or cessation of seizures without excessive sedation ▪ Suppression of arrhythmias ▪ Relief of pain due to neuralgia.

PHOSPHATE/BIPHOSPHATE
(**foss**-fate/bye-**foss**-fate)
Fleet Enema, Phospho-Soda

CLASSIFICATION(S):
Laxative (saline)
Pregnancy Category UK

INDICATIONS
▪ Preparation of the bowel prior to surgery or radiologic studies. May be used intermittently in the treatment of chronic constipation.

ACTION
▪ Osmotically active in the lumen of the GI tract ▪ Produces laxative effect by causing water retention and stimulation of peristalsis ▪ Stimulates motility and inhibits fluid and electrolyte absorption from the small intestine. **Therapeutic Effects:** ▪ Relief of constipation ▪ Emptying of the bowel.

PHARMACOKINETICS
Absorption: 1–20% of rectal administered sodium and phosphate may be absorbed.
Distribution: Distribution not known.
Metabolism and Excretion: Excreted by the kidneys.
Half-life: UK.

CONTRAINDICATIONS AND PRECAUTIONS
Contraindicated in: ▪ Abdominal pain, nausea, or vomiting, especially when associated with fever or other signs of an acute abdomen ▪ Pregnancy (at term) ▪ Renal disease ▪ Severe cardiac disease ▪ Intestinal obstruction.
Use Cautiously in: ▪ Excessive or chronic use (may lead to dependence) ▪ Pregnancy (may cause sodium retention and edema).

ADVERSE REACTIONS AND SIDE EFFECTS*
GI: <u>cramping</u>, <u>nausea</u>.
F and E: sodium retention, hyperphosphatemia, hypocalcemia.

INTERACTIONS
Drug–Drug: ▪ None significant.

---

*<u>Underlines</u> indicate most frequent; **CAPITALS** indicate life-threatening.

ROUTE AND DOSAGE

Each Fleet Enema contains 4.4 g sodium/118 ml. Each 20 ml of Fleet Phospho-Soda oral solution contains 96.4 mEq sodium.

- **PO (Adults):** 20–30 ml Phospho-Soda.
- **PO (Children):** 5–15 ml Phospho-Soda.
- **Rect (Adults and Children >12 yr):** 118 ml Fleet Enema.
- **Rect (Children >2 yr):** ½ of the adult dose.

AVAILABILITY

- **Oral solution:** 18 g sodium phosphate and 48 g sodium biphosphate/100 ml ▪ **Enema:** 7 g sodium phosphate and 19 g sodium biphosphate/118 ml.

TIME/ACTION PROFILE (laxative effect)

	ONSET	PEAK	DURATION
PO	0.5–3 hr	UK	UK
Rect	2–5 min	UK	UK

NURSING IMPLICATIONS

ASSESSMENT

- ▫ Assess patient for fever, abdominal distention, presence of bowel sounds, and usual pattern of bowel function.
- ▫ Assess color, consistency, and amount of stool produced.
- ▪ **Lab Test Considerations:** May cause increased serum sodium and phosphorus levels, decreased serum calcium levels, and acidosis.

POTENTIAL NURSING DIAGNOSES

- ▪ Constipation (indications).
- ▪ Knowledge deficit related to medication regimen (patient/family teaching).

IMPLEMENTATION

- ▪ **General Info:** Do not administer at bedtime or late in the day.
- ▪ **PO:** Administer on an empty stomach for more rapid results. Mix dose in at least ½ glass cold water. May be followed by carbonated beverage or fruit juice to improve flavor.
- ▪ **Rect:** Position patient on left side with knee slightly flexed. Insert pre-lubricated tip about 2 in. into rectum, aiming toward the umbilicus. Gently squeeze bottle until empty. Discontinue if resistance is met, as perforation may occur if contents are forced into rectum.

PATIENT/FAMILY TEACHING

- ▫ Advise patient that laxatives should be used only for short-term therapy. Long-term therapy may cause electrolyte imbalance and dependence.
- ▫ Caution patient on sodium restriction that this product has a high sodium content.
- ▫ Advise patient not to take oral form of this medication within 2 hr of other medications.
- ▫ Encourage patient to use other forms of bowel regulation, such as increasing bulk in the diet, fluid intake, and mobility. Normal bowel habits may vary from 3 times/day to 3 times/wk.
- ▫ Advise patient to notify physician if unrelieved constipation, rectal bleeding, or symptoms of electrolyte imbalance (muscle cramps or pain, weakness, dizziness, and so forth) occur.

EVALUATION

Effectiveness of therapy can be demonstrated by: ▪ Soft, formed bowel movement ▪ Evacuation of the bowel.

PHYSOSTIGMINE

(fi-zoe-**stig**-meen)
Antilerium, Isopto-Eserine

CLASSIFICATION(S):
Cholinergic (anticholinesterase agent), Ophthalmic
Pregnancy Category C (Ophth)

INDICATIONS

- ▪ **IM, IV, SC:** Reversal of CNS effects due to overdose of drugs capable of causing the anticholinergic syndrome, including: ▫ Belladonna or other plant alkaloids ▫ Phenothiazines ▫ Tricyclic antidepressants ▫ Antihistamines (reverses delirium, hallucinations, coma, and some arrhythmias, but not completely effective in reversing cardiac conduction defects or tachycardia) ▪ **Ophth:** As miotic to decrease intraocular pressure in treatment of glaucoma.

ACTION

▪ Inhibits the breakdown of acetylcholine so that it accumulates and has a prolonged effect. Result is generalized cholinergic response, including: ▫ Miosis ▫ Increased tone of intestinal and skeletal musculature ▫ Bronchial and ureteral constriction ▫ Bradycardia ▫ Increased salivation ▫ Lacrimation ▫ Sweating ▫ CNS stimulation. **Therapeutic Effects:** ▪ **IM, IV, SC:** Reversal of anticholinergic excess ▪ **Ophth:** Miosis with decreased intraocular pressure.

PHARMACOKINETICS

Absorption: Readily absorbed from SC and IM sites. Some absorption may occur following ophthalmic use.
Distribution: Widely distributed, crosses the blood–brain barrier.
Metabolism and Excretion: Metabolized by cholinesterases present in many tissues. Small amounts excreted unchanged in the urine.
Half-life: UK.

CONTRAINDICATIONS AND PRECAUTIONS

Contraindicated in: ▪ Hypersensitivity ▪ Hypersensitivity to bisulfites (injection only) ▪ Preparations containing benzyl alcohol should be avoided in newborns ▪ Mechanical obstruction of the GI or GU tract ▪ Pregnancy or lactation (10–20% of newborns will suffer from muscle weakness).
Use Cautiously in: ▪ History of asthma ▪ Ulcer disease ▪ Cardiovascular disease ▪ Epilepsy ▪ Hyperthyroidism ▪ Uveitis or corneal injury (ophth only).

ADVERSE REACTIONS AND SIDE EFFECTS*

CNS: dizziness, weakness, restlessness, hallucinations, SEIZURES.
EENT: miosis, lacrimation; Ophth—

blurred vision, eye pain, eye irritation, brow ache, twitching of eyelids.
Resp: excess respiratory secretions, bronchospasm.
CV: bradycardia, hypotension.
GI: abdominal cramps, nausea, vomiting, diarrhea, excess salivation.
Derm: rash.

INTERACTIONS

Drug–Drug: ▪ Cholinergic effects may be antagonized by other **drugs possessing anticholinergic properties,** including **antihistamines, antidepressants, atropine, haloperidol, phenothiazines, quinidine,** and **disopyramide** ▪ Prolongs action of **depolarizing muscle-relaxing agents (succinylcholine, decamethonium)** ▪ Beneficial ophthalmic effects may be decreased by concurrent **ophthalmic belladonna alkaloids (atropine, scopolamine)** ▪ May decrease the duration of action of **echothiophate** or **isoflurophate** if administered before physostigmine.

ROUTE AND DOSAGE

▪ **IM, IV, (Adults):** 0.5–2 mg initially, then may give 1–4 mg q 20–30 min as symptoms recur.
▪ **IV (Children):** 20 mcg/kg may repeat every 5–10 minutes as needed (up to a total of 2 mg).
▪ **Ophth (Adults and Children):** 1 drop up to 4 times daily or ointment 1–3 times daily.

AVAILABILITY

▪ *Injection:* 1 mg/ml ▪ *Ophthalmic solution:* 0.25%, 0.5% ▪ *Ophthalmic ointment:* 0.25%.

TIME/ACTION PROFILE (SC, IM, IV = systemic cholinergic effects; Ophth = miosis)

	ONSET	PEAK	DURATION
SC	UK	UK	45–60 min*
IM	3–8 min	UK	45–60 min*
IV	3–8 min	UK	45–60 min*
Ophth	1–30 min	UK	12–48 hr

*May be up to 5 hr.

*Underlines indicate most frequent; **CAPITALS** indicate life-threatening.

NURSING IMPLICATIONS

ASSESSMENT

- **General Info:** Monitor pulse, respiratory rate, and blood pressure frequently throughout parenteral administration. Monitor ECG during IV administration.
- **Anticholinergic Excess:** Monitor neurologic status frequently. Institute seizure precautions. Protect patient from self-injury due to CNS effects of overdose.
- **Glaucoma:** Monitor patient for changes in vision, eye irritation, and persistent headache.
- **Toxicity and Overdose:** Overdose is manifested by bradycardia, respiratory distress, seizures, weakness, nausea, vomiting, stomach cramps, diarrhea, diaphoresis, and increased salivation and tearing.
- ◻ Atropine is the antidote.
- ◻ Treatment of overdose includes establishing an airway and supporting ventilation, atropine sulfate 2–4 mg (may be repeated every 3–10 min to control muscarinic effects), pralidoxime chloride 50–100 mg/min (to control neurologic and skeletal muscle effects), and supportive therapy.

POTENTIAL NURSING DIAGNOSES

- Sensory–perceptual alteration: visual (indications, side effects).
- Injury, high risk for (indications).
- Knowledge deficit related to medication regimen (patient/family teaching).

IMPLEMENTATION

- **Direct IV:** Repeated doses may be needed due to short duration of action.
- **Rate:** May be given through Y-site or 3-way stopcock at a rate of 1 mg over 1 min (0.5 mg over 1 min for children). Rapid administration may cause bradycardia; increased salivation, which can lead to respiratory distress; or seizures.

PATIENT/FAMILY TEACHING

- **Anticholinergic Excess:** Explain purpose of medication and need for close monitoring.

- **Ophth:** Instruct patient to take as ordered and not to discontinue without physician's approval. Lifelong therapy may be required. A missed dose of eyedrops should be taken as soon as remembered unless almost time for next dose. If dose of ointment is missed, patient should take it as soon as remembered. If not remembered until next day, patient should wait until usual time for dose.
- ◻ Instruct patient on correct method of application of drops or ointment. (See Appendix H.)
- ◻ Do not touch cap or tip of container to eye, fingers, or any surface.
- ◻ Explain to patient that pupil constriction and temporary stinging and blurring of vision are expected. Physician should be notified if blurred vision and brow ache persist.
- ◻ Caution patient that night vision may be impaired. Advise patient not to drive at night until response to medication is known. To prevent injury at night, patient should use a night light and keep environment uncluttered.
- ◻ Instruct patient to report signs of systemic side effects (sweating, increased salivation, nausea, vomiting, diarrhea, bradycardia, weakness, and respiratory distress).
- ◻ Advise patient of the need for regular eye examinations to monitor intraocular pressure and visual fields.

EVALUATION

Effectiveness of therapy can be demonstrated by: ▪ Reversal of CNS symptoms secondary to anticholinergic excess resulting from drug overdose or ingestion of poisonous plants ▪ Control of elevated intraocular pressure.

PHYTONADIONE

(fye-toe-na-**dye**-one)
AquaMEPHYTON, Konakion,
Mephyton, vitamin K₁

CLASSIFICATION(S):

Vitamin (fat-soluble)
Pregnancy Category UK

INDICATIONS

- Prevention and treatment of hypoprothrombinemia, which may be associated with: □ Excessive doses of oral anticoagulants □ Salicylates □ Certain anti-infective agents □ Nutritional deficiencies □ Prolonged total parenteral nutrition ▪ Prevention of hemorrhagic disease of the newborn.

ACTION

- Required for hepatic synthesis of blood coagulation factors II (prothrombin), VII, IX, and X. **Therapeutic Effect:** ▪ Prevention of bleeding due to hypoprothrombinemia.

PHARMACOKINETICS

Absorption: Well absorbed following oral, IM, or SC administration. Oral absorption requires presence of bile salts. Some vitamin K is produced by bacteria in the GI tract.
Distribution: Crosses the placenta. Does not enter breast milk.
Metabolism and Excretion: Rapidly metabolized by the liver.
Half-life: UK.

CONTRAINDICATIONS AND PRECAUTIONS

Contraindicated in: ▪ Hypersensitivity ▪ Hypersensitivity to benzyl alcohol (AquaMEPHYTON only), phenol, propylene glycol, or polysorbate 80 (Konakion only).
Use Cautiously in: ▪ Impaired liver function.

ADVERSE REACTIONS AND SIDE EFFECTS*

GI: gastric upset, unusual taste.
Derm: rash, urticaria, flushing.
Local: erythema, swelling, pain at injection site.
Misc: hemolytic anemia, kernicterus, hyperbilirubinemia (large doses in very premature infants), allergic reactions.

INTERACTIONS

Drug–Drug: ▪ Large doses will counteract the effect of **oral anticoagulants**

▪ Large doses of **salicylates** or broad-spectrum **anti-infectives** may increase vitamin K requirements ▪ **Cholestyramine, colestipol, mineral oil,** and **sucralfate** may decrease vitamin K absorption.

ROUTE AND DOSAGE

Treatment of Hypoprothrombinemia
- **PO, SC, IM (Adults):** 2.5–10 mg, repeat PO in 12–48 hr if necessary or in 6–8 hr after parenteral dose (up to 25–50 mg).
- **PO, SC, IM (Children):** 5–10 mg.
- **PO, IM, SC (Infants):** 1–2 mg.

Prevention of Hypoprothrombinemia During Total Parenteral Nutrition
- **IM (Adults):** 5–10 mg once weekly.
- **IM (Children):** 2–5 mg once weekly.

Prevention of Hemorrhagic Disease of Newborn
- **SC, IM (Neonates):** 0.5–1 mg, within 1 hr of birth. May be repeated in 6–8 hr (larger doses may be necessary if mother received chronic anticonvulsant therapy).

AVAILABILITY

- *Tablets:* 5 mg ▪ *Injection (aqueous colloid solution):* 2 mg/ml, 10 mg/ml ▪ *Injection (aqueous dispension for IM use only):* 2 mg/ml, 10 mg/ml.

TIME/ACTION PROFILE

	ONSET	PEAK*	DURATION†
PO	6–12 hr	UK	UK
IM, SC	1–2 hr	3–6 hr	12–14 hr

* = Control of hemorrhage.
† = Normal prothrombin time achieved.

NURSING IMPLICATIONS

Assessment

□ Monitor for frank and occult bleeding (guaiac stools, hematest urine and emesis). Monitor pulse and blood pressure frequently; notify physician immediately if symptoms of internal bleeding or hypovolemic shock develop. Inform all personnel of patient's bleeding tendency to prevent

*Underlines indicate most frequent; **CAPITALS** indicate life-threatening.

further trauma. Apply pressure to all venipuncture sites for at least 5 min; avoid unnecessary IM injections.

- **Lab Test Considerations:** Prothrombin time should be monitored prior to and throughout vitamin K therapy to determine response to and need for further therapy.

POTENTIAL NURSING DIAGNOSES

- Nutrition, altered: less than body requirements (indications).
- Tissue perfusion, altered (indications).
- Knowledge deficit related to medication regimen (patient/family teaching).

IMPLEMENTATION

- **General Info:** The parenteral route is preferred for phytonadione therapy, but because of severe hypersensitvity reactions, IV vitamin K is not recommended.
- Administration of whole blood or plasma may also be required in severe bleeding because of the delayed onset of this medication.
- Phytonadione is an antidote for warfarin overdose but does not counteract the anticoagulant activity of heparin.

PATIENT/FAMILY TEACHING

- Instruct patient to take this medication as ordered. If a dose is missed, take as soon as remembered unless almost time for next dose. Notify physician of missed doses.
- Cooking does not destroy substantial amounts of vitamin K. Patient should not drastically alter diet while taking vitamin K. See Appendix K for foods high in vitamin K.
- Caution patient to avoid IM injections and activities leading to injury. Use a soft toothbrush, do not floss, and shave with an electric razor until coagulation defect is corrected.
- Advise patient to report any symptoms of unusual bleeding or bruising (bleeding gums, nosebleed, black tarry stools, hematuria, excessive menstrual flow) to physician.
- Patients receiving vitamin K therapy

should be cautioned not to take over-the-counter medications without advice of physician or pharmacist.
- Advise patient to inform physicians and dentists of the use of this medication prior to treatment or surgery.
- Advise patient to carry identification describing disease process at all times.
- Emphasize the importance of frequent lab tests to monitor coagulation factors.

EVALUATION

Effectiveness of therapy can be demonstrated by: ■ Prevention of spontaneous bleeding or cessation of bleeding in patients with hypoprothrombinemia secondary to impaired intestinal absorption or oral anticoagulant, salicylate, or antibiotic therapy ■ Prevention of hemorrhagic disease in the newborn.

PINDOLOL
(pin-doe-lole)
Visken

CLASSIFICATION(S):
Antihypertensive (beta-adrenergic blocker, nonselective)
Pregnancy Category B

INDICATIONS

■ Used alone or in combination with other agents in the treatment of hypertension. **Unlabeled Uses:** ■ Chronic treatment of angina pectoris ■ Hypertrophic cardiomyopathy ■ Tremors ■ Mitral valve prolapse syndrome.

ACTION

■ Blocks stimulation of beta$_1$ (myocardial) adrenergic receptors and beta$_2$ (pulmonary, vascular, or uterine) receptor sites ■ Possesses mild intrinsic sympathomimetic activity (ISA) which may result in less bradycardia. **Therapeutic Effects:** ■ Decreased heart rate ■ Decreased blood pressure.

PHARMACOKINETICS

Absorption: Well absorbed following oral administration.

Distribution: Moderate penetration of the CNS. Crosses the placenta and enters breast milk.
Metabolism and Excretion: Partially metabolized by the liver, up to 50% excreted unchanged by the kidneys.
Half-life: 3–4 hr.

CONTRAINDICATIONS AND PRECAUTIONS

Contraindicated in: ▪ Uncompensated congestive heart failure ▪ Pulmonary edema ▪ Cardiogenic shock ▪ Bradycardia ▪ Heart block ▪ Pregnancy or lactation (may cause apnea, low Apgar scores, bradycardia, and hypoglycemia in the newborn) ▪ Asthma or COPD.
Use Cautiously in: ▪ Thyrotoxicosis or hypoglycemia (may mask symptoms) ▪ Renal impairment (dosage reduction recommended) ▪ Children (safety not established) ▪ Patients with a history of severe allergic reactions (intensity of reactions may be increased).

ADVERSE REACTIONS AND SIDE EFFECTS*

CNS: fatigue, weakness, depression, insomnia, memory loss, mental changes, nightmares, anxiety, nervousness, dizziness.
CV: BRADYCARDIA, CONGESTIVE HEART FAILURE, PULMONARY EDEMA, peripheral vasoconstriction, hypotension, edema.
EENT: dry eyes, blurred vision.
Resp: bronchospasm, wheezing.
GI: diarrhea, nausea.
GU: impotence, diminished libido.
Derm: rash.
Endo: hyperglycemia, hypoglycemia.
MS: joint pain, arthralgia.

INTERACTIONS

Drug–Drug: ▪ General anesthesia, IV phenytoin, and verapamil may cause additive myocardial depression ▪ Additive bradycardia may occur with concurrent use of cardiac glycosides ▪ Additive hypotension may occur with other antihypertensive agents, acute ingestion of alcohol, and nitrates ▪ Use with

epinephrine, cocaine, amphetamines, ephedrine, norepinephrine, phenylephrine, or pseudophedrine may result in unopposed alpha-adrenergic stimulation, hypertension, or bradycardia ▪ Concurrent thyroid administration may decrease effectiveness ▪ Use with insulin may result in prolonged hypoglycemia ▪ May antagonize beta-adrenergic bronchodilators and decrease effectiveness of theophylline ▪ May also reduce metabolism of theophylline ▪ Avoid concurrent use with MAO inhibitors (hypersensitivity may occur) ▪ NSAIDs may decrease antihypertensive effect ▪ May negate the beneficial beta$_1$ cardiac effects of dopamine or dobutamine.

ROUTE AND DOSAGE

▪ **PO (Adults):** 5 mg bid initially, increase by 10 mg/day at 2–3 wk intervals. Usual dose maintenance is 10–15 mg/day in 2–3 divided doses. Single daily dosing may be used when response is determined (up to 60 mg/day).

AVAILABILITY

▪ *Tablets:* 5 mg, 10 mg.

TIME/ACTION PROFILE
(antihypertensive effect)

	ONSET	PEAK	DURATION
PO	7 days	2 wk	8–24 hr

NURSING IMPLICATIONS

ASSESSMENT

▫ Monitor blood pressure and pulse frequently during period of adjustment and periodically throughout therapy. Confer with physician prior to giving drug if pulse is <50 bpm. Assess for orthostatic hypotension when assisting patient up from supine position.
▫ Monitor intake and output ratios and daily weight. Assess patient routinely for evidence of congestive heart failure (peripheral edema, dyspnea, rales/crackles, fatigue, weight gain, jugular venous distention).

*Underlines indicate most frequent; CAPITALS indicate life-threatening.

- **Lab Test Considerations:** Hepatic and renal function and CBC should be monitored routinely in patients receiving prolonged therapy.
- □ May cause elevations in serum potassium, uric acid, triglyceride and lipoprotein levels, and BUN. May also cause elevated antinuclear antibody (ANA) titers.

POTENTIAL NURSING DIAGNOSES

- Cardiac output, decreased (indications, adverse reactions).
- Knowledge deficit related to medication regimen (patient/family teaching).
- Noncompliance (patient/family teaching).

IMPLEMENTATION

- **PO:** May be administered with food or on an empty stomach. May be crushed and mixed with food or fluid if patient has difficulty swallowing.

PATIENT/FAMILY TEACHING

- □ Instruct patient to take medication exactly as directed, even if feeling well. If a dose is missed, it may be taken as soon as remembered up to 4 hr before next dose. Abrupt withdrawal may precipitate life-threatening arrhythmias, hypertension, and myocardial ischemia.
- □ Teach patient and family how to check pulse and blood pressure. Instruct them to take pulse daily and blood pressure biweekly. Advise patient to withhold dose and contact physician if pulse is <50 bpm or blood pressure changes significantly.
- □ Caution patients to make position changes slowly and to avoid standing in a stationary position for long periods to minimize orthostatic hypotension.
- □ Reinforce need to continue additional therapies for hypertension (weight loss, restricted sodium intake, stress reduction, regular exercise, moderation of alcohol consumption, and cessation of smoking). Pindolol helps control but does not cure hypertension.
- □ Caution patient that this medication

may cause increased sensitivity to cold.
- □ Advise patient to consult physician or pharmacist before taking any over-the-counter drugs, especially cold remedies, concurrently with this medication. Patients should also avoid excessive amounts of coffee, tea, and cola.
- □ May cause dizziness or drowsiness. Caution patient to avoid driving and other activities requiring alertness until response to medication is known.
- □ Diabetic patient should monitor serum glucose closely, especially if weakness, fatigue, or irritability occurs. Pindolol may mask tachycardia and increased blood pressure as signs of hypoglycemia, but sweating and dizziness may still occur.
- □ Instruct patient to inform physician or dentist of this therapy prior to treatment or surgery.
- □ Advise patient to carry identification describing medication regimen at all times.
- □ Instruct patient to notify physician if slow pulse rate, dizziness, depression, or skin rash occurs.

EVALUATION

Effectiveness of therapy can be demonstrated by: ■ Decrease in blood pressure. Hypotensive effects may begin within 7 days, but maximum effect is reached in approximately 2 wk.

PIPECURONIUM
(pip-e-**kyoor**-oh-nee-um)
Arduan

CLASSIFICATION(S):
Neuromuscular blocking agent
(nondepolarizing)
Pregnancy Category C

INDICATIONS

- Production of skeletal muscle paralysis and facilitation of intubation after induction of anesthesia in surgical procedures lasting ≥90 min.

ACTION

■ Prevents neuromuscular transmission by blocking the effect of acetylcholine at the myoneural junction ■ Has no analgesic or anxiolytic effects. **Therapeutic Effect:** ■ Skeletal muscle paralysis.

PHARMACOKINETICS

Absorption: Administered IV only, resulting in complete absorption.
Distribution: Distribution not known.
Metabolism and Excretion: >75% excreted by the kidneys, mostly as unmetabolized drug.
Half-life: 1.7 hr (prolonged in renal impairment).

CONTRAINDICATIONS AND PRECAUTIONS

Contraindicated in: ■ Hypersensitivity to pipecuronium or bromides ■ ICU patients requiring prolonged mechanical ventilation ■ Avoid concurrent use with other nondepolarizing neuromuscular blocking agents ■ Not recommended for use before succinylcholine (may be used following recovery).
Use Cautiously in: ■ Cardiovascular disease, edematous states, elderly patients (delays onset time) ■ Obesity (prolongs duration of paralysis; base dose on ideal body weight) ■ Electrolyte disturbances ■ Myasthenia gravis or myasthenic syndromes (extreme caution; duration may be dangerously prolonged) ■ Patients with renal impairment (dosage reduction recommended if creatinine clearance <80 ml/min) ■ Pregnancy or lactation (safety not established).

ADVERSE REACTIONS AND SIDE EFFECTS*

Most adverse reactions to pipecuronium are extensions of pharmacologic effects.
Resp: apnea, respiratory insufficiency.
CV: hypotension, bradycardia.
MS: muscle weakness.
Misc: allergic reactions.

INTERACTIONS

Drug–Drug: ■ Intensity and duration of paralysis may be prolonged by pretreatment with **aminoglycoside antibiotics, polymyxin B, tetracycline, colistin, clindamycin, lidocaine, magnesium salts, quinidine,** or **procainamide** ■ Additive neuromuscular blockade (prolonged duration and recovery) with **inhalation anesthetics (enflurane, isoflurane, halothane).**

ROUTE AND DOSAGE

Doses are listed for nonobese patients with normal renal function.

■ **IV (Adults):** 70–85 mcg/kg (dosage adjustments required for obesity or renal impairment). If given following recovery from succinlycholine during intubation decrease dose to 50 mcg/kg (70–85 mcg/kg if longer paralysis desired). Additional doses of 10–15 mcg/kg may be required as maintenance (dosage reduction recommended if using concurrent inhalation anesthetics).
■ **IV (Children 1–14 yr):** 57 mcg/kg
■ **IV (Infants 3 mo–1 yr):** 40 mcg/kg.

AVAILABILITY

■ *Injection:* 10 mg/vial.

TIME/ACTION PROFILE

	ONSET	PEAK	DURATION
IV	2.5–3 min	5 min	1–2 hr

NURSING IMPLICATIONS

ASSESSMENT

▫ Assess respiratory status continuously throughout pipecuronium therapy. Pipecuronium should be used only by individuals experienced in endotracheal intubation, and equipment for this procedure should be readily available.
▫ Neuromuscular response to pipecuronium should be monitored with a peripheral nerve stimulator. Paralysis is

---

*Underlines indicate most frequent; **CAPITALS** indicate life-threatening.

initially selective and usually occurs sequentially in the following muscles: levator muscles of eyelids, muscles of mastication, limb muscles, abdominal muscles, muscles of the glottis, intercostal muscles, and the diaphragm. Recovery of muscle function usually occurs in reverse order.

□ Observe the patient for residual muscle weakness and respiratory distress during the recovery period.

■ **Toxicity and Overdose:** If overdose occurs, use peripheral nerve stimulator to determine the degree of neuromuscular blockade. Maintain airway patency and ventilation until recovery of normal respirations occur.

□ Administration of anticholinesterase agents (neostigmine, pyridostigmine) may be used to antagonize the action of pipecuronium once patient has demonstrated some spontaneous recovery from neuromuscular block.

□ Administration of fluids and vasopressors may be necessary to treat severe hypotension or shock.

POTENTIAL NURSING DIAGNOSES
■ Breathing pattern, ineffective (indications).
■ Communication, impaired: verbal (side effects).
■ Fear (side effects).

IMPLEMENTATION
■ **General Info:** Dose is titrated to patient response.
□ Pipecuronium has no effect on consciousness or the pain threshold. Adequate anesthesia should *always* be used when pipecuronium is used as an adjunct to surgical procedures.
□ Store at room temperature.
■ **Direct IV:** Reconstitute with 0.9% NaCl, D5W, D5/0.9% NaCl, LR, Sterile Water for Injection, or Bacteriostatic Water for Injection. Solution reconstituted with bacteriostatic water contains benzyl alcohol and should not be used for newborns; use within 5 days. Solution reconstituted with sterile water or other IV solutions should be refrigerated and used within 24 hr. Do not dilute into

or administer from large volume IV solutions.

PATIENT/FAMILY TEACHING
□ Explain all procedures to patient receiving pipecuronium therapy without anesthesia, as consciousness is not affected by pipecuronium alone.
□ Reassure patient that communication abilities will return as the medication wears off.

EVALUATION
Effectiveness of therapy can be demonstrated by: ■ Adequate suppression of the twitch response when tested with peripheral nerve stimulation and subsequent muscle paralysis.

PIPERACILLIN
(pi-**per**-a-sill-in)
Pipracil

PIPERACILLIN/TAZOBACTAM
(pi-**per**-a-sill-in/tay-zoe-**bak**-tam)
Zosyn

CLASSIFICATION(S):
Anti-infective (extended-spectrum penicillin)
Pregnancy Category B

INDICATIONS

■ *Piperacillin:* Treatment of serious infections due to susceptible organisms, including: □ Skin and skin structure infections □ Bone and joint infections □ Septicemia □ Respiratory tract infections □ Intra-abdominal infections □ Gynecologic and urinary tract infections ■ Combination with an aminoglycoside may be synergistic against *Pseudomonas* ■ Has been combined with other antibiotics in the treatment of infections in immunosuppressed patients ■ Perioperative prophylactic anti-infective in abdominal, genitourinary, and head and neck surgery ■ *Piperacillin/tazobactam:* □ Appendicitis □ Skin and skin structure infections □ Gynecologic infections □ Community-acquired pneumonia caused by piperacillin-resistant, beta-lactamase producing bacteria.

ACTION

- **Piperacillin:** Binds to bacterial cell wall membrane, causing cell death. Spectrum is extended when compared with other penicillins ▪ **Tazobactam:** Inhibits beta-lactamase, an enzyme that can destroy penicillins. **Therapeutic Effect:** ▪ Death of susceptible bacteria. **Spectrum:** ▪ **Piperacillin:** Spectrum similar to penicillin but greatly extended, including several important gram-negative aerobic pathogens, notably: □ *Pseudomonas aeruginosa* □ *Escherichia coli* □ *Proteus mirabilis* □ *Providencia rettgeri* □ *Neisseria gonorrhoeae* ▪ Also active against some anaerobic bacteria, including *Bacteroides* ▪ Not active against penicillinase-producing staphylococci or beta-lactamase–producing *Enterobacteriaceae* ▪ **Piperacillin/tazobactam:** Active against piperacillin-resistant, beta-lactamase producing □ *Bacteroides fragilis* □ *E. coli* □ *Staphylococcus aureus* □ *Haemophilus influenzae*.

PHARMACOKINETICS

Absorption: Piperacillin is well absorbed (80%) from IM sites.
Distribution: Widely distributed. Enters CSF well only when meninges are inflamed. Crosses the placenta and enters breast milk in low concentrations.
Metabolism and Excretion: Piperacillin is mostly (90%) excreted unchanged by the kidneys. 10% excreted in bile. Tazobactam is 80% renally excreted.
Half-life: 0.7–1.3 hr.

CONTRAINDICATIONS AND PRECAUTIONS

Contraindicated in: ▪ Hypersensitivity to penicillins, cephalosporins, or tazobactam.
Use Cautiously in: ▪ Renal impairment (dosage reduction or increased interval recommended if creatinine clearance <40 ml/min) ▪ Pregnancy and lactation (safety not established) ▪ Sodium restriction.

ADVERSE REACTIONS AND SIDE EFFECTS*

Piperacillin
CNS: confusion, lethargy, SEIZURES (high doses).
CV: congestive heart failure, arrhythmias.
Derm: rashes, urticaria.
F and E: hypokalemia, hypernatremia.
GI: nausea, diarrhea, hepatitis.
GU: hematuria (children only), interstitial nephritis.
Hemat: bleeding, bloody dyscrasias, increased bleeding time.
Local: phlebitis at IV site, pain at IM site.
Metab: metabolic alkalosis.
Misc: superinfection, hypersensitivity reactions, including ANAPHYLAXIS and serum sickness.
Piperacillin/Tazobactam
CNS: headache, insomnia, agitation, dizziness.
EENT: rhinitis.
Resp: dyspnea.
CV: chest pain, edema, hypertension.
Derm: rash.
Misc: fever, superinfection.

INTERACTIONS

Drug–Drug: ▪ **Probenecid** decreases renal excretion and increases blood levels ▪ May alter excretion of **lithium** ▪ **Diuretics, glucocorticoids,** or **amphotericin B** may increase the risk of hypokalemia ▪ Additive risk of hepatotoxicity with other **hepatotoxic agents** ▪ May decrease the half-life of **aminoglycosides** (given by different routes) when used concurrently in patients with renal impairment.

ROUTE AND DOSAGE

Contains 1.85 mEq sodium/g of piperacillin.

Piperacillin
- **IM, IV (Adults):** 2–4 g q 4–6 hr; lower doses for uncomplicated urinary tract infections or community

---

*Underlines indicate most frequent; **CAPITALS** indicate life-threatening.

acquired pneumonia. 2 g IM with 1 g probenecid PO 30 min before for uncomplicated gonorrhea.

Piperacillin/Tazobactam
- **IV (Adults):** 3 g piperacillin with 0.375 g tazobactam q 6 hr.

AVAILABILITY

Piperacillin
- *Injection:* 2-g, 3-g, 4-g, 40-g vials.

Piperacillin/Tazobactam
- *Injection:* 2 g piperacillin/0.25 g tazobactam, 3 g piperacillin/0.375 g tazobactam, 4 g piperacillin/0.5 g tazobactam.

TIME/ACTION PROFILE (blood levels)

	ONSET	PEAK
IM	rapid	30–50 min
IV	rapid	end of infusion

NURSING IMPLICATIONS

ASSESSMENT
- Assess patient for infection (vital signs; appearance of wound, sputum, urine, and stool; WBC) at beginning and throughout course of therapy.
- Obtain a history before initiating therapy to determine previous use of and reactions to penicillins or cephalosporins. Persons with a negative history of penicillin sensitivity may still have an allergic response.
- Obtain specimens for culture and sensitivity prior to initiating therapy. First dose may be given before receiving results.
- Observe patient for signs and symptoms of anaphylaxis (rash, pruritus, laryngeal edema, wheezing). Discontinue the drug and notify the physician immediately if these occur. Keep epinephrine, an antihistamine, and resuscitation equipment close by in the event of an anaphylactic reaction.
- **Lab Test Considerations:** Renal and hepatic function, CBC, serum potassium, and bleeding times should be evaluated prior to and routinely throughout course of therapy.

- May cause positive direct Coombs' test results.
- May cause elevated BUN, creatinine, AST (SGOT), ALT (SGPT), serum bilirubin, and LDH.
- *Piperacillin* may cause elevated serum sodium and decreased serum potassium concentrations.
- *Piperacillin/tazobactam* may also cause decreased hemoglobin and hematocrit and thrombocytopenia, eosinophilia, leukopenia, neutropenia, prolonged prothrombin and partial thromboplastin time, and increased alkaline phosphatase. It also may cause proteinuria, hematuria, pyuria, hyperglycemia, decreases in total protein or albumin, and abnormalities in sodium, potassium, and calcium levels.

POTENTIAL NURSING DIAGNOSES
- Infection, high risk for (indications, side effects).
- Knowledge deficit related to medication regimen (patient/family teaching).

IMPLEMENTATION
- **IM:** To constitute for IM use, add 4 ml of Sterile Water, Bacteriostatic Water, 0.9% NaCl for Injection, or 0.5 or 1% lidocaine hydrochloride injection (without epinephrine) to each 2-g vial, 6 ml to each 3-g vial, and 7.8 ml to each 4-g vial for a concentration of 1 g/2.5 ml.
- Inject deep into a well-developed muscle mass and massage well. IM injections should not exceed 2 g at each site.

Piperacillin
- **IV:** The initial reconstitution for IV use is made with at least 5 ml of Sterile Water for Injection, 0.9% NaCl, or bacteriostatic water. Shake well until dissolved. Reconstituted solution is stable for 24 hr at room temperature and 7 days if refrigerated.
- Change IV sites every 48 hr to prevent phlebitis.
- **Direct IV:** Inject slowly, over 3–5 min, to minimize vein irritation.
- **Intermittent Infusion:** Dilute in at

least 50 ml of 0.9% NaCl, D5W, D5/0.9% NaCl, or lactated Ringer's solution.
- **Rate:** Administer over 20–30 min via Y-site injection.
- **Syringe Compatibility:** ▪ heparin.
- **Y-Site Compatibility:** ▪ acyclovir ▪ ciprofloxacin ▪ cyclophosphamide ▪ enalaprilat ▪ esmolol ▪ famotidine ▪ fludarabine ▪ foscarnet ▪ hydromorphone ▪ labetalol ▪ magnesium sulfate ▪ meperidine ▪ morphine ▪ perphenazine ▪ verapamil ▪ zidovudine.
- **Y-Site Incompatibility:** ▪ fluconazole ▪ ondansetron. If aminoglycosides and penicillins must be administered concurrently, administer in separate sites.

Piperacillin/Tazobactam
- **Intermittent Infusion:** Reconstitute with 5 ml of 0.9% NaCl, Sterile or Bacteriostatic Water for Injection, Dextran 6% in Saline, or D5W. Do not use lactated Ringer's solution— incompatible. Shake well until dissolved. Dilute further in at least 50 ml of diluent. Discard any unused solution after 24 hr at room temperature or 48 hr if refrigerated.
- **Rate:** Administer over at least 30 min.

PATIENT/FAMILY TEACHING
▫ Advise patient to report the signs of superinfection (black, furry overgrowth on the tongue; vaginal itching or discharge; loose or foul-smelling stools) and allergy.

EVALUATION
Clinical response can be evaluated by:
▪ Resolution of the signs and symptoms of infection. Length of time for complete resolution depends on the organism and site of infection.

PIRBUTEROL
(peer-**byoo**-ter-ole)
Maxair

CLASSIFICATION(S):
Bronchodilator (beta-adrenergic agonist)
Pregnancy Category C

INDICATIONS
▪ Used as a bronchodilator in reversible airway obstruction due to asthma or COPD.

ACTION
▪ Results in the accumulation of cyclic adenosine monophosphate (cAMP) at beta-adrenergic receptors, producing: ▫ Bronchodilation ▫ CNS and cardiac stimulation ▫ Diuresis ▫ Gastric acid secretion ▪ Relatively selective for beta$_2$ (pulmonary) receptors. **Therapeutic Effect:** ▪ Bronchodilation.

PHARMACOKINETICS
Absorption: Minimal systemic absorption following inhalation.
Distribution: Not known.
Metabolism and Excretion: Metabolized by the liver.
Half-life: 2 hr.

CONTRAINDICATIONS AND PRECAUTIONS
Contraindicated in: ▪ Hypersensitivity to adrenergic amines.
Use Cautiously in: ▪ Cardiac disease ▪ Hypertension ▪ Hyperthyroidism ▪ Diabetes mellitus ▪ Glaucoma ▪ Pregnancy (near term) ▪ Elderly patients (more susceptible to adverse reactions; dosage reduction recommended) ▪ Lactation and children (safety not established) ▪ Excessive use (may lead to tolerance and paradoxical bronchospasm).

ADVERSE REACTIONS AND SIDE EFFECTS*
CNS: <u>nervousness</u>, insomnia, <u>tremor</u>, headache.
EENT: dry mouth.
Resp: cough, paradoxical bronchospasm.
CV: palpitations, tachycardia.
GI: nausea.

---

*<u>Underlines</u> indicate most frequent; **CAPITALS** indicate life-threatening.

INTERACTIONS

Drug–Drug: ▪ Increased risk of adverse cardiovascular effects (hypertension, arrhythmias) with concurrent use of **inhalation anesthetics, cocaine, antidepressants, cardiac glycosides, decongestants, CNS stimulants,** and **vasopressors** ▪ Use with **MAO inhibitors** may lead to hypertensive crisis ▪ **Beta-adrenergic blockers** may decrease effectiveness ▪ Although frequently used in combination with **theophylline-type bronchodilators,** CNS and cardiovascular toxicity may be additive.

ROUTE AND DOSAGE

▪ **Inhalation (Adults and Children >12 yr):** 1–2 inhalations q 4–6 hr, not to exceed 12 inhalations/24 hr.

AVAILABILITY

▪ **Aerosol inhaler:** 200 mcg/spray in 25.6-g canister (≥300 sprays) ▪ **Autoinhaler:** 200 mcg/spray in 14-g canister (≥400 sprays).

TIME/ACTION PROFILE
(bronchodilators)

	ONSET	PEAK	DURATION
Inhaln	5–15 min	60–90 min	4–6 hr

NURSING IMPLICATIONS

ASSESSMENT
□ Assess blood pressure, pulse, respiratory pattern, lung sounds, and character of secretions before administration and during peak of medication.
□ Monitor pulmonary function tests before initiating therapy and periodically throughout course to determine effectiveness of medication.
□ Observe patient for paradoxical bronchospasm (wheezing). If this condition occurs, withhold medication and notify physician immediately.

POTENTIAL NURSING DIAGNOSES
▪ Airway clearance, ineffective (indications).
▪ Knowledge deficit related to medication regimen (patient/family teaching).

IMPLEMENTATION
▪ **Inhalation:** Allow at least 1 min between inhalation of aerosol medications. Have patient rinse mouth with water following each inhalation to decrease dry mouth and throat.

PATIENT/FAMILY TEACHING
□ Instruct patient in the proper use of metered-dose inhaler (see Appendix H). Do not take more than 2 inhalations at one time; allow 1–2 min between inhalations. Wash inhalation assembly at least daily in warm running water.
□ Instruct patient in the proper use of autoinhaler. Remove mouthpiece cover, hold autoinhaler upright, push lever at top to up position, and shake gently. Breathe out normally; put mouthpiece in mouth, and close lips firmly around it. Inhale through mouth with a steady, moderate force to cause a puff of medication to be released. Do not stop when puff is heard and felt, but continue inhaling until full deep breath is taken. Take inhaler away from mouth, hold breath for 10 sec, exhale. Lower top lever, and replace cover. Wait 1 min before taking second breath of pirbuterol. Clean mouthpiece weekly.
□ Caution patient not to exceed recommended dose; may cause adverse effects or loss of effectiveness of medication.
□ Patients using inhalation glucocorticoids and pirbuterol should be advised to use pirbuterol first and allow 5 min to elapse between using other aerosols, unless otherwise directed by physician.
□ Advise patient to contact physician immediately if shortness of breath is not relieved by medication or is accompanied by diaphoresis, dizziness, palpitations, or chest pain.
□ Instruct patient to maintain an adequate fluid intake (2000–3000 ml/day) to help liquefy tenacious secretions.
□ Advise patient to consult physician or pharmacist before taking any over-the-counter medications or alcoholic

beverages concurrently with this therapy.

EVALUATION

Effectiveness of therapy can be demonstrated by: ■ Decrease in bronchoconstriction and bronchospasm □ Increased ease of breathing.

PIROXICAM
(peer-**ox**-i-kam)
{Apo-Piroxicam}, Feldene, {Novopirocam}

CLASSIFICATION(S):
Nonsteroidal anti-inflammatory agent
Pregnancy Category UK

INDICATIONS

■ Management of inflammatory disorders, including: □ Rheumatoid arthritis □ Osteoarthritis.

ACTION

■ Inhibits prostaglandin synthesis. **Therapeutic Effects:** ■ Suppression of pain and inflammation.

PHARMACOKINETICS

Absorption: Well absorbed from the GI tract.
Distribution: Distribution not known. Enters breast milk in small amounts.
Metabolism and Excretion: Mostly metabolized by the liver. Minimal amounts excreted unchanged by the kidneys.
Half-life: 50 hr.

CONTRAINDICATIONS AND PRECAUTIONS

Contraindicated in: ■ Hypersensitivity ■ Cross-sensitivity may exist with other nonsteroidal anti-inflammatory agents, including aspirin ■ Active GI bleeding or ulcer disease ■ Pregnancy.
Use Cautiously in: ■ Severe cardiovascular or hepatic disease ■ History of ulcer disease ■ Lactation or children (safety not established) ■ Renal impairment (dosage reduction recommended).

ADVERSE REACTIONS AND SIDE EFFECTS*

CNS: <u>headache</u>, <u>drowsiness</u>, dizziness.
EENT: blurred vision, tinnitus.
CV: edema.
GI: <u>nausea</u>, <u>dyspepsia</u>, <u>vomiting</u>, diarrhea, constipation, GI BLEEDING, <u>discomfort</u>, HEPATITIS, flatulence, anorexia.
GU: renal failure.
Derm: rashes.
Hemat: blood dyscrasias, prolonged bleeding time.
Misc: allergic reactions, including ANAPHYLAXIS.

INTERACTIONS

Drug–Drug: Concurrent use with **aspirin** decreases piroxicam blood levels and may decrease effectiveness ■ Increased risk of bleeding with **anticoagulants, cefamandole, cefoperazone, cefotetan, heparin, thrombolytic agents, valproic acid,** or **plicamycin** ■ Additive adverse GI side effects with **aspirin, glucocorticoids,** and other **nonsteroidal anti-inflammatory agents** ■ **Probenecid** increases blood levels and may increase toxicity ■ May decrease response to **antihypertensives** or **diuretics** ■ May increase serum levels and risk of toxicity from **lithium** ■ Increased risk of photosensitivity with other **photosensitizing agents** ■ May increase risk of hypoglycemia from **insulin** or **oral hypoglycemic agents** ■ Increased risk of adverse renal effects with **gold compounds, cyclosporine,** or chronic use of **acetaminophen** ■ May increase the risk of hematologic toxicity from **antineoplastic agents** or **radiation therapy**.

ROUTE AND DOSAGE

■ **PO (Adults):** 20 mg/day, may be given as single dose or 2 divided doses.

{} = Available in Canada only.
*<u>Underlines</u> indicate most frequent; **CAPITALS** indicate life-threatening.

AVAILABILITY

▪ *Capsules:* 10 mg, 20 mg ▪ {*Suppositories:* 10 mg, 20 mg}.

TIME/ACTION PROFILE

	ONSET	PEAK	DURATION
PO (analgesic effect)	1 hr	UK	48–72 hr
PO (anti-inflammatory effect)	7–12 days	2–3 wk*	UK

*May take up to 12 wk.

NURSING IMPLICATIONS

ASSESSMENT

▪ **General Info:** Patients who have asthma, aspirin-induced allergy, and nasal polyps are at increased risk for developing hypersensitivity reactions. Monitor for rhinitis, asthma, and urticaria.

▪ **Arthritis:** Assess pain and range of motion prior to and 1–2 hr following administration.

▪ **Lab Test Considerations:** BUN, serum creatinine, CBC, serum potassium, and liver function tests should be evaluated periodically in patients receiving prolonged courses of therapy.

▫ Serum potassium, alkaline phosphatase, LDH, AST (SGOT), and ALT (SGPT) levels may be increased.

▫ Hematocrit, hemoglobin, and uric acid concentrations may be decreased. Blood glucose concentrations may be increased or decreased.

▫ Bleeding time may be prolonged for up to 2 wk following discontinuation of therapy.

POTENTIAL NURSING DIAGNOSES

▪ Pain (indications).
▪ Physical mobility, impaired (indications).
▪ Knowledge deficit related to medication regimen (patient/family teaching).

IMPLEMENTATION

▪ **PO:** Administered with meals or antacids (preferably magnesium-containing or aluminum-containing) to decrease GI irritation.

PATIENT/FAMILY TEACHING

▫ Advise patients to take this medication with a full glass of water and to remain in an upright position for 15–30 min after administration.

▫ Instruct patient to take medication exactly as directed. If a dose is missed, it should be taken as soon as remembered but not if almost time for the next dose. Do not double doses.

▫ This medication may cause drowsiness or dizziness. Advise patient to avoid driving or other activities requiring alertness until response to the medication is known.

▫ Caution patient to avoid the concurrent use of alcohol, aspirin, ibuprofen, acetaminophen, or other over-the-counter medications without consultation with physician or pharmacist.

▫ Advise patient to notify physician or dentist of medication regimen prior to treatment or surgery.

▫ Instruct patient to notify physician if rash, itching, chills, fever, muscle aches, visual disturbances, weight gain, edema, black stools, or persistent headache occurs.

EVALUATION

Effectiveness of therapy can be demonstrated by: ▪ Decreased pain and improved joint mobility. Partial arthritic relief is usually seen within 2 wk, but maximum effectiveness may require up to 12 wk of continuous therapy. Patients who do not respond to one nonsteroidal anti-inflammatory agent may respond to another.

PLASMA PROTEIN FRACTION

(**plaz**-ma **proe**-teen **frak**-shun)
Plasmanate, Plasma-Plex, Plasmatein, Protenate

CLASSIFICATION(S):
Volume expander
Pregnancy Category C

INDICATIONS

- Expansion of plasma volume and maintenance of cardiac output in situations associated with deficiencies in circulatory volume, including: □ Shock □ Hemorrhage □ Burns ■ Temporary replacement therapy in edema associated with low plasma proteins, such as the nephrotic syndrome and end-stage liver disease.

ACTION

- Provides colloidal osmotic pressure (in the form of albumin and globulins) within the intravascular space, causing the shift of water from extravascular tissues back into the intravascular space. **Therapeutic Effect:** ■ Mobilization of fluid from extravascular tissue into intravascular space.

PHARMACOKINETICS

Absorption: Administered IV only, resulting in complete bioavailability.
Distribution: Stays mainly in the intravascular space.
Metabolism and Excretion: UK.
Half-life: UK.

CONTRAINDICATIONS AND PRECAUTIONS

Contraindicated in: ■ Allergic reactions to albumin ■ Severe anemia ■ Congestive heart failure ■ Normal or increased intravascular volume ■ Cardiopulmonary bypass procedures.
Use Cautiously in: ■ Severe hepatic or renal disease ■ Rapid infusion (may cause hypotension or hypertension) ■ Dehydration (additional fluids may be required) ■ Large doses (may cause anemia, requiring transfusion).

ADVERSE REACTIONS AND SIDE EFFECTS*

CNS: headache.
CV: tachycardia, hypotension, vascular overload.
GI: nausea, vomiting, excess salivation.
Derm: erythema, urticaria.
MS: back pain.
Misc: fever, chills, flushing.

INTERACTIONS

Drug–Drug: ■ None significant.

ROUTE AND DOSAGE

Dose is highly individualized and depends on condition being treated. Contains 130–160 mEq sodium/liter. Not to exceed 250 g/24 hr.

Hypovolemia
- **IV (Adults):** 250–500 ml (12.5–25 g protein).
- **IV (Infants and Young Children):** 6.3–33 ml/kg (0.33–1.65 g/kg protein).

Hypoproteinemia
- **IV (Adults):** 1000–1500 ml (50–75 g protein).

AVAILABILITY

- *Injection:* 5% in 50 ml, 250 ml, 500-ml vials.

TIME/ACTION PROFILE
(intravascular volume expansion)

	ONSET	PEAK	DURATION
IV	15–30 min	UK	UK

NURSING IMPLICATIONS

ASSESSMENT

□ Monitor vital signs, CVP, pulmonary capillary wedge pressure (PCWP), and intake and output prior to and frequently throughout therapy. Hypotension may result from too rapid infusion.

□ Assess patient for signs of vascular overload (elevated CVP, elevated PCWP, rales/crackles, dyspnea, hypertension, jugular venous distention) during and following administration.

□ Assess surgical patients for increased bleeding following administration caused by increased blood pressure and circulating blood volume. Plasma protein fraction does not contain clotting factors.

- **Lab Test Considerations:** Monitor hemoglobin, hematocrit, serum protein, and electrolytes throughout course of therapy.

*Underlines indicate most frequent; **CAPITALS** indicate life-threatening.

POTENTIAL NURSING DIAGNOSES
- Cardiac output, decreased (indications).
- Fluid volume deficit (indications).
- Fluid volume excess (side effects).

IMPLEMENTATION
- **General Info:** Administer through a large-gauge (at least 20-G) needle. Use administration set provided by manufacturer.
- ☐ Solution may vary from nearly colorless to straw to brownish. Do not use cloudy solution. Each liter of plasma protein fraction contains 130–160 mEq of sodium. Store at room temperature. Do not administer more than 250 g (5000 ml 5%) in 48 hr.
- ☐ There is no danger of serum hepatitis from plasma protein fraction. Cross-matching is not required.
- ☐ Dehydration should be corrected by additional IV fluids.
- **Intermittent Infusion:** Administer plasma protein fraction undiluted by IV infusion. Infusion must be completed within 4 hr.
- *Rate:* Rate of administration is determined by blood volume, indication, and patient response but should not exceed 10 ml/min, to minimize the possibility of hypotension. As the plasma volume approaches normal, the rate of administration should not exceed 5–8 ml/min. The rate for infants and children should not exceed 5–10 ml/min. Monitor the patient for signs of hypervolemia.
- **Additive Compatibility:** ▪ carbohydrate and electrolyte solutions ▪ whole blood ▪ packed red blood cells ▪ chloramphenicol.
- **Additive Incompatibility:** solutions containing protein hydrolysates ▪ amino acids ▪ alcohol ▪ norepinephrine.

PATIENT/FAMILY TEACHING
- ☐ Explain the rationale for use of this solution to the patient.

EVALUATION
Effectiveness of therapy can be demonstrated by: ▪ Increase in blood pressure and blood volume when used to treat shock ▪ Elevated serum plasma protein in patients with hypoproteinemia.

PLICAMYCIN
(plye-ka-**mye**-sin)
mithramycin, Mithracin

CLASSIFICATION(S):
Antineoplastic (antitumor antibiotic), Electrolyte modifier (hypocalcemic agent)
Pregnancy Category X

INDICATIONS
▪ Treatment of advanced unresponsive testicular carcinoma ▪ Management of hypercalcemia and hypercalciuria associated with malignancy.

ACTION
▪ Forms a complex with DNA that subsequently inhibits RNA synthesis ▪ Antagonizes the action of vitamin D and inhibits the action of parathyroid hormone on osteoclasts. **Therapeutic Effects:** ▪ Death of rapidly replicating cells, particularly malignant ones ▪ Lowering of serum calcium.

PHARMACOKINETICS
Absorption: Administered IV only, resulting in complete bioavailability.
Distribution: Appears to concentrate in the liver, renal tubule, and bone surface. Crosses the blood–brain barrier.
Metabolism and Excretion: Excreted primarily by the kidneys.
Half-life: UK.

CONTRAINDICATIONS AND PRECAUTIONS
Contraindicated in: ▪ Hypersensitivity ▪ Bleeding disorders ▪ Depressed bone-marrow reserve ▪ Hypocalcemia ▪ Severe renal or liver disease ▪ Pregnancy or lactation.

Use Cautiously in: ▪ Patients with childbearing potential ▪ Active infections ▪ Other chronic debilitating illnesses ▪ Renal or hepatic impairment (dosage reduction required) ▪ Children (safety not established).

ADVERSE REACTIONS AND SIDE EFFECTS*

CNS: drowsiness, weakness, lethargy, malaise, headache, depression, nervousness, irritability, dizziness, fatigue.
EENT: epistaxis.
GI: anorexia, nausea, vomiting, stomatitis, diarrhea, hepatitis.
GU: renal failure, gonadal suppression.
Derm: facial flushing, rashes.
F and E: <u>hypocalcemia</u>, hypophosphatemia, hypokalemia, rebound hypercalcemia.
Hemat: BLEEDING, <u>thrombocytopenia</u>, leukopenia, anemia.
Local: phlebitis at IV site.
Misc: fever.

INTERACTIONS

Drug–Drug: ▪ Additive myelosuppression with other **antineoplastic agents** or **radiation therapy** ▪ Increased risk of bleeding with **aspirin, oral anticoagulants, thrombolytic agents, heparin, some cephalosporins, nonsteroidal anti-inflammatory agents, sulfinpyrazone, valproic acid,** or **dextran** ▪ Increased risk of hepatotoxicity with other **hepatotoxic agents** ▪ Increased risk of renal toxicity with other **nephrotoxic agents.**

ROUTE AND DOSAGE

Testicular Tumors
▪ **IV (Adults):** 25–30 mcg/kg once daily for 8–10 days or 25–50 mcg/kg every other day for 8 doses. May be repeated monthly.

Hypercalcemia, Hypercalciuria
▪ **IV (Adults):** 15–25 mcg/kg once daily for 3–4 days, may be repeated after 7 days or 2–3 times weekly.

AVAILABILITY
▪ *Injection:* 2500 mcg/vial.

TIME/ACTION PROFILE

	ONSET	PEAK	DURATION
IV (hematologic effects)	UK	7–10 days	3–4 wk
IV (hypocalcemic effects)	24–48 hr	UK	3–15 days

NURSING IMPLICATIONS

ASSESSMENT

▪ **General Info:** Monitor closely for bleeding (bleeding gums; bruising; petechiae; guaiac stools, urine, and emesis). May begin as epistaxis and progress to severe generalized or GI bleeding. May require blood transfusions, fresh frozen plasma, vitamin K, or aminocaproic acid to control bleeding. Avoid IM injections and rectal temperatures. Apply pressure to venipuncture sites for 10 min.

□ Monitor intake and output, appetite, and nutritional intake. May cause nausea and vomiting. Confer with physician regarding prophylactic use of an antiemetic. Adjust diet as tolerated to help maintain fluid and electrolyte balance and nutritional status.

□ Assess for fever, sore throat, and signs of infection. Notify physician if these symptoms occur.

▪ **Hypercalcemia:** Monitor symptoms of hypercalcemia (nausea, vomiting, anorexia, thirst, weakness, constipation, paralytic ileus, and bradycardia). Observe patient for evidence of hypocalcemia (paresthesia, muscle twitching, laryngospasm, colic, cardiac arrhythmias, and Chvostek's or Trousseau's sign).

▪ **Lab Test Considerations:** Monitor platelet count, prothrombin time, and bleeding time prior to and periodically throughout therapy. Notify physician if platelet count is <150,000/mm^3 or prothrombin time is elevated 4 or more seconds above control.

□ Monitor CBC and differential prior to

---

*Underlines indicate most frequent; **CAPITALS** indicate life-threatening.

and periodically throughout therapy. Notify physician if leukocyte count is <4000/mm³.

□ Monitor serum electrolytes prior to and daily during course of therapy. May cause hypocalcemia, hypokalemia, and hypophosphatemia. Correct electrolyte imbalances before beginning therapy. Calcium and phosphate levels may rebound after therapy.

□ Monitor liver function studies AST [SGOT], ALT [SGPT], LDH, bilirubin) and renal function studies (BUN, creatinine, urinalysis) prior to and periodically throughout therapy to detect hepatotoxicity and nephrotoxicity.

POTENTIAL NURSING DIAGNOSES

- Injury, high risk for (side effects).
- Infection, high risk for (side effects).
- Body image disturbance (side effects).

IMPLEMENTATION

- **General Info:** Solution should be prepared in a biologic cabinet. Wear gloves, gown, and mask while handling medication. Discard equipment in designated containers (see Appendix I).

□ Ensure patency of the IV. If patient complains of discomfort at the IV site or if extravasation occurs, discontinue IV and restart at another site. Extravasation may cause irritation and cellulitis. Apply ice to site to prevent pain and swelling. If swelling occurs, confer with physician regarding application of moderate heat to site.

- **IV:** To reconstitute, add 4.9 ml of Sterile Water for Injection to the 2.5-mg vial of plicamycin to yield a final concentration of 500 mcg/ml. Use immediately after reconstitution.

- **Direct IV:** May be administered undiluted IV push to decrease risk of extravasation.

- *Rate:* Administer over 20–30 min.

- **Intermittent Infusion:** Add to 1000 ml of D5W or 0.9% NaCl.

- *Rate:* Infuse over 4–6 hr. Rapid infusion rate will increase GI side effects.

PATIENT/FAMILY TEACHING

□ Advise patient to notify physician promptly if fever, chills, sore throat, signs of infection, bleeding gums, bruising, petechiae, or blood in urine, stool, or emesis occurs. Caution patient to avoid crowds and persons with known infections. Instruct patient to use soft toothbrush and electric razor. Patients should be cautioned not to drink alcoholic beverages or take products containing aspirin or ibuprofen.

□ Instruct patient to notify physician if weakness, rash, persistent nausea or vomiting, or depression occurs.

□ Instruct patient to inspect oral mucosa for redness and ulceration. If mouth sores occur, advise patient to use sponge brush and rinse mouth with water after eating and drinking. Viscous lidocaine swishes may be used if pain interferes with eating.

□ Advise patient that although fertility may be decreased with plicamycin, contraception should be used during therapy because of potential teratogenic effects on the fetus.

□ Instruct patient not to receive any vaccinations without advice of physician.

□ Emphasize need for periodic lab tests to monitor for side effects.

EVALUATION

Effectiveness of therapy can be demonstrated by: ■ Decrease in size and spread of malignant tissue ■ Normalization of elevated calcium levels in hypercalcemia and hypercalciuria within 24–48 hr.

POLYCARBOPHIL
(pol-i-**kar**-boe-fil)
Equalactin, Fiberall, FiberCon, Mitrolan

CLASSIFICATION(S):
Laxative (bulk-forming agent),
Antidiarrheal
Pregnancy Category UK

INDICATIONS

- Treatment of constipation or diarrhea.

ACTION

- Acts as a bulk laxative by keeping water within the bowel lumen - Acts as an antidiarrheal by taking on water within the bowel lumen to create a formed stool. **Therapeutic Effect:** - Normalization of bowel water content while adding bulk, treating both diarrhea and constipation.

PHARMACOKINETICS

Absorption: Minimal systemic absorption.
Distribution: Distribution not known.
Metabolism and Excretion: Complex plus absorbed water is excreted in the feces.
Half-life: UK.

CONTRAINDICATIONS AND PRECAUTIONS

Contraindicated in: - Hypersensitivity - Abdominal pain - Nausea or vomiting (especially when associated with fever or other signs of acute abdomen) - Serious intra-abdominal adhesions - Dysphagia.
Use Cautiously in: - Pregnancy or lactation (has been used safely).

ADVERSE REACTIONS AND SIDE EFFECTS*

GI: abdominal fullness.

INTERACTIONS

Drug–Drug: - May decrease the absorption of concurrently administered tetracycline.

ROUTE AND DOSAGE

- **PO (Adults):** 1 g 1–4 times daily or as needed, not to exceed 6 g/24 hr.
- **PO (Children 6–12 yr):** 500 mg 1–3 times daily or as needed, not to exceed 3 g/24 hr.
- **PO (Children 2–6 yr):** 500 mg 1–2 times daily, or as needed, not to exceed 1.5 g/24 hr.

AVAILABILITY

- **Tablets:** 500 mg - **Chewable tablets:** 500 mg, 1000 mg.

TIME/ACTION PROFILE (effect on bowel function)

	ONSET	PEAK	DURATION
PO	12–24 hr*	UK	UK

*May take as long as 72 hr.

NURSING IMPLICATIONS

ASSESSMENT

- **General Info:** Assess for fever, nausea, vomiting, abdominal distention, and pain. Notify physician if present. Auscultate bowel sounds. Inquire about patient's usual diet, fluid intake, activity level, and bowel function.
  - Monitor for color, consistency, and amount of stool produced.
- **Diarrhea:** Monitor for signs of dehydration (decreased skin turgor, dry mucous membranes, weight loss, decreased urine output, tachycardia, and hypotension).

POTENTIAL NURSING DIAGNOSES

- Constipation (indications).
- Diarrhea (indications).
- Knowledge deficit related to medication regimen (patient/family teaching).

IMPLEMENTATION

- **General Info:** Administer 1 hr before or 2 hr after tetracycline.
- **Diarrhea:** For treatment of severe diarrhea, dose may be repeated every 30 min. Do not exceed total daily prescribed dose.
- **Constipation:** For treatment of constipation, administer with 8 oz of water or juice.

PATIENT/FAMILY TEACHING

- Encourage patients with constipation to use other forms of bowel regulation, such as increasing bulk in diet, fluid intake, and mobility. Normal bowel habits are individualized and

---

*<u>Underlines</u> indicate most frequent; **CAPITALS** indicate life-threatening.

may vary from 3 times/day to 3 times/wk.

□ Instruct patients with sudden onset of constipation to notify physician, as medical evaluation may be necessary.

□ Instruct patients with diarrhea to notify physician if fever or bloody stools occur or if diarrhea persists or worsens. Discuss need for fluids and diet modifications during episode of diarrhea.

EVALUATION

Effectiveness of therapy can be demonstrated by: ▪ Soft, formed bowel movement. May require 3 days for therapeutic effect to occur.

POLYETHYLENE GLYCOL/ ELECTROLYTE

(po-lee-**eth**-e-leen **glye**-kole/ e-**lek**-troe-lite)
Colovage, Colyte, GoLYTELY, NuLytely, OCL, Peglyte

CLASSIFICATION(S):
Laxative (osmotic)
Pregnancy Category C

INDICATIONS

▪ Bowel cleansing in preparation for GI examination. **Unlabeled Use:** ▪ Treatment of acute iron overdose in children.

ACTION

▪ Polyethylene glycol (PEG) in solution acts as an osmotic agent, drawing water into the lumen of the GI tract. **Therapeutic Effect:** ▪ Evacuation of the GI tract without water or electrolyte imbalance.

PHARMACOKINETICS

Absorption: Ions in the solution are nonabsorbable.
Distribution: Distribution not known.
Metabolism and Excretion: Solution is excreted in fecal contents.
Half-life: UK.

CONTRAINDICATIONS AND PRECAUTIONS

Contraindicated in: ▪ GI obstruction ▪ Gastric retention ▪ Toxic colitis ▪ Megacolon.
Use Cautiously in: ▪ Patients with absent or diminished gag reflex ▪ Unconscious or semicomatose states, in which administration is via nasogastric tube ▪ Barium enema using double-contrast technique (may not allow proper barium coating of mucosa) ▪ Abdominal pain of uncertain cause, particularly if accompanied by fever ▪ Children (safety not established).

ADVERSE REACTIONS AND SIDE EFFECTS*

GI: <u>abdominal fullness</u>, nausea, bloating, cramps, vomiting.

INTERACTIONS

Drug–Drug: ▪ Interferes with the absorption of **orally administered medications** by decreasing transit time. (Do not administer within 1 hr of start of therapy.)

ROUTE AND DOSAGE

▪ **PO (Adults):** 240 ml q 10 min (up to 4 liters) until fecal discharge appears clear and has no solid material. May be given through nasogastric tube at 20–30 ml/min.
▪ **PO (Children):** 25–40 ml/kg/hr until fecal discharge is clear and has no solid material. May also be given through a nasogastric tube.

AVAILABILITY

▪ *Oral solution* ▪ *Powder for oral solution.*

TIME/ACTION PROFILE

	ONSET	PEAK	DURATION
PO	1 hr	UK	4 hr

NURSING IMPLICATIONS

ASSESSMENT

□ Assess patient for abdominal disten-

tion, presence of bowel sounds, and usual pattern of bowel function.
□ Assess color, consistency, and amount of stool produced.
□ Monitor semiconscious or unconscious patients closely for regurgitation when administering via nasogastric tube.

POTENTIAL NURSING DIAGNOSES
- Diarrhea (side effects).
- Knowledge deficit related to medication regimen (patient/family teaching).

IMPLEMENTATION
- **General Info:** Do not add flavorings or additional ingredients to solution prior to administration.
□ Patient should fast for 3–4 hr prior to administration and should never have solid food within 2 hr of administration.
□ Patient should be allowed only clear liquids after administration.
□ May be administered on the morning of the examination as long as time is allotted to drink solution (3 hr) and evacuate bowel (1 additional hr). For barium enema, administer solution early evening (6 PM) prior to exam to allow proper mucosal coating by barium.
- **PO:** Solution may be reconstituted with tap water. Shake vigorously until powder is dissolved.
□ May be administered via nasogastric tube at a rate of 20–30 ml/min.

PATIENT/FAMILY TEACHING
□ Instruct patient to drink 240 ml every 10 min until 4 liters have been consumed or fecal discharge is clear and free of solid matter. Rapidly drinking each 240 ml is preferred over drinking small amounts continuously.

EVALUATION
Effectiveness of therapy can be demonstrated by: - Diarrhea, which cleanses the bowel within 4 hr. The first bowel movement usually occurs within 1 hr of administration.

POLYMYXIN B
(pol-ee-**mix**-in bee)
Aerosporin

CLASSIFICATION(S):
Anti-infective (miscellaneous)
Pregnancy Category UK

INDICATIONS
- **IM, IV:** Treatment of the following serious infections due to susceptible organisms in patients who are unable to tolerate less toxic anti-infectives: □ Urinary tract infections □ Meningitis (requires additional intrathecal administration) □ Septicemia - **Ophth:** Ophthalmic infections - **Top:** Used locally in combination with other anti-infectives in a wide variety of dosage forms for the treatment and prevention of superficial infections.

ACTION
- Binds to bacterial cell wall, resulting in death of the organism. **Therapeutic Effect:** - Bactericidal action. **Spectrum:** - Limited to some gram-negative pathogens that may be resistant to other anti-infectives, including: □ *Haemophilus influenzae* □ *Pseudomonas aeruginosa* □ *Enterobacter aerogenes* □ *Klebsiella pneumoniae* - Not active against *Proteus* or *Neisseria* species.

PHARMACOKINETICS
Absorption: Poorly absorbed following oral administration (up to 10% in neonates). Well absorbed following IM administration. Minimal systemic absorption following topical use.
Distribution: Widely distributed. Does not enter the CNS or cross the placenta.
Metabolism and Excretion: 60% excreted unchanged by the kidneys.
Half-life: 4.3–6 hr (increased in renal impairment).

CONTRAINDICATIONS AND PRECAUTIONS
Contraindicated in: - Hypersensitivity.
Use Cautiously in: - Neuromuscular

diseases, including myasthenia gravis
■ Renal impairment (dosage reduction
recommended) ■ Pregnancy or lactation
(safety not established).

ADVERSE REACTIONS AND SIDE EFFECTS*

CNS: neurotoxicity; IT—headache.
EENT: Ophth—blurred vision, sting-
ing, burning, itching.
Resp: RESPIRATORY PARALYSIS.
GU: nephrotoxicity.
Derm: flushing of the face, rashes;
Top—allergic contact dermatitis.
Local: pain at IM site, phlebitis at IV
site.
MS: IT—stiff neck.
Neuro: neuromuscular blockade.
Misc: fever, hypersensitivity reactions,
including ANAPHYLAXIS, fungal super-
infection.

INTERACTIONS

Drug–Drug: ■ Increased risk of neuromuscular blockade with **general anesthetics** or **neuromuscular blocking
agents, aminoglycoside anti-infectives,
procainamide,** or **quinidine.**

ROUTE AND DOSAGE

1 mg = 10,000 units.

■ **IV (Adults and Children >2 yr):**
15,000–25,000 units/kg/day in divided doses q 12 hr (not to exceed
25,000 units/kg/day).
■ **IM (Adults and Children >2 yr):**
25,000–30,000 units/kg/day in divided doses q 4–6 hr.
■ **IV, IM (Infants):** up to 40,000 units/
kg/day in divided doses.
■ **IT (Adults and Children >2 yr):**
50,000 units/day for 3–4 days, then
every other day for 2 wk after negative CSF cultures and normal CSF
glucose.
■ **Intrathecal (Children <2 yr):**
20,000 units/day for 3–4 days then
25,000 units every other day for 2 wk
after negative CSF cultures and normal CSF glucose; or, 25,000 units
every other day continued for 2 wk

after negative CSF cultures and normal CSF glucose.
■ **Ophth:** 1–3 drops q 1 hr; dosage interval may be increased as response
occurs.

AVAILABILITY

■ *Injection:* 500,000 units/vial ■ *Powder for ophthalmic solution:* 500,000
units/20–50 ml ■ *In combination with:*
neomycin, prednisolone, hydrocortisone, dexamethasone in ophthalmic
preparations. See Appendix A.

TIME/ACTION PROFILE (blood levels)

	ONSET	PEAK
IV	rapid	end of infusion
IM	rapid	within 2 hr

NURSING IMPLICATIONS

ASSESSMENT

▫ Assess patient for infection (vital
signs; appearance of wound, sputum,
urine, and stool; WBC) at beginning
and throughout course of therapy.
▫ Obtain specimens for culture and
sensitivity prior to initiating therapy.
First dose may be given before receiving results.
▫ Monitor intake and output and daily
weight to assess hydration status and
renal function. Notify physician if a
decrease in urine output occurs.
▫ Assess patient for neurotoxic reaction
(irritability, weakness, ataxia, drowsiness, perioral paresthesia, numbness of extremities, blurred vision)
throughout course of therapy. Neurotoxicity is usually associated with
high serum levels.
▫ Assess patient for signs of superinfection (fever, upper respiratory infection, vaginal itching or discharge, increasing malaise, diarrhea). Report
occurrence to physician.
▫ Monitor IV site for thrombophlebitis
throughout therapy.
■ **Lab Test Considerations:** Monitor renal function by urinalysis, specific

gravity, BUN, creatinine, and creatinine clearance prior to and throughout therapy.

POTENTIAL NURSING DIAGNOSES
- Infection, high risk for (indications).
- Injury, high risk for (side effects).

IMPLEMENTATION
- **General Info:** Keep patient well hydrated (1500–2000 ml/day) during therapy.
- **IM:** Reconstitute each 500,000-unit vial with 2 ml of Sterile Water for Injection, 0.9% NaCl, or procaine 1%.
- ☐ IM administration is not routinely recommended because of severe pain at injection site. Administer deep into a well-developed muscle.
- **Intermittent Infusion:** Dilute each 500,000 units in 300–500 ml of D5W. Solution should be refrigerated; discard unused portions after 72 hr.
- ***Rate:*** Infuse slowly over 60–90 min.
- **Y-Site Compatibility:** ▪ esmolol.
- **Additive Compatibility:** ▪ amikacin ▪ colistimethate ▪ diphenhydramine ▪ erythromycin lactobionate ▪ hydrocortisone sodium succinate ▪ kanamycin ▪ methicillin ▪ penicillin G potassium ▪ sodium.
- **Additive Incompatibility:** ▪ amphotericin B ▪ cefazolin ▪ cephalothin ▪ chloramphenicol ▪ heparin ▪ magnesium sulfate ▪ prednisolone sodium phosphate.
- **IT:** Dissolve 500,000 units of polymyxin B in 10 ml of 0.9% NaCl for a concentration of 50,000 units/ml.
- **Ophth:** See Appendix H for administration of ophthalmic preparations.

PATIENT/FAMILY TEACHING
- **IM, IV:** Advise patient to notify physician or nurse if symptoms of superinfection occur.
- **Ophth:** Instruct patient on correct method for instillation of ophthalmic preparation. Solution may cause temporary blurring of vision or burning.
- ☐ Advise patient to notify physician if stinging, burning, or itching becomes pronounced or if redness, irritation, swelling, or pain becomes pronounced or persists.

EVALUATION
Clinical response to therapy can be evaluated by: ▪ Resolution of the signs and symptoms of infection. Length of time for complete resolution depends on the organism and site of infection.

POTASSIUM AND SODIUM PHOSPHATES
(**foss**-fates)

Monobasic Potassium and Sodium Phosphates
K-Phos M.F., K-Phos Neutral, K-Phos No. 2

Potassium and Sodium Phosphates
Uro-KP Neutral, Neutra-Phos

CLASSIFICATION(S):
Electrolyte (phosphate supplement), Urinary acidifier, Antiurolithic
Pregnancy Category C

INDICATIONS

- Treatment and prevention of phosphate depletion in patients who are unable to ingest adequate dietary potassium (potassium and sodium phosphate) ▪ Adjunct therapy of urinary tract infections with methenamine hippurate or mandelate (potassium and sodium phosphates or monobasic potassium phosphate) ▪ Prevention of calcium urinary stones (potassium and sodium phosphates or monobasic potassium phosphate) ▪ Phosphate salts of potassium may be used in hypokalemic patients with metabolic acidosis or coexisting phosphorus deficiency.

ACTION

- Phosphate is present in bone and is involved in energy transfer and carbohydrate metabolism ▪ Serves as a buffer for the excretion of hydrogen ions by the kidneys ▪ Dibasic potassium phosphate is converted in renal tubule to monobasic salt, resulting in urinary acidification, which is required for methenamine hippurate or mandelate to be active as urinary anti-infectives ▪ Acidification of urine increases solubility of calcium, decreasing calcium stone formation. **Therapeutic Effects:** ▪ Replacement of phosphorus in deficiency states ▪ Urinary acidification ▪ Increased efficacy of methenamine ▪ Decreased formation of calcium urinary tract stones.

PHARMACOKINETICS

Absorption: Well absorbed following oral administration. Vitamin D promotes GI absorption of phosphates.
Distribution: Phosphates enter extracellular fluids and are then actively transported to sites of action.
Metabolism and Excretion: Excreted mainly (>90%) by the kidneys.
Half-life: UK.

CONTRAINDICATIONS AND PRECAUTIONS

Contraindicated in: ▪ Hyperkalemia (potassium salts) ▪ Hyperphosphatemia ▪ Hypocalcemia ▪ Severe renal impairment ▪ Untreated Addison's disease (potassium salts) ▪ Severe tissue trauma (potassium salts) ▪ Hyperkalemic familial periodic paralysis (potassium salts).
Use Cautiously in: ▪ Hyperparathyroidism ▪ Cardiac disease ▪ Hypernatremia (sodium phosphate only) ▪ Hypertension (sodium phosphate only) ▪ Renal impairment.

ADVERSE REACTIONS AND SIDE EFFECTS*

Related to hyperphosphatemia, unless indicated.
CNS: listlessness, confusion, weakness.
CV: ARRHYTHMIAS, ECG changes (absent P waves, widening of the QRS complex with biphasic curve), CARDIAC ARREST, hypotension; hyperkalemia—ARRHYTHMIAS, ECG changes (prolonged PR interval, ST segment depression, tall-tented T waves); hypernatremia—edema.
F and E: hypomagnesemia, hyperphosphatemia, hyperkalemia, hypocalcemia, hypernatremia.
GI: diarrhea, nausea, vomiting, abdominal pain.
Local: phlebitis, irritation at IV site.
MS: hypocalcemia—tremors; hyperkalemia—muscle cramps.
Neuro: paresthesias of extremities, flaccid paralysis, heaviness of legs.

INTERACTIONS

Drug–Drug: ▪ Concurrent use of **potassium-sparing diuretics** or **angiotensin converting enzyme (ACE) inhibitors** with potassium phosphates may result in hyperkalemia ▪ Concurrent use of **glucocorticoids** with sodium phosphate may result in hypernatremia ▪ Concurrent administration of **calcium-, magnesium-,** or **aluminum-**containing compounds decreases absorption of phosphates by formation of insoluble complexes ▪ **Vitamin D** enhances the absorption of phosphates.
Drug–Food: ▪ **Oxalates** (in spinach and rhubarb) and **phytates** (in bran and whole grains) may decrease the absorption of phosphates by binding them in the GI tract.

ROUTE AND DOSAGE

Monobasic Potassium and Sodium Phosphates
▪ **PO (Adults and Children >4 yr):** 250 mg (8 mmol) qid; may be increased to 250 mg (8 mmol) q 2 hr (not to exceed 2 g phosphorus/24 hr).
▪ **PO (Children <4 yr):** 200 mg (6.4 mmol) qid.

Potassium and Sodium Phosphates
▪ **PO (Adults and Children >4 yr):** 250 mg (8 mmol) phosphorus qid.
▪ **PO (Children <4 yr):** 200 mg (6.4 mmol) qid.

AVAILABILITY

Monobasic Potassium and Sodium Phosphates
▪ *Tablets for oral solution:* 125.6 mg (4 mmol) phosphorus, 250 mg (8 mmol) phosphorus.

*Underlines indicate most frequent; CAPITALS indicate life-threatening.

Potassium and Sodium Phosphates
■ *Capsules for oral solution:* 250 mg (8 mmol) phosphorus ■ *Tablets for oral solution:* 250 mg (8 mmol) phosphorus ■ *Powder for oral solution:* 250 mg (8 mmol)/75 ml when reconstituted.

TIME/ACTION PROFILE (effects on serum phosphate levels)

	ONSET	PEAK	DURATION
PO	UK	UK	UK

NURSING IMPLICATIONS

ASSESSMENT
□ Assess patient for signs and symptoms of hypokalemia (weakness, fatigue, arrhythmias, presence of U waves on ECG, polyuria, polydipsia), hypophosphatemia (anorexia, weakness, decreased reflexes, bone pain, confusion, blood dyscrasias) throughout course of therapy.
□ Monitor intake and output ratios and daily weight. Report significant discrepancies to physician.
■ **Lab Test Considerations:** Monitor serum phosphate, potassium, sodium, and calcium levels prior to and periodically throughout therapy. Increased phosphate may cause hypocalcemia.
□ Monitor renal function studies prior to and periodically throughout course of therapy.
□ Monitor urinary pH in patients receiving potassium and sodium phosphate as a urinary acidifier.

POTENTIAL NURSING DIAGNOSES
■ Nutrition, altered: less than body requirements (indications).
■ Knowledge deficit related to medication regimen (patient/family teaching).

IMPLEMENTATION
■ **PO:** Tablets should be dissolved in a full glass of water. Capsules should be opened and mixed thoroughly in ⅓ cup of water each. Allow mixture to stand for 2–5 min to ensure it is fully dissolved. Solutions prepared by pharmacy should not be further diluted.
□ Medication should be administered after meals to minimize gastric irritation and laxative effect.
□ Do not administer simultaneously with antacids containing aluminum, magnesium, or calcium.

PATIENT/FAMILY TEACHING
□ Explain to the patient the purpose of the medication and the need to take as directed. If a dose is missed, it should be taken as soon as remembered unless within 1 or 2 hr of the next dose. Explain that the tablets and capsules should not be swallowed whole. Tablets should be dissolved in water; capsules should be opened and the contents mixed in water.
□ Instruct patients in low-sodium diet (see Appendix K).
□ Instruct the patient to promptly report diarrhea, weakness, fatigue, muscle cramps, unexplained weight gain, swelling of lower extremities, shortness of breath, unusual thirst, or tremors.

EVALUATION
Effectiveness of therapy can be demonstrated by: ■ Prevention and correction of serum phosphate and potassium deficiencies ■ Maintenance of acid urine ■ Decreased urine calcium, which prevents formation of renal calculi.

POTASSIUM BICARBONATE/ CITRATE
(poe-**tass**-ee-um bye-kar-boe-nate/**sit**-rate)
Effer-K, K+ Care ET, K-Lyte, Klor-Con/EF

CLASSIFICATION(S):
Electrolyte (potassium supplement)
Pregnancy Category C

INDICATIONS

■ Treatment or prevention of potassium depletion in patients who are unable to ingest adequate dietary potassium.

ACTION

■ Maintains the following cell characteristics: □ Acid-base balance □ Isotonicity □ Electrophysiology ■ Serves as an activator in many enzymatic reactions and is essential to many processes, including: □ Transmission of nerve impulses □ Contraction of cardiac, skeletal, and smooth muscle □ Gastric secretion □ Renal function □ Tissue synthesis □ Carbohydrate metabolism. **Therapeutic Effects:** ■ Replacement in deficiency states ■ Prevention of deficiency.

PHARMACOKINETICS

Absorption: Well absorbed following oral administration of liquid form.
Distribution: Enters extracellular fluid and is then actively transported into cells.
Metabolism and Excretion: Excreted by the kidneys.
Half-life: UK.

CONTRAINDICATIONS AND PRECAUTIONS

Contraindicated in: ■ Hyperkalemia ■ Severe renal impairment ■ Untreated Addison's disease ■ Severe tissue trauma ■ Hyperkalemic familial periodic paralysis.
Use Cautiously in: ■ Cardiac disease ■ Renal impairment.

ADVERSE REACTIONS AND SIDE EFFECTS*

CNS: paresthesias, restlessness, confusion, weakness, paralysis.
CV: <u>arrhythmias</u>, <u>ECG changes</u> (prolonged PR interval, ST segment depression, tall-tented T waves).
GI: <u>nausea</u>, <u>vomiting</u>, <u>diarrhea</u>, <u>abdominal pain</u>, gastric ulceration (tab only).

INTERACTIONS

Drug–Drug: ■ Use with **potassium-sparing diuretics** or **angiotensin converting enzyme (ACE) inhibitors** may lead to hyperkalemia.

ROUTE AND DOSAGE

Potassium chloride contains 10 mEq/g. Potassium citrate contains 9.8 mEq/g.
■ **PO (Adults):** 25–50 mEq 1–2 times daily.

AVAILABILITY

■ *Effervescent tablets:* 20 mEq, 25 mEq
■ *Effervescent tablets/powders in combination with:* potassium gluconate, potassium chloride, and potassium L-lysine. See Appendix A.

TIME/ACTION PROFILE (increase in serum potassium levels)

	ONSET	PEAK	DURATION
PO	UK	1–2 hr	UK

NURSING IMPLICATIONS

ASSESSMENT

□ Assess patient for signs and symptoms of hypokalemia (weakness, fatigue, U wave on ECG, arrhythmias, polyuria, polydipsia) and hyperkalemia (fatigue, muscle weakness, paresthesia, confusion, dyspnea, peaked T waves, depressed ST segments, prolonged QT segments, widened QRS complexes, loss of P waves and cardiac arrhythmias).
■ **Lab Test Considerations:** Monitor serum potassium levels prior to and periodically throughout therapy.
□ Monitor renal function, serum bicarbonate, and pH. Serum magnesium level should be determined in refractory hypokalemia, as hypomagnesemia should be corrected to facilitate effectiveness of potassium replacement. Monitor serum chloride levels, as hypochloremia may occur when chloride is not replaced concurrently with potassium.

POTENTIAL NURSING DIAGNOSES

■ Nutrition, altered: less than body requirements (indications).
■ Knowledge deficit related to medica-

*<u>Underlines</u> indicate most frequent; **CAPITALS** indicate life-threatening.

tion regimen (patient/family teaching).

IMPLEMENTATION

- **PO:** Administer with or after meals to decrease GI irritation.
- Dissolve effervescent tablets and powders in 8 oz cold water or juice. Ensure that effervescent tablet is fully dissolved. Instruct patient to drink slowly.

PATIENT/FAMILY TEACHING

- Explain to patient purpose of the medication and the need to take as directed, especially when concurrent cardiac glycosides or diuretics are ordered. A missed dose should be taken as soon as remembered within 2 hr; if not, return to regular dosage schedule. Do not double dose.
- Emphasize correct method of administration. GI irritation or ulceration may result from insufficient dilution of effervescent.
- Instruct patient to avoid salt substitutes unless approved by physician.
- Advise patient regarding sources of dietary potassium (see Appendix K). Encourage compliance with recommended diet.
- Instruct patient to report promptly dark, tarry, or bloody stools; weakness; unusual fatigue; or tingling of extremities. Physician should be notified if nausea, vomiting, diarrhea, or stomach discomfort persists. Dose may require adjustment.
- Emphasize the importance of regular follow-up examinations to monitor serum levels and monitor progress.

EVALUATION

Effectiveness of therapy can be demonstrated by: ▪ Prevention or treatment of serum potassium depletion.

POTASSIUM CHLORIDE

(poe-**tass**-ee-um **klor**-ide)
Apo-K, Cena-K, Gen-K, K-10, {Kalium Durules}, Kaochlor,

Kaochlor S-F, Kaon Cl, Kato, Kay Ciel, KCl, K-Dur, {K-Long}, K-Lor, Klor-10%, Klor-Con, Klorvess, Klotrix, K-Lyte/Cl Powder, K-Norm, K + Care, K + 10, K-Lease, {K-Long}, K-Tab, Micro-K, LS, {Novolente-K}, Potachlor, Potasalan, Rum-K, Slow-K, Ten-K

CLASSIFICATION(S):
Electrolyte (potassium supplement)
Pregnancy Category C

INDICATIONS

▪ **PO, IV:** Treatment or prevention of potassium depletion in patients who are unable to ingest adequate dietary potassium ▪ **IV:** Treatment of some arrhythmias due to cardiac glycoside toxicity.

ACTION

▪ Maintains the following cell characteristics: □ Acid-base balance □ Isotonicity □ Electrophysiology ▪ Serves as an activator in many enzymatic reactions and is essential to many processes, including: □ Transmission of nerve impulses □ Contraction of cardiac, skeletal, and smooth muscle □ Gastric secretion □ Renal function □ Tissue synthesis □ Carbohydrate metabolism. **Therapeutic Effects:** ▪ Replacement in deficiency states ▪ Prevention of deficiency.

PHARMACOKINETICS

Absorption: Well absorbed following oral administration of liquid form. Absorption is slow but complete from wax matrix extended-release formulations.
Distribution: Enters extracellular fluid and is then actively transported into cells.
Metabolism and Excretion: Excreted by the kidneys.
Half-life: UK.

CONTRAINDICATIONS AND PRECAUTIONS

Contraindicated in: ▪ Hyperkalemia ▪ Severe renal impairment ▪ Untreated Addison's disease ▪ Severe tissue

P

trauma ▪ Hyperkalemic familial periodic paralysis ▪ Known alcohol intolerance (elixirs) ▪ Some products may contain tartrazine (FDC yellow dye #5)—avoid use in patients with aspirin allergy.

Use Cautiously in: ▪ Cardiac disease ▪ Renal impairment ▪ GI hypomotility, including dysphagia or esophageal compression due to left atrial enlargement (tab, enteric-coated tab, extended-release tab or cap) ▪ Diabetes mellitus (liquid products may contain sugar).

ADVERSE REACTIONS AND SIDE EFFECTS*

CNS: paresthesias, restlessness, confusion, weakness, paralysis.

CV: <u>arrhythmias</u>, <u>ECG changes</u> (prolonged PR interval, ST segment depression, tall-tented T waves).

GI: <u>nausea</u>, <u>vomiting</u>, <u>diarrhea</u>, <u>abdominal pain</u>, gastric ulceration (tab only).

Local: irritation at IV site.

INTERACTIONS

Drug–Drug: ▪ Use with **potassium-sparing diuretics** or **angiotensin converting enzyme (ACE) inhibitors** may lead to hyperkalemia ▪ **Anticholinergics** may increase GI mucosal lesions in patients taking wax-matrix potassium chloride preparations.

ROUTE AND DOSAGE

Contains 13.4 mEq potassium/g.

Prevention of Hypokalemia

▪ **PO (Adults):** 16–24 mEq/day in 2–4 divided doses.

Treatment of Hypokalemia

▪ **PO (Adults):** 40–100 mEq/day in 2–4 divided doses.

▪ **PO (Children):** 1–3 mEq/kg/day (15–40 mEq/m²/day) in divided doses.

▪ **IV (Adults with Serum Potassium >2.5 mEq/liter):** up to 200 mEq/day (rate not to exceed 10 mEq/hr).

▪ **IV (Adults with Serum Potassium <2.0 mEq/liter):** up to 400 mEq/day (rate not to exceed 20 mEq/hr).

▪ **IV (Children):** 3 mEq/kg/day (40 mEq/m²/day) as an infusion.

AVAILABILITY

▪ *Oral liquid:* 20 mEq/15 ml, 30 mEq/15 ml, 40 mEq/15 ml ▪ *Powders:* 15 mEq/packet, 20 mEq/packet, 25 mEq/packet ▪ *Controlled-release tablets:* 6.7 mEq, 8 mEq, 10 mEq, 20 mEq ▪ *Controlled-release capsules:* 8 mEq, 10 mEq ▪ *Injection:* 0.1 mEq/ml, 0.4 mEq/ml, 1.5 mEq/ml, 2 mEq/ml ▪ *In combination with:* potassium, bicarbonate, and L-Lysine. See Appendix A.

TIME/ACTION PROFILE (increase in serum potassium levels)

	ONSET	PEAK	DURATION
PO (liquid)	UK	1–2 hr	UK
PO (wax matrix)	UK	30 min	UK
IV	rapid	UK	UK

NURSING IMPLICATIONS

ASSESSMENT

▫ Assess patient for signs and symptoms of hypokalemia (weakness, fatigue, U wave on ECG, arrhythmias, polyuria, polydipsia) and hyperkalemia (see Toxicity and Overdose section).

▫ Monitor pulse, blood pressure, and ECG periodically throughout IV therapy.

▪ **Lab Test Considerations:** Monitor serum potassium levels prior to and periodically throughout therapy.

▫ Monitor renal function, serum bicarbonate, and pH. Serum magnesium level should be determined in refractory hypokalemia; hypomagnesemia should be corrected to facilitate effectiveness of potassium replacement.

▪ **Toxicity and Overdose:** Symptoms of toxicity are those of hyperkalemia (fatigue, muscle weakness, paresthesia, confusion, dyspnea, peaked T waves, depressed ST segments, prolonged QT segments, widened QRS complexes, loss of P waves, and cardiac arrhythmias).

▫ Treatment includes discontinuation of potassium, administration of sodium bicarbonate to correct acidosis,

*<u>Underlines</u> indicate most frequent; **CAPITALS** indicate life-threatening.

dextrose and insulin to facilitate passage of potassium into cells, calcium salts to reverse ECG effects (in patients who are not receiving cardiac glycosides), sodium polystyrene used as an exchange resin, and/or dialysis in patients with impaired renal function.

POTENTIAL NURSING DIAGNOSES

- Nutrition, altered: less than body requirements (indications).
- Knowledge deficit related to medication regimen (patient/family teaching).

IMPLEMENTATION

- PO: Administer with or after meals to decrease GI irritation.
- ▢ Tablets should be administered with full glass of water. Do not chew or crush controlled-release tablets or capsules.
- ▢ Dilute powders and solution in 3–8 oz of cold water or juice. Ensure that effervescent tablet is fully dissolved. Instruct patient to drink slowly.
- IV: Do not administer IM or SC. Avoid extravasation, as severe pain and tissue necrosis may occur.
- Intermittent Infusion: Do not administer undiluted. Each single dose must be diluted and thoroughly mixed in 100–1000 ml of IV solution. Usually limited to 40 mEq/liter of IV solution. In severe hypokalemia may be as concentrated as 80 mEq/liter.
- *Rate:* Infuse at a rate of 10–20 mEq/hr.
- Solution Compatibility: May be diluted in dextrose, saline, Ringer's solution, lactated Ringer's solution, dextrose/saline, dextrose/Ringer's solution, and dextrose/lactated Ringer's solution combinations. Commercially available premixed with many of the above IV solutions.
- Y-Site Compatibility: ▪ acyclovir ▪ aminophylline ▪ ampicillin ▪ amrinone ▪ atropine ▪ betamethasone ▪ calcium gluconate ▪ cephalothin ▪ cephapirin ▪ chlordiazepoxide ▪ chlorpromazine ▪ cyanocobalamin ▪ dexamethasone ▪ digoxin ▪ diphenhydramine ▪ do-

butamine ▪ dopamine ▪ droperidol ▪ droperidol/fentanyl ▪ edrophonium ▪ enalaprilat ▪ epinephrine ▪ esmolol ▪ conjugated estrogens ▪ ethacrynate sodium ▪ famotidine ▪ fentanyl ▪ fludarabine ▪ fluorouracil ▪ furosemide ▪ hydralazine ▪ insulin ▪ isoproterenol ▪ kanamycin ▪ labetalol ▪ lidocaine ▪ magnesium sulfate ▪ menadiol ▪ meperidine ▪ methicillin ▪ methoxamine ▪ methylergonovine ▪ minocycline ▪ morphine ▪ neostigmine ▪ norepinephrine ▪ ondansetron ▪ oxacillin ▪ oxytocin ▪ penicillin G potassium ▪ pentazocine ▪ phytonadione ▪ prednisolone ▪ procaine ▪ prochlorperazine ▪ propranolol ▪ pyridostigmine ▪ sargramostim ▪ scopolamine ▪ sodium bicarbonate ▪ succinylcholine ▪ trimethaphan ▪ trimethobenzamide ▪ zidovudine.
- Y-Site Incompatibility: ▪ diazepam ▪ ergotamine tartrate ▪ phenytoin.
- Additive Compatibility: ▪ aminophylline ▪ bretylium ▪ calcium gluconate ▪ cimetidine ▪ cytarabine ▪ dopamine ▪ heparin ▪ hydrocortisone sodium succinate ▪ isoproterenol ▪ lidocaine ▪ metaraminol ▪ methyldopate ▪ metoclopramide ▪ norepinephrine ▪ phenylephrine ▪ ranitidine ▪ sodium bicarbonate ▪ thiopental ▪ verapamil ▪ vitamin B complex with C.
- Additive Incompatibility: ▪ amphotericin B.

PATIENT/FAMILY TEACHING

- ▢ Explain to patient purpose of the medication and the need to take as directed, especially when concurrent cardiac glycosides or diuretics are taken. A missed dose should be taken as soon as remembered within 2 hr; if not, return to regular dosage schedule. Do not double dose.
- ▢ Emphasize correct method of administration. GI irritation or ulceration may result from chewing entericcoated tablets or insufficient dilution of liquid or powder forms.
- ▢ Controlled-release tablets contain potassium chloride in a wax matrix, which may be expelled in the stool. This is not significant.

□ Instruct patient to avoid salt substitutes unless approved by physician.

□ Advise patient regarding sources of dietary potassium (see Appendix K). Encourage compliance with recommended diet.

□ Instruct patient to report dark, tarry, or bloody stools; weakness; unusual fatigue; or tingling of extremities promptly.

□ Physician should be notified if nausea, vomiting, diarrhea, or stomach discomfort persists. Dosage may require adjustment.

□ Emphasize the importance of regular follow-up examinations to monitor serum levels and to monitor progress.

EVALUATION
Effectiveness of therapy can be demonstrated by: ■ Prevention or treatment of serum potassium depletion.

POTASSIUM GLUCONATE
(poe-**tass**-ee-um **glu**-koe-nate)
Kaon, Kaylixir, K-G Elixir, {Potassium-Rougier}, {Royonate}

CLASSIFICATION(S):
Electrolyte (potassium supplement)
Pregnancy Category C

INDICATIONS
■ Treatment or prevention of potassium depletion in patients who are unable to ingest adequate dietary potassium.

ACTION
■ Maintains the following cell characteristics: □ Acid-base balance □ Isotonicity □ Electrophysiology ■ Serves as an activator in many enzymatic reactions and is essential to many processes, including: □ Transmission of nerve impulses □ Contraction of cardiac, skeletal, and smooth muscle □ Gastric secretion □ Renal function □ Tissue synthesis □ Carbohydrate metabolism. **Therapeu-**tic **Effects:** ■ Replacement in deficiency states ■ Prevention of deficiency.

PHARMACOKINETICS
Absorption: Well absorbed following oral administration.
Distribution: Enters extracellular fluid and is then actively transported into cells.
Metabolism and Excretion: Excreted by the kidneys.
Half-life: UK.

CONTRAINDICATIONS AND PRECAUTIONS
Contraindicated in: ■ Hyperkalemia ■ Severe renal impairment ■ Untreated Addison's disease ■ Severe tissue trauma ■ Hyperkalemic familial periodic paralysis ■ Elixirs may contain alcohol—avoid use in alcohol-intolerant patients ■ Some products may contain tartrazine (FDC yellow dye #5)—avoid use in patients with aspirin allergy.
Use Cautiously in: ■ Cardiac disease ■ Renal impairment ■ Diabetes mellitus (liquid products may contain sugar) ■ GI hypomotility, including dysphagia or esophageal compression due to left atrial enlargement (tablets only).

ADVERSE REACTIONS AND SIDE EFFECTS*
CNS: paresthesias, restlessness, confusion, weakness, paralysis.
CV: arrhythmias, ECG changes (prolonged PR interval, ST segment depression, tall-tented T waves).
GI: nausea, vomiting, diarrhea, abdominal pain, gastric ulceration (tablets only).

INTERACTIONS
Drug–Drug: ■ Use with **potassium-sparing diuretics** or **angiotensin converting enzyme (ACE) inhibitors** may lead to hyperkalemia.

ROUTE AND DOSAGE
Contains 4.3 mEq potassium/g.

{} = Available in Canada only.
*Underlines indicate most frequent; **CAPITALS** indicate life-threatening.

Prevention of Hypokalemia

- PO (Adults): 20 mEq 1–4 times daily (up to 100 mEq/day).
- PO (Children): 2–3 mEq/kg (20–40 mEq/m^2)/day in divided doses.

AVAILABILITY

- *Tablets:* 2 mEq, 5 mEq ▪ *Liquid:* 20 mEq/15 ml ▪ *In combination with:* potassium chloride or potassium citrate. See Appendix A.

TIME/ACTION PROFILE (increase in serum potassium levels)

	ONSET	PEAK	DURATION
PO	UK	1–2 hr	UK

NURSING IMPLICATIONS

ASSESSMENT

- Assess patient for signs and symptoms of hypokalemia (weakness, fatigue, U wave on ECG, arrhythmias, polyuria, polydipsia) and hyperkalemia (fatigue, muscle weakness, paresthesia, confusion, dyspnea, peaked T waves, depressed ST segments, prolonged QT segments, widened QRS complexes, loss of P waves, and cardiac arrhythmias).
- **Lab Test Considerations:** Monitor serum potassium levels prior to and periodically throughout therapy.
- Monitor renal function, serum bicarbonate, and pH. Serum magnesium level should be determined in refractory hypokalemia; hypomagnesemia should be corrected to facilitate effectiveness of potassium replacement. Monitor serum chloride levels; hypochloremia may occur when chloride is not replaced concurrently with potassium.

POTENTIAL NURSING DIAGNOSES

- Nutrition, altered: less than body requirements (indications).
- Knowledge deficit related to medication regimen (patient/family teaching).

IMPLEMENTATION

- **PO:** Administer with or after meals to decrease GI irritation.
- Tablets should be administered with full glass of water. Do not chew or crush.
- Use calibrated measuring device to ensure accurate dosage of elixir. Mix in 120 ml of cold water or juice.

PATIENT/FAMILY TEACHING

- Explain to patient purpose of the medication and the need to take as directed, especially when concurrent cardiac glycosides or diuretics are taken. A missed dose should be taken as soon as remembered within 2 hr; if not, return to regular dosage schedule. Do not double dose.
- Emphasize correct method of administration. GI irritation or ulceration may result from chewing tablets or insufficient dilution of liquid forms.
- Instruct patient to avoid salt substitutes unless approved by physician.
- Advise patient regarding sources of dietary potassium (see Appendix K). Encourage compliance with recommended diet.
- Instruct patient to report dark, tarry, or bloody stools; weakness; unusual fatigue; or tingling of extremities promptly. Physician should be notified if nausea, vomiting, diarrhea, or stomach discomfort persists. Dosage may require adjustment.
- Emphasize the importance of regular follow-up examinations to monitor serum levels and progress.

EVALUATION

Effectiveness of therapy can be demonstrated by: ▪ Prevention or treatment of serum potassium depletion.

POTASSIUM IODIDE

(poe-**tass**-ee-um **eye**-oh-dide)
Iostat, Pima, Thyro-Block, SSKI

CLASSIFICATION(S):
Antithyroid
Pregnancy Category D

INDICATIONS

- Adjunct with other antithyroid drugs in preparation for thyroidectomy ▪ Radiation protectant following administration of radioactive isotopes of iodine or in radiation emergencies.

ACTION

▪ Rapidly inhibits the release and synthesis of thyroid hormones ▪ Decreases the vascularity of the thyroid gland ▪ Prevents thyroidal uptake of radioactive iodine following radiation emergencies. **Therapeutic Effects:** ▪ Control of hyperthyroidism ▪ Decreased bleeding during thyroid surgery ▪ Prevention of thyroid cancers following radiation emergencies.

PHARMACOKINETICS

Absorption: Converted in the GI tract and enters circulation as iodine.
Distribution: Concentrates in the thyroid gland. Crosses the placenta and enters breast milk.
Metabolism and Excretion: Taken up by the thyroid gland.
Half-life: UK.

CONTRAINDICATIONS AND PRECAUTIONS

Contraindicated in: ▪ Hypersensitivity.
Use Cautiously in: ▪ Tuberculosis ▪ Bronchitis ▪ Hyperkalemia ▪ Impaired renal function ▪ Pregnancy and lactation (although iodine has been used safely in pregnancy, thyroid abnormalities in the newborn may be seen).

ADVERSE REACTIONS AND SIDE EFFECTS*

EENT: parotitis.
Derm: acneform eruptions.
Endo: thyroid hyperplasia, hypothyroidism, hyperthyroidism.
GI: gastric irritation, diarrhea.
Misc: hypersensitivity, iodism.

INTERACTIONS

Drug–Drug: ▪ Use with **lithium** may cause additive hypothyroidism ▪ Increases the antithyroid effect of **antithyroid agents (methimazole, propylthiouracil)** ▪ Additive hyperkalemia may result from combined use of potassium

iodide with **potassium-sparing diuretics** or **angiotensin converting enzyme (ACE) inhibitors**.

ROUTE AND DOSAGE

Potassium iodide contains 6 mEq potassium/g; SSKI (saturated solution of potassium iodide) = 1 g iodine/ml; doses expressed in mg of potassium iodide.

Preparation for Thyroidectomy
▪ **PO (Adults and Children):** 250 mg (5 drops of SSKI diluted in liquid) tid for 10 days prior to thyroidectomy, usually given with antithyroid drugs.

Radiation Protectant
▪ **PO (Adults):** 100–150 mg (2–3 drops of SSKI) 24 hr prior to and daily for 3–10 days following exposure to radioactive isotopes of iodine.
▪ **PO (Infants and Children >1 yr):** 130 mg daily for 10 days following exposure to radioactive isotopes of iodine.
▪ **PO (Infants and Children ≤1 yr):** 65 mg daily for 10 days following exposure to radioactive isotopes of iodine.

AVAILABILITY

▪ *Saturated oral solution:* 1 g/ml
▪ *Oral syrup:* 325 mg/5 ml ▪ {*Tablets:* 130 mg}.

TIME/ACTION PROFILE (effects on thyroid function testing)

	ONSET	PEAK	DURATION
PO	24 hr	10–15 days	variable

NURSING IMPLICATIONS

ASSESSMENT
▪ **General Info:** Assess for signs and symptoms of iodism (metallic taste, stomatitis, skin lesions, cold symptoms, severe GI upset). Report these symptoms promptly to physician.
▪ **Hyperthyroidism:** Monitor response symptoms of hyperthyroidism (tachycardia, palpitations, nervousness, insomnia, diaphoresis, heat intolerance, tremors, weight loss).
▪ **Lab Test Considerations:** Monitor

thyroid function tests prior to and periodically during course of therapy.
- ☐ Monitor serum potassium periodically during course of therapy.

POTENTIAL NURSING DIAGNOSES
- Airway clearance, ineffective (indications).
- Knowledge deficit related to medication regimen (patient/family teaching).

IMPLEMENTATION
- **PO:** Mix solution in 8 oz fruit juice, water, or milk. Dissolve tablets in 4 oz water or milk. Administer after meals to minimize GI irritation.
- ☐ Oral solution is normally clear and colorless. Darkening upon standing does not affect potency of drug.
- **Radiation Protectant:** Administer exactly when ordered. In a nuclear emergency 90–99% protection is provided if administered immediately after exposure, 50% protection if administered within 3–4 hr. Protection is limited to the thyroid gland and does not include other effects of radiation exposure.

PATIENT/FAMILY TEACHING
- **Hyperthyroidism:** Instruct patient to take medication exactly as ordered. Missing a dose may precipitate hyperthyroidism. If a dose is missed, take as soon as remembered unless almost time for next dose.
- ☐ Instruct patient to report suspected pregnancy to physician before therapy is initiated.
- ☐ Advise patient to confer with physician regarding avoidance of foods high in iodine (seafood, iodized salt, cabbage, kale, turnips).
- ☐ Advise patient to consult physician or pharmacist prior to using over-the-counter cold remedies. Some cold remedies contain iodide as an expectorant.

EVALUATION
Effectiveness of therapy can be demonstrated by: ▪ Decrease in size and vascularity of the gland prior to thyroid surgery ▪ Protection of the thyroid gland from the effects of radiation.

POTASSIUM PHOSPHATES
(poe-**tass**-ee-um **foss**-fates)
Monobasic Potassium Phosphate
K-Phos Original
Potassium Phosphates
Neutra-Phos-K
Potassium Phosphate

CLASSIFICATION(S):
Electrolyte (phosphate supplement), Urinary acidifier, Antiurolithic
Pregnancy Category C

INDICATIONS
- Treatment and prevention of phosphate depletion in patients who are unable to ingest adequate dietary potassium ▪ Adjunct therapy of urinary tract infections with methenamine hippurate or mandelate (potassium and sodium phosphates or monobasic potassium phosphate) ▪ Prevention of calcium urinary stones (potassium and sodium phosphates or monobasic potassium phosphate) ▪ Phosphate salts of potassium may be used in hypokalemic patients with metabolic acidosis or coexisting phosphorous deficiency.

ACTION
- Phosphate is present in bone and is involved in energy transfer and carbohydrate metabolism ▪ Serves as a buffer for the excretion of hydrogen ions by the kidney ▪ Dibasic potassium phosphate is converted in renal tubule to monobasic salt by hydrogen ions, resulting in urinary acidification ▪ Acidification of urine is required for methenamine hippurate or mandelate to be active as a urinary anti-infective ▪ Acidification of urine increases solubility of calcium, decreasing calcium stone formation. **Therapeutic Effects:** ▪ Replacement of phosphorus in deficiency states ▪ Urinary acidification ▪ Increased efficacy of methenamine ▪ Decreased formation of calcium urinary tract stones.

PHARMACOKINETICS

Absorption: Well absorbed following oral administration. Vitamin D promotes GI absorption of phosphates.

Distribution: Phosphates enter extracellular fluids and are then actively transported to sites of action.

Metabolism and Excretion: Excreted mainly (>90%) by the kidneys.

Half-life: UK.

CONTRAINDICATIONS AND PRECAUTIONS

Contraindicated in: ■ Hyperkalemia ■ Hyperphosphatemia ■ Hypocalcemia ■ Severe renal impairment ■ Untreated Addison's disease ■ Severe tissue trauma ■ Hyperkalemic familial periodic paralysis.

Use Cautiously in: ■ Hyperparathyroidism ■ Cardiac disease ■ Renal impairment.

ADVERSE REACTIONS AND SIDE EFFECTS*

Related to hyperphosphatemia, unless indicated.

CNS: listlessness, confusion, weakness.

CV: ARRHYTHMIAS, ECG changes (absent P waves, widening of the QRS complex with biphasic curve), CARDIAC ARREST, hypotension; hyperkalemia— ARRHYTHMIAS, ECG changes (prolonged PR interval, ST segment depression, tall-tented T waves).

F and E: hypomagnesemia, hyperphosphatemia, hyperkalemia, hypocalcemia.

GI: diarrhea, nausea, vomiting, abdominal pain.

Local: phlebitis, irritation at IV site.

MS: hyperkalemia—muscle cramps; hypercalcemia—tremors.

Neuro: paresthesias of extremities, flaccid paralysis, heaviness of legs.

INTERACTIONS

Drug–Drug: ■ Concurrent use of potassium-sparing diuretics or angiotensin converting enzyme (ACE) inhibitors may result in hyperkalemia ■ Con-

current administration of **calcium-** or **aluminum-**containing compounds decreases absorption of phosphates by formation of insoluble complexes ■ **Vitamin D** enhances the absorption of phosphates.

Drug–Food: ■ **Oxalates** (in spinach and rhubarb) and **phytates** (in bran and whole grains) may decrease the absorption of phosphates by binding them in the GI tract.

ROUTE AND DOSAGE

Monobasic Potassium Phosphate

■ **PO (Adults and Children >4 yr):** 1 g (7.4 mmol) in water qid.
■ **PO (Children <4 yr):** 200 mg (6.4 mmol) in water qid.

Potassium Phosphates

■ **PO (Adults and Children >4 yr):** 1.45 g (8 mmol) qid.
■ **PO (Children <4 yr):** 200 mg (6.4 mmol) phosphorus qid.
■ **IV (Adults):** 10–15 mmol phosphorus/ day as an infusion.
■ **IV (Infants):** 1.5–2 mmol/kg/day phosphorous as an infusion.

AVAILABILITY

Monobasic Potassium Phosphate

■ *Tablets for oral solution:* 500 mg (contains 114 mg or 3.7 mmol phosphorus).

Potassium Phosphates

■ *Capsules for oral solution:* 1.45 g (contains 1.45 g or 8 mmol phosphorus) ■ *Injection:* 93 mg (3 mmol) phosphorus/ml ■ *In combination with:* sodium phosphates.

TIME/ACTION PROFILE (effects on serum phosphate levels)

	ONSET	PEAK	DURATION
PO	UK	UK	UK
IV	rapid (min–hr)	end of infusion	UK

NURSING IMPLICATIONS

Assessment

▫ Assess patient for signs and symp-

---

*Underlines indicate most frequent; CAPITALS indicate life-threatening.

toms of hypokalemia (weakness, fatigue, arrhythmias, presence of U waves on ECG, polyuria, polydipsia) and hypophosphatemia (anorexia, weakness, decreased reflexes, bone pain, confusion, blood dyscrasias) throughout course of therapy.

▫ Monitor pulse, blood pressure, and ECG prior to and periodically throughout IV therapy.

▫ Monitor intake and output ratios and daily weight. Report significant discrepancies to physician.

▪ **Lab Test Considerations:** Monitor serum phosphate, potassium, and calcium levels prior to and periodically throughout therapy. Increased phosphate may cause hypocalcemia.

▫ Monitor renal function studies prior to and periodically throughout course of therapy.

▫ Monitor urinary pH in patients receiving potassium phosphate as a urinary acidifier.

▪ **Toxicity and Overdose:** Symptoms of toxicity are those of hyperkalemia (fatigue, muscle weakness, paresthesia, confusion, dyspnea, peaked T waves, depressed ST segments, prolonged QT segments, widened QRS complexes, loss of P waves, and cardiac arrhythmias) and hyperphosphatemia or hypocalcemia (paresthesia, muscle twitching, laryngospasm, colic, cardiac arrhythmias, or Chvostek's or Trousseau's sign).

▫ Treatment includes discontinuation of infusion, calcium replacement, and lowering serum potassium (dextrose and insulin to facilitate passage of potassium into cells, sodium polystyrene as an exchange resin, and/or dialysis in patients with impaired renal function).

POTENTIAL NURSING DIAGNOSES

▪ Nutrition, altered: less than body requirements (indications).

▪ Knowledge deficit related to medication regimen (patient/family teaching).

IMPLEMENTATION

▪ **PO:** Tablets should be dissolved in a full glass of water. Capsules should be opened and mixed thoroughly in ⅓ cup water each. Allow mixture to stand for 2–5 min to ensure that it is fully dissolved.

▫ Medication should be administered after meals to minimize gastric irritation and laxative effect.

▫ Do not administer simultaneously with antacids containing aluminum, magnesium, or calcium.

▪ **IV:** Administer only in dilute concentration. Common component of total parenteral nutrition. Do not administer IM.

▪ **Continuous Infusion:** Dilute to a concentration no greater than 160 mEq/liter with 0.45% NaCl, 0.9% NaCl, D5W, D10W, D5/0.45% NaCl, D5/0.9% NaCl, or TPN solutions.

▪ *Rate:* Infuse as a continuous infusion at a slow rate.

▪ **Y-Site Compatibility:** ▪ enalaprilat ▪ esmolol ▪ famotidine ▪ labetalol.

▪ **Additive Compatibility:** ▪ magnesium sulfate ▪ metoclopramide ▪ verapamil.

▪ **Solution/Additive Incompatibility:** Ringer's or lactated Ringer's solution, D10/0.9% NaCl, D5/LR, or dobutamine.

PATIENT/FAMILY TEACHING

▫ Explain to patient purpose of the medication and the need to take as directed. If a dose is missed, it should be taken as soon as remembered unless within 1–2 hr of the next dose. Explain that the tablets and capsules should not be swallowed whole. Tablets should be dissolved in water; capsules should be opened and the contents mixed in water.

▫ Instruct the patient to report diarrhea, weakness, fatigue, muscle cramps, or tremors promptly.

EVALUATION

Effectiveness of therapy can be demonstrated by: ▪ Prevention and correction of serum phosphate and potassium deficiencies ▪ Maintenance of acid urine ▪ Decreased urine calcium, which prevents formation of renal calculi.

PRALIDOXIME
(pra-li-**dox**-eem)
Protopam

CLASSIFICATION(S):
Antidote (anticholinesterase poisoning)
Pregnancy Category UK

INDICATIONS

- Early (first 24–36 hr) treatment of organophosphate anticholinesterase insecticide poisoning, usually with atropine and supportive measures, including mechanical ventilation, if necessary ▪ Management of anticholinesterase (neostigmine, pyridostigmine, ambemonium, or nerve gas) overdosage.

ACTION

- Reactivates cholinesterase following poisoning with anticholinesterase agents ▪ May also directly inactivate organophosphates. **Therapeutic Effect:** ▪ Reversal of muscle paralysis following organophosphate poisoning.

PHARMACOKINETICS

Absorption: Variably and incompletely absorbed following oral administration. Well absorbed following IM administration.
Distribution: Widely distributed throughout extracellular water. Does not appear to enter the CNS.
Metabolism and Excretion: 80–90% excreted unchanged by the kidneys.
Half-life: 0.8–2.7 hr.

CONTRAINDICATIONS AND PRECAUTIONS

Contraindicated in: ▪ Hypersensitivity.
Use Cautiously in: ▪ Myasthenia gravis (may precipitate myasthenic crisis) ▪ Renal impairment (dosage reduction required) ▪ Pregnancy, lactation, or children (safety not established) ▪ Efficacy in carbamate insecticide poisoning is not known (may increase toxicity).

ADVERSE REACTIONS AND SIDE EFFECTS*

CNS: dizziness, headache, drowsiness.
EENT: diplopia, blurred vision, impaired accommodation.
Resp: hyperventilation, LARYNGOSPASM.
CV: tachycardia.
GI: nausea.
Derm: rash.
Local: pain at IM site.
MS: muscle weakness, muscle rigidity, neuromuscular blockade.

INTERACTIONS

Drug–Drug: ▪ Avoid concurrent use with **succinylcholine, morphine, aminophylline, theophylline, reserpine,** and **respiratory depressants,** including **barbiturates, opioid analgesics,** and **sedative/hypnotics** in patients with anticholinesterase poisoning.

ROUTE AND DOSAGE
IV route is preferred.

Organophosphate Poisoning
Atropine 2–6 mg IV is given concurrently. If patient is cyanotic, give atropine IM while improving ventilatory status. Atropine is repeated q 5–60 min until toxicity is encountered and is then continued for at least 48 hr.

- **PO (Adults):** In the absence of severe GI, 1–3 g may be given q 5 hr.
- **SC, IM, IV (Adults):** 1–2 g, may be repeated in 1 hr if muscle paralysis is still present or as a continuous IV infusion at 500 mg/hr. If exposure continues, additional doses may be given q 3–8 hr.
- **SC, IM, IV (Children):** 20–40 mg/kg, may be repeated in 1 hr if muscle paralysis is still present. If exposure continues, additional doses may be given q 3–8 hr.

Anticholinesterase Overdose
- **IV (Adults):** 1–2 g, followed by 250 mg q 5 min as needed.

P

---

*Underlines indicate most frequent; **CAPITALS** indicate life-threatening.

AVAILABILITY

▪ **Injection:** 1 g/20-ml vials.

TIME/ACTION PROFILE (plasma levels)

	ONSET	PEAK	DURATION
IM	UK	10–20 min	UK
IV	UK	5–15 min	UK

NURSING IMPLICATIONS

ASSESSMENT

☐ Determine insecticide to which patient was exposed and time of exposure. Therapy should begin as soon as possible within 24 hr. Contact poison control center for complete information on the specific insecticide.

☐ Monitor neuromuscular status prior to and periodically throughout therapy. Document skeletal muscle strength, tidal volume, and vital capacity. Note presence of nicotinic effects of anticholinesterases (twitching, muscle cramps, fasiculations, weakness, pallor, tachycardia, increased blood pressure).

☐ Closely monitor respirations, pulse, and blood pressure. Rapid IV infusion rate may cause tachycardia, laryngospasm, muscle rigidity, and hypertension. Notify physician immediately if hypertension occurs. Physician may order decrease in infusion rate or discontinuation of infusion. Phentolamine may be required to control blood pressure.

▪ **Lab Test Considerations:** May cause elevated AST (SGOT), ALT (SGPT), and CPK levels. These usually return to normal in 2 wk.

POTENTIAL NURSING DIAGNOSES

▪ Injury, high risk for (indications).
▪ Airway clearance, ineffective (indications).

IMPLEMENTATION

▪ **General Info:** Concurrent atropine and supportive measures (suctioning, intubation, and ventilation) may be ordered. Atropine is used to reverse muscarinic effects (bronchoconstriction, dyspnea, cough, increased bronchial secretions, nausea, vomiting, abdominal cramps, diarrhea, increased sweating, salivation, lacrimation, bradycardia, decreased blood pressure, miosis, blurred vision, urinary frequency, incontinence) of anticholinesterases. Pralidoxime is effective only against nicotinic effects.

☐ Dosage may need to be repeated every 3–8 hr if insecticide was ingested; absorption from bowel may continue.

☐ Emergency kit containing pralidoxime, Sterile Water for Injection, 20-ml syringe, needle, and alcohol swab is commercially available for SC, IM, or IV injection.

☐ If dermal exposure has occurred, remove clothing and thoroughly wash hair and skin in sodium bicarbonate or alcohol as soon as possible. Health care workers should wear gloves to prevent self-exposure. Carefully dispose of clothing to prevent contamination of others.

☐ Also available as an auto-injector for nerve gas emergencies.

▪ **SC/IM:** May be administered IM or SC in patients unable to tolerate IV infusion.

▪ **IV:** Reconstitute vial containing 1 g of powdered pralidoxime with 20 ml of Sterile Water for Injection.

▪ **Direct IV:** May be administered undiluted (50 mg/ml) over at least 5 min in patients who cannot tolerate IV infusion (for example, pulmonary edema).

▪ **Intermittent Infusion:** Further dilute in 100 ml of 0.9% NaCl.

▪ **Rate:** Infuse over 15–30 min.

PATIENT/FAMILY TEACHING

☐ Explain purpose of medication to patient.

EVALUATION

Effectiveness of therapy can be demonstrated by: ▪ Reversal of respiratory and skeletal muscle weakness caused by exposure to organophosphate anticholinesterase insecticides or anticholesterase overdose.

PRAVASTATIN
(**pra**-va-sta-tin)
Pravachol

CLASSIFICATION(S):
Lipid-lowering agent
Pregnancy Category X

INDICATIONS
▪ Adjunct to dietary therapy in the management of primary hypercholesterolemia.

ACTION
▪ Inhibits the enzyme (HMG-CoA reductase) responsible for catalyzing an early step in the synthesis of cholesterol. **Therapeutic Effects:** ▪ Lowering of total and low-density lipoprotein (LDL) cholesterol, VLDL cholesterol, and triglycerides ▪ Increased high-density lipoproteins (HDL).

PHARMACOKINETICS
Absorption: Poor absorption following oral administration and rapid hepatic metabolism result in decreased bioavailability (18%).
Distribution: Does not cross the blood–brain barrier. Small amounts appear in breast milk. Enters hepatocytes where action takes place. Remainder of distribution not known.
Metabolism and Excretion: Highly metabolized by the liver. 71% eliminated in the feces. Small amounts (8%) excreted unchanged by the kidneys.
Half-life: 1.8 hr.

CONTRAINDICATIONS AND PRECAUTIONS
Contraindicated in: ▪ Hypersensitivity ▪ Pregnancy or lactation ▪ Active liver disease.
Use Cautiously in: ▪ Women of childbearing age ▪ History of liver disease ▪ Alcoholism ▪ Children <18 yr (safety not established).

ADVERSE REACTIONS AND SIDE EFFECTS*
CNS: headache.

Derm: rashes.
MS: myalgia.

INTERACTIONS
Drug–Drug: ▪ Cholesterol-lowering effect may be additive with **bile acid sequestrants (cholestyramine, colestipol)**, but absorption of pravastatin is decreased if administered concurrently (give 1 hr before or 4 hr after bile acid sequestrant) ▪ Risk of myopathy or rhabdomyolysis may be increased by concurrent **niacin, gemfibrozil, erythromycin,** or **cyclosporine.**

ROUTE AND DOSAGE
▪ **PO (Adults):** 10–20 mg once daily at bedtime may be increased at weekly intervals (up to 40 mg).
▪ **PO (Elderly):** 10 mg once daily at bedtime.

AVAILABILITY
▪ *Tablets:* 10 mg, 20 mg.

TIME/ACTION PROFILE (lipid-lowering effect)

	ONSET	PEAK	DURATION
PO	1 wk	4 wk	UK

NURSING IMPLICATIONS
ASSESSMENT
□ Obtain a diet history, especially in regard to fat consumption.
□ Ophthalmic examinations are recommended prior to and yearly throughout therapy.
▪ **Lab Test Considerations:** Serum cholesterol and triglyceride levels should be evaluated before initiating and periodically throughout course of therapy.
□ Liver function tests, including AST (SGOT), should be monitored prior to and every 6 wk during the first 3 mo of therapy, every 8 wk for the remainder of the first year and then every 6 mo. If AST (SGOT) levels increase to 3 times normal, pravastatin therapy should be discontinued.
□ If patient develops muscle tenderness

*Underlines indicate most frequent; **CAPITALS** indicate life-threatening.

during therapy, CPK levels should be monitored. If CPK levels are markedly increased or myopathy occurs, pravastatin therapy should be discontinued.

POTENTIAL NURSING DIAGNOSES
- Knowledge deficit related to diet and medication regimen (patient/family teaching).
- Noncompliance (patient/family teaching).

IMPLEMENTATION
- PO: Administer once daily at bedtime. May be administered without regard to food.
- If administered in conjunction with bile acid sequestrants (cholestyramine, colestipol), administer pravastatin 1 hr before or at least 4 hr after bile acid sequestrant.

PATIENT/FAMILY TEACHING
- Instruct patient to take medication exactly as directed, not to skip doses or double up on missed doses. Pravastatin helps control but does not cure elevated serum cholesterol levels.
- Advise patient that pravastatin should be used in conjunction with diet restrictions (fat, cholesterol, carbohydrates, alcohol) exercise, and cessation of smoking.
- Instruct patient to notify physician if unexplained muscle pain, tenderness, or weakness occur, especially if accompanied by fever or malaise.
- Instruct female patients to notify physician promptly if pregnancy is planned or suspected.
- Advise patient to notify physician or dentist of medication regimen prior to treatment or surgery.
- Emphasize the importance of follow-up examinations to determine effectiveness and monitor for side effects.

EVALUATION
Effectiveness of therapy can be demonstrated by: ■ Decrease in low-density lipoprotein (LDL), very low-density lipoprotein (VLDL), and total cholesterol levels ■ Increase in high-density lipoprotein levels ■ Decrease in serum triglyceride levels.

PRAZEPAM
(praz-e-pam)
Centrax

CLASSIFICATION(S):
Sedative/hypnotic (benzodiazepine)
Schedule IV
Pregnancy Category UK

INDICATIONS
- Used as an adjunct in the management of anxiety.

ACTION
- Depresses the CNS, probably by potentiating gamma-aminobutyric acid (GABA), an inhibitory neurotransmitter. **Therapeutic Effects:** ■ Sedation ■ Relief of anxiety.

PHARMACOKINETICS
Absorption: Slowly absorbed but is rapidly metabolized following oral administration.
Distribution: Widely distributed. Crosses the blood–brain barrier. Crosses the placenta and enters breast milk.
Metabolism and Excretion: Highly metabolized by the liver and converted to active benzodiazepines (desmethyldiazepam and oxazepam).
Half-life: Oxazepam—5–15 hr; desmethyldiazepam—30–100 hr.

CONTRAINDICATIONS AND PRECAUTIONS
Contraindicated in: ■ Hypersensitivity ■ Cross-sensitivity with other benzodiazepines may exist ■ Comatose patients or those with pre-existing CNS depression ■ Uncontrolled severe pain ■ Narrow-angle glaucoma ■ Pregnancy and lactation.
Use Cautiously in: ■ Hepatic dysfunction ■ Severe renal impairment ■ Patients who may be suicidal or who may have been addicted to drugs previously ■ Elderly or debilitated patients (dosage reduction recommended) ■ Children (safety not established).

ADVERSE REACTIONS AND SIDE EFFECTS*

CNS: <u>dizziness</u>, <u>drowiness</u>, <u>lethargy</u>, hangover, paradoxical excitation, headache.
EENT: blurred vision.
Resp: respiratory depression.
GI: nausea, vomiting, diarrhea, constipation.
Derm: rashes.
Misc: tolerance, psychological dependence, physical dependence.

INTERACTIONS

Drug–Drug: ▪ Additive CNS depression with other **CNS depressants,** including **alcohol, antihistamines, antidepressants, opioid analgesics,** and other **sedative/hypnotics** ▪ Cimetidine, **oral contraceptives, disulfiram, fluoxetine, isoniazid, ketoconazole, metoprolol, propoxyphene, propranolol,** and **valproic acid** may decrease metabolism and increase CNS depression ▪ May decrease the efficacy of **levodopa** ▪ **Rifampin** or **barbiturates** may increase metabolism and decrease effectiveness of prazepam ▪ Sedative effects may be decreased by **theophylline.**

ROUTE AND DOSAGE

▪ **PO (Adults):** 10 mg 3 times daily (range 20–60 mg/day) or give as single bedtime dose of 20–40 mg.
▪ **PO (Elderly or Debilitated Patients):** 10–15 mg/day in divided doses initially.

AVAILABILITY

▪ *Capsules:* 5 mg, 10 mg, 20 mg ▪ *Tablets:* 10 mg.

TIME/ACTION PROFILE (antianxiety effects)

	ONSET	PEAK	DURATION
PO	UK	days–wks	days

NURSING IMPLICATIONS

ASSESSMENT

□ Assess patient for anxiety and level of sedation (ataxia, dizziness, slurred speech) periodically throughout course of therapy.
□ Prolonged high-dose therapy may lead to psychological or physical dependence. Restrict the amount of drug available to patient.
▪ **Lab Test Considerations:** Monitor CBC and liver function tests periodically during prolonged therapy.
□ May cause an increase in serum bilirubin, AST (SGOT), and ALT (SGPT) levels.

POTENTIAL NURSING DIAGNOSES

▪ Anxiety (indications).
▪ Injury, high risk for (side effects).
▪ Knowledge deficit related to medication regimen (patient/family teaching).

IMPLEMENTATION

▪ **PO:** Administer with food if GI irritation becomes a problem.
□ Medication should be tapered at the completion of long-term therapy. Sudden cessation of medication may lead to withdrawal (insomnia, irritability, nervousness, tremors).

PATIENT/FAMILY TEACHING

□ Instruct patient to take prazepam exactly as directed. Do not take more than amount prescribed or increase dose if less effective after a few weeks of therapy. Consult physician prior to adjusting dose or discontinuing.
□ Prazepam may cause drowsiness or dizziness. Caution patient to avoid driving or other activities requiring alertness until response to medication is known.
□ Advise patient to avoid the use of alcohol and to consult physician or pharmacist prior to the use of over-the-counter preparations that contain antihistamines or alcohol.
□ Advise patient to inform physician if pregnancy is planned or suspected.
□ Emphasize the importance of follow-up appointments to monitor progress.

EVALUATION

Effectiveness of therapy can be demonstrated by: ▪ Decreased sense of anxiety □ Increased ability to cope. Maximum

*<u>Underlines</u> indicate most frequent; **CAPITALS** indicate life-threatening.

therapeutic effects are usually seen within 1–2 wk. Effectiveness should be re-evaluated after 4 mo.

PRAZOSIN
(pra-zoe-sin)
Minipress

CLASSIFICATION(S):
Antihypertensive (peripherally acting antiadrenergic)
Pregnancy Category UK

INDICATIONS

- Treatment of mild to moderate hypertension. **Unlabeled Use:** - Management of urinary outflow obstruction in patients with benign prostatic hypertrophy.

ACTION

- Dilates both arteries and veins by blocking postsynaptic alpha$_1$-adrenergic receptors - Decreases contractions in smooth muscle of prostatic capsule. **Therapeutic Effects:** - Lowering of blood pressure - Decreased cardiac preload and afterload - Decreased symptoms of prostatic hypertrophy (urinary urgency, urinary hesitancy, nocturia).

PHARMACOKINETICS

Absorption: 60% absorbed following oral administration.
Distribution: Widely distributed.
Metabolism and Excretion: Extensively metabolized by the liver. Minimal (5–10%) renal excretion of unchanged drug.
Half-life: 2–3 hr.

CONTRAINDICATIONS AND PRECAUTIONS

Contraindicated in: - Hypersensitivity.
Use Cautiously in: - Renal insufficiency (increased sensitivity to effects; dosage reduction may be required) - Pregnancy, lactation, or children (safety not established) - Angina pectoris - When adding diuretics (reduce dose of prazosin).

ADVERSE REACTIONS AND SIDE EFFECTS*

CNS: dizziness, drowsiness, syncope, depression, headache, weakness.
EENT: blurred vision.
CV: first-dose orthostatic hypotension, palpitations, angina, edema.
GI: dry mouth, nausea, vomiting, diarrhea, abdominal cramps.
GU: impotence, priapism.

INTERACTIONS

Drug–Drug: - Additive hypotension with acute ingestion of **alcohol,** other **antihypertensive agents,** or **nitrates** - Antihypertensive effects may be decreased by **nonsteroidal anti-inflammatory agents**.

ROUTE AND DOSAGE

Hypertension
- **PO (Adults):** 1 mg 2–3 times daily initially (give first dose at bedtime). Increase gradually to maintenance dose of 6–15 mg/day in 2–3 divided doses (not to exceed 20–40 mg/day).

Benign Prostatic Hypertrophy
- **PO (Adults):** 1–5 mg twice daily.

AVAILABILITY

- *Capsules:* 1 mg, 2 mg, 5 mg ■ *In combination with:* polythiazide (Minizide). See Appendix A.

TIME/ACTION PROFILE
(antihypertensive effects)

	ONSET	PEAK	DURATION
PO	2 hr	2–4 hr*	10 hr

*Following single dose; maximal antihypertensive effects occur after 3–4 wk of chronic dosing.

NURSING IMPLICATIONS

ASSESSMENT
- Monitor blood pressure and pulse frequently during initial dosage adjustment and periodically throughout course of therapy. Notify physician of significant changes.
- Monitor intake and output ratios and

*Underlines indicate most frequent; **CAPITALS** indicate life-threatening.

daily weight and assess for edema daily, especially at beginning of therapy. Notify physician of weight gain or edema.

- **Lab Test Considerations:** May cause elevated serum sodium levels.

POTENTIAL NURSING DIAGNOSES

- Injury, high risk for (side effects).
- Knowledge deficit related to medication regimen (patient/family teaching).
- Noncompliance (patient/family teaching).

IMPLEMENTATION

- **General Info:** Following initial dose, patient may develop first-dose orthostatic hypotensive reaction, which most frequently occurs 30 min–2 hr after initial dose and may be manifested by dizziness, weakness, lightheadedness, and syncope. Observe patient closely during this period, and take precautions to prevent injury. The first dose may be given at bedtime to minimize this reaction.
- □ Commonly administered concurrently with a thiazide diuretic or a beta-adrenergic blocker.

PATIENT/FAMILY TEACHING

- □ Emphasize the importance of continuing to take this medication, even if feeling well. Instruct patient to take medication at the same time each day. If a dose is missed, take as soon as remembered unless almost time for next dose. Do not double doses.
- □ Encourage patient to comply with additional interventions for hypertension (weight reduction, low-sodium diet, smoking cessation, moderation of alcohol consumption, regular exercise, stress management).
- □ Instruct patient and family on proper technique for blood pressure monitoring. Advise them to check blood pressure at least weekly and to report significant changes to physician.
- □ Prazosin may cause drowsiness or dizziness. Advise patient to avoid driving or other activities requiring alertness until response to medication is known.

- □ Caution patient to avoid sudden changes in position to decrease orthostatic hypotension.
- □ Advise patient to consult physician or pharmacist before taking any cough, cold, or allergy remedies. Patient should also avoid excessive amounts of coffee, tea, or cola.
- □ Emphasize the importance of follow-up visits to determine effectiveness of therapy.

EVALUATION

Effectiveness of therapy can be demonstrated by: ▪ Decrease in blood pressure without appearance of side effects ▪ Decreased symptoms of prostatic hypertrophy.

PREDNISOLONE
(pred-**niss**-oh-lone)
Articulose, Delta-Cortef, Hydeltra-T.B.A., Hydeltrasol, Key-Pred, Nor-Pred T.B.A., Pediapred, Predaject, Predalone, Predalone T.B.A., Predate, Predcor, Predicort, Prednisol, Prelone

CLASSIFICATION(S):
Glucocorticoid (intermediate-acting)
Pregnancy Category UK

INDICATIONS

▪ Used systemically and locally in a wide variety of chronic diseases including: □ Inflammatory □ Allergic □ Hematologic □ Neoplastic □ Autoimmune ▪ Replacement therapy in adrenal insufficiency.

ACTION

▪ Suppresses inflammation and the normal immune response. Has numerous intense metabolic effects ▪ Suppresses adrenal function at chronic doses of 5 mg/day ▪ Has minimal mineralocorticoid (sodium-retaining) activity.
Therapeutic Effects: ▪ Suppression of inflammation and modification of the normal immune response ▪ Replacement therapy in adrenal insufficiency.

PHARMACOKINETICS

Absorption: Well absorbed following oral and IM administration. Chronic high-dose topical application may also lead to systemic absorption. IM acetate salt is long-acting.
Distribution: Widely distributed. Crosses the placenta and probably enters breast milk.
Metabolism and Excretion: Mostly metabolized by the liver and other tissues. Small amounts excreted unchanged by the kidneys.
Half-life: 115–212 min; adrenal suppression lasts 1.25–1.5 days.

CONTRAINDICATIONS AND PRECAUTIONS

Contraindicated in: ▪ Active untreated infections, except for tuberculous meningitis ▪ Lactation (chronic use) ▪ Some products contain bisulfites, alcohol, or phenol and should be avoided in patients with known intolerance to these additives.
Use Cautiously in: ▪ Chronic treatment (will lead to adrenal suppression) ▪ Should never be abruptly discontinued ▪ Supplemental doses may be needed during stress (surgery, infection) ▪ Pregnancy (safety not established) ▪ Children (chronic use will result in decreased growth) ▪ May mask signs of infections (fever, inflammation) ▪ Use lowest possible dose for shortest period of time.

ADVERSE REACTIONS AND SIDE EFFECTS*

CNS: headache, restlessness, psychoses, depression, euphoria, personality changes, increased intracranial pressure (children only).
EENT: cataracts, increased intraocular pressure.
CV: hypertension.
GI: nausea, vomiting, anorexia, peptic ulceration.
Derm: decreased wound healing, petechiae, ecchymoses, fragility, hirsutism, acne.
Endo: adrenal suppression, hyperglycemia.
F and E: hypokalemia, hypokalemic alkalosis, fluid retention (long-term high doses).
Hemat: thromboembolism, thrombophlebitis.
Metab: weight loss, weight gain.
MS: muscle wasting, muscle pain, aseptic necrosis of joints, osteoporosis.
Misc: increased susceptibility to infection, cushingoid appearance (moon face, buffalo hump).

INTERACTIONS

Drug–Drug: ▪ Additive hypokalemia with **diuretics, amphotericin B, mezlocillin, piperacillin,** or **ticarcillin** ▪ Hypokalemia may increase the risk of **cardiac glycoside** toxicity ▪ May increase requirement for **insulin** or **oral hypoglycemic agents** ▪ Increased risk of adverse GI effects with **alcohol, aspirin,** or **nonsteroidal anti-inflammatory agents**.

ROUTE AND DOSAGE

▪ **PO (Adults):** 5–60 mg/day single dose or divided doses (maintenance doses may be given as a single dose or every other day). 200 mg/day for 7 days, then 80 mg every other day for 1 mo for multiple sclerosis.
▪ **PO (Children):** 0.14–2 mg/kg/day in 3–4 divided doses.
▪ **IM, IV (Adults):** 4–60 mg/day.
▪ **IM (Children):** 0.046–2 mg/kg/day as a single dose or 2–3 divided doses.
▪ **Ophth (Adults and Children):** 1 drop q hr initially, then decrease to 2–4 times daily.
▪ **Otic (Adults and Children):** 3–4 drops 2–3 times daily (phosphate).
▪ **IA, IL (Adults):** 2–30 mg (phosphate), 4–40 mg (tebutate), 4–100 mg (acetate) q 3 days–4 wk.

AVAILABILITY

▪ *Tablets:* 5 mg ▪ *Syrup:* 15 mg/5 ml ▪ *Oral liquid:* 5 mg/5 ml ▪ *Prednisolone acetate for suspension for injection (acetate):* 25 mg/ml, 50 mg/ml

*Underlines indicate most frequent; CAPITALS indicate life-threatening.

- *Prednisolone terbutate suspension for injection:* 20 mg/ml ▪ *Prednisolone sodium phosphate solution for injection:* 20 mg/ml ▪ *Ophthalmic solution:* 0.125%, 0.5% ▪ *Ophthalmic suspension:* 0.12%, 0.125%, 1% ▪ *In combination with:* atropine (Mydriaprel). See Appendix A.

TIME/ACTION PROFILE (anti-inflammatory effects)

	ONSET	PEAK	DURATION
PO	1 hr	1–2	1.25–1.5 days
IM (phosphate)	rapid	1 hr	UK
IM (acetate)	slow	UK	up to 4 wk
IV	rapid	1 hr	UK
IA, IL	slow	UK	3 days–4 wk

NURSING IMPLICATIONS

ASSESSMENT

- **General Info:** This drug is indicated for many conditions. Assess involved systems prior to and periodically throughout course of therapy.
- Assess patient for signs of adrenal insufficiency (hypotension, weight loss, weakness, nausea, vomiting, anorexia, lethargy, confusion, restlessness) prior to and periodically throughout course of therapy.
- Monitor intake and output ratios and daily weight. Observe patient for the appearance of peripheral edema, steady weight gain, rales/crackles, or dyspnea. Notify physician should these occur.
- Children should have periodic evaluations of growth.
- **Intra-articular:** Monitor pain, edema, and range of motion of affected joints.
- **Intralesional:** Assess affected area prior to and daily during therapy. Note lesion size and degree of inflammation.
- **Lab Test Considerations:** Patients on prolonged courses of therapy should routinely have hematologic values, serum electrolytes, serum, and urine glucose evaluated. May cause decreased WBC counts. May cause hyperglycemia, especially in persons with diabetes. May cause decreased

serum potassium and calcium and increased serum sodium concentrations.
- Promptly report presence of guaiac-positive stools.
- May increase serum cholesterol and lipid values. May decrease serum protein-bound iodine and thyroxine concentrations.
- Suppresses reactions to skin tests.
- Periodic adrenal function tests may be ordered to assess degree of hypothalamic-pituitary-adrenal (HPA) axis suppression.

POTENTIAL NURSING DIAGNOSES

- Infection, high risk for (side effects).
- Body image disturbance (side effects).
- Knowledge deficit related to medication regimen (patient/family teaching).

IMPLEMENTATION

- **General Info:** If dose is ordered daily or every other day, administer in the morning to coincide with the body's normal secretion of cortisol.
- **PO:** Administer with meals to minimize gastric irritation.
- Use calibrated measuring device to ensure accurate dosage of liquid forms.
- **IM:** Shake suspension well before drawing up. Do not administer suspension IV. IM doses should not be administered when rapid effect is desirable.
- **Direct IV:** Do not use the acetate form of this drug for IV administration.
- *Rate:* Prednisolone sodium phosphate IV may be administered direct IV push at a rate of no more than 10 mg/min.
- **Intermittent Infusion:** May be added to 50–1000 ml of D5W or 0.9% NaCl. Stable for 24 hr.
- *Rate:* Administer infusions at prescribed rate.
- **Y-Site Compatibility:** ▪ potassium chloride ▪ vitamin B complex with C.
- **Additive Compatibility:** ▪ ascorbic acid ▪ cephalothin ▪ cytarabine ▪ erythromycin lactobionate ▪ fluoro-

uracil ▪ heparin ▪ methicillin ▪ penicillin G potassium ▪ penicillin G sodium ▪ vitamin B complex with C.
- **Additive Incompatibility:** ▪ calcium gluceptate ▪ methotrexate ▪ polymyxin B sulfate.
- **Ophth:** See Appendix H for instillation of ophthalmic preparations.

PATIENT/FAMILY TEACHING

□ Instruct patient to take medication exactly as directed. Do not skip doses or double up on missed doses. Stopping the medication suddenly may result in adrenal insufficiency (anorexia, nausea, fatigue, weakness, hypotension, dyspnea, and hypoglycemia). If these signs appear, notify physician immediately. This can be life-threatening.

□ Encourage patients on long-term therapy to eat a diet high in protein, calcium, and potassium and low in sodium and carbohydrates (see Appendix K for foods included).

□ This drug causes immunosuppression and may mask symptoms of infection. Instruct patient to avoid people with known contagious illnesses and to report possible infections.

□ Review side effects with patient. Instruct patient to inform physician promptly if severe abdominal pain or tarry stools occur. Patient should also report unusual swelling, weight gain, tiredness, bone pain, bruising, nonhealing sores, visual disturbances, or behavior changes.

□ Discuss possible effects on body image. Explore coping mechanisms.

□ Instruct patient to inform physician if symptoms of underlying disease return or worsen.

□ Advise patient to carry identification describing disease process and medication regimen in the event of an emergency in which patient cannot relate medical history.

□ Caution patient to avoid vaccinations without consulting physician.

□ Explain need for continued medical follow-up to assess effectiveness and possible side effects of medication. Physician may order periodic lab tests and eye examinations.

EVALUATION

Effectiveness of therapy can be demonstrated by: ▪ Suppression of inflammatory and immune responses in autoimmune disorders, allergic reactions, and organ transplants ▪ Management of symptoms in adrenal insufficiency.

PREDNISONE
(**pred**-ni-sone)
{Apo-Prednisone}, Deltasone, Liquid Pred, Meticorten, Orasone, Panasol, Prednicen-M, Sterapred, {Winpred}

CLASSIFICATIONS(S):
Glucocorticoid (intermediate-acting)
Pregnancy Category UK

INDICATIONS

▪ Used systemically and locally in a wide variety of chronic diseases including: □ Inflammatory □ Allergic □ Hematologic □ Neoplastic □ Autoimmune ▪ Suitable for alternate-day dosing in the management of chronic illness ▪ Replacement therapy in adrenal insufficiency.

ACTION

▪ Suppresses inflammation and the normal immune response ▪ Has numerous intense metabolic effects ▪ Suppresses adrenal function at chronic doses of 5 mg/day ▪ Has minimal mineralocorticoid (sodium-retaining) activity. **Therapeutic Effects:** ▪ Suppression of inflammation and modification of the normal immune response ▪ Replacement therapy in adrenal insufficiency.

PHARMACOKINETICS

Absorption: Well absorbed following oral administration.

Distribution: Widely distributed. Crosses the placenta and probably enters breast milk.

Metabolism and Excretion: Converted by the liver to prednisolone, which is then metabolized by the liver.

Half-life: 3.4–3.8 hr; adrenal suppression lasts 1.25–1.5 days.

CONTRAINDICATIONS AND PRECAUTIONS

Contraindicated in: ▪ Active untreated infections ▪ Lactation (avoid chronic use) ▪ Known alcohol intolerance (some liquid products).

Use Cautiously in: ▪ Chronic treatment (will lead to adrenal suppression) ▪ Should never be abruptly discontinued ▪ Supplemental doses may be needed during stress (surgery, infection) ▪ Pregnancy (safety not established) ▪ Children (chronic use will result in decreased growth) ▪ May mask signs of infections (fever, inflammation) ▪ Use lowest possible dose for shortest period of time.

ADVERSE REACTIONS AND SIDE EFFECTS*

CNS: headache, restlessness, psychoses, depression, euphoria, personality changes, increased intracranial pressure (children only).

EENT: cataracts, increased intraocular pressure.

CV: hypertension.

GI: nausea, vomiting, anorexia, peptic ulceration.

Derm: decreased wound healing, petechiae, ecchymoses, fragility, hirsutism, acne.

Endo: adrenal suppression, hyperglycemia.

F and E: hypokalemia, hypokalemic alkalosis, fluid retention (long-term high doses).

Hemat: thromboembolism, thrombophlebitis.

Metab: weight loss, weight gain.

MS: muscle wasting, muscle pain, aseptic necrosis of joints, osteoporosis.

Misc: increased susceptibility to infection, cushingoid appearance (moon face, buffalo hump).

INTERACTIONS

Drug–Drug: ▪ Additive hypokalemia with **diuretics, amphotericin B, mezlocillin, piperacillin,** or **ticarcillin** ▪ Hypokalemia may increase the risk of **cardiac glycoside** toxicity ▪ May increase requirement for **insulin** or **oral hypoglycemic agents** ▪ Increased risk of adverse GI effects with **alcohol, aspirin,** or **nonsteroidal anti-inflammatory agents**.

ROUTE AND DOSAGE

Maintenance doses may be given once daily or every other day.

▪ **PO (Adults):** 5–60 mg/day single dose or divided doses. For multiple sclerosis, 200 mg/day for 1 wk, then 80 mg every other day for 1 mo.

▪ **PO (Children):** 0.14–2 mg/kg/day in 4 divided doses.

AVAILABILITY

▪ *Tablets:* 1 mg, 2.5 mg, 5 mg, 10 mg, 20 mg, 50 mg ▪ *Oral solution:* 5 mg/5 ml, 5 mg/1 ml ▪ *Syrup:* 5 mg/5 ml.

TIME/ACTION PROFILE (anti-inflammatory effects)

	ONSET	PEAK	DURATION
PO	hr	UK	1.25–1.5 days

NURSING IMPLICATIONS

ASSESSMENT

▫ This drug is indicated for many conditions. Assess involved systems prior to and periodically throughout course of therapy.

▫ Assess patient for signs of adrenal insufficiency (hypotension, weight loss, weakness, nausea, vomiting, anorexia, lethargy, confusion, restlessness) prior to and periodically throughout course of therapy.

---

*Underlines indicate most frequent; **CAPITALS** indicate life-threatening.

▫ Monitor intake and output ratios and daily weight. Observe patient for the appearance of peripheral edema, steady weight gain, rales/crackles, or dyspnea. Notify physician should these occur.

▫ Children should have periodic evaluations of growth.

▪ **Lab Test Considerations:** Patients on prolonged courses of therapy should routinely have hematologic values, serum electrolytes, serum and urine glucose evaluated. May cause decreased WBC counts. May cause hyperglycemia, especially in persons with diabetes. May cause decreased serum potassium and calcium and increased serum sodium concentrations.

▫ Promptly report presence of guaiac-positive stools.

▫ May increase serum cholesterol and lipid values. May decrease serum protein-bound iodine and thyroxine concentrations.

▫ Suppresses reactions to skin tests.

▫ Periodic adrenal function tests may be ordered to assess degree of hypothalamic-pituitary-adrenal (HPA) axis suppression.

POTENTIAL NURSING DIAGNOSES

▪ Infection, high risk for (side effects).

▪ Body image disturbance (side effects).

▪ Knowledge deficit related to medication regimen (patient/family teaching).

IMPLEMENTATION

▪ **General Info:** If dose is ordered daily or every other day, administer in the morning to coincide with the body's normal secretion of cortisol.

▪ **PO:** Administer with meals to minimize gastric irritation.

▫ Use calibrated measuring device to ensure accurate dosage of liquid forms.

PATIENT/FAMILY TEACHING

▫ Instruct patient to take medication exactly as directed. Do not skip doses or double up on missed doses. Stopping the medication suddenly may result in adrenal insufficiency (anorexia, nausea, fatigue, weakness, hypotension, dyspnea, and hypoglycemia). If these signs appear, notify physician immediately. This can be life-threatening.

▫ Encourage patients on long-term therapy to eat a diet high in protein, calcium, and potassium and low in sodium and carbohydrates (see Appendix K for foods included).

▫ This drug causes immunosuppression and may mask symptoms of infection. Instruct patient to avoid people with known contagious illnesses and to report possible infections.

▫ Review side effects with patient. Instruct patient to inform physician promptly if severe abdominal pain or tarry stools occur. Patient should also report unusual swelling, weight gain, tiredness, bone pain, bruising, nonhealing sores, visual disturbances, or behavior changes.

▫ Discuss possible effects on body image. Explore coping mechanisms.

▫ Instruct patient to inform physician if symptoms of underlying disease return or worsen.

▫ Advise patient to carry identification describing disease process and medication regimen in the event of an emergency in which patient cannot relate medical history.

▫ Caution patient to avoid vaccinations without consulting physician.

▫ Explain need for continued medical follow-up to assess effectiveness and possible side effects of medication. Physician may order periodic lab tests and eye examinations.

EVALUATION

Effectiveness of therapy can be demonstrated by: ▪ Suppression of inflammatory and immune responses in autoimmune disorders, allergic reactions, and organ transplants ▪ Management of symptoms in adrenal insufficiency.

PRIMIDONE
(**pri**-mi-done)
{Apo-Primidone}, Myidone,
Mysoline, {Sertan}

CLASSIFICATION(S):
Anticonvulsant
Pregnancy Category UK

INDICATIONS
- Management of tonic-clonic, complex partial, and focal seizures.

ACTION
- Decreases neuron excitability ▪ Increases the threshold of electric stimulation of the motor cortex. **Therapeutic Effect:** ▪ Prevention of seizures.

PHARMACOKINETICS
Absorption: 60–80% absorbed from the GI tract.
Distribution: Widely distributed. Crosses the placenta and enters breast milk.
Metabolism and Excretion: Converted to phenobarbital and another active anticonvulsant compound (PEMA) by the liver.
Half-life: 3–24 hr.

CONTRAINDICATIONS AND PRECAUTIONS
Contraindicated in: ▪ Previous hypersensitivity ▪ Porphyria.
Use Cautiously in: ▪ Severe liver disease (dosage adjustment required) ▪ Pregnancy and lactation (safety not established; may cause hemorrhage in the newborn).

ADVERSE REACTIONS AND SIDE EFFECTS*
CNS: drowsiness, ataxia, vertigo, lethargy, excitement (children).
EENT: visual changes.
Resp: dyspnea.
CV: edema, orthostatic hypotension.
GI: nausea, anorexia, vomiting, hepatitis.

Derm: rashes, alopecia.
Hemat: blood dyscrasias, megaloblastic anemia.
Misc: folic acid deficiency.

INTERACTIONS
Drug–Drug: ▪ Induces liver enzymes and may hasten metabolism and decrease the effectiveness of other drugs metabolized by the liver, including **oral contraceptives, chloramphenicol, acebutolol, propranolol, metoprolol, timolol, doxycycline, glucocorticoids, tricyclic antidepressants, phenothiazines, phenylbutazone,** and **quinidine** ▪ Additive CNS depression with other **CNS depressants,** including **alcohol, antihistamines, opioid analgesics,** and **sedative/hypnotics** ▪ Concurrent use with **phenobarbital** may lead to phenobarbital toxicity.
Drug–Food: ▪ Decreases the absorption of **folic acid.**

ROUTE AND DOSAGE
- **PO (Adults and Children >8 yr):** Initial dose of 100–125 mg hs for 3 days, then 100–125 mg bid for 3 days, then 100–125 mg tid for 3 days, then maintenance dose of 250 mg 3–4 times daily (not to exceed 2 g/day).
- **PO (Children <8 yr):** Initial dose of 50 mg hs for 3 days, then 50 mg bid for next 3 days, 100 mg bid for 3 days, then maintenance dose of 125–250 mg tid (10–25 mg/kg/day).

AVAILABILITY
▪ *Tablets:* 50 mg, 250 mg ▪ *Oral suspension:* 250 mg/5 ml ▪ {*Chewable tablets:* 125 mg}.

TIME/ACTION PROFILE
(anticonvulsant effect)

	ONSET	PEAK	DURATION
PO	4–7 days	7–10 days	8–12 hr

NURSING IMPLICATIONS
ASSESSMENT
▫ Assess location, duration, and char-

acteristics of seizure activity. Institute seizure precautions.

□ Assess patient for allergy to phenobarbital, as it is a primidone metabolite.

□ Assess patient for signs of folic acid deficiency (mental dysfunction, unusual tiredness or weakness, psychiatric disorders, neuropathy, megaloblastic anemia). May be treated with folic acid.

□ CBC and Sequential Multiple Analyzer-12 (SMA-12) tests should be monitored every 6 mon throughout course of therapy. May cause leukopenia and thrombocytopenia. May cause decreased serum bilirubin concentrations.

■ **Toxicity and Overdose:** Serum primidone and phenobarbital (a major metabolite of primidone) levels should be routinely monitored. Therapeutic blood levels for primidone: 5–10 mcg/ml; for phenobarbital: 15–40 mcg/ml.

□ Signs of primidone toxicity include ataxia, lethargy, changes in vision, confusion, and dyspnea.

POTENTIAL NURSING DIAGNOSES
■ Injury, high risk for (indications).
■ Knowledge deficit related to medication regimen (patient/family teaching).

IMPLEMENTATION
■ **General Info:** When switching from alternative anticonvulsant medication to primidone or adding primidone to regimen, increase primidone dose gradually while decreasing or continuing other anticonvulsant dosages to maintain seizure control. The switch to primidone alone should take at least 2 wk. Dosage adjustment is usually done at bedtime.

■ **PO:** May be administered with food to minimize GI irritation. Low initial doses (25 mg twice daily) have been used in patients experiencing nausea and vomiting. Tablets may be crushed and mixed with food or fluids

for patients with difficulty swallowing. Shake liquid preparations well before pouring. Use calibrated measuring device to ensure accurate dosage.

PATIENT/FAMILY TEACHING
□ Instruct patient to take medication every day exactly as directed. If a dose is missed, take as soon as remembered unless within 1 hr of next dose. Abrupt withdrawal may lead to status epilepticus.

□ Primidone may cause drowsiness or dizziness. Caution patient to avoid driving or other activities requiring alertness until response to medication is known. These symptoms usually diminish in frequency and intensity with continued use of the medication. Do not resume driving until physician gives medical clearance based on control of seizure disorder.

□ Caution patient to avoid taking alcohol or other CNS depressants concurrently with this medication.

□ Caution patient to avoid sudden changes in position to decrease orthostatic hypotension.

□ Instruct patient to notify physician or dentist of medication regimen prior to treatment or surgery.

□ Advise patient to carry identification describing medication regimen at all times.

□ Advise patient to notify physician if skin rash, unsteady gait, joint pain, fever, changes in vision, dyspnea, pregnancy, or paradoxical excitement (especially in children or the elderly) occur.

□ Emphasize the importance of routine examinations to monitor progress.

EVALUATION
Effectiveness of therapy can be demonstrated by: ■ Decrease or cessation of seizures without excessive sedation. May require 1 wk or more of therapy before therapeutic response is seen.

PROBENECID
(proe-**ben**-e-sid)
Benemid, {Benuryl}, Probalan

CLASSIFICATION(S):
Antigout agent (uricosuric)
Pregnancy Category UK

INDICATIONS
■ Prevention of recurrences of gouty arthritis ■ Treatment of hyperuricemia secondary to thiazide therapy ■ Used to increase and prolong serum levels of penicillin and related anti-infectives.

ACTION
■ Inhibits renal tubular reabsorption of uric acid, thus promoting its renal excretion. **Therapeutic Effect:** ■ Reduction of serum uric acid levels.

PHARMACOKINETICS
Absorption: Well absorbed following oral administration.
Distribution: Crosses the placenta.
Metabolism and Excretion: Metabolized by the liver. Small amounts (10%) excreted unchanged in the urine.
Half-life: 4–17 hr.

CONTRAINDICATIONS AND PRECAUTIONS
Contraindicated in: ■ Hypersensitivity ■ Chronic high-dose salicylate therapy.
Use Cautiously in: ■ Peptic ulcer ■ Blood dyscrasias ■ Uric acid kidney stones ■ Pregnancy (has been used safely) ■ Renal impairment (dosage reduction recommended). May not be effective if GFRL is 30 ml/min or less.

ADVERSE REACTIONS AND SIDE EFFECTS*
CNS: headache, dizziness.
GI: nausea, vomiting, diarrhea, sore gums, hepatitis, abdominal pain.
GU: urinary frequency, uric acid stones.
Derm: flushing, rashes.
Hemat: anemia, APLASTIC ANEMIA.

INTERACTIONS
Drug–Drug: ■ Increases blood levels of **penicillins, cephalosporins,** and **fluoroquinolones** ■ Blocks excretion and may increase toxicity or effectiveness of **nonsteroidal anti-inflammatory agents, IV acyclovir, methotrexate,** and **nitrofurantoin** ■ Large doses of **aspirin** may decrease uricosuric activity ■ May intensify the effects of **barbiturates, benzodiazepines, clofibrate, dapsone, penicillamine, sulfonylureas, zidovudine,** or **heparin.**

ROUTE AND DOSAGE
Hyperuricemia
■ **PO (Adults):** 250 mg bid for 1 wk, increase to 500 mg bid, then may increase by 500 mg/day every 4 wk (not to exceed 3 g/day).

To Augment Penicillin or Cephalosporin Therapy
■ **PO (Adults):** 500 mg qid.
■ **PO (Children 2–14 yr):** 25 mg/kg initially; then 40 mg/kg/day in 4 divided doses.

Single-Dose Therapy of Gonorrhea
■ **PO (Adults):** 1 g with amoxicillin or penicillin.

AVAILABILITY
■ *Tablets:* 0.5 g ■ *In combination with:* 0.5 mg colchicine (Co/Benenid, Proben-C) and ampicillin (Polycillin PRB, Probampicin). See Appendix A.

TIME/ACTION PROFILE (effects on serum uric acid levels)

	ONSET	PEAK	DURATION
PO	30 min	2–4 hr	8 hr

NURSING IMPLICATIONS
ASSESSMENT
■ **Gout:** Assess involved joints for pain, mobility, and edema throughout course of therapy.
□ Monitor intake and output ratios. Fluids should be encouraged to prevent urate stone formation (2000–3000 ml/

{} = Available in Canada only.
*Underlines indicate most frequent; **CAPITALS** indicate life-threatening.

day). Alkalinization of the urine with sodium bicarbonate, potassium citrate, or acetazolamide may also be ordered for this purpose.

■ **Lab Test Considerations:** May cause false-positive results in copper sulfate urine glucose tests (Clinitest). Use glucose oxidase method (Keto-Diastix, Test-Tape) to monitor urine glucose. CBC, serum uric acid levels, and renal function should be monitored routinely during long-term therapy.

☐ Serum and urine uric acid determinations may be measured periodically when probenecid is used to treat hyperuricemia.

Potential Nursing Diagnoses
■ Pain (indications).
■ Physical mobility, impaired (indications).
■ Knowledge deficit related to medication regimen (patient/family teaching).

IMPLEMENTATION

■ **General Info:** Probenecid therapy is not used to treat gouty arthritis but rather, for prevention. If acute attacks occur during therapy, probenecid is usually continued at full dose along with colchicine or nonsteroidal antiinflammatory agents.

■ **PO:** Administer with food or antacid to minimize gastric irritation.

☐ Gradual dosage reduction should be attempted if uric acid levels remain stable following 6 mo of therapy.

PATIENT/FAMILY TEACHING

☐ Instruct patient to take medication exactly as directed, not to discontinue without consulting physician. Irregular dosage schedules may cause elevation of uric acid levels and precipitate an acute gout attack.

☐ Explain purpose of the medication to patients taking probenecid with penicillin.

☐ Advise patient to follow physician's recommendations regarding weight loss, diet, and alcohol consumption.

☐ Caution patient not to take aspirin or

other salicylates, as they decrease the effects of probenecid.

☐ Instruct patient to report nausea, vomiting, abdominal pain, unusual bleeding or bruising, sore throat, fatigue, malaise, or yellowing of the skin or eyes to physician promptly.

EVALUATION

Therapeutic effects can be demonstrated by: ■ Decrease in pain and swelling in affected joints and subsequent decrease in frequency of gout attacks. May require several months of continuous therapy for maximum effects ■ Decrease in serum uric acid levels ■ Prolonged serum levels of penicillins and other related antibiotics.

PROBUCOL
(**proe**-byoo-kole)
Lorelco

CLASSIFICATION(S):
Lipid-lowering agent
Pregnancy Category B

INDICATIONS
■ Adjunct therapy of primary hypercholesterolemia.

ACTION
■ May decrease transport of cholesterol from intestine or interfere with cholesterol synthesis ■ May also increase fecal excretion of cholesterol and bile acids ■ Lowers high-density lipoprotein (HDL) cholesterol. **Therapeutic Effects:** ■ Lowers serum cholesterol levels ■ Lowers low-density lipoprotein (LDL) cholesterol.

PHARMACOKINETICS
Absorption: Limited and variable absorption following oral administration (2–8%). Absorption is increased by concurrent administration of food.
Distribution: Accumulates in fatty tissue during chronic administration.
Metabolism and Excretion: Appears

to be excreted in feces following biliary elimination.

Half-life: 20 days.

CONTRAINDICATIONS AND PRECAUTIONS

Contraindicated in: ▪ Hypersensitivity ▪ Pregnancy (continue contraception for 6 mo following therapy with probucol) ▪ Lactation ▪ Primary biliary cirrhosis.

Use Cautiously in: ▪ Cardiac arrhythmias ▪ Untreated congestive heart failure ▪ Children (safety not established).

ADVERSE REACTIONS AND SIDE EFFECTS*

CNS: dizziness, headache, insomnia.

EENT: blurred vision, tinnitus, decreased sense of smell, conjunctivitis, lacrimation.

CV: arrhythmias, ECG changes (prolonged QT interval), SUDDEN DEATH.

GI: diarrhea, bloating, flatulence, abdominal pain, nausea, vomiting, indigestion, GI bleeding, decreased taste.

Derm: rashes, pruritus, sweating.

Endo: enlargement of goiter.

Hemat: eosinophilia, anemia, thrombocytopenia.

Neuro: paresthesia, peripheral neuritis.

INTERACTIONS

Drug–Drug: ▪ Increased risk of adverse cardiovascular effects with concurrent use of **tricyclic antidepressants, anticholinergics, group I and III antiarrhythmics, phenothiazines, beta-adrenergic blocking agents, potassium-losing diuretics,** or **cardiac glycosides** ▪ Concurrent use with **clofibrate** may further decrease high-density lipoprotein (HDL) cholesterol.

Drug–Food: ▪ Concurrent administration of **food** increases absorption.

ROUTE AND DOSAGE

▪ **PO (Adults):** 500 mg bid.

AVAILABILITY

▪ *Tablets:* 250 mg, 500 mg.

TIME/ACTION PROFILE (lipid-lowering effects)

	ONSET	PEAK	DURATION
PO	UK	20–50 days	1–3 mo

P

NURSING IMPLICATIONS

ASSESSMENT

▫ Obtain a diet history, especially regarding fat and alcohol consumption.

▪ **Lab Test Considerations:** May cause slight increase in serum bilirubin, blood glucose, BUN, creatine phosphokinase, AST (SGOT), ALT (SGPT), alkaline phosphatase, and uric acid concentrations.

▫ Serum triglyceride and cholesterol levels should be monitored prior to therapy, after 1 mo of therapy, and then every 3–6 mo. Medication should be discontinued if serum triglycerides increase despite low-fat diet.

▫ May decrease hemoglobin, hematocrit, and eosinophil concentrations.

POTENTIAL NURSING DIAGNOSES

▪ Diarrhea (side effects).

▪ Knowledge deficit related to medication regimen (patient/family teaching).

▪ Noncompliance (patient/family teaching).

IMPLEMENTATION

▪ **PO:** Administer with meals to enhance absorption.

PATIENT/FAMILY TEACHING

▫ Instruct patient to take medication as directed. If a dose is missed, take as soon as remembered unless almost time for next dose.

▫ Advise patient that this medication should be used in conjunction with dietary restrictions (fat, cholesterol, carbohydrates, alcohol), exercise, cessation of smoking.

▫ Probucol may occasionally cause dizziness. Avoid driving or other activities requiring coordination until response to medication is known.

*Underlines indicate most frequent; **CAPITALS** indicate life-threatening.

□ Instruct patient to notify physician if abdominal discomfort, nausea, diarrhea, or bloating persists. GI side effects are usually transient.

□ Explain need for medical follow-up to monitor response to therapy and to detect side effects. Patients with a history of cardiac arrhythmias should have periodic ECGs, and therapy should be withdrawn if QT intervals become prolonged or arrhythmias increase.

EVALUATION

Effectiveness of therapy can be demonstrated by: ▪ Decrease in serum cholesterol levels. If a response is not seen within 4 mo, medication is usually discontinued.

PROCAINAMIDE
(proe-**kane**-ah-mide)
Procan SR, Promine, Pronestyl,
Pronestyl-SR

CLASSIFICATION(S):
Antiarrhythmic (group IA)
Pregnancy Category C

INDICATIONS

▪ Treatment of a wide variety of ventricular and atrial arrhythmias, including: □ Atrial premature contractions □ Premature ventricular contractions □ Ventricular tachycardia □ Paroxysmal atrial tachycardia ▪ Maintenance of normal sinus rhythm after conversion from atrial fibrillation or flutter.

ACTION

▪ Decreases myocardial excitability ▪ Slows conduction velocity ▪ May depress myocardial contractility. **Therapeutic Effect:** ▪ Suppression of arrhythmias.

PHARMACOKINETICS

Absorption: Well absorbed (75–90%) following oral and IM administration. Sustained-release oral preparation is more slowly absorbed.

Distribution: Rapidly and widely distributed.
Metabolism and Excretion: Converted by the liver to n-acetylprocainamide (NAPA), an active antiarrhythmic compound. Remainder (40–70%) excreted unchanged by the kidneys.
Half-life: 2.5–4.7 hr (NAPA—7 hr), prolonged in renal impairment.

CONTRAINDICATIONS AND PRECAUTIONS

Contraindicated in: ▪ Hypersensitivity ▪ AV block ▪ Myasthenia gravis ▪ Hypersensitivity to tartrazine (FDC yellow dye #5; present in some oral products).
Use Cautiously in: ▪ Myocardial infarction or cardiac glycoside toxicity ▪ Congestive heart failure, renal or hepatic insufficiency, elderly patients (dosage reduction or increased dosing intervals recommended) ▪ Pregnancy, lactation, or children (safety not established).

ADVERSE REACTIONS AND SIDE EFFECTS*

CNS: confusion, seizures, dizziness.
CV: hypotension, ventricular arrhythmias, asystole, heart block.
GI: nausea, vomiting, bitter taste.
Derm: rashes.
Hemat: leukopenia, thrombocytopenia, AGRANULOCYTOSIS, eosinophilia.
Misc: drug-induced systemic lupus syndrome, fever, chills.

INTERACTIONS

Drug–Drug: ▪ May have additive or antagonistic effects with other **antiarrhythmics** ▪ Additive neurologic toxicity (confusion, seizures) with **lidocaine** ▪ **Antihypertensives** and **nitrates** may potentiate hypotensive effect ▪ Potentiates **neuromuscular blocking agents** ▪ May partially antagonize the therapeutic effects of **anticholinesterase agents** in myasthenia gravis ▪ Increased risk of arrhythmias with **pimozide** ▪ Additive anticholinergic effects with other **drugs possessing anticholinergic properties,** including **antihistamines, antidepres-**

sants, atropine, haloperidol, and phenothiazines ▪ Effects of procainamide
may be increased by **cimetidine, ranitidine, quinidine,** or **trimethoprim**.

ROUTE AND DOSAGE
See infusion rate chart in Appendix D.

▪ **PO, IM (Adults):** 50 mg/kg/day in
divided doses q 3–6 hr (q 6 hr
for sustained-release preparations).
Older patients or those with renal, hepatic, or cardiac insufficiency should
receive lower doses or longer dosing
intervals.
▪ **PO (Children):** 15–50 mg/kg/day in
divided doses q 3–6 hr (up to 4 g/
day)
▪ **IM (Children):** 20–30 mg/kg/day in
divided doses q 4–6 hr (up to 4 g/
day).
▪ **IV (Adults):** 100 mg q 5 min until
arrhythmia is abolished or 500–1000
mg has been given. Wait at least 10
min until further dosing or loading
infusion of 500–600 mg over 25–30
min followed by maintenance infusion of 2–6 mg/min.
▪ **IV (Children):** 3–6 mg/kg over 5 min
followed by 20–80 mcg/kg/min (up to
100 mg/dose or 2 g/day).

AVAILABILITY

▪ *Tablets:* 250 mg, 375 mg, 500 mg
▪ *Sustained-release tablets:* 250 mg,
500 mg, 750 mg, 1000 mg ▪ *Capsules:*
250 mg, 375 mg, 500 mg ▪ *Injection:*
100 mg/ml, 500 mg/ml.

TIME/ACTION PROFILE (anti-
arrhythmic effects)

	ONSET	PEAK	DURATION
PO	30 min	60–90 min	3–4 hr
PO-ER	UK	UK	6 hr
IV	immediate	25–60 min	3–4 hr
IM	10–30 min	15–60 min	3–4 hr

NURSING IMPLICATIONS

ASSESSMENT
□ Monitor ECG, pulse, and blood pressure continuously throughout IV administration. Parameters should be
monitored periodically during oral

administration. IV administration is
usually discontinued if any of the following occur: arrhythmia is resolved,
QRS complex widens by 50%, PR interval is prolonged, blood pressure
drops >15 mmHg, or toxic side effects develop. Patient should remain
supine throughout IV administration
to minimize hypotension.

▪ **Lab Test Considerations:** CBC should
be monitored weekly during the first
3 mo of therapy. May cause decreased
leukocyte, neutrophil, and platelet
counts. Therapy may be discontinued
if leukopenia occurs. Blood counts
usually return to normal within 1 mo
of discontinuation of therapy.
□ Antinuclear antibody (ANA) should
be periodically monitored during prolonged therapy or if symptoms of
lupus-like reaction occur. Therapy is
discontinued if a steady increase in
ANA titer occurs.
□ May cause an increase in AST
(SGOT), ALT (SGPT), alkaline phosphatase, LDH, and bilirubin, and a
positive Coombs' test result.
▪ **Toxicity and Overdose:** Serum procainamide and NAPA levels may be
monitored periodically during dosage
adjustment. Therapeutic blood level
of procainamide is 4–8 mcg/ml.
□ Toxicity may occur with procainamide blood levels of 8–16 mcg/ml
or greater.
□ Signs of toxicity include confusion,
dizziness, drowsiness, decreased urination, nausea, vomiting, and tachyarrhythmias.

POTENTIAL NURSING DIAGNOSES
▪ Cardiac output, decreased (indications).
▪ Knowledge deficit related to medication regimen (patient/family teaching).

IMPLEMENTATION
▪ **General Info:** When converting from
IV to oral dose regimen, allow 3–4 hr
to elapse between last IV dose and
administration of first oral dose.
▪ **PO:** Administer with a full glass of
water on an empty stomach either 1 hr

before or 2 hr after meals for faster absorption. If GI irritation becomes a problem, may be administered with or immediately after meals. Tablets may be crushed and capsules opened and mixed with food or fluids for patients with difficulty swallowing. Do not break, crush, or chew sustained-release tablets (Procan SR, Pronestyl-SR). Wax matrix of sustained-release tablets may be found in stool but is not significant.

- **IM:** Used only when oral and IV routes are not feasible.
- **Direct IV:** Dilute each 100 mg with 10 ml of D5W or Sterile Water for Injection.
- **Rate:** Administer at a rate not to exceed 50 mg/min. Rapid administration may cause ventricular fibrillation or asystole.
- **Intermittent Infusion:** Prepare IV infusion by adding 200 mg–1 g to 50–500 ml of D5W, for a concentration of 2–4 mg/ml. Slight yellow color of solution will not alter potency; do not use when darker than light amber or if solution contains a precipitate.
- **Rate:** Administer initial infusion over 30 min. Maintenance infusion should infuse at 2–6 mg/min to maintain control of arrhythmia. Use infusion pump to ensure accurate dosage (see Appendix D for infusion rate chart).
- **Y-Site Compatibility:** ▪ famotidine ▪ heparin ▪ hydrocortisone sodium succinate ▪ potassium chloride ▪ ranitidine ▪ vitamin B complex with C.
- **Y-Site Incompatibility:** ▪ milrinone.

Patient/Family Teaching

□ Instruct patient to take medication around the clock, exactly as directed, even if feeling well. If a dose is missed, take as soon as remembered within 2 hr (4 hr for sustained-release tablets); omit if remembered later. Do not double doses. Consult physician prior to discontinuing medication, as gradual reduction in dosage may be needed to prevent worsening of condition.

□ Instruct patient or family member on how to take pulse. Advise patient to report changes in pulse rate or rhythm to physician.
□ Procainamide may cause dizziness. Caution patient to avoid driving or other activities requiring alertness until response to medication is known.
□ Advise patient to notify physician immediately if signs of drug-induced lupus syndrome (fever, chills, joint pain or swelling, pain with breathing, skin rash); leukopenia (sore throat, mouth, or gums); or thrombocytopenia (unusual bleeding or bruising) occurs. Medication may be discontinued if these occur.
□ Caution patient not to take over-the-counter medications with procainamide without consulting physician or pharmacist.
□ Advise patient to inform physician or dentist of medication regimen prior to treatment or surgery.
□ Advise patient to carry identification describing disease process and medication regimen at all times.
□ Emphasize the importance of routine follow-up examinations to monitor progress.

EVALUATION
Effectiveness of therapy can be demonstrated by: ▪ Resolution of cardiac arrhythmias without detrimental side effects.

PROCARBAZINE
(proe-**kar**-ba-zeen)
Matulane, {Natulan}

CLASSIFICATION(S):
Antineoplastic (alkylating agent)
Pregnancy Category D

INDICATIONS

▪ In combination with other antineoplastic agents and modalities in the treatment of Hodgkin's disease. **Unlabeled Uses:** ▪ Other lymphomas

■ Brain and lung tumors ■ Multiple myeloma ■ Malignant melanoma ■ Polycythemia vera.

ACTION

■ Appears to inhibit DNA, RNA, and protein synthesis (cell cycle-S phase specific). **Therapeutic Effect:** ■ Death of rapidly replicating cells, particularly malignant ones.

PHARMACOKINETICS

Absorption: Well absorbed following oral administration.
Distribution: Widely distributed. Crosses the blood–brain barrier.
Metabolism and Excretion: Metabolized by the liver.
Half-life: 1 hr.

CONTRAINDICATIONS AND PRECAUTIONS

Contraindicated in: ■ Hypersensitivity ■ Pregnancy or lactation ■ Alcoholism ■ Severe renal or liver impairment ■ Pheochromocytoma ■ Congestive heart failure.
Use Cautiously in: ■ Patients with childbearing potential ■ Infections ■ Decreased bone marrow reserve ■ Other chronic debilitating illnesses ■ Headaches ■ Psychiatric illness ■ Liver impairment ■ Cardiovascular disease.

ADVERSE REACTIONS AND SIDE EFFECTS*

CNS: neuropathy, confusion, depression, psychosis, mania, headache, hallucinations, nightmares, tremor, seizures, syncope, drowsiness, dizziness.
EENT: retinal hemorrhage, nystagmus, photophobia.
Resp: cough, pleural effusions.
CV: edema, tachycardia, hypotension.
GI: nausea, vomiting, anorexia, stomatitis, dry mouth, dysphagia, diarrhea, hepatic dysfunction.
GU: gonadal suppression.
Derm: rashes, pruritus, alopecia, photosensitivity.
Endo: gynecomastia.

Hemat: anemia, leukopenia, thrombocytopenia.
Neuro: neuropathies, paresthesias.
Misc: ascites.

INTERACTIONS

Drug–Drug: ■ Additive CNS depression with other **CNS depressants,** including **alcohol, antidepressants, antihistamines, opioid analgesics,** and **sedative/hypnotics** ■ Disulfiram-like reaction may occur with **alcohol** ■ **Sympathomimetic amines, local anesthetics, levodopa, reserpine, guanethidine, guanadrel, vasoconstrictors,** and **antidepressants** should be avoided, since procarbazine has some MAO inhibitory properties (increased risk of hypertensive reactions) ■ Severe paradoxical reactions may occur with **meperidine** and other **opioid analgesics** (avoid concurrent meperidine—decrease initial dose of other opioid analgesics to 25% of usual dose) ■ Seizure and hyperpyrexia may occur with concurrent use of **MAO inhibitors, tricyclic antidepressants, fluoxetine** (should not be used within 5 wk of fluoxetine), or **carbamazepine** ■ Additive bone marrow depression with other **antineoplastic agents** or **radiation therapy** ■ May potentiate hypoglycemia from **insulin** or **oral hypoglycemic agents.**
Drug–Food: ■ Ingestion of foods high in **tyramine** content (see Appendix K) may result in hypertension ■ Ingestion of foods high in **caffeine** content may result in arrhythmias.

ROUTE AND DOSAGE

■ **PO (Adults):** 2–4 mg/kg/day for 1 wk, then 4–6 mg/kg/day until response is obtained, maintenance dose of 1–2 mg/kg/day.
■ **PO (Children):** 50 mg/m^2/day for 7 days, then 100 mg/m^2/day, maintenance dose of 50 mg/m^2/day.

AVAILABILITY

■ *Capsules:* 50 mg.

---

*Underlines indicate most frequent; **CAPITALS** indicate life-threatening.

TIME/ACTION PROFILE (effects on blood counts)

	ONSET	PEAK	DURATION
PO	14 days	2–8 wk	28 days or more (up to 6 wk)

NURSING IMPLICATIONS

ASSESSMENT

▢ Monitor blood pressure, pulse, and respiratory rate periodically during course of therapy. Notify physician if significant changes occur.

▢ Assess patient's nutritional status (appetite, intake and output ratios, weight, frequency and amount of emesis). Anorexia and weight loss can be decreased by feeding light, frequent meals. Nausea and vomiting can be minimized by administering an antiemetic at least 1 hr prior to receiving medication.

▪ **Lab Test Considerations:** Renal and hepatic function, CBC, and urinalysis should be monitored prior to and routinely throughout course of therapy. Inform physician if WBC <4000/mm^3 or platelet count <100,000/mm^3. The nadir of leukopenia and thrombocytopenia occurs in approximately 4 wk, and recovery usually occurs in about 6 wk. Anemia also may occur.

▢ Closely monitor serum glucose in diabetic patients. Oral hypoglycemics or insulin dosage may need to be reduced, as hypoglycemic effects are enhanced.

▪ **Toxicity and Overdose:** Concurrent ingestion of tyramine-rich foods and many medications may result in life-threatening hypertensive crisis. Signs and symptoms of hypertensive crisis include chest pain, severe headache, nausea and vomiting, photosensitivity, and enlarged pupils. Treatment includes IV phentolamine.

POTENTIAL NURSING DIAGNOSES

▪ Infection, high risk for (adverse reactions).

▪ Nutrition, altered: less than body requirements (adverse reactions).

▪ Knowledge deficit related to medication regimen (patient/family teaching).

IMPLEMENTATION

▪ **PO:** Administer with food or fluids if GI irritation occurs. Confer with pharmacist regarding opening of capsules if patient has difficulty swallowing.

PATIENT/FAMILY TEACHING

▢ Emphasize the need to take medication exactly as directed. If a dose is missed, it should be taken as soon as remembered unless almost time for next dose. Physician should be consulted if vomiting occurs shortly after a dose is taken.

▢ Instruct patient to notify physician promptly if fever, sore throat, signs of infection, bleeding gums, bruising, petechiae, or blood in stool, urine, or emesis occurs. Caution patient to avoid crowds and persons with known infections. Instruct patient to use soft toothbrush and electric razor and to avoid falls. Patient should not receive IM injections or rectal temperatures. Patient should also be cautioned not to drink alcoholic beverages or take medication containing aspirin or ibuprofen, as these may precipitate gastric bleeding.

▢ Caution patient to avoid alcohol, caffeinated beverages, CNS depressants, over-the-counter drugs, and foods or beverages containing tyramine (see Appendix K for foods included) during therapy and for at least 2 wk after therapy has been discontinued, as they may precipitate a hypertensive crisis.

▢ Advise patient that an additional interaction of alcohol with procarbazine is a disulfiram-like reaction (flushing, nausea, vomiting, headache, abdominal cramps).

▢ Instruct patient to inspect oral mucosa for erythema and ulceration. If ulceration occurs, advise patient to use sponge brush and rinse mouth with water after eating and drinking. Viscous lidocaine swishes may be used if mouth pain interferes with eating.

- Medication may cause drowsiness or dizziness. Caution patient to avoid driving or other activities that require alertness until response to medication is known.
- Advise patient that this medication may have teratogenic effects. Contraception should be practiced during therapy and for at least 4 mo after therapy is concluded.
- Discuss the possibility of hair loss with patient. Explore methods of coping.
- Caution patient to use sunscreen and protective clothing to prevent photosensitivity reactions.
- Instruct patient not to receive any vaccinations without advice of physician.
- Advise patient to notify physician or dentist of medication regimen prior to treatment or surgery. This therapy usually should be withdrawn at least 2 wk prior to surgery.
- Emphasize the need for periodic lab tests to monitor for side effects.
- Instruct patient to inform physician if confusion, hallucinations, cough, paresthesia, unsteady gait, severe headache, skin rash, jaundice, or diarrhea occurs.

Evaluation
Effectiveness of therapy can be demonstrated by: ▪ Decrease in size and spread of malignant tissue in Hodgkin's disease.

PROCHLORPERAZINE
(proe-klor-**pair**-a-zeen)
Chlorpazine, Compa-Z, Compazine, Contranzine, {Provazin}, {Stemetil}, Ultrazine

CLASSIFICATION(S):
Antiemetic (phenothiazine),
Antipsychotic
Pregnancy Category UK

INDICATIONS

▪ Management of nausea and vomiting ▪ Treatment of acute and chronic psychoses.

ACTION

▪ Alters the effects of dopamine in the CNS ▪ Possesses significant anticholinergic and alpha-adrenergic blocking activity ▪ Depresses the chemoreceptor trigger zone (CTZ) in the CNS. **Therapeutic Effects:** ▪ Diminished nausea and vomiting ▪ Diminished signs and symptoms of psychoses.

PHARMACOKINETICS

Absorption: Absorption from tablet is variable; may be better with oral liquid formulations. Well absorbed following IM administration.
Distribution: Widely distributed, high concentrations in the CNS. Crosses the placenta and probably enters breast milk.
Metabolism and Excretion: Highly metabolized by the liver and GI mucosa. Converted to some compounds with antipsychotic activity.
Half-life: UK.

CONTRAINDICATIONS AND PRECAUTIONS

Contraindicated in: ▪ Hypersensitivity ▪ Cross-sensitivity with other phenothiazines may exist ▪ Narrow-angle glaucoma ▪ Bone marrow depression ▪ Severe liver or cardiovascular disease ▪ Hypersensitivity to bisulfites or benzyl alcohol (some parenteral products) ▪ Children <2 yr or 9.1 kg.
Use Cautiously in: ▪ Elderly or debilitated patients (dosage reduction recommended) ▪ Pregnancy or lactation (safety not established; may cause adverse reactions in newborns) ▪ Diabetes mellitus ▪ Respiratory disease ▪ Prostatic hypertrophy ▪ CNS tumors ▪ Epilepsy ▪ Intestinal obstruction.

P

ADVERSE REACTIONS AND SIDE EFFECTS*

CNS: sedation, extrapyramidal reactions, tardive dyskinesia, NEUROLEPTIC MALIGNANT SYNDROME.

EENT: dry eyes, blurred vision, lens opacities.

CV: hypotension, tachycardia, ECG changes.

GI: constipation, dry mouth, ileus, anorexia, hepatitis.

GU: urinary retention, pink or reddish-brown discoloration of urine.

Derm: rashes, photosensitivity, pigment changes.

Endo: galactorrhea.

Hemat: AGRANULOCYTOSIS, leukopenia.

Metab: hyperthermia.

Misc: allergic reactions.

INTERACTIONS

Drug–Drug: ▪ Additive hypotension with **antihypertensive agents, nitrates,** or acute ingestion of **alcohol** ▪ Additive CNS depression with other **CNS depressants,** including **alcohol, antidepressants, antihistamines, opioid analgesics, sedative/hypnotics,** or **general anesthetics** ▪ Additive anticholinergic effects with other **drugs possessing anticholinergic properties,** including **antihistamines, antidepressants, atropine, haloperidol,** and other **phenothiazines** ▪ **Lithium** decreases absorption and increases the risk of extrapyramidal reactions ▪ May mask early signs of **lithium** toxicity ▪ Increased risk of agranulocytosis with **antithyroid agents** ▪ Decreases the beneficial effects of **levodopa** ▪ **Antacids** may decrease absorption.

ROUTE AND DOSAGE

Antiemetic, Mild to Moderate Emotional Disturbances

▪ **PO (Adults):** 5–10 mg 3–4 times daily or 15 mg/day as extended-release preparation or 10 mg bid of extended-release preparation (not to exceed 40 mg/day).

▪ **IM (Adults):** 5–10 mg q 3–4 hr (not to exceed 40 mg/day).

▪ **Rect (Adults):** 25 mg bid.

▪ **PO, Rect (Children 18–39 kg):** 2.5 mg tid or 5 mg bid (not to exceed 15 mg/day).

▪ **PO, Rect (Children 14–17 kg):** 2.5 mg 2–3 times daily (not to exceed 10 mg/day).

▪ **PO, Rect (Children 9–13 kg):** 2.5 mg 1–2 times daily (not to exceed 7.5 mg/day).

▪ **IM (Children >2 yr):** 0.13 mg/kg, single dose.

▪ **IV (Adults):** 2.5–10 mg, rate not to exceed 5 mg/min, may be repeated in 30 min; single dose not to exceed 10 mg (not to exceed 40 mg/day).

Psychomotor Agitation, Psychoses

▪ **PO (Adults):** 5–10 mg 3–4 times daily, increased as needed (not to exceed 150 mg/day).

▪ **PO, Rect (Children 2–12 yr):** 2.5 mg 2–3 times daily (not to exceed 10 mg on first day, not to exceed 25 mg/day in children 6–12 yr or 20 mg/day in children 2–5 yr).

▪ **IM (Adults):** 10–20 mg q 2–4 hr as needed initially, then 10–20 mg q 4–6 hr (may give up to q 1 hr; not to exceed 150–200 mg/day).

AVAILABILITY

▪ *Tablets:* 5 mg, 10 mg, 25 mg ▪ *Syrup:* 5 mg/5 ml ▪ *Sustained-release capsules:* 10 mg, 15 mg, 30 mg ▪ *Injection:* 5 mg/ml ▪ *Suppositories:* 2.5 mg, 5 mg, 25 mg.

TIME/ACTION PROFILE (antiemetic effect)

	ONSET	PEAK	DURATION
PO	30–40 min	UK	3–4 hr
PO-ER	30–40 min	UK	10–12 hr
Rect	60 min	UK	3–4 hr
IM	10–20 min	UK	3–4 hr
IV	rapid (min)	UK	3–4 hr

NURSING IMPLICATIONS

ASSESSMENT

▪ **General Info:** Monitor blood pressure (sitting, standing, lying), pulse, and respiratory rate prior to and fre-

*Underlines indicate most frequent; CAPITALS indicate life-threatening.

quently during the period of dosage adjustment.

□ Assess patient for level of sedation following administration.

□ Monitor patient for onset of extrapyramidal side effects (akathisia—restlessness; dystonia—muscle spasms and twisting motions; pseudoparkinsonism—mask facies, rigidity, tremors, drooling, shuffling gait, dysphagia). Notify physician if these symptoms occur, as reduction in dosage or discontinuation of medication may be necessary. Trihexyphenidyl or diphenhydramine may be used to control these symptoms.

□ Monitor for tardive dyskinesia (rhythmic movement of mouth, face, and extremities). Notify physician immediately if these symptoms occur, as these side effects may be irreversible.

□ Monitor for development of neuroleptic malignant syndrome (fever, respiratory distress, tachycardia, convulsions, diaphoresis, hypertension or hypotension, pallor, tiredness). Notify physician immediately if these symptoms occur.

■ **Antiemetic:** Assess patient for nausea and vomiting prior to and 30–60 min following administration.

■ **Antipsychotic:** Monitor patient's mental status (orientation to reality and behavior) prior to and periodically throughout therapy.

□ Observe patient carefully when administering oral medication to ensure that medication is actually taken and not hoarded.

■ **Lab Test Considerations:** CBC and liver function tests should be evaluated periodically throughout course of therapy. May cause blood dyscrasias, especially between wk 4 and 10 of therapy. Hepatotoxicity is more likely to occur between days 14 and 30 of therapy.

□ May cause false-positive or false-negative pregnancy tests and false-positive urine bilirubin test results.

□ May cause increased serum prolactin levels and interfere with gonadorelin test results.

□ May cause Q-wave and T-wave changes in ECG.

POTENTIAL NURSING DIAGNOSES

■ Fluid volume deficit (indications).

■ Thought processes, altered (indications).

■ Knowledge deficit related to medication regimen (patient/family teaching).

IMPLEMENTATION

■ **General Info:** To prevent contact dermatitis avoid getting solution on hands.

□ Phenothiazines should be discontinued 48 hr before and not resumed for 24 hr following metrizamide myelography, as they lower seizure threshold.

■ **PO:** Do not crush or chew sustained-release capsules. Administer with food, milk, or a full glass of water to minimize gastric irritation.

□ Dilute syrup in citrus or chocolate-flavored drinks.

■ **IM:** Do not inject SC. Inject slowly, deep into well-developed muscle. Keep patient recumbent for at least 30 min following injection to minimize hypotensive effects. Slight yellow color will not alter potency. Do not administer solution that is markedly discolored or that contains a precipitate.

■ **Direct IV:** Dilute to a concentration of 1 mg/ml.

■ *Rate:* Administer at a rate of 1 mg/min; not to exceed 5 mg/min.

■ **Intermittent Infusion:** Dilute 20 mg in up to 1 liter dextrose, saline, Ringer's or lactated Ringer's solution, dextrose/saline, dextrose/Ringer's, or lactated Ringer's combinations.

■ **Syringe Incompatibility:** Manufacturer does not recommend mixing prochlorperazine with other medications in syringe.

■ **Y-Site Compatibility:** ■ fluconazole ■ fludarabine ■ heparin ■ hydrocortisone sodium succinate ■ ondansetron ■ potassium chloride ■ sargramostim ■ vitamin B complex with C.

■ **Y-Site Incompatibility:** ■ foscarnet.

- **Additive Compatibility:** ▪ amikacin ▪ ascorbic acid ▪ dexamethasone sodium phosphate ▪ erythromycin lactobionate ▪ ethacrynate sodium ▪ nafcillin ▪ sodium bicarbonate ▪ vitamin B complex with C.
- **Additive Incompatibility:** ▪ amphotericin B ▪ ampicillin ▪ calcium gluceptate ▪ cephalothin ▪ chloramphenicol ▪ chlorothiazide ▪ hydrocortisone sodium succinate ▪ penicillin G sodium.

PATIENT/FAMILY TEACHING

□ Instruct patient to take medication exactly as directed, not to skip doses or double up on missed doses. If a dose is missed, it should be taken as soon as remembered unless almost time for next dose. If more than 2 doses are scheduled each day, missed dose should be taken within about 1 hr of the ordered time. Abrupt withdrawal may lead to gastritis, nausea, vomiting, dizziness, headache, tachycardia, and insomnia.

□ Inform patient of possibility of extrapyramidal symptoms and tardive dyskinesia. Caution patient to report these symptoms immediately to physician.

□ Advise patient to make position changes slowly to minimize orthostatic hypotension.

□ Medication may cause drowsiness. Caution patient to avoid driving or other activities requiring alertness until response to medication is known.

□ Caution patient to avoid taking alcohol or other CNS depressants concurrently with this medication.

□ Advise patient to use sunscreen and protective clothing when exposed to the sun to prevent photosensitivity reactions. Extremes in temperature should also be avoided, as this drug impairs body temperature regulation.

□ Instruct patient to use frequent mouth rinses, good oral hygiene, and sugarless gum or candy to minimize dry mouth. Consult physician or dentist if dry mouth continues >2 wk.

□ Advise patient that increasing bulk and fluids in the diet and exercise may help minimize the constipating effects of this medication.

□ Inform patient that this medication may turn urine pink to reddish-brown.

□ Advise patient to notify physician or dentist of medication regimen prior to treatment or surgery.

□ Instruct patient to notify physician promptly if sore throat, fever, unusual bleeding or bruising, skin rashes, weakness, tremors, visual disturbances, dark-colored urine, or clay-colored stools are noted.

□ Emphasize the importance of routine follow-up examinations to monitor response to medication and detect side effects. Periodic ocular examinations are indicated. Encourage continued participation in psychotherapy as ordered by physician.

EVALUATION

Effectiveness of therapy can be demonstrated by: ▪ Relief of nausea and vomiting ▪ Decrease in excitable, paranoic, or withdrawn behavior when used as an antipsychotic.

PROGESTERONE
(proe-**jess**-te-rone)
Femotrone, Gestrol, Progestaject, {Progestilin}

CLASSIFICATION(S):
Hormone (progestin)
Pregnancy Category D

INDICATIONS

▪ Treatment of secondary amenorrhea and abnormal uterine bleeding caused by hormonal imbalance. **Unlabeled Use:** ▪ Corpus luteum dysfunction.

ACTION

▪ Produces secretory changes in the endometrium: □ Increases in basal body temperature □ Histologic changes in vaginal epithelium □ Relaxation of uterine smooth muscle □ Mammary alveolar tissue growth □ Pituitary inhibition □ Withdrawal bleeding in the presence of estrogen. **Therapeutic Effect:** ▪ Restoration of hormonal balance with control of uterine bleeding.

PHARMACOKINETICS

Absorption: UK.
Distribution: Enters breast milk.
Metabolism and Excretion: UK.
Half-life: UK.

CONTRAINDICATIONS AND PRECAUTIONS

Contraindicated in: ▪ Hypersensitivity ▪ Hypersensitivity to parabens (IM suspension only) ▪ Pregnancy (except corpus luteum dysfunction) ▪ Missed abortion ▪ Thromboembolic disease ▪ Cerebrovascular disease ▪ Severe liver disease ▪ Breast or genital cancer ▪ Porphyria.
Use Cautiously in: ▪ History of liver disease ▪ Renal disease ▪ Cardiovascular disease ▪ Seizure disorders ▪ Mental depression.

ADVERSE REACTIONS AND SIDE EFFECTS*

CNS: depression.
EENT: retinal thrombosis.
CV: THROMBOEMBOLISM, PULMONARY EMBOLISM, thrombophlebitis.
GI: gingival bleeding, hepatitis.
GU: cervical erosions.
Endo: breakthrough bleeding, spotting, amenorrhea, breast tenderness, galactorrhea, changes in menstrual flow.
Derm: rashes, melasma, chloasma.
F and E: edema.
Local: pain, irritation at IM injection site.
Misc: weight gain, weight loss, allergic reactions, including ANAPHYLAXIS and ANGIOEDEMA.

INTERACTIONS

Drug–Drug: ▪ May decrease the effectiveness of **bromocriptine** when used concurrently for galactorrhea/amenorrhea.

ROUTE AND DOSAGE

Secondary Amenorrhea
▪ **IM (Adults):** 50–100 mg (single dose) or 5–10 mg daily for 6–8 days given 8–10 days prior to expected menstrual period.

Abnormal Uterine Bleeding
▪ **IM (Adults):** 50–100 mg (single dose) or 5–10 mg daily for 6 days.

Corpus Luteum Insufficiency
▪ **IM (Adults):** 12.5 mg/day at onset of ovulation for 2 wk (may continue until 11th wk of gestation).

AVAILABILITY

▪ *Injection:* 25 mg/ml, 50 mg/ml, 100 mg/ml.

TIME/ACTION PROFILE

	ONSET	PEAK	DURATION
IM	UK	UK	UK

NURSING IMPLICATIONS

ASSESSMENT
▪ **General Info:** Blood pressure should be monitored periodically throughout therapy.
□ Monitor intake and output ratios and weekly weight. Report significant discrepancies or steady weight gain to physician.
▪ **Amenorrhea:** Assess patient's usual menstrual history. Administration of drug usually begins 8–10 days before anticipated menstruation. Withdrawal bleeding usually occurs 48–72 hr after course of therapy. Therapy should be discontinued if menses occur during injection series.
▪ **Dysfunctional Bleeding:** Monitor pattern and amount of vaginal bleeding (pad count). Bleeding should end by 6th day of therapy. Therapy should be discontinued if menses occur during injection series.
▪ **Lab Test Considerations:** Monitor hepatic function prior to and periodically throughout therapy.
□ May cause increased plasma amino acid and alkaline phosphatase levels.

*Underlines indicate most frequent; **CAPITALS** indicate life-threatening.

□ May decrease pregnanediol excretion concentrations.

□ High doses may increase sodium and chloride excretion.

□ May alter thyroid function test results.

POTENTIAL NURSING DIAGNOSES

■ Sexual dysfunction (indications).

■ Knowledge deficit related to medication regimen (patient/family teaching).

IMPLEMENTATION

■ **IM:** Shake vial before preparing IM dose. Administer deep IM. Rotate sites.

PATIENT/FAMILY TEACHING

□ Advise patient to report signs and symptoms of fluid retention (swelling of ankles and feet, weight gain), thromboembolic disorders (pain, swelling, tenderness in extremities, headache, chest pain, blurred vision), mental depression, or hepatic dysfunction (yellowed skin or eyes, pruritus, dark urine, light-colored stools) to physician.

□ Instruct patient to notify physician if change in vaginal bleeding pattern or spotting occurs.

□ Instruct patient to stop taking medication and notify physician if pregnancy is suspected.

□ Caution patient to use sunscreen and protective clothing to prevent photosensitivity reactions.

□ Advise patient to notify physician or dentist of medication regimen prior to treatment or surgery.

□ Emphasize the importance of routine follow-up physical examinations, including blood pressure; breast, abdomen, and pelvic examinations; and PAP smears.

EVALUATION

Effectiveness of therapy can be demonstrated by: ■ Development of normal cyclic menses.

PROMAZINE
(**proe**-ma-zeen)
Primazine, Prozine, Sparine

CLASSIFICATION(S):
Antipsychotic (phenothiazine)
Pregnancy Category UK

INDICATIONS

■ Treatment of acute and chronic psychoses.

ACTION

■ Alters the effects of dopamine in the CNS ■ Possesses significant anticholinergic and alpha-adrenergic blocking activity. **Therapeutic Effect:** ■ Diminished signs and symptoms of psychoses.

PHARMACOKINETICS

Absorption: Absorption from tablets is variable; may be better with oral liquid formulations. Well absorbed following IM administration.

Distribution: Widely distributed, high concentrations in the CNS. Crosses the placenta and probably enters breast milk.

Metabolism and Excretion: Highly metabolized by the liver and GI mucosa.

Half-life: UK.

CONTRAINDICATIONS AND PRECAUTIONS

Contraindicated in: ■ Hypersensitivity ■ Cross-sensitivity with other phenothiazines may exist ■ Narrow-angle glaucoma ■ Bone marrow depression ■ Severe liver or cardiovascular disease ■ Hypersensitivity to bisulfites or formaldehyde (injection only).

Use Cautiously in: ■ Elderly or debilitated patients (dosage reduction may be required) ■ Pregnancy or lactation (safety not established) ■ Diabetes mellitus ■ Respiratory disease ■ Prostatic hypertrophy ■ CNS tumors ■ Epilepsy ■ Intestinal obstruction.

ADVERSE REACTIONS AND SIDE EFFECTS*

CNS: sedation, extrapyramidal reactions, tardive dyskinesia, NEUROLEPTIC MALIGNANT SYNDROME.
EENT: dry eyes, blurred vision, lens opacities.
CV: hypotension, tachycardia.
GI: constipation, dry mouth, ileus, anorexia, hepatitis.
GU: urinary retention.
Derm: rashes, photosensitivity, pigment changes.
Endo: galactorrhea.
Hemat: AGRANULOCYTOSIS, leukopenia.
Metab: hyperthermia.
Misc: allergic reactions.

INTERACTIONS

Drug–Drug: ■ Additive hypotension with antihypertensive agents, nitrates, or acute ingestion of alcohol ■ Additive CNS depression with other CNS depressants, including alcohol, antihistamines, narcotic analgesics, sedative/hypnotics, or general anesthetics ■ Additive anticholinergic effects with other drugs possessing anticholinergic properties, including antihistamines, antidepressants, atropine, haloperidol, and other phenothiazines ■ Lithium decreases absorption and increases the risk of extrapyramidal reactions ■ May mask early signs of lithium toxicity ■ Decreases beneficial effects of levodopa ■ Increased risk of agranulocytosis with antithyroid agents.

ROUTE AND DOSAGE

Psychoses
■ **PO, IM (Adults):** 10–200 mg q 4–6 hr up to 1000 mg/day.
■ **PO, IM (Children >12 yr):** 10–25 mg q 4–6 hr.

Severe Agitation
■ **IM (Adults):** 50–150 mg initially; if required, additional doses may be given after 30 min up to a total dose of 300 mg, then maintenance dose of 10–200 mg q 4–6 hr as needed (not to exceed 1 g/24 hr).

AVAILABILITY

■ *Tablets:* 25 mg, 50 mg, 100 mg ■ *Injection:* 25 mg/ml, 50 mg/ml.

TIME/ACTION PROFILE
(antipsychotic effects)

	ONSET	PEAK	DURATION
PO	30 min	UK	4–6 hr
IM	within 30 min	UK	UK

NURSING IMPLICATIONS

ASSESSMENT
- Monitor patient's mental status (orientation to reality and behavior) prior to and periodically during therapy.
- Monitor blood pressure (sitting, standing, lying), pulse, and respiratory rate prior to and frequently during the period of dosage adjustment.
- Observe patient carefully when administering oral medication to ensure medication is actually taken and not hoarded.
- Assess patient for level of sedation following administration.
- Monitor patient for onset of extrapyramidal side effects (akathisia—restlessness; dystonia—muscle spasms and twisting motions; pseudoparkinsonism—mask facies, rigidity, tremors, drooling, shuffling gait, dysphagia). Notify physician if these symptoms occur, as reduction in dosage or discontinuation of medication may be necessary. Trihexyphenidyl or diphenhydramine may be used to control these symptoms.
- Monitor for tardive dyskinesia (rhythmic movement of mouth, face, and extremities). Notify physician immediately if these symptoms occur, as these side effects may be irreversible.
- Monitor for development of neuroleptic malignant syndrome (fever, respiratory distress, tachycardia, convulsions, diaphoresis, hypertension or hypotension, pallor, tiredness). Notify physician immediately if these symptoms occur.
- Assess fluid intake and bowel func-

tion. Increased bulk and fluids in the diet help minimize the constipating effects of this medication.

- **Lab Test Considerations:** CBC and liver function tests should be evaluated periodically throughout course of therapy. May cause blood dyscrasias especially between wk 4 and 10 of therapy.

□ May cause false-positive or false-negative pregnancy test results and false-positive urine bilirubin test results.

□ May cause increased serum prolactin levels, thereby interfering with gonadorelin test results.

□ May cause Q-wave and T-wave changes in ECG.

POTENTIAL NURSING DIAGNOSES

- Thought processes, altered (indications).
- Knowledge deficit related to medication regimen (patient/family teaching).
- Noncompliance (patient/family teaching).

IMPLEMENTATION

- **General Info:** To prevent contact dermatitis, avoid getting solution on hands.

□ Phenothiazines should be discontinued 48 hr before and not resumed for 24 hr following metrizamide myelography, as they lower the seizure threshold.

- **PO:** Administer with food, milk, or a full glass of water to minimize gastric irritation.
- **IM:** Do not inject SC. Inject slowly into deep, well-developed muscle. Keep patient recumbent for at least 30 min following injection to minimize hypotensive effects. Slight yellow color will not alter potency. Do not administer solution that is markedly discolored or that contains a precipitate.

PATIENT/FAMILY TEACHING

□ Advise patient to take medication exactly as directed, not to skip doses or double up on missed doses. If a dose is missed, it should be taken as soon as remembered unless almost time for the next dose. If more than 2 doses are scheduled each day, the missed dose should be taken within about 1 hr of the ordered time. Abrupt withdrawal may lead to gastritis, nausea, vomiting, dizziness, headache, tachycardia, and insomnia.

□ Inform patient of possibility of extrapyramidal symptoms, tardive dyskinesia, and neuroleptic malignant syndrome. Caution patient to report these symptoms immediately to physician.

□ Advise patient to make position changes slowly to minimize orthostatic hypotension.

□ Medication may cause drowsiness. Caution patient to avoid driving or other activities requiring alertness until response to medication is known.

□ Caution patient to avoid taking alcohol or other CNS depressants concurrently with this medication.

□ Advise patient to use sunscreen and protective clothing when exposed to the sun to prevent photosensitivity reactions. Extremes in temperature should also be avoided, as this drug impairs body temperature regulation.

□ Instruct patient to use frequent mouth rinses, good oral hygiene, and sugarless gum or candy to minimize dry mouth. Consult physician or dentist if dry mouth continues >2 wk.

□ Advise patient to notify physician or dentist of medication regimen prior to treatment or surgery.

□ Instruct patient to notify physician promptly if sore throat, fever, unusual bleeding or bruising, skin rashes, weakness, tremors, visual disturbances, dark-colored urine, or clay-colored stools are noted.

□ Emphasize the importance of routine follow-up examinations to monitor response to medication and detect side effects. Periodic ocular examinations are indicated. Encourage continued participation in psychotherapy as ordered by physician.

EVALUATION

Effectiveness of therapy can be demon-

strated by: ▪ Decrease in excitable, paranoic, or withdrawn behavior.

PROMETHAZINE
(proe-meth-a-zeen)
Anergan, {Histanil}, Mallergan, Pentazine, Phenameth, Phenazine, Phencen-50, Phenergan, Phenergan Fortis, Phenergan Plain, Phenoject-50, {PMS Promethazine}, Pro-50, Prometh-25, Prometh-50, Prorex, Prothazine Plain, Remsed, V-Gan

CLASSIFICATION(S):
Antihistamine (phenothiazine), Antiemetic, Sedative/hypnotic
Pregnancy Category UK

INDICATIONS

▪ Treatment of various allergic conditions and motion sickness ▪ Preoperative sedation ▪ Treatment and prevention of nausea and vomiting ▪ Adjunct to anesthesia and analgesia.

ACTION

▪ Blocks the effects of histamine ▪ Has inhibitory effect on the chemoreceptor trigger zone in the medulla, resulting in antiemetic properties ▪ Alters the effects of dopamine in the CNS ▪ Possesses significant anticholinergic activity ▪ Produces CNS depression by indirectly decreased stimulation of the CNS reticular system. **Therapeutic Effects:** ▪ Relief of symptoms of histamine excess usually seen in allergic conditions ▪ Diminished nausea or vomiting ▪ Sedation.

PHARMACOKINETICS

Absorption: Well absorbed following oral and IM administration. Rectal administration may be less reliable.
Distribution: Widely distributed. Crosses the blood–brain barrier and the placenta.

Metabolism and Excretion: Metabolized by the liver.
Half-life: UK.

CONTRAINDICATIONS AND PRECAUTIONS

Contraindicated in: ▪ Hypersensitivity ▪ Comatose patients ▪ Prostatic hypertrophy ▪ Bladder neck obstruction ▪ Narrow-angle glaucoma.
Use Cautiously in: ▪ Hypertension ▪ Sleep apnea ▪ Epilepsy ▪ Pregnancy (has been used safely during labor; avoid chronic use during pregnancy) ▪ Lactation (safety not established; may cause drowsiness in infant).

ADVERSE REACTIONS AND SIDE EFFECTS*

CNS: excess sedation, confusion, disorientation, dizziness, fatigue, extrapyramidal reactions, nervousness, insomnia.
CV: tachycardia, bradycardia, hypotension, hypertension.
Derm: rashes, photosensitivity.
EENT: blurred vision, tinnitus, diplopia.
GI: dry mouth, hepatitis, constipation.
Hemat: blood dyscrasias.

INTERACTIONS

Drug–Drug: ▪ Additive CNS depression with other **CNS depressants,** including **alcohol, antianxiety agents,** other **antihistamines, opioid analgesics,** and other **sedative/hypnotics** ▪ Additive anticholinergic effects with other **drugs possessing anticholinergic properties,** including other **antihistamines, antidepressants, atropine, haloperidol,** other **phenothiazines, quinidine,** and **disopyramide.**

ROUTE AND DOSAGE
Allergic Conditions
▪ **PO (Adults):** 25 mg at bedtime or 12.5 mg 4 times daily.
▪ **PO (Children >2 yr):** 25 mg at bed-

time or 5–12.5 mg tid or 0.5 mg/kg at bedtime or 0.125 mg/kg q 4–6 hr.
- **IM, IV, Rect (Adults):** 25 mg, may repeat in 2 hr.

Motion Sickness
- **PO (Adults):** 25 mg 30–60 min prior to departure, may be repeated in 8–12 hr.
- **PO (Children >2 yr):** 12.5–25 mg or 0.5 mg/kg 30–60 min prior to departure, may be given twice daily.

Sedation
- **PO, Rect, IM, IV (Adults):** 25–50 mg.
- **PO, Rect, IM, IV (Children >2 yr):** 10–25 mg or 0.5–1.1 mg/kg.

Sedation During Labor
- **IM, IV (Adults):** 50 mg in early labor; when labor is established, additional doses of 25–75 mg may be given 1–2 times at 4-hr intervals (24-hr dose should not exceed 100 mg).

Antiemetic
- **PO, Rect, IM, IV (Adults):** 10–25 mg q 4 hr as needed.
- **PO, Rect, IM, IV (Children >2 yr):** 0.25–0.5 mg/kg 4–6 times daily.

AVAILABILITY
- **Tablets:** 12.5 mg, 25 mg, 50 mg ▪ **Injection:** 25 mg/ml, 50 mg/ml ▪ **Suppositories:** 12.5 mg, 25 mg, 50 mg ▪ **In combination with:** codeine, dextromethorphan, phenylephrine, and/or pseudoephedrine in a variety of cough and cold preparations. See Appendix A.

TIME/ACTION PROFILE (noted as antihistaminic effects; sedative effects last 2–8 hr)

	ONSET	PEAK	DURATION
PO	20 min	UK	up to 12 hr
IM	20 min	UK	up to 12 hr
Rectal	20 min	UK	up to 12 hr
IV	3–5 min	UK	up to 12 hr

NURSING IMPLICATIONS

Assessment
- **General Info:** Monitor blood pressure, pulse, and respiratory rate frequently in patients receiving IV doses.

▫ Assess patient for level of sedation following administration.
▫ Monitor patient for onset of extrapyramidal side effects (akathisia—restlessness; dystonia—muscle spasms and twisting motions; pseudoparkinsonism—mask facies, rigidity, tremors, drooling, shuffling gait, dysphagia). Notify physician if these symptoms occur.
- **Allergy:** Assess allergy symptoms (rhinitis, conjunctivitis, hives) prior to and periodically throughout course of therapy.
- **Antiemetic:** Assess patient for nausea and vomiting prior to and following administration.
- **Lab Test Considerations:** May cause false-positive or false-negative pregnancy tests.
▫ CBC should be evaluated periodically during chronic therapy, as blood dyscrasias may occur.
▫ May cause increased serum glucose.
▫ May cause false-negative results in skin tests using allergen extracts. Promethazine should be discontinued 72 hr prior to the test.

Potential Nursing Diagnoses
- Fluid volume deficit (indications).
- Injury, high risk for (side effects).
- Knowledge deficit related to medication regimen (patient/family teaching).

Implementation
- **General Info:** When administering promethazine concurrently with opioid analgesics, supervise ambulation closely to prevent injury due to increased sedation.
- **PO:** Administer with food, water, or milk to minimize GI irritation. Tablets may be crushed and mixed with food or fluids for patients with difficulty swallowing.
- **IM:** Administer deep into well-developed muscle. SC administration may cause tissue necrosis.
- **Direct IV:** Doses should not exceed a concentration of 25 mg/ml. Slight yellow color does not alter potency. Do not use if precipitate present.

- *Rate:* Administer each 25 mg slowly, over at least 1 min. Rapid administration may produce a transient fall in blood pressure.
- **Solution Compatibility:** • dextrose • saline • Ringer's or lactated Ringer's solution • dextrose/saline • dextrose/Ringer's • lactated Ringer's combinations.
- **Syringe Compatibility:** • atropine • butorphanol • cimetadine • diphenhydramine • droperidol • fentanyl • glycopyrrolate • hydromorphone • meperidine • metoclopramide • midazolam • pentazocine • ranitidine • scopolamine.
- **Syringe Incompatibility:** • dimenhydrinate • heparin • pentobarbital • thiopental.
- **Y-Site Compatibility:** • fluconazole • fludarabine • ondansetron • sargramostim.
- **Y-Site Incompatibility:** • cefoperazone • foscarnet.

PATIENT/FAMILY TEACHING
- **General Info:** Review dosage schedule with patient. If medication is ordered regularly and a dose is missed, take as soon as remembered unless time for next dose.
- Promethazine may cause drowsiness. Caution patient to avoid driving or other activities requiring alertness until response to medication is known.
- Advise patient that frequent mouth rinses, good oral hygiene, and sugarless gum or candy may decrease dry mouth. Dentist or physician should be notified if dry mouth persists >2 wk.
- Caution patient to use sunscreen and protective clothing to prevent photosensitivity reactions.
- Advise patient to make position changes slowly to minimize orthostatic hypotension. Elderly patients are at increased risk for this side effect.
- Caution patient to avoid concurrent use of alcohol and other CNS depressants with this medication.

- Instruct patient to notify physician if sore throat, fever, jaundice, or uncontrolled movements are noted.
- **Motion Sickness:** When used as prophylaxis for motion sickness, advise patient to take medication at least 30 min and preferably 1–2 hr prior to exposure to conditions that may cause motion sickness.

EVALUATION
Effectiveness of therapy can be demonstrated by: • Relief from allergic symptoms • Prevention of motion sickness • Sedation • Relief from nausea and vomiting.

PROPAFENONE
(proe-**paff**-e-nown)
Rhythmol

CLASSIFICATION(S):
Antiarrhythmic (group IC)
Pregnancy Category C

INDICATIONS
• Treatment of life-threatening ventricular arrhythmias including ventricular tachycardia.

ACTION
• Slows conduction in cardiac tissue by altering transport of ions across cell membranes. **Therapeutic Effect:** • Suppression of ventricular arrhythmias.

PHARMACOKINETICS
Absorption: Although well absorbed following oral administration undergoes rapid hepatic metabolism (bioavailability 3–11%).
Distribution: Distribution not known.
Metabolism and Excretion: Extensively metabolized by the liver, some metabolites have antiarrhythmic activity. >90% of patients are considered extensive metabolizers. Others metabolize propafenone more slowly.
Half-life: 2–10 hr in extensive metabolizers, 10–32 hr in slow metabolizers.

CONTRAINDICATIONS AND PRECAUTIONS

Contraindicated in: ▪ Hypersensitivity ▪ Cardiogenic shock ▪ Conduction disorders including sick-sinus syndrome and AV block (without a pacemaker) ▪ Bradycardia ▪ Severe hypotension ▪ Nonallergic bronchospasm ▪ Electrolyte disturbances ▪ Uncontrolled congestive heart failure.

Use Cautiously in: ▪ Pregnancy, lactation, or children (safety not established) ▪ Severe hepatic or renal impairment (dosage reduction may be necessary) ▪ Elderly patients (lower doses may be necessary).

ADVERSE REACTIONS AND SIDE EFFECTS*

CNS: dizziness, shaking, WEAKNESS.
EENT: blurred vision.
CV: VENTRICULAR ARRHYTHMIAS, SUPRAVENTRICULAR ARRHYTHMIA, conduction disturbances, angina, hypotension, bradycardia.
GI: altered taste, nausea, vomiting, constipation, diarrhea, dry mouth.
Derm: rash.
MS: joint pain.

INTERACTIONS

Drug–Drug: ▪ Increases serum **digoxin** levels by 35–85% (dosage reduction may be required) ▪ Increases blood levels of **metoprolol** and **propranolol** (dosage reduction may be required) ▪ Concurrent use of **local anesthetics** may increase the risk of CNS adverse reactions ▪ May increase the effects of **warfarin** ▪ May increase **cyclosporine** through blood levels and risk of nephrotoxicity ▪ **Rifampin** may decrease serum levels and effectiveness of propafenone.

ROUTE AND DOSAGE

▪ **PO (Adults):** 150 mg q 8 hr, may be gradually increased at 3–4 day intervals as required up to 300 mg q 8 hr.

AVAILABILITY

▪ *Tablets:* 150 mg, 300 mg.

TIME/ACTION PROFILE
(antiarrhythmic effects)

	ONSET	PEAK	DURATION
PO	hrs–days	4–5 days*	hrs

*Chronic dosing.

NURSING IMPLICATIONS

ASSESSMENT

▫ Monitor ECG or Holter monitor prior to and periodically throughout therapy. May cause PR prolongation and QT prolongation.
▫ Monitor blood pressure and pulse periodically throughout therapy.
▫ Monitor intake and output ratios and daily weight. Assess patients for signs of congestive heart failure (peripheral edema, rales/crackles, dyspnea, weight gain, jugular venous distension). May require reduction or discontinuation of therapy.
▪ **Lab Test Considerations:** May cause elevated antinuclear antibody (ANA) titer, which is usually asymptomatic and reversible.
▪ **Toxicity and Overdose:** Signs of toxicity include hypotension, excessive drowsiness, and decreased or abnormal heart rate. Notify physician if these signs occur.

POTENTIAL NURSING DIAGNOSES

▪ Cardiac output, decreased (indications).
▪ Knowledge deficit related to medication regimen (patient/family teaching).

IMPLEMENTATION

▪ **General Info:** Propafenone therapy should be initiated in a hospital with facilities for cardiac rhythm monitoring. Most serious proarrhythmic effects are seen in the first 2 wk of therapy.
▫ Previous antiarrhythmic therapy should be withdrawn 2–5 half-lives before starting propafenone.
▫ Dosage adjustments should be at least 3–4 days apart due to the long half-life of propafenone.

*Underlines indicate most frequent; **CAPITALS** indicate life-threatening.

- Pre-existing hypokalemia or hyperkalemia should be corrected prior to instituting therapy.

PATIENT/FAMILY TEACHING

- Instruct patient to take medication around the clock exactly as directed, even if feeling better. Missed doses should be taken as soon as remembered if within 4 hr; omit if remembered later. Gradual dosage reduction may be necessary.
- Medication may cause dizziness. Caution patient to avoid driving and other activities requiring alertness until response to medication is known.
- Advise patient to notify physician or dentist of medication regimen prior to treatment or surgery.
- Instruct patient to notify physician if fever, sore throat, chills or unusual bleeding or bruising occur or if chest pain, shortness of breath, diaphoresis, palpitations, or visual changes become bothersome.
- Advise patient to carry identification describing disease process and medication regimen at all times.
- Emphasize the importance of follow-up examinations to monitor progress.

EVALUATION

Effectiveness of therapy can be demonstrated by: ▪ Decrease in frequency of ventricular arrhythmias.

PROPANTHELINE
(proe-**pan**-the-leen)
Norpanth, {Probanthel}, Pro-Banthine

CLASSIFICATION(S):
Anticholinergic (antimuscarinic)
Pregnancy Category C

INDICATIONS

▪ Adjunctive therapy in the treatment of peptic ulcer disease. **Unlabeled Use:** Antisecretory or antispasmodic agent.

ACTION

▪ Competitively inhibits the muscarinic action of acetylcholine, resulting in decreased GI secretions. **Therapeutic Effect:** ▪ Reduction of signs and symptoms of peptic ulcer disease.

PHARMACOKINETICS

Absorption: Incompletely absorbed from the GI tract.
Distribution: Distribution not known. Does not cross the blood–brain barrier.
Metabolism and Excretion: Inactivated in the upper small intestine.
Half-life: UK.

CONTRAINDICATIONS AND PRECAUTIONS

Contraindicated in: ▪ Hypersensitivity ▪ Narrow-angle glaucoma ▪ Tachycardia secondary to cardiac insufficiency or thyrotoxicosis ▪ Myasthenia gravis.
Use Cautiously in: ▪ Elderly patients or patients of small stature (dosage reduction required) ▪ Prostatic hypertrophy ▪ Chronic renal, cardiac, or pulmonary disease ▪ Patients who may have intra-abdominal infections ▪ Pregnancy, lactation, or children (safety not established).

ADVERSE REACTIONS AND SIDE EFFECTS*

CNS: drowsiness, confusion, excitement, dizziness.
EENT: blurred vision, mydriasis, photophobia.
CV: palpitations, tachycardia, orthostatic hypotension.
GI: dry mouth, constipation.
GU: urinary hesitancy, urinary retention.
Derm: rash.
Misc: decreased sweating.

INTERACTIONS

Drug–Drug: ▪ Additive anticholinergic effects with other **drugs possessing anticholinergic properties,** including **antihistamines, antidepressants, atropine, haloperidol, phenothiazines,**

quinidine, and **disopyramide** ▪ May alter the absorption of other **orally administered drugs** by slowing motility of the GI tract ▪ **Antacids** and **adsorbent antidiarrheals** decrease the absorption of anticholinergics (avoid taking within 2–3 hr of propantheline) ▪ May increase GI mucosal lesions in patients taking **wax-matrix potassium chloride preparations.**

ROUTE AND DOSAGE

- **PO (Adults):** 15 mg tid, 30 mg hs.
- **PO (Elderly Patients, Patients with Mild Symptoms or Small Stature):** 7.5 mg 3–4 times daily.
- **PO (Children):** *Antisecretory*—1.5 mg/kg/day in 3–4 divided doses. *Antispasmodic*—2–3 mg/kg/day given q 4–6 hr at bedtime.

AVAILABILITY

- **Tablets:** 7.5 mg, 15 mg.

TIME/ACTION PROFILE
(anticholinergic effects)

	ONSET	PEAK	DURATION
PO	30–60 min	2–6 hr	6 hr

NURSING IMPLICATIONS

ASSESSMENT
- □ Assess for abdominal pain prior to and periodically throughout therapy.
- ▪ **Lab Test Considerations:** Antagonizes effects of pentagastrin and histamine during gastric acid secretion test. Avoid administration for 24 hr preceding the test.

POTENTIAL NURSING DIAGNOSES
- ▪ Pain (indications).
- ▪ Constipation (side effects).
- ▪ Knowledge deficit related to medication regimen (patient/family teaching).

IMPLEMENTATION
- ▪ **PO:** Administer 30 min before meals. Bedtime dose should be administered at least 2 hr after last meal of the day.
- □ Do not administer within 1 hr of antacids or antidiarrheal medications.

PATIENT/FAMILY TEACHING
- □ Instruct patient to take medication as directed. If a dose is missed take as soon as remembered unless almost time for next dose. Do not double doses.
- □ May cause drowsiness or blurred vision. Caution patient to avoid driving or other activities requiring alertness until response to medication is known.
- □ Instruct patient that frequent oral rinses, sugarless gum or candy, and good oral hygiene may help relieve dry mouth. Consult physician or dentist regarding use of saliva substitute if dry mouth persists >2 wk.
- □ Advise patient that increasing fluid intake, adding bulk to the diet, and exercise may help alleviate the constipating effects of the drug.
- □ Advise elderly patients to make position changes slowly to minimize the effects of drug-induced orthostatic hypotension.
- □ Caution patient to avoid extremes of temperature. This medication decreases the ability to sweat and may increase the risk of heat stroke.
- □ Instruct patient to notify physician if confusion, excitement, dizziness, rash, difficulty with urination, or eye pain occurs. Physician may order periodic ophthalmic examinations to monitor intraocular pressure, especially in the elderly.

EVALUATION
Effectiveness of therapy can be demonstrated by: ▪ Decrease in GI pain in patients with peptic ulcer disease.

PROPIOMAZINE
(proe-pee-**oh**-ma-zeen)
Largon

CLASSIFICATION(S):
Sedative/hypnotic
(phenothiazine)
Pregnancy Category UK

INDICATIONS

- Used as a sedative preoperatively or during surgery (with opioid analgesics)
- As an adjunct to analgesics in the management of labor.

ACTION

- Alters the effects of dopamine in the CNS. Also has antiemetic and antihistaminic properties. **Therapeutic Effects:**
- Decreased restlessness and apprehension before surgery or during labor.

PHARMACOKINETICS

Absorption: Well absorbed (60%) following IM administration.
Distribution: Distribution not known.
Metabolism and Excretion: Probably metabolized by the liver.
Half-life: IM—10.8 hr; IV—7.7 hr.

CONTRAINDICATIONS AND PRECAUTIONS

Contraindicated in: ▪ Hypersensitivity. Cross-sensitivity with other phenothiazines may occur.
Use Cautiously in: ▪ Patients with underlying CNS depression ▪ First trimester of pregnancy (safety not established).

ADVERSE REACTIONS AND SIDE EFFECTS*

CNS: drowsiness, NEUROLEPTIC MALIGNANT SYNDROME.
CV: hypertension, tachycardia.
GI: dry mouth.

INTERACTIONS

Drug–Drug: ▪ Additive CNS depression with other CNS depressants including **antihistamines, antidepressants, opioid analgesics, benzodiazepines,** and other **sedative/hypnotics** (barbiturate doses should be decreased by at least 50%; opioid analgesics should be decreased by 25–50%).

ROUTE AND DOSAGE

Preoperative Sedation
- IM, IV (Adults): 20–40 mg.

Sedation During Surgery
- IM, IV (Adults): 10–40 mg.

Obstetric Analgesia Adjunct
- IM, IV (Adults): 20–40 mg, may be repeated q 3 hr.

Preoperative, Preanesthetic, Postoperative Sedation
- IM, IV (Children): 0.55–1.1 mg/kg.

AVAILABILITY

- *Injection:* 20 mg/ml.

TIME/ACTION PROFILE (sedation)

	ONSET	PEAK	DURATION
IM	UK	40–60 min	3–6 hr
IV	UK	15–30 min	3–6 hr

NURSING IMPLICATIONS

ASSESSMENT
- ▫ Assess level of anxiety (restlessness, apprehension) throughout therapy.
- ▫ Monitor patient for development of neuroleptic malignant syndrome (fever, respiratory distress, tachycardia, convulsions, diaphoresis, hypertension or hypotension, pallor, tiredness). Notify physician immediately if these symptoms occur.

POTENTIAL NURSING DIAGNOSES
- Anxiety (indications).
- Injury, high risk for (adverse reactions).
- Knowledge deficit related to medication regimen (patient/family teaching).

IMPLEMENTATION
- **General Info:** Do not use solutions that are cloudy or contain a precipitate.
- **Direct IV:** Administer as a bolus. Avoid extravasation, chemical irritation may be severe.
- *Rate:* Administer at a rate of 10 mg/min.
- **Syringe Compatibility:** ▪ atropine ▪ glycopyrrolate ▪ pentazocine.
- **Syringe Incompatibility:** ▪ barbiturates.

---

*Underlines indicate most frequent; **CAPITALS** indicate life-threatening.

PATIENT/FAMILY TEACHING
- Propiomazine causes drowsiness. Caution patient to ask for assistance before ambulation or transfer.
- Inform patient that propiomazine may cause dry mouth.

EVALUATION
Effectiveness of therapy can be determined by: ▪ Decreased restlessness and apprehension before surgery or during labor.

PROPOFOL
(**proe**-poe-fol)
disoprofol, Diprivan

CLASSIFICATION(S):
Anesthetic (general)
Pregnancy Category B

INDICATIONS

▪ Induction of general anesthesia ▪ Maintenance of balanced anesthesia when used with other agents ▪ Initiation and maintenance of monitored anesthesia care (MAC) ▪ Sedation of intubated, mechanically ventilated patients in intensive care units.

ACTION

▪ Short-acting hypnotic. Mechanism of action is unknown ▪ Produces amnesia ▪ Has no analgesic properties. **Therapeutic Effect:** ▪ Induction and maintenance of anesthesia.

PHARMACOKINETICS

Absorption: Administered IV only, resulting in complete absorption.
Distribution: Rapidly and widely distributed. Crosses the blood–brain barrier well. Rapidly redistributed to other tissues. Crosses the placenta and enters breast milk.
Metabolism and Excretion: Rapidly metabolized by the liver.
Half-life: 3–12 hr (blood–brain equilibration half-life 2.9 min).

CONTRAINDICATIONS AND PRECAUTIONS

Contraindicated in: ▪ Hypersensitivity to propofol, soybean oil, egg lecithin, or glycerol ▪ Labor and delivery.
Use Cautiously in: ▪ Cardiovascular disease ▪ Lipid disorders (emulsion may have detrimental effect) ▪ Increased intracranial pressure ▪ Cerebrovascular disorders ▪ Elderly, debilitated, or hypovolemic patients (dosage reduction recommended) ▪ Children or lactation (safety not established).

ADVERSE REACTIONS AND SIDE EFFECTS*

CNS: dizziness, headache.
Resp: APNEA, cough.
CV: bradycardia, hypotension, hypertension.
GI: nausea, vomiting, abdominal cramping, hiccups.
Derm: flushing.
Local: pain, burning, stinging, tingling, numbness, coldness at IV site.
MS: perioperative myoclonia, involuntary muscle movements.
Misc: fever.

INTERACTIONS

Drug–Drug: ▪ Additive CNS and respiratory depression with **alcohol, antihistamines, opioid analgesics,** and **sedative/hypnotics** (dosage reduction may be required).

ROUTE AND DOSAGE

General Anesthesia
▪ **IV (Adults <55 yr):** *Induction—* 2–2.5 mg/kg (40 mg) q 10 sec until induction achieved. *Maintenance—* 100–200 mcg/kg/min. Rates of 150–200 mcg/kg/min are usually required during first 10–15 min after induction, then decreased by 30–50% during first 30 min of maintenance. Rates of 50–100 mcg/kg/min are associated with optimal recovery time. May also be given intermittently in increments of 25–50 mg.
▪ **IV: (Elderly, Debilitated, or Hypo-**

volemic Patients): *Induction*—1–1.5 mg/kg (20 mg) q 10 sec until induction achieved. *Maintenance*—50–100 mcg/kg/min.

Monitored Anesthesia Care (MAC) Sedation

- IV (Adults <55 yr): *Initiation*—100–150 mcg/kg/min infusion or 0.5 mg/kg as slow injection. *Maintenance*—25–75 mg/kg/min infusion or incremental boluses of 10–20 mg.
- IV (Elderly, Debilitated, or ASA III/IV Patients): *Initiation*—Use slower infusion or injection rates. *Maintenance*—20% less than the usual adult infusion dose.

ICU Sedation

- IV (Adults): 5 mg/kg/min for a minimum of 5 min. Additional increments of 5–10 mcg/kg/min over 5–10 min may be given until desired response is obtained. (Range 5–50 mcg/kg/min). Dose should be reassessed every 24 hr.

AVAILABILITY

- *Injection:* 10 mg/ml.

TIME/ACTION PROFILE (loss of consciousness)

	ONSET	PEAK	DURATION*
IV	40 sec	UK	3–5 min

*Time to recovery is 8 min (up to 19 min if opioid analgesics have been used).

NURSING IMPLICATIONS

ASSESSMENT

- Assess respiratory status, pulse, and blood pressure continuously throughout propofol therapy. Propofol should be used only by individuals experienced in endotracheal intubation, and equipment for this procedure should be readily available.
- Assess level of sedation and level of consciousness throughout and following administration.
- **Toxicity and Overdose:** If overdose occurs monitor pulse, respiration, and blood pressure continuously.

Maintain patent airway and assist ventilation as needed. If hypotension occurs, treatment includes IV fluids, repositioning, and vasopressors.

POTENTIAL NURSING DIAGNOSES

- Breathing pattern, ineffective (adverse reaction).
- Injury, high risk for (side effects).
- Knowledge deficit related to medication regimen (patient/family teaching).

IMPLEMENTATION

- **General Info:** Dose is titrated to patient response.
- Propofol has no effect on the pain threshold. Adequate analgesia should *always* be used when propofol is used as an adjunct to surgical procedures.
- **Direct IV:** Shake well before use. If diluted prior to administration, use only D5W and dilute to a concentration not less than 2 mg/ml. Solution is opaque, making detection of contaminates difficult. Do not use if separation of the emulsion is evident. Contains no preservatives; maintain sterile technique and administer immediately after preparation. Discard unused portions and IV lines at the end of procedure or within 6 hr. For ICU sedation discard after 12 hr if administered directly from vial or after 6 hr if transferred to a syringe or other container.
- Frequently causes pain, burning, and stinging at injection site; use larger veins of the forearm, antecubital fossa, or a dedicated IV catheter. Physician may order lidocaine 10–20 mg IV prior to injection to minimize pain.
- **Rate:** Administer over 3–5 min. Titrate to desired level of sedation.
- **Intermittent/Continuous Infusion:** May be administered as an intermittent or continuous infusion (see Route and Dosage for rate). Wake up and assessment of CNS function should be done daily throughout maintenance to determine minimum dose required for sedation. Main-

tain a light level of sedation during these assessments; do not discontinue. Abrupt discontinuation may cause rapid awakening with anxiety, agitation, and resistance to mechanical ventilation.

- **Solution Compatibility:** D5W, LR, D5/LR, D5/0.45% NaCl, or D5/0.2% NaCl.
- **Y-Site Incompatibility:** ▪ blood ▪ plasma.
- **Additive Incompatibility:** Manufacturer does not recommend admixing propofol with other medications.

PATIENT/FAMILY TEACHING

□ Inform patient that this medication will decrease mental recall of the procedure.
□ Medication may cause drowsiness or dizziness. Advise patient to request assistance prior to ambulation and transfer and to avoid driving or other activities requiring alertness for 24 hr following administration.
□ Advise patient to avoid alcohol or other CNS depressants for 24 hr following administration of propofol.

EVALUATION

Effectiveness of therapy can be demonstrated by: ▪ Induction and maintenance of anesthesia □ Amnesia ▪ Sedation in mechanically-ventilated patients in an intensive care setting.

PROPOXYPHENE

(pro-**pox**-i-feen)
Darvon, Darvon-N, Dolene, Doraphen, Doxaphene, {Novopropoxyn}, Profene, Pro-Pox, Propoxycon

PROPOXYPHENE/ACET-AMINOPHEN

Darvocet-N, Dolene AP, Doxapap-N, D-Rex, E-Lor, Genagesic, Pancet, Propacet, Pro-Pox with APAP, Propoxyphene with APAP, Wygesic

PROPOXYPHENE/ASPIRIN/CAFFEINE

Bexophene, Cotanal, Darvon Compound-65, {Darvon-N Compound}, Doraphen Compound, Doxaphene Compound, Margesic A-C, {Novopropoxyn Compound}, Pro-Pox Plus

CLASSIFICATION(S):
Nonopioid analgesic (agonist)
Schedule IV
Pregnancy Category C

INDICATIONS

▪ Management of mild to moderate pain.

ACTION

▪ Binds to opiate receptors in the CNS ▪ Alters the perception of and response to painful stimuli, while producing generalized CNS depression. **Therapeutic Effect:** ▪ Decrease in mild to moderate pain.

PHARMACOKINETICS

Absorption: Well absorbed following oral administration. Napsylate salt is more slowly absorbed.
Distribution: Widely distributed. Probably crosses the placenta. Enters breast milk in small amounts.
Metabolism and Excretion: Mostly metabolized by the liver. Some conversion to morpropoxyphene, a toxic metabolite.
Half-life: 6–12 hr.

CONTRAINDICATIONS AND PRECAUTIONS

Contraindicated in: ▪ Hypersensitivity ▪ Pregnancy or lactation (avoid chronic use) ▪ Children.
Use Cautiously in: ▪ Head trauma ▪ Increased intracranial pressure ▪ Severe renal, hepatic, or pulmonary disease ▪ Hypothyroidism ▪ Adrenal insufficiency ▪ Alcoholism ▪ Elderly or debilitated patients (dosage reduction recommended) ▪ Undiagnosed abdominal pain ▪ Prostatic hypertrophy ▪ Lactation (has been used safely).

{} = Available in Canada only.

ADVERSE REACTIONS AND SIDE EFFECTS*

CNS: dizziness, lightheadedness, headache, weakness, sedation, drowsiness, insomnia, euphoria, dysphoria, paradoxical excitement.
EENT: blurred vision.
CV: hypotension.
GI: nausea, vomiting, abdominal pain, constipation.
Derm: rashes.
Misc: tolerance, physical dependence, psychological dependence.

INTERACTIONS

Drug–Drug: ▪ Use with extreme caution in patients receiving **MAO inhibitors** (may result in unpredictable, severe, and potentially fatal reactions—decrease initial dose to 25% of usual dose) ▪ Additive CNS depression with **alcohol**, **antidepressants**, and **sedative/hypnotics** ▪ **Smoking (nicotine)** increases metabolism and may decrease analgesic effectiveness ▪ Administration of **partial-antagonist opioid analgesics** may precipitate withdrawal in physically dependent patients ▪ **Nalbuphine** or **pentazocine** may decrease analgesic effects.

ROUTE AND DOSAGE

100 mg propoxyphene napsylate = 65 mg propoxyphene hydrochloride.

▪ **PO (Adults):** 65 mg q 4 hr (hydrochloride—Darvon, Dolene) or 100 mg q 4 hr (napsylate—Darvocet-N with acetaminophen, Darvon-N) as needed (not to exceed 390 mg/day as hydrochloride or 600 mg/day as napsylate).

AVAILABILITY

Propoxyphene Hydrochloride
▪ *Capsules:* 65 mg ▪ {*Tablets:* 65 mg}.

Propoxyphene Napsylate
▪ {*Capsules:* 100 mg} ▪ *Tablets:* 50 mg, 100 mg ▪ *Oral suspension:* 50 mg/5 ml.

Propoxyphene Hydrochloride/ Acetaminophen
▪ *Tablets:* propoxyphene 65 mg/acetaminophen 650 mg.

Propoxyphene Napsylate/ Acetaminophen
▪ *Tablets:* propoxyphene 50 mg/acetaminophen 325 mg, propoxyphene 100 mg/acetaminophen 650 mg.

Propoxyphene/Aspirin/Caffeine
▪ *Capsules:* propoxyphene 65 mg, aspirin 389 mg, caffeine 32.4 mg.

TIME/ACTION PROFILE (analgesic effect)

	ONSET	PEAK	DURATION
PO	15–60 min	2–3 hr	4–6 hr

NURSING IMPLICATIONS

ASSESSMENT

▢ Assess type, location, and intensity of pain prior to and 60 min following administration.

▢ Prolonged, high-dose therapy may lead to physical and psychological dependence and tolerance. This should not prevent patient from receiving adequate analgesia. Most patients who receive propoxyphene for medical reasons do not develop psychological dependence. Progressively higher doses may be required to relieve pain with long-term therapy.

▪ **Lab Test Considerations:** May cause elevated serum amylase and lipase levels.

▢ May cause increased AST (SGOT), ALT (SGPT), serum alkaline phosphatase, LDH, and bilirubin concentrations.

▪ **Toxicity and Overdose:** If overdose occurs, naloxone (Narcan) is the antidote.

POTENTIAL NURSING DIAGNOSES

▪ Pain (indications).
▪ Sensory-perceptual alteration: visual, auditory (side effects).
▪ Injury, high risk for (side effects).

IMPLEMENTATION

▪ **General Info:** Explain therapeutic value of medication prior to administration to enhance the analgesic effect.

*Underlines indicate most frequent; **CAPITALS** indicate life-threatening.

□ Regularly administered doses may be more effective than prn administration.

□ Analgesic is more effective if given before pain becomes severe.

□ Coadministration with nonopioid analgesics may have additive analgesic effects and may permit lower opioid doses.

□ Medication should be discontinued gradually after long-term use to prevent withdrawal symptoms.

■ **PO:** Doses may be administered with food or milk to minimize GI irritation.

PATIENT/FAMILY TEACHING

□ Instruct patient on how and when to ask for pain medication.

□ Medication may cause drowsiness or dizziness. Caution patient to avoid driving and other activities requiring alertness until response to the drug is known.

□ Advise patient to make position changes slowly to minimize orthostatic hypotension.

□ Caution patient to avoid concurrent use of alcohol or other CNS depressants with this medication.

□ Encourage patient to turn, cough, and breathe deeply every 2 hr to prevent atelectasis.

□ Advise patient that increased intake of fluids and bulk, increased activity, stool softeners, and laxatives may minimize constipating effects.

EVALUATION

Effectiveness of therapy can be demonstrated by: ■ Decrease in severity of pain without a significant alteration in level of consciousness.

PROPRANOLOL

(proe-**pran**-oh-lole)

{Apo-Propranolol}, {Detensol}, Inderal, Inderal-LA, {Novopranol}

CLASSIFICATION(S):
Antihypertensive, Antianginal, Beta-adrenergic blocker (nonselective), Antiarrhythmic (group II)
Pregnancy Category C

INDICATIONS

■ Treatment of the following: □ Hypertension (alone or with other agents) □ Angina pectoris (alone or with other agents) □ Supraventricular tachyarrhythmias, ventricular tachycardia, and other tachyarrhythmias ■ Symptoms associated with hypertrophic cardiomyopathy (angina, palpitations, syncope) □ Tremors ■ Prevention of myocardial infarction ■ Migraine prophylaxis ■ Management of pheochromocytoma. **Unlabeled Uses:** ■ Management of arrhythmias associated with thyrotoxicosis ■ Treatment of symptoms associated with mitral value prolapse syndrome ■ Adjunct in the management of anxiety.

ACTION

■ Blocks stimulation of beta$_1$ (myocardial) and beta$_2$ (pulmonary, vascular, or uterine) receptor sites. **Therapeutic Effects:** ■ Decreased heart rate ■ Decreased blood pressure ■ Decreased AV conduction.

PHARMACOKINETICS

Absorption: Well absorbed following oral administration. Absorption of sustained-release capsules is slow.
Distribution: Widely distributed. Crosses the blood–brain barrier and the placenta. Enters breast milk.
Metabolism and Excretion: Almost completely metabolized by the liver.
Half-life: 3.4–6 hr.

CONTRAINDICATIONS AND PRECAUTIONS

Contraindicated in: ■ Uncompensated congestive heart failure ■ Pulmonary edema ■ Cardiogenic shock ■ Bradycardia ■ Heart block ■ Hypersensitivity to sulfites (sustained-release only).
Use Cautiously in: ■ Thyrotoxicosis or

{} = Available in Canada only.

hypoglycemia (may mask symptoms) ■ Pregnancy or lactation (may cause apnea, low Apgar scores, bradycardia, and hypoglycemia in the newborn) ■ Do not withdraw abruptly ■ Hepatic impairment (dosage reduction recommended) ■ Children (safety not established) ■ Patients with a history of severe allergic reactions (intensity of reactions may be increased).

ADVERSE REACTIONS AND SIDE EFFECTS*

CNS: <u>fatigue</u>, <u>weakness</u>, <u>depression</u>, memory loss, mental changes, <u>insomnia</u>, drowsiness, confusion, dizziness.
EENT: dry eyes, blurred vision, nasal stuffiness.
Resp: bronchospasm, wheezing.
CV: BRADYCARDIA, CONGESTIVE HEART FAILURE, PULMONARY EDEMA, hypotension, edema.
GI: constipation, <u>diarrhea</u>, <u>nausea</u>, <u>vomiting</u>.
GU: impotence, diminished libido.
Derm: rash.
Endo: hyperglycemia, hypoglycemia.
Misc: <u>Raynaud's phenomenon</u>.

INTERACTIONS

Drug–Drug: ■ **General anesthesia, IV phenytoin,** and **verapamil** may cause additive myocardial depression ■ Additive bradycardia may occur with concurrent use of **cardiac glycosides** ■ Additive hypotension may occur with other **antihypertensive agents,** acute ingestion of **alcohol,** or **nitrates** ■ Concurrent use with **amphetamines, cocaine, ephedrine, epinephrine, norepinephrine, phenylephrine,** or **pseudoephedrine** may result in excess alpha-adrenergic stimulation, hypertension, and bradycardia ■ May negate the beneficial beta$_1$ cardiac effects of **dopamine** or **dobutamine** ■ Use with **insulin** may result in prolonged hypoglycemia ■ May produce hypertension within 14 days of **MAO inhibitor** therapy ■ Concurrent **thyroid** administration may decrease effectiveness ■ **Nonsteroidal anti-inflammatory**

agents may decrease antihypertensive effectiveness ■ May antagonize **beta-adrenergic bronchodilators** ■ **Cimetidine** may decrease metabolism and increase the effects of propranolol ■ May decrease effectiveness of **theophylline** ■ May increase **theophylline** blood levels.

ROUTE AND DOSAGE

Hypertension
■ **PO (Adults):** 40 mg bid initially or 80 mg extended-release preparation, increase at 3–7-day intervals until response is obtained. Usual maintenance dose is 160–480 mg/day in 2 divided doses or 120–160 mg once daily as extended-release preparation. Up to 640 mg/day may be needed. Some patients may need 3 daily doses.

Angina
■ **PO (Adults):** 80–320 mg/day in 2–4 divided doses or 80 mg once daily of extended-release preparation. Increase at 3–7-day intervals until response is obtained.

Tachyarrhythmias
■ **PO (Adults):** 10–30 mg 3–4 times daily.
■ **IV (Adults):** 1–3 mg, may repeat in 2 min if needed; subsequent doses may be repeated q 4 hr.

Myocardial Infarction Prophylaxis
■ **PO (Adults):** 180–240 mg/day in 2–4 divided doses starting 5–21 days after myocardial infarction.

Migraine Prophylaxis
■ **PO (Adults):** 20 mg 4 times daily or 80 mg once daily of extended-release preparation, increase gradually until response is obtained (up to 240 mg/day).

Pheochromocytoma
■ **PO (Adults):** 30–160 mg/day in 3–4 divided doses.

Hypertrophic Cardiomyopathy
■ **PO (Adults):** 20–40 mg 3–4 times daily or 80–160 mg single dose of extended-release preparation.

P

---

*<u>Underlines</u> indicate most frequent; **CAPITALS** indicate life-threatening.

Tremors

- **PO (Adults):** 40 mg twice daily, subsequent dosage adjustments as required (range 120–320 mg/day).

AVAILABILITY

- **Tablets:** 10 mg, 20 mg, 40 mg, 60 mg, 90 mg ▪ **Sustained-release capsules:** 60 mg, 80 mg, 120 mg, 160 mg ▪ **Oral solution:** 4 mg/ml, 8 mg/ml ▪ **Concentrated oral solution:** 80 mg/ml ▪ **Injection:** 1 mg/ml ▪ **In combination with:** hydrochlorothiazide. See Appendix A.

TIME/ACTION PROFILE (PO, PO-ER = antihypertensive effects; IV = antiarrhythmic effects)

	ONSET	PEAK	DURATION
PO	30 min	60–90 min	6–12 hr
PO-ER	UK	6 hr	24 hr
IV	immediate	1 min	4–6 hr

NURSING IMPLICATIONS

Assessment

- **General Info:** Monitor blood pressure and pulse frequently when adjusting dose and periodically throughout therapy. Confer with physician prior to giving drug if pulse <50 bpm. Patients receiving propranolol IV must have continuous ECG monitoring and may have pulmonary capillary wedge pressure (PCWP) or central venous pressure (CVP) monitoring during and for several hours after administration. Assess for orthostatic hypotension when assisting patient up from supine position.
- □ Monitor intake and output ratios and daily weight. Assess patient routinely for evidence of congestive heart failure (peripheral edema, dyspnea, rales/crackles, fatigue, weight gain, jugular venous distension).
- **Angina:** Assess frequency and duration of episodes of chest pain, exercise tolerance, and ECG periodically throughout therapy.
- **Migraine Prophylaxis:** Assess frequency and severity of migraine headaches periodically throughout therapy.
- **Lab Test Considerations:** Hepatic and renal function and CBC should be monitored routinely in patients receiving prolonged therapy.
- □ May cause elevations in serum potassium, uric acid, LDH, glucose, lipoprotein, triglyceride levels, and BUN.

Potential Nursing Diagnoses

- Cardiac output, decreased (indications, adverse reactions).
- Knowledge deficit related to medication regimen (patient/family teaching).
- Noncompliance (patient/family teaching).

Implementation

- **General Info:** Oral and parenteral doses are not interchangeable. Check dose carefully.
- **PO:** Administer medication with meals or immediately after eating. Tablets may be crushed and mixed with food or fluids for patients with difficulty swallowing. Long-acting capsules should be swallowed whole; do not crush, break, or chew.
- **Direct IV:** Administer undiluted or dilute each 1 mg in 10 ml of D5W for injection.
- **Rate:** Administer over at least 1 min.
- **Intermittent Infusion:** May also be diluted for infusion in 50 ml of 0.9% NaCl, D5W, D5/0.45% NaCl, D5/0.9% NaCl, or lactated Ringer's injection.
- **Rate:** Infuse over 10–15 min.
- **Syringe Compatibility:** ▪ amrinone ▪ benzquinamide ▪ milrinone.
- **Y-Site Compatibility:** ▪ amrinone ▪ heparin ▪ hydrocortisone sodium succinate ▪ meperidine ▪ milrinone ▪ morphine ▪ potassium chloride ▪ vitamin B complex with C.
- **Additive Compatibility:** ▪ dobutamine ▪ verapamil.

Patient/Family Teaching

- **General Info:** Instruct patient to take medication exactly as directed, even if feeling well. If dose is missed, it may be taken as soon as remembered, up to 8 hr before next dose. Abrupt withdrawal may precipitate life-threatening arrhythmias, hypertension, or myocardial ischemia.

□ Teach patient and family how to check pulse and blood pressure. Instruct them to take pulse daily and blood pressure at least weekly. Advise patient to withhold dose and contact physician if pulse <50 bpm or blood pressure changes significantly.

□ Reinforce need to continue additional therapies for hypertension (weight loss, restricted sodium intake, stress reduction, regular exercise, moderation of alcohol consumption, smoking cessation). Propranolol helps control but does not cure hypertension.

□ Propranolol may cause drowsiness. Caution patient to avoid driving or other activities that require alertness until response to the drug is known.

□ Caution patient that this medication may cause increased sensitivity to cold.

□ Advise patient to consult physician or pharmacist before taking any over-the-counter drugs concurrently with this medication. Patient should also avoid excessive amounts of coffee, tea, or cola.

□ Diabetic patients should monitor serum glucose closely, especially if weakness, fatigue, or irritability occurs. Propranolol may mask tachycardia and increased blood pressure as signs of hypoglycemia, but sweating and dizziness may still occur.

□ Advise patient to notify physician if slow pulse, dizziness, lightheadedness, confusion, depression, or skin rash occurs.

□ Instruct patient to inform physician or dentist of medication regimen prior to treatment or surgery.

□ Advise patient to carry identification describing medication regimen at all times.

■ **Migraine Prophylaxis:** Caution patient that sharing of this medication may be dangerous.

EVALUATION
Effectiveness of therapy can be demonstrated by: ■ Decrease in blood pressure ■ Decrease in frequency of anginal attacks □ Increase in exercise tolerance □ Reduced ischemic changes in the ECG ■ Decrease in arrhythmias ■ Decrease in frequency and severity of migraine headaches ■ Decrease in tremors.

P

PROPYLTHIOURACIL
(proe-pill-thye-oh-**yoor**-a-sill)
{Propyl-Thyracil}, PTU

CLASSIFICATION(S):
Antithyroid agent
Pregnancy Category D

INDICATIONS
■ Palliative treatment of hyperthyroidism ■ Adjunct in the control of hyperthyroidism in preparation for thyroidectomy or radioactive iodine therapy.

ACTION
■ Inhibits the synthesis of thyroid hormones. **Therapeutic Effect:** ■ Decreased signs and symptoms of hyperthyroidism.

PHARMACOKINETICS
Absorption: Rapidly absorbed from the GI tract.
Distribution: Concentrates in the thyroid gland. Crosses the placenta and enters breast milk in low concentrations.
Metabolism and Excretion: Metabolized by the liver.
Half-life: 1–2 hr.

CONTRAINDICATIONS AND PRECAUTIONS
Contraindicated in: ■ Hypersensitivity.
Use Cautiously in: ■ Decreased bone marrow reserve ■ Pregnancy (may be used safely; however, fetus may develop

thyroid problems) ▪ Lactation (safety not established).

ADVERSE REACTIONS AND SIDE EFFECTS*

CNS: headache, drowsiness, vertigo.
GI: diarrhea, <u>nausea</u>, <u>vomiting</u>, hepatitis, loss of taste.
Derm: <u>rash</u>, urticaria, skin discoloration.
Hemat: AGRANULOCYTOSIS, leukopenia, thrombocytopenia.
MS: arthralgia.
Misc: fever, parotitis, lymphadenopathy.

INTERACTIONS

Drug–Drug: ▪ Additive bone marrow depression with **antineoplastic agents** or **radiation therapy** ▪ Additive antithyroid effects with **lithium, potassium iodide,** or **sodium iodide** ▪ Increased risk of agranulocytosis with **phenothiazines**.

ROUTE AND DOSAGE

▪ **PO (Adults):** 300–900 mg once daily or in 2–4 divided doses (up to 200 mg q 4–6 hr has been used in thyrotoxic crisis). Maintenance dose 50–600 mg/day once daily or in 2–4 divided doses.
▪ **PO (Children >10 yr):** 50–300 mg/day given once daily or in 2–4 divided doses.
▪ **PO (Children 6–10 yr):** 50–150 mg/day given once daily or in 2–4 divided doses.
▪ **PO (Neonates):** 10 mg/kg/day in divided doses.

AVAILABILITY

▪ *Tablets:* 50 mg.

TIME/ACTION PROFILE (effects on clinical thyroid status)

	ONSET	PEAK	DURATION
PO	10–21 days*	6–10 wk	wks

*Effects on serum thyroid hormone concentration may occur within 60 min of a single dose.

NURSING IMPLICATIONS

ASSESSMENT

▢ Monitor response of symptoms of hyperthyroidism or thyrotoxicosis (tachycardia, palpitations, nervousness, insomnia, fever, diaphoresis, heat intolerance, tremors, weight loss, diarrhea).
▢ Assess patient for development of hypothyroidism (intolerance to cold, constipation, dry skin, headache, listlessness, tiredness, or weakness). Dosage adjustment may be required.
▢ Assess patient for skin rash or swelling of cervical lymph nodes. Treatment may be discontinued if this occurs.
▪ **Lab Test Considerations:** Thyroid function studies should be monitored prior to therapy, monthly during initial therapy, and every 2–3 mo throughout therapy.
▢ WBC and differential counts should be monitored periodically throughout course of therapy. Agranulocytosis may develop rapidly and usually occurs during first 2 mo. This necessitates discontinuation of therapy.
▢ May cause increased AST (SGOT), ALT (SGPT), LDH, alkaline phosphatase, serum bilirubin, and prothrombin time.

POTENTIAL NURSING DIAGNOSES

▪ Knowledge deficit related to medication regimen (patient/family teaching).
▪ Noncompliance (patient/family teaching).

IMPLEMENTATION

▪ **General Info:** Can be compounded by pharmacist into enema or suppository.
▪ **PO:** Administer at same time in relation to meals every day. Food may either increase or decrease absorption.

PATIENT/FAMILY TEACHING

▢ Instruct patient to take medication exactly as directed, around the clock. If a dose is missed, take as soon as remembered; take both doses together

---

*Underlines indicate most frequent; **CAPITALS** indicate life-threatening.

if almost time for next dose; check with physician if more than 1 dose is missed. Consult physician prior to discontinuing medication.

□ Instruct patient to monitor weight 2–3 times weekly. Notify physician of significant changes.

□ Medication may cause drowsiness. Caution patient to avoid driving or other activities requiring alertness until response to medication is known.

□ Advise patient to consult physician regarding dietary sources of iodine (iodized salt, shellfish).

□ Advise patient to report sore throat, fever, chills, headache, malaise, weakness, yellowing of eyes or skin, unusual bleeding or bruising, symptoms of hyperthyroidism or hypothyroidism, or rash to physician promptly.

□ Instruct patient to consult physician or pharmacist before taking any over-the-counter medications containing iodine concurrently with this medication.

□ Advise patient to carry identification describing medication regimen at all times and to notify physician or dentist of medication regimen prior to treatment or surgery.

□ Emphasize the importance of routine examinations to monitor progress and to check for side effects.

EVALUATION

Effectiveness of therapy can be demonstrated by: ▪ Decrease in severity of symptoms of hyperthyroidism (lowered pulse rate and weight gain) □ Return of serum thyroid levels to normal. Treatment of 6 mo to several years may be necessary, usually averages 1 yr.

PROTAMINE SULFATE
(proe-ta-meen)

CLASSIFICATION(S):
Antidote (antiheparin agent)
Pregnancy Category C

INDICATIONS

▪ Acute management of severe heparin overdosage ▪ Used to neutralize heparin received during dialysis, cardiopulmonary bypass, and other procedures.

ACTION

▪ A strong base that forms a complex with heparin (an acid). **Therapeutic Effect:** ▪ Inactivation of heparin.

PHARMACOKINETICS

Absorption: Administered IV only, resulting in complete bioavailability.
Distribution: Distribution not known.
Metabolism and Excretion: Metabolic fate not known. Protamine-heparin complex eventually degrades.
Half-life: UK.

CONTRAINDICATIONS AND PRECAUTIONS

Contraindicated in: ▪ Hypersensitivity to protamine or fish ▪ Avoid reconstitution with diluents containing benzyl alcohol if used in neonates.
Use Cautiously in: ▪ Patients who have received previous protamine-containing insulin or vasectomized males (increased risk of hypersensitivity reactions) ▪ Pregnancy, lactation, and children (safety not established).

ADVERSE REACTIONS AND SIDE EFFECTS*

CV: hypertension, hypotension, bradycardia, pulmonary hypertension.
Resp: dyspnea.
GI: nausea, vomiting.
Derm: warmth, flushing.
Hemat: bleeding.
MS: back pain.
Misc: hypersensitivity reactions, including angioedema, pulmonary edema, and ANAPHYLAXIS.

INTERACTIONS

Drug–Drug: ▪ None significant.

ROUTE AND DOSAGE

▪ **IV (Adults and Children):** 1 mg/100 units of heparin. If given >30 min af-

*Underlines indicate most frequent; **CAPITALS** indicate life-threatening.

ter heparin, give 0.5 mg/100 units of heparin. Further doses should be determined by coagulation tests.

AVAILABILITY

- *Injection:* 10 mg/ml.

TIME/ACTION PROFILE (reversal of heparin effect)

	ONSET	PEAK	DURATION
IV	30 sec–1 min	UK	2 hr*

*Depends on body temperature.

NURSING IMPLICATIONS

ASSESSMENT

- ☐ Assess for bleeding and hemorrhage throughout course of therapy. Hemorrhage may recur 8–9 hr after therapy due to rebound effects of heparin. Rebound may occur as late as 18 hr after therapy in patients heparinized for cardiopulmonary bypass.
- ☐ Assess for allergy to fish (salmon), previous reaction to or use of protamine insulin or protamine sulfate. Vasectomized and infertile men also have higher risk of hypersensitivity reaction.
- ☐ Observe patient for signs and symptoms of hypersensitivity reaction (hives, edema, coughing, wheezing). Keep epinephrine, an antihistamine, and resuscitative equipment close by in the event of anaphylaxis.
- ☐ Assess for hypovolemia prior to initiation of therapy. Failure to correct hypovolemia may result in cardiovascular collapse from peripheral vasodilating effects of protamine sulfate.
- **Lab Test Considerations:** Monitor clotting factors, activated clotting time (ACT), activated partial thromboplastin time (aPTT), and thrombin time (TT) 5–15 min after therapy and again as necessary.

POTENTIAL NURSING DIAGNOSES

- Injury, high risk for (indications).
- Tissue perfusion, altered (indications).

IMPLEMENTATION

- **General Info:** Discontinue heparin infusion. In milder cases overdosage may be treated by heparin withdrawal alone.
- ☐ In severe cases, fresh frozen plasma or whole blood may also be required to control bleeding.
- ☐ Dosage varies with type of heparin, route of heparin therapy, and amount of time elapsed since discontinuation of heparin.
- ☐ Do not administer >100 mg in 2 hr without rechecking clotting studies, as protamine sulfate has its own anticoagulant properties.
- **IV:** Reconstitute 50-mg vial with 5 ml Sterile Water for Injection or Bacteriostatic Water for Injection. Reconstitute 250-mg vial with 25 ml. Shake vigorously. Solution reconstituted with Sterile Water for Injection should be discarded after dose is withdrawn. Solution reconstituted with bacteriostatic water is stable for 24 hr when refrigerated.
- **Direct IV:** May be administered slow IV push over 1–3 min.
- **Intermittent Infusion:** May be diluted in D5W or 0.9% NaCl.
- *Rate:* Infuse no faster than 50 mg over 10 min. Rapid infusion rate may result in hypotension, bradycardia, flushing, or feeling of warmth. If these symptoms occur, stop infusion and notify physician.
- **Additive Compatibility:** • cimetidine • verapamil.
- **Additive Incompatibility:** • cephalosporins • penicillins.

PATIENT/FAMILY TEACHING

- ☐ Explain purpose of the medication to patient. Instruct patient to report recurrent bleeding immediately.
- ☐ Advise patient to avoid activities that may result in bleeding (shaving, brushing teeth, receiving injections or rectal temperatures, or ambulation) until risk of hemorrhage has passed.

EVALUATION

Effectiveness of therapy can be demonstrated by: • Control of bleeding • Normalization of clotting factors in heparinized patients.

PSEUDOEPHEDRINE
(soo-doe-e-**fed**-rin)
Allermed, Decofed, DeFed, Dorcol Children's Decongestant, Drixoral Non-Drowsy, Efidac/24, {Eltor 120}, Genafed, Myfedrine, Novafed, PediaCare Infants' Oral Decongestant, Pseudogest, {Robidrine}, Seudotabs, Sinustop Pro, Sudafed, Sufedrin

CLASSIFICATION(S):
Decongestant
Pregnancy Category B

INDICATIONS
▪ Symptomatic management of nasal congestion associated with acute viral upper respiratory tract infections ▪ Used in combination with antihistamines in the management of allergic conditions ▪ Used to open obstructed eustachian tubes in chronic otic inflammation or infection.

ACTION
▪ Stimulates alpha- and beta-adrenergic receptors ▪ Produces vasoconstriction in the respiratory tract mucosa (alpha-adrenergic stimulation) and possibly bronchodilation (beta$_2$-adrenergic stimulation). **Therapeutic Effects:** ▪ Reduction of nasal congestion, hyperemia, and swelling in nasal passages.

PHARMACOKINETICS
Absorption: Well absorbed following oral administration.
Distribution: Appears to enter the CSF. Probably crosses the placenta and enters breast milk.
Metabolism and Excretion: Partially metabolized by the liver. 55–75% excreted unchanged by the kidneys (depends on urine pH).
Half-life: 7 hr (depends on urine pH).

CONTRAINDICATIONS AND PRECAUTIONS
Contraindicated in: ▪ Hypersensitivity to sympathomimetic amines ▪ Hypertension, severe coronary artery disease ▪ Concurrent MAO inhibitor therapy ▪ Known alcohol intolerance (some liquid products).
Use Cautiously in: ▪ Hyperthyroidism ▪ Diabetes mellitus ▪ Prostatic hypertrophy ▪ Ischemic heart disease ▪ Pregnancy or lactation (safety not established) ▪ Glaucoma.

ADVERSE REACTIONS AND SIDE EFFECTS*
CNS: <u>nervousness</u>, excitability, restlessness, weakness, dizziness, insomnia, headache, drowsiness, fear, <u>anxiety</u>, hallucinations, SEIZURES.
CV: CARDIOVASCULAR COLLAPSE, tachycardia, <u>palpitations</u>, hypertension.
GI: <u>anorexia</u>, dry mouth.
GU: dysuria.
Resp: respiratory difficulty.

INTERACTIONS
Drug–Drug: ▪ Additive sympathomimetic effects with other **sympathomimetic agents** ▪ Concurrent use with **MAO inhibitors** may cause hypertensive crisis ▪ Concurrent use with **beta-adrenergic blockers** may result in hypertension or bradycardia ▪ **Drugs that acidify the urine (ammonium chloride)** may decrease effectiveness ▪ **Drugs that alkalinize the urine (sodium bicarbonate, high-dose antacid therapy)** may intensify effectiveness.
Drug–Food: ▪ **Foods that acidify the urine** may decrease effectiveness ▪ **Foods that alkalinize the urine** may intensify effectiveness (see lists in Appendix K).

ROUTE AND DOSAGE
▪ **PO (Adults and Children >12 yr):** 60 mg q 4–6 hr as needed (not to exceed 240 mg/day) or 120 mg of extended-release preparation q 12 hr

---

{} = Available in Canada only.
*<u>Underlines</u> indicate most frequent; **CAPITALS** indicate life-threatening.

or 240 mg extended-release preparation q 24 hr.
- **PO (Children 6–12 yr):** 30 mg q 4–6 hr as needed (not to exceed 120 mg/day) or 4 mg/kg/day or 125 mg/m²/day in 4 divided doses.
- **PO (Children 2–6 yr):** 15 mg q 4–6 hr (not to exceed 60 mg/day) or 4 mg/kg/day or 125 mg/m²/day in 4 divided doses.
- **PO (Children 1–2 yr):** 7 drops (0.2 ml)/kg q 4–6 hr (not to exceed 4 doses/24 hr).
- **PO (Children 3–12 mo):** 3 drops/kg q 4–6 hr (not to exceed 4 doses/24 hr).

AVAILABILITY

- *Tablets:* 30 mg, 60 mg ▪ *Extended-release tablets:* 120 mg ▪ *Capsules:* 60 mg ▪ *Extended-release capsules:* 120 mg, 240 mg ▪ *Syrup:* 30 mg/5 ml ▪ *Oral solution:* 15 mg/5 ml, 30 mg/5 ml ▪ *Drops:* 7.5 mg/0.8 ml (0.8 ml = 1 dropperful) ▪ *In combination with:* antihistamines, acetaminophen, cough suppressants, and expectorants. See Appendix A.

TIME/ACTION PROFILE (decongestant effects)

	ONSET	PEAK	DURATION
PO	30 min	UK	4–8 hr
PO-ER	60 min	UK	12 hr

NURSING IMPLICATIONS

ASSESSMENT
- Assess congestion (nasal, sinus, eustachian tube) prior to and periodically throughout course of therapy.
- Monitor pulse and blood pressure before beginning therapy and periodically throughout therapy.
- Assess lung sounds and character of bronchial secretions. Maintain fluid intake of 1500–2000 ml/day to decrease viscosity of secretions.

POTENTIAL NURSING DIAGNOSES
- Airway clearance, ineffective (indications).

- Knowledge deficit related to medication regimen (patient/family teaching).

IMPLEMENTATION
- **General Info:** Administer pseudoephedrine at least 2 hr before bedtime to minimize insomnia.
- **PO:** Extended-release tablets and capsules should be swallowed whole; do not crush, break, or chew. Contents of the capsule can be mixed with jam or jelly and swallowed without chewing for patients with difficulty swallowing.

PATIENT/FAMILY TEACHING
- Instruct patient to take medication exactly as directed and not to take more than recommended. If a dose is missed, take within 1 hr; if remembered later, omit. Do not double doses.
- Instruct patient to notify physician if nervousness, slow or fast heart rate, breathing difficulties, hallucinations, or seizures occur, as these symptoms may indicate overdosage.
- Instruct patient to contact physician if symptoms do not improve within 7 days or if fever is present.

EVALUATION
Effectiveness of therapy can be demonstrated by: ▪ Decreased nasal, sinus, or eustachian tube congestion.

PSYLLIUM
(**sill**-i-yum)
Cillium, Effer-syllium, Fiberall, Hydrocil, {Karacil}, Konsyl-D, Metamucil, Modane Bulk, Naturacil Caramels, Natural Vegetable, Perdiem Fiber, {Prodiem Plain}, Pro-Lax, Reguloid, Serutan, Sibilin, Syllact, V-Lax

CLASSIFICATION(S):
Laxative (bulk-forming agent)
Pregnancy Category UK

{} = Available in Canada only.

INDICATIONS

■ Management of simple or chronic constipation, particularly if associated with a low-fiber diet ■ Useful in situations where straining should be avoided (after myocardial infarction or rectal surgery, prolonged bedrest) ■ Used in the management of chronic watery diarrhea.

ACTION

■ Combines with water in the intestinal contents to form an emollient gel or viscous solution that promotes peristalsis and reduces transit time. **Therapeutic Effect:** ■ Relief and prevention of constipation.

PHARMACOKINETICS

Absorption: Not absorbed from the GI tract.
Distribution: No distribution occurs.
Metabolism and Excretion: Excreted in feces.
Half-life: UK.

CONTRAINDICATIONS AND PRECAUTIONS

Contraindicated in: ■ Hypersensitivity ■ Abdominal pain, nausea, or vomiting (especially when associated with fever) ■ Serious adhesions ■ Dysphagia.
Use Cautiously in: ■ Some dosage forms contain sugar, aspartame, or excessive sodium and should be avoided in patients on restricted diets ■ Pregnancy and lactation (has been used safely).

ADVERSE REACTIONS AND SIDE EFFECTS*

GI: nausea, vomiting, cramps, intestinal or esophageal obstruction.
Resp: bronchospasm.

INTERACTIONS

Drug–Drug: ■ May decrease the absorption of **oral anticoagulants, salicylates,** or **cardiac glycosides**.

ROUTE AND DOSAGE

■ **PO (Adults):** 1–2 tsp or packets (3–6 g psyllium) in a full glass of liquid 2–3 times daily. Up to 30 g daily in divided doses.
■ **PO (Children >6 yr):** 1 tsp or packet (1.5–3 g psyllium) in ½–1 glass of liquid 2–3 times daily. Up to 15 g daily in divided doses.

AVAILABILITY

■ *Powder:* 3.3–3.5 g/dose or packets ■ *Effervescent powder:* 3–3.5 g/dose or packet ■ *Granules:* 2.5 g/dose ■ *Wafers:* 3.4 g/dose.

TIME/ACTION PROFILE (laxative effect)

	ONSET	PEAK	DURATION
PO	12–24 hr	2–3 days	UK

NURSING IMPLICATIONS

ASSESSMENT

▫ Assess patient for abdominal distention, presence of bowel sounds, and usual pattern of bowel function.
▫ Assess color, consistency, and amount of stool produced.
■ **Lab Test Considerations:** May cause elevated blood glucose levels with prolonged use of preparations containing sugar.

POTENTIAL NURSING DIAGNOSES

■ Constipation (indications).
■ Knowledge deficit related to medication regimen (patient/family teaching).

IMPLEMENTATION

■ **General Info:** Packets are not standardized for volume, but each contains 3–6 g of psyllium.
■ **PO:** Administer with a full glass of water or juice, followed by an additional glass of liquid. Solution should be taken immediately after mixing, as it will congeal. Do not administer without sufficient fluid and do not chew granules.

PATIENT/FAMILY TEACHING

▫ Encourage patient to use other forms of bowel regulation, such as increas-

*Underlines indicate most frequent; **CAPITALS** indicate life-threatening.

ing bulk in the diet, increasing fluid intake, and increasing mobility. Normal bowel habits are individualized and may vary from 3 times/day to 3 times/wk.

□ May be used for long-term management of chronic constipation.

□ Instruct patients with cardiac disease to avoid straining during bowel movements (Valsalva maneuver).

□ Advise patient not to use laxatives when abdominal pain, nausea, vomiting, or fever is present.

EVALUATION

Effectiveness of therapy can be demonstrated by: ■ A soft, formed bowel movement, usually within 12–24 hr. May require 3 days of therapy for results.

PYRAZINAMIDE
(peer-a-**zin**-a-mide)
{PMS Pyrazinamide}, {Tebrazid}

CLASSIFICATION(S):
Antitubercular
Pregnancy Category C

INDICATIONS

■ Used in combination with other agents in the treatment of active tuberculosis.

ACTION

■ Mechanism not known. **Therapeutic Effect:** ■ Bacteriostatic action against susceptible mycobacterium. **Spectrum:** ■ Active only against mycobacterium.

PHARMACOKINETICS

Absorption: Well absorbed following oral administration.
Distribution: Widely distributed. Reaches high concentrations in the CNS (same as plasma). Excreted in breast milk.
Metabolism and Excretion: Mostly metabolized by the liver. Metabolite

(pyrazinoic acid) has antimycobacterial activity. 3–4% excreted unchanged by the kidneys.
Half-life: Pyrazinamide—9.5 hr. Pyrazinoic acid—12 hr. Both are prolonged in renal impairment.

CONTRAINDICATIONS AND PRECAUTIONS

Contraindicated in: ■ Hypersensitivity ■ Cross-sensitivity with ethionamide, isoniazid, niacin, or nicotinic acid may exist ■ Severe liver impairment.
Use Cautiously in: ■ Gout ■ Diabetes mellitus ■ Acute intermittent porphyria ■ Pregnancy (safety not established).

ADVERSE REACTIONS AND SIDE EFFECTS*

GI: HEPATOTOXICITY, nausea, vomiting, diarrhea, anorexia.
GU: dysuria.
Derm: itching, skin rash, photosensitivity, acne.
Hemat: anemia, thrombocytopenia.
Metab: hyperuricemia.
MS: gouty arthritis, arthralgia.

INTERACTIONS

Drug–Drug: ■ None significant.

ROUTE AND DOSAGE

■ **PO (Adults):** 15–30 mg/kg/day as a single dose or divided doses. Up to 60 mg/kg/day has been used in isoniazid-resistant tuberculosis (not to exceed 2 g/day as a single dose or 3 g/day in divided doses). May also be given as 50–70 mg/kg twice weekly.

■ **PO (Children):** 15–30 mg/kg/day as a single dose or in 2 divided doses (up to 1.5 g/day).

AVAILABILITY

■ *Tablets:* 500 mg.

TIME/ACTION PROFILE (blood levels)

	ONSET	PEAK
PO	UK	1–2 hr (4–5 hr*)

*For pyrazinoic acid.

{} = Available in Canada only.
*Underlines indicate most frequent; **CAPITALS** indicate life-threatening.

NURSING IMPLICATIONS

ASSESSMENT

□ Mycobacterial studies and suscepti-bility tests should be performed prior to and periodically throughout ther-apy to detect possible resistance.

■ **Lab Test Considerations:** Hepatic function should be evaluated prior to and every 2–4 wk during therapy. In-creased AST (SGOT) and ALT (SGPT) may not be predictive of clinical hep-atitis and may return to normal levels during treatment. Patients with im-paired liver function should only re-ceive pyrazinamide therapy if crucial to treatment.

□ Monitor serum uric acid concentra-tions during therapy. May cause ele-vations resulting in precipitation of acute gout.

□ May interfere with urine ketone deter-minations.

POTENTIAL NURSING DIAGNOSES

■ Infection, high risk for (indications).

■ Knowledge deficit related to medica-tion regimen (patient/family teach-ing).

■ Noncompliance (patient/family teach-ing).

IMPLEMENTATION

■ **General Info:** May be given concur-rently with isoniazid and/or rifampin.

PATIENT/FAMILY TEACHING

□ Advise patient to take medication ex-actly as directed, not to skip doses or double up on missed doses. Missed doses should be taken as soon as re-membered unless almost time for next dose. Emphasize the importance of continuing therapy even after symp-toms have subsided. Usually requires 2 mo of continuous therapy.

□ Inform diabetic patients that pyra-zinamide may interfere with urine ke-tone measurements.

□ Advise patients to notify physician if no improvement is noticed after 2–3 wk of therapy or if fever, anorexia, malaise, nausea, vomiting, darkened urine, yellowish discoloration of the skin and eyes, pain, or swelling of the joints occurs.

□ Emphasize the importance of regular follow-up examinations to monitor progress and check for side effects.

EVALUATION

Effectiveness of therapy can be demon-strated by: ■ Resolution of signs and symptoms of tuberculosis □ Negative sputum cultures.

PYRIDOSTIGMINE
(peer-id-oh-**stig**-meen)
Mestinon, {Mestinon SR}, Mesti-non Timespan, Regonol

CLASSIFICATION(S):
Cholinergic (anticholinesterase)
Pregnancy Category C

INDICATIONS

■ Used to increase muscle strength in the symptomatic treatment of myasthe-nia gravis ■ Reversal of nondepolarizing neuromuscular blockers.

ACTION

■ Inhibits the breakdown of acetylcho-line and prolongs its effects ■ Effects in-clude: □ Miosis □ Increased intestinal and skeletal muscle tone □ Bronchial and ureteral constriction □ Bradycardia □ Increased salivation □ Lacrimation □ Sweating. **Therapeutic Effects:** ■ Im-proved muscular function in patients with myasthenia gravis ■ Reversal of nondepolarizing neuromuscular block-ing agents.

PHARMACOKINETICS

Absorption: Poorly absorbed following oral administration, necessitating large oral doses as compared to parenteral doses. Extended-release oral prepara-tions release 50% of drug for immedi-ate absorption; remainder is poorly ab-sorbed.

Distribution: Appears to cross the placenta.

Metabolism and Excretion: Metabolized by plasma cholinesterases and the liver.

Half-life: PO—3.7 hr; IV—1.9 hr.

CONTRAINDICATIONS AND PRECAUTIONS

Contraindicated in: ▪ Hypersensitivity to pyridostigmine or bromides ▪ Mechanical obstruction of the GI or GU tract ▪ Known alcohol intolerance (syrup only).

Use Cautiously in: ▪ Pregnancy or lactation (may cause uterine irritability following IV administration near term; 20% of newborns may display transient muscle weakness) ▪ History of asthma ▪ Ulcer disease ▪ Cardiovascular disease ▪ Epilepsy ▪ Hyperthyroidism.

ADVERSE REACTIONS AND SIDE EFFECTS*

CNS: SEIZURES, dizziness, weakness.

EENT: miosis, lacrimation.

Resp: excessive secretions, bronchospasm.

CV: bradycardia, hypotension.

GI: abdominal cramps, nausea, vomiting, diarrhea, excessive salivation.

Derm: sweating, rashes.

INTERACTIONS

Drug–Drug: ▪ Cholinergic effects may be antagonized by other **drugs possessing anticholinergic properties,** including **antihistamines, antidepressants, atropine, haloperidol, phenothiazines, procainamide, quinidine,** or **disopyramide** ▪ Prolongs the action of **depolarizing muscle-relaxing agents (succinylcholine, decamethonium)** ▪ Additive toxicity with other **cholinesterase inhibitors,** including **demecarium, echothiophate,** and **isoflurophate** ▪ Antimyasthenic effects may be decreased by concurrent **guanadrel, guanethidine,** or **trimethophan.**

ROUTE AND DOSAGE

Myasthenia Gravis

▪ **PO (Adults):** 600 mg/day in divided doses (range 60–1500 mg) or 180–540 mg/day given once daily or in 2 divided doses as sustained-release tablets.

▪ **PO (Children):** 7 mg/kg/day in 5–6 divided doses.

▪ **IM, IV (Adults):** 2 mg (¹⁄₃₀ of oral dose); may be repeated q 2–3 hr.

Antidote for Nondepolarizing Neuromuscular Blockers

▪ **IV (Adults):** 10–20 mg; pretreat with 0.6–1.2 mg atropine IV.

AVAILABILITY

▪ *Tablets:* 60 mg ▪ *Sustained-release tablets:* 180 mg ▪ *Syrup:* 60 mg/5 ml ▪ *Injection:* 5 mg/ml.

TIME/ACTION PROFILE (cholinergic effects)

	ONSET	PEAK	DURATION
PO	30–35 min	UK	3–6 hr
PO-SR	30–60 min	UK	6–12 hr
IM	15 min	UK	2–4 hr
IV	2–5 min	UK	2–3 hr

NURSING IMPLICATIONS

ASSESSMENT

▪ **General Info:** Assess pulse, respiratory rate, and blood pressure prior to administration. Notify physician of significant changes in heart rate.

▪ **Myasthenia Gravis:** Assess neuromuscular status, including vital capacity, ptosis, diplopia, chewing, swallowing, hand grasp, and gait prior to administering and at peak effect. Patients with myasthenia gravis may be advised to keep a daily record of their condition and the effects of this medication.

▫ Assess patient for overdosage and underdosage or resistance. Both have similar symptoms (muscle weakness, dyspnea, dysphagia), but symptoms of overdosage usually occur within 1 hr of administration, while symptoms of underdosage occur ≥3 hr after administration. Overdosage (cholinergic crisis) symptoms may also include increased respiratory secretions and

*Underlines indicate most frequent; **CAPITALS** indicate life-threatening.

saliva, bradycardia, nausea, vomiting, cramping, diarrhea, and diaphoresis. A Tensilon test (edrophonium chloride) may be used to differentiate between overdosage and underdosage.

■ **Antidote to Nondepolarizing Neuromuscular Blocking Agents:** Monitor reversal of effect of neuromuscular blocking agents with a peripheral nerve stimulator. Recovery usually occurs consecutively in the following muscles: diaphragm, intercostal muscles, muscles of the glottis, abdominal muscles, limb muscles, muscles of mastication, and levator muscles of eyelids. Closely observe patient for residual muscle weakness and respiratory distress throughout the recovery period. Maintain airway patency and ventilation until recovery of normal respirations occurs.

■ **Toxicity and Overdose:** Atropine is the antidote.

POTENTIAL NURSING DIAGNOSES
■ Physical mobility, impaired (indications).
■ Breathing pattern, ineffective (indications).
■ Knowledge deficit related to medication regimen (patient/family teaching).

IMPLEMENTATION
■ **General Info:** For patients who have difficulty chewing, pyridostigmine may be administered 30 min before meals.
▫ Oral dose is not interchangeable with IV dose. Parenteral form is 30 times more potent.
▫ When used as an antidote to nondepolarizing neuromuscular blocking agents, atropine may be ordered prior to or currently with large doses of pyridostigmine to prevent or to treat bradycardia and other side effects.
■ **PO:** Administer with food or milk to minimize side effects. Sustained-release tablets should be swallowed whole; do not crush, break, or chew. Regular tablets or syrup may be administered with sustained-release

tablets for optimum control of symptoms. Mottled appearance of sustained-release tablet does not affect potency.
■ **Direct IV:** Administer undiluted. Do not add to IV solutions. May be given through Y-site or 3-way stopcock of solution of D5W, 0.9% NaCl, lactated Ringer's solution, D5/Ringer's solution, or D5/LR.
■ *Rate:* For myasthenia gravis, administer each 0.5 mg over 1 min. For reversal of nondepolarizing neuromuscular blocking agents, administer each 5 mg over 1 min.
■ **Syringe Compatibility:** ■ glycopyrrolate.
■ **Y-Site Compatibility:** ■ heparin ■ hydrocortisone sodium succinate ■ potassium chloride ■ vitamin B complex with C.

PATIENT/FAMILY TEACHING
▫ Instruct patient to take medication exactly as directed. Do not skip or double up on missed doses. Patients with a history of dysphagia should have a nonelectric or battery-back-up alarm clock to remind them of exact dose time. Patients with dysphagia may not be able to swallow medication if the dose is not taken exactly on time. Taking dose late may result in myasthenic crisis. Taking dose early may result in cholinergic crisis. Patients with myasthenia gravis must continue this regimen as a lifelong therapy.
▫ Advise patient to carry identification describing disease and medication regimen at all times.
▫ Instruct patient to space activities to avoid fatigue.

EVALUATION
Effectiveness of therapy can be demonstrated by: ■ Relief of ptosis and diplopia; improved chewing, swallowing, extremity strength, and breathing without the appearance of cholinergic symptoms ■ Reversal of nondepolarizing neuromuscular blocking agents in general anesthesia.

PYRIDOXINE
(peer-i-**dox**-een)
Beesix, {Hexa-Betalin}, Nestrex,
Rodex, Vitabee 6, vitamin B₆

CLASSIFICATION(S):
Vitamin (water-soluble)
Pregnancy Category A

INDICATIONS

▪ Treatment and prevention of pyridox-ine deficiency (may be associated with poor nutritional status or chronic debil-itating illnesses) ▪ Treatment and pre-vention of neuropathy, which may de-velop from isoniazid, penicillamine, or hydralazine therapy ▪ Management of isoniazid overdose >10 g.

ACTION

▪ Required for amino acid, carbohy-drate, and lipid metabolism ▪ Used in the transport of amino acids, formation of neurotransmitters, and synthesis of heme. **Therapeutic Effects:** ▪ Prevention of pyridoxine deficiency ▪ Prevention or reversal of neuropathy associated with hydralazine, penicillamine, or isoniazid therapy.

PHARMACOKINETICS

Absorption: Well absorbed from the GI tract.
Distribution: Stored in liver, muscle, and brain. Crosses the placenta and en-ters breast milk.
Metabolism and Excretion: Amounts in excess of requirements are excreted unchanged by the kidneys.
Half-life: 15–20 days.

CONTRAINDICATIONS AND PRECAUTIONS

Contraindicated in: ▪ No known con-traindications.
Use Cautiously in: ▪ Parkinson's dis-ease (treatment with levodopa only) ▪ Pregnancy (chronic ingestion of large doses may produce pyridoxine-depen-dency syndrome in newborn).

ADVERSE REACTIONS AND SIDE EFFECTS*

Adverse reactions listed are seen with excessive doses only.
Neuro: sensory neuropathy.
Misc: pyridoxine-dependency syn-drome.

INTERACTIONS

Drug–Drug: ▪ Interferes with the therapeutic response to **levodopa** ▪ Re-quirements are increased by **isonia-zid, hydralazine, chloramphenicol, peni-cillamine, estrogens,** and **immunosup-pressants.**

ROUTE AND DOSAGE

Dietary/Deficiency Supplementation
▪ **PO (Adults):** 10–20 mg/day for 3 wk, then 2–5 mg/day, up to 10 mg/day during pregnancy.
▪ **PO (Children):** 2.5–10 mg/day for 3 wk, then 2–5 mg/day.

Drug-Induced Deficiency (Cycloserine, Isoniazid, Hydralazine, Penicillamine)— Prevention
▪ **PO (Adults):** 10–50 mg/day (penicil-lamine), 100–300 mg/day (cycloser-ine, hydralazine, or isoniazid).

Drug-Induced Deficiency (Cycloserine, Isoniazid, Hydralazine, Penicillamine)— Treatment
▪ **PO, IM, IV (Adults):** 50–200 mg/day for 3 wk, then 25–100 mg/day.

Drug-Induced Deficiency (Chronic Alcoholism)
▪ **PO (Adults):** 50 mg/day for 2–4 wk, may be continued indefinitely.

Pyridoxine-Dependency Syndrome
▪ **PO (Adults):** 30–600 mg/day initially, then 50 mg/day for life.
▪ **PO, IM, IV (Infants):** 10–100 mg IM, IV initially, followed by PO therapy of 2–100 mg/day, followed by 2–10 mg/day PO for life.
▪ **IM, IV (Adults):** 30–600 mg/day (ini-tial treatment).

{} = Available in Canada only.
*Underlines indicate most frequent; **CAPITALS** indicate life-threatening.

PYRIMETHAMINE 1029

Isoniazid Overdose (> 10 g)

- **IM, IV (Adults):** amount equal to amount of isoniazid ingested given as 4 g IV then 1 g IM q 30 min.

AVAILABILITY

- **Tablets:** 10 mg, 25 mg, 50 mg, 100 mg, 200 mg, 250 mg, 500 mg ▪ **Extended-release tablets:** 100 mg, 150 mg ▪ **Extended-release capsules:** 100 mg, 150 mg ▪ **Injection:** 100 mg/ml ▪ **In combination with:** vitamins, minerals, and trace elements in a variety of multi-vitamin preparations.

TIME/ACTION PROFILE

	ONSET	PEAK	DURATION
PO	UK	UK	UK
IM	UK	UK	UK
IV	UK	UK	UK

NURSING IMPLICATIONS

ASSESSMENT

- Assess patient for signs of vitamin B$_6$ deficiency (anemia, dermatitis, cheilosis, irritability, seizures, nausea, and vomiting) prior to and periodically throughout therapy. Institute seizure precautions in pyridoxine-dependent infants.
- **Lab Test Considerations:** May cause false elevations in urobilinogen concentrations.

POTENTIAL NURSING DIAGNOSES

- Nutrition, altered: less than body requirements (indications).
- Knowledge deficit related to medication regimen (patient/family teaching).

IMPLEMENTATION

- **General Info:** Because of infrequency of single B-vitamin deficiencies, combinations are commonly administered.
- Administration of parenteral vitamin B$_6$ is limited to patients who are NPO or have nausea and vomiting or malabsorption syndromes.
- Protect parenteral solution from light, as decomposition will occur.
- **PO:** Extended-release capsules and tablets should be swallowed whole,

without crushing, breaking, or chewing. For patients unable to swallow capsule, contents of capsules may be mixed with jam or jelly.

- **SC/IM:** Rotate sites; burning or stinging at site may occur.
- **IV:** May be administered direct IV or as infusion in standard IV solutions.
- B$_6$-dependent seizures should cease within 2–3 min of IV administration of pyridoxine.
- **Additive Incompatibility:** ▪ alkaline solutions ▪ erythromycin ▪ iron salts ▪ kanamycin ▪ riboflavin ▪ streptomycin.

PATIENT/FAMILY TEACHING

- Instruct patient to take medication as directed. If a dose is missed, it may be omitted, as an extended period of time is required to become deficient in vitamin B$_6$.
- Encourage patient to comply with physician's diet recommendations. Explain that the best source of vitamins is a well-balanced diet with foods from the 4 basic food groups. Foods high in vitamin B$_6$ include bananas, whole-grain cereals, potatoes, lima beans, and meats.
- Patients self-medicating with vitamin supplements should be cautioned not to exceed RDA (see Appendix L). The effectiveness of megadoses for treatment of various medical conditions is unproven and may cause side effects, such as unsteady gait, numbness in feet, and difficulty with hand coordination.
- Emphasize the importance of follow-up examinations to evaluate progress.

EVALUATION

Effectiveness of therapy may be demonstrated by: ▪ Decrease in the symptoms of vitamin B$_6$ deficiency.

PYRIMETHAMINE
(peer-i-**meth**-a-meen)
Daraprim

INDICATIONS

- Used in combination with other anti-malarials in the treatment of chloro-quine-resistant malaria ▪ Used in combination with a sulfonamide in the treatment of toxoplasmosis. **Unlabeled Use:** ▪ Used in combination with other agents (sulfonamides, dapsone) in the treatment of *Pneumocystis carinii* pneumonia.

ACTION

- Binds to an enzyme in the protozoa, which results in depletion of folic acid. **Therapeutic Effect:** ▪ Death and arrested growth of susceptible organisms (protozoa).

PHARMACOKINETICS

Absorption: Well absorbed following oral administration.

Distribution: Widely distributed with high concentrations achieved in blood cells, kidneys, lungs, liver, and spleen. Some enters CSF (13–26% of serum levels). Crosses the placenta and enters breast milk.

Metabolism and Excretion: Mostly metabolized by the liver. 20–30% excreted unchanged by the kidneys.

Half-life: 4 days (shortened in patients with AIDS).

CONTRAINDICATIONS AND PRECAUTIONS

Contraindicated in: ▪ Hypersensitivity ▪ First 14–16 wk of pregnancy ▪ Megaloblastic anemia due to folate deficiency ▪ Concurrent folate antagonist therapy (due to risk of megaloblastic anemia).

Use Cautiously in: ▪ History of seizures (high doses) ▪ Underlying anemia or bone marrow depression ▪ Impaired liver function ▪ Pregnancy >16 wk (may require concurrent leucovorin) ▪ Lactation (large doses to mother may cause folic and acid deficiency in infant) ▪ G6-PD deficiency.

ADVERSE REACTIONS AND SIDE EFFECTS*

CNS: SEIZURES (high doses), insomnia, headache, lightheadedness, malaise, depression.

Resp: dry throat, pulmonary eosinophilia.

CV: arrhythmias (large doses).

GI: anorexia, nausea, atrophic glossitis (high doses), diarrhea.

GU: hematuria.

Derm: dermatitis, abnormal pigmentation.

Hemat: megaloblastic anemia (high doses), thrombocytopenia, pancytopenia.

Misc: fever.

INTERACTIONS

Drug–Drug: ▪ Increased risk of bone marrow depression with other **bone marrow depressants** including **antineoplastic agents** or **radiation therapy** ▪ Increased risk of megaloblastic anemia with **folate antagonists (methotrexate)**; concurrent use should be avoided.

ROUTE AND DOSAGE

Treatment of Malaria
- **PO (Adults):** 75 mg single dose in combination with other agents.
- **PO (Children):** 1.25 mg/kg single dose in combination with other agents.

Toxoplasmosis (with a Sulfonamide)
- **PO (Adults):** 50–200 mg/day for 1–2 days followed by 25–50 mg/day for 2–6 wk.
- **PO (Children):** 1 mg/kg/day for 1–3 days, then 0.5 mg/kg/day for 4–6 wk.

Toxoplasmosis in AIDS Patients (with a Sulfondiazine or Clindamycin)
- **PO (Adults):** 100–200 mg/day for 1–2 days followed by 50–100 mg/day for 3–6 wk and 25–50 mg/day for life.

*Underlines indicate most frequent; **CAPITALS** indicate life-threatening.

AVAILABILITY

- **Tablets:** 25 mg ▪ **In combination with:** sulfadoxine (Fansidar). See Appendix A.

TIME/ACTION PROFILE (blood levels)

	ONSET	PEAK	DURATION
PO	UK	3 hr	2 wk*

*Suppressive levels.

NURSING IMPLICATIONS

ASSESSMENT

- Assess patient for improvement in signs and symptoms of infection daily throughout course of therapy.
- **Lab Test Considerations:** Monitor CBC and platelet count periodically throughout therapy. May cause decreased WBC and platelet counts.

POTENTIAL NURSING DIAGNOSES

- Infection, high risk for (indications).
- Knowledge deficit related to medication regimen (patient/family teaching).

IMPLEMENTATION

- **PO:** Administer with milk or meals to minimize GI distress.

PATIENT/FAMILY TEACHING

- Instruct patient to take medication exactly as directed and continue full course of therapy, even if feeling better.
- Advise patient to notify physician promptly if sore throat, pallor, purpura, or glossitis occurs. Instruct patients to stop taking pyrimethamine and notify physician immediately at the first sign of a skin rash.
- Emphasize the importance of lab tests at scheduled intervals, especially in patients taking high doses. Tests should not be delayed or missed.

EVALUATION

Effectiveness of therapy can be demonstrated by: ▪ Improvement in signs and symptoms of toxoplasmosis ▪ Improvement in the signs and symptoms of *Pneumocystis carinii* pneumonia.

QUAZEPAM
(**kway**-ze-pam)
Doral

CLASSIFICATION(S):
Sedative/hypotic
(benzodiazepine)
Schedule IV
Pregnancy Category X

Q

INDICATIONS

- Short-term (up to 4 wk) management of insomnia.

ACTION

- Depresses the CNS, probably by potentiating gamma-aminobutyric acid (GABA), an inhibitory neurotransmitter. **Therapeutic Effect:** ▪ Relief of insomnia.

PHARMACOKINETICS

Absorption: Well absorbed following oral administration.
Distribution: >95% bound to plasma proteins.
Metabolism and Excretion: Mostly metabolized by the liver. Two metabolites have CNS depressant activity (2-oxoquazepam and N-desalkylflurazepam).
Half-life: Quazepam—39 hr (increased in elderly); 2-oxoquazepam—39 hr; N-desalkylflurazepam—70–75 hr.

CONTRAINDICATIONS AND PRECAUTIONS

Contraindicated in: ▪ Hypersensitivity ▪ Cross-sensitivity with other benzodiazepines may exist ▪ Pre-existing CNS depression ▪ Severe uncontrolled pain ▪ Narrow-angle glaucoma ▪ Pregnancy or lactation.
Use Cautiously in: ▪ Hepatic dysfunction, elderly, very small or debilitated patients (dosage reduction may be necessary) ▪ Patients who are suicidal or who may have been previously addicted to drugs ▪ Children <18 yr (safety not established).

ADVERSE REACTIONS AND SIDE EFFECTS*

CNS: <u>daytime drowsiness</u>, dizziness, weakness, confusion, hallucinations, trouble sleeping, nervousness, false sense of well-being, headache, slurred speech. **EENT:** blurred vision. **CV:** palpitations. **GI:** dry mouth, abdominal pain, constipation, diarrhea, nausea, vomiting. **GU:** urinary frequency, urinary hesitancy. **Derm:** skin rash, itching. **MS:** muscle spasm. **Neuro:** ataxia, trembling. **Misc:** allergic reactions, changes in libido, physical dependence, psychological dependence.

INTERACTIONS

Drug–Drug: ▪ Additive CNS depression with **alcohol, antihistamines, antidepressants, MAO inhibitors,** other **sedative/hypnotics,** or **opioid analgesics** ▪ **Cimetidine** or **oral contraceptives** may decrease metabolism and increase effects of quazepam ▪ May decrease efficacy of **levodopa** ▪ **Rifampin** or **cigarette smoking** increase metabolism and may decrease effectiveness.

ROUTE AND DOSAGE

▪ **PO (Adults):** 15 mg at bedtime initially, then 7.5–15 mg.
▪ **PO (Elderly or Debilitated Patients):** 15 mg at bedtime for 1–2 nights, then 7.5 mg.

AVAILABILITY

▪ *Tablets:* 7.5 mg, 15 mg.

TIME/ACTION PROFILE (sedation)

	ONSET	PEAK	DURATION
PO	30 min	2 hr	8 hr

NURSING IMPLICATIONS

ASSESSMENT
▫ Assess sleep patterns prior to and periodically throughout course of therapy.
▫ Prolonged therapy may lead to psychological or physical dependence. Restrict amount of drug available to patient, especially if patient is depressed, suicidal, or has a history of addiction.

POTENTIAL NURSING DIAGNOSES
▪ Sleep pattern disturbance (indications).
▪ Injury, high risk for (side effects).
▪ Knowledge deficit related to medication regimen (patient/family teaching).

IMPLEMENTATION
▪ **General Info:** Supervise ambulation and transfer of patients following administration. Remove cigarettes. Side rails should be raised and call bell within reach at all times.

PATIENT/FAMILY TEACHING
▫ Advise patient to take medication exactly as directed. Discuss the importance of preparing environment for sleep (dark room, quiet, avoidance of nicotine and caffeine). Gradual discontinuation may be required following prolonged therapy. May cause disturbed sleep for the first 2 nights following discontinuation of quazepam.
▫ Medication may cause daytime drowsiness. Caution patient to avoid driving and other activities requiring alertness until response to medication is known.
▫ Caution patients to avoid taking alcohol or other CNS depressants concurrently with this medication.
▫ Instruct patient to contact physician immediately if pregnancy is planned or suspected.

EVALUATION
Effectiveness of therapy can be demonstrated by: ▪ Improvement in sleep pattern.

QUINAPRIL
(**kwin**-a-pril)
Accupril

*<u>Underlines</u> indicate most frequent; **CAPITALS** indicate life-threatening.

Q

CLASSIFICATION(S):
Antihypertensive (angiotensin converting enzyme [ACE] inhibitor)
Pregnancy Category C (first trimester), D (second and third trimesters)

INDICATIONS

▪ Alone or in combination with thiazide diuretics in the management of hypertension. **Unlabeled Use:** ▪ In combination with other drugs in the management of congestive heart failure.

ACTION

▪ Prevents the production of angiotensin II, a potent vasoconstrictor that stimulates the production of aldosterone, by blocking its conversion to the active form. Result is systemic vasodilation. **Therapeutic Effect:** ▪ Lowering of blood pressure in hypertensive patients.

PHARMACOKINETICS

Absorption: Well absorbed following oral administration.
Distribution: Distribution not known. Appears to cross the placenta. Small amounts may enter breast milk.
Metabolism and Excretion: UK.
Half-life: UK.

CONTRAINDICATIONS AND PRECAUTIONS

Contraindicated in: ▪ Hypersensitivity ▪ Cross-sensitivity with other ACE inhibitors may exist ▪ Pregnancy or lactation (may cause fetal malformation or death; hypotension, oliguria, or hypokalemia may occur in newborn).
Use Cautiously in: ▪ Renal impairment, hypovolemia, hyponatremia, concurrent diuretic therapy, elderly patients (dosage reduction required if CCr ≤30 ml/min) ▪ Aortic stenosis ▪ Cerebrovascular or cardiac insufficiency ▪ Pregnancy (may cause fetal hypotension, oliguria, renal failure, skull hypoplasia, other fetal abnormalities, and

death; avoid use) ▪ Children (safety not established) ▪ Surgery/anesthesia (hypotension may be exaggerated) ▪ Women with childbearing potential.

ADVERSE REACTIONS AND SIDE EFFECTS*

CNS: headache, dizziness, fatigue, insomnia, weakness.
EENT: ANGIOEDEMA.
Resp: cough.
CV: hypotension, palpitations, chest pain.
GI: nausea, diarrhea.
GU: renal failure, proteinuria, impotence.
Derm: rash.
Hemat: leukopenia, eosinophilia.

INTERACTIONS

Drug–Drug: ▪ Additive or possibly excessive hypotension with other **antihypertensives, diuretics, nitrates,** and acute ingestion of **alcohol** ▪ Hyperkalemia may result with concurrent **potassium supplements, cyclosporine,** or **potassium sparing diuretics** ▪ Antihypertensive response may be blunted by **nonsteroidal anti-inflammatory agents** ▪ Increases blood levels and risk of toxicity from **lithium** ▪ Increased risk of hypersensitivity reaction with **allopurinol** ▪ May decrease absorption of tetracycline (due to magnesium content of tablets) ▪ Incidence of cough may be increased by **capsaicin.**

ROUTE AND DOSAGE

Antihypertensive
▪ **PO (Adults):** 10 mg given once daily. If given with diuretics, initiate therapy with 5 mg once daily (2.5 mg/day in renal impairment). Doses up to 80 mg/day have been used. Larger doses may be divided and given twice daily. Dosage increments should be made at 2-wk intervals.

Congestive Heart Failure
▪ **PO (Adults):** 2.5 mg initially. Maintenance 5–40 mg/day single dose or 2 divided doses.

*Underlines indicate most frequent; **CAPITALS** indicate life-threatening.

AVAILABILITY

- *Tablets:* 5 mg, 10 mg, 20 mg, 40 mg.

TIME/ACTION PROFILE
(antihypertensive effect)

	ONSET	PEAK	DURATION
PO	UK	2–6 hr	12–24 hr

NURSING IMPLICATIONS

ASSESSMENT

- **Hypertension:** Monitor blood pressure and pulse frequently during initial dosage adjustment and periodically throughout course of therapy. Notify physician of significant changes.
- **Congestive Heart Failure:** Monitor weight and assess patient routinely for resolution of fluid overload (peripheral edema, rales/crackles, dyspnea, weight gain, jugular venous distention) if on concurrent diuretic therapy.
- **Lab Test Considerations:** Monitor BUN, creatinine, and electrolyte levels periodically. Serum potassium may be increased, and BUN and creatinine transiently increased while sodium levels may be decreased.
- Monitor CBC periodically during therapy. May cause a decrease in hemoglobin and hematocrit.
- May cause elevated liver enzymes, serum bilirubin, uric acid, and glucose.
- Periodic assessments of urine protein may be ordered because proteinuria and nephrotic syndrome may occur.

POTENTIAL NURSING DIAGNOSES

- Cardiac output, decreased (indications, side effects).
- Knowledge deficit related to medication regimen (patient/family teaching).
- Noncompliance (patient/family teaching).

IMPLEMENTATION

- **PO:** Precipitous drop in blood pressure during first 1–3 hr following first dose may require volume expansion with normal saline but is not normally considered an indication for stopping therapy. Discontinuing diuretic therapy or increasing salt intake 1 wk prior to initiation may decrease risk of hypertension. Monitor closely for at least 1 hr after blood pressure has stabilized. Resume diuretics if blood pressure is not controlled with quinapril.
- Dose is adjusted at 2-wk intervals based on blood pressure response at peak (2–6 hr) and trough (predose) blood levels.

PATIENT/FAMILY TEACHING

- Instruct patient to take quinapril exactly as directed, even if feeling well. Missed doses should be taken as soon as possible but not if almost time for next dose. Do not double doses. Medication controls but does not cure hypertension. Warn patients not to discontinue quinapril therapy unless directed by the physician.
- Encourage patient to comply with additional interventions for hypertension (weight reduction, discontinuation of smoking, moderation of alcohol consumption, regular exercise, and stress management).
- Instruct patient and family on proper technique for blood pressure monitoring. Advise them to check blood pressure at least weekly and report significant changes to physician.
- Caution patient to avoid salt substitutes or foods containing high levels of potassium or sodium unless directed by physician (see Appendix K).
- Caution patient to change positions slowly to minimize orthostatic hypotension, particularly after initial dose. Patients should also be advised that exercising or hot weather may increase hypotensive effects.
- Advise patient to consult physician or pharmacist before taking any over-the-counter medications, especially cold remedies. Patients should also avoid excessive amounts of tea, coffee, or cola.
- May cause dizziness. Caution patient to avoid driving and other activities requiring alertness until response to medication is known.

□ Advise patient to inform physician or dentist of medication regimen prior to treatment or surgery.

□ Instruct patient to notify physician if rash, mouth sores, sore throat, fever, swelling of hands or feet, irregular heartbeat, chest pain, dry cough, swelling of face, eyes, lips, or tongue, or difficulty breathing occurs or if taste impairment or skin rash persist. Persistent dry cough may occur and usually does not subside until medication is discontinued. Consult physician if cough becomes bothersome.

□ Advise patient to notify physician if pregnancy is planned or suspected.

□ Emphasize the importance of follow-up examinations to monitor progress.

EVALUATION
Effectiveness of therapy can be demonstrated by: ▪ Decrease in blood pressure without appearance of side effects ▪ Decrease in the signs and symptoms of congestive heart failure.

QUINIDINE
(**kwin**-i-deen)

quinidine gluconate
Duraquin, Quinaglute, Quinalan

quinidine polygalacturonate
Cardioquin

quinidine sulfate
{Apo-Quinidine}, Cin-Quin, {Novoquinidin}, Quinidex Extentabs, Quinora

CLASSIFICATION(S):
Antiarrhythmic (group IA)
Pregnancy Category C

INDICATIONS
▪ Used in the management of a wide variety of atrial and ventricular arrhythmias, including: □ Atrial premature contractions □ Premature ventricular contractions □ Ventricular tachycardia □ Paroxysmal atrial tachycardia □ Maintenance of normal sinus rhythm after conversion from atrial fibrillation or flutter. **Unlabeled Use:** ▪ Treatment of malaria (IV gluconate only).

ACTION
▪ Decreases myocardial excitability ▪ Slows conduction velocity. **Therapeutic Effect:** ▪ Suppression of arrhythmias.

PHARMACOKINETICS
Absorption: Well absorbed from the GI tract and IM sites. Extended-release quinidine sulfate (Quinidex Extentabs) or gluconate (Duraquin, Quinaglute, Quinalan) oral preparations and polygalacturonate salt are absorbed more slowly following oral administration.
Distribution: Widely distributed. Crosses the placenta and enters breast milk.
Metabolism and Excretion: Metabolized by the liver; 10–30% excreted unchanged by the kidneys.
Half-life: 6–8 hr (increased in congestive heart failure or severe liver impairment).

CONTRAINDICATIONS AND PRECAUTIONS
Contraindicated in: ▪ Hypersensitivity ▪ Conduction defects ▪ Cardiac glycoside toxicity.
Use Cautiously in: ▪ Congestive heart failure or severe liver disease (dosage reduction recommended) ▪ Pregnancy, lactation, or children (safety not established; extended-release preparations should not be used in children).

ADVERSE REACTIONS AND SIDE EFFECTS*
CNS: vertigo, headache, dizziness.
EENT: tinnitus, blurred vision, photophobia, mydriasis, diplopia.
CV: HYPOTENSION, tachycardia, arrhythmias.
GI: diarrhea, nausea, cramping, anorexia, bitter taste, hepatitis.
Derm: rashes.

{} = Available in Canada only.
*Underlines indicate most frequent; **CAPITALS** indicate life-threatening.

Hemat: thrombocytopenia, hemolytic anemia.
Misc: fever.

INTERACTIONS

Drug–Drug: ▪ Increases serum **digoxin** levels and may cause toxicity (dosage reduction recommended) ▪ **Amiodarone** increases quinidine levels and risk of toxicity ▪ **Phenytoin, phenobarbital,** or **rifampin** may increase metabolism and decrease effectiveness ▪ **Cimetidine** and **verapamil** decrease metabolism and may increase blood levels ▪ Potentiates **neuromuscular blocking agents** and **oral anticoagulants** ▪ Additive hypotension with **antihypertensives, nitrates,** and acute ingestion of **alcohol** ▪ May increase **procainamide, propafenone,** or **tricyclic antidepressant** levels and risk of toxicity ▪ May antagonize **anticholinesterase therapy** in patients with myasthenia gravis ▪ **Drugs that alkalinize the urine,** including high-dose **antacid** therapy or **sodium bicarbonate** increase blood levels and the risk of toxicity ▪ Additive anticholinergic effects may occur with **agents having anticholinergic properties** (antihistamines, tricyclic antidepressants).

Drug–Food: ▪ **Foods that alkalinize the urine** (see Appendix K) may increase serum quinidine levels and the risk of toxicity.

ROUTE AND DOSAGE

Quinidine Gluconate
(62% Quinidine)

▪ **PO (Adults):** 324–660 mg q 6–12 hr as extended-release tablets.
▪ **IM (Adults):** 600 mg initially, followed by up to 400 mg q 2 hr.
▪ **IV (Adults):** Infuse at 16 mg/min.

Quinidine Polygalacturonate
(60% Quinidine)

▪ **PO (Adults):** 275–825 mg q 3–4 hr for 3–4 doses then may increase by 137.5–275 mg and repeat 3–4 times until arrhythmia is controlled. Usual maintenance dose is 275 mg q 8–12 hr.

▪ **PO (Children):** 8.25 mg/kg (247.5 mg/m^2) 5 times daily.

Quinidine Sulfate
(83% Quinidine)

Premature Atrial or Ventricular Contractions

▪ **PO (Adults):** 200–300 mg q 6–8 hr or 300–600 mg of extended-release preparation every 8–12 hr maintenance (not to exceed 4 g/day).
▪ **PO (Children):** 6 mg/kg or 180 mg/m^2 5 times daily.

Paroxysmal Atrial Tachycardia

▪ **PO (Adults):** 400–600 mg q 2–3 hr until arrhythmia is terminated, then 200–300 mg q 6–8 hr or 300–600 mg of extended-release preparation every 8–12 hr maintenance (not to exceed 4 g/day).

Conversion of Atrial Fibrillation

▪ **PO (Adults):** 200 mg q 2–3 hr for 5–8 doses, may increase dose daily as needed, then 200–300 mg q 6–8 hr or 300–600 mg of extended-release preparation every 8–12 hr maintenance (not to exceed 4 g/day).

AVAILABILITY

Quinidine Gluconate
▪ *Sustained-release tablets:* 324 mg, 330 mg ▪ *Injection:* 80 mg/ml.

Quinidine Polygalacturonate
▪ *Tablets:* 275 mg.

Quinidine Sulfate
▪ *Tablets:* 200 mg, 300 mg ▪ *Sustained-release tablets:* 300 mg.

TIME/ACTION PROFILE
(antiarrhythmic effects)

	ONSET	PEAK	DURATION
PO (sulfate)	30 min	1–1.5 hr	6–8 hr
PO (sulfate-ER)	UK	4 hr	8–12 hr
PO (gluconate)	UK	3–4 hr	6–8 hr
PO (polygalacturonate)	UK	6 hr	8–12 hr
IM	30 min	30–90 min	6–8 hr
IV	1–5 min	rapid	6–8 hr

NURSING IMPLICATIONS

ASSESSMENT

▫ Monitor ECG, pulse, and blood pressure continuously throughout IV administration. Parameters should be monitored periodically during oral administration. IV administration is usually discontinued if any of the following occur: arrhythmia is resolved, QRS complex widens by 50%, PR or QT intervals are prolonged, frequent ventricular ectopic beats or tachycardia develops. Patient should remain supine throughout IV administration to minimize hypotension.

▪ **Lab Test Considerations:** Hepatic and renal function, CBC, and serum potassium levels should be periodically monitored during prolonged therapy.

▪ **Toxicity and Overdose:** Serum quinidine levels may be monitored periodically during dosage adjustment. Therapeutic serum concentrations are 2–6 mcg/ml. Toxic effects usually occur at concentrations >8 mcg/ml.

▫ Signs and symptoms of toxicity or cinchonism include tinnitus, hearing loss, visual disturbances, headache, nausea, and dizziness. These may occur after a single dose.

▫ Cardiac signs of toxicity include QRS widening, cardiac asystole, ventricular ectopic beats, idioventricular rhythms (ventricular tachycardia, ventricular fibrillation), paradoxical tachycardia, and arterial embolism.

POTENTIAL NURSING DIAGNOSES

▪ Cardiac output, decreased (indications).

▪ Knowledge deficit related to medication regimen (patient/family teaching).

IMPLEMENTATION

▪ **General Info:** A test dose of a single 200-mg quinidine sulfate tablet or 200 mg IM quinidine gluconate may be administered prior to quinidine therapy to check for intolerance.

▫ Higher doses may be required to correct atrial arrhythmias than those required for ventricular arrhythmias.

▪ **PO:** Administer with a full glass of water on an empty stomach either 1 hr before or 2 hr after meals for faster absorption. If GI irritation becomes a problem, may be administered with or immediately after meals. Sustained-release preparations (Quinaglute, Dura-tabs, Quinidex Extentabs, Quinalan) should be swallowed whole; do not break, crush, or chew.

▪ **IV:** Use only clear, colorless solution.

▪ **Intermittent Infusion:** Dilute 800 mg of quinidine gluconate (10 ml) in 50 ml of D5W for injection for a concentration of 16 mg/ml. Solution is stable for 24 hr at room temperature.

▪ *Rate:* Administer quinidine gluconate at a rate not to exceed 1 ml/min. Administer via infusion pump to ensure accurate dose. Rapid administration may cause hypotension.

▪ **Y-Site Compatibility:** ▪ diazepam ▪ milrinone.

▪ **Y-Site Incompatibility:** ▪ furosemide.

PATIENT/FAMILY TEACHING

▫ Instruct patient to take medication around the clock, exactly as directed, even if feeling well. If a dose is missed, take as soon as remembered if within 2 hr; if remembered later, omit. Do not double doses.

▫ Instruct patient or family member on how to take pulse. Advise patient to report changes in pulse rate or rhythm to physician.

▫ Quinidine may cause dizziness or blurred vision. Caution patient to avoid driving or other activities requiring alertness until response to medication is known.

▫ Inform patient that quinidine may cause increased sensitivity to light. Dark glasses may minimize this effect.

▫ Advise patient to inform physician or dentist of medication regimen prior to treatment or surgery.

▫ Instruct patient not to take over-the-counter medications with quinidine without consulting physician or pharmacist.

▫ Advise patient to consult physician if symptoms of cinchonism, rash, or dyspnea occur or if diarrhea is severe or persistent.

▫ Advise patient to carry identification describing disease process and medication regimen at all times.

▫ Emphasize the importance of routine follow-up examinations to monitor progress.

EVALUATION
Effectiveness of therapy can be demonstrated by: ▪ Resolution of cardiac arrhythmias without detrimental side effects.

RAMIPRIL
(**ram**-i-pril)
Altace

CLASSIFICATION(S):
Antihypertensive (angiotensin converting enzyme [ACE] inhibitor)
Pregnancy Category C (first trimester), D (second and third trimesters)

INDICATIONS

▪ Alone or in combination with thiazide diuretics in the management of hypertension.

ACTION

▪ Prevents the production of angiotensin II, a potent vasoconstrictor that stimulates the production of aldosterone, by blocking its conversion to the active form. Result is systemic vasodilation. **Therapeutic Effect:** ▪ Lowering of blood pressure in hypertensive patients.

PHARMACOKINETICS

Absorption: Well absorbed following oral administration.
Distribution: Distribution not known. Appears to cross the placenta. Small amounts may enter breast milk.
Metabolism and Excretion: Mostly metabolized by the liver. Some converted to ramiprilat, an active hypotensive compound.
Half-life: Ramipril—5 hr, ramiprilat—23.5 hr.

CONTRAINDICATIONS AND PRECAUTIONS

Contraindicated in: ▪ Hypersensitivity ▪ Cross-sensitivity with other ACE inhibitors may exist ▪ Pregnancy or lactation (may cause fetal malformation or death; hypotension, oliguria, or hypokalemia may occur in newborn).
Use Cautiously in: ▪ Renal impairment, hypovolemia, concurrent diuretic therapy, hyponatremia, elderly patients (dosage reduction required if serum creatinine >2.5 mg/dl or CCr <40 ml/min/m^2) ▪ Aortic stenosis ▪ Cerebrovascular or cardiac insufficiency ▪ Pregnancy (may cause fetal hypotension, oliguria, renal failure, skull hypoplasia, other fetal abnormalities, and death; avoid use) ▪ Children (safety not established) ▪ Surgery/anesthesia (hypotension may be exaggerated) ▪ Women with childbearing potential.

ADVERSE REACTIONS AND SIDE EFFECTS*

CNS: <u>headache</u>, dizziness, fatigue, insomnia, weakness.
EENT: ANGIOEDEMA.
Resp: <u>cough</u>.
CV: hypotension, palpitations, chest pain.
GI: nausea, diarrhea.
GU: renal failure, proteinuria, impotence.
Derm: rash.
Hemat: leukopenia, eosinophilia.

INTERACTIONS

Drug–Drug: ▪ Additive or possibly excessive hypotension with other **antihypertensives, diuretics, nitrates,** and acute ingestion of **alcohol** ▪ Hyperkalemia may result with concurrent **potassium supplements, cyclosporine,** or **potassium-sparing diuretics** ▪ Antihypertensive response may be blunted by **nonsteroidal anti-inflammatory agents**

---

*<u>Underlines</u> indicate most frequent; **CAPITALS** indicate life-threatening.

- Increases blood levels and risk of toxicity from **lithium** ▪ Increased risk of hypersensitivity reactions with **allopurinol** ▪ Cough may be aggravated by **capsaicin**.

ROUTE AND DOSAGE

- **PO (Adults):** 2.5 mg initially, maintenance 2.5–20 mg/day as a single dose or 2 divided doses. If receiving concurrent diuretics, initial dose should be 1.25 mg (maintenance dose not to exceed 5 mg/day).

AVAILABILITY

- *Capsules:* 1.25 mg, 2.5 mg, 5 mg, 10 mg.

TIME/ACTION PROFILE
(antihypertensive effect)

	ONSET	PEAK	DURATION
PO	1.5–2 hr	6–8 hr	24–72 hr

NURSING IMPLICATIONS

ASSESSMENT

- **Hypertension:** Monitor blood pressure and pulse frequently during initial dosage adjustment and periodically throughout therapy. Notify physician of significant changes.
- **Congestive Heart Failure:** Monitor weight and assess patient routinely for resolution of fluid overload (peripheral edema, rales/crackles, dyspnea, weight gain, jugular venous distension) if on concurrent diuretic therapy.
- **Lab Test Considerations:** Monitor BUN, creatinine, and electrolyte levels periodically. Serum potassium may be increased and BUN and creatinine transiently increased while sodium levels may be decreased.
- Monitor CBC periodically during therapy. May cause a decrease in hemoglobin and hematocrit.
- May cause elevated liver enzymes, serum bilirubin, uric acid, and glucose.
- Periodic assessments of urine protein may be ordered, because proteinuria and nephrotic syndrome may occur.

POTENTIAL NURSING DIAGNOSES

- Cardiac output, decreased (indications, side effects).
- Knowledge deficit related to medication regimen (patient/family teaching).
- Noncompliance (patient/family teaching).

IMPLEMENTATION

- **PO:** Precipitous drop in blood pressure during first 1–3 hr following first dose may require volume expansion with normal saline but is not normally considered an indication for stopping therapy. Discontinuing diuretic therapy or increasing salt intake 1 wk prior to initiation may decrease risk of hypotension. Monitor closely for at least 1 hr after blood pressure has stabilized. Resume diuretics if blood pressure is not controlled with ramipril.

PATIENT/FAMILY TEACHING

- Instruct patient to take ramipril exactly as directed, even if feeling well. Missed doses should be taken as soon as remembered but not if almost time for next dose. Do not double doses. Medication controls but does not cure hypertension. Warn patients not to discontinue ramipril therapy unless directed by the physician.
- Encourage patient to comply with additional interventions for hypertension (weight reduction, smoking cessation, moderation of alcohol consumption, regular exercise, and stress management). Ramipril controls but does not cure hypertension.
- Instruct patient and family on proper technique for blood pressure monitoring. Advise them to check blood pressure at least weekly and report significant changes to physician.
- Caution patient to avoid salt substitutes or foods containing high levels of potassium or sodium unless directed by physician.
- Caution patient to change positions slowly to minimize orthostatic hypotension, particularly after initial dose. Patients should also be advised that

exercising or hot weather may increase hypotensive effects.

□ Advise patient to consult physician or pharmacist before taking any over-the-counter medications, especially cold remedies. Patients should also avoid excessive amounts of tea, coffee, or cola.

□ Ramipril may cause dizziness. Caution patient to avoid driving and other activities requiring alertness until response to medication is known.

□ Advise patient to inform physician or dentist of medication regimen prior to treatment or surgery.

□ Instruct patient to notify physician if rash, mouth sores, sore throat, fever, swelling of hands or feet, irregular heartbeat, chest pain, dry cough, swelling of face, eyes, lips, or tongue, or difficulty breathing occurs or if taste impairment or skin rash persists. Persistent dry cough may occur and usually does not subside until medication is discontinued. Consult physician if cough becomes bothersome.

□ Advise patient to notify physician if pregnancy is planned or suspected.

□ Emphasize the importance of follow-up examinations to monitor progress.

EVALUATION

Effectiveness of therapy can be demonstrated by: ▪ Decrease in blood pressure without appearance of side effects ▪ Decrease in the signs and symptoms of congestive heart failure.

RANITIDINE
(ra-**nit**-ti-deen)
{Apo-Ranitidine}, Zantac,
{Zantac-C}

CLASSIFICATION(S):
Histamine H_2 antagonist,
Antiulcer
Pregnancy Category B

INDICATIONS

▪ Treatment (short-term) and prevention (long-term) of active duodenal ulcers ▪ Short-term treatment of benign gastric ulcers ▪ Management of gastroesophageal reflux disease (GERD) ▪ Treatment of gastric hypersecretory states (Zollinger-Ellison syndrome).

ACTION

▪ Inhibits the action of histamine at the H_2-receptor site located primarily in gastric parietal cells ▪ Inhibits gastric acid secretion. **Therapeutic Effect:** ▪ Healing and prevention of ulcers.

PHARMACOKINETICS

Absorption: Well absorbed following oral and IM administration.

Distribution: Widely distributed. Enters breast milk and probably crosses the placenta. Crosses the blood–brain barrier only in small amounts.

Metabolism and Excretion: Metabolized by the liver, mostly on first pass. 30% eliminated unchanged by the kidneys following oral administration. Up to 70–80% may be eliminated unchanged by the kidneys following parenteral dosing.

Half-life: 1.7–3 hr (increased in renal impairment).

CONTRAINDICATIONS AND PRECAUTIONS

Contraindicated in: ▪ Hypersensitivity. **Use Cautiously in:** ▪ Elderly patients ▪ Renal impairment (increased dose interval recommended if creatinine clearance <50 ml/min) ▪ Hepatic impairment (increased risk of confusion; dosage reduction recommended) ▪ Pregnancy, lactation, or children (safety not established).

ADVERSE REACTIONS AND SIDE EFFECTS*

CNS: confusion, dizziness, headache, malaise, drowsiness.

CV: bradycardia, tachycardia, premature ventricular contractions.

Derm: rashes.
EENT: ocular pain, blurred vision.
Endo: gynecomastia.
GI: nausea, constipation, hepatitis, abdominal pain, diarrhea.
GU: impotence.

INTERACTIONS

Drug–Drug: ▪ **Antacids** may decrease the absorption of ranitidine ▪ **Smoking** may decrease the effectiveness of ranitidine ▪ Reduces absorption of **ketoconazole**.

ROUTE AND DOSAGE

Short-Term Treatment of Active Ulcers
▪ **PO (Adults):** 150 mg bid or 300 mg at bedtime.
▪ **PO (Children):** 2–4 mg/kg twice daily (up to 300 mg/day).
▪ **IM (Adults):** 50 mg q 6–8 hr (up to 400 mg/day).
▪ **IV (Adults):** 50 mg q 6–8 hr or 6.25 mg/hr infusion.
▪ **IV (Children):** 2–4 mg/kg/day given once daily.

Prevention of Duodenal Ulcers
▪ **PO (Adults):** 150 mg once daily, at bedtime.

Management of Gastroesophageal Reflux
▪ **PO (Adults):** 150 mg bid.

Gastric Hypersecretory Conditions (Zollinger-Ellison Syndrome)
▪ **PO (Adults):** 150 mg bid (up to 6 g/day).
▪ **IV (Adults):** 1 mg/kg/hr initially by continuous infusion. Based on gastric acid output after 4 hr, may increase by 0.5 mg/kg/hr up to 2.5 mg/kg/hr.

AVAILABILITY

▪ **Tablets:** 150 mg, 300 mg ▪ {*Capsules:* 150 mg, 300 mg} ▪ *Syrup:* 15 mg/ml ▪ *Injection:* 0.5 mg/ml, 25 mg/ml.

TIME/ACTION PROFILE (inhibition of gastric acid secretion)

	ONSET	PEAK	DURATION
PO	UK	1–3 hr	8–12 hr
IM	UK	15 min	8–12 hr
IV	UK	15 min	8–12 hr

NURSING IMPLICATIONS

ASSESSMENT
▫ Assess patient routinely for epigastric or abdominal pain and frank or occult blood in the stool, emesis, or gastric aspirate.
▫ Assess elderly and severely ill patients routinely for confusion. Notify physician promptly should this occur.
▪ **Lab Test Considerations:** CBC with differential should be monitored periodically throughout therapy.
▫ May cause transient increase in serum transaminase and serum creatinine.
▫ Antagonizes the effects of pentagastrin and histamine during gastric acid secretion test. Avoid administration during the 24 hr preceding the test.
▫ May cause false-negative results for urine protein.
▫ May cause false-negative results in skin tests using allergen extracts. Ranitidine should be discontinued 24 hr prior to the test.

POTENTIAL NURSING DIAGNOSES
▪ Pain (indications).
▪ Knowledge deficit related to medication regimen (patient/family teaching).

IMPLEMENTATION
▪ **PO:** Food does not affect absorption; may be given without regard to meals.
▫ If administering oral doses concurrently with antacids, give at least 1 hr apart.
▪ **Direct IV:** Dilute each 50 mg in 20 ml of 0.9% NaCl or D5W for injection.
▪ **Rate:** Administer over at least 5 min. Rapid administration may cause hypotension and arrhythmias.
▪ **Intermittent Infusion:** Dilute each 50 mg in 100 ml of 0.9% NaCl or D5W. Diluted solution is stable for 48 hr at room temperature. Do not use solution that is discolored or that contains precipitate.
▪ **Rate:** Administer over 15–20 min.
▪ **Continuous Infusion:** Add ranitidine to D5W for a concentration of 150

R

mg/250 ml (no greater than 2.5 mg/ml for Zollinger-Ellison patients).

- **Rate:** Administer at a rate of 6.25 mg/hr. In patients with Zollinger-Ellison syndrome start infusion at 1 mg/kg/hr. If gastric acid output is >10 mEq/hr or patient becomes symptomatic after 4 hr, adjust dose by 0.5 mg/kg/hr increments and remeasure gastric output.
- **Syringe Compatibility:** ▪ atropine ▪ cyclizine ▪ dexamethasone ▪ dimenhydrinate ▪ diphenhydramine ▪ fentanyl ▪ glycopyrrolate ▪ hydromorphone ▪ meperidine ▪ metoclopramide ▪ morphine ▪ nalbuphine ▪ oxymorphone ▪ pentazocine ▪ perphenazine ▪ prochlorperazine ▪ promethazine ▪ scopolamine ▪ thiethylperazine.
- **Syringe Incompatibility:** ▪ hydroxyzine ▪ methotrimeprazine ▪ midazolam ▪ pentobarbital ▪ phenobarbital.
- **Y-Site Compatibility:** ▪ acyclovir ▪ aminophylline ▪ atracurium ▪ bretylium ▪ dobutamine ▪ dopamine ▪ enalaprilat ▪ esmolol ▪ fludarabine ▪ foscarnet ▪ heparin ▪ labetalol ▪ meperidine ▪ morphine ▪ nitroglycerin ▪ ondansetron ▪ pancuronium ▪ procainamide ▪ sargramostim ▪ vecuronium ▪ zidovudine.
- **Additive Compatibility:** ▪ amikacin ▪ chloramphenicol ▪ doxycycline ▪ furosemide ▪ gentamicin ▪ heparin ▪ lidocaine ▪ penicillin G sodium ▪ potassium chloride ▪ ticarcillin ▪ tobramycin ▪ vancomycin.
- **Additive Incompatibility:** ▪ amphotericin B ▪ clindamycin.

PATIENT/FAMILY TEACHING

- ▢ Instruct patient to take medication as directed for the full course of therapy, even if feeling better. If a dose is missed, it should be taken as soon as remembered, but not if almost time for next dose. Do not double doses.
- ▢ Inform patient that smoking interferes with the action of ranitidine. Encourage patient to quit smoking or at least not to smoke after last dose of the day.

- ▢ Ranitidine may cause drowsiness or dizziness. Caution patient to avoid driving or other activities requiring alertness until response to the drug is known.
- ▢ Advise patient to avoid alcohol, products containing aspirin or ibuprofen, and foods that may cause an increase in GI irritation.
- ▢ Advise patient to report onset of black, tarry stools; diarrhea; dizziness; rash; or confusion to physician promptly.

EVALUATION

Effectiveness of therapy can be demonstrated by: ▪ Decrease in abdominal pain ▪ Prevention of gastric irritation and bleeding. Healing of duodenal ulcers can be seen on x-ray examinations or endoscopy. Therapy is continued for at least 6 wk after initial episode ▪ Decrease in symptoms of gastroesophageal reflux disease.

RESERPINE
(re-**ser**-peen)
{Novoreserpine}, {Reserfia}, Serpalan, Serpasil

CLASSIFICATION(S):
Antihypertensive (peripherally acting antiadrenergic)
Pregnancy Category C

INDICATIONS

▪ Used in combination with other antihypertensives (thiazide diuretics) in the management of mild to moderate hypertension.

ACTION

▪ Depletes stores of norepinephrine and inhibits uptake in postganglionic adrenergic nerve endings. **Therapeutic Effect:** ▪ Lowering of blood pressure.

PHARMACOKINETICS

Absorption: 40–50% absorbed following oral administration.

Distribution: Widely distributed. Crosses the placenta and enters breast milk.

Metabolism and Excretion: Metabolized by the liver. At least 50% lost in feces as unabsorbed drug following oral administration. Small amounts excreted unchanged by the kidneys.

Half-life: 11 days.

CONTRAINDICATIONS AND PRECAUTIONS

Contraindicated in: ▪ Hypersensitivity ▪ Active peptic ulcer, ulcerative colitis ▪ Gallstones ▪ Mental depression ▪ Electroconvulsive therapy.

Use Cautiously in: ▪ Cardiac, cerebrovascular, or renal insufficiency ▪ Pregnancy, lactation, or children (safety not established).

ADVERSE REACTIONS AND SIDE EFFECTS*

CNS: <u>drowsiness</u>, <u>fatigue</u>, <u>lethargy</u>, <u>depression</u>, headache, nervousness, anxiety, nightmares.

EENT: <u>nasal stuffiness</u>, miosis, blurred vision, conjunctival congestion.

CV: <u>bradycardia</u>, arrhythmias, angina, edema.

GI: <u>diarrhea</u>, dry mouth, cramps, nausea, vomiting, <u>GI bleeding</u>.

GU: impotence.

Derm: flushing.

Endo: galactorrhea, gynecomastia.

F and E: sodium and water retention.

INTERACTIONS

Drug–Drug: ▪ Additive hypotension with other **antihypertensive agents, nitrates,** or acute ingestion of **alcohol** ▪ Increased risk of arrhythmias with **cardiac glycosides, quinidine, procainamide,** or other **antiarrhythmics** ▪ Excitement and hypertension may result from concurrent **MAO inhibitor** therapy ▪ May decrease the therapeutic response to **ephedrine** or **levodopa** ▪ May increase responsiveness to **direct-acting sympathomimetic amines (dopamine, dobutamine, metaraminol, phenylephrine)** ▪ Additive CNS depression with other **CNS depressants,** including **alcohol, antihistamines, antidepressants, opioid analgesics,** or **sedative/hypnotics** ▪ Effectiveness may be decreased by concurrent nonsteroidal anti-inflammatory agents.

ROUTE AND DOSAGE

▪ **PO (Adults):** 100–250 mcg/day in 1–2 divided doses.
▪ **PO (Children):** 5–20 mcg/kg/day in 1–2 divided doses.

AVAILABILITY

▪ *Tablets:* 0.1 mg, 0.25 mg, 1 mg ▪ *In combination with:* thiazide diuretics and/or hydralazine. See Appendix A.

R

TIME/ACTION PROFILE
(antihypertensive effect)

	ONSET	PEAK	DURATION
PO	several days–3 wk	3–6 wk	1–6 wk

NURSING IMPLICATIONS

ASSESSMENT

▫ Monitor blood pressure and pulse frequently during initial dosage adjustment and periodically throughout course of therapy. Notify physician of significant changes.

▫ Monitor intake and output ratios and daily weight and assess for edema daily, especially at beginning of therapy. Notify physician of weight gain or edema. Reserpine is commonly administered concurrently with diuretics.

▫ Assess patient for depression, early morning insomnia, anorexia, impotence, and self-depreciation. Notify physician promptly if these symptoms develop, as this may necessitate discontinuation of the medication. Mental depression may have an insidious onset and may be severe enough to cause suicide. Risk of depression may persist for several months following discontinuation of therapy.

▪ **Lab Test Considerations:** May cause an increase in serum prolactin concentrations.

*<u>Underlines</u> indicate most frequent; **CAPITALS** indicate life-threatening.

◻ May cause a decrease in urinary catecholamine excretion and urinary vanillylmandelic acid excretion.

POTENTIAL NURSING DIAGNOSES

■ Coping, ineffective individual (side effects).

■ Knowledge deficit related to medication regimen (patient/family teaching).

■ Noncompliance (patient/family teaching).

IMPLEMENTATION

■ PO: Administer with meals or milk to minimize GI irritation.

PATIENT/FAMILY TEACHING

◻ Emphasize the importance of continuing to take this medication, even if feeling well. Instruct patient to take medication at the same time each day. If a dose is missed, omit and return to regular dosage schedule. Do not double doses. Consult physician prior to discontinuing medication.

◻ Encourage patient to comply with additional interventions for hypertension (weight reduction, low-sodium diet, smoking cessation, moderation of alcohol consumption, regular exercise, and stress management). Reserpine helps control but does not cure hypertension.

◻ Instruct patient and family on proper technique for blood pressure monitoring. Advise them to check blood pressure at least weekly and to report significant changes to physician.

◻ Reserpine may cause drowsiness. Advise patient to avoid driving or other activities requiring alertness until response to medication is known.

◻ If dry mouth occurs, frequent mouth rinses, good oral hygiene, or sugarless gum or candy may decrease effect. Notify dentist if dry mouth persists >2 wk.

◻ Caution patient to avoid concurrent use of alcohol or other CNS depressants with this medication.

◻ May cause nasal stuffiness. Advise patient to consult physician or pharmacist before taking any cough, cold, decongestant, or allergy remedies. Patient should also avoid excessive amounts of coffee, tea, or cola.

◻ Advise patient to inform physician or dentist of medication regimen prior to treatment or surgery.

◻ Instruct patient to notify physician promptly if abdominal pain, depression, or change in sleep patterns occurs.

◻ Emphasize the importance of follow-up examinations to monitor progress.

EVALUATION

Effectiveness of therapy can be demonstated by: ■ Decrease in blood pressure without appearance of side effects.

Rh$_o$ (D) IMMUNE GLOBULIN
(arr aych oh dee im-**yoon** glob-yoo-lin)

Rh$_o$ (D) IMMUNE GLOBULIN STANDARD DOSE
Gamulin Rh, HypRho-D, Rhesonativ, RhoGAM

Rh$_o$ (D) GLOBULIN MICRODOSE
HypRho-D Mini-Dose, MICRho-GAM, Mini-Gamulin Rh

CLASSIFICATION(S):
Immune globulin
Pregnancy Category C

INDICATIONS

■ Administered to Rh$_o$(D)-negative patients who have beeen exposed to Rh$_o$(D)-positive blood by: ◻ Delivering an Rh$_o$(D)-positive infant ◻ Miscarrying or aborting an Rh$_o$(D)-positive fetus ◻ Having amniocentesis or intra-abdominal trauma while carrying an Rh$_o$(D)-positive fetus ■ Following accidental transfusion of Rh$_o$(D)-positive blood to an Rh$_o$(D)-negative patient.

ACTION

■ Prevents the production of anti-Rh$_o$(D) antibodies in Rh$_o$(D)-negative patients who have been exposed to Rh$_o$(D)-positive blood. **Therapeutic Effects:** ■ Prevention of antibody response and subsequent prevention of hemolytic disease of the newborn (erythroblastosis fetalis) in future pregnancies of women who have conceived an Rh₀(D)-positive fetus ▪ Prevention of Rh₀(D) sensitization following transfusion accident.

PHARMACOKINETICS

Absorption: Well absorbed from IM sites.
Distribution: Distribution not known.
Metabolism and Excretion: Metabolism and excretion are not known.
Half-life: UK.

CONTRAINDICATIONS AND PRECAUTIONS

Contraindicated in: ▪ Rh₀(D)- or Dᵘ-positive patients ▪ Patients previously sensitized to Rh₀(D) or Dᵘ.
Use Cautiously in: ▪ Patients with previous hypersensitivity reactions to immune globulins or thimerisol.

ADVERSE REACTIONS AND SIDE EFFECTS*

Local: pain at IM site.
Misc: fever.

INTERACTIONS

Drug–Drug: ▪ May decrease antibody response to some **live virus vaccines (measles, mumps, rubella)**.

ROUTE AND DOSAGE

Following Delivery
▪ **IM (Adults):** 1 vial standard dose within 72 hr of delivery.

Prior to Delivery
▪ **IM (Adults):** 1 vial standard dose at 26–28 wk, 1 vial standard dose 72 hr after delivery.

Termination of Pregnancy (<13 wk Gestation)
▪ **IM (Adults):** 1 vial standard dose of *microdose* within 72 hr.

Termination of Pregnancy (>13 wk Gestation)
▪ **IM (Adults):** 1 vial standard dose within 72 hr.

Large Fetal-Maternal Hemorrhage
▪ **IM (Adults):** Packed red blood cell volume of hemorrhage/15 = number of vials of standard dose preparation (round to next whole number of vials).

Transfusion Accident
▪ **IM (Adults):** (Volume of Rh-positive blood administered × Hct of donor blood)/15 = number of vials of standard dose preparation (round to next whole number of vials).

AVAILABILITY
▪ *Injection:* 50 mcg/vial (microdose), 300 mcg/vial (standard dose).

TIME/ACTION PROFILE

	ONSET	PEAK	DURATION
IM	rapid	UK	UK

NURSING IMPLICATIONS

ASSESSMENT
▪ **Lab Test Considerations:** Type and cross-match of mother's and newborn's cord blood must be performed to determine need for medication. Mother must be Rh₀(D)-negative and Dᵘ-negative. Infant must be Rh₀(D)-positive. If there is doubt regarding infant's blood type or if father is Rh₀(D)-positive, medication should be given.
□ An infant born to a woman treated with Rh₀(D) immune globulin antepartum may have a weakly positive direct Coombs' test result on cord or infant blood.

POTENTIAL NURSING DIAGNOSES
▪ Knowledge deficit related to medication regimen (patient/family teaching).

IMPLEMENTATION
▪ **General Info:** Do not give to infant, to Rh₀(D)-positive individual, or to Rh₀(D)-negative individual previously sensitized to the Rh₀(D) antigen. However, there is no more risk than when given to a woman who is not sensitized. When in doubt, administer Rh₀ (D) immune globulin.

R

*Underlines indicate most frequent; **CAPITALS** indicate life-threatening.

- **IM:** Administer into the deltoid muscle. Dose should be given within 3 hr but may be given up to 72 hr after delivery, miscarriage, abortion, or transfusion. Do not administer IV.

PATIENT/FAMILY TEACHING
□ Explain to patient that the purpose of this medication is to protect future $Rh_o(D)$-positive infants.

EVALUATION
Effectiveness of therapy can be demonstrated by: ▪ Prevention of erythroblastosis fetalis in future $Rh_o(D)$-positive infants ▪ Prevention of $Rh_o(D)$ sensitization following transfusion accident.

RIBAVIRIN
(rye-ba-**vye**-rin)
Virazole

CLASSIFICATION(S):
Antiviral
Pregnancy Category X

INDICATIONS
▪ Treatment of severe lower respiratory tract infections caused by the respiratory syncytial virus (RSV) in infants and young children. **Unlabeled Use:** ▪ Early (within 24 hr of symptoms) secondary treatment of influenza A or B in young adults.

ACTION
▪ Inhibits viral DNA and RNA synthesis and subsequent replication ▪ Must be phosphorylated intracellularly to be active. **Therapeutic Effect:** ▪ Virustatic action.

PHARMACOKINETICS
Absorption: Systemic absorption occurs following nasal and oral inhalation.
Distribution: 70% of inhaled drug is deposited in the respiratory tract. Appears to concentrate in the respiratory tract and red blood cells. Enters breast milk.

Metabolism and Excretion: Eliminated from the respiratory tract by distribution across membranes, macrophages, and ciliary motion. Metabolized primarily by the liver.
Half-life: 9.5 hr (40 days in red blood cells).

CONTRAINDICATIONS AND PRECAUTIONS
Contraindicated in: ▪ Hypersensitivity ▪ Women with childbearing potential ▪ Patients receiving mechanically assisted ventilation.
Use Cautiously in: ▪ Underlying anemia ▪ Adults (safety not established).

ADVERSE REACTIONS AND SIDE EFFECTS*
CNS: dizziness, faintness.
CV: CARDIAC ARREST, hypotension.
Derm: rash.
EENT: ocular irritation, erythema of the eyelids, conjunctivitis, photosensitivity, blurred vision.
Hemat: reticulocytosis.

INTERACTIONS
Drug–Drug: ▪ May antagonize the antiviral action of **zidovudine** ▪ May potentiate the hematologic toxicity of **zidovudine** ▪ May increase the risk of **cardiac glycoside** toxicity.

ROUTE AND DOSAGE
- **Inhalation (Infants and Young Children):** 300 ml of 200 mg/ml solution delivered via mist for 12–18 hr/day.

AVAILABILITY
▪ *Powder for reconstitution for aerosol use:* 6 g/vial.

TIME/ACTION PROFILE (blood levels)

	ONSET	PEAK	DURATION
Inhaln	UK	end of inhaln	UK

NURSING IMPLICATIONS
ASSESSMENT
□ Assess patient for infection (vital

---

*<u>Underlines</u> indicate most frequent; **CAPITALS** indicate life-threatening.

signs, sputum, WBC) at beginning and throughout course of therapy.

□ Obtain specimens for culture and sensitivity prior to initiating therapy. First dose may be given before receiving results.

□ Assess respiratory status (lung sounds, quality and rate of respirations) prior to and throughout therapy.

POTENTIAL NURSING DIAGNOSES

- Infection, high risk for (indications, side effects).
- Gas exchange, impaired (indications).
- Knowledge deficit related to medication regimen (patient/family teaching).

IMPLEMENTATION

- **General Info:** Do not administer ribavirin to infants requiring assisted ventilation, because precipitation of the drug in the respiratory equipment may interfere with safe and effective patient ventilation.

□ Ribavirin treatment should begin within the first 3 days of respiratory syncytial virus (RSV) infection to be effective.

- **Inhalation:** Ribavirin aerosol should be administered using the Viratek SPAG model SPAG-2 only. Do not administer via other aerosol-generating devices. Usually administered using an infant oxygen hood attached to the SPAG-2 aerosol generator. Administration by face mask may be used if the oxygen hood cannot be used.

□ Reconstitute ribavirin 6-g vial with preservative-free Sterile Water for Injection or Inhalation. Transfer to clean, sterilized Erlenmeyer flask of the SPAG-2 reservoir and dilute to a final volume of 300 ml. This recommended concentration (20 mg/ml) in the reservoir provides a concentration of aerosol ribavirin of 190 mcg/liter of air over a 12-hr period. Solution should be discarded and replaced every 24 hr.

□ Frequency of aerosol treatments may vary from continuous aerosolization for 3–7 days to aerosolization for a 4-hr period 3 times/day for 3 days.

PATIENT/FAMILY TEACHING

□ Explain the purpose and route of treatment to the patient and parents.

□ Inform patient and parents that ribavirin may cause blurred vision and photosensitivity.

□ Emphasize the importance of receiving ribavirin for the full course of therapy and on a regular or continuous schedule.

EVALUATION

Clinical response can be evaluated by:
- Resolution of the signs and symptoms of respiratory syncytial virus.

R

RIBOFLAVIN
(rye-boe-flay-vin)
vitamin B$_2$

CLASSIFICATION(S):
Vitamin (water-soluble)
Pregnancy Category UK

INDICATIONS

- Treatment and prevention of riboflavin deficiency, which may be associated with poor nutritional status or chronic debilitating illnesses.

ACTION

- Serves as a coenzyme for metabolic reactions involving transfer of hydrogen ions - Necessary for normal red blood cell function. **Therapeutic Effect:** - Replacement in or prevention of deficiency.

PHARMACOKINETICS

Absorption: Well absorbed from the upper GI tract by an active transport process.

Distribution: Widely distributed. Crosses the placenta and enters breast milk.

Metabolism and Excretion: Amounts in excess of requirements are excreted unchanged by the kidneys.

Half-life: 66–84 min.

CONTRAINDICATIONS AND PRECAUTIONS

Contraindicated in: ▪ No known contraindications.
Use Cautiously in: ▪ No known precautions.

ADVERSE REACTIONS AND SIDE EFFECTS*

GU: yellow discoloration of urine (large doses only).

INTERACTIONS

Drug–Drug: ▪ **Phenothiazines, tricyclic antidepressants, probenecid,** and chronic ingestion of **alcohol** increase riboflavin requirements.

ROUTE AND DOSAGE

Treatment of Deficiency
▪ **PO (Adults):** 5–30 mg/day in divided doses for several days, then 1–4 mg/day.
▪ **PO (Children >12 yr):** 3–10 mg/day for several days, then 0.6 mg/1000 calories ingested.

AVAILABILITY

▪ *Tablets:* 10 mg, 25 mg, 50 mg, 100 mg.

TIME/ACTION PROFILE

	ONSET	PEAK	DURATION
PO	UK	UK	UK

NURSING IMPLICATIONS

ASSESSMENT

▫ Assess patient for signs of vitamin B_2 deficiency (dermatoses, stomatitis, ocular inflammation and irritation, photophobia, and cheilosis) prior to and periodically throughout therapy.
▪ **Lab Test Considerations:** May cause false elevations in urobilinogen and urinary catecholamine measurements.

POTENTIAL NURSING DIAGNOSES

▪ Nutrition, altered: less than body requirements (indications).
▪ Knowledge deficit related to medication regimen (patient/family teaching).

IMPLEMENTATION

▪ **General Info:** Because of infrequency of single B-vitamin deficiencies, combinations are commonly administered.

PATIENT/FAMILY TEACHING

▫ Instruct patient to take as directed. If a dose is missed, it may be omitted, as an extended period of time is required to become deficient in riboflavin.
▫ Encourage patient to comply with physician's diet recommendations. Explain that the best source of vitamins is a well-balanced diet with foods from the 4 basic food groups. Foods high in riboflavin include dairy products, enriched flour, nuts, meats, and green leafy vegetables; little is lost from cooking.
▫ Patients self-medicating with vitamin supplements should be cautioned not to exceed RDA (see Appendix L). The effectiveness of megadoses for treatment of various medical conditions is unproven and may cause side effects.
▫ Advise patient to avoid alcoholic beverages, as alcohol impairs the absorption of riboflavin.
▫ Explain to patient that medically insignificant increase in yellow coloration of urine may occur.
▫ Emphasize the importance of follow-up examinations to evaluate progress.

EVALUATION

Effectiveness of therapy can be demonstrated by: ▪ Prevention or decrease in the symptoms of riboflavin deficiency.

RIFABUTIN
(riff-a-**byoo**-tin)
Mycobutin

CLASSIFICATION(S):
Antimycobacterial
Pregnancy Category B

---

*Underlines indicate most frequent; **CAPITALS** indicate life-threatening.

INDICATIONS

■ Used to prevent disseminated *Mycobacterium avium* complex (MAC) disease in patients with advanced human immunodeficiency virus (HIV) infection.

ACTION

■ Appears to inhibit DNA-dependent RNA polymerase in susceptible organisms. **Therapeutic Effect:** ■ Antimycobacterial action against susceptible organisms. **Spectrum:** ■ Active against *Mycobacterium avium* and most strains of *Mycobacterium tuberculosis.*

PHARMACOKINETICS

Absorption: Well absorbed following oral administration (50–85%). Absorption is decreased in HIV-positive patients (20%).
Distribution: Widely distributed to body tissues and fluids.
Metabolism and Excretion: Mostly metabolized by the liver. <5% excreted unchanged by the kidneys.
Half-life: 45 hr.

CONTRAINDICATIONS AND PRECAUTIONS

Contraindicated in: ■ Hypersensitivity. Cross-sensitivity with other rifamycins (rifampin) may occur ■ Active tuberculosis.
Use Cautiously in: ■ Pregnancy, lactation, or children (safety not established).

ADVERSE REACTIONS AND SIDE EFFECTS*

EENT: brown-orange discoloration of tears, ocular disturbances.
Resp: dyspnea.
CV: chest pressure, chest pain.
GI: brown-orange discoloration of saliva, hepatitis, taste disturbance.
GU: brown-orange discoloration of urine.
Derm: rash, skin discoloration.
Hemat: neutropenia, thrombocytopenia, hemolysis.

MS: arthralgia, myositis.
Misc: brown-orange discoloration of body fluids, flu-like syndrome.

INTERACTIONS

Drug–Drug: ■ Increases metabolism and may decrease the effectiveness of other drugs including **glucocorticoids, disopyramide, quinidine, opioid analgesics, oral hypoglycemic agents, oral anticoagulants, estrogens, oral contraceptives, phenytoin, verapamil, fluconazole, quinidine, tocainide, theophylline, zidovudine,** and **chloramphenicol.**

ROUTE AND DOSAGE

■ **PO (Adults):** 300 mg once daily. If GI upset occurs, may give as 150 mg twice daily with food.

AVAILABILITY

■ *Capsules:* 150 mg.

TIME/ACTION PROFILE (blood levels)

	ONSET	PEAK
PO	rapid	2–4 hr

NURSING IMPLICATIONS

ASSESSMENT

□ Monitor patient for signs of active tuberculosis (purified protein derivative [PPD], chest x-ray, sputum culture, blood culture, urine culture, biopsy of suspicious lymph nodes) prior to and throughout therapy. Rifabutin must not be administered to patients with active tuberculosis.
■ **Lab Test Considerations:** Monitor CBC periodically throughout course of therapy. May cause neutropenia and thrombocytopenia.

POTENTIAL NURSING DIAGNOSES

■ Infection, high risk for (indications).
■ Knowledge deficit related to medication regimen (patient/family teaching).
■ Noncompliance (patient/family teaching).

IMPLEMENTATION

■ **PO:** May be administered without regard to meals. High-fat meals slow

*Underlines indicate most frequent; **CAPITALS** indicate life-threatening.

rate but not extent of absorption. May be mixed with foods such as applesauce. If GI upset occurs, administer with food.

PATIENT/FAMILY TEACHING

◻ Advise patient to take medication exactly as directed. Do not skip doses or double up on missed doses. Emphasize the importance of continuing therapy even if asymptomatic.

◻ Advise patient to notify physician promptly if signs and symptoms of neutropenia (sore throat, fever, signs of infection); thrombocytopenia (unusual bleeding or bruising); or hepatitis (yellow eyes and skin, nausea, vomiting, anorexia, unusual tiredness, weakness) occur.

◻ Caution patient to avoid the use of alcohol during this therapy, as this may increase the risk of hepatotoxicity.

◻ Instruct patient to report symptoms of myositis (myalgia, arthralgia) or uveitis (intraocular inflammation) to physician promptly.

◻ Inform patient that saliva, sputum, sweat, tears, urine, and feces may become red-orange to red-brown and that soft contact lenses may become permanently discolored.

◻ Advise patient that this medication has teratogenic properties. Counsel patient to use a nonhormonal form of contraception throughout therapy.

◻ Emphasize the importance of regular follow-up examinations to monitor progress and to check for side effects.

EVALUATION

Effectiveness of therapy can be demonstrated by: ▪ Prevention of disseminated *Mycobacterium avium* complex (MAC) in patients with advanced HIV infection.

RIFAMPIN
(rif-**am**-pin)
Rifadin, Rifampicin, Rimactane,
{Rofact}

CLASSIFICATION(S):
Antitubercular
Pregnancy Category C

INDICATIONS

▪ Used in combination with other agents in the management of active tuberculosis ▪ Used to eliminate carriers of meningococcal disease.

ACTION

▪ Inhibits RNA synthesis by blocking RNA transcription in susceptible organisms. **Therapeutic Effect:** ▪ Bactericidal action against susceptible organisms. **Spectrum:** ▪ Broad spectrum notable for activity against: ◻ *Mycobacteria* ◻ *Staphylococcus aureus* ◻ *Hemophilus influenzae* ◻ *Legionella pneumophila* ◻ *Neisseria meningitidis*.

PHARMACOKINETICS

Absorption: Well absorbed following oral administration.

Distribution: Widely distributed into many body tissues and fluids, including CSF. Crosses the placenta and enters breast milk.

Metabolism and Excretion: Mostly metabolized by the liver. 60% eliminated in the feces via biliary elimination.

Half-life: 3 hr.

CONTRAINDICATIONS AND PRECAUTIONS

Contraindicated in: ▪ Hypersensitivity ▪ Pregnancy or lactation.

Use Cautiously in: ▪ History of liver disease ▪ Concurrent use of other hepatotoxic agents.

ADVERSE REACTIONS AND SIDE EFFECTS*

CNS: headache, drowsiness, confusion, fatigue, ataxia, weakness.

GI: nausea, vomiting, heartburn, abdominal pain, flatulence, diarrhea, hepatitis.

Hemat: hemolytic anemia, thrombocytopenia.

{} = Available in Canada only.

*Underlines indicate most frequent; **CAPITALS** indicate life-threatening.

MS: myalgia, arthralgia.
Misc: flu-like syndrome, <u>red discoloration of all body fluids</u>.

INTERACTIONS

Drug–Drug: ▪ Rifampin stimulates liver enzymes, which may increase metabolism and decrease the effectiveness of other drugs, including **glucocorticoids, disopyramide, quinidine, opioid analgesics, oral hypoglycemic agents, oral anticoagulants, estrogens, phenytoin, verapamil, fluconazole, quinidine, tocainide, theophylline, chloramphenicol,** and **oral contraceptive agents** ▪ Increased risk of hepatotoxicity with other **hepatotoxic agents,** including **alcohol, isoniazid, ketoconazole,** and **miconazole.**

ROUTE AND DOSAGE

Tuberculosis

- **PO, IV (Adults):** 10 mg/kg/day (usual dose 600 mg/day) single dose; may also be given twice weekly.
- **PO, IV (Children):** 10–20 mg/kg/day single dose (not to exceed 600 mg/day).

Asymptomatic Carriers of Meningococcus

- **PO, IV (Adults):** 600 mg q 12 hr for 2 days.
- **PO, IV (Children ≥1 mo):** 10 mg/kg q 12 hr for 2 days.
- **PO (Infants <1 mo):** 5 mg/kg q 12 hr for 2 days.

AVAILABILITY

- **Capsules:** 150 mg, 300 mg ▪ **Injection:** 600 mg/vial.

TIME/ACTION PROFILE (blood levels)

	ONSET	PEAK
PO	rapid	2–4 hr
IV	rapid	end of infusion

NURSING IMPLICATIONS

ASSESSMENT

- Mycobacterial studies and susceptibility tests should be performed prior to and periodically throughout therapy to detect possible resistance.
- Assess lung sounds and character and amount of sputum periodically throughout therapy.
- **Lab Test Considerations:** Hepatic and renal function, CBC, and urinalysis should be evaluated periodically throughout course of therapy.
- May cause increased BUN, AST (SGOT), ALT (SGPT), and serum alkaline phosphatase, bilirubin, and uric acid concentrations.
- May cause false-positive direct Coombs' test results. May interfere with folic acid and vitamin B_{12} assays.

POTENTIAL NURSING DIAGNOSES

- Infection, high risk for (indications).
- Knowledge deficit related to medication regimen (patient/family teaching).
- Noncompliance (patient/family teaching).

IMPLEMENTATION

- **PO:** Administer medication on an empty stomach, at least 1 hr before or 2 hr after meals. If GI irritation becomes a problem, may be administered with food. Antacids may also be taken 1 hr prior to administration. Capsules may be opened and contents mixed with applesauce or jelly for patients with difficulty swallowing.
- Pharmacist can compound a syrup for patients unable to swallow solids.
- **Intermittent Infusion:** Reconstitute 600-mg vial with 10 ml of Sterile Water for Injection and swirl gently to dissolve completely. Dilute further in 500 ml or 100 ml of D5W or 0.9% NaCl. Solution is stable for 24 hr at room temperature.
- **Rate:** Administer solutions diluted in 500 ml over 3 hr and solutions diluted in 100 ml over 30 min.
- **Additive Incompatibility:** Do not admix with other solutions or medications.

PATIENT/FAMILY TEACHING

- Advise patient to take medication

once daily (unless biweekly regimens are used), exactly as directed; not to skip doses or double up on missed doses. Emphasize the importance of continuing therapy even after symptoms have subsided. Course of therapy commonly lasts for 1–2 yr. Patients on short-term prophylactic therapy should also be advised of the importance of compliance with therapy.

□ Advise patient to notify physician promptly if signs and symptoms of hepatitis (yellow eyes and skin, nausea, vomiting, anorexia, unusual tiredness, weakness) or thrombocytopenia (unusual bleeding or bruising) occur.

□ Caution patient to avoid the use of alcohol during this therapy, as this may increase the risk of hepatotoxicity.

□ Instruct patient to report the occurrence of flu-like symptoms (fever, chills, myalgia, headache) promptly.

□ Rifampin may occasionally cause drowsiness. Caution patient to avoid driving or other activities requiring alertness until response to medication is known.

□ Inform patient that saliva, sputum, sweat, tears, urine, and feces may become red-orange to red-brown, and that soft contact lenses may become permanently discolored.

□ Advise patient that this medication has teratogenic properties. Counsel patient to use a nonhormonal form of contraception throughout therapy.

□ Emphasize the importance of regular follow-up examinations to monitor progress and to check for side effects.

EVALUATION

Effectiveness of therapy can be demonstrated by: ▪ Decreased fever and night sweats □ Diminished cough and sputum production □ Negative sputum cultures □ Increased appetite □ Weight gain □ Reduced fatigue □ Sense of well-being in patients with tuberculosis ▪ Prevention of meningococcal meningitis. Prophylactic course is usually short-term.

RIMANTADINE
(ri-**man**-ti-deen)
Flumadine

CLASSIFICATION(S):
Antiviral
Pregnancy Category C

INDICATIONS

▪ Prevention and treatment of influenza A infection in adults ▪ Prevention of influenza A infection in children.

ACTION

▪ Diminishes replication of Influenza A virus by inhibiting uncoating of the virus. **Therapeutic Effects:** ▪ When given prophylactically, prevents the signs and symptoms of Influenza A infection. When administered within 48 hr of influenza-like illness, decreases the duration of fever and other associated symptoms.

PHARMACOKINETICS

Absorption: Appears to be well absorbed following oral administration.
Distribution: Distribution not known.
Metabolism and Excretion: Mostly metabolized by the liver. <25% excreted unchanged in urine.
Half-life: 25 hr (range 13–65 hr). Prolonged in elderly patients and patients with severe hepatic or renal impairment.

CONTRAINDICATIONS AND PRECAUTIONS

Contraindicated in: ▪ Hypersensitivity to rimantadine or amantadine ▪ Lactation.
Use Cautiously in: ▪ Patients with a history of seizures ▪ Elderly patients or patients with severe hepatic or renal disease (dosage reduction recommended if CCr ≤10 ml/min) ▪ Pregnancy (safety not established).

ADVERSE REACTIONS AND SIDE EFFECTS*

CNS: SEIZURES, insomnia, dizziness,

---

*Underlines indicate most frequent; **CAPITALS** indicate life-threatening.

headache, fatigue, impaired concentration, agitation, depression.
EENT: tinnitus.
Resp: dyspnea.
GI: nausea, vomiting, anorexia, dry mouth, abdominal pain, diarrhea, dyspepsia.
Derm: rash.

INTERACTIONS
Drug–Drug: ▪ **Cimetidine, aspirin,** and **acetaminophen** may slightly decrease plasma levels of rimantadine.

ROUTE AND DOSAGE
▪ **PO (Adults and Children >10 yr):** 100 mg twice daily. Elderly patients, patients with severe hepatic or renal impairment (creatinine clearance <10 ml/min) should receive 100 mg daily.
▪ **PO (Children <10 yr):** 5 mg/kg/day as a single dose (not to exceed 150 mg/day).

AVAILABILITY
▪ *Tablets:* 100 mg ▪ *Syrup:* 50 mg/5 ml.

TIME/ACTION PROFILE (blood levels)

	ONSET	PEAK
PO	rapid	6 hr

NURSING IMPLICATIONS
ASSESSMENT
□ Monitor respiratory status (rate, breath sounds, sputum) and temperature periodically. Supportive treatment is indicated if symptoms occur.

POTENTIAL NURSING DIAGNOSES
▪ Infection, high risk for (indications).
▪ Knowledge deficit related to medication regimen (patient/family teaching).

IMPLEMENTATION
▪ **PO:** Do not administer last dose of medication near bedtime, as this drug may produce insomnia in some patients.

PATIENT/FAMILY TEACHING
□ Advise patient to take medication as directed and not to skip doses or double up on missed doses.

□ Rimantadine may cause dizziness. Advise patient to avoid driving or other activities that require alertness until response to the drug is known.
□ Inform patient that frequent mouth rinses, good oral hygiene, and sugarless gum or candy may decrease dry mouth.
□ Advise patient to confer with physician or pharmacist prior to taking over-the-counter medications, especially aspirin or acetaminophen, or drinking alcoholic beverages.
□ Instruct patient and family to notify physician if influenza symptoms occur.

EVALUATION
Effectiveness of therapy can be demonstrated by: ▪ Absence or reduction of influenza A symptoms.

SALIVA SUBSTITUTES
(sa-**lye**-va **sub**-sti-toot)
Moi-Stir, Orex, Salivart, Xero-Lube

CLASSIFICATION(S):
Saliva substitutes
Pregnancy Category UK

INDICATIONS
▪ Management of dry mouth or throat, which may occur as a consequence of:
□ Medications (tricyclic antidepressants, antihistamines, anticholinergics) □ Radiation therapy □ Chemotherapy □ Other illnesses.

ACTION
▪ Composition is similar to saliva
▪ Contains electrolytes in a thickening agent (carboxymethylcellulose). **Therapeutic Effect:** ▪ Relief of dry mouth.

PHARMACOKINETICS
Absorption: Electrolytes may be absorbed through oral mucosa.
Distribution: Distribution not known.
Metabolism and Excretion: Metabolism and excretion not known.
Half-life: UK.

CONTRAINDICATIONS AND PRECAUTIONS

Contraindicated in: ▪ Hypersensitivity to carboxymethylcellulose, parabens, or other components.

Use Cautiously in: ▪ Situations in which absorption of electrolytes may compromise the patient's condition, such as potassium and magnesium in patients with renal failure or sodium in patients with congestive heart failure or hypertension.

ADVERSE REACTIONS AND SIDE EFFECTS*

F and E: excessive absorption of electrolytes.

INTERACTIONS

Drug–Drug: ▪ None significant.

ROUTE AND DOSAGE

▪ **PO (Adults):** Spray or apply to oral mucosa as needed.

AVAILABILITY

▪ **Solution:** in squirt bottle, pump spray, spray can.

TIME/ACTION PROFILE (relief of dry mouth)

	ONSET	PEAK	DURATION
PO	upon application	UK	UK

NURSING IMPLICATIONS

ASSESSMENT

□ Assess patient for xerostomia (dry mouth) or dry throat prior to and periodically throughout therapy.
□ Assess gingiva and oral mucosa for stomatitis.

POTENTIAL NURSING DIAGNOSES

▪ Oral mucous membranes, altered (indications).
▪ Knowledge deficit related to medication regimen (patient/family teaching).

IMPLEMENTATION

▪ **General Info:** Administer as necessary for xerostomia or dry throat.

PATIENT/FAMILY TEACHING

□ Instruct patient to swish saliva substitute around in mouth following spray or application.
□ Advise patient of the importance of good oral hygiene in addition to the use of saliva substitutes.
□ Emphasize the importance of routine dental examinations throughout course of therapy.

EVALUATION

Effectiveness of therapy can be demonstrated by: ▪ Decrease in dry mouth and throat.

SALSALATE
(sal-sa-late)
Amigesic, Argesic-SA, Arthra-G, Dilsalcid, Mono-Gesic, Salflex, salicylsalicylic acid, Salsitab

CLASSIFICATION(S):
Nonopioid analgesic, Nonsteroidal anti-inflammatory agent, Antipyretic
Pregnancy Category C

INDICATIONS

▪ Treatment of mild to moderate pain
▪ Management of inflammatory disorders including: □ Rheumatoid arthritis □ Osteoarthritis ▪ Treatment of fever.

ACTION

▪ Produces analgesia and reduces inflammation by inhibiting the production of prostaglandins ▪ Unlike aspirin, has no effect on platelet function. **Therapeutic Effects:** ▪ Analgesia resulting in reduction of mild to moderate pain ▪ Reduction of inflammation ▪ Reduction of fever.

PHARMACOKINETICS

Absorption: Splits into 2 molecules of salicylic acid following oral administration. Absorbed in the small intestine.
Distribution: Rapidly and widely distributed. Crosses the placenta and enters breast milk.

*Underlines indicate most frequent; CAPITALS indicate life-threatening.

Metabolism and Excretion: Amount excreted unchanged by the kidneys depends on urine pH. As pH increases, amount excreted unchanged increases from 2–3% up to 80%.

Half-life: 2–3 hr for low doses. For larger doses, half-life may increase up to 15–30 hr due to saturation of liver metabolism.

CONTRAINDICATIONS AND PRECAUTIONS

Contraindicated in: ■ Hypersensitivity to aspirin or other nonsteroidal anti-inflammatory agents (less cross-sensitivity than aspirin).

Use Cautiously in: ■ Renal insufficiency (magnesium toxicity may occur) ■ Severe liver impairment ■ Pregnancy (may have adverse effects on fetus and mother) ■ Lactation (safety not established) ■ Children or adolescents with viral infections (may increase the risk of Reye's Syndrome).

ADVERSE REACTIONS AND SIDE EFFECTS*

EENT: tinnitus, hearing loss.

GI: dyspepsia, heartburn, epigastric distress, nausea, vomiting, anorexia, abdominal pain, GI BLEEDING, hepatotoxicity.

Misc: noncardiogenic pulmonary edema; allergic reactions, including ANAPHYLAXIS or LARYNGEAL EDEMA.

INTERACTIONS

Drug–Drug: ■ May enhance the activity of **penicillins, phenytoin, methotrexate, oral hypoglycemic agents, valproic acid,** and **sulfonamides** ■ May antagonize the beneficial effects of **probenecid** or **sulfinpyrazone** ■ **Glucocorticoids** may decrease serum salicylate levels ■ **Urinary acidification** enhances reabsorption and may increase serum salicylate levels ■ **Alkalinization of the urine** or the ingestion of large amounts of **antacids** promotes excretion and decreases serum salicylate levels ■ May blunt the therapeutic response to **diuretics** or **antihypertensives** ■ May

increase the risk of bleeding with **anticoagulants, thrombolytic agents, cefamandole, cefoperazone, cefotetan, valproic acid,** or **plicamycin** (effect less than aspirin) ■ Increased risk of GI irritation with **nonsteroidal anti-inflammatory agents** (effect less than aspirin) ■ Increased risk of ototoxicity with **vancomycin.**

Drug–Food: ■ **Foods capable of acidifying the urine** (see Appendix K) may enhance reabsorption and increase serum salicylate levels.

ROUTE AND DOSAGE

■ **PO (Adults):** 0.5–1 g 2–3 times daily.

AVAILABILITY

■ *Tablets:* 500 mg, 750 mg ■ *Capsules:* 500 mg.

TIME/ACTION PROFILE (analgesia and fever reduction)*

	ONSET	PEAK	DURATION
PO	5–30 min	1–3 hr	3–6 hr

*Antirheumatic effect may take 2–3 wk of chronic dosing.

NURSING IMPLICATIONS

ASSESSMENT

■ **General Info:** Patients who have asthma, allergies, and nasal polyps or who are allergic to tartrazine dyes are at an increased risk for developing hypersensitivity reactions.

■ **Pain:** Assess pain and limitation of movement; note type, location, and intensity prior to and 1–3 hr following administration.

■ **Fever:** Assess fever and note associated signs (diaphoresis, tachycardia, malaise, chills).

■ **Toxicity and Overdose:** Observe patient for the onset of tinnitus, hyperventilation, agitation, mental confusion, lethargy, diarrhea, and sweating. If these symptoms appear, withhold medication and notify physician immediately.

POTENTIAL NURSING DIAGNOSES

■ Pain (indications).

*Underlines indicate most frequent; **CAPITALS** indicate life-threatening.

- Physical mobility, impaired (indications).
- Knowledge deficit related to medication regimen (patient/family teaching).

IMPLEMENTATION
- PO: Administer after meals or with food or an antacid to minimize gastric irritation. Food slows but will not alter the total amount absorbed.

PATIENT/FAMILY TEACHING
□ Instruct patient to take with a full glass of water and to remain in an upright position for 15–30 min after administration.
□ Advise patient to report tinnitus, unusual bleeding of gums, bruising, or black, tarry stools, or fever lasting longer than 3 days.
□ Caution patient to avoid concurrent use of alcohol or ibuprofen with this medication to minimize possible gastric irritation.
□ Advise patients on long-term therapy to inform physician or dentist of medication regimen prior to surgery.
□ Centers for Disease Control warn against giving salicylates to children or adolescents with varicella (chickenpox) or influenza-like or viral illnesses because of a possible association with Reye's syndrome.

EVALUATION
Effectiveness of therapy can be demonstrated by: ▪ Decrease in severity of mild to moderate discomfort ▪ Increased ease of joint movement ▪ Reduction of fever.

SARGRAMOSTIM
(sar-**gram**-oh-stim)
Leukine, Prokine, rhu GM-CSF, recombinant human (granulocyte/macrophage colony stimulating factor)

CLASSIFICATION(S):
Colony stimulating factor
Pregnancy Category C

INDICATIONS
▪ Acceleration of bone marrow recovery following autologous bone marrow transplantation in patients with non-Hodgkin's lymphoma, acute lymphoblastic leukemia, or Hodgkin's disease
▪ Management of bone marrow transplant failure or engraftment delay.

ACTION
▪ Consists of a glycoprotein produced by recombinant DNA technique that is capable of binding to and stimulating the production, division, differentiation, and activation of granulocytes and macrophages. **Therapeutic Effect:** ▪ Accelerated recovery of bone marrow following autologous bone marrow transplantation resulting in decreased risk of infection and other complications.

PHARMACOKINETICS
Absorption: Following IV administration absorption is essentially complete.
Distribution: Distribution not known.
Metabolism and Excretion: Metabolism and excretion not known.
Half-life: UK.

CONTRAINDICATIONS AND PRECAUTIONS
Contraindicated in: ▪ Presence of ≥10% leukemic myeloid blast cells in bone marrow or peripheral blood ▪ Hypersensitivity to GM-CSF, yeast products, or additives (mannitol, tromethamine, or sucrose).
Use Cautiously in: ▪ Pre-existing fluid retention, congestive heart failure, or pulmonary infiltrates ▪ Pre-existing cardiac disease ▪ Myeloid malignancies ▪ Previous extensive radiation or chemotherapy (response may be limited) ▪ Pregnancy (use only if clearly needed) ▪ Lactation or children (safety not established).

ADVERSE REACTIONS AND SIDE EFFECTS*
CNS: weakness, malaise.
Resp: dyspnea.
CV: transient supraventricular tachy-

---

*<u>Underlines</u> indicate most frequent; **CAPITALS** indicate life-threatening.

cardia, peripheral edema, pericardial effusion.
GI: diarrhea.
Derm: rash.
MS: bone pain.
Misc: fever, chills.

INTERACTIONS

Drug–Drug: ▪ **Lithium** or **glucocorticoids** may potentiate myeloproliferative effects of sargramostim (concurrent use should be undertaken cautiously).

ROUTE AND DOSAGE

▪ **IV (Adults):** 250 mcg/m²/day for 14–21 days.

AVAILABILITY

▪ *Powder for injection:* 250 mcg/vial, 500 mcg/vial.

TIME/ACTION PROFILE (noted as effects on blood counts)

	ONSET	PEAK	DURATION
IV	rapid	UK	3–7 days

NURSING IMPLICATIONS

ASSESSMENT

▢ Monitor heart rate, blood pressure, and respiratory status during and immediately following infusion. If dyspnea develops, slow infusion rate by half; may require discontinuation of medication. Assess for peripheral edema daily throughout therapy.

▪ **Lab Test Considerations:** Obtain a CBC and platelet count prior to chemotherapy and twice weekly during therapy to avoid leukocytosis. Monitor absolute neutrophil count (ANC), may increase rapidly. If ANC >20,000/mm³, WBC >50,000/mm³, or platelet count >500,000/mm³, interrupt administration and reduce dose by half. Excessive blood levels usually return to baseline 3–7 days following discontinuation of therapy.

▢ Monitor renal and hepatic function prior to and biweekly throughout therapy in patients with renal or hepatic dysfunction.

POTENTIAL NURSING DIAGNOSES

▪ Infection, high risk for (indications).
▪ Knowledge deficit related to medication regimen (patient/family teaching).

IMPLEMENTATION

▪ **General Info:** Administer 2–4 hr after bone marrow transplant and no earlier than 24 hr following cytotoxic chemotherapy or 12 hr after last dose of radiotherapy.

▢ Refrigerate, but do not freeze powder, reconstituted solution, or diluted solution. Do not shake. Discard if left at room temperature for >6 hr. Vial is for 1 time use only.

▪ **Intermittent Infusion:** Reconstitute with 1 ml of sterile water without preservatives injected toward side of vial. Swirl gently to avoid foaming. Solution should be clear and colorless.

▢ Dilute in 0.9% NaCl. If final concentration is <10 mcg/ml, add a final concentration of 0.1% human albumin to 0.9% NaCl prior to addition of sargramostim to prevent absorption of the components of the drug delivery system. Do not admix with other medications.

▪ *Rate:* Infuse over 2 hr.

▪ **Y-Site Compatibility:** ▪ amikacin ▪ aminophylline ▪ aztreonam ▪ bleomycin ▪ butorphanol ▪ calcium gluconate ▪ carboplatin ▪ carmustine ▪ cefazolin ▪ ceforanide ▪ cefotaxime ▪ cefotetan ▪ ceftizoxime ▪ ceftriaxone ▪ cefuroxime ▪ cimetidine ▪ cisplatin ▪ clindamycin ▪ cyclophosphamide ▪ cytarabine ▪ dacarbazine ▪ dactinomycin ▪ dexamethasone sodium phosphate ▪ diphenhydramine ▪ doxorubicin ▪ doxycycline ▪ droperidol ▪ etoposide ▪ famotidine ▪ floxuridine ▪ fluconazole ▪ fluorouracil ▪ furosemide ▪ gentamicin ▪ heparin ▪ ifosfamide ▪ magnesium sulfate ▪ mannitol ▪ mechlorethamine ▪ meperidine ▪ mesna ▪ methotrexate ▪ metoclopramide ▪ metronidazole ▪ mezlocillin ▪ miconazole ▪ minocycline ▪ mitoxantrone ▪ netilmicin ▪ pentostatin ▪ potassium chloride ▪ prochlorperazine

S

- promethazine ■ ranitidine ■ teniposide ■ ticarcillin ■ ticarcillin/clavulanate ■ trimethoprim/sulfamethoxazole ■ vancomycin ■ vinblastine ■ vincristine ■ zidovudine.
- **Y-Site Incompatibility:** ■ acyclovir ■ ampicillin ■ ampicillin/sulbactam ■ cefonicid ■ cefoperazone ■ ceftazidime ■ chlorpromazine ■ ganciclovir ■ haloperidol ■ hydrocortisone ■ hydromorphone ■ hydroxyzine ■ idarubicin ■ imipenem/cilastatin ■ lorazepam ■ methylprednisolone sodium succinate ■ mitomycin ■ morphine ■ nalbuphine ■ ondansetron ■ piperacillin ■ sodium bicarbonate ■ tobramycin.

PATIENT/FAMILY TEACHING

□ Instruct patient to notify nurse or physician if dyspnea or palpitations occur.

EVALUATION

Effectiveness of therapy can be demonstrated by: ■ Decreased incidence of infection in patients following autologous bone marrow transplantation.

SCOPOLAMINE
(scoe-**pol**-a-meen)
Isopto Hyoscine, Transderm-Scōp, {Transderm-V}, Triptone

CLASSIFICATION(S):
Anticholinergic, Antiemetic, Ophthalmic (mydriatic)
Pregnancy Category C

INDICATIONS

■ **Transdermal:** Prevention of motion sickness ■ **IM, IV, SC:** Preoperatively to produce amnesia and to decrease salivation and excessive respiratory secretions ■ **Ophth:** Mydriatic.

ACTION

■ Inhibits the muscarinic activity of acetylcholine ■ Corrects the imbalance of acetylcholine and norepinephrine in the CNS, which may be responsible for motion sickness. **Therapeutic Effects:** ■ Reduction of nausea and vomiting associated with motion sickness ■ Preoperative amnesia and decreased secretions ■ Mydriasis.

PHARMACOKINETICS

Absorption: Well absorbed following IM, SC, and transdermal administration.
Distribution: Crosses the placenta and blood–brain barrier.
Metabolism and Excretion: Mostly metabolized by the liver.
Half-life: 8 hr.

CONTRAINDICATIONS AND PRECAUTIONS

Contraindicated in: ■ Hypersensitivity ■ Hypersensitivity to bromides (ophthalmic and injection only) ■ Narrow-angle glaucoma ■ Acute hemorrhage ■ Tachycardia secondary to cardiac insufficiency or thyrotoxicosis.
Use Cautiously in: ■ Elderly patients, infants, and children (increased risk of adverse reactions) ■ Possible intestinal obstruction ■ Prostatic hypertrophy ■ Chronic renal, hepatic, pulmonary, or cardiac disease ■ Pregnancy or lactation (safety not established).

ADVERSE REACTIONS AND SIDE EFFECTS*

CNS: drowsiness, confusion.
EENT: blurred vision, mydriasis, photophobia.
CV: palpitations, tachycardia.
GI: dry mouth, constipation.
GU: urinary hesitancy, urinary retention.
Derm: decreased sweating.

INTERACTIONS

Drug–Drug: ■ Additive anticholinergic effects with **antihistamines, antidepressants, quinidine,** or **disopyramide** ■ Additive CNS depression with **alcohol,**

{} = Available in Canada only.
*Underlines indicate most frequent; **CAPITALS** indicate life-threatening.

antidepressants, antihistamines, opioid analgesics, or sedative/hypnotics ▪ May alter the absorption of other **orally administered drugs** by slowing motility of the GI tract ▪ May increase GI mucosal lesions in patients taking oral **wax-matrix potassium chloride preparations.**

ROUTE AND DOSAGE

Prevention of Motion Sickness

- **Transdermal (Adults):** 1.5 mg Transderm-Scōp system delivers 0.5 mg over 72 hr and should be applied at least 4 hr prior to travel. 1.5 mg Transderm-V system (Canadian product) delivers 1 mg over 72 hr and should be applied 12 hr prior to travel.

Parenteral Doses

- **IM, IV, SC (Adults):** *Antiemetic, anticholinergic*—0.3–0.65 mg; *Antisecretory effect*—0.2–0.6 mg; *Amnesic effect*—0.32–0.65 mg; *Sedation*—0.6 mg.
- **IM, IV, SC (Children):** *Antiemetic, anticholinergic*—6 mcg/kg or 0.2 mg/m².
- **IM (Children 8–12 yr):** *Antisecretory*—0.3 mg.
- **IM (Children 3–8 yr):** *Antisecretory*—0.2 mg.
- **IM (Children 7 mo–3 yr):** *Antisecretory*—0.15 mg.
- **IM (Children 4–7 mo):** *Antisecretory*—0.1 mg.

Ophthalmic Use

- **Ophth (Adults):** 1–2 drops 1 hr before refraction, up to 4 times daily for uveitis.
- **Ophth (Children):** 1 drop 2 times daily for 2 days prior to refraction or up to 4 times daily for uveitis.

AVAILABILITY

- ***Transdermal therapeutic system:*** 1.5 mg scopolamine/patch (Transderm-Scōp releases 0.5 mg scopolamine over 3 days; {Transderm-V} releases 1 mg scopolamine over 3 days) ▪ ***Injection:*** 0.3 mg/ml, 0.4 mg/ml, 0.86 mg/ml, 1 mg/ml ▪ ***Ophth solution:*** 0.25%.

TIME/ACTION PROFILE (PO, IM, IV, SC, Transdermal = antiemetic, sedative properties, Ophth = mydriasis)

	ONSET	PEAK	DURATION
PO, IM, SC	30 min	1 hr	4–6 hr
IV	10 min	1 hr	2–4 hr
Transdermal	4 hr	UK	72 hr
Ophth	10–30 min	30–45 min	several days

NURSING IMPLICATIONS

ASSESSMENT

- Assess patient for signs of urinary retention periodically throughout course of therapy.
- Monitor heart rate periodically throughout parenteral therapy.
- Assess patient for pain prior to administration. Scopolamine may act as a stimulant in the presence of pain, producing delirium if used without morphine or meperidine.

POTENTIAL NURSING DIAGNOSES

- Oral mucous membranes, altered (indications, side effects).
- Injury, high risk for (side effects).
- Knowledge deficit related to medication regimen (patient/family teaching).

IMPLEMENTATION

- **Direct IV:** Scopolamine should be diluted with Sterile Water for Injection prior to IV administration. Inject slowly.
- **Syringe Compatibility:** ▪ benzquinamide ▪ butorphanol ▪ chlorpromazine ▪ cimetidine ▪ dimenhydrinate ▪ diphenhydramine ▪ droperidol ▪ fentanyl ▪ hydromorphone ▪ hydroxyzine ▪ meperidine ▪ metoclopramide ▪ midazolam ▪ morphine ▪ nalbuphine ▪ pentazocine ▪ pentobarbital ▪ perphenazine ▪ prochlorperazine ▪ promazine ▪ promethazine ▪ ranitidine ▪ thiopental.
- **Y-Site Compatibility:** ▪ heparin ▪ hydrocortisone sodium succinate ▪ potassium chloride ▪ vitamin B complex with C.

- **Ophth:** See Appendix H for instillation of ophthalmic preparations.

PATIENT/FAMILY TEACHING
- **General Info:** Instruct patient to take medication exactly as directed. If a dose is missed, take as soon as remembered. Do not double doses.
- Medication may cause drowsiness or blurred vision. Caution patient to avoid driving or other activities requiring alertness until response to medication is known.
- Patient should use caution when exercising and in hot weather; overheating may result in heatstroke.
- Advise patient to avoid concurrent use of alcohol and other CNS depressants with this medication.
- Inform patient that frequent mouth rinses, good oral hygiene, and sugarless gum or candy may minimize dry mouth.
- **Transdermal:** Instruct patient on application of transdermal patches. Apply at least 4 hr before exposure to travel to prevent motion sickness. Wash hands and dry thoroughly before and after application. Apply to hairless, clean, dry area behind ear; avoid areas with cuts or irritation. Apply pressure over system to ensure contact with skin. System is effective for 3 days. If system becomes dislodged, replace with a new system on another site behind the ear. System is waterproof and not affected by bathing or showering.
- **Ophth:** Caution patient that this medication may increase sensitivity of eyes to light. Dark glasses may minimize this effect. Notify physician if this lasts longer than 7 days after discontinuation.

EVALUATION
Effectiveness of therapy can be demonstrated by: ■ Decrease in salivation and respiratory secretion preoperatively ■ Postoperative amnesia ■ Prevention of motion sickness ■ Mydriasis.

SECOBARBITAL
(see-koe-**bar**-bi-tal)
{Novosecobarb}, Seconal

CLASSIFICATION(S):
Sedative/hypnotic (barbiturate)
Schedule II
Pregnancy Category C

INDICATIONS

■ Hypnotic agent (short-term use) ■ Preoperative or other sedative ■ Adjunct to regional or spinal anesthesia (IV only).

ACTION

■ Produces all levels of CNS depression. **Therapeutic Effects:** ■ Induction of sleep ■ Sedation.

PHARMACOKINETICS

Absorption: Well absorbed following oral, IM, or rectal administration.
Distribution: Widely distributed, highest concentration in brain and liver. Crosses the placenta; small amounts enter breast milk.
Metabolism and Excretion: Metabolized by the liver.
Half-life: 30 hr.

CONTRAINDICATIONS AND PRECAUTIONS

Contraindicated in: ■ Hypersensitivity ■ Pre-existing CNS depression ■ Uncontrolled severe pain ■ Pregnancy or lactation.
Use Cautiously in: ■ Hepatic or renal impairment ■ Patients who may be suicidal or have been previously addicted to drugs ■ Elderly patients (dosage reduction recommended) ■ Chronic obstructive pulmonary disease ■ Prolonged use (may lead to physical dependence).

ADVERSE REACTIONS AND SIDE EFFECTS*

CNS: drowsiness, lethargy, vertigo, depression, hangover, excitation, delirium.

{} = Available in Canada only.
*Underlines indicate most frequent; **CAPITALS** indicate life-threatening.

Resp: respiratory depression.
GI: nausea, vomiting, diarrhea, constipation.
Derm: rashes, urticaria, photosensitivity.
MS: arthralgia, myalgia.
Neuro: neuralgia.
Misc: hypersensitivity reactions, including ANGIOEDEMA and serum sickness; psychological dependence, physical dependence.

INTERACTIONS

Drug–Drug: ■ Additive CNS depression with other **CNS depressants**, including **alcohol, antihistamines, antidepressants, opioid analgesics,** and other **sedative/hypnotics** ■ **Valproates** may decrease metabolism and increase CNS depression ■ Stimulates hepatic enzymes, which metabolize other drugs, resulting in decreased effectiveness of **oral contraceptives, chloramphenicol, cyclosporine, glucocorticoids, dacarbazine, levothyroxine,** and **quinidine.**

ROUTE AND DOSAGE

Hypnotic
■ **PO (Adults):** 100 mg.
■ **IM (Adults):** 100–200 mg.
■ **IV (Adults):** 50–250 mg.

Preoperative Sedation
■ **PO (Adults):** 100–300 mg 1–2 hr pre-op.
■ **PO (Children):** 2–6 mg/kg 1–2 hr pre-op (not to exceed 100 mg/dose).
■ **IM (Adults):** 1 mg/kg (light sedation) 10–15 min pre-op.
■ **IM (Children):** 4–5 mg/kg 10–15 min pre-op.

AVAILABILITY

■ *Capsules:* 100 mg ■ *Tablets:* 100 mg ■ *Injection:* 50 mg/ml ■ *In combination with:* amobarbital (Tuinal). See Appendix A.

TIME/ACTION PROFILE (hypnotic effect)

	ONSET	PEAK	DURATION
PO	15 min	15–30 min	1–4 hr
IM	UK	7–10 min	1–4 hr

NURSING IMPLICATIONS

ASSESSMENT
□ Assess sleep patterns prior to and periodically throughout course of therapy. Hypnotic doses of secobarbital suppress REM sleep. Patient may experience an increase in dreaming upon discontinuation of medication.
□ Monitor respiratory status, pulse, and blood pressure frequently in patients receiving secobarbital IV. Equipment for resuscitation and artificial ventilation should be readily available.
□ Prolonged therapy may lead to psychological or physical dependence. Restrict amount of drug available to patient, especially if depressed, suicidal, or with a history of addiction.
□ Assess postoperative patients for pain. Secobarbital may increase responsiveness to painful stimuli.

POTENTIAL NURSING DIAGNOSES
■ Sleep pattern disturbance (indications).
■ Injury, high risk for (side effects).
■ Knowledge deficit related to medication regimen (patient/family teaching).

IMPLEMENTATION
■ **General Info:** Supervise ambulation and transfer of patients following administration. Remove cigarettes. Side rails should be raised and call bell within reach at all times.
■ **IM:** Do not administer SC. Injections should be given deep into the gluteal muscle to minimize tissue irritation.
■ **Direct IV:** May be administered undiluted or diluted in Sterile Water for Injection, 0.9% NaCl or Ringer's solution. Do not dilute with lactated Ringer's solution. Do not use solution that is discolored or contains a precipitate.
□ Solution is highly alkaline; avoid extravasation, which may cause tissue damage and necrosis. If extravasation occurs, infiltration with 5% procaine solution into affected area and application of moist heat may be ordered.
■ *Rate:* Administer each 50 mg over at least 1 min. Titrate slowly for de-

S

sired response. Rapid administration may result in respiratory depression, apnea, laryngospasm, bronchospasm, or hypertension.

- **Syringe Incompatibility:** ▪ benzquinamide ▪ cimetidine ▪ glycopyrrolate.

PATIENT/FAMILY TEACHING

□ Advise patient to take medication exactly as directed. Do not increase dose without consulting physician.

□ Discuss the importance of preparing environment for sleep (dark room, quiet, avoidance of nicotine and caffeine).

□ Advise patients on prolonged therapy not to discontinue medication without consulting physician. Abrupt withdrawal may precipitate withdrawal symptoms.

□ Medication may cause daytime drowsiness. Caution patient to avoid driving and other activities requiring alertness until response to medication is known.

□ Caution patient to avoid taking alcohol or other CNS depressants concurrently with this medication.

□ Instruct patient to contact physician immediately if pregnancy is planned or suspected.

EVALUATION

Effectiveness of therapy can be demonstrated by: ▪ Improvement in sleep pattern without excessive daytime sedation. Therapy is usually limited to a 2-wk period ▪ Sedation.

SELEGILINE
(se-**le**-ji-leen)
Eldepryl, SD-Deprenyl

CLASSIFICATION(S):
Antiparkinson agent
Pregnancy Category C

INDICATIONS

- Management of Parkinson's disease with levodopa or levodopa/carbidopa in patients who fail to respond to levodopa/carbidopa alone.

ACTION

- Following conversion by monoamine oxidase to its active form, selegiline inactivates monoamine oxidase by irreversibly binding to it at type B (brain) sites ▪ Inactivation of monoamine oxidase leads to increased amounts of dopamine available in the CNS. **Therapeutic Effect:** ▪ Increased response to levodopa/dopamine therapy in Parkinson's disease.

PHARMACOKINETICS

Absorption: Appears to be well absorbed following oral administration.
Distribution: Widely distributed.
Metabolism and Excretion: Metabolism involves some conversion to amphetamine and methamphetamine. 45% excreted in urine as metabolites.
Half-life: UK.

CONTRAINDICATIONS AND PRECAUTIONS

Contraindicated in: ▪ Hypersensitivity ▪ Concurrent meperidine or opioid analgesic therapy (possible fatal reactions).
Use Cautiously in: ▪ Doses >10 mg/day (increased risk of hypertensive reactions with tyramine-containing foods and some medications).

ADVERSE REACTIONS AND SIDE EFFECTS*

CNS: dizziness, lightheadedness, fainting, confusion, hallucinations, vivid dreams.
GI: <u>nausea</u>, abdominal pain, dry mouth.

INTERACTIONS

Drug–Drug: ▪ May initially increase risk of side effects of **levodopa/carbidopa** (dosage of levodopa/carbidopa may need to be decreased by 10–30%) ▪ Concurrent use with **meperidine** or other **opioid analgesics** may possibly result in a potentially fatal reaction (excitation, sweating, rigidity, and hyper-

---

*<u>Underlines</u> indicate most frequent; **CAPITALS** indicate life-threatening.

tension; or hypotension and coma) ▪ Serotonin syndrome (confusion, agitation, hyperpyrexia, hypertension, seizures) may occur with concurrent use of **fluoxetine** (fluoxetine should be discontinued 5 wk prior to selegiline).

Drug–Food: ▪ Doses >10 mg/day may produce hypertensive reactions with **tyramine-containing foods** (see list in Appendix K).

ROUTE AND DOSAGE

▪ **PO (Adults):** 5 mg bid (with breakfast and lunch).

AVAILABILITY

▪ *Tablets:* 5 mg.

TIME/ACTION PROFILE (onset of beneficial effects in Parkinson's disease)

	ONSET	PEAK	DURATION
PO	2–3 days	UK	UK

NURSING IMPLICATIONS

ASSESSMENT

▫ Assess patient for signs and symptoms of Parkinson's disease (tremor, muscle weakness and rigidity, ataxic gait) prior to and throughout therapy.
▫ Assess blood pressure periodically throughout therapy.

POTENTIAL NURSING DIAGNOSES

▪ Physical mobility, impaired (indications).
▪ Injury, high risk for (indications, side effects).
▪ Knowledge deficit related to medication regimen (patient/family teaching).

IMPLEMENTATION

▪ **General Info:** An attempt to reduce the dose of levodopa/carbidopa by 10–30% may be made after 2–3 days of selegiline therapy.
▪ **PO:** Administer 5-mg tablet with breakfast and lunch.

PATIENT/FAMILY TEACHING

▫ Instruct patient to take medication exactly as directed. Caution patient that taking more than the prescribed dose

may increase side effects and place patient at risk for hypertensive crisis if foods containing tyramine are consumed (see Appendix K).
▫ Inform patient and family of the signs and symptoms of MAO inhibitor-induced hypertensive crisis (severe headache, chest pain, nausea, vomiting, photosensitivity, enlarged pupils). Advise patient to notify physician immediately if severe headache or any other unusual symptom occurs.

EVALUATION

Effectiveness of therapy can be demonstrated by: ▪ Improved response to levodopa/carbidopa in patients with Parkinson's disease.

SENNA
(se-na)
Black-Draught, Dr. Caldwell's Senna Laxative, Fletcher's Castoria, Gentlax, Senexon, Senna Gen, Senokot, SenokotXtra, Senolax, X-Prep Liquid

CLASSIFICATION(S):
Laxative (stimulant)
Pregnancy Category UK

INDICATIONS

▪ Treatment of constipation, particularly when associated with: ▫ Slow transit time ▫ Constipating drugs ▫ Irritable or spastic bowel syndrome ▫ Neurologic constipation.

ACTION

▪ Active components (sennosides) alter water and electrolyte transport in the large intestine, resulting in accumulation of water and increased peristalsis. **Therapeutic Effect:** ▪ Laxative action.

PHARMACOKINETICS

Absorption: Minimally absorbed following oral administration.
Distribution: Distribution not known.
Metabolism and Excretion: Converted

to active laxative compounds by bacteria in the colon.

Half-life: UK.

CONTRAINDICATIONS AND PRECAUTIONS

Contraindicated in: ▪ Hypersensitivity ▪ Abdominal pain of unknown cause, especially if associated with fever ▪ Rectal fissures ▪ Ulcerated hemorrhoids ▪ Known alcohol intolerance (some liquid products).

Use Cautiously in: ▪ Chronic use (may lead to laxative dependence) ▪ Pregnancy or lactation (safety not established) ▪ Possible intestinal obstruction.

ADVERSE REACTIONS AND SIDE EFFECTS*

GI: diarrhea, cramping, nausea.
GU: pink-red or brown-black discoloration of urine.
F and E: electrolyte abnormalities (chronic use or dependence).
Misc: laxative dependence.

INTERACTIONS

Drug–Drug: ▪ May decrease absorption of other **orally administered drugs,** due to decreased transit time.

ROUTE AND DOSAGE

Laxative
▪ **PO (Adults and Children >15 yr):** *Tablets*—374 mg (2 tablets) at bedtime (up to 8 tablets daily); *Granules*—1 tsp at bedtime (up to 4 tsp daily); *Liquid concentrate*—15–30 ml at bedtime; *Syrup*—10–15 ml at bedtime (up to 30 ml daily).
▪ **PO (Children 5–15 yr):** *Liquid concentrate*—10–15 ml at bedtime; *Syrup*—5–10 ml (up to 20 ml daily).
▪ **PO (Children 2–5 yr):** *Liquid concentrate*—5–10 ml at bedtime.
▪ **PO (Children 1–5 yr):** *Syrup*—2.5–5 ml (up to 10 ml daily).
▪ **PO (Children 1 mo–1 yr):** *Syrup*—1.25–2.5 ml (up to 5 ml daily).

Evacuation of Colon Prior to X-rays
▪ **PO (Adults):** 105–157.5 mg of sennosides 12–14 hr prior to exam.

AVAILABILITY

▪ *Tablets:* 187 mg, 217 mg, 374 mg ▪ *Granules:* 326 mg/tsp ▪ *Liquid concentrate:* 33.3 mg/ml ▪ *Syrup:* 218 mg/5 ml ▪ *Suppositories:* 652 mg ▪ *In combination with:* psyllium and docusate. See Appendix A.

TIME/ACTION PROFILE (laxative effect)

	ONSET	PEAK	DURATION
PO	6–12 hr*	UK	3–4 days
Rectal	½–2 hr	UK	UK

*May take as long as 24 hr.

NURSING IMPLICATIONS

ASSESSMENT
▫ Assess patient for abdominal distention, presence of bowel sounds, and usual pattern of bowel function.
▫ Assess color, consistency, and amount of stool produced.

POTENTIAL NURSING DIAGNOSES
▪ Constipation (indications).
▪ Diarrhea (side effects).
▪ Knowledge deficit related to medication regimen (patient/family teaching).

IMPLEMENTATION
▪ **General Info:** When used for constipation due to opioid analgesics, 187 mg of senna may counteract the constipating effects of 120 mg of codeine or its equivalent (see Appendix B for equivalents).
▪ **PO:** Take with a full glass of water. Administer at bedtime for evacuation 6–12 hr later. Administer on an empty stomach for more rapid results.
▫ Shake oral solution well before administering.
▫ Granules should be dissolved or mixed in water or other liquid before administration.

PATIENT/FAMILY TEACHING

▢ Advise patient that laxatives should be used only for short-term therapy. Long-term therapy may cause electrolyte imbalance and dependence.

▢ Encourage patient to use other forms of bowel regulation, such as increasing bulk in the diet, increasing fluid intake, and increasing mobility. Normal bowel habits are individualized and may vary from 3 times/day to 3 times/wk.

▢ Inform patient that this medication may cause a change in urine color to pink, red, violet, yellow, or brown.

▢ Instruct patients with cardiac disease to avoid straining during bowel movements (Valsalva maneuver).

▢ Advise patient not to use laxatives when abdominal pain, nausea, vomiting, or fever are present.

EVALUATION

Effectiveness of therapy can be demonstrated by: ▪ A soft, formed bowel movement.

SERTRALINE
(**ser**-tra-leen)
Zoloft

CLASSIFICATION(S):
Antidepressant
Pregnancy Category B

INDICATIONS

▪ Used in the treatment of depression, often in conjunction with psychotherapy.

ACTION

▪ Inhibits neuronal uptake of serotonin in the CNS, thus potentiating the activity of serotonin. Has little effect on norepinephrine or dopamine. **Therapeutic Effects:** ▪ Antidepressant action.

PHARMACOKINETICS

Absorption: Appears to be well absorbed following oral administration.

Distribution: Distribution is not known.
Metabolism and Excretion: Extensively metabolized by the liver. 14% excreted unchanged in feces.
Half-life: 26 hr.

CONTRAINDICATIONS AND PRECAUTIONS

Contraindicated in: ▪ Hypersensitivity ▪ Concurrent MAO inhibitor therapy (may result in serious, potentially fatal reactions).
Use Cautiously in: ▪ Severe hepatic or renal impairment ▪ Patients with a history of mania ▪ Pregnancy, lactation, or children (safety not established) ▪ Patients at risk of suicide.

ADVERSE REACTIONS AND SIDE EFFECTS*

CNS: <u>headache</u>, <u>dizziness</u>, <u>tremor</u>, <u>insomnia</u>, <u>drowsiness</u>, <u>fatigue</u>, agitation, nervousness, anxiety, yawning, impaired concentration, confusion, weakness.
EENT: rhinitis, pharyngitis, visual abnormalities, tinnitus.
CV: palpitations, chest pain.
GI: <u>dry mouth</u>, <u>nausea</u>, <u>diarrhea</u>, constipation, dyspepsia, vomiting, flatulence, anorexia, abdominal pain, increased appetite, abnormal taste.
GU: <u>male sexual dysfunction</u>, female sexual dysfunction, menstrual disorders, urinary frequency, urinary disorders.
Derm: <u>increased sweating</u>, rash, hot flashes.
MS: myalgia, back pain.
Neuro: paresthesia, hypoesthesia, twitching, hypertonia.
Misc: fever, thirst.

INTERACTIONS

Drug–Drug: ▪ Serious, potentially fatal reactions (hyperthermia, rigidity, myoclonus, autonomic instability, with fluctuating vital signs and extreme agitation, which may proceede to delirium and coma) may occur with concurrent **MAO inhibitor** therapy. MAO inhibitors

S

---

*<u>Underlines</u> indicate most frequent; **CAPITALS** indicate life-threatening.

should be stopped at least 14 days prior to sertraline therapy. Sertraline should be stopped at least 14 days prior to MAO inhibitor therapy ■ Concurrent use with **alcohol** is not recommended ■ May increase the effect of **warfarin**.

ROUTE AND DOSAGE

■ **PO (Adults):** 50 mg/day as a single dose in the morning or evening initially, may be increased at weekly intervals up to 200 mg/day depending on response.

AVAILABILITY

■ *Tablets:* 50 mg, 100 mg ■ {*Capsules:* 50 mg, 100 mg}.

TIME/ACTION PROFILE
(antidepressant effect)

	ONSET	PEAK	DURATION
PO	1–8 wk	UK	UK

NURSING IMPLICATIONS

ASSESSMENT

□ Monitor mood changes. Inform physician if patient demonstrates significant increase in anxiety, nervousness, or insomnia.
□ Assess for suicidal tendencies, especially during early therapy. Restrict amount of drug available to patient.
□ Monitor appetite and nutritional intake. Weigh weekly. Notify physician of significant changes in weight. Adjust diet as tolerated to support nutritional status.
■ **Lab Test Considerations:** Monitor hepatic enzymes and cholesterol periodically during course of therapy. May cause elevated AST (SGOT) and ALT (SGPT). May also cause small increases in total cholesterol and triglycerides.

POTENTIAL NURSING DIAGNOSES

■ Coping, ineffective individual (indications).
■ Injury, high risk for (side effects).
■ Knowledge deficit related to medication regimen (patient/family teaching).

IMPLEMENTATION

■ **PO:** Administer as a single dose in the morning or evening.

PATIENT/FAMILY TEACHING

□ Instruct patient to take sertraline exactly as directed. If a dose is missed, omit dose and return to regular dosing schedule. Do not double doses.
□ May cause drowsiness or dizziness. Caution patient to avoid driving and other activities requiring alertness until response to the drug is known.
□ Advise patient to avoid alcohol or other CNS depressant drugs during therapy and to consult with physician before taking other medications with sertraline.
□ Inform patient that frequent mouth rinses, good oral hygiene, and sugarless gum or candy may minimize dry mouth. If dry mouth persists for more than 2 wk, consult physician or dentist regarding use of saliva substitute.
□ Instruct female patient to inform physician if pregnancy is planned or suspected, or if she is breastfeeding.
□ Advise patient to notify physician if headache, weakness, nausea, anorexia, anxiety, or insomnia persists.
□ Emphasize the importance of follow-up examinations to monitor progress. Encourage patient participation in psychotherapy.

EVALUATION

Effectiveness of therapy can be demonstrated by: ■ Increased sense of well-being □ Renewed interest in surroundings. May require prolonged therapy to obtain antidepressant effects.

SILVER SULFADIAZINE
(sil-ver sul-fa-**dye**-a-zeen)
{Flamazine}, Flint SSD, Silvadene, Thermazene

CLASSIFICATION(S):
Anti-infective (topical)
Pregnancy Category B

INDICATIONS

▪ Prevention and treatment of infection in patients with 2nd- and 3rd-degree burns.

ACTION

▪ Splits to produce bactericidal concentrations of silver and sulfadiazine ▪ Action is at level of cell membrane and cell wall. **Therapeutic Effect:** ▪ Bactericidal action against organisms found in burns. **Spectrum:** ▪ Broad spectrum includes activity against many gram-negative and gram-positive pathogens, some fungi, and anaerobes.

PHARMACOKINETICS

Absorption: Small amounts of silver are systemically absorbed following topical application. Up to 10% of sulfadiazine is absorbed.

Distribution: Distribution not known.

Metabolism and Excretion: Absorbed sulfadiazine is excreted unchanged by the kidneys.

Half-life: UK.

CONTRAINDICATIONS AND PRECAUTIONS

Contraindicated in: ▪ Infants <2 mo (risk of kernicterus) ▪ Pregnancy near term (increased risk of kernicterus in infant) ▪ G6PD deficiency.

Use Cautiously in: ▪ Hypersensitivity to sulfonamides, silver, or parabens ▪ Cross-sensitivity with thiazides, sulfonylurea oral hypoglycemic agents, or carbonic anhydrase inhibitors may exist ▪ Impaired hepatic or renal function ▪ Pregnancy or lactation.

ADVERSE REACTIONS AND SIDE EFFECTS*

GU: crystalluria.
Derm: pain, burning, itching.
Hemat: leukopenia.

INTERACTIONS

Drug–Drug: ▪ Silver may inactivate concurrently applied topical **proteolytic enzymes (fibronolysin, desoxyribonuclease).**

ROUTE AND DOSAGE

▪ **Top (Adults and Children >1 mo):** Apply 1% cream 1–2 times daily in layer 1.5-mm thick.

AVAILABILITY

▪ *Cream:* 10 mg/g.

TIME/ACTION PROFILE (anti-infective action)

	ONSET	PEAK	DURATION
Top	on contact	UK	as long as applied

NURSING IMPLICATIONS

ASSESSMENT

▢ Assess burned tissue for infection (purulent discharge, excessive moisture, odor, and culture results) and sepsis (WBC, fever, or shock) prior to and throughout course of therapy.

▢ Monitor for hypersensitivity reaction (rash, itching, or burning) at and surrounding sites of application.

▪ **Lab Test Considerations:** Monitor renal function studies and CBC periodically when applied to large area, as systemic absorption may cause nephritis and reversible leukopenia. Decrease in neutrophil count is greatest 4 days after initiation of therapy; levels usually normalize after 2–3 days.

POTENTIAL NURSING DIAGNOSES

▪ Infection, high risk for (indications).
▪ Skin integrity, impaired (indications).
▪ Knowledge deficit related to medication regimen (patient/family teaching).

IMPLEMENTATION

▪ **General Info:** Generally applied after cleansing and debriding of burn wound. Premedicate with analgesic.

▪ **Top:** Cream is white; discard if it becomes dark.

▢ Use sterile technique to apply. Cover entire wound at depth of 1.5 mm. Reapply on sites where cream rubs off as a result of patient movement; burn should be coated at all times. Burn may be dressed or kept open, depending upon physician's order.

S

*Underlines indicate most frequent; **CAPITALS** indicate life-threatening.

PATIENT/FAMILY TEACHING
▫ Explain purpose of medication to patient and family. This medication will not stain skin.

EVALUATION
Effectiveness of therapy can be demonstrated by: ▪ Prevention and treatment of infection in 2nd- and 3rd-degree burns. Therapy is continued until burn is healed or skin graft is performed.

SIMETHICONE
(si-**meth**-i-kone)
Extra Strength Gas-X, Flatulex, Gas Relief, Gas-X, Major Con, Mylanta Gas, Mylicon, {Ovol}, Phazyme

CLASSIFICATION(S):
Antiflatulent
Pregnancy Category UK

INDICATIONS
▪ Relief of painful symptoms of excess gas in the GI tract that may occur postoperatively or as a consequence of: ▫ Air swallowing ▫ Dyspepsia ▫ Peptic ulcer ▫ Diverticulitis.

ACTION
▪ Causes the coalescence of gas bubbles ▪ Does not prevent the formation of gas. **Therapeutic Effect:** ▪ Passage of gas through the GI tract by belching or passing flatus.

PHARMACOKINETICS
Absorption: No systemic absorption occurs.
Distribution: Not systemically distributed.
Metabolism and Excretion: Excreted unchanged in the feces.
Half-life: UK.

CONTRAINDICATIONS AND PRECAUTIONS
Contraindicated in: ▪ Not recommended for infant colic.

Use Cautiously in: ▪ Abdominal pain of unknown cause, especially when accompanied by fever.

ADVERSE REACTIONS AND SIDE EFFECTS*
▪ None significant.

INTERACTIONS
Drug–Drug: ▪ None significant.

ROUTE AND DOSAGE
▪ **PO (Adults):** 40–125 mg qid, after meals and at bedtime (up to 500 mg/day).
▪ **PO (Children 2–12 yr):** 40 mg 4 times daily.
▪ **PO (Children <2 yr):** 20 mg 4 times daily (up to 240 mg/day).

AVAILABILITY
▪ **Chewable tablets:** 40 mg, 80 mg, 125 mg ▪ **Tablets:** 60 mg, 90 mg ▪ **Capsules:** 125 mg ▪ **Drops:** 40 mg/0.6 ml ▪ **In combination with:** antacids. See Appendix A.

TIME/ACTION PROFILE (antiflatulent effect)

	ONSET	PEAK	DURATION
PO	immediate	UK	3 hr

NURSING IMPLICATIONS
ASSESSMENT
▫ Assess patient for abdominal pain, distention, and bowel sounds prior to and periodically throughout course of therapy. Frequency of belching and passage of flatus should also be assessed.

POTENTIAL NURSING DIAGNOSES
▪ Pain (indications).
▪ Knowledge deficit related to medication regimen (patient/family teaching).

IMPLEMENTATION
▪ **PO:** Administer after meals and at bedtime for best results. Shake liquid preparations well prior to administration. Chewable tablets should be

---

{} = Available in Canada only.
*<u>Underlines</u> indicate most frequent; **CAPITALS** indicate life-threatening.

chewed thoroughly before swallowing for faster and more complete results.

□ Drops can be mixed with 30 ml of cool water, infant formula, or other liquid. Shake well before using.

PATIENT/FAMILY TEACHING

□ Explain to patient the importance of diet and exercise in the prevention of gas. Also explain that this medication does not prevent the formation of gas.

□ Advise patient to notify physician if symptoms are persistent.

EVALUATION

Effectiveness of therapy can be demonstrated by: ▪ Decrease in abdominal distention and discomfort.

SIMVASTATIN
(sim-va-**stat**-in)
Zocor

CLASSIFICATION(S):
Lipid-lowering agent
Pregnancy Category X

INDICATIONS

▪ Adjunct to dietary therapy in the management of primary hypercholesterolemia.

ACTION

▪ Inhibits the enzyme (HMG-CoA reductase) responsible for catalyzing an early step in the synthesis of cholesterol. **Therapeutic Effect:** ▪ Lowering of total and low-density lipoprotein (LDL) cholesterol and triglycerides ▪ Increased high-density lipoproteins (HDL).

PHARMACOKINETICS

Absorption: 85% absorbed following oral administration, but rapidly metabolized. <5% reaches general circulation. Rapidly hydrolyzed to its active form.

Distribution: Small amounts enter breast milk; remainder of distribution not known.

Metabolism and Excretion: Mostly metabolized by the liver, which is also the site of action. 20% excreted in urine, 70% in feces.

Half-life: UK.

CONTRAINDICATIONS AND PRECAUTIONS

Contraindicated in: ▪ Hypersensitivity ▪ Active liver disease ▪ Pregnancy or lactation.

Use Cautiously in: ▪ Women of childbearing age ▪ Past history of liver disease or alcohol consumption ▪ Patients with risk factors for rhabdomyolysis (severe acute infection; hypertension; major surgery; trauma; severe endocrine, metabolic, or electrolyte disorders, uncontrolled seizures) ▪ Myopathy ▪ Patients <20 yr (safety not established).

ADVERSE REACTIONS AND SIDE EFFECTS*

CNS: headache, weakness.

GI: nausea, diarrhea, abdominal pain, constipation, flatulence, dyspepsia, elevated liver enzymes.

GU: acute renal failure.

MS: myopathy, rhabdomyolysis, arthralgia.

Misc: hypersensitivity reactions.

INTERACTIONS

Drug–Drug: ▪ Risk of rhabdomyolysis is increased by **gemfibrozil**. Avoid concurrent use ▪ **Cyclosporine** also may increase the risk of rhabdomyolysis (decrease initial dose to 5 mg/day, not to exceed 10 mg/day) ▪ Cholesterol-lowering effect may be additive with **bile acid sequestrants (cholestyramine, colestipol)** ▪ Increased risk of myopathy or rhabdomyolysis with concurrent **niacin, erythromycin, gemfibrozil,** or **cyclosporine** ▪ Simvastatin may slightly increase serum **digoxin** levels ▪ May increase the risk of bleeding with **warfarin**.

ROUTE AND DOSAGE

▪ **PO (Adults):** 5–10 mg once daily

---

in the evening (range 5–40 mg/day). Elderly patients, patients with LDL ≤190 mg/dl or patients receiving concurrent cyclopsorine should be started on 5 mg/day. Patients with LDL >190 mg/dl should be started on 10 mg/day. Dosage increments should be made at 4-wk intervals. Patients on concurrent cyclosporine should not receive >10 mg/day.

AVAILABILITY

▪ *Tablets:* 5 mg, 10 mg, 20 mg, 40 mg.

TIME/ACTION PROFILE (lipid-lowering effect)

	ONSET	PEAK	DURATION
PO	2 wk	4–6 wk	UK

NURSING IMPLICATIONS

ASSESSMENT

□ Obtain a diet history, especially in regard to fat consumption.
□ Ophthalmic examinations are recommended prior to and yearly throughout therapy.
▪ **Lab Test Considerations:** Serum cholesterol and triglyceride levels should be evaluated before initiating and periodically throughout course of therapy.
□ Liver function tests, including ALT (SGPT), should be monitored prior to and every 6 wk during the first 3 mo of therapy, every 8 wk for the remainder of the first year, and then every 6 mo. If AST (SGOT) levels increase to 3 times normal, simvastatin therapy should be discontinued.
□ If patient develops muscle tenderness during therapy, CPK levels should be monitored. If CPK levels are markedly increased or myopathy occurs, simvastatin therapy should be discontinued.

POTENTIAL NURSING DIAGNOSES

▪ Knowledge deficit related to diet and medication regimen (patient/family teaching).
▪ Noncompliance (patient/family teaching).

IMPLEMENTATION

▪ **PO:** Administer once daily at bedtime. May be administered without regard to food.

PATIENT/FAMILY TEACHING

□ Instruct patient to take medication exactly as directed, not to skip doses or double up on missed doses. Simvastatin helps control but does not cure elevated serum cholesterol levels.
□ Advise patient that simvastatin should be used in conjunction with diet restrictions (fat, cholesterol, carbohydrates, alcohol); exercise; and cessation of smoking.
□ Instruct patient to notify physician if unexplained muscle pain, tenderness, or weakness occur, especially if accompanied by fever or malaise. Instruct female patients to notify physician promptly if pregnancy is planned or suspected.
□ Advise patient to notify physician or dentist of medication regimen prior to treatment or surgery.
□ Emphasize the importance of follow-up examinations to determine effectiveness and monitor for side effects.

EVALUATION

Effectiveness of therapy can be demonstrated by: ▪ Decrease in low-density lipoprotein (LDL), very low-density lipoprotein (VLDL), and total cholesterol levels ▪ Increase in high-density lipoprotein (HDL) levels ▪ Decrease in serum triglyceride levels.

SODIUM BICARBONATE

(soe-dee-um bye-kar-boe-nate)
Baking Soda, Bellans, Citrocarbonate, Neut, Soda Mint

CLASSIFICATION(S):

Electrolyte modifier (alkalinizing agent), Antacid
Pregnancy Category C

INDICATIONS

▪ **PO, IV:** Management of metabolic acidosis ▪ **PO, IV:** Used to alkalinize urine and promote excretion of certain drugs in overdosage situations (phenobarbital, aspirin) ▪ PO: Antacid.

ACTION

▪ Acts as an alkalinizing agent by releasing bicarbonate ions ▪ Following oral administration, releases bicarbonate, which is capable of neutralizing gastric acid. **Therapeutic Effects:** ▪ Alkalinization ▪ Neutralization of gastric acid.

PHARMACOKINETICS

Absorption: Following oral administration, excess bicarbonate is absorbed and results in metabolic alkalosis and alkaline urine.
Distribution: Widely distributed into extracellular fluid.
Metabolism and Excretion: Sodium and bicarbonate are excreted by the kidneys.
Half-life: UK.

CONTRAINDICATIONS AND PRECAUTIONS

Contraindicated in: ▪ Metabolic or respiratory alkalosis ▪ Hypocalcemia ▪ Excessive chloride loss ▪ As an antidote following ingestion of strong mineral acids ▪ Patients on sodium-restricted diets (oral use as an antacid only) ▪ Renal failure (oral use as an antacid only) ▪ Severe abdominal pain of unknown cause, especially if associated with fever (oral use as an antacid only).
Use Cautiously in: ▪ Congestive heart failure ▪ Renal insufficiency ▪ Concurrent glucocorticoid therapy ▪ Chronic use as an antacid (may cause metabolic alkalosis and possible sodium overload).

ADVERSE REACTIONS AND SIDE EFFECTS*

CV: edema.
F and E: sodium and water retention, metabolic alkalosis, hypernatremia, hypokalemia, hypocalcemia.
GI: PO—gastric distention, flatulence.

Local: irritation at IV site.
Neuro: tetany.

INTERACTIONS

Drug–Drug: ▪ Following oral administration may decrease the absorption of **ketoconazole** ▪ Concurrent use with **calcium-containing antacids** may lead to milk-alkali syndrome ▪ Urinary alkalinization may result in decreased **salicylate** or **barbiturate** blood levels; increased blood levels of **quinidine, mexiletine, flecainide,** or **amphetamines;** increased risk of crystalluria from **fluoroquinolones;** decreased effectiveness of **methenamine.**

ROUTE AND DOSAGE
Contains 12 mEq of sodium/g.

S

Cardiopulmonary Resuscitation
Dose should be determined on the basis of frequent lab assessment.
▪ **IV (Adults, Children, and Neonates):** 1 mEq/kg may repeat 0.5 mEq/kg q 10 min.

Alkalinization of Urine
▪ **PO (Adults):** 48 mEq (4 g) initially. Then 12–24 mEq (1–2 g) q 4 hr (up to 48 mEq q 4 hr) or 1 tsp of powder q 4 hr as needed.
▪ **PO (Children):** 1–10 mEq/kg (12–120 mg/kg) per day in divided doses.
▪ **IV (Adults and Children):** 2–5 mEq/kg.

Antacid
▪ **PO (Adults):** 325 mg–2 g 1–4 times daily or ½ tsp q 2 hr as needed.

Metabolic Acidosis
Dose should be determined on the basis of frequent lab assessment.
▪ **IV (Adults and Children):** 2–5 mEq/kg as a 4–8-hr infusion.

AVAILABILITY

▪ *Oral powder* ▪ *Tablets:* 325 mg, {500 mg}, 520 mg, 650 mg ▪ *Injection:* 4.2% (0.5 mEq/ml), 5% (0.6 mEq/ml), 6.4% (1 mEq/ml) ▪ *Neutralizing additive solution:* 4% (0.48 mEq/ml), 4.2% (0.5 mEq/ml) ▪ *In combination with:* sodium citrate (Citrocarbonate). See Appendix A.

TIME/ACTION PROFILE (PO = antacid effect, IV = alkalinization)

	ONSET	PEAK	DURATION
PO	immediate	30 min	1–3 hr
IV	immediate	rapid	UK

NURSING IMPLICATIONS

ASSESSMENT

□ Assess fluid balance (intake and output, daily weight, edema, lung sounds) throughout therapy. Notify physician if symptoms of fluid overload (hypertension, edema, dyspnea, rales/crackles, frothy sputum) occur.

□ Assess patient for signs of acidosis (disorientation, headache, weakness, dyspnea, hyperventilation), alkalosis (confusion, irritability, paresthesia, tetany, altered breathing pattern), hypernatremia (edema, weight gain, hypertension, tachycardia, fever, flushed skin, mental irritability), or hypokalemia (weakness, fatigue, U wave on ECG, arrhythmias, polyuria, polydipsia) throughout therapy.

□ Observe IV site closely. Avoid extravasation, as tissue irritation or cellulitis may occur. If infiltration occurs, confer with physician regarding warm compresses and infiltration of site with lidocaine or hyaluronidase.

■ **Lab Test Considerations:** Monitor serum sodium, potassium, calcium, bicarbonate concentrations, serum osmolarity, acid/base balance, and renal function prior to and periodically throughout course of therapy.

□ Arterial blood gases (ABGs) should be obtained frequently in emergency situations.

□ Monitor urine pH frequently when used for urinary alkalinization.

□ Antagonizes effects of pentagastrin and histamine during gastric acid secretion test. Avoid administration during the 24 hr preceding the test.

■ **Antacid:** Assess patient for epigastric or abdominal pain and frank or occult

blood in the stool, emesis, or gastric aspirate.

POTENTIAL NURSING DIAGNOSES

■ Gas exchange, impaired (indications).

■ Fluid volume excess (side effects).

■ Knowledge deficit related to medication regimen (patient/family teaching).

IMPLEMENTATION

■ **General Info:** This medication may cause premature dissolution of enteric-coated tablets in the stomach.

■ **PO:** Tablets must be thoroughly chewed and taken with a full glass of water. Effervescent tablets should be completely dissolved before drinking.

□ When used in treatment of peptic ulcers, physician may order administration 1 and 3 hr after meals and at bedtime.

■ **Direct IV:** Administer direct IV push in arrest situation. Use premeasured ampules or prefilled syringes to assure accurate dosage. Dosages should be based on ABG results. Dosage may be repeated every 10 min.

■ *Rate:* May be administered by rapid bolus.

□ Flush IV line before and after administration to prevent incompatible medications used in arrest management from precipitating.

■ **Intermittent/Continuous Infusion:** May be diluted in dextrose, saline, and dextrose/saline combinations.

■ *Rate:* May be administered over 4–8 hr.

■ **Syringe Compatibility:** ■ milrinone ■ pentobarbital.

■ **Syringe Incompatibility:** ■ glycopyrrolate ■ metoclopramide ■ thiopental.

■ **Y-Site Compatibility:** ■ acyclovir ■ famotidine ■ fludarabine ■ insulin ■ morphine ■ potassium chloride ■ tolazoline ■ vitamin B complex with C.

■ **Y-Site Incompatibility:** ■ amrinone ■ calcium chloride ■ sargramostim ■ verapamil.

■ **Additive Compatibility:** ■ amikacin ■ aminophylline ■ amobarbital ■ amphotericin B ▪ calcium chloride ▪ calcium gluceptate ▪ cefoxitin ▪ ceftazidime ▪ cephalothin ▪ cephapirin ▪ chloramphenicol ▪ chlorothiazide ▪ cimetidine ▪ clindamycin ▪ cytarabine ▪ erythromycin ▪ furosemide ▪ heparin ▪ hyaluronidase ▪ hydrocortisone sodium succinate ▪ kanamycin ▪ methotrexate ▪ methyldopate ▪ multivitamins ▪ nafcillin ▪ netilmicin ▪ oxacillin ▪ phenobarbital ▪ phenytoin ▪ phytonadione ▪ potassium chloride ▪ prochlorperazine.

▪ **Additive Incompatibility:** ▪ ascorbic acid ▪ carboplatin ▪ carmustine ▪ cefotaxime ▪ cisplatin ▪ hydromorphone ▪ imipenem cilastatin ▪ isoproterenol ▪ labetalol ▪ levorphanol ▪ magnesium sulfate ▪ methadone ▪ morphine ▪ pentazocine ▪ procaine ▪ secobarbital ▪ streptomycin ▪ vitamin B complex with C. Do not add to Ringer's solution, lactated Ringer's solution, or Ionosol products, as compatibility varies with concentration.

PATIENT/FAMILY TEACHING

▪ **General Info:** Instruct patient to take medication as directed. A missed dose should be taken as soon as remembered unless almost time for next dose.
▫ Review symptoms of electrolyte imbalance with patients on chronic therapy; instruct patient to notify physician if these symptoms occur.
▫ Advise patient not to take milk products concurrently with this medication. Renal calculi or hypercalcemia (milk-alkali syndrome) may result.
▫ Emphasize the importance of regular follow-up examinations to monitor serum electrolyte levels and acid-base balance and to monitor progress.
▪ **Antacid:** Advise patient to avoid routine use of sodium bicarbonate for indigestion. Dyspepsia that persists >2 wk should be evaluated by a physician.
▫ Advise patient on sodium-restricted diet to avoid use of baking soda as a home remedy for indigestion.
▫ Instruct patient to notify physician if

indigestion is accompanied by chest pain, difficulty breathing, or diaphoresis or if stools become dark and tarry.

EVALUATION

Effectiveness of therapy can be demonstrated by: ▪ Increase in urinary pH ▪ Clinical improvement of acidosis ▪ Enhanced excretion of selected overdoses and poisonings ▪ Decreased gastric discomfort.

SODIUM CHLORIDE
(soe-dee-um klor-ide)
Afrin Nasal Mist, Ayr Saline, Breathe Free, Dristan Saline Spray, HuMist Nasal Mist, NaCl, Nasal, Nasal Moist, Ocean, Pretz, Saline X, Salt, SeaMist, Sodium Chloride Nasal

CLASSIFICATION(S):
Electrolyte (replacement solution), Abortifacient
Pregnancy Category UK

INDICATIONS

▪ **IV:** Hydration and provision of sodium chloride in deficiency states ▪ Maintenance of fluid and electrolyte status in situations in which losses may be excessive (excess diuresis or severe salt restriction) ▪ 0.45% ("half-normal saline") solution is most commonly used for hydration and in the treatment of hyperosmolar diabetes ▪ 0.9% ("normal saline") solution is used for: ▫ Replacement ▫ To treat metabolic alkalosis ▫ A priming fluid for hemodialysis ▫ To begin and end blood transfusions ▫ 0.9% and 0.45% may also be used as irrigating solutions ▪ Small volumes of 0.9% sodium chloride (preservative-free or bacteriostatic) are used to reconstitute or dilute other mediations ▪ Hypertonic solution (3%, 5%) may be required in situations in which rapid replacement of sodium is necessary: ▫ Hyponatremia ▫ Hypochloremia ▫ Renal failure ▫ Heart failure. ▪ **PO:** Prevention of or management of volume depletion due to salt restriction or heat prostration when excessive sweating occurs during exposures to high temperatures □ **Nasal:** 0.4–0.75% solutions are used to moisturize dry or irritated nasal mucosa, which may occur as a consequence of colds, allergies, decongestant misuse, intranasal surgery, or other procedures.

ACTION

■ Sodium is a major cation in extracellular fluid and helps maintain water distribution, fluid and electrolyte balance, acid-base equilibrium, and osmotic pressure ■ Chloride is the major anion in extracellular fluid and is involved in maintaining acid-base balance. Solutions of sodium chloride resemble extracellular fluid. **Therapeutic Effects:** ■ **IV, PO:** Replacement in deficiency states and maintenance of homeostasis.

PHARMACOKINETICS

Absorption: Well absorbed following oral administration. Replacement solutions of sodium chloride are administered IV only.
Distribution: Rapidly and widely distributed.
Metabolism and Excretion: Excreted primarily by the kidneys.
Half-life: UK.

CONTRAINDICATIONS AND PRECAUTIONS

Contraindicated in: ■ **IV solution:** □ Hypertonic (3%, 5%) solutions should not be used in patients with elevated, slightly decreased, or normal serum sodium □ Fluid retention or hypernatremia.
Use Cautiously in: ■ **IV:** Patients prone to metabolic, acid-base, or fluid and electrolyte abnormalities, including: □ Geriatric patients □ Those with nasogastric suctioning □ Vomiting □ Diarrhea □ Diuretic therapy □ Glucocorticoid therapy □ Fistulas □ Congestive heart failure □ Severe renal failure □ Severe liver diseases (additional electrolytes may be required) ■ Sodium

chloride preserved with benzyl alcohol should not be used in neonates ■ **PO:** Inadequate hydration (water and other electrolytes must be replaced).

ADVERSE REACTIONS AND SIDE EFFECTS*

CV: edema, congestive heart failure, pulmonary edema.
F and E: hypokalemia, hypervolemia, hypernatremia.
Local: extravasation, irritation at IV site.

INTERACTIONS

Drug–Drug: ■ Excessive amounts of sodium chloride may partially antagonize the effects of **antihypertensive medications** ■ Use with **glucocorticoids** may result in excess sodium retention.

ROUTE AND DOSAGE

0.9% Sodium Chloride (Isotonic)
■ **IV (Adults):** 1 liter (contains 150 mEq sodium per liter) rate and amount determined by condition being treated.

0.45% Sodium Chloride (Hypotonic)
■ **IV (Adults):** 1–2 liter (contains 75 mEq sodium per liter), rate and amount determined by condition being treated.

3%, 5% Sodium Chloride (Hypertonic)
■ **IV (Adults):** 100 ml over 1 hr (3% contains 50 mEq sodium per 100 ml; 5% contains 83.3 mEq sodium per 100 ml).

Oral Replacement
■ **PO (Adults):** 1–2 g 3 times daily.

Nasal Moisturizer
■ **Nasal (Adults and Children):** Use as needed.

AVAILABILITY

■ *IV solutions:* 0.45%, 0.9%, 3%, 5% ■ *In combination with:* dextrose, electrolytes ■ *Diluents:* 0.9% ■ *Concentrate for dilution:* 14.6%, 23.4% ■ *Tablets:* 650 mg, 1 g, 2.25 g ■ *Slow-release tablets:* 600 mg ■ *Nasal solution:* 0.4%, 0.6%, 0.65%, 0.75%.

<u>Underlines</u> indicate most frequent; **CAPITALS indicate life-threatening.*

TIME/ACTION PROFILE (PO, IV = electrolyte effects, intra-amniotic = abortion time)

	ONSET	PEAK	DURATION
PO	UK	UK	UK
IV	rapid (min)	end of infusion	UK
Intra-amniotic	12–24 hr	UK	36 hr

NURSING IMPLICATIONS

ASSESSMENT

□ Assess fluid balance (intake and output, daily weight, edema, lung sounds) throughout course of therapy.

□ Assess patient for symptoms of hyponatremia (headache, tachycardia, lassitude, dry mucous membranes, nausea, vomiting, muscle cramps) or hypernatremia (edema, weight gain, hypertension, tachycardia, fever, flushed skin, mental irritability) throughout therapy. Sodium is measured in relation to its concentration to fluid in the body, and symptoms may change based on patient's hydration status.

▪ **Lab Test Considerations:** Monitor serum sodium, potassium, bicarbonate, and chloride concentrations and acid-base balance periodically for patients receiving prolonged therapy with sodium chloride.

□ Monitor serum osmolarity in patients receiving hypertonic saline solutions.

POTENTIAL NURSING DIAGNOSES

▪ Fluid volume deficit (indications).
▪ Fluid volume excess (side effects).

IMPLEMENTATION

▪ **General Info:** Dosage of sodium chloride depends on patient's age, weight, condition, fluid and electrolyte balance, and acid-base balance.

□ Do not administer bacteriostatic sodium chloride containing benzyl alcohol as a preservative to neonates. This should not be used to reconstitute or to dilute solutions or to flush intravascular cathethers in neonates.

□ Infusion of 0.45% NaCl is hypotonic,

0.9% NaCl is isotonic, and 3% and 5% NaCl are hypertonic.

▪ **Intermittent Infusion:** Administer 3% or 5% NaCl via a large vein and prevent infiltration. After the first 100 ml, sodium, chloride, and bicarbonate concentrations should be re-evaluated to determine the need for further administration.

▪ **Rate:** Rate should not exceed 100 ml/hr.

▪ **Additive Compatibility:** ▪ D5W ▪ D10W ▪ Ringer's and lactated Ringer's injection ▪ dextrose/Ringer's solution combinations ▪ dextrose/lactated Ringer's solution combinations ▪ dextrose/saline combinations ▪ ⅙ M sodium lactate.

PATIENT/FAMILY TEACHING

□ Explain to patient the purpose of the infusion.

EVALUATION

Effectiveness of therapy can be demonstrated by: ▪ Prevention or correction of dehydration ▪ Normalization of serum sodium and chloride levels ▪ Prevention of heat prostration during exposure to high temperatures ▪ Decrease in nasal congestion.

SODIUM CITRATE AND CITRIC ACID
(soe-dee-um sye-trate and sit-rik as-id)
Bicitra, Oracit, Shohl's Solution modified

CLASSIFICATION(S):
Electrolyte modifier (alkalinizing agent), Antiurolithic
Pregnancy Category UK

INDICATIONS

▪ Management of chronic metabolic acidosis associated with chronic renal insufficiency or renal tubular acidosis ▪ Alkalinization of urine ▪ Prevention of cystine and urate urinary calculi ▪ Prevention of aspiration pneumonitis during surgical procedures.

S

ACTION

- Converted to bicarbonate in the body, resulting in increased blood pH • As bicarbonate is renally excreted, urine is also alkalinized, increasing the solubility of cystine and uric acid • Neutralizes gastric acid. **Therapeutic Effects:** • Provision of bicarbonate in metabolic acidosis • Alkalinization of the urine • Prevention of cystine and urate urinary calculi • Prevention of aspiration pneumonitis.

PHARMACOKINETICS

Absorption: Well absorbed following oral administration.

Distribution: Rapidly and widely distributed.

Metabolism and Excretion: Rapidly oxidized to bicarbonate, which is excreted primarily by the kidneys. Small amounts ($<5\%$) excreted unchanged by the lungs.

Half-life: UK.

CONTRAINDICATIONS AND PRECAUTIONS

Contraindicated in: • Severe renal insufficiency • Severe sodium restriction • Congestive heart failure, untreated hypertension, edema, or toxemia of pregnancy.

Use Cautiously in: • Pregnancy or lactation (safety not established).

ADVERSE REACTIONS AND SIDE EFFECTS*

GI: diarrhea.

F and E: fluid overload, hypernatremia (severe renal impairment), metabolic alkalosis (large doses only), hypocalcemia.

MS: tetany.

INTERACTIONS

Drug–Drug: • May partially antagonize the effects of **antihypertensives** • Urinary alkalinization may result in decreased **salicylate** or **barbiturate** blood levels or increased blood levels of **quinidine, flecainide,** or **amphetamines.**

ROUTE AND DOSAGE

Adjust dosage according to urine pH. Contains 1 mEq sodium and 1 mEq bicarbonate/ml solution.

Alkalinizer

- **PO (Adults):** 10–30 ml solution diluted in water qid.
- **PO (Children):** 5–15 ml solution qid.

Antiurolithic

- **PO (Adults):** 10–30 ml solution diluted in water qid.

Neutralization of Gastric Acid

- **PO (Adults):** 15–30 ml solution diluted in 15–30 ml of water.

AVAILABILITY

- *Oral solution:* 500 mg sodium citrate/334 mg citric acid/5 ml (Bicitra), 490 mg sodium citrate/640 mg citric acid/5 ml (Oracit).

TIME/ACTION PROFILE (effects on serum pH)

	ONSET	PEAK	DURATION
PO	rapid (min–hr)	UK	4–6 hr

NURSING IMPLICATIONS

ASSESSMENT

- Assess patient for signs of alkalosis (confusion, irritability, paresthesia, tetany, altered breathing pattern) or hypernatremia (edema, weight gain, hypertension, tachycardia, fever, flushed skin, mental irritability) throughout therapy.
- Monitor patients with renal dysfunction for fluid overload (discrepancy in intake and output, weight gain, edema, rales/crackles, and hypertension).
- **Lab Test Considerations:** Prior to and every 4 mo throughout chronic therapy, monitor hematocrit, hemoglobin, electrolytes, pH, creatinine, urinalysis, and 24-hr urine for citrate.
- Monitor urine pH if used to alkalinize urine.

POTENTIAL NURSING DIAGNOSES

- Knowledge deficit related to medica-

---

*Underlines indicate most frequent; **CAPITALS** indicate life-threatening.

tion regimen (patient/family teaching).

IMPLEMENTATION

- **PO:** Solution is more palatable if chilled. Administer with 30–90 ml of chilled water. Administer 30 min after meals or bedtime snack to minimize saline laxative effect.
- When used as preanesthetic, administer 15–30 ml of sodium citrate with 15–30 ml of chilled water.

PATIENT/FAMILY TEACHING

- Instruct patient to take as directed. Missed doses should be taken within 2 hr. Do not double doses.
- Instruct patients receiving chronic sodium citrate on correct method of monitoring urine pH, maintenance of alkaline urine, and the need to increase fluid intake to 3000 ml/day.
- Advise patients receiving long-term therapy on need to avoid salty foods.

EVALUATION

Effectiveness of therapy can be demonstrated by: ■ Correction of metabolic acidosis ■ Maintenance of alkaline urine with resulting decreased stone formation ■ Buffering the pH of gastric secretions, thereby preventing aspiration pneumonitis associated with intubation and anesthesia.

SODIUM PHOSPHATE
(soe-dee-um **foss**-fate)

CLASSIFICATION(S):
Electrolyte (phosphate supplement)
Pregnancy Category C

INDICATIONS

- Treatment and prevention of phosphate depletion in patients who are unable to ingest adequate dietary phosphates.

ACTION

- Phosphate is present in bone and is involved in energy transfer and carbohydrate metabolism ■ Serves as a buffer for the excretion of hydrogen ions by the kidney. **Therapeutic Effect:** ■ Replacement of phosphorous in deficiency states.

PHARMACOKINETICS

Absorption: Administered IV only, resulting in complete bioavailability.
Distribution: Phosphates enter extracellular fluids and are then actively transported to sites of action.
Metabolism and Excretion: Excreted mainly (>90%) by the kidneys.
Half-life: UK.

CONTRAINDICATIONS AND PRECAUTIONS

Contraindicated in: ■ Hyperphosphatemia ■ Hypocalcemia ■ Severe renal impairment.
Use Cautiously in: ■ Hyperparathyroidism ■ Cardiac disease ■ Hypernatremia ■ Hypertension.

ADVERSE REACTIONS AND SIDE EFFECTS*

Related to hyperphosphatemia, unless indicated.

CNS: listlessness, confusion, weakness.
Resp: hypernatremia—shortness of breath.
CV: ARRHYTHMIAS, ECG changes (absent P waves, widening of the QRS complex with biphasic curve), **CARDIAC ARREST,** hypotension; hypernatremia—edema.
F and E: hypomagnesemia, hyperphosphatemia, hyperkalemia, hypocalcemia, hypernatremia.
GI: diarrhea, nausea, vomiting, abdominal pain.
Local: phlebitis, irritation at IV site.
MS: hypocalcemia—tremors.
Neuro: paresthesias of extremities, flaccid paralysis, heaviness of legs.

INTERACTIONS

Drug–Drug: ■ Concurrent use of **glucocorticoids** with sodium phosphate may result in hypernatremia.

---

*Underlines indicate most frequent; **CAPITALS** indicate life-threatening.

ROUTE AND DOSAGE

- **IV (Adults):** 10–15 mM phosphorus/ liter of parenteral nutrition.
- **IV (Neonates):** 1.5–2 mM/kg/day (infused as part of parenteral nutrition).

AVAILABILITY

- **IV injection for dilution:** 3 mM phosphate and 4 mEq sodium/ml.

TIME/ACTION PROFILE (effects on serum phosphate levels)

	ONSET	PEAK	DURATION
IV	rapid (min–hr)	end of infusion	UK

NURSING IMPLICATIONS

ASSESSMENT

- □ Assess patient for signs and symptoms of hypophosphatemia (anorexia, weakness, decreased reflexes, bone pain, confusion, blood dyscrasias) throughout course of therapy.
- □ Monitor intake and output ratios and daily weight. Report significant discrepancies to physician.
- **Lab Test Considerations:** Monitor serum phosphate, potassium, sodium, and calcium levels prior to and periodically throughout therapy. Increased phosphate may cause hypocalcemia.
- □ Monitor renal function studies prior to and periodically throughout course of therapy.
- **Toxicity and Overdose:** Symptoms of toxicity are those of hyperphosphatemia or hypocalcemia (paresthesia, muscle twitching, laryngospasm, colic, cardiac arrhythmias, Chvostek's or Trousseau's signs) or hypernatremia (thirst, dry flushed skin, fever, tachycardia, hypotension, irritability, decreased urine output).

POTENTIAL NURSING DIAGNOSES

- Nutrition, altered: less than body requirements (indications).
- Knowledge deficit related to medication regimen (patient/family teaching).

IMPLEMENTATION

- **General Info:** Available in oral form in combination with potassium phosphate to acidify urine and to prevent formation of renal calculi.
- **IV:** Administer IV only in dilute concentrations and infuse slowly.
- **Additive Incompatibility:** ▪ calcium ▪ magnesium.

PATIENT/FAMILY TEACHING

- □ Explain purpose of the medication to patient.

EVALUATION

Effectiveness of therapy can be demonstrated by: ▪ Prevention and correction of serum phosphate deficiency.

SODIUM POLYSTYRENE SULFONATE
(**soe**-dee-um po-lee-**stye**-reen **sul**-fon-ate)
Kayexalate, SPS

CLASSIFICATION(S):
Electrolyte modifier (cation exchange resin)
Pregnancy Category C

INDICATIONS

- Treatment of mild to moderate hyperkalemia (if severe, more immediate measures such as sodium bicarbonate IV, calcium or glucose/insulin infusion should be instituted).

ACTION

- Exchanges sodium ions for potassium ions in the intestine (each 1 g is exchanged for 0.5–1 mEq potassium).
Therapeutic Effect: ▪ Reduction of serum potassium levels.

PHARMACOKINETICS

Absorption: Distributed throughout the intestine but is nonabsorbable.
Distribution: Not distributed.
Metabolism and Excretion: Eliminated in the feces.
Half-life: UK.

CONTRAINDICATIONS AND PRECAUTIONS

Contraindicated in: ▪ Life-threatening hyperkalemia (other, more immediate measures should be instituted) ▪ Hypersensitivity to saccharin or parabens (some products) ▪ Ileus ▪ Known alcohol intolerance (suspension only).

Use Cautiously in: ▪ Elderly patients ▪ Congestive heart failure, hypertension, edema ▪ Sodium restriction ▪ Constipation.

ADVERSE REACTIONS AND SIDE EFFECTS*

GI: <u>constipation</u>, <u>fecal impaction</u>, anorexia, nausea, vomiting, gastric irritation.

F and E: hypokalemia, hypocalcemia, sodium retention.

INTERACTIONS

Drug–Drug: ▪ Administration with **calcium** or **magnesium-containing antacids** may decrease resin-exchanging ability and increase risk of systemic alkalosis ▪ Hypokalemia may enhance **cardiac glycoside** toxicity.

ROUTE AND DOSAGE

Each g contains 4.1 mEq sodium.

▪ **PO (Adults):** 15 g 1–4 times daily in water or sorbitol (up to 40 g 4 times daily).
▪ **PO, Rect (Children):** 1 g/kg/dose.
▪ **Rect (Adults):** 25–100 g in 100 ml sorbitol q 6 hr as a retention enema.

AVAILABILITY

▪ *Suspension:* 15 g sodium polystyrene sulfonate with 20 g sorbital/60 ml, 15 g sodium polystyrene sulfonate with 14.1 g sorbital/60 ml ▪ *Powder:* 15 g/4 level tsp.

TIME/ACTION PROFILE (decrease in serum potassium)

	ONSET	PEAK	DURATION
PO	2–12 hr	UK	6–24 hr
Rect	2–12 hr	UK	4–6 hr

NURSING IMPLICATIONS

ASSESSMENT

□ Monitor response of symptoms of hyperkalemia (fatigue, muscle weakness, paresthesia, confusion, dyspnea, peaked T waves, depressed ST segments, prolonged QT segments, widened QRS complexes, loss of P waves, and cardiac arrhythmias). Assess for development of hypokalemia (weakness, fatigue, arrhythmias, flat or inverted T waves, prominent U waves).

□ Monitor intake and output ratios and daily weight. Assess for symptoms of fluid overload (dyspnea, rales/crackles, jugular venous distention, peripheral edema). Physician may order concurrent low-sodium diet in patients with congestive heart failure (see Appendix K for foods included).

□ In patients receiving concurrent cardiac glycosides, assess for symptoms of digitalis toxicity (anorexia, nausea, vomiting, visual disturbances, arrhythmias).

□ Assess abdomen and note character and frequency of stools. Physician may order concurrent sorbitol or laxatives to prevent constipation or impaction. Some products contain sorbitol to prevent constipation. Patient should ideally have 1–2 watery stools each day during course of therapy.

▪ **Lab Test Considerations:** Monitor renal function and electrolytes (especially potassium, sodium, calcium, and magnesium) prior to and periodically throughout therapy. Notify physician when potassium decreases to 4–5 mEq/liter.

POTENTIAL NURSING DIAGNOSES

▪ Constipation, diarrhea (side effects).
▪ Knowledge deficit related to medication regimen (patient/family teaching).

IMPLEMENTATION

▪ **General Info:** Solution is stable for 24 hr when refrigerated.
□ Consult physician regarding discon-

S

---

*<u>Underlines</u> indicate most frequent; **CAPITALS** indicate life-threatening.

tinuation of medications that may increase the serum potassium (ACE inhibitors, potassium-sparing diuretics, potassium supplements, salt substitutes).

- **PO:** An osmotic laxative (sorbitol) is usually administered concurrently to prevent constipation.
- □ For oral administration, add prescribed amount of powder to 3–4 ml water/g of powder. Shake well. Physician may order syrup to improve palatability. Resin cookie or candy recipes are available; discuss with pharmacist or dietician.
- **Retention Enema:** Precede retention enema with cleansing enema. Administer solution via rectal tube or 28 French foley catheter with 30-ml balloon. Insert tube at least 20 cm and tape in place.
- □ For retention enema, add powder to 100 ml of prescribed solution (usually sorbitol or 20% dextrose in water). Shake well to dissolve powder thoroughly; should be of liquid consistency. Position patient on left side and elevate hips on pillow if solution begins to leak. Follow administration of medication with additional 50–100 ml of diluent to ensure administration of complete dose. Encourage patient to retain enema as long as possible, at least 30–60 min.
- □ After retention period irrigate colon with 1–2 liters of non-sodium-containing solution. Y-connector with tubing may be attached to foley or rectal tube; cleansing solution is administered through one port of the Y and allowed to drain by gravity through the other port.

PATIENT/FAMILY TEACHING
- □ Explain purpose and method of administration of medication to patient.
- □ Inform patient of need for frequent lab tests to monitor effectiveness.

EVALUATION
Effectiveness of therapy can be demonstrated by: ▪ Normalization of serum potassium levels.

SOMATROPIN (RECOMBINANT)
(soe-ma-**troe**-pin)
Humatrope

SOMATREM (RECOMBINANT)
(**soe**-ma-trem)
Protropin

CLASSIFICATION(S):
Growth hormone
Pregnancy Category UK

INDICATIONS
▪ Growth failure in children due to deficiency of growth hormone.

ACTION
▪ Produces growth (skeletal and cellular) ▪ Metabolic actions include: □ Increased protein synthesis □ Increased carbohydrate metabolism □ Lipid mobilization □ Retention of sodium, phosphorus, and potassium ▪ Somatropin has the same amino acid sequence as naturally occurring growth hormone; somatrem has one additional amino acid. Both are produced by recombinant DNA techniques. **Therapeutic Effect:** ▪ Increased skeletal growth in children with growth hormone deficiency.

PHARMACOKINETICS
Absorption: Well absorbed following SC or IM administration.
Distribution: Distribution not known.
Metabolism and Excretion: Metabolism and excretion not known.
Half-life: UK.

CONTRAINDICATIONS AND PRECAUTIONS
Contraindicated in: ▪ Closure of epiphyses ▪ Tumors ▪ Hypersensitivity to m-cresol or glycerin (somatropin) or benzyl alcohol (somatrem).
Use Cautiously in: ▪ Growth hormone deficiency due to intracranial lesion ▪ Coexisting adrenocorticotropic hormone (ACTH) deficiency ▪ Thyroid dysfunction.

ADVERSE REACTIONS AND SIDE EFFECTS*

CV: edema.
Endo: hyperglycemia, insulin resistance, hypothyroidism.
Local: pain at injection site.

INTERACTIONS

Drug–Drug: ▪ Excessive **glucocorticoid** use may decrease response to somatropin.

ROUTE AND DOSAGE

Somatropin
▪ **IM, SC (Children):** Up to 0.06 mg/kg (0.16 IU/kg) 3 times weekly.

Somatrem
▪ **IM, SC (Children):** Up to 0.1 mg/kg (0.26 IU/kg) 3 times weekly.

AVAILABILITY

Somatrem
▪ *Powder for injection:* 5 mg (13 IU)/ vial, 10 mg (26 IU)/vial.

Somatropin
▪ *Powder for injection:* {2 mg (5 IU)/ vial}, 5 mg (13 IU)/vial.

TIME/ACTION PROFILE (growth)

	ONSET	PEAK	DURATION
IM, SC	within 3 mo	UK	UK

NURSING IMPLICATIONS

ASSESSMENT

▫ Monitor bone age and height and weight.
▪ **Lab Test Considerations:** Monitor thyroid function prior to and throughout course of therapy. May decrease T_4, radioactive iodine uptake, and thyroxine-binding capacity. Hypothyroidism necessitates concurrent thyroid replacement for growth hormone to be effective.
▫ Monitor blood or urine glucose periodically throughout therapy. Diabetic patients may require increased insulin dose.
▫ Monitor for development of neutraliz-

ing antibodies if growth rate does not exceed 2.5 cm/6 mo.

POTENTIAL NURSING DIAGNOSES

▪ Body image disturbance (indications).
▪ Knowledge deficit related to medication regimen (patient/family teaching).

IMPLEMENTATION

▪ **Somatrem:** Reconstitute 5-mg (10-IU) vial with 10 ml of Bacteriostatic Water for Injection. Do not shake; swirl gently to dissolve. Solution is clear. Discard vial after withdrawing dose.
▪ **Somatropin:** Reconstitute 13-IU vial with 1.5–5 ml of Sterile Water for Injection provided by manufacturer (contains preservative m-cresol). Do not shake; swirl gently to dissolve. Solution is clear. Stable for 14 days when refrigerated.

PATIENT/FAMILY TEACHING

▫ Instruct patient and parents on correct procedure for reconstituting medication, site selection, and technique for IM or SC injection. Review dosage schedule. Somatropin injections should be at least 48 hr apart. Parents should report persistent pain or edema at injection site.
▫ Explain rationale for prohibition of use for increasing athletic performance. Administration to persons without growth hormone deficiency or after epiphyseal closure may result in acromegaly (coarsening of facial features; enlarged hands, feet, and internal organs; increased blood sugars; hypertension).
▫ Emphasize need for regular follow-up with endocrinologist to ensure appropriate growth rate, to evaluate lab work, and to determine bone age by x-ray examination.
▫ Assure parents and child that these dosage forms are synthetic and therefore not capable of transmitting Creutzfeldt-Jakob disease, as was the original somatropin, which was extracted from human cadavers.

*Underlines indicate most frequent; **CAPITALS** indicate life-threatening.

EVALUATION

Clinical response can be evaluated by:
- Child's attainment of adult height in growth failure secondary to pituitary growth hormone deficiency. Therapy is limited to period before closure of epiphyseal plates (approximately up to 14–15 yr in girls, 15–16 yr in boys).

SOTALOL
(soe-ta-lole)
Betapace, {Sotacor}

CLASSIFICATION(S):
Beta-adrenergic blocking agent (nonselective), Antiarrhythmic (group II and III)
Pregnancy Category B

INDICATIONS
- Treatment of life-threatening ventricular arrhythmias such as sustained ventricular tachycardia.

ACTION
- Blocks beta$_1$- and beta$_2$-adrenergic receptors ▪ Lengthens action potential duration in myocardial fibers without affecting conduction ▪ Lowers heart rate and prolongs QTc (QT interval corrected for heart rate) interval with no effect on QRS duration. **Therapeutic Effect:** ▪ Suppression of ventricular arrhythmias.

PHARMACOKINETICS
Absorption: Well absorbed following oral administration.

Distribution: Crosses the placenta and enters breast milk. Remainder of distribution is not known.

Metabolism and Excretion: Eliminated mostly as unchanged drug by the kidneys.

Half-life: 12 hr.

CONTRAINDICATIONS AND PRECAUTIONS
Contraindicated in: ▪ Hypersensitivity

▪ Asthma ▪ Sinus bradycardia ▪ 2nd- or 3rd-degree heart block (unless a functional artificial pacemaker is in place) ▪ Congenital or acquired prolonged QTc interval syndromes ▪ Cardiogenic shock ▪ Uncontrolled congestive heart failure ▪ Sotalol should not be used to treat patients with asymptomatic PVCs.

Use Cautiously in: ▪ Renal impairment (increase dosage interval if creatinine clearance is ≤60 ml/min) ▪ Sick sinus syndrome (may experience sinus pauses or arrest) ▪ Patients with prolonged QTc intervals (>550 msec); hypokalemia; hypomagnesemia; or who require large doses of sotalol (increased risk of proarrhythmic effects) ▪ Acid-base disturbances ▪ Severe or prolonged diarrhea or aggressive diuretic therapy ▪ Recent (10 days) history of myocardial infarction, especially if complicated by left ventricular dysfunction ▪ Patients with diabetes mellitus or thyrotoxicosis (may mask symptoms) ▪ Pregnancy, lactation, or children (safety not established) ▪ Patients with a history of severe allergic reactions (intensity of reactions may be increased).

ADVERSE REACTIONS AND SIDE EFFECTS*
CNS: fatigue, weakness, dizziness, lightheadedness, sleep disturbances, headache, syncope, depression, altered consciousness, anxiety, mood changes.

EENT: visual disturbances.

Resp: dyspnea, asthma.

CV: prolongation of the QTc interval, conduction disturbances, bradycardia, dyspnea, proarrhythmic effects including TORSADES DE POINTES or worsened VENTRICULAR TACHYCARDIA, chest pain, palpitations, edema, vasodilation, hypotension, CONGESTIVE HEART FAILURE, Reynaud's phenomenon, hypertension.

GI: diarrhea, dyspepsia, change in appetite, abdominal pain, flatulence.

GU: sexual dysfunction.

Derm: sweating, rash.

{} = Available in Canada only.
*Underlines indicate most frequent; CAPITALS indicate life-threatening.

MS: extremity pain.
Neuro: paresthesia.
Misc: fever.

INTERACTIONS

Drug–Drug: ▪ Risk of arrhythmias is increased by concurrent **terfenadine, astemizole, phenothiazines,** or **tricyclic antidepressants** ▪ Prolonged refractory period and increased risk of arrhythmias may occur when sotalol is used with **disopyramide, quinidine, procainamide,** or **amiodarone** (avoid concurrent use) ▪ **Digoxin** increases the risk of proarrhythmic effects ▪ Concurrent use with **calcium channel blockers** may increase the risk of conduction disturbances and/or hypotension ▪ Marked hypotension and bradycardia may occur with agents such as **reserpine** or **guanethidine** ▪ Sotalol may alter the requirements for **insulin** or **oral hypoglycemic agents** ▪ The beneficial effects of **beta agonist bronchodilators** or **theophylline** may be antagonized ▪ Excessive hypertension may occur during withdrawal of **clonidine.**

Drug–Food: ▪ Concurrent administration with food decreases absorption by 20%.

ROUTE AND DOSAGE

▪ **PO (Adults):** 80 mg bid initially (range 240–320 mg/day given bid or tid; not to exceed 640 mg/day). Dosage increments should be made at 2–3 day intervals.

AVAILABILITY

▪ *Tablets:* 80-mg tablets, 160-mg tablets, 240-mg tablets.

TIME/ACTION PROFILE
(antiarrhythmic effect)

	ONSET	PEAK	DURATION
PO	hours	2–3 days	UK

NURSING IMPLICATIONS

ASSESSMENT

▫ Monitor ECG continuously during initiation of therapy and dosage adjustment. May cause new or worsened arrhythmias.

▫ Monitor blood pressure and pulse frequently when adjusting dose and periodically throughout therapy. Confer with physician prior to giving drug if pulse <50 bpm. Assess for orthostatic hypotension when assisting patient up from supine position.

▫ Monitor intake and output ratios and daily weight. Assess patient routinely for evidence of congestive heart failure (peripheral edema, dyspnea, rales/crackles, fatigue, weight gain, jugular venous distention).

▪ **Lab Test Considerations:** Monitor serum electroytes. Correct hypokalemia and hypomagnesemia prior to initiating therapy with sotalol.

▫ Hepatic and renal function and CBC should be monitored routinely in patients receiving prolonged therapy.

▫ May cause elevations in serum potassium, uric acid, LDH, glucose, lipoprotein, triglyceride levels, and BUN.

POTENTIAL NURSING DIAGNOSES

▪ Cardiac output, decreased (indications, adverse reactions).

▪ Knowledge deficit related to medication regimen (patient/family teaching).

IMPLEMENTATION

▪ **PO:** Administer medication on an empty stomach, 1 hr before or 2 hr after meals. Administration with food reduces absorption by approximately 20%.

PATIENT/FAMILY TEACHING

▫ Instruct patient to take medication exactly as directed, even if feeling well. Abrupt withdrawal may precipitate life-threatening arrhythmias, hypertension, or myocardial ischemia. Discontinuation should occur slowly over a 1–2 wk period.

▫ Teach patient and family how to check pulse daily. Advise patient to withhold dose and contact physician if pulse <50 bpm.

▫ Sotalol may cause drowsiness or dizziness. Caution patient to avoid driv-

S

ing or other activities that require alertness until response to the drug is known.

□ Caution patient that sotalol may cause increased sensitivity to cold.

□ Advise patient to consult physician or pharmacist before taking any over-the-counter drugs concurrently with this medication. Patient should also avoid excessive amounts of coffee, tea, or cola.

□ Diabetic patients should monitor serum glucose closely, especially if weakness, fatigue, or irritability occurs.

□ Advise patient to notify physician if slow pulse, dizziness, lightheadedness, confusion, depression, or skin rash occurs.

□ Instruct patient to inform physician or dentist of medication regimen prior to treatment or surgery.

□ Advise patient to carry identification describing medication regimen at all times.

EVALUATION
Effectiveness of therapy can be demonstrated by: ■ Decrease in ventricular arrhythmias.

SPECTINOMYCIN
(spek-tin-oh-**mye**-sin)
Trobicin

CLASSIFICATION(S):
Anti-infective (miscellaneous)
Pregnancy Category UK

INDICATIONS

■ Treatment of gonorrhea and gonococcal urethritis, cervicitis, or proctitis in patients who are infected with susceptible strains of *Neisseria gonorrhea*.

ACTION

■ Inhibits bacterial protein synthesis at the level of the 30S ribosome.

Therapeutic Effect: ■ Bactericidal action against susceptible organisms.
Spectrum: ■ Most notable for activity against *Neisseria gonorrhea,* including penicillinase-producing strains (PPNG) ■ Not active against *Treponema pallidum* or *Chlamydia trachomatis.*

PHARMACOKINETICS

Absorption: Rapidly absorbed from IM sites.
Distribution: Distribution not known.
Metabolism and Excretion: Excreted primarily by the kidneys.
Half-life: 1.2–2.8 hr.

CONTRAINDICATIONS AND PRECAUTIONS

Contraindicated in: ■ Hypersensitivity ■ Neonates (diluent contains benzyl alcohol).
Use Cautiously in: Concurrent infection with other sexually transmitted disease (additional anti-infectives may be required) ■ Pregnancy, lactation, or children (safety not established; has been used).

ADVERSE REACTIONS AND SIDE EFFECTS*

CNS: dizziness, headache, nervousness, insomnia.
GI: nausea, vomiting.
Derm: urticaria, transient rashes, pruritus.
Local: <u>pain</u> at IM site.
Misc: hypersensitivity reactions, including ANAPHYLAXIS, chills, fever.

INTERACTIONS

Drug–Drug: ■ None significant.

ROUTE AND DOSAGE

■ **IM (Adults and Children >45 kg):** 2–4 g single dose.
■ **IM (Infants and Children <45 kg):** 40 mg/kg single dose.

AVAILABILITY

■ *Powder for injection:* 2-g vial, 4-g vial.

---

*<u>Underlines</u> indicate most frequent; CAPITALS indicate life-threatening.

TIME/ACTION PROFILE (blood levels)

	ONSET	PEAK
IM	rapid	1 hr

NURSING IMPLICATIONS

ASSESSMENT

- Assess patient for gonorrheal infection (dysuria, urethral discharge, vaginal discharge, perianal discomfort).
- Obtain gram-stain smear and specimens for culture and sensitivity prior to initiating therapy. Dose may be given before receiving results.
- Monitor patients with history of allergies for hypersensitivity reactions (urticaria, wheezing).
- **Lab Test Considerations:** Additional serologic testing for syphilis should be conducted at the time of therapy and again 3 mo later. Spectinomycin does not cure syphilis, but it may mask symptom development.
- When multiple doses are given, increased ALT (SGPT), BUN, and alkaline phosphatase and decreased hemoglobin, hematocrit, and creatinine clearance may occur. Urine output often decreases, but this is not associated with renal toxicity.

POTENTIAL NURSING DIAGNOSES

- Infection, high risk for (indications).
- Knowledge deficit related to safe sex practices (patient/family teaching).

IMPLEMENTATION

- **IM:** Reconstitute 2-g vial with 3.2 ml provided diluent (Bacteriostatic Water with 0.9% benzol alcohol for Injection) and 4-g vial with 6.2 ml diluent. Administer deep into well-developed muscle of dorsogluteal site. The 2-g vial yields 5 ml, which can be injected slowly into one site. The 4-g vial yields 10 ml, which should be divided into two 5-ml injections and administered at separate sites. Suspension is stable for 24 hr.
- Most patients are concurrently infected with chlamydia and should be treated with erythromycin or doxycycline.

PATIENT/FAMILY TEACHING

- Discuss need for all sexual contacts to receive treatment. Patient should abstain from sex until repeat tests confirm resolution of infection. Patient should not share washcloths, towels, or underclothes. Review safe sex practices to prevent reinfection.
- Inform patient that temporary soreness at injection site, nausea, fever, chills, dizziness, and insomnia may occur.
- Explain need for repeat smears or culture and sensitivity tests 1 wk after treatment to ensure effectiveness of treatment.

EVALUATION

Clinical response can be evaluated by:
- Resolution of the signs and symptoms of gonorrheal urethritis □ Recurrence of symptoms is usually indicative of re-exposure, not treatment failure.

S

SPIRONOLACTONE
(speer-oh-no-**lak**-tone)
Aldactone, {Novospiroton}

CLASSIFICATION(S):
Diuretic (potassium-sparing)
Pregnancy Category UK

INDICATIONS

- Most commonly used to counteract potassium loss induced by other diuretics in the management of edema or hypertension ▪ Treatment of hyperaldosteronism.

ACTION

- Acts at distal renal tubule to antagonize the effects of aldosterone, causing excretion of sodium, bicarbonate, and calcium while conserving potassium and hydrogen ions. **Therapeutic Effects:**
- Weak diuretic and antihypertensive effects when compared to other diuretics, but without potassium loss ▪ Counteracts the effects of excessive aldosterone.

{} = Available in Canada only.

PHARMACOKINETICS

Absorption: Well absorbed following oral administration.

Distribution: Crosses the placenta and enters breast milk (canrenone).

Metabolism and Excretion: Converted by the liver to its active diuretic compound (canrenone).

Half-life: 13-24 hr (canrenone).

CONTRAINDICATIONS AND PRECAUTIONS

Contraindicated in: ▪ Hypersensitivity ▪ Hyperkalemia ▪ Renal insufficiency ▪ Pregnancy or lactation ▪ Menstrual abnormalities ▪ Breast enlargement.

Use Cautiously in: ▪ Hepatic dysfunction ▪ Elderly or debilitated patients.

ADVERSE REACTIONS AND SIDE EFFECTS*

CNS: headache, dizziness.

CV: arrhythmias.

GI: <u>nausea</u>, <u>vomiting</u>, <u>anorexia</u>, <u>diarrhea</u>, cramps, constipation, flatulence.

GU: impotence, menstrual irregularities.

Derm: hirsutism, rashes.

Endo: gynecomastia.

F and E: <u>hyperkalemia</u>, hyponatremia, hypochloremia, metabolic acidosis, dehydration.

INTERACTIONS

Drug–Drug: ▪ Additive hypotension with other **antihypertensives, nitrates,** or acute ingestion of **alcohol** ▪ Use with **angiotensin converting enzyme (ACE) inhibitors, cyclosporine,** or **potassium supplements** may lead to hyperkalemia ▪ Decreases **lithium** excretion, may lead to toxicity ▪ **Nonsteroidal anti-inflammatory agents** may decrease the antihypertensive response to spironolactone and increase the risk of adverse renal reactions ▪ May decrease the effect of **anticoagulants.**

Drug–Food: ▪ Ingesting large amounts of **potassium-rich foods** or **salt substitutes** (see list in Appendix K) may lead to hyperkalemia.

ROUTE AND DOSAGE

Edema

▪ **PO (Adults):** 25-400 mg/day in 2-4 divided doses.
▪ **PO (Children):** 1-3 mg/kg/day in single dose or 2-4 divided doses.

Hypertension

▪ **PO (Adults):** 50-200 mg/day in single dose or 2-4 divided doses.
▪ **PO (Children):** 1-3 mg/kg/day in single dose or 2-4 divided doses.

Prevention of Hypokalemia with Potassium-Losing Diuretics

▪ **PO (Adults):** 25-100 mg/day in single dose or 2-4 divided doses.

Primary Hyperaldosteronism

▪ **PO (Adults):** 100-400 mg/day in 2-4 divided doses.

AVAILABILITY

▪ *Tablets:* 25 mg, 50 mg, 100 mg ▪ *In combination with:* hydrochlorothiazide (Aldactazide). See Appendix A.

TIME/ACTION PROFILE (effects on serum potassium)

	ONSET	PEAK	DURATION
PO	1-2 days	5 days	2-3 days

NURSING IMPLICATIONS

ASSESSMENT

▫ Monitor intake and output ratios and daily weight throughout therapy.
▫ If medication is given as an adjunct to antihypertensive therapy, blood pressure and pulse should be evaluated before administering.
▫ Monitor response of signs and symptoms of hypokalemia (weakness, fatigue, U wave on ECG, arrhythmias, polyuria, polydipsia). Assess patient frequently for development of hyperkalemia (fatigue, muscle weakness, paresthesia, confusion, dyspnea, cardiac arrhythmias). Patients who have diabetes mellitus or kidney disease and elderly patients are at increased risk of developing these symptoms.
▫ Periodic ECGs are recommended in patients receiving prolonged therapy.

*Underlines indicate most frequent; CAPITALS indicate life-threatening.

- **Lab Test Considerations:** Serum potassium levels should be evaluated prior to and routinely during course of therapy. Withhold drug and notify physician if patient becomes hyperkalemic.
- ▫ Monitor BUN, serum creatinine, and electrolytes prior to and periodically throughout therapy. May cause increased serum glucose, magnesium, uric acid, BUN, creatinine, potassium, and urinary calcium excretion levels. May also cause decreased sodium levels.
- ▫ May cause false elevations of plasma cortisol concentrations. Spironolactone should be withdrawn 4–7 days before test.

POTENTIAL NURSING DIAGNOSES
- Fluid volume excess (indications).
- Knowledge deficit related to medication regimen (patient/family teaching).

IMPLEMENTATION
- **General Info:** Administer in AM to avoid interrupting sleep pattern.
- **PO:** Administer with food or milk to minimize GI irritation and to increase bioavailability.

PATIENT/FAMILY TEACHING
- **General Info:** Emphasize the importance of continuing to take this medication, even if feeling well. Instruct patient to take medication at the same time each day. If a dose is missed, take as soon as remembered unless almost time for next dose.
- ▫ Caution patient to avoid salt substitutes and foods that contain high levels of potassium or sodium, unless prescribed by physician.
- ▫ May cause dizziness. Caution patient to avoid driving or other activities requiring alertness until response to medication is known.
- ▫ Advise patient to avoid use of over-the-counter medications without consulting with physician or pharmacist.
- ▫ Advise patient to notify physician if muscle weakness or cramps, fatigue, or severe nausea, vomiting, or diarrhea occurs.

- **Hypertension:** Reinforce need to continue additional therapies for hypertension (weight loss, restricted sodium intake, stress reduction, moderation of alcohol intake, regular exercise, and cessation of smoking). Spironolactone helps control but does not cure hypertension.
- ▫ Teach patients on antihypertensive therapy how to check blood pressure weekly.

EVALUATION
Effectiveness of therapy can be demonstrated by: ▪ Prevention of hypokalemia in patients taking diuretics ▪ Treatment of hyperaldosteronism.

STREPTOKINASE
(strep-toe-**kye**-nase)
Kabikinase, Streptase

CLASSIFICATION(S):
Thrombolytic agent
Pregnancy Category C

INDICATIONS
- Treatment of coronary thrombosis associated with acute transmural myocardial infarction ▪ Treatment of: ▫ Recent, severe, or massive deep vein thrombosis ▫ Pulmonary emboli ▫ Arterial embolism ▫ Thrombosis ▪ Management of occluded arteriovenous cannulae.

ACTION
- Directly activates plasminogen, which subsequently dissolves fibrin deposits, including those required for normal hemostasis. **Therapeutic Effects:** ▪ Preservation of left ventricular function after transmural myocardial infarction ▪ Lysis of thrombi or emboli.

PHARMACOKINETICS
Absorption: Administered IV or directly into coronary arteries or cannulae, resulting in immediate and complete bioavailability.
Distribution: Does not cross the placenta.

Metabolism and Excretion: Rapidly cleared from circulation following IV administration by antibodies and the reticuloendothelial system.

Half-life: 23 min (streptokinase/plasmin complex).

CONTRAINDICATIONS AND PRECAUTIONS

Contraindicated in: ▪ Hypersensitivity ▪ Active internal bleeding ▪ Recent (<2 mo) cerebrovascular accident, intracranial or intraspinal surgery, intracranial neoplasm, thoracic surgery ▪ Uncontrolled severe hypertension.

Use Cautiously in: ▪ Pregnancy, lactation, or children (safety not established) ▪ Recent minor trauma or surgery (<2 mo) ▪ Cerebrovascular disease ▪ Diabetic hemorrhagic retinopathy ▪ Recent streptococcal infection ▪ Recent streptokinase therapy ▪ Patients ≥75 yr (increased risk of CNS bleeding) ▪ Arterial emboli originating in the left side of the heart (increased risk of cerebral emboli).

Extreme Caution: ▪ Early postpartum period (10 days) ▪ Patients receiving oral anticoagulant therapy.

ADVERSE REACTIONS AND SIDE EFFECTS*

CV: reperfusion arrhythmias.
EENT: periorbital edema.
Derm: urticaria, flushing.
Hemat: BLEEDING.
Local: phlebitis at IV site.
Misc: fever, hypersensitivity reactions, including ANAPHYLAXIS, bronchospasm.

INTERACTIONS

Drug–Drug: ▪ Concurrent use with other **anticoagulants, cefamandole, cefotetan, plicamycin,** or **agents affecting platelet function,** including **aspirin, nonsteroidal anti-inflammatory agents,** and **dipyridamole** increase the risk of bleeding.

ROUTE AND DOSAGE

Myocardial Infarction
▪ **IV (Adults):** 1,500,000 IU.

▪ **Intracoronary (Adults):** 20,000-IU bolus, followed by 2000 IU/min infusion for 60 min (140,000 IU total dose).

Deep Vein Thrombosis, Pulmonary Emboli, Arterial Embolism, or Thromboses

▪ **IV (Adults):** 250,000-IU loading dose, followed by 100,000 IU/hr for 24 hr for pulmonary emboli, 72 hr for recurrent pulmonary emboli or deep vein thrombosis.

Arteriovenous Cannula Occlusion

▪ **(Adults):** 100,000–250,000 IU into each occluded limb of cannula, clamp for 2 hr, then aspirate.

AVAILABILITY

▪ *Powder for injection:* 250,000 IU/vial, 600,000 IU/vial, 1,500,000 IU/vial.

TIME/ACTION PROFILE (fibrinolysis)

	ONSET	PEAK	DURATION
IV	immediate	rapid	4 hr (up to 12 hr)

NURSING IMPLICATIONS

ASSESSMENT

▪ **General Info:** Monitor vital signs, including temperature, closely during course of therapy.

▫ Assess patient carefully for bleeding every 15 min during the first hour of therapy, every 15–30 min during the next 8 hr, and at least every 4 hr for the duration of therapy. Frank bleeding may occur from invasive sites or body orifices. Internal bleeding may also occur (decreased neurologic status, abdominal pain with coffee ground emesis or black tarry stools, joint pain). If bleeding occurs, stop medication and notify physician immediately.

▫ Inquire about previous reaction to streptokinase therapy. Assess patient for hypersensitivity reaction (rash, dyspnea, fever). If these occur, inform physician promptly. Keep epinephrine, an antihistamine, and resuscitation equipment close by in the event of an anaphylactic reaction.

□ Inquire about recent streptococcal infection. Streptokinase may not be effective if administered between 5 days and 6 mo of a streptococcal infection.

■ **Coronary Thrombosis:** Monitor ECG continuously. Notify physician if significant arrhythmias occur. IV lidocaine or procainamide (Pronestyl) may be ordered prophylactically. Cardiac enzymes should be monitored.

■ **Pulmonary Embolism:** Monitor pulse, blood pressure, hemodynamics, and respiratory status (rate, degree of dyspnea, ABGs).

■ **Deep Vein Thrombosis/Acute Arterial Occlusion:** Observe extremities and palpate pulses of affected extremities every hr. Notify physician immediately if circulatory impairment occurs.

■ **Cannula/Catheter Occlusion:** Monitor ability to aspirate blood as indicator of patency. Ensure that patient exhales and holds breath when connecting and disconnecting IV syringe to prevent air embolism.

■ **Lab Test Considerations:** Hematocrit, hemoglobin, platelet count, prothrombin time, thrombin time, and activated partial thromboplastin time should be evaluated prior to and frequently throughout course of therapy. Bleeding time may be assessed prior to therapy if patient has received platelet aggregation inhibitors.

□ Obtain type and cross-match and have blood available at all times in case of hemorrhage.

■ **Toxicity and Overdose:** If local bleeding occurs, apply pressure to site. If severe or internal bleeding occurs, discontinue infusion. Clotting factors and/or blood volume may be restored through infusions of whole blood, packed red blood cells, fresh frozen plasma, or cryoprecipitate. Do not administer dextran, as it has antiplatelet activity. Aminocaproic acid (Amicar) may be used as an antidote.

POTENTIAL NURSING DIAGNOSES

■ Tissue perfusion, altered (indications).

■ Injury, high risk for (side effects).

IMPLEMENTATION

■ **General Info:** This medication should be used only in settings where hematologic function and clinical response can be adequately monitored.

□ Invasive procedures, such as IM injections or arterial punctures, should be avoided with this therapy. If such procedures must be performed, apply pressure to IV puncture sites for at least 15 min and to arterial puncture sites for at least 30 min.

□ Systemic anticoagulation with heparin is usually begun several hours after the completion of thrombolytic therapy.

□ Acetaminophen may be ordered to control fever.

■ **IV:** Reconstitute with 5 ml of 0.9% NaCl or D5W (direct to sides of vial) and swirl gently; do not shake. Dilute further with 0.9% NaCl for a total volume of 45–500 ml and infuse as directed by physician. Infuse via infusion pump to ensure accurate dosage. Administer through 0.8-micron pore size filter. Use reconstituted solution within 24 hr of preparation.

■ **Y-Site Compatibility:** dobutamine ■ dopamin ■ heparin ■ lidocaine ■ nitroglycerin.

■ **Additive Incompatibility:** Do not admix with any other medication.

■ **Cannula/Catheter Clearance:** IV preparations used for clearing occluded AV cannulas or central lines are mixed with 2 ml of 0.9% NaCl, administered slowly into each occluded limb of cannula, and then clamped for at least 2 hr. Aspirate contents carefully and flush line with 0.9% NaCl.

PATIENT/FAMILY TEACHING

□ Explain purpose of medication. Instruct patient to report hypersensitivity reactions (rash, dyspnea) and bleeding or bruising.

□ Explain need for bedrest and minimal handling during therapy to avoid injury.

EVALUATION

Effectiveness of therapy can be demonstrated by: ▪ Lysis of thrombi and restoration of blood flow ▪ Cannula or catheter patency.

STREPTOMYCIN
(strep-toe-**mye**-sin)

CLASSIFICATION(S):
Anti-infective (aminoglycoside),
Antitubercular
Pregnancy Category UK

INDICATIONS

▪ Combination therapy of active tuberculosis ▪ Streptococcal or enterococcal endocarditis (in combination with a penicillin) ▪ Treatment of tularemia and plague ▪ Use in other situations should be reserved for organisms not sensitive to less toxic anti-infectives or when other contraindications to their use exists.

ACTION

▪ Inhibits protein synthesis in bacteria at the level of the 30S ribosome. **Therapeutic Effect:** ▪ Bactericidal action against susceptible bacteria. **Spectrum:** ▪ Despite activity against many gram-negative pathogens, toxicity precludes its use in most situations ▪ Notable for activity against the following other organisms: ▫ *Mycobacterium tuberculosis* ▫ *Brucella* ▫ *Nocardia* ▫ *Erisypelothrix* ▫ *Pasturella multocida* ▫ *Yersinia pestis* ▪ In the treatment of enterococcal infections, synergy with a penicillin is required.

PHARMACOKINETICS

Absorption: Well absorbed following IM administration.
Distribution: Crosses the placenta. Small amounts enter breast milk. Poor penetration into CSF.
Metabolism and Excretion: Excretion is mainly (>90%) renal.
Half-life: 2–3 hr (increased in renal impairment).

CONTRAINDICATIONS AND PRECAUTIONS

Contraindicated in: ▪ Hypersensitivity ▪ Cross-sensitivity with other aminoglycosides may exist.
Use Cautiously in: ▪ Renal impairment of any kind (dosage reduction required) ▪ Pregnancy (may cause irreversible deafness in newborns) ▪ Lactation (safety not established) ▪ Neuromuscular diseases, such as myasthenia gravis ▪ Elderly patients (dosage reduction recommended).

ADVERSE REACTIONS AND SIDE EFFECTS*

EENT: <u>ototoxicity</u> (vestibular and cochlear).
GU: <u>nephrotoxicity</u>.
Neuro: enhanced neuromuscular blockade.
Misc: hypersensitivity reactions.

INTERACTIONS

Drug–Drug: ▪ May be inactivated by **penicillins** when coadministered to patients with renal insufficiency ▪ Increased risk of respiratory paralysis after **inhalation anesthetics (ether, cyclopropane, halothane,** or **nitrous oxide)** or **neuromusclar blockers (tubocurarine, succinylcholine, decamethonium)** ▪ Increased incidence of ototoxicity with **loop diuretics (ethacrynic acid, bumetanide, furosemide)** ▪ Increased risk of nephrotoxicity with **other nephrotoxic drugs (cisplatin)**.

ROUTE AND DOSAGE

Tuberculosis

▪ **IM (Adults):** 15 mg/kg/day (not to exceed 1 g) or 25–30 mg/kg (not to exceed 1.5 g) 2–3 times weekly.
▪ **IM (Children):** 20–40 mg/kg (not to exceed 1 g)/day or 25–35 mg/kg (not to exceed 1.5 g) 2–3 times weekly.

Other Infections

▪ **IM (Adults):** 1–2 g/day in divided doses q 6–12 hr.
▪ **IM (Children):** 20–40 mg/kg/day in divided doses q 6–12 hr.

---

*<u>Underlines</u> indicate most frequent; **CAPITALS** indicate life-threatening.

AVAILABILITY

▪ **Injection:** 400 mg/ml.

TIME/ACTION PROFILE (blood levels)

	ONSET	PEAK
IM	rapid	1–2 hr

NURSING IMPLICATIONS

ASSESSMENT

▫ Assess patient for infection (vital signs; appearance of wound, sputum, urine, and stool; WBC) at beginning and throughout course of therapy.

▫ Obtain specimens for culture and sensitivity prior to initiating therapy. First dose may be given before receiving results.

▫ Evaluate eighth cranial nerve function by audiometry prior to and throughout course of therapy. Hearing loss is usually in the high-frequency range. Prompt recognition and intervention is essential in preventing permanent damage. Also monitor for vestibular dysfunction (vertigo, ataxia, nausea, vomiting). Eighth cranial nerve dysfunction is associated with persistently elevated peak streptomycin levels. Caloric stimulation tests may also be performed.

▫ Monitor intake and output and daily weight to assess hydration status and renal function.

▫ Assess patient for signs of superinfection (fever, upper respiratory infection, vaginal itching or discharge, increasing malaise, diarrhea). Report to physician.

▪ **Lab Test Considerations:** Monitor renal function by urinalysis, specific gravity, BUN, creatinine, and creatinine clearance prior to and throughout therapy.

▫ May cause increased AST (SGOT), ALT (SGPT), LDH, bilirubin, and serum alkaline phosphatase levels.

▫ May cause decreased serum calcium, magnesium, sodium, and potassium levels.

▪ **Toxicity and Overdose:** Blood levels should be monitored periodically during therapy. Timing of blood levels is important in interpreting results. Draw blood for peak levels 30–60 min after IM injection. Acceptable peak level is 5–25 mcg/ml. Trough levels should not be >5 mcg/ml.

POTENTIAL NURSING DIAGNOSES

▪ Infection, high risk for (indications).
▪ Sensory-perceptual alteration: auditory (side effects).

IMPLEMENTATION

▪ **General Info:** Keep patient well hydrated (1500–2000 ml/day) during therapy.

▫ Solution may vary from colorless to yellow and may darken on exposure to light. This does not affect potency. Do not use solution that contains a precipitate.

▪ **IM:** Reconstitute by adding 4.2–4.5 ml of 0.9% NaCl or Sterile Water for Injection to each 1-g vial for a concentration of 200 mg/ml, or add 3.2–3.5 ml of diluent for a concentration of 250 mg/ml. Add 17 ml of diluent to each 5-g vial for a concentration of 250 mg/ml, or add 6.5 ml for a concentration of 500 mg/ml. Do not administer concentrations >500 mg/ml. Solution is stable for 2–28 days at room temperature or for 14 days if refrigerated, depending on manufacturer.

▫ IM administration should be deep into a well-developed muscle. Alternate injection sites.

▪ **Syringe Incompatibility:** ▪ heparin.

PATIENT/FAMILY TEACHING

▫ Instruct patient to report signs of hypersensitivity, tinnitus, vertigo, or hearing loss.

EVALUATION

Clinical response can be evaluated by:
▪ Resolution of the signs and symptoms of infection. Length of time for complete resolution depends on the organism and site of infection.

STREPTOZOCIN

(strep-toe-**zoe**-sin)
Zanosar

INDICATIONS

■ Management of metastatic islet cell carcinoma of the pancreas. **Unlabeled Uses:** ■ Management of: ▫ Metastatic carcinoid tumor ▫ Hodgkin's disease ▫ Pancreatic adenocarcinoma ▫ Colorectal cancer.

ACTION

■ Inhibits DNA synthesis by cross-linking DNA strands (cell cycle-phase nonspecific). **Therapeutic Effect:** ■ Death of rapidly replicating cells, particularly malignant ones.

PHARMACOKINETICS

Absorption: Administered IV only, resulting in complete bioavailability.
Distribution: Rapidly distributed. High concentrations in liver, pancreas, kidneys, and intestine. Probably crosses the placenta. Active metabolite enters the CSF.
Metabolism and Excretion: Highly metabolized in liver and kidneys. 10–20% excreted unchanged by the kidneys. Small amounts excreted in expired air (5%) and feces (1%).
Half-life: 35–40 min.

CONTRAINDICATIONS AND PRECAUTIONS

Contraindicated in: ■ Hypersensitivity.
Use Cautiously in: ■ Underlying or pre-existing renal disease (dosage reduction recommended) ■ Liver disease ■ Patients with childbearing potential ■ Active infections ■ Decreased bone marrow reserve ■ Other chronic debilitating illnesses ■ Pregnancy, lactation, or children (safety not established).

ADVERSE REACTIONS AND SIDE EFFECTS*

CNS: confusion, lethargy, depression.

GI: <u>nausea</u>, <u>vomiting</u>, HEPATITIS, diarrhea, duodenal ulcer.
GU: proteinuria, <u>nephrotoxicity</u>, gonadal suppression.
F and E: hypophosphatemia.
Hemat: leukopenia, thrombocytopenia, anemia.
Metab: HYPOGLYCEMIA (first dose), hyperglycemia, diabetes.
Local: <u>phlebitis</u> at IV site.
Misc: fever.

INTERACTIONS

Drug–Drug: ■ Additive myelosuppression with other **antineoplastic agents** ■ Increased risk of nephrotoxicity with other **nephrotoxic agents (aminoglycoside antibiotics)** ■ Toxicity may be increased by concurrent **phenytoin** therapy ■ May increase the toxicity of **doxorubicin** ■ May decrease antibody response to **live virus vaccines** and increase the risk of adverse reactions.

ROUTE AND DOSAGE

■ **IV (Adults):** 500 mg/m^2/day for 5 days every 6 wk or 1 g/m^2/wk for 2 wk (not to exceed 1.5 g/m^2/dose).

AVAILABILITY

■ *Powder for injection:* 1 g/vial.

TIME/ACTION PROFILE

	ONSET	PEAK	DURATION
IV	UK	1–2 wk	UK
(effects on blood counts)			
IV	17 days	35 days	UK
(tumor response)			

NURSING IMPLICATIONS

ASSESSMENT

▫ Monitor vital signs prior to and periodically during therapy.
▫ Monitor intake and output and daily weight. Notify physician if significant discrepancies or dependent edema occur, as these may indicate nephrotoxicity. Encourage fluids to 3000 ml/day to reduce risk of renal damage.
▫ Monitor IV site carefully and ensure

patency. Discontinue infusion immediately if severe discomfort, erythema along vein, or infiltration occurs. Streptozocin is a vesicant. Tissue ulceration and necrosis may result from infiltration. Notify physician.

▫ Assess for fever, chills, sore throat, and signs of infection. Notify physician if these symptoms occur.

▫ Monitor platelet count throughout therapy. Assess for bleeding (bleeding gums; bruising; petechiae; guaiac stools, urine, and emesis). If thrombocytopenia occurs, avoid IM injections and rectal temperatures and apply pressure to venipuncture sites for 10 min.

▫ Monitor hydration status, appetite, and nutritional intake. Severe, protracted nausea and vomiting may occur 1–4 hr after beginning infusion. Nausea and vomiting may worsen with subsequent doses. Administration of an antiemetic and adjusting diet as tolerated may help maintain fluid and electrolyte balance and nutritional status.

▫ Anemia may occur. Monitor for increased fatigue, dyspnea, and orthostatic hypotension.

▪ **Lab Test Considerations:** Monitor renal status prior to and frequently throughout therapy and for 4 wk after course of therapy. Nephrotoxicity is common and may be manifested by elevated BUN and creatinine, decreased creatinine clearance, and presence of protein in urine. Reduction or discontinuation of streptozocin may allow reversal of renal damage.

▫ Monitor for hepatotoxicity, evidenced by increased AST (SGOT), ALT (SGPT), LDH, serum bilirubin, and alkaline phosphatase or decreased serum albumen at least weekly.

▫ Monitor serum glucose prior to and after initial dose and periodically during therapy.

▫ Monitor serum uric acid prior to and periodically throughout therapy.

▫ Monitor CBC and differential prior to and weekly throughout therapy.

Notify physician of significant decreases.

POTENTIAL NURSING DIAGNOSES
▪ Infection, high risk for (side effects).
▪ Fluid volume, deficit: high risk for (side effects).
▪ Knowledge deficit related to medication regimen (patient/family teaching).

IMPLEMENTATION
▪ **General Info:** IV dextrose should be immediately available, as hypoglycemia may occur in response to initial dose.
▫ Solution is pale gold. Do not use if dark brown. Stable for 12 hr at room temperature, 96 hr at 2–8°C.
▫ Solution should be prepared in a biologic cabinet. Wear gloves, gown, and mask while handling medication. Discard equipment in designated containers (see Appendix I).
▪ **IV:** Reconstitute vial with 9.5 ml of D5W or 0.9% NaCl, for a concentration of 100 mg/ml. May be further diluted in 10–200 ml of D5W or 0.9% NaCl. Do not admix.
▪ *Rate:* Infuse over 10–15 min. Slower infusion rates (45–60 min) have been used to decrease venous irritation. May also be infused over 6 hr.

PATIENT/FAMILY TEACHING
▫ Instruct patient to notify nurse immediately if pain or redness develops at IV site.
▫ Instruct patient to notify nurse immediately if symptoms of hypoglycemia occur (anxiety, chills, cold sweats, confusion, cool pale skin, difficulty in concentration, drowsiness, excessive hunger, headache, irritability, nausea, nervousness, shakiness, unusual tiredness, or weakness).
▫ Instruct patient to notify physician if decreased urine output, swelling of lower extremities, yellowing of skin, fever, chills, sore throat, signs of infection, bleeding gums, bruising, petechiae, or blood in urine, stool, or emesis occurs. Caution patient to avoid crowds and persons with known infections. Instruct patient to

use soft toothbrush and electric razor. Patient should be cautioned not to drink alcoholic beverages or take products containing aspirin or ibuprofen.

□ This drug may cause gonadal suppression; however, patient should still practice birth control. Advise patient to inform physician immediately if pregnancy is suspected.

□ Instruct patient not to receive any vaccinations without advice of physician.

□ Advise patient of need for medical follow-up and frequent lab tests.

EVALUATION

Effectiveness of therapy can be demonstrated by: ■ Decrease in size and spread of tumor.

STRONG IODINE SOLUTION (LUGOL'S SOLUTION)
(eye-oh-dine)

CLASSIFICATION(S):
Antithyroid
Pregnancy Category C

INDICATIONS

■ Adjunct with other antithyroid drugs in preparation for thyroidectomy.

ACTION

■ Rapidly inhibits the release and synthesis of thyroid hormones ■ Decreases the vascularity of the thyroid gland. **Therapeutic Effects:** ■ Control of hyperthyroidism ■ Decreased bleeding during thyroid surgery.

PHARMACOKINETICS

Absorption: Converted in the GI tract and enters the circulation as iodine.
Distribution: Concentrates in the thyroid gland. Crosses the placenta and enters breast milk.
Metabolism and Excretion: Taken up by the thyroid gland.
Half-life: UK.

CONTRAINDICATIONS AND PRECAUTIONS

Contraindicated in: ■ Hypersensitivity.
Use Cautiously in: ■ Tuberculosis ■ Bronchitis ■ Hyperkalemia ■ Impaired renal function ■ Pregnancy and lactation (thyroid abnormalities may be seen in the newborn).

ADVERSE REACTIONS AND SIDE EFFECTS*

Derm: acneform eruptions.
Endo: thyroid hyperplasia, hypothyroidism, hyperthyroidism.
GI: GI irritation, diarrhea.
Misc: hypersensitivity, iodism.

INTERACTIONS

Drug–Drug: ■ Use with **lithium** may cause additive hypothyroidism ■ Increases the antithyroid effect of **antithyroid agents (methimazole, propylthiouracil)** ■ Additive hyperkalemia may result from combined use of potassium iodide with **potassium-sparing diuretics, potassium supplements,** or **angiotensin converting enzyme (ACE) inhibitors.**

ROUTE AND DOSAGE

Preparation for Thyroidectomy
■ PO (Adults and Children): Strong iodine solution 0.1–0.3 ml (3–5 drops) tid.

AVAILABILITY

■ *Oral solution:* 50 mg iodine plus 100 mg potassium iodide/ml.

TIME/ACTION PROFILE (effects on thyroid function testing)

	ONSET	PEAK	DURATION
PO	24 hr	10–15 days	variable

NURSING IMPLICATIONS

ASSESSMENT

□ Assess for signs and symptoms of iodism (metallic taste, stomatitis, skin lesions, cold symptoms, severe GI upset). Report these symptoms to physician promptly.

*Underlines indicate most frequent; **CAPITALS** indicate life-threatening.

□ Monitor response symptoms of hyperthyroidism (tachycardia, palpitations, nervousness, insomnia, diaphoresis, heat intolerance, tremors, weight loss).

□ Monitor for hypersensitivity reaction (rash, pruritus, laryngeal edema, wheezing). Discontinue drug and notify physician immediately if these occur.

▪ **Lab Test Considerations:** Monitor thyroid function tests prior to and periodically during course of therapy.

□ Monitor serum potassium periodically during course of therapy.

POTENTIAL NURSING DIAGNOSES

▪ Knowledge deficit related to medication regimen (patient/family teaching).

IMPLEMENTATION

▪ **PO:** Mix solution in a glass of fruit juice. Administer after meals to minimize GI irritation.

□ Solution is normally clear and colorless. Darkening upon standing does not affect potency of drug.

PATIENT/FAMILY TEACHING

▪ **Hyperthyroidism:** Instruct patient to take medication exactly as directed. Missing a dose may precipitate hyperthyroidism.

□ Instruct patient to report suspected pregnancy to physician before therapy is initiated.

□ Advise patient to confer with physician regarding avoidance of foods high in iodine (seafood, iodized salt, cabbage, kale, turnips).

□ Advise patient to consult physician or pharmacist prior to using over-the-counter cold remedies. Some cold remedies use iodide as an expectorant.

EVALUATION

Effectiveness of therapy can be demonstrated by: ▪ Decrease in size and vascularity of the gland prior to thyroid surgery. Use of iodides in the treatment of hyperthyroidism is usually limited to 2 wk.

STRONTIUM-89 CHLORIDE
(stron-tee-um)
Metastron

CLASSIFICATION(S):
Radiopharmaceutical
Pregnancy Category D

INDICATIONS

▪ Management of bone pain in patients with painful skeletal metastases.

ACTION

▪ Preferentially taken up by bone tumors and metastatic bone lesions, where selective irradiation takes place. **Therapeutic Effect:** ▪ Decreased pain from boney metastases. Due to delayed onset, adequate analgesia should be provided until effects of strontium are evident.

PHARMACOKINETICS

Absorption: IV administration results in complete bioavailability.

Distribution: Taken up and is selectively retained by metastatic bone lesions.

Metabolism and Excretion: 67% excreted in urine, 33% in feces.

Half-life: (physical half-life) 50.5 days.

CONTRAINDICATIONS AND PRECAUTIONS

Contraindicated in: ▪ Lactation ▪ Pregnancy.

Use Cautiously in: ▪ Women with childbearing potential ▪ Children <18 yr (safety not established) ▪ Patients with platelet counts <60,000 mm^3 or WBCs <2400 mm^3 ▪ Diminished bone marrow reserve or other chronic debilitating illness ▪ Patients with a life expectancy <1–3 wk.

ADVERSE REACTIONS AND SIDE EFFECTS*

Hemat: neutropenia, thrombocytopenia, anemia.

MS: transient increase in bone pain.

S

---

*Underlines indicate most frequent; **CAPITALS** indicate life-threatening.

INTERACTIONS

Drug–Drug: ▪ Additive bone marrow toxicity with **antineoplastic agents** or **radiation therapy**.

ROUTE AND DOSAGE

▪ **IV (Adults):** 148 MBq, 4 mCi or 1.5–2.2 MBq/kg, 40–60 mCi/kg, not to be repeated any sooner than 90 days.

AVAILABILITY

▪ **Radioactive injection:** 10.9–22.6 mg/ml (148 MBq, 4 mCi) in 10-ml vials.

TIME/ACTION PROFILE (pain relief)

	ONSET	PEAK	DURATION
IV	7–20 days	variable	variable

NURSING IMPLICATIONS

ASSESSMENT

□ Assess pain (intensity, location) periodically throughout therapy. Patient may experience a transient increase in bone pain for 2–3 days beginning 2–3 days after administration. This is normal, and increasing analgesic doses may be required. Pain should begin to diminish after 1–2 wk or longer and may allow for reduction or discontinuation of analgesics. Effects may continue for several months.

▪ **Lab Test Considerations:** Monitor hematologic parameters (WBC, platelets) at least once every other week during therapy. Platelets are usually decreased 30% from preadministration levels. The nadir of thrombocytopenia is 12–16 wk. Leukopenia may also occur. Recovery to preadministration levels usually occurs within 6 mo.

POTENTIAL NURSING DIAGNOSES

▪ Pain (indications).
▪ Knowledge deficit related to medication regimen (patient/family teaching).

IMPLEMENTATION

▪ **General Info:** Should be administered only by physicians trained and experienced in the safe use and administration of radiopharmaceuticals who have been approved by the appropriate governmental agency to license the use of radionuclides.

□ Perform urinary catheterization on incontinent patients prior to administration to minimize the risk of radioactive contamination of clothing, bed linen, and the patient's environment.

▪ **Direct IV:** Administered by slow injection over 1–2 min. A flushing sensation may be experienced following a rapid (<30 sec) injection.

PATIENT/FAMILY TEACHING

□ Instruct patient to continue taking pain medication until strontium-89 becomes effective. Physician may then advise patient to gradually decrease analgesics.

□ Advise patient that no change in eating or drinking is necessary. Alcohol and caffeine need not be avoided unless advised by physician.

□ Strontium-89 is present in the blood and urine for 1 wk following injection. Caution patient to take the following precautions for the first week: (1) Use a normal toilet rather than a urinal if possible; flush twice; (2) Wipe up any spilled urine with a tissue and flush it away; (3) Always wash hands after using the toilet; (4) Immediately wash any linen or clothes that become stained with urine or blood. Wash them separately from other clothes and rinse thoroughly; (5) If any urine collection device is used, follow the instructions on its use; (6) Wash away any spilled blood if a cut occurs.

□ Instruct patient to notify any health care practitioner or caregiver of strontium-89 therapy prior to treatment.

□ Advise patient to contact physician if the effects of strontium-89 decrease and pain returns.

□ Emphasize the importance of periodic blood tests.

EVALUATION

Effectiveness of therapy can be determined by: ▪ Decrease in pain due to bony metastases. Repeat administration is based on patient's response to therapy, current symptoms, and hematologic status. Repeat doses are not recommended at intervals of <90 days.

SUCCIMER
(sux-i-mer)
Chemet

CLASSIFICATION(S):
Antidote (lead chelator)
Pregnancy Category C

INDICATIONS
- Treatment of lead poisoning in children with blood lead levels >45 mcg/dl.

ACTION
- Forms a water-soluble compound with lead allowing urinary elimination of excessive amounts of lead. **Therapeutic Effect:** - Decreased blood lead levels and decreased target organ damage in lead poisoning.

PHARMACOKINETICS
Absorption: Rapidly but variably absorbed following oral administration.
Distribution: Distribution not known.
Metabolism and Excretion: Extensively metabolized. 10% excreted unchanged by the kidneys.
Half-life: 2 days.

CONTRAINDICATIONS AND PRECAUTIONS
Contraindicated in: - Hypersensitivity or allergy to succimer - Lactation (should be discouraged during succimer therapy).
Use Cautiously in: - Pregnancy or children <1 yr (safety not established) - Renal failure (chelates are not dialyzable).

ADVERSE REACTIONS AND SIDE EFFECTS*
CNS: headache, drowsiness, dizziness.
EENT: cloudy film in eye, plugged ears, otitis media, watery eyes.
Resp: sore throat, rhinorrhea, nasal congestion, cough.

CV: arrhythmias.
GI: <u>nausea</u>, <u>vomiting</u>, diarrhea, anorexia, hemorrhoidal symptoms, metallic taste, elevated liver function tests, abdominal cramps.
GU: oliguria, voiding difficulty, proteinuria.
Derm: rashes, mucocutaneous eruptions, pruritus.
Hemat: thrombocytosis, eosinophilia.
MS: back, rib, flank pain; leg pain.
Neuro: paresthesia, sensorimotor neuropathy.
Misc: chills, fever, flu-like syndrome, moniliasis.

INTERACTIONS
Drug–Drug: - Not recommended for use with other **chelating agents**.

ROUTE AND DOSAGE
- **PO (Adults and Children):** 10 mg/kg (350 mg/m^2) q 8 hr for 5 days, then reduce to 10 mg/kg (350 mg/m^2) q 12 hr for 2 more wk. Repeated courses should follow a 2-wk rest period.

AVAILABILITY
- **Capsules:** 100 mg.

TIME/ACTION PROFILE (urinary lead excretion)

	ONSET	PEAK	DURATION
PO	within 2 hr	2–4 hr	8–12 hr

NURSING IMPLICATIONS
ASSESSMENT
- Assess patient and family members for evidence of lead poisoning prior to and frequently throughout course of therapy. Acute lead poisoning is characterized by a metallic taste, colicky abdominal pain, vomiting, diarrhea, oliguria, and coma. Symptoms of chronic poisoning vary with severity and include anorexia, a blue-black line along the gums, intermittent vomiting, paresthesia, encephalopathy, seizures, and coma.
- Monitor strict intake and output and daily weight. Notify physician of

*<u>Underlines</u> indicate most frequent; **CAPITALS** indicate life-threatening.

any discrepancies. Patients undergoing succimer therapy should be adequately hydrated.

□ Monitor neurologic status closely (level of consciousness, pupil response, movement). Notify physician immediately of any changes.

□ Monitor patient for signs of allergic or other mucocutaneous reactions, especially during repeated courses of succimer therapy.

■ **Lab Test Considerations:** Monitor blood and urine lead levels prior to and periodically throughout therapy. After therapy, monitor patients for rebound of blood levels at least once weekly until stable. Succimer is indicated for treatment of blood lead levels of >45 mcg/dl.

□ May cause elevated serum transaminases, alkaline phosphatase, and cholesterol; monitor prior to and at least weekly during therapy.

□ May interfere with serum and urine lab tests.

POTENTIAL NURSING DIAGNOSES

■ Injury, high risk for: poisoning (indications, patient/family teaching).

■ Home maintenance management, impaired (indications).

■ Knowledge deficit related to medication regimen (patient/family teaching).

IMPLEMENTATION

■ **General Info:** Coadministration of succimer with other chelation agents is not recommended. Patients who have received EDTA or BAL may receive subsequent therapy with succimer after 4 wk.

□ Course of treatment lasts 19 days. Doses are administered every 8 hr for 5 days and then every 12 hr for 14 days. Unless blood levels indicate prompt treatment is needed, a minimum of 2 wk between courses is recommended.

■ **PO:** If patient is unable to swallow the capsule, open capsule and sprinkle medicated beads on a small amount of soft food or place in a spoon and follow with a fruit drink.

PATIENT/FAMILY TEACHING

□ Discuss need for follow-up appointments to monitor lead levels. Additional treatments may be necessary.

□ Instruct patient to drink adequate fluids throughout therapy.

□ Advise patient to notify physician if rash occurs.

□ Consult public health department regarding potential sources of lead poisoning in the home, workplace, and recreational areas. Chelation therapy cannot be used as prophylaxis for lead poisoning.

EVALUATION

Effectiveness of therapy can be demonstrated by: ■ Decrease in symptoms of lead poisoning □ Decrease in blood lead levels to below 45 mcg/dl although the normal upper limit is 29 mcg/dl.

SUCCINYLCHOLINE
(sux-sin-il-**koe**-leen)
Anectine, Quelicin, Sucostrin, Suxamethonium

CLASSIFICATION(S):
Neuromuscular blocking agent (depolarizing)
Pregnancy Category UK

INDICATIONS

■ Used after induction of anesthesia in surgical procedures to produce skeletal muscle paralysis.

ACTION

■ Prevents neuromuscular transmission by blocking the effect of acetylcholine at the myoneural junction ■ Has agonist activity initially, producing fasciculation ■ Causes the release of histamine ■ Has no analgesic or anxiolytic effects. **Therapeutic Effect:** ■ Skeletal muscle paralysis.

PHARMACOKINETICS

Absorption: Well absorbed following deep IM administration.
Distribution: Widely distributed into

extracellular fluid. Crosses the placenta in small amounts.

Metabolism and Excretion: 90% metabolized by pseudocholinesterase in plasma. 10% excreted unchanged by the kidneys.

Half-life: UK.

CONTRAINDICATIONS AND PRECAUTIONS

Contraindicated in: ▪ Hypersensitivity to succinylcholine or parabens ▪ Plasma pseudocholinesterase deficiency ▪ Children and neonates (continuous infusions).

Use Cautiously in: ▪ History of malignant hyperthermia ▪ History of pulmonary disease, renal or liver impairment ▪ Elderly or debilitated patients ▪ Glaucoma ▪ Electrolyte disturbances ▪ Patients receiving cardiac glycosides ▪ Fractures or muscular spasm ▪ Myasthenia gravis or myasthenic syndromes ▪ Has been used in pregnant women undergoing cesarean section ▪ Neonates and children (increased risk of malignant hyperthermia).

ADVERSE REACTIONS AND SIDE EFFECTS*

Most adverse reactions to succinylcholine are extensions of pharmacologic effects.

CV: hypotension, arrhythmias.

Resp: bronchospasm, apnea.

F and E: hyperkalemia.

MS: muscle fasciculation.

Misc: MALIGNANT HYPERTHERMIA.

INTERACTIONS

Drug–Drug: ▪ Concurrent administration of **cholinesterase inhibitors (ecothiophate, isofluorophate,** and **demecarium eyedrops)** reduces pseudocholinesterase activity and intensifies paralysis ▪ Intensity and duration of paralysis may be prolonged by pretreatment with **general anesthesia, aminoglycoside antibiotics, polymyxin B, colistin, clindamycin, lidocaine, quinidine, procainamide, beta-adrenergic**

blocking agents, potassium-losing diuretics, and **magnesium**.

ROUTE AND DOSAGE

IV route is preferred, but deep IM injection may be used in children and patients without vascular access.

Test Dose
▪ **IV (Adults):** 5–10 mg (0.1 mg/kg), then assess respiratory function.

Short Procedures
▪ **IV (Adults):** 0.6 mg/kg (range 0.3–1.1 mg/kg); additional doses depend on response.
▪ **IV (Children):** 1–2 mg/kg; additional doses depend on response.

Prolonged Procedures
▪ **IV (Adults):** 2.5 mg/min infusion (range 0.5–10 mg/min) or 0.6 mg/kg (range 0.3–1.1 mg/kg) initially, then 0.04–0.07 mg/kg as necessary.

Intramuscular Dosing
▪ **IM (Adults):** 2.5–4 mg/kg (total dose not to exceed 150 mg).
▪ **IM (Children):** Up to 2.5 mg/kg (total dose not to exceed 150 mg).

AVAILABILITY

▪ *Injection:* 20 mg/ml, 50 mg/ml, 100 mg/ml ▪ *Powder for injection:* 100 mg/vial ▪ *Powder for infusion:* 500 mg/vial, 1 g/vial.

TIME/ACTION PROFILE (skeletal muscle paralysis)

	ONSET	PEAK	DURATION
IM	up to 3 min	UK	10–30 min
IV	0.5–1 min	1–2 min	4–10 min

NURSING IMPLICATIONS

ASSESSMENT

▫ Assess respiratory status continuously throughout use of succinylcholine. Succinylcholine should be used only by individuals experienced in endotracheal intubation, and equipment for this procedure should be immediately available.

▫ Monitor neuromuscular response to succinylcholine with a peripheral

S

nerve stimulator intraoperatively. Paralysis is initially selective and usually occurs consecutively in the following muscles: levator muscles of eyelids, muscles of mastication, limb muscles, abdominal muscles, muscles of the glottis, intercostal muscles, and the diaphragm.

□ Monitor ECG, heart rate, and blood pressure throughout use of succinylcholine.

□ Assess patient for history of malignant hyperthermia prior to administration. Monitor for signs of malignant hyperthermia (tachycardia, tachypnea, hypercarbia, jaw muscle spasm, lack of laryngeal relaxation, hyperthermia) throughout administration.

□ Observe patient for residual muscle weakness and respiratory distress during the recovery period.

▪ **Lab Test Considerations:** May cause hyperkalemia, especially in patients with severe trauma, burns, or neurologic disorders.

▪ **Toxicity and Overdose:** If overdose occurs, use peripheral nerve stimulator to determine degree of neuromuscular blockade. Maintain airway patency and ventilation until recovery of normal respirations occurs.

POTENTIAL NURSING DIAGNOSES
▪ Breathing pattern, ineffective (indications).
▪ Communication, impaired verbal (side effects).

IMPLEMENTATION
▪ **General Info:** Succinylcholine has no effect on consciousness or the pain threshold. Adequate anesthesia should *always* be used when succinylcholine is used as an adjunct to surgical procedures or when painful procedures are performed. Benzodiazepines and/or analgesics should be administered concurrently when prolonged succinylcholine therapy is used for ventilator patients, as patient is awake and able to feel all sensations.

□ If eyes remain open throughout prolonged administration, protect corneas with artificial tears.

□ To prevent excessive salivation, patients may be premedicated with atropine or scopolamine.

□ A small dose of a nondepolarizing agent may be used prior to succinylcholine to decrease the severity of muscle fasciculations.

▪ **IM:** If IM route is used, administer deep into the deltoid muscle.

▪ **IV:** A test dose of 5–10 mg or 0.1 mg/kg may be administered to determine patient's sensitivity and recovery time.

▪ **Direct IV:** Usual adult dose is administered over 10–30 sec. Dose is titrated to patient response.

▪ **Continuous Infusion:** Dilute as a 0.1–0.2% solution (1–2 mg/ml) in dextrose/Ringer's or lactated Ringer's combinations, dextrose/saline combinations, 0.45% NaCl, 0.9% NaCl, D5W, D10W, Ringer's or lactated Ringer's injection. Solution is stable for 24 hr at room temperature. Administer only clear solutions. Discard any unused solution.

▪ *Rate:* Administer at a rate of 0.5–10 mg/min. Titrate dose to patient response and degree of relaxation required.

▪ **Syringe Compatibility:** ▪ heparin.

▪ **Y-Site Compatibility:** ▪ potassium chloride ▪ vitamin B complex with C.

▪ **Additive Compatibility:** ▪ amikacin ▪ cephapirin ▪ meperidine ▪ morphine ▪ scopolamine.

▪ **Additive Incompatibility:** ▪ barbiturates ▪ nafcillin ▪ sodium bicarbonate.

PATIENT/FAMILY TEACHING
□ Explain all procedures to patient receiving succinylcholine therapy without anesthesia, as consciousness is not affected by succinylcholine alone. Provide emotional support.

□ Reassure patient that communication abilities will return as the medication wears off.

EVALUATION

Effectiveness of therapy can be demonstrated by: ■ Adequate suppression of the twitch response when tested with peripheral nerve stimulation with subsequent muscle paralysis.

SUCRALFATE
(soo-**kral**-fate)
Carafate, {Sulcrate}

CLASSIFICATION(S):
Antiulcer agent (protectant)
Pregnancy Category B

INDICATIONS

■ Short-term management of duodenal ulcers ■ Maintenance (preventive) therapy of duodenal ulcer. **Unlabeled Uses:** ■ Management of gastric ulcer or gastroesophageal reflux ■ Prevention of aspirin-induced gastric mucosal injury due to high-dose aspirin or nonsteroidal anti-inflammatory agents in patients with rheumatoid arthritis.

ACTION

■ Reacts with gastric acid to form a thick paste, which selectively adheres to the ulcer surface. **Therapeutic Effect:** ■ Protection of ulcers, with subsequent healing.

PHARMACOKINETICS

Absorption: Systemic absorption is minimal (<5%).
Distribution: Distribution not known.
Metabolism and Excretion: >90% is eliminated in the feces.
Half-life: 6–20 hr.

CONTRAINDICATIONS AND PRECAUTIONS

Contraindicated in: ■ Hypersensitivity. **Use Cautiously in:** ■ Children (safety not established).

ADVERSE REACTIONS AND SIDE EFFECTS*

CNS: dizziness, vertigo, sleepiness.

GI: constipation, diarrhea, nausea, gastric discomfort, indigestion, dry mouth.
Derm: rashes, pruritus.

INTERACTIONS

Drug–Drug: ■ May decrease the absorption of **phenytoin, fat-soluble vitamins,** or **tetracycline** ■ Concurrent **antacids** decrease the effectiveness of sucralfate ■ Decreases absorption of **fluoroquinolones** (avoid concurrent use).

ROUTE AND DOSAGE

Treatment of Ulcers
■ **PO (Adults):** 1 g qid, 1 hr before meals and at bedtime.

Prevention of Ulcers
■ **PO (Adults):** 1 g twice daily 1 hr before a meal.

Gastroesophageal Reflux
■ **PO (Adults):** 1 g qid, 1 hr before meals and at bedtime.
■ **PO (Children):** 500 mg–1 g qid, 1 hr before meals and at bedtime.

AVAILABILITY

■ *Tablets:* 1 g ■ {*Oral suspension:* 500 mg/5 ml}.

TIME/ACTION PROFILE (mucosal protectant effect)

	ONSET	PEAK	DURATION
PO	30 min	UK	5 hr

NURSING IMPLICATIONS

ASSESSMENT

□ Assess patient routinely for abdominal pain and frank or occult blood in the stool.

POTENTIAL NURSING DIAGNOSES

■ Pain (indications).
■ Constipation (side effects).
■ Knowledge deficit related to medication regimen (patient/family teaching).

IMPLEMENTATION

■ **PO:** Administer on an empty stomach, 1 hr before meals and at bedtime. Do not crush or chew tablets. If nasogas-

{} = Available in Canada only.

*Underlines indicate most frequent; **CAPITALS** indicate life-threatening.

tric administration is required, consult pharmacist for diluent, as sucralfate is relatively insoluble and may form a bezoar.

◻ If antacids are also prescribed, do not administer within 30 min before or 1 hr after sucralfate dosage.

PATIENT/FAMILY TEACHING

◻ Advise patient to continue with course of therapy for 4–8 wk, even if feeling better, to ensure ulcer healing. If a dose is missed, take as soon as remembered unless almost time for next dose; do not double doses.

◻ Advise patient that increase in fluid intake, dietary bulk, and exercise may prevent drug-induced constipation.

◻ Inform patient that cessation of smoking may help prevent recurrence of duodenal ulcers.

◻ Emphasize the importance of routine examinations to monitor progress.

EVALUATION

Effectiveness of therapy can be demonstrated by: ▪ Decrease in abdominal pain ◻ Healing of duodenal ulcers, seen by x-ray examination and endoscopy.

SUFENTANIL
(soo-**fen**-ta-nil)
Sufenta

CLASSIFICATION(S):
Opioid analgesic (agonist)
Schedule II
Pregnancy Category C

INDICATIONS

▪ Analgesic adjunct when given in the maintenance of balanced anesthesia with barbiturate/nitrous oxide/oxygen ▪ Analgesic administered by continuous IV infusion with nitrous oxide/oxygen while maintaining general anesthesia ▪ Primary induction of anesthesia with 100% oxygen in major surgical procedures.

ACTION

▪ Binds to opiate receptors in the CNS, altering the response to and perception of pain and causing generalized CNS depression. **Therapeutic Effects:** ▪ Decreased intensity of moderate to severe pain ▪ Anesthesia.

PHARMACOKINETICS

Absorption: Following IV administration absorption is essentially complete.
Distribution: Does not readily penetrate adipose tissue. Crosses the placenta, enters breast milk.
Metabolism and Excretion: Mostly metabolized by the liver. Some metabolism in small intestine.
Half-life: 2.7 hr (increased during cardiopulmonary bypass).

CONTRAINDICATIONS AND PRECAUTIONS

Contraindicated in: ▪ Hypersensitivity ▪ Known intolerance.
Use Cautiously in: ▪ Elderly patients ▪ Debilitated or severely ill patients ▪ Diabetic patients ▪ Severe pulmonary disease ▪ Hepatic disease ▪ CNS tumors ▪ Increased intracranial pressure ▪ Head trauma ▪ Adrenal insufficiency ▪ Undiagnosed abdominal pain ▪ Hypothyroidism ▪ Alcoholism ▪ Cardiac disease (arrhythmias) ▪ Pregnancy (has been used in women undergoing cesarean section—drowsiness may occur in infant) ▪ Lactation (safety not established).

ADVERSE REACTIONS AND SIDE EFFECTS*

CNS: dizziness, sleepiness, drowsiness.
EENT: blurred vision.
Resp: apnea, postoperative respiratory depression.
CV: bradycardia, tachycardia, hypotension, hypertension, arrhythmias.
GI: nausea, vomiting.
Derm: itching, erythema.
MS: thoracic muscle rigidity, intraoperative muscle movement.
Misc: chills.

*Underlines indicate most frequent; **CAPITALS** indicate life-threatening.

INTERACTIONS

Drug–Drug: ▪ Concurrent use of **alcohol, antihistamines, antidepressants,** or **sedative/hypnotics** results in additive CNS depression ▪ **MAO inhibitors** should be avoided for 14 days prior to use ▪ **Cimetidine** or **erythromycin** may prolong duration of recovery ▪ Concurrent use of **benzodiazepines** may increase the risk of hypotension ▪ **Nalbuphine** or **pentazocine** may decrease response to sufentanil.

ROUTE AND DOSAGE

Low-Dose Anesthesia Adjunct
▪ **IV (Adults):** 0.5–1 mcg/kg initially, supplemental doses of 10–25 mcg may be given as needed (not to exceed 1 mcg/kg/hr when administered with nitrous oxide and oxygen).

Moderate-Dose Anesthesia Adjunct
▪ **IV (Adults):** 2–8 mcg/kg initially, supplemental doses of 10–50 mcg may be given as needed (not to exceed 1 mcg/kg/hr when administered with nitrous oxide and oxygen).

Primary Anesthesia (with 100% Oxygen)
▪ **IV (Adults):** 8–30 mcg/kg initially, supplemental doses of 25–50 mcg may be given as needed.
▪ **IV (Children):** *Cardiovascular surgery*—10–25 mcg/kg initially, followed by maintenance doses of up to 25–50 mcg.

AVAILABILITY
▪ *Injection:* 50 mcg/ml.

TIME/ACTION PROFILE (analgesia)

	ONSET	PEAK	DURATION
IV	within 1 min	UK	5 min

NURSING IMPLICATIONS

ASSESSMENT
▢ Monitor respiratory rate and blood pressure frequently throughout course of therapy. Notify physician of significant changes immediately. The respiratory depressant effects of sufentanil last longer than the analgesic effects. Subsequent opioid doses should be reduced by ¼–⅓ of the usually recommended dose. Monitor closely.
▪ **Lab Test Considerations:** May cause elevated serum amylase and lipase concentrations.
▪ **Toxicity and Overdose:** If overdose occurs, naloxone (Narcan) is the antidote.

POTENTIAL NURSING DIAGNOSES
▪ Pain (indications).
▪ Breathing pattern, ineffective (adverse reactions).
▪ Injury, high risk for (side effects).

IMPLEMENTATION
▪ **General Info:** Benzodiazepines may be administered prior to administration of sufentanil to reduce the induction dose requirements and to decrease the time until loss of consciousness. This combination may increase the risk of hypotension.
▢ Opioid antagonist, oxygen, and resuscitative equipment should be readily available during the administration of sufentanil.
▪ **Direct IV:** Slow IV administration may reduce the incidence or severity of muscle rigidity, bradycardia, or hypotension.
▪ *Rate:* Administer slowly, over at least 1–2 min.
▪ **Continuous Infusion:** When used as a primary anesthetic agent, a continuous infusion of sufentanil may be administered with or following the initial loading dose to provide immediate and sustained effects throughout a prolonged surgical procedure.

PATIENT/FAMILY TEACHING
▢ Caution patient to make position changes slowly to minimize orthostatic hypotension.
▢ Medication causes dizziness and drowsiness. Advise patient to call for assistance during ambulation and transfer, and to avoid driving or other activities requiring alertness for at least 24 hr after administration of sufentanil following outpatient surgery and until response to medication is known.

□ Instruct patient to avoid alcohol or other CNS depressants for 24 hr after administration of sufentanil following outpatient surgery.

EVALUATION

Effectiveness of therapy can be demonstrated by: ■ General quiescence □ Reduced motor activity □ Pronounced analgesia.

SULFAMETHOXAZOLE
(sul-fa-meth-**ox**-a-zole)
{Apo-Sulfamethoxazole}, Gantanol, Gantanol DS

CLASSIFICATION(S):
Anti-infective (sulfonamide)
Pregnancy Category C

INDICATIONS

■ Treatment of: □ Urinary tract infections □ Nocardiosis □ Toxoplasmosis and malaria (in combination with other anti-infectives).

ACTION

■ Interferes with bacterial folic acid synthesis. **Therapeutic Effect:** ■ Bacteriostatic action against susceptible bacteria. **Spectrum:** ■ Notable for activity against some gram-positive pathogens, including: □ Streptococci and staphylococci □ *Clostridium perfringens* □ *Clostridium tetani* □ *Nocardia aster-oides* ■ Active against some gram-negative pathogens, including: □ *Enterobacter* □ *Escherichia coli* □ *Klebsiella* □ *Proteus mirabilis* □ *Proteus vulgaris* □ *Salmonella* □ *Shigella*.

PHARMACOKINETICS

Absorption: Well absorbed following oral administration.
Distribution: Widely distributed. Crosses the placenta and enters breast milk.
Metabolism and Excretion: Mostly metabolized by the liver. 20% excreted unchanged by the kidneys.
Half-life: 7–12 hr.

CONTRAINDICATIONS AND PRECAUTIONS

Contraindicated in: ■ Hypersensitivity ■ Glucose-6-phosphate dehydrogenase (G6PD deficiency) ■ Porphyria ■ Pregnancy or lactation ■ Infants <2 mo (unless treating congenital toxoplasmosis).
Use Cautiously in: ■ Severe renal or hepatic impairment.

ADVERSE REACTIONS AND SIDE EFFECTS*

CNS: dizziness, ataxia, depression, confusion, psychosis, ataxia, drowsiness, restlessness.
GI: anorexia, nausea, vomiting, hepatitis.
GU: crystalluria.
Derm: rashes, exfoliative dermatitis, photosensitivity.
Hemat: APLASTIC ANEMIA, thrombocytopenia, AGRANULOCYTOSIS, eosinophilia.
Neuro: peripheral neuropathy.
Misc: superinfection, fever, hypersensitivity reactions, including STEVENS-JOHNSON SYNDROME and serum sickness.

INTERACTIONS

Drug–Drug: ■ May enhance the action and increase the risk of toxicity from **oral hypoglycemic agents, phenytoin, methotrexate, anticoagulants,** or **zidovudine** ■ Concurrent use with **methenamine** may increase the risk of crystalluria ■ Increased risk of drug-induced hepatitis with other **hepatotoxic agents**.

ROUTE AND DOSAGE

■ **PO (Adults):** 2 g initially, then 1 g q 8–12 hr.
■ **PO (Children >2 mo):** 50–60 mg/kg initially (not to exceed 2 g), then 25–30 mg/kg q 12 hr (not to exceed 75 mg/kg/day).

AVAILABILITY

- **Tablets:** 500 mg ▪ **Oral suspension:** 500 mg/5 ml ▪ **In combination with:** trimethoprim (see Trimethoprim/Sulfamethoxazole monograph) and phenazopyridine (Azo-Gantanol). See Appendix A.

TIME/ACTION PROFILE (blood levels)

	ONSET	PEAK
PO	1 hr	2 hr

NURSING IMPLICATIONS

ASSESSMENT

- Assess patient for infection (vital signs, appearance of wound, sputum, urine, and stool; WBC) at beginning and throughout course of therapy.
- Obtain specimens for culture and sensitivity prior to initiating therapy. First dose may be given before receiving results.
- Assess patient for allergy to sulfonamides.
- Monitor intake and output ratios. Fluid intake should be sufficient to maintain a urine output of at least 1200–1500 ml daily to prevent crystalluria and stone formation.
- **Lab Test Considerations:** Monitor CBC and urinalysis periodically throughout therapy.
- May produce elevated serum bilirubin, creatinine, and alkaline phosphatase concentrations.

POTENTIAL NURSING DIAGNOSES

- Infection, high risk for (indications, side effects).
- Knowledge deficit related to medication regimen (patient/family teaching).
- Noncompliance related to medication regimen (patient/family teaching).

IMPLEMENTATION

- **PO:** Administer around the clock on an empty stomach, at least 1 hr before or 2 hr after meals, with a full glass of water. Tablets may be crushed and taken with fluid of patient's choice for

patients with difficulty swallowing. Use calibrated measuring device for liquid preparations.

PATIENT/FAMILY TEACHING

- Instruct patient to take medication around the clock and to finish the drug completely as directed, even if feeling better. If a dose is missed, it should be taken as soon as remembered. Advise patient that sharing of this medication may be dangerous.
- May cause dizziness. Caution patient to avoid driving or other activities requiring alertness until response to medication is known.
- Caution patient to use sunscreen and protective clothing to prevent photosensitivity reactions.
- Advise patient to notify physician if skin rash, sore throat, fever, mouth sores, or unusual bleeding or bruising occurs.
- Instruct patient to notify physician if symptoms do not improve within a few days. Emphasize the importance of follow-up examinations to monitor progress and side effects.

EVALUATION

Clinical response can be evaluated by:
- Resolution of the signs and symptoms of infection. Length of time for complete resolution depends on the organism and site of infection.

SULFASALAZINE
(sul-fa-**sal**-a-zeen)
Azulfidine, {PMS Sulfasalazine}, {Salazopyrin}, S.A.S.-500

CLASSIFICATION(S):
Anti-infective (sulfonamide), Gastrointestinal (anti-inflammatory)
Pregnancy Category B

INDICATIONS

- Used with other treatment modalities (glucocorticoids, diet) in the management of ulcerative colitis.

{} = Available in Canada only.

ACTION

- May have mild local antibacterial and anti-inflammatory properties in the colon. **Therapeutic Effect:** - Reduction in symptoms of ulcerative colitis.

PHARMACOKINETICS

Absorption: 10–15% absorbed following oral administration.
Distribution: Widely distributed. Crosses the placenta and enters breast milk.
Metabolism and Excretion: Split by intestinal bacteria into sulfapyridine and 5-aminosalicylic acid. Some of absorbed sulfasalazine is excreted by bile back into intestine. 15% excreted unchanged by the kidneys. Sulfapyridine also excreted mostly by the kidneys.
Half-life: 6 hr.

CONTRAINDICATIONS AND PRECAUTIONS

Contraindicated in: - Hypersensitivity reactions to sulfonamides or salicylates
- Cross-sensitivity with furosemide, sulfonylurea hypoglycemic agents, or carbonic anhydrase inhibitors may exist - G6PD deficiency - Urinary tract or intestinal obstruction - Children <2 yr
- Porphyria.
Use Cautiously in: - Severe hepatic or renal impairment - Pregnancy (has been used safely) - Lactation (safety not established).

ADVERSE REACTIONS AND SIDE EFFECTS*

CNS: headache, dizziness, ataxia, depression, confusion, psychosis, drowsiness, restlessness.
Resp: pneumonitis.
GI: anorexia, nausea, diarrhea, vomiting, hepatitis.
GU: crystalluria, oligospermia, infertility, orange-yellow discoloration of urine.
Derm: rashes, yellow discoloration, exfoliative dermatitis, photosenstivity.
Hemat: megaloblastic anemia, APLASTIC ANEMIA, thrombocytopenia, AGRANULOCYTOSIS, eosinophilia.

Neuro: peripheral neuropathy.
Misc: fever, hypersensitivity reactions, including STEVENS-JOHNSON SYNDROME and serum sickness.

INTERACTIONS

Drug–Drug: - May enhance the action and increase the risk of toxicity from **oral hypoglycemic agents, phenytoin, methotrexate, zidovudine,** or **oral anticoagulants** - Increased risk of drug-induced hepatitis with other **hepatotoxic agents** - Increased risk of crystalluria with **methenamine.**
Drug–Food: - May decrease **iron** and **folic acid** absorption.

ROUTE AND DOSAGE

- **PO (Adults):** 3–4 g/day in 3–4 divided doses initially, then 500 mg 4 times daily as maintenance.
- **PO (Children >2 yr):** 40–60 mg/kg/day in 3–6 divided doses, initially, maintenance dose of 30 mg/kg/day in 4 divided doses (not to exceed 2 g/day).

AVAILABILITY

- *Tablets:* 500 mg - *Enteric-coated tablets:* 500 mg - *Oral suspension:* 250 mg/5 ml.

TIME/ACTION PROFILE (blood levels)

	ONSET	PEAK
PO	1 hr	1.5–6 hr

NURSING IMPLICATIONS

ASSESSMENT

- ▢ Assess frequency, quantity, and consistency of stools and abdominal pain at beginning and throughout course of therapy.
- ▢ Assess patient for allergy to sulfonamides and salicylates.
- ▢ Monitor intake and output ratios. Fluid intake should be sufficient to maintain a urine output of at least 1200–1500 ml daily to prevent crystalluria and stone formation.
- ▢ Proctoscopy and sigmoidoscopy may be required periodically during treat-

*Underlines indicate most frequent; **CAPITALS** indicate life-threatening.

ment to determine patient response and dosage adjustments.

- **Lab Test Considerations:** Monitor CBC prior to and monthly during prolonged therapy. Discontinue sulfasalazine if blood dyscrasias occur.
- □ Monitor urinalysis prior to and periodically throughout therapy for crystalluria and urinary cell calculi formation.

POTENTIAL NURSING DIAGNOSES

- Pain (indications).
- Diarrhea (indications).
- Knowledge deficit related to medication regimen (patient/family teaching).

IMPLEMENTATION

- **General Info:** Varying dosing regimens may be used to minimize GI side effects.
- **PO:** Administer after meals or with food to minimize GI irritation, with a full glass of water. Do not crush or chew enteric-coated tablets. Shake oral suspension well prior to administration. Use a calibrated measuring device to measure liquid preparations.

PATIENT/FAMILY TEACHING

- □ Instruct patient to take medication as directed, even if feeling better. If a dose is missed, it should be taken as soon as remembered unless almost time for next dose.
- □ May cause dizziness. Caution patient to avoid driving or other activities that require alertness until response to medication is known.
- □ Caution patient to use sunscreen and protective clothing to prevent photosensitivity reactions.
- □ Inform patient that this medication may cause orange-yellow discoloration of urine and skin, which is not significant. May permanently stain contact lenses yellow.
- □ Advise patient to notify physician if skin rash, sore throat, fever, mouth sores, or unusual bleeding or bruising occurs.

- □ Instruct patient to notify physician if symptoms do not improve after 1–2 mo of therapy.

EVALUATION

Clinical response can be evaluated by:
- Decrease in diarrhea and abdominal pain □ Return to normal bowel habits in inflammatory bowel disease.

SULFINPYRAZONE
(sul-fin-**peer**-a-zone)
{Antazone}, Antiple, {Anturan}, Anturane, {Apo-Sulfinpyrazone}, {Novopyrazone}

CLASSIFICATION(S):
Antigout agent (uricosuric)
Pregnancy Category UK

S

INDICATIONS

- Management (long-term) of gout. **Unlabeled Use:** ▪ Used as an antiplatelet agent in the prevention of myocardial infarction.

ACTION

- Decreases serum uric acid levels by decreasing renal reabsorption and subsequently increasing urinary excretion ▪ Decreases platelet aggregation ▪ Increases platelet survival. **Therapeutic Effect:** ▪ Prevention of gouty attacks by keeping serum uric acid levels lowered.

PHARMACOKINETICS

Absorption: Well absorbed following oral administration.

Distribution: Distribution to tissues not known.

Metabolism and Excretion: Mostly metabolized by the liver. Converted to compounds with uricosuric (parahydroxy-sulfinpyrazone) and antiplatelet activity (sulfide metabolite).

Half-life: 3 hr (1 hr for parahydroxy-sulfinpyrazone, up to 13 hr for sulfide metabolite).

CONTRAINDICATIONS AND PRECAUTIONS

Contraindicated in: ▪ Hypersensitivity ▪ Cross-sensitivity with oxyphenbutazone and phenylbutazone may exist.
Use Cautiously in: ▪ History of blood dyscrasias ▪ GI bleeding ▪ History of kidney stones ▪ Neoplastic disease or radiation therapy (increased risk of uric acid stone formation) ▪ Acute attacks of gout.

ADVERSE REACTIONS AND SIDE EFFECTS*

GI: GI bleeding, <u>nausea</u>, <u>vomiting</u>, abdominal pain.
GU: uric acid kidney stones.
Derm: <u>rashes</u>.
Hemat: blood dyscrasias.
Misc: fever.

INTERACTIONS

Drug–Drug: ▪ Concurrent use of **antineoplastic agents** (increased risk of uric acid kidney stones) ▪ Increased risk of bleeding with **aspirin, other nonsteroidal anti-inflammatory agents, anticoagulants, cefamandole, cefoperazone, cefotetan, plicamycin, valproic acid,** or **thrombolytic agents** ▪ Decreases blood levels and may decrease effectiveness of **nitrofurantoin, theophylline,** or **verapamil** ▪ Uricosuric effect may be decreased by **salicylates** or **niacin.**

ROUTE AND DOSAGE

Hypouricemic
▪ **PO (Adults):** 100–200 mg bid, increased up to 800 mg/day in 2 divided doses.

AVAILABILITY

▪ *Capsules:* 100 mg ▪ *Tablets:* 100 mg, {200 mg}.

TIME/ACTION PROFILE
(hypouricemic effects)

	ONSET	PEAK	DURATION
PO	UK	UK	4–10 hr

NURSING IMPLICATIONS

ASSESSMENT

▪ **Gout:** Assess involved joints for pain, mobility, and edema throughout course of therapy.
▫ Monitor intake and output ratios. Fluids should be encouraged to prevent urate stone formation (2000–3000 ml/day). Alkalinization of the urine with sodium bicarbonate, potassium citrate, or acetazolamide may also be ordered for this purpose.
▪ **Lab Test Considerations:** CBC, serum uric acid levels, and renal function should be monitored routinely during long-term therapy.
▫ Serum and urine uric acid determinations may be measured periodically when sulfinpyrazone is used to treat hyperuricemia.

POTENTIAL NURSING DIAGNOSES
▪ Pain (indications).
▪ Physical mobility, impaired (indications).
▪ Knowledge deficit related to medication regimen (patient/family teaching).

IMPLEMENTATION
▪ **General Info:** Sulfinpyrazone therapy is not used to treat gouty arthritis but rather, to prevent it. If acute attacks occur during therapy, sulfinpyrazone is usually continued at full dose along with treatment with colchicine or nonsteroidal anti-inflammatory agents.
▫ Initiation of sulfinpyrazone therapy should not occur within 2–3 wk of an acute gout attack.
▪ **PO:** Administer with food or antacid to minimize gastric irritation.

PATIENT/FAMILY TEACHING
▫ Instruct patient to take medication exactly as directed, and not to discontinue without consulting physician. Irregular dosage schedules may cause elevation of uric acid levels and precipitate an acute gout attack. Missed doses should be taken as

---

*<u>Underlines</u> indicate most frequent; **CAPITALS** indicate life-threatening.

soon as remembered, unless almost time for next dose.
- ☐ Advise patient to follow physician's recommendations regarding weight loss, diet, and alcohol consumption.
- ☐ Caution patient not to take aspirin or other salicylates, as they decrease the effects of sulfinpyrazone.
- ☐ Instruct patient to report rash, nausea, vomiting, abdominal pain, unusual bleeding or bruising, sore throat, fatigue, or fever to physician promptly.

EVALUATION
Effectiveness of therapy can be demonstrated by: ▪ Decrease in pain and swelling in affected joints and subsequent decrease in frequency of gout attacks. May require several months of continuous therapy for maximum effects ▪ Prevention of myocardial infarction.

SULFISOXAZOLE
(sul-fi-**sox**-a-zole)
Gantrisin, {Novosoxazole}

CLASSIFICATION(S):
Anti-infective (sulfonamide)
Pregnancy Category C

INDICATIONS
▪ PO: Treatment of urinary tract infections, nocardiosis, and, in combination with other anti-infectives, malaria, and pelvic inflammatory disease in prepubertal adolescents ▪ Ophth: Treatment of superficial eye infections ▪ PO, Ophth: Treatment of trachoma and other chlamydial eye infections. **Unlabeled Use:** ▪ Prevention of recurrent otitis media.

ACTION
▪ Interferes with bacterial folic acid synthesis. **Therapeutic Effect:** ▪ Bacteriostatic action against susceptible bacteria. **Spectrum:** ▪ Notable for activity against some gram-positive pathogens,

including: ☐ Streptococci and staphylococci ☐ *Clostridium perfringens* ☐ *Clostridium tetani* ☐ *Nocardia aster-oides* ▪ Active against some gram-negative pathogens, including: ☐ *Enterobacter* ☐ *Escherichia coli* ☐ *Klebsiella* ☐ *Proteus mirabilis* ☐ *Proteus vulgaris* ☐ *Salmonella* ☐ *Shigella.*

PHARMACOKINETICS
Absorption: Well absorbed following oral administration.
Distribution: Widely distributed. Crosses the placenta and enters breast milk.
Metabolism and Excretion: Mostly metabolized by the liver.
Half-life: 5–8 hr.

CONTRAINDICATIONS AND PRECAUTIONS
Contraindicated in: ▪ Hypersensitivity to sulfonamides ▪ Cross-sensitivity with furosemide, thiazides, sulfonylurea oral hypoglycemic agents, or carbonic anhydrase inhibitors may exist ▪ Porphyria ▪ Pregnancy or lactation ▪ Glucose-6-phosphate dehydrogenase (G6PD) deficiency ▪ Known alcohol intolerance (oral suspension only).
Use Cautiously in: ▪ Severe renal or hepatic impairment.

ADVERSE REACTIONS AND SIDE EFFECTS*
CNS: dizziness, ataxia, depression, confusion, psychosis, drowsiness, restlessness.
GI: anorexia, nausea, vomiting, hepatitis.
GU: crystalluria.
Derm: rashes, exfoliative dermatitis, photosensitivity.
Hemat: APLASTIC ANEMIA, thrombocytopenia, AGRANULOCYTOSIS, eosinophilia.
Neuro: peripheral neuropathy.
Misc: fever, superinfection, hypersensitivity reactions, including STEVENS-JOHNSON SYNDROME and serum sickness.

{} = Available in Canada only.
*Underlines indicate most frequent; **CAPITALS** indicate life-threatening.

INTERACTIONS

Drug–Drug: ▪ May enhance the action and increase the risk of toxicity from **oral hypoglycemic agents, methotrexate, phenytoin, zidovudine,** or **oral anticoagulants** ▪ Increased risk of crystalluria with **methenamine** ▪ Increased risk of drug-induced hepatitis with other **hepatotoxic agents** ▪ Ophthalmic form is incompatible with **silver nitrate** or **mild silver protein**.

ROUTE AND DOSAGE

▪ **PO (Adults):** 2–4 g initially, then 4–8 g/day in divided doses q 4–6 hr (not to exceed 12 g/day).
▪ **PO (Children >2 mo):** 75 mg/kg initially, then 150 mg/kg/day in divided doses q 4–6 hr (not to exceed 6 g/day).
▪ **Ophth (Adults):** 1 drop 3 or more times daily, may increase interval as infection resolves.

AVAILABILITY

▪ *Tablets:* 500 mg ▪ *Oral suspension:* 500 mg/5 ml ▪ *Oral syrup:* 500 mg/5 ml ▪ *Opthalmic solution:* 4%.

TIME/ACTION PROFILE (blood levels)

	ONSET	PEAK
PO	1 hr	2–4 hr
Ophth	UK	UK

NURSING IMPLICATIONS

ASSESSMENT
▫ Assess patient for infection (vital signs; appearance of wound, sputum, urine, and stool; WBC; earache) at beginning and throughout course of therapy.
▫ Obtain specimens for culture and sensitivity prior to intiating therapy. First dose may be given before receiving results.
▫ Assess patient for allergy to sulfonamides.
▫ Monitor intake and output ratios. Fluid intake should be sufficient to maintain a urine output of at least 1200–1500 ml daily to prevent crystalluria and stone formation.

▪ **Lab Test Considerations:** Monitor CBC prior to and monthly during prolonged therapy. Therapy should be discontinued if blood dyscrasias occur.
▫ Monitor urinalysis prior to and periodically throughout therapy for crystalluria and formation of urinary calculi.

POTENTIAL NURSING DIAGNOSES
▪ Infection, high risk for (indications, side effects).
▪ Knowledge deficit related to medication regimen (patient/family teaching).
▪ Noncompliance related to medication regimen (patient/family teaching).

IMPLEMENTATION
▪ **PO:** Administer around the clock on an empty stomach, at least 1 hr before or 2 hr after meals, with a full glass of water. Tablets may be crushed and taken with liquids for patients with difficulty swallowing. Use calibrated measuring device for liquid preparations.
▪ **Ophth:** See Appendix H for instillation of ophthalmic preparations.

PATIENT/FAMILY TEACHING
▪ **General Info:** Instruct patient to take medication around the clock and to finish the drug completely as directed, even if feeling better. If a dose is missed, it should be taken as soon as remembered unless almost time for next dose. Advise patient that sharing of this medication may be dangerous.
▫ May cause dizziness. Caution patient to avoid driving and other activities requiring alertness until response to medication is known.
▫ Caution patient to use sunscreen and protective clothing to prevent photosensitivity reactions.
▫ Advise patient to notify physician if skin rash, sore throat, fever, mouth sores, or unusual bleeding or bruising occurs.
▫ Instruct patient to notify physician if symptoms do not improve within a few days. Emphasize the importance

of follow-up examinations to monitor blood counts.
- **Ophth:** Instruct patient in correct technique for instillation of ophthalmic preparations.
  □ Advise patient that stinging or burning may occur after instillation of ophthalmic preparations.
  □ Ophthalmic ointment may cause blurred vision. Caution patient to avoid driving or other activities requiring visual acuity until response to medication is known.

EVALUATION
Clinical response can be evaluated by:
- Resolution of the signs and symptoms of infection. Length of time for complete resolution depends on the organism and site of infection.

SULINDAC
(**soo**-lin-dak)
{Apo-Sulin}, Clinoril, {Novo-Sundac}

CLASSIFICATION(S):
Nonsteroidal anti-inflammatory agent
Pregnancy Category UK

INDICATIONS
- Management of inflammatory disorders, including: □ Rheumatoid arthritis □ Osteoarthritis □ Acute gouty arthritis □ Bursitis.

ACTION
- Inhibits prostaglandin synthesis.
Therapeutic Effects: - Suppression of pain and inflammation.

PHARMACOKINETICS
Absorption: Well absorbed from the GI tract following oral administration.
Distribution: Distribution not known. Enters breast milk in small amounts.
Metabolism and Excretion: Converted by the liver to active drug. Minimal amounts excreted unchanged by the kidneys.
Half-life: 7.8 hr (16.4 hr for active metabolite).

CONTRAINDICATIONS AND PRECAUTIONS
Contraindicated in: - Hypersensitivity - Cross-sensitivity may exist with other nonsteroidal anti-inflammatory agents, including aspirin - Active GI bleeding or ulcer disease - Pregnancy.
Use Cautiously in: - Severe cardiovascular, renal, or hepatic disease (dosage modification recommended) - History of ulcer disease - Lactation or children (safety not established).

ADVERSE REACTIONS AND SIDE EFFECTS*
CNS: <u>headache</u>, drowsiness, <u>dizziness</u>.
CV: edema.
EENT: blurred vision, tinnitus.
GI: <u>nausea</u>, <u>dyspepsia</u>, <u>vomiting</u>, <u>diarrhea</u>, <u>constipation</u>, GI BLEEDING, <u>discomfort</u>, HEPATITIS, flatulence, anorexia, diarrhea, pancreatitis.
GU: renal failure.
Derm: <u>rashes</u>, photosensitivity.
Hemat: blood dyscrasias, prolonged bleeding time.
Misc: Allergic reactions, including hypersensitivity syndrome and ANAPHYLAXIS.

INTERACTIONS
Drug–Drug: - Concurrent use of **aspirin** may decrease effectiveness - Increased risk of bleeding with **anticoagulants, thrombolytic agents, cefamandole, cefoperazone, cefotetan, valproic acid,** or **plicamycin** - Additive adverse GI side effects with **aspirin, glucocorticoids,** and other **nonsteroidal anti-inflammatory agents** - May decrease response to **antihypertensives** or **diuretics** - May increase serum levels and risk of toxicity from **lithium** - May increase the risk of hematologic toxicity from **antineoplastic agents** or **radiation therapy** - Increased risk of adverse

S

{} = Available in Canada only.
*<u>Underlines</u> indicate most frequent; **CAPITALS** indicate life-threatening.

renal effects with **gold compounds, cyclosporine,** or chronic use of **acetaminophen** ▪ **Antacids** decrease blood levels and decrease effectiveness of sulindac ▪ Increased risk of photosensitivity reactions with other **photosensitizing medications** ▪ Increased risk of hypoglycemia with **insulin** or **oral hypoglycemic agents**.

ROUTE AND DOSAGE

▪ **PO (Adults):** 150–200 mg bid (not to exceed 400 mg/day).

AVAILABILITY

▪ *Tablets:* 150 mg, 200 mg.

TIME/ACTION PROFILE

	ONSET	PEAK	DURATION
PO (analgesic)	1–2 days	UK	UK
PO (anti-inflammatory)	few days–1 wk	2 wk or more	UK

NURSING IMPLICATIONS

ASSESSMENT

□ Patients who have asthma, aspirin-induced allergy, and nasal polyps are at increased risk for developing hypersensitivity reactions. Monitor for rhinitis, asthma, and urticaria.

□ Assess pain and range of movement prior to and after 1–2 wk of therapy.

▪ **Lab Test Considerations:** BUN, serum creatinine, CBC, and liver function tests should be evaluated periodically in patients receiving prolonged courses of therapy.

□ Serum potassium, glucose, alkaline phosphatase, AST (SGOT), and ALT (SGPT) may show increased levels.

□ Bleeding time may be prolonged for 1 day following discontinuation of therapy.

POTENTIAL NURSING DIAGNOSES

▪ Pain (indications).

▪ Physical mobility, impaired (indications).

▪ Knowledge deficit related to medication regimen (patient/family teaching).

IMPLEMENTATION

▪ **PO:** May be administered with food, milk, or antacids to decrease GI irritation. Food slows but does not reduce the extent of absorption. Tablets may be crushed and mixed with fluids or food.

PATIENT/FAMILY TEACHING

□ Advise patient to take this medication with a full glass of water and to remain in an upright position for 15–30 min after administration.

□ Instruct patient to take medication exactly as directed. If a dose is missed, it should be taken as soon as remembered but not if almost time for the next dose. Do not double doses.

□ May cause dizziness. Advise patient to avoid driving or other activities requiring alertness until response to the medication is known.

□ Caution patient to avoid concurrent use of alcohol, aspirin, ibuprofen, acetaminophen, or other over-the-counter medications without consulting physician or pharmacist.

□ Advise patient to notify physician or dentist of medication regimen prior to treatment or surgery.

□ Advise patient to use sunscreen and protective clothing to prevent photosensitivity reactions.

□ Instruct patient to notify physician if rash, itching, weight gain, edema, black stools, or persistent headache occurs.

EVALUATION

Effectiveness of therapy can be demonstrated by: ▪ Decreased pain and improved joint mobility. Partial arthritic relief may be seen within 7 days, but maximum effectiveness may require 2–3 wk of continuous therapy. Patients who do not respond to one nonsteroidal anti-inflammatory agent may respond to another.

SUMATRIPTAN

(soo-ma-**trip**-tan)
Imitrex

CLASSIFICATION(S):
Antimigraine
Pregnancy Category C

INDICATIONS

■ Acute treatment of migraine attacks.

ACTION

■ Acts as a selective agonist at specific vascular serotonin receptor sites, causing vasoconstriction in large intracranial arteries. **Therapeutic Effect:** ■ Relief of acute attacks of migraine.

PHARMACOKINETICS

Absorption: Well absorbed (97%) following SC administration.
Distribution: Does not cross the blood–brain barrier. Remainder of distribution not known.
Metabolism and Excretion: Metabolized by the liver.
Half-life: 2 hr.

CONTRAINDICATIONS AND PRECAUTIONS

Contraindicated in: ■ Hypersensitivity ■ Patients with ischemic heart disease or signs and symptoms of ishemic heart disease, Prinzmetal's angina, or uncontrolled hypertension.
Use Cautiously in: ■ Patients with any history of cardiovascular disease ■ Patients with childbearing potential ■ Pregnancy, lactation, or children <18 yr (safety not established).

ADVERSE REACTIONS AND SIDE EFFECTS*

CNS: <u>dizziness</u>, <u>vertigo</u>, feeling of heaviness, feeling of tightness, strange feeling, tight feeling in head, drowsiness, headache, anxiety, malaise, fatigue, weakness.
EENT: throat discomfort, nasal sinus discomfort, alterations in vision.
CV: transient hypertension, chest tightness, chest pressure, coronary vasospasm, angina, ECG changes.
GI: abdominal discomfort, dysphagia.
Derm: <u>tingling</u>, <u>warm sensation</u>, burning sensation, cool sensation, flushing.
Local: <u>injection site reaction</u>.
MS: neck pain, neck stiffness, myalgia, muscle cramps, jaw discomfort.
Neuro: numbness.

INTERACTIONS

Drug–Drug: ■ The risk of vasospastic reactions may be increased by concurrent use of **ergotamine** (avoid use of ergotamine and sumatriptan within 24 hr of each other).

ROUTE AND DOSAGE

■ **SC (Adults):** 6 mg, may repeat after 1 hr (not to exceed 12 mg in 24 hr).

AVAILABILITY

■ *Injection:* 6 mg/0.5 ml unit-of-use syringes, 0.6 mg/0.5 ml single-use vials, SELFdose injection kit (containing 2 unit-of-use syringes and instructions).

TIME/ACTION PROFILE (relief of migraine)

	ONSET	PEAK	DURATION
SC	30 min	up to 2 hr	up to 24 hr

NURSING IMPLICATIONS

ASSESSMENT

▫ Assess pain location, intensity, and duration and associated symptoms (photophobia, phonophobia, nausea, vomiting) during migraine attack.
▫ Give initial dose in physician's office to patients with potential for coronary artery disease (CAD) (postmenopausal women, men over 40 years, patients with risk factors for CAD [hypertension, hypercholesterolemia, obesity, diabetes, smokers, family history]). Monitor blood pressure prior to and for 1 hr following initial injection. If angina occurs, monitor ECG for ischemic changes.

POTENTIAL NURSING DIAGNOSES

■ Pain (indications).
■ Knowledge deficit related to medication regimen (patient/family teaching).

<u>Underlines</u> indicate most frequent; **CAPITALS indicate life-threatening.*

IMPLEMENTATION

- **SC:** Administer as a single injection just below the skin.

PATIENT/FAMILY TEACHING

☐ Instruct patient on the proper technique for loading, administering, and discarding the auto-injector. Patient information pamphlet is provided. Instructional video is available from the manufacturer.

☐ Inform patient that sumatriptan should only be used during a migraine attack. It is meant to be used for relief of migraine attacks but not to prevent or reduce the number of attacks.

☐ Instruct patient to administer sumatriptan as soon as symptoms of a migraine attack appear, but it may be administered any time during an attack. If migraine symptoms return, a second injection may be used. Allow at least 1 hr between doses, and do not use more than 2 injections in any 24-hr period.

☐ Caution patient not to use sumatriptan if she is pregnant, suspects she is pregnant, or plans to become pregnant. Adequate contraception should be used during therapy.

☐ Advise patient to notify physician prior to next dose of sumatriptan if pain or tightness in the chest occurs during use. If pain is severe or does not subside, notify physician immediately. If wheezing; heart throbbing; swelling of eyelids, face, or lips; skin rash; skin lumps; or hives occurs, notify physician immediately and do not take more sumatriptan without physician's approval. If feelings of tingling, heat, flushing, heaviness, pressure, drowsiness, dizziness, tiredness, or sickness develop discuss with physician at next visit.

☐ Sumatriptan may cause dizziness or drowsiness. Caution patient to avoid driving or other activities requiring alertness until response to medication is known.

☐ Inform patient that pain or redness at the injection site usually lasts less than 1 hr.

EVALUATION

Effectiveness of therapy can be determined by: ▪ Relief of migraine attack.

TACRINE
(**tak**-rin)
Cognex

CLASSIFICATION(S):
Cholinesterase inhibitor
(reversible)
Pregnancy Category C

INDICATIONS

▪ Management of mild to moderate dementia associated with Alzheimer's disease.

ACTION

▪ Increases levels of acetylcholine in the CNS by inhibiting its breakdown. **Therapeutic Effect:** ▪ Improved cognitive function in patients with mild to moderate Alzheimer's disease. Does not affect the course of the disease.

PHARMACOKINETICS

Absorption: Rapidly absorbed following oral administration, although bioavailability is low (17%).
Distribution: Distribution not known.
Metabolism and Excretion: Highly metabolized by the liver.
Half-life: 2–4 hr.

CONTRAINDICATIONS AND PRECAUTIONS

Contraindicated in: ▪ Hypersensitivity to tacrine or other acridines ▪ Jaundice associated with previous courses of tacrine therapy.
Use Cautiously in: ▪ Patients with a history or risk of GI bleeding, including current therapy with nonsteroidal anti-inflammatory agents.

ADVERSE REACTIONS AND SIDE EFFECTS*

CNS: dizziness, headache.

---

*Underlines indicate most frequent; **CAPITALS** indicate life-threatening.

CV: bradycardia.

GI: GI bleeding, nausea, vomiting, diarrhea, ALT elevations, dyspepsia, anorexia.

INTERACTIONS

Drug–Drug: ▪ Increases **theophylline** levels and risk of toxicity (blood level monitoring recommended, dosage reduction may be required) ▪ Potentiates the effects of **succinylcholine** (increases neuromuscular blockade) during anesthesia ▪ May potentiate the action of **cholinergic agents** (bethanechol) ▪ **Cigarette smoking** decreases blood levels of tacrine ▪ **Cimetidine** increases tacrine levels ▪ May interfere with the action of **anticholinergic agents.**

Drug–Food: Food decreases absorption of tacrine by 30–40%.

ROUTE AND DOSAGE

▪ **PO (Adults):** 10 mg qid for 6 wk. If ALT remains unchanged, increase dose to 20 mg qid. Further increments may be made at 6-wk intervals as tolerated, up to 160 mg/day.

AVAILABILITY

▪ *Capsules:* 10 mg, 20 mg, 30 mg, 40 mg.

TIME/ACTION PROFILE (improvement in cognitive function)

	ONSET	PEAK	DURATION
PO	within 6 wk	18–24 wk	UK

NURSING IMPLICATIONS

ASSESSMENT

□ Assess cognitive function (memory, attention, reasoning, language, ability to perform simple tasks) periodically throughout therapy.
□ Monitor heart rate periodically during therapy. May cause bradycardia.
▪ **Lab Test Considerations:** May cause ALT (SGPT) elevations; monitor levels weekly for at least the first 18 wk of therapy and then every 3 mo throughout therapy. Weekly monitoring should be resumed for at least 6 wk after any dose increase. If ALT (SGPT) levels are <3 times the upper limit of normal, continue dose titration; if levels are >3 to <5 times the upper limit of normal, decrease the dose of tacrine by 40 mg/day, and resume dose titration when ALT (SGPT) returns to normal. Tacrine should be discontinued if ALT (SGPT) levels are >5 times the upper limit of normal. Levels usually return to normal 4–6 wk after discontinuation of therapy.
□ Tacrine should be permanently discontinued and a new trial should not be attempted in patients with clinical jaundice and a total bilirubin >3 mg/dl.

POTENTIAL NURSING DIAGNOSES

▪ Thought processes, altered (indications).
▪ Injury, high risk for (indications).
▪ Knowledge deficit related to medication regimen (patient/family teaching).

IMPLEMENTATION

▪ **PO:** Administer at regular intervals between meals. If GI upset occurs, may be administered with meals; however, plasma levels may be reduced by 30–40%.

PATIENT/FAMILY TEACHING

□ Emphasize the importance of taking tacrine at regular intervals as directed. Abrupt discontinuation of doses of >80 mg/day may cause a decline in cognitive function and behavioral disturbances.
□ Advise patient and caregiver to notify physician if nausea, vomiting, diarrhea, rash, jaundice, or changes in the color of the stool occur.

EVALUATION

Clinical response to therapy can be determined by: ▪ Improvement in cognitive function (memory, attention, reasoning, language, ability to perform simple tasks) in patients with Alzheimer's disease.

TAMOXIFEN
(ta-**mox**-i-fen)
Nolvadex, {Nolvadex-D}, {Novo-
Tamoxifen}, {Tamofen},
{Tamone}

CLASSIFICATION(S):
Antineoplastic (estrogen blocker)
Pregnancy Category D

INDICATIONS

▪ Adjuvant therapy of breast cancer following surgery and radiation (delays
recurrence) ▪ Palliative or adjunctive
treatment of advanced breast cancer.

ACTION

▪ Competes with estrogen for binding
sites in breast and other tissues ▪ Reduces DNA synthesis and estrogen response. **Therapeutic Effect:** ▪ Suppression of tumor growth.

PHARMACOKINETICS

Absorption: Absorbed following oral
administration.
Distribution: Distribution not known.
Metabolism and Excretion: Mostly
metabolized by the liver. Slowly eliminated in the feces. Minimal amounts excreted in the urine.
Half-life: 7 days.

CONTRAINDICATIONS AND
PRECAUTIONS

Contraindicated in: ▪ Hypersensitivity
▪ Pregnancy or lactation.
Use Cautiously in: ▪ Women with
childbearing potential ▪ Decreased
bone marrow reserve.

ADVERSE REACTIONS AND SIDE
EFFECTS*

CNS: confusion, depression, headache,
weakness.
CV: edema.
EENT: blurred vision.
GI: nausea, vomiting.
GU: vaginal bleeding.
Derm: photosensitivity.

F and E: hypercalcemia.
Hemat: thrombocytopenia, leukopenia.
Metab: hot flashes.
MS: bone pain.
Misc: tumor flare.

INTERACTIONS

Drug–Drug: ▪ **Estrogens** will decrease
the effectiveness of concurrently administered tamoxifen.

ROUTE AND DOSAGE

▪ **PO (Adults):** 10–20 mg twice daily.

AVAILABILITY

▪ *Tablets:* 10 mg, 20 mg ▪ {*Enteric-
coated tablets:* 20 mg}.

TIME/ACTION PROFILE (tumor
response)

	ONSET	PEAK	DURATION
PO	4–10 wk	several mo	UK

NURSING IMPLICATIONS

ASSESSMENT

▫ Assess for an increase in bone or
tumor pain. Confer with physician
regarding analgesics. This transient
pain usually resolves despite continued therapy.
▪ **Lab Test Considerations:** Monitor
CBC, platelets, and calcium levels
prior to and throughout course of
therapy. May cause transient hypercalcemia in patients with metastases
to the bone. An estrogen receptor as-
say should be assessed prior to initiation of therapy.

POTENTIAL NURSING DIAGNOSES

▪ Knowledge deficit related to medication regimen (patient/family teaching).

IMPLEMENTATION

▪ **PO:** Administer with food or fluids
if GI irritation becomes a problem.
Consult physician if patient vomits
shortly after administration of medication to determine need for repeat
dose.

{} = Available in Canada only.
*Underlines indicate most frequent; **CAPITALS** indicate life-threatening.

□ Do not crush, break, or chew enteric-coated tablet.

PATIENT/FAMILY TEACHING

□ Instruct patient to take medication exactly as directed. If a dose is missed, it should be omitted.

□ If skin lesions are present, inform patient that lesions may temporarily increase in size and number and may have increased erythema.

□ Advise patient to report bone pain to physician promptly. This pain may be severe. Inform patient that this may be an indication of the drug's effectiveness and will resolve over time. Analgesics should be ordered to control pain.

□ Instruct patient to monitor weight weekly. Weight gain or peripheral edema should be reported to physician.

□ This medication may induce ovulation and may have teratogenic properties. Advise patient to use a non-hormonal method of contraception during and for 1 mo after the course of therapy.

□ Caution patient to wear sunscreen and protective clothing to prevent photosensitivity reactions.

□ Advise patient that medication may cause hot flashes. Notify physician if these become bothersome.

□ Instruct patient to notify physician promptly if swelling, shortness of breath, weakness, or blurred vision occurs. Patient should also report vaginal bleeding or confusion.

EVALUATION

Effectiveness of therapy can be demonstrated by: ▪ Decrease in the size or spread of breast cancer. Observable effects of therapy may not be seen for 4–10 wk after initiation.

TEMAZEPAM
(tem-**az**-a-pam)
Razepam, Restoril

CLASSIFICATION(S):
Sedative/hypnotic (benzodiazepine)
Schedule IV
Pregnancy Category X

INDICATIONS

▪ Management of insomnia (short-term).

ACTION

▪ Acts at many levels in the CNS, producing generalized depression ▪ Effects may be mediated by gamma-aminobutyric acid (GABA), an inhibitory neurotransmitter. **Therapeutic Effect:** ▪ Relief of insomnia.

PHARMACOKINETICS

Absorption: Well absorbed following oral administration.

Distribution: Widely distributed, crosses blood–brain barrier. Probably crosses the placenta and enters breast milk. Accumulation of drug occurs with chronic dosing.

Metabolism and Excretion: Metabolized by the liver.

Half-life: 10–20 hr.

CONTRAINDICATIONS AND PRECAUTIONS

Contraindicated in: ▪ Hypersensitivity ▪ Cross-sensitivity with other benzodiazepines may exist ▪ Pre-existing CNS depression ▪ Severe uncontrolled pain ▪ Narrow-angle glaucoma ▪ Pregnancy or lactation.

Use Cautiously in: ▪ Pre-existing hepatic dysfunction ▪ Patients who may be suicidal or have been addicted to drugs previously ▪ Elderly or debilitated patients (dosage reduction recommended).

ADVERSE REACTIONS AND SIDE EFFECTS*

CNS: dizziness, drowsiness, lethargy, hangover, paradoxical excitation.
EENT: blurred vision.
GI: nausea, vomiting, diarrhea, constipation.

---

*Underlines indicate most frequent; **CAPITALS** indicate life-threatening.

Derm: rashes.
Misc: tolerance, psychological dependence, physical dependence.

INTERACTIONS

Drug–Drug: ▪ Additive CNS depression with **alcohol, antidepressants, antihistamines, opioid analgesics,** and other **sedative/hypnotics** ▪ May decrease efficacy of **levodopa** ▪ **Rifampin** or **smoking** increase metabolism and may decrease effectiveness of temazepam ▪ **Probenecid** may prolong the effects of temazepam ▪ Sedative effects may be antagonized by **theopylline.**

ROUTE AND DOSAGE

▪ **PO (Adults):** 15 mg at bedtime (up to 30 mg).
▪ **PO (Elderly or Debilitated Patients):** 7.5 mg at bedtime initially.

AVAILABILITY

▪ *Tablets:* 15 mg, 30 mg ▪ *Capsules:* 7.5 mg, 15 mg, 30 mg.

TIME/ACTION PROFILE (sedation)

	ONSET	PEAK	DURATION
PO	30 min	2–3 hr	UK

NURSING IMPLICATIONS

ASSESSMENT
▫ Assess sleep patterns prior to and periodically throughout course of therapy.
▫ Prolonged high-dose therapy may lead to psychological or physical dependence. Restrict amount of drug available to patient, especially if patient is depressed or suicidal or has a history of addiction.

POTENTIAL NURSING DIAGNOSES
▪ Sleep pattern disturbance (indications).
▪ Injury, high risk for (side effects).
▪ Knowledge deficit related to medication regimen (patient/family teaching).

IMPLEMENTATION
▪ **PO:** Administer with food if GI irritation becomes a problem.

PATIENT/FAMILY TEACHING
▫ Instruct patient to take temazepam exactly as directed. Discuss the importance of preparing environment for sleep (dark room, quiet, avoidance of nicotine and caffeine). If less effective after a few weeks, consult physician; do not increase dose.
▫ May cause daytime drowsiness or dizziness. Caution patient to avoid driving or other activities requiring alertness until response to medication is known.
▫ Advise patient to avoid the use of alcohol and other CNS depressants and to consult the physician or pharmacist prior to the use of over-the-counter preparations that contain antihistamines or alcohol.
▫ Advise patient to inform physician if pregnancy is planned or suspected.
▫ Emphasize the importance of follow-up appointments to monitor progress.

EVALUATION
Effectiveness of therapy can be demonstrated by: ▪ Improvement in sleep habits, which may not be noticeable until the third day of therapy.

TENIPOSIDE
(ten-i-poe-side)
Vumon, VM-26

CLASSIFICATION(S):
Antineoplastic agent (podophyllotoxin derivative)
Pregnancy Category D

INDICATIONS

▪ Used in combination with other agents for induction therapy for refractory acute lymphoblastic leukemia in children.

ACTION

▪ Damages DNA prior to mitosis (cycle-dependent and phase specific). **Therapeutic Effects:** ▪ Death of rapidly replicating cells, particularly malignant ones.

PHARMACOKINETICS

Absorption: IV administration results in complete bioavailability.

Distribution: Limited distribution into the CSF.

Metabolism and Excretion: 44% excreted by the kidneys. 10% or less is eliminated in feces.

Half-life: 5 hr.

CONTRAINDICATIONS AND PRECAUTIONS

Contraindicated in: ▪ Hypersensitivity ▪ Known intolerance to castor oil, alcohol, or benzyl alcohol ▪ Pregnancy or lactation ▪ Preparations containing benzyl alcohol should be avoided in newborns.

Use Cautiously in: ▪ Patients with Down's syndrome (more susceptible to the myelosuppressive effects). Initial dose of first course of therapy should be reduced by 50% ▪ Patients with hepatic impairment, childbearing potential, active infections, decreased bone marrow reserve or other chronic debilitating illnesses.

ADVERSE REACTIONS AND SIDE EFFECTS*

CNS: acute CNS depression, transient cortical blindness.

CV: hypotension.

GI: nausea, vomiting, mucositis, diarrhea.

Derm: alopecia, rashes.

Endo: gonadal suppression.

Hemat: leukopenia, thrombocytopenia, anemia.

Local: phlebitis at IV site.

Neuro: peripheral neurotoxicity.

Misc: allergic reactions, including ANAPHYLAXIS, fever.

INTERACTIONS

Drug–Drug: ▪ Myelosuppression may be increased by **sodium salicylate, tolbutamide, sulfamethizole,** other **antineoplastic agents,** or **radiation therapy**.

ROUTE AND DOSAGE

Several regimens have been used. These are examples.

▪ **IV (Children):** Teniposide 165 mg/m^2 in combination with cytarabine 300 mg/m^2 twice weekly for 8–9 doses. Another regimen uses teniposide 250 mg/m^2 in combination with vincristine 1.5 mg/m^2 weekly for 4–8 wk with prednisone 40 mg/m^2/day for 28 days.

AVAILABILITY

▪ *Injection:* 10 mg/ml in 5-ml ampules.

TIME/ACTION PROFILE (effects on blood counts)

	ONSET	PEAK	DURATION
IV	UK	UK	UK

NURSING IMPLICATIONS

ASSESSMENT

▫ Monitor blood pressure prior to and every 15 min during infusion. If hypotension occurs, stop infusion and notify physician. After stabilizing blood pressure with IV fluids and supportive measures, infusion may be resumed at slower rate.

▫ Monitor for hypersensitivity reaction (fever, chills, pruritus, urticaria, bronchospasm, tachycardia, hypotension). If these occur, stop infusion and notify physician. Keep epinephrine, antihistamine, and resuscitative equipment close by in the event of an anaphylactic reaction.

▫ Assess for fever, chills, sore throat, and signs of infection. Notify physician if these symptoms occur.

▫ Assess for bleeding (bleeding gums, bruising, petechiae, guaiac test stools, urine, and emesis). Avoid IM injections and rectal temperatures. Apply pressure to venipuncture sites for 10 min.

▫ Monitor intake and output, appetite, and nutritional intake. Teniposide causes nausea and vomiting in 30% of patients. Confer with physician regarding prophylactic use of an antiemetic. Adjust diet as tolerated to help maintain fluid and electrolyte balance and nutritional status.

*Underlines indicate most frequent; **CAPITALS** indicate life-threatening.

- **Lab Test Considerations:** Monitor CBC and differential prior to and periodically throughout therapy. Notify physician if the leukocyte count is less than 1000/mm³ or the platelet count is less than 75,000/mm³. Therapy may be discontinued if platelet count is less than 50,000/mm³ or absolute neutrophil count is less than 500/mm³.
- □ Monitor liver function studies (AST [SGOT], ALT [SGPT], LDH, bilirubin) and renal function studies (BUN, creatinine) prior to and periodically throughout therapy to detect hepatotoxicity and nephrotoxicity.
- □ May cause increased uric acid. Monitor levels periodically during therapy.

POTENTIAL NURSING DIAGNOSES
- Injury, high risk for (side effects).
- Infection, high risk for (side effects).
- Knowledge deficit related to medication regimen (patient/family teaching).

IMPLEMENTATION
- **General Info:** Avoid contact with skin. Use Luer-Lok tubing to prevent accidental leakage. If contact with skin occurs, immediately wash skin with soap and water.
- □ Solution should be prepared in a biologic cabinet. Wear gloves, gown, and mask while handling medication. Discard equipment in designated containers (see Appendix I).
- **Intermittent Infusion:** Dilute with D5W or 0.9% NaCl for a final concentration of 0.1, 0.2, 0.4, or 1 mg/ml. Solution must be prepared and administered in nonplastic equipment to prevent cracking of plastic and possible drug leakage. Glass or polyolefin plastic bags or containers should be used; PVC containers are not recommended. Concentrations of 1 mg/ml should be administered within 4 hr of dilution. Diluted solutions are stable for 24 hr at room temperature.
- **Rate:** Administer over 30–60 min or longer. Do not give by rapid infusion; may result in hypotension.
- **Y-Site/Additive Incompatibility:** ▪ hep-

arin. Flush IV line with D5W or 0.9% NaCl only. Do not admix or administer via Y-site with other medications or solutions.

PATIENT/FAMILY TEACHING
- □ Advise patient to notify physician if fever, chills, sore throat, signs of infection, bleeding gums, bruising, petechiae, or blood in urine, stool, or emesis occurs. Caution patient to avoid crowds and persons with known infections. Instruct patient to use soft toothbrush and electric razor.
- □ Patient should be cautioned not to drink alcoholic beverages or take products containing aspirin or ibuprofen.
- □ Instruct patient to notify physician if abdominal pain, yellow skin, weakness, paresthesia, or gait disturbances occur.
- □ Instruct patient to inspect oral mucosa for redness and ulceration. If mouth sores occur, advise patient to use sponge brush and rinse mouth with water after eating and drinking.
- □ Discuss with patient the possibility of hair loss. Explore coping strategies.
- □ Advise patient to use a nonhormonal method of contraception throughout therapy.
- □ Instruct patient not to receive any vaccinations without advice of physician.
- □ Emphasize the need for periodic lab tests to monitor for side effects.

EVALUATION
Effectiveness of therapy can be demonstrated by: ▪ Improvement of hematologic status in leukemias.

TERAZOSIN
(ter-**ay**-zoe-sin)
Hytrin

CLASSIFICATION(S):
Antihypertensive (peripherally acting antiadrenergic)
Pregnancy Category C

INDICATIONS

- Treatment of mild to moderate hypertension (alone or with other agents, such as diuretics) ▪ Management of outflow obstruction in patients with prostatic hypertrophy.

ACTION

- Dilates both arteries and veins by blocking postsynaptic alpha$_1$-adrenergic receptors ▪ Decreases contractions in smooth muscle of the prostatic capsule. **Therapeutic Effects:** ▪ Lowering of blood pressure ▪ Decreased symptoms of prostatic hypertrophy (urinary urgency, hesitancy, nocturia).

PHARMACOKINETICS

Absorption: Well absorbed following oral administration.
Distribution: Distribution not known.
Metabolism and Excretion: 50% metabolized by the liver. 10% excreted unchanged by the kidneys. 20% excreted unchanged in feces. 40% eliminated in bile.
Half-life: 12 hr.

CONTRAINDICATIONS AND PRECAUTIONS

Contraindicated in: ▪ Hypersensitivity.
Use Cautiously in: ▪ Pregnancy, lactation, or children (safety not established).

ADVERSE REACTIONS AND SIDE EFFECTS*

CNS: <u>dizziness</u>, nervousness, somnolence, <u>weakness</u>, <u>headache</u>.
CV: palpitations, hypotension, tachycardia, arrhythmias, chest pain.
Derm: pruritus, first dose orthostatic hypotensive reaction.
EENT: <u>nasal congestion</u>, blurred vision, conjunctivitis, sinusitis.
F and E: peripheral edema, fever.
GI: <u>nausea</u>, vomiting, diarrhea, dry mouth, abdominal pain.
GU: impotence, urinary frequency.
Metab: weight gain.
MS: extremity pain, back pain, arthralgia.

Neuro: paresthesia.
Resp: dyspnea.

INTERACTIONS

Drug–Drug: ▪ Additive hypotension with other **antihypertensive agents,** acute ingestion of **alcohol,** or **nitrates** ▪ **Nonsteroidal anti-inflammatory agents, sympathomimetics,** or **estrogens** may decrease the effects of antihypertensive therapy.

ROUTE AND DOSAGE

The first dose should be taken at bedtime.

Hypertension

- **PO (Adults):** 1 mg initially, then slowly increase up to 5 mg/day; may be given as single dose or in 2 divided doses (not to exceed 20 mg/day).

Benign Prostatic Hypertrophy

- **PO (Adults):** 1 mg at bedtime, gradually may be increased up to 5–10 mg/day.

AVAILABILITY

- *Tablets:* 1 mg, 2 mg, 5 mg, 10 mg.

TIME/ACTION PROFILE
(antihypertensive effects)

	ONSET*	PEAK†	DURATION*
PO	15 min	6–8 wk	24 hr

*After single dose.
†After multiple oral dosing.

NURSING IMPLICATIONS

ASSESSMENT

- ☐ Monitor blood pressure (lying and standing) and pulse frequently during initial dosage adjustment and periodically throughout course of therapy. Notify physician of significant changes.
- ☐ Assess patient for first dose orthostatic reaction and syncope. May occur 30 min–2 hr following initial dose and occasionally thereafter. Incidence may be dose-related. Volume-depleted or sodium-restricted patients may be more sensitive to this effect.

*<u>Underlines</u> indicate most frequent; **CAPITALS** indicate life-threatening.

□ Monitor intake and output ratios and daily weight; assess for edema daily, especially at beginning of therapy.

POTENTIAL NURSING DIAGNOSES

- Injury, high risk for (side effects).
- Knowledge deficit related to medication regimen (patient/family teaching).
- Noncompliance (patient/family teaching).

IMPLEMENTATION

- **General Info:** May be used in combination with diuretic or beta-adrenergic blocker to minimize sodium and water retention. If these are added to terazosin therapy, reduce dose of terazosin initially and titrate to effect.
- **PO:** Administer daily dose at bedtime. If necessary, dosage may be increased to twice daily.

PATIENT/FAMILY TEACHING

□ Emphasize the importance of continuing to take this medication as directed, even if feeling well. Medication controls but does not cure hypertension. Instruct patient to take medication at the same time each day. If a dose is missed, take as soon as remembered. If not remembered until next day, do not take; do not double doses.

□ Encourage patient to comply with additional interventions for hypertension (weight reduction, low-sodium diet, smoking cessation, moderation of alcohol consumption, regular exercise, and stress management). Instruct patient and family on proper technique for blood pressure monitoring. Advise them to check blood pressure at least weekly and to report significant changes to physician.

□ Advise patient to weigh self twice weekly and assess feet and ankles for fluid retention.

□ Terazosin may cause dizziness or drowsiness. Advise patient to avoid driving or other activities requiring alertness until response to the medication is known.

□ Caution patient to avoid sudden changes in position to decrease ortho-static hypotension. Alcohol, CNS depressants, standing for long periods, hot showers, and exercising in hot weather should be avoided because of enhanced orthostatic effects.

□ Advise patient to consult physician or pharmacist before taking any cough, cold, or allergy remedies. Patient should also avoid excessive amounts of tea, coffee, and cola.

□ Instruct patient to notify physician or dentist of medication regimen prior to any surgery.

□ Advise patient to notify physician if frequent dizziness or fainting or swelling of feet or lower legs occurs.

□ Emphasize the importance of follow-up examinations to evaluate effectiveness of medication.

EVALUATION

Effectiveness of therapy can be demonstrated by: ■ Decrease in blood pressure without appearance of side effects ■ Decreased symptoms of prostate by pertrophy.

TERBUTALINE
(ter-**byoo**-ta-leen)
Brethaire, Brethine, Bricanyl

CLASSIFICATION(S):
Bronchodilator (beta-adrenergic agonist)
Pregnancy Category B

INDICATIONS

■ Used as a bronchodilator in reversible airway obstruction due to asthma or COPD. **Unlabeled Use:** ■ Prevention and treatment of preterm labor (tocolytic).

ACTION

■ A beta-adrenergic agonist that results in the accumulation of cyclic adenosine monophosphate (cAMP) ■ Results of increased levels of cAMP at beta-adrenergic receptors include: □ Bronchodilation □ CNS and cardiac stimulation □ Diuresis □ Gastric acid secretion ■ Relatively selective for beta$_2$ (pulmonary) recep-

tors. **Therapeutic Effect:** ■ Bronchodilation.

PHARMACOKINETICS

Absorption: 35–50% absorbed following oral administration, but rapidly
undergoes first-pass metabolism. Well
absorbed following SC administration.
Minimal absorption following inhalation.
Distribution: Distribution not known.
Enters breast milk.
Metabolism and Excretion: Partially
metabolized by the liver. 60% excreted
unchanged by the kidneys following SC
administration.
Half-life: UK.

CONTRAINDICTIONS AND PRECAUTIONS

Contraindicated in: ■ Hypersensitivity
to adrenergic amines or any ingredients
in preparations (fluorocarbon propellant in inhaler).
Use Cautiously in: ■ Elderly patients
(more susceptible to adverse reactions; may require dosage reduction)
■ Pregnancy, lactation, or children <12
yr (safety not established—has been
used during pregnancy, but may cause
hypokalemia, hypoglycemia, or pulmonary edema in the mother and hypoglycemia in the newborn) ■ Cardiac disease ■ Hypertension ■ Hyperthyroidism
■ Diabetes mellitus ■ Glaucoma ■ Pregnancy near term ■ Excessive use of inhalers (may lead to tolerance and paradoxical bronchospasm).

ADVERSE REACTIONS AND SIDE EFFECTS*

CNS: <u>nervousness</u>, <u>restlessness</u>, in-
somnia, <u>tremor</u>, headache, anxiety.
CV: hypertension, arrhythmias, angina,
tachycardia, palpitations, PULMONARY
EDEMA (maternal—during tocolysis).
GI: nausea, vomiting.
F and E: hypokalemia (during tocolysis
in mother).

INTERACTIONS

Drug–Drug: ■ Additive adrenergic effects with other **adrenergic (sympatho-**
mimetic) agents, including **deconges-**
tants and **vasopressors** ■ Use with **MAO**
inhibitors may lead to hypertensive
crisis ■ **Beta-adrenergic blockers** may
block therapeutic effect.

ROUTE AND DOSAGE

Bronchodilation

- **PO (Adults and Children >15 yr):**
  2.5–5 mg tid, at 6-hr intervals (not to
  exceed 15 mg/24 hr).
- **PO (Children 12–15 yr):** 2.5 mg tid, at
  6-hr intervals.
- **SC (Adults):** 250 mcg, may repeat in
  15–30 min (not to exceed 500 mcg in 4
  hr).
- **Inhalation (Adults and Children >12**
  yr): 1–2 inhalations q 4–6 hr.

Tocolysis (Arrest of Preterm Labor)

- **PO (Adults):** 2.5 mg q 4–6 hr until delivery.
- **SC (Adults):** 250 mcg q hr until contractions stop.
- **IV (Adults):** 10 mcg/min infusion, increase by 5 mcg/min q 10 min until
  contractions stop (not to exceed 80
  mcg/min). After contractions have
  stopped for 30 min, decrease infusion
  rate to lowest effective amount and
  maintain for 4–8 hr.

AVAILABILITY

- *Tablets:* 2.5 mg, 5 mg ■ *Aerosol for*
  inhalation: 0.2 mg/puff in 10.5-g can
  (≥300 puffs) ■ *Injection:* 1 mg/ml.

TIME/ACTION PROFILE (bronchodilation)

	ONSET	PEAK	DURATION
PO	30 min	1–2 hr	4–8 hr
SC	15 min	30–60 min	1.5–4 hr
Inhaln	5–30 min	1–2 hr	3–6 hr

NURSING IMPLICATIONS

ASSESSMENT

- **Bronchospasm:** Assess blood pressure, pulse, respiratory pattern, lung
  sounds, and character of secretions
  prior to and after treatment. Cardiovascular effects are increased with
  parenteral use.

*Underlines indicate most frequent; **CAPITALS** indicate life-threatening.

▫ Observe patient for drug tolerance and rebound bronchospasm.

▪ **Preterm Labor:** Monitor maternal pulse and blood pressure, frequency and duration of contractions, and fetal heart rate. Notify physician if contractions persist or increase in frequency or duration or if symptoms of maternal or fetal distress occur. Maternal side effects include tachycardia, palpitations, tremor, anxiety, and headache.

▫ Assess maternal respiratory status for symptoms of pulmonary edema (increased rate, dyspnea, rales/crackles, frothy sputum).

▫ Monitor mother and neonate for symptoms of hypoglycemia (anxiety, chills, cold sweats, confusion, cool pale skin, difficulty in concentration, drowsiness, excessive hunger, headache, irritability, nausea, nervousness, rapid pulse, shakiness, unusual tiredness or weakness) and mother for hypokalemia (weakness, fatigue, U wave on ECG, arrhythmias).

▪ **Lab Test Considerations:** Monitor maternal serum glucose and electrolytes. May cause hypokalemia and hypoglycemia. Monitor neonate's serum glucose, as hypoglycemia may also occur in neonate.

POTENTIAL NURSING DIAGNOSES

▪ Airway clearance, ineffective (indications).

▪ Knowledge deficit related to medication regimen (patient/family teaching).

▪ Noncompliance (patient/family teaching).

IMPLEMENTATION

▪ **PO:** Tablet may be crushed and mixed with food or fluids for patients with difficulty swallowing.

▪ **SC:** Administer SC injections in lateral deltoid area. Do not use solution if discolored.

▪ **IV:** Use infusion pump to ensure accurate dosage. Begin infusion at 10 mcg/min. Increase dosage by 5 mcg every 10 min until contractions cease.

Maximum dose is 80 mcg/min. Begin to taper dose in 5-mcg decrements after a 30–60 min contraction-free period is attained. Switch to oral dosage form after patient is contraction-free 4–8 hr on the lowest effective dose.

▪ **Syringe Compatibility:** ▪ doxapram.

▪ **Y-Site Compatibility:** ▪ insulin.

▪ **Solution/Additive Compatibility:** May be diluted in D5W, 0.9% NaCl, or 0.45% NaCl. Compatible with aminophylline.

▪ **Additive Incompatibility:** ▪ bleomycin.

PATIENT/FAMILY TEACHING

▪ **Bronchospasm:** Instruct patient to take medication exactly as directed. If a dose is missed, take if remembered within 1 hr, otherwise do not take; do not double doses. Taking more often than prescribed may lead to tolerance.

▫ Advise patient to maintain adequate fluid intake to help liquify tenacious secretions.

▫ Advise patient to consult physician if respiratory symptoms are not relieved or worsen after treatment. Patient should also inform physician if chest pain, headache, severe dizziness, palpitations, nervousness, or weakness occurs.

▪ **Metered-dose Inhaler:** Instruct patient on correct use of inhaler (see Appendix H).

▫ Patients taking inhalation glucocorticoids concurrently with terbutaline should be advised to take terbutaline first and allow 15 min to elapse between using the 2 aerosols, unless directed by physician.

▪ **Preterm Labor:** Physician should be notified immediately if labor resumes or significant side effects occur.

EVALUATION

Effectiveness of therapy can be demonstrated by: ▪ Decrease in bronchoconstriction and bronchospasm ▫ Increase in ease of breathing ▪ Control of preterm labor in a fetus of 20–36 wk gestational age.

TERFENADINE
(ter-**fen**-i-deen)
Seldane

CLASSIFICATION(S):
Antihistamine
Pregnancy Category C

INDICATIONS
- Symptomatic relief of allergic symptoms caused by histamine release, including nasal allergies and allergic dermatoses.

ACTION
- Blocks the effects of histamine. **Therapeutic Effect:** - Relief of symptoms associated with histamine excess usually seen in allergic conditions.

PHARMACOKINETICS
Absorption: Rapidly and completely absorbed following oral administration.
Distribution: Distribution not known. Appears to have minimal penetration of the blood–brain barrier.
Metabolism and Excretion: Mostly metabolized by the liver. Eliminated mostly in the feces, via biliary excretion.
Half-life: 16–23 hr.

CONTRAINDICATIONS AND PRECAUTIONS
Contraindicated in: - Hypersensitivity.
Use Cautiously in: - Prostatic hypertrophy - Narrow-angle glaucoma - Pregnancy, lactation, or children <12 yr (safety not established) - Cardiovascular disease.

ADVERSE REACTIONS AND SIDE EFFECTS*
CNS: drowsiness, sedation, headache, dizziness, nervousness, weakness.
CV: palpitations, tachycardia.
EENT: visual disturbances.
GI: nausea, vomiting, abdominal pain, diarrhea, constipaiton, dry mouth, dry lips.

Derm: rashes, dry skin.
MS: musculoskeletal pain.
Misc: allergic reactions.

INTERACTIONS
Drug–Drug: - Additive CNS depression with other **CNS depressants**, including **alcohol, antidepressants, opioid analgesics**, and **sedative/hypnotics** - Additive anticholinergic effects with other **drugs possessing anticholinergic properties**, including **antidepressants, atropine, haloperidol, phenothiazines, quinidine**, and **disopyramide** - Increased risk of serious arrhythmias with **azole antifungals** (fluconazole, itraconazole, ketoconazole, miconazole) or **erythromycin**. Similar risk may occur with **azithromycin** or **clarithromycin**.

ROUTE AND DOSAGE
- **PO (Adults and Children ≥12 yr):** 60 mg twice daily.
- **PO (Children 6–12 yr):** 30–60 mg twice daily.
- **PO (Children 3–6 yr):** 15 mg twice daily.

AVAILABILITY
- *Tablets:* 60 mg, {120 mg} - {*Oral suspension:* 6 mg/ml} - *In combination with:* pseudoephedrine (Seldane-D). See Appendix A.

TIME/ACTION PROFILE
(antihistaminic effects)

	ONSET	PEAK	DURATION
PO	1–2 hr	3–6 hr	6–12 hr

NURSING IMPLICATIONS
ASSESSMENT
- Assess allergy symptoms (rhinitis, conjunctivitis, hives) prior to and periodically throughout course of therapy.
- Assess lung sounds and character of bronchial secretions. Maintain fluid intake of 1500–2000 ml/day to decrease viscosity of secretions.
- **Lab Test Considerations:** Will cause false-negative reactions on allergy

*Underlines indicate most frequent; **CAPITALS** indicate life-threatening.

skin tests; discontinue 3 days prior to testing.

POTENTIAL NURSING DIAGNOSES

- Airway clearance, ineffective (indications).
- Injury, high risk for (adverse reactions).
- Knowledge deficit related to medication regimen (patient/family teaching).

IMPLEMENTATION

- **PO:** Administer with food or milk to decrease GI irritation.

PATIENT/FAMILY TEACHING

- Instruct patient to take medication as directed. If a dose is missed, take as soon as remembered unless almost time for next dose.
- Inform patient that drug may cause drowsiness, although it is less likely to occur than with other antihistamines. Avoid driving or other activities requiring alertness until response to drug is known.
- Instruct patient to contact physician if symptoms persists.

EVALUATION

Effectivness of therapy can be demonstrated by: ■ Decrease in allergic symptoms.

TESTOSTERONE
(tess-**toss**-te-rone)

TESTOSTERONE BASE
Andro, Andronaq, Histerone, {Malogen}, Testamone, Testaqua, Testoject

TESTOSTERONE CYPIONATE
Andro-Cyp, Andronaq-LA, Andronate, dep Andro, Depotest, Duratest, T-Cypionate, Testa-C, Testred, Testoject-LA, Cypionate, Virilon IM

TESTOSTERONE ENANTHATE
Andro LA, Andropository, Andryl, Delatest, Delatestryl, Durathate, Everone, {Malogex}, Testone LA, Testrin-PA

TESTOSTERONE PROPIONATE
{Malogen}, Testex

CLASSIFICATION(S):
Hormone (androgen)
Schedule III
Pregnancy Category X

INDICATIONS

■ Treatment of hypogonadism in androgen-deficient males ■ Treatment of delayed puberty in males ■ Palliative treatment of androgen-responsive breast cancer.

ACTION

- Responsible for the normal growth and development of male sex organs
- Maintenance of male secondary sex characteristics: □ Growth and maturation of the prostatic, seminal vesicles, penis, scrotum □ Development of male hair distribution □ Vocal cord thickening □ Alterations in body musculature and fat distribution. **Therapeutic Effects:** ■ Correction of hormone deficiency in male hypogonadism □ Initiation of male puberty ■ Suppression of tumor growth in some forms of breast cancer.

PHARMACOKINETICS

Absorption: Well absorbed from IM sites. Cypionate, decanoate, propionate, and enanthate salts are absorbed slowly.
Distribution: Probably crosses the placenta and enters breast milk.
Metabolism and Excretion: Metabolized by the liver.
Half-life: Base—10–100 min; cypionate—8 days.

CONTRAINDICATIONS AND PRECAUTIONS

Contraindicated in: ■ Hypersensitivity ■ Pregnancy and lactation ■ Male patients with breast or prostate cancer ■ Hypercalcemia ■ Severe liver, renal, or cardiac disease.
Use Cautiously in: ■ Diabetes mellitus

- Coronary artery disease ▪ History of liver disease ▪ Prepubertal males.

ADVERSE REACTIONS AND SIDE EFFECTS*

CV: edema.
GI: nausea, vomiting, changes in appetite, hepatitis.
GU: bladder irritability, prostatic enlargement, menstrual irregularities.
EENT: deepening of voice.
Endo: females—clitoral enlargement, change in libido, decreased breast size; males—acne, priapism, facial hair, oligospermia, impotence, gynecomastia.
F and E: hypercalcemia.
Local: pain at injection site.

INTERACTIONS

Drug–Drug: ▪ Decreases metabolism and may enhance the action of **oral anticoagulants**, **oral hypoglycemic agents**, and **glucocorticoids** ▪ May also enhance the effect of **insulin** ▪ Additive hepatotoxicity with other **hepatotoxic agents**.

ROUTE AND DOSAGE

Replacement Therapy
- **IM (Adults):** 25–50 mg 2–3 times/wk (base or propionate) or 50–400 mg q 2–4 wk (enanthate or cypionate).

Delayed Male Puberty
- **IM (Adolescents):** Up to 100 mg/mo for up to 6 mo.

Palliative Management of Breast Cancer
- **IM (Adults):** 50–100 mg 3 times/wk (propionate or base) or 200–400 mg q 2–4 wk (cypionate or enanthate).

AVAILABILITY

▪ *Sterile testosterone suspension for injection (base):* 25 mg/ml, 50 mg/ml, 100 mg/ml ▪ *Testosterone cypionate injection:* 100 mg/ml, 200 mg/ml ▪ *Testosterone enanthate injection:* 100 mg/ml, 200 mg/ml ▪ *Testosterone propionate injection:* 50 mg/ml, 100 mg/ml ▪ *In combination with:* estradiol. See Appendix A.

TIME/ACTION PROFILE (androgenic effects)*

	ONSET	PEAK	DURATION
IM—base	UK	UK	1–3 days
IM—cypionate	UK	UK	2–4 wk
IM—enanthate	UK	UK	2–4 wk
IM—propionate	UK	UK	1–3 days

*Response is highly variable among individuals; may take months.

NURSING IMPLICATIONS

Assessment

- **General Info:** Monitor intake and output ratios, weigh patient twice weekly, and assess patient for edema. Notify physician of significant changes indicative of fluid retention.
- **Males:** Monitor for precocious puberty in boys (acne, darkening of skin, development of male secondary sex characteristics—increase in penis size, frequent erections, growth of body hair).
  - Monitor for breast enlargement, persistent erections, and increased urge to urinate in men. Monitor for difficulty urinating in elderly men, as prostate enlargement may occur.
- **Females:** Assess for virilism (deepening of voice, unusual hair growth or loss, clitoral enlargement, acne, menstrual irregularity).
  - In women with metastatic breast cancer, monitor for symptoms of hypercalcemia (nausea, vomiting, constipation, lethargy, loss of muscle tone, thirst, polyuria).
- **Lab Test Considerations:** Monitor hemoglobin and hematocrit periodically throughout course of therapy; may cause polycythemia.
  - Monitor hepatic function tests and serum cholesterol levels periodically throughout course of therapy. May cause increased AST (SGOT), increased or decreased cholesterol lev-

T

els, and suppression of clotting factors II, V, VII, and X.

□ Monitor serum and urine calcium levels and serum alkaline phosphatase concentrations in metastatic cancer.

□ May alter results of fasting blood sugar, glucose tolerance tests, thyroid function tests, and metyrapone tests. Decreased creatine and creatinine clearance may last up to 2 wk following discontinuation of therapy. Serum chloride, potassium, phosphate, and sodium levels may be increased.

□ May cause increased levels in 24-hr urine tests for 17-ketosteroid concentrations.

POTENTIAL NURSING DIAGNOSES

■ Sexual dysfunction (indications, side effects).

■ Knowledge deficit related to medication regimen (patient/family teaching).

IMPLEMENTATION

■ **General Info:** Range-of-motion exercises should be done with all bedridden patients to prevent mobilization of calcium from the bone.

■ **IM:** Administer IM deep into gluteal muscle. Crystals may form at low temperatures; warming and shaking vial will redissolve crystals. Use of a wet syringe or needle will cause a cloudy solution but will not affect potency.

PATIENT/FAMILY TEACHING

□ Advise patient to report the following signs and symptoms to physician promptly: in male patients, priapism (sustained and often painful erections) or gynecomastia; in female patients, virilism (which may be reversible if medication is stopped as soon as changes are noticed); hypercalcemia (nausea, vomiting, constipation, and weakness); edema (unexpected weight gain, swelling of feet); hepatitis (yellowing of skin or eyes and abdominal pain); or unusual bleeding or bruising.

□ Explain rationale for prohibition of use for increasing athletic performance. Testosterone is neither safe nor effective for this use and has a potential risk of serious side effects.

□ Instruct patient to notify physician immediately if pregnancy is planned or suspected.

□ Advise diabetic patients to monitor blood or urine closely for alterations in blood sugar concentrations.

□ Emphasize the importance of regular follow-up physical examinations, lab tests, and x-ray examinations to monitor progress.

□ Radiologic bone age determinations should be evaluated every 6 mo in prepubertal children to determine rate of bone maturation and effects on epiphyseal centers.

EVALUATION

Effectiveness of therapy can be demonstrated by: ■ Resolution of the signs of androgen deficiency without side effects ■ Decrease in the size and spread of breast malignancy in postmenopausal women. In antineoplastic therapy, response may require 3 mo of therapy; if signs of disease progression appear, therapy should be discontinued.

TETRACYCLINE
(te-tra-**sye**-kleen)
Achromycin, Alatet, {Apo-Tetra}, Nor-tet, {Novotetra}, {Nu-Tetra}, Panmycin, Robitet, Sumycin, Teline, Tetracap, Tetracyn, Tetralan, Topicycline

CLASSIFICATION(S):
Anti-infective (tetracycline)
Pregnancy Category UK

INDICATIONS

■ **PO:** Treatment of various infections due to unusual organisms, including: □ *Mycoplasma* □ *Chlamydia* □ *Rickettsia* ■ **PO:** Treatment of gonorrhea and syphilis in penicillin-allergic patients ■ **PO, Top:** Treatment of acne ■ Prevention of exacerbations of chronic bronchitis ■ **Ophth:** Treatment of superficial eye infections and trachoma ▪ **Ophth:** Prevention of ophthalmia neonatorum ▪ **Top:** Treatment and prophylaxis of superficial skin infections.

ACTION

▪ Inhibits bacterial protein synthesis at the level of the 30S bacterial ribosome. **Therapeutic Effect:** ▪ Bacteriostatic action against susceptible bacteria. **Spectrum:** ▪ Includes activity against some gram-positive pathogens: □ *Bacillus antracis* □ *Clostridium perfringens* □ *Clostridium tetani* □ *Listeria monocytogenes* □ *Nocardia* □ *Propionibacterium acnes* □ *Actinomyces isrealii* ▪ Active against some gram-negative pathogens: □ *Hemophilus influenzae* □ *Legionella pneumophila* □ *Yersinia entercolitica* □ *Yersinia pestis* □ *Neisseria gonorrhoeae* □ *Neisseria meningitidis.*

PHARMACOKINETICS

Absorption: 60–80% absorbed following oral administration.
Distribution: Widely distributed, some penetration into CSF. Crosses the placenta and enters breast milk.
Metabolism and Excretion: Excreted mostly unchanged by the kidneys.
Half-life: 6–12 hr.

CONTRAINDICATIONS AND PRECAUTIONS

Contraindicated in: ▪ Hypersensitivity ▪ Hypersensitivity to bisulfites (some products) ▪ Children <8 yr (permanent staining of teeth) ▪ Pregnancy (risk of permanent staining of teeth in infant if used during last half of pregnancy) ▪ Lactation ▪ Known alcohol intolerance (topical solution only).
Use Cautiously in: ▪ Cachectic or debilitated patients ▪ Hepatic or renal disease.

ADVERSE REACTIONS AND SIDE EFFECTS*

GI: <u>nausea</u>, <u>vomiting</u>, <u>diarrhea</u>, pancreatitis, esophagitis.
Derm: rashes, photosensitivity.

Hemat: blood dyscrasias.
Misc: superinfection, hypersensitivity reactions.

INTERACTIONS

Drug–Drug: ▪ May enhance the effect of **oral anticoagulants** ▪ May decrease the effectiveness of **oral contraceptives** ▪ **Antacids, calcium, iron,** and **magnesium** form insoluble compounds (chelates) and decrease absorption of tetracycline ▪ **Sucralfate** may bind to tetracycline and prevent its absorption from the GI tract ▪ **Cholestyramine** or **colestipol** decrease oral absorption of tetracyclines.
Drug–Food: ▪ **Calcium** in foods or **dairy products** decreases absorption by forming insoluble compounds (chelates).

ROUTE AND DOSAGE

▪ **PO (Adults):** 1–2 g/day in divided doses every 6–12 hr (small doses of 125–500 mg/day for chronic treatment of acne).
▪ **PO (Children >8 yr):** 25–50 mg/kg/day in divided doses every 6–12 hr.
▪ **Ophth (Adults and Children):** Thin strip of ointment q 2–4 hr or 1 drop of suspension q 6–12 hr (may be used more frequently); single dose used for prevention of ophthalmia neonatorum.
▪ **Top (Adults and Children >8 yr):** Ointment 1–2 times daily for superficial skin infections or solution applied twice daily for acne.

AVAILABILITY

▪ *Tablets:* 250 mg, 500 mg ▪ *Capsules:* 100 mg, 250 mg, 500 mg ▪ *Oral suspension:* 125 mg/5 ml ▪ *Topical solution:* 2.2 mg/ml ▪ *Ophthalmic suspension:* 10 mg/ml ▪ *Ophthalmic ointment:* 10 mg/g.

TIME/ACTION PROFILE (blood levels)

	ONSET	PEAK
PO	1–2 hr	2–4 hr

*<u>Underlines</u> indicate most frequent; **CAPITALS** indicate life-threatening.

NURSING IMPLICATIONS

ASSESSMENT

- Assess patient for infection (vital signs; appearance of wound, sputum, urine, and stool; WBC) at beginning and throughout course of therapy.
- Obtain specimens for culture and sensitivity prior to initiating therapy. First dose may be given before receiving results.
- **Lab Test Considerations:** Renal and hepatic functions and CBC should be monitored periodically during long-term therapy.
- May cause increased BUN, AST (SGOT), ALT (SGPT), serum alkaline phosphatase, bilirubin, and amylase concentrations.
- May cause false elevations in urinary catecholamine levels.

POTENTIAL NURSING DIAGNOSES

- Infection, high risk for (indications, side effects).
- Knowledge deficit related to medication regimen (patient/family teaching).
- Noncompliance related to medication regimen (patient/family teaching).

IMPLEMENTATION

- **General Info:** May cause yellow-brown discoloration and softening of teeth and bones if administered prenatally or during early childhood. Not recommended for children younger than 8 yr.
- **PO:** Administer around the clock. Administer at least 1 hr before or 2 hr after meals. Take with a full glass of liquid and at least 1 hr before going to bed to avoid esophageal ulceration. Use calibrated measuring device for liquid preparations. Shake liquid preparations well. Do not administer within 1–3 hr of other medications.
- Avoid administration of milk, calcium, antacids, magnesium-containing medications, or iron supplements within 1–3 hr of tetracycline.
- **Ophth:** See Appendix H for instillation of ophthalmic preparations.
- **Top:** Apply to entire affected area.

PATIENT/FAMILY TEACHING

- **General Info:** Instruct patient to take medication around the clock and to finish the drug completely as directed, even if feeling better. Avoid taking milk, antacids, calcium, magnesium-containing medications, and iron supplements within 1–3 hr of tetracycline. Advise patient that sharing of this medication may be dangerous.
- Caution patient to use sunscreen and protective clothing to prevent photosensitivity reactions.
- Advise patient to report the signs of superinfection (black, furry overgrowth on the tongue, vaginal itching or discharge, loose or foul-smelling stools) and allergy.
- Instruct patient to notify physician if symptoms do not improve.
- Caution patient to discard outdated or decomposed tetracyclines, as they may be toxic.
- **Ophth:** Instruct patient on correct technique for instillation of ophthalmic preparations. Caution patient not to allow tip of container to come in contact with eye, fingers, or any other surface.
- Ophthalmic preparations may cause blurred vision. Caution patient to avoid driving or other activities requiring visual acuity until response to medication is known.
- **Top:** Instruct patient in correct technique for application of solution or ointment. Advise patient to avoid frequent washing of affected area and to wait at least 1 hr before applying other topical acne preparations.
- Advise patient that topical preparations may stain clothing and may cause slight yellowing of skin.
- Instruct patient to consult physician if no improvement in lesions with 2 wk of treatment with ointment or 6–8 wk with solution.

EVALUATION

Clinical response can be evaluated by:
- Resolution of the signs and symptoms of infection. Length of time for complete resolution depends on the organism

and site of infection ▪ Decrease in acne lesions.

THEOPHYLLINE
(thee-off-i-lin)
Accurbron, Aerolate, Aquaphyllin, Asmalix, Bronkodyl, Elixomin, Elixophyllin, Lanophyllin, Lixolin, {Pulmophylline}, Slophyllin Syrup, Synophylate, Theoclear, Theolair, Theon, Theophyl, Theostat

THEOPHYLLINE EXTENDED RELEASE
Aerolate, Constant-T, Elixophyllin SR, LaBID, Quibron-T/SR, Respbid, Slo-bid Gyrocaps, Slophyllin Gyrocaps, Sustaire, T-Phyl, Theo-24, Theobid Duracap, Theobid Jr. Duracap, Theochron, Theoclear LA, Theoclear LA Cenules, Theo-Dur, Theo-Dur Sprinkle, Theolair-SR, Theophyl-SR, Theospan-SR, Theo-Sav, Theo-Time, Theovent Long-Acting, Uniphyl

CLASSIFICATION(S):
Bronchodilator (phosphodiesterase inhibitor)
Pregnancy Category C

INDICATIONS
▪ Bronchodilator in reversible airway obstruction due to asthma or COPD. **Unlabeled Use:** ▪ Respiratory and myocardial stimulant in apnea of infancy.

ACTION
▪ Inhibits phosphodiesterase, producing increased tissue concentrations of cyclic adenosine monophosphate (cAMP) ▪ Increased levels of cAMP result in: □ Bronchodilation □ CNS and cardiac stimulation □ Diuresis □ Gastric acid secretion. **Therapeutic Effect:** ▪ Bronchodilation.

PHARMACOKINETICS
Absorption: Well absorbed from oral dosage forms. Absorption from extended-release dosage forms is slow but complete.
Distribution: Widely distributed. Crosses the placenta. Breast milk concentrations 70% of plasma levels.
Metabolism and Excretion: Mostly metabolized by the liver to caffeine, which may accumulate in neonates. Metabolites are renally excreted.
Half-life: 3–13 hr. Increased in the elderly (>60 yr), neonates, and patients with CHF or liver disease. Shortened in cigarette smokers and children.

CONTRAINDICATIONS AND PRECAUTIONS
Contraindicated in: ▪ Uncontrolled arrhythmias ▪ Hyperthyroidism ▪ Known alcohol intolerance (some oral liquids). **Use Cautiously in:** ▪ Elderly patients >60 yr (dosage reduction required) ▪ CHF, cor pulmonale, or liver disease (dosage reduction required) ▪ Cigarette smokers (larger doses may be required) ▪ Pregnancy (has been used safely) ▪ Children <6 yr (avoid sustained-release preparations) ▪ Obese patients (dose should be based on ideal body weight).

ADVERSE REACTIONS AND SIDE EFFECTS*
CNS: nervousness, anxiety, headache, insomnia, SEIZURES.
CV: tachycardia, palpitations, arrhythmias, angina pectoris.
GI: nausea, vomiting, anorexia, cramps.
Neuro: tremor.

INTERACTIONS
Drug–Drug: ▪ Additive CV and CNS side effects with **adrenergic (sympathomimetic) agents** ▪ May decrease the therapeutic effect of **lithium ▪ Smoking, phenobarbital, rifampin, phenytoin** and **ketoconazole** increase metabolism

and may decrease effectiveness ■ **Erythromycin, beta-adrenergic blockers, influenza vaccination, cimetidine, oral contraceptives, glucocorticoids, disulfiram, interferon, mexiletine, fluoroquinolones, thiabendazole, tacrine,** and large doses of **allopurinol** decrease metabolism and may lead to toxicity ■ Increased risk of arrhythmias with **halothane** ■ **Isoniazid, carbamazepine,** or **loop diuretics** may increase or decrease theophylline levels.

Drug-Food: ■ Additive adverse reactions may occur with excessive ingestion of **xanthine (caffeine)-containing food** or **beverages**. Excess consumption of **charcoal-broiled beef** may decrease effectiveness.

ROUTE AND DOSAGE

Initial or loading doses are required only in patients who have not received theophylline in any form recently. Theophylline serum levels should be used to assess all regimens.

Bronchodilator

- **PO (Adults):** 5 mg/kg initially; then in *otherwise healthy nonsmoking adults*—3 mg/kg q 8 hr; *young adult smokers*—3 mg/kg q 6 hr; *patients >60 yr or patients with cor pulmonale*—2 mg/kg q 8 hr; *patients with congestive heart failure or liver disease*—1–2 mg/kg q 12 hr (daily dose may be divided and given as extended-release dosage forms q 12–24 hr). Dose should not exceed 13 mg/kg/day or 900 mg, whichever is less.

- **PO (Children 9–16 yr):** 5 mg/kg initially, followed by 12 mg/kg/day in divided doses q 6 hr (daily dose may be divided and given q 8–24 hr as extended-release forms). Dose should not exceed 20 mg/kg/day in patients 9–12 yr or 18 mg/kg/day in patients 12–16 yr or 900 mg, whichever is less.

- **PO (Children 1–9 yr):** 5 mg/kg initially, followed by 4 mg/kg q 6 hr (not to exceed 24 mg/kg/day or 900 mg, whichever is less).

- **PO (Infants 6 mo–1 yr):** [(0.2 × age in weeks) + 5] × kg = 24-hr dose (in mg). Give in divided doses q 6 hr.

- **PO (Infants up to 6 mo):** [(0.2 × age in weeks) + 5] × kg = 24-hr dose (in mg). Give in divided doses q 8 hr.

- **PO (Premature Infants >24 days old):** 1.5 mg/kg q 12 hr.

- **PO (Premature Infants ≤24 days old):** 1 mg/kg q 12 hr.

- **IV (Adults):** 5 mg/kg initially over 20–30 min initially, then in *otherwise healthy nonsmoking adults*—0.43 mg/kg/hr; *young adult smokers*—0.7 mg/kg/hr; *patients >60 yr or patients with cor pulmonale*—0.26 mg/kg/hr; *patients with congestive heart failure or liver disease*—0.2 mg/kg/hr. Maintenance infusion rates may be decreased after 12 hr.

- **IV (Children 12–16 yr):** 5 mg/kg initially, then in *nonsmokers*—0.5 mg/kg/hr; *smokers*—0.7 mg/kg/hr.

- **IV (Children 9–12 yr):** 5 mg/kg initially, then 0.7 mg/kg/hr.

- **IV (Children 1–9 yr):** 5 mg/kg initially, then 0.8 mg/kg/hr.

- **IV (Children up to 1 yr):** 5 mg/kg initially, then dose in mg/kg/hr = (0.008) (age in weeks) + 0.21.

Respiratory Stimulant

- **PO (Neonates):** 5 mg/kg initially, then 2 mg/kg/day in 2 divided doses.

- **IV (Neonates):** 5 mg/kg initially, then 1–1.5 mg/kg q 12 hr.

AVAILABILITY

■ *Immediate-release tablets:* 100 mg, 125 mg, 200 mg, 250 mg, 300 mg ■ *Immediate-release capsules:* 100 mg, 200 mg ■ *Timed-release tablets:* 100 mg, 200 mg, 250 mg, 300 mg, 400 mg, 450 mg ■ *Timed-release capsules:* 50 mg, 65 mg, 75 mg, 100 mg, 125 mg, 130 mg, 200 mg, 250 mg, 260 mg, 300 mg ■ *Syrup:* 80 mg/15 ml, 150 mg/15 ml ■ *Elixir:* 80 mg/15 ml ■ *Oral solution:* 80 mg/15 ml, 150 mg/15 ml ■ *Injection (with dextrose):* 0.8 mg/ml 1.6 mg/ml, 3.2 mg/ml, 4 mg/ml ■ *In combination with:* guaifenesin, potassium iodide, iodinated glycerol, and epinephrine. See Appendix A.

TIME/ACTION PROFILE
(bronchodilation)

	ONSET*	PEAK	DURATION
PO	rapid	1–2 hr	6 hr
PO-ER	delayed	4–8 hr	8–24 hr
IV	rapid	end of infusion	6–8 hr

*If a loading dose has been given.

NURSING IMPLICATIONS

ASSESSMENT

◻ Assess blood pressure, pulse, and respiratory status (rate, lung sounds, use of accessory muscles) prior to and throughout course of therapy. Ensure that oxygen therapy is correctly instituted.

◻ Monitor intake and output ratios for an increase in diuresis or fluid overload due to volume of medication.

◻ Patients with a history of cardiovascular problems should be monitored for ECG changes.

▪ **Lab Test Considerations:** Monitor ABGs and serum electrolytes prior to and periodically throughout therapy.

▪ **Toxicity and Overdose:** Monitor drug levels routinely. Peak levels should be evaluated 15–30 min after IV loading dose, 1–2 hr after rapid-acting forms, and 4–12 hr after extended-release forms. Therapeutic plasma levels range is 10–20 mcg/ml. Drug levels >20 mcg/ml are associated with toxicity. Caffeine ingestion may falsely elevate drug concentration levels.

◻ Observe patient closely for the appearance of progressive theophylline toxicity (anorexia, nausea, vomiting, restlessness, insomnia, tachycardia, arrhythmias, seizures). Notify physician immediately if these symptoms occur.

POTENTIAL NURSING DIAGNOSES

▪ Airway clearance, ineffective (indications).

▪ Activity intolerance (indications).

▪ Knowledge deficit related to medication regimen (patient/family teaching).

IMPLEMENTATION

▪ **General Info:** Give these medications around the clock. Once-a-day doses should be administered in the morning.

◻ Do not refrigerate elixirs, solutions, syrups, or suspensions, as crystals may form. Crystals should dissolve when liquid is warmed to room temperature.

◻ Wait at least 4 hr after discontinuing IV therapy to begin immediate-release oral dosage; for extended-release oral dosage form, administer first oral dose at time of IV discontinuation.

▪ **PO:** Administer with a full glass of water or food to minimize GI irritation. Food slows but does not reduce the extent of absorption. Use calibrated measuring device to ensure accurate dose of liquid preparations.

◻ Do not crush enteric-coated or timed-release tablets or capsules.

▪ **Continuous Infusion:** IV theophylline and 5% dextrose is packed in a moisture-barrier overwrap. Remove immediately before administration and squeeze bag to check for leaks. Discard if solution is not clear.

▪ *Loading Dose:* Administer over 20–30 min. If patient has had another form of theophylline prior to loading dose, serum theophylline level should be obtained and loading dose proportionately reduced.

▪ *Rate:* Do not exceed 20 mg/min. Rapid administration may cause hypotension, arrhythmias, syncope, and death. Infusion rate may be increased after 12 hr. Administer via infusion pump to ensure accurate dosage. Monitor ECG continuously, as tachyarrythmias may occur.

▪ **Y-Site Compatibility:** ▪ acyclovir ▪ famotidine.

▪ **Y-Site Incompatibility:** ▪ hetastarch.

▪ **Additive Compatibility:** ▪ methylprednisolone.

▪ **Additive Incompatibility:** ▪ ascorbic acid ▪ erythromycin glucceptate ▪ meperidine ▪ methicillin ▪ morphine ∎ penicillin G ∎ phenobarbital ∎ phenytoin ∎ vancomycin.

PATIENT/FAMILY TEACHING
□ Emphasize the importance of taking only the prescribed dose at the prescribed time intervals. Missed doses should be taken as soon as remembered or omitted if close to next dose.
□ Encourage patient to drink adequate liquids (2000 ml/day minimum) to decrease the viscosity of airway secretions.
□ Advise patient not to take any over-the-counter cough, cold, or breathing preparations without consulting physician or pharmacist. These medications may increase side effects and cause arrhythmias.
□ Advise patient to minimize intake of xanthine-containing foods or beverages (cola, coffee, chocolate) and not to eat charcoal-broiled foods daily.
□ Instruct patient not to change brands or dosage forms without consulting physician.
□ Encourage patient not to smoke. Instruct patient to inform physician if smoking pattern changes, as dosage adjustment may be necessary.
□ Advise patient to contact physician promptly if usual dose of medication fails to produce the desired results, symptoms worsen after treatment, or toxic effects occur.
□ Emphasize the importance of having serum levels routinely tested every 6–12 mo.

EVALUATION
Effectiveness of therapy can be demonstrated by: ∎ Increased ease in breathing □ Clearing of lung fields on auscultation ∎ Effective respiratory patterns in neonatal apnea.

THIAMINE
(thye-a-min)
Betalin S, {Betaxin}, {Bewon}, Biamine, vitamin B₁

CLASSIFICATION(S):
Vitamin (water-soluble)
Pregnancy Category A

INDICATIONS
∎ Treatment of thiamine deficiencies (beriberi) ∎ Prevention of Wernicke's encephalopathy ∎ Dietary supplement in patients with GI disease, alcoholism, or cirrhosis.

ACTION
∎ Required for carbohydrate metabolism. **Therapeutic Effect:** ∎ Replacement in deficiency states.

PHARMACOKINETICS
Absorption: Well absorbed from the GI tract by an active process. Excessive amounts are not absorbed completely. Also well absorbed from IM sites.
Distribution: Widely distributed. Enters breast milk.
Metabolism and Excretion: Metabolized by the liver. Excess amounts are excreted unchanged by the kidneys.
Half-life: UK.

CONTRAINDICATIONS AND PRECAUTIONS
Contraindicated in: ∎ Hypersensitivity ∎ Known alcohol intolerance (elixir only).
Use Cautiously in: ∎ Wernicke's encephalopathy (condition may be worsened unless glucose is administered before thiamine).

ADVERSE REACTIONS AND SIDE EFFECTS*
Adverse reactions and side effects are extremely rare and are usually associated with IV administration or extremely large doses.
CNS: weakness, restlessness.
EENT: tightness of the throat.
CV: hypotension, VASCULAR COLLAPSE, vasodilation.
Resp: respiratory distress, pulmonary edema.

{} = Available in Canada only.
*Underlines indicate most frequent; **CAPITALS** indicate life-threatening.

GI: nausea, GI bleeding.
Derm: warmth, tingling, pruritus, urticaria, sweating, cyanosis.
Misc: angioedema.

INTERACTIONS
Drug–Drug: ▪ May enchance **neuromuscular blocking agents**.

ROUTE AND DOSAGE
Thiamine Deficiency (Beriberi)
▪ **PO (Adults):** 5–10 mg 3 times daily.
▪ **PO (Children):** 10–50 mg/day in divided doses.
▪ **IM, IV (Adults):** 5–100 mg tid.
▪ **IM, IV (Children):** 10–25 mg/day.

Alcohol-Induced Deficiency
▪ **PO (Adults):** 40 mg/day.

Dietary Supplement
▪ **PO (Adults):** 1–2 mg/day.
▪ **PO (Children):** 0.5–1 mg/day.
▪ **PO (Infants):** 0.3–0.5 mg/day.

AVAILABILITY
▪ *Tablets:* 50 mg, 100 mg, 250 mg, 500 mg ▪ *Enteric-coated tablets:* 20 mg ▪ {*Elixir:* 250 mcg/5 ml} ▪ *Injection:* 100 mg/ml ▪ *In combination with:* other vitamins, minerals, and trace elements in multi-vitamin preparations.

TIME/ACTION PROFILE (time for symptoms of deficiency—edema and heart failure—to resolve; confusion and psychosis take longer to respond)

	ONSET	PEAK	DURATION
PO	hr	days	days–wk
IM	hr	days	days–wk
IV	hr	days	days–wk

NURSING IMPLICATIONS
ASSESSMENT
▫ Assess patient for signs and symptoms of thiamine deficiency (anorexia, GI distress, irritability, palpitations, tachycardia, edema, paresthesia, muscle weakness and pain, depression, memory loss, confusion, psychosis, visual disturbances, elevated serum pyruvic acid levels).
▫ Assess patient's nutritional status

(diet, weight) prior to and throughout course of therapy.
▫ Monitor patients receiving IV thiamine for anaphylaxis (wheezing, urticaria, edema).
▪ **Lab Test Considerations:** May interfere with certain methods of testing serum theophylline, uric acid, and urobilinogen concentrations.

POTENTIAL NURSING DIAGNOSES
▪ Nutrition, altered: less than body requirements (indications).
▪ Knowledge deficit related to diet and medication regimen (patient/family teaching).

IMPLEMENTATION
▪ **General Info:** Because of infrequency of single B-vitamin deficiencies, combinations are commonly administered.
▪ **IM, IV:** Parenteral administration is reserved for patients in whom oral administration is not feasible.
▪ **IM:** Administration may cause tenderness and induration at injection site. Cool compresses may decrease discomfort.
▪ **IV:** Sensitivity reactions and deaths have occurred from IV administration. An intradermal test dose is recommended in patients with suspected sensitivity. Monitor site for erythema and induration.
▪ **Direct IV:** Administer undiluted each 100 mg over at least 5 min.
▪ **Continuous Infusion:** May be diluted in dextrose/Ringer's or lactated Ringer's combinations, dextrose/saline combinations, D5W, D10W, Ringer's and lactated Ringer's injection, 0.9% NaCl, or 0.45% NaCl and is usually administered with other vitamins.
▪ **Y-Site Compatibility:** ▪ famotidine.
▪ **Additive Incompatibility:** ▪ barbiturates ▪ solutions with neutral or alkaline pH, such as carbonates, bicarbonates, citrates, and acetates ▪ erythromycin ▪ kanamycin ▪ streptomycin.

PATIENT/FAMILY TEACHING
▫ Encourage patient to comply with physician's dietary recommenda-

T

tions. Explain that the best source of vitamins is a well-balanced diet with foods from the 4 basic food groups.

▫ Teach patient that foods high in thiamine include cereals (whole grain and enriched), meats (especially pork), and fresh vegetables; loss is variable during cooking.

▫ Caution patients self-medicating with vitamin supplements not to exceed RDA (see Appendix L). The effectiveness of megadoses of vitamins for treatment of various medical conditions is unproven and may cause side effects.

EVALUATION

Effectiveness of therapy can be demonstrated by: ▪ Prevention of or decrease in the signs and symptoms of vitamin B_1 deficiency ▫ Decrease in the symptoms of neuritis, ocular signs, ataxia, edema, and heart failure may be seen within hours of administration and may disappear within a few days ▫ Confusion and psychosis may take longer to respond and may persist if nerve damage has occurred.

THIETHYLPERAZINE
(thye-eth-il-**per**-a-zeen)
Norzine, Torecan

CLASSIFICATION(S):
Antiemetic (phenothiazine)
Pregnancy Category UK

INDICATIONS

▪ Management of nausea and vomiting.

ACTION

▪ Alters the effects of dopamine in the CNS ▪ Depresses the chemoreceptive trigger zone (CTZ) and vomiting center in the CNS. **Therapeutic Effect:** ▪ Diminished nausea and vomiting.

PHARMACOKINETICS

Absorption: Well absorbed following oral, rectal, or IM administration.
Distribution: Widely distributed, high concentrations in the CNS. Crosses the placenta and probably enters breast milk.
Metabolism and Excretion: Highly metabolized by the liver and GI mucosa.
Half-life: UK.

CONTRAINDICATIONS AND PRECAUTIONS

Contraindicated in: ▪ Hypersensitivity ▪ Hypersensitivity to bisulfites (IM) ▪ Hypersensitivity to aspirin or tartrazine (tab) ▪ Cross-sensitivity with other phenothiazines may exist ▪ Narrow-angle glaucoma ▪ Bone marrow depression ▪ Severe liver or cardiovascular disease ▪ Pregnancy ▪ Children <12 yr.
Use Cautiously in: ▪ Elderly or debilitated patients (dosage reduction recommended) ▪ Lactation (safety not established) ▪ Diabetes mellitus ▪ Respiratory disease ▪ Prostatic hypertrophy ▪ CNS tumors ▪ Epilepsy ▪ Intestinal obstruction.

ADVERSE REACTIONS AND SIDE EFFECTS*

CNS: sedation, extrapyramidal reactions, tardive dyskinesia, restlessness, headache, cerebral vascular spasm, NEUROLEPTIC MALIGNANT SYNDROME.
EENT: dry eyes, blurred vision, lens opacities, tinnitus.
CV: hypotension (following IM use), peripheral edema.
Derm: rashes, photosensitivity, pigment changes.
Endo: galactorrhea.
GI: constipation, dry mouth, ileus, anorexia, hepatitis, altered taste.
GU: urinary retention.
Hemat: AGRANULOCYTOSIS, leukopenia.
Metab: hyperthermia.
Neuro: trigeminal neuralgia.
Misc: allergic reactions.

INTERACTIONS

Drug–Drug: ▪ Additive hypotension with **antihypertensive agents,** acute ingestion of **alcohol,** or **nitrates** ▪ Additive CNS depression with other

---

*Underlines indicate most frequent; **CAPITALS** indicate life-threatening.

CNS depressants, including alcohol, antihistamines, opioid analgesics, sedative/hypnotics, or general anesthetics ▪ Additive anticholinergic effects with other drugs possessing anticholinergic properties, including antihistamines, antidepressants, atropine, disopyramide, haloperidol, and other phenothiazines ▪ May decrease the beneficial effects of levodopa ▪ May block alpha-adrenergic effects of epinephrine resulting in severe hypotension and tachycardia.

ROUTE AND DOSAGE
▪ PO, IM, Rect (Adults): 10 mg 1–3 times daily.

AVAILABILITY
▪ *Tablets:* 10 mg ▪ *Suppositories:* 10 mg ▪ *Injection:* 5 mg/ml.

TIME/ACTION PROFILE (antiemetic effect)

	ONSET	PEAK	DURATION
PO	30 min	UK	4 hr
IM	UK	UK	UK
Rectal	UK	UK	UK

NURSING IMPLICATIONS

ASSESSMENT
□ Assess patient for nausea and vomiting prior to and 30–60 min following administration.
□ Monitor blood pressure (sitting, standing, lying), pulse, and respiratory rate prior to and frequently during initial therapy.
□ Assess patient for level of sedation following administration.
□ Assess urine output for possible urinary retention.
□ Observe patient carefully for extrapyramidal symptoms (akathisia—restlessness; dystonia—muscle spasms and twisting motions; pseudoparkinsonism—mask facies, rigidity, tremors, drooling, shuffling gait dysphagia). Notify physician if these symptoms occur, as reduction in dose or discontinuation of medication may be necessary. Trihexyphenidyl or di-

phenhydramine may be used to control these symptoms.
□ Monitor for tardive dyskinesia (rhythmic movement of mouth, face, and extremities). Notify physician immediately if these symptoms occur, as these side effects may be irreversible.
□ Monitor for development of neuroleptic malignant syndrome (fever, respiratory distress, tachycardia, convulsions, diaphoresis, hypertension or hypotension, pallor, tiredness). Notify physician immediately if these symptoms occur.
▪ Lab Test Considerations: CBC and liver function tests should be evaluated periodically throughout course of prolonged therapy.
□ May cause false-positive or false-negative pregnancy tests.

POTENTIAL NURSING DIAGNOSES
▪ Fluid volume deficit (indications).
▪ Injury, high risk for (side effects).
▪ Knowledge deficit related to medication regimen (patient/family teaching).

IMPLEMENTATION
▪ IM: Inject slowly into deep, well-developed muscle. Administer only clear, colorless solution. Keep patient recumbent for at least 60 min following injection to minimize hypotensive effects.
□ Do not administer IV, may cause severe hypotension.

PATIENT/FAMILY TEACHING
□ Advise patient to make position changes slowly to minimize orthostatic hypotension.
□ Medication may cause drowsiness. Caution patient to avoid driving or other activities requiring alertness until response to medication is known.
□ Caution patient to avoid taking alcohol or other CNS depressants concurrently with this medication.
□ Inform patient of possibility of extrapyramidal symptoms and tardive dyskinesia. Caution patient to report these symptoms immediately to physician.
□ Advise patient to use sunscreen and

protective clothing when exposed to the sun to prevent photosensitivity reactions. Extremes in temperature should also be avoided, as this drug impairs body temperature regulation.

☐ Instruct patient to use frequent mouth rinses, good oral hygiene, and sugarless gum or candy to minimize dry mouth. Consult physician or dentist if dry mouth continues >2 wk.

☐ Advise patient that increasing bulk and fluids in the diet and exercise may help minimize the constipating effects of this medication.

☐ Instruct patient to notify physician promptly if sore throat, fever, unusual bleeding or bruising, skin rashes, weakness, tremors, visual disturbances, dark-colored urine, or clay-colored stools are noted.

☐ Patients on prolonged therapy should have periodic lab tests and ocular examinations.

EVALUATION
Effectiveness of therapy can be demonstrated by: ▪ Relief of nausea and vomiting.

THIOGUANINE
(thye-oh-**gwon**-een)
6-thioguanine, {Lanvis}

CLASSIFICATION(S):
Antineoplastic (antimetabolite)
Pregnancy Category UK

INDICATIONS

▪ Used in combination chemotherapeutic regimens to induce remission in acute myelogenous leukemia ▪ Has also been used alone or in combination with other agents in the treatment of acute lymphocytic leukemia and chronic myelogenous leukemia.

ACTION

▪ Incorporated into DNA and RNA, subsequently disrupting synthesis (cell cycle—S-phase specific). **Therapeutic Effects:** ▪ Death of rapidly replicating cells, especially malignant ones ▪ Immunosuppressive properties.

PHARMACOKINETICS

Absorption: Variable and incomplete (30%) following oral administration.
Distribution: Probably does not enter the CSF. Crosses the placenta.
Metabolism and Excretion: Highly metabolized by the liver.
Half-life: 11 hr.

CONTRAINDICATIONS AND PRECAUTIONS

Contraindicated in: ▪ Hypersensitivity ▪ Pregnancy or lactation ▪ Severe liver disease.
Use Cautiously in: ▪ Patients with childbearing potential ▪ Infections ▪ Decreased bone marrow reserve ▪ Other chronic debilitating illnesses.

ADVERSE REACTIONS AND SIDE EFFECTS*

EENT: loss of vibratory sense.
GI: jaundice, hepatotoxicity, nausea, vomiting, stomatitis, diarrhea.
GU: gonadal suppression.
Derm: rash, dermatitis.
Hemat: leukopenia, thrombocytopenia, anemia.
Metab: hyperuricemia.
Neuro: unsteady gait.

INTERACTIONS

Drug–Drug: ▪ Additive bone marrow depression with other **antineoplastic agents** or **radiation therapy** ▪ May decrease antibody response to **live virus vaccines** and increase the risk of adverse reactions.

ROUTE AND DOSAGE
Many other protocols are used.
Induction
▪ **PO (Adults and Children):** 2 mg/kg (75–100 mg/m²) per day, rounded off to nearest 20 mg given as single dose. After 4 wk may increase to 3 mg/kg.

Maintenance Dosage

- **PO (Adults and Children):** 2–3 mg/kg (100 mg/m^2) per day.

AVAILABILITY

- *Tablets:* 40 mg.

TIME/ACTION PROFILE (effect on blood counts)

	ONSET	PEAK	DURATION
PO	7–10 days	14 days	21 days

NURSING IMPLICATIONS

ASSESSMENT

- Assess for fever, chills, sore throat, and signs of infection. Notify physician if these symptoms occur.
- Monitor platelet count throughout therapy. Assess for bleeding (bleeding gums, bruising, petechiae, guaiac stools, urine, and emesis). If thrombocytopenia occurs, avoid IM injections and rectal temperatures and apply pressure to venipuncture sites for 10 min.
- Monitor intake and output, appetite, and nutritional intake. Administration of an antiemetic and adjusting diet as tolerated may help maintain fluid and electrolyte balance and nutritional status.
- Anemia may occur. Monitor for increased fatigue, dyspnea, and orthostatic hypotension.
- Monitor for symptoms of gout (increased uric acid, joint pain, edema). Encourage patient to drink at least 2 liters of fluid/day. Physician may order allopurinol or alkalinization of urine to decrease uric acid levels.
- **Lab Test Considerations:** Monitor CBC and differential at least weekly, daily in patients with elevated leukocyte counts. Bone marrow suppression usually occurs in 2–4 wk, but rapid decrease in leukocyte count may occur in 1–2 wk. Notify physician of any rapid or severe drop in blood counts, as therapy may need to be withheld until values stabilize. Bone marrow aspiration may be required

to detect thioguanine-induced hypoplasia.
- Monitor for increased uric acid, creatinine, and BUN.
- Monitor for hepatotoxicity evidenced by increased AST (SGOT), ALT (SGPT), LDH, serum bilirubin, and alkaline phosphatase.

POTENTIAL NURSING DIAGNOSES

- Infection, high risk for (side effects).
- Injury, high risk for (side effects).
- Knowledge deficit related to medication regimen (patient/family teaching).

IMPLEMENTATION

- **PO:** Administer daily dose at bedtime. May also be divided into 2 doses and given 12 hr apart.
- If patient has difficulty swallowing tablets, confer with pharmacist regarding preparation of syrup.

PATIENT/FAMILY TEACHING

- Instruct patient to take thioguanine exactly as directed, even if nausea and vomiting occur. If vomiting occurs shortly after dose is taken, consult physician. Take combinations of drugs at prescribed times. If a dose is missed, do not take at all.
- Instruct patient to notify physician if decreased urine output, swelling of lower extremities, yellowing of skin, nausea, vomiting, severe diarrhea, mouth sores, fever, chills, sore throat, signs of infection, bleeding gums, bruising, petechiae, or blood in urine, stool, or emesis occurs.
- Caution patient to avoid crowds and persons with known infections. Instruct patient to use soft toothbrush and electric razor. Caution patient not to drink alcoholic beverages or take products containing aspirin or ibuprofen.
- This medication may cause gonadal suppression; however, patient should still use birth control. Advise patient to inform physician immediately if pregnancy is suspected.
- Instruct patient to inspect oral mucosa for redness and ulceration. If ul-

ceration occurs, advise patient to use sponge brush and rinse mouth with water after eating and drinking. Physician may order viscous lidocaine swishes if pain interferes with eating.

□ Instruct patient not to receive any vaccinations without advice of physician.

□ Advise patient of need for medical follow-up and frequent lab tests.

EVALUATION
Effectiveness of therapy can be demonstrated by: ▪ Induction of remission in patients with leukemia.

THIOPENTAL
(thye-oh-**pen**-tal)
Pentothal

CLASSIFICATION(S):
Anesthetic (barbiturate), Anticonvulsant
Schedule III
Pregnancy Category C

INDICATIONS

▪ Used to provide an unconscious state as part of balanced anesthesia in combination with muscle relaxants and/or analgesics during short surgical procedures ▪ Treatment of seizures in patients with increased intracranial pressure ▪ Part of narcoanalysis or narcosynthesis in psychiatric patients.
Unlabeled Use: ▪ Management of increased intracranial pressure.

ACTION

▪ Produces all levels of CNS depression: □ Depresses the sensory cortex □ Decreases motor activity □ Alters cerebellar function □ Inhibits transmission in the nervous system ▪ Raises the seizure threshold. **Therapeutic Effects:** ▪ Induction of sleep and anesthesia without analgesia (short-acting) ▪ Decreased seizure activity ▪ Lowering of intracranial pressure.

PHARMACOKINETICS

Absorption: Readily absorbed from the rectal mucosa.
Distribution: Rapidly distributed to the CNS, then redistributed to viscera (liver, kidneys, heart), then to muscle, and finally to fat. Crosses the placenta readily. Small amounts enter breast milk.
Metabolism and Excretion: Mostly metabolized by the liver. Small amounts are converted to pentobarbital.
Half-life: 12 hr (increased in obese patients and in pregnant patients at term).

CONTRAINDICATIONS AND PRECAUTIONS

Contraindicated in: ▪ Hypersensitivity ▪ Porphyria ▪ Status asthmaticus ▪ Inflammatory rectal or lower bowel conditions or patients undergoing rectal surgery (rectal form only).
Use Cautiously in: ▪ Severe cardiovascular disease, shock, or hypotension ▪ Myxedema ▪ Addison's disease ▪ Increased intracranial pressure ▪ Liver disease ▪ Renal disease ▪ Myasthenia gravis ▪ Pregnancy or lactation (safety not established) ▪ Middle-aged, elderly, or debilitated patients (dosage reduction may be required) ▪ Repeated use (tolerance may develop) ▪ Repeated doses, large doses, or prolonged infusion in 24-hr period (increased risk of excessive somnolence, respiratory or circulatory depression—dosage reduction required).

ADVERSE REACTIONS AND SIDE EFFECTS*

CNS: emergence delirium, headache, prolonged somnolence.
EENT: salivation.
Resp: respiratory depression, APNEA, laryngospasm, bronchospasm, hiccoughs, sneezing, coughing.
CV: hypotension, myocardial depression, arrhythmias.
GI: rectal irritation (after rectal administration), nausea, vomiting.
Derm: erythema, pruritus, urticaria, rashes.

*Underlines indicate most frequent; **CAPITALS** indicate life-threatening.

Local: pain, phlebitis at IV site.
MS: skeletal muscle hyperactivity.
Misc: allergic reactions, including ANAPHYLAXIS, shivering.

INTERACTIONS

Drug–Drug: Additive CNS depression with other **CNS depressants,** including **alcohol, antihistamines, antidepressants, opioid analgesics,** and **sedative/hypnotics** ▪ Increased risk of hypotension with **antihypertensives, diuretics,** or **ketamine.**

ROUTE AND DOSAGE

Dosages must be carefully titrated by patient response.

Test Dose
▪ IV (Adults): 25–75 mg.

Anesthesia
▪ IV (Adults): 50–100 mg initially, followed by 50–100 mg as needed or 3–5 mg/kg as a single dose.
▪ IV (Children): 3–5 mg/kg initially, followed by 1 mg/kg as needed.

Anticonvulsant
▪ IV (Adults): 50–125 mg.

Preanesthetic Sedation (basal anesthesia)
▪ Rect (Adults and Children): 30 mg/kg.

Narcoanalysis
▪ IV (Adults): 100 mg/min until patient becomes confused.

Basal Narcosis
▪ Rect (Adults and Children): Up to 9 mg/kg, not to exceed 1–1.5 g in children weighing more than 34 kg or 3–4 g in adults weighing 90 kg or more.

Increased Intracranial Pressure
▪ IV (Adults): 1.5–3.5 mg/kg as needed.

AVAILABILITY

▪ *Injection:* 250 mg, 400 mg, 500 mg, 1 g ▪ *Rectal suspension:* 400 mg/g.

TIME/ACTION PROFILE (anesthetic effects)

	ONSET	PEAK	DURATION
IV	30–60 sec	UK	10–30 min
Rect	8–10 min	UK	UK

NURSING IMPLICATIONS

ASSESSMENT
▪ **General Info:** Assess blood pressure, ECG, heart rate, and respiratory status continuously throughout thiopental therapy. Monitor for apnea immediately after IV injection, especially in the presence of opioid premedication.
▫ Monitor IV site carefully. Extravasation may cause pain, swelling, ulceration, and necrosis. Intra-arterial injection may cause arteritis, vasospasm, edema, thrombosis, and gangrene of the extremity.
▪ **Increased Intracranial Pressure:** Assess level of consciousness and intracranial pressure before and throughout therapy.
▪ **Toxicity and Overdose:** Monitor for signs of overdose, which may occur from too rapid injections (drop in blood pressure, possibly to shock levels) or excessive or repeated injections (respiratory distress, laryngospasm, apnea).

POTENTIAL NURSING DIAGNOSES
▪ Breathing pattern, ineffective (side effects).
▪ Injury, high risk for (side effects).

IMPLEMENTATION
▪ **General Info:** Thiopental should be used only by individuals qualified to administer anesthesia and experienced in endotracheal intubation. Equipment for this procedure should be immediately available.
▫ Administer premedication with anticholinergics (atropine, glycopyrrolate) to decrease mucus secretions. Opioids may be administered preoperatively because of the lack of analgesic effects of thiopental. Administer preoperative medications so peak effects are attained shortly before induction of anesthesia. Administer muscle relaxants separately.
▫ Concurrent use of nitrous oxide 67% decreases the requirements for thiopental by ⅔.
▪ **Rect:** May be administered as a rectal suspension. Do not exert excessive pressure on plunger, to prevent over-

dose. Use a new applicator for each repeat administration. Unless fecal impaction is present, cleansing enema is not usually required prior to administration of rectal thiopental.
- **IV:** Dilute thiopental with Sterile Water for Injection, D5W, or 0.9% NaCl. Solution should be freshly prepared and used within 24 hr of reconstitution. Refrigerate and keep tightly sealed. Do not administer solution containing a precipitate.
- **Direct IV:** A test dose of 25–75 mg (1–3 ml of a 2.5% solution) may be administered to determine tolerance or unusual sensitivity to thiopental. Observe patient for at least 60 sec.
- □ When thiopental is used as the sole anesthetic agent, small repeated doses of 2 or 2.5% concentration may be used to maintain desired level of anesthesia.
- **Rate:** Administer slowly. Rapid administration may cause overdose.
- **Continuous Infusion:** Solutions of 0.2–0.4% have been administered by continuous infusion to maintain anesthesia when thiopental is the sole agent. May be diluted in solution with D5/0.45% NaCl, D5W, multiple electrolyte solutions, 0.45% NaCl, 0.9% NaCl, and ⅙ M sodium lactate.
- **Syringe Compatibility:** ▪ aminophylline ▪ hydrocortisone sodium succinate ▪ neostigmine ▪ pentobarbital ▪ scopolamine ▪ tubocurarine.
- **Syringe Incompatibility:** ▪ benzquinamide ▪ chlorpromazine ▪ dimenhydrinate ▪ diphenhydramine ▪ ephedrine ▪ glycopyrrolate ▪ meperidine ▪ morphine ▪ pentazocine ▪ prochlorperazine ▪ promethazine ▪ propiomazine.
- **Additive Compatibility:** ▪ chloramphenicol ▪ hydrocortisone sodium succinate ▪ pentobarbital ▪ potassium chloride.
- **Additive Incompatibility:** ▪ amikacin ▪ cephapirin ▪ chlorpromazine ▪ codeine ▪ dimenhydrinate ▪ diphenhydramine ▪ hydromorphone ▪ regular

insulin ▪ levorphanol ▪ meperidine ▪ methadone ▪ morphine ▪ penicillin G potassium ▪ prochlorperazine ▪ promazine ▪ promethazine ▪ succinylcholine ▪ dextrose/Ringer's or lactated Ringer's injection combinations ▪ D10/0.9% NaCl, D10W ▪ Ringer's and lactated Ringer's injection.

PATIENT/FAMILY TEACHING
- □ Thiopental may cause psychomotor impairment for 24 hr following administration. Caution patient to avoid driving or other activities requiring alertness for 24 hr.
- □ Advise patient to avoid use of alcohol or other CNS depressants for 24 hr following anesthesia, unless directed by physician or dentist.

EVALUATION
Effectiveness of therapy can be demonstrated by: ▪ Loss of consciousness and maintenance of desired level of anesthesia.

THIORIDAZINE
(thye-oh-**rid**-a-zeen)
{Apo-Thioridazine}, Mellaril, Mellaril S, {Novo-Ridazine}, {PMS Thioridazine}

CLASSIFICATION(S):
Antipsychotic (phenothiazine)
Pregnancy Category UK

INDICATIONS
- ▪ Treatment of acute and chronic psychoses ▪ Management of depression/anxiety ▪ Treatment of severe behavioral problems in children.

ACTION
- ▪ Alters the effects of dopamine in the CNS ▪ Possesses significant anticholinergic and alpha-adrenergic blocking activity. **Therapeutic Effect:** ▪ Diminished signs and symptoms of psychoses.

PHARMACOKINETICS
Absorption: Absorption from tablets is

{} = Available in Canada only.

variable; may be better with oral liquid formulations.

Distribution: Widely distributed, high concentrations in the CNS. Crosses the placenta and enters breast milk.

Metabolism and Excretion: Highly metabolized by the liver and GI mucosa.

Half-life: UK.

CONTRAINDICATIONS AND PRECAUTIONS

Contraindicated in: ▪ Hypersensitivity ▪ Cross-sensitivity with other phenothiazines may exist ▪ Narrow-angle glaucoma ▪ Bone marrow depression ▪ Severe liver or cardiovascular disease ▫ Known alcohol intolerance (concentrate only).

Use Cautiously in: ▪ Elderly or debilitated patients ▪ Pregnancy or lactation (safety not established) ▪ Diabetes mellitus ▪ Respiratory disease ▪ Prostatic hypertrophy ▪ CNS tumors ▪ Epilepsy ▪ Intestinal obstruction.

ADVERSE REACTIONS AND SIDE EFFECTS*

CNS: sedation, extrapyramidal reactions, tardive dyskinesia, NEUROLEPTIC MALIGNANT SYNDROME.

EENT: dry eyes, blurred vision, lens opacities.

CV: hypotension, tachycardia.

GI: constipation, dry mouth, ileus, anorexia, hepatitis.

GU: urinary retention.

Derm: rashes, photosensitivity, pigment changes.

Endo: galactorrhea.

Hemat: AGRANULOCYTOSIS, leukopenia.

Metab: hyperthermia.

Misc: allergic reactions.

INTERACTIONS

Drug–Drug: ▪ Additive hypotension with other **antihypertensive agents,** **nitrates,** and acute ingestion of **alcohol** ▪ Additive CNS depression with other **CNS depressants,** including **alcohol, antihistamines, opioid analgesics, sedative/hypnotics,** and **general anes-**thetics ▪ Additive anticholinergic effects with other **drugs possessing anticholinergic properties,** including **antihistamines, antidepressants, atropine, haloperidol,** other **phenothiazines,** and **disopyramide** ▪ **Lithium** decreases blood levels of thioridazine ▪ Thioridazine may mask early signs of **lithium** toxicity and increases the risk of extrapyramidal reactions ▪ Increased risk of agranulocytosis with **antithyroid agents** ▪ Concurrent use with **epinephrine** may result in severe hypotension and tachycardia ▪ May decrease the effectiveness of **levodopa.**

ROUTE AND DOSAGE

Psychoses
▪ **PO (Adults and Children >12 yr):** 50–100 mg tid initially, maintenance 10–200 mg qid up to 800 mg/day.

Depressive Neuroses with Anxiety, Fears, Depression; Anxiety in the Elderly
▪ **PO (Adults):** 25 mg tid (range of 20–200 mg/day).

Behavioral Problems in Children
▪ **PO (Children >2 yr):** 0.25–3 mg/kg/day in 2–3 divided doses (10–25 mg 2–3 times daily).

AVAILABILITY

▪ *Tablets:* 10 mg, 15 mg, 25 mg, 50 mg, 100 mg, 150 mg, 200 mg ▪ *Oral suspension:* {10 mg/5 ml}, 25 mg/5 ml, 100 mg/5 ml ▪ *Concentrated oral solution:* ▪ 30 mg/ml, 100 mg/ml.

TIME/ACTION PROFILE
(antipsychotic effects)

	ONSET	PEAK	DURATION
PO	UK	UK	8–12 hr

NURSING IMPLICATIONS

ASSESSMENT
▫ Assess mental status (orientation, mood, behavior) and degree of anxiety prior to and periodically throughout therapy.

---

*Underlines indicate most frequent; **CAPITALS** indicate life-threatening.

□ Monitor blood pressure (sitting, standing, lying), pulse, and respiratory rate prior to and frequently during the period of dosage adjustment.

□ Observe patient carefully when administering medication to ensure that medication is actually taken and not hoarded.

□ Assess patient for level of sedation following administration.

□ Monitor intake and output ratios and daily weight. Notify physician if significant discrepancies occur.

□ Observe patient carefully for extrapyramidal symptoms (akathisia—restlessness; dystonia—muscle spasms and twisting motions; pseudoparkinsonism—mask facies pill-rolling motions, drooling, tremors, rigidity, shuffling gait). Notify physician if these symptoms occur, as reduction of dose or discontinuation of medication may be necessary. Trihexyphenidyl or diphenhydramine may be used to control these symptoms.

□ Monitor for tardive dyskinesia (uncontrolled movements of face, mouth, tongue, or jaw and involuntary movements of extremities). Notify physician immediately at the onset of these symptoms, as they may be irreversible.

□ Monitor for development of neuroleptic malignant syndrome (fever, respiratory distress, tachycardia, convulsions, diaphoresis, hypertension or hypotension, pallor, tiredness). Notify physician immediately if these symptoms occur.

■ **Lab Test Considerations:** CBC and liver function tests should be evaluated periodically throughout course of therapy. May cause blood dyscrasias, especially between weeks 4 and 10 of therapy.

□ May cause false-positive or false-negative pregnancy tests and false-positive urine bilirubin test results.

□ May cause increased serum prolactin levels, thereby interfering with gonadorelin test results.

□ May cause Q wave and T wave changes in ECG.

POTENTIAL NURSING DIAGNOSES
■ Coping, ineffective individual (indications).
■ Thought processes, altered (indications).
■ Knowledge deficit related to medication regimen (patient/family teaching).

IMPLEMENTATION
■ **General Info:** To prevent contact dermatitis, avoid getting solution on hands.

□ Phenothiazines should be discontinued 48 hr before and not resumed for 24 hr following metrizamide myelography, as they lower the seizure threshold.

■ **PO:** Administer with food, milk, or a full glass of water to minimize gastric irritation.

□ Dilute concentrate in 120 ml of distilled or acidified tap water or fruit juice just prior to administration.

PATIENT/FAMILY TEACHING
□ Advise patient to take medication exactly as directed, not to skip doses or double up on missed doses. If a dose is missed, it should be taken as soon as remembered unless almost time for the next dose. If more than 2 doses are scheduled each day, the missed dose should be taken within 1 hr of the scheduled time.

□ Abrupt withdrawal may cause gastritis, nausea, vomiting, dizziness, headache, tachycardia, and insomnia.

□ May cause drowsiness. Caution patient to avoid driving or other activities requiring alertness until response to medication is known.

□ Advise patient to use sunscreen and protective clothing when exposed to the sun to prevent photosensitivity reactions. Extremes in temperature should also be avoided, as this drug impairs body temperature regulation.

□ Instruct patient to use frequent mouth rinses, good oral hygiene, and sugarless gum or candy to minimize dry mouth. Consult physician or dentist if dry mouth continues >2 wk.

□ Advise patient that increasing activity

and bulk and fluids in the diet help minimize the constipating effects of this medication.

☐ Caution patient to avoid taking alcohol or other CNS depressants concurrently with this medication.

☐ Advise patient to notify physician or dentist of medication regimen prior to treatment or surgery.

☐ Instruct patient to notify physician promptly if sore throat, fever, unusual bleeding or bruising, skin rashes, weakness, tremors, visual disturbances, difficulty urinating, dark-colored urine, or clay-colored stools are noted.

☐ Emphasize the importance of routine follow-up examinations to monitor response to medication and to detect side effects. Periodic ocular examinations are indicated. Encourage continued participation in psychotherapy as ordered by physician.

EVALUATION

Effectiveness of therapy can be demonstrated by: ▪ Decrease in excitable, paranoic, or withdrawn behavior ▪ Decrease in anxiety associated with depression.

THIOTEPA
(thye-oh-**tep**-a)

CLASSIFICATION(S):
Antineoplastic (alkylating agent)
Pregnancy Category UK

INDICATIONS

▪ **Bladder Instillation:** Management or prophylaxis of superficial tumors of the bladder following local resection ▪ **IV:** Palliative treatment for breast and ovarian cancer ▪ **Intracavitary Instillation:** Prevention of recurrent malignant effusions in pleura, pericardium, or peritoneum.

ACTION

▪ Disrupts protein, DNA, and RNA synthesis by cross-linking strands of DNA and RNA (cell cycle-phase nonspecific). **Therapeutic Effects:** ▪ Death of rapidly replicating cells, particularly malignant ones ▪ Has immunosuppressive properties.

PHARMACOKINETICS

Absorption: Variably absorbed following instillation (10–100%).
Distribution: Distribution not known.
Metabolism and Excretion: Extensively metabolized.
Half-life: UK.

CONTRAINDICATIONS AND PRECAUTIONS

Contraindicated in: ▪ Hypersensitivity ▪ Pregnancy or lactation.
Use Cautiously in: ▪ Patients with childbearing potential ▪ Active infections ▪ Decreased bone marrow reserve ▪ Other chronic debilitating illnesses ▪ Severe hepatic or renal disease.

ADVERSE REACTIONS AND SIDE EFFECTS*

CNS: headache, dizziness.
EENT: tightness of the throat.
GI: nausea, anorexia, vomiting, stomatitis.
GU: gonadal suppression.
Derm: alopecia, rash, pruritus, hives.
Hemat: thrombocytopenia, leukopenia, anemia.
Local: pain at IV site, pain at site of intracavitary instillation.
Metab: hyperuricemia.
Misc: fever, allergic reactions.

INTERACTIONS

Drug–Drug: ▪ Additive bone marrow depression with other **antineoplastic agents** or **radiation therapy** ▪ May prolong apnea after **succinylcholine** ▪ May decrease antibody response to **live virus vaccines** and increase the risk of adverse reactions.

ROUTE AND DOSAGE

Bladder Instillation
▪ **Intravesical (Adults):** 30–60 mg re-

T

---

*Underlines indicate most frequent; **CAPITALS** indicate life-threatening.

tained for 2 hr weekly for 4 wk, then monthly.

Palliative Therapy of Breast, Ovarian Cancer

▪ **IV (Adults):** 300–400 mcg/kg q 1–4 wk or 200 mcg/kg daily for 4–5 days q 2–4 wk.

Malignant Effusions

▪ **Intracavitary (Adults):** 600–800 mcg/kg q 1–4 wk (range 70–800 mcg/kg).

AVAILABILITY

▪ *Injection:* 15 mg/vial.

TIME/ACTION PROFILE (noted as effects on blood counts; effects after intracavitary administration are highly variable)

	ONSET	PEAK	DURATION
IV	10 days (up to 30 days)	14 days	21 days

NURSING IMPLICATIONS

ASSESSMENT

▫ Monitor vital signs prior to and periodically during therapy.

▫ Assess for fever, chills, sore throat, and signs of infection. Notify physician if these symptoms occur.

▫ Monitor platelet count throughout therapy. Assess for bleeding (bleeding gums, bruising, petechiae, guaiac stools, urine, and emesis). Avoid IM injections and rectal temperatures. Apply pressure to venipuncture sites for 10 min.

▫ Monitor intake and output, appetite, and nutritional intake. Assess for nausea, vomiting, and anorexia. Administration of an antiemetic and adjusting diet as tolerated may help maintain fluid and electrolyte balance and nutritional status.

▫ Anemia may occur. Monitor for increased fatigue, dyspnea, and orthostatic hypotension.

▫ Monitor for symptoms of gout (increased uric acid, joint pain, edema). Encourage patient to drink at least 2 liters of fluids/day. Allopurinol or al-

kalinization of urine may be used to decrease uric acid levels.

▪ **Lab Test Considerations:** Monitor CBC and differential prior to and weekly throughout therapy and for at least 3 wk after therapy. The nadir of leukopenia occurs after 10–14 days, although it may be delayed up to 1 mo. Notify physician if platelet count $<150,000/mm^3$ or leukocyte count $<3000/mm^3$.

▫ Monitor for increased AST (SGOT), ALT (SGPT), LDH, serum bilirubin, uric acid, creatinine, and BUN.

POTENTIAL NURSING DIAGNOSES

▪ Infection, high risk for (side effects).

▪ Injury, high risk for (side effects).

▪ Knowledge deficit related to medication regimen (patient/family teaching).

IMPLEMENTATION

▪ **General Info:** Safe for IM or SC administration.

▫ Solution is clear to slightly opaque. Do not use solution that is cloudy or that contains precipitate. Stable for 5 days if refrigerated after reconstitution.

▫ Solution should be prepared in a biologic cabinet. Wear gloves, gown, and mask while handling medication. Discard equipment in designated containers (see Appendix I).

▫ Reconstitute 15 mg of powder with 1.5 ml of Sterile Water for Injection. This concentration is suitable for intratumor injection. May be further diluted for other routes.

▫ May be administered by physician via several routes.

▪ **Intracavitary:** Reconstitute solution. Thiotepa is instilled via tube that was used to drain the effusion.

▪ **Bladder Instillation:** Limit fluids per physician's order for 8–12 hr prior to treatment. Reconstitute solution. Mix 60 mg with 30–60 ml of sterile water and instill in bladder via Foley catheter. Reposition patient every 15 min to allow maximal contact of solution with tumors. Solution should be retained for 2 hr. The lesser amount of solution (30 ml) is usually reserved for patients unable to hold 60 ml.

- **Direct IV:** Following reconstitution, may be administered undiluted over 1–3 min.
- **Intermittent Infusion:** Dilute further in 50–100 ml of 0.9% NaCl, D5W, dextrose/saline combinations, Ringer's or lactated Ringer's solution.
- **Syringe Compatibility:** procaine HCl 2% or epinephrine 1:1000.

PATIENT/FAMILY TEACHING

□ Instruct patients receiving thiotepa via Foley catheter to notify physician if hematuria or dysuria occurs.

□ Instruct patient to notify physician if fever, chills, sore throat, signs of infection, bleeding gums, bruising, petechiae, or blood in urine, stool, or emesis occurs. Caution patient to avoid crowds and persons with known infections. Instruct patient to use soft toothbrush and electric razor. Caution patient not to drink alcoholic beverages or take products containing aspirin or ibuprofen.

□ Instruct patient to inspect oral mucosa for redness and ulceration. If ulceration occurs, advise patient to use sponge brush and rinse mouth with water after eating and drinking. Physician may order viscous lidocaine swishes if pain interferes with eating.

□ This drug may cause gonadal suppression; however, patient should still use birth control. Advise patient to inform physician immediately if pregnancy is suspected.

□ Discuss possibility of hair loss with patient. Explore methods of coping.

□ Instruct patient not to receive any vaccinations without advice of physician.

□ Advise patient of need for medical follow-up and frequent lab tests.

EVALUATION

Effectiveness of therapy can be demonstrated by: ▪ Decrease in size and spread of malignant tissue.

THIOTHIXENE
(thye-oh-**thix**-een)
Navane

CLASSIFICATION(S):
Antipsychotic (thioxanthene)
Pregnancy Category UK

INDICATIONS

- Management of psychoses, especially in withdrawn, apathetic schizophrenic patients and patients suffering from delusions and hallucinations.

ACTION

- Alters the effect of dopamine in the CNS. **Therapeutic Effect:** ▪ Diminished signs and symptoms of psychoses.

PHARMACOKINETICS

Absorption: Well absorbed following oral and IM administration.
Distribution: Widely distributed. Crosses the placenta.
Metabolism and Excretion: Mainly metabolized by the liver.
Half-life: 30 hr.

CONTRAINDICATIONS AND PRECAUTIONS

Contraindicated in: ▪ Hypersensitivity ▪ Cross-sensitivity with other phenothiazines may exist ▪ Narrow-angle glaucoma ▪ Bone marrow depression ▪ Severe liver or cardiac disease.

Use Cautiously in: ▪ Elderly or debilitated patients (dosage reduction may be required) ▪ Diabetes mellitus ▪ Respiratory disease ▪ Prostatic hypertrophy ▪ CNS tumors ▪ Epilepsy ▪ Intestinal obstruction ▪ Pregnancy, lactation, or children (safety not established).

ADVERSE REACTIONS AND SIDE EFFECTS*

CNS: sedation, extrapyramidal reactions, tardive dyskinesia, NEUROLEPTIC MALIGNANT SYNDROME.
EENT: dry eyes, blurred vision, lens opacities.
CV: hypotension, tachycardia.

---

*Underlines indicate most frequent; **CAPITALS** indicate life-threatening.

GI: constipation, dry mouth, ileus, anorexia, hepatitis, nausea.
GU: urinary retention.
Derm: rashes, photosensitivity, pigment changes.
Endo: galactorrhea.
Hemat: leukopenia, leukocytosis.
Metab: hyperpyrexia.
Misc: allergic reactions.

INTERACTIONS

Drug–Drug: ▪ Additive hypotension with **antihypertensive agents,** acute ingestion of **alcohol,** and **nitrates** ▪ Additive CNS depression with other **CNS depressants,** including **alcohol, antihistamines, antidepressants, opioidanalgesics,** and **sedative/hypnotics** ▪ Additive anticholinergic effects with other **drugs having anticholinergic properties,** including **antihistamines, antidepressants, quinidine,** or **disopyramide** ▪ May decrease the effectiveness of **levodopa** ▪ Increased risk of cardiac effects with **quinidine.**

ROUTE AND DOSAGE

▪ **PO (Adults):** 2 mg tid or 5 mg bid (not to exceed 60 mg/day).
▪ **IM (Adults):** 4 mg 2–4 times daily (not to exceed 30 mg/day).

AVAILABILITY

▪ *Capsules:* 1 mg, 2 mg, 5 mg, 10 mg, 20 mg ▪ *Concentrated oral solution:* 5 mg/ml ▪ *Injection:* 2 mg/ml, 5 mg/ml.

TIME/ACTION PROFILE
(antipsychotic effects)

	ONSET	PEAK	DURATION
PO	day–wk	UK	UK
IM	1–6 hr	UK	UK

NURSING IMPLICATIONS

ASSESSMENT

□ Monitor patient's mental status (delusions, hallucinations, and behavior) prior to and periodically throughout therapy.
□ Observe patient carefully when administering oral medication to ensure that medication is actually taken and not hoarded.

□ Assess patient for level of sedation following administration.
□ Monitor patient for onset of extrapyramidal side effects (akathisia—restlessness; dystonia—muscle spasms and twisting motions; pseudoparkinsonism—mask facies, rigidity, tremors, drooling, shuffling gait, dysphagia). Notify physician if these symptoms occur, as reduction in dosage or discontinuation of medication may be necessary. Trihexyphenidyl or diphenhydramine may be used to control these symptoms.
□ Monitor for tardive dyskinesia (rhythmic movement of mouth, face, and extremities). Notify physician immediately if these symptoms occur, as these side effects may be irreversible.
□ Monitor for development of neuroleptic malignant syndrome (fever, respiratory distress, tachycardia, convulsions, diaphoresis, hypertension or hypotension, pallor, tiredness). Notify physician immediately if these symptoms occur.
▪ **Lab Test Considerations:** Thiothixene increases serum prolactin levels and lowers serum uric acid levels.
□ Monitor CBC and differential prior to and periodically throughout therapy. Risk of leukopenia is highest between weeks 4 and 10 of therapy.
□ Monitor liver function studies prior to and periodically during therapy. Risk of hepatotoxicity is greatest 2–4 wk after beginning therapy.

POTENTIAL NURSING DIAGNOSES

▪ Thought processes, altered (indications).
▪ Injury, high risk for (side effects).
▪ Knowledge deficit related to medication regimen (patient/family teaching).

IMPLEMENTATION

▪ **General Info:** All forms of solution may cause dermatitis; avoid skin contact.
□ Thiothixene lowers the seizure threshold; institute seizure precautions for patients with history of seizure disorder and discontinue thiothixene 48

hr before and do not resume for 24 hr following metrizamide myelography.

- **PO:** Administer capsules with food or milk to decrease gastric irritation.
□ Dilute oral solution with 240 ml of milk, juice, carbonated drink, or soup to decrease gastric irritation. Measure dose with provided dropper.
- **IM:** Dilute each 10-mg vial with 2.2 ml of Sterile Water for Injection, for a concentration of 5 mg/ml. Administer deep into well-developed muscle.

PATIENT/FAMILY TEACHING

□ Instruct patients receiving parenteral thiothixene to remain supine for 30 min after administration. Position changes should be made slowly.
□ Instruct patient on need to take medication exactly as directed. If a dose is missed, it should be taken as soon as remembered until 2 hr before next dose. Do not double doses. Patients on long-term high-dose therapy may need dose tapered to avoid withdrawal symptoms (dyskinesia, tremors, dizziness, nausea, and vomiting).
□ Instruct patients receiving oral solution on correct method of measuring dose with provided dropper.
□ Drowsiness may occur. Caution patient to avoid driving or other activities requiring alertness until response to medication is known.
□ Inform patient of possibility of extrapyramidal symptoms and tardive dyskinesia. Caution patient to report these symptoms immediately to physician.
□ Advise patient that frequent mouth rinses, good oral hygiene, and sugarless gum or candy may decrease mouth dryness. Physician or dentist should be notified if dryness persists >2 wk.
□ Advise patient that increasing bulk and fluids in the diet and exercise may help minimize the constipating effects of this medication.
□ Caution patient to use sunscreen and protective clothing to prevent photosensitivity reactions.
□ Caution patient to avoid concurrent use of alcohol, other CNS depressants, and over-the-counter medications without prior physician approval.
□ Caution patient to avoid exercising in hot weather and taking very hot baths, as this drug impairs temperature regulation.
□ Instruct patient to notify physician promptly if sore throat, fever, skin rashes or discoloration, weakness, tremors, or visual disturbances are noted.
□ Advise patient to notify physician or dentist of medication regimen prior to treatment or surgery.
□ Emphasize the importance of continued medical follow-up for psychotherapy, eye examinations, and laboratory tests.

EVALUATION

Effectiveness of therapy can be demonstrated by: ▪ Decrease in psychotic ideation.

T

THYROID
(thye-royd)
Armour Thyroid, S-P-T, Thyrar, Thyroid Strong

CLASSIFICATION(S):
Hormone (thyroid)
Pregnancy Category A

INDICATIONS

▪ Replacement or substitution therapy in diminished or absent thyroid function of many causes ▪ Treatment of some types of thyroid cancer.

ACTION

▪ Principal effect is increasing metabolic rate of body tissues: □ Promotes gluconeogenesis □ Increases utilization and mobilization of glycogen stores □ Stimulates protein synthesis □ Promotes cell growth and differentiation □ Aids in the development of the brain and CNS ▪ Contains T_3 (triiodothyronine) and T_4 (thyroxine) activity. **Thera-**

peutic Effects: ▪ Replacement in deficiency states with restoration of normal hormonal balance ▪ Suppression of thyrotropin-dependent thyroid cancers.

PHARMACOKINETICS

Absorption: Well absorbed from the GI tract following oral administration.

Distribution: Distributed into most body tissues. Thyroid hormones do not readily cross the placenta; minimal amounts enter breast milk.

Metabolism and Excretion: Metabolized by the liver and other tissues. Undergoes enterohepatic recirculation. Excreted in the feces via the bile.

Half-life: T_3 (liothyronine)—1–2 days; T_4 (thyroxine)—6–7 days.

CONTRAINDICATIONS AND PRECAUTIONS

Contraindicated in: ▪ Hypersensitivity ▪ Recent myocardial infarction ▪ Thyrotoxicosis. Products are from animal sources (beef, pork) and should be avoided in patients with known hypersensitivity.

Use Cautiously in: ▪ Cardiovascular disease ▪ Severe renal insufficiency ▪ Uncorrected adrenocortical disorders ▪ Elderly and myxedematous patients (extremely sensitive to thyroid hormones; initial dosage should be markedly reduced).

ADVERSE REACTIONS AND SIDE EFFECTS*

CNS: <u>irritability</u>, <u>insomnia</u>, <u>nervousness</u>, headache.

CV: <u>tachycardia</u>, <u>arrhythmias</u>, increased cardiac output, angina pectoris, increased blood pressure, CARDIOVASCULAR COLLAPSE, hypotension.

GI: diarrhea, cramps, vomiting.

Derm: increased sweating, hair loss (in children).

Endo: menstrual irregularities.

Metab: <u>weight loss</u>, heat intolerance.

MS: accelerated bone maturation in children.

INTERACTIONS

Drug–Drug: ▪ **Cholestyramine** or **colestipol** decrease oral absorption ▪ May alter the effectiveness of **oral anticoagulants** ▪ May cause an increase in the requirement for **insulin** or **oral hypoglycemic agents** in diabetics ▪ Additive cardiovascular effects with **adrenergic agents (sympathomimetics)** ▪ May decrease response to **beta-adrenergic blockers**.

ROUTE AND DOSAGE

1 gr = 60 mg and is equivalent to 100 mcg or less of levothyroxine (T_4) or 25 mcg of liothyronine (T_3).

- ▪ **PO (Adults):** 30–60 mg/day increase at monthly intervals (usual dose 60–120 mg/day). In adults with severe hypothyroidism or cardiovascular disease, initiate therapy with 15 mg/day. In elderly patients, begin with 7.5–15 mg/day.
- ▪ **PO (Children >12 yr):** more than 90 mg/day (1.2–1.8 mg/kg/day).
- ▪ **PO (Children 6–12 yr):** 60–90 mg/day (2.4–3 mg/kg/day).
- ▪ **PO (Children 1–5 yr):** 45–60 mg/day (3–3.6 mg/kg/day).
- ▪ **PO (Children 6–12 mo):** 30–45 mg/day (3.6–4.8 mg/kg/day).
- ▪ **PO (Infants):** 15–30 mg/day (4.8–6 mg/kg/day).

AVAILABILITY

▪ *Tablets:* 15 mg, 30 mg, 60 mg, 90 mg, 120 mg ▪ *Strong tablets:* 30 mg, 60 mg, 120 mg, 180 mg—these are 50% stronger than thyroid USP ▪ *Strong tablets (sugar coated):* 30 mg, 60 mg, 120 mg, 180 mg (these are 50% more potent than thyroid) ▪ *Tablets (bovine):* 30 mg, 60 mg, 120 mg ▪ *Capsules (pork):* 60 mg, 90 mg, 120mg, 180 mg.

TIME/ACTION PROFILE (effects on thyroid function tests)

	ONSET	PEAK	DURATION
PO	days–wk	1–3 wk	days–wk

*<u>Underlines</u> indicate most frequent; **CAPITALS** indicate life-threatening.

NURSING IMPLICATIONS

ASSESSMENT

- **General Info:** Assess apical pulse and blood pressure prior to and periodically during therapy. Observe patient for signs of myocardial ischemia and tachyarrhythmias.
- Monitor for symptoms of hyperthyroidism (tachycardia, chest pain, nervousness, insomnia, diaphoresis, tremors, weight loss).
- **Children:** Monitor bone age, height and weight, and psychomotor development.
- **Lab Test Considerations:** Thyroid function tests should be monitored prior to and throughout therapy.
- Monitor blood and urine glucose in diabetics; insulin or oral hypoglycemic dose may need to be increased.

POTENTIAL NURSING DIAGNOSES

- Knowledge deficit related to medication regimen (patient/family teaching).

IMPLEMENTATION

- **PO:** Administer as a single dose, preferably before breakfast to prevent insomnia.

PATIENT/FAMILY TEACHING

- **General Info:** Instruct patient to take medication exactly as directed, at the same time each day. If a dose is missed, take as soon as remembered unless almost time for next dose. If more than 2 or 3 doses are missed, notify physician. Do not discontinue without consulting physician.
- Instruct patient and family on correct technique for checking pulse. Dose should be withheld and physician notified if resting pulse is >100 beats/min.
- Explain to patient that thyroid does not cure hypothyroidism, it provides a replacement hormone; therapy may be lifelong.
- Caution patient not to change brands of this medication, as this may effect drug potency.
- Advise patient to notify physician if headache, nervousness, diarrhea, excessive sweating, heat intolerance, chest pain, increased pulse rate, palpitations, or any unusual symptoms occur.
- Caution patient to avoid taking other medications concurrently with thyroid, without consulting physician or pharmacist.
- Instruct patient to inform physician or dentist of thyroid therapy prior to treatment or surgery.
- Emphasize importance of follow-up examinations to monitor effectiveness of therapy. Thyroid function tests are performed at least yearly.
- **Children:** Discuss with parents need for routine follow-up studies to ensure correct development. Inform parents that partial hair loss may be experienced by children on thyroid therapy. This is usually temporary.

EVALUATION

Clinical response can be evaluated by:
- Resolution of symptoms of hypothyroidism. Response includes: □ Diuresis □ Weight loss □ Increased sense of well-being □ Increased energy, pulse rate, appetite, psychomotor activity □ Normalization of skin texture and hair □ Correction of constipation □ Increased T_3 and T_4 levels. Sleeping pulse and basal morning temperature may be used to determine effectiveness ■ In children, effectiveness of therapy is determined by: □ Appropriate physical and psychomotor development.

T

TICARCILLIN
(tye-kar-**sil**-in)
Ticar

CLASSIFICATION(S):
Anti-infective (extended-spectrum penicillin)
Pregnancy Category UK

INDICATIONS

- Treatment of serious infections due to susceptible organisms including:
- Skin and skin structure infections

▢ Bone and joint infections ▢ Septicemia ▢ Respiratory tract infections ▢ Intra-abdominal ▢ Gynecologic ▢ Urinary tract infections ▪ Combination with an aminoglycoside may be synergistic against *Pseudomonas* ▪ Has been combined with other anti-infectives in the treatment of infections in immunosuppressed patients.

ACTION

▪ Binds to bacterial cell wall membrane, causing cell death. **Therapeutic Effects:** ▪ Bactericidal action against susceptible bacteria ▪ Spectrum is extended, compared to other penicillins. **Spectrum:** ▪ Similar to penicillin but greatly extended to include several important gram-negative aerobic pathogens, notably: ▢ *Pseudomonas aeruginosa* ▢ *Escherichia coli* ▢ *Proteus mirabilis* ▢ *Providencia rettgeri* ▪ Active against some anaerobic bacteria, including *Bacteroides* ▪ Not active against penicillinase-producing staphylococci or beta-lactamase–producing Enterobacteriaceae.

PHARMACOKINETICS

Absorption: Well absorbed following IM administration.

Distribution: Widely distributed. Enters CSF well only when meninges are inflammed. Crosses the placenta and enters breast milk in low concentrations.

Metabolism and Excretion: 10% metabolized by the liver, 90% excreted unchanged by the kidneys.

Half-life: 0.9–1.3 hr (increased in renal impairment).

CONTRAINDICATIONS AND PRECAUTIONS

Contraindicated in: ▪ Hypersensitivity to penicillins or cephalosporins.

Use Cautiously in: ▪ Renal impairment (dosage reduction and/or increased interval required if creatinine clearance <60 ml/min) ▪ Pregnancy and lactation (safety not established)

▪ History of hypersensitivity ▪ Severe liver disease.

ADVERSE REACTIONS AND SIDE EFFECTS*

CNS: confusion, lethargy, SEIZURES (high doses).

CV: congestive heart failure, arrhythmias.

GI: nausea, diarrhea.

GU: hematuria (children only).

Derm: rashes, urticaria.

F and E: hypokalemia, hypernatremia.

Hemat: bleeding, blood dyscrasias, increased bleeding time.

Local: phlebitis.

Metab: metabolic alkalosis.

Misc: superinfection, hypersensitivity reactions, including ANAPHYLAXIS and serum sickness.

INTERACTIONS

Drug–Drug: ▪ **Probenecid** decreases renal excretion and increases blood levels ▪ May alter excretion of **lithium** ▪ **Diuretics, glucocorticoids,** or **amphotericin B** may increase the risk of hypokalemia ▪ Hypokalemia increases the risk of **cardiac glycoside** toxicity.

ROUTE AND DOSAGE

Contains 5.2 mEq sodium/g.

Serious Infections

▪ **IV (Adults and Children >40 kg):** 3 g q 3–6 hr (150–300 mg/kg/day in divided doses).

▪ **IV (Children <40 kg):** 200–300 mg/kg/day in divided doses q 4–6 hr.

▪ **IM, IV (Neonates >2 kg and >7 days):** 100 mg/kg q 8 hr.

▪ **IM, IV (Neonates >2 kg and <7 days):** 75 mg/kg q 8 hr.

▪ **IM, IV (Neonates <2 kg and >7 days):** 75 mg/kg q 8 hr.

▪ **IM, IV (Neonates <2 kg and <7 days):** 75 mg/kg q 12 hr.

Uncomplicated Urinary Tract Infections

▪ **IM, IV (Adults and Children >40 kg):** 1 g q 6 hr.

▪ **IM, IV (Children <40 kg):** 50–100 mg/kg/day in divided doses q 6–8 hr.

---

*Underlines indicate most frequent; CAPITALS indicate life-threatening.

AVAILABILITY

- **Injection:** 1-g, 3-g, 6-g, 20-g, 30-g vials ▪ **In combination with:** clavulanate. See Ticarcillin/Clavulate monograph.

TIME/ACTION PROFILE (blood levels)

	ONSET	PEAK
IM	rapid	30–75 min
IV	rapid	end of infusion

NURSING IMPLICATIONS

ASSESSMENT

- ▫ Assess patient for infection (vital signs; appearance of wound, sputum, urine, and stool; WBC) at beginning and throughout course of therapy.
- ▫ Obtain a history before initiating therapy to determine previous use of and reactions to penicillins or cephalosporins. Persons with a negative history of penicillin sensitivity may still have an allergic response.
- ▫ Obtain specimens for culture and sensitivity prior to initiating therapy. First dose may be given before receiving results.
- ▫ Observe patient for signs and symptoms of anaphylaxis (rash, pruritus, laryngeal edema, wheezing). Discontinue drug and notify physician immediately if these occur. Keep epinephrine, an antihistamine, and resuscitation equipment close by in the event of an anaphylactic reaction.
- ▪ **Lab Test Considerations:** Renal and hepatic function, CBC, serum potassium, and bleeding times should be evaluated prior to and routinely throughout course of therapy.
- ▫ May cause false-positive urine protein testing and increased BUN, creatinine, AST (SGOT), ALT (SGPT), serum bilirubin, alkaline phosphatase, LDH, and uric acid levels. May also cause increased bleeding time.
- ▫ May cause hypernatremia and hypokalemia with high doses.

POTENTIAL NURSING DIAGNOSES

- ▪ Infection, high risk for (indications, side effects).
- ▪ Knowledge deficit related to medica-

tion regimen (patient/family teaching).

IMPLEMENTATION

- ▪ **IM:** Reconstitute 1-g vial with 2 ml of Sterile Water or Bacteriostatic Water for Injection or 1% lidocaine hydrochloride injection (without epinephrine), for a concentration of 1 g/2.5 ml.
- ▫ Inject deep into a well-developed muscle mass, to minimize discomfort, and massage well. IM injections should not exceed 2 g at each site.
- ▪ **IV:** Change IV sites every 48 hr to prevent phlebitis.
- ▫ Add at least 4 ml of Sterile Water for Injection to each 1-g vial. Further dilute to at least 20 ml with 0.9% NaCl, D5W, Ringer's or lactated Ringer's solution. Solution is stable for 48 hr at room temperature, 14 days if refrigerated.
- ▪ **Direct IV:** Administer as slowly as possible to minimize vein irritation. Do not administer concentrations >50 mg/ml.
- ▪ **Intermittent Infusion:** Dilute further for a concentration of 10–100 mg/ml.
- ▪ **Rate:** Administer over 30 min–2 hr, 10–20 min in neonates.
- ▪ **Y-Site Compatibility:** ▪ acyclovir ▪ cyclophosphamide ▪ famotidine ▪ fludarabine ▪ hydromorphone ▪ magnesium sulfate ▪ meperidine ▪ morphine ▪ ondansetron ▪ perphenazine ▪ sargramostim ▪ verapamil.
- ▪ **Y-Site Incompatibility:** ▪ fluconazole. If aminoglycosides and penicillins must be administered concurrently, administer in separate sites.
- ▪ **Additive Compatibility:** ▪ ranitidine.

PATIENT/FAMILY TEACHING

- ▫ Advise patient to report the signs of superinfection (black, furry overgrowth on the tongue, vaginal itching or discharge, loose or foul-smelling stools) and allergy.

EVALUATION

Clinical response can be evaluated by:
- ▪ Resolution of the signs and symptoms of infection. Length of time for complete resolution depends on the organism and site of infection.

T

TICARCILLIN/CLAVU-LANATE
(tye-kar-**sil**-in/klav-yoo-**la**-nate)
Timentin

CLASSIFICATION(S):
Anti-infective (extended-spectrum penicillin)
Pregnancy Category B

INDICATIONS

- Treatment of serious infections due to susceptible organisms including: □ Skin and skin structure infections □ Bone and joint infections □ Septicemia □ Respiratory tract infections □ Intra-abdominal infections □ Gynecologic infections □ Urinary tract infections ▪ Combination with an aminoglycoside may be synergistic against *Pseudomonas* ▪ Has been combined with other anti-infectives in the treatment of infections in immunosuppressed patients.

ACTION

- Binds to bacterial cell wall membrane, causing cell death ▪ Addition of clavulanate enhances resistance to beta-lactamase, an enzyme produced by bacteria capable of inactivating some penicillins. **Therapeutic Effect:** ▪ Bactericidal action against susceptible bacteria ▪ Spectrum is extended compared to other penicillins. **Spectrum:** ▪ Similar to penicillin but greatly extended to include several important gram-negative aerobic pathogens, notably: □ *Pseudomonas aeruginosa* □ *Escherichia coli* □ *Proteus mirabilis* □ *Providencia rettgeri* ▪ Active against some anaerobic bacteria, including *Bacteroides* ▪ Not active against penicillinase-producing staphylococci or beta-lactamase producing Enterobacteriaceae.

PHARMACOKINETICS

Absorption: Administered IV only, resulting in complete bioavailability.
Distribution: Widely distributed. Enters CSF well only when meninges are inflamed. Crosses the placenta and

enters breast milk in low concentrations.
Metabolism and Excretion: 10% of ticarcillin is metabolized by the liver, 90% excreted unchanged by the kidneys. Clavulanate is metabolized by the liver.
Half-life: Ticarcillin—0.9–1.3 hr (increased in renal impairment); clavulanate—1.1–1.5 hr.

CONTRAINDICATIONS AND PRECAUTIONS

Contraindicated in: ▪ Hypersensitivity to penicillins or cephalosporins.
Use Cautiously in: ▪ Renal impairment (dosage reduction and/or increased interval required if creatinine clearance <60 ml/min) ▪ Pregnancy and lactation (safety not established) ▪ History of hypersensitivity ▪ Severe liver disease.

ADVERSE REACTIONS AND SIDE EFFECTS*

CNS: confusion, lethargy, SEIZURES (high doses).
CV: congestive heart failure, arrhythmias.
GI: nausea, diarrhea.
GU: hematuria (children only).
Derm: rashes, urticaria.
F and E: hypokalemia, hypernatremia.
Hemat: bleeding, blood dyscrasias, increased bleeding time.
Local: phlebitis.
Metab: metabolic alkalosis.
Misc: superinfection, hypersensitivity reactions, including ANAPHYLAXIS and serum sickness.

INTERACTIONS

Drug–Drug: ▪ Probenecid decreases renal excretion and increases blood levels ▪ May alter excretion of **lithium** ▪ **Diuretics, glucocorticords,** or **amphotericin B** may increase the risk of hypokalemia ▪ Hypokalemia increases the risk of **cardiac glycoside** toxicity.

ROUTE AND DOSAGE

Ticarcillin contains 4.75 mEq sodium/g (6.2 mEq/g if premixed); ticarcillin/

---

*Underlines indicate most frequent; **CAPITALS** indicate life-threatening.

clavulanate contains 0.15 mEq potassium/100 mg clavulanate. 3 g ticarcillin plus 100 mg clavulanate labeled as 3.1 g combined potency.
- **IV (Adults >60 kg):** 3.1 g q q 4–6 hr.
- **IV (Children >12 yr and Adults <60 kg):** 200–300 mg/kg/day of ticarcillin equivalent in divided doses q 4–6 hr.

AVAILABILITY
- *Injection:* 3 g ticarcillin with 0.1 g clavulanic acid/vial.

TIME/ACTION PROFILE (blood levels)

	ONSET	PEAK
IV	rapid	end of infusion

NURSING IMPLICATIONS
ASSESSMENT
- Assess patient for infection (vital signs; appearance of wound, sputum, urine, and stool; WBC) at beginning and throughout course of therapy.
- Obtain a history before initiating therapy to determine previous use of and reactions to penicillins or cephalosporins. Persons with a negative history of penicillin sensitivity may still have an allergic response.
- Obtain specimens for culture and sensitivity prior to initiating therapy. First dose may be given before receiving results.
- Observe patient for signs and symptoms of anaphylaxis (rash, pruritus, laryngeal edema, wheezing). Discontinue drug and notify physician immediately if these occur. Keep epinephrine, an antihistamine, and resuscitation equipment close by in the event of an anaphylactic reaction.
- **Lab Test Considerations:** Renal and hepatic function, CBC, serum potassium, and bleeding times should be evaluated prior to and routinely throughout course of therapy.
- May cause false-positive urine protein testing and increased BUN, creatinine, AST (SGOT), ALT (SGPT), serum bilirubin, alkaline phosphatase,

LDH, and uric acid levels. May also cause increased bleeding time.
- May cause hypernatremia and hypokalemia with high doses.

POTENTIAL NURSING DIAGNOSES
- Infection, high risk for (indications, side effects).
- Knowledge deficit related to medication regimen (patient/family teaching).

IMPLEMENTATION
- **Intermittent Infusion:** Change IV sites every 48 hr to prevent phlebitis.
- Add 13 ml of Sterile Water or 0.9% NaCl for Injection to each 3.1-g vial, to provide a concentration of ticarcillin 200 mg/ml and clavulanic acid 6.7 mg/ml. Further dilute in 0.9% NaCl, D5W, or Ringer's or lactated Ringer's solution. Stable for 6 hr at room temperature, 72 hr if refrigerated.
- **Rate:** Administer over 30 min via Y-site or direct IV.
- **Y-Site Incompatibility:** If Y-site is used, temporarily discontinue primary infusion during ticarcillin/clavulanate administration.

PATIENT/FAMILY TEACHING
- Advise patient to report the signs of superinfection (black, furry overgrowth on the tongue, vaginal itching or discharge, loose or foul-smelling stools) and allergy.

EVALUATION
Clinical response can be evaluated by:
- Resolution of the signs and symptoms of infection. Length of time for complete resolution depends on the organism and site of infection.

TICLOPIDINE
(tye-**cloe**-pi-deen)
Ticlid

CLASSIFICATION(S):
Platelet aggregation inhibitor
Pregnancy Category B

INDICATIONS
- Prevention of stroke in patients who

have had a completed thrombotic stroke or precursors to stroke who are unable to tolerate aspirin.

ACTION

- Inhibits platelet aggregation by altering the function of platelet membranes
- Prolongs bleeding time. **Therapeutic Effect:** ▪ Decreased incidence of stroke in high risk patients.

PHARMACOKINETICS

Absorption: Well absorbed (>80%) following oral administration.

Distribution: Distribution not known.

Metabolism and Excretion: Extensively metabolized by the liver. Minimal excretion of unchanged drug by the kidneys.

Half-life: Single dose—12.6 hr; multiple dosing—4–5 days.

CONTRAINDICATIONS AND PRECAUTIONS

Contraindicated in: ▪ Hypersensitivity ▪ Bleeding disorders ▪ Active bleeding ▪ Severe liver disease.

Use Cautiously in: ▪ Pregnancy, lactation, or children <18 yr (safety not established) ▪ Risk of bleeding (trauma, surgery, history of ulcer disease) ▪ Renal or hepatic impairment (dosage adjustments may be necessary) ▪ Elderly patients (increased sensitivity).

ADVERSE REACTIONS AND SIDE EFFECTS*

CNS: headache, weakness, dizziness.

EENT: epistaxis, tinnitus.

GI: diarrhea, nausea, vomiting, GI fullness, GI pain, anorexia, abnormal liver function tests.

GU: hematuria.

Derm: urticaria, rashes, ecchymoses, pruritus.

Hemat: neutropenia, INTRACEREBRAL BLEEDING, bleeding, thrombocytopenia.

Metab: hypertriglyceridemia, hypercholesterolemia.

INTERACTIONS

Drug–Drug: ▪ **Aspirin** potentiates the effect of ticlopidine on platelets (concurrent use not recommended) ▪ **Cimetidine** decreases metabolism of ticlopidine and may increase the risk of toxicity ▪ Ticlopidine decreases metabolism of **theophylline** and may increase the risk of toxicity.

Drug–Food: ▪ Absorption of ticlopidine is increased by taking with **food**.

ROUTE AND DOSAGE

- **PO (Adults):** 250 mg bid with food.

AVAILABILITY

- *Tablets:* 250 mg.

TIME/ACTION PROFILE (effect on platelet function)

	ONSET	PEAK	DURATION
PO	within 4 days	8–11 days	2 wk

NURSING IMPLICATIONS

ASSESSMENT

□ Assess patient for symptoms of stroke periodically throughout therapy.

▪ **Lab Test Considerations:** Causes prolonged bleeding time, which is time- and dose-dependent.

□ Monitor CBC with differential every 2 wk from the second week to the end of the third month of therapy; more frequently if absolute neutrophil count (ANC) is declining or <30% of baseline. If neutropenia occurs, ticlopidine should be discontinued. Neutrophil counts usually return to normal within 1–3 wk of discontinuation of therapy. After the first 3 months of therapy, CBC's need to be obtained only for patients with signs and symptoms of infection.

□ May cause thrombocytopenia. If platelet count is <80,000/mm^3, discontinue ticlopidine.

□ May cause increased serum total cholesterol and triglyceride levels. Levels usually increase 8–10% within the first month and persist at that level.

□ May cause elevated alkaline phosphatase, AST (SGOT), and ALT

*Underlines indicate most frequent; **CAPITALS** indicate life-threatening.

(SGPT), levels during the first 4 mo of therapy.
- **Toxicity and Overdose:** Prolonged bleeding time is normalized within 2 hr after administration of IV methylprednisolone. May also use platelet transfusions to reverse effects of ticlopidine on bleeding time.

POTENTIAL NURSING DIAGNOSES
- Injury, high risk for (indications, side effects).
- Knowledge deficit related to medication regimen (patient/family teaching).

IMPLEMENTATION
- **PO:** Administer with food or immediately after eating to minimize GI discomfort and increase absorption.

PATIENT/FAMILY TEACHING
- Instruct patient to take medication exactly as directed.
- Advise patient to notify physician promptly if fever, chills, sore throat, unusual bleeding or bruising, severe or persistent diarrhea, skin rash, jaundice, dark-colored urine, or light-colored stools occur.
- Advise patient to notify physician or dentist of medication regimen prior to treatment or surgery. Medication may need to be discontinued 10–14 days prior to surgery.
- Emphasize the importance of routine lab tests to monitor for side effects.

EVALUATION
Effectiveness of therapy can be demonstrated by: ▪ Prevention of stroke.

TIMOLOL
(tim-oh-lole)
{Apo-Timol}, Blocadren, Timoptic

CLASSIFICATION(S):
Beta-adrenergic blocker (nonselective), Antihypertensive, Ophthalmic (antiglaucoma)
Pregnancy Category C

INDICATIONS
- **PO:** □ Used alone or in combination with other agents in the treatment of hypertension □ Prevention of myocardial infarction □ Migraine headache prophylaxis ▪ **Ophth:** Treatment of glaucoma and other forms of elevated intraocular pressure. **Unlabeled Uses:** ▪ Management of: □ Chronic stable angina pectoris □ Tachyarrhythmias □ Hypertrophic cardiomyopathy □ Pheochromocytoma □ Thyrotoxicosis □ Anxiety □ Tremor □ Mitral valve prolapse.

ACTION
- Blocks stimulation of beta$_1$ (myocardial) and beta$_2$ (pulmonary, vascular, or uterine) receptor sites. **Therapeutic Effects:** ▪ Decreased blood pressure ▪ Prevention of myocardial infarction ▪ Decreased intraocular pressure ▪ Prevention of migraine headaches.

PHARMACOKINETICS
Absorption: Well absorbed following oral administration. Some absorption may occur following ophthalmic use.
Distribution: Distribution not known. Enters breast milk.
Metabolism and Excretion: Extensively metabolized by the liver.
Half-life: 3–4 hr.

CONTRAINDICATIONS AND PRECAUTIONS
Contraindicated in: ▪ Uncompensated congestive heart failure ▪ Pulmonary edema ▪ Cardiogenic shock ▪ Bradycardia or heart block ▪ Children (safety not established).
Use Cautiously in: ▪ Thyrotoxicosis or hypoglycemia (may mask symptoms) ▪ Hepatic impairment (dosage reduction may be required) ▪ Pregnancy or lactation (may cause apnea, low Apgar scores, bradycardia, and hypoglycemia in the newborn) ▪ Ophthalmic use (systemic reactions may occur) ▪ Patients with a history of severe allergic reactions (intensity of reactions may be increased).

{} = Available in Canada only.

ADVERSE REACTIONS AND SIDE EFFECTS*

CNS: <u>fatigue</u>, <u>weakness</u>, <u>depression</u>, memory loss, mental changes, <u>insomnia</u>, dizziness.

CV: BRADYCARDIA, CONGESTIVE HEART FAILURE, PULMONARY EDEMA, hypotension, edema, <u>peripheral vasoconstriction</u>.

EENT: dry eyes, blurred vision, nasal stuffiness.

Resp: bronchospasm, wheezing.

GI: constipation, <u>diarrhea</u>, <u>nausea</u>, <u>vomiting</u>.

GU: impotence, diminished libido.

Derm: rash.

Endo: hyperglycemia, hypoglycemia.

INTERACTIONS

Drug–Drug: ▪ General anesthesia, IV phenytoin, and verapamil may cause additive myocardial depression ▪ Additive bradycardia may occur with concurrent use of cardiac glycosides ▪ Additive hypotension may occur with other antihypertensive agents, acute ingestion of alcohol, or nitrates ▪ Concurrent use with amphetamines, cocaine, ephedrine, epinephrine, norepinephrine, phenylephrine, or pseudoephedrine may result in excess alpha-adrenergic stimulation, hypertension, and bradycardia ▪ May negate the beneficial beta$_1$ cardiac effects of dopamine or dobutamine ▪ Use with insulin may result in prolonged hypoglycemia ▪ May produce hypertension within 14 days of MAO inhibitor therapy ▪ Nonsteroidal anti-inflammatory agents may decrease antihypertensive effectiveness ▪ Cimetidine may decrease metabolism and increase effects of timolol ▪ May decrease effects of beta-adrenergic bronchodilators or theophylline.

ROUTE AND DOSAGE

Hypertension

▪ PO (Adults): 10 mg twice daily (usual dose 20–40 mg/day, up to 60 mg/day).

Prevention of Myocardial Infarction

▪ PO (Adults): 10 mg bid started within 1–4 wk after myocardial infarction.

Migraine Prophylaxis

▪ PO (Adults): 10 mg twice daily initially, may be given as 20 mg once daily; up to 30 mg/day, as 20 mg in morning and 10 mg in evening.

Glaucoma

▪ Ophth (Adults): 1 drop 1–2 times daily.

▪ Ophth (Children): 1 drop of 0.25% solution 1–2 times daily.

AVAILABILITY

▪ *Tablets:* 5 mg, 10 mg, 20 mg ▪ *Ophthalmic solution:* 0.25%, 0.5% ▪ *In combination with:* hydrochlorthiazide (Timolide). See Appendix A.

TIME/ACTION PROFILE
(PO = antihypertensive effect; Ophth = effect on intraocular pressure)

	ONSET	PEAK	DURATION
PO	UK	1–2 hr*	12–24 hr
Ophth	15–30 min	1–5 hr	24 hr

*Maximal antihypertensive effects may take several weeks.

NURSING IMPLICATIONS

ASSESSMENT

▪ **General Info:** Monitor blood pressure and pulse frequently during period of adjustment and periodically throughout therapy. Confer with physician prior to giving drug if pulse is <50 bpm. Assess for orthostatic hypotension when assisting patient up from supine position.

▫ Monitor intake and output ratios and daily weight. Assess patient routinely for evidence of congestive heart failure (peripheral edema, dyspnea, rales/crackles, fatigue, weight gain).

▪ **Ophth:** Intraocular pressure should be monitored periodically during initial therapy and after approximately 4 wk of ophthalmic therapy.

▪ **Lab Test Considerations:** May cause elevations in serum potassium, uric acid, triglyceride, lipoprotein, LDH, alkaline phosphatase levels, and BUN levels.

*<u>Underlines</u> indicate most frequent; CAPITALS indicate life-threatening.

□ Hepatic and renal function and CBC should be monitored routinely in patients receiving prolonged therapy.

POTENTIAL NURSING DIAGNOSES
- Cardiac output, decreased (indications, adverse reactions).
- Knowledge deficit related to medication regimen (patient/family teaching).
- Noncompliance (patient/family teaching).

IMPLEMENTATION
- PO: May be administered without regard to meals. May be crushed and mixed with food or fluid if patient has difficulty swallowing.
- Ophth: See Appendix H for instillation of ophthalmic preparations.

PATIENT/FAMILY TEACHING
- General Info: Instruct patient to take medication exactly as directed, even if feeling well. If a dose is missed it may be taken as soon as remembered up to 4 hr before next dose. Abrupt withdrawal may precipitate life-threatening arrhythmias, hypertension, or myocardial ischemia.
□ Teach patient and family how to check pulse and blood pressure with all dosage forms. Instruct them to take pulse daily and blood pressure at least weekly. Advise patient to withhold dose and contact physician if pulse is <50 bpm or blood pressure changes significantly.
□ Reinforce need to continue additional therapies for hypertension (weight loss, restricted sodium intake, stress reduction, regular exercise, moderation of alcohol consumption, cessation of smoking). Timolol controls but does not cure hypertension.
□ Caution patient that this medication may cause increased sensitivity to cold.
□ Advise patient to consult physician or pharmacist before taking any over-the-counter drugs, especially cold remedies, concurrently with this medication. Patient should also avoid excessive amounts of coffee, tea, and cola.

□ Diabetics should monitor serum glucose closely, especially if weakness, fatigue, or irritability occurs. May mask tachycardia and increase in blood pressure as signs of hypoglycemia, but dizziness and sweating may still occur.
□ Instruct patient to inform physician or dentist of this therapy prior to treatment or surgery.
□ Advise patient to carry identification describing medication regimen at all times.
□ Instruct patient to notify physician if irregular heartbeats, dizziness, depression, or skin rash occur.
- Ophth: Instruct patient on correct technique for administration of ophthalmic solution. Emphasize the importance of not touching tip of container to eye, finger, or any other surface and of preventing systemic absorption by placing pressure on the inner canthus.

EVALUATION
Effectiveness of therapy can be demonstrated by: ■ Decrease in blood pressure ■ Prevention of myocardial reinfarction ■ Decreased intraocular pressure ■ Prevention of migraine headaches.

TOBRAMYCIN
(toe-bra-**mye**-sin)
Nebcin, Tobrex

CLASSIFICATION(S):
Anti-infective (aminoglycoside)
Pregnancy Category D

INDICATIONS

■ IM, IV: Treatment of serious gram-negative bacillary infections and infections due to staphylococci when penicillins or other less toxic drugs are contraindicated or resistance to gentamicin has occurred ■ IM, IV: Treatment of the following infections due to susceptible organisms: □ Bone infections □ CNS infections □ Respiratory tract infections □ Skin and soft tissue infections □ Abdominal infections □ Complicated urinary tract infections □ Endocarditis □ Septicemia ■ **Ophth:** Treatment of superficial eye infections.

ACTION

■ Inhibits protein synthesis in bacteria at the level of the 30S bacterial ribosome. **Therapeutic Effect:** ■ Bactericidal action against susceptible bacteria. **Spectrum:** ■ Notable for activity against important gram-negative pathogens, where resistance to gentamicin has occurred, including: □ *Pseudomonas aeruginosa* □ *Klebsiella pneumoniae* □ *Escherichia coli* □ *Proteus* □ *Serratia* □ *Acenitobacter* ■ Treatment of enterococcal infections requires synergy with a penicillin.

PHARMACOKINETICS

Absorption: Well absorbed after IM administration. Minimal absorption following topical administration.

Distribution: Widely distributed in extracellular fluids following IM or IV administration. Crosses the placenta. Poor penetration into CSF.

Metabolism and Excretion: Excretion is mainly renal (>90%). Dosage adjustments are required for any decrease in renal function. Minimal amounts metabolized by the liver.

Half-life: 2–3 hr (increased in renal impairment).

CONTRAINDICATIONS AND PRECAUTIONS

Contraindicated in: ■ Hypersensitivity ■ Cross-sensitivity with other aminoglycosides may exist.

Use Cautiously in: ■ Renal impairment of any kind (dosage adjustments required if creatinine clearance <70 ml/min) ■ Pregnancy (may cause congenital deafness) ■ Lactation (safety not established) ■ Neuromuscular diseases, such as myasthenia gravis ■ Obese patients (dose should be based on ideal body weight).

ADVERSE REACTIONS AND SIDE EFFECTS*

EENT: ototoxicity (vestibular and cochlear), ocular stinging or burning (ophth).

GU: nephrotoxicity.

Neuro: enhanced neuromuscular blockade.

Misc: hypersensitivity reactions.

INTERACTIONS

Drug–Drug: ■ Inactivated by **penicillins** when coadministered to patients with renal insufficiency ■ Possible respiratory paralysis after **inhalation anesthetics (ether, cyclopropane, halothane,** or **nitrous oxide)** or **neuromuscular blockers (tubocurarine, succinylcholine, decamethonium)** ■ Increased incidence of ototoxicity with **loop diuretics (bumetanide, furosemide)** ■ Increased incidence of nephrotoxicity with other **nephrotoxic drugs (cisplatin).**

ROUTE AND DOSAGE

All doses after initial loading dose should be determined by renal function/blood levels.

■ **IM, IV (Adults):** 0.75–1.25 mg/kg q 6 hr or 1–1.7 mg/kg q 8 hr (up to 8 mg/kg/day in divided doses).

■ **IM, IV (Older Infants and Children):** 1.5–1.9 mg/kg q 6 hr or 2–2.5 mg/kg q 8–16 hr.

■ **IM, IV (Premature or Full-Term Neonates <7 days):** up to 2 mg/kg q 12–24 hr.

■ **Ophth (Adults and Children):** 1 cm ribbon of ointment 2–3 times daily (q 3–4 hr for severe infections) or 1–2 drops of solution q 4 hr (q 30–60 min for severe infections).

AVAILABILITY

■ *Injection:* 10 mg/ml, 30 mg/ml, 40 mg/ml ■ *Ophthalmic solution:* 3 mg/ml ■ *Ophthalmic ointment:* 3 mg/g ■ *In combination with:* dexamethasone (TobraDex). See Appendix A.

TIME/ACTION PROFILE (blood levels)

	ONSET	PEAK
IM	rapid	30–90 min
IV	rapid	end of infusion
Ophth oint	rapid	UK
Ophth soln	rapid	UK

NURSING IMPLICATIONS

ASSESSMENT

□ Assess patient for infection (vital signs; appearance of wound, sputum, urine, and stool; WBC) at beginning and throughout course of therapy.

□ Obtain specimens for culture and sensitivity prior to initiating therapy. First dose may be given before receiving results.

□ Evaluate eighth cranial nerve function by audiometry prior to and throughout course of therapy. Hearing loss is usually in the high-frequency range. Prompt recognition and intervention is essential in preventing permanent damage. Also monitor for vestibular dysfunction (vertigo, ataxia, nausea, vomiting). Eighth cranial dysfunction is usually associated with persistently elevated peak tobramycin levels.

□ Monitor intake and output and daily weight to assess hydration status and renal function.

□ Assess patient for signs of superinfection (fever, upper respiratory infection, vaginal itching or discharge, increasing malaise, diarrhea). Report to physician.

■ **Lab Test Considerations:** Monitor renal function by urinalysis, specific gravity, BUN, creatinine, and creatinine clearance prior to and throughout therapy.

□ May cause increased AST (SGOT), ALT (SGPT), LDH, bilirubin, and serum alkaline phosphatase levels.

□ May cause decreased serum calcium, magnesium, sodium, and potassium levels.

■ **Toxicity and Overdose:** Blood levels should be monitored periodically during therapy. Timing of blood levels is important in interpreting results. Draw blood for peak levels 30–60 min after IM injection and immediately after IV infusion is completed. Trough levels should be drawn just prior to next dose. Acceptable peak level is 4–10 mcg/ml; trough level should not be >2 mcg/ml.

POTENTIAL NURSING DIAGNOSES

■ Infection, high risk for (indications).

■ Sensory-perceptual alteration: auditory (side effects).

IMPLEMENTATION

■ **General Info:** Keep patient well-hydrated (1500–2000 ml/day) during therapy.

■ **IM:** Administer deep into a well-developed muscle. SC administration is not recommended and may be painful.

■ **Intermittent Infusion:** Dilute each dose of tobramycin in 50–200 ml of D5W, D10W, D5/0.9% NaCl, 0.9% NaCl, Ringer's or lactated Ringer's solution to provide a concentration not >1 mg/ml (0.1%). Pediatric doses may be diluted in proportionately smaller amounts. Stable for 24 hr at room temperature, 96 hr if refrigerated. Also available in commercially mixed piggyback injections.

■ **Rate:** Infuse slowly, over 30–60 min in both adult and pediatric patients. Flush IV line with D5W or 0.9% NaCl following administration.

■ **Syringe Incompatibility:** ■ cefamandole ■ clindamycin ■ heparin.

■ **Y-Site Compatibility:** ■ acyclovir ■ ciprofloxacin ■ cyclophosphamide ■ enalaprilat ■ esmolol ■ fluconazole ■ fludarabine ■ foscarnet ■ furosemide ■ hydromorphone ■ insulin ■ labetalol ■ magnesium sulfate ■ meperidine ■ morphine ■ perphenazine ■ tolazoline ■ zidovudine.

■ **Y-Site Incompatibility:** ■ heparin ■ hetastarch ■ sargramostim. If aminoglycosides and cephalosporins or penicillins must be administered concurrently, administer in separate sites.

■ **Additive Incompatibility:** Manufac-

turer recommends that tobramycin not be admixed with other drugs.
- **Ophth:** Do not touch tip of container to eye, fingers, or any other surface. See Appendix H for instillation of ophthalmic preparations.

PATIENT/FAMILY TEACHING
- **General Info:** Instruct patient to report signs of hypersensitivity, tinnitus, vertigo, or hearing loss.
- **Ophth:** Patients with ophthalmic infections should be advised to avoid wearing contact lenses until infection is resolved and physician approves.

EVALUATION
Clinical response can be evaluated by:
- Resolution of the signs and symptoms of infection. Length of time for complete resolution depends on organism and site of infection.

TOCAINIDE
(toe-**kay**-nide)
Tonocard

CLASSIFICATION(S):
Antiarrhythmic (group IB)
Pregnancy Category C

INDICATIONS
- Treatment of life-threatening ventricular arrhythmias including multifocal and unifocal premature ventricular contractions and ventricular tachycardia.

ACTION
- Suppresses automaticity of conduction tissue and spontaneous depolarization of the ventricles during diastole
- Has little or no effect on heart rate.
Therapeutic Effect: ▪ Suppression of arrhythmias.

PHARMACOKINETICS
Absorption: Well absorbed following oral administration.
Distribution: Widely distributed. Crosses the blood–brain barrier.
Metabolism and Excretion: Partially

metabolized by the liver. 30–50% excreted unchanged by the kidneys.
Half-life: 11–23 hr.

CONTRAINDICATIONS AND PRECAUTIONS
Contraindicated in: ▪ Hypersensitivity ▪ Advanced heart block.
Use Cautiously in: ▪ Congestive heart failure ▪ Hepatic or renal impairment (dosage reduction recommended) ▪ Pregnancy, lactation, or children (safety not established).

ADVERSE REACTIONS AND SIDE EFFECTS*
CNS: lightheadedness, vertigo, tremor, headache, hallucinations, changes in mood, restlessness, sedation, SEIZURES, coma, depression, paranoia, dizziness.
EENT: blurred vision, tinnitus, thirst.
Resp: pneumonia, pulmonary fibrosis.
CV: hypotension, tachycardia, bradycardia, palpitations, congestive heart failure, arrhythmias, angina, conduction disturbances, hypertension, SINUS ARREST.
GI: nausea, vomiting, anorexia, diarrhea, constipation, dyspepsia, dysphagia, abdominal discomfort, hepatitis.
GU: urinary retention.
Derm: rashes, sweating, flushing, alopecia.
Hemat: AGRANULOCYTOSIS, LEUKOPENIA, NEUTROPENIA, THROMBOCYTOPENIA.
MS: arthralgia, myalgia.
Neuro: myasthenia gravis, numbness.

INTERACTIONS
Drug–Drug: ▪ Additive cardiac effects with other **antiarrhythmics** ▪ Concurrent use with **beta-adrenergic blocking agents** may precipitate congestive heart failure ▪ **Cimetidine** or **rifampin** may decrease blood levels of tocainide.

ROUTE AND DOSAGE
- **PO (Adults):** 400 mg q 8 hr initially; usual maintenance dose 1.2–1.8 g/day in divided doses q 8 hr (up to

---

*Underlines indicate most frequent; **CAPITALS** indicate life-threatening.

2.4 g/day may be used). Dosing twice daily may be used in some patients.

AVAILABILITY

▪ *Tablets:* 400 mg, 600 mg.

TIME/ACTION PROFILE
(antiarrhythmic effects)

	ONSET	PEAK	DURATION
PO	30–60 min	0.5–2 hr	8–12 hr

NURSING IMPLICATIONS

ASSESSMENT

□ ECG, pulse, and blood pressure should be monitored prior to and periodically throughout therapy.

□ Assess lungs periodically throughout therapy. Notify physician if cough, wheezing, or shortness of breath occurs. Chest x-rays should also be evaluated if signs of pulmonary complications occur.

▪ **Lab Test Considerations:** CBC, WBC with differential and platelet counts should be monitored weekly during the first 3 mo of therapy and frequently thereafter. Blood counts should be performed promptly if patient develops signs of infection (fever, chills, sore throat, stomatitis), bleeding or bruising. Leukopenia, agranulocytosis, and thrombocytopenia usually occur after 2–12 wk of therapy and return to normal 1 mo after discontinuation.

POTENTIAL NURSING DIAGNOSES

▪ Cardiac output, decreased (indications).
▪ Knowledge deficit related to medication regimen (patient/family teaching).

IMPLEMENTATION

▪ **PO:** Administer with food or milk to minimize GI irritation.

PATIENT/FAMILY TEACHING

□ Instruct patient to take medication around the clock, exactly as directed, even if feeling well. If a dose is missed, take as soon as remembered if within 4 hr; do not take if remembered later. Do not double doses.

Consult with physician prior to discontinuing medication, as gradual reduction in dosage may be needed to prevent worsening of condition.

□ Instruct patient or family member on how to take pulse. Advise patient to report changes in pulse rate or rhythm to physician.

□ Tocainide may cause dizziness or lightheadedness. Caution patient to avoid driving or other activities requiring alertness until response to medication is known.

□ Advise patient to inform physician or dentist of medication regimen prior to treatment or surgery.

□ Advise patient to carry identification describing disease process and medication regimen at all times.

□ Instruct patient to notify physician if trembling, shaking, fever, chills, sore throat, ulcers in the mouth, unusual bleeding or bruising, dyspnea, cough, wheezing, or palpitations occur. Physician should also be notified if nausea, vomiting, or diarrhea becomes severe.

□ Emphasize the importance of routine follow-up examinations to monitor progress.

EVALUATION

Effectiveness of therapy can be demonstrated by: ▪ Resolution of ventricular arrhythmias without detrimental side effects.

TOLAZOLINE
(tole-**az**-oh-leen)
Priscoline

CLASSIFICATION(S):
Antihypertensive
(miscellaneous)
Pregnancy Category UK

INDICATIONS

▪ Treatment of pulmonary hypertension in newborns when oxygenation cannot be provided by other methods (oxygen therapy, mechanical ventilation).

ACTION

- Direct-acting vasodilator • Also causes vasodilation by alpha-adrenergic blockade. **Therapeutic Effects:** ▪ Decreased pulmonary arterial pressure ▪ Decreased vascular resistance.

PHARMACOKINETICS

Absorption: Administered IV only, resulting in complete bioavailability.
Distribution: Distribution not known.
Metabolism and Excretion: Excreted mostly unchanged by the kidneys.
Half-life: 3–10 hr (neonates).

CONTRAINDICATIONS AND PRECAUTIONS

Contraindicated in: ▪ Hypotension.
Use Cautiously in: ▪ Acidosis ▪ Mitral stenosis (paradoxical response may occur) ▪ Gastritis or history of GI bleeding ▪ Renal impairment (dosage reduction may be necessary if urine output is <0.9 ml/kg/hr).

ADVERSE REACTIONS AND SIDE EFFECTS*

EENT: mydriasis.
CV: hypotension, tachycardia, SHOCK.
GI: GI BLEEDING, diarrhea, nausea, vomiting.
GU: acute oliguric renal failure.
Derm: flushing, piloerection.
F and E: hypochloremic alkalosis.
Hemat: thrombocytopenia.

INTERACTIONS

Drug–Drug: ▪ Concurrent use with **epinephrine** or **norepinephrine** may result in initial hypotension, followed by rebound hypertension ▪ May antagonize the vasopressor effects of **dopamine, ephedrine, metaraminol, methoxamine,** or **phenylephrine.**

ROUTE AND DOSAGE

- **IV (Newborns):** 1–2 mg/kg initially, then 0.2 mg/kg/hr for each 1 mg/kg loading dose. Initial dose may be repeated.

AVAILABILITY

▪ *Injection:* 25 mg/ml.

TIME/ACTION PROFILE (vascular response)

	ONSET	PEAK	DURATION
IV	30 min	UK	UK

NURSING IMPLICATIONS

ASSESSMENT

- Monitor arterial blood pressure, ECG, and heart rate routinely throughout administration. Tolazoline should be discontinued if systolic blood pressure cannot be maintained at >40–50 mmHg.
- Monitor pulmonary artery pressure (PAP) and pulmonary capillary wedge pressure (PCWP) frequently throughout administration.
- Monitor intake and output and daily weight throughout therapy.
- Assess patient for bleeding, bruising, petechiae, or blood in stools, urine, or emesis throughout therapy.
- **Lab Test Considerations:** Monitor arterial blood gases (ABGs), CBC, and serum electrolytes, especially potassium and chloride, routinely throughout therapy. If hypochloremic metabolic acidosis occurs, wean patient from tolazoline and administer potassium and chloride.
- Hematest gastric aspirate periodically to determine GI bleeding.
- **Toxicity and Overdose:** If profound hypotension occurs, keep patient's head low and administer IV fluids. Do not administer epinephrine or norepinephrine, as further hypotension followed by rebound hypertension may occur. Dopamine may be infused simultaneously with tolazoline if IV fluids fail to maintain blood pressure.

POTENTIAL NURSING DIAGNOSES

- Tissue perfusion, altered (indications).
- Gas exchange, impaired (indications).

---

*Underlines indicate most frequent; **CAPITALS** indicate life-threatening.

- Knowledge deficit related to medication regimen (patient/family teaching).

IMPLEMENTATION

- **General Info:** Administer only in a neonatal intensive care area equipped to provide trained personnel and respiratory support.
- Antacids may be ordered prior to therapy to minimize GI bleeding.
- **Direct IV:** Administer initial dose undiluted over 10 min via scalp vein. May also be infused into any vein that drains into the superior vena cava to maximize delivery to the pulmonary artery. Follow with maintenance infusion. Initial bolus may be repeated during infusion if needed.
- **Continuous Infusion:** May be diluted in D5W, D10W, 0.45% NaCl, 0.9% NaCl, Ringer's or lactated Ringer's solution, dextrose/saline combinations, dextrose/Ringer's or lactated Ringer's combinations. Do not use diluents containing benzyl alcohol for neonates; fatal reaction may occur.
- Administer via infusion pump for accurate dosage.
- **Y-Site Compatibility:** ■ aminophylline ■ ampicillin ■ calcium gluconate ■ cefotaxime ■ cimetidine ■ dobutamine ■ dopamine ■ furosemide ■ gentamicin ■ phytonadione ■ sodium bicarbonate ■ tobramycin ■ vancomycin.
- **Y-Site Incompatibility:** ■ indomethacin.

PATIENT/FAMILY TEACHING

- Explain purpose of medication to parents. Provide emotional support.

EVALUATION

Effectiveness of therapy can be determined by: ■ Decrease in pulmonary artery pressure and vascular resistance. Response should be seen within 30 min of initial dose.

TOLMETIN
(tole-met-in)
Tolectin, Tolectin DS

CLASSIFICATION(S):
Nonsteroidal anti-inflammatory agent
Pregnancy Category C

INDICATIONS

- Management of inflammatory disorders including: □ Rheumatoid arthritis □ Juvenile rheumatoid arthritis □ Osteoarthritis.

ACTION

- Inhibits prostaglandin synthesis. **Therapeutic Effects:** ■ Suppression of pain and inflammation.

PHARMACOKINETICS

Absorption: Well absorbed from the GI tract following oral administration.
Distribution: Distribution not known.
Metabolism and Excretion: Mostly metabolized by the liver. 20% excreted unchanged by the kidneys.
Half-life: 1 hr.

CONTRAINDICATIONS AND PRECAUTIONS

Contraindicated in: ■ Hypersensitivity ■ Cross-sensitivity may exist with other nonsteroidal anti-inflammatory agents, including aspirin ■ Active GI bleeding or ulcer disease ■ Pregnancy.
Use Cautiously in: ■ Severe cardiovascular, renal, or hepatic disease ■ History of ulcer disease ■ Lactation (safety not established) ■ Severe hepatic or renal impairment (dosage reduction recommended).

ADVERSE REACTIONS AND SIDE EFFECTS*

CNS: headache, drowsiness, dizziness, sleep disturbances, depression.
EENT: visual disturbances, tinnitus.
CV: edema, hypertension.
GI: nausea, dyspepsia, vomiting, diarrhea, constipation, GI BLEEDING, discomfort, flatulence, HEPATITIS.
GU: renal failure.
Derm: rashes.
Hemat: prolonged bleeding time.
MS: muscle weakness.

*Underlines indicate most frequent; **CAPITALS** indicate life-threatening.

Misc: allergic reactions, including ANA-PHYLAXIS.

INTERACTIONS

Drug–Drug: ▪ Increased risk of bleeding with **anticoagulants, cefamandole, cefoperazone, cefotetan, thrombolytic agents,** or **plicamycin** ▪ Additive adverse GI side effects with **aspirin, glucocorticoids,** and other **nonsteroidal anti-inflammatory agents** ▪ May decrease response to **antihypertensives** or **diuretics** ▪ May increase serum levels and risk of toxicity from **lithium** ▪ May increase the risk of hematologic toxicity from **antineoplastic agents** or **radiation therapy** ▪ Increased risk of adverse renal effects with **gold compounds, cyclosporine,** or chronic use of **acetaminophen** ▪ May increase the risk of hypoglycemia from **insulin** or **oral hypoglycemic agents.**

ROUTE AND DOSAGE

▪ **PO (Adults):** 400 mg 3 times daily initially (range 600–1800 mg/day in 3–4 divided doses, not to exceed 2000 mg/day).
▪ **PO (Children >2 yr):** 20 mg/kg initially (range 15–30 mg/kg/day in 3–4 divided doses, not to exceed 30 mg/kg/day).

AVAILABILITY

▪ *Tablets:* 200 mg, 600 mg ▪ *Capsules:* 400 mg.

TIME/ACTION PROFILE (anti-inflammatory effects)

	ONSET	PEAK	DURATION
PO	within 7 days	1–2 wk	UK

NURSING IMPLICATIONS

ASSESSMENT

▢ Patients who have asthma, aspirin-induced allergy, and nasal polyps are at increased risk for developing hypersensitivity reactions. Monitor for rhinitis, asthma, and urticaria.
▢ Assess pain and range of motion prior to and weekly during therapy.
▪ **Lab Test Considerations:** BUN, serum creatinine, CBC, and liver function tests should be evaluated periodically in patients receiving prolonged courses of therapy.
▢ Serum potassium, BUN, AST (SGOT) and ALT (SGPT) may show increased levels.
▢ Hemoglobin and hematocrit may be decreased. Bleeding time may be prolonged for up to 2 days after discontinuation.
▢ May cause false-positive results for urinary protein.

POTENTIAL NURSING DIAGNOSES

▪ Pain (indications).
▪ Physical mobility, impaired (indications).
▪ Knowledge deficit related to medication regimen (patient/family teaching).

IMPLEMENTATION

▪ **PO:** May be administered with food, milk, or antacids to decrease GI irritation. Food slows but does not reduce the extent of absorption. Tablets may be crushed and capsules opened and mixed with fluids or food.

PATIENT/FAMILY TEACHING

▢ Advise patient to take this medication with a full glass of water and to remain in an upright position for 15–30 min after administration.
▢ Instruct patient to take medication exactly as directed. If a dose is missed, it should be taken as soon as remembered but not if almost time for the next dose. Do not double doses.
▢ This medication may cause drowsiness or dizziness. Advise patient to avoid driving or other activities requiring alertness until response to medication is known.
▢ Caution patient to avoid the concurrent use of alcohol, aspirin, ibuprofen, acetaminophen, or other over-the-counter medications without consulting physician.
▢ Instruct patient to notify physician if rash, itching, muscle aches, visual disturbances, weight gain, edema, black stools, or persistent headache occurs.

□ Advise patient to inform physician or dentist of medication regimen prior to treatment or surgery.

EVALUATION
Effectiveness of therapy can be demonstrated by: ■ Decrease in pain □ Improved joint mobility. Partial arthritic relief is usually seen within 7 days, but maximum effectiveness may require 1–2 wk of continuous therapy. Patients who do not respond to one nonsteroidal antiinflammatory agent may respond to another.

TOPICAL ANTIFUNGALS

amphotericin b
(am-foe-**ter**-i-sin B)
Fungizone

ciclopirox
(sye-kloe-**peer**-ox)
Loprox

clioquinol
(klye-oh-**kwin**-ole)
Iodochlorhydroyquin, Vioform

clotrimazole
(kloe-**trye**-ma-zole)
{Canesten}, {Clotrimaderm}, Lotrimin, Lotrimin AF, Mycelex, Mycelex OTC, {Myclo}, {Neozol}

econazole
(ee-**kon**-a-zole)
Spectazole

haloprogin
(hal-oh-**proe**-jin)
Halotex

ketoconazole
(kee-toe-**kon**-a-zole)
Nizoral

miconazole
(mye-**kon**-a-zole)
Micatin, Monistat-Derm

naftifine
(**naff**-ti-feen)
Naftin

nystatin
(nye-**stat**-in)
Mycostatin, {Nodostine}, Nilstat, {Nyoderm}, Nystex

oxiconazole
(ox-i-**kon**-a-zole)
Oxistat

sulconazole
(sul-**kon**-a-zole)
Exelderm

terbinafine
(ter-**bin**-a-feen)
Lamisil

tolnaftate
(tol-**naff**-tate)
Adsorbine Antifungal, Adsorbine Jr. Antifungal, Aftate, Desenex Spray, Genaspor, NP-27, Quinsana Plus, Tinactin, Ting, Zeasorb-AF

triacetin
(trye-a-**seet**-in)
Fungoid, Ony-Clear Nail

undecylenic acid
(un-de-**sill**-enn-ik **as**-id)
Breezee Mist Aerosol, Caldesene, Cruex, Decylenes, Desenex Cream, Desenex Foam, Desenex Powder, Desenex Powder Aerosol, Pedi-Dri, Pedi-Pro Phicon F

Pregnancy Category B (ciclopirox, clotrimazole, haloprogin, naftifine, oxiconazole, terbinafine); C (econazole, ketoconazole)

INDICATIONS

■ Treatment of a variety of cutaneous fungal infections, including cutaneous candidiasis, *tinea pedis* (athlete's foot), *tinea cruris* (jock itch), *tinea corporis* (ringworm), and *tinea versicolor*. Undecyclenic acid is used only for tinea infections. Amphotericin B is used only for candidal infections (newer agents may be more effective).

ACTION

■ Nystatin, clotrimazole, econazole, miconazole, and tioconazole effect the synthesis of the fungal cell wall allowing leakage of cellular contents. Undecylenic acid also contains zinc undecylenate, which acts as an astringent. Some

T

agents (triacetin) also have antibacterial properties. **Therapeutic Effects:**
- Fungistatic or fungicidal action depending on agent and concentration with resultant decrease in symptoms of fungal infection.

PHARMACOKINETICS

Absorption: Most agents are minimally, if at all, absorbed through intact skin. Clioquinol is rapidly and extensively absorbed and may affect thyroid function.

Distribution: Distribution following topical administration not known. Action is primarily local.

Metabolism and Excretion: Metabolism and excretion not known following local application.

Half-life: ciclipirox—1.7 hr; miconazole—24.1 hr (terminal).

CONTRAINDICATIONS AND PRECAUTIONS

Contraindicated in: - Hypersensitivity to active ingredients, additives, preservatives, or bases - Some products contain alcohol or bisulfites and should be avoided in patients with known intolerance - Clioquinol contains iodine and should not be used in patients with known hypersensitivity.

Use Cautiously in: - Pregnancy, lactation, or children (safety not established—ciclopirox, haloprogin, naftifine, terbinafine, undecylenic acid) - Nail and scalp infections (may require additional systemic therapy).

ADVERSE REACTIONS AND SIDE EFFECTS*

Local: burning, itching stinging, redness, local hypersensitivity reactions.

INTERACTIONS

Drug–Drug: - If sufficient ketoconazole is absorbed through skin, it may increase the cardiotoxicity of **terfenadine** or nephrotoxicity of **cyclosporine**.

ROUTE AND DOSAGE

Amphotericin B
- **Topical (Adults):** Apply cream, lotion, or ointment 2–4 times daily for 1–4 wk.

Ciclopirox
- **Topical (Adults):** Apply cream or lotion twice daily for 2 wk.

Clioquinol
- **Topical (Adults):** Apply 2–3 times daily. Not to be used for >7 days.

Clotrimazole
- **Topical (Adults):** Apply cream, solution, or lotion twice daily for 1–4 wk.

Econazole
- **Topical (Adults):** Apply cream once daily for *tinea pedis, tinea cruris,* or *tinea versicolor.* Apply twice daily for cutaneous candidiasis. Use for 2–4 wk.

Haloprogin
- **Topical (Adults):** Apply daily for 2–4 wk.

Ketoconazole
- **Topical (Adults):** Apply cream once daily for cutaneous candidiasis or twice daily for seborrheic dermatitis. For dandruff, use shampoo twice weekly (wait 3 days between treatments) for 4 wk, then intermittently.

Miconazole
- **Topical (Adults):** Apply cream, powder, or spray twice daily (once daily for tinea versicolor) for up to 1 mo.

Naftifine
- **Topical (Adults):** Apply cream once daily or gel twice daily.

Nystatin
- **Topical (Adults and Children):** Apply cream, ointment, or powder 2–3 times daily until healing is complete.

Oxiconazole
- **Topical (Adults):** Apply cream or lotion 1–2 times daily for 2 wk–1 mo.

Sulconazole
- **Topical (Adults):** Apply 1–2 times daily (twice daily for *tinea pedis*).

Terbinafine
- **Topical (Adults):** Apply twice daily for *tinea pedis* (athlete's foot) or 1–2 times daily for *tinea cruris* (jock itch)

*Underlines indicate most frequent; **CAPITALS** indicate life-threatening.

or *tinea corporis* (ringworm) for 1–4 wk.

Tolnaftate
- **Topical (Adults):** Apply twice daily for 2–3 wk.

Triacetin
- **Topical (Adults):** Apply cream or solution 3 times daily or tincture twice daily. Use spray as directed.

Undecylenic Acid
- **Topical (Adults):** Apply as needed/directed.

AVAILABILITY

Amphotericin B
- *Cream:* 3% ▪ *Lotion:* 3% ▪ *Ointment:* 3%.

Ciclopirox
- *Cream:* 1% ▪ *Lotion:* 1%.

Clioquinol
- *Cream:* 3% ▪ *Ointment:* 3% ▪ *In combination with:* hydrocortisone (Vioform-HC). See Appendix A.

Clotrimazole
- *Cream:* 1% ▪ *Solution:* 1% ▪ *Lotion:* 1% ▪ *In combination with:* betamethasone (Lotrisone). See Appendix A.

Econazole
- *Cream:* 1%.

Haloprogin
- *Cream:* 1% ▪ *Solution:* 1%.

Ketoconazole
- *Cream:* 2% ▪ *Shampoo:* 2%.

Miconazole
- *Cream:* 2% ▪ *Powder:* 2% ▪ *Aerosol powder:* 2% ▪ *Spray:* 2%.

Naftifine
- *Cream:* 1% ▪ *Gel:* 1%.

Nystatin
- *Cream:* 100,000 units/g ▪ *Ointment:* 100,000 units/g ▪ *Powder:* 100,000 units/g ▪ *In combination with:* triamcinolone (Mycigen II, Mycolog-II, Myci-Triacet II, Mytrex). See Appendix A.

Oxiconazole
- *Cream:* 1% ▪ *Lotion:* 1%.

Sulconazole
- *Cream:* 1% ▪ *Solution:* 1%.

Terbinafine
- *Cream:* 1%.

Tolnaftate
- *Cream:* 1% ▪ *Solution:* 1% ▪ *Gel:* 1% ▪ *Powder:* 1% ▪ *Spray powder:* 1% ▪ *Spray liquid:* 1%.

Triacetin
- *Solution* ▪ *Tincture* ▪ *Cream* ▪ *Aerosol spray* ▪ *In combination with:* hydrocortisone (Fugoid-HC). See Appendix A.

Undecylenic acid
- *Cream:* 8%, 20% ▪ *Ointment:* 22% ▪ *Powder:* 10%, 15%, 19% ▪ *Foam:* 10% ▪ *Soap:* 97.5 g/bar.

TIME/ACTION PROFILE (resolution of symptoms/lesions)

	ONSET	PEAK
ciclopirox	within 1st wk	UK
clotrimazole	within 1st wk	UK
miconazole	2–3 days	2 wk
triacetin	within 1st wk	UK

NURSING IMPLICATIONS

ASSESSMENT
- ▫ Inspect involved areas of skin and mucous membranes prior to and frequently throughout course of therapy. Increased skin irritation may indicate need to discontinue medication.

POTENTIAL NURSING DIAGNOSES
- ▪ Skin integrity, impaired (indications).
- ▪ Infection, high risk for (indications).
- ▪ Knowledge deficit related to medication regimen (patient/family teaching).

IMPLEMENTATION
- ▪ **General Info:** Consult physician for proper cleansing technique prior to applying medication.
- ▫ Choice of vehicle is based on use. Ointments, creams, and liquids are used as primary therapy. Lotion is usually preferred in intertriginous areas; if cream is used, apply sparingly to avoid maceration. Powders are usually used as adjunctive ther-

apy but may be used as primary therapy for mild conditions.

- **Topical:** Apply small amount to cover affected area completely. Avoid the use of occlusive wrappings or dressings unless directed by physician.

- **Ketoconazole shampoo:** Moisten hair and scalp thoroughly with water. Apply sufficient shampoo to produce enough lather to wash scalp and hair and gently massage it over the entire scalp area for approximately 1 min. Rinse hair thoroughly with warm water. Repeat process, leaving shampoo on hair for an additional 3 min. After the second shampoo, rinse and dry hair with towel or warm air flow. Shampoo twice a week for 4 wk with at least 3 days between each shampooing and then intermittently as needed to maintain control.

- **Triacetin:** For spray products, shake well. Dry affected areas prior to spraying. Spray onto affected nails, holding actuator down 1–2 sec.

PATIENT/FAMILY TEACHING

- ☐ Instruct patient to apply medication as directed for full course of therapy, even if feeling better. Emphasize the importance of avoiding the eyes.
- ☐ Caution patient that some products may stain fabric, skin, or hair. Check label information. Fabrics stained from cream or lotion can usually be cleaned by handwashing with soap and warm water; stains from ointments can usually be removed with standard cleaning fluids.
- ☐ Patients with athlete's foot should be taught to wear well-fitting, ventilated shoes and to change shoes and socks at least once a day.
- ☐ Advise patient to report increased skin irritation or lack of response to therapy to physician.

EVALUATION

Effectiveness of therapy can be demonstrated by: ▪ Decrease in skin irritation and resolution of infection. Early relief of symptoms may be seen in 2–3 days. For Candida, *tinea cruris,* and *tinea corporis,* 2 wk are needed, and for *tinea pedis,* therapeutic response may take 3–4 wk.

TOPICAL GLUCOCORTICOIDS

alclometasone
(al-kloe-**met**-a-sone)
Aclovate

amcinonide
(am-**sin**-oh-nide)
Cyclocort

betamethasone
(bay-ta-**meth**-a-sone)
Alphatrex, {Beben}, {Betacort}, Betaderm, Betatrex, Beta-Val, Betmethacort, {Betnovate}, {Celestoderm}, Dermabet, Diprolene, Diprosone, {Ectosonel}, Maxivate, {Metaderm}, {Novobetamet}, Psorion, Uticort, Valisone, Valnac

clobetasol
(kloe-**bay**-ta-sol)
{Dermovate}, Temovate

clocortolone
(kloe-**kore**-toe-lone)
Cloderm

desonide
(**dess**-oh-nide)
DesOwen, Tridesilon

desoximetasone
(dess-ox-i-**met**-a-sone)
Topicort

dexamethasone
(dex-a-**meth**-a-sone)
Aeroseb-Dex, Decaderm, Decaspray

diflorasone
(dye-**flor**-a-sone)
Florone, Maxiflor, Psorcon

fluocinolone
(floo-oh-**sin**-oh-lone)
Bio-Syn, Derma-Smoothe/FS, Fluocet, {Fluoderm}, {Fluolar}, Fluonid, {Fluonide}, Flurosyn, FS Shampoo, Synalar, {Synamol}, Synemol

fluocinonide
(floo-oh-**sin**-oh-nide)
Fluocin, Licon, {Lidemol}, Lidex,
{Lyderm}, {Topsyn}, Vasoderm

flurandrenolide
(floor-an-**dren**-oh-lide)
Cordran, {Drenison}

fluticasone
(floo-**tik**-a-sone)
Cutivate

halcinonide
(hal-**sin**-oh-nide)
Halog

halobetasol
(hal-oh-**bay**-ta-sol)
Ultravate

hydrocortisone
(hye-droe-**kor**-ti-sone)
Acitocort, Aeroseb-HC, Ala-Cort,
Allercort, Alphaderm, Anusol
HC, Bactine, {Barriere-HC}, Cal-
deCORT Anti-Itch, Carmol HC,
Cetacort, {Cortacet}, Cortaid,
{Cortate}, Cort-Dome, {Cortef},
Corticaine, {Corticreme}, Corti-
fair, Cortizone, {Cortoderm}, Cor-
tril, Delcort, Dermacort, Demi-
Cort, Dermtex HC, {Emo-Cort},
Epifoam, FoilleCort, Gly-Cort,
Gynecort, Hi-Cor, Hycort, {Hy-
derm}, Hydro-Tex, Hytone, Lacti-
Care-HC, Lanacort, Lemoderm,
Locoid, My Cort, 9-1-1, {Novoehy-
drocort}, NutracortPharm, Phar-
macort, Pentacort, Rederm, Rhu-
licortS-T Cort, Synacort, {Sarna
HC}, Texa-Cort, {Unicort},
Westcort

mometasone
(moe-**met**-a-sone)
Elocon

prednicarbate
(pred-ni-**kar**-bate)
Dermatop

triamcinolone
(trye-am-**sin**-oh-lone)
Aristocort, Flutex, Kenac, Kenalog, Kenonel, {Triaderm}, {Tria-
nide}, Triderm, Trymex

Pregnancy Category C

INDICATIONS
▪ Used in the management of a wide variety of allergic/immunologic reactions.

ACTION
▪ Supresses normal immune response
and inflammation. If systemically absorbed for prolonged periods of time
may produce adrenal suppression.
Therapeutic Effects: ▪ Suppression of
dermatologic inflammation and immune processes.

PHARMACOKINETICS
Absorption: Minimal if used as directed. Prolonged use on large surface
areas or large amounts applied will produce systemic absorption and adrenal
suppression.
Distribution: Remains primarily at site
of action, unless applied to large areas
or in large amounts.
Metabolism and Excretion: Not
known following topical administration.
Half-life: UK.

CONTRAINDICATIONS AND PRECAUTIONS
Contraindicated in: ▪ Hypersensitivity
or known intolerance to glucocorticoid
or components of vehicles (ointment or
cream base, preservative, alcohol) ▪ Untreated bacterial or viral infections.
Use Cautiously in: ▪ Pregnancy, lactation, or children (chronic high-dose usage may result in adrenal suppression
in mother, growth suppression in children; children may be more susceptible
to adrenal and growth suppression)
▪ Use cautiously in patients with
hepatic dysfunction ▪ Clobetasol not
recommended for use in children <12
yr ▪ Desoximetasone not recommended
in children <10 yr.

ADVERSE REACTIONS AND SIDE EFFECTS*
Local: burning, irritation, edema, hypopigmentation, maceration, hypertrichosis, perioral dermatitis, allergic
contact dermatitis, secondary infection,

*Underlines indicate most frequent; **CAPITALS** indicate life-threatening.

dryness, folliculitis, atrophy, miliaria, striae, hypersensitivity reactions. **Misc:** adrenal suppression.

INTERACTIONS
Drug–Drug: ▪ None significant.

ROUTE AND DOSAGE
▪ **Top (Adults and Children):** Apply 1–6 times daily (depends on product, preparation, and condition being treated).

AVAILABILITY
Alclometasone
▪ *Cream:* 0.05% ▪ *Ointment:* 0.05%.

Amcinonide
▪ *Cream:* 0.1% ▪ *Lotion:* 0.1% ▪ *Ointment:* 0.1%.

Betamethasone
▪ *Cream:* 0.01%, 0.025%, 0.05%, 0.1% ▪ *Gel:* 0.25%, 0.05% ▪ *Lotion:* 0.1%, 0.25%, 0.05% ▪ *Ointment:* 0.25%, 0.05%, 0.1% ▪ *Spray:* 0.1%.

Clobetasol
▪ *Cream:* 0.05% ▪ *Ointment:* 0.05% ▪ *Scalp solution:* 0.05%.

Clocortolone
▪ *Cream:* 0.1%.

Desonide
▪ *Cream:* 0.05% ▪ *Ointment:* 0.05% ▪ *Lotion:* 0.05%.

Desoximetasone
▪ *Cream:* 0.25%, 0.05% ▪ *Gel:* 0.05% ▪ *Ointment:* 0.25%.

Dexamethasone
▪ *Cream:* 1% ▪ *Spray:* 0.01%, 0.04%.

Diflorasone
▪ *Cream:* 0.05% ▪ *Ointment:* 0.05%.

Fluocinolone
▪ *Cream:* 0.01%, 0.02%, 0.025% ▪ *Ointment:* 0.025% ▪ *Solution:* 0.01% ▪ *Shampoo:* 0.01% ▪ *Oil:* 0.01%.

Fluocinonide
▪ *Cream:* 0.05 ▪ *Gel:* 0.05% ▪ *Ointment:* 0.05% ▪ *Solution:* 0.05%.

Flurandrenolide
▪ *Cream:* 0.025%, 0.05% ▪ *Ointment:* 0.025%, 0.05% ▪ *Lotion:* 0.05% ▪ *Tape:* 4 mcg/m².

Fluticasone
▪ *Cream:* 0.05% ▪ *Ointment:* 0.005%.

Halcinonide
▪ *Cream:* 0.025%, 0.1% ▪ *Ointment:* 0.1% ▪ *Solution:* 0.1%.

Halobetasol
▪ *Cream:* 0.05% ▪ *Cream:* 0.05%.

Hydrocortisone
▪ *Cream:* 0.5%, 1%, 2.5% ▪ *Gel:* 0.5%, 1% ▪ *Ointment:* 0.5%, 1% ▪ *Lotion:* 0.25%, 0.5%, 1%, 2%, 2.5% ▪ *Solution:* 1% ▪ *Spray:* 0.5%, 1%.

Mometasone
▪ *Cream:* 0.1% ▪ *Ointment:* 0.1% ▪ *Lotion:* 0.1%.

Prednicarbate
▪ *Cream:* 0.1%.

Triamcinolone
▪ *Cream:* 0.025%, 0.1%, 0.5% ▪ *Ointment:* 0.025, 0.1%, 0.5% ▪ *Lotion:* 0.025%, 0.1% ▪ *Spray:* 2 sec/spray ▪ *In combination with:* acetic acid, antifungals, anti-infectives, antihistamines, urea and benzoyl peroxide in various otic and topical preparations. See Appendix A.

TIME/ACTION PROFILE (response depends on condition being treated)

	ONSET	PEAK	DURATION
Topical	min–hr	hr–days	hr–days

NURSING IMPLICATIONS
ASSESSMENT
▫ Assess affected skin prior to and daily during therapy. Note degree of inflammation and pruritus. Notify physician if symptoms of infection (increased pain, erythema, purulent exudate) develop.
▪ **Lab Test Considerations:** Periodic adrenal function tests may be ordered to assess degree of hypothalamic-pituitary-adrenal (HPA) axis suppression in chronic topical therapy. Children and patients with dose applied to a large area or using an occlusive dressing are at highest risk for HPA suppression.

POTENTIAL NURSING DIAGNOSES

- Skin integrity, impairment (indications).
- Infection, high risk for (side effects).
- Knowledge deficit related to medication regimen (patient/family teaching).

IMPLEMENTATION

- **General Info:** Choice of vehicle depends on site and type of lesion. Ointments are more occlusive and preferred for dry scaly lesions. Creams should be used on oozing or intertriginous areas where the occlusive action of ointments might cause folliculitis or maceration. Creams may be preferred for esthetic reasons even though they may be more drying to skin than ointments. Gels, aerosols, lotions, and solutions are useful in hairy areas.
- **Topical:** Apply *ointments, creams,* or *gels* sparingly as a thin film to clean, slightly moist skin. Wear gloves. Apply occlusive dressing only if specified by physician.
- Apply *lotion, solution,* or *gel* to hair by parting hair and applying a small amount to affected area. Rub in gently. Protect area from washing, clothing, or rubbing until medication has dried. Hair may be washed as usual but not right after applying medication.
- Use *aerosols* by shaking well and spraying on affected area, holding container 3–6 in. away. Spray for about 2 sec to cover an area the size of a hand. Do not inhale. If spraying near face, cover eyes.

PATIENT/FAMILY TEACHING

- Instruct patient on correct technique of medication administration. Emphasize importance of avoiding the eyes. If a dose is missed, it should be applied as soon as remembered unless almost time for the next dose. Do not double doses.
- Caution patient to use only as directed. Avoid using cosmetics, bandages, dressings, or other skin products over the treated area unless directed by physician.
- Advise parents of pediatric patients not to apply tight fitting diapers or plastic pants on a child treated in the diaper area; these garments work like an occlusive dressing and may cause more of the drug to be absorbed into the child's body.
- Instruct patient to inform physician if symptoms of underlying disease return or worsen or if symptoms of infection develop.

EVALUATION

Effectiveness of therapy can be demonstrated by: ▪ Resolution of skin inflammation, pruritus, or other dermatologic conditions.

TOPICAL/MUCOSAL ANESTHETICS

benzocaine
(**ben**-zoe-kane)
Americaine, Americaine Anesthetic Lubricant, Americaine Hemorrhoidal, Anbesol Maximum Strength, Baby Anbesol, Baby Orajel, Baby Orajel Nighttime Formula, Benzocol, Benzodent, Children's Chloraseptic, Chloraseptic Cool Mint Flavor, {Dentocaine}, Hurricaine, Orabase-O, Orajel, Rid-a-Pain, {Sabex Teething Syrup}, Spec-T, T-Caine, Tyrobenz Maximum Strength Orajel

butamben
(byoo-**tam**-ben)
Butesin Picrate

dibucaine
(**dye**-byoo-kane)
Nupercainal

dyclonine
(**dye**-klon-een)
Children's Sucrets, Dyclone, Sucrets Maximum Strength, Sucrets Wild Cherry Regular Strength

lidocaine
(**lye**-doe-kane)
Xylocaine, Xylocaine Viscous

pramoxime
(pra-**mox**-een)
Fleet Relief, Prax, ProctoFoam/
nonsteroid, Tronolane, Tro-
nothane

tetracaine
(**tet**-ra-kane)
Pontocaine, {Supracaine}

**Pregnancy Category B (lido-
caine); C (dyclonine, tetracaine)**

INDICATIONS

▪ **Topical:** Relief of pruritus or pain
associated with minor skin disorders
including burns, abrasions, bruises, in-
sect stings/bites, dermatitis, hemorrhoids, or other forms of skin irritation
▪ *Mucosal:* Provides local anesthesia to
mucosal surfaces prior to instrumenta-
tion, minor procedures, or endoscopy.
Decreases irritation due to minor
mouth/throat conditions including sore
throat, gingivitis, stomatitis, or teething. Also used to suppress the gag reflex during endoscopy or intubation.

ACTION

▪ Inhibits initiation and conduction of
sensory nerve impulses. **Therapeutic
Effect:** ▪ Local anesthesia with subsequent loss of sensation or relief of pain
and/or pruritus.

PHARMACOKINETICS

Absorption: Benzocaine is poorly absorbed through intact skin. Other
agents may be readily absorbed. Degree
of absorption increases with surface
area; presence of lesions, cuts, or abrasions; and amount of agent applied.
Distribution: Distribution not known.
Metabolism and Excretion: Ester-type
(PABA derivatives, benzocaine, butamben, tetracaine) are metabolized by
plasma and liver cholinesterases. Small
amounts of amide-type agents (dibucaine and lidocaine) that may be absorbed are mostly metabolized by the
liver. Some metabolites of lidocaine are
active.
Half-life: UK.

CONTRAINDICATIONS AND
PRECAUTIONS

Contraindicated in: ▪ Hypersensitivity. Cross-sensitivity may occur among
related agents (amide types—dibucaine, lidocaine, ester types—benzocaine, butamben, tetracaine) ▪ Hypersensitivity to any components of
preparations including stabilizers, colorants, or bases ▪ Active, untreated infection of affected area ▪ Not to be used
in the eye ▪ Some products contain alcohol and should be avoided in patients
with known alcohol intolerance ▪ Topical benzocaine products should not be
used in children <2 yr.
Use Cautiously in: ▪ Large or severely
abraded areas of skin or mucous membrane ▪ Prolonged use (not recommended) ▪ Elderly or debilitated patients (increased risk of toxicity; use
smaller doses) ▪ Children (increased
risk of systemic toxicity, safety not established for some products, benzocaine may cause methemoglobinemia;
use smaller doses).

ADVERSE REACTIONS AND SIDE
EFFECTS*

Derm: *topical use*—contact dermatitis, urticaria, edema, burning stinging,
tenderness, irritation.
EENT: *mucosal use*—decreased or absent gag reflex.
Misc: allergic reactions, including
ANAPHYLAXIS.

INTERACTIONS

Drug–Drug: ▪ Toxicity of ester-type
agents may be increased by concurrent
use of **cholinesterase inhibitors** ▪ If
large amounts of lidocaine are absorbed, its metabolism may be de-

---

*Underlines indicate most frequent; CAPITALS indicate life-threatening.

creased by **beta-adrenergic blockers** or **cimetidine**.

ROUTE AND DOSAGE

Benzocaine

- **Topical/Mucosal (Adults and Children):** Apply cream, ointment, topical solutions, or dental/oral products as needed. Lozenges may be used hourly (not to exceed 12 lozenges/day). Rectal products may be used twice daily.

Butamben

- **Topical (Adults):** Apply as needed.

Dibucaine

- **Topical (Adults and Children):** Apply as needed (not to exceed 30 g/day in adults or 7.5 g as cream or 15 g as ointment/day in children). Rectal dosage forms may be used twice daily.

Dyclonine

- **Topical/Mucosal (Adults):** 2- or 3-mg lozenge may be dissolved in the mouth q 2 hr, or solution may be used 4 times daily. For anesthetizing mucosal surfaces, up to 200 mg in solution may be used.
- **Topical/Mucosal (Children >3 yr):** 1.2 mg lozenge may be dissolved in mouth q 2 hr.

Lidocaine

- **Topical (Adults):** Apply as needed (not to exceed 35 g/day as cream).
- **Mucosal (Adults):** For anesthetizing oral surfaces, 20 mg as 2 sprays/quadrant (not to exceed 30 mg/quadrant) may be used. 15 ml of the viscous solution may be used q 3 hr for oral or pharyngeal pain. For anesthetizing the female urethra, 3–5 ml of the jelly or 20 mg as 2% solution may be used. For anesthetizing the male urethra, 5–10 ml of the jelly or 5–15 ml of 2% solution may be used before catheterization or 30 ml of jelly prior to cystoscopy or similar procedures. Topical solutions may be used to anesthetize mucous membranes of the larynx, trachea, or esophagus.

Pramoxine

- **Topical/Mucosal (Adults):** Topical products may be used q 3 hr as needed. Rectal products may be used up to 5 times daily.

Tetracaine

- **Topical/Mucosal (Adults):** Apply cream as needed (not to exceed 28.35 g/day). Topical solutions may be used to anesthetize mucous membranes of the larynx, trachea, or esophagus.

AVAILABILITY

Benzocaine

- ***Cream:*** 5% ■ ***Ointment:*** 5%, 20% ■ ***Topical solution:*** 20% ■ ***Dental ointment:*** 20% ■ ***Dental paste:*** 20% ■ ***Jelly:*** 7.5%, 10%, 20% ■ ***Gel:*** 20% ■ ***Lozenges:*** 5 mg, 6 mg, 10 mg ■ ***Aerosol solution:*** 20% ■ ***Rectal ointment:*** 20% ■ ***In combination with:*** menthol (Dermoplast), butamben, and tetracaine (Cetacaine). See Appendix A.

Butamben

- ***Ointment:*** 1% ■ ***In combination with:*** benzocaine and tetracaine (Cetacaine).

Dibucaine

- ***Cream:*** 0.5% ■ ***Ointment:*** 1% ■ ***Rectal ointment:*** 1%.

Dyclonine

- ***Lozenges:*** 1.2 mg, 2 mg, 3 mg ■ ***Oral topical solution:*** 0.1% ■ ***Topical solution:*** 0.5%, 1%.

Lidocaine

- ***Topical aerosol:*** 10% ■ ***Oral topical solution (viscous lidocaine):*** 5% ■ ***Jelly:*** 2% ■ ***Ointment:*** 2.5%, 5%.

Pramoxine

- ***Cream:*** 1% ■ ***Rectal aerosol foam:*** 1% ■ ***Rectal cream:*** 1% ■ ***Rectal ointment:*** 1% ■ ***Rectal suppositories:*** 1% ■ ***In combination with:*** menthol (Pramagel). See Appendix A.

Tetracaine

- ***Cream:*** 1% ■ ***Topical solution:*** 2% ■ *{**Topical aerosol solution:*** 700 mcg/spray} butamben and tetracaine (Cetacaine) ■ ***In combination with:*** menthol (Pontocaine Ointment), butamben, and benzocaine (Cetacaine).

TIME/ACTION PROFILE (mucosal anesthetic effects)

	ONSET	PEAK	DURATION
benzocaine	about 1 min	UK	15–20 min
butamben	UK	UK	UK
dibucaine	within 15 min	UK	2–4 hr
dyclonine	up to 10 min	UK	60 min
lidocaine	within 2–5 min	UK	10–60 min*
pramoxine	3–5 min	UK	UK
tetracaine	3–10 min†	UK	30–60 min

*Depends on dosage form and site of application.
†Onset is slower following topical use.

NURSING IMPLICATIONS

ASSESSMENT

▢ Assess type, location, and intensity of pain prior to and a few minutes after administration of anesthetic.

▢ Assess integrity of involved skin and mucous membranes prior to and periodically throughout course of therapy. Notify physician if signs of infection or irritation develop.

POTENTIAL NURSING DIAGNOSES

■ Pain (indications).

■ Knowledge deficit related to medication regimen (patient/family teaching).

IMPLEMENTATION

■ **Topical:** Alcohol-free preparation is available for teething pain in babies. Apply to gums by rubbing gel on with fingers or cotton swab.

■ **Throat Spray:** Ensure that gag reflex is intact before allowing patient to drink or eat.

PATIENT/FAMILY TEACHING

■ **General Info:** Instruct patient on correct application technique. Emphasize need to avoid contact with eyes.

▢ Advise patient to discontinue use if erythema, rash, or irritation at site of administration occurs.

▢ Advise adults using liquid form around the mouth to avoid smoking until solution is dry.

■ **Teething Gel:** Instruct patients to notify pediatrician if pain is excessive or prolonged. Advise parents to avoid feeding immediately after application to prevent choking from diminished gag reflex.

■ **Lozenge:** Instruct patient to suck on lozenge and allow it to slowly dissolve. Consult physician if throat pain persists more than 2 days. Avoid use in young children because of danger of choking.

EVALUATION

Effectiveness of therapy can be demonstrated by: ■ Temporary relief of discomfort associated with minor irritations of skin or mucous membranes ■ Temporary local anesthesia of mucosal surfaces.

TOPICAL/NASAL DECONGESTANTS

desoxyephedrine
(des-oxy-e-**fed**-rin)
Vicks Inhaler

ephedrine
(e-**fed**-rin)
Kondon's Nasal Jelly, Pretz-D, Vicks Vatronol

epinephrine
(ep-i-**neff**-rin)
Adrenalin

naphazoline
(naff-a-**zoe**-leen)
Privine

oxymetazoline
(ox-i-met-**az**-oh-leen)
Afrin, Allerest 12 Hour Nasal, Chlorphed-LA, Dristan Long Acting, Duramist Plus, 4-Way Long Lasting Nasal, Genasal, Nasal Relief, Neo-Synephrine 12 Hour, Nostrilla, NTZ Long Acting Nasal, 12 Hour Sinarest, Sinex Long-Acting, Twice-A-Day

phenylephrine
(fen-ill-**eff**-rin)
Alconefrin 12, Children's Nostril, Neo-Synephrine, Sinex

propylhexadrine
(proe-pil-**hex**-a-dreen)
Benzedrex Inhaler

tetrahydrozoline
(tet-ra-hye-**dro**-zoe-leen)
Tyzine

xylometazoline
(zye-loe-met-**a**-zoe-leen)
Otrivin

Pregnancy Category C (tetrahydrozoline)

INDICATIONS

- Relief of nasal congestion that may accompany colds, allergies, or sinusitis
- Adjunctive therapy of otitis media.

ACTION

- Stimulate alpha-adrenergic receptors in vascular smooth muscle resulting in local vasoconstriction. This effect shrinks swollen mucous membranes and increases drainage. **Therapeutic Effect:** - Decreased nasal congestion.

PHARMACOKINETICS

Absorption: Although systemic absorption is minimal, repeated use of large doses may lead to systemic side effects.
Distribution: Action is primarily local. Remainder of distribution is not known.
Metabolism and Excretion: Epinephrine is taken up by adrenergic nerve endings and metabolized by enzymes (catechol-O-methyl transferase and monoamine oxidase) in the liver and other tissues. Phenylephrine is metabolized in the liver and intestine by monoamine oxidase. Propylhexadrine is metabolized by the liver.
Half-life: Ephedrine—3–6 hr (depending on urine pH).

CONTRAINDICATIONS AND PRECAUTIONS

Contraindicated in: - Hypersensitivity or known intolerance to active ingredients, additives, solutions, or preservatives (may contain bisulfites, thimerosal, aromatics, or chlorobutanol).
Use Cautiously in: - Patients with cardiovascular disease, hypertension, diabetes mellitus, or hyperthyroidism.

ADVERSE REACTIONS AND SIDE EFFECTS*

CNS: headache, lightheadedness, nervousness, insomnia.
EENT: rebound nasal congestion, nasal burning, stinging or dryness, sneezing.
CV: tachycardia.
Neuro: trembling.

INTERACTIONS

Drug–Drug: - Epinephrine may decrease the effectiveness of **insulin** or **oral hypoglycemic agents** - Concurrent use of epinephrine with **beta blockers** may result in initial hypertension followed by bradycardia - Increased risk of arrhythmias with **theophylline** - Therapeutic effects may be decreased by **agents that acidify the urine**, while toxicity may be increased by **agents that alkalinize urine** - Vasopressor effects of epinephrine may be increased by **guanethidine, reserpine,** or **tricyclic antidepressants,** while pressor effects of ephedrine are decreased - May decrease the effectiveness of **guanethidine** - Effectiveness may be decreased by concurrent **phenothiazines** - Severe reactions (hypertension, hyperpyrexia, headache) may occur when ephedrine is used with **monoamine oxidase inhibitors** - Vasopressor response may be increased by **methyldopa** - **Furazolidone** may increase the vasopressor effects of ephedrine.

ROUTE AND DOSAGE

Desoxyephedrine
- **Nasal Inhalation (Adults and Children ≥6 yr):** 1–2 inhalations in each nostril no more frequently than q 2 hr (not to be used for >7 days).

Ephedrine
- **Intranasal (Adults):** *Drops*—Fill product dropper to upper level. Apply in each nostril not more frequently than q 4 hr.

T

- **Intranasal (Children 6–12 yr):** *Drops*—Fill product dropper to lower level. Apply in each nostril not more frequently than q 4 hr.

Epinephrine
- **Intranasal (Adults and Children ≥6 yr):** Apply with swab or as drops or spray as needed.

Naphazoline
- **Intranasal (Adults and Children ≥12 yr):** 1–2 drops/sprays not more frequently than q 6 hr.

Oxymetazoline
- **Intranasal (Adults and Children ≥6 yr):** 2–3 drops/sprays (0.05% solution) twice daily or q 12 hr.
- **Intranasal (Children 2–5 yr):** 2–3 drops (0.025% solution) in each nostril twice daily, morning and evening.

Phenylephrine
- **Intranasal (Adults and Children ≥12 yr):** 2–3 drops/sprays of 0.25–0.5% solution in each nostril no more frequently than q 3–4 hr or 2–3 drops/sprays of 1% solution in each nostril no more frequently than q 4 hr.
- **Intranasal (Children 6–11 yr):** 2–3 drops/sprays of 0.25% solution in each nostril q 3–4 hr.
- **Intranasal (Infants >6 mo):** 1–2 drops of 0.16% solution in each nostril q 3 hr.

Propylhexadrine
- **Intranasal (Adults and Children ≥6 yr):** 1–2 inhalations in each nostril no more frequently than q 2 hr (not to be used for >3 days).

Tetrahydrozoline
- **Intranasal (Adults and Children ≥6 yr):** 2–4 drops of 0.1% solution q 3–4 hr as needed or 3–4 sprays in each nostril q 4 hr as needed.
- **Intranasal (Children 2–6 yr):** 2–3 drops of 0.05% solution in each nostril q 4–6 hr as needed.

Xylometazoline
- **Intranasal (Adults and Children ≥12 yr):** 2–3 drops/sprays of 0.1% solution in each nostril q 8–10 hr.
- **Intranasal (Children 2–12 yr):** 2–3 drops of 0.05% solution in each nostril q 8–10 hr.

AVAILABILITY

Desoxyephedrine
- **Nasal inhaler:** 50 mg/inhaler.

Ephedrine
- **Nasal spray:** 0.25% **Nasal drops:** 0.5% **Nasal jelly:** 1%.

Epinephrine
- **Nasal solution:** 0.1%.

Naphazoline
- **Nasal solution:** 0.05%.

Oxymetazoline
- **Nasal solution:** 0.025%, 0.05%.

Phenylephrine
- **Nasal solution:** 0.125%, 0.16%, 0.25%, 0.5%, 1%.

Propylhexadrine
- **Nasal inhaler:** 250 mg/inhaler.

Tetrahydrozoline
- **Nasal solution:** 0.05%, 0.1%.

Xylometazoline
- **Nasal drops:** 0.05%, 0.1% **Nasal spray:** 0.1%.

TIME/ACTION PROFILE (local vasoconstriction)

	ONSET	PEAK	DURATION
desoxy-ephedrine	UK	UK	UK
ephedrine	UK	UK	6 hr
epineph-rine	within 5 min	UK	UK
naphazo-line	within 10 min	UK	2–6 hr
oxymetazo-line	within 5–10 min	UK	5–12 hr
phenyleph-rine	rapid	UK	30 min–4 hr
propylhexa-drine	within 0.5–5 min	UK	0.5–2 hr
tetrahydro-zoline	within min	UK	4–8 hr
xylometazo-line	within 5–10 min	UK	5–6 hr

NURSING IMPLICATIONS

ASSESSMENT
- **General Info:** Monitor patient for signs of systemic side effects (in-

creased pulse, blood pressure, and blood sugar in diabetic patients). Notify physician if these symptoms occur.

- **Rhinitis:** Assess severity of nasal congestion prior to and periodically throughout course of therapy.

POTENTIAL NURSING DIAGNOSES

- Airway clearance, ineffective (indications).
- Knowledge deficit related to medication regimen (patient/family teaching).

IMPLEMENTATION

- **Nasal Solution:** Squeeze bulb until dropper contains correct amount of medication. Tilt head back and place 2 drops of solution into 1 nostril. Tilt head forward and turn head to the opposite side and inhale through the nostril. Repeat the process with the other side.
- **Nasal Spray:** Keep head upright and squeeze bottle prescribed number of times briskly while sniffing through nostril.
- **Nasal Inhalers:** Warm inhaler in the hand before use. Wipe the inhaler after each use.

PATIENT/FAMILY TEACHING

- **General Info:** Instruct patient to avoid known allergens.
- **Nasal:** Emphasize need to take only as directed. Rebound congestion may occur if used too frequently or for prolonged duration (longer than 3–5 days).
- Instruct patient not to share the container with other patients. Do not allow the tip of the container to touch the nasal passage. Discard medication when no longer required.
- Advise patient that a mild transient stinging sensation may occur following application, but it often disappears after a few applications.
- Instruct patient to contact physician if no improvement is seen within 7 days, if symptoms are accompanied by a high fever, or if condition worsens. Also, notify physician if insom-

nia, weakness, dizziness, tremor, or irregular heartbeat occurs.

EVALUATION
Effectiveness of therapy can be demonstrated by: - Decrease in nasal congestion.

TRACE METAL ADDITIVE
Concentrated Multiple Trace Element, ConTE-PAK-4, M.T.E.-4, M.T.E.-4 Concentrated, M.T.E.-5, M.T.E.-5 Concentrated, M.T.E.-6, M.T.E.-6 Concentrated, M.T.E.-7, MulTE-PAK-4, MulTE-PAK-5, Multiple Trace Element, Multiple Trace Element Neonatal, Multiple Trace Element Pediatric, Neotrace 4, PedTE-PAK-4, Pedtrace-4, P.T.E.-4, P.T.E.-5

CLASSIFICATION(S):
Nutritional supplement
Pregnancy Category C

T

INDICATIONS

- Administered as a component in total parenteral nutrition (TPN, parenteral hyperalimentation) - May contain any or all of the following: □ Chromium □ Copper □ Iodine □ Manganese □ Molybdenum □ Selenium □ Zinc.

ACTION

- Trace metals serve as cofactors or catalysts for numerous diverse homeostatic processes. **Therapeutic Effect:** - Replacement in deficiency states when oral ingestion is not feasible.

PHARMACOKINETICS

Absorption: Administered IV only, resulting in complete bioavailability.
Distribution: Widely distributed.
Metabolism and Excretion: Excretion depends on individual trace element.
Half-life: UK.

CONTRAINDICATIONS AND PRECAUTIONS

Contraindicated in: - Hypersensitivity

to iodine (iodine-containing products only).

Use Cautiously in: ▪ Pregnancy or lactation ▪ Nasogastric suction, fistula drainage, prolonged vomiting or diarrhea (may increase requirements) ▪ Renal impairment or biliary obstruction (may increase risk of toxicity) ▪ Isolated trace element deficiency (other additives may be excessive—use only those required).

ADVERSE REACTIONS AND SIDE EFFECTS*

Listed for individual trace metals— usually associated with toxicity.
Chromium: nausea, vomiting, GI ulceration, renal damage, hepatic damage, SEIZURES, COMA.
Copper: behavioral changes, weakness, diarrhea, photophobia, peripheral edema, progressive marasmus.
Iodine: metallic taste, sore mouth, increased salivation, runny nose, sneezing, headache, swelling of eyelids, parotitis, acneform skin lesions.
Manganese: irritability, speech difficulties, gait disturbances, headache, anorexia, impotence, apathy.
Molybdenum: gout-like syndrome.
Selenium: hair loss, weak nails, mental depression, nervousness, vomiting, garlic-like breath, garlic-like sweat, metallic taste, GI discomfort.
Zinc: toxicitiy poorly defined but may include hypothermia, blurred vision, loss of consciousness, tachycardia, pulmonary edema, jaundice, oliguria, hypotension, vomiting.

INTERACTIONS

Drug–Drug: ▪ None significant in replacement doses.

ROUTE AND DOSAGE

▪ **IV (Adults and Children):** Amount necessary to maintain normal trace element levels.

AVAILABILITY

All must be diluted in large-volume parenterals prior to use ▪ *Injection:* Each ml contains 0.85–4 mcg chromium, 0.1–0.4 mg copper, 0.025–0.16 manganese, and 0.5–1.5 mg zinc. Some products also contain iodide, selenium, and molybdenum. ▪ *Concentrated injection:* Each ml contains 10 mcg chromium, 1 mg copper, 0.5 mg manganese, and 5 mg zinc. Some products also contain iodide and selenium.

TIME/ACTION PROFILE (replacement)

	ONSET	PEAK	DURATION
IV	rapid	UK	UK

NURSING IMPLICATIONS

ASSESSMENT

▫ Assess nutritional status by 24-hr recall prior to therapy.
▫ Monitor patient for signs and symptoms of trace metal deficiencies prior to and throughout therapy, as follows:
▫ *Chromium:* glucose intolerance, ataxia, peripheral neuropathy, confusion.
▫ *Copper:* leukopenia, neutropenia, anemia, iron deficiency, skeletal abnormalities, defective tissue formation.
▫ *Iodine:* impaired thyroid function, goiter, cretinism.
▫ *Manganese:* nausea, vomiting, weight loss, dermatitis, changes in hair.
▫ *Molybdenum:* tachycardia, tachypnea, headache, night blindness, nausea, vomiting, edema, lethargy, disorientation, coma, hypouricemia, hypouricosuria.
▫ *Selenium:* cardiomyopathy, muscle pain, kwashiorkor, Kershan disease.
▫ *Zinc:* diarrhea, apathy, depression, anorexia, hypogonadism, growth retardation, anemia, hepatosplenomegaly, impaired wound healing, decreased sense of taste and smell.
▪ **Lab Test Considerations:** Serum trace metal concentrations should be monitored periodically throughout TPN therapy.

*Underlines indicate most frequent; CAPITALS indicate life-threatening.

POTENTIAL NURSING DIAGNOSES

- Nutrition, altered: less than body requirements (indications).
- Knowledge deficit related to medication regimen (patient/family teaching).

IMPLEMENTATION

- **IV:** Solution usually does not contain preservatives; discard unused portion.
- **Continuous Infusion:** Must be diluted prior to administration. Dilute each dose in at least 1 liter of IV solution.
  □ Administer at prescribed rate for TPN infusion.
- **Additive Compatibility:** Usually compatible with other trace metals, electrolytes, and dextrose/amino acid combinations used for TPN.

PATIENT/FAMILY TEACHING

□ Explain purpose of infusion of TPN and components to patient.

EVALUATION

Effectiveness of therapy can be demonstrated by: ▪ Prevention or treatment of trace metal deficiencies.

TRAZADONE
(**traz**-oh-done)
Desyrel, Trazon, Trialodine

CLASSIFICATION(S):
Antidepressant (miscellaneous)
Pregnancy Category C

INDICATIONS

▪ Treatment of major depression often in conjunction with psychotherapy. **Unlabeled Use:** ▪ Management of chronic pain syndromes, including diabetic neuropathy.

ACTION

▪ Alters the effects of serotonin in the CNS. **Therapeutic Effect:** ▪ Antidepressant action, which may develop only over several weeks.

PHARMACOKINETICS

Absorption: Well absorbed following oral administration.
Distribution: Widely distributed.
Metabolism and Excretion: Extensively metabolized by the liver. Minimal excretion of unchanged drug by the kidneys.
Half-life: 5–9 hr.

CONTRAINDICATIONS AND PRECAUTIONS

Contraindicated in: ▪ Hypersensitivity ▪ Recovery period following myocardial infarction ▪ Concurrent electroconvulsive therapy.
Use Cautiously in: ▪ Cardiovascular disease ▪ Suicidal behavior ▪ Pregnancy, lactation, or children (safety not established) ▪ Severe hepatic or renal disease (dosage reduction recommended) ▪ Elderly patients (initial dosage reduction recommended).

ADVERSE REACTIONS AND SIDE EFFECTS*

CNS: <u>drowsiness</u>, dizziness, lightheadedness, fatigue, weakness, insomnia, confusion, hallucinations, slurred speech, nightmares, syncope, headache.
EENT: blurred vision, tinnitus.
CV: <u>hypotension</u>, chest pain, tachycardia, arrhythmias, palpitations, hypertension.
GI: <u>dry mouth</u>, constipation, nausea, vomiting, bad taste, flatulence, diarrhea, excess salivation.
GU: urinary frequency, impotence, priapism, hematuria.
Derm: rashes.
Hemat: anemia, leukopenia.
MS: myalgia.
Neuro: tremor.

INTERACTIONS

Drug–Drug: ▪ May increase **digoxin** or **phenytoin** serum levels ▪ Additive CNS depression with other **CNS depressants** including **alcohol, antihistamines, opioid analgesics,** and **sedative/hypnotics** ▪ Additive hypotension with **antihyper-**

*<u>Underlines</u> indicate most frequent; **CAPITALS** indicate life-threatening.

tensive agents, acute ingestion of **alcohol,** or **nitrates.**

ROUTE AND DOSAGE

- **PO (Adults):** 150 mg/day in 3 divided doses, increase by 50 mg/day q 3–4 days until desired response (not to exceed 400 mg/day in outpatients or 600 mg/day in hospitalized patients).
- **PO (Children 6–18 yr):** 1.5–2 mg/kg/day in divided doses. May be increased q 3–4 days up to 6 mg/kg/day.
- **PO (Elderly Patients):** 75 mg/day in divided doses initially.

AVAILABILITY

- ***Tablets:*** 50 mg, 100 mg, 150 mg, 300 mg.

TIME/ACTION PROFILE
(antidepressant effect)

	ONSET	PEAK	DURATION
PO	1–2 wk	2–4 wk	wks

NURSING IMPLICATIONS

ASSESSMENT

- Assess mental status and mood changes frequently. Assess for suicidal tendencies, especially during early therapy. Restrict amount of drug available to patient.
- Monitor blood pressure and pulse rate prior to and during initial therapy. Patients with pre-existing cardiac disease should have ECGs monitored prior to and periodically during therapy to detect arrhythmias.
- **Lab Test Considerations:** Assess CBC and renal and hepatic function prior to and periodically during therapy. Slight, clinically insignificant decrease in leukocyte and neutrophil counts may occur.

POTENTIAL NURSING DIAGNOSES

- Coping, ineffective individual (indications).
- Knowledge deficit related to medication regimen (patient/family teaching).

IMPLEMENTATION

- **PO:** Administer with or immediately

after meals to minimize side effects (nausea, dizziness) and allow maximum absorption of trazadone. A larger portion of the total daily dose may be given at bedtime to decrease daytime drowsiness and dizziness.

PATIENT/FAMILY TEACHING

- Instruct patient to take medication exactly as directed. If a dose is missed, take as soon as remembered, not taking if within 4 hr of next scheduled dose; do not double doses. Consult physician prior to discontinuing medication; gradual dosage reduction is necessary to prevent aggravation of condition.
- Trazadone may cause drowsiness and blurred vision. Caution patient to avoid driving and other activities requiring alertness until response to drug is known.
- Caution patient to make position changes slowly to minimize orthostatic hypotension.
- Advise patient to avoid concurrent use of alcohol or other CNS depressant drugs.
- Inform patient that frequent rinses, good oral hygiene, and sugarless candy or gum may diminish dry mouth. Physician or dentist should be notified if this persists >2 wk. An increase in fluid intake, fiber, and exercise may prevent constipation.
- Advise patient to notify physician or dentist of medication regimen prior to treatment or surgery.
- Instruct patient to notify physician if priapism, irregular heartbeat, fainting, confusion, skin rash, or tremors occur. If dry mouth, nausea and vomiting, dizziness, headache, muscle aches, constipation, or diarrhea becomes pronounced, physician should be notified.
- Emphasize the importance of follow-up examinations to evaluate progress.

EVALUATION

Effectiveness of therapy can be demonstrated by: ■ Resolution of depression □ Increased sense of well-being □ Renewed interest in surroundings □ Increased appetite □ Improved energy level □ Improved sleep ■ Decrease in severity of pain in chronic pain syndromes. Therapeutic effects are usually seen within 1 wk, although 4 wk may be required to obtain significant therapeutic results.

TRETINOIN
(tret-i-noyn)
Retin-A, {Stieva-A}, vitamin A acid

CLASSIFICATION(S):
Antiacne agent
Pregnancy Category C

INDICATIONS
■ Management of acne vulgaris.

ACTION
■ Decreases the formation of microcomedomes and stimulates turnover of follicular epithelium. **Therapeutic Effects:** Decreases acne formation with improved skin appearance.

PHARMACOKINETICS
Absorption: Small amount of systemic absorption occurs with limited surface area application.
Distribution: UK.
Metabolism and Excretion: >5% of dose applied to skin is excreted in urine.
Half-life: UK.

CONTRAINDICATIONS AND PRECAUTIONS
Contraindicated in: ■ Hypersensitivity to tretinoin or any components in the formulation ■ Known alcohol intolerance (gel and liquid only).
Use Cautiously in: ■ Areas around the mouth, eyes, angles of the nose, or other mucous membranes ■ Pregnancy, lactation, or children (safe use not established).

ADVERSE REACTIONS AND SIDE EFFECTS*
Derm: photosensitivity, redness, blistering, edema, crusting, hyperpigmentation, hypopigmentation.

INTERACTIONS
Drug–Drug: ■ Concurrent use with **keratolytic agents** (benzoyl peroxide, salicylic acid, sulfur, or resorcinol) increases the risk of excessive skin irritation ■ Increased risk of photosensitivity with other **photosensitizing agents** ■ Risk of irritation may be increased by other **topical skin-care products** (aftershave, cover-up, make-up, perfumes, colognes) ■ Increases absorption of **topical minoxidil**

ROUTE AND DOSAGE
■ **Topical (Adults and Adolescents):** Apply once daily at bedtime.

AVAILABILITY
■ *Cream:* 0.05%, 0.01% ■ *Gel:* 0.025%, 0.01% ■ *Liquid:* 0.05%.

TIME/ACTION PROFILE (improved skin appearance)

	ONSET	PEAK	DURATION
topical	2–3 wk	6 wk	UK

NURSING IMPLICATIONS

ASSESSMENT
□ Assess skin prior to and periodically during therapy. Note number and severity of cysts, degree of skin dryness, erythema, and itching. Response to frequency of application and dosage concentration is variable and should be closely monitored. Transient worsening of acne may occur at initiation of therapy. This may be due to the effects of tretinoin on deep, previously undetected lesions and is not a reason to discontinue therapy.

POTENTIAL NURSING DIAGNOSES
■ Skin integrity, impaired (indications, side effects).

T

{} = Available in Canada only.
*<u>Underlines</u> indicate most frequent; **CAPITALS** indicate life-threatening.

- Body image disturbance (indications).
- Knowledge deficit related to medication regimen (patient/family teaching).

IMPLEMENTATION

- **Topical:** Tretinoin should be applied once a day before bedtime. Cover the entire area lightly. Wash hands immediately after application.
- **Liquid:** Apply with fingertip, gauze pad, or cotton swab. Do not saturate gauze pad or cotton swab to the extent that medication runs on to unaffected area.
- **Gel:** Excessive application results in "pilling" of gel, which minimizes overapplication of tretinoin.
- May induce severe local edema and peeling at the site of application. If this occurs, tretinoin may be used less frequently, or discontinued temporarily or completely.

PATIENT/FAMILY TEACHING

- Instruct patient to take or apply tretinoin exactly as directed. Application may cause a transient feeling of warmth and a slight stinging. Avoid application near eyes, mouth, angle of the nose, and mucous membranes. Do not apply excessive amounts, as this may cause redness, peeling, or discomfort and will not improve results.
- Explain to patient that a temporary worsening of acne may occur at beginning of therapy.
- Advise patient to consult with physician before using other acne preparations while using tretinoin. Normal use of cosmetics is permissible, but area to be treated must be thoroughly cleansed prior to application. Medicated or abrasive soaps or cleansers, soaps and cosmetics that have a strong drying effect, and products that have a high concentration of alcohol, astringents, spices, or lime also may worsen dry skin.
- Caution patient to use sunscreens and protective clothing to prevent photosensitivity reactions. Physician should be consulted about sunscreen, as some sunscreens may worsen acne. Patients should be taught to minimize exposure to sunlight and sunlamps, and if sunburned to cease tretinoin treatment until fully recovered. Other weather extremes (wind, cold) also may be irritating to skin.

EVALUATION

Effectiveness of therapy can be demonstrated by: ▪ Decrease in the number and severity of cysts in severe acne. Therapeutic results are usually seen in 2–3 wk but may require 6 wk for optimal results. Once results are satisfactory, maintain therapy with less frequent applications or other dosage forms.

TRIAMCINOLONE
(trye-am-**sin**-oh-lone)
Azmacort, Aristocort, Aristospan, Articulose L.A., Cenocort A, Cinonide, Kenac, Kenacort, Kenaject, Kenalog, Kenonel, Nasacort, Tac-3, Tramacort, Triaderm, Triam-A, Triam-Forte, Triamolone, Triamonide, Tri-Kort, Trilog, Trilone, Tristoject

CLASSIFICATION(S):
Glucocorticoid (intermediate-acting), Anti-inflammatory agent

Pregnancy Category UK

INDICATIONS

▪ Used systemically and locally in a wide variety of □ Chronic inflammatory diseases □ Allergic diseases □ Hematologic diseases □ Neoplastic diseases □ Autoimmune diseases ▪ Not suitable for alternate-day therapy.

ACTION

▪ Suppresses inflammation and the normal immune response ▪ Has numerous intense metabolic effects ▪ Suppresses adrenal function at chronic doses of 4 mg/day ▪ Practically devoid of mineralocorticoid (sodium-retaining) activity. **Therapeutic Effects:** ▪ Suppression of inflammation ▪ Modification of the normal immune response.

PHARMACOKINETICS

Absorption: Well absorbed following oral and IM administration. IM acetonide and diacetate salts are long-acting.
Distribution: Widely distributed. Crosses the placenta and probably enters breast milk.
Metabolism and Excretion: Mostly metabolized by the liver and other tissues. Small amounts excreted unchanged by the kidneys.
Half-life: 200 + min; adrenal suppression lasts 2.25 days.

CONTRAINDICATIONS AND PRECAUTIONS

Contraindicated in: ▪ Active untreated infections ▪ Lactation (avoid chronic use) ▪ Known alcohol intolerance (inhaler and some topical products).
Use Cautiously in: ▪ Chronic treatment (will lead to adrenal suppression) ▪ Stress (surgery, infection—supplemental doses required) ▪ Chronic use in children (will result in decreased growth) ▪ May mask signs of infections (fever, inflammation) ▪ Children <12 yr (intranasal—safety not established).

ADVERSE REACTIONS AND SIDE EFFECTS*

CNS: headache, restlessness, psychoses, fatigue, depression, euphoria, personality changes; increased intracranial pressure (children only).
EENT: cataracts, increased intraocular pressure; Intranasal—nasal irritation, dry mucous membranes, nasosinus congestion, throat discomfort, sneezing, epistaxis.
CV: hypertension.
GI: nausea, vomiting, anorexia, PEPTIC ULCERATION.
Endo: adrenal suppression, hyperglycemia.
Derm: decreased wound healing, petechiae, ecchymoses, fragility, hirsutism, acne.
F and E: hypokalemia, hypokalemic alkalosis, fluid retention (long-term high doses).
Hemat: thromboembolism, thrombophlebitis.
Metab: weight loss, weight gain.
MS: muscle wasting, muscle pain, aseptic necrosis of joints, osteoporosis.
Misc: increased susceptibility to infection, cushingoid appearance (moon face, buffalo hump).

INTERACTIONS

Drug–Drug: ▪ Additive hypokalemia with **diuretics, amphotericin B, azlocillin, carbenicillin, mezlocillin, piperacillin,** or **ticarcillin** ▪ Hypokalemia may increase the risk of **cardiac glycoside** toxicity ▪ May increase requirement for **insulin** or **hypoglycemic agents** ▪ Increased risk of adverse GI effects with **nonsteroidal anti-inflammatory agents, alcohol,** or **aspirin.**

ROUTE AND DOSAGE

Adrenocortical Insufficiency
▪ **PO (Adults):** 4–12 mg/day as a single dose or 2–4 divided doses.
▪ **PO (Children):** 117 mcg/kg/day (3.3 mg/m²/day) as a single dose or divided dose.

Other Uses
▪ **PO (Adults):** 4–48 mg/day as a single dose or 2–4 divided doses (up to 60 mg/day).
▪ **PO (Children):** 416 mcg–1.7 mg/kg/day (12.5–50 mg/m²/day) as a single dose or divided doses.
▪ **IM (Adults):** 40–80 mg q 4 wk as acetonide suspension or 40 mg weekly as diacetate suspension.
▪ **IM (Children):** 40 mg q 4 wk or 30–200 mcg/kg (1–6.25 mg/m²) given q 1–7 days as acetonide suspension or 40 mg weekly as diacetate suspension.
▪ **Intra-articular (Adults):** 2.5–15 mg as acetonide suspension or 3–48 mg q 1–8 wk as diacetate suspension or 2–20 mg q 3–4 wk as hexacetonide suspension.
▪ **Intralesional (Adults):** 1 mg q 7 days or longer as acetonide suspension or 3–48 mg q 1–8 wk as diacetate sus-

T

*Underlines indicate most frequent; **CAPITALS** indicate life-threatening.

pension *or* 0.5 mg/square in. of affected skin as the hexacetonide suspension.

- **Inhalation (Adults):** 2 sprays 3–4 times daily (up to 12–16 sprays/day).
- **Inhalation (Children 6–12 yr):** 1–2 sprays 3–4 times daily (not to exceed 12 sprays/day).
- **Nasal Inhalation (Adults):** 2 sprays in each nostril once daily (up to 2 sprays in each nostril twice daily or 1 spray in each nostril 4 times daily).

AVAILABILITY

- *Tablets:* 1 mg, 2 mg, 4 mg, 8 mg, 16 mg • *Oral syrup:* 2 mg/5 ml, 4.85 mg/5 ml • *Suspension for injection (acetonide):* 3 mg/ml, 10 mg/ml, 40 mg/ml • *Suspension for injection (diacetate):* 25 mg/ml, 40 mg/ml • *Suspension for injection (hexacetonide):* 5 mg/ml, 20 mg/ml • *Inhalation:* 100 mcg/spray in a 20-g canister (240 sprays) • *Intranasal inhalation:* 55 mcg/spray in 15-mg canister (100 sprays/canister).

TIME/ACTION PROFILE (anti-inflammatory activity)

	ONSET	PEAK	DURATION
PO	UK	1–2 hr	2.25 days
IM— acetonide	24–48 hr	UK	1–6 wk
IM— diacetate	slow	UK	4 days–4 wk
IA— acetonide	UK	UK	several wk
IA— diacetate	UK	UK	1–8 wk
IA— hexacetonide	UK	UK	3–4 wk
Inhalation	1–2 wk	UK	UK
Intranasal	hrs–days	2–3 wk	UK

NURSING IMPLICATIONS

ASSESSMENT

- ☐ This drug is indicated for many conditions. Assess involved systems prior to and periodically throughout course of therapy.
- ☐ Assess patient for signs of adrenal insufficiency (hypotension, weight loss, weakness, nausea, vomiting, anorexia, lethargy, confusion, restlessness) prior to and periodically throughout course of therapy.
- ☐ Monitor intake and output ratios and daily weights. Observe patient for the appearance of peripheral edema, steady weight gain, rales/crackles, or dyspnea. Notify physician should these occur.
- ☐ Children should have periodic evaluations of growth.
- **Lab Test Considerations:** Patients on prolonged courses of therapy should routinely have hematologic values, serum electrolytes, serum, and urine glucose evaluated. May cause decreased WBC counts. May cause hyperglycemia, especially in persons with diabetes. May decrease serum potassium and calcium and increase serum sodium concentrations.
- ☐ Promptly report presence of guaiac-positive stools.
- ☐ May suppress reactions to allergy skin tests.
- ☐ Periodic adrenal function tests may be ordered to assess degree of hypothalamic-pituitary-adrenal axis suppression.

POTENTIAL NURSING DIAGNOSES

- Infection, high risk for (side effects).
- Knowledge deficit related to medication regimen (patient/family teaching).
- Body image disturbance (side effects).

IMPLEMENTATION

- **General Info:** Administer daily dose in the morning to coincide with the body's normal secretion of cortisol.
- **PO:** Administer with meals to minimize gastric irritation. Tablets may be crushed and administered with food or fluids for patients with difficulty swallowing. Use calibrated measuring device to ensure accurate dosage of liquid forms.
- **IM:** Shake suspension well before drawing up. Administer IM deep into well-developed muscle. Do not administer triamcinolone IV.
- **Top:** Wear gloves when applying topical medications.

- **Nasal Spray:** Patients also using topical decongestant should be given decongestant 5–15 min before triamcinolone. Instruct patient to blow nose gently if unable to breathe freely through nasal passages before medication administration.

PATIENT/FAMILY TEACHING
- **General Info:** Instruct patient to take medication exactly as directed, not to skip or double up on missed doses. Stopping the medication suddenly may result in adrenal insufficiency (anorexia, nausea, fatigue, weakness, hypotension, dyspnea, and hypoglycemia). If these signs appear notify physician immediately. This can be life-threatening.
- Encourage patients on long-term therapy to eat a diet high in protein, calcium, and potassium and low in sodium and carbohydrates (see Appendix K for foods included).
- This drug causes immunosuppression and may mask symptoms of infection. Instruct patient to avoid people with known contagious illnesses and to report possible infections immediately.
- Review side effects with patient. Instruct patient to inform physician promptly if severe abdominal pain or tarry stools occur. Patient should also report unusual swelling, weight gain, tiredness, bone pain, bruising, nonhealing sores, visual disturbances, or behavior changes.
- Instruct patient to inform physician if symptoms of underlying disease return or worsen.
- Discuss possible effects on body image. Explore coping mechanisms.
- Advise patient to carry identification in the event of an emergency in which patient cannot relate medical history.
- Caution patient to avoid vaccinations without consulting physician.
- Explain need for continued medical follow-up to assess effectiveness and possible side effects of medication. Physician may order periodic lab tests and eye examinations.

- **Top:** Instruct patient on correct technique of administration. Apply topical preparations to skin that is clean and slightly moist. Use occlusive dressing only if ordered by physician; may enhance absorption of medication. Apply with cotton-tipped applicator. Avoid contact with eyes.
- **Inhalation:** Instruct patient in the use of metered-dose inhaler (see Appendix H).
- **Nasal Spray:** Instruct patient in correct technique for administering nasal spray (see Appendix H). Warn patient that temporary nasal stinging may occur.
- Instruct patient to notify physician if symptoms do not improve within 1 mo or if nasal discharge becomes purulent.

EVALUATION
Effectiveness of therapy can be demonstrated by: - Suppression of the inflammatory and immune responses in autoimmune disorders, allergic reactions, and neoplasms.

TRIAMTERENE
(trye-**am**-ter-een)
Dyrenium

CLASSIFICATION(S):
Diuretic (potassium-sparing)
Pregnancy Category C

INDICATIONS
- Most commonly used to counteract potassium loss induced by other diuretics in the management of edema or hypertension.

ACTION
- Acts at distal tubule, causing excretion of sodium, bicarbonate, and calcium while conserving potassium and hydrogen ions. **Therapeutic Effects:**
- Weak diuretic and antihypertensive response compared to other diuretics
- Conservation of potassium.

PHARMACOKINETICS

Absorption: Absorption varies greatly among individuals.
Distribution: Widely distributed.
Metabolism and Excretion: Partially metabolized by the liver. Some excretion of unchanged drug.
Half-life: 100–150 min.

CONTRAINDICATIONS AND PRECAUTIONS

Contraindicated in: ▪ Hypersensitivity ▪ Renal impairment ▪ Pregnancy or lactation ▪ Hyperkalemia.
Use Cautiously in: ▪ Impaired hepatic function ▪ Hyperuricemia ▪ History of nephrolithiasis ▪ Children (safety not established).

ADVERSE REACTIONS AND SIDE EFFECTS*

CNS: dizziness, weakness, headache.
CV: hypotension.
GI: nausea, vomiting, diarrhea.
GU: nephrolithiasis, bluish discoloration of urine.
Derm: rashes, photosensitivity.
F and E: HYPERKALEMIA, hyponatremia.
Hemat: megaloblastic anemia, blood dyscrasias.
MS: muscle cramps.
Misc: hypersensitivity reactions.

INTERACTIONS

Drug–Drug: ▪ Additive hypotension with other **antihypertensives,** acute ingestion of **alcohol,** or **nitrates** ▪ Use with **angiotensin converting enzyme (ACE) inhibitors, cyclosporine,** or **potassium supplements** may lead to hyperkalemia ▪ Decreases **lithium** excretion, may lead to toxicity ▪ Increases levels of **amantadine** ▪ Effects increased by **cimetidine** ▪ Increased risk of nephrotoxicity with **indomethacin.**
Drug–Food: ▪ Ingestion of **foods high in potassium content** (see list in Appendix K) may lead to hyperkalemia.

ROUTE AND DOSAGE

▪ **PO (Adults):** 25–200 mg/day single dose or divided doses.

AVAILABILITY

▪ *Capsules:* 50 mg, 100 mg ▪ {*Tablets:* 50 mg, 100 mg} ▪ *In combination with:* hydrochlorothiazide, {Apo-Triazide}, Dyazide, Maxzide, {Novo-Triamzide}. See Appendix A.

TIME/ACTION PROFILE (potassium-sparing effects)

	ONSET	PEAK	DURATION
PO	2 hr	6–8 hr	12–16 hr

NURSING IMPLICATIONS

ASSESSMENT

▫ Monitor intake and output ratios and daily weight throughout therapy. Assess for peripheral edema and auscultate lungs for rales/crackles periodically during therapy.
▫ Assess patient routinely for signs of hyperkalemia (fatigue, muscle weakness, paresthesia, confusion, dyspnea, cardiac arrhythmias). Patients who have diabetes mellitus or kidney disease and elderly patients are at increased risk of developing these symptoms.
▫ Periodic ECGs are recommended in patients receiving prolonged therapy.
▪ **Lab Test Considerations:** Serum potassium levels should be evaluated prior to and routinely during therapy. Withhold drug and notify physician if patient becomes hyperkalemic.
▫ Monitor BUN, serum creatinine, and electrolytes prior to and periodically throughout therapy. CBC and platelet count should also be monitored periodically throughout therapy. May cause increased serum glucose, magnesium, uric acid, BUN, creatinine, potassium, and urinary calcium excretion levels. May also cause decreased sodium levels.

---

*Underlines indicate most frequent; CAPITALS indicate life-threatening.

POTENTIAL NURSING DIAGNOSES
- Fluid volume excess (indications).
- Knowledge deficit related to medication regimen (patient/family teaching).

IMPLEMENTATION
- **General Info:** Available in combination with hydrochlorothiazide (Dyazide, Maxzide). Capsules (Dyazide) are not bioequivalent to tablets (Maxzide). When changing brands, dosage may need to be adjusted.
- Administer in the morning to avoid interrupting sleep pattern.
- **PO:** Administer with food or milk to minimize GI irritation and increase bioavailability. Capsules may be opened and contents mixed with food or fluids for patients with difficulty swallowing.

PATIENT/FAMILY TEACHING
- Emphasize the importance of continuing to take this medication even if feeling better. Instruct patient to take medication at the same time each day. If a dose is missed, take as soon as remembered unless almost time for next dose. Do not double doses.
- Caution patients to avoid salt substitutes and foods that contain high levels of potassium or sodium, unless physician specifically prescribes them (see Appendix K).
- Advise patient to use sunscreen and protective clothing to prevent photosensitivity reactions.
- May cause dizziness. Caution patient to avoid driving or other activities requiring alertness until response to medication is known.
- Advise patient to avoid use of over-the-counter medications without first consulting with physician or pharmacist.
- Inform patient that triamterene may cause bluish-colored urine.
- Advise patient to notify physician if muscle cramps, fever, sore throat, mouth sores, unusual bleeding or bruising, fatigue, weakness or severe nausea, vomiting, or diarrhea occurs.

EVALUATION
Effectiveness of therapy can be demonstrated by: ▪ Increase in diuresis and a decrease in edema while maintaining serum potassium levels in acceptable ranges.

TRIAZOLAM
(trye-**az**-oh-lam)
{Apo-Triazo}, Halcion, {Novo-triolam}, {Nu-Triazo}

CLASSIFICATION(S):
Sedative/hypnotic (benzodiazepine)
Schedule IV
Pregnancy Category X

INDICATIONS
▪ Short-term management of insomnia.

ACTION
▪ Acts at many levels in the CNS, producing generalized depression ▪ Effects may be mediated by gamma aminobutyric acid (GABA), an inhibitory neurotransmitter. **Therapeutic Effect:** ▪ Relief of insomnia.

PHARMACOKINETICS
Absorption: Well absorbed following oral administration.
Distribution: Widely distributed, crosses blood–brain barrier. Probably crosses the placenta and enters breast milk.
Metabolism and Excretion: Metabolized by the liver.
Half-life: 1.6–5.4 hr.

CONTRAINDICATIONS AND PRECAUTIONS
Contraindicated in: ▪ Hypersensitivity ▪ Cross-sensitivity with other benzodiazepines may exist ▪ Pre-existing CNS depression ▪ Uncontrolled severe pain ▪ Pregnancy, lactation, or children.
Use Cautiously in: ▪ Pre-existing hepatic dysfunction (dosage reduction

{} = Available in Canada only.

recommended) ▪ Patients who may be suicidal or have been addicted to drugs previously ▪ Elderly or debilitated patients (dosage reduction recommended).

ADVERSE REACTIONS AND SIDE EFFECTS*

CNS: dizziness, drowsiness, lethargy, hangover, paradoxical excitation, confusion, mental depression, headache, anterograde amnesia.
Derm: rashes.
EENT: blurred vision.
GI: nausea, vomiting, diarrhea, constipation.
Misc: tolerance, psychological dependence, physical dependence.

INTERACTIONS

Drug–Drug: ▪ Additive CNS depression with **alcohol, antidepressants, antihistamines,** and **opioid analgesics** ▪ May decrease effectiveness of **levodopa** ▪ May increase toxicity of **zidovudine** ▪ **Isoniazid** may decrease excretion and increase effects of triazolam ▪ **Cimetidine** or **erythromycin** may decrease metabolism and enhance actions of triazolam ▪ Sedative effects may be decreased by **theophylline**.

ROUTE AND DOSAGE

▪ **PO (Adults):** 125–250 mcg (up to 500 mcg) at bedtime.
▪ **PO (Elderly or Debilitated Patients):** 125 mcg at bedtime initially, may be increased as needed.

AVAILABILITY

▪ *Tablet:* 0.125 mg, 0.25 mg.

TIME/ACTION PROFILE (sedation)

	ONSET	PEAK	DURATION
PO	15–30 min	3 days*	UK

*Maximum hypnotic response.

NURSING IMPLICATIONS

ASSESSMENT

□ Assess sleep patterns prior to and periodically throughout therapy.

□ Prolonged high-dose therapy may lead to psychological or physical dependence. Restrict the amount of drug available to patient, especially if patient is depressed, suicidal, or has a history of addiction.

POTENTIAL NURSING DIAGNOSES

▪ Sleep pattern disturbance (indications).
▪ Injury, high risk for (side effects).
▪ Knowledge deficit related to medication regimen (patient/family teaching).

IMPLEMENTATION

▪ **PO:** Administer with food if GI irritation becomes a problem.

PATIENT/FAMILY TEACHING

□ Instruct patient to take triazolam exactly as directed. Discuss the importance of preparing environment for sleep (dark room, quiet, avoidance of nicotine and caffeine). If less effective after a few weeks, consult physician; do not increase dose.

□ May cause daytime drowsiness or dizziness. Caution patient to avoid driving or other activities requiring alertness until response to medication is known.

□ Advise patient to avoid the use of alcohol and other CNS depressants and to consult physician or pharmacist prior to using over-the-counter preparations that contain antihistamines or alcohol.

□ Advise patient to inform physican if pregnancy is planned or suspected or if confusion, depression, or persistent headaches occur. Instruct family or caregiver to notify physician if personality changes occur.

□ Instruct patient to notify physician if an increase in daytime anxiety occurs. May occur after as few as 10 days of therapy. May require discontinuation of triazolam.

□ Emphasize the importance of follow-up appointments to monitor progress.

EVALUATION

Effectiveness of therapy can be demon-

---

*Underlines indicate most frequent; **CAPITALS** indicate life-threatening.

strated by: ▪ Improvement in sleep patterns, which may not be noticeable until the third day of therapy.

TRIFLUOPERAZINE
(trye-floo-oh-**pair**-a-zeen)
{Apo-Trifluoperazine}, {Novo-Flurazine}, {Solazine}, Stelazine, {Terfluzine}

CLASSIFICATION(S):
Antipsychotic (phenothiazine)
Pregnancy Category UK

INDICATIONS
▪ Treatment of acute and chronic psychoses ▪ Adjunct in the management of anxiety when safer agents are contraindicated.

ACTION
▪ Alters the effects of dopamine in the CNS ▪ Possesses significant anticholinergic and alpha-adrenergic blocking activity. **Therapeutic Effect:** ▪ Diminished signs and symptoms of psychoses.

PHARMACOKINETICS
Absorption: Absorption from tablets is variable; may be better with oral liquid formulations. Well absorbed following IM administration.
Distribution: Widely distributed, high concentrations in the CNS. Crosses the placenta and enters breast milk.
Metabolism and Excretion: Highly metabolized by the liver.
Half-life: UK.

CONTRAINDICATIONS AND PRECAUTIONS
Contraindicated in: ▪ Hypersensitivity ▪ Cross-sensitivity with other phenothiazines may exist ▪ Hypersensitivity to bisulfites (oral concentrate only) ▪ Narrow-angle glaucoma ▪ Bone marrow depression ▪ Severe liver or cardiovascular disease.
Use Cautiously in: ▪ Elderly or debilitated patients (dosage reduction recommended) ▪ Pregnancy or lactation (safety not established; may cause adverse effects in the newborn) ▪ Diabetes mellitus ▪ Respiratory disease ▪ Prostatic hypertrophy ▪ CNS tumors ▪ Epilepsy ▪ Intestinal obstruction.

ADVERSE REACTIONS AND SIDE EFFECTS*
CNS: <u>sedation</u>, <u>extrapyramidal reactions</u>, tardive dyskinesia, NEUROLEPTIC MALIGNANT SYNDROME.
EENT: dry eyes, blurred vision, lens opacities.
CV: hypotension, tachycardia.
GI: <u>constipation</u>, dry mouth, ileus, anorexia, hepatitis.
GU: urinary retention.
Derm: rashes, <u>photosensitivity</u>, pigment changes.
Endo: galactorrhea.
Hemat: AGRANULOCYTOSIS, leukopenia.
Metab: hyperthermia.
Misc: allergic reactions.

INTERACTIONS
Drug–Drug: ▪ Additive hypotension with **antihypertensive agents**, acute ingestion of **alcohol**, or **nitrates** ▪ Additive CNS depression with other **CNS depressants**, including **alcohol**, **antihistamines**, **opioid analgesics**, **sedative/hypnotics**, and **general anesthetics** ▪ Additive anticholinergic effects with other **drugs having anticholinergic properties**, including **antihistamines**, **antidepressants**, other **phenothiazines**, **quinidine**, and **disopyramide** ▪ Acute encephalopathy may occur with **lithium** ▪ May decrease the effectiveness of **levodopa** ▪ Increased risk of agranulocytosis with **antithyroid drugs** ▪ Lithium decreases absorption and may increase risk of extrapyramidal reactions.

ROUTE AND DOSAGE
Psychoses
▪ **PO (Adults):** 2–5 mg bid (up to 40 mg/day).

- **PO (Children 6–12 yr):** 1 mg once or twice daily (up to 15 mg/day).
- **IM (Adults):** 1–2 mg q 4–6 hr (up to 10 mg/day).
- **IM (Children):** 1 mg once or twice daily.

Anxiety

- **PO (Adults):** 1–2 mg bid (not to exceed 6 mg/day or more than 12 wk).

AVAILABILITY

- *Tablets:* 1 mg, 2 mg, 5 mg, 10 mg
- *Oral concentrate:* 10 mg/ml ■ *Injection:* 2 mg/ml.

TIME/ACTION PROFILE
(antipsychotic effects)

	ONSET	PEAK	DURATION
PO	UK	UK	12–24 hr
IM	UK	UK	4–6 hr

NURSING IMPLICATIONS

ASSESSMENT

- Assess mental status (orientation, mood, behavior) and degree of anxiety prior to and periodically throughout therapy.
- Monitor blood pressure (sitting, standing, lying), pulse, and respiratory rate prior to and frequently during the period of dosage adjustment.
- Observe patient carefully when administering medication to ensure that medication is actually taken and not hoarded.
- Monitor intake and output ratios and daily weight. Notify physician if significant discrepancies occur.
- Monitor patient for onset of extrapyramidal side effects (akathisia—restlessness; dystonia—muscle spasms and twisting motions; pseudoparkinsonism—mask facies, rigidity, tremors, drooling, shuffling gait, dysphagia). Notify physician if these symptoms occur, as reduction in dosage or discontinuation of medication may be necessary. Physician may also order trihexyphenidyl or diphanhydramine to control these symptoms.
- Monitor for tardive dyskinesia (rhythmic movement of mouth, face, and extremities). Notify physician immediately if these symptoms occur, as these side effects may be irreversible.
- Monitor for development of neuroleptic malignant syndrome (fever, respiratory distress, tachycardia, convulsions, diaphoresis, hypertension or hypotension, pallor, tiredness). Notify physician immediately if these symptoms occur.
- **Lab Test Considerations:** CBC and liver function tests should be evaluated periodically throughout course of therapy. May cause blood dyscrasias, especially between weeks 4 and 10 of therapy.
- May cause false-positive or false-negative pregnancy tests and false-positive urine bilirubin test results.
- May cause increased serum prolactin levels, thereby interfering with gonadorelin test results.
- May cause Q wave and T wave changes in ECG.

POTENTIAL NURSING DIAGNOSES

- Coping, ineffective individual (indications).
- Thought processes, altered (indications).
- Knowledge deficit related to medication regimen (patient/family teaching).

IMPLEMENTATION

- **General Info:** To prevent contact dermatitis, avoid getting solution on hands.
- Phenothiazines should be discontinued 48 hr before and not resumed for 24 hr following metrizamide myelography, as they lower the seizure threshold.
- Solution may be slightly yellow. Do not use if solution is brown or contains a precipitate. Protect from light.
- **PO:** Administer oral doses with food, water, or milk to minimize GI irritation. Tablets may be crushed and mixed with food or fluids for patients with difficulty swallowing.
- Dilute concentrate just prior to administration, in at least 120 ml of tomato or fruit juice, milk, carbonated

beverage, coffee, tea, or water. Semi-solid foods (soups, puddings) may also be used.

- **IM:** Administer deep into well-developed muscle. SC administration may cause tissue necrosis. Keep patient recumbent for at least 30 min following injection to minimize hypotensive effects.

PATIENT/FAMILY TEACHING

□ Advise patient to take medication exactly as directed, not to skip doses or double up on missed doses. If a dose is missed it should be taken as soon as remembered unless almost time for the next dose. If more than 2 doses are scheduled each day, the missed dose should be taken within about 1 hr of the ordered time.

□ Abrupt withdrawal may lead to gastritis, nausea, vomiting, dizziness, headache, tachycardia, and insomnia.

□ May cause drowsiness. Caution patient to avoid driving or other activities requiring alertness until response to medication is known.

□ Advise patient to make position changes slowly to minimize orthostatic hypotension.

□ Advise patient to use sunscreen and protective clothing when exposed to the sun to prevent photosensitivity reactions. Extremes in temperature should also be avoided, as this drug impairs body temperature regulation.

□ Caution patient to avoid taking alcohol or other CNS depressants concurrently with this medication.

□ Instruct patient to use frequent mouth rinses, good oral hygiene, and sugarless gum or candy to minimize dry mouth. Consult physician or dentist if dry mouth continues >2 wk.

□ Advise patient that increasing activity and bulk and fluids in the diet helps minimize the constipating effects of this medication.

□ Advise patient to notify physician or dentist of medication regimen prior to treatment or surgery.

□ Instruct patient to notify physician promptly if sore throat, fever, unusual bleeding or bruising, skin rashes, weakness, tremors, visual disturbances, difficulty urinating, dark-colored urine, or clay-colored stools are noted.

□ Emphasize the importance of routine follow-up examinations to monitor response to medication and detect side effects. Periodic ocular examinations are indicated. Encourage continued participation in psychotherapy as ordered by physician.

EVALUATION

Effectiveness of therapy can be demonstrated by: ■ Decrease in excitable, paranoic, or withdrawn behavior ■ Decrease in anxiety associated with depression. Therapeutic effects of oral doses may not be seen for 2–3 wk.

TRIHEXYPHENIDYL
(trye-hex-ee-**fen**-i-dill)
Apo-Trihex, Artane, {Novo-hexidyl}, Trihexane, Tri-hexy

CLASSIFICATION(S):
Antiparkinson (anticholinergic)
Pregnancy Category C

INDICATIONS

■ Adjunct in the management of parkinsonian syndrome due to many causes, including drug-induced parkinsonism.

ACTION

■ Inhibits the action of acetylcholine, resulting in: □ Decreased sweating and salivation □ Mydriasis (pupillary dilation) □ Increased heart rate ■ Also has spasmolytic action on smooth muscle ■ Inhibits cerebral motor centers and blocks efferent impulses. **Therapeutic Effect:** ■ Diminished signs and symptoms of parkinsonian syndrome (tremors, rigidity).

PHARMACOKINETICS

Absorption: Well absorbed following oral administration.
Distribution: Distribution not known.
Metabolism and Excretion: Metabolism and excretion not known.
Half-life: UK.

CONTRAINDICATIONS AND PRECAUTIONS

Contraindicated in: ▪ Hypersensitivity ▪ Narrow-angle glaucoma ▪ Acute hemorrhage ▪ Tachycardia secondary to cardiac insufficiency ▪ Thyrotoxicosis ▪ Known alcohol intolerance (elixir only).

Use Cautiously in: ▪ Elderly and very young patients (increased risk of adverse reactions) ▪ Intestinal obstruction or infection ▪ Prostatic hypertrophy ▪ Chronic renal, hepatic, pulmonary, or cardiac disease ▪ Pregnancy or lactation (safety not established).

ADVERSE REACTIONS AND SIDE EFFECTS*

CNS: <u>dizziness</u>, <u>nervousness</u>, drowsiness, weakness, headache, confusion.
EENT: <u>blurred vision</u>, <u>mydriasis</u>.
CV: tachycardia, orthostatic hypotension.
GI: <u>dry mouth</u>, <u>nausea</u>, constipation, vomiting.
GU: urinary hesitancy, urinary retention.
Derm: decreased sweating.

INTERACTIONS

Drug–Drug: ▪ Additive anticholinergic effects with other **drugs having anticholinergic properties,** including **phenothiazines, tricyclic antidepressants, quinidine,** and **disopyramide** ▪ Additive CNS depression with other **CNS depressants,** including **alcohol, antihistamines, opioid analgesics,** and **sedative/hypnotics** ▪ Anticholinergics may alter the absorption of other **orally administered drugs** by slowing motility of the GI tract ▪ **Antacids** may decrease absorption ▪ May increase GI mucosal lesions in patients taking oral **wax-matrix potassium chloride preparations.**

ROUTE AND DOSAGE

▪ **PO (Adults):** 1–2 mg/day initially, increase by 2 mg q 3–5 days. Usual maintenance dose is 5–15 mg/day in 3–4 divided doses. Extended-release (Artane Sequels) preparations may be given q 12 hr after daily dose has been determined using conventional tablets or liquid.

AVAILABILITY

▪ *Tablets:* 2 mg, 5 mg ▪ *Elixir:* 2 mg/5 ml ▪ *Extended-release capsules:* 5 mg.

TIME/ACTION PROFILE
(antiparkinson effects)

	ONSET	PEAK	DURATION
PO	1 hr	2–3 hr	6–12 hr
PO-ER	UK	UK	12–24 hr

NURSING IMPLICATIONS

ASSESSMENT

▫ Assess parkinsonian and extrapyramidal symptoms (akinesia, rigidity, tremors, pill rolling, mask facies, shuffling gait, muscle spasms, twisting motions, and drooling) prior to and throughout course of therapy.

▫ Patients with mental illness are at risk of developing exaggerated symptoms of their disorder during early therapy with this medication. Withhold drug and notify physician if significant behavioral changes occur.

POTENTIAL NURSING DIAGNOSES

▪ Physical mobility, impaired (indications).
▪ Injury, high risk for (indications).
▪ Knowledge deficit related to medication regimen (patient/family teaching).

IMPLEMENTATION

▪ **General Info:** Extended-release capsules are not used until dosage is established with shorter-acting forms.

- **PO:** Usually administered after meals. May be administered before meals if patient suffers from dry mouth or with meals if gastric distress is a problem. Extended-release capsules should be swallowed whole; do not break, crush, or chew. Use calibrated measuring device to ensure accurate dosage of elixir.

PATIENT/FAMILY TEACHING

□ Instruct patient to take this drug exactly as directed. If a dose is missed, take as soon as remembered, unless next scheduled dose is within 2 hr; do not double doses.

□ Medication should be tapered gradually when discontinuing or a withdrawal reaction may occur (anxiety, tachycardia, insomnia, return of parkinsonian or extrapyramidal symptoms).

□ May cause drowsiness or dizziness. Advise patient to avoid driving or other activities that require alertness until response to medication is known.

□ Caution patient to make position changes slowly to minimize orthostatic hypotension.

□ Instruct patient that frequent rinsing of mouth, good oral hygiene, and sugarless gum or candy may decrease mouth dryness. Patient should notify physician if dryness persists (saliva substitutes may be used). Also notify dentist if dryness interferes with use of dentures.

□ Advise patient to consult physician or pharmacist prior to taking over-the-counter medications, especially cold remedies, or drinking alcoholic beverages.

□ Caution patient that this medication decreases perspiration. Overheating may occur during hot weather. Patient should remain indoors, in an air-conditioned environment, during hot weather.

□ Advise patient to increase activity and bulk and fluid in diet to minimize constipating effects of medication.

□ Advise patient to notify physician if confusion, rash, urinary retention, severe constipation, or visual changes occur.

EVALUATION

Effectiveness of therapy can be demonstrated by: ■ Resolution of parkinsonian signs and symptoms ■ Resolution of drug-induced extrapyramidal symptoms.

TRIMETHAPHAN
(trye-**meth**-a-fan)
Arfonad

CLASSIFICATION(S):
Antihypertensive (ganglionic blocker)
Pregnancy Category D

INDICATIONS

■ Rapid reduction of blood pressure in the management of hypertensive emergencies ■ Particularly useful in lowering blood pressure in patients with acute aortic dissection ■ Controlled hypotension in patients undergoing head and neck surgery.

ACTION

■ Blocks nerve transmission at sympathetic and autonomic ganglia ■ Produces vasodilation and histamine release ■ Increases peripheral blood flow and decreases blood pressure. **Therapeutic Effect:** ■ Decreased blood pressure.

PHARMACOKINETICS

Absorption: Administered IV only, resulting in complete bioavailability.
Distribution: Crosses the placenta.
Metabolism and Excretion: Mainly excreted unchanged by the kidneys. Small amounts may be metabolized by pseudocholinesterase.
Half-life: UK.

CONTRAINDICATIONS AND PRECAUTIONS

Contraindicated in: ■ Hypersensitivity ■ Anemia ■ Hypovolemia ■ Shock ■ Asphyxia ▪ Glaucoma ▪ Respiratory insufficiency ▪ Pregnancy.

Use Cautiously in: ▪ Patients with allergies ▪ Elderly or debilitated patients (increased sensitivity to effects) ▪ Children ▪ Cardiovascular disease ▪ Degenerative CNS disease ▪ Diabetes mellitus ▪ Addison's disease ▪ Safety in lactation not established ▪ Hepatic or renal impairment.

ADVERSE REACTIONS AND SIDE EFFECTS*

CNS: weakness, restlessness.
EENT: cycloplegia, mydriasis.
Resp: apnea, RESPIRATORY ARREST (large doses only).
CV: hypotension, tachycardia, angina.
GI: anorexia, nausea, vomiting, dry mouth, ileus (if therapy >48 hr).
GU: urinary retention.
Derm: urticaria, itching.
Misc: tachyphylaxis.

INTERACTIONS

Drug–Drug: ▪ Additive hypotension with other **antihypertensives, nitrates, diuretics, anesthetics,** or **procainamide** ▪ May prolong neuromuscular blockade from **succinylcholine** or **tubocurarine**.

ROUTE AND DOSAGE

Severe Hypertension, Hypertensive Emergencies

▪ **IV (Adults):** 500 mcg–1 mg/min initially, may be increased gradually to achieve desired response (range 1–5 mg/min).
▪ **IV (Children):** 50–150 mcg/kg/min, rate determined by response.

Aortic Dissection

▪ **IV (Adults):** 1–4 mg/min initially, increased as needed to maintain systolic blood pressure of 100–120 mm Hg.

Controlled Hypotension During Anesthesia

▪ **IV (Adults):** 3–4 mg/min initially followed by 300 mcg–6 mg/min infusion.

AVAILABILITY

▪ *Injection:* 50 mg/ml.

TIME/ACTION PROFILE
(antihypertensive effect)

	ONSET	PEAK	DURATION
IV	immediate	UK	10–15 min

NURSING IMPLICATIONS

ASSESSMENT

▫ Monitor blood pressure, pulse, and respirations at least every 5 min during initial adjustment of dosage and at least every 15 min throughout course of therapy. Titrate infusion rate according to physician's parameters. Patients with cardiac history should be monitored with continuous ECG.
▫ Monitor intake and output ratios and weight and assess for edema, jugular vein distension, dyspnea, and rales/crackles, especially in patients with pulmonary edema.
▫ Monitor patients with any allergy history closely for development of tachyphylaxis, because of the effect on histamine release.
▫ Pupil examination will be inaccurate because of mydriatic (dilating) effect.
▫ Monitor for nausea and vomiting; protect airway in patients with diminished level of consciousness. Monitor abdominal status (distention, bowel sounds) in patients on therapy >48 hr, as ileus may occur.
▪ **Lab Test Considerations:** May cause slightly decreased serum potassium and may prevent surgically induced elevation in serum glucose.
▪ **Toxicity and Overdose:** Toxicity is manifested by severe hypotension. Stop infusion, inform physician, and administer vasopressors.

POTENTIAL NURSING DIAGNOSES

▪ Cardiac output, altered (indications).
▪ Tissue perfusion, altered (side effects).

*Underlines indicate most frequent; **CAPITALS** indicate life-threatening.

IMPLEMENTATION

- **IV:** Refrigerate prior to reconstitution. Prepare solution immediately prior to use. IV stable for 24 hr after reconstitution.
- **Continuous Infusion:** Dilute 500-mg (10-ml) vial in 500 ml of D5W, 0.9% NaCl, or Ringer's solution, for a final concentration of 1 mg/ml.
- *Rate:* Infusion rate must be regulated by IV pump or controller and titrated to patient's blood pressure.
- **Y-Site Compatibility:** ▪ heparin ▪ hydrocortisone ▪ potassium chloride.
- **Additive Incompatibility:** Admixture is not recommended with any medication.

PATIENT/FAMILY TEACHING

- ▢ Explain purpose of medication to patient.
- ▢ Instruct alert patients to remain supine throughout course of therapy to prevent orthostatic hypotension.

EVALUATION

Effectiveness of therapy can be demonstrated by: ▪ Short-term control of blood pressure in hypertensive crisis ▪ Control of intraoperative hypotension.

TRIMETHOBENZAMIDE

(trye-meth-oh-**ben**-za-mide)
Arrestin, Benzacot, Brogan, Stemetic, T-Gen, Tebamide, Tegamide, Ticon, Tigan, Tiject-20, Triban, Tribenzagan, Trimazide

CLASSIFICATION(S):
Antiemetic *(miscellaneous)*
Pregnancy Category UK

INDICATIONS

▪ Management of mild to moderate nausea and vomiting.

ACTION

▪ Inhibits emetic stimulation of the chemoreceptor trigger zone in the medulla. **Therapeutic Effect:** ▪ Decreased nausea and vomiting.

PHARMACOKINETICS

Absorption: Absorption following oral, IM, and rectal administration.
Distribution: Distribution not known.
Metabolism and Excretion: Metabolism and excretion not known. Appears to be mostly metabolized by the liver.
Half-life: UK.

CONTRAINDICATIONS AND PRECAUTIONS

Contraindicated in: ▪ Hypersensitivity ▪ Hypersensitivity to benzocaine (suppositories only) ▪ Premature or newborn infants.
Use Cautiously in: ▪ Pregnancy or lactation (safety not established) ▪ Children who may have a viral illness (may increase risk of Reye's syndrome).

ADVERSE REACTIONS AND SIDE EFFECTS*

CNS: <u>drowsiness</u>, extrapyramidal reactions, depression, SEIZURES, coma.
CV: <u>hypotension</u>.
GI: diarrhea, hepatitis.
Derm: rashes.
Hemat: blood dyscrasias.
Local: <u>pain</u>, stinging, burning, or redness at IM injection site, <u>rectal irritation</u> (suppositories).

INTERACTIONS

Drug–Drug: ▪ Additive CNS depression with other **CNS depressants,** including **alcohol, antidepressants, antihistamines, opioid analgesics,** and **sedative/hypnotics.**

ROUTE AND DOSAGE

- **PO (Adults):** 250 mg 3–4 times daily.
- **PO (Children 15–45 kg):** 100–200 mg 3–4 times daily as needed.
- **IM, Rect (Adults):** 200 mg 3–4 times daily as needed.
- **Rect (Children 15–45 kg):** 100–200 mg 3–4 times daily as needed.
- **Rect (Children <15 kg):** 100 mg 3–4 times daily as needed.

AVAILABILITY

- *Capsules:* 100 mg, 250 mg ▪ *Suppos-*

T

---

*<u>Underlines</u> indicate most frequent; **CAPITALS** indicate life-threatening.

itories: 100 mg, 200 mg ▪ *Injection:* 100 mg/ml.

TIME/ACTION PROFILE (antiemetic effect)

	ONSET	PEAK	DURATION
PO	10–40 min	UK	3–4 hr
IM	15–35 min	UK	2–3 hr
Rect	10–40 min	UK	3–4 hr

NURSING IMPLICATIONS

ASSESSMENT

▫ Assess patient for nausea and vomiting prior to and 30–60 min following administration.

▫ Assess blood pressure for hypotension following parenteral administration.

POTENTIAL NURSING DIAGNOSES

▪ Fluid volume deficit (indications).

▪ Injury, high risk for (side effects).

▪ Knowledge deficit related to medication regimen (patient/family teaching).

IMPLEMENTATION

▪ **PO:** Capsules can be opened and contents mixed with food or fluids for patients with difficulty swallowing.

▪ **IM:** Inject deep into well-developed muscle mass to minimize tissue irritation.

▪ **Syringe Compatibility:** ▪ glycopyrrolate ▪ hydromorphone ▪ midazolam ▪ nalbuphine.

▪ **Y-Site Compatibility:** ▪ heparin ▪ hydrocortisone sodium succinate ▪ potassium chloride ▪ vitamin B complex with C.

PATIENT/FAMILY TEACHING

▫ Instruct patient to take medication exactly as directed. Missed doses should be taken as soon as remembered, unless almost time for next dose; do not double doses.

▫ Advise patient to make position changes slowly to minimize orthostatic hypotension following parenteral doses.

▫ May cause drowsiness. Caution patient to avoid driving or other activities requiring alertness until response to medication is known.

▫ Caution patient to avoid taking alcohol or other CNS depressants concurrently with this medication.

▫ Instruct patient to notify physician promptly if sore throat, fever, unusual weakness or tiredness, tremors, or yellowing of the skin and eyes occurs.

EVALUATION

Effectiveness of therapy can be demonstrated by: ▪ Prevention and relief of nausea and vomiting.

TRIMETHOPRIM
(trye-**meth**-oh-prim)
Proloprim, Trimpex

CLASSIFICATION(S):
Anti-infective (miscellaneous)
Pregnancy Category C

INDICATIONS

▪ Treatment of uncomplicated urinary tract infections. **Unlabeled Uses:** ▪ Prophylaxis of chronic recurrent urinary tract infections ▪ With dapsone in the management of mild to moderate *Pneumocystis carinii* pneumonia (PCP).

ACTION

▪ Interferes with bacterial folic acid synthesis. **Therapeutic Effect:** ▪ Bactericidal action against susceptible organisms. **Spectrum:** ▪ Some gram-positive pathogens, including: ▫ *Streptococcus pneumoniae* ▫ Group A beta-hemolytic streptococci ▫ Some staphylococci and *Enterococcus* ▪ Gram-negative spectrum includes the following Enterobacteriaceae: ▫ *Acinetobacter* ▫ *Citrobacter* ▫ *Enterobacter* ▫ *Escherichia coli* ▫ *Klebsiella pneumoniae* ▫ *Proteus mirabilis* ▫ *Salmonella* ▫ *Shigella* ▪ Other strains of *Proteus,* some *Providencia;* some *Serratia* and *Pneumocystis carinii* are also susceptible.

PHARMACOKINETICS

Absorption: Well absorbed following oral administration.

Distribution: Widely distributed. Crosses the placenta and is distributed into breast milk in high concentrations. **Metabolism and Excretion:** 80% excreted unchanged in the urine. 20% metabolized by the liver.
Half-life: 8–11 hr (increased in renal impairment).

CONTRAINDICATIONS AND PRECAUTIONS

Contraindicated in: ▪ Hypersensitivity ▪ Megaloblastic anemia secondary to folate deficiency.
Use Cautiously in: ▪ Renal impairment (dosage reduction required if creatinine clearance ≤30 ml/min) ▪ Pregnancy, lactation, or children <12 yr (safety not established) ▪ Debilitated patients ▪ Severe hepatic impairment ▪ Folate deficiency.

ADVERSE REACTIONS AND SIDE EFFECTS*

GI: epigastric discomfort, nausea, vomiting, glossitis, altered taste, hepatitis.
Derm: rash, pruritus.
Hemat: neutropenia, thrombocytopenia, megaloblastic anemia.
Misc: fever.

INTERACTIONS

Drug–Drug: ▪ Increased risk of folate deficiency when used with **phenytoin** or **methotrexate** ▪ Increased risk of bone marrow depression when used with **antineoplastic agents** or **radiation therapy** ▪ **Rifampin** may decrease effectiveness by increasing elimination.

ROUTE AND DOSAGE

Treatment of Urinary Tract Infections
▪ **PO (Adults):** 100 mg q 12 hr or 200 mg as a single daily dose.

Prophylaxis of Chronic Urinary Tract Infections
▪ **PO (Adults):** 100 mg/day (single dose).

Pneumocystis Carinii Pneumonia
▪ **PO (Adults):** 20 mg/kg/day with 100 mg dapsone daily for 21 days.

AVAILABILITY

▪ *Tablets:* 100 mg, 200 mg ▪ *In combination with:* sulfamethoxazole. See Trimethoprim/Sulfamethoxazole monograph.

TIME/ACTION PROFILE (blood levels)

	ONSET	PEAK
PO	rapid	1–4 hr

NURSING IMPLICATIONS

ASSESSMENT
□ Assess patient for urinary tract infection (fever, cloudy urine, frequency, urgency, pain and burning on urination) or other signs of infection at beginning and throughout therapy.
□ Obtain specimens for culture and sensitivity prior to initiating therapy. First dose may be given before receiving results.
□ Monitor intake and output ratios. Fluid intake should be sufficient to maintain urine output of at least 1200–1500 ml daily.
▪ **Lab Test Considerations:** May produce elevated serum bilirubin, creatinine, BUN, AST (SGOT), and ALT (SGPT).
□ Monitor CBC and urinalysis periodically throughout therapy. Therapy should be discontinued if blood dyscrasias occur.

POTENTIAL NURSING DIAGNOSES
▪ Infection, high risk for (indications, side effects).
▪ Knowledge deficit related to medication regimen (patient/family teaching).

IMPLEMENTATION
▪ **PO:** Administer on an empty stomach, at least 1 hr before or 2 hr after meals, with a full glass of water. May be administered with food if GI irritation occurs.

PATIENT/FAMILY TEACHING
□ Instruct patient to take medication and to finish medication completely as directed, even if feeling better. If a

*Underlines indicate most frequent; **CAPITALS** indicate life-threatening.

dose is missed, it should be taken as soon as remembered, with subsequent doses spaced evenly apart. Advise patient that sharing of this medication may be dangerous.

□ Advise patient to notify physician if skin rash, sore throat, fever, mouth sores, or unusual bleeding or bruising occurs. Leucovorin (folinic acid) may be administered if folic acid deficiency occurs.

□ Instruct patient to notify physician if symptoms do not improve.

□ Emphasize the importance of routine follow-up examinations to evaluate progress.

EVALUATION

Clinical response can be evaluated by:
■ Resolution of the signs and symptoms of infection. Therapy is usually required for 10–14 days for resolution of urinary tract infection ■ Decreased incidence of urinary tract infections during prophylactic therapy.

TRIMETHOPRIM/SULFA-METHOXAZOLE

(trye-**meth**-oh-prim/sul-fa-meth-**ox**-a-zole)
{Apo-Sulfatrim}, {Apo-Sulfatrim DS}, Bactrim, Bactrim DS, Cotrim, Cotrim DS, {Novotrimel}, {Novotrimel DS}, {Nu-Cotrimox}, {Nu-Cotrimox DS}, {Roubac}, Septra, Septra DS, SMZ/TMP, Sulfomethoprim, Sulfamethoprim DS, Sulfaprim, Sulfaprim DS, Sulfatrim, Sulfatrim DS, Sulfoxaprim,Sulfoxaprim DS, TMP/SMX, TMP/SMZ, Triazole, Triazole DS, Trimeth-Sulfa, Trisulfam, Uroplus

CLASSIFICATION(S):
Anti-infective (sulfonamide)
Pregnancy Category C

INDICATIONS

■ Treatment of the following infections due to susceptible organisms: bronchi-

tis, *Shigella* enteritis, otitis media, *Pneumocystis carinii* pneumonia, urinary tract infections ■ Treatment of traveler's diarrhea. **Unlabeled Uses:** ■ Biliary tract infections, osteomyelitis, burn and wound infections, chlamydial infections, endocarditis, gonorrhea, intra-abdominal infections, nocardiosis, rheumatic fever prophylaxis, sinusitis, eradication of meningococcal carriers, prophylaxis of urinary tract infections and as an alternative agent in the treatment of chancroid ■ Prevention of bacterial infections in immunosuppressed patients ■ Prevention of *Pneumocystis carinii* pneumonia in HIV-positive patients.

ACTION

■ Combination inhibits the metabolism of folic acid in bacteria at two different points. **Therapeutic Effect:** ■ Bactericidal action against susceptible bacteria. **Spectrum:** ■ Active against many strains of gram-positive aerobic pathogens including □ *Streptococcus pneumoniae* □ *Staphylococcus aureus,* group A beta-hemolytic streptococci □ Nocardia □ Enterococcus ■ Has activity against many aerobic gram-negative pathogens, such as □ *Acinetobacter* □ *Enterobacter* □ *Klebsiella pneumoniae* □ *Escherichia coli* □ *Proteus mirabilis* □ *Shigella* □ *Hemophilus influenzae* (including ampicillin-resistant strains) ■ *Pneumocystis carinii* (a protozoa) ■ Not active against *Pseudomonas aeruginosa.*

PHARMACOKINETICS

Absorption: Well absorbed from the GI tract.
Distribution: Widely distributed. Crosses the blood–brain barrier and placenta and enters breast milk.
Metabolism and Excretion: Some metabolism by the liver (20%), remainder excreted unchanged by the kidneys.
Half-life: *trimethoprim*—8–11 hr, *sulfamethoxazole*—7–12 hr.

CONTRAINDICATIONS AND PRECAUTIONS

Contraindicated in: ▪ Hypersensitivity to sulfonamides or trimethoprim ▪ Megaloblastic anemia secondary to folate deficiency ▪ Pregnancy, lactation, or children <2 mo ▪ Severe renal impairment.

Use Cautiously in: ▪ Impaired hepatic or renal function (dosage reduction required if creatinine clearance <30 ml/min) ▪ HIV-positive patients (increased incidence of adverse reactions).

ADVERSE REACTIONS AND SIDE EFFECTS*

CNS: headache, insomnia, fatigue, depression, hallucinations.

GI: nausea, vomiting, stomatitis, diarrhea, HEPATIC NECROSIS.

GU: crystalluria.

Derm: rashes, TOXIC EPIDERMAL NECROLYSIS, photosensitivity.

Hemat: APLASTIC ANEMIA, AGRANULOCYTOSIS, leukopenia, thrombocytopenia, megaloblastic anemia, hemolytic anemia.

Local: phlebitis at IV site.

Misc: allergic reactions including STEVENS JOHNSON SYNDROME, ERYTHEMA MUTIFORME, fever.

INTERACTIONS

Drug–Drug: ▪ May increase half-life, decrease clearance, and exaggerate folic acid deficiency caused by **phenytoin** ▪ May enhance the effects of **oral hypoglycemic agents** and **oral anticoagulants** ▪ May increase the toxicity of **methotrexate** ▪ Increases the risk of thrombocytopenia from **thiazide diuretics** (elderly patients) ▪ Decreases efficacy of **cyclosporine** and increases risk of nephrotoxicity.

ROUTE AND DOSAGE

(TMP = trimethoprim; SMZ = sulfamethoxazole)

Bacterial Infections

▪ **PO (Adults):** 160 mg TMP/800 mg SMZ q 12 hr.

▪ **PO (Children >2 mo):** 4–6 mg/kg TMP/20–30 mg/kg SMZ q 12 hr.

▪ **IV (Adults and Children >2 mo):** 8–10 mg/kg TMP/40–50 mg/kg SMZ daily in divided doses q 6–12 hr.

Pneumocyctis Carinii Pneumonia (Treatment)

▪ **PO (Adults and Children >2 mo):** 3.75–5 mg/kg TMP/18.75–25 mg SMZ q 6 hr.

▪ **IV (Adults and Children >2 mo):** 15–20 mg/kg TMP/75–100 mg/kg SMZ daily in divided doses q 6–8 hr.

Pneumocystis Carinii Pneumonia (Prevention)

▪ **PO (Adults):** 160 mg TMP/800 mg SMZ daily (may also be given 3 times weekly).

▪ **PO (Children >1 mo):** 150 mg/m^2 TMP/375 mg/m^2 SMZ daily as a single dose or in divided doses (may also be given 3 times weekly).

AVAILABILITY

▪ **Tablets:** {20 mg TMP, 100 mg SMZ}, 80 mg TMP/400 mg SMZ, 160 mg TMP/800 mg SMZ ▪ **Suspension:** 40 mg TMP/200 mg SMZ per 5 ml ▪ **Injection:** 80 mg TMP/400 mg SMZ per 5 ml.

TIME/ACTION PROFILE (blood levels)

	ONSET	PEAK
PO	rapid	2–4 hr
IV	rapid	end of infusion

NURSING IMPLICATIONS

ASSESSMENT

◻ Assess patient for infection (vital signs; appearance of wound, sputum, urine, and stool; WBC) at beginning and throughout course of therapy.

◻ Obtain specimens for culture and sensitivity prior to initiating therapy. First dose may be given before receiving results.

◻ Inspect IV site frequently. Phlebitis is common.

◻ Assess patient for allergy to sulfonamides.

*Underlines indicate most frequent; **CAPITALS** indicate life-threatening.

□ Monitor intake and output ratios. Fluid intake should be sufficient to maintain a urine output of at least 1200–1500 ml daily to prevent crystalluria and stone formation.

■ **Lab Test Considerations:** Monitor CBC and urinalysis periodically throughout therapy.

□ May produce elevated serum bilirubin, creatinine, and alkaline phosphatase.

POTENTIAL NURSING DIAGNOSES

■ Infection, high risk for (indications, side effects).

■ Knowledge deficit related to medication regimen (patient/family teaching).

■ Noncompliance related to medication regimen (patient/family teaching).

IMPLEMENTATION

■ **General Info:** Do not administer medication IM.

■ **PO:** Administer around the clock on an empty stomach at least 1 hr before or 2 hr after meals, with a full glass of water. Use calibrated measuring device for liquid preparations.

■ **Intermittent Infusion:** Dilute each 5-ml ampule with 125 ml of D5W. May reduce diluent to 75 ml if fluid restriction required. Do not use if solution is cloudy or contains a precipitate. Solution is stable for 6 hr in standard dilution and 2 hr in fluid-restricted dilution at room temperature. Do not refrigerate.

■ *Rate:* Infuse over 60–90 min. Do not administer rapidly or by bolus injection.

■ **Syringe Compatibility:** ■ heparin.

■ **Y-Site Compatibility:** ■ acyclovir ■ atracurium ■ cyclophosphamide ■ enalaprilat ■ esmolol ■ fludarabine ■ hydromorphone ■ labetalol ■ magnesium sulfate ■ meperidine ■ morphine ■ pancuronium ■ perphenazine ■ sargramostim ■ vecuronium ■ zidovudine.

■ **Additive Incompatibility:** Manufacturer recommends that no other medication or solution be admixed with trimethoprim/sulfamethoxazole.

PATIENT/FAMILY TEACHING

□ Instruct patient to take medication around the clock and to finish the drug completely as directed, even if feeling well. If a dose is missed, it should be taken as soon as remembered. Advise patient that sharing of this medication may be dangerous.

□ Caution patient to use sunscreen and protective clothing to prevent photosensitivity reactions.

□ Advise patient to notify physician if skin rash, sore throat, fever, mouth sores, or unusual bleeding or bruising occurs.

□ Instruct patient to notify physician if symptoms do not improve within a few days.

■ **Home Care Issues:** Instruct family or caregiver on dilution, rate, and administration of drug and proper care of IV equipment.

EVALUATION

Clinical response to therapy can be evaluated by: ■ Resolution of the signs and symptoms of infection. Length of time for complete resolution depends on organism and site of infection.

TRIPROLIDINE
(trye-**proe**-li-deen)
Actidil, Alleract, Myidyl

CLASSIFICATION(S):
Antihistamine
Pregnancy Category B

INDICATIONS

■ Symptomatic relief of allergic symptoms caused by histamine release
■ Most useful in the management of nasal allergies and allergic dermatoses.

ACTION

■ Blocks the effects of histamine. **Therapeutic Effect:** ■ Relief of symptoms associated with histamine excess usually seen in allergic conditions.

PHARMACOKINETICS

Absorption: Well absorbed following oral administration.

Distribution: Widely distributed. Minimal amounts excreted in breast milk. Crosses the blood–brain barrier.
Metabolism and Excretion: Extensively metabolized by the liver.
Half-life: 5 hr.

CONTRAINDICATIONS AND PRECAUTIONS

Contraindicated in: ▪ Hypersensitivity ▪ Acute attacks of asthma ▪ Lactation ▪ Known alcohol intolerance (some liquids).
Use Cautiously in: ▪ Elderly patients (increased risk of adverse reactions) ▪ Narrow-angle glaucoma ▪ Liver disease ▪ Pregnancy (safety not established) ▪ Prostatic hypertrophy.

ADVERSE REACTIONS AND SIDE EFFECTS*

CNS: <u>drowsiness</u>, <u>sedation</u>, excitation (in children), dizziness.
EENT: <u>blurred vision</u>.
CV: hypotension, <u>hypertension</u>, palpitations, arrhythmias.
GI: <u>dry mouth</u>, constipation.
GU: urinary hesitancy, retention.

INTERACTIONS

Drug–Drug: ▪ Additive CNS depression with other **CNS depressants,** including **alcohol, opioid analgesics,** and **sedative/hypnotics** ▪ Additive anticholinergic effects with other **drugs possessing anticholinergic properties,** including **antidepressants, atropine, haloperidol, phenothiazines, quinidine,** and **disopyramide** ▪ **MAO inhibitors** intensify and prolong the anticholinergic effects of antihistamines.

ROUTE AND DOSAGE

▪ **PO (Adults):** 2.5 mg q 4–6 hr (not to exceed 10 mg/24 hr).
▪ **PO (Children 6–12 yr):** 1.25 mg q 6–8 hr (not to exceed 5 mg/24 hr).
▪ **PO (Children 4–6 yr):** 937 mcg q 6–8 hr (not to exceed 3.75 mg/24 hr).
▪ **PO (Children 2–4 yr):** 625 mcg q 6–8 hr (not to exceed 2.5 mg/24 hr).
▪ **PO (Children 4 mo–2 yr):** 312 mcg q 6–8 hr (not to exceed 1.25 mg/24 hr).

AVAILABILITY

▪ *Tablets:* 2.5 mg ▪ *Syrup:* 1.25 mg/5 ml ▪ *In combination with:* pseudoephedrine (Actigen, Actifed, Allerfrim, Allerphed, Aprodone, Triafed, Triofed, Triposed). See Appendix A.

TIME/ACTION PROFILE
(antihistaminic effects)

	ONSET	PEAK	DURATION
PO	15–60 min	1–2 hr	6–8 hr*

*Up to 12 hr with extended-release preparations.

NURSING IMPLICATIONS

Assessment
▫ Assess allergy symptoms (rhinitis, conjunctivitis, hives) prior to and periodically throughout therapy.
▫ Assess lung sounds and character of bronchial secretions. Maintain fluid intake of 1500–2000 ml/day to decrease viscosity of secretions.
▪ **Lab Test Considerations:** May cause false-negative reactions on allergy skin tests; discontinue 3 days prior to testing.

Potential Nursing Diagnoses
▪ Airway clearance, ineffective (indications).
▪ Injury, high risk for (adverse reactions).
▪ Knowledge deficit related to medication regimen (patient/family teaching).

Implementation
▪ **PO:** Administer oral doses with food or milk to decrease GI irritation. Use calibrated measuring device to ensure accurate dose of syrup.

Patient/Family Teaching
▫ If a dose is missed, it should be taken as soon as remembered unless almost time for next dose.
▫ Instruct patient to contact physician if symptoms persist.
▫ Triprolidine may cause drowsiness. Caution patient to avoid driving or other activities requiring alertness until response to drug is known.

*<u>Underlines</u> indicate most frequent; **CAPITALS** indicate life-threatening.

□ Caution patient against using alcohol or other CNS depressants concurrently with this drug.
□ Advise patient that good oral hygiene, frequent mouth rinses, and sugarless gum or candy may help relieve mouth dryness. Physician or dentist should be notified if mouth dryness persists >2 wk.

EVALUATION

Effectiveness of therapy can be demonstrated by: ▪ Decrease in allergic symptoms.

TUBOCURARINE
(too-boh-**cure**-a-reen)
{Tubarine}

CLASSIFICATION(S):
Neuromuscular blocking agent (nondepolarizing)
Pregnancy Category C

INDICATIONS

▪ Production of skeletal muscle paralysis after induction of anesthesia in surgical procedures ▪ Used during mechanical ventilation to improve pulmonary compliance ▪ Adjunct to electroconvulsive therapy ▪ Diagnostic agent in myasthenia gravis.

ACTION

▪ Prevents neuromuscular transmission by blocking the effect of acetylcholine at the myoneural junction ▪ Has no anxiolytic or analgesic effects. **Therapeutic Effect:** ▪ Skeletal muscle paralysis.

PHARMACOKINETICS

Absorption: Although well absorbed following IM administration, effect is delayed as compared to IV administration.
Distribution: Extensively distributed and subsequently redistributed to various tissue compartments. Saturation of compartments occurs, explaining pro-

longed duration of action following repeated doses.
Metabolism and Excretion: 30–75% excreted unchanged by the kidneys. 11% excreted in bile. Small amounts are metabolized by the liver.
Half-life: 2 hr.

CONTRAINDICATIONS AND PRECAUTIONS

Contraindicated in: ▪ Hypersensitivity to tubocurarine ▪ Some products contain chlorobutanol, benzyl alcohol, or bisulfite (avoid use in patients with hypersensitivity to these ingredients).
Use Cautiously in: ▪ History of pulmonary disease, renal or liver impairment ▪ Elderly or debilitated patients ▪ Electrolyte disturbances ▪ Myasthenia gravis or myasthenic syndromes.

ADVERSE REACTIONS AND SIDE EFFECTS*

CV: hypotension, arrhythmias.
EENT: excess salivation.
Resp: bronchospasm, APNEA.
GI: decreased GI tone, decreased GI motility.
MS: muscle weakness.
Misc: allergic reactions.

INTERACTIONS

Drug–Drug: ▪ Intensity and duration of paralysis may be prolonged by pretreatment with **succinylcholine, general anesthesia, aminoglycoside antibiotics, polymyxin B, colistin, clindamycin, lidocaine, quinidine, procainamide, beta-adrenergic blocking agents, potassium-losing diuretics,** and **magnesium** ▪ Dosage should be reduced by ⅔ if concurrent **ether** is used, ⅓ if **methoxyflurane** is used, and ⅙ if **halothane** or **cyclopropane** is used ▪ **Doxapram** masks residual effects.

ROUTE AND DOSAGE

Preferred route is IV, but IM may be used in infants or other patients without venous access.

{} = Available in Canada only.
*Underlines indicate most frequent; **CAPITALS** indicate life-threatening.

Adjunct to General Anesthesia

- **IM, IV (Adults):** 6–9 mg initially, followed by 3–4.5 mg after 3–5 min if needed. Additional doses of 3 mg (0.165 mg/kg) may be given as need is determined.
- **IV (Infants and Children):** 500–600 mcg/kg.
- **IV (Neonates–4 wk):** 250–500 mcg/kg initially, then additional increments of ⅕–⅙ of initial dose may be given.

Adjunct to Electroconvulsive Therapy

- **IV (Adults):** 165 mcg/kg (initial doses should be 3 mg less than calculated dose).

Aid to Mechanical Ventilation

- **IV (Adults):** 1 mg (16.5 mcg/kg), subsequent doses may be given as necessary.

Diagnoses of Myasthenia Gravis

- **IV (Adults):** 4–33 mcg/kg. Profound myasthenic symptoms may occur.

AVAILABILITY

- *Injection:* 3 mg (20 units)/ml.

TIME/ACTION PROFILE (skeletal muscle paralysis)

	ONSET	PEAK	DURATION*
IV	1 min	2–5 min	20–90 min
IM	15–25 min	UK	UK

*Duration increases with repeated doses.

NURSING IMPLICATIONS

ASSESSMENT

- ◻ Assess respiratory status continuously throughout use of tubocurarine. Notify physician of significant changes immediately.
- ◻ Neuromuscular response to tubocurarine should be monitored intraoperatively with a peripheral nerve stimulator. Paralysis is intially selective and usually occurs consecutively in the following muscles: levator muscles of eyelids, muscles of mastication, limb muscles, abdominal muscles, muscles of the glottis, intercostal muscles, and the diaphragm. Recovery of

muscle function usually occurs in reverse order.
- ◻ Monitor ECG, heart rate, and blood pressure throughout use of tubocurarine.
- ◻ Observe patient for residual weakness and respiratory distress during the recovery period.
- **Toxicity and Overdose:** If overdose occurs, use peripheral nerve stimulator to determine the degree of neuromuscular blockade. Maintain airway patency and ventilation until recovery of normal respiration occurs.
- ◻ Administer anticholinesterase agents (edrophonium, neostigmine, pyridostigmine) to antagonize the action of tubocurarine. Atropine is usually administered prior to or concurrently with anticholinesterase agents to counteract the muscarinic effects.
- ◻ Administration of fluids and vasopressors may be necessary to treat severe hypotension or shock.

POTENTIAL NURSING DIAGNOSES

- Breathing pattern, ineffective (indications).
- Communication, impaired verbal (side effects).
- Fear (patient/family teaching).

IMPLEMENTATION

- **General Info:** Tubocurarine should be used only by individuals experienced in endotracheal intubation, and equipment for this procedure should be immediately available.
- ◻ Tubocurarine has no effect on consciousness or the pain threshold. Adequate anesthesia should *always* be used when tubocurarine is used as an adjunct to surgical procedures or when painful procedures are performed. Benzodiazepines and/or analgesics should be administered concurrently when prolonged tubocurarine therapy is used for ventilator patients, as patient is awake and able to feel all sensations.
- ◻ If eyes remain open throughout prolonged administration, protect corneas with artificial tears.

- **Direct IV:** Administer IV dose undiluted over 1–1.5 min. Rapid injection or large doses cause histamine release, resulting in hypotension and bronchospasm. Titrate dose to patient response.
- **Syringe Compatibility:** ▪ pentobarbital ▪ thiopental.
- **Solution Compatibility:** ▪ dextrose in Ringer's or lactated Ringer's combinations ▪ dextrose in saline combinations ▪ D5W ▪ D10W ▪ 0.45% NaCl ▪ 0.9% NaCl ▪ Ringer's and lactated Ringer's injection.
- **Additive Incompatibility:** Incompatible with most barbiturates, sodium bicarbonate, and trimethaphan.

PATIENT/FAMILY TEACHING
- ▢ Explain all procedures to patient receiving tubocurarine therapy without anesthesia, as consciousness is not affected by tubocurarine alone. Provide emotional support.
- ▢ Reassure patient that communication abilities will return as the medication wears off.

EVALUATION
Effectiveness of therapy can be demonstrated by: ▪ Adequate suppression of the twitch response when tested with peripheral nerve stimulation and subsequent muscle paralysis ▪ Diagnosis of myasthenia gravis.

UROKINASE
(yoor-oh-**kye**-nase)
Abbokinase, Abbokinase Open-Cath

CLASSIFICATION(S):
Thrombolytic agent
Pregnancy Category B

INDICATIONS

▪ Treatment of acute, massive pulmonary emboli ▪ Lysis of coronary artery thrombi ▪ Management of occluded IV catheters.

ACTION

▪ Directly activates plasminogen. **Therapeutic Effect:** ▪ Lysis of thrombi or emboli.

PHARMACOKINETICS

Absorption: Administered IV only, resulting in complete bioavailability.
Distribution: Distribution not known.
Metabolism and Excretion: Metabolized by the liver.
Half-life: 10–20 min.

CONTRAINDICATIONS AND PRECAUTIONS

Contraindicated in: ▪ Hypersensitivity ▪ Active internal bleeding ▪ Recent (<2 mo) cerebrovascular accident ▪ Intracranial or intraspinal surgery or intracranial neoplasm.
Use Cautiously in: ▪ Recent (<2 mo) minor trauma or surgery ▪ Patients who are at risk of left heart thrombus ▪ Cerebrovascular disease ▪ Diabetic hemorrhagic retinopathy ▪ Pregnancy, lactation, or children (safety not established) ▪ Elderly patients (increased risk of intracranial bleeding).

ADVERSE REACTIONS AND SIDE EFFECTS*

Resp: bronchospasm.
Derm: rash.
Hemat: BLEEDING.
Misc: fever, hypersensitivity reactions, including ANAPHYLAXIS.

INTERACTIONS

Drug–Drug: ▪ Concurrent use with other **anticoagulants, cefamandole, cefotetan, plicamycin,** or **agents affecting platelet function,** including **aspirin, nonsteroidal anti-inflammatory agents, valproic acid,** or **dipyridamole** increases the risk of bleeding.

ROUTE AND DOSAGE

Lysis of Coronary Thrombi, Myocardial Infarction
- **Intracoronary (Adults):** 6000 IU/min for up to 2 hr (preceded by 2500–10,000 units of heparin IV).

*Underlines indicate most frequent; **CAPITALS** indicate life-threatening.

Pulmonary Emboli, Deep Vein Thrombosis

- **IV (Adults):** 4400 IU/kg loading dose over 10 min followed by 4400 IU/kg/hr for 12 hr.

Occluded IV Catheters

- **Into Catheter (Adults):** 1–1.8 ml of 5000 IU/ml solution injected into catheter, then aspirated; may repeat q 5 min for 30 min; if no result, may cap and leave in catheter for 30–60 min, then aspirate.

AVAILABILITY

- *Injection:* 250,000 IU/5-ml vial, 5000 IU/1-ml vial.

TIME/ACTION PROFILE (thrombolysis)

	ONSET	PEAK	DURATION
IV	immediate	rapid	up to 12 hr

NURSING IMPLICATIONS

ASSESSMENT

- ☐ Monitor vital signs, including temperature, closely during therapy.
- ☐ Assess patient carefully for bleeding every 15 min during the first hour of therapy, every 15–30 min during the next 8 hr, and at least every 4 hr for the duration of therapy. Frank bleeding may occur from invasive sites or body orifices. Internal bleeding may also occur (decreased neurologic status, abdominal pain with coffee ground emesis or black tarry stools, joint pain). If bleeding occurs, stop medication and notify physician immediately.
- ☐ Inquire about previous reaction to urokinase therapy. Assess patient for hypersensitivity reaction (rash, dyspnea) or fever. If these occur, inform physician promptly. Keep epinephrine, an antihistamine, and resuscitation equipment close by in the event of an anaphylactic reaction.
- **Coronary Thrombosis:** Monitor ECG continuously. Notify physician if significant arrhythmias occur. IV lido-caine or procainamide (Pronestyl) may be ordered prophylactically. Cardiac enzymes should be monitored.
- **Pulmonary Embolism:** Monitor pulse, blood pressure, hemodynamics, and respiratory status (rate, degree of dyspnea, ABGs).
- **Deep Vein Thrombosis/Acute Arterial Occlusion:** Observe extremities and palpate pulses of affected extremities every hour. Notify physician immediately if circulatory impairment occurs.
- **Cannula/Catheter Occlusion:** Assess ability to aspirate blood as indicator of patency. Ensure that patient exhales and holds breath when connecting and disconnecting IV syringe, to prevent air embolism.
- **Lab Test Considerations:** Hematocrit, hemoglobin, platelet count, prothrombin time, thrombin time, and activated partial thromboplastin time should be evaluated prior to and frequently throughout course of therapy. Bleeding time may be assessed prior to therapy if patient has received platelet aggregation inhibitors.
- ☐ Obtain type and cross-match and have blood available at all times in case of hemorrhage.
- **Toxicity and Overdose:** If local bleeding occurs, apply pressure to site. If severe or internal bleeding occurs, discontinue infusion. Clotting factors and/or blood volume may be restored through infusions of whole blood, packed red blood cells, fresh frozen plasma, or cryoprecipitate. Do not administer dextran, as it has antiplatelet activity. Aminocaproic acid (Amicar) may be used as an antidote.

POTENTIAL NURSING DIAGNOSES

- Tissue perfusion, altered (indications).
- Injury, high risk for (side effects).

IMPLEMENTATION

- **General Info:** This medication should be used only in settings in which hematologic function and clinical response can be adequately monitored.

□ Invasive procedures, such as IM injections or arterial punctures, should be avoided with this therapy. If such procedures must be performed, apply pressure to IV puncture sites for at least 15 min and to arterial puncture sites for at least 30 min.

□ Systemic anticoagulation with heparin is usually begun several hours after the completion of thrombolytic therapy.

▪ **Intermittent Infusion:** Reconstitute each vial with 5.2 ml of Sterile Water for Injection without preservatives (direct to sides of vial) and swirl gently; do not shake. Dilute further with 190 ml of 0.9% NaCl or D5W. Use reconstituted solution immediately after preparation.

▪ *Rate:* Infuse as directed by physician through a 0.22- or 0.45-micron filter. Administer via infusion pump to ensure accurate dosage.

▪ **Additive Incompatibility:** Manufacturer recommends not admixing with any medications.

▪ **Cannula/Catheter Clearance:** Add 1 ml of the previously reconstituted drug to 9 ml of Sterile Water for Injection without preservatives. Inject 1 ml slowly and gently into occluded cannula, and then clamp for 5 min. Aspirate contents carefully to remove clot. If unsuccessful, reclamp for 5 min. Repeat aspiration every 5 min until clot clears or for 30 min. If still unsuccessful, clamp for 30–60 min and attempt to aspirate again. A second dose of urokinase may be needed.

□ Available in a dual-chamber vial, which reconstitutes to 5000 IU/ml concentration for clearance of occluded cannulae and catheters.

PATIENT/FAMILY TEACHING

□ Explain purpose of medication to patient. Instruct patient to report hypersensitivity reactions (rash, dyspnea), bleeding or bruising.

□ Explain need for bed rest and minimal handling during therapy to avoid injury.

EVALUATION
Effectiveness of therapy can be demonstrated by: ▪ Lysis of thrombi and restoration of blood flow ▪ Cannula or catheter patency.

VAGINAL ANTIFUNGALS

butoconazole
(**byoo**-toe-kon-a-zole)
Femstat

clotrimazole
(kloe-**trye**-ma-zole)
{Canesten}, Gyne-Lotrimin, Mycelex G, Mycelex Twin Pak, {Myclo}

miconazole
(mye-**kon**-a-zole)
Monistat, Monistat 3, Monistat 7, Monistat Dual Pak

nystatin
(nye-**stat**-in)
Mycostatin, Nilstat, {Nadostine}, {Nyoderm}, O-V Statin

terconazole
(ter-**kon**-a-zole)
Terazol

tioconazole
(tye-oh-**kon**-a-zole)
{Gyne-Trosyd}, Vagistat

Pregnancy Category A (nystatin), B (clotrimazole), C (butoconazole, terconazole, tioconazole)

INDICATIONS

▪ Treatment of vulvovaginal candidiasis.

ACTION

▪ Damage fungal cell membrane, allowing leakage of cellular contents. Not active against bacteria. **Therapeutic Effects:** ▪ Inhibited growth/death of susceptible Candida with decrease in accompanying symptoms of vulvovaginitis (vaginal burning, itching, discharge).

{} = Available in Canada only.

PHARMACOKINETICS

Absorption: Nystatin, miconazole, and ticonazole are minimally absorbed. 5.5% of butoconazole is absorbed, 3–10% of clotrimazole, 5–15% of terconazole following intravaginal administration.
Distribution: Distribution not known.
Metabolism and Excretion: Small amounts of clotrimazole absorbed are rapidly metabolized.
Half-life: miconazole 20–25 hr (following parenteral administration).

CONTRAINDICATIONS AND PRECAUTIONS

Contraindicated in: ▪ Hypersensitivity to active ingredients, additives, preservatives or other components in preparations ▪ Butoconazole is contraindicated in the first trimester of pregnancy ▪ Lactation (except terconazole).
Use Cautiously in: ▪ Patients with recurrent vulvovaginal yeast infections (may represent chronic illness requiring other interventions) ▪ Lactation (safe use not established for terconazole).

ADVERSE REACTIONS AND SIDE EFFECTS*

CNS: *terconazole*—headache.
Local: irritation, sensitization, vulvovaginal burning.
Misc: hypersensitivity reactions, *terconazole*—body pain.

INTERACTIONS

Drug–Drug: ▪ None significant.

ROUTE AND DOSAGE

Butoconazole
▪ **Vaginal Cream (Adults and Adolescents):** 1 applicatorful (5 g) at bedtime for 3–6 days.

Clotrimazole
▪ **Vaginal Tablets (Adults and Adolescents):** 100 mg (one 100-mg vaginal tablet) at bedtime for 7 nights *or* 200 mg (two 100-mg vaginal tablets) at bedtime for 3 nights *or* 500 mg (one 500-mg vaginal tablet) as a single bedtime dose.
▪ **Vaginal Cream (Adults and Adolescents):** 1 applicatorful (5 g) at bedtime for 7–14 days.

Miconazole
▪ **Vaginal Tablets (Adults and Adolescents):** one 200-mg suppository at bedtime for 3 days or one 100-mg suppository at bedtime for 7 days.
▪ **Vaginal Cream (Adults and Adolescents):** 1 applicatorful at bedtime for 7 days.

Nystatin
▪ **Vaginal Tablets (Adults and Adolescents):** 100,000 units (1 tablet) daily for 2 wk.

Terconazole
▪ **Vaginal Cream (Adults and Adolescents):** 1 applicatorful (5 g) at bedtime for 7 days.

Tioconazole
▪ **Vaginal Ointment (Adults and Adolescents):** 1 applicatorful (4.6 g) at bedtime as a single dose.

AVAILABILITY

Butoconazole
▪ *Vaginal cream:* 2%.

Clotrimazole
▪ *Vaginal tablets:* 100 mg, 500 mg
▪ *Vaginal cream:* 1%.

Miconazole
▪ *Vaginal cream:* 2% ▪ *Vaginal lotion:* 2% ▪ *Vaginal suppositories.*

Nystatin
▪ *Vaginal tablets:* 100,000 units.

Terconazole
▪ *Vaginal cream:* 0.4%.

Tioconazole
▪ *Vaginal ointment:* 6.5%.

TIME/ACTION PROFILE

	ONSET	PEAK
butoconazole vaginal	rapid	UK
clotrimazole vaginal	rapid	UK
nystatin vaginal	rapid	UK
terconazole vaginal	rapid	UK
tioconazole vaginal	rapid	UK

*Underlines indicate most frequent; **CAPITALS** indicate life-threatening.

NURSING IMPLICATIONS

ASSESSMENT

◻ Inspect involved areas of skin and mucous membranes prior to and frequently throughout course of therapy. Increased skin irritation may indicate need to discontinue medication.

POTENTIAL NURSING DIAGNOSES

- Infection, high risk for (indications).
- Skin integrity, impaired (indications).
- Knowledge deficit related to medication regimen (patient/family teaching).

IMPLEMENTATION

- **General Info:** Consult physician for proper cleansing technique prior to applying medication. Sitz baths and vaginal douches may be ordered concurrently with this therapy.
- **Vag:** Applicators are supplied for vaginal administration.

PATIENT/FAMILY TEACHING

- **Vag:** Instruct patient to apply medication as directed for full course of therapy, even if feeling better. Therapy should be continued during menstrual period.
- ◻ Instruct patient on proper use of vaginal applicator. Medication should be inserted high into the vagina at bedtime. Instruct patient to remain recumbent for at least 30 min following insertion. Advise use of sanitary napkins to prevent staining of clothing or bedding.
- ◻ Advise patient to consult physician regarding douching and intercourse during therapy. Vaginal medication may cause minor skin irritation in sexual partner. Advise patient to refrain from sexual conduct during therapy or have male partner wear a condom.
- ◻ Advise patient to report to physician increased skin irritation or lack of response to therapy.

EVALUATION

Clinical response to therapy can be evaluated by: ▪ Decrease in skin irritation and vaginal discomfort. Therapeutic response is usually seen after 1 wk. Diagnosis should be reconfirmed with smears or cultures prior to a second course of therapy to rule out other pathogens associated with vulvovaginitis. Recurrent vaginal infections may be a sign of systemic illness.

VALPROIC ACID
(val-**pro**-ik **as**-id)
Dalpro, Depakene, Deproic, Myproic Acid

DIVALPROEX SODIUM
(dye-val-**pro**-ex **soe**-dee-um)
Depakote, {Epival}

CLASSIFICATION(S):
Anticonvulsant
Pregnancy Category D

INDICATIONS

▪ Treatment of simple and complex absence seizures. **Unlabeled Uses:** ▪ Treatment of partial seizures with complex symptomatology ▪ Myoclonic seizures ▪ Tonic-clonic seizures.

ACTION

▪ Increases levels of gamma aminobutyric acid (GABA), an inhibitory neurotransmitter in the CNS. **Therapeutic Effect:** ▪ Suppression of absence seizures.

PHARMACOKINETICS

Absorption: Well absorbed from the GI tract following oral administration. Divalproex is enteric-coated and absorption is delayed by 1 hr.

Distribution: Rapidly distributed into plasma and extracellular water. Crosses blood–brain barrier and placenta and enters breast milk.

Metabolism and Excretion: Mostly metabolized by the liver, minimal amounts excreted unchanged in the urine.

Half-life: 5–20 hr.

CONTRAINDICATIONS AND PRECAUTIONS

Contraindicated in: ▪ Hypersensitivity ▪ Hepatic impairment.

Use Cautiously in: ▪ Bleeding disorders ▪ Pregnancy and lactation (safety not established) ▪ History of liver disease ▪ Organic brain disease ▪ Bone marrow depression ▪ Renal impairment ▪ Children (increased risk of hepatotoxicity).

ADVERSE REACTIONS AND SIDE EFFECTS*

CNS: drowsiness, sedation, headache, dizziness, ataxia, confusion.
EENT: visual disturbances.
GI: nausea, vomiting, indigestion, HEPATOTOXICITY, pancreatitis, hypersalivation, anorexia, increased appetite, diarrhea, constipation.
Derm: rashes.
Hemat: prolonged bleeding time, leukopenia, thrombocytopenia.
Metab: hyperammonemia.
Neuro: paresthesia.

INTERACTIONS

Drug–Drug: ▪ Increased risk of bleeding with **antiplatelet agents** (including **aspirin** and **nonsteroidal anti-inflammatory agents**), **cefamandole, cefoperazone, cefotetan, heparin, thrombolytic agents,** or **warfarin** ▪ Decreases the metabolism of **barbiturates** and **primidone,** increasing risk of toxicity ▪ Additive CNS depression with other **CNS depressants,** including **alcohol, antihistamines, antidepressants, opioid analgesics, MAO inhibitors,** and **sedative/hypnotics** ▪ May increase or decrease the effects and toxicity of **phenytoin** ▪ **MAO inhibitors** and other **antidepressants** may lower seizure threshold and decrease effectiveness of valproates ▪ **Carbamazepine** may decrease valproic acid blood levels ▪ Valproic acid may increase toxicity of **carbamazepine** ▪ **Felbamate** increases valproic acid blood levels.

ROUTE AND DOSAGE
Doses expressed in mg of valproic acid.

▪ **PO (Adults and Children):** Initial dose of 15 mg/kg/day, increase by 5–10 mg/kg/day at weekly intervals until therapeutic levels are reached (not to exceed 60 mg/kg/day). When daily dosage exceeds 250 mg, give in 2 divided doses.

AVAILABILITY

Valproic Acid
▪ *Capsules:* 250 mg.
Sodium Valproate
▪ *Syrup:* 250 mg/5 ml.
Divalproex Sodium
▪ *Delayed-release tablets:* 125 mg, 250 mg, 500 mg ▪ *Sprinkle capsules:* 125 mg.

TIME/ACTION PROFILE
(onset = anticonvulsant effect; peak = blood levels)

	ONSET	PEAK	DURATION
PO— liquid	2–4 days	15–120 min	24 hr
PO— capsules	2–4 days	1–4 hr	24 hr
PO— enteric-coated tab	2–4 days	3–5 hr	24 hr

NURSING IMPLICATIONS

ASSESSMENT
▫ Assess location, duration, and characteristics of seizure activity. Institute seizure precautions.
▪ **Lab Test Considerations:** Monitor CBC prior to and periodically throughout therapy. May cause leukopenia and thrombocytopenia.
▫ Monitor hepatic function (LDH, AST [SGOT], ALT [SGPT], and bilirubin) prior to and periodically throughout course of therapy. May cause hepatotoxicity; monitor closely, especially during initial 6 mo of therapy.
▫ May interfere with accuracy of thyroid function tests.

*Underlines indicate most frequent; **CAPITALS** indicate life-threatening.

- May cause false-positive results in urine ketone tests.
- **Toxicity and Overdose:** Therapeutic serum levels range from 50–100 mcg/ml. However, a good correlation between daily dose, serum level, and therapeutic effects has not been established.

POTENTIAL NURSING DIAGNOSES
- Injury, high risk for (indications).
- Knowledge deficit related to medication regimen (patient/family teaching).

IMPLEMENTATION
- **General Info:** Single daily doses are usually administered at bedtime because of sedation.
- **PO:** Administer with or immediately after meals to minimize GI irritation. Swallow capsules and enteric-coated tablets whole; do not break or chew, as this will cause irritation of the mouth or throat. Do not administer tablets with milk, to prevent premature dissolution. Delayed release divalproex sodium may cause less GI irritation than valproic acid capsules.
- Shake liquid preparations well before pouring. Use calibrated measuring device to ensure accurate dosage. Syrup may be mixed with food or other liquids to improve taste.
- Sprinkle capsules may be swallowed whole or opened and the entire capsule contents sprinkled on a teaspoonful of soft food (applesauce, pudding). Swallow drug/food mixture immediately; do not chew. Do not store for future use.
- To convert from valproic acid to divalproex sodium, initiate divalproex sodium at same total daily dose and dosing schedule as valproic acid. Once patient is stabilized on divalproex sodium, administration 2–3 times daily may be attempted.

PATIENT/FAMILY TEACHING
- Instruct patient to take medication exactly as directed. If a dose is missed on a once-a-day schedule it should be taken as soon as remembered that day. If on a multiple-dose schedule, take within 6 hr of the scheduled time; then space remaining doses throughout the remainder of the day. Abrupt withdrawal may lead to status epilepticus.
- May cause drowsiness or dizziness. Caution patient to avoid driving or other activities requiring alertness until effects of medication are known.
- Caution patient to avoid taking alcohol, CNS depressants, or over-the-counter medications concurrently with valproates without consulting physician or pharmacist.
- Instruct patient to notify physician or dentist of medication regimen prior to treatment or surgery.
- Advise patient to carry identification describing medication regimen at all times.
- Advise patient to notify physician if anorexia, severe nausea and vomiting, yellow skin or eyes, fever, sore throat, malaise, weakness, facial edema, lethargy, unusual bleeding or bruising, pregnancy, or loss of seizure control occurs. Children <2 yr of age are especially at risk for fatal hepatotoxicity.
- Emphasize the importance of routine examinations to monitor progress.

EVALUATION
Effectiveness of therapy can be demonstrated by: ■ Decrease or cessation of seizures without excessive sedation.

VANCOMYCIN
(van-koe-**mye**-sin)
Vancocin

CLASSIFICATION(S):
Anti-infective (miscellaneous)
Pregnancy Category C

INDICATIONS

- **IV:** Treatment of potentially life-threatening infections when less toxic anti-infectives are contraindicated. Particularly useful in staphylococcal infections, including: □ Endocarditis □ Osteomyelitis □ Pneumonia □ Septicemia

□ Soft tissue infections in patients who have allergies to penicillin or its derivatives or where sensitivity testing demonstrates resistance to methicillin ▪ **PO:** Treatment of pseudomembranous colitis due to *Clostridium difficile* ▪ **IV:** Part of endocarditis prophylaxis in high-risk patients who are allergic to penicillin.

ACTION

▪ Binds to bacterial cell wall, resulting in cell death. **Therapeutic Effect:** ▪ Bactericidal action against susceptible organisms. **Spectrum:** ▪ Active against gram-positive pathogens, including: □ Staphylococci (including methicillin-resistant strains of *Staphylococcus aureus*) □ Group A beta-hemolytic streptococci □ *Streptococcus pneumoniae* □ *Corynebacterium* □ *Clostridium*.

PHARMACOKINETICS

Absorption: Poorly absorbed from the GI tract.
Distribution: Widely distributed. Some penetration (20–30%) of CSF. Crosses placenta.
Metabolism and Excretion: Oral doses excreted primarily in the feces. IV vancomycin eliminated almost entirely by the kidneys.
Half-life: 6 hr (increased in renal impairment).

CONTRAINDICATIONS AND PRECAUTIONS

Contraindicated in: ▪ Hypersensitivity.
Use Cautiously in: ▪ Renal impairment (dosage reduction required if CCr ≤80 ml/min) ▪ Pregnancy and lactation (safety not established) ▪ Hearing impairment ▪ Intestinal obstruction or inflammation (increased systemic absorption when given orally).

ADVERSE REACTIONS AND SIDE EFFECTS*

Associated with IV administration unless otherwise indicated.
EENT: IV and PO—ototoxicity.

CV: hypotension.
GI: nausea, PO—vomiting, unpleasant taste.
GU: nephrotoxicity.
Derm: rashes.
Hemat: leukopenia, eosinophilia.
Local: phlebitis.
MS: back and neck pain.
Misc: hypersensitivity reactions, including ANAPHYLAXIS; fever, chills, red man syndrome, superinfection.

INTERACTIONS

Drug–Drug: ▪ May cause additive ototoxicity and nephrotoxicity with other **ototoxic** and **nephrotoxic drugs** (**aspirin, aminoglycosides, cyclosporine, cisplatin, loop diuretics**) ▪ May enhance neuromuscular blockade from **nondepolarizing neuromuscular blockers** ▪ Increased risk of histamine flush when used with **anesthetics** in children.

ROUTE AND DOSAGE

Serious Systemic Infections

▪ **IV (Adults):** 500 mg (7.5 mg/kg) q 6 hr or 1 g (15 mg/kg) q 12 hr (up to 3–4 g/day).
▪ **IV (Children):** 40 mg/kg/day in divided doses q 6–12 hr.
▪ **IV (Neonates 1 wk–1 mo):** 15 mg/kg initially, then 10 mg/kg q 8 hr.
▪ **IV (Neonates <1 wk):** 15 mg/kg initially, then 10 mg/kg q 12 hr.

Endocarditis Prophylaxis in Penicillin-Allergic Patients

▪ **IV (Adults and Adolescents):** 1 g single dose 1 hr preprocedure.
▪ **IV (Children):** 20 mg/kg single dose 1 hr preprocedure.

Pseudomembranous Colitis

▪ **PO (Adults):** 0.5–2 g/day in divided doses q 6–8 hr.
▪ **PO (Children):** 40 mg/kg/day in divided doses q 6–8 hr (not to exceed 2 g/day).
▪ **PO (Neonates):** 10 mg/kg/day in divided doses.

AVAILABILITY

▪ *Capsules:* 125 mg, 250 mg ▪ *Oral so-*

V

*Underlines indicate most frequent; **CAPITALS** indicate life-threatening.

lution: 500 mg/5 ml ▪ *Injection:* 500 mg, 1-g, 5-g, 10-g vials.

TIME/ACTION PROFILE (blood levels)

	ONSET	PEAK
IV	rapid	end of infusion

NURSING IMPLICATIONS

ASSESSMENT

▢ Assess patient for infection (vital signs; appearance of wound, sputum, urine, and stool; WBC) at beginning and throughout course of therapy.

▢ Obtain specimens for culture and sensitivity prior to initiating therapy. First dose may be given before receiving results.

▢ Monitor IV site closely. Vancomycin is irritating to tissues and causes necrosis and severe pain with extravasation. Rotate infusion site.

▢ Monitor blood pressure throughout IV infusion.

▢ Evaluate eighth cranial nerve function by audiometry and serum vancomycin levels prior to and throughout course of therapy in patients with borderline renal function or those over 60 years of age. Prompt recognition and intervention is essential in preventing permanent damage.

▢ Monitor intake and output ratios and daily weight. Cloudy or pink urine may be a sign of nephrotoxicity.

▢ Assess patient for signs of superinfection (black, furry overgrowth on tongue, vaginal itching or discharge, loose or foul-smelling stools). Report occurrence to physician.

▪ **Pseudomembranous Colitis:** Assess bowel status (bowel sounds, frequency and consistency of stools, presence of blood in stools) throughout therapy.

▪ **Lab Test Considerations:** Monitor for casts, albumin, or cells in the urine or decreased specific gravity, CBC, and renal function periodically throughout course of therapy.

▢ May cause increased BUN levels.

▪ **Toxicity and Overdose:** Peak serum vancomycin levels should not exceed 5–40 mcg/ml. Trough concentrations should not exceed 5–10 mcg/ml.

POTENTIAL NURSING DIAGNOSES

▪ Infection, high risk for (indications).

▪ Sensory-perceptual alteration: auditory (side effects).

▪ Knowledge deficit related to medication regimen (patient/family teaching).

IMPLEMENTATION

▪ **PO:** Use calibrated measuring device for liquid preparations. IV dosage form may be diluted in 30 ml of water for oral or nasogastric tube administration. Resulting solution has a bitter, unpleasant taste. Stable for 14 days if refrigerated.

▪ **Intermittent Infusion:** Dilute each 500-mg vial with 10 ml of Sterile Water for Injection. Dilute further with 100–200 ml of 0.9% NaCl, D5W, D10W, or lactated Ringer's solution. Solution is stable for 14 days after initial reconstitution if refrigerated. After further dilution, solution is stable for 96 hr if refrigerated.

▪ **Rate:** Administer over 60 min. Do not administer rapidly or as a bolus to minimize risk of thrombophlebitis, hypotension, and red man or red neck syndrome (sudden severe hypotension, flushing and/or maculopapular rash of face, neck, chest, upper extremities). Thrombophlebitis can be minimized by using dilute solutions of 2.5–5 mg/ml and rotating sites.

▪ **Continuous Infusion:** Should be used only if intermittent infusion is not feasible.

▪ **Rate:** May also be prepared as a continuous infusion with 1–2 g in sufficient volume to infuse over 24 hr.

▪ **Syringe Incompatibility:** ▪ heparin.

▪ **Y-Site Compatibility:** ▪ acyclovir ▪ atracurium ▪ cyclophosphamide ▪ enalaprilat ▪ esmolol ▪ fluconazole ▪ fludarabine ▪ hydromorphone ▪ insulin ▪ labetalol ▪ magnesium sulfate ▪ meperidine ▪ methotrexate ▪ morphine ▪ ondansetron ▪ pancuronium ▪ perphenazine ▪ sargramostim ▪ tolazoline ▪ vecuronium ▪ zidovudine.

- **Y-Site Incompatibility:** ▪ foscarnet.
- **Additive Compatibility:** ▪ amikacin ▪ calcium gluconate ▪ cimetidine ▪ dimenhydrinate ▪ hydrocortisone sodium succinate ▪ potassium chloride ▪ ranitidine ▪ vitamin B complex with C.
- **Additive Incompatibility:** ▪ chloramphenicol ▪ chlorothiazide ▪ dexamethasone ▪ methicillin.

PATIENT/FAMILY TEACHING

□ Advise patients on oral vancomycin to take exactly as directed. Missed doses should be taken as soon as remembered, unless almost time for next dose; do not double doses.
□ Instruct patient to report signs of hypersensitivity, tinnitus, vertigo, or hearing loss.
□ Advise patient to notify physician if no improvement is seen in a few days.
□ Patients with a history of rheumatic heart disease or valve replacement need to be taught the importance of using antimicrobial prophylaxis prior to invasive dental or medical procedures.

EVALUATION

Clinical response can be evaluated by:
▪ Resolution of the signs and symptoms of infection. Length of time for complete resolution depends on organism and site of infection ▪ Endocarditis prophylaxis.

VASOPRESSIN
(vay-soe-**press**-in)
Pitressin, {Pressyn}

CLASSIFICATION(S):
Hormone (antidiuretic)
Pregnancy Category UK

INDICATIONS
▪ Treatment of central diabetes insipidus due to deficient antidiuretic hormone.

ACTION
▪ Alters the permeability of the renal collecting ducts, allowing reabsorption of water ▪ Direct stimulant effect on musculature of the GI tract. **Therapeutic Effect:** ▪ Decreased urine output and increased urine osmolality in diabetes insipidus.

PHARMACOKINETICS
Absorption: IM absorption may be unpredictable.
Distribution: Widely distributed throughout extracellular fluid.
Metabolism and Excretion: Rapidly degraded by the liver and kidneys. Small amounts (<5%) excreted unchanged by the kidneys.
Half-life: 10–20 min.

CONTRAINDICATIONS AND PRECAUTIONS
Contraindicated in: ▪ Chronic renal failure with increased BUN ▪ Hypersensitivity to beef or pork proteins.
Use Cautiously in: ▪ Perioperative polyuria (increased sensitivity to vasopressin) ▪ Comatose patients ▪ Seizures ▪ Migraine headaches ▪ Asthma ▪ Heart failure ▪ Cardiovascular disease ▪ Elderly patients and children (increased sensitivity to vasopressin) ▪ Renal impairment.

ADVERSE REACTIONS AND SIDE EFFECTS*
CNS: dizziness, "pounding" sensation in head.
CV: chest pain, MYOCARDIAL INFARCTION, angina.
GI: abdominal cramps, belching, diarrhea, nausea, vomiting, flatulence, heartburn.
Derm: sweating, paleness, perioral blanching.
Neuro: trembling.
Misc: water intoxication (high doses only), fever, allergic reactions.

INTERACTIONS
Drug–Drug: ▪ Antidiuretic effect may

be decreased by concurrent administration of **alcohol, lithium, demeclocycline, heparin,** or **norepinephrine** ▪ Antidiuretic effect may be increased by concurrent administration of **carbamazepine, chlorpropamide, clofibrate,** or **fludrocortisone** ▪ Vasopressor effect may be increased by concurrent administration of **ganglionic blocking agents.**

ROUTE AND DOSAGE

- ▪ **IM, SC (Adults):** 5–10 units 2–3 times daily.
- ▪ **IM, SC (Children):** 2.5–10 units 3–4 times daily.

AVAILABILITY

- ▪ *Injection:* 20 units/ml.

TIME/ACTION PROFILE (antidiuretic effect)

	ONSET	PEAK	DURATION
IM	UK	UK	2–8 hr

NURSING IMPLICATIONS

ASSESSMENT

- ▪ **General Info:** Monitor ECG periodically throughout therapy.
- ▪ **Diabetes Insipidus:** Monitor urine osmolality and urine volume frequently to determine effects of medication. Assess patient for symptoms of dehydration (excessive thirst, dry skin and mucous membranes, tachycardia, poor skin turgor). Weigh patient daily, monitor intake and output, and assess for edema.
- ▪ **Lab Test Considerations:** Monitor urine specific gravity throughout course of therapy.
- □ Monitor serum electrolyte concentrations periodically throughout therapy.
- ▪ **Toxicity and Overdose:** Signs and symptoms of water intoxication include confusion, drowsiness, headache, weight gain, difficulty urinating, seizures, and coma.
- □ Treatment of overdose includes water restriction and temporary discontinuation of vasopressin until polyuria occurs. If symptoms are severe, administration of mannitol, hypertonic dextrose, urea, and/or furosemide may be used.

POTENTIAL NURSING DIAGNOSES

- ▪ Fluid volume deficit (indications).
- ▪ Fluid volume excess (adverse reactions).
- ▪ Knowledge deficit related to medication regimen (patient/family teaching).

IMPLEMENTATION

- ▪ **General Info:** Aqueous vasopressin injection may be administered SC or IM for diabetes insipidus.
- □ Administer 1–2 glasses of water at the time of administration to minimize side effects (blanching of skin, abdominal cramps, nausea).

PATIENT/FAMILY TEACHING

- □ Instruct patient to take medication exactly as directed. Do not use more than the prescribed amount. Missed doses should be taken as soon as remembered, unless almost time for next dose.
- □ Advise patient to drink 1–2 glasses of water at the time of administration to minimize side effects (blanching of skin, abdominal cramps, nausea). Inform patient that these side effects are not serious and usually disappear in a few minutes.
- □ Caution patient to avoid concurrent use of alcohol while taking vasopressin.
- □ Patients with diabetes insipidus should carry identification describing disease process and medication regimen at all times.

EVALUATION

Effectiveness of therapy can be demonstrated by: ▪ Decrease in urine volume □ Relief of polydipsia □ Increased urine osmolality in patients with central diabetes insipidus.

VECURONIUM
(ve-kure-**oh**-nee-yum)
Norcuron

INDICATIONS

• Production of skeletal muscle paralysis and facilitation of intubation after induction of anesthesia in surgical procedures • Used during mechanical ventilation to increase pulmonary compliance.

ACTION

• Prevents neuromuscular transmission by blocking the effect of acetylcholine at the myoneural junction • Has no analgesic or anxiolytic effects. **Therapeutic Effect:** • Skeletal muscle paralysis.

PHARMACOKINETICS

Absorption: Administered IV only, resulting in complete bioavailability.

Distribution: Rapidly distributed in extracellular fluid. Minimal penetration of the CNS.

Metabolism and Excretion: Some metabolism by the liver (20%), with conversion to at least one active metabolite. 35% excreted unchanged by the kidneys.

Half-life: 81–80 min (decreased near term in pregnant patients, increased in patients with hepatic impairment).

CONTRAINDICATIONS AND PRECAUTIONS

Contraindicated in: • Hypersensitivity to vecuronium or bromides • Neonates (if product contains benzyl alcohol).

Use Cautiously in: • Patients with any history of pulmonary or cardiovascular disease or renal or liver impairment • Elderly or debilitated patients • Electrolyte disturbances • Myasthenia gravis or myasthenic syndromes (extreme caution) • Pregnancy or lactation (safety not established) • Infants <7 wk (safety not established) • Children 7 wk–1 yr (increased sensitivity resulting in prolonged recovery time).

ADVERSE REACTIONS AND SIDE EFFECTS*

Most adverse reactions to vecuronium are extensions of pharmacologic effects.

Resp: APNEA, respiratory insufficiency.
MS: muscle weakness.
Misc: allergic reactions.

INTERACTIONS

Drug–Drug: • Intensity and duration of paralysis may be prolonged by pretreatment with **succinylcholine, general anesthesia, aminoglycoside antibiotics, polymyxin B, colistin, clindamycin, lidocaine, quinidine, procainamide, beta-adrenergic blocking agents, potassium-losing diuretics,** and **magnesium** • Additive neuromuscular blockade with **inhalation anesthetics**—decrease vecuronium dose by 15% when used with **enflurane** or **isoflurane,** and decrease dose of anesthetic by 30–50%.

ROUTE AND DOSAGE

• **IV (Adults and Children >10 yr):** 80–100 mcg/kg for intubation. 60–85 mcg/kg if given after steady-state anesthesia achieved or 40–60 mcg/kg after succinylcholine-assisted intubation and anesthesia (wait for disappearance of succinylcholine effects) or 50–60 mcg/kg during balanced anesthesia. Up to 150–280 mcg/kg has been used in some patients. Then maintenance dose of 10–15 mcg/kg 25–40 min after initial dose, then q 12–15 min as needed or as a continuous infusion at 1 mcg/kg/min (range 0.8–1.2 mcg/kg/min).

AVAILABILITY

• *Injection:* 10-mg vial.

TIME/ACTION PROFILE (skeletal muscle paralysis)

	ONSET	PEAK	DURATION
IV	1 min	3–5 min	15–25 min

NURSING IMPLICATIONS

ASSESSMENT

□ Assess respiratory status continuously throughout use of vecuronium. Notify physician of significant changes immediately.

□ Neuromuscular response to vecuronium should be monitored intraoperatively with a peripheral nerve stimulator. Paralysis is initially selective and usually occurs consecutively in the following muscles: levator muscles of eyelids, muscles of mastication, limb muscles, abdominal muscles, muscles of the glottis, intercostal muscles, and the diaphragm. Recovery of muscle function usually occurs in reverse order.

□ Monitor ECG, heart rate, and blood pressure throughout use of vecuronium.

□ Observe patient for residual muscle weakness and respiratory distress during the recovery period.

■ **Toxicity and Overdose:** If overdose occurs use peripheral nerve stimulator to determine the degree of neuromuscular blockade. Maintain airway patency and ventilation until recovery of normal respiration occurs.

□ Administer anticholinesterase agents (edrophonium, neostigmine, pyridostigmine) to antagonize the action of vecuronium. Atropine is usually administered prior to or concurrently with anticholinesterase agents to counteract the muscarinic effects.

□ Administration of fluids and vasopressors may be necessary to treat severe hypotension or shock.

POTENTIAL NURSING DIAGNOSES

■ Breathing pattern, ineffective (indications).

■ Communication, impaired verbal (side effects).

■ Fear (patient/family teaching).

IMPLEMENTATION

■ **General Info:** Vecuronium should be used only by individuals experienced in endotracheal intubation, and equipment for this procedure should be immediately available.

□ Vecuronium has no effect on consciousness or the pain threshold. Adequate anesthesia should *always* be used when vecuronium is used as an adjunct to surgical procedures or when painful procedures are performed. Benzodiazepines and/or analgesics should be administered concurrently when prolonged vecuronium therapy is used for ventilator patients, as patient is awake and able to feel all sensations.

□ If eyes remain open throughout prolonged administration, protect corneas with artificial tears.

■ **IV:** Reconstitute vecuronium with bacteriostatic water (may be provided by manufacturer), D5W, 0.9% NaCl, D5/0.9% NaCl, or lactated Ringer's injection. Solution reconstituted with bacteriostatic water is stable if refrigerated for 5 days. If other diluents are used, solution is stable for 24 hr if refrigerated. Discard all unused solution.

■ **Direct IV:** Reconstitute each dose in 5–10 ml. Titrate dose according to patient response.

■ **Continuous Infusion:** Dilute vecuronium to a concentration of 10–20 mg/100 ml.

■ *Rate:* Titrate rate of infusion according to patient response.

■ **Syringe/Y-Site Incompatibility:** Incompatible in syringe or via Y-site injection with most barbiturates.

■ **Y-Site Compatibility:** ■ aminophylline ■ cefazolin ■ cefuroxime ■ cimetidine ■ dopamine ■ epinephrine ■ esmolol ■ fentanyl ■ gentamicin ■ heparin ■ hydrocortisone sodium succinate ■ isoproterenol ■ lorazepam ■ midazolam ■ morphine ■ nitroglycerin ■ nitroprusside ■ ranitidine ■ trimethoprim/sulfamethoxazole ■ vancomycin.

PATIENT/FAMILY TEACHING

□ Explain all procedures to patient receiving vecuronium therapy without anesthesia, as consciousness is not affected by vecuronium alone. Provide emotional support.

□ Reassure patient that communication abilities will return as the medication wears off.

EVALUATION
Effectiveness of therapy can be demonstrated by: ▪ Adequate suppression of the twitch response when tested with peripheral nerve stimulation and subsequent muscle paralysis.

VERAPAMIL
(ver-**ap**-a-mil)
Calan, Calan SR, Isoptin, Isoptin SR, Verelan

CLASSIFICATION(S):
Calcium channel blocker, Antianginal, Antihypertensive, Antiarrhythmic (group IV), Coronary vasodilator
Pregnancy Category C

INDICATIONS

▪ **PO:** Treatment of angina pectoris
▪ **PO:** Management of hypertension
▪ **PO, IV:** Control of supraventricular tachyarrhythmias and rapid ventricular rates in atrial flutter or fibrillation. **Unlabeled Uses:** ▪ Relief of ventricular outflow obstruction in the management of hypertrophic cardiomyopathy ▪ Prevention of migraine headaches.

ACTION

▪ Inhibits calcium transport into myocardial and vascular smooth muscle cells, resulting in inhibition of excitation-contraction coupling and subsequent contraction ▪ Decreases SA and AV conduction and prolongs the AV node refractory periods in cardiac conduction tissue. **Therapeutic Effects:** ▪ Coronary vasodilation, resulting in decreased frequency and severity of angina pectoris ▪ Decreased blood pressure ▪ Suppression of supraventricular tachyarrhythmias.

PHARMACOKINETICS

Absorption: Well absorbed following oral administration.

Distribution: Distribution not known. Small amounts enter breast milk.
Metabolism and Excretion: Mostly metabolized by the liver, much of it on first pass through the liver.
Half-life: 4.5–12 hr.

CONTRAINDICATIONS AND PRECAUTIONS

Contraindicated in: ▪ Hypersensitivity ▪ Sinus bradycardia ▪ Advanced heart block ▪ Severe congestive heart failure.
Use Cautiously in: ▪ Liver disease or elderly patients (dosage reduction recommended) ▪ Pregnancy, lactation, or children (safety not established) ▪ Hypertrophic cardiomyopathy (when accompanied by paroxysmal nocturnal dyspnea, orthopnea, left ventricular obstruction, SA node dysfunction, heart block, or elevated pulmonary wedge pressure) ▪ Congestive heart failure ▪ Sick-sinus syndrome ▪ Duchenne's muscular dystrophy (may precipitate respiratory muscle failure).

ADVERSE REACTIONS AND SIDE EFFECTS*

CNS: dizziness, headache, fatigue.
CV: bradycardia, hypotension, edema, heart block, congestive heart failure, SINUS ARREST, ASYSTOLE.
GI: constipation, nausea, abdominal discomfort.
Resp: pulmonary edema.

INTERACTIONS

Drug–Drug: ▪ Increases serum digoxin levels and may cause toxicity ▪ Increased risk of bradycardia, congestive heart failure, and arrhythmias when used with **beta-adrenergic blocking agents** or **disopyramide** ▪ Additive hypotension with **antihypertensive agents,** acute ingestion of **alcohol, nitrates,** or **quinidine** ▪ Decreases effectiveness of oral **rifampin** ▪ Increases muscle relaxant effects of **nondepolarizing neuromuscular blockers** ▪ Coadministration with **calcium** and **vitamin D** may result in decreased effectivenes of verapamil ▪ May increase or decrease

V

lithium blood levels ▪ Verapamil may decrease metabolism of and increase risk of toxicity from **carbamazepine, cyclosporine, prazosin,** or **quinidine** ▪ Increases anesthetic effect of **etodimate** ▪ Severe hypotension may occur with **fentanyl** ▪ May increase risk of toxicity from **theophylline**.

ROUTE AND DOSAGE

- **PO (Adults):** 80–120 mg 3 times daily, increased in daily or weekly intervals as needed; initial dose of 40 mg 3 times daily in patients with hepatic impairment, poor left ventricular function, or the elderly, or 120–240 mg/day as a single dose of extended-release preparation increased in daily or weekly intervals as needed (range 240–480 mg/day).
- **PO (Children):** 4–8 mg/kg/day in divided doses.
- **IV (Adults):** 5–10 mg (75–150 mg/kg) over 2 min, may repeat 10 mg in 30 min.
- **IV (Children 1–16 yr):** 100–300 mcg/kg over 2 min (with ECG monitoring), may repeat in 30 min. Initial dose not to exceed 5 mg, repeat dose not to exceed 10 mg.
- **IV (Children <1 yr):** 100–200 mcg/kg over 2 min (with ECG monitoring), may repeat in 30 min.

AVAILABILITY

▪ *Tablets:* 40 mg, 80 mg, 120 mg ▪ *Sustained-release tablets:* 120 mg, 180 mg, 240 mg ▪ *Sustained-release capsules:* 120 mg, 180 mg, 240 mg ▪ *Injection:* 2.5 mg/ml.

TIME/ACTION PROFILE
(cardiovascular effects)

	ONSET	PEAK	DURATION
PO	1–2 hr	30–90 min*	3–7 hr
PO-SR	UK	5–7 hr	24 hr
IV	1–5 min†	3–5 min	2 hr†

*Single dose; effects from multiple doses may not be evident for 24–48 hr.
†Antiarrhythmic effects; hemodynamic effects begin 3–5 min following injection and persist for 10–20 min.

NURSING IMPLICATIONS

ASSESSMENT

- **General Info:** Monitor blood pressure and pulse before and frequently during parenteral administration and periodically throughout therapy.
- ☐ Monitor intake and output ratios and daily weight. Assess patient for signs of congestive heart failure (peripheral edema, rales/crackles, dyspnea, weight gain, jugular venous distention).
- ☐ Patients receiving cardiac glycosides concurrently with verapamil should have routine serum digitalis levels and be monitored for signs and symptoms of cardiac glycoside toxicity.
- ☐ Monitor ECG periodically in patients receiving long-term therapy.
- **Angina:** Assess location, duration, intensity, and precipitating factors of patient's anginal pain.
- **Arrhythmias:** ECG should be monitored continuously during IV administration. Notify physician of symptomatic bradycardia or prolonged hypotension promptly. Emergency equipment and medication should be available.
- **Lab Test Considerations:** May cause elevated alkaline phosphatase, CPK, LDH, AST (SGOT), and ALT (SGPT) levels.

POTENTIAL NURSING DIAGNOSES

- Cardiac output, decreased (indications).
- Pain (indications).
- Knowledge deficit related to medication regimen (patient/family teaching).

IMPLEMENTATION

- **PO:** Administer with meals or milk to minimize gastric irritation.
- ☐ Sustained-release tablets should be swallowed whole or broken in half; do not crush or chew.
- **IV:** Patients should remain recumbent for at least 1 hr following IV administration to minimize hypotensive effects.
- **Direct IV:** Administer IV undiluted

VIDARABINE 1221

through Y-site or 3-way stopcock over 2 min for each single dose. Administer over 3 min in elderly patients.

- **Syringe Compatibility:** ▪ amrinone ▪ heparin ▪ milrinone.
- **Y-Site Compatibility:** ▪ amrinone ▪ dobutamine ▪ dopamine ▪ famotidine ▪ hydralazine ▪ meperidine ▪ methicillin ▪ milrinone ▪ penicillin G potassium ▪ piperacillin ▪ ticarcillin.
- **Y-Site Incompatibility:** ▪ albumin ▪ ampicillin ▪ mezlocillin ▪ nafcillin ▪ oxacillin ▪ sodium bicarbonate.

PATIENT/FAMILY TEACHING

- **General Info:** Advise patient to take medication exactly as directed, even if feeling well. Missed doses should be taken as soon as remembered, unless almost time for next dose; do not double doses. Do not discontinue therapy without consulting physician, as gradual dosage reduction may be necessary.
- □ Instruct patient or family members to take pulse each day before taking verapamil. Advise patient to notify physician if pulse is irregular or <50 bpm.
- □ Caution patient to make position changes slowly to minimize orthostatic hypotension.
- □ Verapamil may cause dizziness. Advise patient to avoid driving or other activities requiring alertness until response to the medication is known.
- □ Instruct patient to avoid concurrent use of alcohol or over-the-counter medications without consulting physician or pharmacist.
- □ Instruct patient to notify physician if headache is severe or persistent.
- **Angina:** Instruct patients on concurrent nitrate therapy to continue taking both medications as ordered and using SL nitroglycerin as needed for anginal attacks.
- □ Advise patient to contact physician if chest pain worsens or does not improve after therapy or is accompanied by diaphoresis or shortness of breath, or if severe, persistent headache occurs.

- □ Advise patient to discuss activity limitations with physician.
- **Hypertension:** Instruct patient and family on correct method for monitoring blood pressure weekly. Advise patient to notify physician if significant changes occur.
- □ Encourage patient to comply with additional interventions for hypertension (low-sodium diet, regular exercise, weight reduction, stress management, moderation of alcohol consumption, discontinuation of smoking). Verapamil controls but does not cure hypertension.

EVALUATION

Effectiveness of therapy can be demonstrated by: ▪ Decrease in frequency and severity of anginal attacks □ Decreased need for nitrate therapy □ Increase in activity tolerance and sense of well-being ▪ Decrease in blood pressure to normal limits ▪ Resolution and prevention of supraventricular tachyarrhythmias.

VIDARABINE
(vye-**dare**-a-been)
adenine arabinoside, Ara-A, Vira-A

V

CLASSIFICATION(S):
Antiviral
Pregnancy Category C

INDICATIONS

▪ **IV:** Treatment of □ Herpes simplex encephalitis □ Serious herpes simplex infections in neonates □ Herpes zoster due to reactivated varicella-zoster in immunosuppressed patients ▪ **Ophth:** Treatment of herpes simplex keratitis and keratoconjunctivitis. **Unlabeled Use:** ▪ Treatment of varicella-zoster infections in immunosuppressed patients.

ACTION

▪ Appears to inhibit viral DNA synthesis. **Therapeutic Effect:** ▪ Decreased viral replication.

PHARMACOKINETICS

Absorption: Complete bioavailability follows IV administration. No apparent systemic absorption following ophthalmic administration.

Distribution: Widely distributed. Crosses the blood–brain barrier well.

Metabolism and Excretion: 75–90% converted to another active antiviral compound (ara-HX). Both are excreted by the kidneys.

Half-life: Vidarabine—1.5 hr; ara-HX—3.3 hr (both increased in renal impairment).

CONTRAINDICATIONS AND PRECAUTIONS

Contraindicated in: ▪ Hypersensitivity. **Use Cautiously in:** ▪ Impaired renal function (dosage reduction required) ▪ Impaired hepatic function ▪ Patients susceptible to fluid overload or cerebral edema.

ADVERSE REACTIONS AND SIDE EFFECTS*

CNS: malaise, weakness, tremors, ataxia, hallucinations, psychoses, confusion, headache, encephalopathy.

Derm: pruritus, rash.

EENT: Ophth—ocular burning, itching, irritation, blurred vision, photophobia.

F and E: hyponatremia, fluid overload.

GI: <u>nausea</u>, <u>vomiting</u>, <u>anorexia</u>, <u>weight loss</u>, diarrhea, <u>GI bleeding</u>, hepatitis.

Hemat: anemia, leukopenia, thrombocytopenia.

Local: phlebitis at IV site.

INTERACTIONS

Drug–Drug: ▪ Concurrent use with **allopurinol** may increase the risk of adverse reactions (tremors, anemia, nausea, pain, and pruritus).

ROUTE AND DOSAGE

Herpes Simplex Encephalitis

▪ **IV (Adults and Children):** 15 mg/kg/day for 10 days.

Herpes Simplex Keratitis or Keratoconjunctivitis

▪ **Ophth (Adults and Children):** Instill ointment in lower conjunctival sac 5 times daily (q 3 hr), decreased to twice daily when healing has occurred.

Herpes Zoster in Immunosuppressed Patients

▪ **IV (Adults and Children):** 10 mg/kg/day for 5 days.

Herpes Simplex Virus Infections in Neonates

▪ **IV (Neonates):** 15 mg/kg/day for 10 days.

AVAILABILITY

▪ *Suspension for injection:* 200 mg/ml in 5-ml vials ▪ *Ophthalmic ointment:* 3%.

TIME/ACTION PROFILE (blood levels)

	ONSET	PEAK	DURATION
IV	rapid	end of infusion	UK

NURSING IMPLICATIONS

ASSESSMENT

▪ **Ophth:** Assess eye lesions prior to and daily during therapy.

▪ **Encephalitis:** Assess level of consciousness and neurologic status frequently throughout therapy.

▫ Assess patient for fluid overload (rales/crackles, dyspnea, weight gain, peripheral edema, jugular venous distention) during IV infusions.

▪ **Lab Test Considerations:** May cause elevation of AST (SGOT) and total bilirubin.

▫ Monitor CBC, WBC, and platelet count periodically throughout therapy.

▫ May cause decreased leukocytes, platelets, reticulocytes, hemoglobin, and hematocrit. These effects are usually reversible 3–5 days after discontinuation of therapy.

POTENTIAL NURSING DIAGNOSES

▪ Infection, high risk for (indications).

---

*Underlines indicate most frequent; **CAPITALS** indicate life-threatening.

- Skin integrity, impaired (indications).
- Knowledge deficit related to medication regimen (patient/family teaching).

IMPLEMENTATION
- **Intermittent Infusion:** Any IV solution is suitable as a diluent, except for blood products or protein solution. Prewarm the IV solution to 35–40°C (95–100°F) to facilitate dilution of the suspension. Shake until completely clear and in solution. Use an in-line filter (0.45-micron pore size or smaller) for final filtration. Dilute just prior to administration and use within 48 hr. Do not refrigerate solution.
  □ For adults, dilute each 1 mg of vidarabine in 2.22 ml of solution (450 mg requires 1 liter). Depending on dose, may require more than 1 liter of solution.
  □ For neonates, dilute each 200 mg (1 ml) of vidarabine in 9 ml of 0.9% NaCl or Sterile Water for Injection, for a concentration of 20 mg/ml. Withdraw dose from diluted suspension and dilute further in minimum volume (2.22 ml IV fluid per mg of vidarabine).
- **Rate:** Administer total daily dose for both adults and neonates over 12–24 hr using an infusion pump for accurate rate regulation.

PATIENT/FAMILY TEACHING
- **Ophth:** Instruct patient on correct application technique for ophthalmic vidarabine (see Appendix H).
  □ Instruct patient to instill vidarabine as directed and not to use more frequently or longer than directed. Missed doses should be instilled as soon as remembered, unless almost time for next dose. Advise patient not to discontinue use of ointment without consulting physician. Patient should also contact physician if no improvement is seen in 7 days, condition worsens, or pain, burning, or irritation of the eye occurs.

  □ Ointment may cause blurred vision. Caution patient to avoid driving or other activities requiring visual acuity until vision has cleared.
  □ Advise patient to wear dark glasses and avoid bright lights to prevent photophobic reactions.
  □ Patients with ophthalmic infections should be advised to avoid wearing contact lenses until the infection is resolved and physician approves.
  □ Emphasize the importance of follow-up ophthalmic examinations to determine progress.

EVALUATION
Effectiveness of therapy can be demonstrated by: ■ Re-epithelialization of the cornea in herpetic keratitis. Treatment is not usually continued for more than 21 days or 3–5 days after healing has occurred, except in chronic cases or infections that are difficult to cure ■ Resolution of the signs and symptoms of herpetic encephalitis.

VINBLASTINE
(vin-**blass**-teen)
Alkaban-AQ, Velban, {Velbe}, Velsar

CLASSIFICATION(S):
Antineoplastic agent (vinca alkaloid)
Pregnancy Category UK

INDICATIONS
■ Combination chemotherapy of: □ Lymphomas □ Nonseminomatous testicular carcinoma □ Advanced breast cancer □ Other tumors.

ACTION
■ Binds to proteins of mitotic spindle, causing metaphase arrest. Cell replication is stopped as a result (cell cycle-specific for M phase). **Therapeutic Effects:** ■ Death of rapidly replicating cells, particularly malignant ones ■ Has immunosuppressive properties.

PHARMACOKINETICS

Absorption: Administered IV only, resulting in complete bioavailability.
Distribution: Does not cross the blood-brain barrier well.
Metabolism and Excretion: Converted by the liver to an active antineoplastic compound. Excreted in the feces via biliary excretion, some renal elimination.
Half-life: 24 hr.

CONTRAINDICATIONS AND PRECAUTIONS

Contraindicated in: ▪ Hypersensitivity ▪ Pregnancy or lactation.
Use Cautiously in: ▪ Patients with childbearing potential ▪ Infections ▪ Decreased bone marrow reserve ▪ Other chronic debilitating illnesses ▪ Patients with impaired hepatic function (decrease dose by 50% if serum bilirubin >3 mg/dl).

ADVERSE REACTIONS AND SIDE EFFECTS*

CNS: neurotoxicity, depression, weakness, seizures.
Resp: BRONCHOSPASM.
GI: nausea, vomiting, anorexia, diarrhea, stomatitis, constipation.
GU: gonadal suppression.
Derm: dermatitis, vesiculation, alopecia.
Hemat: anemia, leukopenia, thrombocytopenia.
Local: phlebitis at IV site.
Metab: hyperuricemia.
Neuro: peripheral neuropathy, paresthesia, neuritis.

INTERACTIONS

Drug–Drug: ▪ Additive bone marrow depression with other **antineoplastic agents** or **radiation therapy** ▪ Bronchospasm may occur in patients who have been previously treated with **mitomycin** ▪ May decrease antibody response to **live virus vaccines** and increase the risk of adverse reactions.

ROUTE AND DOSAGE

Doses may vary greatly depending on tumor, schedule, condition of patient, and blood counts.
▪ **IV (Adults):** 3.7 mg/m^2 (100 mcg/kg), single dose; increase at weekly intervals as tolerated by 1.8 mg/m^2 (50 mcg/kg) to a maximum of 18.5 mg/m^2 (usual dose is 5.5–7.4 mg/m^2). Maintenance dose 10 mg 1–2 times monthly or one increment less than last dose q 7–14 days.
▪ **IV (Children):** 2.5 mg/m^2, single dose; increase as tolerated at weekly intervals by 1.25 mg/m^2 to a maximum of 7.5 mg/m^2. Maintenance dose is 1 increment less than last dose q 7–14 days.

AVAILABILITY

▪ *Injection:* 10-mg vials.

TIME/ACTION PROFILE (effects on white blood cell counts)

	ONSET	PEAK	DURATION
IV	5–7 days	10 days	7–14 days

NURSING IMPLICATIONS

ASSESSMENT

▢ Monitor blood pressure, pulse, and respiratory rate during course of therapy. Notify physician immediately if respiratory distress occurs. Bronchospasm can be life-threatening and may occur at time of infusion or several hours later.
▢ Assess for fever, sore throat, and signs of infection. Notify physician if these symptoms occur.
▢ Assess for bleeding (bleeding gums, bruising, petechiae, guaiac stools, urine, and emesis). Avoid IM injections and rectal temperatures. Apply pressure to venipuncture sites for 10 min.
▢ May cause nausea and vomiting. Monitor intake and output, appetite, and nutritional intake. Confer with physician regarding prophylactic use of an antiemetic. Adjust diet as tolerated.
▢ Assess injection site frequently for

*Underlines indicate most frequent; **CAPITALS** indicate life-threatening.

redness, irritation, or inflammation. If extravasation occurs infusion must be stopped and restarted elsewhere to avoid damage to SC tissue. Standard treatment includes application of heat.

□ Monitor for symptoms of gout (increased uric acid, joint pain, edema). Encourage patient to drink at least 2 liters of fluid per day. Physician may order allopurinol or alkalinization of urine to decrease uric acid levels.

□ Anemia may occur. Monitor for increased fatigue and dyspnea.

■ **Lab Test Considerations:** Monitor CBC prior to and routinely throughout course of therapy. Notify physician if WBC <2000; subsequent doses are usually withheld until WBC is at least 4000. The nadir of leukopenia occurs in 5–10 days and recovery usually occurs 7–14 days later. Thrombocytopenia may also occur in patients who have received radiation or other chemotherapy agents.

□ Monitor liver function studies (AST [SGOT], ALT [SGPT], LDH, bilirubin) and renal function studies (BUN, creatinine) prior to and periodically throughout therapy.

□ May cause increased uric acid. Monitor periodically during therapy.

POTENTIAL NURSING DIAGNOSES

■ Infection, high risk for (adverse reactions).
■ Nutrition, altered: less than body requirements (adverse reactions).
■ Knowledge deficit related to medication regimen (patient/family teaching).

IMPLEMENTATION

■ **General Info:** Solution should be prepared in a biologic cabinet. Wear gloves, gown, and mask while handling medication. Discard IV equipment in specially designated containers (see Appendix I).

■ **Direct IV:** Dilute each 10 mg with 10 ml of 0.9% NaCl for injection with phenol or benzyl alcohol. Reconstituted medication is stable for 30 days if refrigerated.

■ *Rate:* Administer each single dose over 1 min through Y-site injection or 3-way stopcock of a free-flowing infusion of 0.9% NaCl or D5W.

■ **Intermittent Infusion:** May be further diluted with 50–100 ml of 0.9% NaCl.

■ *Rate:* Administer over 15–30 min. Administering medication over a longer period or with more diluent may increase irritation of vein.

■ **Syringe Compatibility:** ■ bleomycin ■ cisplatin ■ cyclophosphamide ■ droperidol ■ fluorouracil ■ leucovorin calcium ■ methotrexate ■ metoclopramide ■ mitomycin ■ vincristine.

■ **Y-Site Compatibility:** ■ bleomycin ■ cisplatin ■ cyclophosphamide ■ doxorubicin ■ droperidol ■ fludarabine ■ fluorouracil ■ heparin ■ leucovorin calcium ■ methotrexate ■ metoclopramide ■ mitomycin ■ ondansetron ■ sargramostim ■ vincristine.

■ **Y-Site Incompatibility:** ■ furosemide.

PATIENT/FAMILY TEACHING

□ Advise patient to notify physician if fever, chills, sore throat, signs of infection, bleeding gums, bruising, petechiae, or blood in urine, stool, or emesis occurs. Caution patient to avoid crowds and persons with known infections. Instruct patient to use soft toothbrush and electric razor. Caution patient not to drink alcoholic beverages or take products containing aspirin or ibuprofen.

□ Instruct patient to inspect oral mucosa for redness and ulceration. If ulceration occurs advise patient to avoid spicy foods, use sponge brush, and rinse mouth with water after eating and drinking. Viscous lidocaine swishes may be used if mouth pain interferes with eating.

□ Instruct patient to report symptoms of neurotoxicity (paresthesia, pain, difficulty walking, persistent constipation).

□ Advise patient that this medication may have teratogenic effects. Contraception should be used during and for at least 2 mon after therapy is concluded.

□ Discuss with patient the possibility of hair loss. Explore coping strategies.

□ Instruct patient not to receive any vaccinations without advice of physician.

□ Emphasize need for periodic lab tests to monitor for side effects.

EVALUATION

Effectiveness of therapy can be demonstrated by: ■ Regression of malignancy without the appearance of detrimental side effects.

VINCRISTINE
(vin-**kriss**-teen)
Oncovin, Vincasar PFS

CLASSIFICATION(S):
Antineoplastic agent (vinca alkaloid)
Pregnancy Category D

INDICATIONS

■ Used alone and in combination with other treatment modalities (antineoplastic agents, surgery, or radiation therapy) in the treatment of: □ Hodgkin's disease □ Leukemias □ Neuroblastoma □ Malignant lymphomas □ Rhabdomyosarcoma □ Wilms' tumor □ Other tumors.

ACTION

■ Binds to proteins of mitotic spindle, causing metaphase arrest ■ Cell replication is stopped as a result (cell cycle-specific for M phase) ■ Has little or no effect on bone marrow. **Therapeutic Effects:** ■ Death of rapidly replicating cells, particularly malignant ones ■ Has immunosuppressive properties.

PHARMACOKINETICS

Absorption: Administered IV only, resulting in complete bioavailability.
Distribution: Rapidly and widely distributed.
Metabolism and Excretion: Metabolized by the liver and eliminated in the feces via biliary excretion.
Half-life: 10.5–37.5 hr.

CONTRAINDICATIONS AND PRECAUTIONS

Contraindicated in: ■ Hypersensitivity ■ Pregnancy or lactation.
Use Cautiously in: ■ Patients with childbearing potential ■ Infections ■ Decreased bone marrow reserve ■ Other chronic debilitating illnesses ■ Hepatic impairment (dosage reduction recommended if serum bilirubin >3 mg/dl).

ADVERSE REACTIONS AND SIDE EFFECTS*

CNS: mental status changes, depression, agitation, insomnia.
Resp: bronchospasm.
GI: nausea, vomiting, anorexia, stomatitis, constipation, ileus, abdominal cramps.
GU: urinary retention, nocturia, oliguria, gonadal suppression.
Derm: alopecia.
Endo: syndrome of inappropriate secretion of antidiuretic hormone (SIADH).
Hemat: anemia, leukopenia, thrombocytopenia (mild and brief).
Local: phlebitis at IV site.
Metab: hyperuricemia.
Neuro: neurotoxicity (ascending peripheral neuropathy).

INTERACTIONS

Drug–Drug: ■ Bronchospasm may occur in patients who have been previously treated with **mitomycin** ■ **L-asparaginase** may decrease hepatic metabolism of vincristine (give vincristine 12–24 hr prior to asparaginase) ■ May decrease antibody response to **live virus vaccines** and increase the risk of adverse reactions.

ROUTE AND DOSAGE

Many other protocols are used.

■ **IV (Adults):** 10–30 mcg/kg (0.4–1.4 mg/m^2), may repeat weekly (not to exceed 2 mg each dose).
■ **IV (Children >10 kg):** 1.5–2 mg/m^2 single dose, may repeat weekly.
■ **IV (Children <10 kg):** 50 mcg/kg single dose, may repeat weekly.

*Underlines indicate most frequent; **CAPITALS** indicate life-threatening.

AVAILABILITY

- *Injection:* 1 mg/ml in 1-ml, 2-ml, 5-ml vials.

TIME/ACTION PROFILE (effects on blood counts, which are usually mild)

	ONSET	PEAK	DURATION
IV	UK	UK	7 days

NURSING IMPLICATIONS

ASSESSMENT

- ◻ Monitor blood pressure, pulse, and respiratory rate during course of therapy. Notify physician of significant changes.
- ◻ Monitor neurologic status. Assess for paresthesia (numbness, tingling, pain); loss of deep tendon reflexes (Achilles reflex is usually first involved); weakness (wrist or foot drop, gait disturbances); cranial nerve palsies (jaw pain, hoarseness, ptosis, visual changes); autonomic dysfunction (ileus, difficulty voiding, orthostatic hypotension; impaired sweating); and CNS dysfunction (decreased level of consciousness, agitation, hallucinations). Notify physician if these symptoms develop, as they may persist for months.
- ◻ Monitor intake and output ratios and weight; inform physician if significant discrepancies occur. Decreased urine output with concurrent hyponatremia may indicate SIADH, which usually responds to fluid restriction.
- ◻ Assess infusion site frequently for redness, irritation, or inflammation. If extravasation occurs, infusion must be stopped and restarted elsewhere to avoid damage to SC tissue. Standard treatment includes application of heat and local injection of hyaluronidase.
- ◻ Assess nutritional status. An antiemetic may be ordered to minimize nausea and vomiting.
- ◻ Monitor for symptoms of gout (increased uric acid, joint pain, edema). Encourage patient to drink at least 2 liters of fluid per day. Physician may order allopurinol or alkalinization of urine to decrease uric acid levels.
- **Lab Test Considerations:** Monitor CBC prior to and periodically throughout course of therapy. May cause slight leukopenia 4 days after therapy, which resolves within 7 days. Platelet count may increase or decrease.
- ◻ Monitor liver function studies (AST [SGOT], ALT [SGPT], LDH, bilirubin) and renal function studies (BUN, creatinine) prior to and periodically throughout therapy.
- ◻ May cause increased uric acid. Monitor periodically during therapy.

POTENTIAL NURSING DIAGNOSES

- Injury, high risk for (adverse reactions).
- Nutrition, altered: less than body requirements (adverse reactions).
- Knowledge deficit related to medication regimen (patient/family teaching).

IMPLEMENTATION

- **General Info:** Solution should be prepared in a biologic cabinet. Wear gloves, gown, and mask while handling medication. Discard IV equipment in specially designated containers (see Appendix I).
- ◻ Do not administer SC, IM, or IT. Intrathecal administration is fatal.
- **Direct IV:** Manufacturer does not recommend dilution in solutions that alter the pH; mix only with 0.9% NaCl or D5W.
- **Rate:** Administer each dose direct IV push over 1 min through Y-site injection or 3-way stopcock of a free-flowing infusion of 0.9% NaCl or D5W.
- **Syringe Compatibility:** ▪ bleomycin ▪ cisplatin ▪ cyclophosphamide ▪ doxapram ▪ doxorubicin ▪ droperidol ▪ fluorouracil ▪ heparin ▪ leucovorin calcium ▪ methotrexate ▪ metoclopramide ▪ mitomycin ▪ vinblastine.
- **Syringe Incompatibility:** ▪ furosemide.
- **Y-Site Compatibility:** ▪ bleomycin ▪ cisplatin ▪ cyclophosphamide ▪ doxorubicin ▪ droperidol ▪ fludarabine

- fluorouracil ▪ heparin ▪ leucovorin calcium ▪ methotrexate ▪ metoclopramide ▪ mitomycin ▪ ondansetron ▪ sargramostim ▪ vinblastine.
- **Y-Site Incompatibility:** ▪ furosemide.

PATIENT/FAMILY TEACHING

▢ Instruct patient to report symptoms of neurotoxicity (paresthesia, pain, difficulty walking, persistent constipation).

▢ Inform patient that increased fluid intake, dietary fiber, and exercise may minimize constipation. Physician may order stool softeners or laxatives. Patient should inform physician if severe constipation or abdominal discomfort occurs, as this may be a sign of neuropathy.

▢ Advise patient to notify physician if fever, chills, sore throat, signs of infection, bleeding gums, bruising, petechiae; blood in urine, stool, or emesis; or mouth sores occur. Caution patient to avoid crowds and persons with known infections.

▢ Advise patient that this medication may have teratogenic effects. Contraception should be used during and for at least 2 mo after therapy is concluded.

▢ Discuss with patient the possibility of hair loss. Explore coping strategies.

▢ Instruct patient not to receive any vaccinations without advice of physician.

▢ Emphasize need for periodic lab tests to monitor for side effects.

EVALUATION
Effectiveness of therapy can be demonstrated by: ▪ Regression of malignancy without the appearance of detrimental side effects.

VITAMIN A
(vye-ta-min A)
Aquasol A, Del-Vi-A

CLASSIFICATION(S):
Vitamin (fat-soluble)
Pregnancy Category X

INDICATIONS

▪ Treatment and prevention of deficiency states ▪ Prevention of vitamin A deficiency in patients who have fat malabsorption or are taking bile acid sequestrants.

ACTION

▪ Serves as a cofactor in many biochemical processes ▪ Necessary for growth, bone development, vision, reproduction and integrity of mucosal and epithelial surfaces, and formation of visual pigment. **Therapeutic Effects:** ▪ Resolution of signs of deficiency ▪ Prevention of deficiency.

PHARMACOKINETICS

Absorption: GI absorption requires bile acids, fat, lipase, and protein. Aqueous preparations are absorbed more readily than emulsions.
Distribution: Stored primarily in the liver (2-yr supply), small amounts stored in kidneys and lungs. Does not cross the placenta but enters breast milk.
Metabolism and Excretion: Mostly metabolized by the liver.
Half-life: UK.

CONTRAINDICATIONS AND PRECAUTIONS

Contraindicated in: ▪ Hypervitaminosis A ▪ Malabsorption (oral products) ▪ Hypersensitivity to ingredients in preparations (chlorobutanol, polysorbate 80, butylated hydroxyanisole, butylated hydroxytoluene).
Use Cautiously in: ▪ Lactation (supplements to infant necessary) ▪ Pregnancy (avoid amounts greater than RDA; see Appendix L) ▪ Severely impaired renal function.

ADVERSE REACTIONS AND SIDE EFFECTS*

Misc: hypervitaminosis A syndrome.

INTERACTIONS

Drug–Drug: ▪ **Cholestyramine, colestipol,** and **mineral oil** decrease absorp-

---

*Underlines indicate most frequent; CAPITALS indicate life-threatening.

tion of vitamin A ▪ **Oral contraceptives** increase plasma levels of vitamin A.

ROUTE AND DOSAGE

- **PO (Adults):** 100,000 units/day for 3 days, then 25,000–50,000 units/day for 14 days. If xerophthalmia is present, dose is 25,000–50,000 units/day.
- **PO (Children 1–8 yr):** 10,000 units/kg/day for 5 days, then 17,000–35,000 units/day for 10 days. If xerophthalmia is present, dose is 5000 units/kg/day for 5 days, then IM vitamin A is added to regimen.
- **PO (Children <1 yr):** 10,000 units/kg/day for 5 days, then 7500–15,000 units/day for 10 days.
- **IM (Adults):** 50,000–100,000 units/day for 3 days, then 50,000 units/day for 2 wk.
- **IM (Children 1–8 yr):** 5000–35,000 units/day for 10 days.
- **IM (Children <1 yr):** 5000–15,000 units/day for 10 days.
- **IV (Adults and Children):** Infused as part of TPN in amounts required to meet nutritional needs (in parenteral multivitamin preparations).

AVAILABILITY

- *Capsules:* 10,000 units, 25,000 units, 50,000 units ▪ *Tablets:* 10,000 units, 25,000 units, 50,000 units ▪ *Oral solution:* 5000 units/0.1 ml ▪ *Injection:* 50,000 units/ml.

TIME/ACTION PROFILE

	ONSET	PEAK	DURATION
PO	UK	UK	UK
IM	UK	UK	UK

NURSING IMPLICATIONS

Assessment

- Assess patient for signs of vitamin A deficiency (night blindness; frequent eye, ear, sinus, and GU infections; dry mucous membranes; rough scaly skin with goose pimple-like lesions; photophobia; and dry eyes) prior to and periodically throughout therapy.
- Assess nutritional status through 24-hr diet recall. Determine frequency of consumption of vitamin A-rich foods.
- **Lab Test Considerations:** Chronic toxicity may cause increased blood glucose, calcium, BUN, cholesterol, and triglyceride levels.
- Plasma vitamin A and carotene levels may be evaluated prior to therapy to determine vitamin A deficiency.
- With high doses, erythrocyte and leukocyte counts may be decreased and erythrocyte sedimentation rate (ESR) and prothrombin time (PT) may be increased.

Potential Nursing Diagnoses

- Nutrition, altered: less than body requirements (indications).
- Knowledge deficit related to medication regimen (patient/family teaching).

Implementation

- **PO:** Administer with or after meals.
- Solution may be dropped directly into mouth or mixed with cereal, fruit juice, or other food. Use calibrated dropper supplied by manufacturer to measure solution accurately.
- **IM:** Parenteral administration is indicated only when oral administration is not possible (because of malabsorption, NPO status, or vomiting or when ocular damage is severe).
- Do not administer vitamin A intravenously, because of the risk of anaphylactic shock and death.

Patient/Family Teaching

- Instruct patient to take medication as directed. If a dose is missed it should be omitted, as fat-soluble vitamins are stored in the body for long periods.
- Encourage patient to comply with physician's diet recommendations. Explain that the best source of vitamins is a well-balanced diet with foods from the 4 basic food groups.
- Foods high in vitamin A include liver, fish liver oils, egg yolks, yellow-orange fruits and vegetables, dark green leafy vegetables, whole milk, vitamin A-fortified skim milk, butter,

and margarine. Ordinary cooking does not destroy vitamin A, but frozen foods loose 5–10% during storage for 12 mo.

□ Patients self-medicating with vitamin supplements should be cautioned not to exceed RDA (see Appendix L). The effectiveness of megadoses for treatment of various medical conditions is unproven, and this may cause side effects and toxicity.

□ Review symptoms of hypervitaminosis A syndrome (headaches, bulging fontanelles in infants, irritability, yellow-orange discoloration of skin, drying and desquamation of skin and lips, hair loss, anorexia, vomiting, joint and bone pain). Instruct patient to report these promptly to physician.

□ Advise patient that mineral oil may interfere with the absorption of fat-soluble vitamins and should not be used concurrently.

□ Emphasize the importance of follow-up examinations to evaluate progress. Ophthalmologic examinations may be required prior to and periodically throughout therapy.

EVALUATION
Effectiveness of therapy can be demonstrated by: ▪ Prevention of or decrease in the symptoms of vitamin A deficiency.

VITAMIN B COMPLEX WITH VITAMIN C

Oral
Albee-T, Bee-T-Vites, B Complex + C, Beminal 500, C-B Time, High Potency, N-Vites, Probec-T, Stresscaps, Sublingual B Total Liquid, Surbex with C, Surbu-Gen-T, Superplex-T, Surplex-T

Parenteral
Key Plex, Neurodep, Vicam

CLASSIFICATION(S):
Vitamin (water-soluble)
Pregnancy Category UK

INDICATIONS
▪ Treatment and prevention of vitamin deficiencies.

ACTION
▪ Contains B-complex vitamins (B_1, B_2, B_3, B_5, B_6, B_{12}) and vitamin C, a diverse group of compounds necessary for normal growth and development that act as coenzymes or catalysts in numerous metabolic processes. **Therapeutic Effect:** ▪ Replacement of vitamins in patients who are deficient or at risk of deficiency.

PHARMACOKINETICS
Absorption: Well absorbed following oral administration. Some absorptive processes require cofactors (B_{12}).
Distribution: Widely distributed, crosses the placenta and enters breast milk.
Metabolism and Excretion: Utilized in various biologic processes. Excess amounts are excreted unchanged by the kidneys.
Half-life: UK.

CONTRAINDICATIONS AND PRECAUTIONS
Contraindicated in: ▪ Hypersensitivity to ingredients in preparations (benzyl alcohol, parabens, bisulfites, tartrazine).

ADVERSE REACTIONS AND SIDE EFFECTS*
In recommended doses, adverse reactions are extremely rare.
Misc: allergic reactions to preservatives, ANAPHYLAXIS (thiamine).

INTERACTIONS
Drug–Drug: ▪ Large amounts of vitamin B_6 may interfere with the beneficial effect of **levodopa**.

ROUTE AND DOSAGE
▪ **PO, IV (Adults and Children):** Amount sufficient to meet RDA for age group (see Table in Appendix L).

---

*Underlines indicate most frequent; **CAPITALS** indicate life-threatening.

AVAILABILITY

■ *Tablets, capsules, sublingual liquid:* contain vitamins B$_1$ (5–50 mg); B$_2$ (1.7–50 mg); B$_3$ (20–150 mg); B$_5$ (10–100 mg); B$_6$ (2.5–10 mg); vitamin B$_{12}$ (50–1000 mcg); and vitamin C (50–600 mg) per tablet, capsule, or ml ■ *In combination with:* folic acid, biotin, chromium, soy protein, brewers yeast, potassium, manganese, and zinc in multivitamin/mineral products ■ *Injection:* contains vitamin B$_1$ (50 mg); B$_2$ (5 mg); B$_3$ (125 mg); B$_5$ (6 mg); B$_{12}$ (1000 mcg); and vitamin C (50 mg/ml).

TIME/ACTION PROFILE

	ONSET	PEAK	DURATION
PO	UK	UK	UK

NURSING IMPLICATIONS

ASSESSMENT

□ Assess patient for signs of vitamin deficiency prior to and periodically throughout therapy. Assess nutritional status through 24-hr diet recall. Determine frequency of consumption of vitamin-rich foods. Therapy is limited to periods of high physiologic stress when patient is not able to ingest adequate vitamins orally.

□ Monitor patient for anaphylaxis (wheezing, urticaria, edema): contains thiamine.

POTENTIAL NURSING DIAGNOSES

■ Nutrition, altered: less than body requirements (indications).

■ Knowledge deficit related to medication regimen (patient/family teaching).

IMPLEMENTATION

■ **PO:** Available in capsule and tablet form.

■ **Continuous Infusion:** Usually administered as part of a large volume parenteral admixture.

PATIENT/FAMILY TEACHING

◻ Encourage patient to comply with physician's diet recommendations. Explain that the best source of vitamins is a well-balanced diet with foods from the 4 basic food groups.

EVALUATION

Effectiveness of therapy can be demonstrated by: ■ Prevention of or decrease in the symptoms of vitamin deficiencies.

VITAMIN B$_{12}$ PREPARATIONS

cyanocobalamin
(sye-an-oh-koe-**bal**-a-min)
{Anacobin}, {Bedoz}, Cobex, Crystamine, Crysti-12, Cynaoject, Cyomin, Rubesol-1000, {Rubion}, Rubramin PC

hydroxocobalamin
(hye-drox-oh-koe-**bal**-a-min)
vitamin B$_{12}$, {Acti-B$_{12}$}, Alphamine, Hydrobexan, HydroCobex, Hydro-Crysti-12, LA-12

CLASSIFICATION(S):
Vitamin (water-soluble), Antianemic
Pregnancy Category C

INDICATIONS

■ Treatment and prevention of vitamin B$_{12}$ deficiency ■ Treatment of pernicious anemia ■ Used diagnostically as part of the Schilling Test.

ACTION

■ A necessary coenzyme for many metabolic processes including fat and carbohydrate metabolism and protein synthesis ■ Required for the formation of red blood cells. **Therapeutic Effects:** ■ Correction of manifestations of pernicious anemia (megaloblastic indices, GI lesions, and neurologic damage) ■ Prevention of vitamin B$_{12}$ deficiency.

PHARMACOKINETICS

Absorption: Absorption from the GI tract requires intrinsic factor and calcium. Well absorbed following IM and SC administration.

V

Distribution: Stored in the liver. Crosses the placenta and enters breast milk.

Metabolism and Excretion: Excess amounts are eliminated unchanged in the urine.

Half-life: 6 days (400 days in liver).

CONTRAINDICATIONS AND PRECAUTIONS

Contraindicated in: ▪ Hypersensitivity ▪ Hereditary optic nerve atrophy (accelerates nerve damage) ▪ Avoid using benzyl alcohol–containing preparations in premature infants (associated with fatal "gasping syndrome").

Use Cautiously in: ▪ Cardiac disease ▪ Uremia, folic acid deficiency, concurrent infection, iron deficiency (response to B$_{12}$ will be impaired).

ADVERSE REACTIONS AND SIDE EFFECTS*

CV: peripheral vascular thrombosis.

GI: diarrhea.

Derm: itching, swelling of the body, urticaria.

F and E: hypokalemia.

Local: pain at IM site.

Misc: hypersensitivity reactions including ANAPHYLAXIS.

INTERACTIONS

Drug–Drug: ▪ Chloramphenicol and antineoplastic agents may decrease the hematologic response to vitamin B$_{12}$ ▪ Aminoglycosides, colchicine, extended-release potassium supplements, anticonvulsants, cimetidine, excess intake of alcohol, or vitamin C may decrease oral absorption of vitamin B$_{12}$.

ROUTE AND DOSAGE

Cyanocobalamin
▪ **PO (Adults):** 1–25 mcg/day.
▪ **PO (Children >1 yr):** 1 mcg/day.
▪ **PO (Children <1 yr):** 0.3 mcg/day.
▪ **IM, SC (Adults):** 100 mcg/day for 6–7 days, then 100 mcg every other day for 7 more doses, then 100 mcg q 3–4 days for 2–3 more weeks initially, then 100–200 mcg every month.

"Flushing" dose for Shilling Test is 1000 mcg.
▪ **IM, SC (Children):** 30–50 mcg/day for 2 weeks or more (total dose 1–5 mg) initially, then 100 mcg monthly.

Hydroxocobalamin
▪ **IM, SC (Adults):** 30–50 mcg/day (up to 100 mcg/day) for 5–10 days, then 100–200 mcg monthly. "Flushing" dose for Shilling Test is 1000 mcg.
▪ **IM, SC (Children):** 30–50 mcg/day for 2 or more weeks (total dose of 1–5 mg), then 100 mcg monthly.

AVAILABILITY

Cyanocobalamin
▪ *Tablets:* 25 mcg, 50 mcg, 100 mcg, 250 mcg, 500 mcg, 1000 mcg ▪ *Injection:* 30 mcg/ml, 100 mcg/ml, 1000 mcg/ml.

Hydroxocobalamin
▪ *Injection:* 100 mcg/ml, 1000 mcg/ml.

TIME/ACTION PROFILE
(reticulocytosis)

	ONSET	PEAK	DURATION
cyanoco-balamin IM, SC	UK	3–10 days	UK
hydroxoco-balamin IM, SC	UK	3–10 days	UK

NURSING IMPLICATIONS

ASSESSMENT
▫ Assess patient for signs of vitamim B$_{12}$ deficiency (pallor, neuropathy, psychosis, red inflamed tongue) prior to and periodically throughout therapy.
▪ **Lab Test Considerations:** Monitor plasma folic acid levels, reticulocyte count, and plasma vitamin B$_{12}$ levels prior to and between the fifth and seventh day of therapy with cyanocobalamin and between the 3rd and 10th day of therapy with hydroxocobalamin. Patients receiving vitamin B$_{12}$ for megaloblastic anemia should have serum potassium level evaluated

for hypokalemia during the first 48 hr of treatment.

POTENTIAL NURSING DIAGNOSES
- Nutrition, altered: less than body requirements (indications).
- Activity intolerance (indications).
- Knowledge deficit related to medication regimen (patient/family teaching).

IMPLEMENTATION
- **General Info:** Usually administered in combination with other vitamins, as solitary vitamin B deficiencies are rare.
- Administration of vitamin B_{12} by the oral route is useful only for nutritional deficiencies. Patients with small bowel disease, malabsorption syndrome, or gastric or ileal resections require parenteral administration.
- **PO:** Administer with meals to increase absorption.
- May be mixed with fruit juices. Administer immediately after mixing, as ascorbic acid alters stability.
- **IV:** IV route is not recommended; however, cyanocobalamin may be admixed in TPN solutions.
- **Y-Site Compatibility:** ▪ heparin ▪ hydrocortisone sodium succinate ▪ potassium chloride
- **Additive/Solution   Compatibility:** ▪ dextrose/Ringer's or lactated Ringer's combinations ▪ dextrose/saline combinations ▪ D5W ▪ D10W ▪ 0.45% NaCl ▪ 0.9% NaCl ▪ Ringer's or lactated Ringer's solution ▪ ascorbic acid ▪ vitamin B complex with C.

PATIENT/FAMILY TEACHING
- Encourage patient to comply with diet recommendations of physician. Explain that the best source of vitamins is a well-balanced diet with foods from the 4 basic food groups.
- Foods high in vitamin B_{12} include meats, seafood, egg yolk, and fermented cheeses; little vitamins are lost with ordinary cooking.
- Patients self-medicating with vitamin supplements should be cautioned not to exceed RDA (see Appendix L). The

effectiveness of megadoses for treatment of various medical conditions is unproven and may cause side effects.
- Inform patients of the lifelong need for vitamin B_{12} replacement following gastrectomy or ileal resection.
- Emphasize the importance of follow-up examinations to evaluate progress.

EVALUATION
Effectiveness of therapy can be demonstrated by: ▪ Resolution of the symptoms of vitamin B_{12} deficiency □ Increase in reticulocyte count.

VITAMIN E
(vye-ta-min E)
alphatocopherol, Amino-Opti-E, Aquasol E, Chew-E, E-200, E-400, E-1000, E-Complex-600, E-Vitamin, Eprolin, Pheryl-E, Vita Plus E, Vite E, Vitec

CLASSIFICATION(S):
Vitamin (fat-soluble)
Pregnancy Category UK

INDICATIONS
- **PO:** Used as a dietary supplement
- **PO:** Used in low-birth-weight infants to prevent and treat hemolysis due to vitamin E deficiency ▪ **Top:** Treatment of irritated, chapped, or dry skin.

ACTION
- Prevents the oxidation (antioxidant) of other substances ▪ Protects red blood cell membranes against hemolysis, especially in low-birth-weight neonates. **Therapeutic Effects:** ▪ Prevention and treatment of deficiency in high-risk patients.

PHARMACOKINETICS
Absorption: 20–80% absorbed following oral administration. Absorption requires fat and bile salts.
Distribution: Widely   distributed, stored in adipose tissue (4-yr supply).
Metabolism and Excretion: Metabolized by the liver, excreted in bile.
Half-life: UK.

CONTRAINDICATIONS AND PRECAUTIONS

Contraindicated in: ▪ Hypersensitivity to ingredients in preparations (parabens, propylene, glycol).

Use Cautiously in: ▪ Anemia due to iron deficiency ▪ Low-birth-weight infants (oral administration may cause necrotizing enterocolitis) ▪ Vitamin K deficiency (may increase risk of bleeding).

ADVERSE REACTIONS AND SIDE EFFECTS*

Seen primarily with large doses over long periods of time.

CNS: fatigue, weakness, headache.
EENT: blurred vision.
GI: necrotizing enterocolitis (oral administration in low-birth-weight infants), nausea, diarrhea, cramps.
Derm: rash.
Endo: gonadal dysfunction.

INTERACTIONS

Drug–Drug: ▪ **Cholestyramine, colestipol, mineral oil,** and **sucralfate** decrease absorption ▪ May decrease hematologic response to **iron supplements** ▪ May increase the risk of bleeding with **warfarin.**

ROUTE AND DOSAGE

Prevention of Deficiency
▪ **PO (Adults):** 30 units/day.

Treatment of Deficiency
▪ **PO (Adults):** 60–75 units/day.
▪ **PO (Children):** 1 unit/kg/day.

Topical
▪ **Top (Adults and Children):** Apply to affected areas as needed.

AVAILABILITY

▪ *Capsules:* 100 units, 200 units, 400 units, 600 units, {800 units}, 1000 units ▪ *Oral solution:* 50 units/ml ▪ *Tablets:* 100 units, 200 units, 400 units ▪ *Chewable tablets:* 400 units ▪ *Ointment* ▪ *Cream* ▪ *Lotion* ▪ *Oil*.

TIME/ACTION PROFILE

	ONSET	PEAK	DURATION
PO	UK	UK	UK

NURSING IMPLICATIONS

ASSESSMENT

▫ Assess patient for signs of vitamin E deficiency (neonates—irritability, edema, hemolytic anemia, creatinuria; adults/children (rare)—muscle weakness, ceroid deposits, anemia, creatinuria) prior to and periodically throughout therapy.

▫ Assess nutritional status through 24-hr diet recall. Determine frequency of consumption of vitamin E-rich foods.

▪ **Lab Test Considerations:** Large doses may increase cholesterol, triglyceride, and CPK levels.

POTENTIAL NURSING DIAGNOSES

▪ Nutrition, altered: less than body requirements (indications).
▪ Knowledge deficit related to medication regimen (patient/family teaching).

IMPLEMENTATION

▪ **PO:** Administer with or after meals.
▫ Chewable tablets should be chewed well or crushed before swallowing. Solution may be dropped directly into mouth or mixed with cereal, fruit juice, or other food. Use calibrated dropper supplied by manufacturer to measure solution accurately.

PATIENT/FAMILY TEACHING

▫ Instruct patient to take medication as directed. If a dose is missed it should be omitted, as fat-soluble vitamins are stored in the body for long periods.

▫ Encourage patient to comply with physician's diet recommendations. Explain that the best source of vitamins is a well-balanced diet with foods from the 4 basic food groups.

▫ Foods high in vitamin E include vegetable oils, wheat germ, whole grain cereals, egg yolk, and liver. Vitamin E

---

*Underlines indicate most frequent; **CAPITALS** indicate life-threatening.

content is not markedly affected by cooking.

□ Patients self-medicating with vitamin supplements should be cautioned not to exceed RDA (see Appendix L). The effectiveness of megadoses for treatment of various medical conditions is unproven and this may cause side effects and toxicity.

□ Review symptoms of overdosage (blurred vision, flu-like symptoms, headache, breast enlargement). Instruct patient to report these promptly to physician.

□ Mineral oil may interfere with the absorption of fat-soluble vitamins and should not be used concurrently.

EVALUATION
Effectiveness of therapy can be demonstrated by: ■ Prevention of or decrease in the symptoms of vitamin E deficiency ■ Control of dry or chapped skin.

WARFARIN
(**war**-fa-rin)
Coumadin, Sofarin, {Warfilone}

CLASSIFICATION(S):
Anticoagulant
Pregnancy Category UK

INDICATIONS
■ Prophylaxis and treatment of: □ Venous thrombosis □ Pulmonary embolism □ Atrial fibrillation with embolization ■ Adjunct in the treatment of coronary occlusion ■ Prevention of thrombus formation and embolization after prosthetic valve placement.

ACTION
■ Interferes with hepatic synthesis of vitamin K-dependent clotting factors (II, VII, IX, and X). **Therapeutic Effect:** ■ Prevention of thromboembolic events.

PHARMACOKINETICS
Absorption: Well absorbed from the GI tract following oral administration.

Distribution: Crosses the placenta but does not enter breast milk.
Metabolism and Excretion: Metabolized by the liver.
Half-life: 0.5–3 days.

CONTRAINDICATIONS AND PRECAUTIONS
Contraindicated in: ■ Pregnancy ■ Uncontrolled bleeding ■ Open wounds ■ Active ulcer disease ■ Malignancy ■ Recent brain, eye, or spinal cord injury or surgery ■ Severe liver disease ■ Uncontrolled hypertension.
Use Cautiously in: ■ Patients with history of ulcer or liver disease ■ History of poor compliance ■ Women with childbearing potential.

ADVERSE REACTIONS AND SIDE EFFECTS*
GI: nausea, cramps.
Derm: dermal necrosis.
Hemat: BLEEDING.
Misc: fever.

INTERACTIONS
Drug–Drug: ■ Androgens, cefamandole, cefoperazone, cefotetan, chloral hydrate, chloramphenicol, disulfiram, metronidazole, moxalactam, plicamycin, streptokinase, urokinase, sulfonamides, quinidine, nonsteroidal anti-inflammatory agents, valproates, and **aspirin** may increase the response to warfarin and increase the risk of bleeding ■ Alcohol, barbiturates, and **oral contraceptives containing estrogen** may decrease the anticoagulant response to warfarin.
Drug–Food: ■ Ingestion of large quantities of **foods high in vitamin K content** (see list in Appendix K) may antagonize the anticoagulant effect of warfarin.

ROUTE AND DOSAGE
■ **PO (Adults):** 10 mg/day for 2–4 days, then adjust daily dose by results of prothrombin time (range 2–10 mg/day). Initiate therapy with lower doses in elderly or debilitated patients.

{} = Available in Canada only.
*Underlines indicate most frequent; **CAPITALS** indicate life-threatening.

AVAILABILITY

- **Tablets:** 1 mg, 2 mg, 2.5 mg, 5 mg, 7.5 mg, 10 mg.

TIME/ACTION PROFILE (effects on coagulation tests)

	ONSET	PEAK	DURATION
PO	several hrs	0.5–3 days	2–5 days

NURSING IMPLICATIONS

ASSESSMENT

- Assess patient for signs of bleeding and hemorrhage (bleeding gums, nose bleed, unusual bruising, tarry black stools, hematuria, fall in hematocrit or blood pressure, guaiac-positive stools, urine, or nasogastric aspirate). Notify physician if these occur.
- Assess patient for evidence of additional or increased thrombosis. Symptoms will depend on area of involvement.
- **Lab Test Considerations:** Prothrombin time (PT) and other clotting factors should be monitored frequently during therapy. Therapeutic PT ranges from 1.5–2.0 times greater than control. Notify physician if significant discrepancies occur.
- Hepatic function and CBC should be monitored prior to and periodically throughout course of therapy.
- Stool and urine should be monitored for occult blood prior to and periodically throughout course of therapy.
- **Toxicity and Overdose:** Withholding 1 or more doses of medication is usually sufficient if PT is excessively prolonged or minor bleeding occurs. If overdose occurs or anticoagulation needs to be immediately reversed, the antidote is vitamin K (phytonadione, AquaMEPHYTON). Administration of whole blood or plasma also may be required in severe bleeding because of the delayed onset of vitamin K.

POTENTIAL NURSING DIAGNOSES

- Tissue perfusion, altered (indications).
- Injury, high risk for (side effects).
- Knowledge deficit related to medication regimen (patient/family teaching).

IMPLEMENTATION

- **General Info:** Administer medication at same time each day.
- Protect injectable form from light.
- **PO:** Medication requires 3–5 days to reach effective levels. It is usually begun while patient is still on IV heparin.
- Do not interchange brands; potencies may not be equivalent.

PATIENT/FAMILY TEACHING

- Instruct patient to take medication exactly as directed. If a dose is missed it should be taken as soon as remembered that day. Do not double doses. Physician should be informed of missed doses at time of check-up or lab tests.
- Review foods high in vitamin K (see Appendix K). Patient should have consistent limited intake of these foods, as vitamin K is the antidote for warfarin, and alternating intake of these foods will cause PT levels to fluctuate.
- Caution patient to avoid IM injections and activities leading to injury. Instruct patient to use a soft toothbrush, not to floss, and to shave with an electric razor during warfarin therapy. Advise patient that venipunctures and injection sites require application of pressure to prevent bleeding or hematoma formation.
- Advise patient to report any symptoms of unusual bleeding or bruising (bleeding gums, nose bleed, black tarry stools, hematuria, excessive menstrual flow). Notify physician if these occur.
- Instruct patient not to take alcohol over-the-counter medications, especially those containing aspirin or ibuprofen, without advice of physician or pharmacist.
- Emphasize the importance of frequent lab tests to monitor coagulation factors.
- Instruct patient to carry identification

describing medication regimen at all times and to inform all health care personnel caring for patient of anticoagulant therapy prior to lab tests, treatment, or surgery.

EVALUATION
Clinical respone can be evaluated by:
- Prolonged PT (1.3–2.0 times the control, may vary with indication) without signs of hemorrhage.

ZALCITABINE
(zal-**site**-a-been)
HIVID, dideoxycitidine, ddC

CLASSIFICATION(S):
Antiviral
Pregnancy Category C

INDICATIONS
- Used in combination with zidovudine in the management of adult HIV-positive patients who have advanced disease (CD4 count ≤300 cells/mm^3) and are clinically or immunologically deteriorating.

ACTION
- Following intracellular conversion to its active form, it inhibits viral DNA synthesis and subsequent viral replication. **Therapeutic Effects:** ■ Slows the progression of HIV disease ■ Improves CD4 cell count.

PHARMACOKINETICS
Absorption: Well absorbed following oral administration (80%).
Distribution: Distributes into intracellular fluid. Crosses the blood–brain barrier. Remainder of distribution not known.
Metabolism and Excretion: 70% excreted by the kidneys.
Half-life: 2 hr.

CONTRAINDICATIONS AND PRECAUTIONS
Contraindicated in: ■ Hypersensitivity.
Use Cautiously in: ■ Patients with re-

nal impairment (dosage modification recommended if creatinine clearance is <40 ml/min) ■ Patients with any signs of peripheral neuropathy (zalcitabine should be briefly discontinued and restarted at 50% of the previous dose if improvement occurs) ■ Pre-existing liver disease or history of alcohol abuse (increased risk of liver function abnormalities) ■ History of pancreatitis or hypertriglyceridemia ■ Safe use in pregnancy, lactation, or children has not been established.

ADVERSE REACTIONS AND SIDE EFFECTS*
CNS: headache, dizziness, fatigue, confusion, impaired concentration.
EENT: pharyngitis.
CV: CARDIOMYOPATHY, CONGESTIVE HEART FAILURE, chest pain.
GI: PANCREATITIS, esophageal ulcerations, oral ulcers, nausea, dysphagia, anorexia, abdominal pain, vomiting, diarrhea, elevated liver enzymes.
Derm: rash, pruritus, dermatitis.
Hemat: neutropenia, leukopenia.
MS: myalgia, arthralgia.
Neuro: peripheral neuropathy.
Misc: weight loss, hypersensitivity reactions.

INTERACTIONS
Drug–Drug: ■ Risk of neuropathy is increased by concurrent use of other **drugs causing neuropathy** (chloramphenicol, cisplatin, disulfiram, ethiomide, glutethimide, gold, hydralazine, iodoquinol, isoniazid, metronidazole, nitrofurantoin, phenytoin, ribavirin, vincristine) ■ Concurrent use with **didanosine** is not recommended ■ Risk of pancreatitis is increased by concurrent use of other **drugs causing pancreatitis** (alcohol, asparaginase, azathioprine, estrogens, furosemide, methyldopa, nitrofurantoin, pentamidine, sulfonamides, tetracyclines, thiazide diuretics, valproic acid) ■ **Aminoglycoside anti-infectives, amphotericin B,** and **foscarnet** may increase the risk of toxicity

Z

Underlines indicate most frequent; CAPITALS indicate life-threatening.

from zalcitabine by decreasing its elimination.

Drug–Food: ■ Food decreases absorption.

ROUTE AND DOSAGE

- **PO (Adults):** 0.75 mg zalcitabine in combination with 200 mg zidovudine every 8 hr. No dose adjustment required for patients weighing >30 kg.

AVAILABILITY

- *Tablets:* 0.375 mg, 0.75 mg.

TIME/ACTION PROFILE (blood levels)

	ONSET	PEAK
PO	rapid	1–2 hr

NURSING IMPLICATIONS

ASSESSMENT

- Assess patient for change in severity of symptoms of acquired immunodeficiency syndrome (AIDS) and for symptoms of opportunistic infections throughout therapy.
- Monitor patient for signs and symptoms of peripheral neuropathy. Zalcitabine should be discontinued when moderate discomfort from numbness, tingling, burning or pain of the extremities, loss of a previously present Achilles tendon reflex, or any related symptoms occurs, especially if symptoms last longer than 3 days and are bilateral. If zalcitabine is not stopped promptly, peripheral neuropathy may progress to severe pain and may be potentially irreversible. Neuropathy may progress despite discontinuation of zalcitabine but usually is slowly reversible with prompt discontinuation. If peripheral neuropathy improves to very mild symptoms, zalcitabine may be reintroduced at 50% of the regular dose.
- Monitor patients for symptoms of pancreatitis (nausea, vomiting, abdominal pain) throughout therapy. If these symptoms or associated lab test signs occur, discontinue zalcitabine, as fatalities have occurred.
- **Lab Test Considerations:** Monitor CD4 levels prior to and periodically throughout therapy.
- Monitor serum amylase, lipase, triglyceride, and calcium throughout therapy. Rising serum amylase, lipase, and triglyceride and decreasing calcium levels may indicate pancreatitis. Assess baseline in patients with a prior history of pancreatitis or increased amylase, those on parenteral nutrition, or those with a history of ethanol abuse. Zalcitabine should be discontinued if serum amylase is elevated by 1.5–2 times the normal limits.
- Monitor CBC and liver function studies prior to and periodically during therapy. May cause leukopenia and anemia and increase in AST (SGOT), ALT (SGPT), and alkaline phosphatase levels.

POTENTIAL NURSING DIAGNOSES

- Infection, high risk for (indications, side effects).
- Knowledge deficit related to medication regimen (patient/family teaching).

IMPLEMENTATION

- **PO:** Administer on an empty stomach, 1 hr before and 2 hr after meals for maximum absorption. Administer every 8 hr around the clock.

PATIENT/FAMILY TEACHING

- Instruct patient to take zalcitabine exactly as directed, around the clock. Emphasize the importance of compliance with therapy, not taking more than the prescribed amount, and not discontinuing without consulting physician. Missed doses should be taken as soon as remembered, unless almost time for next dose; do not double doses.
- Inform patient that zalcitabine does not cure AIDS and does not reduce the risk of transmission of HIV to others through sexual contact or blood contamination. Caution patient to avoid sexual contact, use a condom, and avoid sharing needles or donating blood to prevent spreading the AIDS virus to others.

□ Instruct patient to notify physician promptly if signs of peripheral neuropathy or pancreatitis occur.

□ Advise women with child-bearing potential to use a nonhormonal method of contraception throughout therapy.

□ Advise patient not to take other medications without consulting physician or pharmacist.

□ Emphasize the importance of regular follow-up examinations and blood tests to determine progress and monitor for side effects.

EVALUATION

Effectiveness of therapy can be demonstrated by: ▪ Improvement in CD4 levels in patients with advanced HIV infection.

ZIDOVUDINE
(zye-**doe**-vue-deen)
{Apo-Zidovudine}, azidothymidine, AZT, {Novo-AZT}, Retrovir

CLASSIFICATION(S):
Antiviral
Pregnancy Category C

INDICATIONS

▪ Management of human immunodeficiency virus (HIV) and AIDS infection.

ACTION

▪ Following intracellular conversion to its active form, inhibits viral RNA synthesis by inhibiting the enzyme DNA polymerase (reverse transcriptase) ▪ Prevents viral replication. **Therapeutic Effects:** ▪ Virustatic action against selected retroviruses ▪ Not curative, but may slow the progression or decrease the severity of the disease and its associated sequelae.

PHARMACOKINETICS

Absorption: Well absorbed following oral administration.
Distribution: Widely distributed. En-

ters the CNS. Probably crosses the placenta.
Metabolism and Excretion: Mostly (75%) metabolized by the liver. 15–20% excreted unchanged by the kidneys.
Half-life: 1 hr.

CONTRAINDICATIONS AND PRECAUTIONS

Contraindicated in: ▪ Hypersensitivity ▪ Lactation.
Use Cautiously in: ▪ Decreased bone marrow reserve (dosage reduction required for anemia or granulocytopenia) ▪ Severe hepatic or renal disease (dosage modification may be required) ▪ Pregnancy or children (safety not established).

ADVERSE REACTIONS AND SIDE EFFECTS*

CNS: headache, weakness, malaise, somnolence, restlessness, insomnia, anxiety, confusion, depression, decreased mental acuity, dizziness, fainting.
GI: nausea, abdominal pain, diarrhea, dyspepsia, anorexia, vomiting, hepatitis.
Derm: nail pigmentation.
Hemat: anemia, granulocytopenia, thrombocytosis.
MS: back pain, myalgia.
Neuro: tremor.

INTERACTIONS

Drug–Drug: ▪ Additive bone marrow depression with other **agents having bone-marrow-depressing properties (antineoplastic agents** or **radiation therapy)** or **ganciclovir** ▪ Additive neurotoxicity may occur with **acyclovir** ▪ Toxicity may be increased by concurrent administration of **probenecid** ▪ Zidovudine levels are decreased by **clarithromycin.**

ROUTE AND DOSAGE

Symptomatic HIV Infection
▪ **PO (Adults and Children >13 yr):** 100 mg q 4 hr (600 mg/day).

Z

{} = Available in Canada only.
*Underlines indicate most frequent; **CAPITALS** indicate life-threatening.

- **PO (Children 3 mo–12 yr):** 180 mg/m^2 every 6 hr (not to exceed 200 mg q 6 hr).
- **IV (Adults and Adolescents):** 1–2 mg/kg infused over 1 hr q 4 hr. Change to oral therapy as soon as possible.
- **IV (Children):** 120 mg/m^2 q 6 hr (not to exceed 160 mg/dose).

Asymptomatic HIV Infection
- **PO (Adults):** 100 mg q 4 hr while awake (500 mg/day).

AVAILABILITY
- *Capsules:* 100 mg ▪ *Oral syrup:* 50 mg/5 ml ▪ *Injection:* 200 mg/20 ml.

TIME/ACTION PROFILE (blood levels)

	ONSET	PEAK	DURATION
PO	UK	0.5–1.5 hr	UK
IV	rapid	end of infusion	UK

NURSING IMPLICATIONS

ASSESSMENT
- ☐ Assess patient for change in severity of symptoms of acquired immunodeficiency syndrome (AIDS) and for symptoms of opportunistic infections throughout therapy.
- ▪ **Lab Test Considerations:** Monitor CBC every 2 wk during the first 8 wk of therapy in patients with advanced HIV disease and decrease to every 4 wk after the first 2 mo if zidovudine is well tolerated, or monthly during the first 3 mo and every 3 mo thereafter unless indicated in patients who are asymptomatic or have early symptoms. Commonly causes granulocytopenia and anemia. Anemia may occur 2–4 wk after initiation of therapy. Anemia may respond to epoetin alpha administration. Granulocytopenia usually occurs after 6–8 wk of therapy. Dosage reduction, discontinuation of therapy, or blood transfusions should be considered if hemoglobin is <7.5 g/dl or reduction of >25% from baseline and/or granulocyte count is <750/mm^3 or reduction of >50% from baseline. Therapy may be gradually resumed when bone marrow recovery is evident.

POTENTIAL NURSING DIAGNOSES
- ▪ Infection, high risk for (indications, side effects).
- ▪ Knowledge deficit related to medication regimen (patient/family teaching).

IMPLEMENTATION
- ▪ **General Info:** Administer capsules every 4 hr around the clock.
- ▪ **IV:** Patient should receive the IV infusion only until oral therapy can be administered.
- ▪ **Intermittent Infusion:** Remove the calculated dose from the vial and dilute with D5W for a concentration of <4 mg/ml. Stable for 24 hr at room temperature or 48 hr if refrigerated.
- ▪ *Rate:* Infuse at a constant rate over 1 hr. Avoid rapid infusion or bolus injection.
- ▪ **Y-Site Compatibility:** ▪ acyclovir ▪ amikacin ▪ amphotericin B ▪ aztreonam ▪ ceftazidine ▪ ceftriaxone ▪ cimetidine ▪ clindamycin ▪ dexamethasone ▪ dobutamine ▪ dopamine ▪ erythromycin lactobionate ▪ fluconazole ▪ fludarabine ▪ gentamicin ▪ heparin ▪ imipenem/cilastatin ▪ lorazepam ▪ metoclopramide ▪ morphine ▪ nafcillin ▪ ondansetron ▪ oxacillin ▪ pentamidine ▪ phenylephrine ▪ piperacillin ▪ potassium chloride ▪ ranitidine ▪ sargramostim ▪ tobramycin ▪ trimethoprim-sulfamethoxazole ▪ vancomycin.
- ▪ **Additive Incompatibility:** blood products or protein solutions.

PATIENT/FAMILY TEACHING
- ☐ Instruct patient to take zidovudine exactly as directed, around the clock, even if sleep is interrupted. Emphasize the importance of compliance with therapy, not taking more than the prescribed amount, and not discontinuing without consulting physician. Missed doses should be taken as soon as remembered, unless almost time for next dose; do not double doses.
- ☐ Instruct patient that zidovudine should not be shared with others.
- ☐ Zidovudine may cause dizziness or

fainting. Caution patient to avoid driving or other activities requiring alertness until response to medication is known.

☐ Inform patient that zidovudine does not cure AIDS and does not reduce the risk of transmission of HIV to others through sexual contact or blood contamination. Caution patient to avoid sexual contact, use a condom, and avoid sharing needles or donating blood to prevent spreading the AIDS virus to others.

☐ Instruct patient to notify physician promptly if fever, sore throat, or signs of infection occur. Caution patient to avoid crowds and persons with known infections. Instruct patient to use soft toothbrush, to use caution when using toothpicks or dental floss, and to have dental work done prior to therapy or deferred until blood counts return to normal.

☐ Advise patient to avoid taking any over-the-counter medications without consulting physician or pharmacist.

☐ Emphasize the importance of regular follow-up examinations and blood counts to determine progress and monitor for side effects.

EVALUATION
Effectiveness of therapy can be demonstrated by: ▪ Delayed progression of AIDS, and decreased opportunistic infections in patients with human immunodeficiency virus (HIV).

ZINC SULFATE
(zink **sul**-fate)
Orazinc, {PMS Egozinc}, Verazinc, Zin 15, Zinc 220, Zinca-Pak, Zincate, Zinkaps

CLASSIFICATION(S):
Nutritional supplement (trace metal)
Pregnancy Category UK

INDICATIONS
▪ Replacement and supplementation therapy in patients who are at risk for zinc deficiency, including patients on long-term parenteral nutrition. **Unlabeled Use:** ▪ Management of impaired wound healing due to zinc deficiency.

ACTION
▪ Serves as a cofactor for many enzymatic reactions ▪ Required for normal growth and tissue repair, wound healing, and senses of taste and smell. **Therapeutic Effect:** ▪ Replacement in deficiency states.

PHARMACOKINETICS
Absorption: Poorly absorbed from the GI tract (20–30%).
Distribution: Widely distributed. Concentrates in muscle, bone, skin, kidney, liver, pancreas, retina, prostate, red blood cells, and white blood cells.
Metabolism and Excretion: 90% excreted in feces, remainder lost in urine and sweat.
Half-life: UK.

CONTRAINDICATIONS AND PRECAUTIONS
Contraindicated in: ▪ Hypersensitivity or allergy to any components in formulation ▪ Pregnancy or lactation (supplemental amounts greater than RDA for pregnant or lactating patients; see list in Appendix L) ▪ Preparations containing benzyl alcohol should not be used in neonates.
Use Cautiously in: ▪ Renal failure.

ADVERSE REACTIONS AND SIDE EFFECTS*
GI: nausea, vomiting, gastric irritation (oral use only).

INTERACTIONS
Drug–Drug: ▪ Oral zinc may decrease the absorption of **tetracyclines** or **fluoroquinolones**.
Drug–Food: ▪ Caffeine, dairy prod-

Z

{} = Available in Canada only.
*<u>Underlines</u> indicate most frequent; **CAPITALS** indicate life-threatening.

ucts, and **bran** may decrease the absorption of orally administered zinc.

ROUTE AND DOSAGE

RDA = 15 mg. Doses expressed in mg elemental zinc unless otherwise noted. Zinc sulfate contains 23% zinc.

Dietary Supplement
- **PO (Adults):** 25–50 mg/day.

IV Nutritional Supplementation— Metabolically Stable Patients
- **IV (Adults):** 2.5–4 mg/day, additional 2 mg/day in acute catabolic states.
- **IV (Infants and Children ≤5 yr):** 100 mcg/kg/day.
- **IV (Premature Infants <1500 g and up to 3 kg):** 300 mcg/kg/day.

Metabolically Stable Adults with Small Bowel Fluid Losses
- **IV (Adults):** Additional 12.2 mg/liter TPN solution.

AVAILABILITY

- **Tablets:** 66 mg, 110 mg ▪ **Capsules:** 220 mg ▪ **Injection:** 1 mg/ml, 5 mg/ml.

TIME/ACTION PROFILE

	ONSET	PEAK	DURATION
PO	UK	UK	UK
IV	UK	UK	UK

NURSING IMPLICATIONS

Assessment
- ☐ Monitor progression of symptoms of zinc deficiency (impaired wound healing, growth retardation, decreased sense of taste, decreased sense of smell) throughout course of therapy.
- ▪ **Lab Test Considerations:** Serum zinc levels may not accurately reflect zinc deficiency.

Potential Nursing Diagnoses
- ▪ Nutrition, altered: less than body requirements (indications).
- ▪ Knowledge deficit related to medication regimen (patient/family teaching).

Implementation
- ▪ **PO:** Administer oral doses with food

to decrease gastric irritation. Administration with caffeine, dairy products, or bran may impair absorption.
- ▪ **IV:** Zinc is often included as a trace mineral in total parenteral nutrition solution prepared by pharmacist.

Patient/Family Teaching
- ☐ Encourage patient to comply with physician's diet recommendations. Explain that the best source of vitamins is a well-balanced diet with foods from the 4 basic food groups. Foods high in zinc include seafood, organ meats, and wheat germ.
- ☐ Patients self-medicating with vitamin supplements should be cautioned not to exceed RDA (see Appendix L). The effectiveness of megadoses for treatment of various medical conditions is unproven and may cause side effects.
- ☐ Instruct patients receiving oral zinc to notify physician if severe nausea or vomiting, abdominal pain, or tarry stools occur.
- ☐ Emphasize the importance of follow-up examinations to evaluate progress.

Evaluation
Effectiveness of therapy can be demonstrated by: ▪ Improved wound healing ☐ Improved senses of taste or smell. 6–8 wk of therapy may be required before full effect is seen.

ZOLPIDEM
(**zole**-pi-dem)
Ambien

CLASSIFICATION(S):
Hypnotic (nonbenzodiazepine)
Pregnancy Category B

INDICATIONS

- ▪ Used in the short-term treatment of insomnia.

ACTION

- ▪ Produces CNS depression by binding to gamma-aminobutyric acid (GABA)

receptors ▪ Has no analgesic properties.
Therapeutic Effects: ▪ Sedation and induction of sleep.

PHARMACOKINETICS

Absorption: Rapidly absorbed following oral administration.
Distribution: Enters breast milk. Remainder of distribution not known.
Metabolism and Excretion: Converted to inactive metabolites, which are excreted by the kidneys.
Half-life: 2.5–2.6 hr (increased in elderly patients and patients with hepatic impairment).

CONTRAINDICATIONS AND PRECAUTIONS

Contraindicated in: ▪ Hypersensitivity.
Use Cautiously in: ▪ Patients with a history of previous psychiatric illness, suicide attempt, drug or alcohol dependency ▪ Elderly patients and patients with impaired hepatic function (initial dosage reduction recommended) ▪ Patients with pulmonary disease.

ADVERSE REACTIONS AND SIDE EFFECTS*

CNS: daytime drowsiness, dizziness, amnesia, "drugged" feeling.
GI: nausea, vomiting, diarrhea.
Misc: hypersensitivity reactions.

INTERACTIONS

Drug–Drug: ▪ Additive CNS depression may occur with concurrent use of other **sedative/hypnotic agents, tricyclic antidepressants, opioid analgesics,** or **antihistamines.**
Drug–Food: Food decreases and delays absorption.

ROUTE AND DOSAGE

▪ **PO (Adults):** 10 mg at bedtime. Elderly or debilitated patients or patients with hepatic impairment should be started on 5 mg.

AVAILABILITY

▪ *Tablets:* 5 mg, 10 mg.

TIME/ACTION PROFILE (sedation)

	ONSET	PEAK	DURATION
PO	UK	UK	UK

NURSING IMPLICATIONS

ASSESSMENT

□ Assess metal status, sleep patterns, and potential for abuse prior to administering this medication. Prolonged use of greater than 7–10 days may lead to physical and psychological dependence. Limit amount of drug available to the patient.
□ Assess alertness at time of peak effect. Notify physician if desired sedation does not occur.
□ Assess patient for pain. Medicate as needed. Untreated pain decreases sedative effects.

POTENTIAL NURSING DIAGNOSES

▪ Sleep pattern disturbance (indications).
▪ Injury, high risk for (side effects).
▪ Knowledge deficit related to medication regimen (patient/family teaching).

IMPLEMENTATION

▪ **General Info:** Before administering, reduce external stimuli and provide comfort measures to increase effectiveness of medication.
□ Protect patient from injury. Place bed side rails up. Assist with ambulation. Remove cigarettes from patients with hypnotic dose.
▪ **PO:** Tablets should be swallowed whole with a full glass of water. For faster onset of sleep, do not administer with or immediately after a meal.

PATIENT/FAMILY TEACHING

□ Instruct patient to take zolpidem exactly as directed. Do not take more than the amount prescribed because of the habit-forming potential. Not recommended for use longer than 7–10 days. If used for 2 wk or longer, abrupt withdrawal may result in fatigue, nausea, flushing, lightheaded-

Z

Underlines indicate most frequent; **CAPITALS indicate life-threatening.*

ness, uncontrolled crying, vomiting, GI upset, panic attack, or nervousness.

▫ May cause daytime drowsiness or dizziness. Advise patient to avoid driving or other activities requiring alertness until response to this medication is known.

▫ Caution patient to avoid concurrent use of alcohol or other CNS depressants.

EVALUATION

Effectiveness of therapy can be demonstrated by: ▪ Relief of insomnia.

APPENDIX CONTENTS

APPENDIX A
Commonly Used Combination Drugs

The drugs listed in this section are in alphabetical order according to trade names. Following each trade name are the generic names of the active ingredients contained in each preparation. For information on these drugs, look up each generic name in the combination, listed separately in the *Drug Guide*. For specific doses and inert ingredients, see drug label.

Actifed—pseudoephedrine/triprolidine
Actifed Sinus Daytime—pseudoephedrine/acetaminophen
Actifed Sinus Nightime—pseudoephedrine/diphenhydramine/acetaminophen
Advil Cold & Sinus—pseudoephedrine/ibuprofen
Alazide—hydrochlorothiazide/spironolactone
Aldactazide—hydrochlorothiazide/spironolactone
Aldoclor—methyldopa/chlorothiazide
Aldoril—hydrochlorothiazide/methyldopa
Alka-Seltzer—citric acid/sodium bicarbonate/potassium bicarbonate
Alka-Seltzer Advanced Formula—sodium bicarbonate/calcium bicarbonate/acetaminophen/citric acid/potassium bicarbonate
Alka-Seltzer Plus Cold & Cough Tablets—phenylpropanolamine/chlorpheniramine/dextromethorphan/aspirin
Alka-Seltzer Plus Cold Medicine—chlorpheniramine/phenylpropanolamine/aspirin
Alka-Seltzer Plus Night-Time Cold Tablets—phenylpropanolamine/brompheniramine/dextromethorphan/aspirin
Alka-Seltzer with Aspirin—sodium bicarbonate/citric acid/aspirin
All-Nite Cold Formula Liquid—pseudoephedrine/doxylamine/dextromethorphan/acetaminophen
Allerest 12 Hour—phenylpropanolamine/chlorpheniramine
Alodopa—hydrochlorothiazide/methyldopa
Amacodone—acetaminophen/hydrocodone
Amaphen #3—acetaminophen/butalbital/caffeine/codeine
Ambenyl Cough Syrup—codeine/bromodiphenhydramine/alcohol
Amesec—ephedrine/theophylline
Anacin—aspirin/caffeine
Anacin Maximum Strength—aspirin/caffeine
Anacin PM (Aspirin Free)—diphenhydramine/acetaminophen
Anaplex HD—hydrocodone/phenylephrine/chlorpheniramine
Anaplex Liquid—chlorpheniramine/pseudoephedrine
Anatuss Syrup—guaifenesin/dextromethorphan/phenylpropanolamine
Anatuss Tablets—guaifenesin/dextromethorphan/phenylpropanolamine/acetaminophen
Anexsia—hydrocodone/acetaminophen
Antrocol—atropine/phenobarbital
Apresazide—hydralazine/hydrochlorothiazide
Apresoline-Esidrix—hydralazine/hydrochlorothiazide
Aprodine Syrup—pseudoephedrine/triprolidine
Aquaphor Antibiotic Ointment—polymyxin B/bacitracin zinc
Aralen Phosphate with Primaquine Phosphate Tablets—chloroquine/primaquine
Arthritis Pain Formula—aspirin/aluminum hydroxide/magnesium hydroxide
Ascriptin—aspirin/aluminum hydroxide/magnesium hydroxide/calcium carbonate
Ascriptin A/D—acetylsalicylic acid/magnesium hydroxide/aluminum hydroxide/calcium carbonate

Augmentin—amoxicillin/clavulanic acid
Azo Gantanol—sulfamethoxazole/phenazopyridine
Azo Gantrisin—sulfisoxazole/phenazopyridine
B and O Supprettes—belladonna extract/opium
B-A-C #3—aspirin/butalbital/caffeine/codeine
Bacticort Ophthalmic—hydrocortisone/neomycin/polymyxin B
Bactrim—trimethoprim/sulfamethoxazole
Bancap HC—acetaminophen/hydrocodone
Banex Capsules—guaifenesin/phenylpropanolamine/phenylephrine
Banex-LA Tablets—guaifenesin/phenylpropanolamine
Bayer Children's Cough Syrup—dextromethorphan/phenylpropanolamine
Bayer Select Maximum Strength Headache—acetaminophen/caffeine
Bayer Select Maximum Strength Menstrual—acetaminophen/pamabrom
Bayer Select Maximum Strength Night Time Pain Relief—acetaminophen/diphen-
    hydramine
Bayer Select Maximum Strength Sinus Pain Relief—acetaminophen/pseudo-
    ephedrine
Bellergal-S—ergotamine/phenobarbital/bellafoline
Benadryl Decongestant—diphenhydramine/pseudoephedrine
Benylin Decongestant Liquid—diphenhydramine/pseudoephedrine/alcohol
Benylin Expectorant Liquid—guaifenesin/dextromethorphan/alcohol
Blephamide Ophthalmic—prednisolone/sulfacetamide
Bromfed Capsules and Tablets—brompheniramine/pseudoephedrine
Bromo Seltzer—sodium bicarbonate/acetaminophen/citric acid
Bromophen T.D.—brompheniramine/phenylephrine/phenylpropanolamine
Bronkaid Tablets—ephedrine/theophylline/guaifenesin
Bronkolixir—theophylline/ephedrine/guaifenesin/phenobarbital
Bufferin—aspirin/calcium carbonate/magnesium oxide/magnesium carbonate
Bufferin AF Nite Time—acetaminophen/diphenhydramine/simcthicone
Cafatine PB—ergotamine/caffeine/alkaloids of belladonna/sodium pentobarbital
Cafergot—ergotamine/caffeine
Caladryl Lotion—diphenhydramine/calamine/camphor/alcohol
Calcet—elemental calcium/vitamin D
Calcidrine Syrup—codeine/calcium iodide
Cam-Ap-Es—hydralazine/hydrochlorothiazide/reserpine
Camalox—aluminum hydroxide/magnesium hydroxide/calcium carbonate
Capozide—hydrochlorothiazide/captopril
Cetacaine—benzocaine/tetracaine/butyl aminobenzoate
Cetapred Ophthalmic—prednisolone/sodium sulfacetamide
Cheracol Syrup—codeine/guaifenesin
Cherapas—hydralazine/hydrochlorothiazide/reserpine
Chlor-Trimeton 12 Hour Relief—pseudoephedrine/chlorpheniramine
Chlor-Trimeton Decongestant—pseudoephedrine/chlorpheniramine
Chloromycetin Hydrocortisone Ophthalmic—hydrocortisone/chloramphenicol
Chloroserpine—chlorothiazide/reserpine
Clindex—chlordiazepoxide/clidinium
Clinoxide—chlordiazepoxide/clidinium
Clipoxide—chlordiazepoxide/clidinium
Clysodrast—bisacodyl/tannic acid
Co-Apap—pseudoephedrine/chlorpheniramine/dextromethorphan/acetaminophen
Co-Gesic—acetaminophen/hydrocodone
Co-Trimoxazole—trimethoprim/sulfamethoxazole
CoAdvil—ibuprofen/pseudoephedrine

Codamine—hydrocodone/phenylpropanolamine
Codehist DH Elixir—pseudoephedrine/chlorpheniramine/codeine
Codiclear DH Syrup—hydrocodone/guaifenesin
Codimal DH—hydrocodone/phenylephrine/pyrilamine
Codimal Expectorant—guaifenesin/phenylpropanolamine
Codimal LA—chlorpheniramine/pseudoephedrine
Codimal PH—codeine/phenylephrine/pyrilamine
Col-Probenecid—probenecid/colchicine
Colabid—probenecid/colchicine
ColBENEMID—probenecid/colchicine
Coldrine—pseudoephedrine/acetaminophen
Coly-Mycin S Otic—hydrocortisone/neomycin/colistin/thonzonium bromide
Combipres—chlorthalidone/clonidine
Comhist—phenylephrine/chlorpheniramine/phenyltoloxamine
Comtrex—chlorpheniramine/acetaminophen/dextromethorphan/pseudoephedrine
Comtrex-Allergy-Sinus—chlorpheniramine/acetaminophen/pseudoephedrine
Comtrex Liqui-Gels—acetaminophen/phenylpropanolamine/chlorpheniramine/
    dextromethorphan
Congess—guaifenesin/pseudoephedrine
Congestac—guaifenesin/pseudoephedrine
Contac Cough Formula Liquid—dextromethorphan/guaifenesin
Contac Cough & Sore Throat Formula—dextromethorphan/guaifenesin/acetamino-
    phen
Contac Day Cold and Flu—pseudoephedrine/dextromethorphan
Contac 12 Hour—phenylpropanolamine/chlorpheniramine
Contac Jr. Non-Drowsy Cold Liquid—pseudoephedrine/dextromethorphan/acet-
    aminophen
Contac Night Cold and Flu—pseudoephedrine/diphenhydramine/dextromethor-
    phan
Contac Nighttime Cold—pseudoephedrine/doxylamine succinate/dextromethor-
    phan/acetaminophen/alcohol
Contac Non-Drowsy Formula Sinus—pseudoephedrine/acetaminophen
Contac Severe Cold—phenylpropanolamine/chlorpheniramine/dextromethorphan/
    acetaminophen
Contac Severe Cold and Flu Hot Medicine—pseudoephedrine/chlorpheniramine/
    dextromethorphan/acetaminophen
Cope—aspirin/caffeine/magnesium hydroxide/aluminum hydroxide
Cordran-N—flurandrenolide/neomycin
Coricidin—chlorpheniramine/acetaminophen
Coricidin 'D'—phenylpropanolamine/chlorpheniramine/acetaminophen
Correctol—docusate sodium/phenolphthalein
Cortisporin Ophthalmic/Otic—neomycin/polymyxin B/hydrocortisone
Cortisporin Topical—bacitracin zinc/neomycin/polymyxin B/hydrocortisone
Corzide—nadolol/bendroflumethiazide
CoTylenol Cold Formula—chlorpheniramine/acetaminophen/pseudoephedrine/
    dextromethorphan
Cyclomydril—cyclopentolate/phenylephrine
D-S-S Plus—docusate sodium/casanthranol
Dallergy—chlorpheniramine/phenylephrine/methscopolamine
Dallergy-D—pseudoephedrine/chlorpheniramine
Damacet-P—hydrocodone/acetaminophen
Damason-P—hydrocodone/aspirin/caffeine
Darvocet-N 100—propoxyphene-N/acetaminophen

DayCare—guaifenesin/dextromethorphan/pseudoephedrine/acetaminophen
Deconamine SR—pseudoephedrine/chlorpheniramine
Deconsal II—pseudoephedrine/guaifenesin
Demazin—phenylpropanolamine/chlorpheniramine
Demerol APAP—acetaminophen/meperidine
Demi-Regroton—chlorthalidone/reserpine
Demulen—ethinyl estradiol/ethynodiol diacetate
Dexacidin Ophthalmic—dexamethasone/neomycin/polymyxin B
Dexasporin Ophthalmic—dexamethasone/neomycin/polymyxin B
Di-Gel—aluminum hydroxide/magnesium hydroxide/simethicone
Di-Gel Advanced Formula—magnesium hydroxide/calcium carbonate/simethicone
Dialose Plus Tablets—docusate potassium/phenolphthalein sodium
Dieutrim T.D. Capsules—benzocaine/phenylpropanolamine/carboxymethyl-
  cellulose
Dihistine DH—pseudoephedrine/chlorpheniramine/codeine
Dilantin with Phenobarbital Kapseals—phenytoin/phenobarbital
Dilaudid Cough Syrup—guaifenesin/hydromorphone
Dilor-G—dyphylline/guaifenesin
Dimetane Decongestant—brompheniramine/phenylephrine
Dimetapp—brompheniramine/phenylpropanolamine
Dimetapp Cold & Flu—phenylpropanolamine/brompheniramine/acetaminophen
Dimetapp Sinus—pseudoephedrine/ibuprofen
Diupres—chlorothiazide/reserpine
Diurese-R—reserpine/trichlormethiazide
Diurigen with Reserpine—reserpine/chlorothiazide
Diutensin-R—methyclothiazide/reserpine
Doan's PM Extra Strength—magnesium salicylate/diphenhydramine HCl
Dolacet C-3—hydrocodone/acetaminophen
Donnagel—kaolin/pectin/atropine/hyoscyamine/scopolamine
Donnatal—phenobarbital/hyoscyamine/atropine/scopolamine
Donnazyme—pancreatin/lipase/protease/amylase
Doxidan—docusate calcium/phenolphthalein
Dristan—phenylephrine/chlorpheniramine/acetaminophen
Dristan Allergy—pseudoephedrine/brompheniramine
Dristan Cold + Flu—acetaminophen/pseudoephedrine/chlorpheniramine/dextro-
  methorphan
Dristan Cold Multi-Symptom—acetaminophen/pseudoephedrine/bromphenir-
  amine
Drixoral Plus—pseudoephedrine/dexbrompheniramine/acetaminophen
Drixoral Tablet—pseudoephedrine/dexbrompheniramine
DT—diphtheria toxoid/tetanus toxoid
DTP—diphtheria toxoid/tetanus toxoid/pertussis
Duo-Medihaler—phenylephrine/isoproterenol
Duratuss—guaifenesin/pseudoephedrine
Duratuss HD—guaifenesin/hydrocodone/pseudoephedrine
Dura-Vent—phenylpropanolamine/guaifenesin
Dura-Vent/A—phenylpropanolamine/chlorpheniramine
Dura-Vent/DA—phenylephrine/chlorpheniramine/methscopolamine
Dyazide—hydrochlorothiazide/triamterene
E-Pilo—epinephrine bitartrate/pilocarpine
Elase—fibrinolysin/desoxyribonuclease
Elase-Chloromycetin Ointment—fibrinolysin/desoxyribonuclease/chloramphenicol
Elixophyllin-GG—guaifenesin/theophylline

Empirin #2, #3, #4—aspirin/codeine phosphate
Endal HD—chlorpheniramine/hydrocodone/phenylephrine
Enlon-Plus—atropine/endrophonium
Enovid—mestranol/norethynodrel
Entazyme—pancreatin/lipase/protease/amylase
Entex—phenylephrine/phenylpropanolamine/guaifenesin
Entex LA—phenylpropanolamine/guaifenesin
Epifoam Aerosol Foam—hydrocortisone/pramoxine
Equagesic—aspirin/meprobamate
Equazine M—aspirin/meprobamate
Eryzole—erythromycin/sulfisoxazole
Esimil—guanethidine/hydrochlorothiazide
Etrafon—perphenazine/amitriptyline
Ex-Lax Extra Gentle—docusate sodium/phenolphthalein
Excedrin Extra Strength—aspirin/acetaminophen/caffeine
Excedrin P.M. Aspirin Free Tablets and Caplets—acetaminophen/diphen-
    hydramine citrate
Excedrin Sinus—pseudoephedrine/acetaminophen
Fedahist—pseudoephedrine/chlorpheniramine
Feen-A-Mint Dual Formula—docusate sodium/phenolphthalein
Femcaps—acetaminophen/caffeine/ephedrine/atropine
Fergon Plus—ferrous gluconate/ascorbic acid
Ferro-Sequels—docusate sodium/ferrous fumarate
Fiogesic—phenylpropanolamine/pyrilamine/pheniramine/calcium carbaspirin
Fioricet with codeine—acetaminophen/butalbital/caffeine/codeine
Fiorinal—aspirin/caffeine/butalbital
Fiorinal #1, #2, #3—aspirin/caffeine/butalbital/codeine
FML-S Ophthalmic—flurometholone/sulfacetamide
4-Way Fast Acting Original—phenylephrine/naphazoline/pyrilamine
Gaviscon Liquid—aluminum hydroxide/magnesium carbonate
Gaviscon Tablets—aluminum hydroxide/magnesium trisilicate/alginic acid/
    sodium bicarbonate
Gelusil—aluminum hydroxide/magnesium hydroxide/simethicone
Genatuss DM Syrup—guaifenesin/dextromethorphan/alcohol
Granulex—trypsin/Balsam Peru/castor oil
H.H.R. Tablets—hydralazine/hydrochlorothiazide/reserpine
Halotussin-DM—guaifenesin/dextromethorphan/alcohol
Head and Chest Cold Medicine—guaifenesin/phenylpropanolamine
Hemorrhoidal HC—hydrocortisone acetate/bismuth/benzyl/benzoate/balsam peru/
    zinc oxide
Hexatussin—chlorpheniramine/hydrocodone/phenindamine/phenylephrine/
    pyrilamine
Histafed C Cough Syrup—pseudoephedrine/triprolidine/codeine
Histafed LA—chlorpheniramine/pseudoephedrine
Histamic—chlorpheniramine/phenylephrine/phenylpropanolamine/phenyl-
    toloxamine
Humibid DM—dextromethorphan/guaifenesin
Hyco-Pap—acetaminophen/hydrocodone
Hycodan—hydrocodone/homatropine
Hycomine Compound—chlorpheniramine/acetaminophen/phenylephrine/hydro-
    codone/caffeine
Hycomine Syrup—hydrocodone/phenylpropanolamine
Hycotuss Expectorant—guaifenesin/hydrocodone/alcohol

Hydrazide—hydralazine/hydrochlorothiazide
Hydro-Serp—hydrochlorothiazide/reserpine
Hydrocet—hydrocodone/acetaminophen
Hydrogesic—hydrocodone/acetaminophen
Hydropine—hydroflumethiazide/reserpine
Hydropres-50—hydrochlorothiazide/reserpine
Hydroserpine—hydrochlorothiazide/reserpine
Hydrosine—hydrochlorothiazide/reserpine
Iberet Filmtab—ferrous sulfate/ascorbic acid/calcium pantothenate/B–complex
  vitamins
Iberet Liquid—ferrous sulfate/ascorbic acid/dexpanthenol/B–complex vitamins
Ilopan-choline—dexpanthenol/choline
Inderide—hydrochlorothiazide/propranolol
Iophen-C—iodinated glycerol/codeine
Iophen-DM—iodinated glycerol/dextromethorphan
Kank-a—benzocaine/benzoin compound/cetylpyridium/castor oil
Kapectolin PG—kaolin/pectin/atropine/hyoscyamine/hyoscine/powdered opium/
  alcohol
Kondremul with Phenolphthalein—phenolphthalein/mineral oil/Irish moss
Lactinex—L. acidophilus/L bulgaricus
Levsin w/Phenobarbital—hyoscyamine/phenobarbital
Librax—chlordiazepoxide/clindinium
Lida-Mantel-HC Cream—hydrocortisone/lidocaine
Lidox—chlordiazepoxide/clidinium
Limbitrol—chlordiazepoxide/amitriptyline
Lo/Ovral—ethinyl estradiol/norgestrel
Lopressor HCT—hydrochlorothiazide/metoprolol
Lorcet—acetaminophen/hydrocodone
Lortab—acetaminophen/hydrocodone
Lortab ASA—aspirin/hydrocodone
Lotensin HCT—hydrochlorothiazide/benazepril
Lotrisone—betamethasone/clotrimazole
Lufyllin-EPG—ephedrine/dyphylline/guaifenesin/phenobarbital
Lufyllin-GG—dyphylline/guaifenesin
M-M-R II—mixture of 3 viruses: measles/mumps/rubella
M-R-Vax II—mixture of 2 viruses: measles/rubella
Maalox Plus—aluminum hydroxide/magnesium hydroxide/simethicone
Maalox Tablets—aluminum hydroxide/magnesium hydroxide
Mallopres—hydrochlorothiazide/reserpine
Marax—ephedrine/theophylline/hydroxyzine
Maxitrol Ophthalmic—neomycin/dexamethasone/polymyxin B
Maxzide—hydrochlorothiazide/triamterene
Medi-Flu Liquid—pseudoephedrine/chlorpheniramine/dextromethorphan/acet-
  aminophen
Medipain 5—hydrocodone/acetaminophen
Menrium—chlordiazepoxide/esterified estrogens
Mepergan—meperidine/promethazine
Meprobamate Compound—aspirin/meprobamate
Meprogesic Q—aspirin/meprobamate
Metatensin—reserpine/trichlormethiazide
Metimyd Ophthalmic—prednisolone/sodium sulfacetamide
Midol Maximum Strength Multi System Menstrual—acetaminophen/pamabrom/
  pyrilamine

Midol Multi-Symptom—acetaminophen/pyrilamine
Midol Original Formula—cinnamedrine/aspirin/caffeine
Midol, Teen—acetaminophen/pamabrom
Midrin—isometheptene/acetaminophen/dichloralphenazone
Minizide—prazosin/polythiazide
Modane Plus—docusate sodium/phenolphthalein
Moduretic—hydrochlorothiazide/amiloride
Myapap with Codeine Elixir—codeine/acetaminophen
Mycolog II—triamcinolone acetonide/nystatin
Mylanta—aluminum hydroxide/magnesium hydroxide/simethicone
Mylanta Gelcaps—calcium carbonate/magnesium carbonate
Naldecon—chlorpheniramine/phenylephrine/phenylpropanolamine/phenyl-
    toloxamine
Naldecon CX Liquid—guaifenesin/phenylpropanolamine/codeine
Naldecon DX Syrup—guaifenesin/dextromethorphan/phenylpropanolamine
Naldecon EX Syrup—guaifenesin/phenylpropanolamine
Naquival—reserpine/trichlormethiazide
Nasatab LA—guaifenesin/pseudoephedrine
Neocortef Topical—hydrocortisone acetate/neomycin
NeoDecadron—neomycin/dexamethasone
Neosporin Cream—polymyxin B/neomycin
Neosporin GU Irrigant—neomycin/polymyxin B
Neosporin Ophthalmic Ointment—polymyxin B/neomycin/bacitracin
Neosporin Ophthalmic Solution—polymyxin B/neomycin/gramicidin
Neosporin Plus Cream—polymyxin B/neomycin/lidocaine
Neosporin Topical Ointment—neomycin/bacitracin zinc/polymyxin B
Nephrox—aluminum hydroxide/mineral oil
Nolamine—phenylpropanolamine/chlorpheniramine/phenindamine
Norcet—hydrocodone/acetaminophen
Norgesic—orphenadrine/caffeine/aspirin
Normozide—labetalol/hydrochlorothiazide
Novafed A—chlorpheniramine/pseudoephedrine
Novahistine DH—chlorpheniramine/pseudoephedrine/codeine
Novahistine DMX—guaifenesin/dextromethorphan/pseudoephedrine
Novahistine Expectorant—guaifenesin/pseudoephedrine/codeine
NyQuil Children's Allergy/Head Cold—pseudoephedrine/chlorpheniramine
NyQuil Hot Therapy—acetaminophen/pseudoephedrine/dextromethorphan/doxyl-
    amine
NyQuil Nighttime Cold/Flu Medicine—pseudoephedrine/doxylamine/
    dextromethorphan/alcohol (may contain tartrazine)
Nytime Cold Medicine—pseudoephedrine/doxylamine/dextromethorphan/acet-
    aminophen/alcohol
Octicair Otic—hydrocortisone/neomycin/polymyxin B
Ocu-Cort—hydrocortisone/bacitracin/neomycin/polymyxin B
Ocu-Lone-C—prednisolone acetate/sodium sulfacetamide
Ocu-Spor B—neomycin/bacitracin/polymyxin B
Ocu-Spor-G—neomycin/gramicidin/polymyxin B
Ocu-Trol—neomycin/dexamethasone/polymyxin B
Ocumycin—bacitracin/polymyxin B
Ophthocort—hydrocortisone acetate/chloramphenicol/polymyxin B
Optimyd—prednisolone acetate/sodium sulfacetamide
Ornade—phenylpropanolamine/chlorpheniramine
Orphengesic—orphenadrine/aspirin/caffeine

Ortho-Novum 7/7/7—norethindrone/ethinyl estradiol (3 phases)
Otocort—hydrocortisone/neomycin/polymyxin B
P-A-C Tablets—aspirin/caffeine (contains tartrazine)
P-V-Tussin Tablets—guaifenesin/hydrocodone/phenindamine
Pamprin—acetaminophen/pamabrom/pyrilamine
Panacet 5/500—hydrocodone/acetaminophen
Panasal 5/500—hydrocodone/aspirin
Papadeine #3, #4—codeine/acetaminophen
Parapectolin—kaolin/pectin/paregoric
Pedia Care Cold-Allergy—pseudoephedrine/chlorpheniramine
Pedia Care Cough-Cold Formula—pseudoephedrine/chlorpheniramine/dextro-
    methorphan
Pedia Care NightRest Liquid—pseudoephedrine/chlorpheniramine/dextromethor-
    phan
Pediacof—codeine/phenylephrine/chlorpheniramine/potassium iodide/
    alcohol
Pediazole—erythromycin/sulfisoxazole
Percocet—oxycodone/acetaminophen
Percogesic—phenyltoloxamine/acetaminophen
Perdiem Granules—senna/psyllium
Peri-Colace—docusate sodium/casanthranol
Pertussin AM Liquid—dextromethorphan/pseudoephedrine/guaifenesin
Phenaphen #2, #3, #4—acetaminophen/codeine
Phenergan VC—phenylephrine/promethazine
Phenergan-D Tablets—pseudoephedrine/promethazine
Pherazine DM—dextromethorphan/promethazine/alcohol
Phillips' LaxCaps—docusate sodium/phenolphthalein
PMB—conjugated estrogens/meprobamate
Polaramine Expectorant—guaifenesin/dexchlorpheniramine/pseudoephedrine
Poly-Histine—pheniramine/pyrilamine/phenyltoloxamine/alcohol
Poly-Histine CS—phenylpropanolamine/brompheniramine/codeine
Poly-Histine DM—brompheniramine/phenylpropanolamine/dextromethorphan
Poly-Pred Ophthalmic Suspension—prednisolone acetate/neomycin/polymyxin B
Polycillin-PRB—ampicillin/probenecid
Polycitra—potassium citrate/sodium citrate/citric acid
Polysporin—polymyxin B/bacitracin
Polytrim Ophthalmic—polymyxin B/trimethoprim
Premsyn PMS—acetaminophen/pamabrom/pyrilamine
Primatene—theophylline/ephedrine
Primatene Dual Action—theophylline/ephedrine/guaifenesin
Primaxin—imipenen/cilistatin sodium
Prinzide—lisinopril/hydrochlorothiazide
Probampacin—ampicillin/probenecid
Proben-C—probenecid/colchicine
Procto-Foam HC Aerosol Foam—hydrocortisone/pramoxine
Propacet 100—propoxyphene-N/acetaminophen
Propain HC—hydrocodone/acetaminophen
Pseudo-Chlor—pseudoephedrine/chlorpheniramine
Pseudogest Plus—pseudoephedrine/chlorpheniramine
Quadrinal Tablets—ephedrine/theophylline/potassium iodide/phenobarbital
Quelidrine Cough Syrup—dextromethorphan/phenylephrine/ephedrine/chlorphen-
    iramine/ammonium chloride/ipecac
Quibron—guaifenesin/theophylline

Quiet Night Liquid—pseudoephedrine/doxylamine/dextromethorphan/acetaminophen

R&C Shampoo—pyrethins/piperonyl butoxide

Rauzide—bendroflumethiazide/powdered rauwolfia serpentina

Regroton—chlorthalidone/reserpine

Regulace—docusate sodium/casanthranol

Renese-R—polythiazide/reserpine

Respaire-60 SR—guaifenesin/pseudoephedrine

RID Shampoo—pyrethins/piperonyl butoxide

Rid-A-Pain with Codeine—codeine/aspirin/acetaminophen/caffeine/salicylamide

Rifamate—isoniazid/rifampin

Riopan Plus—magaldrate/simethicone

Robaxisal—aspirin/methocarbamol

Robitussin A-C Syrup—codeine/guaifenesin/alcohol

Robitussin-CF Syrup—guaifenesin/dextromethorphan/phenylpropanolamine/alcohol

Robitussin Cough and Cold—dextromethorphan/pseudoephedrine

Robitussin-DAC—codeine/guaifenesin/pseudoephedrine/alcohol

Robitussin-DM Syrup—guaifenesin/dextromethorphan

Robitussin Night Relief Liquid—dextromethorphan/pyrilamine/phenylephrine/acetaminophen

Robitussin-PE—guaifenesin/pseudoephedrine/alcohol

Rolaids Sodium Free Tablets—magnesium hydroxide/calcium carbonate

Rondec—pseudoephedrine/carbinoxamine

Ru-Tuss DE Tablets—pseudoephedrine/guaifenesin

Ru-Tuss Expectorant—guaifenesin/pseudoephedrine/dextromethorphan/alcohol

Ru-Tuss Tablets—phenylephrine/phenylpropanolamine/chlorpheniramine/hyoscyamine/atropine/scopolamine

Ru-Tuss II Capsules—phenylpropanolamine/chlorpheniramine

Ru-Tuss with Hydrocodone—hydrocodone/phenylephrine/pyrilamine/pheniramine/phenylpropanolamine/alcohol

Ryna—pseudoephedrine/chlorpheniramine

Ryna-C—pseudoephedrine/chlorpheniramine/codeine

Rynatan—phenylephrine/chlorpheniramine/pyrilamine

Rynatuss—ephedrine/carbetapentane/chlorpheniramine/phenylephrine

Salazide—reserpine/hydroflumethiazide

Salutensin—reserpine/hydroflumethiazide

Scot-Tussin Original 5-Action Liquid—phenylephrine/pheniramine/sodium citrate/sodium salicylate/caffeine citrate

Sedapap #3—acetaminophen/butalbital/codeine

Seldane-D—terfenadine/pseudoephedrine

Senokot-S—standardized senna concentrate/docusate sodium

Septra—trimethoprim/sulfamethoxazole

Ser-A-Gen—hydralazine/hydrochlorothiazide/reserpine

Ser-Ap-Es—hydralazine/hydrochlorothiazide/reserpine

Seralazide—hydrochlorothiazide/reserpine/hydralazine

Serathide—hydralazine/hydrochlorothiazide/reserpine

Serpazide—hydralazine/hydrochlorothiazide/reserpine

Sinarest No Drowsiness Tablets—pseudoephedrine/acetaminophen

Sine-Aid—pseudoephedrine/acetaminophen

Sine-Off Maximum Strength Allergy/Sinus Caplets—pseudoephedrine/chlorpheniramine/acetaminophen

Sine-Off Maximum Strength No Drowsiness Formula Caplets—pseudoephedrine/
acetaminophen
Sinemet—carbidopa/levodopa
Sinutab Maximum Strength—acetaminophen/chlorpheniramine/pseudoephedrine
Slo-Phyllin GG Capsules—guaifenesin/theophylline
Soma Compound—aspirin/carisoprodol
Spirozide—hydrochlorothiazide/spironolactone
St. Joseph Cold Tablets for Children—phenylpropanolamine/acetaminophen
Sudafed Cough Syrup—guaifenesin/dextromethorphan/pseudoephedrine
Sudafed Plus Tablets—pseudoephedrine/chlorpheniramine
Sulphrin Ophthalmic Ointment—prednisolone acetate/sodium sulfacetamide
Sulpred—prednisolone acetate/sulfacetamide
Sultrin Triple Sulfa Vaginal—sulfathiazole/sulfacetamide/sulfabenzamide/urea
Synalgos DC—aspirin/caffeine/dihydrocodeine
T.E.H. Compound—ephedrine/theophylline/hydroxyzine
T-Gesic—hydrocodone/acetaminophen
Talacen—acetaminophen/pentazocine
Talwin Compound—aspirin/pentazocine
Talwin NX—pentazocine/naloxone
Tavist-D—clemastine/phenylpropanolamine
Tedral—ephedrine/theophylline/phenobarbital
Tedrigen—ephedrine/theophylline/phenobarbital
Tenoretic—chlorthalidone/atenolol
Terphan Elixir—dextromethorphan/terpin hydrate
Terra-Cortril Suspension—hydrocortisone acetate/oxytetracycline
Terramycin with Polymyxin B Sulfate Ophthalmic Ointment—polymyxin B/oxytetra-
cycline
Theodrine—ephedrine/theophylline/phenobarbital
TheraFlu Flu and Cold Medicine—pseudoephedrine/chlorpheniramine/acetamino-
phen
TheraFlu Flu, Cold & Cough Medicine—pseudoephedrine/chlorpheniramine/
dextromethorphan/acetaminophen
Thiosulfil-A—sulfamethizole/phenazopyridine
Timentin—ticarcillin/clavulanic acid
Timolide—hydrochlorothiazide/timolol
TMP-SMZ—trimethoprim/sulfamethoxazole
TobraDex Ophthalmic—dexamethasone/tobramycin
Trandate HCT—hydrochlorothiazide/labetalol
Tri-Hydroserpine—hydralazine/hydrochlorothiazide/reserpine
Tri-Levlen—levo-norgestrel/ethinyl estradiol
Triacin-C Cough Syrup—codeine/pseudoephedrine/triprolidine
Triaminic—pyrilamine/pheniramine/phenylpropanolamine
Triaminic Allergy—phenylpropanolamine/chlorpheniramine
Triaminic-DM—dextromethorphan/phenylpropanolamine
Triaminic Expectorant—guaifenesin/phenylpropanolamine
Triaminic Expectorant DH—guaifenesin/hydrocodone/phenylpropanolamine/
pheniramine/pyrilamine/alcohol
Triaminic Nite Light Liquid—pseudoephedrine/chlorpheniramine/dextro-
methorphan
Triaminic TR Tablets—phenylpropanolamine/pyrilamine/pheniramine
Triaminicol—phenylpropanolamine/chlorpheniramine/dextromethorphan
Triavil—perphenazine/amitriptyline

Trigesic—aspirin/caffeine/acetaminophen
Trimedine—dextromethorphan/chlorpheniramine/phenylephrine
Triminol Cough Syrup—dextromethorphan/chlorpheniramine/phenylpropanol-
   amine
Trinalin Repetabs—azatadine maleate/pseudoephedrine
Triphasil—levonorgestrel/ethinyl estradiol
Triple Antibiotic Ophthalmic—polymyxin B/neomycin/bacitracin
Tuinal—amobarbital/secobarbital
Tums Liquid Extra Strength with Simethicone—simethicone/calcium carbonate
Tums Plus—simethicone/calcium carbonate
Tuss-Ornade—phenylpropanolamine/caramiphen
Tussi-Organidin—codeine/iodinated glycerol
Tussi-Organidin DM—iodinated glycerol/dextromethorphan
Tussionex—chlorpheniramine/hydrocodone (as polistirex)
Ty-Cold Tablets—pseudoephedrine/chlorpheniramine/dextromethorphan/acet-
   aminophen
Ty-Tab #3, #4 Tablets—codeine/acetaminophen
Tylenol #1, #2, #3, #4—acetaminophen/codeine
Tylenol Children's Cold Multi-Symptom Plus Cough—acetaminophen/dextromet-
   horphan/chlorpheniramine/pseudoephedrine
Tylenol Cold Effervescent—phenylpropanolamine/chlorpheniramine/acetamino-
   phen
Tylenol Cold & Flu Medication—acetaminophen/chlorpheniramine/
   pseudoephedrine/dextromethorphan
Tylenol Cold and Flu No Drowsiness Formula—acetaminophen/pseudoephedrine/
   dextromethorphan
Tylenol Cold Multi-Symptom—acetaminophen/chlorpheniramine/pseudo-
   ephedrine/dextromethorphan
Tylenol Maximum Strength Allergy Sinus—acetaminophen/chlorpheniramine/
   pseudoephedrine
Tylenol Maximum Strength Sinus Tablets—pseudoephedrine/acetaminophen
Tylenol No Drowsiness Cold—pseudoephedrine/dextromethorphan/acetamino-
   phen
Tylenol PM—acetaminophen/diphenhydramine
Tylox—oxycodone/acetaminophen
Unasyn—ampicillin/sulbactam
Unipres—hydralazine/hydrochlorothiazide/reserpine
Urised—methenamine/phenyl salicylate/atropine/hyoscyamine/benzoic acid/
   methylene blue
Vanex HD—chlorpheniramine/hydrocodone/phenylephrine
Vanquish—aspirin/acetaminophen/caffeine/aluminum hydroxide/magnesium
   hydroxide
Vaseretic—enalapril/hydrochlorothiazide
Vasocidin Ophthalmic—prednisolone/sulfacetamide
Veltap Elixir—brompheniramine/phenylephrine/phenylpropanolamine/alcohol
Vicks Children's NyQuil Allergy/Head Cold Liquid—pseudoephedrine/chlor-
   pheniramine
Vicks Cough Silencers—dextromethorphan/benzocaine
Vicks DayQuil—dextromethorphan/pseudoephedrine/acetaminophen/guaifenesin
Vicks Formula 44—dextromethorphan/chlorpheniramine/alcohol
Vicks Formula 44D Liquid—dextromethorphan/pseudoephedrine/guaifenesin
Vicks Formula 44M Cough and Cold Liquid—dextromethorphan/pseudoephedrine/
   chlorpheniramine/acetaminophen

Vicodin—acetaminophen/hydrocodone
Vioform-Hydrocortisone—clioquinol/hydrocortisone
Visine Extra—polyethylene glycol 400/tetrahydrozoline
Wigraine—ergotamine/caffeine
Zestoretic—lisinopril/hydrochlorothiazide
Ziac—bisoprolol/hydrochlorothiazide
Zydone—hydrocodone/acetaminophen

APPENDIX B
Equianalgesic Tables

OPIOID ANALGESICS COMMONLY USED FOR SEVERE PAIN

Equianalgesic doses are equivalent to 10 mg of IM morphine (i.e., morphine 10 mg IM = meperidine 75 mg IM = oxycodone 30 mg PO).

NAME	EQUIANALGESIC DOSE (mg)		STARTING ORAL DOSE		COMMENTS	PRECAUTIONS AND CONTRAINDICATIONS
	ORAL	PARENTERAL*	ADULTS (mg)	CHILDREN (mg/kg)		
Morphine	30†	10	15–30	0.3	Standard of comparison for opioid analgesics; sustained-release preparations (MS Contin, Oramorph-SR) release drug over 8–12 hr.	For all opioids, caution in patients with impaired ventilation, bronchial asthma, increased intracranial pressure, liver failure.
Hydromorphone (Dilaudid)	7.5	1.5	4–8	0.06	Slightly shorter duration than morphine.	
Oxycodone	30	—	15–30	0.3		
Methadone (Dolophine)	20	10	5–10	0.2	Good oral potency; long plasma half-life (24–36 hr).	Accumulates with repetitive dosing, causing excessive sedation (on days 2–5).
Levorphanol (Levo-Dromoman)	4	2	2–4	0.04	Long plasma half-life (12–16 hr).	Accumulates on days 2–3.
Fentanyl	—	0.1	—	—	Transdermal fentanyl (Duragesic) 25–50 mcg/hr roughly equivalent to 30 mg sustained-release morphine q 8 hr.	Because of skin reservoir of drug, 12-hr delay in onset and offset of transdermal patch; fever increases rate of absorption.
Oxymorphone (Numorphan)	—	1	—	—	5 mg rectal suppository = 5 mg morphine IM.	Like IM morphine.
Meperidine (Demerol)	300	75	Not recommended	—	Slightly shorter acting than morphine.	Normeperidine (toxic metabolite) accumulates with repetitive dosing, causing CNS excitation; avoid in patients with impaired renal function or who are receiving monoamine oxidase inhibitors, irritating to tissues with repeated IM injection.

Opioid Agonist-Antagonists

Nalbuphine (Nubain)	—	10	—	—	Not available orally; not scheduled under Controlled Substances Act.	Incidence of psychotomimetic effects lower than with pentazocine; may precipitate withdrawal in opioid-dependent patients.
Butorphanol (Stadol)	—	2	—	—	Like nalbuphine.	Like nalbuphine.
Dezocine (Dalgan)	—	10	—	—	Like nalbuphine.	May precipitate withdrawal in opioid-dependent patients; SC injection irritating.
Buprenorphine (Buprenex)	—	0.4	—	—	Not available orally; sublingual preparation not yet in US; less abuse liability than morphine; does not produce psychotomimetic effects.	May precipitate withdrawal in opioid-dependent patients; not readily reversed by naloxone; avoid in labor.

*These are standard IM doses for acute pain in adults and also may be used to convert doses for IV infusions and repeated small IV boluses. For single IV boluses, use half the IM dose. IV doses for children >6 mo = parenteral equianalgesic dose × weight (kg)/100.

†Some experts argue that 60 mg of oral morphine is the more accurate equivalent dose and suggest caution in converting patients from high doses of oral morphine to other drugs if the 30-mg equivalent is used.

FENTANYL TRANSDERMAL DOSE BASED ON DAILY MORPHINE EQUIVALENCE DOSE*

ORAL 24-HR MORPHINE (mg/day)	IM 24-HR MORPHINE (mg/day)	FENTANYL TRANSDERMAL (mcg/hr)
45–134	8–22	25
135–224	23–37	50
225–314	38–52	75
315–404	53–67	100
405–494	68–82	125
495–584	83–97	150
585–674	98–112	175
675–764	113–127	200
765–854	128–142	225
855–944	143–157	250
945–1034	158–172	275
1035–1124	173–187	300

*A 10-mg IM or 60-mg oral dose of morphine every 4 hr for 24 hr (total of 60 mg/day IM or 360 mg/day oral) was considered approximately equivalent to fentanyl transdermal 100 mcg/hr.

OPIOID ANALGESICS COMMONLY USED FOR MILD TO MODERATE PAIN

NAME	STARTING DOSE* ADULTS (mg)	STARTING DOSE* CHILDREN (mg/kg)	COMMENTS	PRECAUTIONS AND CONTRAINDICATIONS
Morphine-like Agonists				
Codeine	30–60	0.5–1	Many preparations include combination: with nonopioid analgesics.†	Caution in patients with impaired ventilation, bronchial asthma, increased intracranial pressure, liver failure.
Oxycodone	5	0.1	Shorter acting; many preparations include acetaminophen, which limits dose to 12 tabs/day.†	Same as for codeine.
Meperidine (Demerol)	50	NR‡	Shorter acting; biotransformed to normeperidine, a toxic metabolite.	Normeperidine accumulates with repetitive dosing, causing CNS excitation; avoid in patients with impaired renal function or who are receiving monoamine oxidase inhibitors; avoid any chronic use.
Propoxyphene (Darvon)	65–130	NR	Weak analgesic; many preparations include nonopioid analgesics; biotransformed to potentially toxic metabolite (norpropoxyphene).	Propoxyphene and metabolite accumulate with repetitive dosing; overdose complicated by convulsions.
Mixed Agonist-Antagonist				
Pentazocine (Talwin)	50	NR	Some preparations include naloxone to discourage parenteral abuse.	May cause psychotomimetic effects; may precipitate withdrawal in opioid-dependent patients.

*Starting doses are approximately equianalgesic to aspirin 650 mg (adults) or 10–15 mg/kg (children). The optimal dose for each patient is determined by titration.
†In children, opioid-acetaminophen formulations must not exceed the maximum safe dose of acetaminophen, 90 mg/kg/day.
‡NR = not recommended.

Adapted from American Pain Society, Principles of Analgesic Use in the Treatment of Acute Pain and Cancer Pain, ed 3, 1992.

APPENDIX C
Schedules of Controlled Substances

Classes or schedules are determined by the Drug Enforcement Agency (DEA), which is an arm of the United States Justice Department, and are based on the potential for abuse and dependence liability (physical and psychological) of the medication. Some states may have stricter prescription regulations.

Schedule I (C-I): Potential for abuse is so high as to be unacceptable. May be used for research with appropriate limitations. Examples are LSD and heroin.

Schedule II (C-II): High potential for abuse and extreme liability for physical and psychological dependence (amphetamines, opioid analgesics, dronabinol, certain barbiturates). Outpatient prescriptions must be in writing. In emergencies, telephone orders may be acceptable if a written prescription is provided within 72 hr. No refills are allowed.

Schedule II Drugs Included in *Davis's Drug Guide for Nurses*

alfentanil	meperidine
amobarbital	methadone
codeine (single entity; solid dosage form or injectable)	methylphenidate
	morphine
dronabinol	oxycodone
droperidol/fentanyl	oxymorphone
fentanyl	pentobarbital (oral and parenteral)
glutethimide	secobarbital (oral and parenteral)
hydromorphone	sufentanil
levorphanol	

Schedule III (C-III): Intermediate potential for abuse (less than C-II) and intermediate liability for physical and psychological dependence (certain nonbarbiturate sedatives, certain nonamphetamine CNS stimulants, and limited dosages of certain opioid analgesics). Outpatient prescriptions can be refilled 5 times within 6 mo from date of issue if authorized by prescriber. Telephone orders are acceptable.

Schedule III Drugs Included in *Davis's Drug Guide for Nurses*

anabolic steroids (testosterone, nandrolone)
butalbital compound (in combination with nonopioid analgesics)
codeine (in combination with nonopioid analgesics; solid oral dosage forms)
hydrocodone (in combination with nonopioid analgesics)
pentobarbital (rectal)
thiopental

Schedule IV (C-IV): Less abuse potential than Schedule III with minimal liability for physical or psychological dependence (certain sedative/hypnotics, certain antianxiety agents, some barbiturates, benzodiazepines, chloral hydrate, pentazocine, and propoxyphene). Outpatient prescriptions can be refilled 5 times within 6 mo from date of issue if authorized by prescriber. Telephone orders are acceptable.

Schedule IV Drugs Included in *Davis's Drug Guide for Nurses*

alprazolam	codeine (elixir or oral suspension with acetaminophen)
chloral hydrate	
chlordiazepoxide	diazepam
clonazepam	difenoxin/atropine
clorazepate	estazolam

flurazepam
halazepam
lorazepam
meprobamate
midazolam
oxazepam
pemoline
pentazocine

phenobarbital
prazepam
propoxyphene
quazepam
temazepam
triazolam
zolpidem

Schedule V (C-V): Minimal abuse potential. Number of outpatients refills determined by prescriber. Some products (cough suppressants with small amounts of codeine, and antidiarrheals containing paregoric) may be available without prescription to patients >18 yr of age.

Schedule V Drugs Included in *Davis's Drug Guide for Nurses*
buprenorphine
codeine (in cough preparations; <10 mg/5 ml or dosage unit)
diphenoxylate/atropine

Infusion Rate Tables

ALTEPLASE (Activase)

Dilution: 20-mg vial with 20 ml diluent or 50-mg vial with 50 ml diluent = 1 mg/ml.

Alteplase 1 mg/ml pt >65 kg	dose (vol) *first hr**	dose (vol) *second hr*	dose (vol) *third hr*
	60 mg (60 ml)	20 mg (20 ml)	20 mg (20 ml)

Alteplase 1 mg/ml pt <65 kg	dose (mg/kg) *first hr†*	dose (mg/kg) *second hr*	dose (mg/kg) *third hr*
	0.75 mg/kg	0.25 mg/kg	0.25 mg/kg

* Give 6–10 mg (6–10 ml) as a bolus over first 1–2 min.
† 0.075–0.125 mg/kg of this given as a bolus over the first 1–2 min.

AMINOPHYLLINE

Dilution: 250 mg in 250 ml or 500 mg in 500 ml or 1000 mg in 1000 ml = 1 mg/ml.
Loading dose in patients who have not received aminophylline in preceding 24 hr = 5.6 mg/kg (5.6 ml/kg) of above dilution administered over 20 min.

Aminophylline Infusion Rates (ml/hr)
Concentration = 1 mg/ml

Dose	Patient Weight					
	50 kg	60 kg	70 kg	80 kg	90 kg	100 kg
loading dose (mg)*	280 mg	336 mg	392 mg	448 mg	504 mg	560 mg
0.9 mg/kg/hr	45 ml/hr	54 ml/hr	63 ml/hr	72 ml/hr	81 ml/hr	90 ml/hr
0.8 mg/kg/hr	40 ml/hr	48 ml/hr	56 ml/hr	64 ml/hr	72 ml/hr	80 ml/hr
0.7 mg/kg/hr	35 ml/hr	42 ml/hr	49 ml/hr	56 ml/hr	63 ml/hr	70 ml/hr
0.6 mg/kg/hr	30 ml/hr	36 ml/hr	42 ml/hr	48 ml/hr	54 ml/hr	60 ml/hr
0.5 mg/kg/hr	25 ml/hr	30 ml/hr	35 ml/hr	40 ml/hr	45 ml/hr	50 ml/hr
0.4 mg/kg/hr	20 ml/hr	24 ml/hr	28 ml/hr	32 ml/hr	36 ml/hr	40 ml/hr
0.3 mg/kg/hr	15 ml/hr	18 ml/hr	21 ml/hr	24 ml/hr	27 ml/hr	30 ml/hr
0.2 mg/kg/hr	10 ml/hr	12 ml/hr	14 ml/hr	16 ml/hr	18 ml/hr	20 ml/hr
0.1 mg/kg/hr	5 ml/hr	6 ml/hr	7 ml/hr	8 ml/hr	9 ml/hr	10 ml/hr

*Loading dose administered over 20 min.

AMRINONE (Inocor)

Dilution: 100 mg/100 ml = 1 mg/ml.
Dilute with 0.45% or 0.9% sodium chloride.
Loading dose: 0.75 mg/kg (0.75 ml/kg) over 2–3 min.
To calculate infusion rate (ml/min), multiply patient's weight (kg) by dose in ml/kg/min.
To calculate infusion rate (ml/hr), multiply patient's weight (kg) by dose in mg/kg/min × 60.

Amrinone Infusion Rates
(ml/hr)
Concentration = 1 mg/ml

Patient Weight

Dose	50 kg	60 kg	70 kg	80 kg	90 kg	100 kg
loading dose (mg)*	37.5 mg	45 mg	52.5 mg	60 mg	67.5 mg	75 mg
5 mcg/kg/min	15 ml/hr	18 ml/hr	21 ml/hr	24 ml/hr	27 ml/hr	30 ml/hr
6 mcg/kg/min	18 ml/hr	21.6 ml/hr	25.5 ml/hr	28.8 ml/hr	32.4 ml/hr	36 ml/hr
7 mcg/kg/min	21 ml/hr	25.2 ml/hr	29.4 ml/hr	33.6 ml/hr	37.8 ml/hr	42 ml/hr
8 mcg/kg/min	24 ml/hr	28.8 ml/hr	33.6 ml/hr	38.4 ml/hr	43.2 ml/hr	48 ml/hr
9 mcg/kg/min	27 ml/hr	32.4 ml/hr	37.8 ml/hr	43.2 ml/hr	48.6 ml/hr	54 ml/hr
10 mcg/kg/min	30 ml/hr	36 ml/hr	42 ml/hr	48 ml/hr	54 ml/hr	60 ml/hr

* Given over 2–3 min.

BRETYLIUM (Bretylol)

A. For life-threatening ventricular arrhythmias: (V Fib. or hemodynamically unstable V Tach).
Administer 5 mg/kg (0.1 ml/kg) of *undiluted* drug by rapid IV injection. *Undiluted* drug
concentration = 50 mg/1 ml.

Rapid IV Injection of Undiluted Bretylium
Doses given in volume of undiluted bretylium injection
50 mg/1 ml

Patient Weight

Dose	50 kg	60 kg	70 kg	80 kg	90 kg	100 kg
5 mg/kg	5 ml	6 ml	7 ml	8 ml	9 ml	10 ml

B. For other ventricular arrhythmias: Dilution: 2 g/500 ml = 4 mg/ml. Administer as 5–10 mg/kg
(1.25–2.5 ml/kg) IV over 10–30 min, may be repeated q 6 hr or administered as a continuous
infusion at 1–2 mg/min.

Bretylium Intermittent Infusion Rates
Volume of diluted bretylium
to infuse over 10–30 min
Concentration = 4 mg/ml

Patient Weight

Dose	50 kg	60 kg	70 kg	80 kg	90 kg	100 kg
5 mg/kg	62.5 ml	75 ml	87.5 ml	100 ml	112.5 ml	125 ml
6 mg/kg	75 ml	90 ml	105 ml	120 ml	135 ml	150 ml
7 mg/kg	87.5 ml	105 ml	122.5 ml	140 ml	157.5 ml	175 ml
8 mg/kg	100 ml	120 ml	140 ml	160 ml	180 ml	200 ml
9 mg/kg	112.5 ml	135 ml	157.5 ml	180 ml	202.5 ml	225 ml
10 mg/kg	125 ml	150 ml	175 ml	200 ml	225 ml	250 ml

Bretylium Continuous Infusion Rates
Concentration = 4 mg/ml

Dose mg/min	Dose ml/hr
1.0 mg/min	15 ml/hr
1.5 mg/min	23 ml/hr
2.0 mg/min	30 ml/hr

DOBUTAMINE (Dobutrex)

Dilution: May be prepared as 250 mg/1000 ml = 250 mcg/ml.
500 mg/1000 ml = 500 mcg/ml.
1000 mg/1000 ml = 1000 mcg/ml.
To calculate infusion rate (ml/min), multiply patient's weight (kg) by dose in ml/kg/min.
To calculate infusion rate (ml/hr), multiply patient's weight (kg) by dose in ml/kg/min × 60.

Dobutamine Infusion Rates (ml/hr)
Concentration = 250 mcg/ml

Patient Weight

Dose	50 kg	60 kg	70 kg	80 kg	90 kg	100 kg
2.5 mcg/kg/min	30 ml/hr	36 ml/hr	42 ml/hr	48 ml/hr	54 ml/hr	60 ml/hr
5 mcg/kg/min	60 ml/hr	72 ml/hr	84 ml/hr	96 ml/hr	108 ml/hr	120 ml/hr
7.5 mcg/kg/min	90 ml/hr	108 ml/hr	126 ml/hr	144 ml/hr	162 ml/hr	180 ml/hr
10 mcg/kg/min	120 ml/hr	144 ml/hr	168 ml/hr	192 ml/hr	216 ml/hr	240 ml/hr

Dobutamine Infusion Rates (ml/hr)
Concentration = 500 mcg/ml

Patient Weight

Dose	50 kg	60 kg	70 kg	80 kg	90 kg	100 kg
2.5 mcg/kg/min	15 ml/hr	18 ml/hr	21 ml/hr	24 ml/hr	22.5 ml/hr	30 ml/hr
5 mcg/kg/min	30 ml/hr	36 ml/hr	42 ml/hr	48 ml/hr	54 ml/hr	60 ml/hr
7.5 mcg/kg/min	45 ml/hr	54 ml/hr	63 ml/hr	72 ml/hr	81 ml/hr	90 ml/hr
10 mcg/kg/min	60 ml/hr	72 ml/hr	84 ml/hr	96 ml/hr	108 ml/hr	120 ml/hr

Dobutamine Infusion Rates (ml/hr)
Concentration = 1000 mcg/ml

Patient Weight

Dose	50 kg	60 kg	70 kg	80 kg	90 kg	100 kg
2.5 mcg/kg/min	7.5 ml/hr	9 ml/hr	10.5 ml/hr	12 ml/hr	11.3 ml/hr	15 ml/hr
5 mcg/kg/min	15 ml/hr	18 ml/hr	21 ml/hr	24 ml/hr	27 ml/hr	30 ml/hr
7.5 mcg/kg/min	22.3 ml/hr	27 ml/hr	31.5 ml/hr	36 ml/hr	40.5 ml/hr	45 ml/hr
10 mcg/kg/min	30 ml/hr	36 ml/hr	41 ml/hr	48 ml/hr	54 ml/hr	60 ml/hr

DOPAMINE (Intropin)

Dilution: May be prepared as 200 mg/500 ml = 400 mcg/ml.
400 mg/500 ml = 800 mcg/ml.
800 mg/500 ml = 1600 mcg/ml†.
To calculate infusion rate (ml/min), multiply patient's weight (kg) by dose in ml/kg/min.
To calculate infusion rate (ml/hr), multiply patient's weight (kg) by dose in ml/kg/min × 60.

Dopamine Infusion Rates (ml/hr)
400 mcg/ml Concentration

Patient Weight

Dose	50 kg	60 kg	70 kg	80 kg	90 kg	100 kg
2 mcg/kg/min	15 ml/hr	18 ml/hr	21 ml/hr	24 ml/hr	27 ml/hr	30 ml/hr
5 mcg/kg/min	37.5 ml/hr	45 ml/hr	52.5 ml/hr	60 ml/hr	67.5 ml/hr	75 ml/hr
10 mcg/kg/min	75 ml/hr	90 ml/hr	105 ml/hr	120 ml/hr	135 ml/hr	150 ml/hr
20 mcg/kg/min	150 ml/hr	180 ml/hr	210 ml/hr	240 ml/hr	270 ml/hr	300 ml/hr
30 mcg/kg/min	225 ml/hr	270 ml/hr	315 ml/hr	360 ml/hr	405 ml/hr	450 ml/hr
40 mcg/kg/min	300 ml/hr	360 ml/hr	420 ml/hr	480 ml/hr	540 ml/hr	600 ml/hr
50 mcg/kg/min	375 ml/hr	450 ml/hr	525 ml/hr	600 ml/hr	675 ml/hr	750 ml/hr

Dopamine Infusion Rates (ml/hr)
800 mcg/ml Concentration

Patient Weight

Dose	50 kg	60 kg	70 kg	80 kg	90 kg	100 kg
2 mcg/kg/min	7.5 ml/hr	9 ml/hr	10.5 ml/hr	12 ml/hr	13.5 ml/hr	15 ml/hr
5 mcg/kg/min	18.8 ml/hr	22.5 ml/hr	26.3 ml/hr	30 ml/hr	33.8 ml/hr	37.5 ml/hr
10 mcg/kg/min	37.5 ml/hr	45 ml/hr	52.5 ml/hr	60 ml/hr	67.5 ml/hr	75 ml/hr
20 mcg/kg/min	75 ml/hr	90 ml/hr	105 ml/hr	120 ml/hr	135 ml/hr	150 ml/hr
30 mcg/kg/min	112.5 ml/hr	135 ml/hr	157.5 ml/hr	180 ml/hr	202.5 ml/hr	225 ml/hr
40 mcg/kg/min	150 ml/hr	180 ml/hr	210 ml/hr	240 ml/hr	270 ml/hr	300 ml/hr
50 mcg/kg/min	187.5 ml/hr	225 ml/hr	262.5 ml/hr	300 ml/hr	337.5 ml/hr	375 ml/hr

Dopamine Infusion Rates (ml/hr)
1600 mcg/ml Concentration*

Patient Weight

Dose	50 kg	60 kg	70 kg	80 kg	90 kg	100 kg
2 mcg/kg/min	3.8 ml/hr	4.5 ml/hr	5.3 ml/hr	6 ml/hr	6.8 ml/hr	7.5 ml/hr
5 mcg/kg/min	9.4 ml/hr	11.2 ml/hr	13.1 ml/hr	15.0 ml/hr	16.9 ml/hr	18.7 ml/hr
10 mcg/kg/min	18.8 ml/hr	22.5 ml/hr	26.3 ml/hr	30 ml/hr	33.8 ml/hr	37.5 ml/hr
20 mcg/kg/min	37.5 ml/hr	45 ml/hr	52.5 ml/hr	60 ml/hr	67.5 ml/hr	75 ml/hr
30 mcg/kg/min	56.3 ml/hr	67.5 ml/hr	78.8 ml/hr	90 ml/hr	101.3 ml/hr	112.5 ml/hr
40 mcg/kg/min	75 ml/hr	90 ml/hr	105 ml/hr	120 ml/hr	135 ml/hr	150 ml/hr
50 mcg/kg/min	93.8 ml/hr	112.5 ml/hr	131.3 ml/hr	150 ml/hr	168.8 ml/hr	187.5 ml/hr

* Appropriate concentration for patients with fluid restriction.

EPINEPHRINE

Dilution: 1 mg/250 ml = 4 mcg/ml.

Epinephrine Infusion Rates (ml/hr)
Concentration = 4 mcg/ml

Dose (mcg/ml)	Dose (ml/hr)
1 mcg/min	15 ml/hr
2 mcg/min	30 ml/hr
3 mcg/min	45 ml/hr
4 mcg/min	60 ml/hr

ESMOLOL (Brevibloc)

Dilution: 5 g/500 ml = 10 mg/ml.
Loading regimen = 500 mcg/kg (0.05 ml/kg) loading dose over 1 min, followed by 50 mcg/kg/min (0.005 ml/kg/min) infusion over 4 min. If no response, repeat loading dose over 1 min and increase infusion rate to 100 mcg/kg/min for 4–10 min. If no response, loading dose may be repeated before increasing infusion rates in 50 mcg/kg/min increments.

Esmolol Infusion Rates
Concentration = 10 mg/ml

Patient Weight

Dose	50 kg	60 kg	70 kg	80 kg	90 kg	100 kg
loading dose (ml)*	2.5 ml	3 ml	3.5 ml	4 ml	4.5 ml	5 ml
50 mcg/kg/min	15 ml/hr	18 ml/hr	21 ml/hr	24 ml/hr	27 ml/hr	30 ml/hr
75 mcg/kg/min	22.5 ml/hr	27 ml/hr	31.5 ml/hr	36 ml/hr	40.5 ml/hr	45 ml/hr
100 mcg/kg/min	30 ml/hr	36 ml/hr	42 ml/hr	48 ml/hr	54 ml/hr	60 ml/hr
125 mcg/kg/min	37.5 ml/hr	45 ml/hr	52.5 ml/hr	60 ml/hr	67.5 ml/hr	75 ml/hr
150 mcg/kg/min	38 ml/hr	54 ml/hr	63 ml/hr	72 ml/hr	81 ml/hr	90 ml/hr
175 mcg/kg/min	52.5 ml/hr	63 ml/hr	73.5 ml/hr	84 ml/hr	94.5 ml/hr	105 ml/hr
200 mcg/kg/min	60 ml/hr	72 ml/hr	84 ml/hr	96 ml/hr	108 ml/hr	120 ml/hr

* Loading dose given over 1 min.

HEPARIN

Dilution: 20,000 units/1000 ml = 20 units/ml.
Loading dose: 1000–2000 units as a bolus.

Heparin Infusion Rates (ml/hr)
Concentration = 20 units/ml

Dose (units/hr)	Dose (ml/hr)
500 units/hr	25 ml/hr
750 units/hr	37.5 ml/hr
1000 units/hr	50 ml/hr
1250 units/hr	62.5 ml/hr
1500 units/hr	75 ml/hr
1750 units/hr	87.5 ml/hr
2000 units/hr	100 ml/hr

ISOPROTERENOL (Isuprel)

Dilution: 2 mg/500 ml.

Isoproterenol Infusion Rates (ml/hr)
Concentration = 4 mcg/ml

Dose (mcg/min)	Dose (ml/hr)
2 mcg/min	30 ml/hr
5 mcg/min	75 ml/hr
10 mcg/min	150 ml/hr
15 mcg/min	225 ml/hr
20 mcg/min	300 ml/hr

LIDOCAINE (Xylocaine)

Dilution: May be prepared as 1 g/1000 ml = 1 mg/ml.
2 g/1000 ml = 2 mg/ml.
4 g/1000 ml = 4 mg/ml.
8 g/1000 ml = 8 mg/ml.
Loading dose: 50–100 mg at 25–50 mg/min.

Lidocaine Infusion Rates (ml/hr)

Dose (mg/min)	1 mg/ml concentration	2 mg/ml concentration	4 mg/ml concentration	8 mg/ml concentration
1 mg/min	60 ml/hr	30 ml/hr	15 ml/hr	7.5 ml/hr
2 mg/min	120 ml/hr	60 ml/hr	30 ml/hr	15 ml/hr
3 mg/min	180 ml/hr	90 ml/hr	45 ml/hr	22.5 ml/hr
4 mg/min	240 ml/hr	120 ml/hr	60 ml/hr	30 ml/hr

MILRINONE

Loading dose: 50 mcg/kg given over 10 min.

Milrinone Infusion Rates (ml/hr)

Patient Weight

Dose	50 kg	60 kg	70 kg	80 kg	90 kg	100 kg
loading dose (mg)	2.5 mg	3.0 mg	3.5 mg	4.0 mg	4.5 mg	5.0 mg

Milrinone Infusion Rates (ml/hr)
Concentration = 100 mcg/ml

Patient Weight

Dose	50 kg	60 kg	70 kg	80 kg	90 kg	100 kg
0.375 mcg/kg/min	11 ml/hr	13.2 ml/hr	15.4 ml/hr	17.6 ml/hr	19.8 ml/hr	22.0 ml/hr
0.400 mcg/kg/min	12 ml/hr	14.4 ml/hr	16.8 ml/hr	19.2 ml/hr	21.6 ml/hr	24.0 ml/hr
0.500 mcg/kg/min	15.0 ml/hr	18.0 ml/hr	21.0 ml/hr	24.0 ml/hr	27.0 ml/hr	30.0 ml/hr
0.600 mcg/kg/min	18.0 ml/hr	21.6 ml/hr	25.2 ml/hr	28.8 ml/hr	32.4 ml/hr	36.0 ml/hr
0.700 mcg/kg/min	21.0 ml/hr	25.2 ml/hr	29.4 ml/hr	33.6 ml/hr	37.8 ml/hr	42.0 ml/hr
0.750 mcg/kg/min	22.5 ml/hr	27.0 ml/hr	31.5 ml/hr	36.0 ml/hr	40.5 ml/hr	45.0 ml/hr

Concentration = 150 mcg/ml

Patient Weight

Dose	50 kg	60 kg	70 kg	80 kg	90 kg	100 kg
0.375 mcg/kg/min	7.5 ml/hr	9.0 ml/hr	10.5 ml/hr	12.0 ml/hr	13.4 ml/hr	15.0 ml/hr
0.400 mcg/kg/min	8.0 ml/hr	9.6 ml/hr	11.2 ml/hr	12.8 ml/hr	14.4 ml/hr	16.0 ml/hr
0.500 mcg/kg/min	10.0 ml/hr	12.0 ml/hr	14.0 ml/hr	16.0 ml/hr	18.0 ml/hr	20.0 ml/hr
0.600 mcg/kg/min	12.0 ml/hr	14.4 ml/hr	16.8 ml/hr	19.2 ml/hr	21.6 ml/hr	24.0 ml/hr
0.700 mcg/kg/min	14.0 ml/hr	16.8 ml/hr	19.6 ml/hr	22.4 ml/hr	25.2 ml/hr	28.0 ml/hr
0.750 mcg/kg/min	15.0 ml/hr	18.0 ml/hr	21.0 ml/hr	24.0 ml/hr	27.0 ml/hr	30.0 ml/hr

Concentration = 200 mcg/ml

Patient Weight

Dose	50 kg	60 kg	70 kg	80 kg	90 kg	100 kg
0.375 mcg/kg/min	5.5 ml/hr	6.6 ml/hr	7.7 ml/hr	8.8 ml/hr	9.9 ml/hr	11.1 ml/hr
0.400 mcg/kg/min	6.0 ml/hr	7.2 ml/hr	8.4 ml/hr	9.6 ml/hr	10.8 ml/hr	12.0 ml/hr
0.500 mcg/kg/min	7.5 ml/hr	9.0 ml/hr	10.5 ml/hr	12.0 ml/hr	13.5 ml/hr	15.0 ml/hr
0.600 mcg/kg/min	9.0 ml/hr	10.8 ml/hr	12.6 ml/hr	14.4 ml/hr	16.2 ml/hr	18.0 ml/hr
0.700 mcg/kg/min	10.5 ml/hr	12.6 ml/hr	14.7 ml/hr	16.8 ml/hr	18.9 ml/hr	21.0 ml/hr
0.750 mcg/kg/min	11.0 ml/hr	13.5 ml/hr	15.4 ml/hr	17.6 ml/hr	19.8 ml/hr	22.0 ml/hr

---

NITROGLYCERIN (Nitro-bid, Nitrol, Nitrostat, Tridil)

Dilution: May be prepared as 5 mg/100 ml (25 mg/500 ml, 50 mg/1000 ml) = 50 mcg/ml.
25 mg/250 ml (50 mg/500 ml, 100 mg/1000 ml) = 100 mcg/ml.
50 mg/250 ml (100 mg/500 ml, 200 mg/1000 ml = 200 mcg/ml.

Note that different products are available in different concentrated solutions and should be used with appropriate infusion tubing. Changes in tubing may result in altered response to a given dose.

Nitroglycerin Infusion Rates (ml/hr)

Dose (mcg/min)	50 mcg/ml concentration	100 mcg/ml concentration	200 mcg/ml concentration
2.5 mcg/min	3 ml/hr	1.5 ml/hr	0.75 ml/hr
5 mcg/min	6 ml/hr	3 ml/hr	1.5 ml/hr
10 mcg/min	12 ml/hr	6 ml/hr	3 ml/hr
15 mcg/min	18 ml/hr	9 ml/hr	4.5 ml/hr
20 mcg/min	24 ml/hr	12 ml/hr	6 ml/hr
30 mcg/min	36 ml/hr	18 ml/hr	9 ml/hr
40 mcg/min	48 ml/hr	24 ml/hr	12 ml/hr
50 mcg/min	60 ml/hr	30 ml/hr	15 ml/hr
60 mcg/min	72 ml/hr	36 ml/hr	18 ml/hr

NITROPRUSSIDE (Nipride, Nitropress)

Dilution: May be prepared as 50 mg/1000 ml = 50 mcg/ml.
100 mg/1000 ml = 100 mg/ml.
200 mg/1000 ml = 200 mcg/ml.

To calculate infusion rate (ml/min), multiply patient's weight (kg) by dose in ml/kg/min.
To calculate infusion rate (ml/hr), multiply patient's weight (kg) by dose in ml/kg/min × 60.
Dosing range: 0.3 mcg/kg/min–10 mcg/kg/min.

Nitroprusside Infusion Rates (ml/kg/min)

Dose (mcg/kg/min)	50 mcg/ml concentration	100 mcg/ml concentration	200 mcg/ml concentration
0.3 mcg/kg/min	0.006 ml/kg/min	—	—
0.5 mcg/kg/min	0.01 ml/kg/min	—	—
1 mcg/kg/min	0.02 ml/kg/min	0.01 ml/kg/min	—
2 mcg/kg/min	0.04 ml/kg/min	0.02 ml/kg/min	0.01 ml/kg/min
3 mcg/kg/min	0.06 ml/kg/min	0.03 ml/kg/min	0.015 ml/kg/min
4 mcg/kg/min	0.08 ml/kg/min	0.04 ml/kg/min	0.02 ml/kg/min
5 mcg/kg/min	0.1 ml/kg/min	0.05 ml/kg/min	0.025 ml/kg/min
6 mcg/kg/min	0.12 ml/kg/min	0.06 ml/kg/min	0.03 ml/kg/min
7 mcg/kg/min	0.14 ml/kg/min	0.07 ml/kg/min	0.035 ml/kg/min
8 mcg/kg/min	0.16 ml/kg/min	0.08 ml/kg/min	0.04 ml/kg/min
9 mcg/kg/min	0.18 ml/kg/min	0.09 ml/kg/min	0.045 ml/kg/min
10 mcg/kg/min	0.2 ml/kg/min	0.1 ml/kg/min	0.05 ml/kg/min

Nitroprusside Infusion Rates (ml/hr)
50 mcg/ml Concentration

Patient Weight

Dose	50 kg	60 kg	70 kg	80 kg	90 kg	100 kg
0.3 mcg/kg/min	18 ml/hr	22 ml/hr	25 ml/hr	29 ml/hr	32 ml/hr	36 ml/hr
0.5 mcg/kg/min	30 ml/hr	36 ml/hr	42 ml/hr	48 ml/hr	54 ml/hr	60 ml/hr
1 mcg/kg/min	60 ml/hr	72 ml/hr	84 ml/hr	96 ml/hr	108 ml/hr	120 ml/hr
2 mcg/kg/min	120 ml/hr	144 ml/hr	168 ml/hr	192 ml/hr	216 ml/hr	240 ml/hr
3 mcg/kg/min	180 ml/hr	216 ml/hr	252 ml/hr	288 ml/hr	324 ml/hr	360 ml/hr
4 mcg/kg/min	240 ml/hr	288 ml/hr	336 ml/hr	384 ml/hr	432 ml/hr	480 ml/hr
5 mcg/kg/min	300 ml/hr	360 ml/hr	420 ml/hr	480 ml/hr	540 ml/hr	600 ml/hr
6 mcg/kg/min	360 ml/hr	432 ml/hr	504 ml/hr	576 ml/hr	648 ml/hr	720 ml/hr
7 mcg/kg/min	420 ml/hr	504 ml/hr	588 ml/hr	672 ml/hr	756 ml/hr	840 ml/hr
8 mcg/kg/min	480 ml/hr	576 ml/hr	672 ml/hr	768 ml/hr	864 ml/hr	960 ml/hr
9 mcg/kg/min	540 ml/hr	648 ml/hr	672 ml/hr	864 ml/hr	972 ml/hr	1080 ml/hr
10 mcg/kg/min	600 ml/hr	720 ml/hr	840 ml/hr	960 ml/hr	1080 ml/hr	1200 ml/hr

Nitroprusside Infusion Rates (ml/hr)
100 mcg/ml Concentration

Patient Weight

Dose	50 kg	60 kg	70 kg	80 kg	90 kg	100 kg
0.3 mcg/kg/min	9 ml/hr	11 ml/hr	13 ml/hr	14 ml/hr	16 ml/hr	18 ml/hr
0.5 mcg/kg/min	15 ml/hr	18 ml/hr	21 ml/hr	24 ml/hr	27 ml/hr	30 ml/hr
1 mcg/kg/min	30 ml/hr	36 ml/hr	42 ml/hr	48 ml/hr	54 ml/hr	60 ml/hr
2 mcg/kg/min	60 ml/hr	72 ml/hr	84 ml/hr	96 ml/hr	108 ml/hr	120 ml/hr
3 mcg/kg/min	90 ml/hr	108 ml/hr	126 ml/hr	144 ml/hr	162 ml/hr	180 ml/hr
4 mcg/kg/min	120 ml/hr	144 ml/hr	168 ml/hr	192 ml/hr	216 ml/hr	240 ml/hr
5 mcg/kg/min	150 ml/hr	180 ml/hr	210 ml/hr	240 ml/hr	270 ml/hr	300 ml/hr
6 mcg/kg/min	180 ml/hr	216 ml/hr	252 ml/hr	288 ml/hr	324 ml/hr	360 ml/hr
7 mcg/kg/min	210 ml/hr	252 ml/hr	294 ml/hr	336 ml/hr	378 ml/hr	420 ml/hr
8 mcg/kg/min	240 ml/hr	288 ml/hr	336 ml/hr	384 ml/hr	432 ml/hr	480 ml/hr
9 mcg/kg/min	270 ml/hr	324 ml/hr	336 ml/hr	432 ml/hr	486 ml/hr	540 ml/hr
10 mcg/kg/min	300 ml/hr	360 ml/hr	420 ml/hr	480 ml/hr	540 ml/hr	600 ml/hr

Nitroprusside Infusion Rates (ml/hr)
200 mcg/ml Concentration

Patient Weight

Dose	50 kg	60 kg	70 kg	80 kg	90 kg	100 kg
0.3 mcg/kg/min	5 ml/hr	5 ml/hr	6 ml/hr	7 ml/hr	8 ml/hr	9 ml/hr
0.5 mcg/kg/min	7.5 ml/hr	9 ml/hr	10.5 ml/hr	12 ml/hr	13.5 ml/hr	15 ml/hr
1 mcg/kg/min	15 ml/hr	18 ml/hr	21 ml/hr	24 ml/hr	27 ml/hr	30 ml/hr
2 mcg/kg/min	30 ml/hr	36 ml/hr	42 ml/hr	48 ml/hr	54 ml/hr	60 ml/hr
3 mcg/kg/min	45 ml/hr	54 ml/hr	63 ml/hr	72 ml/hr	81 ml/hr	90 ml/hr
4 mcg/kg/min	60 ml/hr	72 ml/hr	84 ml/hr	96 ml/hr	108 ml/hr	120 ml/hr
5 mcg/kg/min	75 ml/hr	90 ml/hr	105 ml/hr	120 ml/hr	135 ml/hr	150 ml/hr
6 mcg/kg/min	90 ml/hr	108 ml/hr	126 ml/hr	144 ml/hr	162 ml/hr	180 ml/hr
7 mcg/kg/min	105 ml/hr	126 ml/hr	147 ml/hr	168 ml/hr	189 ml/hr	210 ml/hr
8 mcg/kg/min	120 ml/hr	144 ml/hr	168 ml/hr	192 ml/hr	216 ml/hr	240 ml/hr
9 mcg/kg/min	135 ml/hr	162 ml/hr	168 ml/hr	216 ml/hr	243 ml/hr	270 ml/hr
10 mcg/kg/min	150 ml/hr	180 ml/hr	210 ml/hr	240 ml/hr	270 ml/hr	300 ml/hr

NOREPINEPHRINE (Levophed)

Dilution: May be prepared as 1 mg/250 ml = 4 mcg/ml.
To calculate infusion rate (ml/hr), multiply infusion rate in ml/min × 60.

Norepinephrine Infusion Rates (ml/hr)
Concentration = 4 mcg/ml

Dose (mcg/min)	Dose (ml/hr)
8 mcg/min	120 ml/hr
9 mcg/min	135 ml/hr
10 mcg/min	150 ml/hr
11 mcg/min	165 ml/hr
12 mcg/min	180 ml/hr

PHENYLEPHRINE (Neo-Synephrine)

Dilution: 10 mg/500 ml = 20 mcg/ml.

Phenylephrine Infusion Rates (ml/hr)
Concentration = 20 mcg/ml

Dose (mg/min)	Dose (ml/hr)
0.04 mg/min	120 ml/hr
0.06 mg/min	180 ml/hr
0.08 mg/min	240 ml/hr
0.10 mg/min	300 ml/hr
0.12 mg/min	360 ml/hr
0.14 mg/min	420 ml/hr
0.16 mg/min	480 ml/hr
0.18 mg/min	540 ml/hr

PROCAINAMIDE (Pronestyl)

Dilution: May be prepared as 1000 mg/500 ml = 2 mg/ml.
Loading dose: 50–100 mg q 5 min until arrhythmia is controlled; adverse reaction occurs, or 500 mg has been given, *or* 500–600 mg as a loading infusion over 25–30 min.

Procainamide Infusion Rates (ml/hr)
Concentration = 2 mg/ml

Dose (mg/min)	Dose (ml/hr)
1 mg/min	30 ml/hr
2 mg/min	60 ml/hr
3 mg/min	90 ml/hr
4 mg/min	120 ml/hr
5 mg/min	150 ml/hr
6 mg/min	180 ml/hr

APPENDIX E
Food and Drug Administration Pregnancy Categories

Category A
As demonstrated by studies that are adequate and well controlled, no risk to the fetus in the first trimester has been shown. In addition, there does not appear to be risk in the second or third trimester.

Category B
Studies in animals may or may not have shown risk. If risk has been shown in animals, no risk has been shown in human studies. If risk has not been seen in animals, there are insufficient data in pregnant women.

Category C
Adverse effects have been demonstrated in animals, but there are insufficient data in pregnant women. In certain clinical situations, the benefits of use of the medication could outweigh possible risks.

Category D
Based on information collected in clinical investigations or postmarketing surveillance, human fetal risk has been demonstrated. In certain clinical situations, the benefits of use of the medication could outweigh possible risks.

Category X
Human fetal risk has been clearly documented in human studies, animal studies, clinical investigation, or postmarketing surveillance. Possible risks to the fetus outweigh potential benefits to the pregnant woman. Avoid use during pregnancy.

APPENDIX F
Formulas Helpful for Calculating Doses

Ratio and Proportion

A ratio is the same as a fraction and can be expressed as a fraction (½) or in the algebraic form (1 : 2). This relationship is stated as *one is to two.*

A proportion is an equation of equal fractions or ratios.

$$\frac{1}{2} = \frac{4}{8}$$

To calculate doses, begin each proportion with the two known values, for example, 15 grains = 1 gram (known equivalent) or 10 milligrams = 2 milliliters (dosage available) on one side of the equation. Next, make certain that the units of measure on the opposite side of the equation are the same as the units of the known values and are placed on the same level of the equation.

Problem A:
$$\frac{15\,gr}{1\,g} = \frac{10\,gr}{x\,g}$$

Problem B:
$$\frac{10\,mg}{2\,ml} = \frac{5\,mg}{x\,ml}$$

Once the proportion is set up correctly, cross-multiply the opposing values of the proportion.

Problem A:
$$\frac{15\,gr}{1\,g} \diagdown\!\!\!\!\diagup \frac{10\,gr}{x\,g}$$

$$15x = 10$$

Problem B:
$$\frac{10\,mg}{2\,ml} \diagdown\!\!\!\!\diagup \frac{5\,mg}{x\,ml}$$

$$10x = 10$$

Next, divide each side of the equation by the number with the x to determine the answer. Then, add the unit of measure corresponding to x in the original equation.

Problem A:
$$\frac{15x}{15} = \frac{10}{15}$$

$$x = \frac{2}{3} \text{ or } 0.6\,g$$

Problem B:
$$\frac{10x}{10} = \frac{10}{10}$$

$$x = 1\,ml$$

Calculation of IV Drip Rate
To calculate the drip rate for an intravenous infusion, 3 values are needed:

I. The amount of solution and corresponding time for infusion. May be ordered as:

1000 ml over 8 hr

or

125 ml/hr

II. The equivalent in time to convert hours to minutes.

1 hr = 60 min

III. The drop factor or number of drops that equal 1 ml of fluid. (This information can be found on the IV tubing box.)

10 gtt = 1 ml

Set up the problem by placing each of the three values in a proportion.

$$\frac{125 \text{ ml}}{1 \text{ hr}} \times \frac{1 \text{ hr}}{60 \text{ min}} \times \frac{10 \text{ gtt}}{1 \text{ ml}}$$

Numbers and units of measure can be canceled out from the upper and lower levels of this equation.

The numbers cancel, leaving:

$$\frac{125 \text{ ml}}{1 \text{ hr}} \times \frac{1 \text{ hr}}{60 \text{ min}} \times \frac{10 \text{ gtt}}{1 \text{ ml}}$$

The units cancel, leaving:

$$\frac{125 \text{ ml}}{1 \text{ hr}} \times \frac{1 \text{ hr}}{6 \text{ min}} \times \frac{1 \text{ gtt}}{1 \text{ ml}}$$

Next, multiply each level across and divide the numerator by the denominator for the answer.

$$\frac{125 \text{ ml}}{1 \text{ hr}} \times \frac{1 \text{ hr}}{6 \text{ min}} \times \frac{1 \text{ gtt}}{1 \text{ ml}} = \frac{125 \text{ gtt}}{6 \text{ min}}$$

$$125 \div 6 = 20.8 \text{ or } 21 \text{ gtt/min}$$

To calculate creatinine clearance (Ccr) in adults from serum creatinine:

Male: $Ccr = \frac{\text{weight (kg)} \times (140 - \text{age})}{72 \times \text{serum creatinine (mg/dl)}}$

Female: $Ccr = 0.85 \times$ calculation for males

To calculate ideal body weight (kg) in adults:

Male = 50 kg + 2.3 kg (each inch >5 ft)
Female = 45.5 kg + 2.3 kg (each inch >5 ft)

To calculate body surface area (BSA) in adults and children:

1. *Dubois method:*

    SA $(cm^2) = $ wt $(kg)^{0.425} \times$ ht $(cm)^{0.725} \times 71.84$

    SA $(m^2) = K \times \sqrt[3]{wt^2\,(kg)}$ (common K value 0.1 for
    toddlers, 0.103 for neonates)

2. *Simplified method:*

    BSA $(m^2) = \sqrt{\dfrac{ht\,(cm) \times wt\,(kg)}{3600}}$

APPENDIX G
Body Surface Area Nomograms

ESTIMATING BODY SURFACE AREA IN CHILDREN

For pediatric patients of average size, body surface area may be estimated with the scale on the left. Match weight to corresponding surface area. For other pediatric patients, use the scale on the right. Lay a straightedge on the correct height and weight points for your patient, and observe the point where it intersects on the surface area scale at center.

FOR CHILDREN OF NORMAL HEIGHT AND WEIGHT

NOMOGRAM FOR OTHER CHILDREN

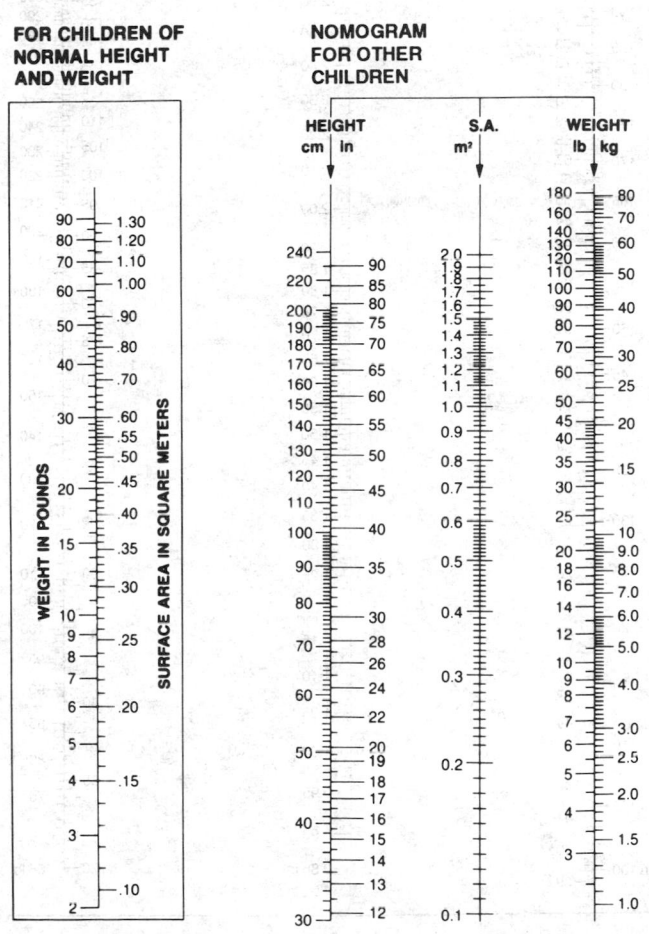

From Nelson Text Book of Pediatrics, ed 14. WB Saunders, Philadelphia, 1992, with permission.

1277

ESTIMATING BODY SURFACE AREA IN ADULTS

Use a straightedge to connect the patient's height in the left-hand column to weight in the right-hand column. The intersection of this line with the center scale estimates the body surface area.

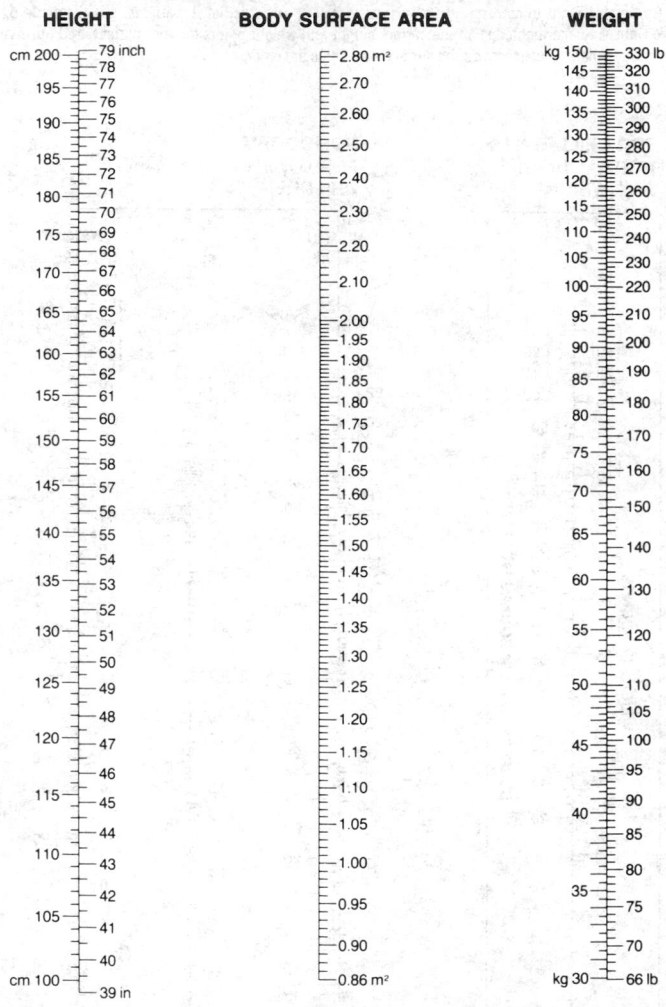

HEIGHT	BODY SURFACE AREA	WEIGHT

APPENDIX H
Administration Techniques

Subcutaneous Injection Sites

Administration of Ophthalmic Medications

For instillation of ophthalmic solutions, instruct patient to lie down or tilt head back and look at ceiling. Pull down on lower lid, creating a small pocket, and instill solution into pocket. With systemically acting drugs apply pressure to the inner canthus for 1–2 min to minimize systemic absorption. Instruct patient to gently close eye. Wait 5 min before instilling second drop or any other ophthalmic solutions.

For instillation of ophthalmic ointment, instruct patient to hold tube in hand for several minutes to warm. Squeeze a small amount of ointment (¼–½ in.) inside lower lid. Instruct patient to close eye gently and roll eyeball around in all directions with eye closed. Wait 10 min before instilling any other ophthalmic ointments.

Do not touch cap or tip of container to eye, fingers, or any surface.

Administration of Medications with Metered-dose Inhalers

Instruct patient on the proper use of the metered-dose inhaler. There are 3 methods of using a metered-dose inhaler. Shake inhaler well. (1) Take a drink of water to moisten the throat; place the inhaler mouthpiece 2 finger-widths away from mouth; tilt head back slightly. While activating the inhaler, take a slow deep breath for 3–5 sec, hold the breath for 10 sec and breathe out slowly. (2) Exhale and close lips firmly around mouthpiece. Administer during second half of inhalation, and hold breath for as long as possible to ensure deep instillation of medication. (3) Use a spacer. Consult physician to determine method desired prior to instruction. Allow 1–2 min between inhalations. Rinse mouth with water or mouthwash after each use to minimize dry mouth and hoarseness. Wash inhalation assembly at least daily in warm running water.

Administration of Nasal Sprays: Clear nasal passages of secretions prior to use. If nasal passages are blocked, use a decongestant immediately prior to use to ensure adequate penetration of the spray. Keep head upright. Breathe in through nose during administration. Sniff hard for a few minutes after administration.

Intramuscular Injection Sites

Deltoid site

Dorsogluteal site

Ventrogluteal site

Vastus lateralis site

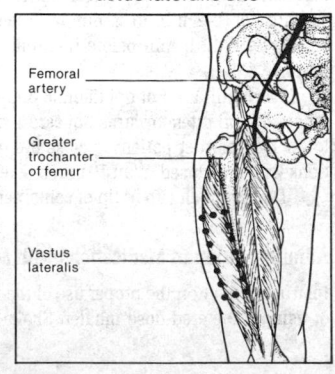

APPENDIX I
Recommendations for the Safe Handling of Cytotoxic (Antineoplastic) Drugs*

Introduction

Cytotoxic drugs are toxic compounds and are known to have carcinogenic, mutagenic and/or teratogenic potential. With direct contact they may cause irritation to the skin, eyes, and mucous membranes and ulceration and necrosis of tissue. The toxicity of cytotoxic drugs dictates that the exposure of health care personnel to these drugs should be minimized. At the same time, the requirement for maintenance of aseptic conditions must be satisfied.

Potential Routes of Exposure

The following information reviews the routes through which exposure may occur and presents recommendations for the safe handling of parenteral cytotoxic drugs by pharmacists, nurses, physicians and other personnel who participate in the preparation and administration of these drugs to patients. These guidelines apply in any setting in which cytotoxic drugs are prepared—including pharmacies, nursing units, clinics, physicians' offices, and the home health care environment. The primary routes of exposure during the preparation and administration phases are through the inhalation of aerosolized drug or by direct skin contact.

During drug preparation, a variety of manipulations are performed that may result in aerosol generation, spraying, and splattering. Examples of these manipulations include the withdrawal of needles from drug vials, the use of syringes and needles or filter straws for drug transfer, the opening of ampules, and the expulsion of air from the syringe when measuring the precise volume of a drug. Pharmaceutical practice calls for the use of aseptic techniques and a sterile environment. Many pharmacies provide this sterile environment by using a horizontal laminar flow work bench. However, while this type of unit provides product protection, it may expose the operator and the other room occupants to aerosols generated during drug preparation procedures. Therefore, a Class II laminar flow (vertical) biologic safety cabinet that provides both product and operator protection is needed for the preparation of cytotoxic drugs. This is accomplished by filtering incoming and exhaust air through a high-efficiency particulate air (HEPA) filter. It should be noted that the filters are not effective for volatile materials because they do not capture vapors and gases. Personnel should be familiar with the capabilities, limitations and proper use of the biologic safety cabinet selected.

During administration (clearing air from a syringe or infusion line) and leakage at tubing, syringe, or stopcock connections should be avoided to prevent opportunities for accidental skin contact and aerosol generation. Dispose of syringes and unclipped needles into a leakproof and puncture-resistant container.

The disposal of cytotoxic drugs and trace contaminated materials (e.g., gloves, gowns, needles, syringes, vials) presents a possible source of exposure to pharmacists, nurses, and physicians as well as to ancillary personnel, especially the housekeeping staff. Excreta from patients receiving cytotoxic drug therapy may contain high concentrations of the drug. All personnel should be aware of this source of potential exposure and should take appropriate precautions as established by your hospital or clinic to avoid accidental contact.

The potential risks to pharmacists, nurses, and physicians from repeated con-

*Produced by the NIH Division of Safety and the NIH Clinical Center Pharmacy Department and Cancer Nursing Service. NIH Publication No. 92-2621.

tact with parenteral cytotoxic drugs can be effectively controlled by using a combination of specific containment equipment and certain work techniques, which are described in the recommendations sections. For the most part, the techniques are merely an extension of good work practices by health care and ancillary personnel and are similar in principle and practice to *Universal Precautions*. These may be supplemented as deemed appropriate for the work being performed. By using these precautions, personnel are better able to minimize possible exposure to cytotoxic drugs.

Recommended Practices for Personnel Preparing Cytotoxic Drugs

Professionally accepted standards concerning the aseptic preparation of parenteral products should be followed. Only properly trained personnel should handle cytotoxic drugs.

Training sessions should be offered to new professionals as well as to technical and housekeeping personnel who may come in contact with these drugs. Safe handling should be the focus of such training.

PART 1

All procedures involved in the preparation of cytotoxic drugs should be performed in a Class II, Type A, or Type B laminar flow biologic safety cabinet. The cabinet exhaust should be discharged to the outdoors in order to eliminate the exposure of personnel to drugs that may volatilize after retention on filters of the cabinet. The **cabinet of choice** is a **Class II, Type B,** which discharges exhaust to the outdoors and can be obtained with a bag-in/bag-out filter to protect the peronnel servicing the cabinet and to facilitate disposal.

PART 2

Alternatively, a **Class II, Type A** cabinet can be equipped with a canopy or thimble unit that exhausts to the outdoors. For detailed information about the design, capabilities and limitations of various types of biologic safety cabinets, refer to the National Sanitation Foundation Standard 49.

The work surface of the safety cabinet should be covered with plastic-backed absorbent paper. This will reduce the potential for dispersion of droplets and spills and facilitate cleanup. This paper should be changed after any overt spill and at the end of each work shift.

Personnel preparing the drugs should wear unpowdered latex surgical gloves and a disposable gown with elastic or knit cuffs. Gloves should be changed regularly and immediately if torn or punctured. Protective clothing should not be worn outside of the drug preparation area. Overtly contaminated gowns require immediate removal and replacement. In case of skin contact with any cytotoxic drug, thoroughly wash the affected area with soap and water. However, do not abrade the skin by using a scrub brush. Flush the affected eye(s), while holding back the eyelid(s), with copious amounts of water for at least 15 minutes. Then seek medical evaluation by a physician.

Vials containing drugs requiring reconstitution should be vented to reduce the internal pressure with a venting device using a 0.22 micron hydrophobic filter or other appropriate means such as a chemotherapy dispensing pin. This reduces the probability of spraying and spillage.

If a chemotherapy dispensing pin is not used, a sterile alcohol pad should be carefully placed around the needle and vial top during withdrawal from the septum.

The external surfaces contaminated with a drug should be wiped clean with an alcohol pad prior to transfer or transport.

When opening the glass ampule, wrap it and then snap it at the break point using an alcohol pad to reduce the possibility of injury and to contain the aerosol produced. Use a 5 micron filter needle or straw when removing the drug solution.

Syringes and IV bottles containing cytotoxic drugs should be labeled and dated. Before these items leave the preparation area, an additional label reading, **"Caution—Chemotherapy, Dispose of Properly"** is recommended.

After completing the drug preparation process, wipe down the interior of the safety cabinet with water (for injection or irrigation) followed by 70% alcohol using disposable towels. All wastes are considered contaminated and should be disposed of properly.

Contaminated needles and syringes, IV tubing, butterfly clips, and so on, should be disposed of intact to prevent aerosol generation and injury. **Do not recap needles.** Place these items in a puncture-resistant container along with any contaminated bottles, vials, gloves, absorbent paper, disposable gowns, gauze, and other waste. The container should then be placed in a box labeled, **"Cytotoxic waste only,"** sealed and disposed of according to Federal, state, and local requirements. Linen contaminated with drugs, patient excreta, or body fluids should be handled separately.

Hands should be washed between glove changes and after glove removal.

Cytotoxic drugs are categorized as regulated wastes and therefore, should be disposed of according to Federal, state, and local requirements.

Recommended Practices for Personnel Administering Parenteral Cytotoxic Drugs

Some cytotoxic drugs are excreted from patients in high concentrations. Personnel should be knowledgeable regarding which drugs fit this description and take care to avoid skin contact and to minimize aerosol generation. When disposing of excreta from patients, all personnel should wear gowns and latex surgical gloves.

A protective outer garment such as a closed-front surgical-type gown with knit cuffs should be worn. Gowns may be of the disposable or washable variety.

Disposable latex surgical gloves should be worn during those procedures in which exposure to the drugs may result and when handling patient body fluids or excreta. When bubbles are removed from syringes or IV tubing, an alcohol pad should be placed carefully over the tip of such items in order to collect any of the cytotoxic drugs that may be inadvertently discharged. Discard gloves after each use and wash hands.

Contaminated needles and syringes and IV apparatus should be disposed of intact into a labeled, puncture-resistant container in order to minimize aerosol generation and risk of injury. **Do not recap needles.** The container, as well as other contaminated materials, should be placed in a box labeled, **"Cytotoxic waste only."** Linen overtly contaminated with any cytotoxic agent or excreta from a patient within 48 hr following drug administration may be safely handled by using the procedures prescribed for isolation cases. For example, place the contaminated articles in a "yellow" cloth bag lined with a water-soluble plastic bag and then place into the washing machine. Linen without overt contamination can be handled by routine laundering procedures.

In case of skin contact with any cytotoxic drug, thoroughly wash the affected area with soap and water. However, do not abrade the skin by using a scrub brush. Flush the affected eye(s), while holding back the eyelid(s), with copious amounts of water for at least 15 minutes. Then seek medical evaluation by a physician. Always wash hands after removing gloves.

Normal Values of Common Laboratory Tests

SERUM TESTS

HEMATOLOGIC	MALE	FEMALE
Hemoglobin	13.5–18 g/dl	12–16 g/dl
Hematocrit	40–54%	38–47%
Red blood cells (RBC)	4.6–6.2 million/mm^3	4.2–5.4 million/mm^3
Leukocytes (WBC)	5,000–10,000/mm^3	
Neutrophils	54–75% (3,000–7,500/mm^3)	
Bands	3–8% (150–700/mm^3)	
Eosinophils	1–4% (50–400/mm^3)	
Basophils	0–1% (25–100/mm^3)	
Monocytes	2–8% (100–500/mm^3)	
Lymphocytes	25–40% (1,500–4,500/mm^3)	
T-lymphocytes	60–80% of lymphocytes	
B-lymphocytes	10–20% of lymphocytes	
Platelets	150,000–450,000/mm^3	
Prothrombin time (PT)	9.6–11.8 sec	9.5–11.3 sec
Partial thromboplastin time (PTT)	30–45 sec	
Bleeding time (duke)	1–3 min	
(ivy)	3–6 min	
(template)	3–6 min	
Clotting time (Lee-White)	4–8 min	

CHEMISTRY	MALE	FEMALE
Sodium	135–145 mEq/L	
Potassium	3.5–5.0 mEq/L	
Chloride	95–105 mEq/L	
Bicarbonate (HCO$_3$)	19–25 mEq/L	
Total calcium	9–11 mg/dl or 4.5–5.5 mEq/L	
Ionized calcium	4.2–5.4 mg/dl or 2.1–2.6 mEq/L	
Phosphorous/phosphate	2.4–4.7 mg/dl	
Magnesium	1.8–3.0 mg/dl or 1.5–2.5 mEq/L	
Glucose	70–110 mg/dl	
Osmolality	285–310 mOsm/kg	

HEPATIC	MALE	FEMALE
AST (SGOT)	8–46 U/L	7–34 U/L
ALT (SGPT)	10–30 IU/ml	
Total bilirubin	0.3–1.2 mg/dl	
Conjugated bilirubin	0.0–0.2 mg/dl	
Unconjugated (indirect) bilirubin	0.2–0.8 mg/dl	
Alkaline phosphatase	20–90 U/L	

RENAL	MALE	FEMALE
BUN	6–20 mg/dl	
Creatinine	0.6–1.3 mg/dl	0.5–1.0 mg/dl
Uric acid	4.0–8.5 mg/dl	2.7–7.3 mg/dl

ARTERIAL BLOOD GASES	MALE	FEMALE
pH	7.35–7.45	
pO$_2$	80–100 mmHg	
pCO$_2$	35–45 mmHg	
O$_2$ Saturation	95–97%	
Base excess	$+2-(-2)$	
Bicarbonate (HCO$_3$)	22–26 mEq/L	

URINE TESTS

URINE	MALE	FEMALE
pH	4.5–8.0	
Specific gravity	1.010–1.025	

APPENDIX K
Dietary Guidelines for Food Sources

Potassium-Rich Foods

avocados	grapefruit	oranges	rhubarb
bananas	lima beans	peaches	sunflower seeds
broccoli	nuts	potatoes	spinach
cantaloupe	navy beans	prunes	tomatoes
dried fruits			

Sodium-Rich Foods

baking mixes (pancakes, muffins)	canned soups	Parmesan cheese
	canned spaghetti sauce	pickles
barbecue sauce	cured meats	potato salad
buttermilk	dry onion soup mix	pretzels, potato chips
butter/margarine	"fast" foods	sauerkraut
canned chili	macaroni and cheese	tomato ketchup
canned seafood	microwave dinners	TV dinners

Calcium-Rich Foods

bok choy	cream soups	oysters
broccoli	milk and dairy products	spinach
canned salmon/sardines	molasses (blackstrap)	tofu
clams		

Vitamin K-Rich Foods

asparagus	cabbage	fish	rice
beans	cauliflower	milk	spinach
broccoli	cheeses	mustard greens	turnips
brussel sprouts	collards	pork	yogurt

Low-Sodium Foods

baked or broiled poultry	grits (not instant)	potatoes
	honey	puffed wheat and rice
canned pumpkin	jams and jellies	red kidney and lima beans
cooked turnips	lean meats	sherbet
egg yolk	low-calorie mayonnaise	unsalted nuts
fresh vegetables	macaroons	whiskey
fruit		

Foods that Acidify Urine

cheeses	fish	meats	poultry
cranberries	grains (breads and cereals)	plums	prunes
eggs			

Foods that Alkalinize Urine

all fruits except cranberries, prunes, plums	all vegetables	milk

Foods Containing Tyramine

aged cheeses
avocados
bananas
beer
caffeine-containing beverages
chocolate
fermented sausage (bologna, salami, pepperoni)

liver
over-ripe fruit
red wine
smoked or pickled fish
yeasts
yogurt

Iron-Rich Foods

cereals
dried beans and peas

dried fruit
leafy-green vegetables

lean red meats
organ meats

Vitamin D-Rich Foods

breads
cereals

fish
fish liver oils

fortified milk

APPENDIX L
Recommended Dietary Allowances (RDAs),[a] revised 1989

AGE (YEARS) AND SEX GROUP	WEIGHT[b]		HEIGHT[b]		PROTEIN	VITAMIN A	FAT-SOLUBLE VITAMINS		
	kg	lb	cm	in	gm	µg RE[c]	VITAMIN D[d] µg	VITAMIN E mg α-TE[e]	VITAMIN K µg
Infants									
0.0–0.5	6	13	60	24	13	375	7.5	3	5
0.5–1.0	9	20	71	28	14	375	10	4	10
Children									
1–3	13	29	90	35	16	400	10	6	15
4–6	20	44	112	44	24	500	10	7	20
7–10	28	62	132	52	28	700	10	7	30
Males									
11–14	45	99	157	62	45	1000	10	10	45
15–18	66	145	176	69	59	1000	10	10	65
19–24	72	160	177	70	58	1000	10	10	70
25–50	79	174	176	70	63	1000	5	10	80
51+	77	170	173	68	63	1000	5	10	80
Females									
11–14	46	101	157	62	46	800	10	8	45
15–18	55	120	163	64	44	800	10	8	55
19–24	58	128	164	65	46	800	10	8	60
25–50	63	138	163	64	50	800	5	8	65
51+	65	143	160	63	50	800	5	8	65
Pregnant					60	800	10	10	65
Lactating									
first 6 mo					65	1300	10	12	65
second 6 mo					62	1200	10	11	65

RECOMMENDED DIETARY ALLOWANCES (RDAs),[a] REVISED 1989 (CONTINUED)

AGE (YEARS) AND SEX GROUP	WATER-SOLUBLE VITAMINS							MINERALS						
	VITAMIN C	THIA-MIN	RIBO-FLAVIN	NIACIN	VITAMIN B_6	FOLATE	VITAMIN B_{12}	CAL-CIUM	PHOS-PHORUS	MAG-NESIUM	IRON	ZINC	IODINE	SELE-NIUM
	mg	mg		mg NE[f]	mg	µg				mg			µg	
Infants														
0.0–0.5	30	0.3	0.4	5	0.3	25	0.3	400	300	40	6	5	40	10
0.5–1.0	35	0.4	0.5	6	0.6	35	0.5	600	500	60	10	5	50	15
Children														
1–3	40	0.7	0.8	9	1.0	50	0.7	800	800	80	10	10	70	20
4–6	45	0.9	1.1	12	1.1	75	1.0	800	800	120	10	10	90	20
7–10	45	1.0	1.2	13	1.4	100	1.4	800	800	170	10	10	120	30
Males														
11–14	50	1.3	1.5	17	1.7	150	2.0	1200	1200	270	12	15	150	40
15–18	60	1.5	1.8	20	2.0	200	2.0	1200	1200	400	12	15	150	50
19–24	60	1.5	1.7	19	2.0	200	2.0	1200	1200	350	10	15	150	70
25–50	60	1.5	1.7	19	2.0	200	2.0	800	800	350	10	15	150	70
51+	60	1.2	1.4	15	2.0	200	2.0	800	800	350	10	15	150	70

RECOMMENDED DIETARY ALLOWANCES (RDAs),[a] REVISED 1989 (CONTINUED)

AGE (YEARS) AND SEX GROUP	WATER-SOLUBLE VITAMINS							MINERALS						
	VITAMIN C	THIAMIN	RIBOFLAVIN	NIACIN	VITAMIN B$_6$	FOLATE	VITAMIN B$_{12}$	CALCIUM	PHOSPHORUS	MAGNESIUM	IRON	ZINC	IODINE	SELENIUM
	mg	mg		mg NE[f]	mg	µg	µg	mg					µg	
Females														
11–14	50	1.1	1.3	15	1.4	150	2.0	1200	1200	280	15	12	150	45
15–18	60	1.1	1.3	15	1.5	180	2.0	1200	1200	300	15	12	150	50
19–24	60	1.1	1.3	15	1.6	180	2.0	1200	1200	280	15	12	150	55
25–50	60	1.1	1.3	15	1.6	180	2.0	800	800	280	15	12	150	55
51+	60	1.0	1.2	13	1.6	180	2.0	800	800	280	10	12	150	55
Pregnant	70	1.5	1.6	17	2.2	400	2.2	1200	1200	320	30	15	175	65
Lactating														
first 6 mo	95	1.6	1.8	20	2.1	280	2.6	1200	1200	355	15	19	200	75
second 6 mo	90	1.6	1.7	20	2.1	260	2.6	1200	1200	340	15	16	200	75

[a] The allowances, expressed as average daily intakes over time, are intended to provide for individual variations among most normal persons as they live in the United States under usual environmental stresses. Diets should be based on a variety of common foods in order to provide other nutrients for which human requirements have been less well defined. See text for detailed discussion of allowances and of nutrients not tabulated.

[b] Weights and heights of Reference Adults are actual medians for the US population of the designated age, as reported by NHANES II. The median weights and heights of those under 19 yr of age were taken from Hamill PVV, Drizd, TA, Johnson, CL, Reed, RB, Roche, AF, and Moore, WM: Physical growth. National Center for Health Statistics Percentiles. Am J Clin Nutr 32:607, 1979. The use of these figures does not imply that the height-to-weight ratios are ideal.

[c] Retinol equivalents. 1 retinol equivalent = 1 µg retinol or 6 µg β-carotene. See text for calculation of vitamin A activity of diets as retinol equivalents.

[d] As cholecalciferol. 10 µg cholecalciferol = 400 IU of vitamin D.

[e] α-Tocopherol equivalents. 1 mg d-α tocopherol = 1 α-TE. See text for variation in allowances and calculation of vitamin E activity of the diet as α-tocopherol equivalents.

[f] NE (niacin equivalent) is equal to 1 mg of niacin or 60 mg of dietary tryptophan.

Electrolyte Equivalents and Caloric Values of Commonly Used Large-Volume Parenterals

	mEq/LITER							CALORIES/ LITER
	Na	K	Ca	Mg	Cl	Acetate	Lactate	
Solution								
D5W	—	—	—	—	—	—	—	170
D10W	—	—	—	—	—	—	—	340
0.9% NaCl	154	—	—	—	154	—	—	—
D5/0.9% NaCl	154	—	—	—	154	—	—	170
D5/0.45% NaCl	77	—	—	—	77	—	—	170
D5/0.2% NaCl	38.5	—	—	—	38.5	—	—	170
D5/LR	130	4	3	—	109	—	28	170–180
D5/Ringer's	147.5	4	4	—	156	—	—	170
LR	130	4	3	—	109	—	28	9
Ringer's Injection	147	4	4	—	156	—	—	—

D5W = 5% dextrose in water.
D10W = 10% dextrose in water.
0.9% NaCl = 0.9% sodium chloride = normal saline.
D5/0.9% NaCl = 5% dextrose in water with 0.9% sodium chloride = D5 with normal saline.
D5/0.45% NaCl = 5% dextrose in water with 0.45% sodium chloride = D5 with half normal saline.
D5/0.2% NaCl = 5% dextrose in water with 0.2% sodium chloride = D5 with quarter normal saline.
D5/LR = 5% dextrose in water with lactated Ringer's solution.
D5/Ringer's = 5% dextrose in water with Ringer's solution.
LR = Lactated Ringer's solution.

APPENDIX N
Routine Pediatric and Adult Immunizations

ROUTINE PEDIATRIC IMMUNIZATIONS

GENERIC NAME (BRAND NAMES)	ROUTE AND DOSAGE	CONTRAINDICATIONS AND PRECAUTIONS	ADVERSE REACTIONS/ SIDE EFFECTS	NOTES
DTwP–Diphtheria toxoid, tetanus toxoid, and whole-cell pertussis vaccine (Tri-Immunol)	0.5 ml IM at 2 mo, 4 mo, and 6 mo	Acute infection, immunosuppressive therapy, previous CNS damage or convulsions.	Redness, tenderness, induration at injection site, fever, malaise, myalgia, urticaria, hypotension, neurologic reactions, allergic reactions.	If unusual reactions occur, individual components may be given as separate injections. Tetanus booster should be repeated every 10 yrs.
DTaP Diptheria toxoid, tetanus toxoid, and acellular pertussis vaccine (Acel-Imune, Tripedia)	0.5 m IM at 15 mo (Tripedia) or 17 mo (Acel-Imune) and booster at 4–7 yr (either product)	Acute infection, immunosuppressive therapy, previous CNS damage or convulsions.	Same as for DTwP, but incidence is less.	Use only for 4th and 5th doses of primary DTP immunization; 1st three doses of primary immunization series should be with DTwP product.
Trivalent oral polio vaccine (Orimune)	0.5 ml PO at 2 mo, 4 mo, 15–18 mo and booster at 4–6 yr	Vomiting, diarrhea, allergy to streptomycin or neomycin, acute illness, immunosuppression.	Vaccine-associated paralysis.	Additional dose may be given at 6 mo.
Measles, mumps, and rubella vaccines (M-M-R II)	Single dose SC at 15 mo	Allergy to egg or neomycin. Active infection. Immunosuppression.	Burning, stinging, pain at injection site, arthritis/arthralgia (40%), fever, encephalitis, allergic reactions.	If usual reactions occur, individual components may be given as separate injections. In adults unimmunized against measles, 2 doses of measles vaccine 0.5 ml SC (Attenuvax) may be given 2 mo apart; if previously immunized give a single dose. In adults unimmunized against rubella, a single dose of rubella vaccine 0.5 ml SC (Meruvax II) may be given.

Vaccine	Dosage	Contraindications	Side Effects	Comments
Hemophilus b conjugate vaccine (Hib-TITER, Pedvax-HIB, ProHIBit)	Infants 2–6 mo old: 0.5 ml IM HibTITER at 2, 4, 6 mo. Infants 7–11 mo old: 2 doses 0.5 ml IM HibTITER 2 mo apart. Infants 12–14 mo old: single 0.5 ml IM dose of HibTITER. Children 15 mo–5 yr: single dose of 0.5 ml IM PedvaxHIB or ProHIBit.	Allergy to diphtheria toxoid or thimerisol.	Induration, erythema tenderness at injection site, fever.	(ProHIBit only for single immunization in children 15–59 mo, HibTITER not for this use.)
DTwP-HIB Diphtheria and tetanus toxoids and whole-cell pertussis and Hemcphilus b conjugate vaccine (Tetramune)	0.5 ml IM at 2 mo, 4 mo, 6 mo, and 15–18 mo	Allergy to diphtheria toxicol or thimerisol, acute infection, immunosuppressive therapy, previous CNS damage or convulsions.	Induration, erythema tenderness at injection site, fever, malaise, myalgia, urticaria, hypotension, neurologic reactions, allergic reactions.	Alternative to separate injections for first 3–4 doses of primary immunization series.
Hepatitis B Vaccine (Engerix-B, Recombivax HB)	Children 0–10 yr: 0.5 ml IM Engerix-B or 0.25 ml IM Recombivax HB at 0, 1, and 6 mo. Children 11–19 yr: 1 ml IM Engerix-B or 0.5 ml IM Recombivax HB. Infants born to HBsAg-positive mothers: 0.5 ml IM Recombivax HB at 0, 1, and 6 mo, preceded by hepatitis B immune globulin	Hypersensitivity to thimerisol (Recombivax) or yeast (both products).	Local soreness	In high-risk patients 0–10 yr, 0.5 ml IM Engerix-B at 0, 1, 2 and 12 mo may be given, and in children >10 yr, Engerix-B 1 ml IM at 0, 1, 2, and 12 mo may be given.

ROUTINE PEDIATRIC IMMUNIZATIONS (CONTINUED)

Nursing Implications:

ASSESSMENT

- Assess previous immunization history and history of hypersensitivity.

POTENTIAL NURSING DIAGNOSES

- Infection, high risk for (indications)
- Knowledge deficit related to medication regimen (patient/family teaching).

IMPLEMENTATION

- Measles, mumps, and rubella vaccine, trivalent oral polio virus vaccine, and diphtheria toxoid, tetanus toxoid, and pertussis vaccine may be given concomitantly.
- Administer each immunization by appropriate route: □ PO: Polio □ SC: measles, mumps, rubella □ IM: diphtheria, tetanus toxoid, pertussis.

PATIENT/FAMILY TEACHING

- Inform parent of potential and reportable side effects of immunization. Physician should be notified if patient develops fever over 39.4°C (103°F); difficulty breathing; hives; itching; swelling of eyes, face, or inside of nose; sudden, severe tiredness or weakness; or convulsions occur.
- Review next scheduled immunization with parent.

EVALUATION

Effectiveness of therapy can be demonstrated by: ■ Prevention of diseases through active immunity.

ROUTINE ADULT IMMUNIZATIONS

GENERIC NAME (BRAND NAMES)	INDICATIONS	DOSAGE/ROUTE	CONTRAINDICATIONS	ADVERSE REACTIONS/SIDE EFFECTS
Hepatitis B vaccine (Engerix-B, Recombivax HB, Recombivax HB Dialysis Formulation)	High-risk patients, health care workers	3 doses of 0.5 ml IM, given at 0, 1, and 6 mo. Dialysis patients should receive special formulation (40 mcg surface antigen/ml)	Hypersensitivity to thimerisol (Recombivax) or yeast.	Local soreness.
Influenza vaccine (Flu-Imune, Fluogen, Fluzone, Influenza virus vaccine [trivalent])	Everyone >65 yr, high-risk patients, health care workers	0.5 ml IM every year (new strain developed yearly)	Allergy to eggs, egg protein, chickens, bisulfites, or thimerisol.	Fever, chills, myalgia, malaise.

1294

Vaccine	Recipients	Dose	Contraindications	Side Effects
Measles vaccine (Attenuvax)	Unimmunized patients born after 1956	2 doses 0.5 ml SC at least 1 mo apart	Pregnancy, immunosuppression, allergy to eggs, egg protein, chickens, neomycin.	Low-grade fever.
	Patients previously immunized with single dose (for college entry, health care workers, or foreign travel)	1 dose 0.5 ml SC		
Pneumococcal vaccine, polyvalent (Pneumovax 23, Pnu-Imune 23)	Everyone >65 yr, high-risk patients	0.5 ml IM	Hypersensitivity to pheno- or thimerisol.	Local soreness.
Rubella vaccine (Menvax II)	Unimmunized young women, health care workers	0.5 ml SC	Pregnancy, immunosuppression, allergy to neomycin.	Low-grade fever, lymphadenopathy, sore throat, arthralgia, and arthritis are common in nonimmune adults.
Tetanus-diphtheria (Adult Td)	Unimmunized	2 doses 0.5 ml IM 1–2 mo apart, then a 3rd dose 6–12 mo later	Hypersensitivity to previous dose or to thimerisol; previous neurologic reaction.	Local pain and swelling.
	Everyone	Booster every 10 yr		

ACTIVITY/REST
Activity intolerance
Activity intolerance, high risk for
Disuse syndrome, high risk for
Diversional activity deficit
Fatigue
Sleep pattern disturbance

CIRCULATION
Cardiac output, decreased
Dysreflexia
Tissue perfusion, altered (specify):
cerebral, cardiopulmonary, renal,
gastrointestinal, peripheral

EGO INTEGRITY
Adjustment, impaired
Anxiety (specify level)
Body image disturbance
Coping, defensive
Coping, ineffective individual
Decisional conflict (specify)
Denial, ineffective
Fear
Grieving, anticipatory
Grieving, dysfunctional
Hopelessness
Personal identity disturbance
Post-trauma response
Powerlessness
Rape-trauma syndrome
Rape-trauma syndrome: compound re-
action
Rape-trauma syndrome: silent reaction
Self-esteem, chronic low
Self-esteem disturbance
Self-esteem, situational low
Spiritual distress

ELIMINATION
Bowel incontinence
Constipation
Constipation, colonic
Constipation, perceived
Diarrhea
Incontinence, functional
Incontinence, reflex
Incontinence, stress
Incontinence, total
Incontinence, urge

Urinary elimination, altered patterns of
Urinary retention [acute/chronic]

FOOD/FLUID
Breastfeeding, effective
Breastfeeding, ineffective
Breastfeeding, interrupted
Feeding pattern, ineffective infant
Fluid volume deficit [active loss]
Fluid volume deficit [regulatory failure]
Fluid volume deficit, high risk for
Fluid volume excess
Nutrition, altered: less than body re-
quirements
Nutrition, altered: more than body re-
quirements
Nutrition, altered: high risk for more
than body requirements
Oral mucous membranes, altered
Swallowing, impaired

HYGIENE
Self-care deficit: feeding, bathing/hy-
giene, dressing/grooming, toileting

NEUROSENSORY
Peripheral neurovascular dysfunction,
high risk for
Sensory-perceptual alterations (spec-
ify): visual, auditory, kinesthetic,
gustatory, tactile, olfactory
Thought processes, altered
Unilateral neglect

PAIN/COMFORT
Pain [acute]
Pain, chronic

RESPIRATION
Airway clearance, ineffective
Aspiration, high risk for
Breathing pattern, ineffective
Gas exchange, impaired
Ventilation, spontaneous: inability to
sustain
Ventilatory weaning response, dysfunc-
tional

SAFETY
Body temperature, altered, high risk for
Health maintenance, altered

Home maintenance management, impaired
Hyperthermia
Hypothermia
Infection, high risk for
Injury, high risk for
Physical mobility, impaired
Poisoning, high risk for
Protection, altered
Self-multilation, high risk for
Skin integrity, impaired
Skin integrity, impaired, high risk for
Suffocation, high risk for
Thermoregulation, ineffective
Tissue integrity, impaired
Trauma, high risk for
Violence, high risk for: directed at self/others

SEXUALITY (COMPONENT OF EGO INTEGRITY AND SOCIAL INTERACTION)
Sexual dysfunction
Sexuality patterns, altered

SOCIAL INTERACTION
Caregiver role strain
Caregiver role strain, high risk for
Communication, impaired verbal
Family coping, compromised
Family coping, disabling
Family coping, potential for growth
Family processes, altered
Parental role conflict
Parenting, altered
Parenting, altered, high risk for
Relocation stress sydrome
Role performance, altered
Social interaction, impaired
Social isolation

TEACHING/LEARNING
Growth and development, altered
Health-seeking behaviors (specify)
Knowledge deficit [learning need] (specify)
Noncompliance [compliance, altered] (specify)
Therapeutic regimen (individuals), ineffective management of

APPENDIX P
Recent Drug Release Update

NEW DRUGS

GENERIC NAME (BRAND NAME)	CLASSIFICATION	USE(S)	DOSE	FDA APPROVAL STATUS
cefipime (Maxipime)	Anti-infective (cephalosporin)	Infections due to susceptible organisms	IM, IV (Adults): 1–2 g q 8–12 hr*	Submitted for FDA approval
cladribine (Leustatin)	Antineoplastic agent	Hairy cell leukemia	IV (Adults): 0.09 mg/kg/day for 7 days	Approved 2/93
dornase alfa (Pulmozyme)	DNA enzyme (recombinant human)	Cystic fibrosis	Inhalation (Adults and Children >5 yr): 2.5 mg once daily	Approved 12/93
fenofibrate (Lipidil)	Lipid-lowering agent	Hypertriglyceridemia	PO (Adults): 100 mg/day initially	Approved by FDA
fluvastatin (Lescol)	Lipid-lowering agent	Hypercholesterolemia	PO (Adults): 20 mg at bedtime	Approved by FDA
fluvoxamine (Luvox)	Antipsychotic	Obsessive-compulsive disorder	PO (Adults): 50–300 mg/day*	Recommended for FDA approval
gabapentin (Neurontin)	Anticonvulsant	Partial seizures	PO (Adults): 900–1800 mg/day in 3 divided doses	Approved by FDA
granisetron (Kytril)	Antiemetic	Prevention of nausea and vomiting from chemotherapy	IV (Adults): 10 mcg/kg over 5 min given 30 min prior to chemotherapy	Approved by FDA
lamotrigine (Lamictal)	Anticonvulsant	Partial seizures	PO (Adults and Children >12 yr): 100–700 mg/day in 2 divided doses*	Recommended for FDA approval
levocabastine (Livostin)	Ophthalmic antihistamine	Seasonal allergic conjunctivitis	Ophth (Adults): 1 drop 4 times daily for up to 2 wk	Approved 12/93
levomethadyl (ORLAAM)	Opioid agonist	Treatment of heroin addiction	PO (Adults): 60–90 mg 3 times weekly (maintenance)	Approved 6/93

Drug	Classification	Indication	Dosage	Status
lodoxamide (Alomide)	Mast cell stabilizer	Vernal keratoconjunctivitis, vernal conjunctivitis, vernal keratitis	Ophth (Adults and Children >2 yr): 1–2 drops 4 times daily for up to 3 mo	Approved 9/93
masoprocol (Actinex)	Topical antineoplastic	Multiple actinic keratoses	Topical (Adults): Apply twice daily for 28 days	Approved 9/92
perindopril (Aceon)	Antihypertensive	Essential hypertension	PO (Adults): 4–8 mg/day	Approved by FDA
risperidone (Risperdal)	Antipsychotic	Psychotic disorders	PO (Adults): 1 mg twice daily initially, up to 4–6 mg/day	Approved by FDA
salmeterol (Serevent)	Bronchodilator	Reversible airway disease	Inhalation (Adults): 50–100 mcg twice daily*	Recommended for FDA approval
trimetrexate (Neutrexin)	Antiprotozoal	Moderate to severe *Pneumocystis carinii* pneumonia	IV (Adults): 45 mg/m^2/day for 21 days with concurrent leucovorin for 24 days	Approved 12/93
varicella vaccine (Varivex)	Live attenuated vaccine	Prevention of chickenpox	SC (Children): 0.5 ml	Recommended for FDA approval
venlafaxine (Effexor)	Antidepressant	Depression	PO (Adults): 75–375 mg/day in 3 divided doses*	Approved by FDA

RECENT DRUG RELEASE UPDATE (CONTINUED)

NEW DOSAGE FORMS

GENERIC NAME (BRAND NAME)	CLASSIFICATION	USE(S)	DOSE	FDA APPROVAL STATUS
diclofenac immediate-release tablets (Cataflam)	Nonsteroidal anti-inflammatory agent	Analgesia and primary dysmenorrhea, osteoarthritis, rheumatoid arthritis, ankylosing spondylitis	PO (Adults): 100–200 mg/day in 3–4 divided doses	Approved by FDA
fentanyl oral transmucosal (Fentanyl Oralet)	Opioid analgesic	Anesthetic premedication, anesthesia, monitored anesthesia care	PO (Adults >50 mg): 400 mcg PO (Elderly): 2.5–5 mcg/kg PO (Children): 5–15 mcg/kg	Approved 12/93
mupirocin nasal (Bactroban)	Anti-infective	Decreases carrier state of *Staphylococcus aureus*	Nasal: Up to 4 times daily*	Submitted for FDA approval
sucralfate suspension (Carafate)	Antiulcer	Short-term management of duodenal ulcer	PO (Adults): 1 g 4 times daily	Approved by FDA
testosterone scrotal patch (Testoderm)	Androgenic hormone	Testosterone deficiency	Transdermal (Adults): 4–6 mg/day	Approved 10/93
timolol ophthalmic gel (Timoptic-XE)	Antiglaucoma	Ocular hypertension, open-angle glaucoma	Ophth (Adults): Apply once daily	Approved by FDA

NEW INDICATIONS

clarithromycin (Biaxin)	Anti-infective	Disseminated mycobacterial infections due to *Mycobacterium avium* and *Mycobacterium intracellulare*	PO (Adults): 500 mg bid PO (Children): 7.5 mg/kg bid (not to exceed 500 mg bid)	Approved by FDA
goserelin (Zoladex)	Gonadotropin-releasing hormone	Endometriosis	Implant (Adults): 3.6 mg q 28 days	Approved 6/93
immune globulin IV (Gamimune N)	Immune globulin	Reduces infections and graft-versus-host disease in bone marrow transplant patients	IV (Adults): 500 mg/kg/day for 5 days starting 1 wk before transplant then weekly for 13 wk	Approved by FDA
immune globulin IV (Gamimune N)	Immune globulin	Prevents bacterial infections in HIV-infected children	IV (Children): 400 mg/kg q 28 days	Approved by FDA
naproxen sodium tablets (Aleve)	Nonsteroidal anti-inflammatory agent	Nonprescription analgesic/antipyretic	PO (Adults 12–65 yr): 600 mg/day in divided doses q 8–12 hr PO (Adults >65 yr): 400 mg/day in divided doses q 12 hr	Approved by FDA
propofol (Diprivan)	General anesthetic	Pediatric anesthesia	IV (Children >3 yr): *Induction*—2.5–3.5 mg/kg over 20–30 sec *Maintenance*—7.5–18 mg/kg/hr	Approved 12/93
quinapril (Accupril)	Angiotensin-converting enzyme inhibitor	Congestive heart failure	PO (Adults): 10–40 mg/day in 2 divided doses	Approved 12/93
somatropin (Nutropin HGH)	Recombinant growth hormone	Prevention of growth failure in children with chronic renal insufficiency	SC (Children): 50 mcg/kg/day	Approved 12/93
zidovudine (Retrovir)	Antiviral	Decreases incidence of HIV infection in infants born to HIV-infected women	*Antepartum*—PO (Adults): 500 mg/day *Intrapartum*—IV (Adults): 2 mg/kg initially, then 1 mg/kg/hr while in labor *Postpartum*—PO (Infants): 2 mg/kg q 6 hr for 6 wk	Dose used in phase III randomized placebo-controlled trial to evaluate the efficacy, safety, and tolerance of oral AZT in pregnant HIV-infected women and infants[†]

*Pending final FDA approval.
[†]Conducted by National Institutes of Allergy and Infectious Disease—AIDS Clinical Trial Group (Study #026).

APPENDIX Q
Sample FDA MedWatch Form

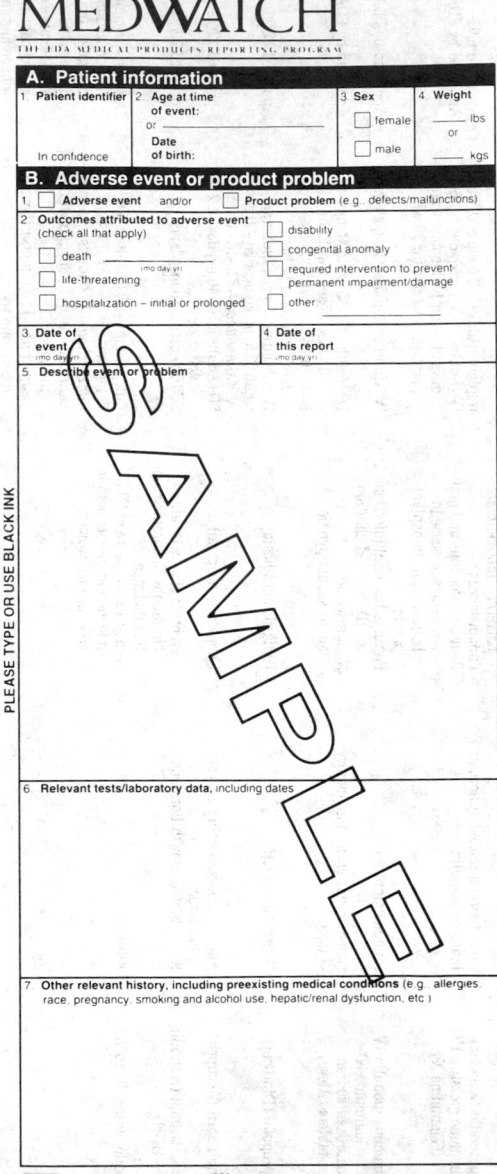

PLEASE TYPE OR USE BLACK INK

MEDWATCH
THE FDA MEDICAL PRODUCTS REPORTING PROGRAM

A. Patient information

1 Patient identifier	2 Age at time of event: or Date of birth:	3 Sex	4 Weight
In confidence		☐ female ☐ male	___ lbs or ___ kgs

B. Adverse event or product problem

1. ☐ Adverse event and/or ☐ Product problem (e.g. defects/malfunctions)

2. Outcomes attributed to adverse event (check all that apply)
   - ☐ death ___ (mo day yr)
   - ☐ life-threatening
   - ☐ hospitalization – initial or prolonged
   - ☐ disability
   - ☐ congenital anomaly
   - ☐ required intervention to prevent permanent impairment/damage
   - ☐ other: ___

3. Date of event (mo day yr)	4 Date of this report (mo day yr)

5. Describe event or problem

6. Relevant tests/laboratory data, including dates

7. Other relevant history, including preexisting medical conditions (e.g. allergies, race, pregnancy, smoking and alcohol use, hepatic/renal dysfunction, etc.)

Mail to: MEDWATCH
5600 Fishers Lane
Rockville, MD 20852-9787

or FAX to:
1-800-FDA-0178

FDA Form 3500 (6/93)

1302

C. Suspect medication(s)

1. Name (give labeled strength & mfr/labeler, if known)

#1

#2

2. Dose, frequency & route used

#1

#2

3. Therapy dates (if unknown, give duration)
(from/to (or best estimate))

#1

#2

4. Diagnosis for use (indication)

#1

#2

5. Event abated after use stopped or dose reduced

#1 ☐ yes ☐ no ☐ doesn't apply

#2 ☐ yes ☐ no ☐ doesn't apply

6. Lot # (if known)

#

#2

7. Exp. date (if known)

#1

#2

8. Event reappeared after reintroduction

#1 ☐ yes ☐ no ☐ doesn't apply

#2 ☐ yes ☐ no ☐ doesn't apply

9. NDC # (for product problems only)

— —

10. Concomitant medical products and therapy dates (exclude treatment of event)

D. Suspect medical device

1. Brand name

2. Type of device

3. Manufacturer name & address

4. Operator of device
☐ health professional
☐ lay user/patient
☐ other

5. Expiration date (mo/day/yr)

6.
model #

catalog #

serial #

lot #

other #

7. If implanted, give date (mo/day/yr)

8. If explanted, give date (mo/day/yr)

9. Device available for evaluation? (Do not send to FDA)
☐ yes ☐ no ☐ returned to manufacturer on _____ (mo/day/yr)

10. Concomitant medical products and therapy dates (exclude treatment of event)

E. Reporter (see confidentiality section on back)

1. Name, address & phone #

2. Health professional?
☐ yes ☐ no

3. Occupation

4. Also reported to
☐ manufacturer
☐ user facility
☐ distributor

5. If you do NOT want your identity disclosed to the manufacturer, place an " X " in this box. ☐

Mail to: MEDWATCH
5600 Fishers Lane
Rockville, MD 20852-9787

or FAX to:
1-800-FDA-0178

FDA Form 3500 (6/93)

1303

BIBLIOGRAPHY

American Hospital Formulary Service: Drug Information 93. American Society of Hospital Pharmacists, Bethesda, 1993.

Cella, JH and Watson, J: Nurse's Manual of Laboratory Tests, FA Davis, Philadelphia, 1989.

Doenges, ME and Moorhouse, MF: Nurse's Pocket Guide: Nursing Diagnoses with Interventions, ed 4. FA Davis, Philadelphia, 1993.

Facts and Comparisons. JB Lippincott, St. Louis, 1994.

Fischbach, FT: A Manual of Laboratory Diagnostic Tests, ed 3. JB Lippincott, Philadelphia, 1988.

Mathewson-Kuhn, M: Pharmacotherapeutics: A Nursing Process Approach, ed 2. FA Davis, Philadelphia, 1991.

Physicians' Desk Reference (PDR). Medical Economics, Oradell, 1993.

Trissel, LA: Supplement to Handbook of Injectable Drugs, ed 7. American Society of Hospital Pharmacists, Bethesda, 1992.

USP Dispensing Information (USP-DI): Drug Information for the Health Care Provider, volume I. United States Pharmacopeial Convention, Rockville, ed 14, 1994.

USP Dispensing Information (USP-DI): Advice for the Patient, volume II. United States Pharmacopeial Convention, Rockville, ed 14, 1994.

Whitney, E and Boyle, M: Understanding Nutrition, ed 3. West Publishing Company, St. Paul, 1984.

NOTES

NOTES

NOTES

COMPREHENSIVE INDEX*
generic/Trade/CLASSIFICATION

*Entries for **generic** names appear in **boldface type**, trade names appear in regular type, CLASSIFICATIONS appear in BOLDFACE SMALL CAPS, and *Combination drugs* appear in *italics*. A "C" and a **boldface** page number following a generic name identify the page in the "Classification" section on which that drug is listed.

*Entries for **generic** names appear in **boldface type,** trade names appear in regular type, CLASSIFICATIONS appear in BOLDFACE SMALL CAPS, and *Combination drugs* appear in *italics*. A "C" and a **boldface** page number following a generic name identify the page in the "Classification" section on which that drug is listed.

*Entries for **generic** names appear in **boldface type,** trade names appear in regular type, CLASSIFICATIONS appear in BOLDFACE SMALL CAPS, and *Combination drugs* appear in *italics.* A "C" and a **boldface** page number following a generic name identify the page in the "Classification" section on which that drug is listed.

*Entries for **generic** names appear in **boldface type,** trade names appear in regular type, CLASSIFICATIONS appear in BOLDFACE SMALL CAPS, and *Combination drugs* appear in *italics*. A "C" and a **boldface** page number following a generic name identify the page in the "Classification" section on which that drug is listed.

*Entries for **generic** names appear in **boldface type,** trade names appear in regular type, CLASSIFICATIONS appear in BOLDFACE SMALL CAPS, and *Combination drugs* appear in *italics.* A "C" and a **boldface** page number following a generic name identify the page in the "Classification" section on which that drug is listed.

*Entries for **generic** names appear in **boldface type,** trade names appear in regular type, **CLASSIFICATIONS** appear in **BOLDFACE SMALL CAPS,** and *Combination drugs* appear in *italics*. A "C" and a **boldface** page number following a generic name identify the page in the "Classification" section on which that drug is listed.

*Entries for **generic** names appear in **boldface type,** trade names appear in regular type, CLASSIFICATIONS appear in BOLDFACE SMALL CAPS, and *Combination drugs* appear in *italics.* A "C" and a **boldface** page number following a generic name identify the page in the "Classification" section on which that drug is listed.

*Entries for **generic** names appear in **boldface type,** trade names appear in regular type, CLASSIFICATIONS appear in BOLDFACE SMALL CAPS, and *Combination drugs* appear in *italics*. A "C" and a **boldface** page number following a generic name identify the page in the "Classification" section on which that drug is listed.

*Entries for **generic** names appear in **boldface type,** trade names appear in regular type, CLASSIFICATIONS appear in BOLDFACE SMALL CAPS, and *Combination drugs* appear in *italics.* A "C" and a **boldface** page number following a generic name identify the page in the "Classification" section on which that drug is listed.

*Entries for **generic** names appear in **boldface type,** trade names appear in regular type, CLASSIFICATIONS appear in BOLDFACE SMALL CAPS, and *Combination drugs* appear in *italics*. A "C" and a **boldface** page number following a generic name identify the page in the "Classification" section on which that drug is listed.

---

*Entries for **generic** names appear in **boldface type**, trade names appear in regular type, CLASSIFICATIONS appear in BOLDFACE SMALL CAPS, and *Combination drugs* appear in *italics*. A "C" and a **boldface** page number following a generic name identify the page in the "Classification" section on which that drug is listed.

*Entries for **generic** names appear in **boldface type,** trade names appear in regular type, CLASSIFICATIONS appear in BOLDFACE SMALL CAPS, and *Combination drugs* appear in *italics*. A "C" and a **boldface** page number following a generic name identify the page in the "Classification" section on which that drug is listed.

*Entries for **generic** names appear in **boldface type,** trade names appear in regular type, CLASSIFICATIONS appear in BOLDFACE SMALL CAPS, and *Combination drugs* appear in *italics.* A "C" and a **boldface** page number following a generic name identify the page in the "Classification" section on which that drug is listed.

*Entries for **generic** names appear in **boldface type,** trade names appear in regular type, CLASSIFICATIONS appear in BOLDFACE SMALL CAPS, and *Combination drugs* appear in *italics*. A "C" and a **boldface** page number following a generic name identify the page in the "Classification" section on which that drug is listed.

---

*Entries for **generic** names appear in **boldface type,** trade names appear in regular type, CLASSIFICATIONS appear in BOLDFACE SMALL CAPS, and *Combination drugs* appear in *italics*. A "C" and a **boldface** page number following a generic name identify the page in the "Classification" section on which that drug is listed.

*Entries for **generic** names appear in **boldface type,** trade names appear in regular type, CLASSIFICATIONS appear in BOLDFACE SMALL CAPS, and *Combination drugs* appear in *italics*. A "C" and a **boldface** page number following a generic name identify the page in the "Classification" section on which that drug is listed.

*Entries for **generic** names appear in **boldface type,** trade names appear in regular type, CLASSIFICATIONS appear in BOLDFACE SMALL CAPS, and *Combination drugs* appear in *italics*. A "C" and a **boldface** page number following a generic name identify the page in the "Classification" section on which that drug is listed.

*Entries for **generic** names appear in **boldface type,** trade names appear in regular type, CLASSIFICATIONS appear in BOLDFACE SMALL CAPS, and *Combination drugs* appear in *italics*. A "C" and a **boldface** page number following a generic name identify the page in the "Classification" section on which that drug is listed.

*Entries for **generic** names appear in **boldface type**, trade names appear in regular type, CLASSIFICATIONS appear in BOLDFACE SMALL CAPS, and *Combination drugs* appear in *italics*. A "C" and a **boldface** page number following a generic name identify the page in the "Classification" section on which that drug is listed.

---

*Entries for **generic** names appear in **boldface type,** trade names appear in regular type, **CLASSIFICATIONS** appear in **BOLDFACE SMALL CAPS,** and *Combination drugs* appear in *italics*. A "C" and a **boldface** page number following a generic name identify the page in the "Classification" section on which that drug is listed.

NOTES

NOTES

NOTES

NOTES

NOTES